Orthopaedics: A Study Guide
Spivak, Di Cesare, Feldman, Koval, Rokito, and Zuckerman

Errata

After this book went to press, the publisher learned of the following errors in the text. The publisher regrets any inconvenience this may cause and apologizes for these errors. **Boldface** indicates the text that is correct; where no boldface is apparent the content is significantly altered.

p. 98: *The legend for Fig. 17-3 should read:*

Figure 17-3
Extensor mechanism, **dorsal** view (see text for details). [Reproduced with permission from Coons MS, Green SM: Boutonniere deformity. *Hand Clin* 1995; 11(3):388,389.]

p. 103: *Right-hand column, first paragraph, first sentence should read:*

The lumbosacral plexus provides innervation to the lower extremities and consists of the ventral rami of spinal nerves T12-S3 (Fig. 18-2).

Right-hand column, fourth paragraph, first sentence should read:

The lateral femoral cutaneous nerve (**L2-3**) runs parallel to the iliacus muscle before it passes under the inguinal ligament, medial to the anterior superior iliac spine.

p. 146: *Left-hand column, sixth paragraph, second sentence should read:*

Weakness in this muscle often presents with scapular winging and may be secondary to a long thoracic nerve injury **(Fig. 23-1)**.

Left-hand column, eighth paragraph, last sentence should read:

This may or may not be accompanied by pain (Fig. 23-**2**).

Right-hand column, second complete paragraph, last sentence should read:

The presence of a sulcus sign signifies inferior capsular laxity but not necessarily instability (Fig. 23-**3**).

p. 147: *Left-hand column, first complete paragraph, last two sentences should read:*

In addition, a lidocaine subacromial injection test can further elicit the diagnosis of impingement **(Fig. 23-4)**. Improvement of symptoms post-injection (a positive test) supports the diagnosis of rotator cuff pathology, while a negative test leads the physician to look elsewhere for the etiology of the patient's symptoms.

p. 253: *Right-hand column, second complete paragraph, fourth sentence should read:*

Histologically, the cap consists of hyaline cartilage covered by thin fibrous peri**chondrium**.

p. 254: *Left-hand column, second paragraph, last two sentences should read:*

Excision of an osteochondroma must be done at the base of the stalk and include the cap and peri**chondrium**. Care should be taken to avoid disrupting the cap and perichondrium.

p. 258: *Left-hand column, first paragraph, third sentence should read:*

Most lesions occur in the pelvis, followed by the **femur** and proximal humerus.

p. 263: *Left-hand column, first paragraph, fourth sentence should read:*

The tumor may also be found in the **skull and vertebrae. In the long bones, it tends to appear in the diaphyseal region**.

p. 268: *Right-hand column, fourth complete sentence should read:*

The femur, pelvis, humerus, vertebrae, and tibia are the most frequent sites of involvement, respectively.

p. 348: *Table 54-1 should have an additional entry at the bottom:*

Cervical angina

p. 471: *An updated version of Table 72-8 follows:*

--- Table 72-8 ---

Guidelines of American Burn Association for Transfer of Patients to Burn Unit

1. Third degree burns in any age group
2. Second degree burns greater that 10 percent total body surface area (TBSA)
3. Burn patients with concomitant trauma (e.g., fractures) where burn injury poses greatest risk to morbidity/mortality
4. Burns that may result in cosmetic or functional disability, and burns of face, hands, feet, eyes, ears, genitalia, perineum, or major joints
5. High voltage electrical injury, including lightning injury
6. Inhalation injury or associated trauma
7. Chemical burns
8. Burns in patients with disease that would affect management, recovery, or their chances of dying
9. Burned children in hospitals without qualified pediatric care
10. Burn injury in patients with special social, emotional, or long-term rehabilitation

SOURCE: Reproduced and modified with permission from American Burn Association, 1999, Chicago.

p. 771: *Left-hand column, second complete paragraph, second sentence and an insert should read:*

It is **typically** transmitted as an autosomal dominant disorder, but is not clinically apparent at birth. Autosomal recessive inheritance has been reported, as well as gonadal mosaicism.

p. 772: *Right-hand column, second paragraph should read:*

The Conradi-Hünermann type of chondrodysplasia punctata is transmitted **as an X-linked dominant disorder,** but there is variable clinical expression. **It is usually fatal in males.**

Right-hand column, third paragraph, last sentence should read:

The skin is dry and scaling, with linear striations**, referred to as ichthyosis**.

Right-hand column, second primary heading and following paragraph should read:

CHONDRODYSPLASIA PUNCTATA: X-LINKED RECESSIVE TYPE

The X-linked **recessive** type of chondrodysplasia punctata contributes about 25 percent of the cases of chondrodysplasia punctata.

p. 773: *Left-hand column, fifth paragraph, second sentence should read:*

Hypoplastic scapulae **may** also **be** a feature, **as may the presence of fused capitate and hamate bones.**

p. 769: *The following table, which constitutes a summary of the material covered in Chap. 131 was omitted:*

—————— *Table 131-1* ——————

Skeletal Dysplasias

Dysplasia and Inheritance	Clinical Features	Radiographic Features
Achondroplasia, AD/SM	Distinctive facies, trident hand, spine abnormalities, rhizomelic shortening, height=123–130 cm; most common dysplasia	Decreased interpedicular distance, small foramen magnum
Hypochondroplasia, AD/SM	Normal face, taller than achondroplast, height=132–147 cm	Normal vertebrae
Diastrophic dysplasia, AR	Perioral fullness, cleft palate, "cauliflower ear," resistant clubfoot, height=86–120 cm; more common in Finland	Shortened ulna/fibula; saucer-shaped femoral heads, C2-3 subluxation
Pseudoachondroplasia, AD/AR/GM	Normal face and cranium, otherwise similar to achondroplasia, C1-2 instability, height=82–130 cm	Irregular femoral epiphyses, platyspondyly with anterior beaking, no decrease in interpedicular distance
SED Congenita, AD/SM	Flat midface, cleft palate, hypertelorism, myopia and retinal detachment, C1-2 instability, height=84–128 cm	Delay in ossification centers, vertebral bodies flatten → kyphosis, premature osteoarthritis
SED Tarda, XR	Presents in late childhood/adolescence, most above 3d percentile in height, premature osteoarthritis, height=130–155 cm	Epiphyseal involvement proximal joints, premature osteoarthritis, bilateral flattening hips—resembles LCP disease
Multiple epiphyseal dysplasia, AD/AR/SM	Present at age 5–10 years, most above 3d percentile in height, severe hip osteoarthritis, height=135–150 cm	Bilateral epiphyseal involvement of hips, knees, and ankles, bilateral femoral heads—resembles LCP disease
Metaphyseal chondrodysplasia		
McKusick type (Cartilage-hair hypoplasia), AR	Distal overgrowth of fibulas, sparse, light-colored hair, height=110–140 cm; Amish population	Metaphyseal involvement
Schmid type, AD/SM	Bowleg is usual presentation at 2 years of age, height=130–160 cm; confused with vitamin-D resistant rickets	Metaphyseal involvement
Chondrodysplasia punctata		
Conradi-Hünermann type, XD/SM	Asymmetric shortening of limb, ichthyosis, cataracts, alopecia; usually lethal in males	Multiple punctate calcifications in vertebral column and epiphyses of long bones in infancy
X-linked recessive type, XR	Hypoplasia of distal phalanges	Dumbbell-shaped humeri w/punctate stippling in infancy
Rhizomelic type, AR	Recurrent infections → death in 1st year	Vertebral column spared
Chondroectodermal dysplasia (Ellis-van Creveld Syndrome), AR	Mesomelic dwarfism; postaxial polydactyly, congenital heart disease, height=110–155 cm; Amish population	Fused capitate and hamate bones, hypoplastic scapulae, CDH, scoliosis
Campomelic dysplasia, AD/GM	Flat facies, saber tibias, resistant clubfoot, cleft palate, micrognathia; mostly female patients (XY females)	Hypoplastic scapulae
Mucopolysaccharidoses		
Hurler's (MP-IH), AR	Coarse facies, umbilical hernia, hepatosplenomegaly, mental retardation, corneal clouding; dermatan sulfate and heparan sulfate in urine	Enlarged sella turcica, beaked vertebrae, T-L kyphosis, claw-hand deformity, C1-2 instability
Hunter's (MP-II), XR	Same as above, but less severe, height=105–140 cm; dermatan sulfate and heparan sulfate in urine	Same as above
Morquio's (MP-IV), AR	No mental retardation; C1-2 instability, height=80–120 cm; keratan sulfate in urine	Bullet-shaped metacarpals

NOTE: AD, autosomal dominant; AR, autosomal recessive; SM, spontaneous mutation; XR, X-linked recessive; XD, X-linked dominant; SED, Spondyloepiphyseal dysplasia; LCP, Legg-Calvé-Perthes disease; GM, gonadal mosaicism; CDH, congenital dislocation of hip

ORTHOPAEDICS
A Study Guide

ORTHOPAEDICS
A Study Guide

Jeffrey M. Spivak, M.D.

Paul E. Di Cesare, M.D.

David S. Feldman, M.D.

Kenneth J. Koval, M.D.

Andrew S. Rokito, M.D.

Joseph D. Zuckerman, M.D.

All with
The Hospital for Joint Diseases Orthopaedic Institute
and the New York University School of Medicine

McGraw-Hill
Health Professions Division

New York St. Louis San Francisco Auckland Bogotá Caracas Lisbon London Madrid
Mexico City Milan Montreal New Delhi San Juan Singapore Sydney Tokyo Toronto

McGraw-Hill

A Division of The McGraw·Hill Companies

ORTHOPAEDICS: A Study Guide

1234567890 DOCDOC 99

ISBN 0-07-060355-3

This book was set in Times Roman by York Graphics, Inc.
The editors were Martin Wonsiewicz and Steven Melvin;
the production supervisor was Helene G. Landers.
The text and cover were designed by Marsha Cohen/Parallelogram.
The index was prepared by Alexandra Nickerson.

R.R. Donnelley and Sons Company, Inc., was the printer and binder.

**Cataloging-in-Publication Data is on file for this title at the Library of
Congress**

To my wife Melanie and my children Amanda and Russell, who fill my thoughts during the many hours at work and ensure my well being and confirm my sense of purpose when I'm home.—J. M. S.

To my wife Beth and daughters Atara, Emily, and Tali for their love, patience, and understanding.—D. S. F.

To my lovely wife Mary and fantastic children Courtney and Michael who are so supportive and understanding.—K. J. K.

For my wife and best friend Susan and for our daughters Ariel, Shelby, and Lindsay.
And for my parents.—A. S. R.

For my loving and understanding wife Pamela and sons Casey, Scott, and Dean.—P. E. Di C.

To the residents and faculty of the NYU-HJD Department of Orthopaedic Surgery—in recognition of your hardwork, determination, and commitment to excellence.—J. D. Z.

CONTENTS

PART III   PHYSICAL EXAMINATION

PART IV   DIAGNOSTIC TESTING

**SECTION 7:
ORTHOPAEDIC INFECTIONS**

**SECTION 8:
SPORTS MEDICINE/ARTHROSCOPY**

PART VI   RELATED TOPICS

CONTRIBUTORS

Gina B. Aharonoff, M.P.H.
Assistant Director
Geriatric Hip Fracture Research Group
NYU–HJD Department of Orthopaedic Surgery
New York, New York

Donna J. Astion, M.D.
Associate Chief
Foot and Ankle Service
NYU–HJD Department of Orthopaedic Surgery
New York, New York
and
Instructor in Orthopaedic Surgery
New York University School of Medicine

Dan Atar, M.D.
Chairman, Orthopedic Department
Soroka Medical Center
Ben Gurion University
Beersheva, Israel
and
Clinical Associate Professor of Orthopaedic Surgery
New York University School of Medicine

Ann E. Barr, Ph.D., P.T.
Consultant
Occupational and Industrial Orthopaedic Center
NYU–HJD Department of Orthopaedic Surgery
New York, New York
and
Assistant Professor
Department of Physical Therapy
College of Allied Health Professions
Temple University
Philadelphia, Pennsylvania

Javier Beltran, M.D.
Chairman
Department of Radiology
The Hospital for Joint Diseases
New York, New York

John A. Bendo, M.D.
Director
Clinical Research—Spine Center
NYU–HJD Department of Orthopaedic Surgery
New York, New York
and
Clinical Instructor in Orthopaedic Surgery
New York University School of Medicine
New York, New York

Aleksandar Berić, M.D., D.Sc.
Director
Clinical Neurophysiology Service
The Hospital for Joint Diseases
New York, New York
and
Associate Professor of Neurology
New York University School of Medicine
New York, New York

Ralph L. Bernstein, M.D.
Chairman
Department of Anesthesiology
The Hospital for Joint Diseases
New York, New York
and
Professor of Clinical Anesthesiology
New York University School of Medicine
New York, New York

Norman C. Blumenthal, Ph.D.
Associate Director of Research
Bioengineering Laboratory
The Hospital for Joint Diseases
New York, New York

Paul M. Brisson, M.D., F.R.C.S. (C)
Attending Orthopaedic Surgeon
NYU–HJD Department of Orthopaedic Surgery
New York, New York

Omar E. Burschtin, M.D.
Division of Pulmonary and Critical Care Medicine
Department of Medicine
New York University Medical Center
New York, New York
and
Clinical Instructor in Medicine
New York University School of Medicine
New York, New York

James W. Cahill, M.D.
Consultant
Sports Medicine Service
NYU–HJD Department of Orthopaedic Surgery
New York, New York
and
Associate Attending Orthopaedic Surgeon
Department of Orthopaedic Surgery
University of Medicine and Dentistry of New Jersey
Hackensak, New Jersey

Donald J. Cally, M.D.
Consultant
Spine Service

NYU–HJD Department of Orthopaedic Surgery
New York, New York
and
Attending Orthopaedic Surgeon
Albany Memorial Hospital
Albany, New York

Gail S. Chorney, M.D.
Associate Chief
Pediatric Orthopaedic Surgery
NYU-HJD Department of Orthopaedic Surgery
New York, New York
and
Assistant Professor of Orthopaedic Surgery
New York University School of Medicine
New York, New York

Matthew S. Coons, M.D.
Consultant, Hand Service
NYU–HJD Department of Orthopaedic Surgery
New York, New York
and
Attending Orthopaedic Surgeon
West Hudson Hospital
Kearny, New Jersey

Frances Cuomo, M.D.
Chief, Shoulder Service
NYU-HJD Department of Orthopaedic Surgery
New York, New York
and
Associate Professor of Orthopaedic Surgery
New York University School of Medicine
New York, New York

Allan J. Dayan, M.D.
Attending Orthopaedic Surgeon
NYU-HJD Department of Orthopaedic Surgery
New York, New York
and
Clinical Instructor in Orthopaedic Surgery,
New York University School of Medicine
New York, New York

Paul E. Di Cesare, M.D., F.A.C.S.
Director, Musculoskeletal Research Center
NYU-HJD Department of Orthopaedic Surgery
New York, New York
and
Assistant Professor of Orthopaedic Surgery
New York University School of Medicine
New York, New York

Werner K. Doyle, M.D.
Attending Neurosurgeon
Department of Functional and Stereotactic Neurosurgery
The Hospital for Joint Diseases
New York, New York
and
Assistant Professor of Clinical Neurosurgery
New York University School of Medicine
New York, New York

Yosef Eidelman, M.D.[†]
Attending Surgeon
Department of Plastic and Reconstructive Surgery
Jacobi Medical Center
Bronx, New York
and
Instructor in Surgery
New York University School of Medicine
New York, New York
[†]deceased

Stephen J. Eshman, M.D., F.A.C.S.
Consultant, Hand Service
NYU–HJD Department of Orthopaedic Surgery
New York, New York
and
Attending Orthopaedic Surgeon
Arlington Hospital
Arlington, Virginia

David S. Feldman, M.D.
Chief, Pediatric Orthopaedics Service
NYU-HJD Department of Orthopaedic Surgery
New York, New York
and
Assistant Professor of Orthopaedic Surgery
New York University School of Medicine
New York, New York

Jo Ellen Finkel, M.D.
Department of Radiology
The Hospital for Joint Diseases
New York, New York
and
Assistant Professor of Clinical Radiology
New York University School of Medicine
New York, New York

Victor H. Frankel, KNO, M.D., Ph.D.
President
The Hospital for Joint Diseases
New York University Medical Center
New York, New York
and
Professor of Orthopaedic Surgery
New York University School of Medicine
New York, New York

Sally R. Frenkel, Ph.D.
Research Scientist
Coordinator, Chondrocyte Transplantation Laboratory
Musculoskeletal Research Center
NYU-HJD Department of Orthopaedic Surgery
New York, New York
and
Assistant Research Professor of Orthopaedic Surgery and Cell
  Biology
New York University School of Medicine
New York, New York

Gerard J. Girasole, M.D.
Consultant
Spine Service

NYU-HJD Department of Orthopaedic Surgery
New York, New York
and
Attending Orthopaedic Surgeon
Saint Vincent's Medical Center
Bridgeport, Connecticut

Vladimir Golyakhovsky, M.D., Ph.D.

Attending Orthopaedic Surgeon
NYU-HJD Department of Orthopaedic Surgery
New York, New York
and
Associate Professor of Orthopaedic Surgery
New York University School of Medicine
New York, New York

Alfred D. Grant, M.D.

Director
Center for Neuromuscular and Developmental Disorders
and
Director
New York Ilizarov Center for Limb Lengthening and
Reconstruction
NYU-HJD Department of Orthopaedic Surgery
New York, New York
and
Clinical Professor of Orthopaedic Surgery
New York University School of Medicine
New York, New York

Steven M. Green, M.D.

Associate Chief
Hand Service
NYU-HJD Department of Orthopaedic Surgery
New York, New York
and
Clinical Associate Professor of Orthopaedic Surgery
New York University School of Medicine
New York, New York

John C. Grew, Ph.D.

Consultant
Musculoskeletal Research Center
NYU-HJD Department of Orthopaedic Surgery
New York, New York
and
Assistant Professor
Department of Biology
New Jersey City University
Jersey City, New Jersey

Stephane Grijseels, M.D.

Consultant
Department of Radiology
The Hospital for Joint Diseases
New York, New York
and
Department of Radiology
University of Missippi Medical Center
Jackson, Mississippi

Paul Gusmorino, M.D.

Medical Director
The Pain Center

The Hospital for Joint Diseases
New York, New York
and
Clinical Assistant Professor of Psychiatry
New York University School of Medicine
New York, New York

Kathleen A. Haines, M.D.

Director
Pediatric Rheumatology
The Hospital for Joint Diseases
New York, New York
and
Associate Professor of Clinical Pediatrics and Medicine
New York University School of Medicine
New York, New York

Brian Hainline, M.D.

Attending Neurologist
Department of Neurosciences
The Hospital for Joint Diseases
New York, New York
and
Clinical Associate Professor of Neurology
New York University School of Medicine
New York, New York

Andrew Harrison, M.D.

Consultant
Sports Medicine Service
NYU-HJD Department of Orthopaedic Surgery
New York, New York
and
Director
Central New Jersey Sports Medicine and Orthopaedic Center
Lakewood, New Jersey

Rudi N. Hiebert, B.Sc.

Research Associate and Interim Director
Epidemiology Unit
NYU-HJD Department of Orthopaedic Surgery
New York, New York

Christina M. Hift, M.D.

Infectious Disease Consultant
Pediatric Rheumatology Consultant
The Hospital for Joint Diseases
New York, New York
and
Clinical Assistant Professor of Pediatrics
Albert Einstein College of Medicine
Bronx, New York

Neal L. Hochwald, M.D.

Consultant
Hand Service
NYU-HJD Department of Orthopaedic Surgery
New York, New York
and
Attending Orthopaedic Surgeon
Huntington Hospital
Huntington, New York

John T. Hughes, M.D.
Attending Neurologist
Department of Neurosciences
The Hospital for Joint Diseases
New York, New York
and
Director
Department of Neurology
Our Lady of Mercy Medical Center
Bronx, New York
and
Assistant Professor of Neurology
New York University School of Medicine
New York, New York

Samuel Kenan, M.D.
Chief
Orthopaedic Oncology Service
NYU-HJD Department of Orthopaedic Surgery
New York, New York
and
Professor of Clinical Orthopaedics
New York University School of Medicine
New York, New York

William L. King, M.D.
Attending Orthopaedic Surgeon
Hand Service
NYU-HJD Department of Orthopaedic Surgery
New York, New York
and
Clinical Instructor in Orthopaedic Surgery
New York University School of Medicine
New York, New York

Kenneth J. Koval, M.D.
Chief
Fracture Service
NYU-HJD Department of Orthopaedic Surgery
New York, New York
and
Associate Professor of Orthopaedic Surgery
New York University School of Medicine
New York, New York

Paul L. Kuflik, M.D.
Attending Orthopaedic Surgeon
NYU-HJD Department of Orthopaedic Surgery
New York, New York
and
Attending Orthopaedic Surgeon
Beth Israel Medical Center
New York, New York

Frederick J. Kummer, Ph.D.
Associate Director
Musculoskeletal Research Center
NYU-HJD Department of Orthopaedic Surgery
New York, New York

and
Research Professor of Orthopaedic Surgery
New York University School of Medicine
New York, New York

Wallace B. Lehman, M.D., F.A.C.S.
Chief
Pediatric Orthopaedic Surgery
NYU-HJD Department of Orthopaedic Surgery
New York, New York
and
Professor of Clinical Orthopaedic Surgery
New York University School of Medicine
New York, New York

Salvatore Robert Lenzo, M.D.
Attending Orthopaedic Surgeon
Hand Service
NYU-HJD Department of Orthopaedic Surgery
New York, New York
and
Clinical Assistant Professor of Orthopaedic Surgery
New York University School of Medicine
New York, New York

Lynn J. Letko, M.D.
Consultant
Spine Service
NYU-HJD Department of Orthopaedic Surgery
New York, New York
and
Attending Orthopaedic Surgeon
Princeton Medical Center
Princeton New Jersey

Jess H. Lonner, M.D.
Consultant
Foot and Ankle Service
Consultant
Oncology Service
NYU-HJD Department of Orthopaedic Surgery
New York, New York
and
Attending Orthopaedic Surgeon
PENN Orthopaedic Institute
Philadelphia, Pennsylvania
and
Assistant Professor of Orthopaedic Surgery
University of Pennsylvania School of Medicine
Philadelphia, Pennsylvania

Howard J. Luks, M.D.
Consultant, Sports Medicine Service
NYU-HJD Department of Orthopaedic Surgery
New York, New York
and
Chief of Sports Medicine and Arthroscopy
Department of Orthopaedic Surgery
Westchester County Medical Center
Valhalla, New York

and
Instructor
New York Medical College
Valhalla, New York

Patrick A. Meere, M.D., F.R.C.S. (C)
Attending Orthopaedic Surgeon
NYU-HJD Department of Orthopaedic Surgery
New York, New York
and
Chairman, Department of Orthopaedic Surgery
The Brooklyn Hospital Center
Brooklyn, New York
and
Clinical Assistant Professor of Orthopaedic Surgery
New York University School of Medicine
New York, New York

David S. Menche, M.D.
Attending Orthopaedic Surgeon
Sports Medicine Service
The Hospital for Joint Diseases
New York, New York
and
Assistant Professor of Clinical Orthopaedic Surgery
New York University School of Medicine
New York, New York

John W. Michael, M.Ed., C.P.O., F.A.A.O.P., F.I.S.P.O
Director of Technical and Professional Services
Otto Bock USA
and
Instructor, Century College
Minneapolis, Minnesota
and
Prosthetic-Orthotic Consultant
Northwestern University Prosthetic Orthotic Center
Chicago, Illinois
and
University of Texas Health Science Center
Dallas, Texas
and
California State University
Dominguez Hills, California

Ellen S. Moran, M.S.
Genetic Counselor, Center for Neuromuscular and Developmental
   Disorders
NYU-HJD Department of Orthopaedic Surgery
New York, New York

Ronald Moskovich, M.D., F.R.C.S.
Associate Chief, Spine Service
NYU-HJD Department of Orthopaedic Surgery
New York, New York
and
Assistant Professor of Orthopaedic Surgery
New York University School of Medicine
New York, New York

Michael G. Neuwirth, M.D.
Attending Orthopaedic Surgeon
NYU-HJD Department of Orthopaedic Surgery
New York, New York
and
Attending Orthopaedic Surgeon
Beth Israel Medical Center
New York, New York

Nissim Ohana, M.D.
Consultant, Spine Service
NYU-HJD Department of Orthopaedic Surgery
New York, New York
and
Clinical Instructor in Orthopaedic Surgery
Ben Gurion University Medical School
Beersheva, Israel

Jennifer O'Sulllivan Pogue, M.D.
Consultant, Hand Service
NYU-HJD Department of Orthopaedic Surgery
New York, New York
and
Staff Physician
Stamford Hospital
Stamford, Connecticut

Nader Paksima, D.O.
Attending Orthopaedic Surgeon, Hand Service
NYU-HJD Department of Orthopaedic Surgery
New York, New York
and
Director of Upper Extremity, Hand, and Microvascular Surgery
Jamaica Hospital Medical Center
Jamaica, New York

Francis Rockland Pelham, M.D.
Attending Surgeon, Hand Service
NYU-HJD Department of Orthopaedic Surgery
New York, New York
and
Clinical Instructor of Plastic and Reconstructive Surgery
The Albert Einstein College of Medicine
Bronx, New York

Geoffrey I. Phillips, M.D.
Consultant, Sports Medicine Service
NYU-HJD Department of Orthopaedic Surgery
New York, New York
and
Associate Physician
Department of Orthopaedic Surgery
Kaiser Permanente
Walnut Creek, California

Mark I. Pitman, M.D.
Chief, Sports Medicine Service
NYU-HJD Department of Orthopaedic Surgery
New York, New York
and

Clinical Associate Professor of Orthopaedic Surgery
New York University School of Medicine
New York, New York

Martin A. Posner, M.D.
Chief, Hand Service
NYU-HJD Department of Orthopaedic Surgery
New York, New York
and
Clinical Professor of Orthopaedic Surgery
New York University School of Medicine
New York, New York

Paula J. Rackoff, M.D.
Attending Rheumatologist
Beth Israel Medical Center
New York, New York

Kamshad Raiszadeh, M.D.
Consultant, Spine Service
NYU-HJD Department of Orthopaedic Surgery
New York, New York
and
Attending Orthopaedic Surgeon
Sharp Memorial Hospital
San Diego, California
and
Clinical Instructor
Department of Orthopaedic Surgery
University of California
San Diego School Medicine
San Diego, California

John L. Ricci, Ph.D.
Consultant, Musculoskeletal Research Center
NYU-HJD Department of Orthopaedic Surgery
New York, New York
and
Associate Professor
Department of Orthopaedics
University of Medicine and Dentistry of New Jersey—New Jersey
  Medical School
Newark, New Jersey

Andrew S. Rokito, M.D.
Assistant Chief, Shoulder Service
Associate Chief, Sports Medicine Service
NYU-HJD Department of Orthopaedic Surgery
New York, New York
and
Assistant Professor of Orthopaedic Surgery
New York University School of Medicine
New York, New York

William N. Rom, M.D., M.P.H.
Director, Division of Pulmonary and Critical Care Medicine
Department of Medicine
New York University Medical Center
New York, New York
and
Professor of Medicine and Environmental Medicine

New York University School of Medicine
New York, New York

Andrew D. Rosenberg, M.D.
Vice Chairman, Department of Anesthesiology
The Hospital for Joint Diseases
New York, New York
and
Associate Professor of Clinical Anesthesiology
New York University School of Medicine
New York, New York

Zehava Sadka Rosenberg, M.D.
Department of Radiology
The Hospital for Joint Diseases
New York, New York
and
Associate Professor of Clinical Radiology
New York University School of Medicine
New York, New York

Jose Santiago Figueroa, M.D.
Consultant, Hand Service
NYU-HJD Department of Orthopaedic Surgery
New York, New York
and
Chief, Hand Service
San Juan City Hospital
Puerto Rico Medical Center
San Juan, Puerto Rico
and
Professor of Orthopaedics Ad Honorem
University of Puerto Rico School of Medicine
San Juan, Puerto Rico

Myles Rubin Samotin, M.D.
Consultant, Foot and Ankle Service
NYU-HJD Department of Orthopaedic Surgery
New York, New York
and
Attending Orthopaedic Surgeon
Naples Community Hospital
Naples, Florida

Norman Y. Schoenberg, M.D.
Department of Radiology
Hospital for Joint Diseases
New York, New York
and
Assistant Professor of Clinical Radiology
New York University School of Medicine
New York, New York

Amaryllis J. Scott, M.D.
Consultant, Shoulder Service
NYU-HJD Department of Orthopaedic Surgery
New York, New York
and
Attending Orthopaedic Surgeon
Holy Family Hospital
Spokane, Washington

Steven Shankman, M.D.
Vice Chairman, Department of Radiology
The Hospital for Joint Diseases
New York, New York

Steven C. Sheskier, M.D.
Attending, Foot and Ankle Service
NYU-HJD Department of Orthopaedic Surgery
New York, New York

Lester Silver, M.D.
Attending, Hand Service
NYU-HJD Department of Orthopaedic Surgery
New York, New York
and
Chief, Division of Plastic Surgery
Mount Sinai Medical Center
New York, New York
and
Professor of Plastic Surgery
Mount Sinai School of Medicine
New York, New York

Jordan A. Simon, M.D.
Fellow, Musculoskeletal Research Center
NYU-HJD Department of Orthopaedic Surgery
New York, New York

Mary Louise Skovron, Ph.D.
Consultant, Epidemiology Unit
NYU-HJD Department of Orthopaedic Surgery
New York, New York
and
Adjunct Assistant Professor of Environmental Medicine
New York University School of Medicine
New York, New York

Mark F. Sloane, M.D.
Attending, Division of Pulmonary and Critical Care
Department of Medicine
New York University Medical Center
New York, New York
and
Clinical Assistant Professor of Medicine
New York University School of Medicine
New York, New York

Jeffrey M. Spivak, M.D.
Director, Spine Center
NYU-HJD Department of Orthopaedic Surgery
New York, New York
and
Assistant Professor of Orthopaedic Surgery
New York University School of Medicine
New York, New York

David J. Steiger, M.D.
Director, Intensive Care Unit
The Hospital for Joint Diseases
New York, New York
and
Assistant Professor of Medicine
New York University School of Medicine
New York, New York

Linda Stehling, M.D.
Medical Consultant
Scottsdale, Arizona

German C. Steiner, M.D.
Chairman, Department of Pathology and Laboratory Medicine
Hospital for Joint Diseases
New York, New York
and
Professor of Surgical Pathology
New York University School of Medicine
New York, New York

Steven A. Stuchin, M.D.
Director, Orthopaedic Surgery Services
Assistant Chief, Hand Service
NYU-HJD Department of Orthopaedic Surgery
New York, New York
and
Associate Professor of Clinical Orthopaedic Surgery
New York University School of Medicine
New York, New York

Brian C. Toolan, M.D.
Consultant, Foot and Ankle Service
Consultant, Oncology Service
NYU-HJD Department of Orthopaedic Surgery
New York, New York
and
Attending Orthopaedic Surgeon
Section of Orthopaedic Surgery and Rehabilitative Medicine
Department of Surgery
The University of Chicago Medical Center
Chicago, Illinois
and
Assistant Professor of Orthopaedic Surgery
The University of Chicago School of Medicine
Chicago, Illinois

Stanley Wallach, M.D.
Director, Endocrinology and the Osteoporosis Center
The Hospital for Joint Diseases
New York, New York
and
Clincial Professor of Medicine
New York University School of Medicine
New York, New York

Daniel W. Wilen, M.D.
Attending Orthopaedic Surgeon
NYU-HJD Department of Orthopaedic Surgery
New York, New York

Jamie R. Wisser, M.D.
Attending Orthopaedic Surgeon, Hand Service
NYU-HJD Department of Orthopaedic Surgery
New York, New York

Daniel S. Zapson, M.D.
Consultant, Sports Medicine Service
NYU-HJD Department of Orthopaedic Surgery
New York, New York
and
Staff Physician

Fallon Clinic
Worcester, Massachusetts

Joseph D. Zuckerman, M.D.
Chairman
NYU-HJD Department of Orthopaedic Surgery
New York, New York
and
Walter A.L. Thompson Professor of Orthopaedic Surgery
New York University School of Medicine
New York, New York

Numerous general texts of orthopaedic surgery and musculoskeletal medicine already exist. One may ask then, why another?

Of the existing textbooks, many are large multivolume tomes providing extensive detail and far-reaching discussion. Readers seeking a basic and tightly structured understanding of orthopaedics must be prepared to spend time searching and sifting through copious amounts of information. At the very least, these texts are problematic as review guides. The second type of orthopaedic text is extremely condensed, written almost completely in outline form. These books assume significant prior knowledge on the part of the reader; the dense concentration of facts and relative lack of explanatory information can obscure supportive concepts and create ambiguity, particularly for those topics with which the reader is most unfamiliar.

Our general text was conceived to fill the void between these two textbook formats. As such, the editors have strived to create a structured text basic and descriptive enough to be used as a learning guide for medical students and residents, and concise and comprehensive enough for residents, fellows, and attendings to use for review of specific topics or musculoskeletal medicine in general. The book will also serve as a useful reference for nonorthopaedists involved in musculoskeletal medicine, including rheumatologists, internists, neurologists, physiatrists, chiropractic physicians, and physical therapists.

This book is divided into six parts. Part I deals with the basic scientific processes of orthopaedics, both biological and biomechanical. Parts II and III describe the anatomy, surgical approaches, and physical exam of the musculoskeletal system, using a regional anatomic approach. Part IV details the various methods of diagnostic testing for dysfunction of the musculoskeletal system. Part V, the bulk of the book, deals with clinical orthopaedic disorders, including neoplastic, degenerative, traumatic, and infectious conditions. Subspecialties such as oncology, spine, sports medicine, hand, foot and ankle, and pediatric orthopaedics are grouped separately. A full section on orthopaedic rehabilitation is included as well. Part VI includes related topics such as rheumatology, metabolic bone disease, pain management, and medical considerations in the orthopaedic patient.

Just as the fields of musculoskeletal medicine and orthopaedic surgery have become subspecialized, the 90 author-contributors to this book reflect expert subspecialists in their respective fields. While the majority may be orthopaedic surgeons, the authors also include experts in the fields of basic science, bioengineering, prosthetics and orthotics, orthopaedic radiology, neurology, rheumatology, critical care, pain management, and epidemiology. All of the authors are currently affiliated with the Hospital for Joint Diseases Orthopaedic Institute or were affiliated at some point during their training or career.

ACKNOWLEDGMENTS

A text of this size and complexity cannot be completed without the help of many additional nonauthor contributors. These are the true "unsung heroes" of this book, and deserve our acknowledgments and sincere thanks.

Members of the resident staff assisted in the preparation of manuscripts for a number of the authors. We thank them all, including Michael C. Schwartz, M.D., a senior resident instrumental in assisting D. S. Menche, M.D., in his chapters.

Library assistance, critical for most texts, was provided by both Arthur Strange at New York University and especially Claudia Lascar at the Hospital for Joint Diseases. Excellent photographic work was provided by Frank J. Martucci and his assistant Duane E. Harris.

A special thanks to our artist, Hugh Nachamie, who spent much extra time for little in return, seemingly thriving on the satisfaction of a job well done. We also acknowledge the efforts of his assistant, Elliot Friedman.

Technical assistance, including electronic file manipulation, computer scanning, and some editorial work was provided by William S. Green, who deserves our appreciation and thanks.

Special recognition is due to Baynon McDowell, our Hospital for Joint Diseases–based assistant in the Department of Orthopaedic Surgery. Coordinating a large, multicontributor effort such as this text is clearly a full-time job. It was accomplished with apparent ease by Baynon due to her extraordinary organizational abilities, attention to detail, and dedication to the entire project. Large problems were never insurmountable, and minor problems were never too insignificant. This book could not have been completed without her skill and effort.

ORTHOPAEDICS
A Study Guide

Chapter 1

MUSCULOSKELETAL EMBRYOLOGY

Sally R. Frenkel

The skeletal system develops from the mesodermal germ layer, arising from embryonic connective tissue, or mesenchyme. Mesenchymal cells are pluripotent; that is, they may differentiate along any of several different pathways, and form fibroblasts, chondroblasts, or osteoblasts.

DEVELOPMENT OF BONE AND CARTILAGE

Most bones first appear as condensations of mesenchymal cells that form hyaline cartilage templates (Fig. 1-1). These templates become ossified by endochondral ossification. Some bones develop in mesenchyme by intramembranous bone formation without a cartilaginous stage. Condensations of mesenchyme are apparent in embryos of approximately five weeks of age. The mesenchymal cells proliferate and differentiate, and are referred to as chondroblasts. They deposit collagen or elastic fibers in the matrix, the organic intercellular substance. Three types of cartilage are produced: hyaline, elastic, and fibrocartilage. Hyaline cartilage is the type found at articular surfaces. Elastic cartilage provides flexible support to the external ear and parts of the larynx. Fibrocartilage is a component of menisci and intervertebral discs.

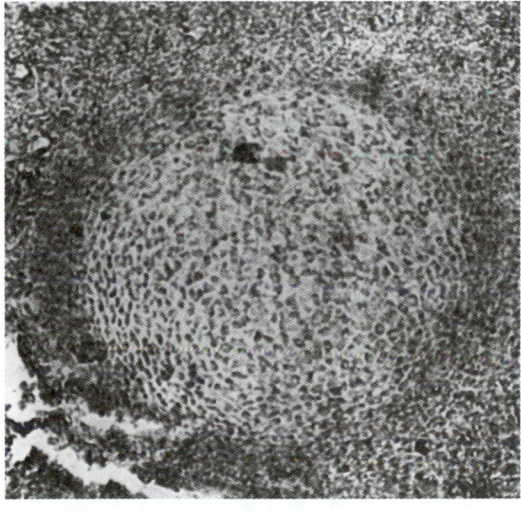

A

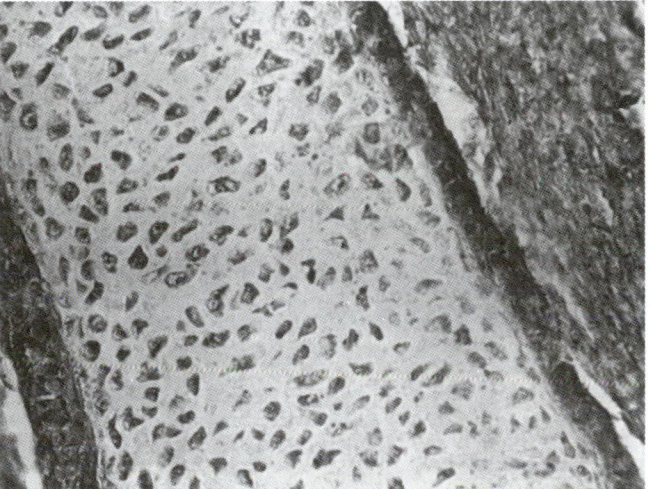

B

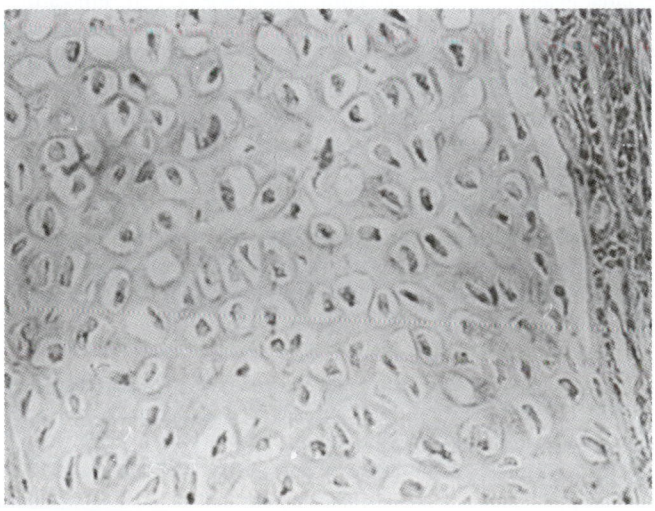

C

Figure 1-1
Photomicrograph showing early bone development in a chick embryo. ×100, immunoperoxidase stain. *A.* Mesenchymal condensation appears on day 6. *B.* By day 7.5, chondrogenic cells have elongated to form the anlage of the future bone. *C.* On day 9, lacunae are visible surrounding the maturing cells.

1

INTRAMEMBRANOUS OSSIFICATION

This type of bone formation occurs in mesenchyme, without an intervening cartilage primordium. The mesenchyme is invaded by vasculature; subsequently, some cells differentiate into osteoblasts and deposit osteoid, a "prebone" tissue. Osteoblasts then secrete calcium phosphate into the osteoid. Osteoblasts become encased in the calcifying matrix; mature cells are termed osteocytes.

Newly formed bone is arranged in thin splinters or spicules. The spicules organize into lamellae, or layers. Concentric lamellae are organized around blood vessels, forming Haversian systems, or osteons. New layers continue to be added, forming plates of compact bone on the surfaces. Between the plates, remaining spicules are called spongy bone. Between spongy bone spicules, the mesenchyme differentiates into bone marrow. A population of cells known as osteoclasts absorb bone. Throughout life, bone is continually remodeled, as osteoclasts resorb bone while osteoblasts deposit new bone. The rate of new bone formation slows with aging.

Ossification in the embryo relies on the maternal supply of calcium and phosphorus. Pregnant women are advised to maintain adequate intake of these elements in order to preserve their own bones and teeth; otherwise the mineral reserves will be used by the developing embryonic skeleton.

ENDOCHONDRAL OSSIFICATION

This type of bone formation occurs via the ossification of a cartilaginous template. In a long bone a primary ossification center appears in the diaphysis, or shaft. The chondrocytes at this site hypertrophy, the matrix becomes invested with calcium phosphate, and the cells die. The perichondrium surrounding the diaphysis is converted to a periosteum, as a thin layer of bone is deposited. Invasion of blood vessels into the bone contributes to the breakdown of the cartilage. Cells migrating with the vasculature differentiate into bone marrow with its blood-forming precursor cells, or into osteoblasts that deposit bone matrix on the spicules of calcified cartilage. From the primary ossification center, this process continues outward toward the epiphyses, or ends of the bone.

Bone lengthening occurs at the diaphyseal-epiphyseal junction (Fig. 1-2). Although the diaphyses of most long bones are ossified to a large extent by the time of birth, most epiphyses are still cartilaginous.

Secondary ossification centers appear in the epiphyses during early childhood. The epiphyseal cartilage cells hypertrophy, with concurrent invasion of blood vessels. A narrow region termed the epiphyseal plate or growth plate remains cartilaginous until growth of the bone is fully completed, usually before the age of twenty.

The cartilaginous portion of the growth plate is divided into the reserve or resting zone, the proliferative zone, and the hypertrophic zone (Fig. 1-3). Cells in the reserve zone store lipids and other materials to serve as nutrients. The function of the proliferative zone, as the name implies, is proliferation and also production of matrix components. Proliferation of these cells results in longitudinal growth of bone. The very large cells of the hypertrophic zone are responsible for calcification of the matrix, ultimately resulting in the conversion of cartilage to bone.

Deposition of bone at the periosteal surface and absorption on the medullary (marrow cavity) surface causes an increase in the thickness of the bone. This remodeling of bone continues throughout adulthood.

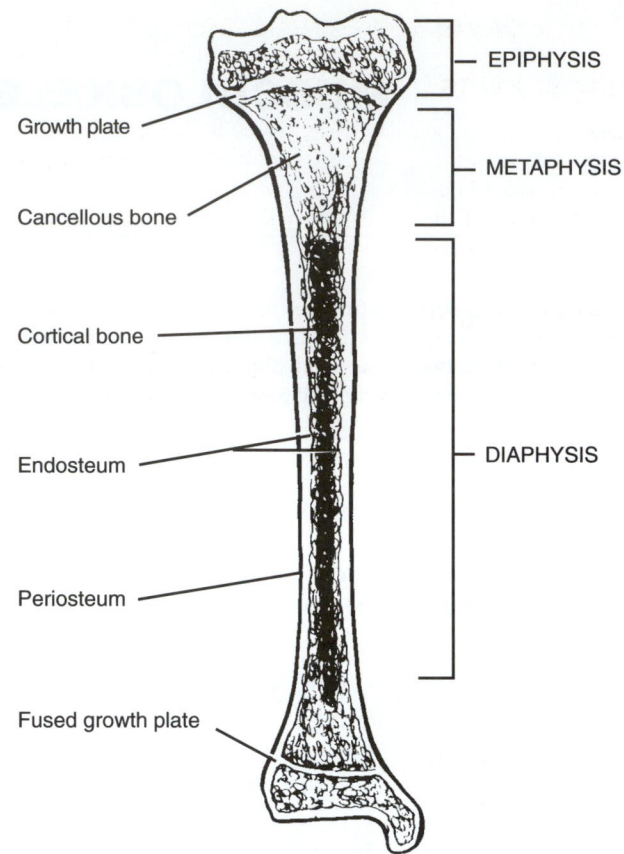

Figure 1-2
Schematic diagram of a tibia. The interior of a typical long bone showing the growing proximal end with a growth plate and a distal end with the epiphysis fused to the metaphysis. [Reproduced and modified with permission from Jee WSS: The skeletal tissues. In Weiss L (ed): *Histology*, 5th ed. New York: Elsevier Biomedical; 1983. © 1992, Leon Weiss, M.D.]

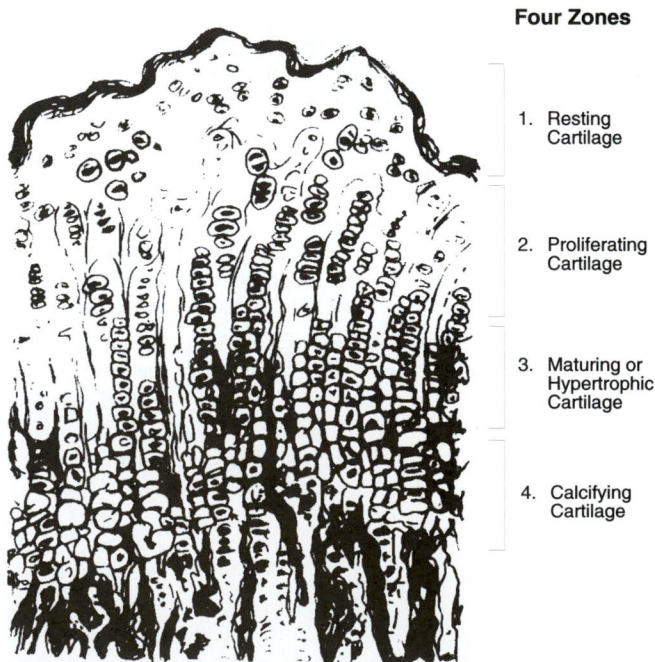

Figure 1-3
Illustration of epiphyseal plate. Four zones associated with endochondral ossification are highlighted.

DEVELOPMENT OF JOINTS

SYNOVIAL JOINTS

Mesenchyme between the developing bones differentiates into the intraarticular ligaments and joint capsule. It also forms the synovial membrane, which lines and secretes lubricant for the articular cartilage at the ends of the bones and lines the joint capsule interior. Examples of this type of joint are the knee and elbow.

CARTILAGINOUS JOINTS

The mesenchyme between the developing bones differentiates into hyaline cartilage, such as in the costochondral joints; or fibrocartilage, as with the symphysis pubis. Hyaline cartilage caps the bones of the joint.

FIBROUS JOINTS

The mesenchyme between the bones differentiates into dense fibrous connective tissue, as is found in the sutures of the skull.

THE AXIAL SKELETON

The axial skeleton includes the vertebral column, the twelve pairs of ribs, the sternum, and the skull.

DEVELOPMENT OF THE VERTEBRAL COLUMN

The embryonic structure that will form the future spinal cord is the neural tube. Adjacent to the notochord and neural tube, two columns of mesoderm form. The segmental somites arise from these mesodermal columns, beginning at about 20 days of embryonic development. Each somite is composed of mesenchymal cells, and differentiates into two structures, the sclerotome and the dermatomyotome. Sclerotomal cells will surround the notochord and the neural tube, and form the primordia of the vertebrae and the ribs. Mesenchyme surrounding the neural tube will form the vertebral arch, while cells surrounding the notochord form the centrum and, later, the body of the vertebrae. This "surrounding" is not strictly due to migration of cells around the neural structures, but is rather the result of their changing positions relative to each other as growth and elongation of the embryo continues. Cells of the sclerotome give rise to ligaments associated with the vertebral column, as well as to the intervertebral discs. The dermatomyotome gives rise to the dermis of the skin and to the dorsal musculature.

The somites that will form the vertebrae are segmental structures; the pathway of the spinal nerves that emerge from the spinal cord to innervate peripheral structures would therefore be blocked by the developing vertebrae. To avoid this, the somite becomes divided in half, at the potential point through which the nerve must pass. The inferior half of one somite will subsequently fuse with the superior half of its caudal neighbor. The vertebrae are thus formed by parts of two adjacent vertebrae (Fig. 1-4).

The notochord degenerates within the newly forming vertebral bodies. Between the vertebrae, notochord remnants give rise to the soft, gelatinous nucleus pulposus of the intervertebral disc, that will become surrounded by the tough, fibrous anulus fibrosus.

During the sixth week, the mesenchymal vertebrae begin differentiation into cartilaginous primordia. Ossification will follow during week 8, and continue through early adulthood.

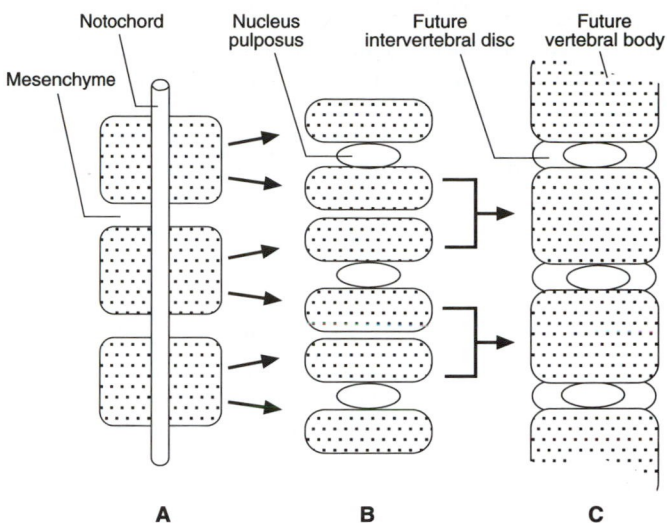

Figure 1-4
Development of vertebral column at different stages. *A.* At week 4, sclerotomic segments are divided by intersegmental tissue. *B.* Caudal aspect of one sclerotome intrudes into the intersegmental mesenchyme and fuses with the cranial half of the sclerotome below (*see arrows in A, B*). *C.* The vertebral bodies are made of the upper and lower aspects of two adjacent sclerotomes plus the intersegmental tissue.

The halves of the vertebral arch fuse by age five. At approximately the time of puberty, secondary ossification centers appear; these centers fuse with the rest of the vertebra at about 25 years.

The normal complement of vertebrae includes seven cervical, twelve thoracic, five lumbar, and five sacral vertebrae. An extra or absent vertebra in one segment of the column may be compensated for by an absent or extra vertebra in an adjacent segment; for example, eleven thoracic vertebrae with six lumbar vertebrae.

DEVELOPMENT OF RIBS AND STERNUM

The ribs develop from small processes on the thoracic vertebrae, referred to as costal processes. Two sternal bands develop in the body wall, independently of the developing ribs. These bands become cartilaginous, and become attached to the first six costal cartilages. The plates fuse in the midline to form the manubrium, body, and xiphoid process. Centers of ossification appear before birth. The center for the xiphoid process appears during childhood.

MALFORMATIONS OF THE AXIAL SKELETON

Klippel-Feil Syndrome

This syndrome is also known as brevicollis. It is characterized by short neck, low hairline, and limited neck movements. The syndrome is characterized radiographically by one or more block vertebrae (failure of segmentation) resulting in the short neck and limited motion. Klippel-Feil syndrome may be associated with other congenital anomalies, as well as vertebral anomalies in the other regions of the spine.

Spina Bifida

This condition results from failure of fusion of the vertebral arch. One or several vertebrae may be affected. The meninges and/or the spinal cord may herniate through the vertebral defect, with possible severe neurological symptoms. A fairly benign variety of this condition is spina bifida occulta, in which the patient is asymptomatic. The skin over the spinal defect is normal, and the only evidence (other than radiographic) may be a dimple or tuft of hair overlying the defective vertebra.

Spina bifida is associated with a deficiency of folic acid in the maternal diet. It can be diagnosed during pregnancy by means of amniocentesis. A fetus with spina bifida will cause an elevated level of alpha-fetoprotein in the amniotic fluid. Recently, a test for alpha-fetoprotein in maternal serum has been developed.

Accessory Ribs

An extra rib in the lumbar region is the most common type, and causes no symptoms. However, a cervical rib, which is attached to the seventh cervical vertebra, may compress the brachial plexus or the subclavian vessels, resulting in thoracic outlet syndrome (Fig. 1-5*A*).

Congenital Scoliosis

Anomalies in vertebral development cause congenital scoliosis. These anomalies may be classified as failures of formation or failures of segmentation. Failure of appearance of one of the chondrification centers in the vertebra and subsequent failure of half of the vertebra to form results in a hemivertebra; if there is a partial failure of formation, the result is a wedge vertebra (Fig. 1-5*B*). Failures of segmentation may be unilateral or bilateral. Unilateral failure of segmentation causes the formation of an unsegmented bar, which has no growth potential; the opposite side therefore produces a progressive curve. If the failure of segmentation is bilateral, the result is a block vertebra (Fig. 1-6).

Skull Malformations

These abnormalities may be minor, or major and life-threatening. With large defects, there is often herniation of the meninges and/or

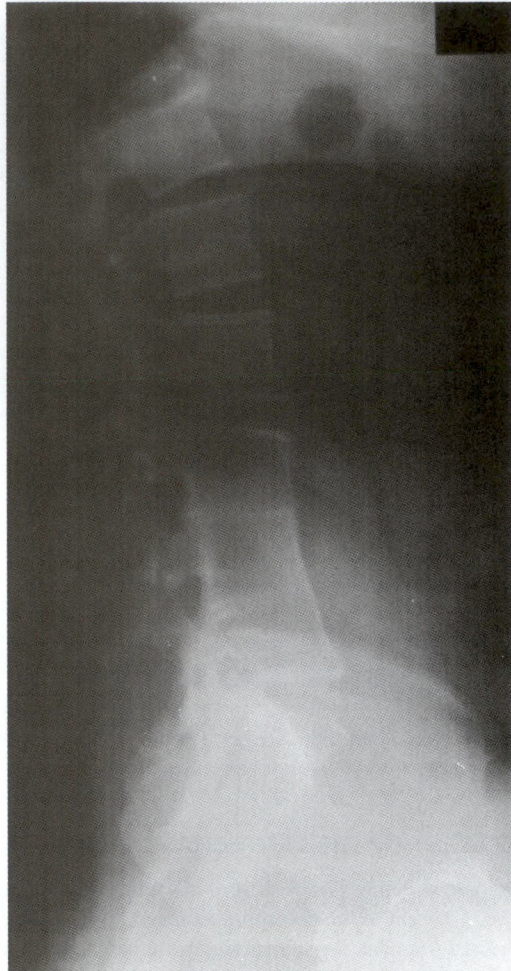

Figure 1-6
Radiograph, block vertebrae—L3–L5.

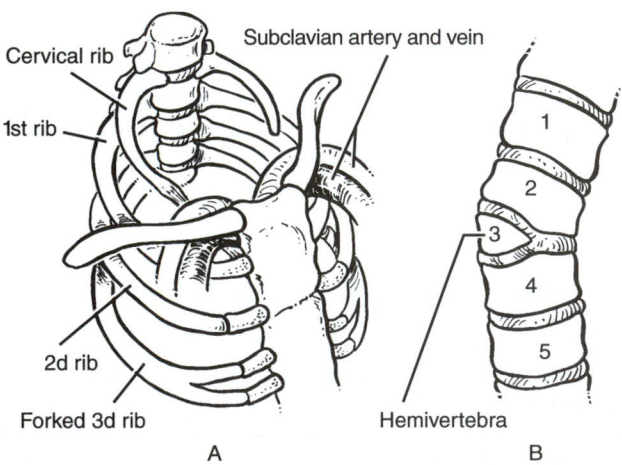

A   B

Figure 1-5
Drawings of vertebral and rib abnormalities. *A*. Cervical and forked ribs. Observe that the left cervical rib has a fibrous band passing posterior to the subclavian vessels and attaching to the sternum. It is very likely that this condition produced neurovascular changes in the left upper limb. *B*. Anterior view of the vertebral column showing a hemivertebra (half vertebra). The right half of the third thoracic vertebra is absent. Note the associated lateral curvature, or scoliosis, of the vertebral column (spine). (Reproduced with permission from Moore, KL: The articular and skeletal systems. In: *The Developing Human,* 5th ed. Philadelphia: Saunders, 1993:364.)

the brain. *Acrania* or *cranioschisis* is a nearly absent cranial vault; the brain is a mass of undifferentiated nervous tissue. This is often associated with major vertebral column defects.

LIMBS

Limbs arise as buds or outpocketings that become visible early in the fifth week of development. Each bud consists of a mesenchymal bar derived from the mesoderm, covered by a layer of ectoderm, the apical ectodermal ridge (AER). This ridge has an inductive influence on the underlying mesenchyme. The section of the mesenchymal bar adjacent to the AER will form the bones and connective tissues of the limb; further away from the AER, cells will differentiate into cartilage and muscle. The most proximal portion of the future limb develops first, followed in order by the more distal parts, with the hands and feet the last to develop. The lower limb develops approximately two days later than the upper limb.

By the sixth week cartilage templates of the limb bones are recognizable. Primary ossification centers are present by week twelve of development, in the midshaft region of the future bone. Ossification proceeds toward the ends of the bone; the ends are referred to as the epiphyses. In the phalanges, only one end of the bone has a growth plate, or epiphyseal plate. In vertebrae there may be several primary and secondary centers of ossification. When the epiphyseal plates have ossified, no further longitudinal growth is possible. A growth plate located at the site of a tendon attachment is known as an apophysis; apophyses do not contribute to longitudinal bone growth.

During week 7, rotation of the limbs occurs. The upper limb rotates 90 degrees laterally so that the flexor muscles lie in the anterior compartment, and extensors lie on the lateral and posterior surface; the thumbs become lateral. The lower limb rotates in the opposite direction, 90 degrees medially. The big toe becomes medial; the extensors lie anteriorly and the flexors posteriorly.

At 16 weeks, the distal-most portion of the limb buds will form the hand and foot plates. These plates are separated from the rest of the limb by a circular constriction. Another constriction divides the rest of the limb into upper and lower parts, so that the parts of the future extremity become recognizable. To form the digits of the hand and foot, programmed cell death (apoptosis) must occur in the AER. The death of these cells separates the ridge into the five future fingers or toes. The development of each finger is now subject to induction by its own AER.

LIMB ANOMALIES

Amelia, Meromelia, and Micromelia

Amelia is the absence of an entire bone, or of an entire extremity. A less severe form of this disorder is *meromelia,* in which the hand or foot may develop, but is attached to the trunk by a small, defective bone. *Micromelia* is the occurrence of an abnormally short segment in a limb. Among the causes of such defects are teratogenic agents such as the drug thalidomide, formerly prescribed as a sleeping pill and antinauseant. An unusually high incidence of limb malformations (described above) occurring at the time thalidomide was introduced led to the discovery that its use in pregnant women caused missing or abnormal limbs, as well as other developmental defects. The drug was subsequently removed from the market. Thalidomide is currently being reexamined as a possible antirheumatic agent.

Polydactyly

Polydactyly is the presence of extra digits in the hands or feet. The extra digit may not have appropriate innervation, or may function normally. Extra digits usually occur bilaterally, while a missing digit more often affects one side only.

Syndactyly

Syndactyly is a condition that results when programmed cell death does not occur properly in the hands or feet. Some tissue may remain in between the digits, causing a "webbed" appearance or actual fusion of the adjacent digits.

Lobster Claw

Lobster claw occurs when there is an abnormal space between the second and fourth metacarpal bones. The third metacarpal and phalangeal bones are usually absent, and on either side of the missing finger the remaining two bones are fused, giving the hand a clawlike appearance.

Club Foot

Club foot deformity occurs when the sole of the foot turns inward, and the foot is adducted and plantar flexed. It occurs more frequently in males, and may be hereditary. A possible cause of this defect may be the position of the fetus's legs during pregnancy.

Developmental Dislocation of the Hip

Developmental dislocation of the hip (formerly known as congenital dislocation of the hip) occurs more frequently in females. This condition is the result of an underdevelopment of the acetabulum and head of the femur. It is frequently associated with breech delivery; it is possible that fetal development in the breech position may contribute to defective hip development.

SYSTEMIC SKELETAL ABNORMALITIES

ACHONDROPLASIA

Achondroplasia is caused by a disturbance of the endochondral ossification in the epiphyseal plates of the long bones, resulting in *dwarfism.* While the head is of normal size, upper and lower limbs are very short. Mental development is usually unaffected. The defect is in the epiphyseal proliferative zone; where chondrocyte proliferation is sharply decreased, and matrix production is consequently lessened as well. This results in decreased longitudinal growth. Formation of membranous bone is normal.

ACROMEGALY

Acromegaly is a disorder of the pituitary gland which affects skeletal development. This condition is caused by congenital hyperactivity of the pituitary, and causes enlargement of the face, hands, and feet. It may also result in an overall unusual growth of the body, known as giantism.

OSTEOPETROSIS

Osteopetrosis is also known as marble bone disease or Albers-Schönberg disease. It occurs when osteoclasts do not resorb bone. The growth plate is normal, but the calcified cartilage is not absorbed or removed. Some bone is laid down on the cartilage, but it fails to mature.

SUGGESTED READING

Carlson BM: *Human Embryology and Developmental Biology,* 2d ed. St. Louis: Mosby; 1998.

Moore KL, Persand TVN Shiota K: *Color Atlas of Clinical Embryology.* Philadelphia: Saunders; 1994.

Moore KL: *The Developing Human,* 5th ed. Philadelphia: Saunders; 1993.

Sadler TW: *Langman's Medical Embryology,* 7th ed. Baltimore: Williams & Wilkins; 1995.

Chapter 2

GENERAL JOINT ANATOMY AND PHYSIOLOGY

Paul E. Di Cesare

The human skeleton is connected by a variety of coaptations collectively known as arthroses or joints. Joints can be subclassified as either synovial (cavitated) or nonsynovial (solid; fibrous or cartilaginous). Examples of nonsynovial fibrous joints are the cranial junctions (sutures or suture joints) where bone is connected to bone by collagenous ligament that is continuous with the periosteum. Nonsynovial cartilaginous joints are either synchondroses or symphyses. Examples of synchondrodial joints include epiphyseal plates and the multiplex connections of the pelvis where bone is connected to bone by hyaline growth cartilage. These joints usually undergo bony union (synostosis) when developmental growth ceases. In symphysial joints, bones are connected to hyaline cartilage with intervening fibrocartilaginous discs and are represented by the symphyses pubis and vertebrae. In synovial or cavitated joints, motion is enhanced through connections between surfaces of endochondral bone, hyaline cartilage, synovial membranes, capsules and ligaments. Also known as diarthrodial joints, they are represented by joints such as the knee and hip and are further classified on the basis of their degrees of freedom of motion and shape.

Diarthrodial joints consist of subchondral bone that is lined by hyaline articular cartilage and enclosed by a strong fibrous capsule lined by synovial tissue. These two linings are bathed in synovial fluid and constitute the boundaries of the joint cavity. In some joints (e.g., knee) intraarticular meniscus (fibrocartilage) are also present and are important in load dispersion to the subchondral bone. The functions of the articular cartilage is to provide a lining that protects the subchondral bone, to more evenly distribute and transfer the mechanical forces to the subchondral bone, to provide for joint congruity, and to provide a low friction surface to facilitate movement of the joint. Under normal condition the articular cartilage has little wear despite seeing forces that may be 5 to 10 times the body weight.

DEVELOPMENT OF DIARTHRODIAL JOINTS

At an early stage of development, a condensed mesenchyme forms to separate the cartilaginous anlage of the bones on either side of the joint (Fig. 2-1). This is followed by the formation of small fluid-filled clefts that are the precursors of the synovial cavity. The clefts later join together to form the synovial cavity that is lined by the developing synovium and joint capsule. The articular cartilage is formed by a layer of cells at the end of the epiphyseal growth plate and it is not until closure of the growth plate at maturity that the fully differentiated structure is realized. The area of exposed cartilage to the synovium lacks a perichondrial layer on the joint surface and as a result can only undergo interstitial growth.

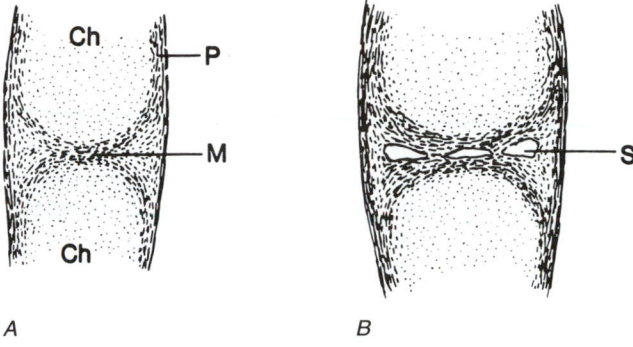

A   *B*

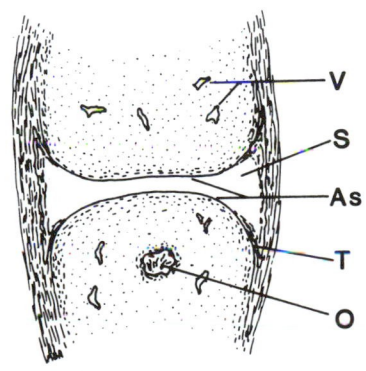

C

Figure 2-1

Sequence of changes during early development of a diarthrodial joint. (*A*) Two skeletal primordia in early stage of chondrogenesis (Ch), separated by intervening condensed mesenchyme (M), and surrounded by developing perichondrium (P). (*B*) Small clefts, precursors of the synovial cavity (S), have developed in the mesenchyme between the cartilaginous primordia. (*C*) Clefts have coalesced to form the synovial cavity (S), lined by developing synovium and surrounded by the developing joint capsule. The articular surfaces (As) are exposed, but at the peripheral transitional region (T), the cartilage is still covered by a perichondrium. Within the cartilaginous epiphyses are vascular canals (V) and an epiphyseal center of ossification (O) in early stage of formation. Note that the change in size of the diagrams does not accurately portray the extent of actual growth in the joint. [Reproduced with permission from Aydelotte MB, Kuettner KE: Heterogeneity of articular chondrocytes and cartilage matrix. In Woessner JF Jr., Howell DS (eds): *Joint Cartilage Degradation: Basic and Clinical Aspects* (Series editor: Furst DE). New York: Marcel Dekker; 1993:41.]

COMPOSITION

STRUCTURE

Articular cartilage is composed of chondrocytes interspersed within an extracellular matrix that makes up approximately 95 percent of the tissue by volume. The cartilage extracellular matrix is produced, organized, and maintained by the chondrocytes. Adult articular cartilage has been classified by a zonal organization based upon histological sections made perpendicular to the articular surface (Fig. 2-2). The descriptive classification uses subjective criteria such as collagen orientation, proteoglycan distribution, and chondrocyte organization at different depths from the articular surface. Zone I is the superficial zone that lies adjacent to the joint cavity and comprises approximately 5 to 10 percent of the matrix volume. It is characterized by uniform, tangentially aligned collagen fibers, discoidal chondrocytes, and low proteoglycan content. Zone II, the intermediate, transitional, or middle layer comprises 40 to 45 percent of the matrix volume. It is characterized by a network of obliquely oriented collagen fibrils, round or spherical cells, and a marked proteoglycan content. Zone III, the deep or radial layer, comprises 40 to 45 percent of the matrix volume. It is characterized by radially aligned collagen fibers, rounded cells often arranged in columns, and high proteoglycan content. Zone IV, the calcified cartilage layer, comprises 5 to 10 percent of the matrix volume. It is characterized by radial aligned collagen fibers, rounded chondrocytes within a calcified matrix, with high concentration of calcium salts and low to absent proteoglycans. The upper boundary of zone IV is the tidemark and the lower boundary the cement line that was formed during ossification of the growth plate at skeletal maturity. The tidemark is present on histological sections only after decalcification consists of proteins and lipids without proteoglycans. The tidemark is a relatively smooth, undulating interface that can vary with age or disease. The extracellular matrix in any zone in mature cartilage is also characterized as pericellular, territorial, or interterritorial matrices based upon its closeness to the chondrocytes. Each of these regions has a different biochemical composition. The pericellular matrix is a thin layer of proteoglycans and noncollagenous proteins that completely surrounds the chondrocytes. The territorial matrix is characterized by a thin layer of collagen fibrils arranged in a distinct fibrillar network that surrounds the pericellular matrix. The largest matrix region, the interterritorial matrix, consists of the matrix between the territorial matrices and contains large collagen fibrils and abundant proteoglycans.

Chondrocytes were once believed to exist in an empty space or lacuna. This has been clearly shown to be an artifact of routine fixation and staining for light microscopy. Instead, chondrocytes are now considered to exist as a chondron—the chondron being the chondrocyte, "lacuna" space, and "perilacunar" rim. The chondron is believed to be a true microanatomical unit of adult articular cartilage.

CHEMISTRY

The extracellular matrix of articular cartilage is assembled by specific molecular interactions to form a highly differentiated connective tissue matrix that is responsible for the tissue's biomechanical and physical properties. The main components of the extracellular matrix are collagens, proteoglycans, and noncollagenous proteins. The predominant collagen molecule of all hyaline cartilages is type II collagen, making up 95 percent of the total collagen weight. Its fibrils form a three-dimensional network that is stabilized by both covalent intra- and intermolecular crosslinks. Trifunctional hydroxypyridinium cross-links are a specific intermolecular crosslink that is prevalent in adult articular cartilage. The collagen fibrillar network acts both as a structural framework to provide mechanical support to the tissue and as a binding surface for molecules involved in mediating either matrix-matrix or cell-matrix interactions. There have been a number of cartilage disorders that have been linked to defects or deficiencies of type II collagen. These include achondrogenesis, type II achondrogenesis-hypochondrogenesis, spondyloepiphyseal dysplasia, Stickler syndrome, familial osteoarthritis with mild chondroplasia, and Kniest dysplasia. Cartilage also contains collagen types V, VI, IX, X, XI, XII, and XIV. Collagen IX comprises approximately 1 to 2 percent of the total collagen of adult articular cartilage and consists of three collagenous and four noncollagenous domains. Type IX collagen is localized on the surface of major collagen fibrils and is believed to limit fiber diameter, prevent fibril-fibril interactions, and may also mediate the connection of type II collagen to the matrix proteoglycans. Types V and XI (previously known as $1\alpha 2\alpha 3\alpha$)

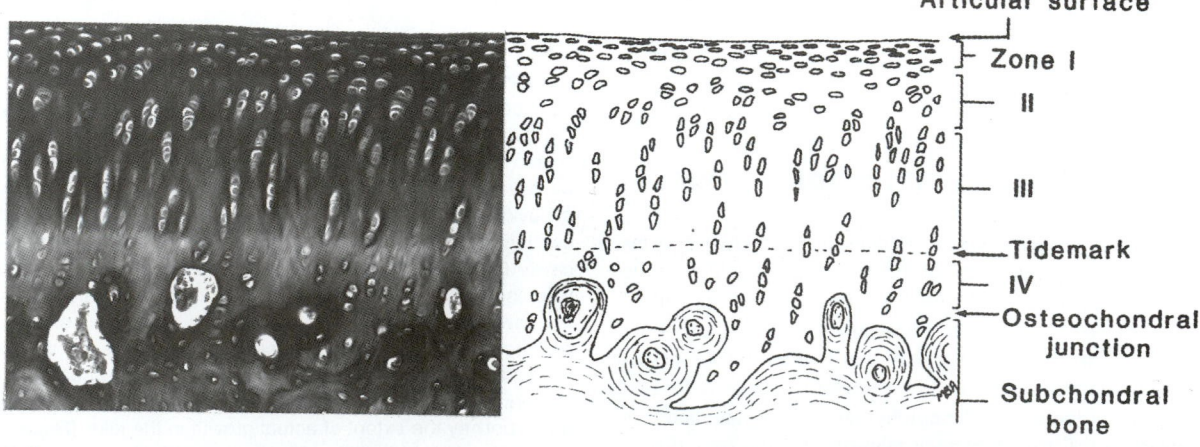

Figure 2-2
Vertical section through the articular cartilage and subchondral bone of canine femoral condyle, showing the four zones of the cartilage, the tidemark, osteochondral junction, and subchondral bone. These regions are also represented diagrammatically on right. (Section of canine femur, stained Mallory-Heidenham, x 170. Photo and illustration courtesy of J.M. Williams, Ph.D., Department of Anatomy, Rush-Presbyterian-St. Luke's Medical Center, Chicago, with permission). [Previously published in Woessner JF Jr., Howell DS (eds): *Joint Cartilage Degradation: Basic and Clinical Aspects.* New York: Marcel Dekker; 1993: chap 2:43.]

collagen make up approximately 3 percent of the total collagen and appear to be a subclass of fibril-forming collagens. Collagen X is interesting in that it is expressed in cartilage in a topographical and developmentally regulated manner (localized in the deep calcified zone), in particular the epiphyseal growth plate, and may play a role in the mineralization process. Collagen VI shows a topographical distribution to the pericellular matrix and may facilitate cell-matrix interactions; it comprises approximately 1 percent of the total cartilage collagen. Type XII and XIV collagens are structurally related molecules with large noncollagenous domains present only in small amounts in articular cartilage with unknown function.

Proteoglycans are complex multidomain molecules that are composed of a protein core to which are bound polysaccharide (glycosaminoglycan) side chains. The large aggregating proteoglycan in articular cartilage (also known as aggrecan) makes up 80 to 90 percent of all cartilage proteoglycans. Aggrecan consists of a core protein with multiple glycosaminoglycan side chains covalently attached. Sequence analysis together with molecular electron microscopy has demonstrated that the core protein consists of three globular (G1, G2, and G3) and two extended domains (Fig. 2-3). The last N-terminal globular domain (G1) interacts with the hyaluronic acid and is stabilized by link protein to form the aggregate structure (Fig. 2-4). This type of domain structure is also seen in aggregating proteoglycans from several other types of connective tissue matrix. An extended molecular domain exists between the G1 and G2 domains. In the extended domain between the G2 and G3 globular domains is a keratan sulfate attachment region that contains up to 30 keratan sulfate side chains followed by a chondroitin sulfate attachment region containing up to 100 chondroitin sulfate side chains. Proteoglycan structure influences the tissue's mechanical properties, however, and is variable due to differences in keratan sulfate and chondroitin sulfate chain length, protein core length, and extent of aggregation structure within the cartilage matrix. The proteoglycans affect the cartilage's mechanical and physical properties such as compressive stiffness, sheer stiffness, osmotic pressure, and regulation of hydration. Cartilage also contains at least four other small homologous proteoglycans that do not aggregate; biglycan, decorin, fibromodulin, and lumican. These small proteoglycans are also present in a variety of other connective tissues (i.e., tendon) in addition to cartilage. Biglycan and decorin both contain dermatan sulfate side chains whereas both fibromodulin and lumican contain keratan sulfate side chains. Both decorin and fibromodulin appear to bind to collagen and may modulate fibril formation. The function of biglycan and lumican are not known. There are several noncollagenous proteins found in the extracellular cartilage matrix that may play critical roles in both the biological and physical properties of the cartilage. Most of these proteins have been found in other connective tissues, but several are most concentrated in articular cartilage with distinctive distributions within the cartilage. Cartilage oligomeric matrix protein (COMP), a member of the thrombospondin family, is a pentameric multidomain protein that may be important in mediating both cell-matrix and matrix-matrix interactions. Immunolocalization of COMP in human articular cartilage reveals a temporal and spatial change in distribution from a predominately pericellular localization in fetal cartilage to a predominately interterritorial localization in normal adult cartilage. Thrombospondin 1 is also present in smaller amounts in articular cartilage than COMP and in other tissues has been shown to be important in mediating cell-matrix interactions. Fibronectin is present in both normal and osteoarthritic cartilage with greater amounts in the later. Fibronectin can mediate cell-matrix interactions as well as interact with other constituents of the extracellular matrix. Matrix-gla protein is found in articular cartilage and may be involved in calcium phosphate precipitation in the deep mineralized zone of the cartilage. Chondrocalcin (also known as collagen II carboxyl-terminal peptide) is the C-terminal propeptide of type II collagen formed from the cleavage of procollagen II, and may play a role in mineralization by binding hydroxyapatite crystals. Two other abundant extracellular matrix proteins are a 58-kDa protein and a 36-kDa protein, both unnamed, that appear to mediate chondrocyte attachment.

Lipids located both in the chondrocytes and matrix constitute 1 percent or less of the weight of the cartilage. Matrix vesicles have been observed at all cartilaginous zones but their function is not known. The remaining composition of the cartilage tissue includes water (60 to 85 percent by weight) and inorganic salts.

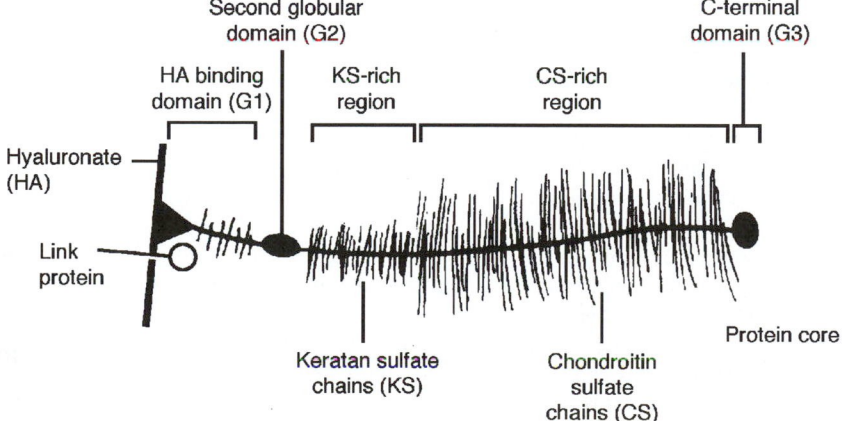

Figure 2-3

A schematic diagram of the aggrecan molecule and its binding to hyaluronate. The protein core has several globular domains (G1, G2, and G3), with other regions containing the keratan sulfate and chondroitin sulfate glycosaminoglycan chains. The N-terminal G1 domain is able to bind specifically to hyaluronate. This binding is stabilized by link protein. [Reproduced with permission from Mankin HJ, Mow VC, Buckwalter JA, et al: Form and function of articular cartilage In Simon SR, Wilson J (eds): *Orthopaedic Basic Science*. Rosemont, IL: American Academy of Orthopaedic Surgeons; 1994:9.]

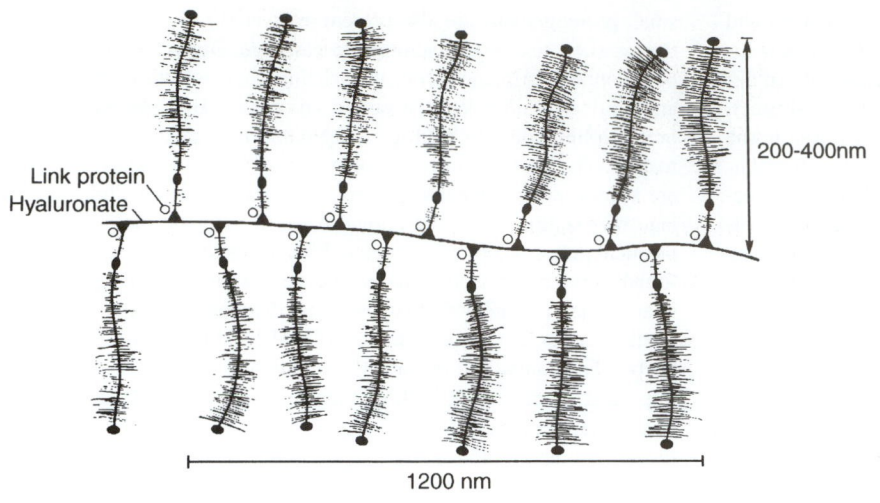

Link protein
Hyaluronate

200-400nm

1200 nm

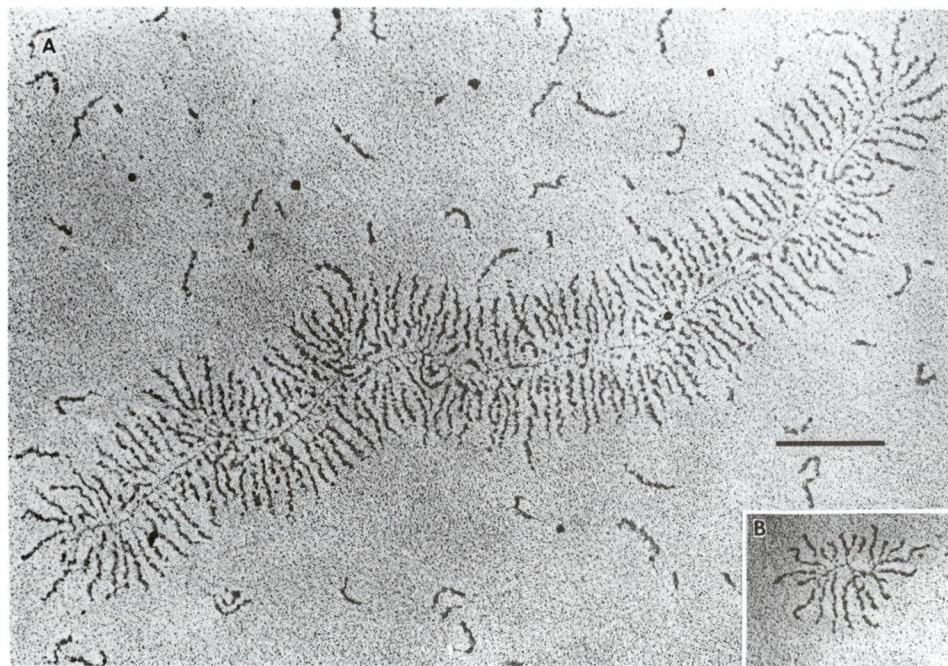

Figure 2-4

Top: A diagram of the aggrecan molecules arranged as a proteoglycan aggregate. Many aggrecan molecules can bind to a chain of hyaluronate, forming macromolecular complexes that effectively are immobilized within the collagen network. *Bottom*: Electron micrographs of bovine articular cartilage proteoglycan aggregates from (*A*) skeletally immature calf and (*B*) skeletally mature steer. These show the aggregates to consist of a central hyaluronic acid filament and multiple attached monomers (bar = 500μm). [Top illustration reproduced with permission from Mankin HJ, Mow VC, Buckwalter JA, Iannotti JP, Ratcliffe A: Form and function of articular cartilage. In Simon SR (ed): *Orthopaedic Basic Science*. Rosemont, IL: American Academy of Orthopaedic Surgeons; 1994: p. 10. Bottom photo and inset printed with permission from Buckwalter JA, Kuettner KE, Thonar E J-M: Age-related changes in articular cartilage proteoglycans: Electron microscopic studies. *J Orthop Res* 1985:254.]

METABOLISM OF ARTICULAR CARTILAGE

Chondrocytes exist within a specialized microenvironment, the territorial matrix, without cell-to-cell contact. Cartilage is also avascular, aneural, and alymphatic, and as a result each individual cell is responsible for the metabolism of the extracellular matrix in its immediate vicinity. Under normal circumstances chondrocyte metabolism is therefore influenced by cytokines, its pericellular matrix, and mechanical forces. A vast array of proteolytic enzymes produced by periarticular cells and chondrocytes serve to degrade the cartilage elements to effect matrix turnover. There are four classes of proteinases that are found within the matrix that may be involved with the degradation of cartilage based upon their catalytic mechanism: serine, cysteine, apartic, and metalloproteinases. Chondrocytes depend upon diffusion of small molecules for nutrition and communication. Generally the lower one-third of the cartilage is supplied by diffusion from the subchondral bone and the upper two-thirds from diffusion from the synovial fluid. As a result, chondrocytes tend to

exist with lower oxygen levels, higher carbon dioxide levels, and at a lower pH than other cells. There is a normal turnover of the extracellular matrix of the cartilage controlled by the chondrocytes. Proteoglycans are degraded and released from the matrix by limited proteolytic cleavage. Aggrecan is degraded by an "aggrecanase" that cleaves the protein core between the G1 and G2 molecular domains thereby disrupting the aggregate structure. Proteoglycan fragments can then be further degraded by other proteases and can then released from the matrix into the synovial fluid. Collagen turnover is by a slower rate, probably mediated by metalloproteinases. Metalloproteinases depend on divalent cations for their activity. Regulation of metalloproteinases activity is controlled both by their activation and inhibition. Metalloproteinases are synthesized as latent enzymes that require enzymatic modifications to become active.

The active enzymes can also then be inhibited irreversibly by a specific inhibitors produced by the chondrocytes [i.e., tissue inhibitor of metalloproteinases (TIMP) with the net activity related to the amount of each within the tissue]. Little is known about the matrix

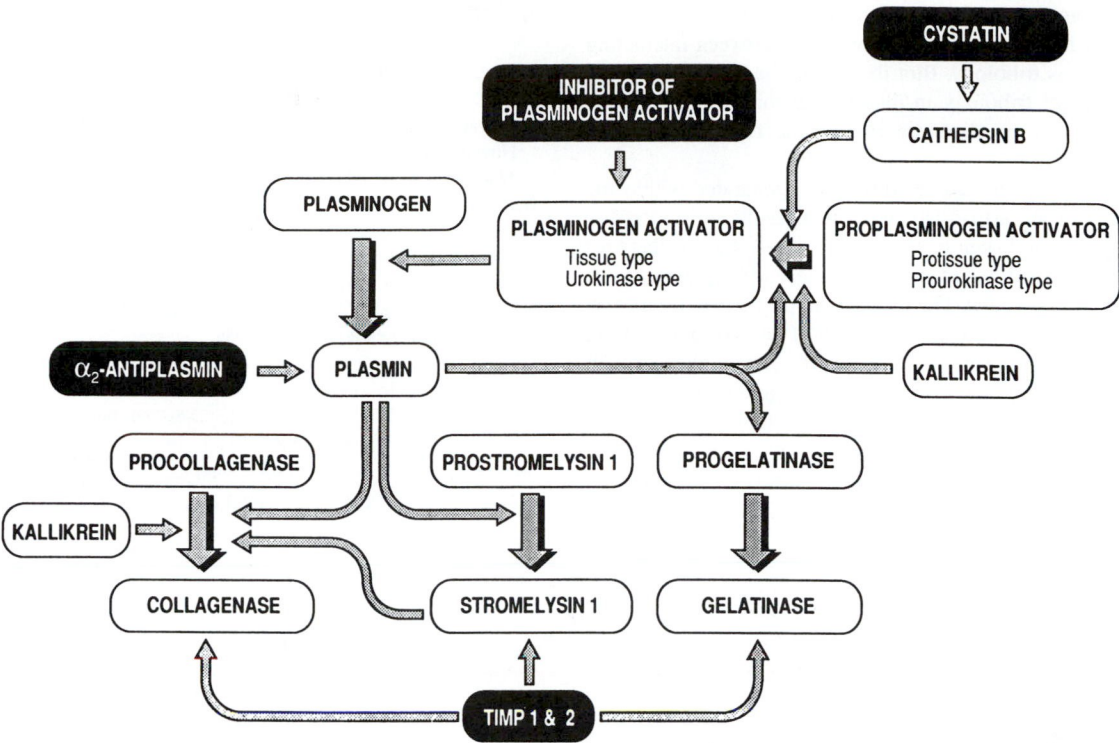

Figure 2-5
Activators and inhibitors of the most important proteinases in cartilage. (Reproduced with permission from Mow VC, Ratcliffe A: Cartilage and diarthrodial joints as paradigms for hierarchical materials and structures. *Biomaterials* 1992;13:82. Courtesy of AR Poole, Montreal, Canada.)

turnover of the noncollagenous proteins. A schematic diagram of the most well-characterized proteinases with their activators and inhibitors is in the diagram of Fig. 2-5.

DEGRADATION

It is generally believed that the degradation of the extracellular matrix in osteoarthritis occurs through different processes than that in rheumatoid arthritis. In osteoarthritis, mechanical stresses on aging cartilage are believed to induce an altered chondrocyte metabolic response leading to loss of cartilage. The cartilage is thought to be degraded initially from within by endogenous factors and later by mechanical forces as the physical properties of the cartilage are altered. Repair efforts by the chondrocytes are often represented by the appearance of chondrocyte clusters or clones and the presence of fibrocartilage. In rheumatoid arthritis, erosion of the cartilage is believed to be caused from outside the cartilage both by the proliferating synovial pannus and by degradative enzymes released into the synovial fluid by periarticular cells. However, soluble mediators such as cytokines produced by periarticular cells can also diffuse to the chondrocytes and induce a metabolic imbalance. Recent evidence has also implicated cytokines, synthesized by the chondrocytes, to have profound effects on chondrocyte matrix homeostasis by either an autocrine or paracrine manner.

SYNOVIAL MEMBRANE AND FLUID

The synovial membrane is a highly vascularized tissue that is composed of type A phagocytic cells, type B secretory cells, and undif-

ferentiated precursor cells that serve a reservoir of the differentiated lining cells. The type A phagocytic cells function to remove debris from the synovial fluid and are noted to contain prominent Golgi apparatuses, vacuoles, lysosomes, with an abundant cytoskeletal network for active phagocytosis. The periarticular lymphatic system also is involved with removal of large macromolecules from the synovial fluid. The type B secretory cells appear fibroblast-like, contain a large rough endoplasmic reticulum and are important in secreting molecules important for joint lubrication and nutrition in addition to degradative enzymes and cytokines. Synovial fluid is a highly viscous liquid secreted by the synovium. In the healthy human knee joint 1 to 5 ml of fluid are usually present. The synovial membrane lacks a basement membrane and contains fenestrated capillaries. As a result the synovial fluid is a dialysate of blood plasma and contains, in addition, hyaluronate that is secreted by the type B cells. The synovial fluid acts to provide joint lubrication by decreasing the frictional coefficient at both the cartilage-cartilage and cartilage-synovium interfaces and as a source of nutrients to the articular cartilage. The composition of synovial fluid typically has an identical glucose and electrolyte concentration to plasma.

BIOMECHANICS

Articular cartilage of diarthrodial joints must function under high loads for many years. In order to sustain the tissue's integrity, articular cartilage is a biphasic material consisting of both a solid and liquid phase. Cartilage is a porous and permeable material consisting of between 65 to 85 percent water based upon total tissue weight. The mechanical functions of cartilage are to minimize contact stresses by deforming, to increase contact areas and decrease point loading, and to contribute to joint lubrication to minimize joint friction and wear.

The science of friction, wear, and lubrication between interacting surfaces is known as tribology. Biotribology is the term used to describe that branch of tribology in diarthrodial joints. The biphasic properties of articular cartilage are responsible for the functional properties of the joint.

Tensile, shear, and compressive stresses are generated within the articular cartilage when a load is applied that results in fluid efflux and tissue deformation. When that load is removed, the cartilage regains its initial composition and structure by reabsorbing the exudate fluid by interstitial fluid flow. The mechanical properties of biphasic creep and stress-relaxation are a direct result of the movement of the interstitial fluid and as a result allow the cartilage to withstand both high and frequent joint loading. Articular cartilage also exhibits viscoelastic properties due to the movement of the long-chained molecules (collagen and proteoglycans) contained within the matrix. It is both the movement of interstitial fluid and the deformation of the viscoelastic matrix that are responsible for the mechanical behavior of the cartilage.

SUGGESTED READINGS

Adolphe M (ed): *Biological Regulation of the Chondrocytes*. Boca Raton, FL: CRC Press; 1992.

Buckwalter JA, Mow VC: Cartilage repair in osteoarthritis. In Moskowitz RW, Howell DS, Goldberg VM, Mankin HJ, (eds): *Osteoarthritis, Diagnosis and Management,* 2d ed. Philadelphia: WB Saunders; 1992:71.

Buckwalter JA, Mow VC, Ratcliffe A: Restoration of injured or degenerated articular cartilage. *J Amer Acad Ortho Surg* 1994; 2:192.

Heinegård D, Oldberg A: Structure and biology of cartilage and bone matrix noncollagenous macromolecules. *FASEB J* 1989; 3:2042.

Nordin M, Frankel VH: *Basic Biomechanics of the Musculoskeletal System*. Philadelphia: Lea & Febiger; 1989.

Simon SR (ed): *Orthopaedic Basic Science.* Rosemont, IL: American Academy of Orthopaedic Surgeons; 1994.

Woessner JF Jr: Matrix metalloproteinases and their inhibitors in connective tissue remodeling. *FASEB J* 1991; 5:2145.

Woessner JF Jr, Howell DS (eds): *Joint Cartilage Degradation: Basic and Clinical Aspects.* New York: Marcel Dekker; 1993.

Chapter 3

TISSUE ANATOMY

John L. Ricci

Tendon, ligament, cartilage, and bone are the main structural tissues that are routinely encountered in orthopaedic medicine. A basic knowledge of the structure of these tissues is essential for an understanding of their mechanical properties, healing characteristics, and surgical repair. This chapter represents a concise survey of the important structural characteristics of these tissues.

TENDON AND LIGAMENT

Tendons and ligaments are similar in composition, in microstructure, and in function. They both serve as the supporting cables of the body in an environment of high tensile forces. While tendons connect skeletal muscles to bone, and ligaments connect bone to bone (and support viscera), they are both dense connective tissue structures that consist largely of directionally oriented, high tensile-strength collagen. For the purposes of this chapter they will be discussed together and their differences will be contrasted.

The *microstructure and composition* of tendons and ligaments are similar. On a microscopic scale they both consist of an extracellular matrix (ECM) of unidirectionally oriented collagen sparsely populated by long, spindle-shaped fibroblasts (in some cases referred to as fibrocytes) positioned between collagen bundles (Fig. 3–1). They are largely type I collagen (with small amounts of type III), with tendons consisting of 86 percent (dry weight) collagen and ligaments

consisting of 70 percent (dry weight) collagen. There are small amounts (less than 1 percent) of elastin in tendon and ligament, with the exception of flaval and nuchal ligaments of the spine. In these specialized structures elastin is the primary structural element. Other components include proteoglycans, cells, lipids (mostly from cell membranes), and cell attachment proteins related to cell-ECM interaction.

The *collagen structural organization* of tendons and ligaments is similar. Both are mostly type I collagen, which consists of two $\alpha_1(I)$, and one $\alpha_2(I)$ polypeptide chains in a right-handed triple-helix, held together by hydrogen and covalent bonds. On a microfibril level, referred to as quaternary structure, these collagen molecules are arranged in a quarter-stagger arrangement which gives collagen its characteristic banding pattern and allows alignment between charged amino acids, providing high strength and stability. Groups of microfibrils form subfibrils and fibrils, with fibrils forming a composite with glycoproteins and water, interspersed with fibroblasts, forming fascicles (Fig. 3–2). Within fascicles in tendons the collagen components are unidirectionally oriented, and fascicles are held together by loose connective tissue, called endotenon, which contains blood vessels, lymphatics, and nerves. In ligaments the collagen often has a less unidirectional organization and sometimes forms a woven pattern. The endotenon also permits longitudinal movement of individual fascicles when tensile forces are applied to the structure. The connective tissue surrounding groups of fascicles, and/or the entire structure, is referred to as the epitenon. In the case of tendons the fascicles may be arranged in parallel fashion, while in ligaments they may be arranged in more complex spiral or woven patterns.

Histologically, the parallel orientation of collagen in tendons and ligaments can best be observed using polarized light, which also shows another unique characteristic of this type of tissue—its crimp pattern (Fig. 3–3). Crimp refers to a discrete, regular, wavy pattern in the collagenous structure that imparts mechanical properties and will be discussed elsewhere.

Gliding tendons, like the flexor tendons of the hand, are enclosed by a tendon sheath with discrete parietal (the inside surface of the sheath) and visceral (the epitenon or outside layer of the tendon) synovium layers, which provide synovial fluid for lubrication and nutrition. This sheath directs the movement of the tendon, and in areas where the tendon makes a sharp bend the sheath is sometimes thickened into a pulley-like structure. In these areas, where the tendon is exposed to high compressive stresses, regions of tendon take on a cartilage-like appearance. These tendons, sometimes referred to as avascular tendons, receive vascular access only through vincula—small, loose, flexible strips of connective tissue that connect with the mesotenon and paratenon, the loose connective tissues around the sheath. These tendons are thought to receive nutrient partly by diffusion through the synovial fluid in the tendon sheath.

Vascular tendons and ligaments are not enclosed in a sheath. They are surrounded by a loose connective tissue paratenon which is di-

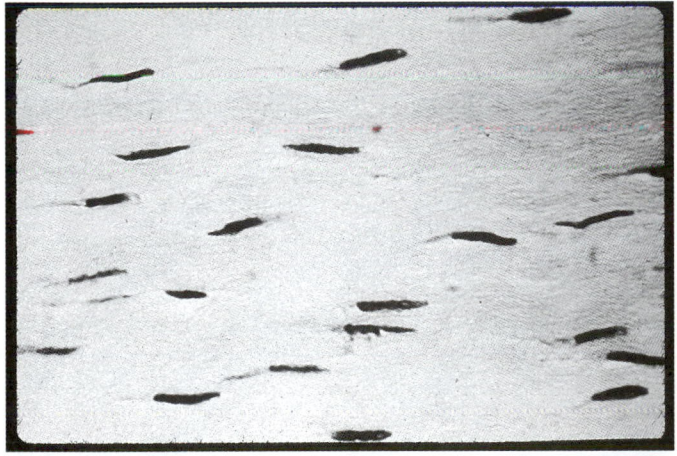

Figure 3-1
Photomicrograph of a longitudinal section of a human flexor tendon showing the spindle-shaped fibroblasts (H&E, X250). [Reproduced with permission from Woo SL-Y, An K-N, Arnoczky DVM, et al: Anatomy, biology, and biomechanics of tendon, ligament, and meniscus. In Simon SR (ed): *Orthopaedic Basic Science.* Rosemont, IL: American Academy of Orthopaedic Surgeons; 1994:47.]

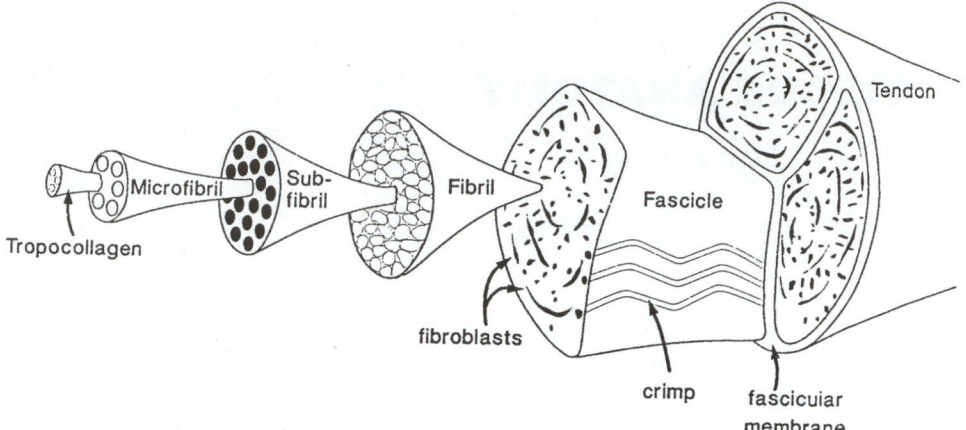

Figure 3-2
Schematic representation of the microarchitecture of a tendon. [Reproduced adapted illustration with permission from Woo SL-Y, An K-N, Arnoczky DVM, et al: Anatomy, biology, and biomechanics of tendon, ligament, and meniscus. In Simon SR (ed): *Orthopaedic Basic Science*. Rosemont, IL: American Academy of Orthopaedic Surgeons; 1994:49. From Kastelic J, Baer E: Deformation in tendon collagen. In Vincent JFV, Currey JD (eds): *The Mechanical Properties of Biologic Materials*. Cambridge, Cambridge University Press, 1980: 397–435.]

rectly connected to the epitenon and provides vascular access from many points. Inside the tendon or ligament these vessels anastomose to form a longitudinal system of capillaries that run through the endotenon tissues.

Attachments of tendon and ligament to bone represent a small (less than 1 mm) transitional region where two types of tissue with different structural and mechanical properties merge. Two types of insertions have been described that differ in morphology but contain common elements. Direct insertions are more morphologically distinct but are less prevalent. They contain superficial fibers that join with the periosteum and deep fibers that have four morphological phases: ligament, fibrocartilage, mineralized fibrocartilage, and bone. Indirect insertions have less distinct zones and usually show predominantly superficial fibers with only a few deep fibers. These insertions have abundant Sharpey fibers which secure the bone to the periosteum.

CARTILAGE

Articular cartilage is the body's bearing surface and has unique properties that provide diarthrodial joints with extraordinary wear-resistance, low-friction, lubrication, shock absorption, and load transfer characteristics. It consists primarily of an avascular ECM made up predominately of water, proteoglycans, collagens, and a few other components, with a sparse population of dispersed chondrocytes.

Water makes up 65 to 80 percent of the wet weight of cartilage. It strongly interacts with proteoglycan, and is moved through the molecular pores of the ECM by compressive forces. This provides nutrient transport, lubrication, and the viscoelastic and compressive properties unique to cartilage.

Proteoglycans are complex macromolecules that consist of an unbranched hyaluronate core linked to extended polysaccharide (glycosaminoglycan) chains. Eighty to 90 percent of proteoglycans in cartilage are large aggregated molecules, referred to as aggrecans. They consist of long hyaluronate cores with attached keratan sulfate and chondroitin sulfate polysaccharides. The compressive properties of cartilage result, in large part, from the interaction of water, Ca^{2+}, and Na^+, with the carboxyl (COOH) and sulfate (SO_4) groups present on all glycosaminoglycans. In the presence of water these groups become ionized (COO^- and SO_3^-) and use Ca^{2+} and Na^+ to maintain electroneutrality. These ions provide Donnan osmotic pressure, and close packing of proteoglycans provides strong charge-to-charge repulsion forces—with the two effects providing the swelling pressure of cartilage that gives it its compressive properties.

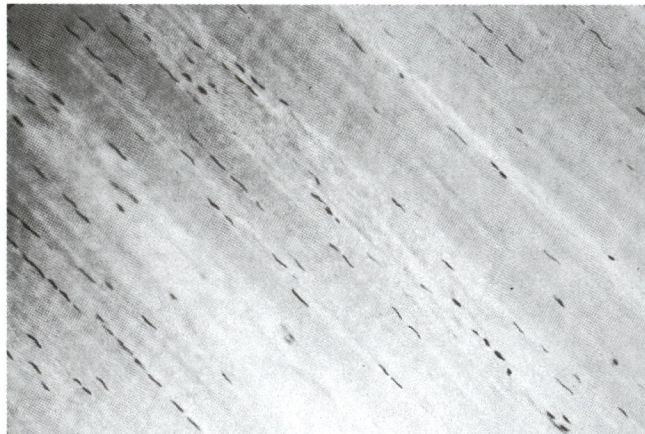

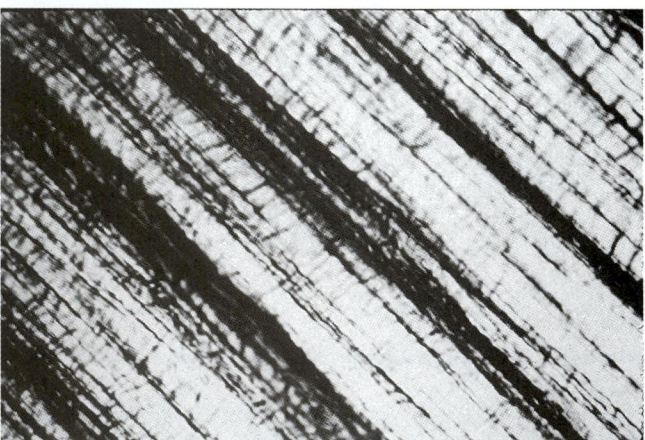

Figure 3-3
Photomicrograph of a longitudinal section of a human flexor tendon. Note the parallel rows of fibroblasts lying between the collagen bundles *(left)*. Photomicrograph of same section under polarized light microscopy, illustrating the parallel, longitudinally arranged collagen bundles *(right)* (H&E, X100). [Reproduced with permission from Woo SL-Y, An K-N, Arnoczky DVM, et al: Anatomy, biology, and biomechanics of tendon, ligament, and meniscus. In Simon SR (ed): *Orthopaedic Basic Science*. Rosemont, IL: American Academy of Orthopaedic Surgeons; 1994:49.]

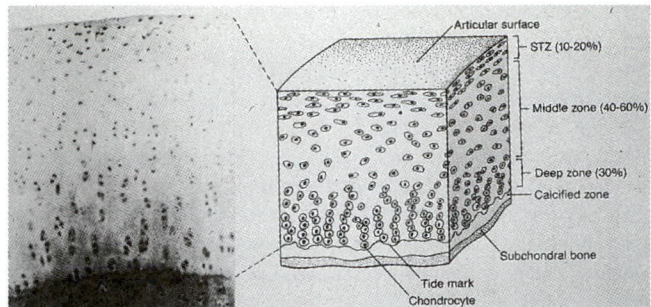

Figure 3-4
Histologic section of normal adult articular cartilage showing even Safranin O staining and distribution of chondrocytes *(left)*. Schematic diagram of chondrocyte organization in the three major zones of the uncalcified cartilage, the tidemark, and the subchondral bone *(right)*. [Reproduced with permission from Mow VC, Proctor CS, Kelly MA: Biomechanics of articular cartilage. In Nordin M, Frankel VH (eds): *Basic Biomechanics of the Musculoskeletal System,* 2d ed. Philadelphia: Lea & Febiger; 1989:32.]

Collagen makes up 10 to 20 percent of the wet weight of cartilage. The main collagen component of cartilage is type II collagen, which is a triple-helical structure consisting of three α_2 (I) chains, with smaller amounts of types V, VI, IX, X, and XI collagen present in various distributions. The type II collagen is in the form of very small fibers (10 to 100 nm, much smaller than those in tendon or bone) that are intra- and intermolecularly cross-linked to form a three-dimensional matrix. This matrix traps proteoglycan aggregates and provides tensile properties.

Other matrix components in cartilage include small amounts of lipids (1 percent or less) that are found in cell membranes as well as the ECM, and non-collagenous proteins.

Cartilage structure varies locally according to depth and can be divided into four zones (Fig. 3–4): the superficial zone (at the articular surface), the middle or transitional one, the deep zone, and the zone of calcification (at the subchondral bone junction). Amounts of proteoglycan, collagen, and water vary according to zone.

In the *superficial zone* (the uppermost 10 to 20 percent) the collagen is oriented parallel to the surface, the cells are elongated parallel to the collagen, the proteoglycan content is lowest, and the collagen and water content (80 percent wet weight) are highest. In the *transitional zone* (40 to 60 percent) the cells are more rounded and the collagen fibers are relatively large and randomly oriented. The *deep zone* (30 percent) has the lowest water content (65 percent wet weight), the highest proteoglycan concentration, and spherical cells arranged in columnar arrays. The *zone of calcification* represents the border between cartilage and subchondral bone. It consists of ECM containing hydroxyapatite mineral with small pyknotic cells. In histological preparations a wavy line, referred to as the tidemark, is the uppermost border of mineralization and divides the zone of calcification from the deep zone.

BONE

Bone is a mineralized connective that exists in a number of functional forms. It is a dynamic and well-organized tissue that has amazing compressive and tensile properties resulting from its ECM, which is largely a composite of collagen and hydroxyapatite mineral. An accurate analogy exists between the properties of bone and steel-reinforced concrete. In both materials high-tensile-strength reinforcing fibers or rods provide tensile strength, while the surrounding mineral matrix provides compressive properties.

Two microscopic forms of bone exist: woven and lamellar. Woven bone is usually a temporary structure. It is found in the embryo and in newborns, in fracture callus, and in growing bone. As a long-term structure it is only found in pathological bone in situations where rapid growth and turnover are occurring.

Structurally, it consists of disoriented collagen fibers, varied levels of mineralization, and large numbers of randomly oriented cells (Fig. 3–5). Because of the random orientation of collagen in woven bone, its mechanical properties are isotropic.

Lamellar bone is the end result of remodeling of woven bone in infants, fracture callus, and growing bone. It is a much more ordered and mature structure that consists of discrete layers of heavily mineralized oriented collagen (Fig. 3–5). Because of its highly organized nature, it is anisotropic; its mechanical properties depend on its orientation relative to applied forces. It is found in several forms and named according to its three-dimensional structure.

On a structural level, woven and lamellar bone form two main types of structures: trabecular and cortical bone (Fig. 3–6).

Trabecular bone, which is also referred to as spongy or cancellous bone, is a porous three-dimensional structure consisting of branched beams and plates. It has one-quarter of the mass of cortical bone, and because of its high surface area it can remodel very rapidly. When this type of bone forms or heals it initially consists of thin trabeculae of woven bone which then remodel to a trabecular pattern of lamellar bone. These structures are subjected to complex stresses and strains and remodel accordingly, usually forming structures aligned according to compressive stress patterns.

Cortical bone, in humans, is found as the shell around all bones. It can bear high bending and torsional forces as well as compressive forces. It forms the diaphysis in all long bones and the covering of all other bones. In many cases it exists as a thin shell of only a few lamellae. In small animals like rats and mice all cortical bone consists of layers of lamellar bone called compact bone. In these situations the bone lives by diffusion of nutrients from outside the lamellae—no internal vessels are required. In large animals that experience rapid growth, thick bones require internal vessels. In these situations plexiform bone is often observed, which has layers of lamellar and woven bone, with vessels found in the woven layer.

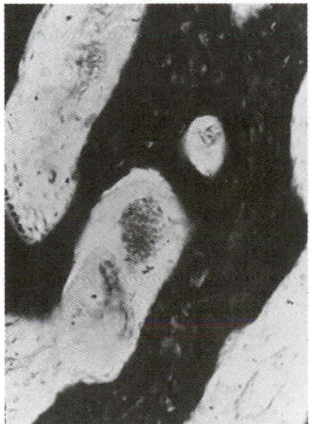
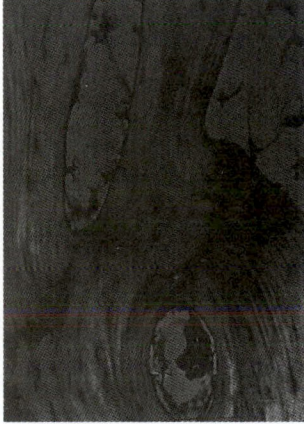

Figure 3-5
Photomicrographs of woven and lamellar bone. [Reproduced with permission from Kaplan FS, Hayes WC, Keaveny TM, et al: Form and function of bone. In Simon SR (ed): *Orthopaedic Basic Science.* Rosemont, IL: American Academy of Orthopaedic Surgeons; 1994:130.]

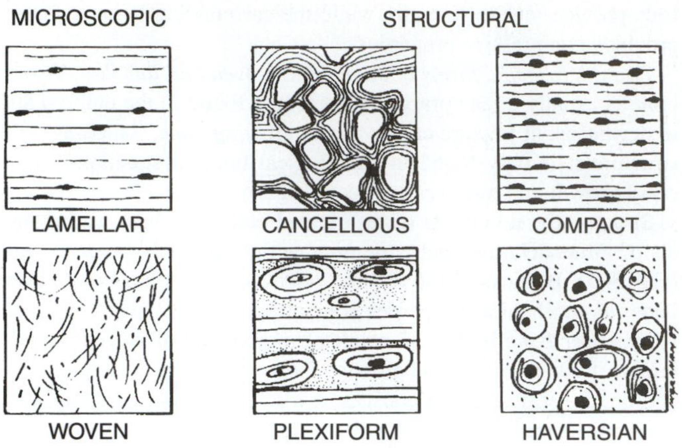

Figure 3-6
Diagrams of types of bones. [Reproduced with permission from Kaplan FS, Hayes WC, Keaveny TM, et al: Form and function of bone. In Simon SR (ed): *Orthopaedic Basic Science.* Rosemont, IL: American Academy of Orthopaedic Surgeons; 1994:129.]

Haversian bone is the thick form of cortical bone found in humans. It is a complex form of lamellae consisting of bone layered around neurovascular channels. Individual units consisting of layers of bone around a single neurovascular channel are called osteons. They are in the form of cylinders that branch and anastomose with the vessels, which are in a central canal in the osteon. Osteons are composed of circumferential lamellae, with interstitial lamellae filling the spaces between osteons. Osteons are nearly always oriented parallel to the long axis of bones, and bone has its strongest mechanical properties parallel to these osteons.

The central canals of osteons are most often filled with capillaries that originate from the principal nutrient arteries; however, lymph vessels are sometimes seen in osteons, and nerves are also present. The vessels in osteons form a complex network arising from nutrient arteries, which supply thick, dense bone with nutrition.

Osteoblasts, osteocytes, and osteoclasts are the cells responsible respectively for formation, maintenance, and resorption of bone. The terms osteoblast and osteocyte refer to functional definitions of the same mesenchymally derived cell type: if the cell is actively producing bone, it is referred to as an osteoblast; if it is an essentially quiescent cell that is trapped in a bone matrix, it is referred to as an osteocyte.

Osteoblasts by definition are bone-forming cells. Since bone formation (and resorption as well) are surface phenomenon, osteoblasts are always found on the surfaces of the lamellae of trabecular bone or haversian bone, or on the surface of woven bone. These cells are usually seen as a group forming a discrete layer on the surface of a bone lamellae. Histologically, they are seen as a layer of osteoid, a combination of cells and incompletely mineralized bone matrix. Usually, these cells are polarized, forming cuboidal or columnar layers of cells, in which the cells are oriented with the nucleus at the end of the cell opposite where the new bone is forming. These cells are histologically basophilic, and in transmission electron microscopy preparations show abundant amounts of rough endoplasmic reticulum (for protein synthesis), Golgi apparatus (for secretion of these proteins), mitochondria, and cytoskeleton elements. These cells produce type I collagen, are responsive to parathyroid hormone (PTH), and produce osteocalcin when stimulated by 1,25-dihydroxy-vitamin D.

Osteocytes are osteoblasts that are buried in bone matrix and have reduced their synthetic activity. They have a higher nucleus-to-cytoplasmic ratio (less cytoplasm, rough endoplasmic reticulum, and Golgi apparatus) and are usually found within and between bone lamellae, oriented to the lamellae and to the long axis of osteons. They have extensive cell processes that extend through canaliculi—tiny canals through the mineral structure of the bone—and form a communication network with other osteoblasts and with the central canals of osteons. This network allows nutrient and metabolite exchange between the osteoblasts and the vessels of the central canal, as well as cell to cell communication. The system is thought to allow the osteoblast to help regulate calcium metabolism through interaction with the crystals of the mineral structure. This system of communication is also thought to allow bone to respond to mechanical strain. Considering that bone responds to cyclic strain on a very precise level (actually a microstrain level), this network of interconnected cells must be very sensitive to small changes in the state of the ECM.

Osteoclasts are a unique type of highly specialized cells that are responsible for resorption of bone during remodeling. They represent a large (20 to 100 μm in diameter), multinucleated cell that is derived in bone marrow from hematopoietic precursors—the same cells that give rise to similar macrophages, such as multinucleate foreign body giant cells. However, in contrast to these macrophages, osteoclasts are specialized to produce tartrate-resistant acid phosphatase, and they actively resorb bone and express specialized cell surface markers. Morphologically, aside from their multinucleate structure, they are distinctive in that they are polarized and often show a structure referred to as a ruffled or brush border adjacent to the resorptive surface. This structure is a specialized region of infolded cell membrane with high surface area adjacent to numerous channels, vesicles, and synthetic machinery in the cell cytoplasm. Areas of the ruffled membrane attach to bone through integrins, resorb the mineral of bone through production of hydrogen ions to produce a restricted area of low pH, and also resorb the organic components of the ECM through proteolytic acid and enzyme digestion.

Bone matrix consists of a composite of minerals and proteins with water, cells, and other macromolecules. The main components can be divided into organic and inorganic phases. Minerals generally comprises 60 to 70 percent of the tissue, water 5 to 8 percent, and the rest is organic. Most of the inorganic component is collagen (90 percent), with 5 percent being noncollagenous proteins.

The inorganic phase of bone consists of hydroxyapatite, $Ca_{10}(PO_4)_6(OH)_2$, a biological analogue of a naturally occurring mineral. In bone, it consists of extremely small, platelike crystals, 20 to 80 nm long and 2 to 5 nm thick, that contain impurities which influence the crystal structure. These apatite crystals usually contain impurities, such as carbonate, sodium, potassium, magnesium, and citrate. They may also contain fluoride, strontium, aluminum, and other impurities that reflect dietary and environmental exposure. These impurities strongly influence the stability of the apatite—some, like fluoride, are used intentionally to stabilize apatite and make it more resistant to degradation.

The organic phase of bone consists largely (90 percent) of type I collagen, which forms a randomly oriented matrix in woven bone and a highly ordered, layered structure in lamellar bone. This collagen, like that of tendon and ligament, consists of two α_1 (I), and one α_2 (I) polypeptide chains in a right-handed triple helix. These 300 nm-long molecules are parallel-aligned in a quarter-stagger arrangement which leaves gaps between the ends of the molecules. Non-collagenous proteins are often found in these gaps, and mineralization is thought to commence here.

Non-collagenous proteins in bone consist of bone sialoproteins like osteopontin and osteonectin, proteins containing g-carboxyglutamic acids, such as osteocalcin, proteoglycans, and bone morphogenic proteins (BMPs).

SUGGESTED READINGS

Amiel D, Frank C, Harwood F, et al: Tendons and ligaments: A morphological and biochemical comparison. *J Orthop Res* 1984; 1:257.

Boskey AL: Mineral-matrix interactions in bone and cartilage. *Clin Orthop* 1992; 281:244.

Buckwalter JA, Hunziker EB: Articular cartilage biology and morphology. In Mow VC, Ratcliffe A (eds): *Structure and Function of Articular Cartilage.* Boca Raton: CRC Press; 1993.

Buckwalter JA, Glimcher MJ, Cooper RR, et al: Bone Biology. Part I: Structure, blood supply, cells, matrix, and mineralization. Part II: Formation, form, remodeling, and regulation of cell function (Instructional Course Lecture). *J Bone Joint Surg [Am]* 1995; 77:1256-1275, 1276-1289.

Burks RT: Gross anatomy. In Daniel DM, Akeson WH, O'Connor JJ (eds): *Knee Ligaments: Structure, Function, Injury, and Repair.* New York: Raven Press; 1990:59-76.

Daniel DM, Akeson WH, O'Connor JJ (eds): *Knee Ligaments: Structure, Function, Injury, and Repair.* New York: Raven Press; 1990.

Hall BK (ed): *Bone. Volume 1: The Osteoblast and Osteocyte.* Caldwell, NJ: Telford Press; 1989.

Hall BK (ed): *Bone. Volume 2: The Osteoclast.* Boca Raton, FL: CRC Press; 1991.

Hall BK (ed): *Bone. Volume 3: Bone Matrix and Bone Specific Products.* Boca Raton, FL: CRC Press; 1991.

Hall BK (ed): *Bone. Volume 4: Bone Metabolism and Mineralization.* Boca Raton, FL: CRC Press; 1991.

Mow VC, Ratcliffe A (eds): *Structure and Function of Articular Cartilage.* Boca Raton, FL: CRC Press; 1993.

Mow VC, Ratcliffe A, Poole AR: Cartilage and diarthrodial joints as paradigms for hierarchical materials and structures. *Biomaterials* 1992; 13:67.

Muller W: *The Knee: Form, Function, and Ligament Reconstruction.* Berlin: Springer-Verlag; 1983.

Schenk RK, Eggli PS, Hunziker EB: Articular cartilage morphology. In Kuettner KE, Schleyerbach R, Hascall VC (eds): *Articular Cartilage Biochemistry.* New York: Raven Press; 1986:3.

Simon SR (ed): *Orthopaedic Basic Science.* Rosemont, IL: American Academy of Orthopaedic Surgeons; 1994.

Woo SL-Y, Buckwalter JA (eds): *Injury and Repair of the Musculoskeletal Soft Tissues* (AAOS/NIAMS Workshop, 1987). Park Ridge, IL: American Academy of Orthopaedic Surgeons; 1988.

Chapter 4

BONE METABOLISM

Norman C. Blumenthal

CALCIUM

Bone serves as a reservoir for over 99 percent of the body's calcium. Calcium is also important in muscle and nerve function, in the clotting mechanism, and many other areas. Plasma calcium is about equally free and bound (usually to albumin). It is absorbed from the gut (duodenum) via active transport (ATP and calcium-binding protein required) that is regulated by $1,25\text{-}(OH)_2$ vitamin D_3, and also absorbed by passive diffusion (jejunum). It is 98 percent reabsorbed by the kidney (60 percent in proximal tubule). The dietary requirement of calcium is about 900 mg/day; it increases to about 1500 mg/day for adolescents, in pregnancy, and in postmenopausal females, and to about 2000 mg/day for lactating females. Most people have a positive calcium balance in their first three decades of life and a negative balance after the fourth decade. About 400 mg of calcium is released from bone on a daily basis. Calcium may be excreted in stool. Hypercalcemia can lead to hyperreflexia and convulsions. Hypocalcemia leads to somnolence and areflexia.

PHOSPHATE

Besides being a key component of bone mineral, phosphate has an important role in enzyme systems and molecular interactions (metabolite and buffer). Approximately 85 percent of the body's phosphate stores are in bone. Plasma phosphate is mostly in the unbound form, and is reabsorbed by the kidney (also in the proximal tubule). Dietary intake of phosphate is usually adequate; daily requirement is 1000 to 1500 mg/day. It may excrete in urine.

BONE FORMATION AND REMODELING

In the mature skeleton, bone undergoes a continuous process of resorption and formation known as remodeling. Bone remodeling occurs at multiple localized sites throughout the skeleton, and it is tightly regulated at the tissue and cellular levels such that net skeletal mineral balance is maintained. Remodeling provides a mechanism whereby the skeleton can accommodate to the physical, metabolic, and hormonal stresses applied to it.

The remodeling cycle begins locally at the tissue level with the removal of discrete amounts of older, fully mineralized bone. This is achieved by osteoclasts which adhere to the surface of bone and remove its mineral and collagenous matrix components. In cortical bone, cell-mediated bone resorption produces haversian canals that course through the surrounding mineralized tissue. In cancellous bone, osteoclastic resorption results in shallow erosions along the surfaces of bony trabeculae that are called resorption bays or Howship's lacunae. A period of cellular quiescence follows the completion of localized osteoclastic activity during the remodeling cycle; subsequently, osteoblasts migrate to areas of previous osteoclastic bone resorption.

Osteoblasts deposit new collagen, which then becomes infused with calcium phosphate mineral. Normally, the volume of mineralized tissue formed during the skeletal remodeling cycle is sufficient to replace virtually all bone that was previously removed by osteoclasts; thus, skeletal mineral balance is achieved, and bone mass is maintained. The term coupling is commonly used to describe the physiologic equilibrium between bone resorption and bone formation.

Factors, such as parathyroid hormone (PTH), prostaglandins, and various cytokines, promote the resorption of bone by increasing the cellular activity of individual osteoclasts, by increasing the number of osteoclasts, or both. These changes, if sustained, ultimately produce a new steady state of increased skeletal remodeling since bone formation increases with bone resorption through the mechanism of coupling. Mineralized bone formation may not fully compensate for persistently high levels of resorption activity under conditions of increased bone turnover, however, and this imbalance can reduce the bone mineral content and bone mass over time. Such is the case in primary hyperparathyroidism.

Mineralized bone formation during skeletal remodeling can be divided into two discrete but closely integrated components: the initial deposition of an unmineralized collagenous bone matrix, or osteoid; and the subsequent calcification of this matrix. Osteoblasts migrate to sites of previous bone resorption, and these cells synthesize procollagen. Procollagen is extruded from the cell and undergoes cleavage at the carboxy- and amino- terminal ends of the molecule. Extracellular collagen is deposited along the surface of bone where it undergoes extensive inter- and intramolecular crosslinkage during its incorporation into the developing osteoid seam. Before mineralization can begin, osteoid must undergo a number of important biochemical changes that require several days to complete. The interval between the initial deposition of newly formed bone collagen and the onset of mineralization is known as the mineralization lag time. This variable is a measure of the rate at which osteoid matures.

As newly formed osteoid undergoes maturation, osteoblasts deposit additional collagen along the advancing edge of the osteoid seam. The growing osteoid seam consists, therefore, of immature, newly synthesized collagen both at and near the surface and more fully mature collagen deeper within it. The mineralization front, also termed the zone of initial mineralization, is the site where calcification begins in fully mature collagen, at the junction between the osteoid seam and adjacent mineralized bone. This is the site where calcification begins in collagen that has fully matured. Adequate mineralization requires sufficient concentrations of calcium and phosphorus in the surrounding biological fluids and a collagenous matrix that has completed the biochemical changes required for calcification. The deposition of mineral within osteoid normally proceeds toward the surface at an average linear rate similar to that at which new collagen is laid down by osteoblasts located at the advancing edge of the osteoid seam. Consequently, the width of an individual osteoid seam is determined by the relative rates at which collagen and mineral are deposited within it.

The dynamic events outlined above can be evaluated at the tissue and cellular levels using the technique of quantitative bone histomorphometry. Factors that delay the onset of calcification within newly formed osteoid such as hypocalcemia or hypophosphatemia result in classic histologic osteomalacia, a pathologic condition in which osteoid is not fully mineralized. Osteoid seams are widened, the volume of osteoid is increased, and the mineralization lag time is prolonged. Similar changes are seen in conditions where the rate of collagen maturation is reduced by inhibitors of collagen crosslinkage. Osteoid accumulates in bone because the deposition of mineral within the osteoid seam proceeds more slowly than the formation of collagen along the osteoid surface. Although the absolute rates of mineral deposition and collagen synthesis are diminished in osteomalacia, the overall rate of mineralized bone formation must be less than the rate of collagen synthesis, in order for the volume of osteoid to increase and for overt histologic osteomalacia to develop.

In contrast to osteomalacia, skeletal disorders that are characterized by primary reductions in bone collagen synthesis do not produce osteoid accumulation if the maturation of collagen is not delayed, or if the mineralization of osteoid is not impaired. In both diabetes and caloric deprivation, bone formation is reduced as a consequence of primary reductions in bone collagen synthesis. The respective rates of mineral and collagen deposition are diminished to a similar degree in these two conditions, and histologic evaluations of bone reveal normal or decreased amounts of osteoid. The width of osteoid seams is also normal or reduced, and these findings differ markedly from those of classic osteomalacia. Because the histologic features by light microscopy are frequently unremarkable in conditions where bone formation and turnover are low in the absence of defective mineralization, the diagnosis of these disorders is based primarily upon measurements of mineralized bone formation using the technique of double tetracycline labeling. Tetracycline binds to the mineral portion of bone, which will fluoresce under excitation. The fluorescent band corresponds to the time of tetracycline administration.

MECHANISMS OF BONE MINERALIZATION

There is at present no unified theory of the mechanism of bone mineralization. There are many, seemingly diverse, experiments which show that a number of individual chemical processes accompany the deposition of mineral in the organic matrix of bone.

The mechanisms proposed for the infusion of the organic matrix of hard tissues with apatite mineral fall into three general categories: (a) raising the supersaturation in localized volumes to levels that would cause spontaneous precipitation, (b) providing substances which create nucleating sites or remove barriers to these sites and (c) removing or neutralizing bone mineral inhibitor. All these mechanisms may take place separately or simultaneously, as well as intracellularly and/or extracellularly.

Most of the studies on the control of bone mineral formation have been on the role of certain molecular species, both nucleators and inhibitors, found in the regions of active calcification. The following have been proposed as nucleation substrates for hard tissue hydroxyapatite formation: collagen, g-carboxyglutamate-containing proteins, phosphoproteins, glycoproteins, calcium-acidic phospholipid-phosphate complexes, and proteolipids. All these materials are present in bone and/or other normal and pathological mineral tissue. Some of these have been shown to nucleate hydroxyapatite in vivo, while others have only been shown to bind calcium ions.

The initial mineral deposits in the organic matrix of bone are shown by electron microscopy to be at discrete sites in, or on, the collagen fibrils. The phosphoproteins may play a structural and/or regulatory role in the calcifying organic matrix by providing an epitaxial substrate for apatite nucleation. There are a variety of phosphoproteins in calcifying tissue which may have multiple roles including providing a substrate for apatite nucleation, and controlling the size, shape, and orientation of these crystals. The exact role of the phosphoproteins found in calcifying tissues remains to be elucidated. However, the high concentration of these phosphoproteins at the mineralization front in calcified tissue suggests that this material must be involved, in a way yet to be determined, in the process of mineral deposition.

A number of biologically relevant chemical species slow down or inhibit direct hydroxyapatite precipitation, or the transformation of amorphous calcium phosphate to crystalline hydroxyapatite related to bone mineral. Mg^{+2} in high enough concentration (Mg^{+2}/Ca molar ratio >0.2) will prevent apatite formation. The pyrophosphate ion is a well known inhibitor of apatite as are its biologically relevant analogs ATP and ADP. A number of synthetic analogs of diphosphonic acid also prevent apatite formation.

Proteoglycans are believed to be involved in the regulation of cartilage and bone mineralization, by acting as inhibitors of mineral deposition. Cartilage is of the order of 25 to 60 mg proteoglycan per ml of gel. Past work has indicated that proteoglycan must be removed or modified for cartilage to mineralize. Small concentrations of this proteoglycan will delay but not prevent apatite formation. The proteoglycan subunit (monomer) is less effective than the aggregate but is still a potent apatite inhibitor. Both aggregate and subunit retard but do not prevent the transformation of amorphous calcium phosphate to crystalline hydroxyapatite.

ALUMINUM-INDUCED OSTEOMALACIA

The accumulation of aluminum in tissues has been implicated in the pathogenesis of several clinical disorders of the musculoskeletal, central nervous, and hematologic systems. Early clinical reports suggested that aluminum deposition in the brain was related to the development of a progressive and lethal encephalopathy in patients receiving maintenance hemodialysis. Many patients with the syndrome of dialysis encephalopathy, or dialysis dementia, also exhibited clinical manifestations of a severe form of osteomalacia characterized by recurrent fractures and progressive muscle weakness. This disorder was usually refractory to treatment with active vitamin D sterols, and several clinical and biochemical features distinguished it from other types of renal osteodystrophy. Subsequent investigations documented that patients with concurrent manifestations of dialysis-associated osteomalacia and encephalopathy had extensive deposits of aluminum in bone. Water that contained aluminum and that was used for the preparation of hemodialysis solutions was the predominant source of aluminum loading in these patients.

The widespread use of reverse osmosis for water purification in dialysis facilities has substantially reduced the incidence of dialysis encephalopathy, but aluminum-related bone disease remains a substantial clinical problem. Some 25 to 30 percent of patients undergoing regular dialysis have evidence of aluminum deposition in bone. Such patients are at risk for aluminum accumulation in tissues due to the continued therapeutic use of aluminum-containing, phosphate-binding antacids that are given to control hyperphosphatemia and secondary hyperparathyroidism. Although aluminum is poorly absorbed from the gastrointestinal tract, large quantities of these agents are administered on a daily basis. Since excretion represents the major route of elimination for aluminum, amounts transported by the gut cannot be excreted by the kidney in subjects with advanced renal failure. Consequently, enterally absorbed aluminum accumulates in plasma and in tissues, and only limited quantities are removed by conventional dialysis because of the extensive tissue and protein binding of aluminum.

The majority of cases of aluminum-related bone disease have been identified in patients undergoing maintenance dialysis. However, additional observations both in adults and in pediatric patients indicate that aluminum accumulation in skeletal tissue can produce metabolic bone disease in subjects with normal renal function inadvertently given repeated parenteral loads of aluminum via nutrition solutions contaminated with aluminum. Other intravenous solutions also contain aluminum, and their therapeutic use may lead to substantial aluminum loading, particularly in neonates and premature infants.

Several histopathologic lesions have been described in patients with evidence of aluminum deposition in bone. Osteomalacia is the most common aluminum-related skeletal disorder, but variant forms such as the aplastic lesion of renal osteodystrophy also occur. The bone biopsy findings in osteomalacia and aplastic bone share certain histologic and dynamic features when evaluated using quantitative histomorphometry, but they differ substantially in several important respects. For example, aluminum-related osteomalacia is characterized by an excess of unmineralized bone collagen, or osteoid, whereas the amount of osteoid is normal or diminished in the aplastic lesion of aluminum-related bone disease. These observations suggest that the skeletal manifestations of aluminum toxicity are not uniform, and data from both clinical and experimental studies indicate that aluminum loading adversely affects bone formation and turnover by several different mechanisms.

The specific pathways by which aluminum disrupts the metabolism of bone at the tissue and cellular levels have yet to be fully characterized, and the role of aluminum as a modifier of systemic factors that modulate bone formation and turnover remains to be clarified.

For further reading on aluminum-induced osteomalacia, see Blumenthal and Posner (1984), Blumenthal (1985), and de Broe and Coburn (1990).

CALCIUM-PHOSPHATE METABOLISM

Calcium and phosphate metabolism is affected by an elaborate interplay of hormones and even the levels of the metabolites themselves. The hormones each affect processes of the gut mucosa, kidney, and bone (Table 4–1). Feedback mechanisms play an important role in the regulation of plasma levels of calcium and phosphate (Fig. 4–1). Peak bone mass usually occurs in the second or third decade and is greater in men and in blacks. After this peak, bone loss occurs at a rate of 0.3 to 0.5 percent per year (2 to 3 percent per year for untreated females during the 6th through 10th years after menopause).

Parathyroid hormone (PTH) is an 84-amino acid peptide made and secreted from chief cells in the four parathyroid glands; PTH helps upregulate plasma calcium. Its release is activated via a b_2 receptor in the parathyroid gland. Decreased calcium levels in the extracellular fluid stimulate release of PTH. PTH may also have a role in bone loss in the aged. Its actions on bone, gut, and the kidney are outlined in Table 4–1.

Vitamin D_3 is a naturally occurring steroid that is activated by ultraviolet irradiation from sunlight or utilized from dietary intake (vitamin D_2). It is hydroxylated to the 25 (OH)-vitamin D_3 form in the liver, and is hydroxylated a second time in the kidney. Conversion to the 1,25-$(OH)_2$-vitamin D_3 form activates the hormone, whereas conversion to the 24,25-$(OH)_2$-vitamin D_3 form inactivates it. The active form acts to increase plasma calcium and phosphate concentrations (Table 4–1).

Calcitonin is a 32-amino acid peptide hormone made by clear (C) cells in parafollicles of the thyroid gland; this hormone also has a limited role in calcium regulation. Increased calcium levels in the extracellular milieu cause its secretion. Calcitonin may also have a physiologic role in fracture healing and the treatment of osteoporosis. Its role, still not fully known, is to decrease plasma calcium by its actions on the bone, the kidney, and the gut mucosa (Table 4–1).

The following hormones also have an effect on bone metabolism:

1. Estrogen—Prevents bone loss by inhibiting resorption. Supplementation is helpful in postmenopausal women, but only if it is

---

Table 4-1

Hormone Actions in Calcium-phosphate Metabolism

Hormone	Bone	Kidney	Gut
PTH	Mobilizes calcium and phosphate Releases osteocytic perilacunar stores (fast) Increases osteocyte number and activity (slow)	Increases resorption of calcium (cAMP required) Increases excretion of phosphate Stimulates 1,25-$(OH)_2$ vitamin D_3 (calcitnol) production	Increases absorption (through vitamin D_3)
1,23-D_3	Promotion and mobilization of calcium Increases osteocyte number and activity	Increases phosphate + calcium resorption Encourages production of 24,25-$(OH)_2$-vitamin D_3	Promotes calcium and phosphate absorption Acts by inducing calcium-binding protein
Calcitonin	Decreases osteoclastic (and osteocytic) resorption (Osteoclasts lose ruffled border and clear zone)	Decreases resorption of calcium and phosphate Increases secretion of electrolytes	Decreases secretion of acid

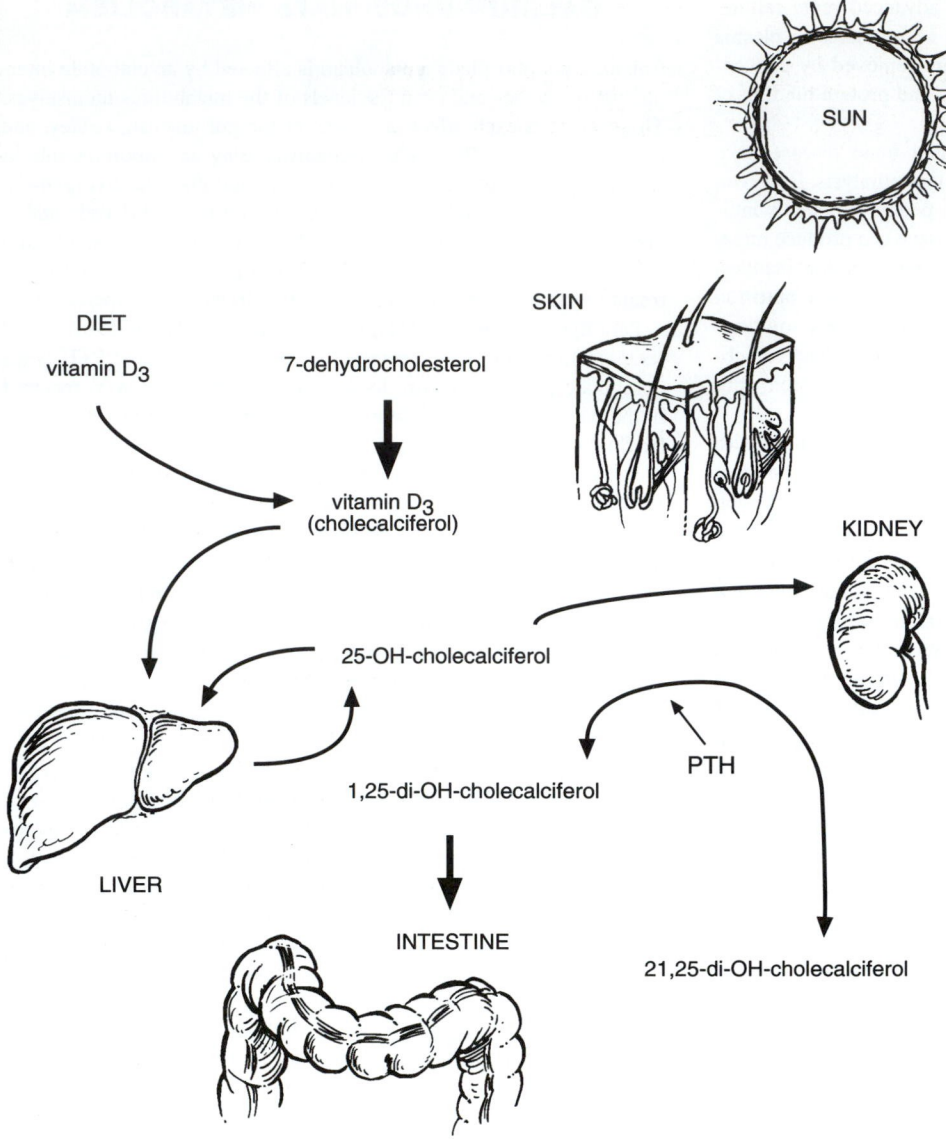

SUN

DIET

vitamin D₃

7-dehydrocholesterol

SKIN

vitamin D₃
(cholecalciferol)

KIDNEY

25-OH-cholecalciferol

1,25-di-OH-cholecalciferol

PTH

LIVER

INTESTINE

21,25-di-OH-cholecalciferol

Figure 4-1
Schematic of vitamin D metabolism. [Reproduced with permission from Kaplan FS et al: Form and function of bone. In: Simon SR (ed): *Orthopaedic Basic Science*. Rosemont, IL: American Academy of Orthopaedic Surgeons; 1994:165.]

started within the first 5 to 10 years after the onset of menopause. The risk of endometrial cancer for patients taking estrogen is reduced when it is combined with cyclic progestin therapy.

2. Corticosteroids—Increase bone loss [decrease gut absorption by decreasing binding proteins, and decrease bone formation (cancellous bone more affected than cortical bone) through inhibition of collagen synthesis]. Adverse effects with therapy may be reduced with alternate-day therapy.

3. Thyroid Hormones—Affect bone resorption more than bone formation, leading to osteoporosis. Large (thyroid-suppressive) doses of thyroxine can lead to osteoporosis.

4. Growth Hormone—Causes a positive calcium balance by increasing gut absorption more than its increase in urinary excretion. Insulin and somatomedins participate in this effect.

5. Growth Factors—TGF, PDGF, and monolymphokines have a role in bone and cartilage repair.

SUGGESTED READINGS

Betts F, Blumenthal NC, Posner AS: Bone mineralization. *J Crystal Growth.* 1981; 53:63.

Blumenthal NC: Binding of aluminum to hydroxyapatite and amorphous calcium phosphate as a model for aluminum associated osteomalacia. In: Butler WT (ed): *The Chemistry and Biology of Mineralized Tissues* (Proceedings of the Second International Conference on the Chemistry and Biology of Mineralized Tissues, Alabama, Sept. 9–14). Birmingham, AL: EBSCO Media; 1985:385.

Blumenthal NC, Posner AS: In vitro model of aluminum induced osteomalacia: inhibition of hydroxyapatite formation and growth. *Calc Tiss Int.* 1984; 36:439.

Buckwalter JA, Glimcher MJ, Cooper RR, et al: Part I: Structure, blood supply, cells, matrix, and mineralization (instructional course lecture). *J Bone Joint Surg [Am]* 1995; 8:1256.

Buckwalter JA, Glimcher MJ, Cooper RR, et al. Bone biology. Part II: Formation, form, remodeling, and regulation of cell function (instructional course lecture). *J Bone Joint Surg [Am]* 1995; 8:1276.

De Broe ME, Coburn JW (eds): *Aluminum and Renal Failure.* Boston: Kluwer Academic Publishers; 1990.

Posner AS, Betts F, Blumenthal NC: Chemistry and structure of precipitated hydroxyapatites. In Nriagu JO, Moore PB (eds): *Phosphate Minerals.* New York: Springer-Verlag; 1984:330.

Slavkin H, Price P (eds): *Chemistry and Biology of Mineralized Tissues.* New York: Excerpta Medica; 1992.

Chapter 5

FRACTURE HEALING AND BONE GRAFTING

Sally R. Frenkel and Kenneth J. Koval

FRACTURE HEALING

The repair of bone fracture includes the processes of inflammation, repair, and remodeling; however, the type of healing varies depending on the method of treatment. With closed treatment, endochondral healing with periosteal bridging callus formation occurs; in rigid-fixation treatment, where there is mechanical immobilization and near-anatomic reduction, primary bone healing (osteonal) without visible callus formation occurs.

The initial healing responses to fracture are localized hemorrhage and clot formation by damaged blood vessels. An inflammatory reaction follows secondary to a chemotactic phase, and typically includes: local reactions with morphologic changes, destruction and/or removal of foreign or injurious materials, several or all of the classic responses or signs of healing (redness, warmth, swelling, and pain), and sometimes inhibited or loss of function. No one sign is always present during the inflammatory phase. Perichondral ossification follows when endosteum and periosteum adjacent to the fracture proliferate osteoprogenitor cells, forming a primary soft callus of hyaline cartilage within several days to two weeks; later, a medullary (hard) callus supplements the bridging soft callus. Radiographically, callus is typically evident when a widening of the fracture gap occurs due to osteoclastic resorption and with the disappearance of the fracture line as the fibrocartilage template mineralizes. The degree of fracture immobilization is indirectly proportional to the amount of callus formed.

In contrast, direct or primary bone healing is without callus formation, and is fundamentally a process of bone remodeling. It requires stable fixation. The injured tissue releases activating substances shortly following fracture that permit an ingrowth of blood vessels and mesenchymal cells. Osteoblasts then differentiate, and osteoid (new bone) is laid down onto those surfaces of bone that are exposed. These become areas of lamellar bone (parallel layers in cancellous bone; concentric layers in compact bone). Nonlamellar, also known as woven (reticular) bone, will initially fill gaps in excess of 200 μm and is later replaced by lamellar bone. Small defects usually demonstrate healing within several weeks, followed by Haversian remodeling and restoration of original bony architecture.

Bone repair may be significantly affected by favorable or unfavorable conditions. An important factor for healing is the preservation of the blood supply; excessive soft-tissue stripping should therefore be avoided. The environment is another factor which modulates the repair process; hormones have impact on osteoblastic and osteoclastic activity (Table 5-1). Successful restoration of osseous morphology and internal architecture is conditional on the remodeling process. Normal muscle contraction and weightbearing, with their attendant stresses at the site of the healing fracture, lead to restoration of the normal architecture (initially, internal and secondarily, external configuration) and function over several years (Wolff's law).

Long-term remodeling for significant fractures may take up to 7 years. The repopulation of marrow is indicative of complete fracture healing.

Fractures that can be expected to have a good healing response include those that: are within cancellous bone; have an adequate blood supply; have minimum soft tissue injury; do not have a hematoma; do not have an associated infection; and have good apposition for spiral, oblique, or impacted fractures.

BONE GRAFTING

Bone grafting, attempted as far back as the 1600s and first successfully undertaken in the early 1800s, is today one of the most useful and dependable reconstructive surgical procedures available to the orthopaedic surgeon. It is variously estimated that upwards of a quarter-million bone-grafting procedures are performed in the United States annually. Bone grafting is performed in a wide range of clinical situations: fusions; correction of discontinuities due to congenital or traumatic deformity, especially fracture nonunions; and augmentation of sites of resection for tumor.

While the fundamental techniques of bone grafting have been established for decades, in recent years orthopaedic researchers have equipped the surgeon with a variety of exciting alternatives. New developments include the fabrication of novel biomaterials for use as bone substitutes and the isolation of such materials as growth factors to aid in bone ingrowth and new bone formation. As a result, bone

Table 5-1

The Effect of Hormones on Healing

Hormone	Effect on Healing	Mechanism
Glucocorticoids	(−)	Decreased callus proliferation
Calcitonin	(+)	Decreased osteoclastic activity
Thyroid hormone	(+)	Increases rate of bone remodeling
Parathyroid hormone	(+)	Increases rate of bone remodeling
Growth hormone	(+)	Increases amount of callus

grafts are now viewed as biological structures, not mere scaffold material.

Several factors influence the outcome of a bone grafting procedure, including the donor material, the host site, and surgical technique.

TYPES OF GRAFT

Graft tissue harvested from and implanted into the same individual is termed *autogenous* (or *autogenic*), the graft is called an *autograft*. *Allogeneic* tissue refers to tissue harvested from another individual of the same species; the graft is called an *allograft*. Autogenous bone is almost always used as a fresh graft. Allografts are typically fresh-frozen, lyophilized (freeze-dried), or chemically sterilized after harvesting, a process that both decreases the immunogenicity of these tissues and renders all their cells unviable.

Both autogenous and allogeneic cancellous and cortical bone, and to a lesser extent corticocancellous bone and bone marrow, are commonly employed as donor material (Fig. 5-1). Osteochondral segments and demineralized bone matrix are special types of allografts, and use is also made of such materials as bone morphogenetic protein, hydroxyapatite, ceramics, polymers, and composites.

There are advantages and disadvantages to using various types of bone for grafting. The demands of the clinical setting usually dictate the choice (Table 5-2). In a strictly biological sense, autogenous cancellous bone is the ideal material for a graft, and as such it is the most frequent source of graft material. Cancellous bone is more amenable to revascularization than is cortical bone, and as a result it has a greater potential for osteoinduction (the process of promoting growth of new bone). Cortical bone heals at a slower rate, but has good potential for osteoconduction (the process of promoting bone ingrowth) and superior mechanical properties (Table 5-2).

All autografts have the advantage of precluding the risk of immune reaction or transplanting infectious agents. Practical and mechanical considerations may argue in favor of using allografts in many clinical situations, as they comprise a virtually unlimited supply of structurally sound graft material in any size and shape. Moreover, their use may preclude a second invasive procedure for the purpose of harvesting an autograft, with its attendant risks and drawbacks. The main disadvantages of allografts—immunogenicity and, to a somewhat lesser extent, the risk of transmitting pathogens—have been largely overcome in recent years by advances in the processing and storage of harvested bone. Because viral transmission nevertheless remains a real if small risk, it is incumbent upon the surgeon to be thoroughly familiar with the issues involved, including the reliability of any given tissue bank.

The implications of the differences in types of donor material will become clear in the following discussions of biological process of incorporation of bone graft into the host site and the mechanical considerations that govern (or do not govern) choice of material.

BIOLOGICAL MECHANISM OF BONE INCORPORATION

Incorporation of a bone graft is a dynamic process involving the biological and structural properties of both the transplanted material and

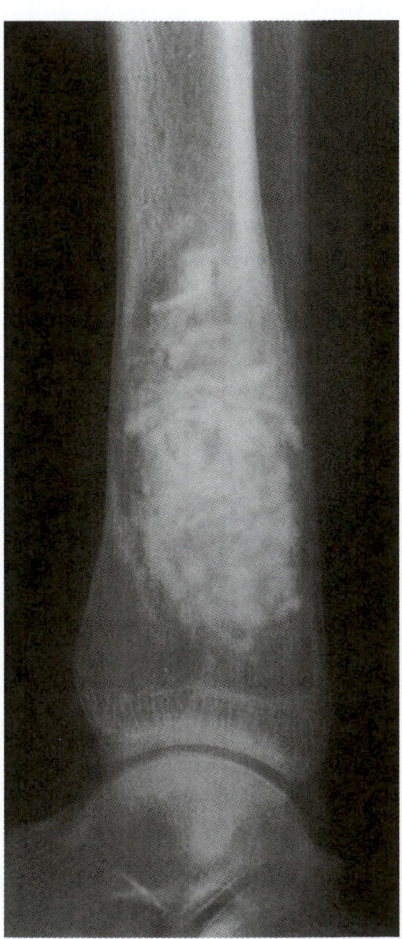
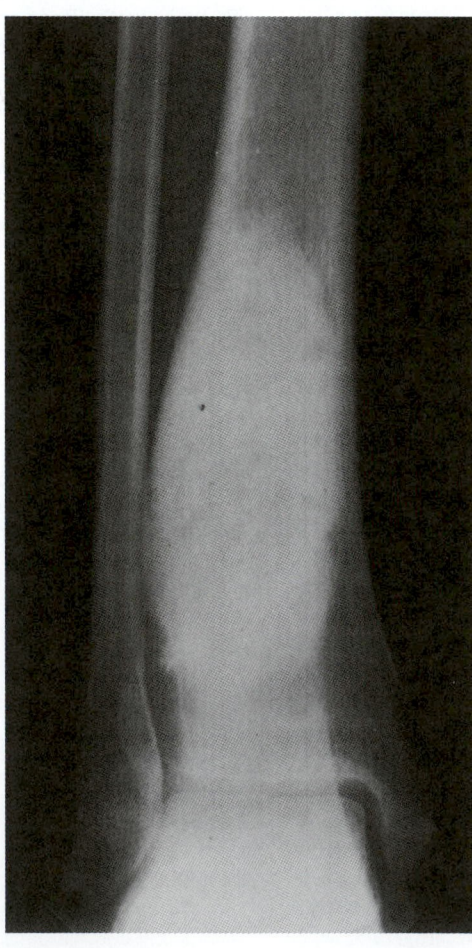

A   *B*

Figure 5-1
A. A 12-year-old female with non-ossifying fibroma of distal tibia treated by curettage and bank bone graft. *B*. One year later, the bone graft is fully incorporated.

Table 5-2

Properties of Bone Grafts by Type and Source

	Source			
	Autograft		**Allograft**	
	Cancellous	**Cortical**	**Cancellous**	**Cortical**
Donor site	Most common (for vascularized grafts): • Iliac crest • Fibula Other sites: • Rib—for anterior spine fusion			
Advantages	• Significant osteogenic, osteoconductive, osteoinductive potential • Amenable to revascularization • Not immunogenic; no risk of acquired infection	• Less osteogenic, osteoconductive, osteoinductive potential • Can provide structural support • Not immunogenic; no risk of acquired infection	• Second surgical exposure obviated • Virtually unlimited in size, amount, quality, type, and shape	• Can provide structural support • Slow incorporation via creeping substitution
Disadvantages	• Second surgical exposure required to obtain graft, with attendant risks, including loss of mechanical integrity • Limited available amount • Limited available shape • Limited in size, amount, quality, type, and shape	• Resists revascularization, remodeling	• Virtually no osteogenic, osteoconductive, osteoinductive potential (due to lack of live cells)[a] • Immunogenic; carries risk of acquired infection • Expensive to harvest, etc.	• May fatigue and fail under cyclic loading

[a] Specially processed osteochondral tissue may retain viable cells

---

the host bed into which it is placed. This process, and hence the ultimate fate of a bone graft, thus varies significantly depending on whether the donor material is autogenous or allogeneic in origin and on whether it is cancellous or cortical bone.

Cancellous Bone

Incorporation of any graft comprises an initial inflammatory response followed by the longer-term process of vascular invasion, new bone formation, and remodeling. This four-stage process applies to all graft materials, but varies significantly depending on the types of bone used. For autogenous cancellous bone, this sequence proceeds as follows:

Phase 1: The initial phase, during and immediately following surgery, is characterized by an inflammatory process similar to that in trauma, including formation of a fibrin clot. Vascularization, attended by mobilization of immature mesenchymal cells at the host-donor interface, begins as early as two to three days.

Phase 2: By 6 to 8 weeks postimplantation, vascular ingrowth is well under way, accompanied by invasion of progenitor mesenchymal cells.

Phase 3: The period from 2 to 6 months is characterized by formation of new bone on donor trabeculae and trabecular osteoclastic resorption ("creeping substitution").

Phase 4: Beginning around month 6, mechanical forces (in accordance with Wolff's law) induce adaptive trabecular remodeling and reorientation, which eventually results in the pattern of normal bone. This phase is usually complete by one year after surgery.

Allogeneic cancellous bone elicits a somewhat different response: the process of incorporation takes approximately twice as long and is less satisfactory. Animal studies have revealed that after the initial, phase 1 events (inflammation and clot formation) the fibrin clot breaks down, probably due to an antigenic immune response, resulting in persistent inflammation, delayed osteoclastic resorption and new bone formation, and ultimately delayed or incomplete graft incorporation.

Cortical Bone

Incorporation of cortical autografts, like that of cancellous allografts, takes about twice as long as cancellous autografts. The primary reason is that cortical bone's greater density presents a formidable barrier to revascularization. As a result, creeping substitution, which in a cancellous autograft proceeds concurrently with osteoinduction, is the dominant phase 3 process in cortical graft, and only subsequently does osteoblastic new bone formation take place. Cortical material thus experiences incomplete substitution with viable bone.

Incorporation of cortical allografts is similar to that of autograft material, but due to immunogenic factors, creeping substitution (phase 3) proceeds even more slowly.

Corticocancellous Bone

Corticocancellous bone, as the name suggests, contains portions of both cortical and cancellous bone, and to some extent it combines the benefits of both: an environment for revascularization as well as mechanical strength. As a graft, it incorporates much as does cancellous bone.

Vascularized Grafts

Vascularized grafts—specifically, autografts—were first successfully applied in the mid-1970s, and their use, especially to correct large osseous defects, has increased markedly since then. Because successful incorporation of a graft into host bone is positively correlated with extent and rate of revascularization, the rate of incorporation of vascularized graft material in phase 2 and phase 3 is significantly accelerated.

FUNCTION

Choice of surgical procedure and material used for bone grafting varies according to the site of grafting and the function the graft is expected to perform. The means of filling a small defect are much different from those used to add significant mechanical support.

STRUCTURAL SUPPORT FOR MECHANICAL LOADING

Major structural grafts—those that are expected to aid in weight-bearing or provide some other mechanical function—require rigid, well-contoured attachment to the host bone to ensure both superior contact and stability. (In turn, mechanical loading is most often essential in the process of remodeling that ensures long-term fixation.)

Grafts that must resist mechanical loads are typically held in place using Kirschner wires, screws, and/or bolts. Especially when cancellous bone is used as an onlay or for fusion, rigid fixation is required to bridge the discontinuity and fix a graft in place.

Because large sections of bone usually cannot be supplied from autogenous components, structural grafts are almost always allografts; the exception is when a vascularized graft is required or when autograft bone can be mobilized with little or no morbidity such as from an excised femoral head during total hip replacement.

BENDING AND ROTATION

Onlay and inlay bone grafts and bone stents are occasionally useful for internal fixation where the mechanical loading is primarily in bending and/or rotation (Fig. 5-2), although this application of bone grafting has largely been replaced by the use of fracture fixation hardware, including devices fabricated from bioabsorbable materials. Onlay grafts of avascular cortical bone, for example, while they exhibit little or no osteoinductive activity and are slow to revascularize and respond to remodeling, nevertheless incorporate well in selected situations, such as in long bone fractures.

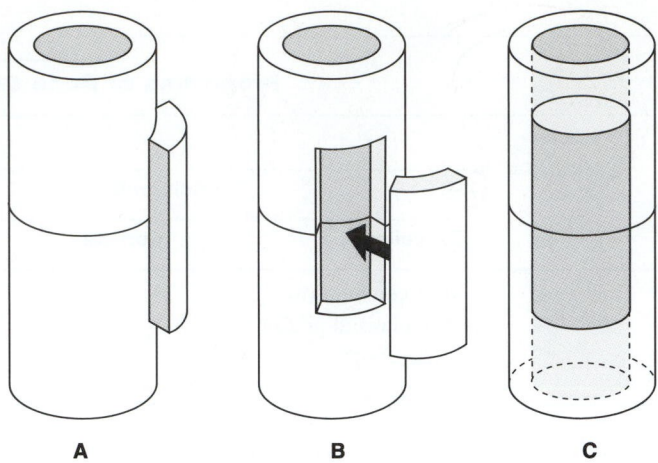

Figure 5-2
Onlay (*A*), inlay (*B*), and stent (*C*) grafts. [Reproduced with permission from Muschler GF, Lane JM: Orthopaedic surgery. In Habal MB, Reddi AH (eds): *Bone Grafts and Bone Substitutes.* Philadelphia: WB Saunders; 1992:383.

COMPRESSION

Strut grafts are appropriate in settings where the mechanical loading is primarily compressive, as in the spine and hip. Healing bone adjacent to or surrounding a strut limits the critical mechanical demands placed on the strut to the time of incorporation of the neighboring bone, usually 8 to 20 weeks.

COMPLEX LOADING

Replacement of an entire bone or a significant portion of bone represents a complex situation in which short- and long-term mechanical integrity depends on several mechanical and biological variables, including the strength of the replacement material, the loading demands at the graft site, and the rate and extent of ensuing revascularization, osteoconduction, and remodeling.

In terms of biocompatibility, vascularized autogenous bone would be preferable for this application. Bone from the standard donor sites (Fig. 5-3), however—iliac crests, ribs, and fibulae—is generally mechanically insufficient when implanted but will hypertrophy in response to mechanical loading. Even when internal fixation is used for rigid stabilization to shield the grafted area from mechanical load, the graft eventually becomes the principal source of structural stability. Most grafting for bone replacement therefore utilizes allograft bone, with a somewhat greater success rate.

Specific techniques employed in such situations are as follows:

- *Segmental replacement.* These grafts, used to replace an entire segment of bone between two adjacent joints (but not the articular surfaces), may consist of either allograft bone or vascularized fibulae (Fig. 5-4). While screws may be used for fixation, the minimum number to guarantee osteosynthesis is recommended in order to avoid stress risers that may lead to fracture—a consideration that again favors the use of allograft segments.
- *Bone transport via external fixation.* Although not bone grafting in the technical sense, the system devised by G. A. Ilizarov nevertheless achieves the goals of grafting for such conditions as nonunion by an ingenious process of osteotomy and controlled distraction. (For extended discussion, see Chap. 12.)

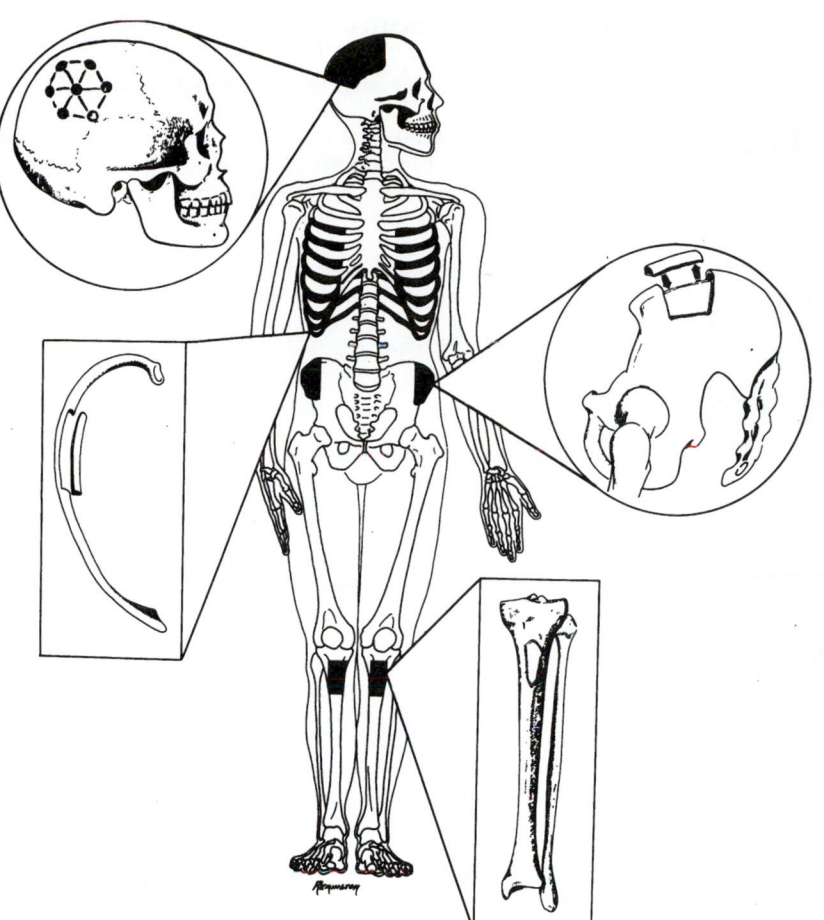

Figure 5-3
Bone graft donor sites. Reproduced as modified with permission from Habal MB. Craniofacial surgery. In Habal MB, Reddi AH (eds): *Bone Grafts and Bone Substitutes.* Philadelphia: WB Saunders; 1992:318. (From Habal MB: Bone graft and bone substitute. Biology and clinical applications. *Plastic Surgery Education Foundation/ Instructional Courses.* St. Louis: Mosby Year-Book; 1990; 3:280.

- *Bone blocks.* Blocks of bone from various sites are typically used as replacement material in an open cavity in mechanically uncompromised bone.
- *Periprosthetic grafts.* Where bone stock is insufficient to accommodate a standard implant, as in total hip or knee replacement, and use of a custom prosthesis is deemed too expensive or otherwise inadvisable, autogenous or (for larger defects) allograft bone can be utilized as grafting material. This approach has both advantages (e.g., the bone graft can be customized to conform to conventional implant design) and disadvantages, the most significant being the uncertainty of long-term mechanical integrity.

DEFECT CORRECTION

In situations where a graft material is not required to bear significant mechanical loading, for example, when the aim is to fill a cavitary defect, pieces of bone (e.g., chips, strips, "matchsticks") are laid on or into the graft site; in some cases, they may be set in place using a bone tap. Biosynthetic materials, sometimes incorporating growth factors, are increasingly being used for this purpose.

Particulate bone, consisting of chips of indeterminate small size, is typically used to fill discontinuity defects, especially those that are mechanically reinforced by some other device. Further down the scale of finer consistency is bone slurry, consisting of cortical or corticocancellous particles approximately 100 to 250 μm in diameter, and bone paste (often mixed with blood and such other components as collagen). They provide a matrix for vascularization and thus facilitate healing and remodeling.

Demineralized bone matrix (DBM), which can be considered a special type of bone allograft material, is used in a variety of clinical settings. After undergoing the demineralization process, the DBM apparently retains its osteoinductive capacity and is rendered less antigenic as well.

Biosynthetic materials, sometimes incorporating growth factors, are increasingly being used for this purpose. These include ceramics, various polymers, and calcium sulfate hemihydrate, whose healing ability may be augmented by the admixture of any of several bone morphogenetic proteins or other growth factors.

Hydroxyapatite (HA) and tricalcium phosphate are the most common ceramics. Both materials are available as solid or porous blocks, chips, or granules. In general, tricalcium phosphate is resorbed a few months after implantation, whereas high-density crystalline HA tends to degrade more slowly, over a matter of years.

Although it does not involve bone grafting as such, the repair of articular surface defects falls squarely within the province of the orthopaedist. Unlike other musculoskeletal components, harvested chondrocytes can be processed to retain their viability. Because hyaline cartilage is for all practical purposes avascular, however, these allografts are particularly resistant to satisfactory regeneration. To compensate, researchers have attempted a variety of strategies, such as incorporating cartilage cells within a collagen matrix and adding growth factors to their preparations.

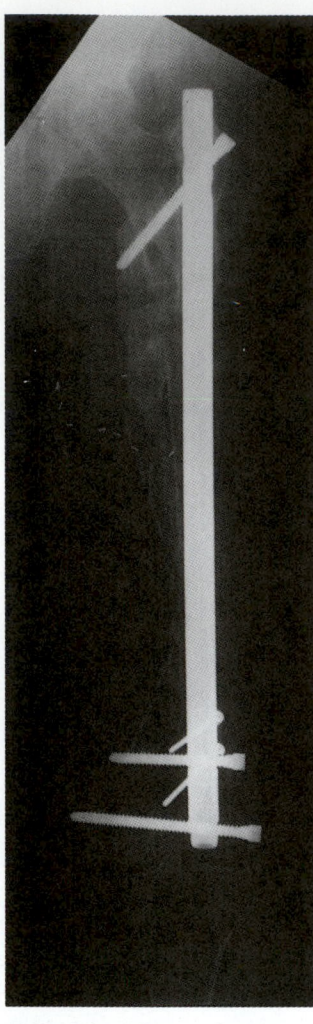
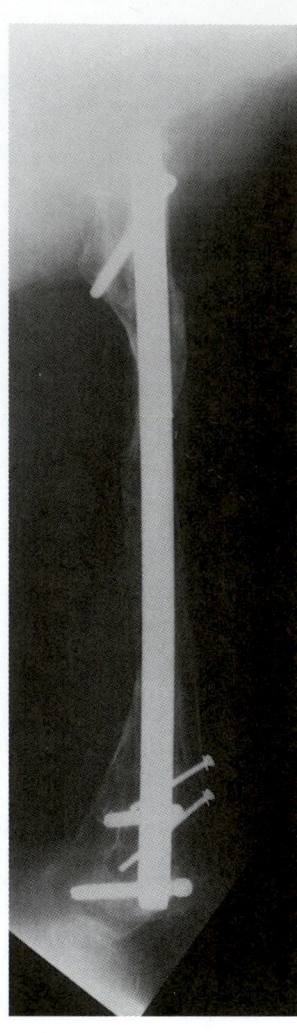

A   *B*

Figure 5-4
Segmental replacement for osteomyelitis using a delayed vascularized fibular graft and autogenous cancellous graft. *A.* AP. *B.* Lateral.

SUGGESTED READINGS

Einhorn TA: Enhancement of fracture healing. *J Bone Joint Surg [Am] 1995;* 77:940.

Esterhai JL Jr, Gristina AG, Poss R (eds): *Musculoskeletal Infection* (1990 symposium supported by AAOS/NIAMSD). Park Ridge, IL: American Academy of Orthopaedic Surgeons; 1992.

Habal MB, Reddi AH (eds). *Bone Grafts and Bone Substitutes.* Philadelphia: WB Saunders; 1992.

Schenk RK: Biology of fracture repair. In Browner BD, Jupiter JB, Levine AM, et al (eds). *Skeletal Trauma,* 2d ed. Philadelphia: WB Saunders; 1998:50–73.

Chapter 6

SOFT TISSUE REPAIR

Sally R. Frenkel and John C. Grew

The soft tissues associated with the skeleton each respond differently to injury. Consequently, a variety of techniques are used to effect repair of such injuries.

ARTICULAR CARTILAGE

Articular cartilage is an avascular tissue whose matrix endows it with unique biomechanical properties, allowing it to withstand forces normally transmitted across joints. The matrix architecture is determined principally by the arrangement of its type II collagen fibers and the associated proteoglycans, which provide the tissue with its mechanical strength and allow it to retain from 60 to 80 percent water within the matrix. Cartilage cells, or chondrocytes, are responsible for the secretion and maintenance of these and other matrix components (other collagens, large and small glycosaminoglycans, etc.). Acute injury or slower arthritic degeneration of cartilage affects both the composition of the matrix macromolecules and their distribution in the matrix, thereby reducing the tensile strength and compressibility of the tissue. Cartilage may be progressively lost from the articular surface and the subchondral bone may be exposed, with accompanying pain and loss of function.

The repair response of articular cartilage varies with the depth of the injury. If limited to the cartilage layer, the damaged tissue will become necrotic, and little if any regeneration is likely to occur; this may be ascribed to the avascular nature of the tissue. There may also be deterioration in the adjacent healthy tissue. If the subchondral bony plate is penetrated, the access to the bone's blood supply allows limited repair in the form of fibrous tissue or fibrocartilage, which is usually mechanically inadequate and temporary. The structural, biochemical, and mechanical differences between the fibrocartilage and the tissue normally found on the articular surface will probably cause this neocartilage to erode over a period of time, ranging from a few months to several years.

To restore pain-free function to a damaged articular surface, many techniques have attempted to induce regeneration of the hyaline cartilage. The ideal regenerate would be fully integrated with the adjacent host cartilage and the subchondral bone; a poorly reconstituted subchondral plate appears to predispose the overlying tissue to accelerated deterioration. The type and quantity of collagens and proteoglycans should be as close to that of normal tissue as possible, to allow the repair to have the mechanical and biochemical properties necessary at the articular surface, such as compressibility, strength, resistance to shear, and creation of a low-friction articulation. Current surgical treatment for damaged cartilage may consist of debridement or removal of loose flaps or pieces of cartilage, abrasion/burr arthroplasty at the site of the lesion, or subchondral drilling (Fig. 6-1).

Shaving or abrasion of a fibrillated articular surface may relieve symptoms and reduce locking of the joint; however, this procedure may also result in necrosis of the adjacent tissue and further fibrillation. Drilling into the subchondral bone induces the growth of fibrocartilage. A clot will form at the site, and precursor cells (presumably

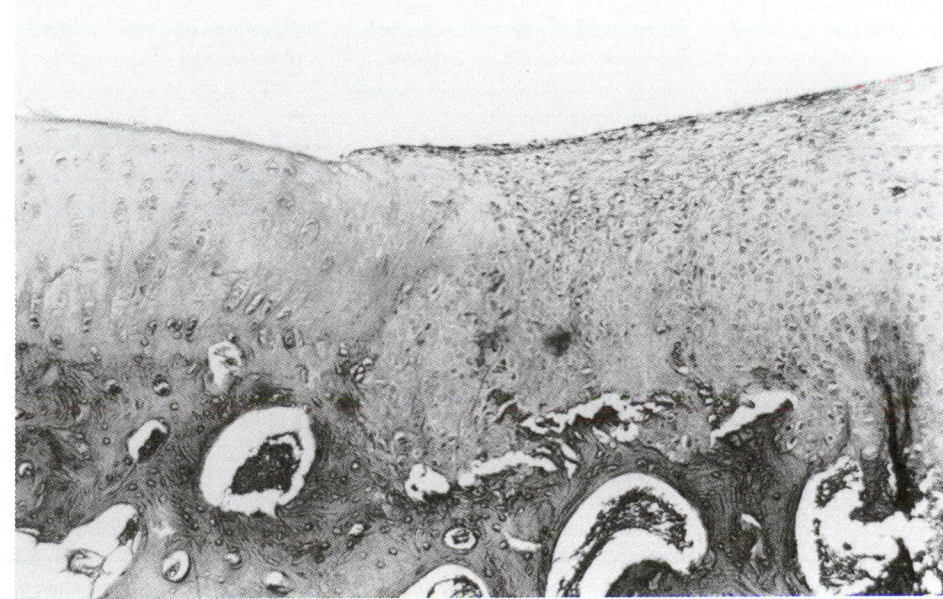

Figure 6-1
Cartilage repair 6 weeks after subchondral drilling in a rabbit. Native tissue is on the left, repair on the right. Repair is very cellular and disorganized, but surface is smooth and tissues are well-bonded to each other.

from the bone marrow and possibly the synovium) will migrate into the site. These cells will produce a matrix more fibrous than the normal surface, and the tissue will often fill the drill hole and spread onto the exposed bony surface. Although this tissue may provide relief from symptoms for some time, it often ultimately deteriorates due to the inability of the fibrocartilage to maintain the mechanical and chemical properties at the surface that normal hyaline cartilage would possess. Another recently developed method which may stimulate clot formation and subsequent repair is the treatment of the lesion and adjacent surface with mild enzyme solutions, to partially degrade the matrix proteoglycans. Long-term studies of this treatment are not yet available.

Some studies report that for small lesions which penetrate the bone, a regimen of continuous passive motion (CPM) following surgical treatment may improve the quality of the repair tissue, and render it longer-lasting. CPM does not appear to have any advantage for the repair of injuries which are limited to the cartilage layer. Periosteal, perichondrial, and osteochondral grafting have all been attempted with varying degrees of success. Periosteum and perichondrium possess a cambium layer that contains precursor cells that can be induced to differentiate into chondrocytes. Unlike osteochondral grafts, these cell sources have the advantage of being autologous and readily available. However, the durability of the repair tissue formed by such grafting has not been established.

Osteochondral allografts have been used with varying degrees of success; a properly fitted frozen allograft has a 70 to 85 percent chance of success. However, these grafts often undergo a slow deterioration. The degeneration may be ascribed to joint incongruity or immunogenicity of the graft.

An experimental technique undergoing active investigation is the transplantation of chondrocytes or chondrogenic cells of periosteal, perichondrial, or mesenchymal origin. A recent clinical study utilized a biopsy of autologous chondrocytes subjected to cell culture and reimplantation of the expanded population of cells at the defect site under a sutured periosteal flap. A hyaline-like repair tissue was observed; however, the investigators did not determine whether repair resulted from implanted chondrocytes or from periosteal cells. Several investigators have applied tissue engineering concepts to use of a variety of biomaterials to design chondrocyte-seeded implants for articular cartilage repair. A successful engineered biomaterial implant for articular cartilage repair must (1) provide a scaffold that will support chondrocytes, maintain their phenotype, and encourage normal metabolism; (2) prevent fibrocartilage formation; (3) retain its structural properties at the surgical site until endogenous tissue ingrowth occurs; and (4) resorb without adverse effect after adequate repair. Among the devices tested are demineralized bone (with perichondrium), polylactic acid matrices, polyglycolic acid matrices, hydroxyapatite/Dacron composites, fibrin, collagen gels, and collagen fiber matrices. Many of these implants have succeeded in effecting a hyaline-appearing repair of the created defect for varying lengths of time. In some cases, the repair may be accompanied by fibrocartilage formation. The performance of these implants may be improved by augmentation with growth factors (GF), which stimulate chondrocyte proliferation and/or matrix deposition. GFs being evaluated include transforming GF, insulin-like GF, fibroblast GF, and bone morphogenetic protein.

TENDON

Tendons attach muscle to bone. Like cartilage, tendons have a matrix whose chief components are type I collagen and proteoglycan. The collagen fibers are arranged in parallel longitudinal bundles, with the vascular and nerve supplies traveling in the surrounding loose connective tissue. The geometry of the fiber arrangement is responsible for the tensile strength of the tendon.

Depending on their function, tendons may be enclosed by a sheath or by a loose connective tissue paratenon. The sheath allows tendons to bend at sharp angles, as is necessary in the hand flexors. Where such bending does not occur, a paratenon surrounds the tendon.

Tendons may be avulsed from their bony insertions, or may be transected. When transected, a tendon first undergoes an inflammatory response at the wound site. If a paratenon is present, its fibroblasts will migrate into the area between the cut ends of the tendon and form granulation tissue. The fibroblasts will synthesize collagen, whose fibrils will at first be oriented perpendicular to the tendon's long axis. Over time, the lines of stress on the tendon will cause the collagen fibers to become oriented parallel to the long axis. The large tendon/scar callus which forms will remodel slowly, with the tensile strength of the tendon increasing as the callus size decreases and its collagen becomes more organized. If no stress is placed on the tendon, remodeling will not occur. Directional stress stimulates secretion of collagen and crosslinking of fibers, resulting in increasing strength. At approximately five months after injury, the scar has a close histological resemblance to the normal tendon.

In sheathed tendons, it appears that cells from the cut tendon ends or from the sheath may contribute to the scar; the source of the bridging callus is an unresolved question.

SURGICAL REPAIR

For successful exogenous and endogenous tendon repair and restoration of full tendon function, the most important factor is the ability of the surgical technique to achieve and maintain the closest apposition possible between the severed ends of the tendon. This is dependent upon the strength of the suture material and its susceptibility to viscoelastic creep, and the strength of the suture technique and type of knotting. Any surgical technique must take care to preserve the vascular supply to the tendon or risk a less successful repair. Postoperatively, a regimen of passive mobilization appears to reduce and possibly prevent the most serious complication of repair, the formation of adhesions. Passive mobilization also improves the early strength of the tendon. An extremely important contributory factor to the success of a repair is the extent of the injury to surrounding structures, including crush injuries of the soft tissue and fractures. Predictably, repair of a tendon with minor damage to the surrounding tissue bed has a far better outcome than repair in more complex injury situations.

Avulsion of a tendinous insertion is most often a sports-related injury. If surgical treatment is required, this treatment usually consists of reattachment to the bone with nonabsorbable staples, sutures, and screws with spiked washers.

LIGAMENT

Ligaments connect bone to bone, and may be extra- or intraarticular. As in tendons, the cellular component is the fibroblast, with type I collagen being the most important structural element in the extracellular matrix. However, the collagen in tendons is more highly organized than in ligaments. Also present in the matrix are a high percentage of water (60 to 70 percent of the wet weight), type III collagen, proteoglycans, fibronectin, and small amounts of elastin. The mechanoreceptors and free nerve endings present in ligaments may assist in joint stabilization.

When an extraarticular ligament is injured, a fibrin clot will form between the torn ends, and fibroblasts will proliferate and secrete matrix components. The earliest repair tissue contains an increased percentage of type III collagen, which over time remodels to contain more type I collagen. As crosslinks form between the type I collagen fibrils, the tensile strength of the repair increases. As is the case with tendons, applied stress is important in the remodeling of the repair tissue. The remodeling may take a year or longer to be complete.

SURGICAL REPAIR

Ligaments within the joint, such as the cruciates, do not have the ability to repair themselves to the extent that extraarticular ligaments have. For extraarticular ligaments, surgical repair may not provide a significant advantage over self-repair. However, surgery is often necessary in repair of cruciate ligament tears, whether with synthetic or biological graft materials.

Tendons are frequently used as autograft material, with one of the most thoroughly tested autografts being the bone-patellar tendon-bone complex. Allografts must be processed to render them sterile; this is generally achieved through sterile harvest and freezing cobalt irradiation or ethylene oxide gas sterilization. Either of these procedures may alter the mechanical properties of the graft, as may storage of the graft by freezing. Allografts have a higher failure rate than do autografts. The position of insertion and initial tension on the graft during repair are important determinants of the mechanical strength of the replacement.

Ligament shortening due to contraction following injury may limit joint motion; in cases of ligament "stretch," laxity may be a persistent problem. Absence of stress on the ligament leads to shortening; studies indicate that this shortening may be prevented by application of artificial stress-generated electrical potentials, simulating those normally produced by mechanical loading of the ligament.

PERIPHERAL NERVE

Peripheral nerves are frequently damaged during musculoskeletal injuries of the extremities, where nerves of various sizes are closely apposed to appendicular long bones and joint spaces. In some cases, such as carpal tunnel and thoracic outlet syndromes, anatomical constraints and repeated movement conspire to irritate or compress nerves without overt trauma. A fortunate feature of many nerve injuries is their self-limiting nature: resultant pain limits further involvement and facilitates more rapid recovery from injury.

Traumatic nerve injury is currently classified by histopathological criteria, rather than by source or mode of injury. In first degree injury, also called neurapraxia, there is conductivity loss at the site of lesion without degeneration of affected fibers. Thus, sensory and motor functions may be temporarily impaired, but recovery is usually complete. Local factors are important in first degree injuries; for example, epineural density often protects smaller sensory fibers better than larger motor fibers. Hence, motor impairment is typically more frequent and longer lasting than sensory impairment.

Second degree nerve injury, known as axonotmesis, results in complete severing of nerve fibers at the point of injury. This interruption of axonal continuity results in short-term loss of sensory and motor functions. The long-term outcome of second degree injury can still, however, be favorable, depending upon the magnitude and geometry of the trauma. The key feature of this level of injury is the integrity of the endoneurium and perineurium. Classical Wallerian degeneration of severed fibers follows the trauma, accompanied by muscular atrophy. Some sensory and motor function returns subsequently as damaged fibers reestablish sensory and motor connections distal to the site of injury, extending processes through the remaining neurilemma.

Third-, fourth-, and fifth-degree nerve injuries, collectively known as neurotmesis, results from complete severing of nerve fibers at the point of injury with accompanying damage to endoneurium, perineurium, and epineurium, respectively. These injuries all involve loss of sensory and motor functions. Interruption of axonal integrity is followed by Wallerian degeneration, retrograde axonal degeneration, depletion of Nissl substance from the cell body (chromatolysis), loss of function, and muscle atrophy. Prognosis and recovery vary in proportion to the level of damage to surrounding connective tissues. Surgery is frequently required to realign severed fibers, fascicles, and trunks. Spontaneous axonal regeneration infrequently occurs when perineurium and epineurium are interrupted, and this is often nonproductive.

Injury, inflammation, and fibrosis exacerbate functional loss and complicate regeneration of nerve fibers, following even mild injuries. Skeletal displacement and edema may impinge upon nerves, deforming them and causing local ischemia. Fibrosis and adhesions impair conduction and produce progressive irritation.

Mode of injury plays a role in the overall outcome of an injury and its repair. Compression injuries of nerve are the most common type, especially among nontraumatic injuries. This may be due to the high level of sensitivity of nerves to compression, of both traumatic and inflammatory origin. Examples of this sensitivity are the extremely debilitating effects of radiculopathies and the entrapment neuropathies.

Stretching injuries, which do in extreme cases produce high-degree injury, are less likely to do so than compression injury, due to an inherent slackness of peripheral nerve tissue. In the relaxed state, nerves tend to follow an undulating course and are capable of elongating and sliding within their perineurial tubes, attaining 120 to 130 percent of their original length. Forcible displacement of a joint, or prolonged fixation of a limb may supersede these tolerances and cause injury, particularly at a joint at risk of trauma. Compression injury-type tissue changes are seen during and after stretch injury, such as fiber deformation, ischemia, and edema. Severing of fibers and connective tissue sheaths occur with increasing stretching distance.

The regeneration and repair of nerve depend ultimately on the degree of injury to the surrounding layers of connective tissue. Wallerian degeneration may be effectively reversed by regeneration of processes distal to the site of injury. However, neurons are incapable of dividing and migrating, and regeneration must draw solely upon the existing neuron pool (Fig. 6-2A). Within days after a second or higher-degree injury, the distal process degenerates, followed by its neurilemmacyte (Schwann cell) sheath (Fig. 6-2B). Inflammatory cells phagocytose this debris. At the same time, the nucleus becomes acentrically positioned and chromatolysis occurs. After 2 to 3 weeks, the severed fiber regenerates itself, along a path established by newly formed neurilemmacytes which organize themselves into a dense cord retracing the previous pathway (Fig. 6-2C and D). These newly formed processes are neurofilament-rich and vesicle-poor, compared to nontraumatized fibers, and possess additional collateral endings. Should the severed proximal and distal fibers be misaligned following trauma (Fig. 6-2E), the regenerated endings may come to innervate mismatched end structures (e.g., a motor fiber may regenerate along a sensory pathway). Neurilemmacytes are believed to control and coordinate the regeneration of nerve fibers, but little is known about how they do so. A number of soluble and membrane-bound factors produced by inflammatory cells, neurilemmacytes, and connective tissue cells certainly contribute to the regenerative activities of neuron processes and neurilemmacytes.

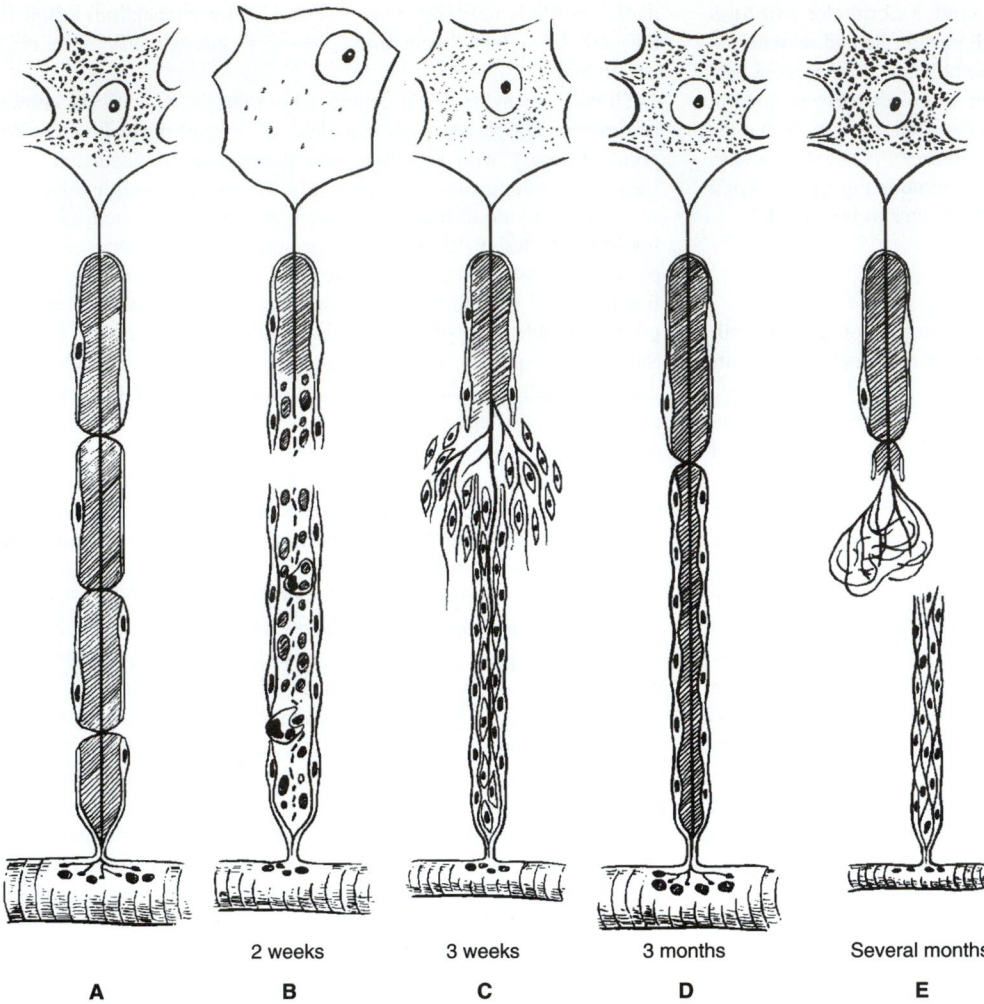

2 weeks · 3 weeks · 3 months · Several months

A · B · C · D · E

Figure 6-2
Sequence of events in the regeneration of an injured nerve fiber (see text for explanation). (Reproduced with permission from: Junquirea LC, Carneiro J, Kelley RO: Nerve tissue and the nervous system. In: *Basic Histology,* 8th ed. Norwalk, CT: Appleton-Lange; 1995: 179. Adapted from Willis RA, Willis AT: Injury and repair of nervous tissue. In: *Principles of Pathology and Bacteriology,* 3d ed. London: Butterworths; 1972:33.)

SKELETAL MUSCLE

Muscle injury is commonly classified and treated according to the mode of trauma. Injured muscle tissue becomes inflamed and edematous, and is infiltrated by leukocytes which phagocytose necrotic muscle tissue and provide soluble mediators of regeneration such as fibroblast growth factor (FGF) and prostaglandins. These factors act on the connective tissue elements and satellite cell populations of injured muscle to effect the coordinated regeneration of both its contractile (muscle) and elastic (connective tissue) components. Regeneration of muscle tissue depends on reestablishing a patent blood supply to provide inflammatory cells and soluble mediators of myoblast activity. These and other factors, such as agrin, a protein situated in the muscle cell membrane (sarcolemma), undoubtedly also contribute regenerative signals to nerve endings damaged by the trauma.

The prognosis for laceration and transection injuries in muscle depends on the completeness of separation and the realignment of separated ends, particularly with regard to the reestablishment of blood flow. Most necrotic change at the site of laceration and transection injuries results from ischemia which accompanies local vascular damage. Dense fibrotic tissue is often deposited to rejoin the severed ends of transected muscles, with reduced tensile strength and contractile force following healing.

Stretch and contraction injuries initially disrupt the sarcomeric myofilament array and rupture the sarcotubules and sarcolemma of the myofiber. Later changes include alterations in mitochondrial morphology and enzyme activity. The myotendinous and osteotendinous junctions are more prone to tear injury upon stretch than either muscle or tendon tissue, particularly during unaccustomed exercise when muscle and tendon are used to absorb shock or force. The regeneration process and its outcome in stretch and contraction injuries vary with the extent of fiber tearing and the intensity of inflammation induced by the trauma.

Regeneration of atrophied muscle involves replenishment of the contractile myofilament proteins lost during the period of disuse or immobilization rather than on mitotic cell division. Thus, protein synthetic activities within the myofiber contribute to the repair of disuse injury. Additionally, insulin sensitivity of the muscle gradually increases and regains its original level, in proportion to insulin receptor density in the sarcolemma. Soluble factors such as growth hormone (somatotropin), testosterone, and corticosteroids promote these cellular activities. Exertion-induced damage to individual fibers and their sarcolemmae appear to cause the muscle soreness and cramping which often follows unaccustomed exercise. Inflammation and the resultant cellular responses to inflammatory mediators may contribute to the reversal of cellular damage. Recovery is generally independent of all factors except rest.

Mature skeletal muscle fibers are post-mitotic cells which are ordinarily incapable of dividing in an adult human. Skeletal muscle fibers are formed in the embryo by the fusion of uninucleate myoblasts into multinucleate syncitiae which we recognize as the familiar skeletal muscle fibers. A small number myoblasts persists, however, in adult muscle tissue as quiescent stem cells (satellite cells) that respond to injury or stimuli such as FGF by proliferating and fusing to form additional myofibers. Experiments have demonstrated that the basal lamina of muscle fibers, especially at neuromuscular junctions, contain hormone-like signals which direct the independent regeneration of injured muscle and nerve endings to reestablish neuromuscular connections. Agrin directs the reappearance of acetylcholine receptors at neuromuscular junctions in regenerating skeletal muscle.

BLOOD VESSELS

Vascular damage during orthopaedic injury includes trauma to local extramedullary blood vessels, intracortical osteonic (Haversian) vessels, and intramedullary bone marrow. In all cases, inflammatory mediators and other soluble factors play critical roles in the generation of new blood vessels (neovascularization), as does tissue hypoxia. Moreover, the removal and replacement of necrotic bone is ultimately dependent on the regeneration of associated blood vessels, just as the initial stages of osteogenesis depend on vascularization of embryonic connective tissues and infiltration by primitive marrow elements.

The chemical mediators involved in the interrelated fracture repair and vascular regeneration processes are diverse and have many sources. Factors influencing the revascularization of injured tissues include: FGF, vascular endothelial growth factor, transforming growth factors α and β, tumor necrosis factor α, platelet-derived growth factor, interleukin-8, α-interferon, cartilage-derived inhibitor, and thrombospondin. These are provided by platelets and a number of cell and tissue types, including fibroblasts, macrophages, and skeletal muscle and bone cells. The targets of these factors include fibroblasts, pericytes, vascular endothelial cells, and smooth muscle fibers. Bone cells, additionally, may respond to signals elaborated by regenerating fibroblasts, pericytes, vascular endothelial cells, and smooth muscle fibers.

Blood vessels initially develop by the proliferation and differentiation of vascular endothelial cells, with nonendothelial components developing later. New capillaries sprout from a continuous endothelial cell layer first by mitosis and later by formation of large vacuoles which fuse with those of neighboring cells to form a lumen. The direction of sprouting is guided by a pseudopod which extends laterally in intimate contact with basement membrane laminin and connective tissue ligands, probably in response to chemoattractant signals or oxygen concentration. Pericytes become associated with new capillaries shortly after endothelial cells have established a lumen, apparently developing under the influence of transforming growth factor β. Pericytes, in turn, produce osteonectin, which is believed to drive osteogenesis accompanying vascularization at sites of bone repair.

Vessels which are severed during trauma may anastomose by alignment of their severed ends and extension of new capillary sprouts. Osteonic vessels are similarly revascularized by ingrowth of capillary sprouts, and these may additionally anastomose with surviving vessels. Connective tissues and smooth muscle develop circumferentially after regeneration of the endothelium, probably in response to soluble factors such as FGF and insoluble basement membrane and fiber ligands.

SUGGESTED READINGS

Alberts B, Bray D, Lewis J, et al: Cell junctions, cell adhesions, and the extracellular matrix. In: *Molecular Biology of the Cell*, 3d ed. New York: Garland; 1994:992–993.

Alberts B, Bray D, Lewis J, et al: Differentiated cells and the maintenance of tissues. In: *Molecular Biology of the Cell*, 3d ed. New York: Garland; 1994:1152–1154.

Bischoff R: Proliferation of muscle satellite cells on intact myofibers in culture. *Dev Biol* 1986; 115:129.

Bodine SC, Lieber RL: Peripheral nerve physiology, anatomy, and pathology. In: Simon SR (ed): *Orthopaedic Basic Science*. Rosemont, IL: American Academy of Orthopaedic Surgeons; 1994:325.

Burden SJ: The extracellular matrix and subsynaptic sarcolemma at nerve-muscle synapses. In Saltpeter MM (ed): *The Vertebrate Neuromuscular Junction*. New York: AR Liss; 1987.

Darnell JE, Lodish HF, Baltimore D: Multicellularity: Cell-cell and cell-matrix interaction. In: *Molecular Cell Biology*, 3d ed. New York: Scientific American Books; 1995:1185–1187.

Friedman MJ, Ferkel RD (eds): *Prosthetic Ligament Reconstruction of the Knee*. Philadelphia: WB Saunders; 1988.

Insall JN: Intra-articular surgery for degenerative arthritis of the knee. *J Bone Joint Surg Br* 1967; 49:211.

Johnson LL: Arthroscopic abrasion arthroplasty: historical and pathologic perspective—present status. *Arthroscopy* 1986; 2(1):54.

Jones EG: The nervous tissue. In Weiss L (ed): *Cell and Tissue Biology. A Textbook of Histology*, 6th ed. Baltimore: Urban & Schwarzenberg; 1988; chap 9:277.

Pachence JM, Frenkel SR, Lin H: Development of a tissue analog for cartilage repair. In Cima L, Ron E (eds): *Tissue Inducing Biomaterials*. Pittsburgh: Materials Research Society Press; 1992:125.

Potenza AD: Concepts of tendon healing and repair. In: *Symposium on Tendon Surgery in the Hand* (American Academy of Orthopaedic Surgeons, March 1974, Philadelphia; monograph). St. Louis: Mosby, 1975.

Schor AM, Canfield AE, Sutton AB, et al: Pericyte differentiation. *Clin Orthop* 1995; 313:81.

Sunderland S, Bradley KC: Stress–strain phenomena in human peripheral nerve trunks. *Brain* 1961; 84:102.

Sunderland S: A classification of peripheral nerve injuries producing loss of function. *Brain* 1951; 74:491.

Terzis JK, Skoulis TG: Injury of nerve tissue during stretching. In Brighton CT, Friedlaender GE, Lane JM (eds): *Bone Formation and Repair*. Rosemont, IL: American Academy of Orthopaedic Surgeons; 1994:421.

Toolan BC, Frenkel SR, Pachence JM, et al: Effects of growth-factor-enhanced culture on a chondrocyte-collagen implant for cartilage repair. *J Biomed Mater Res* 1996; 31:273.

Chapter 7

BASIC BIOMECHANICS

Frederick J. Kummer

STATICS AND DYNAMICS

When all of the forces acting on a body sum to zero, the body is said to be in equilibrium—the so-called static state. When the forces are not in equilibrium, a dynamic state may exist and accelerations are produced resulting in motion. A study of statics is useful in determining the loads on joints. For a biomechanical analysis, a force is depicted as a vector that is represented by an arrow defining the direction that the force acts by its orientation and the magnitude of the force by its length. A force acting at a distance from the center of a body creates a moment ($M = F \times d$). The result of several forces acting on a body can then be determined by simple mathematical or geometrical manipulation of the force vectors. In single-leg stance, the force on the hip joint is produced primarily from two sources: the superincumbent body weight, which is equivalent to approximately 85 percent of the total body weight, and the abductor muscle, which contracts to keep the pelvis level (Fig. 7-1). Because this is a static situation, the sum of the moments about the center of the hip is equal to zero ($\Sigma M = 0$); thus, the downward moment created by the remaining body weight acting along the distance from the center of mass of the body to the hip center is balanced by the upward moment created by the abductors acting through the distance from the greater trochanter to the center of the hip. The contraction of the abductor muscle produces a force of about two times body weight, so that when the two forces are added, the resultant force on the head of the femur is approximately three times body weight.

Dynamic studies enable the determination of the forces present during accelerations and motion. The relationship between torque, which is a force acting at a distance from the center of rotation, and acceleration of the limb is important. To walk faster, increased accelerations are required, so an increased torque must be developed. Since the torque about a joint is equal to the acting forces times the distance to the joint, and this distance is constant, the forces must necessarily increase.

By analyzing motion, the accelerations producing it can be determined. The motion of the knee and the force of the knee joint during normal level walking are illustrated in Fig. 7-2. Note that three force peaks are present during stance phase. They are due to the various muscle activities. Just after heel strike, the joint reaction force ranges from two to three times the body weight and is associated with contraction of the hamstring muscles, which have a decelerating and stabilizing effect on the knee. During knee flexion in the middle of the stance phase, the joint reaction force is approximately two times the body weight and is associated with contraction of the quadriceps muscle, which acts to prevent buckling of the knee during stance phase, or flexion. The third peak joint reaction force occurs during the late stance phase just before toe-off. This force ranges from two to four times the body weight, varying among the subjects tested, and is associated with contractions of the gastrocnemius muscle. In the late swing phase, contraction of the hamstring muscles results in a joint reaction force approximately equal to body weight. This demonstrates that a large force is applied across the joint even though the foot may not be in contact with the floor. These force patterns may change with velocity. As the velocity increases, the forces necessary to produce accelerations usually increase. For example, slow walking demonstrates a different force pattern from nominal walking. Non-weight-bearing crutch walking does not eliminate the joint forces

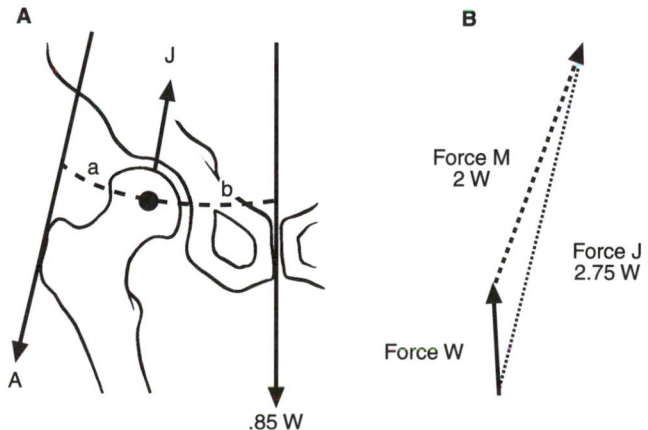

Figure 7-1
Forces acting on the hip joint during standing on one leg. The moment of the body ($0.85\ W \times b$) is equal to the abductor moment ($A \times a$). Summing the body and abductor forces produces the load on the femoral head.

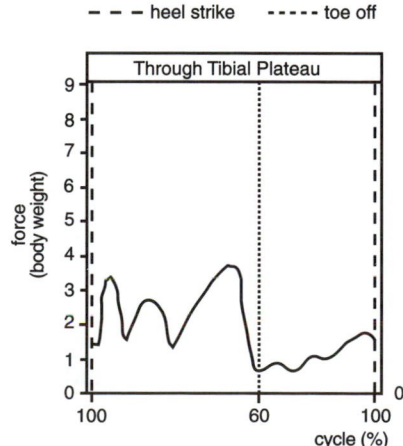

Figure 7-2
Forces and motion of the knee during level walking.

caused by muscle action accelerating and decelerating the protected limb.

BASIC MECHANICS

To develop an understanding of the internal effect of forces, it is necessary to study the loads on the structure and the resultant deformation. The principal loading situations are tension, compression, shear bending, and torsion. If load is applied to a structure such as a whole bone, a load-deformation curve can be developed as the loads are increased, and the deformations increase (Fig. 7-3). Three parameters for determining the strength of a structure are reflected on the load-deformation curve:

- The load that the structure can sustain before failing
- The deformation that it can sustain before failing
- The energy that it can store before failing

The strength in terms of load and deformation, or ultimate strength, is indicated on the curve by the ultimate failure point. The strength in terms of energy storage is indicated by the size of the area under the entire curve. The larger the area is, the greater the energy stored in the structure as the load is applied. The stiffness of the structure is indicated by the slope of the curve in the elastic region. The steeper the slope, the stiffer is the material. The load-deformation curve is useful for determining the mechanical properties of whole structures such as a whole bone, an entire ligament or tendon, or a surgical implant. This knowledge is helpful in the study of fracture behavior and repair, the response of a structure to physical stress, or the effect of various treatment programs.

Characterizing a bone or other structure, in terms of the material that composes it independent of its geometry, requires standardization of the testing conditions and the size and shape of the test specimens. Such standardized testing is useful for comparing the mechanical properties of two or more materials, such as the relative strength of bone and tendon tissue or the relative stiffness of various materials used in prosthetic implants. An exact unit of measurement can be used when standardized samples are tested, that is, the load per unit of area of the sample (stress), and the amount of deformation in terms of the percentage of change in the sample's dimensions (strain). The curve generated is a stress-strain curve, and the slope of this curve is the modulus of elasticity. Metals have a high modulus, bone is approximately an order of magnitude lower, and most polymers and biologic materials are at least a further order of magnitude lower. Stress is the load, or force, per unit area that develops on the cross

section of a structure in response to externally applied loads. The three units most commonly used for measuring stress in standardized samples are newtons per centimeter squared (N/cm^2); newtons per meter squared, or pascals (Pa); and meganewtons per meter squared, or megapascals (MPa). The stress on a perpendicular plane of a cylinder under tension and compression, and the stress on a shear plane are illustrated in Fig. 7-4.

Strain is the deformation (relative change in dimension) that develops within a structure in response to externally applied loads. The two basic types of strain are linear strain, which causes a change in the length of the specimen, and shear strain, which causes a change in the angular relationships within the structure. Linear strain is measured as the amount of linear deformation (lengthening or shortening) of the sample divided by the sample's original length. It is a non dimensional parameter expressed as a percentage (for example, centimeter per centimeter). Shear strain is measured as the amount of angular change with respect to a perpendicular reference angle lying in the plane of interest in the sample.

Biologic tissues have different stress-strain relationships depending on their composition. In the case of the soft tissues, made up of collagen and elastin fibers, the curve has a characteristic toe portion, and, as the force increases, becomes much stiffer. Cartilage, under tension loading, exhibits a similar type of stress-strain relationship. Biologic tissues also exhibit properties that are not found in structural material, such as stainless steel; they are anisotropic, exhibiting differing mechanical behavior as a function of test direction, so that the stress-strain behavior of a bone sample, for instance, depends on its orientation in relation to the long axis of the bone from which it is taken.

Another property that tissue may exhibit is viscoelasticity, which is time-dependent behavior under load. Cartilage under a constant compressive stress shows a creep response (a continuing lengthening or shortening over time), because of exudation of fluid from the sample, until an equilibrium is reached. If a constant deformation is applied to the cartilage, the phenomenon of stress relaxation occurs in which the stress slowly decreases as a function of time. Collagenous connective tissues also demonstrate viscoelasticity. It is evident that the duration of the contact pressure is of great importance. For exam-

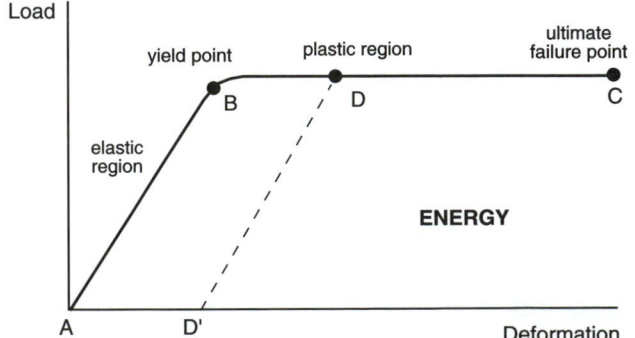

Figure 7-3
Load-deformation curve for an idealized material.

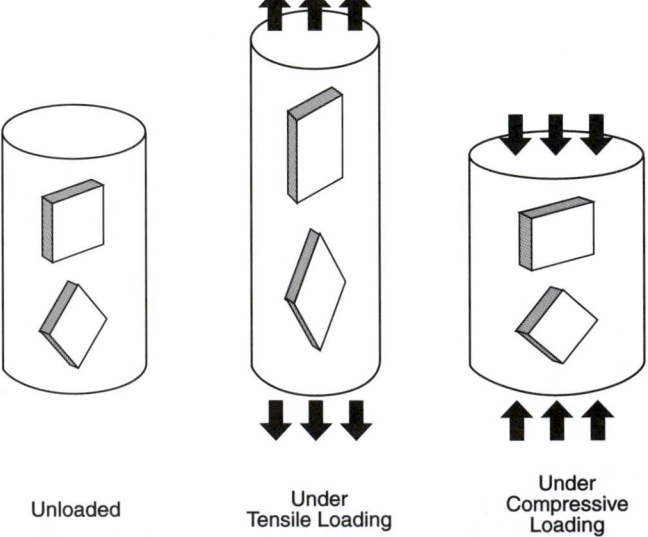

Figure 7-4
State of strain under tension and compression loading. *Block rectangles* represent a unit tensile and shear (45 degrees) element in the unloaded state.

ple, it has been demonstrated that this tissue, under tension loading, exhibits a time-dependent stretch; that is, the material will continue to stretch as a constant load is applied for measurable periods of time. This reaction to the load comprises four well-defined regions. As the load is applied, there is an area of immediate elastic deformation; if the load is taken off immediately, the material recoils elastically back to its original size. If, however, the load is left on, the material continues to stretch. This stretching tends to reach a limiting or steady-state value. If the load is allowed to remain for an appreciable period of time and is then removed, there is an immediate elastic recoil toward the material's original dimension. Return to the original dimension does not always occur if plastic deformation takes place. These responses to prolonged loading are typical of the response shown by materials classified as viscoelastic. Load relaxation and creep phenomena are found in ligaments and tendons. Knowledge of this time-dependent behavior is useful in overcoming contractures. Bone also exhibits viscoelastic, time-dependent behavior. As the loading or strain rate increases, the stress-strain curve also changes, becoming steeper in the elastic region to level off at higher values of stress. This effect is present in bone tissue or whole bone and determines the fracture patterns resulting from various types of injuries, for example, high speed or low speed.

A complex state of stress and strain can be described as a result of combined simple loading conditions in tension, compression, and shear. If a joint structure is placed under compressive loading, compressive stresses and strains will result on certain planes, while tension and shear stresses and strains occur in other directions.

A change in normal kinematics resulting in an altered state of stress or strain in a joint is one of the mechanisms leading to degenerative arthritis. A meniscal tear converts the knee joint from a three-dimensional joint to a planar joint by blocking normal tibial rotation. As a result of this restriction to motion, the instant center is displaced from its normal position. Forcing the joint to rotate about an abnormal instant center is similar to forcing a door to rotate about a bent hinge: the door jamb or the door will be worn down. This same process occurs in any joint that is forced to revolve about an abnormal instant center. Distraction may cause stretching of the ligaments. Compression may cause articular surface wear and an abnormal stress distribution in the articulating surfaces.

This altered stress distribution may occur, not only in the contact areas of the cartilage, but also adjacent to and beneath this area. A localized resorption reaction can occur in the region of altered stress and strain, sometimes followed by osteophyte formation. Even small mechanical changes can induce biologic processes that result in de-

generative arthritis. Caution should be exerted in exercising joints that display kinematic abnormalities on physical examination.

JOINT LUBRICATION

Human joints are exposed to a great variation of loading conditions. There can be high-impact, short-duration loads, such as in running; moderately low loads with a prolonged loading time, such as in standing; and low loads with rapid motion in the swing phase of walking. Over a lifetime, there is relatively little wear in the joints, indicating a very superior lubricating system. There are two types of lubrication. One is boundary lubrication, which is due to a single layer (monolayer) of lubricant adsorbed on each bearing surface. In the case of joints, boundary lubrication is achieved by a macromolecular monolayer attached to each articular surface. These layers carry loads and are effective in reducing friction. The second type of lubrication—fluid film lubrication—produces a greater bearing surface separation, and is due to a thin film of lubricant (Fig. 7-5). The pressure developed in the lubricating fluid carries the loads. In engineering materials, such as steel and bronze, the thickness and extent of the fluid film as well as its load-bearing capacity do not depend on the bearing materials. The lubricating characteristics depend on the physical properties, such as joint fluid viscosity, the shape of the gap between the two bearing surfaces, and the velocity of the relative surface motion. In the human joint, the bearing materials, such as the articular cartilage, are not rigid and have much lower modules of elasticity. Elastohydrodynamic lubrication therefore also occurs. As the joint surfaces move and pressure is developed, the fluid pressure deforms the surfaces. This changes the film geometry by increasing the surface area and shape of contact; thus, there is less chance of the lubricant escaping from between the bearing surfaces, and a longer lasting film is generated. This results in lower stresses on the cartilage.

In the joints, a mixed mode of lubrication occurs, with the joint surface loads being sustained by fluid film pressures in areas of noncontact and by boundary lubrication in areas of contact. In addition, cartilaginous joint surfaces differ from typical engineering bearings in that the cartilage is filled with fluid and is porous and permeable; surfaces can exude a lubricating fluid. As the joint moves and the surfaces slide, fluid is exuded in front of and beneath the leading half of the load. Once the peak stresses decrease, fluid is reabsorbed back into the cartilage, and it returns to its original dimensions. The viscosity of a lubricating fluid is very important. Synovial fluid undergoes large changes in viscosity both with changes in temperature (i.e.,

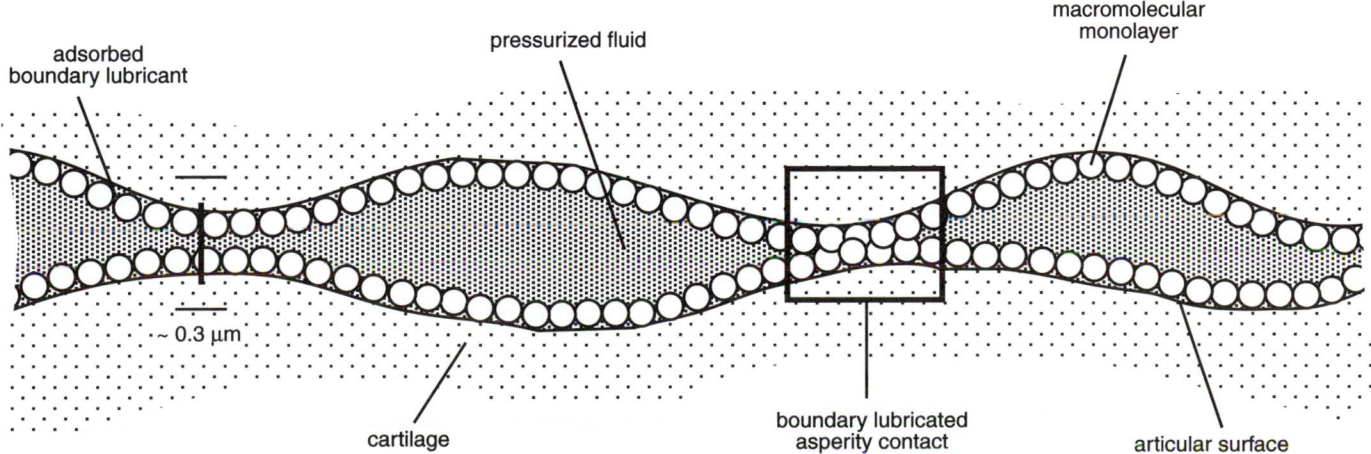

Figure 7-5
Schematic of various aspects of articular cartilage lubrication.

it is a Newtonian fluid) and with changes in velocity gradient (i.e., its thixotropic viscosity decreases as shear rate increases). For very fast velocities, a thinner, less-viscous lubricating film is desirable. If a joint effusion is present, the thixotropic properties of the synovial fluid may be compromised, resulting in reduced lubrication and subsequent wear of the joint surfaces.

SUGGESTED READINGS

Burstein AH, Wright TM: *Fundamentals of Orthopaedic Biomechanics.* Baltimore, Williams and Wilkins; 1994.

Chaffin DB, Andersson G: *Occupational Biomechanics.* 2d ed. New York: John Wiley and Sons; 1991.

Fung YC: *Biomechanics: Mechanical Properties of Living Tissues.* 2d ed. New York: Springer-Verlag, 1993.

Gozna ER, Harrington IJ, Evans DC: *Biomechanics of Musculoskeletal Injury.* Baltimore: Williams and Wilkins; 1982.

Mow VC, Hayes WC, (eds): *Basic Orthopaedic Biomechanics.* New York: Raven; 1991.

Nordin M, Frankel, VH, (eds): *Basic Biomechanics of the Skeletal System.* 2d ed. Philadelphia: Lea and Febiger; 1989.

Ozkaya N, Nordin M: *Fundamentals of Biomechanics: Equilibrium, Motion and Deformation.* New York: Van Nostrand Reinhold; 1991.

Radin EL, (ed): *Practical Biomechanics for the Orthopedic Surgeon.* 2d ed. New York: Churchill Livingstone; 1992.

Valenta J, (ed): *Biomechanics.* New York: Elsevier Science; 1993.

Winter DA, (ed): *Biomechanics and Motor Control of Human Movement.* 2d ed. New York: John Wiley and Sons; 1990.

Chapter 8

TISSUE MECHANICAL PROPERTIES

John L. Ricci

The mechanical properties of tendon and ligament, cartilage, and bone differ greatly. All of these tissues are complex structures consisting of composites of structural proteins and other materials. Under optimal conditions of age and health their properties are perfectly suited to their purposes.

All biological tissues are *viscoelastic*. This term implies that their mechanical properties are rate-dependent—that is, when a tissue is exposed to mechanical force, its response depends on the rate at which the force is applied.

TENDON AND LIGAMENT

GENERAL PROPERTIES

Tendons and ligaments function as flexible cables that the body uses to connect dynamic structures like muscles and organs, and rigid structures like bone. Such a purpose requires that these tissues have shock-absorbing capabilities, and that they be very strong in tension.

These tissues consist largely of longitudinally-aligned type I collagen—which gives them their great tensile strength. A stress/strain curve of a typical tendon or ligament (Fig. 8–1) shows three distinct regions. The first region, characterized by high strain at low stress, is referred to as the *toe region* of the curve. Here the collagen aligns parallel to the direction of loading and loses its crimp pattern under low load. This feature is relatively small in tendon and ligament because most of the collagen is already oriented parallel to the direction of loading. The toe region gives tendon and ligament its shock-absorbing capability. The second region of the curve is the *linear*

(straight) *region*. Here the slope of the curve is higher than in the toe region and represents the elastic modulus of the material. In the third region (*yield and failure region*) the plot plateaus and curves downward or abruptly drops as permanent stretching and failure of the structure occurs. The main parameters obtained from this curve are the elastic modulus (from the linear region), the ultimate tensile strength (maximum load) or the maximum stress (based on maximum load and cross-sectional area), ultimate strain (based on deformation to failure), and strain energy density to failure (the area under the curve). Elastic strain recovery of tendons is 90 to 96 percent after loading and unloading, indicating that they do not waste much energy during normal activity.

ANATOMIC LOCATION, AGE, AND EXERCISE

The effects of anatomic location can be seen when comparing properties of the flexor tendons of the digits (Fig. 8–2). The tendons of the little finger have significantly lower modulus of elasticity than the index, ring, and middle finger, with the middle finger having the highest modulus. While all of these tendons have similar ultimate strains, the middle finger tends to have a higher ultimate strain than the other three.

Age has effects on all regions of the stress-strain curves of tendons and ligaments. Age-related decrease in crimp angle of collagen results in a smaller toe region. Modulus increases until skeletal maturity and remains constant after. At early age a long failure region with near-zero modulus is observed, while at older ages this yield plateau is not as evident. Ultimate stress and strain increase with age until maturity.

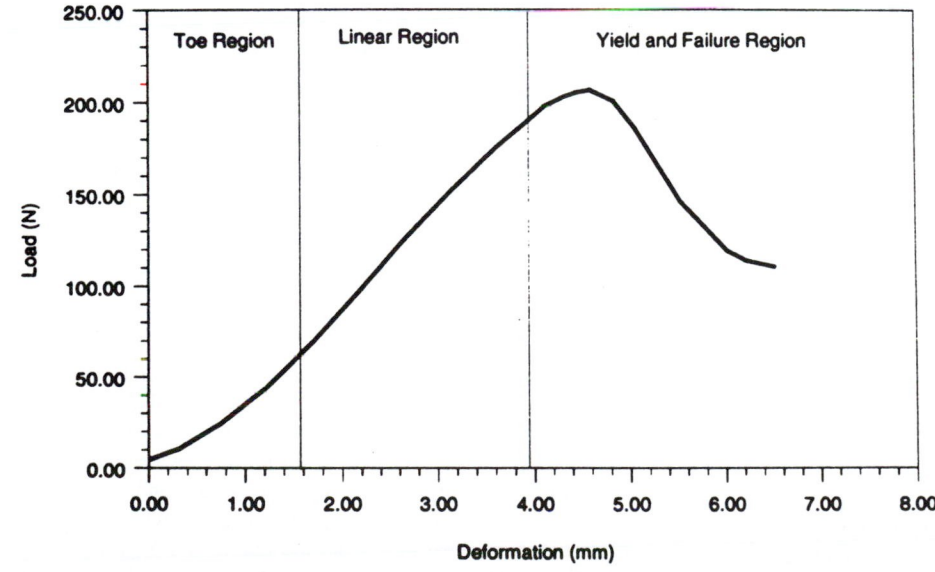

Figure 8-1
Basic stress-strain or load-deformation curve for tendon. [Reproduced with permission from Woo SL-Y, An K-N, Arnoczky DVM, et al: Anatomy, biology, and biomechanics of tendon, ligament, and meniscus. In Simon SR (ed): *Orthopaedic Basic Science.* Rosemont, IL: American Academy of Orthopaedic Surgeons; 1994:51.]

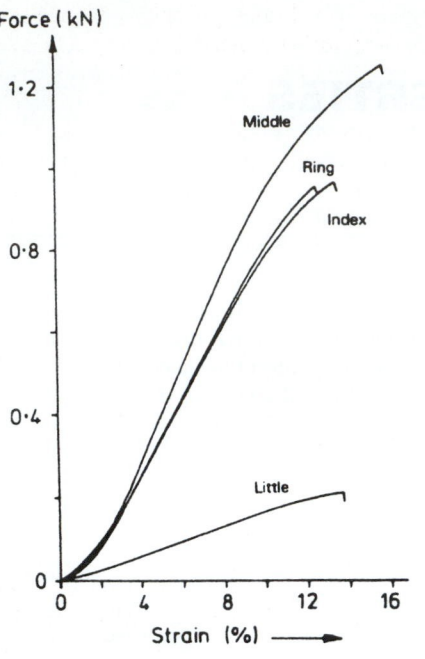

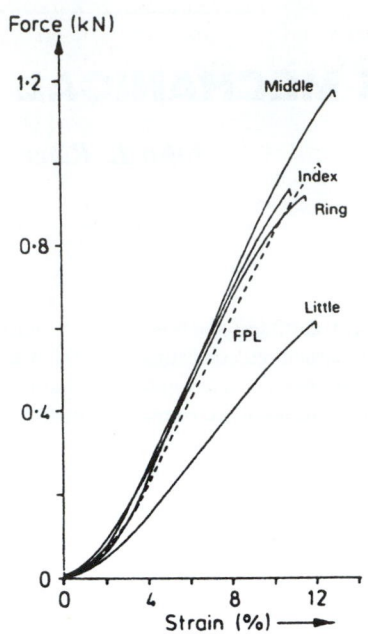

Figure 8-2

(*Left*) Mean tensile behavior of tendons of flexor digitorum superficialis. (*Right*) Mean tensile behavior of tendons of flexor digitorum profundus and flexor pollicis longus. (Reproduced with permission from Pring DJ, Amis AA, Coombs RRH: The mechanical properties of human flexor tendons in relation to artificial tendons. *J Hand Surg [Br]* 1985; 10:335.)

Exercise increases the weight, stiffness, and ultimate tensile strength of tendons. Conversely, immobility compromises the properties of tendons and ligaments. Specifically, collagen synthesis can be enhanced by exercise, and crimp angle and length may also be influenced. Exercised tendons show higher percentages of thick collagen fibrils, which can survive greater tensile forces due to more extensive cross-linking.

Viscoelasticity of these tissues means that their properties depend on the amount, rate, and history of force application. They exhibit creep (increase in strain, over time, when constant force is applied), stress relaxation (decrease in stress, over time, when a constant strain is applied), and hysteresis (difference in loading and unloading curves

due to energy loss). The result of these properties is that during cyclic loading the stress-strain curve shifts to the right (Fig. 8–3)—these structures become less stiff (lower modulus of elongation) and show higher strains after a number of exercise cycles. This has important implications for isometric muscle contraction, where the length of the muscle-tendon unit remains constant but the tendon elongates allowing the muscle to shorten and decrease fatigue. The viscoelastic properties of these structures also mean that higher strain rates (increased elongation speed) result in increased modulus of elasticity (stiffness).

Mechanical properties of human tendon and ligament can be summarized as follows: Human tendon has an elastic modulus of 1.2 to 1.8 GPa, ultimate tensile strength of 50 to 105 MPa, and ultimate strains of 9 to 35 percent. Young human anterior cruciate ligaments and medial collateral ligaments fail at reported ultimate loads of 340 to 2200 N, and at stiffnesses of approximately 220 to 240 N/mm (GPa).

CARTILAGE

Cartilage is the composite material the body uses as a bearing surface. It lines the bone surfaces in synovial joints, acting as a low-friction, lubricated surface and shock absorber. It is subject to high static and cyclic loading over several decades. Functionally it is a composite of collagen fibrils (reinforcement) in a hydrated proteoglycan matrix. The mechanical properties of the cartilage result from the unique interaction of these components with water and ions from body fluids.

BIPHASIC BEHAVIOR OF CARTILAGE

The mechanical properties of cartilage can be best understood if it is viewed as a biphasic material consisting of solid and liquid phases. The solid phase is a soft, porous, permeable matrix consisting mainly of collagen and proteoglycan. The liquid phase is water (and ions) forming 65 to 80 percent of the total tissue weight and residing in the pore structure of the solid matrix. The unique mechanical properties of cartilage arise partially from the interaction of water, ions, and proteoglycan which provide a swelling pressure. This is caused by proteoglycans trapped in the collagen matrix, which imbibe wa-

Figure 8-3

During cyclic loading of tendon, the stress-strain curve gradually shifts to the right. Usually, after 10 cycles, the curves become quite repeatable and steady. [Woo SL-Y, An K-N, Arnoczky DVM, et al: Anatomy, biology, and biomechanics of tendon, ligament, and meniscus. In Simon SR (ed): *Orthopaedic Basic Science*. Rosemont, IL: American Academy of Orthopaedic Surgeons; 1994:52.]

ter and swell. Since they are trapped in a strong matrix and can only swell to one-fifth of their normal free solution volume, the result is swelling pressure—caused by water-proteoglycan interaction and resisted by the tensile properties of the collagenous matrix. The physico-chemical reason for this swelling pressure results from the charged nature of the proteoglycan component. The proteoglycans contains SO_3^- and COO^- groups spaced at 10 to 15 angstrom intervals. To maintain electroneutrality these negative charges must interact with positive charges from electrolyte ions in solution. The concentration of these charges requires that total ion concentration in the proteoglycan be greater than that in the external bathing solution. The swelling pressure caused by these ions is known as the *Donnan osmotic pressure*. The close spacing of these charged groups fixed on the proteoglycan molecules also causes charge-to-charge repulsion forces that contribute to the swelling pressure, which generate a chemical expansion stress. Total swelling pressure is the sum of the Donnan osmotic pressure and the chemical expansion stress, which is counteracted by the stress generated in the solid matrix. Specifically, this resistance is known as the elastic stiffness or *bulk modulus* of the solid matrix. Total swelling pressure has been calculated to be 0.1 to 0.25 MPa in cartilage equilibrated in physiologic saline.

Damage to the collagen or proteoglycan components of the matrix can seriously compromise the mechanical properties of cartilage. Damage to the collagen matrix will result in swelling (gain in volume from water uptake), and loss of proteoglycan can also result in swelling because more space is available for water and proteoglycan expansion. Even subtle changes in this interaction between the two phases of this matrix can result in significant mechanical properties changes. For example, during early osteoarthritic changes, increase in cartilage hydration is a routine finding.

Along with swelling pressure, frictional resistance to interstitial flow provides cartilage with much of its viscoelastic properties. Functionally this means that, when a pressure gradient is applied to cartilage, water is capable of flowing through the matrix—in the same way that water flows through a sponge when the sponge is compressed. Resistance to this flow is based on a number of factors, including porosity, that can be expressed as a permeability coefficient (or inversely as a diffusive drag coefficient). Cartilage shows a very large drag coefficient—indicating that high pressures are required to move water through cartilage.

Cartilage permeability is nonlinear. That is, as cartilage is compressed, its permeability is reduced. This is based on reduction in water content and porosity as well as increased negative charge density.

VISCOELASTIC PROPERTIES OF CARTILAGE

Articular cartilage exhibits time-dependent behavior when loaded or deformed. In cartilage there are both flow-dependent and flow-independent mechanisms for this behavior. Behavior of cartilage under compression is best described as flow-dependent, while shear behavior is best described as flow-independent. Tensile properties are a combination of the two.

Flow-Dependent Viscoelasticity

When a constant compressive stress is applied to cartilage, deformation will increase with time (it will exhibit creep behavior) until an equilibrium is reached. It will also exhibit stress-relaxation—when deformed to a constant strain, stress will relax over time to an equilibrium value. This behavior is based on fluid flow and pressurization. When a constant load is applied to cartilage—resulting in creep—fluid flow results in gradual, nonlinear, transfer of load from the fluid phase to the solid phase. In human cartilage this typically

takes from 2.8 to 5.6 h depending on loading conditions. Human cartilage exhibits a range of compression characteristics depending on location and other factors. Its compressive aggregate modulus has been reported to range from 0.4 to 1.5 MPa. Cartilage exhibits a Poisson's ratio (a measure of how much a material expands, or bulges, when compressed or contracts when stretched) ranging from 0.0 to 0.1 in humans and up to 0.4 in animals. Because of its long equilibrium time, cartilage is almost never at equilibrium under normal loading conditions. Thus, fluid pressure is the main load-bearing mechanism in cartilage.

Flow-Independent Viscoelastic Shear Properties

The flow-independent viscoelastic properties of cartilage can be demonstrated under pure shear conditions—when no fluid flow is induced. This is done by shearing the tissue in such a way that volume remains constant. When this is done, the predominant contributor to the shear properties are the randomly-oriented collagen fibers of the middle and deep zones. The shear modulus of human cartilage has been shown to range from 0.05 to 0.30 MPa.

Shear stress can cause damage in cartilage through compression, and in particular during blunt trauma, because of the rigid fixation of cartilage to subchondral bone. During compression, cartilage will deform and spread laterally (as will any material with a Poisson's ration other than zero) causing stresses and strains within the material that may cause damage, as well as shearing of the cartilage from the subchondral bone.

TENSILE PROPERTIES

Tensile experiments on articular cartilage show that both the solid matrix (flow-independent) and fluid flow through the matrix (flow-dependent and caused by change in volume) contribute to its viscoelastic properties. If these tests are conducted at extremely slow rates or at equilibrium, the tensile response of the solid matrix can be tested independent of these viscoelastic mechanisms. A typical stress-strain curve produced in this way shows a toe region followed by a linear response region (Fig. 8–4). The toe region is produced by alignment of the collagenous elements (similar to tendon or ligament),

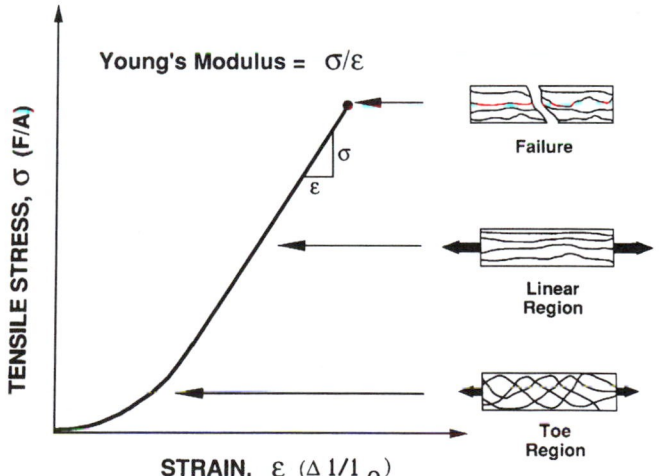

Figure 8-4

Representation of how the collagen network in a fibrous composite material such as articular cartilage might function during tension. [Reproduced with permission from Buckwalter JA, Mow VC: Cartilage repair in osteoarthritis. In Moskowitz RW, Howell DS, Goldberg VM, et al (eds): *Osteoarthritis: Diagnosis and Medical/Surgical Management*, 2d ed. Philadelphia, WB Saunders; 1992: 80.]

and the linear response indicates the tensile modulus, which ranges from 5 to 50 MPa in humans. This response depends on sample location, with superficial zone samples showing higher stiffness because of collagen content and orientation.

BONE

Bones form a network of structural elements that form the main rigid support framework of the body. Bone material itself is an anisotropic composite that is capable of repairing itself and remodeling its structure over time in response to its environment. Environmental factors that influence bone remodeling include its mechanical environment (exercise or disuse), certain hormones, metabolic conditions, and pharmaceutical agents. Remodeling of bone is an adaptive phenomenon that maintains structural integrity through maintenance of a biomechanical homeostasis. This is apparent in fracture healing, increase in bone density with exercise, and changes in long bone cross-sectional area to compensate for age-related decrease in density.

BASIC MATERIAL PROPERTIES

The material properties of bone vary greatly depending on the type of bone, the orientation of its microstructure, and the test parameters. A typical stress-strain plot for cortical bone (Fig. 8–5) in tension shows three regions—a linear region from which the elastic (Young's) modulus is obtained, a yield region which produces the yield strength, and a post-yield region which ends in the fracture point and produces the ultimate strength. Note that there is no toe region in the plot, as is seen in tensile tests of tendon, ligament, and cartilage. Similar plots are generated in compression tests and torsional tests, where the bone is twisted about its longitudinal axis. Torsional tests generate a stress-strain curves where the stress is shear stress and the strain is shear

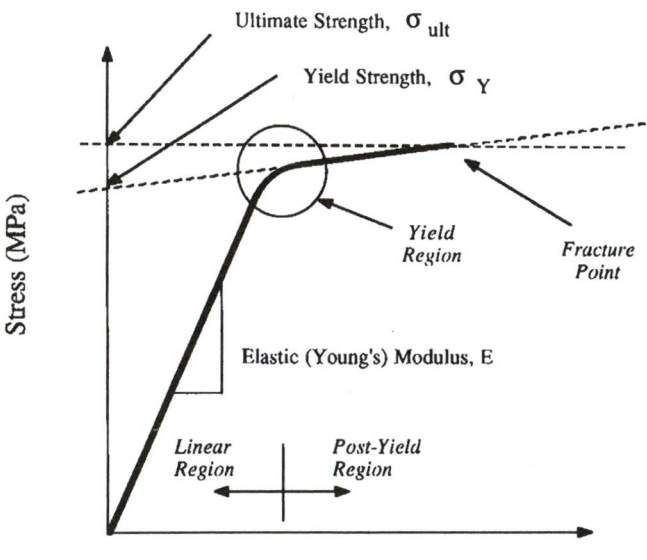

Figure 8-5
Typical stress-strain plot for cortical bone in tension, showing the linear, yield, and post-yield regions. Note that the yield and ultimate strengths are similar. [Reproduced with permission from Keaveny TM, Hayes WC: Mechanical properties of cortical and trabecular bone. In Hall BK (ed): *Bone. Volume 7: Bone Growth—B*. Boca Raton, FL: CRC Press; 1993:290.]

strain. The resultant shear modulus is analogous to the Young's modulus.

The above represent single tests to failure. Fatigue testing—where bone is subjected to multiple low amplitude loading cycles—represents a very different test environment.

As with the soft tissues discussed above, bone is viscoelastic and all test results are dependent on rate and history of loading.

Cortical and trabecular bone differ greatly in porosity (apparent density) and microstructure. Cortical bone—defined as bone with less than 30 percent porosity—typically has an apparent density of 1.85 g/cm^3 while trabecular bone has an apparent density of 0.30 g/cm^3. Trabecular bone varies in density much more than cortical bone, and its mechanical properties are very sensitive to this variation.

Architectural differences also contribute to the mechanical properties differences of cortical and trabecular bone. While cortical bone is a solid structure with typically 10 percent porosity from Haversian and Volkmann's canals, as well as cell lacunae and canaliculi, trabecular bone is not a solid structure but a network of interconnected rods and plates akin to an open-cell foam. The predominant orientation of this network depends on the direction of the forces applied to the bone according to Wolff's Law.

Elastic behavior of bone depends on material orientation, and can be described using the Young's modulus and Poisson's ratio. Cortical bone is sometimes described as transversely isotropic. This means that cortical bone has one set of properties when tested parallel to the axis of the osteons, and another when tested perpendicular to them. This is a type of anisotropic behavior. As opposed to an isotropic material which has a single Young's modulus, cortical bone in its longitudinal direction (parallel to the osteonal structure) shows a Young's modulus approximately 1.5 times that in the transverse direction. Trabecular bone can show widely varying Young's moduli (up to an order of magnitude difference) depending on apparent density and the predominant orientation of the trabecular structure.

Typical isotropic engineering materials like metals show Poisson's ratios of approximately 0.3, and can range from 0.0 to 0.5. Cortical bone has a relatively high Poisson's ratio of approximately 0.6.

Trabecular bone shows an entirely different behavior than cortical bone with respect to Poisson's ratio. Because of its open cell foam arrangement of interconnecting rods, compression causes bending of these rods on a microstructural level even if the specimen is in pure compression. The deformation behavior of this type of structure therefore depends on the microstructural arrangement of the trabeculae. Poisson's ratios for open cell foams vary greatly and are often nearly zero or even negative numbers (these materials contract when compressed). Poisson's ratios for trabecular bone have been reported in the range of 0.06 to 0.95.

Strength of cortical bone depends on its loading direction relative to its osteonal structure as well as the type of test. Bone is typically stronger in compression than in tension or torsion. Typical tensile and compressive strengths for cortical bone in the longitudinal direction are in the range of 130 MPa and 190 MPa, respectively. In the transverse direction tensile and compressive strengths are approximately 50 MPa and 130 MPa, respectively. Typical Young's modulus for cortical bone is in the range of 17,000 MPa (or 17 GPa).

Young's modulus of trabecular bone ranges from approximately 10 MPa to 9650 MPa depending on site, age, and type of test. In general, the upper end of this range represents high apparent density trabecular bone found in areas of the cranium, subchondral plates, and vertebral body endplates. In general, trabecular bone is much less stiff than cortical bone. Because of the open cell foam arrangement of trabecular bone, the relationship between its modulus and its apparent density is best described by a power function (with an exponent of 2) that, in real terms means that small changes in density result in

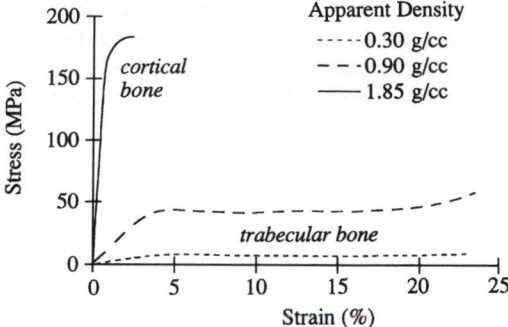

Figure 8-6
Example of typical compressive stress-strain behaviors of trabecular and cortical bone for different apparent densities. [Reproduced with permission from Keaveny TM, Hayes WC: Mechanical properties of cortical and trabecular bone. In Hall BK (ed): *Bone. Volume 7: Bone Growth—B*. Boca Raton, FL: CRC Press; 1993:326.]

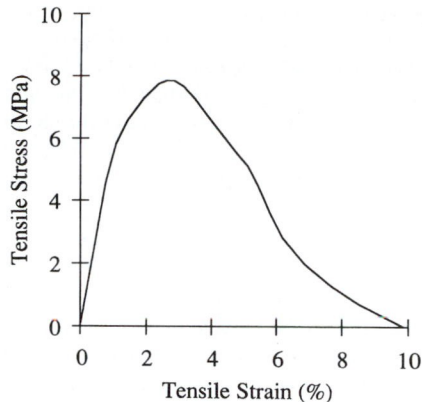

Figure 8-8
Tensile stress-strain behavior of trabecular bone. Compare this with the compressive behavior in Fig. 8–6. (Reproduced with permission from Gibson LJ, Ashby MF: *Cellular Solids: Structure and Properties*. New York: Pergamon Press, 1988.)

large changes in modulus. In elderly cadaveric vertebrae, for instance, a 25 percent reduction in apparent density results in a 56 percent decrease in modulus. Predominant orientation of the structural elements of trabecular bone also determines strength and modulus, and the uniaxial properties of trabecular bone differ greatly in compression versus tension. In compression, the stress-strain curve for trabecular bone shows three regions (Fig. 8–6). In the first (linear) region the individual trabeculae bend and compress, while in the second region failure occurs from a combination of trabecular fracture and buckling. Within this region trabecular bone can undergo very high strain. In the third region the sample stiffens and the trabeculae compress to form a more solid structure.

This is very different behavior than that shown by cortical bone in compression (Fig. 8–7). Its yield strength and ultimate strength are very close. Thus when cortical bone is loaded to its yield point it is very close to fracture, while trabecular bone can support considerable load and can sustain high strains well past its yield point.

In tension, while cortical bone again shows close yield strength and ultimate strength values, trabecular bone shows very different behavior than that seen in compression. While the linear region of the

stress-strain curve (Fig. 8–8) is similar to that seen in compression, after the yield point is reached the trabecular bone can support less and less tension as more and more trabeculae fracture.

Thus the compressive and tensile properties of cortical and trabecular bone can be summarized as follows: Cortical bone is a much stiffer material than trabecular bone; it is relatively ductile in tension in the longitudinal direction and brittle in transverse loading. In the longitudinal direction, its ultimate strains are higher than its yield strains in both tension and compression—making it a tough material which can absorb large amounts of energy before fracture.

Trabecular bone seems designed to carry compressive loads. It is a relatively low-density material that can withstand significant compressive forces, even post-yield, and can sustain high strains without transferring them to surrounding bone.

VISCOELASTIC BEHAVIOR

Cortical bone shows typical viscoelastic behavior in that its modulus and ultimate strength increase as a function of strain rate—bone is stronger during more strenuous activity. At strain rates produced during normal activities—which vary by an order of magnitude from 0.001 (slow walking) to 0.03 (running), modulus increases by 15 percent. Cortical bone strength is 20 percent higher during a brisk walk than during a slow walk. At the much higher strain rates (greater than 0.1 per second) that are seen during impact trauma, bone is considerably more brittle than during normal activities.

Cortical bone also displays creep behavior. If exposed to constant stress, it will deform slowly over time. If loaded to certain levels (that are below yield and ultimate strengths) for enough time, creep fracture will occur. The time required for this type of failure decreases as stress increases. If the stresses are removed before failure, permanent deformation can be induced in the bone.

Trabecular bone also shows strain rate dependence, although the relationship between strain rates and increases in modulus and strength are not as dramatic as those seen in cortical bone and are not as well understood. A 100-fold increase in strain rate from 0.001 (slow walking) to 0.1 (impact trauma) only causes a 30 percent increase in both modulus and strength. Bone marrow also has an effect on trabecular bone's load-carrying capacity—but only at very high strain rates. This is probably due to restriction of the flow of marrow elements through intertrabecular spaces at high strain rates.

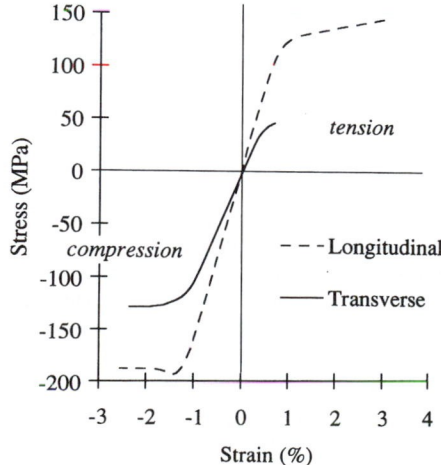

Figure 8-7
Stress-strain plots for human cortical bone for tensile and compressive loading. Data are shown for both longitudinal and transverse loading directions. (Reproduced with permission from Gibson LJ, Ashby MF: *Cellular Solids: Structure and Properties*. New York: Pergamon Press, 1988.)

AGE EFFECTS

Both cortical and trabecular bone show progressive deterioration with age in humans. In cortical bone the longitudinal modulus and tensile strengths of the human femoral diaphysis has been shown to decrease by about 2 percent per decade after age 20. This results in significant reduction in energy absorption (area under the stress-strain curve)—increasing fracture risk 7 percent per decade. Cortical bone loses stiffness and strength, and becomes more brittle, with age.

Trabecular bone loses density and changes architecture with age. It has been shown that trabecular bone in the lumbar spine decreases in density approximately 50 percent between ages 20 and 80. This decrease in density causes massive reductions in the material properties of this bone because of the power function relationship between bone density and properties. The change in architecture results in thinner, longer trabeculae that are fewer in number and more likely to buckle under load. The absolute loss of trabecular numbers is thought to be irreversible since bone can only remodel at existing surfaces. Much if this loss of bone is categorized as senile osteoporosis (seen in both males and females) and postmenopausal osteoporosis (seen in a relatively small number of females).

FATIGUE PROPERTIES

During normal activity, human bone is exposed to cyclic loading. In most cases cyclic loading does not cause damage to bone, but if certain stress levels and load cycles are exceeded, damage in the form of microcracks can occur in both cortical and trabecular bone. These microcracks can accumulate and compromise bone strength. They also probably stimulate bone remodeling on a microstructural level, and it is easy to understand how age-related reduction in remodeling and bone turnover can allow this type of damage to accumulate, resulting in spontaneous fractures.

In general, fatigue life of bone correlates better with strain than stress. Small numbers of cycles with high strains or large numbers of cycles at low strain can cause fatigue fracture—as long as the damage accumulates faster than it can be repaired. It is important to recognize that fatigue fracture, like creep fracture, can occur at levels lower than observed yield and ultimate strengths.

In real numbers, 5000 cycles of loading correspond to the number of steps in 10 miles of running, while one million cycles corresponds to 1000 miles. Fatigue data on human bones suggests that a total running distance of less than 1000 miles can cause fatigue fracture in human cortical bone. This correlates with stress fractures observed in military recruits undergoing strenuous training.

Fatigue fracture in bone correlates to three stages—crack initiation which results in a small decrease in bone stiffness, crack growth (propagation) which results in further degradation of stiffness, and final fracture, during which stiffness is rapidly lost along with the ability to support load.

The location, shape, and extent of crack formation is a function of bone architecture (with Haversian canals and other voids acting as initiators), and magnitude and sign (compression or tension) of applied loads. Bone attempts to repair these cracks and remodel to reduce stresses around the cracks. How well bone repairs these initial cracks is extremely important in reducing damage accumulation and

preventing the second stage. During the second stage these cracks tend to run together and propagate along weak interfaces such as between osteons. This causes some osteons to debond, changing the direction of crack propagation from perpendicular to parallel to the loading direction, and effectively stopping crack progression. If these cracks continue to propagate and coalesce to the point that the weak interfaces can no longer contain them, then the third stage results in rapid reduction in mechanical properties and in failure.

SUGGESTED READINGS

Betsch DF, Baer E: Structure and mechanical properties of rat tail tendon. *Biorheology* 1980; 17:83.

Buckwalter JA, Glimcher MJ, Cooper RR, et al: Bone biology. Part I: Structure, blood supply, cells, matrix, and mineralization. Part II: Formation, form, remodeling, and regulation of cell function (Instructional Course Lecture). *J Bone Joint Surg [Am]* 1995; 77;1256–1275, 1276–1289.

Cohen RE, Hooley CJ, McCrum NG: Viscoelastic creep of collagenous tissue. *J Biomech* 1976; 9:175.

Cowin SC: *Bone Mechanics.* Boca Raton, FL: CRC Press; 1989.

Fung YC: *Biomechanics: Mechanical Properties of Living Tissues.* New York: Springer-Verlag, 1981.

Fung YC: Stress-strain-history relations of soft tissue in simple elongation. In Fung YC, Perrone N, Anliker M (eds): *Biomechanics: Its Foundations and Objectives.* Englewood Cliffs: Prentice Hall; 1972:181–208.

Hubbard RP, Chun KJ: Mechanical responses of tendons to repeated extensions and wait periods. *J Biomech Eng* 1988; 110:11.

Mow VC, Hayes WC (eds): *Basic Orthopaedic Biomechanics,* 2d ed. New York: Lippincott-Raven, 1997.

Mow VC, Setton LA, Ratcliffe A, et al: Structure-function relationships for articular cartilage and effects of joint instability and trauma on cartilage function. In Brandt KD (ed): *Cartilage Changes in Osteoarthritis.* Indianapolis: Indiana University School of Medicine; 1990:22–42.

Mow VC, Zhu W, Ratcliffe A: Structure and function of articular cartilage and meniscus. In Mow VC, Hayes WC (eds): *Basic Orthopacdic Biomechanics.* New York: Raven Press; 1991:143–198.

Noyes FR, DeLucas JL, Torvik PJ: Biomechanics of anterior cruciate ligament failure: An analysis of strain-rate sensitivity and mechanisms of failure in primates. *J Bone Joint Surg [Am]* 1974; 56:236.

Noyes FR: Functional properties of knee ligaments and alterations induced by immobilization: A correlative biomechanical and histological study in primates. *Clin Orthop* 1977; 123:210.

Pring DJ, Amis AA, Coombs RR: The mechanical properties of human flexor tendons in relation to artificial tendons. *J Hand Surg [Br]* 1985; 10:331.

Simon SR (ed): *Orthopaedic Basic Science.* American Academy of Orthopaedic Surgeons, 1994.

Stockwell RA: Structure and function of the chondrocyte under mechanical loading. In Helminen HJ (ed*): Joint Loading: Biology and Health of Articular Structures.* Bristol, UK: Wright-Butterworth Scientific; 1992:126.

Woo SL-Y, Gomez MA, Woo YK, et al: Mechanical properties of tendons and ligaments: II. The relationships of immobilization and exercise on tissue remodeling. *Biorheology* 1982; 19:397.

Woo SL-Y, Peterson RH, Ohland KJ, et al: The effects of strain rate on the properties of the medial collateral ligament in skeletally immature and mature rabbits: A biomechanical and histological study. *J Orthop Res* 1990; 8:712.

Woo SL-Y: Mechanical properties of tendons and ligaments: I. Quasi-static and nonlinear viscoelastic properties. *Biorheology* 1982; 19:385.

Chapter 9

IMPLANT BIOMATERIALS

Frederick J. Kummer

There are a variety of metal, plastic, and ceramic biomaterials used in orthopaedics. Each has characteristic mechanical properties and in vivo stability that determine its efficacy for a particular application. How these materials are fabricated, the specific design in which they are used, and the clinical environment in which they are placed determine their success or failure as an implant biomaterial (Table 9-1).

METALS

The three basic metals used for implants are stainless steels, cobalt-based alloys, and titanium alloys; specifically, the majority of trauma devices are fabricated from 316L stainless steel and joint implants from Co–Cr–Mo or Ti–6Al–4V alloys. In general, stainless steels are the easiest to fabricate, Co-based alloys are the most wear resistant, and titanium alloys are the most biocompatible. Titanium alloys have approximately one-half the modulus of elasticity of stainless steels and cobalt-based alloys which means equivalent devices made from titanium alloys are twice as flexible and will transfer higher stress to bone.

Metallic implants are fabricated in three basic ways: (1) machining in which the implant is cut, milled, or drilled to the desired configuration, (2) casting where the implant is formed from molten metal poured in a mold, or (3) forging where the implant is shaped, either hot or cold, by a series of deformations such as bending or hammering.

The final properties of the implant are determined by the inherent mechanical properties of the metal, and are affected by the processing technique, in combination with aspects of the implant design such as size or thickness and the presence of stress risers such as holes or reduced sections. The two most important material mechanical properties for an implant are yield stress and fatigue strength; in general, forged metals are superior to cast metals.

Implant metals are corrosion resistant due to the presence of a passive outer film. With stainless steel, this layer can break down in constrained interstices, such as between a plate and screw, causing localized corrosion—termed crevice corrosion. Release of metal ions from corrosion, wear, or fretting, particularly Cr or Ni, has been suggested as a cause of metal sensitivity. Small particles (with a high surface area available for ion release) from wear have been implicated as one cause of osteolysis.

POLYMERS

The two main orthopaedic polymers are ultra-high-molecular-weight (UHMW) polyethylene and acrylic bone cement. Polyethylene is used for the articulating surfaces of joint implants, and is fabricated by machining or molding. Its mechanical properties are determined primarily by the molecular weight and distribution. Its wear resistance is deleteriously affected by inclusions, the presence of internal defects, and oxidation which can be altered by the sterilization

---

Table 9-1

Mechanical Properties of Biomaterials

	Ultimate Strength (MPa)	Modulus (GPa)	Elongation (%)
Metals			
Co–Cr alloy			
Cast	600	220	8
Forged	950	220	15
Stainless steel (cold-worked)	850	210	10
Ti–6Al–4V	900	110	15
Polymers			
Ultra-high-molecular-weight polyethylene	35	0.5	400
Bone cement (PMMA)	20	2.0	2–4
Ceramic			
Alumina	300	350	<2
Biological			
Cortical bone	100–150	10–15	~4
Tendon; ligament	20–35	2.0–4.0	10–25

method (e.g., gamma irradiation). Wear is also a factor of design in which the aspects of the congruency of bearing surfaces determine localized stresses within the polyethylene. Attempts to improve the wear properties of polyethylene such as carbon fiber reinforcement and processing to modify the polymer structure have been largely unsuccessful. Wear and resulting debris particles of polyethylene are thought to be the major cause of osteolysis. There have been increasing concerns about the effects of polyethylene wear debris leading to implant loosening due to localized inflammatory processes causing bone resorption. Recent studies have shown that there is significant variation in polyethylene quality (molecular weight, inclusions, defects) and that this variation is directly associated with clinical wear behavior. The current use of gamma irradiation for sterilization appears to promote deterioration of the mechanical properties of polyethylene due to continued internal oxidation of the free radicals created and to molecular weight and crystallinity changes; as a result, some manufacturers instead use ethylene oxide for sterilization. A new (extended-chain) polyethylene has recently been clinically introduced that is processed by a treatment of heat and pressure; laboratory tests indicate that it has somewhat improved mechanical properties and wear resistance. There is some concern that its increased stiffness can lead to higher subsurface stresses in the polyethylene, and there is evidence that its clinical wear performance has been decreased.

Bone cements consist of a prepolymerized acrylic component which is incorporated in acrylic monomer polymerized with an initiator such as benzoyl peroxide; a radiopaque agent such as $BaSO_4$ is often added. Available bone cements vary with respect to their viscosity and setting behavior which is affected by how they are handled; cooling decreases viscosity and increases setting time. Handling also causes internal defects such as pores or laminations, which decrease the mechanical strength of the cement by acting as stress risers. Vacuum mixing or centrifuging can minimize these defects. Appropriate powdered antibiotics can be added up to 10 percent by weight for infected cases without significantly affecting mechanical properties of the cement. Mechanical mixing techniques, such as vibration, result in improved mechanical properties (compressive strength, shear strength, and modulus of elasticity) as compared to manual mixing techniques. Centrifugation improves static mechanical strength of bone cement as compared to hand mixing, but has no significant effect on low-cycle fatigue strength.

Chemical modifications, such as the use of butyl methacrylate, decrease the brittleness of methylmethacrylate and improve resistance to fatigue crack propagation; additions of water or various low-molecular-weight polyethylenes can reduce the polymerization temperature, but deleteriously affect mechanical properties. Reinforced cement composites formed by the addition of metal, polymer, or ceramic fibers have been shown to increase mechanical properties, particularly fatigue strength. However, they increase viscosity of the cement, which creates difficulties in filling and in the penetration of the cement into bone.

Bioceramics such as HA particles and bone chips have been added to cement to improve biocompatibility and promote bone approximation and fixation. Due to coating of these additions by the cement during mixing, however, their utility appears minimal.

BIODEGRADABLE POLYMERS

One new area of orthopaedic biomaterials is the use of biodegradable polymers. Materials such as polylactic acid polymers (PLA), polyglycolic acid polymers (PGA), polycaprolactate, and various polypeptides have been extensively studied in animal experiments. PLA-PGA copolymers have been clinically used for low-demand fracture fixa-

tion devices (e.g., malleolar screws and K-wires). These polymers are based on repeat units of naturally occurring proteins or carbohydrates that reoccur when broken down in the body by enzymatic or hydrolytic processes. Most of these polymers lack the strength for weight-bearing applications. Reinforcement with glass or carbon fibers (composites), increased device geometries (e.g., 50 percent thicker plates), and processing techniques such as extrusion that orients the polymer chains to increase strength and stiffness have been proposed as strengthening methods. Ideally, the biodegradable material should have sufficient strength to stabilize the fracture (osteotomy) during healing, degrade to prevent stress shielding, and finally completely disappear. There has been some recent concern with PGA and PLA for this application; during hydrolytic degradation, low molecular weight fragments form which decrease local pH. Some clinical results have shown pain and cyst formation at approximately one year.

Another potential use of these biodegradable polymers is as carriers of antibiotics and growth factors to achieve their localized, controlled release. By control of the types and characteristics of the polymers used, several substances can be released at various times or rates making this a potential system for release of growth factors. This has been experimentally used in bulk forms and as coatings on metallic implants. One particular application is PLA polymer coatings containing antibiotics and/or silver compounds on cementless prostheses for use in infected cases. Composites of biopolymers such as purified collagen with bioceramics (e.g., hydroxyapatite or hydroxyapatite alone) have been proposed as bone defect fillers. These materials have been used both in the powdered and bulk form and do not have some of the potential problems associated with allograft materials. Solid ceramic grafts tend to be brittle and take a long time to resorb and be replaced by bone; porous grafts are more readily resorbed but lack appreciable mechanical strength. A recent area of orthopaedic polymeric development is the use of biodegradable implants such as pins or screws for trauma applications. Materials such as PLA, PGA, and various polypeptides have been used; however, their relatively low mechanical strength has precluded their use in weightbearing applications and some materials have demonstrated untoward tissue reactions.

CERAMICS

The two major uses of ceramic biomaterials in orthopedics are for bearing applications and biocompatible coatings for implant fixation. Alumina and zirconia have been mostly used for femoral heads articulating against ceramic or polyethylene acetabular components. They exhibit very low wear rates and excellent biocompatibility, but due to the nature of ceramics, can fail by brittle fracture or become subject to third-body wear in ceramic-on-ceramic articulations. One difficulty with ceramics is joining them to a metal implant; taper fits are most common, but can produce deleterious, internal tensile hoop stresses in the ceramic.

Clinical data reveal that the use of a ceramic (Al_2O_3) head articulating against polyethylene results in lower wear of the acetabular component than does a metal head. Several long-term studies from Sweden have demonstrated approximately 50 percent less volumetric wear of the polyethylene. Laboratory experiments have demonstrated that zirconia (Th- or Y-dispersed) femoral heads, currently offered by several implant manufacturers, exhibit wear resistance and mechanical properties superior to those of alumina heads due to the zirconia's finer grain size.

Clinical series of alumina-alumina articulating surfaces in total hip arthroplasties have yielded excellent results, with few failures related to wear or to loosening due to wear debris. However, ceramic-ceramic articulations have exhibited severe wear when improper device placement leads to high surface stresses, because the ceramic is brittle and prone to local fragmentation of the alumina, resulting in third-body wear.

Although hydroxyapatite coatings for enhancement of initial device stabilization by bone ingrowth continue to be used clinically, some questions as to their long-term stability have arisen due to coating delamination and/or osteoclastic resorption. Commercially available coatings are applied by plasma spraying and vary with respect to thickness, porosity, chemical composition, and crystallinity. A canine transcortical plug push-out study confirmed the superior shear strength of a 50-μm-thick coating over a 200-μm coating. However, it has been argued that an implant will remain stable if the coating is resorbed, but not if the coating delaminates. Less biologically stable ceramics such as tricalcium phosphate coatings have been used to enhance initial bone ongrowth.

Both hydroxyapatite and tricalcium phosphate coatings have been applied to porous metallic implants to enhance bone ingrowth and initial fixation. In one study in rabbits, use of both ceramic coatings resulted in improved implant perimeter bone contact and a higher amount of bone ingrown into the implant pores. Partially and completely resorbable calcium phosphate cements have been proposed to address some of the shortcomings of acrylic cements. Some of these new cements harden in a manner analogous to plaster of Paris; others incorporate a polyacrylic acid similar to glass-ionomer dental cements. They use an aqueous base and exhibit no appreciable exotherm during hardening, and as a result should minimize adverse biological response. Their major problem is achieving adequate mechanical tensile strength for weight-bearing applications. The most promising current applications are for filling of osseous defects and consolidation of fracture fragments. Clinical studies are in progress for the treatment of Colles' fractures.

Hydroxyapatite ceramic is being used as bone graft substitute or extender in a variety of clinical settings, including tumors, trauma, spinal fusion, and repair of autologous bone graft sites. It can be used as granules combined with autograft, biodegradable polymers or ceramics, or as a structural block graft (usually porous). In one study of 60 benign bone tumors treated by curettage and block calcium hydroxyapatite ceramic implantation, the ceramic was found to become well incorporated in almost all cases; late biopsies in several cases showed significant bone ingrowth into the ceramic pore structure.

SUGGESTED READINGS

Ducheyne P, Hastings GW (eds): *Metal and Ceramic Biomaterials.* Boca Raton, FL: CRC; 1984.

Mears DC: *Materials and Orthopaedic Surgery.* Baltimore: Williams & Wilkins; 1979.

Park JB, Lakes RS: *Biomaterials: An Introduction,* 2d ed. New York: Plenum; 1992.

von Recum AF (ed): *Handbook of Biomaterials Evaluation: Scientific, Technical, and Clinical Testing of Implant Materials.* New York: Macmillan; 1986.

Williams DF: *Biocompatibility of Orthopedic Implants.* Boca Raton, FL: CRC; 1982.

Yettram AL: *Material Properties and Stress Analysis in Biomechanics.* Manchester: Manchester University Press (St. Martin's Press, NY); 1989.

Chapter 10

JOINT BIOMECHANICS

Frederick J. Kummer

Victor H. Frankel

Purposeful motion is a requirement for life. Loss of motion results in degradation of function, disability, and ultimately, an inability to perform the activities necessary for daily living. Biomechanics is the study of biologic systems, utilizing engineering science and methodology. It enables analysis of body motion and the forces to produce that motion. *Kinematics* is the branch of biomechanics concerned with motion of a body without reference to force or mass, and can be assessed at several different levels: gross motion of joints, motion during specific activities, motion necessary for the general activities of daily living, and, finally, joint surface motion.

The determination of a patient's joint motion and its deviation from normal joint motion is a classic, physical examination procedure, well known and important to those who treat the locomotor system. It is thus necessary to appreciate the normal range of motion (ROM) needed for activities of daily living (Table 10-1).

MOTION ANALYSIS

A common reason for a patient to seek orthopaedic care for the musculoskeletal system is difficulty with gait. The study of normal gait serves as an introduction to the study of joint biomechanics. Progression of the body during gait requires the displacement of the center of gravity of the body, which in turn requires energy expenditure. There are three types of energy: *potential energy* is the energy stored in a body through to its elevation above the ground, *strain*

Table 10-1

Mean Values for Maximum Hip Motion in Three Planes during Common Activities

Activity	Plane of Motion	Recorded Value (degrees)
Tying shoe with foot on the floor	Sagittal	124
	Frontal	19
	Transverse	15
Tying shoe with feet across opposite thigh	Sagittal	110
	Frontal	23
	Transverse	33
Sitting down on chair and rising from sitting	Sagittal	104
	Frontal	20
	Transverse	17
Stooping to obtain object on floor	Sagittal	117
	Frontal	21
	Transverse	18
Squatting	Sagittal	122
	Frontal	28
	Transverse	26
Ascending stairs	Sagittal	67
	Frontal	16
	Transverse	18
Descending stairs	Sagittal	36

energy is the energy stored in the muscles and bone of the body due to contraction and deformation, and *kinetic energy* is the energy possessed by a moving mass and is equal to one-half the mass times the velocity squared. The energy level is constant if no work is done, as in the example of an ideal, simple pendulum where the loss of potential energy as it swings down is exactly compensated for by its gain in kinetic energy. If the energy level is not constant, work must be done to produce the change in energy level. This situation occurs during gait. The kinetic and potential energy levels for the different segments of the lower extremity are not constant. The difference in energy is made up by the work done by the muscles at the joints; forward displacement of the body results, but a large part of the energy is dissipated in the rotations of the segments. In pathologic gait situations, or situations in which external supports are used, more energy is expended in gait. This is an important consideration where gait is desired, but general health conditions mean that excess energy requirements will have a deleterious effect. Energy expenditure during gait of a patient with arthritic joints can rise easily by 50 percent.

Disorders of the hip, knee, and ankle will prevent some or all of these energy-saving mechanisms from operating so that more effort is required for gait. For the rheumatologist managing a patient with both joint and systemic problems, minimizing energy expenditure during gait is an important goal.

JOINTS AND RANGE OF MOTION

There are several basic types of joints, the hinge and ball-and-socket being the most common as represented by the knee and elbow and by the hip and shoulder, respectively. The knee and elbow are not strictly hinge joints, as both accommodate a degree of rotation and translation that is necessary for proper function. Early knee prostheses designs were a simple hinge, and most were loosened by the forces created by motion during normal activity. Motion is constrained by the shape of the articulation and by the surrounding osseous architecture and soft tissues such as the ligaments and capsule. The amount of motion (or ROM) is important in the diagnoses of clinical problems and also serves as an objective factor to evaluate treatment. Prosthetic replacements of joints will recover most of the motion lost by disease and enable patients to perform activities of daily living. As seen in Table 10-1, ROM is usually defined in three planes of activity: sagittal (flexion–extension), frontal (abduction-adduction), and transverse (internal–external rotation).

JOINT LAXITY AND STABILITY

When the limbs are acted upon by forces or moments, the joints normally respond by moving in some manner and are only restricted by the small frictional forces of soft tissue viscoelasticity. Nonphysiologic loads are resisted by joint congruency and ligamentous structure. Laxity of a joint is the amount of looseness or play in a specific direction, whereas stability of a joint in a particular position is affected by muscle forces and gravity.

When joints are loaded, loads are transmitted by the cartilage and underlying bone which deform to increase contact area, and this reduces the contact stresses that, if excessive (high magnitudes and/or number of applications), can lead to degeneration of the joint surfaces. This factor is also important in prosthetic replacements where high contact stresses can lead to wear and loosening due to the biologic response to wear particles. Contact areas have been extensively studied for most joints; the main determinants are the amount of load and joint position.

Joint laxity is also influenced by joint position because of the orientation of the supporting ligaments. For example, anterior and posterior drawer tests in the intact knee depend on the cruciate ligaments, which act in an opposing manner.

JOINT SURFACE MOTION

During motion, the surfaces of the joint accelerate over each other in a reciprocal manner as the joint goes from flexion to extension. A technique for studying surface joint motion is to study the center of rotation of the joint. The distal humerus forms an almost perfect cylinder. As the olecranon rotates about the distal humerus, in effect it does so about a simple axis of rotation. The surface motion at any particular point on the surface is perpendicular to the line which connects that point to the center of rotation. In the case of the distal humerus, the joint motion is always tangent to the joint surface. In the case of the knee joint, though, with its changing curvature of radius, the instant center of rotation must move as the joint goes from flexion to extension, in order to keep the joint surfaces moving parallel to each other (Fig. 10-1). If the center of rotation for a particular ROM is displaced due to an arthritic process or to an interarticular injury, the normal gliding will be altered, and the joint may be distracted or compressed. If the center of rotation is on the surface, there is no sliding friction because only rolling occurs. Rotation of a joint about an abnormal center of rotation causes joint surface damage, and can lead to cartilage degeneration.

KINEMATICS

Kinematics is the branch of biomechanics that describes the motion of a body under the action of given force. Accelerations are necessary for motion, and the body generates these accelerations through the forces produced by muscle contractions. In a simple model of a limb, the muscle is attached distally to the limb's axis of rotation, and

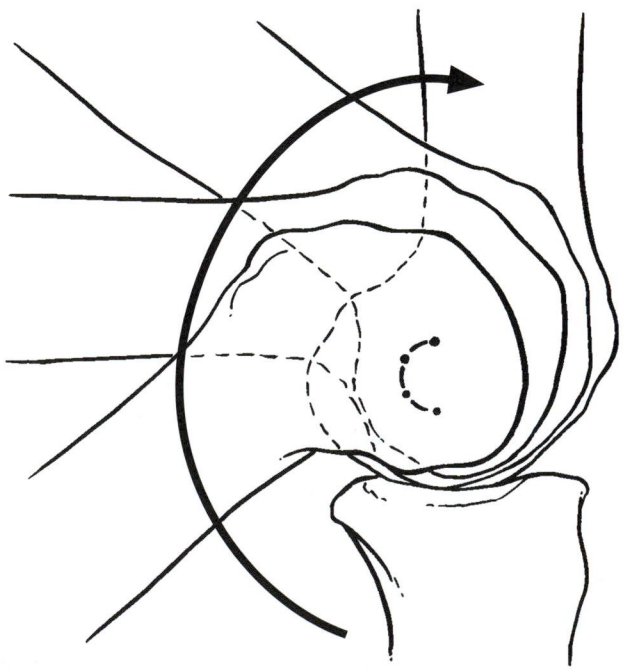

Figure 10-1
Instant center pattern in normal knee.

its contraction produces a torque about that axis. A torque, or moment, is the product of a force and a distance. The torque (is related to the acceleration (A) by the expression $T = I \times A$. The mass moment of inertia (I) is a function, not only of the mass, but of the distribution of the mass about an axis.

Muscle forces have both an external effect and an internal effect. The external effect of the force produces a joint torque that results in an acceleration with concomitant motions: force, torque, acceleration, and motion. The internal effect of the force produces both deformation of the joint surfaces and internal stresses and strains within the cartilage and underlying bone.

SUMMARY

Biomechanics utilizes engineering science to describe functions of the body. It enables one to understand the relationship between forces and motion and between motion and forces. The biologic portion of biomechanics must not be overlooked. Biologic processes that may be influenced by forces must be studied with a knowledge of not only the magnitude and direction of the forces, but also their rate of application. Disuse osteoporosis may result from the application of less than normal forces. Fatigue fractures result from the application of increased forces. Joint wear and subsequent degenerative arthritis may result from a change in both the magnitude and direction of the forces on an injured joint. An understanding of the basic concepts of biomechanics is necessary for dealing with the musculoskeletal system.

SUGGESTED READINGS

Donatelli R, Wolf SL (eds): *The Biomechanics of the Foot and Ankle.* Philadelphia: FA Davis; 1990.

Goel VK, Weinstein JN (eds): *Biomechanics of the Spine: Clinical and Surgical Perspective.* Boca Raton: CRC; 1990.

LeVeau BF, Williams M: *Williams & Lissner's Biomechanics of Human Motion,* 3d ed. Philadelphia: WB Saunders; 1992.

Maquet PGJ: *Biomechanics of the Knee with Application to the Pathogenesis and the Surgical Treatment of Osteoarthritis.* Berlin: Springer-Verlag; 1976.

Pauwels F: *Biomechanics of the Normal and Diseased Hip: Theoretical Foundation, Techniques and Results of Treatment: An Atlas.* Berlin: Springer-Verlag; 1976.

Payne CB: *Biomechanics of the Foot and Related Pathology.* Riccarton, New Zealand: Podiatry Associates; 1982.

Vaughan CL, Murphy GN, DuToit LL (eds): *Biomechanics of Human Gait: An Annotated Bibliography,* 2d ed. Champaign, IL: Human Kinetics; 1987 [*Electronic format—two 3.5-inch diskettes:* Vaughan CL, Besser MP, Sussman KA, et al, (eds): *Biomechanics of Human Gait: An Electronic Bibliography,* 2d ed. Champaign, IL: Human Kinetics; 1992].

White AA, Panjabi MM (eds): *Clinical Biomechanics of the Spine.* 2d ed. Philadelphia: Lippincott; 1990.

Chapter 11

IMPLANT BIOMECHANICS

Frederick J. Kummer

Implant devices can be divided into two main categories: fracture-fixation devices intended to stabilize a fracture mechanically and osteotomy and joint replacements intended as a substitute for a diseased or damaged joint. A number of biomechanical principles are associated with their design and surgical application that affect clinical efficacy and survival.

FIXATION DEVICES

The design and use of fixation devices relies initially on an understanding of bone healing and the loads and forces to which the device is subjected. The basic AO* principle is rigid internal fixation achieved by compression of bone surfaces through the use of an appropriate device and its correct surgical application. Currently, there is controversy over whether completely rigid fixation is the optimal condition for bone healing. Although gross motion between two or more bone fragments usually leads to nonunion and fibrocartilage tissue formation, there is a low level of displacement (micromotion) that appears advantageous to healing by providing a mechanical signal that stimulates the biologic repair processes. However, the optimal frequency, waveform, and total number of cycles of this signal are uncertain and are being investigated. There is also concern for the process of stress shielding that occurs when the fixation device carries most or all of the mechanical load, and thus promotes localized osseous resorption owing to the resultant unloading of the bone around the device. Much of the initial osteopenia seen beneath fracture plates, however, is due to vascular disruption.

Bone healing in the presence of a gap with minimal movement passes through several stages of repair with a concomitant increase in mechanical strength: hematoma and inflammation, callus formation, replacement by woven bone, and, finally, remodeling into lamellar or trabecular bone (Fig. 11-1). With direct bone apposition and compression, or in the case of a rigidly fixed, small gap, more rapid healing occurs because the initial repair stages are eliminated or minimized. The local strain in the healing region (change in gap size divided by the original gap size) determines the nature of the tissues formed.

The other important factor for healing is adequate blood supply. This necessitates the surgeon preserving the vascular supply of the bone (e.g., periosteum) and providing conditions for early revascularization by careful operative technique (e.g., soft tissue preservation). Numerous studies have demonstrated that there is a direct relationship between the quantity and quality of microvascular structures in the healing region and the rate of formation and mechanical properties of the new bone.

FIXATION DEVICES AND METHODS

Wires, staples, pins, plates, and screws are the common implant devices used to achieve fixation and may be made of stainless steel

*AO/ASIF. Arbeitsgemeinschaft Osteosynthesefragen/Association for the Study of Internal Fixation.

(316L), titanium (or Ti-6A1-4V), and sometimes of cobalt–chromium alloy. There is recent interest and clinical application for the use of biodegradable polymers such as polylactic acid for these applications although these materials were first proposed over 20 years ago. There also continues to be research into the use of various glues and adhesives for bone fixation. Each material has advantages and disadvantages such as strength, modulus (stiffness), corrosion resistance, and ease of imaging magnetic resonance imaging and computer-assisted tomography).

Wire fixation used as cerclage or a bone suture is a common application; in both cases, multiple wires are required to provide stable, three-dimensional fixation. This necessitates achieving equal tension during tightening, because loosening at one or more sites can provide a locus for motion and possible nonunion or cause malpositioning. Problems with wire fixation include the necessity and surgical complexity of making a bone hole and passing the wire, breakage during tightening or later due to fatigue (cyclic loading), and cut-through of

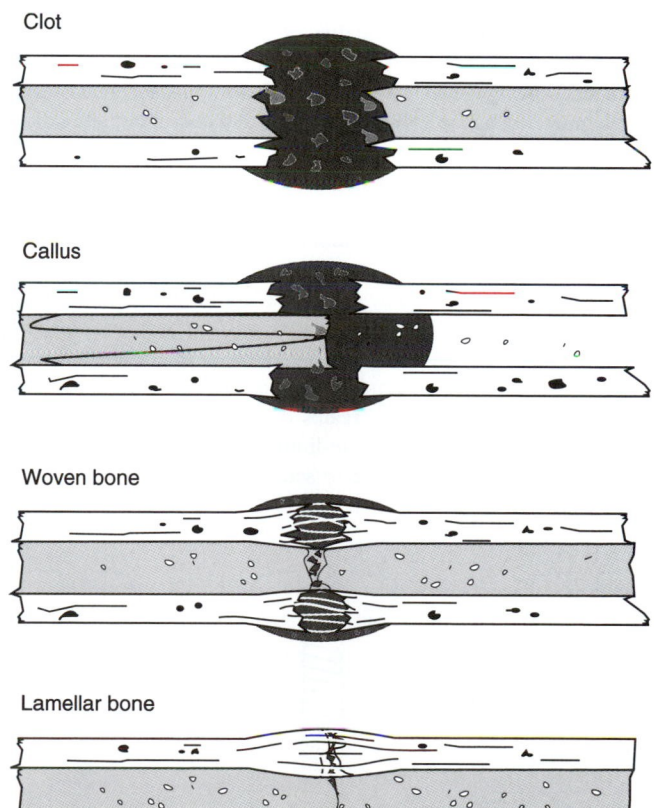

Clot

Callus

Woven bone

Lamellar bone

Figure 11-1
Stages of bone healing.

the bone. For cerclage applications, there is concern about compromise of the periosteal blood supply and resulting increased healing time required for revascularization.

Some recent developments are wire tensioning/twisting instruments and the use of crimping systems to avoid the problems with twisting or knot tying. Also, there are nonmetallic-oriented polymers (Spectra: Dupont; Wilmington, DE.) which do not stretch like traditional suture materials and that can be used with a suture anchor system to eliminate the difficulty of looping a suture through bone.

Staples alone usually do not provide sufficient mechanical stability for permanent fixation, and their use often requires predrilling holes for the staple legs; pneumatically driven staples can be used to tack fragments rapidly prior to a more rigid fixation, but need careful control of the insertion driving force to prevent untoward damage to the bone. Some staple designs have been developed that can affect compression during insertion, such as prebent staple legs or fabrication from nitenol (an alloy that changes shape when heated to body temperature).

Kirschner wires are normally used to hold fragments prior to rigid fixation and for percutaneous pinning but, in general, lack sufficient mechanical stability for their use as primary fixation. At least two should be used for each bone fragment and, to prevent "pistoning" of the fragment, they should not be inserted in a parallel manner. Threaded pins provide additional stability because they minimize sliding of the bone fragments, but their removal is more difficult. Occasionally, pinning is used in combination with suture looped around the pin ends. This "tension band" technique provides significantly increased mechanical stability.

The major intrinsic factors that influence screw-holding power are outer thread diameter, configuration, and length; extrinsic factors are bone quality, type, and orientation of screw insertion and driving torque. The two basic types of screws are cortical and cancellous, which are distinguished by their thread design; cancellous screws have a greater distance between adjacent threads (pitch) and ratio of outer thread diameter to body diameter (Fig. 11-2). The inherent holding power of a screw is a function of the outer thread diameter times the length of its threads within the bone. When used to hold two bone fragments together, screws commonly are used in a lag modality in which the proximal portion of the screw remains free within one fragment (either by using a screw design having no proximal threads or by enlargement of the hole in the proximal fragment, which should require the use of a washer under the screw head for adequate support). Insertion torque determines the force with which bone fragments are held together and creates the friction that prevents their motion. Control of torque (torque-limiting screwdriver) is important to prevent stripping of the bone or screw head failure.

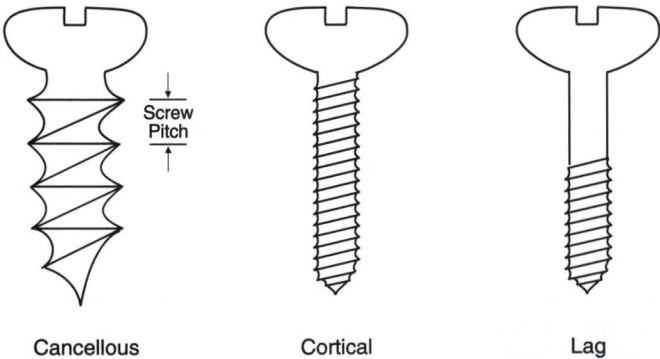

Figure 11-2
Types of bone screws.

Cancellous   Cortical   Lag

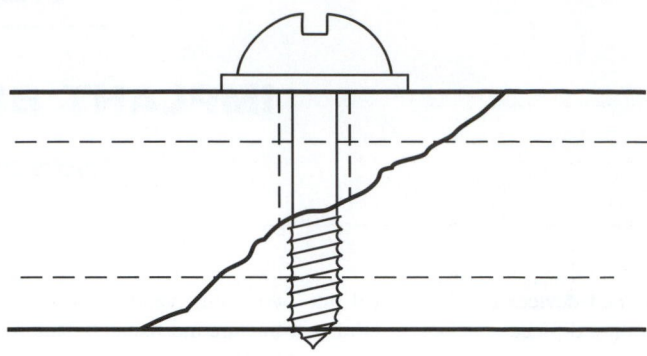

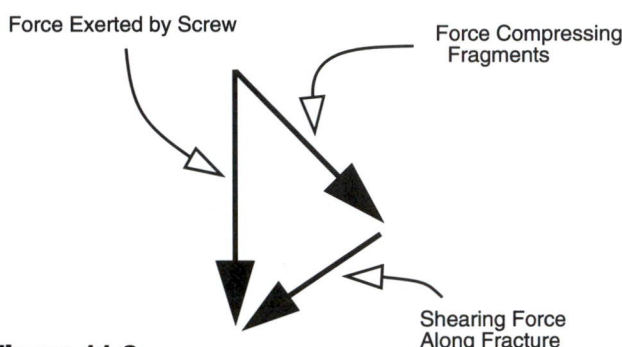

Figure 11-3
Lag screw fixation and forces on the fracture.

Force Exerted by Screw

Force Compressing Fragments

Shearing Force Along Fracture

Anatomic constraints or surgical exposure may prevent screws from being inserted perpendicularly to the bone axis. In addition, the orientation of the ends of bone fragments is not always perpendicular to the screw axis. In these cases, the holding power of the screw is decreased, and a shear component of the holding force is created that acts to destabilize alignment (Fig. 11-3). Pretapping of the screws is usually not necessary and has been shown to have minimal effect on their holding ability; many screws are self-tapping owing to a modification to the design of the leading threads. Usually, two or more screws are required for function, although one screw has been suggested for some applications if sufficient interfragment approximation can be achieved to create adequate friction between the bone surfaces for stability.

The quality of bone also determines screw-holding ability; cortical bone is approximately ten times stronger than cancellous bone. The thickness of the cortex and degree of osteopenia (bone density) are thus critical for fixation strength and influence the number of screws required for adequate stability. Using screws in a bicortical manner appreciably increases the strength of fixation.

Anatomic constraints limit the number or size of screws that can be applied in a given region. As a result, screws are often combined with plates in order to achieve adequate stability and increased strength of fixation. The optimal site for a single plate application is on the side of the bone subjected to tension; usually two plates are applied to achieve better fixation stability. Owing to anatomic constraints such as soft tissue thickness, sometimes thinner plates are used, for example, for forearm fracture stabilization, but these plates are sufficiently stiff (function of width times height squared) to prevent undesired fracture motion caused by bending loads. Screws should be inserted with a torque driver and the tightness of all screws rechecked; if this is not done, one screw may bear most of the load and possibly fail. Some plates use a specially designed screw hole

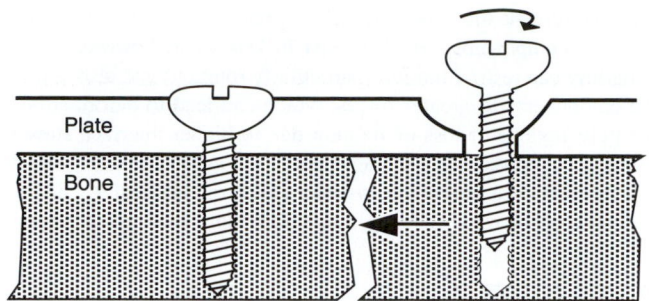

Figure 11-4
Bone plate hole designed to compress fracture.

slot that is countersunk to accommodate the screw head, which is off-set in order to obtain interfragmentary compression as the screw is tightened (Fig. 11-4). An alternative solution is to pre-bend the plate before application so that, when tightened, the bone fragments are approximated as the plate straightens. Some new plate designs use threaded holes to engage the screw so that bicortical screw insertion is not as essential for maximum fixation stability.

Plates can also be used to span gaps created by severe fractures or tumor surgery and are frequently used with bone grafts for this application. Unless the graft is exactly sized, the plate will bear the entire load across the defect. The bending moment on the plate–screw fixation linearly increases with defect size, and necessitates adequate stabilization, particularly at the more highly loaded, proximal end, where at least three screws are needed. Multiple-holed plates enable selection of the best osseous sites for screw purchase and should permit anchoring of the graft by at least two additional screws.

The major surgical considerations for the use of plates are the requirements of a larger exposure and the possibility of periosteal blood supply compromise (some plate designs have inferior feet or ridges to minimize this possibility). There is also interest in polymeric plates that would be more flexible in order to achieve a greater degree of micromotion that could be advantageous to bone healing and minimize stress shielding.

Hip fracture devices can be applied internally or externally, the most common external device being a side plate affixed to the femur and supporting an internal, sliding lag screw through the neck across the fracture. The relationship of biomechanical forces borne by the device and by the bone (load bearing–load sharing) influence fracture healing and device survival. An important factor is the ability of the device to slide to consolidate the fracture during healing. Internal devices for fixation are usually intramedullary (IM) nails and, in comparison to external devices, are subject to fewer forces because of their location closer to the neutral bending axis of the bone. Their size is critical because their bending stiffness is proportional to the diameter cubed, for torsion to the fourth power. This is why one large nail provides more stable fixation than multiple smaller rods. Size, amount of curvature, and the amount of reaming are also important because the stability of the fixation relies on load transfer to the bone; distal and proximal screws often are used to increase torsional stability. Bending of the nail caused by insertion in a curved medullary cavity can make insertion of these distal screws difficult.

External fixation devices are also used for fracture stabilization; multiple transcutaneous pins are inserted into the bone and stabilized with an external bar(s) or ring. Factors that influence stability are the number, diameter, orientation, and length of pins and their orientation with respect to the fracture or osteotomy; however, these factors are subject to surgical considerations.

SPINAL IMPLANTS

Spinal implants used for deformity correction or fixation consist of various combinations of rods or plates with different means of attachment such as hooks, screws, and wires. The junctions between these components are often the site of failure of fixation. A specific problem for spinal implants is that the size and location of appropriate sites for attachment are limited. This is important because these devices are subject to appreciable forces during flexion and extension of the neck and torso, and failure at the device–bone interface can occur. As a result, fixation is often applied both anteriorly and posteriorly.

SURGICAL FACTORS

A number of factors determine the optimal fixation method for a specific application. First are mechanical considerations—specifically the types (tension, bending, and/or torsion) and magnitude of forces to which the fixation will be subjected and whether these forces will be cyclic, requiring additional strength of fixation to account for possible fatigue of the supporting bone. The second factor is the bone quality, which determines the strength available to support the fixation device. Other factors are related to surgical and anatomic considerations, for example, the exposure (possible scarring and vascular compromise) and whether the device will fit adequately within the soft tissues and if neurovascular structures are at risk.

Fixation strength can be evaluated by laboratory testing of actual implants in cadaver bone. One difficulty of such testing is to simulate adequately in the test model the complex *in vivo* forces to which the device or fixation technique is subjected. Another difficulty is to simulate the biologic repair processes that would act to stabilize the fixation. Cadaver studies can also determine the anatomic structures at risk. The other major method to evaluate the efficacy of a particular fixation method is clinical trials. Care must be taken, though, to adopt the appropriate techniques to quantify data and to design the trial (number of patients and adequate follow-up) so that the many variables can be properly statistically analyzed.

JOINT IMPLANTS

The clinical objective of total joint prostheses is to replace a diseased or damaged joint with an artificial construct of metal and plastic that duplicates the biomechanics of a normal joint and provides the patient with long-term, pain-free ability for activities of daily living. The design of total joint prostheses has been one of evolution with input from clinical results and laboratory studies. For example, the early knee prosthetics had a fixed hinge with no capability for rotation and thus did not duplicate normal knee motion and kinematics, and as a result demonstrated unacceptable wear and loosening.

TOTAL HIP REPLACEMENT AND ENDOPROSTHESES

Total hip replacement is one of the more successful orthopaedic procedures. The current state of the art is a stem fixed without bone cement using a hydroxyapatite or porous ingrowth coating, a modular head (metal surface processed to improve wear or ceramic), and a modular acetabular component consisting of a metal shell with a polyethylene insert designed to minimize polyethylene wear. However, excellent clinical results have been obtained with a monolithic cemented stem and a cemented all-polyethylene acetabulum. For cemented stems, designs having round corners and a broad medial surface have improved stress transferred to the cement without stress concentration. The most important issue is polyethylene wear and biologic response to wear debris leading to loosening. Improved polyethylene quality and assembly designs are one current method of reducing this problem. Ceramic-on-ceramic and metal-on-metal articulations are being investigated. Laboratory studies have shown that a 26- to 28-mm head is a compromise between the volumetric wear seen with 32-mm heads and the linear wear seen with 22-mm heads. There is concern that modularity can lead to corrosion at the taper junction and limit the range of motion. This concern about modular devices has recently increased because of findings from examinations of removed implants. Although modularity enables surgeons to achieve optimal fit intraoperatively and minimizes device inventory, factors such as corrosion (galvanic or crevice) at the interfaces resulting in release of metallic ions and/or micromotion leading to increased debris production have been clinically demonstrated and have been the subject of numerous laboratory studies. Many manufacturers have responded by narrowing the tolerances of the modular fit to minimize the possibility of creating a crevice between the components, developing better locking methods, and improving instrumentation for component assembly prior to implantation. Surgically, it is critical to ensure that the junctions are clean and dry before assembly.

Hemiarthroplasty is a common treatment of hip fractures in the elderly. Appropriate head sizing is critical for device longevity. The use of bipolar prostheses in which there are two articulations (prosthesis head within the inner acetabular shell and between the outer acetabular shell and the patient's acetabulum) have demonstrated improved range of motion in the laboratory but not clinically.

KNEE IMPLANTS

The current designs of total knees have demonstrated excellent long-term clinical success. Unicondylar implants have had less-impressive results. These designs attempt to duplicate the anatomy of the normal knee and rely somewhat on soft tissue structures for stabilization. The design of the articulation also affects stability and wear. The more congruent the articulation, the greater is the area of contact between components, which results in less wear; however, greater congruity can restrict motion (particularly rotation) and also subjects the components to greater forces, which can lead to deformation of the polyethylene or loss of fixation due to higher interface stresses. Some knee replacements are designed to accommodate soft tissue deficiencies, such as loss of the posterior collateral ligament. Again there is a trade-off between stability, range of motion, and implant stresses.

OTHER JOINTS

Replacements of the ankle, elbow, and shoulder are also available. Difficulties in device fixation, particularly in the talus and the glenoid, where small areas of bone lead to high interfacial stresses between the prosthesis and fixation, have created problems with device longevity. Maintenance of adequate soft tissue structures is important for unconstrained designs particularly in the elbow and shoulder; as in the knee, constrained designs can lead to loosening of implant fixation due to high interface stresses.

SUGGESTED READINGS

Benzel EC: *Biomechanics of Spine Stabilization.* New York: McGraw-Hill; 1995.

Ducheyne P, Hastings GW (eds): *Functional Behavior of Orthopedic Biomaterials,* Boca Raton, FL: CRC; 1984, vols 1,2.

Ghista DN (ed): *Biomedical Engineering and Instrumentation,* vol 7, *Biomechanics of Medical Devices.* New York: Marcel Dekker; 1981.

Maquet PGJ, Pauwels F: *Biomechanics of the Hip: As Applied to Osteoarthritis and Related Conditions.* Berlin: Springer-Verlag; 1985.

Tencer AF, Johnson KD: *Biomechanics in Orthopedic Trauma: Bone Fracture and Fixation.* London, Martin Dunitz; 1994.

Vincent JF (ed): *Practical Approach,* vol. 105, *Biomechanics-Materials: A Practical Approach.* Oxford: IRL at Oxford University Press; 1992.

Chapter 12

BASICS OF THE ILIZAROV METHOD

Vladimir Golyakhovsky

BIOLOGY

Introduced by the Russian Professor G. A. Ilizarov, between 1950 and the 1960s, the method of distractional osteogenesis is based on the tension-stress effect of a gradual forceful motion applied to bone fragments by a stable circular external fixator. Ilizarov was the first to observe that under influence of this force at a particular rate and frequency, the motion of distraction produces a new growth of virtually all the local tissues involved—including bone, muscle, tendon, fascia, vessel wall, intercalary growth of existing nerve trunks, new nerve fibers, and the skin. With continual and gradual distraction, new bone formation occurs by intramembranous ossification and develops parallel to the applied force. Local neovascularization is a principal force responsible for all tissue neogenesis. An increase in local and regional vascularity helps to provide an adequate and sufficient blood supply.

For development of the bone collagen columns, that is, of the lengthening, deposited along lines of the mechanical stress of distraction, the first and most important condition is preservation of local blood circulation. Normally, two-thirds of the cortical blood supply comes from the nutrient artery located in the bone marrow. The periosteal arterioles provide one third of the blood supply. In the case of any bone destruction, with partial or complete bone marrow interruption, the periosteal arterioles begin to increase and extend their function as the main source of the cortex blood supply. Therefore, in order to optimize the anatomic and physiologic conditions for new bone formation, the preservation of both endosteal and periosteal blood supply is of great importance.

BIOMECHANICS

Three fundamental principles govern the biomechanical environment of the Ilizarov method.

1. Utilization of multiplanar circular fixator enables multidirectional bone transfixation (transosseous osteosynthesis), which brings maximum stability of the fragments when the Ilizarov fixator rings are connected to the bone fragments and to each other, the resultant frame actually replicates the cylindrical shape of the tubular cortical bone shell, with a greater diameter.

   The Ilizarov circular fixator possesses some of the most optimal biomechanical characteristics for bone distraction, compression, and fracture healing. In comparison to the conventional uni- and biplanar large-pin fixators, it maintains axial elasticity and much higher stiffness to bending when the bone is loaded.

2. Utilization of the smooth, nonthreaded K-wires of small diameter (1.8 mm and 1.5 mm), under tension between 100 to 130 kg, introduced multidirectionally, brings firm stability of each bone fragment. Introduction of the olive-type stoppers (a wire with a rounded bulge that becomes seated against the bone), adds to the bone stability and to the frame position stability itself.

In addition, the restricted elasticity of the tensioned K-wires allows for cyclic micromotion at the site of osteotomy or fracture. This has long been considered to be stimulatory to bone healing. Restricted elasticity of the tensioned K-wires was shown to activate the piezoelectric phenomena in the cells of bone marrow, in compact bone, and in the newly developed regenerate. If the tissues are stimulated by the elastic micromotion, the nerve impulses are activated, and help control the passage of electrically charged ions through the cells activating their ion channels.

Dr. Ilizarov considered this mechanism to be an analog to the mechanism of the fetal growth plate activity, and coined the term "tension stress" to reflect the essential dynamics of the technique. The exact mechanism of existing elastic micromotion-cellular development is not completely known.

3. Introduction of a technique of corticotomy (or compactectomy), that is a circumferential transection of the cortex of tubular bone (femur, tibia, humerus) without cutting into the bone marrow and periosteum, was also developed by Dr. Ilizarov. As opposed to a wide-open osteotomy which cuts through the vasculature, the goal of the corticotomy is to preserve local and regional blood circulation. This elegant and intricate surgical technique is performed through a small skin incision (1.0 to 2.0 cm). Location of the incision must be at a site where the bone is located close to the skin in order to control the direction of bone transection more precisely. Periosteum separation and cleavage of the site of the initial bone cut must be avoided. This protects the periosteal arterioles from distraction and prevents hypoplastic bone regeneration of the section of the cut. With a narrow osteotome (1/4 in.), cautious but firm blows of the mallet are applied in a fan-shaped manner, directing the osteotome tip laterally and medially without extracting it. Depending on the shape of the bone cross-section, transection is directed alternately along the medial and lateral cortex walls. At this point the tapping is ceased and the osteotome handle is turned alternately with pliers, with its position at the farthest medial and lateral transection corners. Usually, there is already a microcleft in the posterior wall cortex, and the cracking sound of its divergence should be the sign of the completed corticotomy. If correctly performed, this technique provokes almost no bleeding from the wound. It is strongly recommended that the bone be cut only with the fixator already in place in order to be able to keep osteotomized fragments in steady position.

   Depending on the goal of treatment in a particular patient, the corticotomy can be performed at one level (monofocal) or two levels (bifocal) on the same bone. In general, the monofocal corticotomy is indicated for (1) lengthening up to 5 cm; (2) bone fragment transportation up to 5 to 7 cm; (3) stimulation of local and regional blood circulation in the limb for generation of osteogenesis without significant bone lengthening (e.g., in pseudoarthrosis or nonunion); and (4) gradual correction of bone deformity.

TECHNIQUE OF BONE DISTRACTION

Distraction is used for bone lengthening (primarily), for correction of bone deformities, for bone segment transport (replacing bone grafting), as a stimulus for nonunion healing, as a stimulus for neovascularization, and for contracture correction. Three parameters of distractional forces produce the full effect of distraction: speed, rhythm and distribution of them along the bone circumference.

The optimal speed for lengthening is 1 mm/day and the optimal rhythm of distraction is four times per day. Therefore, there must be four distraction adjustments daily at intervals of 6 h, with each adjustment being 0.25 mm, or one-fourth of the threaded rods pitch. The speed and rhythm of distraction are adjustable. In some cases they can be increased (up to 1.5 mm/day, by the six 0.25 mm/turn). In others they can be reduced (to 0.5 mm/day, by the two 0.25 mm/turn). The motor forces in both situations, however, must be distributed evenly on the moving bone fragment circumference. The optimal distribution of distraction forces is four points of application with 90-degree angles between them.

There are two ways to perform distraction. The first is by applying two #10 wrenches simultaneously to the nuts attached to the fixator's ring. The first wrench is used to loosen the nut farthest from the distraction site; the second is used to tighten the opposing nut. When both nuts are adjusted one-quarter of a full turn, a distraction of 0.25 mm is achieved. The second and most reliable method of distraction is achieved by using the graduated telescopic rod, which has a rotating head with a ratchet mechanism. One-quarter of the turn corresponds to 0.25 mm of distraction.

TECHNIQUE OF BONE COMPRESSION

Compression is used in treatment of bone nonunion (primarily), correction of bone deformities, bone segment transport, arthrodesis (fusion) technique, and reversing distraction in case of hypoplastic bone regenerate development. In most situations compression is produced in the same manner as distraction, but in the opposite direction. The same three parameters of operation affect compression: speed, rhythm, and distribution of forces on the bone circumference. The same techniques used to produce distraction also are applicable to compression. The chief indication for reduction of the compression speed and rhythm is severe pain at the site of compression, which can be a reflection of neurovascular deficiency.

FRAME ASSEMBLAGE

In constructing any type of Ilizarov frame, the major considerations are:

1. The stability of the fixation of the frame to the bone
2. The prevention of gross bone fragment motion
3. The ability to manipulate bone and to perform necessary fragment movements such as straightening, bending, distraction, compression, rotation, or a combination of these movements.

There are two methods of Ilizarov frame construction. The first is to construct the required frame in advance, assembling all the parts with consideration of existing deformities, and then placing the sterilized frame as a whole over the limb during surgery, and transfixing the rings to the bone with the K-wires (Fig. 12-1). The main advantages of the frame preassembly are that it saves time during the sur-

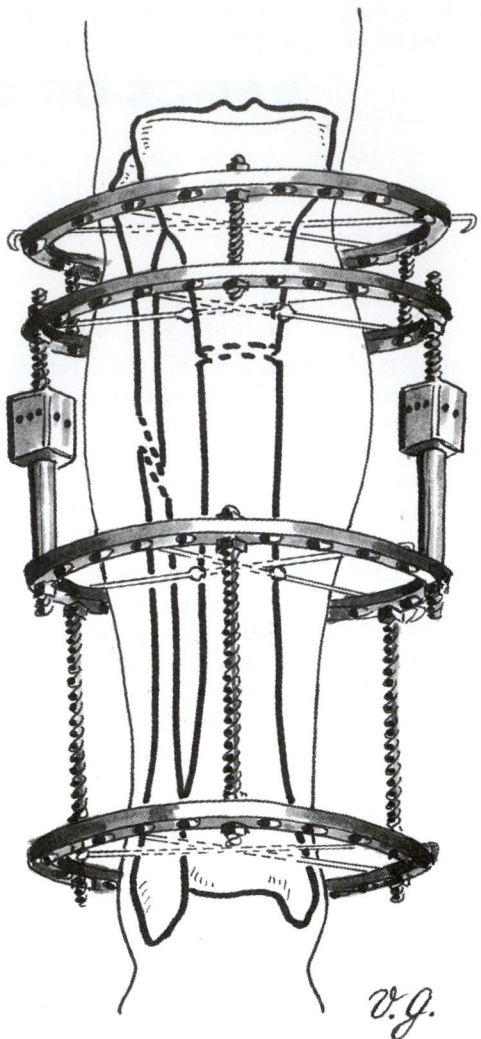

Figure 12-1
The preassembled four-ring Ilizarov frame is transfixed to the tibia and fibula. Interrupted lines represent the sides of the osteotomy (corticotomy) for the purpose of lengthening.

gical procedure and gives the surgeon the latitude to try some component variations. The disadvantage is that it may require adjustments, because it is impossible to foresee all necessary modifications, especially in complicated cases and if the surgeon lacks experience in frame assembly.

The second method is to construct the frame during surgery, assembling it piece-by-piece over the limb. To do this the K-wires first have to be introduced into the bone, then the rings and other parts connected to them, until the entire frame is built. The chief advantage of this method is that it affords a surgeon greater experience in practical frame construction details and may help the surgeon avoid having to make corrections during the procedure. The primary disadvantage is that piece-by-piece frame assembly requires a great deal of time, adding to an already lengthy procedure. Once the physician has adequate experience in the Ilizarov technique, the use of a preassembled frame is more advantageous.

The position of the rings determine their function in the frame. The main, proximal frame-supporting ring is stationary and always located at the base of the frame. It bears the weight of the entire construct. In the femoral frame it is replaced by the supporting arch; in the humeral frame it is replaced by the half ring with extremities.

The stabilizing frame supporting ring can be stationary or movable, depending on the frame purpose and is always located most distally.

The pusher-puller ring is a movable ring used for the application of distraction-compression forces. It is always located distal to the fracture-osteotomy-nonunion site. Depending on frame size, there may be two pusher-puller rings acting simultaneously or in opposite directions.

The reference ring is a medially positioned ring and used as a reference for the supporting rings or pusher-puller rings; it can be stationary or movable, depending on location.

Choice of ring level determines distribution of the forces applied to the ring. The choice of the ring inclination determines the direction of the forces applied to each ring. At any chosen level, each ring has to be set in a position of correct inclination with regard to the bone axis. In most cases the ring inclination is perpendicular to the bone segment-fragment at this level. During bone lengthening, muscle tension can cause a deviation in the distracted bone fragment. This possible influence must be taken into account when setting the inclination of the proximal main supporting ring to ensure prevention of development of deformity. To prevent this, 5 to 7 degrees of recurvature and varus positioning of the main supporting ring will bring correct direction of distraction.

The space between skin and ring, as a rule, should be at least 3 cm (two-fingers breadth rule) circumferentially. This gap is important to protect the skin and soft tissues if swelling occurs, to allow for bolt and nut manipulation, and to permit wire tract care during the duration of the treatment. In the lower extremity, a four-ring Ilizarov fixator frame is most commonly used. In some cases, however, it may be necessary to apply up to six rings. In the upper extremity, a two- or three-ring Ilizarov frame is usually sufficient.

HINGES

The Ilizarov fixator is a versatile device. Unlike other fixators, it can be used to treat virtually any type of deformity. This is possible because the hinged-rings are able to secure and establish the exact angulation essential for correction of a deformity. Subsequently, the hinges are used as pivotal (rotation) point components for necessary straightening. The position, orientation, and number of hinges are critical factors for deformity correction. Used in combination with distraction-compression devices (graduated telescopic rods), the hinges make it possible to gradually correct deformities with simultaneous transformation of the bone and soft tissues. The advantages of using hinges are: they constrain motion in a specific plane or planes; they provide a specific fulcrum for calculation and control of specific correction of angulation or displacement; and they provide biologic adaptation of tissues to new desired positioning.

Ilizarov hinges are assembled easily from standard parts connected by the bolts and nuts, and attached to the threaded rods, which in turn, are attached to the rings. Several important parameters must be considered in hinge positioning:

1. The two rings to which hinges are attached must be strictly perpendicular to their bone fragments; they must either start perpendicularly and end angulated, or vice versa.
2. The two hinges located at the opposite sides of deformity usually are required for stability.
3. The hinge rotation axis must be situated on the horizontal level of the deformity apex. If two hinges are used, both must be on that level.

4. It is critically important that hinges of the same plane are oriented along the same plane as the deformity.
5. Movement of the axis of rotation of hinges to concave or convex sides of a deformity produces corresponding compression or distraction of the fragments.
6. The positioning of the hinges can be used to achieve different types of deformity correction, such as opening wedge, distraction, compression, translation, and derotation.

A two-axis hinge consists of a single unit that permits rotation around two orthogonal axes. These hinges are used for the simultaneous correction of two concurrent types of deformity. Although they make it possible to shift a bone fragment in two directions, they are limited by the restricted ability of the distraction-compression devices to act in both directions simultaneously.

SEGMENTAL BONE TRANSPORT FOR LARGE BONE LOSS AND SEVERE INFECTION

Ilizarov introduced a new technique of bone transport following corticotomy that consists of sliding a bone fragment internally to fill a defect and thus regenerate bone. The bone transport technique eliminates the need for bone grafting, simultaneously restores a bony defect, eliminates limb shortening, corrects deformity, improves the condition of the local soft tissues, and increases local and regional blood circulation. The three types of bone transport technique are external, internal, and combined external-internal. They differ in the way the bone fragments are transfixed to the frame and how they are "transported" to the intended site. The external technique is indicated for combined bone loss replacement (not greater than 5 cm) with correction of deformities and with limb lengthening (Fig. 12-2A). The internal technique is indicated for large bone loss (up to 15 cm) replacement without deformity correction or limb lengthening [for example, if a large tibial defect coexists with an intact fibula (Fig. 12-2B)]. The combined technique is indicated mainly in cases of major bone loss (more than 10 cm) together with limb deformities, deep soft tissue scars, and local blood supply insufficiency.

INDICATION FOR ILIZAROV FRACTURE TREATMENT

Application of the Ilizarov method is appropriate in many fracture settings including: complex open and closed fractures of long bones, shaft or supracondylar fractures (displaced, transverse, spiral, butterfly, and segmental); intraarticular fractures (dislocation, condylar with displacement); comminuted fractures (unstable, with bone loss or segmental defect); compound fractures (with soft tissue loss, with compartmental syndrome); and grade C-3 fractures.

FIXATOR REMOVAL AND COMPLICATIONS OF ILIZAROV TECHNIQUE

Treatment with the Ilizarov technique consists of five stages: (1) the fixator application and a latency period of 4 to 7 days; (2) a period of distraction/compression of 1 to 5 months (depending on the case); (3) a period of immobility and fixation of the bone position (this usually takes almost twice as long as distraction-compression); (4) 15 to 20 days of frame dynamization consisting of loosening the nuts of

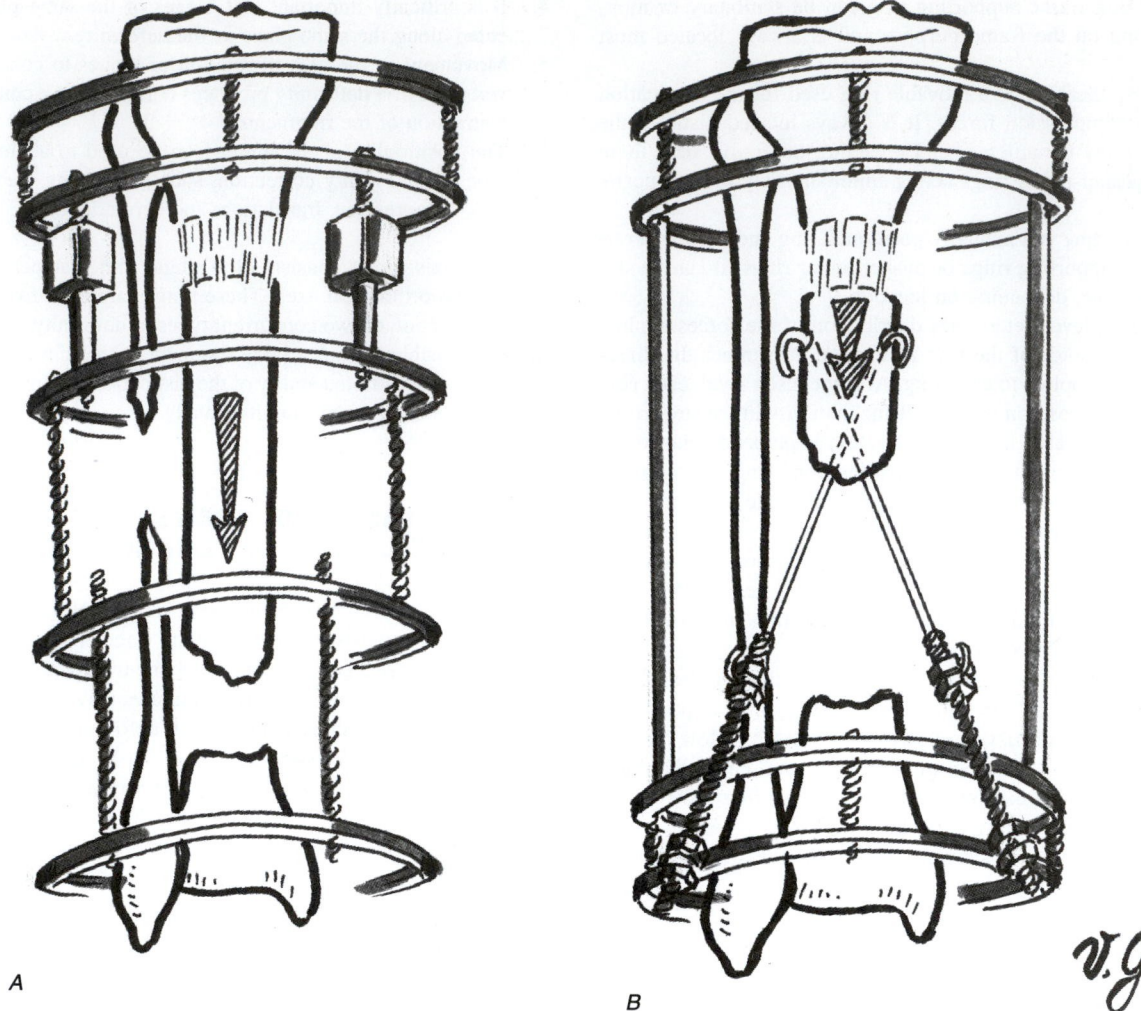

A

B

v.g.

Figure 12-2
External (*A*) and internal (*B*) bone transport techniques for bone loss treatment. The arrows show the direction of the bone fragment motion.

the sites of the connecting rod attachments; and (5) fixator removal and period of immobilization with a cast or brace. This is usually for 2 to 3 weeks and not compulsory (depends on the case).

Before fixator removal, the quality of healing and/or the newly formed bone can be evaluated radiographically. Tomographic evaluation of regenerate quality is also recommended. Because metallic materials interfere with the CT image, they have to be replaced temporarily with nonmetal connectors (improvised from the fiberglass rolls) at the time of the procedure. It is also possible to evaluate regenerate sonographically. Also prior to fixator removal, the tension of all K-wires must be released before they are cut. The rings must be separated by removing the connectors and taken off one by one. Concomitant clinical evaluation of the regenerate or healing of the bone must be done at this time.

Many complications may arise during the long course of treatment with the Ilizarov technique. Most, however, are preventable or correctable and will not interfere with successful results of treatment. They are: (1) general, due to the method; (2) specific, related to technique; and (3) inflammatory. Complications due to method or technique

are related to application of the fixator and may become apparent soon after the procedure is performed. These are: pin tract infections (superficial or deep), vessel injury, and joint contracture. Their incidence averages approximately 10 to 15 percent, depending on the surgeon's experience. However, some complications may not develop until after the patient has been discharged from the hospital. These include: persistent pain, restriction of joint motion, temporary nerve palsy, bone fragment deviation, and bone regenerate deformity. These occur in approximately 5 to 10 percent of cases. Thus it is important to see the patient in the office or clinic soon after discharge and at least once every three to four weeks during treatment.

SUGGESTED READINGS

Bianchi Maiocchi A, Aronoson J (eds): *Operative Principles of Ilizarov: Fracture Treatment, Non-union Osteomyelitis, Lengthening, Deformity Correction.* Baltimore: William & Wilkins, 1991.

Fauro C, Merloz P: *Transfixation: Atlas of Anatomical Sections for the External Fixation of Limbs.* New York: Springer-Verlag, 1987.

Golyakhovsky V, Frankel VH: *Operative Manual of Ilizarov Techniques:* St. Louis: Mosby Desk Yearbook; 1993.

Green SA (ed): Basic Ilizarov techniques. *Tech Orthop* 1990; 5:4.

Green SA: *Complications of External Skeletal Fixation.* Springfield, IL: Charles C Thomas; 1981.

Ilizarov GA: The tension-stress effect on the genesis and growth of tissues: Part I: The influence of stability of fixation and soft-tissue preservation. *Clin Orthop* 1989; 238:249.

Ilizarov GA: The tension-stress effect on the genesis and growth of tissues: Part II: The influence of rate and frequency of distraction. *Clin Orthop* 1990; 239:263.

Ilizarov GA: *Transosseous Osteosynthesis: Theoretical and Clinical Aspects of the Regeneration and Growth of Tissue.* New York: Springer-Verlag; 1991.

Lehman WB (ed): *Operating Room Guide to Cross Sectional Anatomy of the Extremities and Pelvis.* New York: Raven; 1989.

Paley D: Current techniques of limb lengthening. *J Pediatr Orthop* 1988; 8:73.

Chapter 13

SPINE

Kamshad Raiszadeh and Jeffrey M. Spivak

BASIC ANATOMY

OSTEOLOGY

The cervical spine contains seven vertebrae and is lordotic in the sagittal plane. The vertebral body width increases, proceeding caudally. Important palpable anterior neck skin surface landmarks for vertebral level include the mandible (C2–3), hyoid bone (C3), thyroid cartilage (C4–5), and cricoid cartilage (C6).

The atlas (C1) has no vertebral body; this embryologic element joins with the axis (C2) as the dens, or odontoid process. The atlas has concave superior and inferior facets, and a rudimentary spinous process called the posterior tubercle. The anterior arch of the atlas lies in front of and articulates with the dens (Fig. 13–1). The third through sixth cervical vertebrae are considered "typical," with short bifid spinous processes and transverse processes having anterior and posterior tubercles, with a gutter in between. C7 is transitional, having only a posterior tubercle as its trans-verse process and a long spinous process (vertebra prominens), which is not bifid.

In the subaxial cervical spine, the nerve roots exit the neural foramina between the vertebral bodies and the posterolateral lateral masses, and are best visualized on oblique radiographs. The superior and inferior borders of the foramen are the pedicles. The posterolateral border is the anterior surface of the superior articular process. The anteromedial border is the uncovertebral joint (a.k.a. neurocentral joint or joint of Luschka), which is a synovial joint that develops at ages 9 to 12 as a fissuring of the posterolateral annulus fibrosis.

The thoracic spine consists of 12 vertebrae. Generally, the vertebral bodies increase caudally in width even though T1–T3 may be smaller than C7. Unique features of the thoracic vertebrae include costal facets on all 12 vertebral bodies and an anterior facet on the transverse processes of T1–T9. The first thoracic vertebra contains a large and prominent spinous process.

The lumbar spine consists of five vertebrae, and the sacrum is made up of five vertebral segments, with some variability as to the sacral-

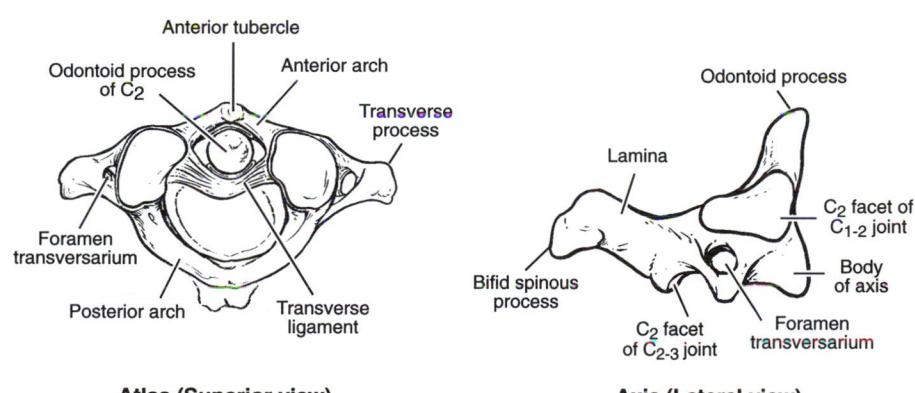

Atlas (Superior view)

Axis (Lateral view)

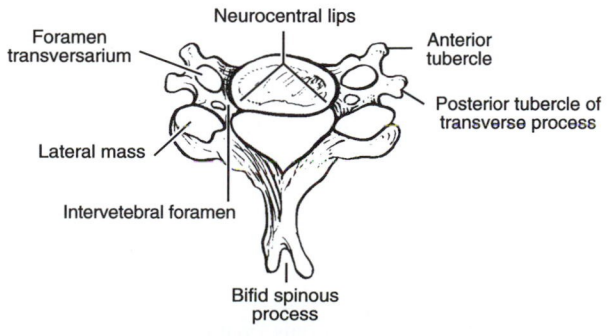

Typical cervical vertebra (Superior view)

Figure 13-1
Cervical osteology.

ization of L5 (more common) or the lumbarization of S1. The lumbar vertebral bodies are larger than those of the thoracic vertebrae and increase in size from L1 to L5. Mamillary processes project posteriorly and laterally from the caudal aspect of the superior articular facet. The transverse processes are thin and long, with the exception of the fifth lumbar vertebra.

Vertebral alignment is generally straight when viewed coronally, but a normal series of lordotic and kyphotic curves are observed in the sagittal plane. Primary kyphotic curves are maintained in the thoracic and sacral regions into adulthood, but the cervical and lumbar spine regions develop secondary lordotic curves in response to sitting and standing postures. Normally, the cervical spine is aligned in 15 to 25 degrees of lordosis. Normal thoracic kyphosis is 20 to 50 degrees, and typical lumbar lordosis is 45 to 60 degrees. The apex of the thoracic kyphosis is typically around T7, and the apex of the lumbar lordosis is typically at L3. Two-thirds of the lumbar lordosis occurs from L4 to the sacrum. In contrast to thoracic kyphosis, which occurs mainly from slight wedging of the vertebral bodies, most of the lumbar lordosis occurs in the disc spaces.

Neutral sagittal balance is defined as the sagittal vertical axis (a plumb line dropped from the C7 vertebral body) intersecting the posterior superior corner of the S1 vertebral body. The sacral inclination or slope (angle between the plumb line and a line drawn parallel to the back of the proximal sacrum) is approximately 50 degrees.

The orientation of the facet joints is a major factor in the range of motion at each level of the spine. The typical cervical (C2–C7) facet joints are oriented 45 degrees in the sagittal plane and 0 degrees in the coronal plane. At each facet joint, the superior articular process (of the caudal vertebra) is positioned anterior and inferior to the inferior articular process (of the cranial vertebra). Half of the cervical rotation occurs at the C1–2 level, and half of the cervical flexion–extension occurs at the occiput-C1 level. Smaller amounts of flexion–extension, rotation, and lateral bend occur segmentally from C2 to C7.

The orientation of the thoracic facets is very close to the coronal plane and about 60 degrees from horizontal in the sagittal plane. This orientation allows motion in the coronal plane (lateral bend) and around the sagittal axis (rotation) and transverse axis (flexion–extension), limited mainly by the constraints of the rib cage. The orientation of the pedicles is angled approximately 20 degrees caudal in the sagittal plane.

The lumbar facets are oriented mainly in the sagittal plane. This anatomic constraint dictates the plane of major motion of the lumbar spine, which is flexion–extension. Rotational motion is minimal, resisted by this facet orientation. For each lumbar facet joint, the superior articular process (of the caudal vertebra) is lateral and anterior to the inferior articular process (from the cephalad vertebra). The anatomic axis of the lumbar pedicles is gradually more medially directed (from posterior to anterior) from L1 to L5, with L5 being approximately 30 degrees medially directed. Sagittally, the pedicles are oriented perpendicular to the long axis of the vertebral bodies (parallel to the vertebral end plates).

LIGAMENTS

Specialized ligaments at the atlanto-occipital level include the two articular capsules (anterior and posterior) and the tectorial membrane, which is the cephalad extension of the posterior longitudinal ligament. Specialized ligamentous attachments to the dens include the centrally located apical ligament, the paired alar or "check" ligaments (which run obliquely from the tip of the dens to occiput), and the longitudinal and vertical bands of the cruciform ligament. At the atlantoaxial level, the transverse ligament is the major stabilizer. It extends from one lateral mass of C1 to the other, posterior to the dens

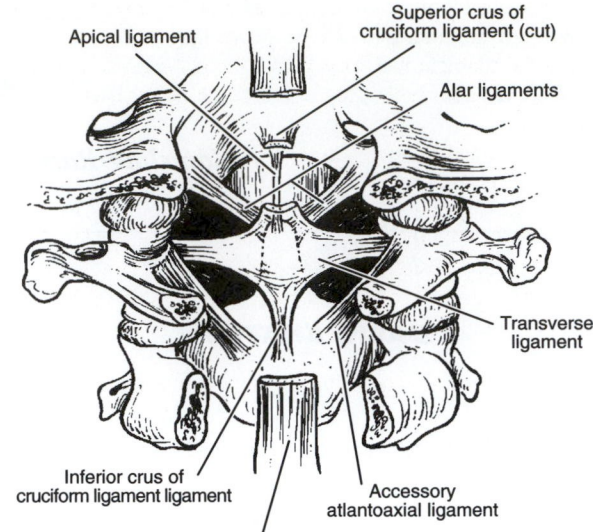

A

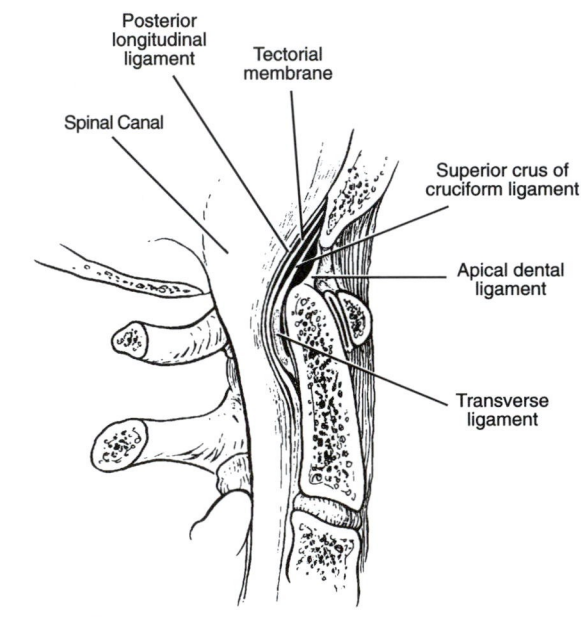

B

Figure 13-2
Cervical ligamentous supports. *A.* Occipital—C2 articulations, posterior cut-away view. *B.* Lateral cut-away view. [Reproduced with permission from Scheider PL, Dzenis PE, Kahanovitz N: Spinal trauma. In Zuckerman JD (ed): *Orthopaedic Injuries in the Elderly*. Baltimore: Urban & Schwartzenberg; 1990:215.]

(Fig. 13–2). The lateral band of the cruciform ligament also contributes to the stability of this level.

In the subaxial cervical spine, the vertebral bodies are bound together by the stronger anterior longitudinal ligament (ALL) and the weaker posterior longitudinal ligament (PLL). The ligamentum flavum, which is a strong, yellow, elastic ligament connecting the laminae, runs from the anterior surface of the cephalad lamina to the posterior surface of the caudal lamina. Supraspinous and interspinous ligaments lie dorsal to or in between the spinous processes, respectively. The supraspinous ligament is in continuity with the ligamentum nuchae, which runs from C7 to the occiput and acts as a posterior tension band to maintain an upright neck position.

Ligamentous support in the posterior thoracic spine consists mainly of the facet joint capsules, supraspinous and interspinous ligaments, and ligamentum flavum. Specialized ligamentous supports involve the rib articulations. Strong radiate ligaments connect the rib head and the thoracic vertebral body. The rib head is also attached to the thoracic transverse processes via the strong costotransverse ligaments.

Similarly named ligamentous supports exist in the lumbar spine. The ALL is thickest medially and thins at the periphery. Separate fibers extend from one to five vertebral levels. The weaker PPL is an hourglass shape with the wider (yet thinner) sections located over the discs. The typical posterolateral disc herniation occurs at the lateral aspect of these expansions. The ligamentum flavum lies between the lamina, coursing from the midportion of the anterior aspect of the superior lamina to the cephalad edge of the inferior lamina. The supraspinous and interspinous ligaments provide support, and the intertransverse ligaments run between adjacent transverse processes but contribute little to overall spinal stability. The specialized iliolumbar ligaments are stout ligaments that connect the transverse processes of L5, and sometimes L4, with the posterior ilium. Avulsion fractures of these transverse processes can occur in conjunction with an unstable vertical shear pelvic fracture.

The intervertebral discs are fibrocartilaginous. The outer annulus is composed of multiple lamellar layers with alternating obliquely oriented fibers comprised mainly of type I collagen. The central nucleus pulposus is more gelatinous in consistency, made primarily of type II collagen. The distinction between the annulus and nucleus becomes less apparent as one ages.

MUSCLES

The most superficial muscle of the anterior neck is the platysma [cranial nerve (CN) VII innervated]. Deeper to the platysma, the stylohyoid and digastric muscles (CN XII) are situated cephalad to the hyoid bone, and the "strap" muscles are caudal. The strap muscle group includes the sternohyoid and omohyoid superficially, and the thyrohyoid and sternothyroid deep. All are innervated by the ansa cervicalis. The sternocleidomastoid (CN XI and ansa cervicalis) runs obliquely across the neck. Originating at the mastoid process of the skull, the muscle splits into a sternal head and clavicular head for attachment. Its motion is to bend the neck to the ipsilateral side and rotate the head to the contralateral side.

The prevertebral musculature includes the longus colli, longus capitus, and rectus capitus anterior and lateralis. More laterally are situated the scalene muscles (scalenus anterior, medius, and posterior).

The most superficial layer of the posterior spinal musculature is the trapezius muscle, innervated by the spinal accessory nerve, and the latissimus dorsi and lumbodorsal fascia, innervated by the thoracodorsal nerve. The intermediate muscle layer includes the splenius capitus, semispinalis capitus, longissimus capitus, and splenius cervicis in the cervical region, and the sacrospinalis system (spinalis, longissimus, and iliocostalis) in the thoracolumbar region. All of these muscles are segmentally innervated.

The deep posterior neck muscles of the upper cervical spine form the borders of the suboccipital triangle. The three muscular borders include the superior and inferior heads of the obliquus capitis muscle and the rectus capitus posterior major muscle. The contents of the suboccipital triangle include the vertebral artery and the posterior ramus of the first cervical nerve. The greater occipital nerve is located superficial to the suboccipital triangle.

The deep muscles of the thoracolumbar spine include the broad semispinalis and multifidus and the shorter intertransversarii, rotators, and interspinalis muscles. In the thoracic spine, the deep muscles are sagittally oriented in cross section, with the rotators overlying the lamina. This is in contrast to the lumbar spine, where the short rotator muscles are coronally oriented and the multifidus directly overlies the spinous process and lamina.

BLOOD SUPPLY

The vertebral arteries, which are the first branches of the subclavian arteries, contribute only 10 to 15 percent of the cerebral blood flow and yet are the major blood supply to greater than 90 percent of the cervical spinal cord, nerve roots, vertebrae, and supporting tissues. The vertebral artery ascends through the transverse foramina of C1–C6 (anterior to and not through C7), accompanied by the descending vertebral vein (which *does* travel through the C7 transverse foramen as well). Its path in the transverse foramina is anterior to the lateral masses. After passing through the foramen of the transverse process of the atlas, the vertebral artery travels medially along the cephalad surface of the posterior arch of C1 in the sulcus of the vertebral artery. Along the cephalad surface of C1, the vertebral artery stays at least 1.5 cm lateral from the midline, making this a safe lateral margin for dissection of tissues off the superior aspect of the posterior arch of C1. Following this path along C1, the vertebral arteries then ascend through the foramen magnum where they contribute to the circle of Willis.

Radicular arteries (medullary feeders) that arise from the vertebral artery supply the single anterior median and paired posterior spinal arteries throughout the length of the cervical spinal cord. There is no significant collateral connection between these two systems. The majority of the spinal cord (up to 85 percent) throughout its length is supplied by branches of the anterior spinal artery. On average, there are eight medullary feeders to the anterior spinal artery and 12 to the posterior spinal arteries throughout the length of the spinal cord. The most consistent cervical medullary feeder is at the C5–6 level. The intracranial blood supply from the basilar artery anastomoses with the anterior spinal artery, supplying the spinal cord variably up to the C4 level.

The posterior radicular arteries are much smaller and more frequent in their segmental occurrence, but their contribution to the cervical cord blood supply is much less critical. These segmental arteries are at each vertebral level and supply the vertebral bodies, nerve roots, and surrounding tissues. Of importance is the blood supply to the odontoid process, via the bilateral posterior ascending arteries that join at the level of the tip of the odontoid to form the apical arcade. The apical arcade also receives a contribution from the meningeal artery, a branch of the occipital artery.

In the thoracic spine, the blood supply to the spinal cord is through branches of the posterior intercostal arteries. The intercostal arteries arise segmentally from the aorta and divide into an anterior branch, which courses along the undersurface of the rib, and a posterior branch. The posterior branch reaches the spinal cord via the interspinal foramen and anastomoses with the anterior spinal artery. These posterior segmental arteries are variable in number and size. At least two and at most 16 spinal branches have been noted, all of which approach the spinal cord at different levels and contribute to its blood supply. The artery of Adamkiewicz, which is the largest of these radicular arteries, originates from a left posterior intercostal artery in 80% percent of cases, most commonly at the ninth to 11th thoracic vertebral level. The artery of Adamkiewicz by itself is not sufficient to supply the caudal segments of the spinal cord alone; there are actually several medullary feeder arteries at different levels that are important for maintaining the spinal cord supply.

There is a critical blood supply zone in the thoracic spine. The number and size of cervical and lumbar medullary radicular arteries exceed that in the area of the thoracic cord, resulting in a "watershed" region. This "critical supply zone" of the spinal cord generally lies between the fourth and ninth thoracic vertebrae, and operative measures in this zone require careful dissection. During the anterior approach, the segmental arteries should be divided as far anteriorly as possible, and the vessels should be dissected free in the posterior direction over only a short distance so as not to disrupt the arterial arcades that join the segmental arteries outside and within the vertebral canal. To avoid damage to the spinal artery branches, electrocautery should not be used in the vicinity of the intervertebral foramen.

NEURAL ANATOMY

In the cross section of the spinal cord shown in Fig. 13–3, note the topographic orientation of the lateral corticospinal tract and dorsal column. Dorsal roots and ganglia (sensory) and the ventral roots (motor) converge to form the spinal nerve, which is extradural as it approaches the intervertebral foramen. The dura becomes the epineurium surrounding the spinal nerve. After exiting the foramen, the dorsal primary ramus that supplies the muscles and skin of the neck and back emerges. The ventral rami supply the anteromedial trunk and limbs. The cervical nerve roots 1 to 7 exit the spinal canal above the named vertebral body and pedicle, while the C8 root exits in the C7–T1 interspace. Thoracic nerve roots exit below the named pedicle, in the lower portion of the named vertebral body. In the lumbar spine, the nerve root (e.g., L4) is formed at and traverses the respective disc space (i.e., L3–4) above the named vertebral body (i.e., L4) and exits the respective foramen under the pedicle (of L4). Herniated disks will usually impinge upon the traversing nerve root. After exiting the foramen, the spinal nerve delivers the dorsal primary rami that supply the muscles of the back, while the ventral rami supply the limbs.

The spinal cord ends caudally at the level of the L1–2 disc space most commonly. The lowest portion of the spinal cord is known as the conus medullaris, which is generally at the level of L1 anatomically but controls sacral cord function and is responsible for lower parasympathetic control over bowel and bladder function and erection in males. The nerve roots below the level of the conus are known as the cauda equina and include all lumbar, sacral, and coccygeal root function.

The cervical sympathetic chain, which lies anterior to the lateral masses and prevertebral fascia covering the longus colli, extends from C2 caudally with three cervical ganglionic enlargements: the superior ganglion (C2–3 level), the middle ganglion (C6 level), and the inferior ganglion (frequently fused with first thoracic or stellate ganglion).

The diaphragm is innervated by the phrenic nerve (C2–C4). Its innervation, as well as its blood supply, arise centrally. During the thoracoabdominal approach, therefore, the diaphragm is transected within 2 cm from its rib insertions to avoid damaging the phrenic vessels and branches of the phrenic nerve.

The sensation of the face and top of head are supplied by the divisions of the fifth cranial (trigeminal) nerve. The occipital region and upper neck are supplied by C2, while the lower neck is supplied by C3. The nipples are at the T4 dermatomal level, while the umbilicus is at the T10 level. The only thoracic level reflex is the abdominal reflex, which is sensitive for cord pathology, such as a syrinx.

The functions of the lower cervical and lumbar roots are listed in Table 13–1.

APPLIED ANATOMY OF THE NECK

The fascial layers of the anterior neck are divided into superficial and deep layers (Fig. 13–4). The superficial fascia invests the platysma. The deep fascia has three layers: superficial, middle, and deep. The superficial layer invests the sternocleidomastoid and trapezius. The middle layer is the pretracheal fascia, which invests the strap muscles, trachea, esophagus, and thyroid. This fascia is continuous with the lateral margin of the carotid sheath. The deep layer is the prevertebral fascia, which invests the posterior paracervical and anterior prevertebral musculature.

The anterior aspect of the neck can be divided by the sternocleidomastoid into the posterior and anterior triangles (Fig. 13–5). The posterior triangle borders are the trapezius, sternocleidomastoid, and middle third of clavicle. The inferior belly of the omohyoid further divides this space into subclavian (lower) and occipital (upper) triangles.

The anterior triangle is bounded by the sternocleidomastoid, the anterior median line of the neck, and lower border of mandible. It is further subdivided into the submandibular, carotid, and muscular triangles. The posterior belly of the digastric separates the carotid from the submandibular triangles; the superior belly of the omohyoid separates the carotid from the muscular triangles. The standard anterior approach to the midcervical spine is done through the muscular triangle (see below).

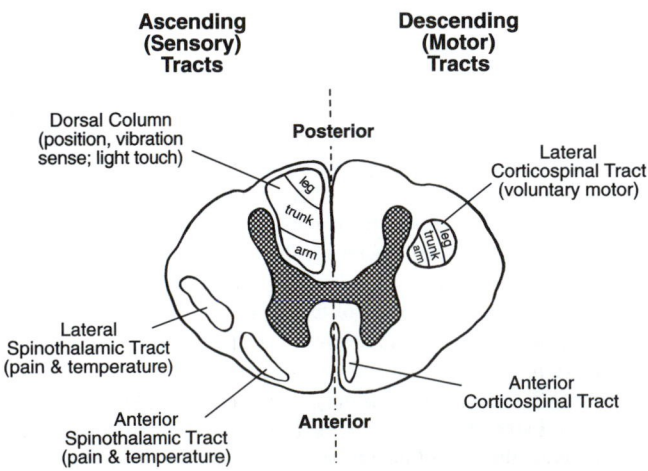

Figure 13-3
Cross section of the spinal cord—cervical region.

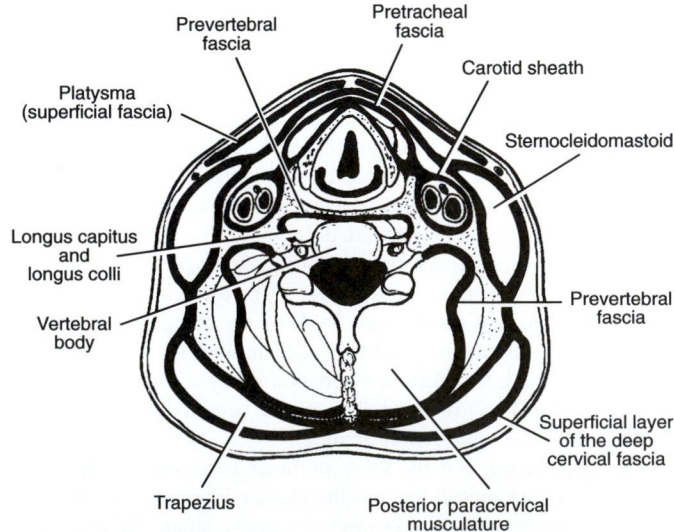

Figure 13-4
Fascial layers of the neck.

Table 13-1

Functions of the Cervical and Lumbar Nerves by Spinal Level

Root	Reflex	Muscles	Sensation
C5	Biceps	Deltoid/biceps	Lateral arm (deltoid patch)
C6	Brachioradialis	Wrist extension	Radial forearm
	Biceps		Thumb
C7	Triceps	Wrist flexors	Middle finger
		Finger extensions	
		Triceps (elbow ext.)	
C8		Finger flexion	Little finger
		Hand intrinsics	Ulnar forearm
T1		Hand intrinsics	Medial arm
L1		Internal oblique,	Posterolateral buttocks
		Transverse abdominis	Inguinal area above pubis
L2	Cremaster	Hip adductors	Prox ant. med. thigh
		Hip flexors	
L3		Hip adductors	Lateral thigh
		Hip flexors	
L4	Quadriceps	Quadriceps	Medial leg and foot
		Tibialis anterior	
L5		EHL	1st web space, dorsal foot
		Foot inversion	
		(Tib Post)	
S1	Achilles	FHL, gastrocsoleus	Lateral foot
		Peroneus longus/brevis	

The recurrent laryngeal nerve, coming from the vagus nerve, courses on the left side around the aortic arch before ascending toward the larynx between the trachea and the esophagus. On the right side, the nerve ascends superior to the aortic arch, making it more vulnerable to injury during an anterior surgical approach.

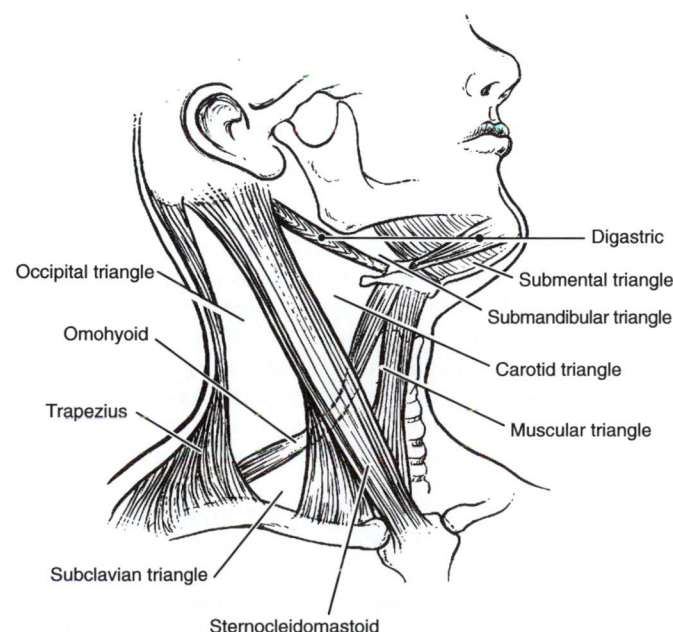

Figure 13-5
Triangles of the neck.

Labels: Occipital triangle, Omohyoid, Trapezius, Subclavian triangle, Sternocleidomastoid, Digastric, Submental triangle, Submandibular triangle, Carotid triangle, Muscular triangle

SURGICAL APPROACHES

CERVICAL SPINE

Transoropharyngeal Approach

The main indication for this approach is for direct decompression of the C1–2 complex due to fixed anterior spinal cord compression, most commonly seen in rheumatoid disease with fixed subluxation. Tumors of the dens, osteomyelitis, os odontoideum, and dens pseudoarthrosis represent additional indications. In this approach, surgery is performed in an area colonized by bacteria, making postoperative infection more likely. The use of oral disinfection and topical antibiotics applied before wound closure and in the perioperative period helps to minimize this problem. The approach may be facilitated by first performing a tracheostomy, but this is not necessary in most cases.

Special retractors are used to hold down the tongue and to pull up the soft palate. The posterior pharyngeal wall is incised, the incision extending from the easily palpable anterior tubercle of the atlas to the level of C2 or C3. The long muscles of the neck are divided longitudinally in the midline and subperiosteally elevated laterally, which brings into view the anterior tubercle and lateral mass of the atlas and the body of the axis. Once exposed, the anterior arch of C1 and the underlying dens can be resected using a power burr. It is recommended that the anterior dura be exposed to assure complete decompression.

During the subperiosteal muscle elevation, the atlas may be exposed to a maximum of 2 cm lateral to the midline, but the C2 and C3 vertebrae should not be exposed by more than 1 cm because of risk of injury to the vertebral artery. The vertebral artery is at particular risk at the inferior border of C2. Also, lateral to the lateral mass of the atlas, the elevator may penetrate the retromandibular fossa, and injuries to CN IX and XII may result.

Anterior Approach to C3–T1

Approach from either side is possible and is a matter of surgeon's preference; right-handed surgeons generally prefer the right-sided approach. Because of the irregular and higher course of the recurrent laryngeal nerve on the right side, a left-sided approach is considered by some to be safer for exposures of C6–T1.

The patient is positioned in the supine position. Skeletal tong traction is optional, allowing for maximal externally applied cervical traction. An extension moment may also be applied through the use of a cervical head halter. This apparatus, however, may interfere with approaches and exposure of the C3–C5 region, especially in patients with relatively short necks. A pad is placed between the scapulae, and the head is rotated slightly toward the opposite side of the approach. The shoulders can be positioned caudally by using strips of adhesive tape applied over the acromion process.

The choice of location for the skin incision is based on the surface anatomy previously described. Location may be confirmed by x-ray with a skin marker. A transverse incision following Langer's lines is used, preferably in an existing neck skinfold. The incision extends from the midline to the medial border of the sternocleidomastoid. Generally, this transverse incision can be mobilized to expose almost the entire cervical spine. For a broad exposure of multiple levels, a longitudinal incision along the anterior border of the sternocleidomastoid muscle may be used.

Following the incision, the platysma is most commonly divided transversely. The superior and inferior aspects of the platysma are undermined with care to maintain a bloodless field. The superficial cervical fascia is then divided longitudinally at the anterior border of the sternocleidomastoid. Again, strict hemostasis is maintained by ligation or cautery of coursing cervical veins. The superior belly of the omohyoid muscle runs transversely at the level of C6–7 and, if it lies within the area of interest, is isolated and transected. The carotid pulse is then palpated, and dissection is continued medial to the carotid sheath, bluntly dividing the middle layer of the deep cervical (pretracheal) fascia longitudinally. The contents of the carotid sheath (common carotid artery, internal jugular vein, and vagus nerve) are retracted laterally while the strap musculature (sternohyoid and sternothyroid) and visceral structures (trachea, larynx, esophagus, and thyroid) are retracted medially. The anterior surface of the spine, including the paired longus colli muscles, is palpated. The deep cervical (prevertebral) fascia is then longitudinally incised in the midline, taking care to retract the esophagus medially. As a rule, the prominent transverse process of the sixth cervical vertebra (carotid or Chassaignac's tubercle) is palpable lateral to the longus colli muscle. In 10 percent of cases, however, the seventh cervical vertebra may also have a prominent transverse process if the vertebral artery enters the foramen at C7. An intraoperative lateral radiograph is always done to confirm the correct level by using a spinal needle (bent in a "Z" configuration to avoid unwanted deep needle penetration) in the intervertebral disk.

Exposure of the lower cervical spine may necessitate ligation of the inferior thyroid artery. If exposure above C4 is required, the superior thyroid artery and vein often need to be ligated and transected. When exposing more proximal segments of the cervical spine, the lingual artery and facial artery (both arising from external carotid) may be ligated if necessary. The superior laryngeal nerve runs beneath the lingual and facial arteries to pass into the larynx. The hypoglossal nerve comes from the cranial side and turns medially anterior to the external carotid artery. Both of these nerves need to be protected during high cervical dissection.

Posterior Approach to the Cervical Spine

The patient is placed in the prone position, with padding under the chest and head. After shaving of the hair in the operative field, a midline longitudinal incision is made. The cervical fascia is incised and the nuchal ligament (bloodless plane) is divided longitudinally to the tips of the spinous processes. By using a combination of diathermy and elevator subperiosteal dissection, the short rotator and multifidus muscles are stripped from the spinous process and articular processes. For exposure of the occiput, the attaching musculature (trapezius and semispinalis capitus) is separated using a T-shaped dissection. The posterior tubercle of the atlas is palpated, and the overlying musculature is detached using an elevator or diathermy. The superior surface of the posterior arch of the atlas can be safely exposed for about 1.5 cm bilaterally; further lateral dissection risks damage to the vertebral arteries. More laterally, between the atlas and axis, the posterior branch of the second spinal nerve arises. In rheumatoid arthritis, the posterior arch of the atlas is very thin and can be injured by excessive dissector pressure.

THORACIC SPINE

Transthoracic Approach to T4–T11

The spine can be approached by either a right-sided or a left-sided thoracotomy. If the pathology does not dictate the use of one side, a right-sided thoracotomy is generally preferred because of the presence of the aorta and the heart on the left. The right side is also the usual convexity of the scoliotic curve, and thoracotomy for scoliosis is generally performed on the side of the convexity.

The patient is positioned in a lateral decubitus position. Good extension can be obtained by slightly flexing the operating table at the level of the incision. As a rule, the approach is made two ribs higher than the center of the lesion or the apex of the scoliotic curve, because it is easier to dissect caudally along the lower rib than cephalad due to the descending course of the ribs. A curvilinear incision is made above the selected rib or interspace. It begins 4 finger breadths lateral to the spinous processes and may be extended as far as the costochondral junction. The latissimus dorsi muscle is divided transversely to its fibers and in line with the incision. The nerve supply to the latissimus dorsi is from superior (thoracodorsal nerve), so its transection should be limited to only the most inferior portion needed. The rib level can be checked by passing a hand anterior to the latissimus below the scapula and counting off the ribs starting cranially; the first rib usually cannot be palpated. Anteriorly, the serratus anterior is exposed and transected again as far caudally as possible to spare the long thoracic nerve approaching from a superior direction. If a rib is to be resected during the approach, its periosteum is divided and complete exposure of the rib with a rib stripper follows. The rib is then transected first lateral to the costotransverse articulation and then medial to the costochondral border. The parietal pleura of the thoracic cavity is now opened in the bed of the resected rib. If no rib is to be resected, dissection proceeds along the superior border of the inferior rib of the desired interspace, to avoid injury to the neurovascular bundles traveling along the inferior rib surface. A thoracotomy spreader is used to open the thoracic cavity. The lung is retracted anteriorly, and the vertebrae are exposed. The parietal pleura overlying the vertebrae is incised longitudinally, exposing the vertebrae, discs, and segmental vessels at the midbody level. There are variations in the azygos and hemiazygos veins, but the vertebrae can usually be accessed by a median division of the intercostal veins without violating the longitudinal systems. It is often not always necessary to divide the segmental vessels in the thoracic spine if only disc space releases are needed. In this case, the parietal pleura can be divided in line with the disc and a peanut or blunt Hohmann retractor used anteriorly to protect the contralateral structures while the disk is resected, leaving the segmental vessels over the bodies intact.

Closure of the thoracotomy is accomplished by first placing a chest tube. Nonabsorbable sutures are placed around the ribs, with the suture being placed through drill holes in the inferior rib to avoid injury to the intercostal vessels. A rib approximator is then applied and the sutures tied. A running suture is used to reapproximate the intercostal musculature, followed repair of the anterior serratus and latissimus dorsi muscles.

Transpleural–Retroperitoneal Approach to the Thoracolumbar Junction

Exposure of the thoracolumbar junction is possible by using either a right-sided or a left-sided approach, but a left-sided approach is preferable for anatomic reasons. A right-sided approach is hampered by the liver and by the fragile inferior vena cava. Again, in cases of scoliosis, entry on the convex side of the curvature is the rule.

The patient is placed in a right lateral decubitus position. The skin incision is located over the ninth or tenth rib. It begins posteriorly near the posterior axillary line and follows the rib as far as the costal cartilage, continuing obliquely to the upper and middle abdomen, depending on the distal extent needed. Using diathermy, the muscle (latissimus dorsi, serratus, and external oblique) overlying the tenth rib is incised down to the bone. Attention is directed toward first dissection of the subphrenic region. The internal oblique and transverse abdominis muscles are split. The peritoneum becomes visible and is retracted medially from the lateral abdominal wall. This retroperitoneal dissection is carried down until the psoas muscle becomes visible, and the peritoneum is stripped from the inferior surface of the diaphragm. Next, attention is directed to the supraphrenic region where the periosteum of the tenth rib is transected with electrocautery along its entire length. The rib is dissected in line with the intercostal muscle fiber insertions (posterior to anterior along the cranial border, and anterior to posterior along the caudal border) and then removed by transection at the costochondral margin and posteriorly. The costal cartilage is divided longitudinally to serve as a marker for later wound closure. The chest cavity is then entered in the bed of the tenth rib, and the lung retracted superiorly. The diaphragm is now exposed both superiorly and inferiorly, and is transected under direct vision about 2 cm from its rib insertion posteriorly to the spine. Marking sutures are placed at regular intervals to allow for a better reapproximation of the diaphragm during repair.

The crus of the diaphragm is then divided, taking care to protect the greater splanchnic nerve and sympathetic trunk. The retroperitoneal space is bluntly developed and the parietal pleura incised along the long axis of the spine. Segmental vessels are transected between ligatures. Exposure of the vertebrae follows, always beginning over the intervertebral disks where no segmental vessels are found. The sympathetic trunk is retracted laterally and the psoas muscle is stripped off the intervertebral disks as far posteriorly as the pedicle and intervertebral foramen.

Costotransversectomy to T3–T10

Costotransversectomy, which affords a posterolateral approach to the thoracic vertebrae and discs, is indicated for biopsy of the thoracic vertebrae and discs or anterior decompression of the thoracic spinal canal, as in disc herniations and thoracic fractures. More commonly, however, anterior thoracic decompression is done via a more directly anterior thoracotomy approach. Costotransversectomy for biopsy is common for diagnosis of infection and tumor of the thoracic spine.

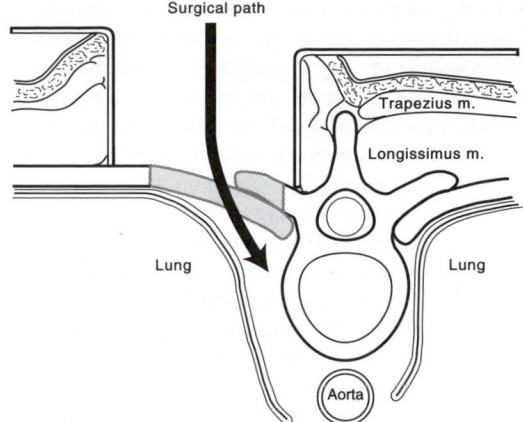

Figure 13-6
Operative path for costotransversectomy.

The approach may be made from either side, with the patient in a prone or semilateral position. The semilateral position, with the operative side elevated, provides a better anterior view. For approaches to the upper thoracic spine, the arm is maximally elevated to move the scapula as far superior and lateral as possible. A paramedian or curvilinear (apex lateral) skin incision is most commonly used, centered on the level of interest. The trapezius muscle is incised in line with the incision, isolating the lateral edge of the paraspinal muscles and elevating them medially to expose the transverse processes, lateral lamina, and costovertebral articulations (Fig. 13-6). The ribs of concern are subperiosteally elevated as described for the thoracotomy approach, with care taken to maintain the parietal pleura intact. Exposure of the rib is carried from the costotransverse articulation to the desired length laterally (about 10 cm). The rib is divided laterally, and its medial articulation with the transverse process is exposed as far as the lamina. The transverse process is excised at its base, and the laterally separated rib is removed by subperiosteally stripping as far medially as the costovertebral articulation, followed by rotating the rib free from its costovertebral joint capsule. The parietal pleura is then bluntly dissected anteriorly off the disc space and vertebrae, maintained anterior, and protected using a ribbon or similar retractor. Care should be taken during the exposure to avoid damaging the segmental vessels and nerve running along the inferior border of the rib being removed. For larger exposures, however, one or more neurovascular bundles can be ligated and transected. The segmental nerves starting at T6 innervate the abdominal muscles and should be preserved if possible. In general, disc space and/or vertebral biopsy can be done with excision of a single rib. Commonly for decompression, however, three adjacent ribs may need to be resected. Wound closure is accomplished by reapproximation of divided musculature in layers. A chest tube is not used unless the parietal pleura has been violated (check positive-pressure breathing prior to wound closure.)

Costotransversectomy can also be done using a midline approach, with wide elevation of the paraspinal musculature over the transverse processes. The longissimus may need to be transversely dissected and retracted superiorly and inferiorly at the level of the pathology in question. This midline approach may be more useful a more limited biopsy exposure and when the anterior spinal work is combined with posterior instrumentation for stabilization.

Midline Posterior Approach

The patient is placed in the prone position, with appropriate anterior padding with padded posts or laminectomy rolls. The abdomen is maintained off pressure to avoid venous congestion, which can increase venous bleeding during surgery. The skin incision is made down to the fascia at the appropriate level. In children, the cartilaginous spinous process apophyses are split in the midline whereas, in adults, the fascia is released from both sides of the spinous processes by cautery. The deep dissection is carried out subperiosteally out to the transverse processes, usually starting on the concave side in scoliosis cases. The deep musculature of the thoracic spine originates laterally and caudally, inserting on the lamina and transverse processes more medially and cephalad. This makes the deep dissection most easily accomplished in a caudal to cephalad direction. Bleeding is controlled by electrocautery and packing. If spinal fusion is planned, the joint capsules and cartilage of the appropriate facets are removed by using curettes, rongeurs, and gouges, taking care to coagulate the facet bleeders.

LUMBAR SPINE

Retroperitoneal Approach to L2–Sacrum

The lumbar spine approaches can be made from the right or the left side. The side of approach may be determined by the underlying disease (e.g., scoliotic component or tumor expansion); otherwise, a left-sided approach should be chosen, because of the presence of the aorta on the left, which is easier to work with surgically than is the inferior vena cava on the right. The patient is placed in a right lateral decubitus position or may be positioned in a "floppy lateral" position. The right leg is flexed at the hip and knee. All pressure sites should be well cushioned.

If a higher lumbar exposure is required (e.g., L2), it is advantageous to expose subperiosteally and resect the 12th rib. The skin incision continues along the 12th rib before running obliquely and anteriorly toward the rectus sheath, approximately 3 finger breadths above away from the iliac crest. Depending on the distal exposure, the incision may be extended caudally to the lateral border of the rectus sheath. The latissimus dorsi is dissected transversely to the direction of its fibers and the external oblique parallel to its fibers. Deeper dissections is accomplished by dividing the posterior serratus muscle in the posterior incision area and the internal oblique and transversus abdominis more anteriorly.

After division through the deep abdominal muscle, the retroperitoneal space is entered. The kidney and ureter are retracted medially, bringing the quadratus lumborum muscle into view. The periosteum over the 12th rib is incised, and the distal portion of the rib is resected. Care should be taken to avoid inadvertent opening of the pleural cavity. The periosteum of the rib bed is transected near the midline, and the cranial half, together with the diaphragm insertion, is retracted superiorly. Care is also taken to protect the 11th and 12th intercostal nerves.

To expose the vertebrae, the retroperitoneal tissue over the lumbar spine is split longitudinally with the sympathetic trunk maintained laterally. The segmental vessels are exposed at the level of the vertebral bodies and transected. The vertebral bodies and intervertebral disks are then accessible.

Pararectal Retroperitoneal Approach to L3–Sacrum

The patient is placed in the supine position with the hips and knees flexed about 30 degrees and the hip abducted 15 degrees. The hip flexion is necessary to relax the psoas muscle and iliac vessels so that the lower lumbar spine can be more easily exposed anterolaterally. The skin incision is made in a curved line over the lateral border of the rectus muscle, from 2 to 3 finger breadths above the umbilicus to 3 finger breadths above the pubic symphysis. A longitudinal para-

median incision can also be used. The approach may be made from either side; if a choice exists, the left side is preferable since the common iliac vein lies medial to the artery and thus does not need to be mobilized as far.

The approach through or around the rectus abdominis muscle can be handled in a number of ways. In one technique, the lateral border of the rectus is identified and the anterior sheath incised. The superficial epigastric vessels are ligated. The inferior end of the incision runs medial to the superficial inguinal ring and therefore has to turn medially, following the outline of the rectus muscle. The preperitoneal space is entered after incision of the posterior layer of the rectus sheath (unless the rectus is incised precisely at the union of the anterior and posterior layers). Care should be taken to elevate the lateral border of the muscle to avoid injuring the peritoneum. Behind the posterior layer of the rectus sheath, the inferior epigastric vessels are exposed at the caudal border of the incision and are ligated if the lumbosacral junction is to be exposed. In another technique, the rectus muscle is retracted laterally after longitudinal incision of the anterior rectus fascia about 4 finger breadths from the midline. The preperitoneal space is entered below the arcuate ligament, which can be incised longitudinally to expose above the lumbosacral junction. Once the rectus is retracted and the retroperitoneal space entered, the parietal peritoneum is retracted medially from the lateral abdominal wall by using a swab on a stick and digital dissection. The psoas muscle with the overlying genitofemoral nerve is identified, as is the common iliac artery and vein in the retroperitoneal fatty tissue. At the inferior margin of L4, the ureter accompanied by the testicular vessels cross the common iliac artery from lateral to mediocaudal. Coursing above the aortic bifurcation is the superior hypogastric plexus, which fans out anteriorly to the promontory. The plexus should be preserved because it carries sympathetic supply to the genitourinary system, and injury to it may lead to retrograde ejaculation.

For exposure off the lower lumbar spine, the psoas muscle is retracted laterally, exposing the segmental vessels and the ascending lumbar vein. These are exposed and ligated as needed. For exposure of the sacral promontory or the anterior side of the sacrum, the dissection proceeds anterior to the common iliac vessels. Ligation of the middle sacral vessels anterior to the promontory provides exposure of the L5-S1 disc in the midline. For wider exposure of the anterior sacrum, the internal iliac vessels are ligated bilaterally from close to their origin from the common iliac artery and vein. This allows the common iliac artery and vein mobility for further lateral retraction, exposing the first and second anterior sacral foramina.

Transperitoneal Approach to L4–S1

The patient is placed in the supine position, with a roll under the lumbar spine. The operating table is angled to produce hyperlordosis, which facilitates access to the promontory. The skin incision may be made in the midline or as a "Pfannenstiel" transverse incision 2 to 3 finger breadths above the symphysis. The linea alba is exposed and transected in the midline. The underlying peritoneum is then elevated and split longitudinally.

The wound is separated with large laparotomy hooks and the greater omentum retracted superiorly. The mesocolon on the right and left sides is also retracted with moist sponges, and the sigmoid is retracted inferiorly with a spatula. The posterior peritoneal layer is then incised in the midline. Care is taken to avoid injury to the branches of the retroperitoneal superior hypogastric plexus; electrocautery is avoided, if possible. The peritoneum is bilaterally mobilized laterally by blunt dissection. The layer of fat and connective tissue covering the retroperitoneal vessels is bluntly opened over the right common iliac artery to the right of the midline. The tissue overlying the aortic bifurcation, which includes the superior hypogastric plexus, is now bluntly dissected free of the bifurcation toward the left in one layer. The promontory is now visible. The middle sacral artery and the not always present vein are then ligated. Vessel loops may aid in mobilization of the aorta and common iliac arteries. Clear access to the sacrum and L5–S1 is now possible. The L4–5 disk can be exposed by careful dissection and retraction of the vena cava and common iliac veins. In the case of a deeply localized aortic bifurcation or deep venous confluence, dissection between the aorta and the vena cava may be advantageous for exposure of the L4–5 and even L3–4. In this case, the aorta is retracted to the left after ligation of the fourth lumbar vascular bundle, and the vena cava is dissected toward the right.

Posterior Midline Approach to the Lumbar Spine

The posterior approach to the lumbar spine is carried out in the same way as just described for the thoracic spine, except that dissection is generally performed caudally, because the deepest musculature traverses from lamina laterally to more caudal spinous processes medially, making deeper subperiosteal muscle dissection more easily accomplished from cephalad to caudal. The facets are oriented sagittally compared to the coronally positioned thoracic facets. Care must be taken to identify cases of spina bifida so that dissection does not inadvertently enter the vertebral canal. The dissection is carried out in cases of fusion to the transverse processes.

Paraspinal Approach (Wiltse)

The principle indication for this approach is spondylolisthesis in an adolescent. A longitudinal midline incision is made, and the skin and subcutaneous tissue are mobilized laterally on both sides. The lumbar fascia is incised lengthwise approximately 2 cm lateral to the spinous process. At this region, there is a natural groove between the multifidus and the longissimus/iliocostalis muscles. This plane is relatively avascular and leads to the L4–5 facet. After separation of the muscle groups, retractors are placed, and distal dissection is carried out by diathermy through the increasingly flat multifidus muscle to the L5–S1 joint and sacral alae. The sacral alae, the lateral aspect of the L5–S1 facet joint, and the transverse process of L5 are all exposed subperiosteally. Care is taken to avoid injuring the L4–5 facet

articulation or damaging the L5 nerve root with deep dissection between the sacral alae and L5 transverse process.

Limited Open Approach for Laminotomy and Intervertebral Disk Removal

The patient is generally positioned in the kneeling position, and the site of the incision is identified by x-ray verification of a spinal needle. A small 2-cm incision is made, and the lumbar fascia is maximally opened on the affected side of the spinous process. Subperiosteal dissection is performed out to the facet joint, taking care to preserve the joint capsule.

The spinal canal is then entered by either curetting the ligamentum flavum from the superior aspect of the inferior lamina, or by sharp incision of the flavum. Kerrison rongeurs are used to complete the removal of ligamentum flavum and appropriate amount of bone. Atraumatic blunt dissection is used to expose the dura and involved nerve root. The nerve root is most easily identified as it courses medial to its similarly named pedicle on the way to its intervertebral foramen.

SUGGESTED READINGS

AANS Publications Committee: *Surgical Exposure of the Spine: an Extensile Approach.* Park Ridge, IL: American Association of Neurological Surgeons, 1995.

An HS: *Principles and Techniques in Spine Surgery.* Baltimore: Williams & Wilkins, 1997.

Bridwell KH, Dewald RL (eds): *The Textbook of Spinal Surgery,* 2d ed. Philadelphia: Lippincott-Raven, 1997.

Frymoyer JW (ed): *The Adult Spine: Principles and Practice,* 2d ed. Philadelphia: Lippincott-Raven, 1997.

Hoppenfeld S: The spine, in *Surgical Exposures in Orthopaedics: The Anatomic Approach,* 2d ed. Philadelphia: JB Lippincott; 1994:chap 6.

Lehman RM, Grunwerg B, Hall T: Anterior approach to the cervicothoracic junction: an anatomic dissection. *J Spinal Disorders* 1997; 10:33.

Rothman RH, Simeone FA (eds): *The Spine,* 4th ed. Philadelphia: WB Saunders, 1998.

Trindade AM, Antunes JL: Anterior approaches to non-traumatic lesions of the thoracic spine. *Adv Tech Standards Neurosurg* 1997; 23:205.

Chapter 14

BRACHIAL PLEXUS

Andrew S. Rokito

OVERVIEW

The brachial plexus is derived from the ventral primary rami of C5 to T1. It emerges between the anterior and middle scalene muscles, passes posterior to the clavicle, and extends into the axilla.

The plexus is composed of five *roots* (C5 to T1, although there may also be C4 and T2 contributions), three *trunks* (superior, middle, and inferior), six *divisions* (three anterior and three posterior), three *cords* (lateral, posterior, and medial), and multiple *branches* (Fig. 14–1).

There are four preclavicular branches originating from the roots and upper trunk: long thoracic (C5, 6, 7), dorsal scapular (C5), suprascapular (C5, 6), and the nerve to the subclavius (C5, 6). Seven postclavicular branches arise from the cords: lateral pectoral (C5, 6, 7), medial pectoral (C8, T1), medial brachial cutaneous (T1), medial antebrachial cutaneous (C8, T1), upper subscapular (C5, 6), thoracodorsal (C6, 7, 8), and lower subscapular (C5, 6). There are five postclavicular terminal branches: musculocutaneous (C5, 6, 7), axillary (C5, 6), radial (C5, 6, 7, 8, T1), median (C5, 6, 7, 8, T1), and ulnar (C7, C8, T1).

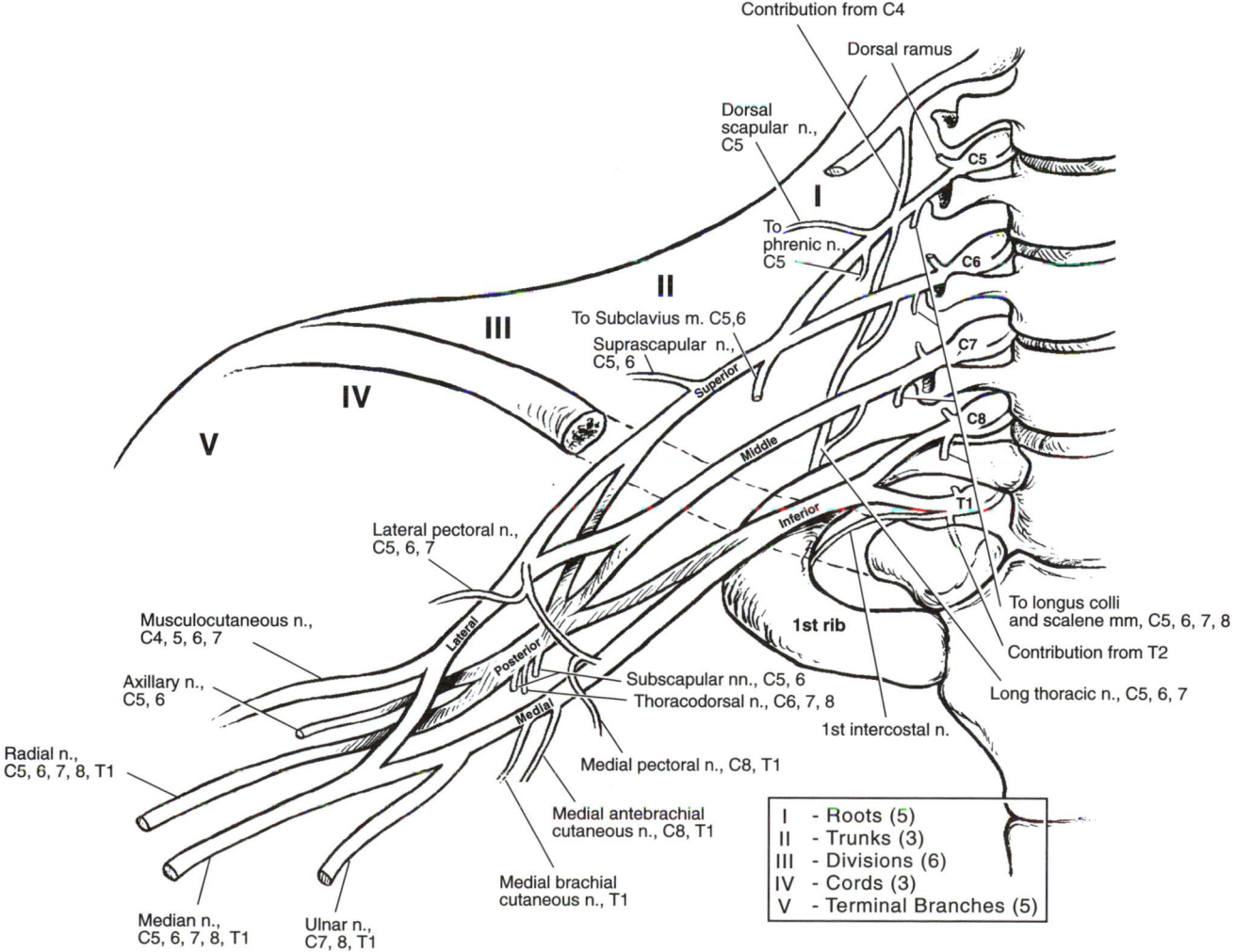

Figure 14-1
Right brachial plexus.

Table 14-1

Division of Subclavian Artery

Part	Branches	Course/Misc.
1	Superior Thoracic	Serratus anterior
		Pectoralis major
2	Thoracoacromial	Deltoid
		Acromial
		Pectoralis
		Clavicular
		branches
	Lateral Thoracic	Serratus anterior
3	Subscapular	Thoracodorsal and
		circumflex
		scapular branches
		(triangular space)
	Anterior circumflex	Humeral head
	humeral	
	Posterior circumflex	Quadrangular space
	humeral	

VESSELS

The subclavian artery originates from the aortic arch on the left side and the brachiocephalic trunk on the right. It emerges between the anterior and middle scalenes with the brachial plexus and becomes the axillary artery as it passes over the first rib. The axillary artery can be thought of as having three parts—medial, posterior, and lateral—based on its relationship to the pectoralis minor. The number of branches arising from each part corresponds to the number of that part (Table 14–1).

SURGICAL APPROACH

The patient is placed in the supine, semi-sitting position. An oblique incision is made at the midportion of the posterior border of the sternocleidomastoid, carried distally and medially, and curved horizontally just below the clavicle. It can be extended distally into the deltopectoral groove, if necessary. The platysma is divided in line with the skin incision and the external jugular vein, located posterior to the sternocleidomastoid, is either retracted medially or ligated. The brachial plexus lies directly under the vein, between the anterior and middle scalenes, deep to the fascia. The spinal accessory nerve lies superficially in the apex of the wound and must be protected. The suprascapular vessels, located inferiorly near the clavicle, are also usually ligated as are the transverse cervical vessels which cross the plexus in the posterior triangle. The omohyoid muscle crosses the plexus obliquely and is divided and repaired later.

The clavicle is subperiosteally exposed. The middle third is osteomized and removed and the trapezius and pectoralis major are reflected superiorly and inferiorly, respectively. The subclavius muscle is also released and reflected. The entire brachial plexus and axillary artery are now exposed. Stabilization of the clavicle with internal fixation is performed at the end of the procedure. Due to the extensive soft tissue dissection and poor medullary blood supply of the clavicle, this procedure does carry a significant risk of nonunion.

SUGGESTED READING

Millesi H: Brachial plexus injuries. In Jupiter JB, Flynn EJ (eds): *Flynn's Hand Surgery,* 4th ed. Baltimore: Williams & Wilkins; 1991:460.
Netter FH: Part I: Anatomy, physiology, and metabolic disorders. Brachial plexus. In *The Ciba Collection of Medical Illustrations,* vol 8. Summit, NJ: Ciba-Geigy; 1991:28–29.

Chapter 15

SHOULDER, HUMERUS, ELBOW, AND FOREARM

Jordan A. Simon, James W. Cahill, and Andrew S. Rokito

SHOULDER

ANATOMY OF THE SHOULDER

The shoulder is comprised of three mobile joints: the glenohumeral, scapulothoracic, and the acromioclavicular joint. The combined motion of these three articulations allows for the extreme mobility of the shoulder.

Osteology

The scapula is a flat bone, shaped like an inverted triangle. The scapular spine divides the dorsal surface into the supraspinatus fossa and infraspinatus fossa. The acromion is the lateral expansion of the scapular spine which articulates with the lateral edge of the clavicle at the acromioclavicular joint. The coracoid process is a hook-shaped anterior projection of the scapula, located medial to the glenoid. The coracoid serves as the attachment point for several muscles and ligaments. The glenoid fossa faces laterally and slightly anterior. The supraglenoid and infraglenoid tubercles provide attachment points for the long head of the biceps and triceps muscles, respectively. The glenoid is relatively shallow and deepened by the surrounding fibrocartilaginous glenoid labrum. The scapular notch, located on the superior aspect of the scapula and medial to the glenoid neck, is bounded superiorly by the transverse scapular ligament.

Articulations

The scapulothoracic joint lies between the subscapularis and the serratus anterior. There is no bony articulation. The scapula is supported posteriorly by the attachment of the levator scapulae, rhomboideus major and minor to the medial border of the scapula, and the trapezius muscle to the scapular spine. The clavicle acts as a strut anteriorly through the acromioclavicular joint and the coracoclavicular ligaments. The scapulothoracic joint allows three degrees of freedom: protraction/retraction, elevation/depression, and rotation.

The glenohumeral joint is a shallow ball and socket joint. The fibrous glenohumeral joint capsule is reinforced by the superior, middle, and inferior glenohumeral ligaments which attach the glenoid lip to the anatomic neck of the humerus. The inferior glenohumeral ligament is the strongest of the three. Dynamic stability of the glenohumeral joint is provided by the muscles of the rotator cuff: the supraspinatus, infraspinatus, teres minor, and subscapularis. The tendon of the long head of the biceps passes over the humeral head, acting as a depressor during abduction. It is located intracapsular but extrasynovial. The coracoacromial arch, composed of the acromion posteriorly and the coracoacromial ligament anteriorly, separates the rotator cuff muscles from the overlying deltoid.

The acromioclavicular joint contains an articular disc as well as a thin capsule. The articulation is reinforced by the capsule which provides anterior/posterior support and coracoclavicular ligaments, the conoid and trapezoid ligaments which resist vertical forces. The motion at this articulation is primarily a gliding motion.

Bursae

The subacromial bursa is located between the supraspinatus tendon and the inferior surface of the acromion. This often communicates with the subdeltoid bursa, located between the humeral head and overlying deltoid insertion. Communication of these bursae with the joint capsule is indicative of a rotator cuff tear. The subscapularis bursa communicates with the joint capsule in the normal shoulder.

Musculature of the Shoulder Girdle

The scapula is supported by muscles originating from the thoracic vertebrae, the thoracic cage posteriorly, and the base of the skull anteriorly (Fig. 15-1). The combined action of these muscles provides control for rotation, protraction/retraction, and elevation/depression of the scapula. The muscles which cross the glenohumeral joint provide abduction/adduction and flexor/extension of the arm.

Vascular Anatomy

The subclavian artery passes posterior to the clavicle and becomes the axillary artery as it passes lateral to the first rib. The axillary artery is divided into three parts based on its relationship to the pectoralis minor muscle.

The first part of the axillary artery, proximal to the pectoralis minor, gives off one major branch: the supreme thoracic artery supplying the upper thorax.

The second part, posterior to the pectoralis minor, gives off two major branches: the thoracoacromial artery and the long thoracic artery. The acromial branch of the thoracoacromial artery lies within the coracoacromial ligament. The long thoracic artery lies superficial to the serratus anterior, supplying this muscle.

The third part of the axillary artery, lateral to the pectoralis minor, sends off three branches before becoming the brachial artery: the subscapular artery, the posterior humeral circumflex artery, and the anterior humeral circumflex artery.

Nerves

The brachial plexus surrounds the axillary artery on the medial side of the coracobrachialis and short head of the biceps as they insert onto the coracoid process. Care should be taken to remain lateral to these landmarks to avoid damage to the nearby neurovascular structures. The suprascapular nerve (C4-C6) branches from the upper trunk

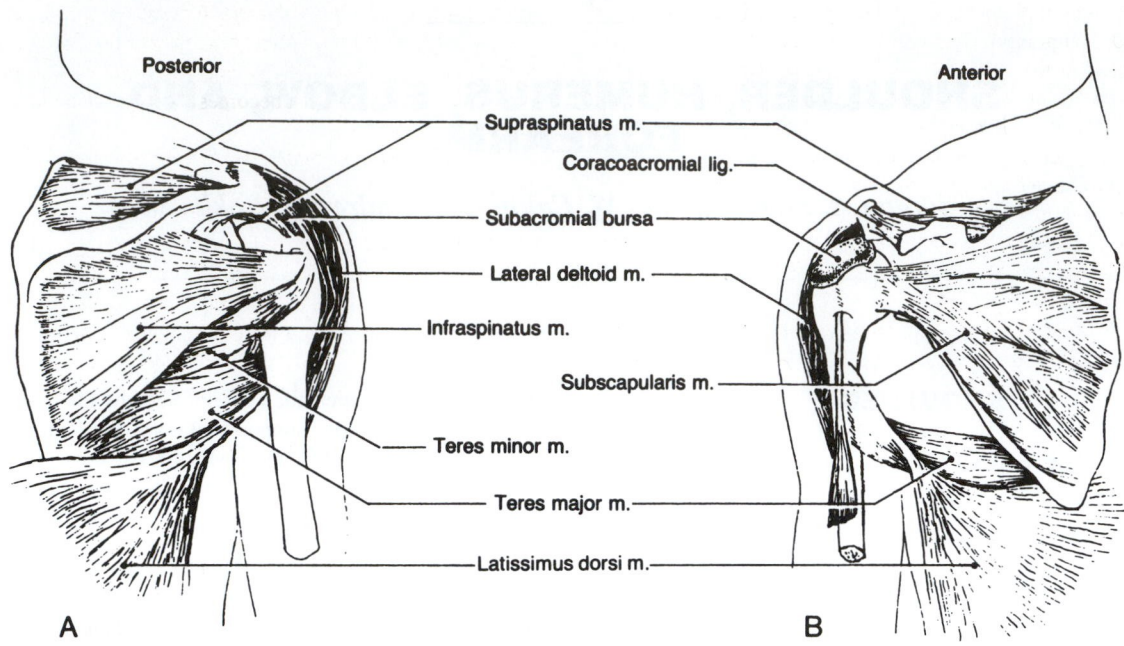

Figure 15-1
A. Posterior muscles of the right rotator cuff. The supraspinatus, infraspinatus, and teres minor are shown. *B.* Anterior muscles of the right rotator cuff. The supraspinatus and subscapularis are shown. (Reproduced by permission from April EW: Shoulder region. In *The National Medical Series for Independent Study: Anatomy,* 2d ed. New York: John Wiley & Sons; 1990:52.)

of the brachial plexus and passes through the suprascapular notch, under the transverse scapular ligament, to innervate the supraspinatus and infraspinatus muscles. The axillary nerve passes through the quadrangular space and around the posterior humerus to innervate the deltoid and the teres minor muscles.

SURGICAL APPROACHES TO THE SHOULDER

Anterior Approach to the Shoulder

There are two possible incisions that can be used for the anterior approach to the shoulder. The deltopectoral incision is made along the deltopectoral groove, beginning just above the coracoid process. Although this provides good exposure, the scar created is commonly broad and obvious. An axillary incision may alternatively be made along the anterior axillary fold with the arm abducted and externally rotated to provide a more cosmetic scar.

The superficial dissection is carried out through the interval between the deltoid (axillary nerve) and the pectoralis major (medial and lateral pectoral nerves). The cephalic vein should be protected during this approach; however, if damaged, it may be ligated without significant complications. The deep dissection requires medial retraction of the coracobrachialis and short head of the biceps to expose the underlying tendon of the subscapularis muscle. This may require osteotomy of the coracoid, although inferior traction should be avoided to prevent neurapraxia of the musculocutaneous nerve. All dissection should remain lateral to these muscles to protect the axillary artery and brachial plexus from injury. The subscapularis tendon is divided 1.5 cm proximal to its insertion on the lesser tuberosity. External rotation of the arm during division brings the field away from the axillary nerve within the quadrangular space, minimizing the risk of injury. The location of the incision in the anterior joint capsule is determined by the specific procedure being performed.

Proximal extension to expose the brachial plexus and axillary artery

involves proximal extension of the incision over the midportion of the clavicle and osteotomy. Distal extension may be carried out via an anterolateral approach to the humerus.

Anterolateral Approach to the Shoulder

A transverse incision is made from the anterolateral edge of the acromion to the lateral border of the coracoid. The fascia over the deltoid is dissected and the deltoid is split in line with its fibers for 5 cm. A stay suture is placed at the inferior border of the incision to prevent propagation and damage to the axillary nerve. The acromioclavicular joint and anterior edge of the acromion are exposed by detachment of the origin of the deltoid. The coracoacromial ligament may be resected to reveal the supraspinatus bursa and tendon. The acromial branch of the thoracoacromial artery lies within this ligament and will cause excessive bleeding if not cauterized. Proximal or distal extension of this approach is not recommended.

Lateral Approach to the Shoulder

A 5 cm longitudinal incision is made from the anterolateral margin of the acromion distally over the lateral margin of the arm. The deltoid is split for 5 cm from the edge of the acromion and a stay suture is placed to prevent further separation of the deltoid fibers and damage to the axillary nerve. The greater tuberosity with the insertion of the supraspinatus tendon will be apparent at this point. Manipulation of the arm will allow visualization of the rotator. Distal extension is impossible. Proximal extension may be accomplished by extension of the incision over the supraspinatus fossa and incision of the trapezius.

Posterior Approach to the Shoulder

An incision is made from the posterior margin of the acromion along the length of the scapular spine. The deltoid is released from the scapular spine and the plane between the deltoid (axillary nerve) and the infraspinatus (suprascapular nerve) is located. Deep dissection is carried out between the infraspinatus (suprascapular nerve) and the teres minor (axillary nerve). Retraction within this plane reveals the posterior joint capsule, glenoid rim, and glenoid neck. Care must be taken to remain superior to the teres minor as dissection inferior to this muscle may damage the axillary nerve or posterior humeral circumflex artery within the quadrangular space. Medial retraction of the infraspinatus must also be limited to prevent stretching of the suprascapular nerve as it travels from the supraspinatus fossa to infraspinatus fossa.

The exposure may be enlarged distally by incision of the infraspinatus tendon 1 cm from its insertion on the greater tuberosity.

HUMERUS

ANATOMY OF THE HUMERUS

Osteology

The humerus is the largest bone of the upper extremity. Bony landmarks include the greater tuberosity, lesser tuberosity, and deltoid tubercle which serve as muscular attachment points. Proximally, the humerus is divided into two distinct regions: the anatomic and surgical neck. The surgical neck is located distal to the greater and lesser tuberosities. The shaft of the humerus contains two significant grooves that are of anatomic importance. Proximally, the bicipital groove is situated between the two tuberosities. The tendon of the long head of the biceps muscle is located in this groove. More distally in the midportion of the humeral shaft on its posterior aspect lies a groove for the radial nerve. Distally, the humerus flares into medial and lateral epicondyles.

Musculature

The muscular anatomy of the brachium can be divided into flexor and extensor compartments. The flexor muscles include the biceps, brachii, coracobrachialis, and brachialis. The extensor compartment consists of the triceps muscle. The triceps muscle is divided into the long head, lateral head, and medial head. (Table 15-1).

Nerves

Four major nerves traverse the brachium: the musculocutaneous nerve, the radial nerve, the median nerve, and the ulnar nerve.

The musculocutaneous nerve is formed from the lateral cord of the brachial plexus. It pierces the coracobrachialis 5 to 8 cm distal to the coracoid and then branches to supply this muscle, the biceps, and the brachialis. More distally, it becomes the lateral antebrachial cutaneous nerve of the forearm.

The radial nerve is formed from the posterior cord of the brachial plexus and spirals around the humerus from medial to lateral while supplying the triceps muscles. Laterally, it emerges between the brachialis and brachioradialis anterior to the lateral epicondyle.

The median nerve arises from the medial and lateral cords of the brachial plexus and accompanies the brachial artery along the upper extremity, crossing from medial to lateral as it traverses distally. The median nerve does not innervate any of the muscles present in the humeral region. It does, however, send some branches to the elbow joint.

The ulnar nerve is a continuation of the medial cord of the brachial plexus and remains medial to the brachial artery. Distally, the nerve courses posterior to the medial epicondyle of the humerus. Like the median nerve, it gives off no branches to the brachial musculature but does send some branches to the elbow joint.

The cutaneous nerves arise directly from the brachial plexus and consist of the medial, lateral, and dorsal brachial cutaneous nerves. Proximally, the axillary nerve supplies the cutaneous region overlying the deltoid muscle in the mid portion.

Vascular Anatomy

The brachial artery runs medially with the median nerve under the biceps brachii muscle. The profunda brachii artery runs with the radial nerve to supply the triceps muscle. The brachial artery bifurcates after giving off anastomotic branches to the elbow joint to become the radial and ulnar arteries.

SURGICAL APPROACHES TO THE HUMERUS

The Anterior Approach to the Humerus

The incision begins at the coracoid process extending in line with the deltopectoral groove and extending along the lateral border of the biceps brachii muscle. The incision should be continued distally as far as needed but should stop approximately 5 cm above the flexion crease of the elbow. Proximally, the internervous plane lies between the deltoid muscle (axillary nerve) and the pectoralis major (medial and lateral pectoral nerves). This muscular interval is developed dis-

---

Table 15-1

Muscles of the Arm

Muscle	Origin	Insertion	Action	Innervation
Coracobrachialis	Coracoid	Mid. humerus (medial)	Flexion, Adduction	Musculocutaneous
Biceps	Coracoid (SH) Supraglenoid (LH)	Radial tuberosity	Supination, Flexion	Musculocutaneous
Brachialis	Anterior humerus	Ulnar tuberosity (anterior)	Flexes forearm	Musculocutaneous and radial
Triceps	Infraglenoid (LH) Post. humerus (lat H) Post. humerus (MH)	Olecranon	Extends forearm	Radial

NOTE: SH, short head; LH, long head; lat H, lateral head; MH, medial head.
SOURCE: Reproduced with permission by Miller MD: Anatomy. In: *Review of Orthopaedics*. Philadelphia: WB Saunders; 1992:310.

tally to the level of the deltoid tuberosity and to the insertion of the pectoralis major into the lateral lip of the bicipital groove. The shaft of the humerus is exposed by incising the periosteum longitudinally just lateral to the insertion of the tendon of the pectoralis major. The incision is continued proximally, taking care to stay lateral to the tendon of the long head of the biceps. The anterior circumflex humeral artery traverses the field from medial to lateral at this level and should be cauterized or ligated. Distally, the plane lies between the medial fibers of the brachialis (musculocutaneous nerve) and the lateral fibers of the brachialis (radial nerve). The interval between the biceps brachii and the brachialis is identified and developed until the anterior aspect of the brachialis muscle is visible. Care must be taken to identify and protect the musculocutaneous nerve deep to the biceps brachii. The fibers of the brachialis muscle are split longitudinally, exposing the underlying humeral shaft.

The approach can be extended proximally by extension to an anterior approach to the shoulder. However, the approach cannot be extended distally.

Anterolateral Approach to the Distal Humerus

The incision begins approximately 10 cm proximal to the flexion crease of the elbow and extends distally along the lateral border of the biceps brachii to just above the flexion crease.

The lateral cutaneous nerve of the forearm can be identified in the distal aspect of exposure. The interval between brachialis (radial nerve, lateral innervation) and brachioradialis (radial nerve) is identified after medial retraction of the biceps muscle. The radial nerve is identified distally between the two muscles and traced proximally until it pierces the lateral intermuscular septum. With the radial nerve protected, the periosteum along the lateral border of the brachialis muscle is incised to expose the humeral shaft.

Proximal extension is accomplished by developing the plane between the brachialis medially (radial nerve) and the lateral head of the triceps (radial nerve) posterolaterally. Distally, the approach may be extended into an anterior approach of the elbow.

The Posterior Approach to the Humerus

A longitudinal incision extends from the olecranon fossa to an area approximately 8 cm below the level of the acromion, just short of the spiral groove containing the radial nerve. The two superficial heads of the triceps muscle, lateral and long, are split bluntly in the proximal portion of the dissection and sharply where they fuse to form a common tendon. As the lateral head of the triceps muscle is retracted, the profunda brachii artery and the radial nerve must be identified as they emerge from the hiatus of the lateral intermuscular septum and traced into the spiral groove. The medial head of the triceps is incised down to bone. The dissection must remain subperiosteal to avoid damaging the ulnar nerve which pierces the medial intermuscular septum as it passes from anterior to posterior in the lower third of the arm.

Extension of the approach proximally is not possible above the level of the spiral groove. Distally, the approach is easily extended over the olecranon and onto the proximal ulna.

Lateral Approach to the Distal Humerus

The incision is made from a point 4 to 6 cm proximal to the lateral epicondyle to the level of the epicondyle. The plane between the brachioradialis (radial nerve) and the triceps muscle (radial nerve) is developed and carried down through periosteum. Dissection is then continued subperiosteally, anteriorly, and posteriorly to expose the distal

humerus. The common extensor origin may be incised and subperiosteally dissected if further exposure of the lateral epicondyle is needed. The radial nerve remains safe with this approach provided the approach is not extended proximally.

Proximal extension is not possible because the radial nerve crosses the proposed line of dissection. Distally, the approach may be extended to the radial head by using the internervous plane between the anconeus (radial nerve) and the extensor carpi ulnaris (posterior interosseous nerve).

ELBOW

ANATOMY OF THE ELBOW

The elbow joint is composed of three articulations: the ulnohumeral, radiohumeral, and proximal radioulnar joints. The bony architecture is strengthened by the supporting ligamentous structures to create a mobile joint with great stability.

Osteology

The triangular distal humerus is classically viewed as being composed of two bony columns supporting the central trochlea. The lateral column includes the lateral epicondyle and terminates at the capitellum. The medial column terminates at the medial epicondyle. The spool-shaped trochlea is located between the columns with its axis in 4 to 8 degrees of valgus and 3 to 8 degrees of internal rotation with respect to the humeral shaft. The rotational axis of the capitellum lies 12 to 15 mm anterior to the axis of the humeral shaft in line with the trochlear axis. Proximal to the trochlea are the coronoid fossa anteriorly and olecranon fossa posteriorly, separated from each other by a thin shell of bone. The flared proximal ulna is known as the olecranon which articulates with the trochlea at the semilunar notch. The anterior lip of the olecranon is known as the coronoid process. The radial notch lies lateral to the coronoid process and provides the ulnar contribution to the proximal radioulnar joint. The proximal radius is composed of the concave, disc-shaped radial head with its short, narrow neck. The radial head, as well as the radial notch, semilunar notch, trochlea, and capitellum, is covered with articular cartilage.

Five centers of ossification within the elbow appear at characteristic ages (Table 15-2).

Articulations

The ulnohumeral articulation is characterized as a ginglymus or hinge joint which has one degree of freedom: flexion/extension. It is reinforced by the fan-shaped ulnar collateral ligament which is divided into anterior, middle, and posterior bands. Stability is enhanced by the congruence of the articular surfaces. The radiohumeral articulation is a trochoid or pivot joint which allows flexion/extension as well

Table 15-2	
Five Centers of Ossification in the Elbow	
Capitellum	2 years
Radial head	4 years
Medial epicondyle	5 years
Trochlea	7 years
Lateral epicondyle	9 years

as rotation of the radius. It is reinforced by the lateral collateral ligament which is formed by a condensation of the joint capsule and also comprised of three bands. The proximal radioulnar joint has one degree of freedom which permits pronation/supination about an axis joining the proximal and distal radioulnar articulations. It is reinforced by the annular ligament which originates on the anterior lip of the radial notch of the proximal ulna, wraps around the radial head and neck, and inserts on the posterior lip of the radial notch. The elbow joint capsule surrounds these three articulations. Distention of the capsule with intracapsular fractures will cause the posterior fat pad, located within the olecranon fossa, to become visible on x-ray. The anterior fat pad, located in the coronoid fossa, may be visible in normal elbows.

Musculature

The medial epicondyle acts as the origin for the flexor muscles of the forearm: the flexor carpi radialis, flexor carpi ulnaris, palmaris longus, and flexor digitorum superficialis. The lateral epicondyle provides the origin of the extensor muscles: the extensor carpi radialis longus and brevis, extensor carpi ulnaris, and extensor digiti minimi as well as the anconeus and supinator muscles.

Vascular Anatomy

There is a complex collateral circulation around the elbow with the largest vessel, the brachial artery, located deep to the bicipital aponeurosis, superficial to the brachialis muscle, and medial to the biceps tendon. In the cubital fossa, the brachial artery bifurcates to form the radial and ulnar arteries. The profunda brachii artery also contributes collateral vessels around the elbow and provides branches to perfuse the posterior forearm.

Nerves

The radial, ulnar, and median nerves pass around the elbow joint as they travel to innervate the muscles of the forearm. The median nerve passes through the antecubital fossa anterior to the medial epicondyle, deep to the bicipital aponeurosis, and lies medial to the brachial artery in 82 percent of the population. The radial nerve passes anterior to the lateral epicondyle, between the brachialis and brachioradialis muscles as it enters the forearm. The ulnar nerve passes posterior to the medial epicondyle within the ulnar groove.

SURGICAL APPROACHES TO THE ELBOW

Posterior Approach to the Elbow

A longitudinal incision is made 5 cm proximal to the tip of the olecranon and continued distally, curving laterally over the tip of the olecranon and then back medially over the subcutaneous surface of the ulna. The deep fascia is incised in the midline, and the ulnar nerve is exposed and protected within the ulnar groove.

A transverse or chevron osteotomy is made about 2 cm distal to the tip of the olecranon, passing through the midportion of the semilunar notch of the ulna. The proximal fragment is freed of medial and lateral soft tissue attachments and retracted proximally to expose the distal humeral articulations. Alternatively, the triceps tendon may be split and the olecranon left intact. Stripping of soft tissue along the humeral shaft should be limited to the distal quarter to prevent damage to the radial nerve. Anterior neurovascular structures are protected by flexion of the elbow during dissection and strict subperiosteal dissection.

Proximal extension is not advised in order to prevent damage to the radial nerve. Distal extension can be accomplished via extension along the subcutaneous border of the ulna.

Medial Approach to the Elbow

An 8 to 10 cm incision is made on the medial aspect of the elbow, centered over the medial epicondyle. The ulnar nerve should be exposed initially and protected during dissection. The plane between the pronator teres (median nerve) and the brachialis (musculocutaneous nerve) is identified. The median nerve enters the pronator teres near the midline and is retracted inferiorly as the pronator is retracted medially away from the underlying brachialis muscle. A drill hole may be made in the medial epicondyle to facilitate fixation later. An osteotomy of the medial epicondyle is performed and the fragment is retracted distally. Proximal dissection is continued in the interval between the brachialis (musculocutaneous nerve) and triceps (radial nerve) muscles. Incision of the medial collateral ligament and joint capsule exposes the medial aspect of the elbow joint.

Proximal extension is carried out in the plane between the brachialis and triceps to expose the distal humeral shaft. Distal extension is not possible as distal retraction of the medial epicondyle with its attached muscles may lead to stretching of the median nerve.

Anterior Approach to the Elbow

A serpentine incision is made from 5 cm proximal to the flexion crease, medial to the insertion of the biceps tendon, and continued along the medial border of the brachioradialis muscle for 5 cm.

The lateral cutaneous nerve of the forearm (musculocutaneous nerve) emerges about the interval between the brachialis muscle and biceps tendon and may be located along the subcutaneous border of the forearm. The bicipital aponeurosis is incised and reflected laterally. The brachial vein and median nerve can be identified medial to the brachial artery. The radial nerve is identified running between the brachialis and brachioradialis proximally before entering the substance of the supinator muscle at the arcade of Frohse.

There is no useful proximal or distal extension for this approach.

Anterolateral Approach to the Elbow

The incision is started 5 cm proximal to the flexion crease on the lateral border of the biceps muscle, and extended distally over the medial border of the brachioradialis muscle. The lateral cutaneous nerve of the forearm should be protected. The radial nerve is identified proximally between the brachialis (musculocutaneous nerve) and brachioradialis (radial nerve) muscles. The plane between the brachioradialis (radial nerve) and pronator teres (median nerve) is developed distally.

The radiocapitellar joint is exposed by incising the anterior joint capsule between the radial nerve and brachialis muscle. With the forearm supinated, the supinator muscle can be dissected off the radius to expose the radial neck and proximal third of the shaft (Fig. 15-2).

Proximal extension is accomplished by developing the plane between the brachialis and triceps muscles. Distal extension is accomplished via continuation as described in the section below on the anterior approach to the radius.

Posterolateral Approach to the Radial Head (Kocher Approach)

A 5 cm longitudinal incision is centered directly over the radial head. The interval between the extensor carpi ulnaris (posterior interosseous

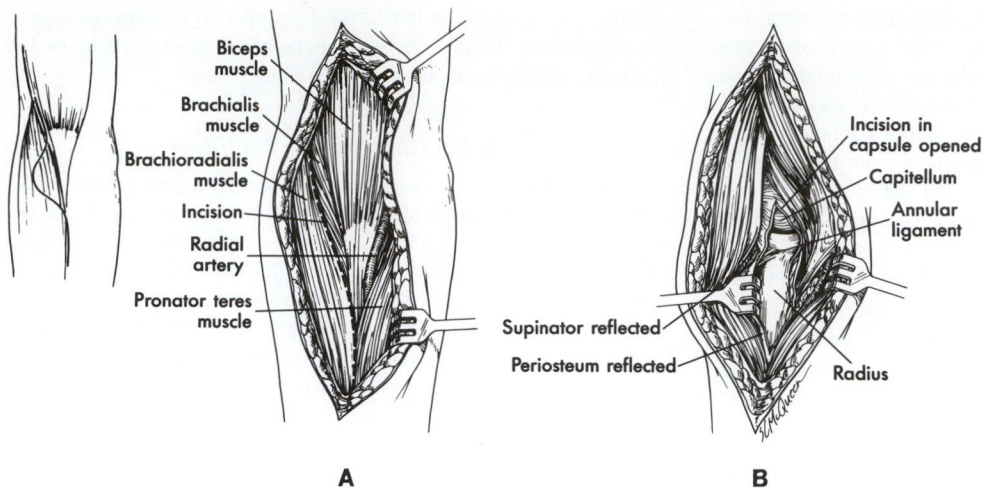

A

B

Figure 15-2
Modified Henry anterolateral approach to elbow joint. A. Fascia incised to expose interval between brachioradialis laterally and biceps and brachialis proximally and pronator distally. B. With reflection of supinator muscle and supination of the forearm, the capitellum and proximal radius are exposed. [Reproduced and modified (intervening operative steps excluded) by permission from Crenshaw AH Jr: Surgical techniques and approaches. In Canale ST (ed): *Campbell's Operative Orthopaedics,* 9th ed. St. Louis: Mosby; 1998:131.]

nerve) and anconeus (radial nerve) is identified distally, and the plane is developed proximally to the lateral humeral epicondyle. Pronation of the forearm at this point will protect the posterior interosseous nerve. The joint capsule is incised to reveal the radiocapitellar joint and annular ligament. Dissection should not proceed distal to the annular ligament to prevent damage to the posterior interosseous nerve.

Limited proximal extension can be accomplished through dissection along the lateral supracondylar ridge to better expose the capitellum. There is no useful distal extension.

FOREARM

ANATOMY OF THE FOREARM

Osteology

The forearm is composed of the radius and ulna. The radial head articulates proximally with the capitellum of the humerus. The radial head is a flattened disc-shaped structure covered by articular cartilage. Just distal to the radial head, the bicipital tuberosity lies on the anteromedial surface of the radial neck. The shaft of the radius curves gently with a lateral convexity. The distal radius flares at the metaphyseal region to form a broad articular surface composed of the lunate and scaphoid fossae with the radial styloid located laterally. Lister's tubercle is palpable on the dorsal surface of the distal radius between the groove for the extensor carpi radialis longus and brevis and the extensor pollicis longus tendons. The proximal ulna is well described above in the section on elbow osteology. The shaft of the ulna is triangular in cross section. Distally, the ulna becomes narrow and terminates at the ulnar head and styloid process.

Articulations

The proximal radioulnar articulation is well described in the section on elbow anatomy. The distal radioulnar joint is reinforced by the interosseous membrane of the forearm. The distal radius articulates with the proximal row of the carpus, while the distal ulna is separated from the lunate and triquetral bones by the triangular fibrocartilage complex (TFCC). The TFCC is composed of an articular disc with supporting ligaments. See details in the section on anatomy of the wrist.

Musculature

The muscles of the forearm may be divided into the volar flexors and dorsal extensors. Both the volar and dorsal groups are further divided into superficial and deep layers (Table 15-3).

Vascular Anatomy

The radial artery and ulnar artery arise at the bifurcation of the brachial artery within the cubital fossa. The radial artery crosses deep to the bicipital aponeurosis and passes superficial to the pronator teres. The radial artery continues deep to the brachioradialis and lies between this muscle and the flexor carpi radialis as it enters the wrist region. The radial recurrent artery is a proximal branch which runs anterior to the lateral humeral epicondyle to form an anastomosis with the radial collateral branch of the profunda brachii artery. The ulnar artery passes deep to the pronator teres muscle and lies between the flexor digitorum superficialis and profundus proximally. Distally, the artery lies on the flexor digitorum profundus, between the flexor carpi ulnaris and flexor digitorum superficialis. Anterior and posterior ulnar recurrent arteries branch proximally and lie anterior and posterior to the medial epicondyle, respectively. The common interosseous artery branches from the ulnar artery in the proximal forearm. This bifurcates almost immediately to form the anterior and posterior interosseous arteries. These two arteries join again at the wrist as the anterior interosseous artery passes through the interosseous membrane. Deep veins accompany the corresponding arteries. Superficial veins include the basilic vein on the dorsal ulnar surface of the forearm, the median antebrachial vein lies on the anterior aspect of the forearm, and the distal extension of the cephalic vein radially.

Nerves

The radial nerve enters the forearm volar to the lateral humeral epicondyle, running between the brachialis and brachioradialis muscles. The radial nerve innervates the anconeus and mobile wad of three (brachioradialis, extensor carpi radialis longus, and brevis) before bifurcating to form the superficial radial nerve and the posterior interosseous nerve. The posterior interosseous nerve enters the substance of the supinator muscle and eventually lies immediately dorsal to the interosseous membrane. It supplies all the extensor muscles except the mobile wad of three as described above. The superficial radial nerve provides cutaneous sensation to the dorsal radial surface of the hand after exiting the forearm between the extensor carpi radialis longus and brachioradialis muscles.

The median nerve exits the antecubital fossa medial to the brachial artery and continues into the forearm where it splits the two heads of the pronator teres muscle and runs distally between the flexor digitorum superficialis and profundus muscles. The median nerve supplies all the superficial flexors of the forearm except the flexor carpi

Table 15-3

Muscles of the Forearm

Muscle	Origin	Insertion	Action	Innervation
Superficial Flexors				
Pronator teres (PT)	Med. epicondyle & coronoid	Mid. lat. radius	Pronate, flex forearm	Median
Flexor carpi radialis (FCR)	Med. epicondyle	2d & 3d metacarpal bases	Flex wrist	Median
Palmaris longus (PL)	Med. epicondyle	Palmar aponeurosis	Flex wrest	Median
Flexor carpi ulnaris (FCU)	Med. epicondyle & post. ulna	Pisiform	Flex wrist	Ulnar
Flexor digitorum superficialis (FDS)	Med. epicondyle & ant. radius	Base of middle phalanges	Flex PIP	Median
Deep Flexors				
Flexor digitorum profundus (FDP)	Ant. & med. ulna	Base of distal phalanges	Flex DIP	Median-ant. interosseous/ and Ulnar
Flexor pollicis longus (FPL)	Ant. & lat. radius	Base of distal phalanges	Flex IP, thumb	Median-ant. interosseous
Pronator Quadratus (PQ)	Distal ulna	Volar radius	Pronate hand	Median-ant. interosseous
Superficial Extensors				
Brachioradialis (BR)	Lat. supracondylar humerus	Lat. distal radius	Flex forearm	Radial
Ext. carpi radialis longus (ECRL)	Lat. supracondylar humerus	2d metacarpal base	Extend wrist	Radial
Ext. carpi radialis brevis (ECRB)	Lat. epicondyle of humerus	3d metacarpal base	Extend wrist	Radial
Anconeus	Lat. epicondyle of humerus	Proximal dorsal ulna	Extend forearm	Radial
Extensor digitorum (ED)	Lat. epicondyle of humerus	Extensor aponeurosis	Extend digits	Radial-post. interosseous
Extensor ditigi minimi (EDM)	Common extensor tendon	Small finger extensor carpi ulnaris	Extend small finger	Radial-post. interosseous
Ext. carpi ulnaris (ECU)	Lat. epicondyle of humerus	5th metacarpal base	Extend/Adduct hand	Radial-post. interosseous
Deep Extensors				
Supinator	Lat. epicondyle of humerus, ulna	Dorsolateral radius	Supinate forearm	Radial-post. interosseous
Abductor pollicis longus (APL)	Dorsal ulna/Radius	1st metacarpal base	Abduct thumb, extend	Radial-post interosseous
Extensor pollicis brevis (EPB)	Dorsal radius	Thumb proximal phalanx base	Extend thumb MCP	Radial-post. interosseous
Extensor pollicis longus (EPL)	Dorsolateral ulna	Thumb dorsal phalanx base	Extend thumb IP	Radial-post. interosseous
Extensor indicis proprius (EIP)	Dorsolateral ulna	Index finger extensor apparatus (ulnarly)	Extend index finger	Radial-post. interosseous

SOURCE: Reproduced with permission from Miller MD: Anatomy. In: *Review of Orthopaedics*. Philadelphia: WB Saunders; 1992: 318.

ulnaris. The anterior interosseous nerve is given off as the median nerve enters the pronator teres and innervates the deep flexors of the forearm (flexor pollicis longus, flexor digitorum profundus to the index and middle fingers, and the pronator quadratus).

The ulnar nerve enters the forearm between the two heads of the flexor carpi ulnaris muscle. It runs distally between the flexor carpi ulnaris and flexor digitorum profundus. In the forearm, the ulnar nerve innervates the flexor carpi ulnaris and the ulnar half of the flexor digitorum profundus. At the wrist, it enters the hand through Guyon's canal.

SURGICAL APPROACHES TO THE FOREARM

Anterior Approach to the Radius (of Henry)

The incision is made along a line running from just lateral to the biceps tendon to the radial styloid. The exact location and length of the incision depends on the length of bone to be exposed.

Proximal third: The deep fascia of the forearm is incised taking care not to damage the lateral antebrachial cutaneous nerve overlying the brachioradialis. The plane between the medial border of the brachioradialis (radial nerve) and pronator teres (median nerve) is developed. With the arm fully supinated, the insertion of the supinator muscle is evident on the anterior aspect of the radius. The insertion should be incised and the muscle stripped subperiosteally from the shaft of the radius. As the muscle is retracted laterally, the posterior interosseous nerve is protected. Care should be taken to avoid placing retractors on the posterior aspect of the radial neck as the posterior interosseous nerve may contact the bone at this point and be damaged by a poorly placed retractor.

Middle third: The middle third of the radius is exposed by developing the plane between the brachioradialis (radial nerve) and pronator teres (median nerve). As the arm is pronated, the insertion of the pronator teres on the lateral aspect of the radius is brought into the surgical field. The insertion is incised and the muscle stripped subperiosteally and retracted medially. The origin of the flexor digitorum superficialis may also be stripped from the anterior aspect of the radius.

Distal third: The plane between the brachioradialis (radial nerve) and the flexor carpi radialis (median nerve) is developed. The superficial radial nerve and radial artery lie deep to the brachioradialis muscle. With the arm partially supinated, the origin of the pronator quadratus and flexor pollicis longus may be incised and the muscles stripped subperiosteally and retracted medially.

Posterior Approach to the Radius

The incision is made along a line joining the lateral humeral epicondyle to the ulnar margin of Lister's tubercle. The length and location of the incision are dictated by the area to be exposed.

Proximal third: After incision of the deep fascia, dissection is carried out in the plane between the extensor carpi radialis brevis (radial nerve) and the extensor digitorum communis (posterior interosseous nerve). The supinator muscle will be evident overlying the dorsal aspect of the radius. The posterior interosseous nerve emerges from the substance of the supinator 1 cm proximal to its distal border. The supinator is incised to free the nerve, with care taken to preserve branches to the supinator itself. The arm is fully supinated and the supinator muscle detached at its insertion to expose the proximal third of the radius.

Middle third: After dissection between the extensor carpi radialis brevis and extensor digitorum communis superficially, the abductor pollicis longus and extensor pollicis brevis can be seen covering the middle third of the radius. These muscles may be separated from the underlying bone and retracted proximally or medially to allow exposure to the underlying bone.

Distal third: Superficial dissection is carried out between the extensor carpi radialis brevis and extensor digitorum communis. The distal third of the radius is exposed by incision of the periosteum distal to the distal margin of the extensor pollicis brevis.

Approach to the Shaft of the Ulna

A longitudinal incision is made over the subcutaneous border of the ulna in the area of interest. The interval between the flexor carpi ulnaris (ulnar nerve) and extensor carpi ulnaris (posterior interosseous nerve) is most easily identified in the distal aspect of the incision. Dissection is carried down to bone and the ulna is exposed subperiosteally. Proximally, the plane between the anconeus (radial nerve) and flexor carpi ulnaris (ulnar nerve) may be developed to expose the olecranon. Care must be taken to remain in the subperiosteal plane to avoid damage to the ulnar nerve and artery which lie deep to the flexor carpi ulnaris.

This approach may be extended proximally by extension into a posterior approach to the elbow and humerus.

APPENDIX

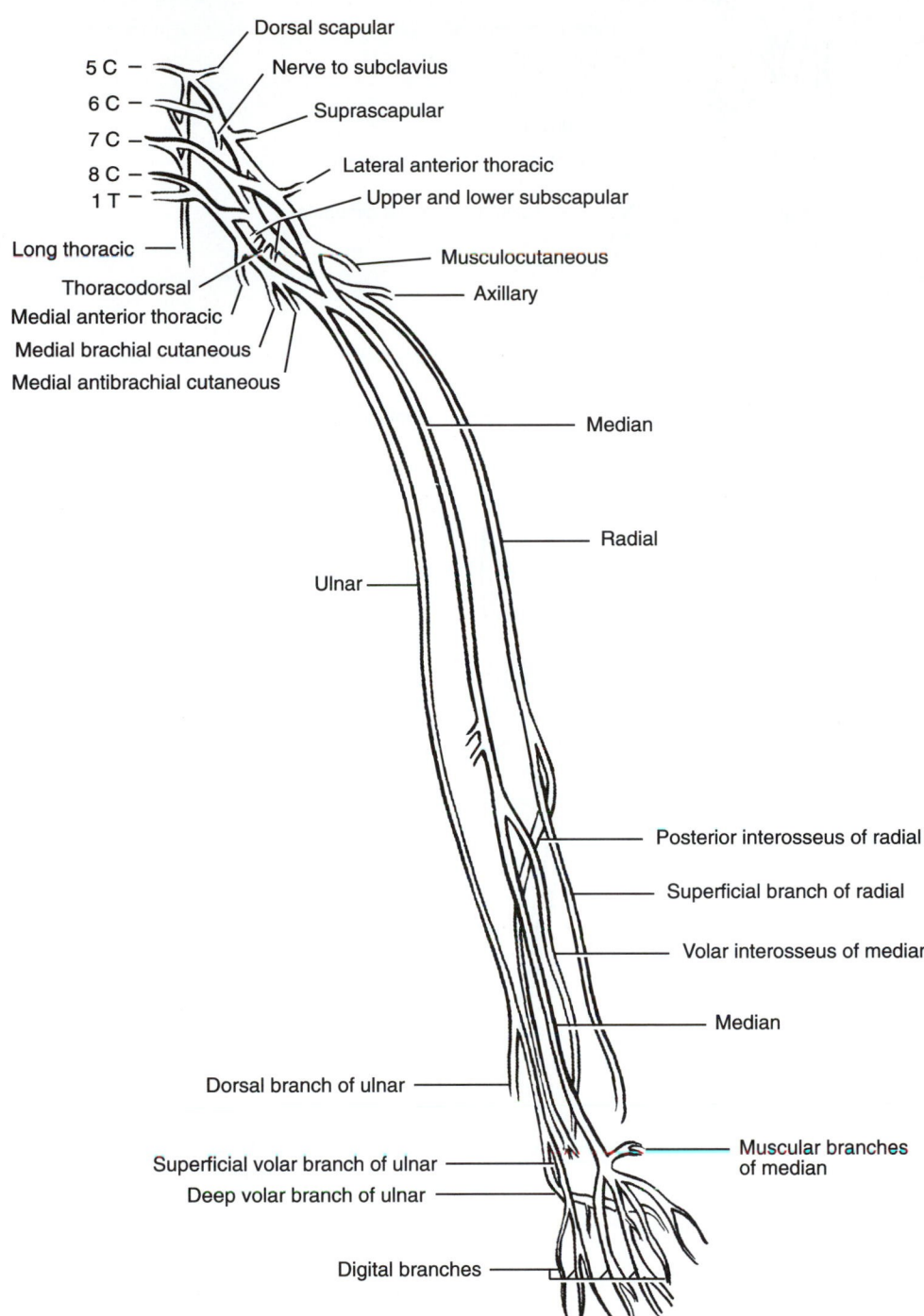

Figure 15-3

Nerves of the upper extremity. [Reproduced and modified with permission from Warfel JH: *The Extremities*, 4th ed. Philadelphia: Lea & Febiger (now Lippincott Williams & Wilkins); 1981:113.]

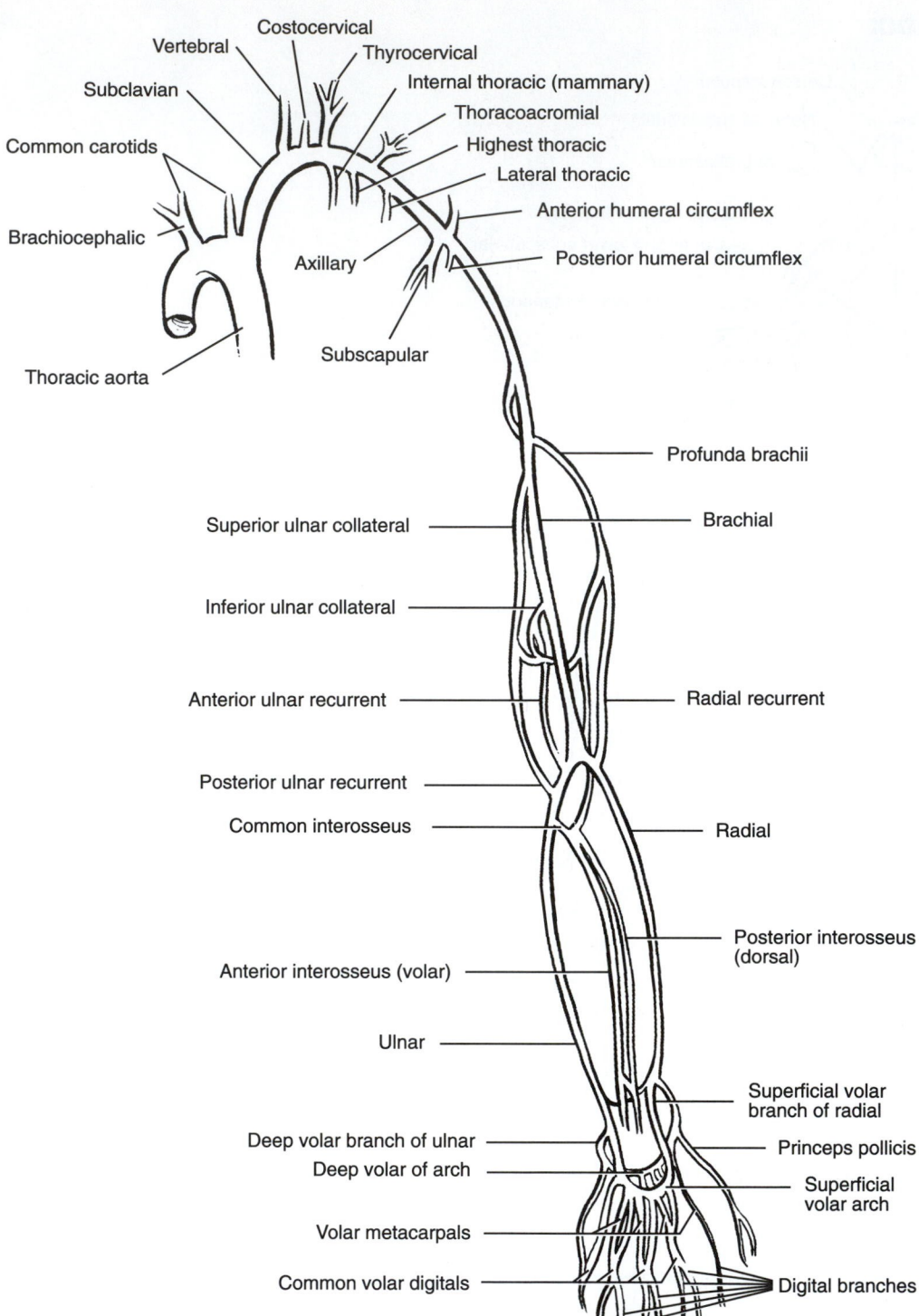

Figure 15-4
Arteries of the upper extremity. [Reproduced and modified with permission from Warfel JH: *The Extremities*, 4th ed. Philadelphia: Lea & Febiger (now Lippincott Williams & Wilkins); 1981:114.]

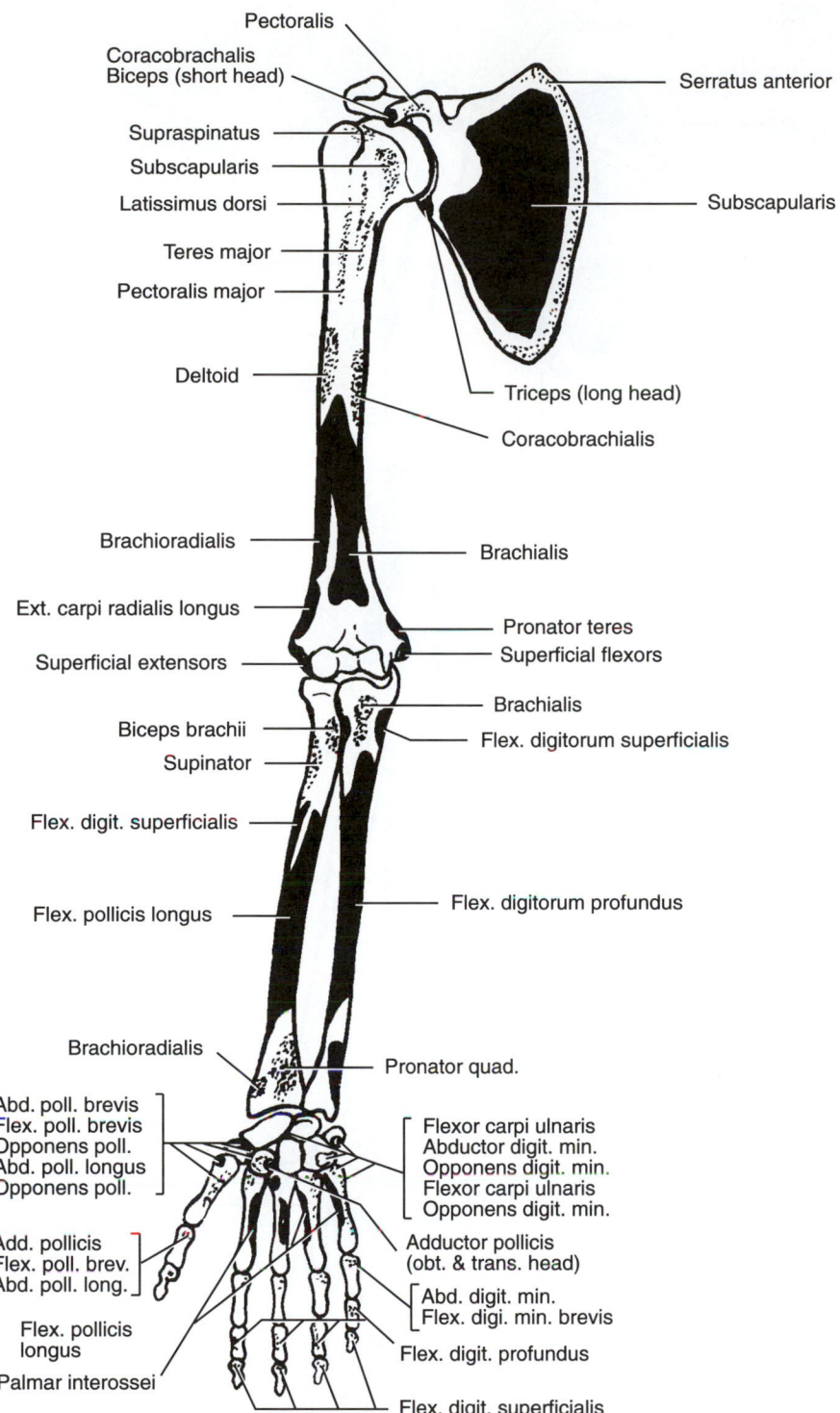

Figure 15-5
Muscles of the upper right extremity (anterior). [Reproduced and modified with permission from Warfel JH: *The Extremities*, 4th ed. Philadelphia: Lea & Febiger (now Lippincott Williams & Wilkins); 1981:117.]

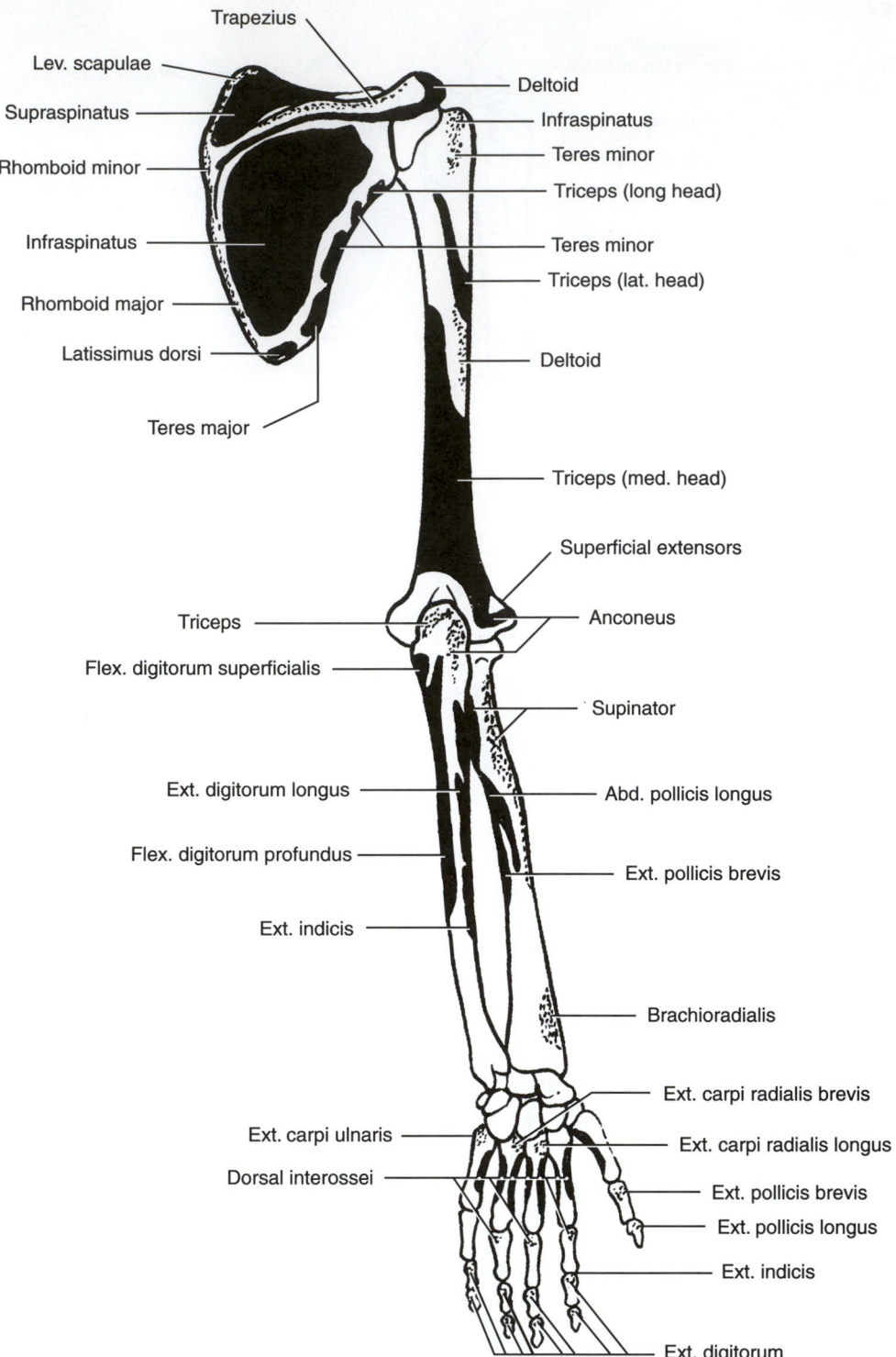

Figure 15-6
Muscles of the upper right extremity (posterior). [Reproduced and modified with permission from Warfel JH: *The Extremities*, 4th ed. Philadelphia: Lea & Febiger (now Lippincott Williams & Wilkins); 1981:118.]

SUGGESTED READINGS

April EW: Part II. Upper extremity. In: *The National Medical Series for Independent Study: Clinical Anatomy,* 3d ed. Baltimore: Williams & Wilkins; 1996:47.

Crenshaw AH Jr: Surgical techniques and approaches. In Canale ST (ed): *Campbell's Operative Orthopaedics,* vol 1, 9th ed. St. Louis: Mosby; 1998: 111–133.

Hoppenfeld S, de Boer P: The elbow. In: *Surgical Exposures in Orthopaedics: The Anatomic Approach,* 2d ed. Philadelphia: JB Lippincott; 1994:83.

Hoppenfeld S, de Boer P: The forearm. In: *Surgical Exposures in Orthopaedics: The Anatomic Approach,* 2d ed. Philadelphia: JB Lippincott; 1994:117.

Hoppenfeld S, de Boer P: The humerus. In: *Surgical Exposures in Orthopaedics: The Anatomic Approach*, 2d ed. Philadelphia: JB Lippincott; 1994:51

Hoppenfeld S, de Boer P: The shoulder. In: *Surgical Exposures in Orthopaedics: The Anatomic Approach*, 2d ed. Philadelphia: JB Lippincott; 1994:1

Rosen H: The treatment of nonunions and pseudarthroses of the humeral shaft. *Orthop Clin North Am* 1990; 21:737–738.

Chapter 16

WRIST

Jennifer O'Sullivan Pogue

The wrist comprises the area of the upper extremity that extends from a transverse line drawn between the head of the ulna and the radial styloid, to a transverse line drawn from the base of the thumb. Within this small area are eight carpal bones, five metacarpal bases, a complex system of ligaments, nine tendons, the three major nerves of the hand with their branches, the distal radius and ulna, complex arterial and venous systems, and the accompanying soft tissues.

SOFT TISSUES

The soft tissues of the wrist encase and protect the underlying complex anatomy. The skin on the palmar surface is thicker, callused, and fixed to the deeper structures via a denser fascia whose fiber bundles adhere to the skin to form the flexion creases. The dorsal skin, in contrast, is thinner, more elastic and mobile, and only loosely attached to underlying structures due to a thinner, looser, underlying fascia. There is very little subcutaneous fat in the hand. The fascia is continuous with the fascia of the hand and arm.

Beneath the soft tissues and tendons, the wrist joint is surrounded by a capsule of connective tissue. On the dorsum of the wrist, the capsule is thin and pliable and does not contribute any stability to the wrist. On the volar side of the wrist, however, the capsule includes the radiocarpal ligaments, which are the main stabilizing ligaments of the wrist. These ligaments on the volar surface must be preserved in surgery.

EXTENSOR TENDONS

The extensor tendons pass across the wrist encased in fascial compartments formed by a thickened fascial band called the extensor retinaculum (Fig. 16-1). The retinaculum acts as a pulley for the extensor tendons, preventing them from bowstringing as they are pulled across the joint. The retinaculum has a supratendinous layer from which vertical septa arise that extend to insert into the radius. In doing so, six separate fascial compartments are formed.

The first compartment contains the abductor pollicis longus and extensor pollicis brevis; the second contains the extensor carpi radialis

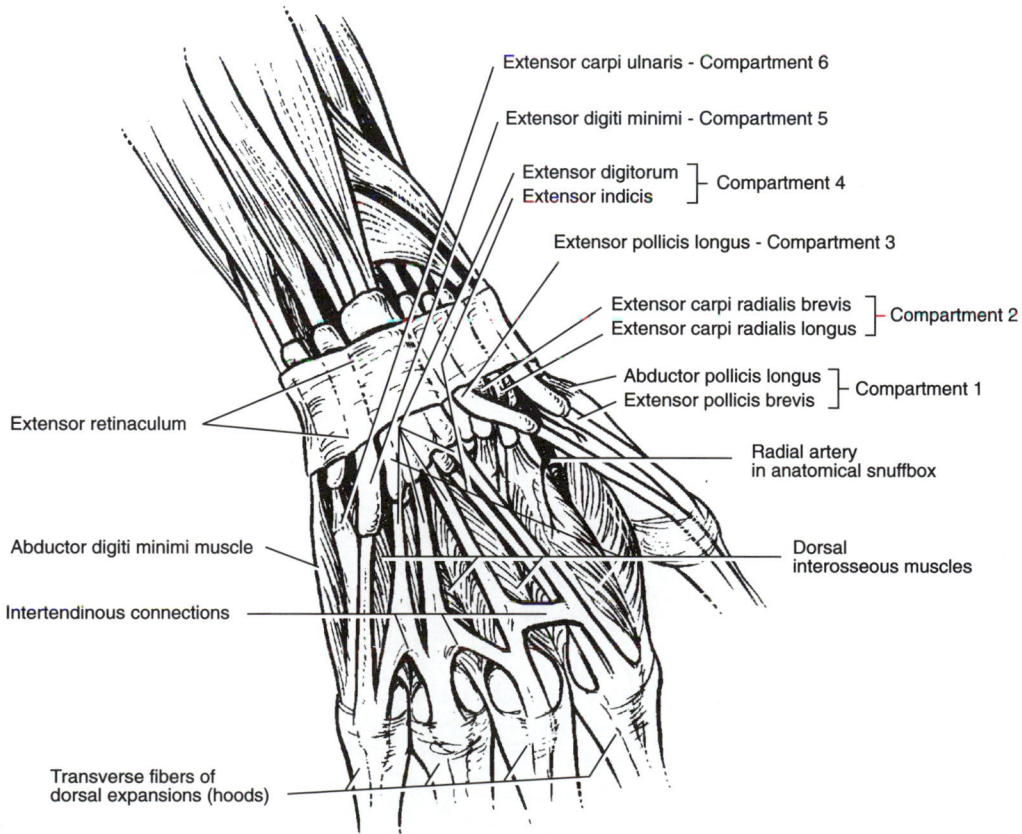

Figure 16-1
Extensor tendons.

Extensor carpi ulnaris - Compartment 6
Extensor digiti minimi - Compartment 5
Extensor digitorum
Extensor indicis } Compartment 4
Extensor pollicis longus - Compartment 3
Extensor carpi radialis brevis
Extensor carpi radialis longus } Compartment 2
Abductor pollicis longus
Extensor pollicis brevis } Compartment 1
Radial artery in anatomical snuffbox
Dorsal interosseous muscles
Extensor retinaculum
Abductor digiti minimi muscle
Intertendinous connections
Transverse fibers of dorsal expansions (hoods)

longus and brevis; the third contains the extensor pollicis longus; the fourth contains the extensor digitorum and the extensor indicis proprius; the fifth contains the extensor digiti minimi; and the sixth contains the extensor carpi ulnaris.

FLEXOR TENDONS

The extrinsic flexors to the fingers and thumb pass through the carpal tunnel to insert distally in the phalanges. The palmaris longus passes superficial to the flexor retinaculum, spanning out into an aponeurosis known as the superficial palmar fascia that covers the palm. Its tendon is absent in 10 to 15 percent of people.

The extrinsic flexors and extensors balance each other, further stabilizing the wrist. The extensor carpi ulnaris counteracts the extensor carpi radialis brevis and abductor pollicis longus; the extensor carpi radialis longus and extensor carpi radialis brevis counteract the flexor carpi ulnaris, flexor digitorum profundi, and flexor digitorum superficiali; and the extensor digitorum communis and extensor indicis proprius counteract the flexor carpi radialis and flexor pollicis longus.

CARPAL TUNNEL

On the flexor surface of the carpus is the carpal tunnel, through which pass nine tendons and one nerve (Fig. 16-2). The carpal bones are shaped like a "U" to form the floor of the tunnel. The transverse carpal ligament (flexor retinaculum) forms the roof. The transverse carpal ligament is a thick fibrous ligament that extends from the tuberosity of the scaphoid to the trapezium, the pisiform, the triquetrum, and the hook of the hamate.

The carpal tunnel contains the flexors digitorum profundus and superficialis to the fingers, the flexor pollicis longus, and the median nerve. The structures within the canal are arranged in four layers. The median nerve is most superficial, lying just deep and parallel to the palmaris longus tendon. Lying in two layers beneath the median nerve are the flexor superficialis tendons, with the ring and middle finger tendons lying more superficial to the index and little finger tendons. Along the floor of the canal are the four flexor profundus tendons to the fingers. The flexor pollicis longus runs along the radial side of the tunnel at the same depth as the profundus tendons. In 10 percent

of people, a persistent median artery travels alongside the median nerve through the canal.

GUYON'S CANAL

Guyon's canal is a triangular canal on the ulnar side of the wrist through which the ulnar artery and nerve pass. The roof is formed by the volar carpal ligament and adjoining flexor carpi ulnaris insertion. The lateral wall is formed by the hook of the hamate and the transverse carpal ligament insertion. The medial wall is formed by the pisohamate ligament and pisiform. The floor is formed by the transverse carpal ligament. No tendons pass through this canal. Guyon's canal is often the location of ulnar neuropathies and ulnar artery aneurysms.

NERVES

The *median nerve* travels deep to and within the fascia of the flexor digitorum superficialis in the forearm to enter the wrist through the carpal tunnel (Fig. 16-3). A palmar cutaneous branch is given off 5 cm proximal to the wrist and travels superficial to the transverse carpal ligament along the ulnar side of the flexor carpi radialis to supply sensation to the thenar eminence. The median nerve gives off a motor branch to the thenar eminence prior to passing distally into the hand where it supplies sensation to the radial 3-1/2 digits. In most cases, it is given off distal to the transverse carpal ligament and then travels in retrograde fashion to supply the thenar eminence. Variations include branching of the motor branch proximal to or within the carpal canal, piercing of the branch through the transverse carpal ligament, and accessory branches of the motor nerve.

The *ulnar nerve* travels with the ulnar artery in the forearm beneath the flexor carpi ulnaris. At the distal third of the forearm, a dorsal sensory branch is given off that travels between the flexor carpi ulnaris and ulna to emerge on the dorsal aspect of the wrist to supply sensation to the ulnar base of the hand. The main trunk of the ulnar nerve continues distally and radial to the flexor carpi ulnaris and enters the wrist through Guyon's canal, where it divides into superficial and deep branches. The superficial branch continues through the canal, supplying the palmaris brevis and the skin of the ulnar

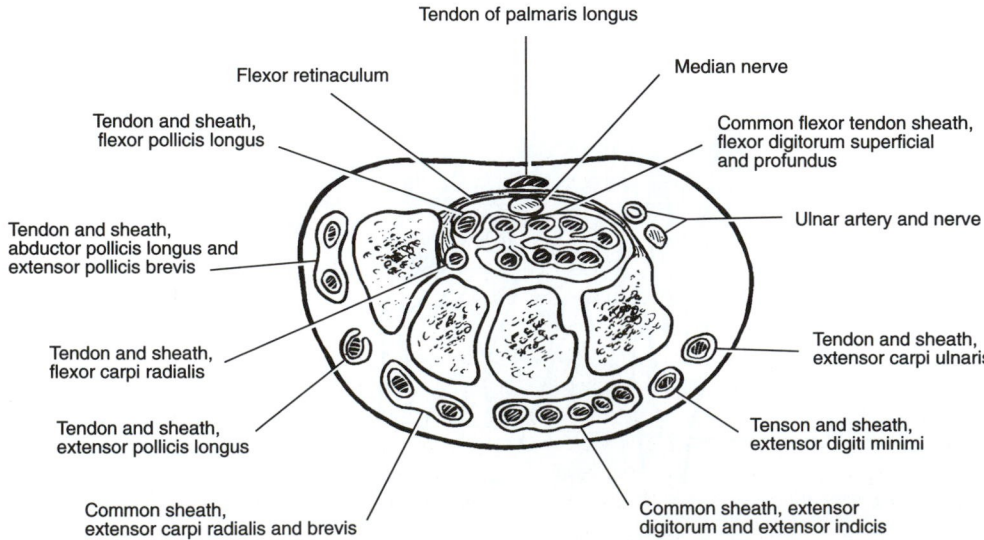

Tendon of palmaris longus

Flexor retinaculum

Median nerve

Tendon and sheath, flexor pollicis longus

Common flexor tendon sheath, flexor digitorum superficial and profundus

Tendon and sheath, abductor pollicis longus and extensor pollicis brevis

Ulnar artery and nerve

Tendon and sheath, flexor carpi radialis

Tendon and sheath, extensor carpi ulnaris

Tendon and sheath, extensor pollicis longus

Tenson and sheath, extensor digiti minimi

Common sheath, extensor carpi radialis and brevis

Common sheath, extensor digitorum and extensor indicis

Figure 16-2
Carpal tunnel. (Reproduced and modified with permission from Jenkins DB: *Hollinshead's Functional Anatomy of the Limbs and Back*, 6th ed. Philadelphia: WB Saunders; 1991:162.)

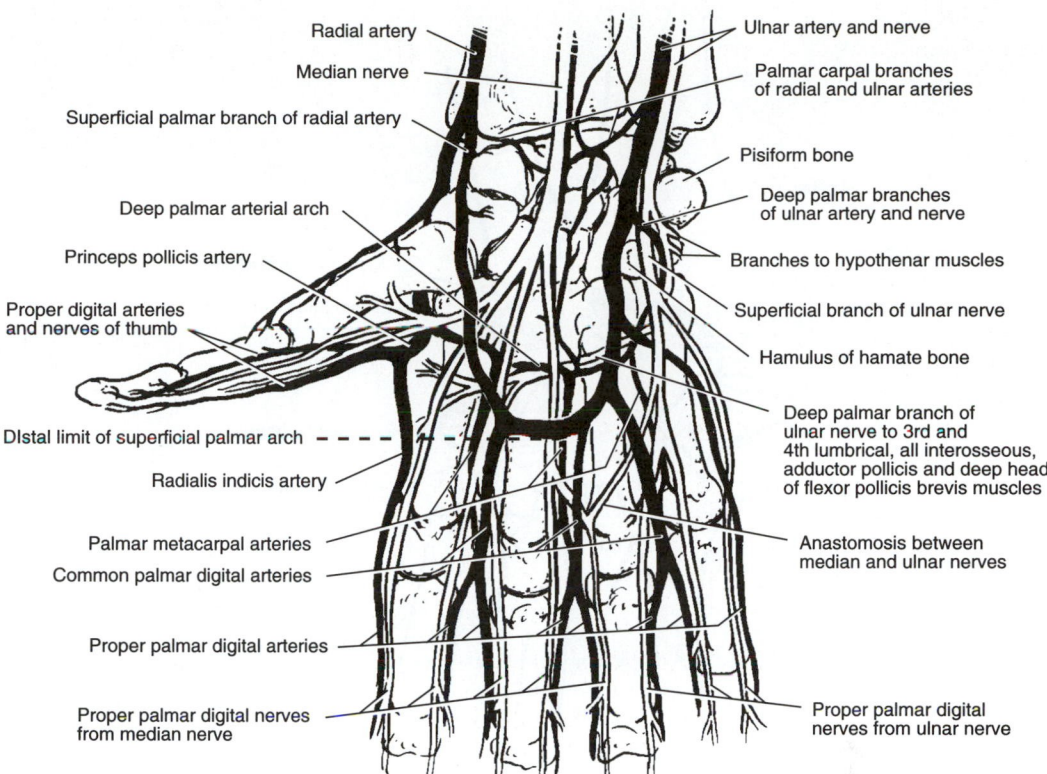

Radial artery
Median nerve
Superficial palmar branch of radial artery
Deep palmar arterial arch
Princeps pollicis artery
Proper digital arteries and nerves of thumb
Distal limit of superficial palmar arch
Radialis indicis artery
Palmar metacarpal arteries
Common palmar digital arteries
Proper palmar digital arteries
Proper palmar digital nerves from median nerve

Ulnar artery and nerve
Palmar carpal branches of radial and ulnar arteries
Pisiform bone
Deep palmar branches of ulnar artery and nerve
Branches to hypothenar muscles
Superficial branch of ulnar nerve
Hamulus of hamate bone
Deep palmar branch of ulnar nerve to 3rd and 4th lumbrical, all interosseous, adductor pollicis and deep head of flexor pollicis brevis muscles
Anastomosis between median and ulnar nerves
Proper palmar digital nerves from ulnar nerve

Figure 16-3
Arteries and nerves of the wrist. (Reproduced and modified with permission from Netter FH: Arteries and nerves of hand: Palmar views. In: *Atlas of Human Anatomy.* Summit, NJ: CIBA-Geigy; 1989:439. Copyright 1989. Novartis. Reprinted with permission from the *Atlas of Human Anatomy,* illustrated by Frank H. Netter, M.D. All rights reserved.)

1-1/2 digits. The deep branch leaves the main trunk opposite the pisiform and passes between the origins of the abductor digiti minimi and flexor digiti minimi brevis muscles to supply the interosseous muscles, the ulnar two lumbricals, and the adductor muscle to the index finger.

Only the sensory branch of the *radial nerve* extends distally to the wrist and hand. After traveling in the distal forearm with the radial artery, usually beneath the brachioradialis muscle, the sensory nerve branch travels dorsally and pierces the deep fascia of the distal forearm, where it divides into two or more branches that travel superficially to supply sensory innervation to the dorsoradial side of the hand. The deep motor branch of the radial nerve becomes the posterior interosseous nerve that is found in the wrist on the interosseous membrane between the third and fourth extensor compartments, where it serves as an articular branch.

VASCULATURE

The radial artery travels into the wrist deep to the abductor pollicis longus and extensor pollicis brevis (Fig. 16-3). It then passes through the anatomic snuff-box deep to the extensor pollicis longus through the interval between the first and second metacarpal bases to form the deep palmar arterial arch. Prior to this, it gives off branches to the thumb and a dorsal arch named the dorsal carpal rete. The dorsal carpal rete is further formed by the terminal posterior branch of the anterior interosseous artery and the ulnar artery. This arch gives off three dorsal metacarpal arteries, which supply the dorsal branches to the fingers and which also anastomose with perforating branches from the deep palmar arch.

The ulnar artery travels with the ulnar nerve deep to the flexor carpi ulnaris in the forearm. It then crosses the wrist anterior to the flexor retinaculum and travels distally, first branching to the hy-

pothenar muscles and then forming the superficial palmar arch. The superficial palmar arch lies just superficial to the tendons and gives off palmar branches, which supply the digits. The superficial palmar arch lies at a line drawn from the outstretched thumb. The deep palmar arch, which is just distal to the superficial arch and lies deep to the tendons, sends penetrating branches through the interosseous spaces to supply the dorsum of the hand. The palm is supplied by branches of the superficial and deep palmar arterial arches. Blood is supplied to individual bones of the carpus through ligamentous attachments. The veins on the palmar aspect drain mainly to the dorsal venous network via penetrating branches. The dorsal network drains toward either the ulnar (basilic) or the radial (cephalic) veins, both of which then travel in their respective directions to the volar surface of the forearm. The lymphatic drainage follows the dorsal venous drainage.

BONES AND SPECIALIZED JOINTS

Multiple articulations occur between the 15 bones in the wrist, making the wrist among the most complex structures of the musculoskeletal system (Fig. 16-4). Specifically, these articulations include the radioulnar, radiocarpal, intercarpal, midcarpal, and carpometacarpal joints. The segment of bones between the metacarpals and forearm is the carpus, which contains eight carpal bones arranged in two rows, between which is the midcarpal joint. The proximal row of the carpus contains the triquetrum, the lunate, and the proximal pole of the scaphoid. The distal row contains the trapezium, the trapezoid, the capitate, the hamate, and the distal portion of the scaphoid. Each carpal bone is unique, contributing to the complex alignment, stability, and mobility of the wrist.

The *scaphoid* extends across both the proximal and distal carpal rows, acting as a link for the midcarpal joint. The scaphoid articu-

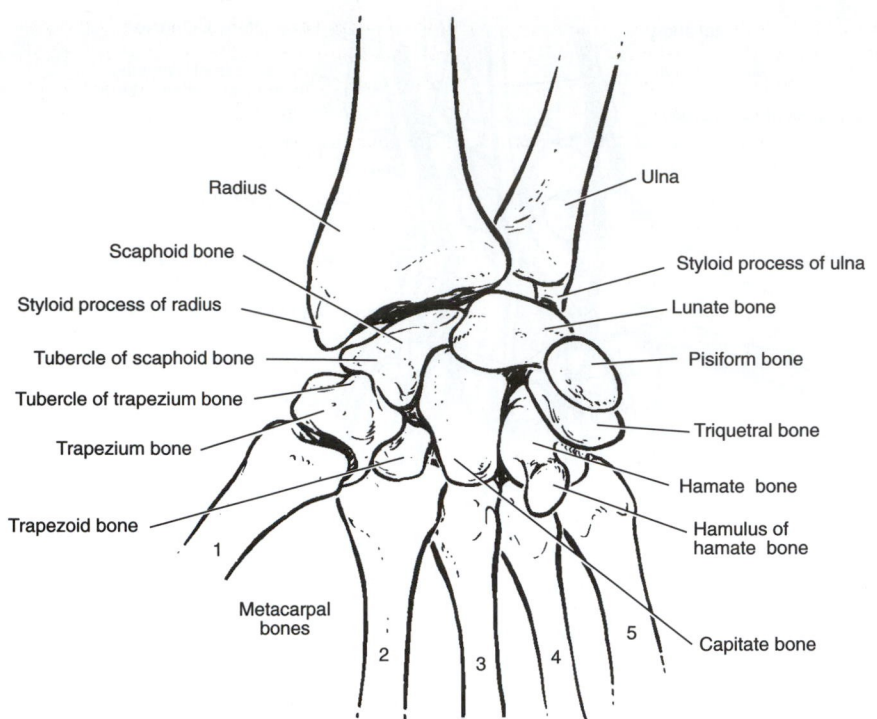

Figure 16-4
Bones of the wrist.

lates with the radius, the lunate, the capitate, the trapezium, and the trapezoid. Due to its many articulations, most of the scaphoid's surface is covered with cartilage. This leaves only a narrow area of bone for attaching ligaments that supply it with blood from branches of the radial artery. The distal two-thirds of the scaphoid has a much more reliable blood supply than the proximal pole.

The central location of the *lunate* and its many ligamentous attachments make it one of the most important contributors of stability and mobility to the wrist. It is a wedge-shaped bone with a wider palmar surface than its dorsal surface and therefore tends to rotate dorsally with ligamentous instability. The lunate is often subject to load stresses that may cause avascular necrosis because of its central location between the radius and the capitate.

The *triquetrum* is a wedge-shaped bone that articulates with the lunate, the hamate, and the pisiform. The *pisiform* sits on the palmar surface of the triquetrum within the tendon of the flexor carpi ulnaris. Since it is a sesamoid bone, it does not contribute to the mobility of the wrist.

The *trapezoid* is the smallest of the metacarpal bones and articulates with the second metacarpal, the scaphoid, the trapezium, and the capitate.

The *trapezium* articulates with the first and second metacarpals, the trapezoid, and the scaphoid. Its articulation with the first metacarpal has the characteristics of a saddle joint. This articulation is also known as the basal joint.

The *capitate* is the largest of the carpal bones and, in a normally aligned wrist, lies in line with the third metacarpal, lunate, and radius. It articulates with the third and fourth metacarpals, the trapezoid, lunate, scaphoid, and hamate.

The *hamate* articulates with the fourth and fifth metacarpals, the lunate, the triquetrum, and the capitate. Its articulations with the metacarpals are saddle shaped. On the volar surface protrudes a hook, or hamulus, which provides insertion sites for the flexor retinaculum and the flexor carpi ulnaris tendon via the pisohamate ligament.

The bases of the *metacarpals* articulate with each other and with the distal row of carpal bones. The articulations between the bases of the second and third metacarpals are fixed and immobile, while the saddle-like articulations of the fourth and fifth metacarpal bases allow some degree of motion. The first metacarpal has the greatest mobility at its carpometacarpal joint. The *first metacarpal* differs from the others in that it is shorter, broader, flatter, more mobile, and separated from the other metacarpals by a wider intermetacarpal distance.

The first carpometacarpal joint is also known as the *basal joint*. As a saddle joint articulating with the trapezium, it allows for stability during motion in the flexion–extension and adduction–abduction planes during motion. The capsule and ligaments of the joint limit movements at their extremes; but otherwise the capsule is loose, allowing the metacarpal base to ride up on the trapezium for greater rotation. The joint is most stable in adduction because in this position the most convex part of the trapezial surface fits into the deepest part of the metacarpal base. In contrast, during abduction, these two surfaces are pulled away from each other, allowing the flatter anterolateral surfaces to slide on each other. The basal joint is further stabilized by the anterior oblique (or volar or ulnar) ligament, which extends from the volar tubercle on the trapezium to the metacarpal beak. There is also a posterior oblique ligament that extends from the dorsal tubercle of the trapezium to the metacarpal beak.

On the volar surface of the *first metacarpophalangeal joint* is the palmar plate, which extends between the two bones, but is most firmly attached to the metacarpal. It contains two sesamoid bones that also articulate with the first metacarpal head. The flexor pollicis longus passes between these two sesamoids before entering the flexor sheath of the thumb. Collateral ligaments stabilize the joint, extending between the metacarpal head and the base of the proximal phalanx, and attaching to the palmar plate. These lie deep to the overlying dorsal hood expansion. Mobility of this joint may vary considerably between people.

The *distal radius* articulates with the radial carpus, bearing 80 percent of the axial load of the wrist. It begins at the radial metaphyseal flare, approximately 2 cm proximal to its articulating surface. It contains two concave fossas distally for articulation with the scaphoid and lunate at the radiocarpal joint. The scaphoid fossa is triangular with its apex forming the radial styloid. The radial styloid often has a groove through which passes the abductor pollicis longus tendon. Just ulnar and dorsal to the radial styloid arises a longitudinal prominence, Lister's tubercle, which acts as a fulcrum for the extensor pollicis longus tendon. The lunate fossa is separated from the scaphoid fossa by a small ridge into which inserts the triangular fibrocartilage. The distal radius also has one concave surface ulnarly, which is called the sigmoid notch, for articulation with the ulna. The convex dorsal aspect of the distal radius acts as a fulcrum for the extensor tendons that pass over it.

The *distal ulna* or ulna head articulates with the ulnar carpus and the radius. Projecting distally and ulnarly off the head is the ulnar styloid. Just proximal to the styloid is an area with multiple vascular foramina upon which attach the ulnar collateral ligament and the triangular fibrocartilage. The ulnar collateral ligament extends from the ulnar styloid to the triquetrum. The triangular fibrocartilage is a thick fibrocartilaginous disc that extends from the distal articular surface of the ulna, to the distal edge of the sigmoid notch, to the ulna styloid process. The *distal radioulnar joint* (DRUJ) consists of the articulation of the ulna and radius at the sigmoid notch, and the proximal surface of the triangular fibrocartilage complex (TFCC). The DRUJ is stabilized by the TFCC, the extensor carpi ulnaris (ECU), the pronator quadratus, and the distal interosseous membrane. The DRUJ is a diarthrodial joint that enables rotatory movement. In pronation and supination, the radius can rotate around the relatively fixed ulna up to 150 degrees in a dorsovolar arc. During this rotation the ulna translocates 8 to 9 degrees in the radioulnar plane within the notch. The semicylindrical pocket shape of the sigmoid notch contributes stability to the joint. A weak capsule is formed by transverse fibers between the volar and dorsal surfaces of the radius and ulna. The dorsal ligaments of the sigmoid notch tighten during pronation, and the volar ligaments tighten during supination, maintaining the ulna within the notch.

The *triangular fibrocartilage complex* or TFCC, which is the stabilizing complex for the distal radioulnar and ulnocarpal joints, maintains correct alignment between the radius, ulna, and carpus. It is located at the distal articular surface of the ulna and consists of the triangular fibrocartilage, the ulnar collateral ligament, the volar and dorsal radioulnar ligaments, the meniscus homologue, the ECU tendon sheath, the ulnolunate ligament, and the ulnotriquetral ligament. A hyaline articular disc in the center of the TFCC represents the meniscus homologue and cushions the lunate and triquetrum from forces transmitted to the ulna through the triangular fibrocartilage disc and capsule, respectively. Because it absorbs axial load and ulnar stress to the wrist, the TFCC is subject to acute tears and degenerative perforations. Furthermore, because the central portion of the TFCC is avascular, it tends to heal poorly.

LIGAMENTS

The major ligaments of the wrist are intracapsular (Fig. 16-5). The volar ligaments, which stabilize against hyperextension, are more substantial than the dorsal ones, both physically and functionally. The ligaments are further distinguished as either extrinsic or intrinsic. The extrinsic ligaments extend beyond the carpus to the radius or metacarpals, whereas the intrinsic ligaments originate and insert within the carpus.

The intrinsic ligaments are of three types: short, medium, and long. The carpal bones are stabilized by palmar and dorsal interosseous ligaments. A ligament extends from the scaphoid to the capitate to the trapezium to form the V-shaped deltoid ligament. Dorsally, a ligament extends from the triquetrum to the scaphoid and trapezium. The dorsal extrinsic system extends from the dorsal distal radius to the lunate, triquetrum, and scaphoid. The volar extrinsic system consists of the radial collateral ligament, the palmar radiocarpal ligaments, and the ulnocarpal complex.

The volar intrinsic and extrinsic carpal ligament systems interact to control radial and ulnar deviation of the wrist. Together, they form

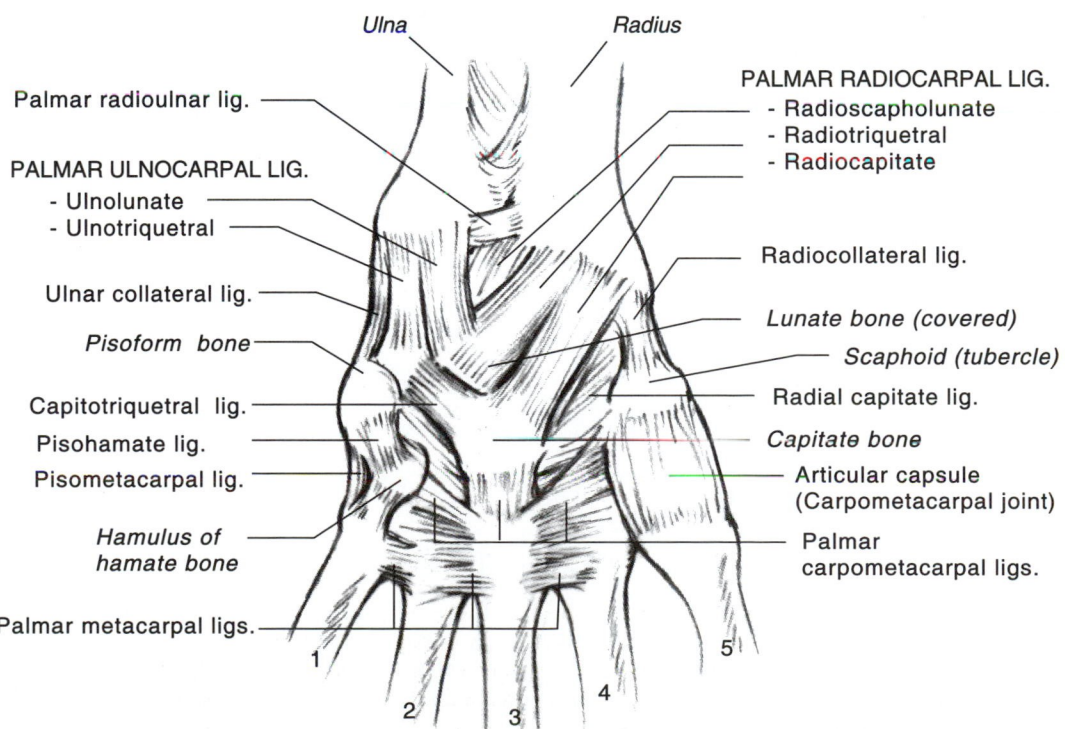

Figure 16-5
Palmar ligaments.

a double V-shaped configuration. The more proximal V is composed of the ulnolunate ligament and the radiolunate ligament, with the apex of the V at the lunate. The distal V is made up of the palmar intercarpal ligament that spans the triquetrum to the capitate to the scaphoid, with the apex at the capitate. Between these two V's is a space of potential weakness known as the space of Poirier. As the wrist deviates in an ulnar or radial direction, the V-shaped ligaments are put on stretch differentially, check-reigning movements of the lunate and capitate, and thus imposing stability to the wrist.

SURGICAL APPROACHES

If surgery is required to address injury or disease, an understanding of the surgical approaches to the wrist will help direct the surgeon in choosing the best approach for a particular procedure. Skin incisions may be made on either the palmar or the dorsal aspects of the wrist. Generally, palmar incisions should parallel preexisting skin creases and not cross the joint creases or the wrist at right angles, to avoid subsequent hypertrophic scars or contractures. For smaller lesions, transverse incisions may provide a more aesthetic scar, but the surgeon must anticipate the possibility of needing to extend the incision if necessary. Z-plasties and flaps can be used where needed, but care must be taken not to close flaps or skin edges under tension. With all incisions, one must be careful not to injure the major sensory nerve branches; longitudinal veins should be preserved where possible. Once through the skin, the deeper incisions are usually made parallel to the tendons or major neurovascular bundles. It is not necessary and usually contraindicated to close the wrist capsule, but all supporting ligamentous structures should be respected and repaired where possible. Single-layer skin closures are sufficient.

A volar approach is the best exposure to the flexor tendons and the median and ulnar nerves. The carpal tunnel is usually approached by an incision parallel to the thenar crease, in line with the third interosseous space, where the ring finger points upon flexion to the proximal palm. The incision is extended longitudinally through the transverse carpal ligament to expose the underlying canal, median nerve, and tendons. The ulnar nerve and artery may be approached proximally by an incision parallel to the radial border of the flexor carpi ulnaris. Retraction of this tendon will reveal the underlying nerve and artery. Distally, an incision along the radial aspect of the hypothenar eminence, extending through the volar carpal ligament, will open Guyon's canal through which both structures pass.

The dorsal wrist may be approached with a longitudinal incision through the skin, followed by a transverse or "T" incision through the wrist capsule. Curved or S-shaped skin incisions may be used, but may have more problems with healing in compromised patients. The wrist capsule is incised to allow exposure of the underlying pathology usually by entering the dorsal wrist between the third and fourth extensor compartments. This will allow access to the distal radius and dorsal radiocarpal joint. The bones of the wrist, particularly the metacarpals, are usually approached dorsally by longitudinal incisions.

The scaphoid may be accessed either volarly or dorsally. The volar incision, which is made on the ulnar side of the wrist between the radial artery and the flexor carpi radialis, is extended longitudinally through the deep fascia, the proximal edge of the flexor retinaculum, and the wrist capsule to expose the scaphoid. A volar approach minimizes disruption of the scaphoid's blood supply. Proximal extension of this incision will expose the distal radius and the radial styloid lying beneath the pronator quadratus. The scaphoid may also be approached through a dorsoradial incision. An incision over the snuffbox, between the extensor pollicis longus and brevis muscles, should adequately expose it. Care must be taken not to injure the sensory branches of the radial nerve that run superficial to the tendons. Retraction of the extensor carpi radialis longus ulnarly and the branch of the radial artery volarly, and incision of the wrist capsule, will reveal the radioscaphoid joint.

The basal joint may be accessed through a hockey-stick or curvilinear incision that begins over the radial aspect of the carpometacarpal joint and curves palmar and ulnar. A small transverse incision through the proximal palmar skin crease over the metacarpophalangeal joint is used to correct trigger thumb.

SUGGESTED READINGS

Green DP (ed): *Operative Hand Surgery,* 4th ed. New York: Churchill Livingstone; 1998.

Hollinshead WH, Rosse C: *Textbook of Anatomy,* 4th ed. Philadelphia: Harper and Row; 1985.

Hoppenfeld S, de Boer P: *Surgical Exposures in Orthopaedics: The Anatomic Approach.* Philadelphia: JB Lippincott; 1994.

Netter FH: *Atlas of Human Anatomy.* Summit, NJ: Ciba-Geigy; 1989.

Stuchin SA: Wrist anatomy. *Hand Clin* 1992; 8:603.

Taleisnik J: *Wrist,* 2d ed. New York: Churchill Livingstone; 1998.

Williams R: *Contemporary Extensile Exposure in Orthopaedic Surgery.* Baltimore: Williams & Wilkins; 1997.

Chapter 17

HAND

Matthew S. Coons

HAND ANATOMY

The hand is exquisitely designed. Its function is completely dependent upon its anatomy.

BONES

The bones of the hand consist of the metacarpals and phalanges. There are five metacarpals, all of which have growth plates located distally at the neck, except for the thumb, which has its growth plate at the base. There are three phalanges for each of the fingers, except for the thumb which has two phalanges. The growth plates for the phalanges are located proximally. The function of the hand is based on two fixed units. The first fixed unit consists of the distal carpal row, which provides the fixed transverse arch. The second unit provides the fixed longitudinal arch and consists of the second and third metacarpals.

JOINTS

The metacarpal phalangeal joints are ellipsoid joints. Each has a volar plate which prevents recurvatum. The volar plate is strong distally and "dove tails," anchoring proximally.

Collateral ligaments are important for lateral stability of the metacarpal phalangeal joints. The collateral ligaments are loose when the joint is extended. The cam-effect of the collateral ligaments causes the ligaments to tighten with metacarpal phalangeal flexion. Deep transverse metacarpal ligaments also exist at this joint.

The interphalangeal joints are hinge joints. A volar plate and collateral ligaments are also present at these joints.

MUSCLES

The muscles of the hand are either extrinsic, with the muscle bellies in the forearm, or intrinsic, with the origins and the insertions of muscles within the hand.

There are three muscle forearm compartments. The first compartment, or the anterior compartment, consists of the flexor/pronator muscles and is arranged in three layers from superficial to deep. The superficial layer of the anterior compartment consists of the flexor carpi radialis (FCR) muscle, the palmaris longus (PL) muscle, and the flexor carpi ulnaris (FCU) muscle, in addition to the pronator teres (PT). The intermediate layer consists of the flexor digitorum superficialis muscle (FDS). The deep layer includes both the flexor digitorum profundus (FDP) muscle and the flexor pollicis longus (FPL) muscle.

The second, posterior, compartment consists of the extensor muscles in the forearm. The third compartment of the forearm is the lateral compartment, sometimes called the "mobile wad." The muscles in the lateral compartment include the brachioradialis muscle, the extensor carpi radialis longus (ECRL), and the extensor carpi radialis brevis (ECRB).

EXTRINSIC MUSCLES

Flexor System

There are three wrist flexors: the flexor carpi radialis, the palmaris longus, and the flexor carpi ulnaris muscles. The flexor carpi radialis inserts into the volar base of the index metacarpal. The palmaris longus, which is missing in 10 to 15 percent of the population, inserts into the palmar fascia. The flexor carpi ulnaris inserts onto the pisiform.

The finger flexors include the flexor digitorum superficialis, the flexor digitorum profundus, and the flexor pollicis longus in the thumb. The flexor digitorum superficialis inserts into the base of the middle phalanx and flexes the proximal interphalangeal joint (PIP). The flexor digitorum profundus tendon inserts onto the base of the distal phalanx. This flexes the distal interphalangeal joint (DIP) and contributes to the flexion of the PIP. The flexor pollicis longus inserts onto the base of the distal phalanx of the thumb and flexes the interphalangeal joint of the thumb. At the level of the palm, the flexor digitorum profundus is dorsal to the flexor digitorum superficialis. The flexor digitorum superficialis splits at Camper's chiasm, and the flexor digitorum profundus passes through the chiasm to lie in a volar position at the digital level.

The flexors pass through the carpal tunnel. The transverse carpal ligament comprises the volar roof of the carpal tunnel. The transverse carpal ligament is anchored to the scaphoid and the trapezius on the medial aspect and to the hamate and the pisiform on the ulnar side. The contents of the carpal tunnel consist of 9 tendons and one nerve: the four flexor digitorum superficialis tendons, the four flexor digitorum profundus tendons, the flexor pollicis longus tendon, and the median nerve.

At the digital level, the flexor tendons travel in a fibroosseous canal (the flexor tendon sheath), which consists of a series of pulleys to prevent bow-stringing of the flexor tendons. There are five annular (A) pulleys and three cruciate (C) pulleys (See Fig. 17-1). The A2 and A4 pulleys are the most critical for optimal function of the digits and overlie the proximal phalanx and middle phalanx, respectively.

The thumb has three pulleys, two annular and one oblique, the order of which from proximal to distal is A1, O, A2. The oblique is the critical pulley of the thumb.

The blood supply to the flexor tendons are from the vincula (folds of mesotenon with the incorporated vessel on the dorsal surface of the tendons). There are four vincula per digit, one long and one short for each tendon. The nutrition to heal a transected flexor tendon comes from both its blood supply and the synovial fluid within the flexor tendon sheath.

The five zones of flexor tendon injuries consist of the following: Zone one (I) is that portion of the digit distal to the flexor digitorum superficialis insertion. Zone two (II) is from the flexor digitorum superficialis insertion to the origin of the A1 pulley. Historically, this

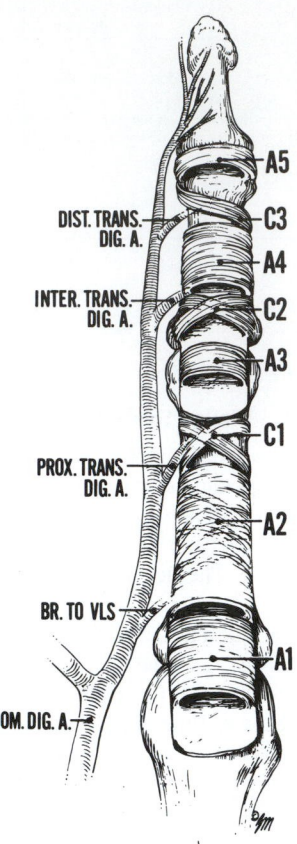

DIST. TRANS. DIG. A.

INTER. TRANS. DIG. A.

PROX. TRANS. DIG. A.

BR. TO VLS

COM. DIG. A.

A5
C3
A4
C2
A3
C1
A2
A1

Figure 17-1
Annular pulleys and cruciate pulleys. (Reproduced with permission from Schneider LH, Hunter JM: Flexor tendons—late reconstruction. In Green DP (ed): *Operative Hand Surgery*. New York: Churchill Livingstone; 1993:1894.)

zone was termed by Bunnell as "No man's land." Zone three (III) is from the A1 pulley to the distal transverse carpal ligament. Zone four (IV) is within the carpal tunnel and Zone five (V) is proximal to the carpal tunnel.

The five zones of thumb injury consist of: Zone one (I) at the level of the flexor pollicis longus insertion and distal, Zone two (II) from the flexor pollicis longus insertion to the neck of the metacarpal, Zone three (III) at the thenar muscle level, Zone four (IV) within the carpal tunnel, and Zone five (V) area proximal to the carpal tunnel.

INTRINSIC MUSCLES

The intrinsic muscles of the hand consist of the thenar muscles, the hypothenar muscles, the lumbricals, and the dorsal and volar interossei muscles. Their actions, innervations, origins and insertions are summarized in Table 17-1 and Fig. 17-2.

EXTENSOR SYSTEM

The extensors are arranged in six compartments on the dorsum of the hand and are numbered from radial to ulnar. The first dorsal compartment consists of the abductor pollicis longus (APL) and the extensor pollicis brevis (EPB). The abductor pollicis longus inserts onto the dorsal base of the thumb metacarpal. The extensor pollicis brevis inserts onto the dorsal base of the proximal phalanx of the thumb.

The second compartment consists of the extensor carpi radialis longus and the extensor carpi radialis brevis. The ECRL inserts onto the dorsal base of the index metacarpal. The ECRB inserts into the base of the middle metacarpal. The ECRB is termed a "true," or primary, wrist extensor since it has a central pull with no radial or ulnar deviation as the ECRL and the ECU have, respectively.

The third dorsal compartment consists of the extensor pollicis longus (EPL). The extensor pollicis longus inserts into the distal

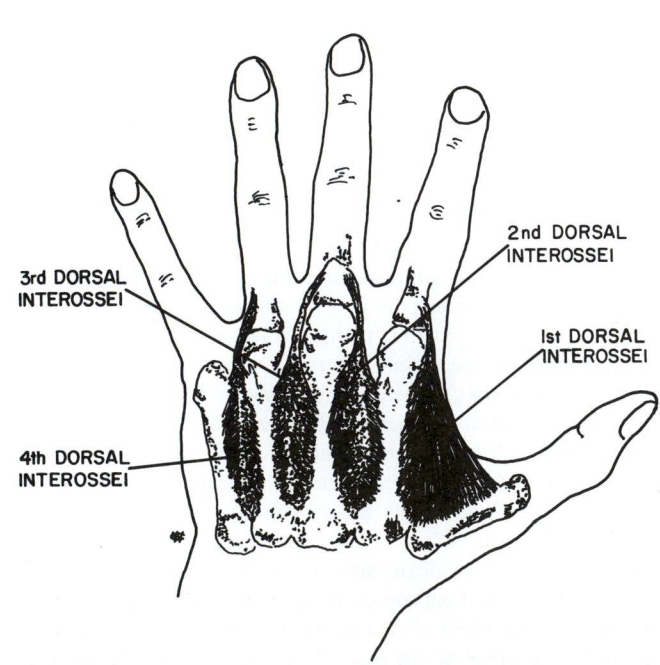

3rd DORSAL INTEROSSEI

2nd DORSAL INTEROSSEI

1st DORSAL INTEROSSEI

4th DORSAL INTEROSSEI

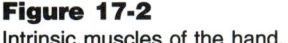

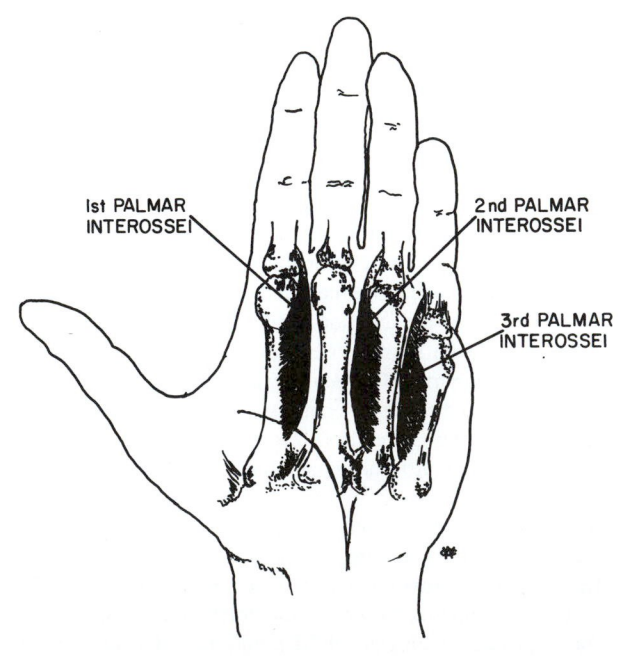

1st PALMAR INTEROSSEI

2nd PALMAR INTEROSSEI

3rd PALMAR INTEROSSEI

Figure 17-2
Intrinsic muscles of the hand.

Table 17-1

Muscles of the Hand

Muscle	Action	Innervation		Origin	Insertion
Thenar muscles					
Abductor pollicis brevis (APB)	Thumb abduction	Median		Trapezoid, scaphoid	Radial base proximal phalanx
Opponens pollicis	Abducts, flex medial rotation	Median		Trapezium	Thumb metacarpal
Flexor pollicis brevis (FPB)	Flex MCP	Superficial Head– Median/deep head –ulnar		Trapezium, capitate	Radial base proximal phalanx
Adductor pollicis (AP)	Thumb adduction	Ulnar		Capitate, 2d/3d metacarpal	Ulnar base proximal phalanx
Hypothenar muscles					
Palmaris brevis (PB)	Skin retraction	Ulnar		TCL, palmar aponeurosis	Ulnar palm
Abductor digiti minimi (ADM)	Small finger abduction	Ulnar		Pisiform	Ulnar base proximal phalanx
Flexor digiti minimi brevis (FDMB)	Flex MCP	Ulnar		Hamate, TCL	Ulnar bone proximal phalanx
Opponens digiti minimi (ODM)	Abduct, flex, lat. rotation	Ulnar		Hamate, TCL	V. metacarpal
Intrinsic muscles					
Lumbrical	Extend PIP	Median Ulnar	Index long Ring small	Radial aspect FDP tendon	Lateral bands
Dorsal interosseous (DIO)	Abduct, flex MCP	Ulnar		Metacarpals	Base prox. phalanx, extensor apparatus
Volar interosseous (VIO)	Adduct, flex MCP	Ulnar		Metacarpals	Base prox. phalanx, extensor apparatus

Source: Reproduced and modified with permission from Miller MD: *Review of Orthopaedics*. Philadelphia: WB Saunders; 1992:325.

---

phalanx of the thumb. The tendon passes ulnar to Lister's tubercle at the radius.

The fourth dorsal compartment consists of the extensor digiti communis and the extensor indicis proprius. The extensor digiti communis are the primary extensor tendons to the digits. The extensor indicis proprius is ulnar to the extensor digiti communis and provides independent extension to the index digit.

The fifth dorsal compartment consists of the extensor digiti minimi. This gives independent extension to the small digit.

The sixth dorsal compartment consists of the extensor carpi ulnaris (ECU). The ECU inserts at the dorsal base of the fifth metacarpal.

The anatomic snuff box is the depression at the dorsal thumb-metacarpal base, bounded by the first and third dorsal compartments.

The extensor mechanism of the digits consists of tendons and a retinacular system. The central slips insert at the dorsal base of the middle phalanx. The lateral bands converge at the dorsal base of the distal phalanx. The lateral bands are held together dorsally by the triangular ligament. The transverse retinacular ligament originates from the PIP volar plate and inserts into the lateral band. The transverse retinacular ligaments stabilize the lateral bands and limit their dorsal migration with joint extension. The oblique retinacular ligaments (ORL) originate from the flexor sheath and proximal phalanx volar to the PIP joint axis. The oblique retinacular ligaments gradually ascend dorsally to insert onto the distal phalanx, dorsal base with the terminal extensor tendons. The coordinated movements between the PIP and DIP form a dynamic tenodesis (Fig. 17-3).

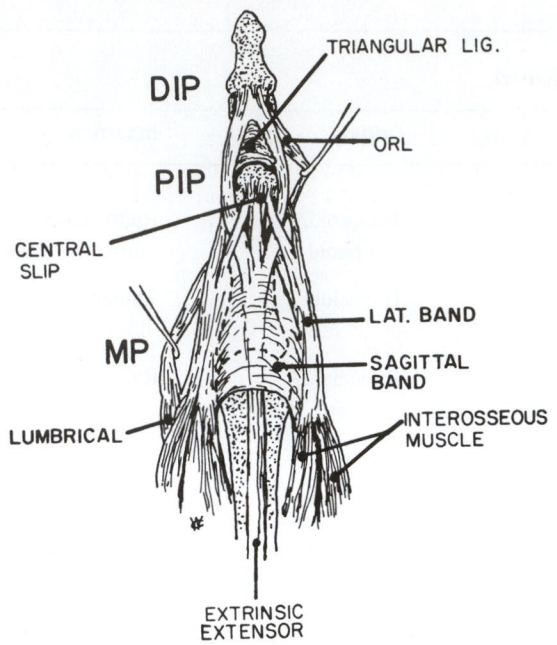

Figure 17-3
Extensor mechanism, lateral view (see text for details). (Reproduced with permission from Coons MS, Green SM: Boutonniere deformity. *Hand Clin* 1995; 11(3):388,389.)

The metacarpal phalangeal joint is flexed by the interosseus muscles and the lumbrical muscle. It is extended by the extensor digiti communis in conjunction with the sagittal band.

The proximal interphalangeal joint is flexed by the flexor digitorum superficialis and flexor digitorum profundus. The PIP joint is extended via the lumbrical at the lateral band contribution and the extensor digiti communis at its central slip.

The DIP joint is flexed by the flexor digitorum profundus and extended by the extensor digitorum communis at its terminal insertion and the oblique retinacular ligament.

The flexion arc of the normal digits equals the sum of the metacarpal phalangeal, proximal interphalangeal, and distal interphalangeal flexions. The normal flexion arc is 290 degrees. The metacarpal phalangeal joint flexion is usually 90 degrees, which consists of 31 percent of the flexion arc. The PIP joint usually flexes 120 degrees, which constitutes 41 percent of the flexion arc, and the DIP flexes 80 degrees, which consists of 28 percent of the flexion arc.

ARTERIAL BLOOD SUPPLY

The ulnar artery is the main contributor to the superficial palmar arch, which is distal to the deep arch. The ulnar artery gives rise to the common digital arteries which supply the ulnar three web spaces.

The radial artery is the main contributor to the deep palmar arch, which supplies the radial digital artery of the index digit and supplies the princeps pollicis artery, which provides blood to the thumb.

The complete arches, which are codominant, are present in only approximately 30 percent of patients. The common digital arteries are volar to the nerves in the palm. Proper digital arteries are dorsal to the digital nerves in the digit.

NERVES

The median nerve passes through the carpal tunnel. The palmar cutaneous branch of the median nerve innervates the thenar skin; its deep muscle branch innervates the thenar muscles. The median nerve also supplies the abductor pollicis brevis muscle, the opponens pollicis, and the superficial head of the flexor pollicis brevis muscle, as well as the lumbricals to the index and middle digits and sensation to the radial 3-1/2 digits. Proximal to the carpal tunnel, the median nerve lies between the palmaris longus and the flexor carpi radialis tendons.

The ulnar nerve passes through Guyon's canal. The superficial branch innervates the skin and the palmaris brevis muscle. The deep branch innervates the intrinsic muscles. The intrinsic muscles which the ulnar nerve innervates are the adductor pollicis, the deep head of the flexor pollicis brevis, the hypothenar muscles (the palmaris brevis, the abductor digiti minimi, the flexor digiti minimi brevis, the opponens digiti minimi), and the lumbrical to the ring and small digits. Both the dorsal and volar interossei are also innervated by the ulnar nerve. In addition, the ulnar nerve supplies sensation to the ulnar 1-1/2 digits.

The radial nerve has no motor function or innervation of intrinsic muscles. It does supply sensation to the dorsal aspect of the hand and the proximal portions of the radial 3-1/2 digits.

NAILS

Complete longitudinal regrowth of the nail takes between 70 and 160 days at a rate of 0.1 mm per day. When a subungual hematoma is greater than 25 percent of a nail bed surface, the nail should be removed for evaluation of the nail bed and possible repair. Fifty percent of nailbed lacerations are associated with distal phalanx fractures. The lunula is at the junction of the intermediate (germinal) and ventral (sterile) matrix. The nail bed (matrix) is all soft tissue below the nail plate which promotes nail generation and migration (Fig. 17-4).

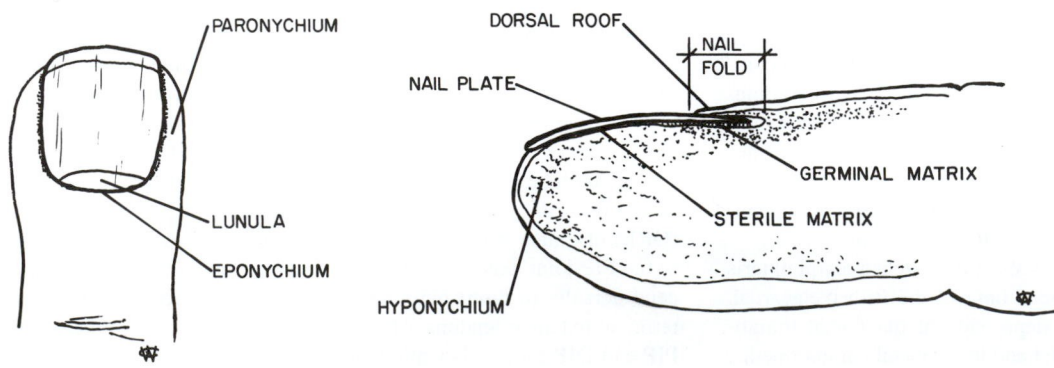

Figure 17-4
Anatomy of the nail and nail bed.

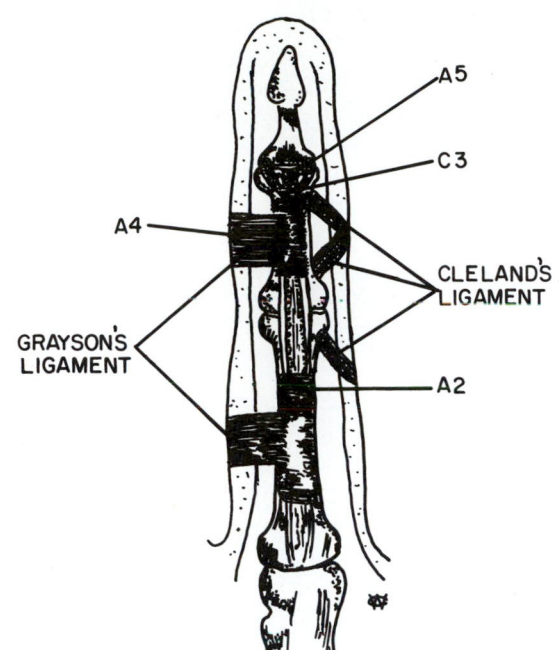

Figure 17-5
Ligaments of the digit. Grayson's ligament is adhered to annular pullies A2 and A4.

SURGICAL APPROACHES TO THE DIGITS

A midlateral approach to the digits is planned by making an incision at the apex of the interphalangeal creases with the PIP and DIP joints maximally flexed. The line that connects these midlateral marks is the incision line. The neurovascular bundle is volar to this incision.

The zig zag (Brunner) volar (palmar approach) incision connects the flexion creases at its lateral extent. This incision does not cross the flexion crease at right angles, eliminating contractures across the joints. This allows a good approach to the flexor sheath. To reach the neurovascular bundle, Grayson's ligaments must be cut. Cleland's and Grayson's ligaments are lateral ligaments which envelop the neurovascular bundles. Cleland's ligaments are dorsal (C for ceiling) and Grayson's ligaments are volar (G for ground) (Fig. 17-5).

SUGGESTED READINGS

Berger RA: General anatomy. In Cooney WP (ed): *The Wrist*. St. Louis: CV Mosby; 1998:32.

Berger RA: Ligament anatomy. In Cooney WP (ed): *The Wrist*. St. Louis: CV Mosby; 1998:73.

Bogumill GP: Anatomy of the wrist. In Lichtman DM, Alexander AH (eds): *Anatomy of the Wrist and Its Disorders*. Philadelphia: Saunders; 1998:19.

Chase RA: Anatomy and kinesiology of the hand. In Hunter JM, Schneider LH, Mackin EJ, et al (eds): *Rehabilitation of the Hand*, 3d ed. Philadelphia: CV Mosby; 1990:13.

Cooney WP: Vascular and neurologic anatomy of the wrist. In Cooney WP (ed): *The Wrist*. St. Louis: CV Mosby; 1998:106.

Garcia-Elias M, Dobyns JH: Bones and joints. In Cooney WP (ed): *The Wrist*. St. Louis: CV Mosby; 1998:61.

Green DP (ed): *Operative Hand Surgery*, 3d ed. New York: Churchhill Livingstone; 1993.

Spinner M (ed): *Kaplan's Functional and Surgical Anatomy of the Hand*, 3d ed. Philadelphia: JB Lippincott; 1984.

Chapter 18

PELVIS, ACETABULUM, AND LUMBAR PLEXUS

Kenneth J. Koval

ANATOMY

PELVIS OSSEOUS

The pelvis is a ringlike structure formed by two innominate bones and the sacrum. Each innominate bone is further composed of three smaller bones, the ishium, ilium, and pubis (developmentally, three primary ossification centers), all of which appear between 2 and 6 months of age and fuse by age 15 years. The sacrum is an inverted pyramid-type structure formed by five-fused vertebrae and wedged in between the two hip bones. Superiorly, the sacrum articulates with the facets of vertebra L5 and its intervebral disc. Laterally, it articulates with the auricular surfaces of the ilia to form bilateral synovial joints. The two hemipelvii are joined posteriorly at the sacroiliac joint and anteriorly at the pubic symphysis.

The pelvis is divided into two anatomical regions, the true and false pelves, by a plane (plane of the pelvic brim) which lies across the pelvis and passes through the promontory of the sacrum, the iliopectineal line (arcuate line), and the upper margin of the symphysis pubis. The false pelvis lies above the iliopectineal line, is bordered posteriorly and laterally by the ilia, has no anterior bony components, and forms part of the boundary of the abdomen proper containing the iliacus muscle and the abdominal contents. The true pelvis lies below and behind the iliopectineal line, has more complete bony walls (part of the ilium, ischium, pubis, sacrum, and coccyx), and contains the lower part of the abdomen (below and behind the lower aspect of the abdomen proper). The floor of the true pelvis is formed by the coccyx, levator ani muscles, the urethra, urinary bladder, rectum, and the vagina.

PELVIS JOINTS

The pelvis has three joints, the sacroiliac, the symphysis pubis, and the sacrococcygeal symphysis. The upper part of the sacroiliac joint is fibrous, receives most of the weight of the body, and transmits that weight to the hip bones; the lower aspect of the joint is synovial, providing the articulation between the sacrum and ilia. While it allows virtually no movement, the sacroiliac joint does provide resilience when weight is transferred to it from the sacrum. The symphysis pubis joins the two pubic bones. Each pubic bone is covered with hyaline cartilage, and the two are joined by fibrocartilage. Ligaments, fibers crossing from the fibrocartilage pad, the external oblique aponeuroses, and tendons of the recti abdominis muscles secure the joint. Movement of the symphysis pubis joint is slight, but will increase during pregnancy, allowing delivery of the fetus. The sacrococcygeal symphysis corresponds to the joints and ligaments of the other vertebral bodies, and also may be more freely moveable during pregnancy. The joints between the other coccygeal vertebrae are symphyses, fused in the male at an early age, but not in the female until the later years.

LIGAMENTOUS

The pelvis, without its considerable ligamentous support, lacks intrinsic osseous stability. It is the ligamentous structures that enable the critical vertical and rotational stability of the pelvis. The posterior sacroiliac ligaments, crossing the cleft between the tuberosity of the ileum and the sacral tuberosity (Fig. 18-1), are the strongest ligaments of the body, and are divided into long and short components. The short components provide rotational stability and the long ligaments vertical stability. The anterior sacroiliac ligaments, while they provide support, are not as strong as their posterior counterparts. The sacrospinous ligaments, which attach the lateral margins of sacrum and coccyx to the ischial spine, divide the pelvic floor into the greater and lesser sciatic foramen and resist rotational forces of the pelvis. The thick sacrotuberous ligaments connect the posterolateral sacrum to the ischial tuberosity, and provide additional vertical and rotational stability. Lastly, the iliolumbar ligaments pass from the iliac crest to the transverse process of the L4-5 vertebra. These ligaments resist anterior translation of the spine over the sacrum.

MUSCULATURE

The iliac crest provides sites of attachment for the abdominal oblique, transversus abdominis, quadratus lumborum, and gluteus maximus muscles. The anterior superior iliac spine is the site of origin for the sartorius and tensor fasciae latae muscle. One head of the rectus femoris originates from the inner ilium (ant. inferior spine); the other originates from the acetabular rim (posteriorly). The inner ilium is the site of attachment for the iliacus muscle, and the outer ilium, the attachment for the gluteus minimus and medius muscles. The obturator foramen is the site of attachment for the obturator muscles, the inferior pubic rami the site for the adductor muscles, and the ischial tuberosity the site for the hamstrings. The inner wall of the sacrum serves as attachment for the piriformis.

VASCULATURE

Within the pelvis, the aorta bifurcates into the common iliac arteries at L4, which pass anterior to the equivalent bifurcation of the inferior vena cava (L4-5); these vessels further divide into the internal and external vessels at the level of the sacral ala.

The external iliac vessels pass along the pectineal line (medial border of the psoas major) and under the inquinal ligament, supplying the psoas major and nearby lymph nodes. The inferior epigastric and deep iliac circumflex vessels branch off the external iliac vessels just proximal to the inguinal ligament and before the external iliac vessels enter the femoral canal to become the femoral vessels in the thigh.

The internal iliac vessels branch into anterior and posterior components at the S1 level. The two terminal branches of the anterior component are the internal pudendal artery (smaller terminal), supplying the external genitalia and the inferior gluteal artery (larger

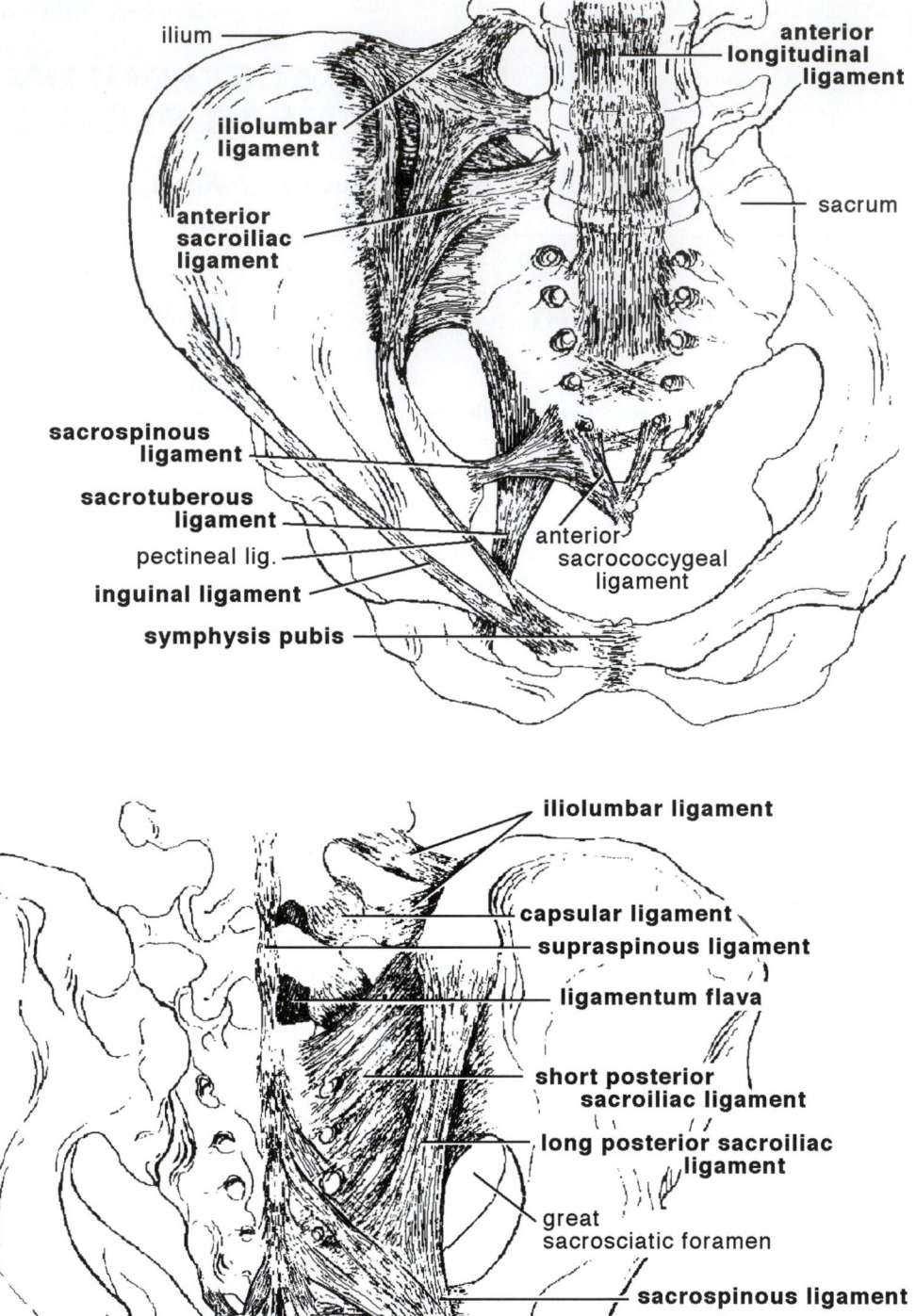

Figure 18-1
Ligaments of pelvis. (*Top*) Anterior view and (*bottom*) posterior view. [Reproduced with permission from Crouch JE: The vertebral column. In: *Functional Human Anatomy*. Philadelphia: Lea & Febiger (now Lippincott Williams and Wilkins); 1965:149.]

terminal) supplying mainly the buttock and the thigh (gluteus maximus, obdurator internus, gemelli, quadratus femoris, and parts of the hamstrings). The anterior division of the internal iliac vessels are also the blood supply for the pelvic viscera. The superior gluteal artery, the continuation of the posterior component of the internal iliac artery, supplies the piriformis and obturator internus within the pelvis and then passes through the greater sciatic notch where it divides into superficial and deep branches. The superficial branch supplies the gluteus maximus and the deep branch the gluteus medius and minimus muscles.

ACETABULUM

The acetabulum is a deep cuplike receptacle that faces forward, downward, and laterally, and receives the head of the femur. It is often described as being comprised of an anterior and posterior column. The anterior column includes the rim of the iliac wing, the brim of the pelvis, the anterior wall of the acetabulum, and the superior pubic ramus. The posterior column is described as including the ischium, the ischial tuberosity, and the posterior wall of the acetabulum. The superior and posterior walls of the acetabulum are thicker than the anterior wall, and the inferior wall, also called the acetabular notch, is deficient. The fossa is filled with adipose tissue and is encosed in a synovial membrane. From the medial aspect of the acetabulum, the ligamentum teres, along with some fibers of the transverse ligament, extend laterally to the fovea capitis of the head of the femur; the function of the ligament seems mainly to provide nutrient vessels to the femur head.

LUMBOSACRAL PLEXUS

The lumbosacral plexus provides innervation to the lower extremities and consists of the ventral rami of spinal nerves T12-S1 (Fig. 18-2). The plexus lies across two muscles: the lumbar component is on the anterior part of the iliopsoas and the sacral is on the piriformis.

The ilioinguinal and iliohypogastric nerves (T12-L1) pass around the abdominal wall to innervate the skin of the groin area.

The genitofemoral nerve (L1-2) travels through the psoas muscle to supply sensation to the anteromedial thigh and scrotum. This nerve also controls the cremasteric reflex.

The lateral femoral cutaneous nerve (L1-2) runs parallel to the iliacus muscle before it passes under the inguinal ligament, medial to the anterior superior iliac spine. It provides sensory innervation to the anterolateral thigh.

The femoral nerve (L2-4) runs within the fascia of the iliopsoas and, before it leaves the pelvis, under the inguinal ligament lateral to

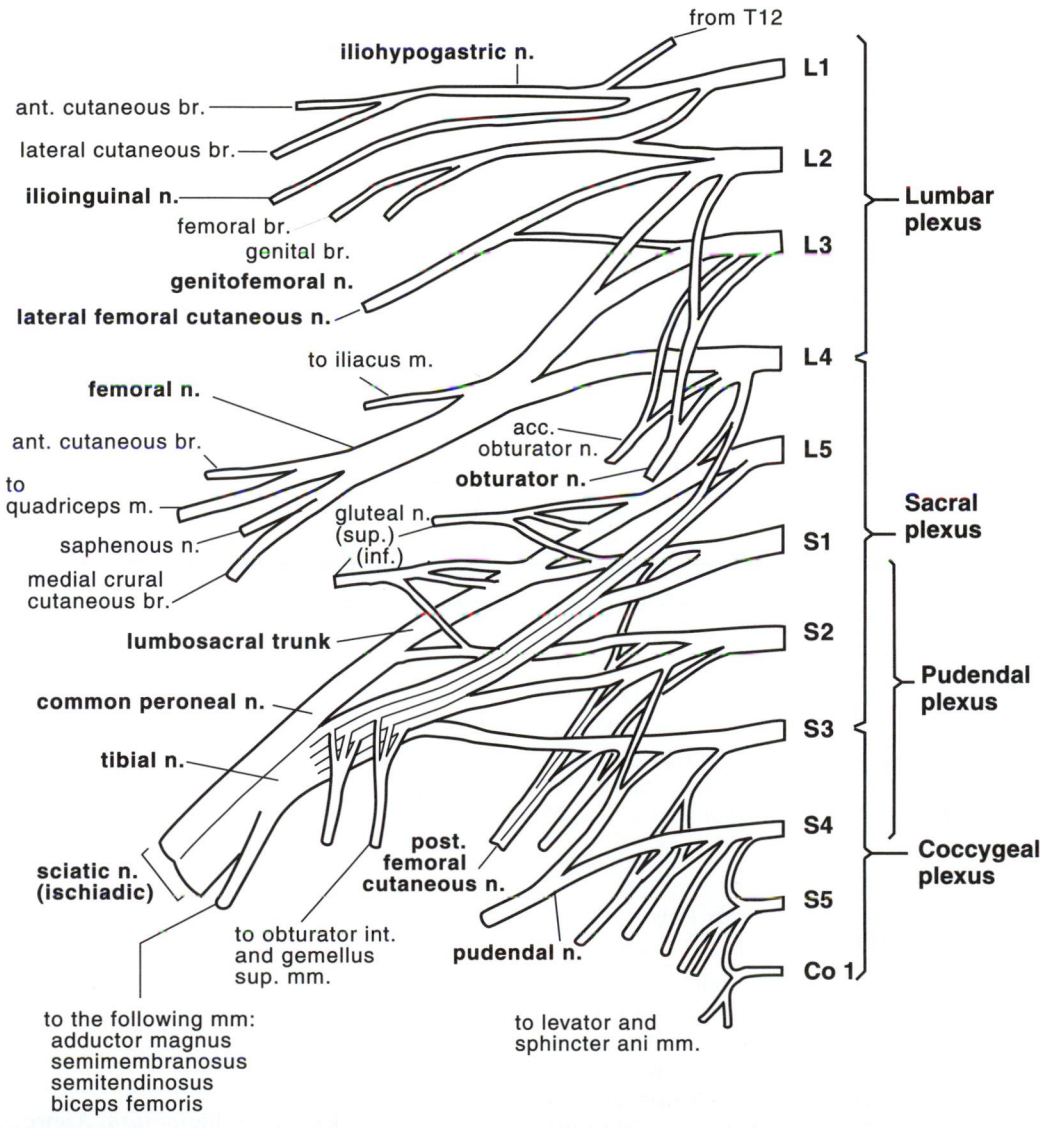

Figure 18-2
Nerves of the lumbar, sacral, and coccygeal plexuses. (Reproduced and modified with permission from Crouch JE: Spinal nerves. In: *Functional Human Anatomy.* Philadelphia: Lea and Febiger (now Lippincott, Williams & Wilkins); 1965:513.)

the femoral artery. It has both sensory (anterior thigh and medial leg) as well as motor (knee extensors) components.

The obturator nerve (L2-4) courses over the medial aspect of the psoas muscle, then onto the obturator membrane, and finally exits the pelvis via the obturator foramen. It supplies sensory innervation to the medial aspect of the thigh and motor innervation to the adductors of the thigh.

At the lumbosacral trunk (L4-5), the lumbar and sacral components of the plexus are joined.

The superior gluteal nerve (L4-S1), with its associated artery, passes through the greater sciatic notch, above the piriformis muscle. This nerve provides a motor component to the gluteus medius and minimus as well as to the tensor fasciae latae.

The inferior gluteal nerve (L5-S2) travels through the greater sciatic notch (below the piriformis) to supply the gluteus maximus.

The sciatic nerve (L4-S3) also passes through the greater sciatic notch to supply sensory nerves to the leg below the knee and motor nerves to the posterior compartment of the thigh and all compartments of the leg.

The pudendal nerve (S2-S4) exits the pelvis via the greater sciatic notch and reenters the pelvis through the lesser sciatic notch to provide cutaneous, sensory innervation to the genital organs and perineum.

SURGICAL APPROACHES TO THE PELVIS AND ACETABULUM

PELVIS

Anterior Approach to the Symphysis Pubis

For an anterior approach to the symphysis pubis, the patient is placed in a supine position. A transverse incision is made 2 cm proximal to the symphysis pubis or a vertical incision is made in the mid-line. The linea alba is identified and split longitudinally, separating the rectus abdominis muscles. Beneath the abdominal wall is the peritoneal fat proximally, and the bladder distally. Periosteal elevation of the superior aspect of the symphysis pubis completes the exposure. To expose the superior pubic rami, a Hohmann retractor can be used to displace the abdominal muscles laterally.

Anterior Approach to the Posterior Pelvis

The patient is placed supine for an anterior approach to the posterior pelvis. The incision is started just proximal to the anterior superior iliac spine and continued posteriorly approximately two-thirds around the iliac crest. The periosteum is incised and the abdominal musculature is released. The iliacus is dissected from the internal iliac fossa to expose the anterior sacroiliac joint and the sacrum. The L5 nerve root is at risk during this approach as it passes over the sacral ala.

Posterior Approach to the Posterior Pelvis

In this posterior approach, the patient is placed in a prone or a lateral position. A vertical incision is made two centimeters lateral to the posterior superior iliac spine. The subcutaneous tissues are retracted and the gluteus maximus is reflected subperiosteally. The origin of the gluteus maximus is detached from the sacrum and the iliac crest, exposing the multifidus and erector spinae muscles. Mobilization of the piriformis muscle exposes the greater sciatic notch and the posterior sacroiliac joint. One can visualize the posterior sacral lamina by elevating the multifidus muscles. The major risk with this approach is wound healing complications.

ACETABULUM

Kocher-Langenbeck Approach

The Kocher-Langenbeck approach exposes the posterior column of the acetabulum. The patient is placed in a prone or lateral position. An incision is made 5 cm lateral to the posterior superior iliac spine, and extended distally over the greater trochanter and the lateral thigh. The iliotibial band is incised and the fibers of the gluteus maximus dissected; the insertion of the gluteus maximus is then tagged and transected. The sciatic nerve is identified on the posterior aspect of the quadratus femoris. Care should be taken to gently retract the sciatic nerve keeping the hip extended and knee flexed to minimize tension on the nerve. The short external rotators are identified, tagged, and incised at their trochanteric insertions; they are then traced to the lesser and greater sciatic notches. The ischium is dissected subperiosteally to the origin of the hamstrings; the gluteus medius and minimus are also dissected subperiosteally off the posterior and lateral ilium. A greater trochanteric osteotomy may be performed to allow for greater exposure. The structures at risk with this approach are the sciatic nerve, and the superior gluteal artery and vein.

Ilioinguinal Approach

The ilioinguinal approach is used to access the anterior column and inner aspect of the innominate bone. The patient is placed in a supine position. The incision is started two finger breadths proximal to the symphysis pubis, is advanced laterally to the anterior superior iliac spine and continued along the iliac crest posteriorly. The periosteum of the superior and inner aspects of the ilium is dissected to release the insertions of the abdominal wall musculature and iliacus. This dissection is carried to the sacroiliac joint. The first abdominal layer encountered is the external oblique aponeurosis and external sheath of the rectus abdominis, which are incised and reflected distally to unroof the inguinal canal. The spermatic cord or round ligament is then identified as is the ilioinguinal nerve; a Penrose drain is placed around both structures. The inguinal ligament is then incised in line with the direction of its fibers, which releases the transversalis fascia medially and the origins of the transversus abdominis and internal oblique laterally. Care must be taken to avoid the external iliac vessels, the femoral sheath and the lateral femoral cutaneous nerve deep to the inguinal ligament. The conjoined tendon is also released from its insertion to the pubis (medial to the transversalis fascia) and a portion of the rectus abdominis insertion is transected. The iliopectineal fascia divides the psoas muscle and femoral nerve from the femoral artery and vein. This fascial layer can now be incised, allowing access to the true pelvis. Penrose drains are placed around the psoas muscle and femoral vessels. One must confirm the presence or lack of an anomalous obturator artery, the corona mortise, which may be difficult to control if incised.

There are three *windows* which allow visualization of the entire anterior column and superior pubic ramus. The first window provides access to internal iliac fossa, the anterior sacroiliac joint, and the pelvic brim. The second window is obtained by retracting the iliopsoas muscle laterally and the great vessels medially and exposes the pelvic brim, from the anterior sacroiliac joint to the pectineal eminence, and the quadrilateral region. The third window, medial to the great vessels, exposes the superior pubic ramus and the symphysis pubis.

Extended Iliofemoral Approach

The extended iliofemoral approach provides exposure to both acetabular columns simultaneously. The patient is positioned laterally. The incision starts at the posterior superior iliac spine, continues around the iliac crest to the anterior superior iliac spine, and then turns anterolaterally down the thigh. The periosteum is sharply incised over the iliac crest releasing the gluteal musculature and the tensor fasciae latae. The fascia lata is incised over the anterolateral thigh, exposing the tensor fasciae latae muscle which is retracted to reveal the rectus femoris. The fascial layer between the tensor fasciae latae and rectus femoris is incised longitudinally. A second fascial layer separates the rectus femoris from the vastus lateralis and it is also incised. Beneath this layer are the lateral femoral circumflex vessels which are clamped and ligated. The gluteal muscles are elevated from the iliac wing posterior and distal to expose the greater sciatic notch. The tendons to the gluteus medius and minimus are identified at their insertion into the greater trochanter, tagged and transsected, leaving a cuff of tissue for later reattachment. The short external rotator muscles of the thigh, the gemelli and obturator internus, are identified and incised at their trochanteric insertions. The reflected head of the rectus femoris is excised to better expose the hip capsule and a capsulotomy is performed. The inner aspect of the ilium can be accessed by detachment of the abdominal muscles, the sartorius, and the inguinal ligament, and periosteal reflection of the iliacus muscle; one must avoid, however, devascularization of the anterior column.

SUGGESTED READINGS

Crenshaw AH Jr: Surgical techniques and approaches. In Canale ST (ed): *Campbell's Operative Orthopaedics*, 9th ed. St. Louis: Mosby; 1998: 96–110.

Hoppenfeld S: The hip and acetabulum. In: *Surgical Exposures in Orthopaedics: The Anatomic Approach*, 2d ed. Philadelphia: JB Lippincott; 1994:323.

Hoppenfeld S: The pelvis. In: *Surgical Exposures in Orthopaedics: The Anatomic Approach*, 2d ed. Philadelphia: JB Lippincott; 1994:303.

Hoppenfeld S: The spine. In: *Surgical Exposures in Orthopaedics: The Anatomic Approach*, 2d ed. Philadelphia: JB Lippincott; 1994:215.

Kellam JF, Browner JD: Fractures of the pelvic ring. In Browner BD, Jupiter JB, Levine AM, et al (eds): *Skeletal Trauma*, 2d ed. Philadelphia: WB Saunders; 1998:1117.

Letournel E, Judet R: *Fractures of the Acetabulum*, 2d ed. Berlin: Springer-Verlag; 1993.

Leventhal MR: Spinal anatomy and surgical approaches. In Canale St (ed): *Campbell's Operative Orthopaedics*, 9th ed. St. Louis: Mosby; 1998:2681.

Matta JM: *Surgical Approaches to Fractures of the Acetabulum and Pelvis.* Los Angeles: Joel M. Matta, MD; 1989.

Olson SA, Matta JM: Surgical treatment of acetabulum fractures. In Browner BD, Jupiter JB, Levine AM, et al (eds): *Skeletal Trauma*, 2d. Philadelphia: WB Saunders; 1998:1181.

Chapter 19

HIP, THIGH, KNEE, AND LEG

Paul E. Di Cesare

HIP

ANATOMY

The hip joint is formed by the spheroid head of the femur and the deep socket of the acetabulum. Movement of the hip joint is generally characterized as extension, flexion, abduction, adduction, and internal and external rotation. The cup of the acetabulum is extended and, therefore, deepened by an added rim of tissue, the fibrocartilaginous labrum, which extends across the acetabular notch as the transverse acetabular ligament. The hip capsule is attached to the labrum and transverse acetabular ligament of the acetabulum, to the medial side of the greater trochanter of the femur, to the intertrochanteric line anteriorly, to a site immediately superior and medial to the lesser trochanter and, finally, to the neck of the femur posteriorly.

Three prominent ligaments (the iliofemoral, ischiofemoral, and pubofemoral) and one minor ligament (the zona orbicularis) of the hip joint conjoin with the joint capsule. The iliofemoral or "Y" ligament of Bigelow, which is the largest and most important hip capsule ligament, extends from the anterior inferior iliac spine across the anterior hip joint to attach to the anterior aspect of the greater trochanter and the intertrochanteric line as an inverted "Y." The ischiofemoral ligament extends from the ischium body at and inferior to the acetabulum, and extends horizontally across the posterior aspect of the hip capsule to insert at the base of the posterosuperior neck of the femur. The pubofemoral ligament originates from the body of the pubis and crosses anterior to the hip joint to insert into the lower aspect of the femoral neck and the lower limb of the iliofemoral ligament. The zona orbicularis, which is the fourth and least prominent ligament and is covered by the other ligaments, consists of circular fibers that encircle the capsule at the femoral neck. Inside the hip capsule, and extending from the acetabular fossa and transverse acetabular ligament to the fovea of the femoral head, is the ligament of the head (ligamentum teres) surrounded by synovium.

Innervation of the hip joint varies, depending on joint area, and may include branches of the femoral nerve (anteriorly); anterior–inferior branches of the obturator nerve; occasionally, the accessory obturator nerve; and a branch from either the nerve to the quadratus femoris or the superior gluteal nerve posteriorly.

The blood supply of the femoral head and neck is complex and has important orthopaedic implications (Fig. 19-1). The medial and lateral circumflex arteries send branches that anastomose to form an extracapsular arterial ring at the base of the femoral neck. Coming off the arterial ring, the ascending cervical arteries, also known as the capsular or retinacular arteries, pierce the joint capsule and run along the neck of the femur, deep to the synovial membrane.

The four main retinacular arteries—anterior, medial, posterior, and lateral—are named for their position relative to the femoral neck. The lateral retinacular artery is the most important for blood supply to the femoral head and neck, the majority of the blood supply in the adult originating from the medial femoral circumflex artery. The retinacu-

lar arteries may also send small branches to supply the metaphysis of the femoral neck. The retinacular vessels again anastomose at the margin of the articular cartilage to form the subsynovial intra-articular ring. Small epiphyseal arterial branches then pierce and supply blood to the femoral head. The artery of the ligamentum teres is a branch of the posterior division of the obturator artery or a branch from the medial circumflex artery and supplies blood to a small area of bone adjacent to the fovea of the femoral head, but is clinically important only in children.

The femoral triangle, which is located in the anterior proximal thigh, is formed by the inguinal ligament proximally, the sartorius laterally, and the medial border of the adductor longus medially. The iliopsoas and pectineus muscle make up the floor. Contained within the femoral triangle from lateral to medial are the femoral nerve, artery, and vein, which enter the femoral triangle deep to the inguinal ligament and exit distally, deep to the sartorius muscle. Within the femoral triangle, the femoral artery (also called the superficial femoral artery) gives off the profunda femoris artery from its posterolateral side. The two largest tributaries of the profunda femoris artery are the medial and lateral femoral circumflex arteries. The lateral femoral circumflex artery originates from the lateral side of the profunda femoris artery to run laterally across the iliopsoas muscle and then deep to the sartorius and rectus femoris, where it divides into an ascending, a descending, and a transverse branch. The medial femoral circumflex artery originates from the medial or posteromedial side of the profunda femoris artery and runs posteriorly between the iliopsoas and pectineus muscles. The cruciate or crucial anastomosis, located at the inferior margin of the quadratus femoris muscle, is formed by a descending branch of the inferior gluteal artery, the first perforating branch of the profunda femoral artery, and the medial and lateral circumflex arteries. The superficial femoral artery continues in the thigh within the adductor canal, separated from the profunda femoral vessel by the adductor longus muscle. The femoral artery then passes from medial to posterior in the thigh through a tendinous hiatus in the adductor magnus (Hunter's canal), becoming the popliteal artery.

The acetabulum is formed by three separate bones—the ilium, the ischium, and the pubis—that fuse at approximately 15 years of age. The ilium becomes the superior part, the pubis forms the anterior part, and the ischium forms the posteroinferior aspect of the acetabulum. The acetabulum is positioned at approximately 45 degrees from the floor when standing and is anteverted. The inferior wall of the acetabulum is incomplete and is referred to as the acetabular or cotyloid fossa.

SURGICAL APPROACHES OF THE HIP

There are five basic approaches to expose and enter the hip joint: anterior, anterolateral, posterior, lateral, and medial. The keys to each approach are the different muscular intervals surrounding the hip joint that are used.

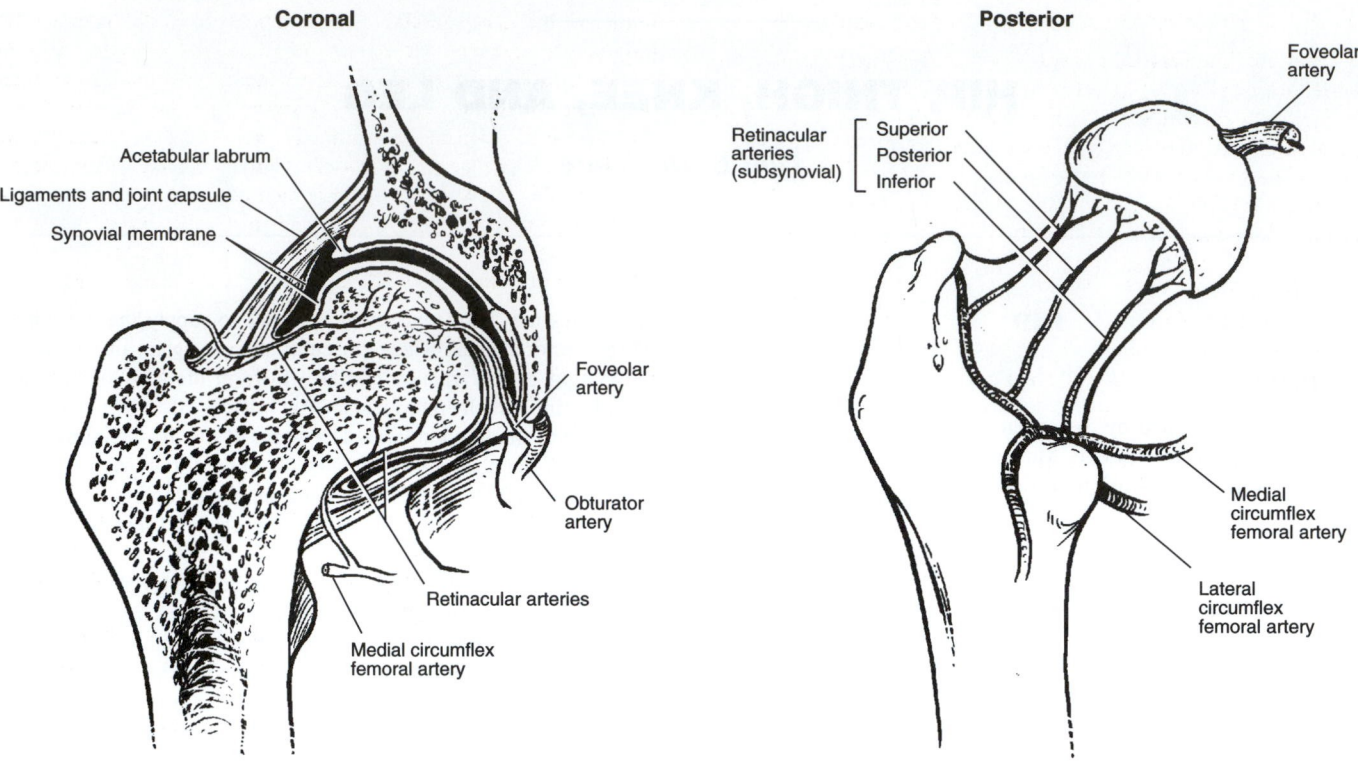

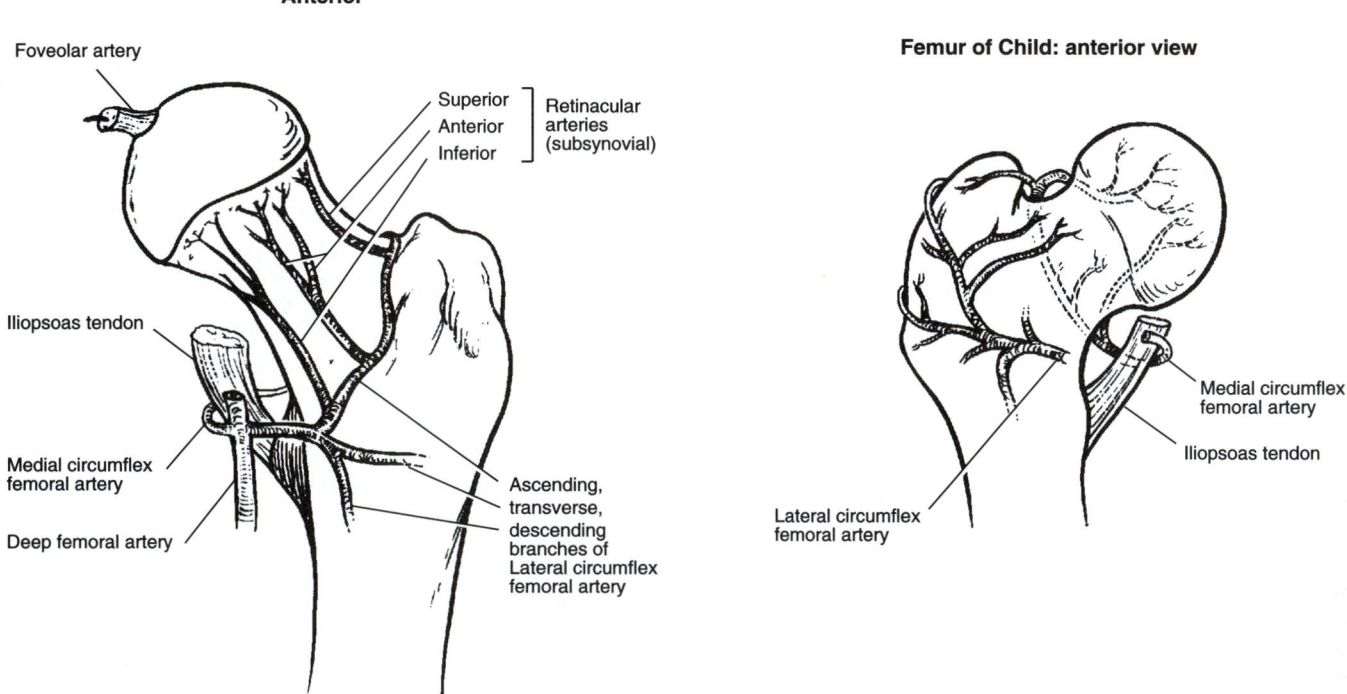

Figure 19-1

Arteries of the femoral head and neck in the adult and child. (Copyright 1989. Novartis. Reprinted with permission from the *Atlas of Human Anatomy,* illustrated by Frank H. Netter, M.D. All rights reserved.)

Anterior Approach (Smith-Peterson)

By using the internervous interval between the tensor fasciae latae (superior gluteal nerve) and the sartorius (femoral nerve), the anterior approach exposes both the hip joint and the ilium. The anterior approach is used most often for open reduction of the developmentally dysplastic hip (when the head is located anterosuperior to the anatomic acetabulum), synovial biopsies, hip arthrodesis, tumor excision, and, on rare occasion, for total joint or hemiarthroplasty. The most proximal aspect of the approach may also gain exposure for open reduction and internal fixation of some pelvic fractures or for certain pelvic osteotomies.

With the patient supine, the skin incision traces from the anterior half of the iliac crest distally to the anterior superior iliac spine and then curves distally for another 10 cm toward the lateral side of the patella. This approach takes advantage of two internervous planes: a superficial internervous plane between the sartorius (femoral nerve) and the tensor fasciae latae (superior gluteal nerve) and a deep internervous plane between the rectus femoris (femoral nerve) and the gluteus medius (superior gluteal nerve). For the superficial dissection, care must be taken to find and retract medially the lateral femoral cutaneous nerve. The deep fascia on the medial side of the tensor fasciae latae is then opened, as is the ascending branch of the lateral femoral circumflex artery that runs across the interval between the two muscles.

The deep dissection uses the internervous interval between the rectus femoris (femoral nerve) and the gluteus medius (superior gluteal nerve). Both heads (direct and reflected) of the rectus femoris are then detached from the superior lip of the acetabulum and anterior capsule of the hip joint. The rectus femoris is retracted medially and the gluteus medius laterally. The iliopsoas, which is often partly attached to the inferior aspect of the hip joint capsule as it approaches the lesser trochanter, is then released from the capsule and retracted medially. With the limb in adduction and external rotation, a capsulotomy is performed. The hip can then be dislocated by external rotation and adduction.

For surgery on the pelvis, one can detach the origins of the tensor fasciae latae and the sartorius, and then detach the origins of the gluteus medius and minimus from the outer wing of the ilium by blunt dissection. The femoral nerve and vessels can be at risk if the surgical dissection is out of plane or if extreme retraction is used.

Anterolateral Approach (Watson-Jones)

The anterolateral approach uses the intramuscular interval between the tensor fasciae latae and the gluteus medius; both muscles are innervated by the superior gluteal nerve. The anterolateral approach is the approach used most commonly for revision and in some primary total joint replacements because it allows for a wide exposure of both the acetabulum and proximal femur and canal. This approach is also useful for open reduction and internal fixation of femoral neck fractures and for synovial biopsy of the hip. The hip abductors are released most commonly by a trochanteric osteotomy or, occasionally, by detaching the anterior part of the gluteus medius and the gluteus minimus tendons from the greater trochanter.

The patient is positioned in either the lateral or supine position, with the operative extremity flexed about 30 degrees and adducted. The midpoint of a 15-cm straight, longitudinal incision is centered on the tip of the greater trochanter and extended in both directions parallel to the femur. Since there is no internervous plane for this approach, care should be taken not to develop a plane up to the muscle origins on the ilium because the superior gluteal nerve enters the tensor fasciae latae very close to its origin. The deep fascia of the thigh is then incised in line with the skin incision just posterior to the

border of the tensor fasciae latae to expose the vastus lateralis distally and the gluteus medius more proximally. An interval between the tensor fasciae latae and the gluteus medius is developed by blunt dissection. Next, the branches of the superior gluteal artery that cross the interval between the tensor fasciae latae and the gluteus medius are ligated. The gluteus medius can then be retracted from the hip joint capsule. The vastus lateralis is then detached from its origin at the vastus lateralis ridge on the femur and reflected inferiorly for approximately 1 to 2 cm. One can now osteotomize the greater trochanter or detach the abductors from the greater trochanter. The trochanter is osteotomized, beginning just distal to the vastus lateralis ridge, by using either an oscillating saw, Gigli saw, or osteotomes in a flat or chevron manner. The greater trochanter is reflected toward the superior aspect of the incision.

Alternatively, one can dissect free the anterior portion of the gluteus medius and the gluteus minimus tendons from the greater trochanter. Following removal of the reflected head of the rectus femoris from its attachments on the joint capsule and anterior rim of the acetabulum, the hip joint capsule can be opened. The psoas tendon also may attach to the hip joint capsule and may need to be dissected free to improve exposure.

Care must be taken to avoid the femoral neurovascular bundle that is located anterior to the psoas. Within the femoral triangle, the femoral nerve is most lateral and can be injured by excessive medial retraction, causing a compression neurapraxia. The femoral artery and vein (more superficial) and the profunda femoris artery (more deep) are located anterior to the iliopsoas muscle and are at risk from incorrectly placed retractors that penetrate the iliopsoas. The anterior capsule of the hip joint is incised with a longitudinal incision. After capsulotomy, the hip can be dislocated anteriorly by hip external rotation.

Posterior Approach (Southern or Moore)

The posterior approach uses the interval created by splitting the gluteus maximus (single largest muscle in the body) and therefore avoids removing the hip abductors. There is no true internervous plane in this approach since the gluteus maximus is split in the line of its fibers. The gluteus maximus receives its innervation from the inferior gluteal nerve that enters the muscle medial and superior to the muscle split and is therefore not significantly denervated during the approach. The gluteus maximus also has a dual arterial supply from both the superior and the inferior gluteal arteries. The posterior approach is useful primarily for hemiarthroplasty, but is also used for primary or revision total hip arthroplasty, open reduction and internal fixation of posterior acetabular fractures, drainage of infected hip joints, removal of loose bodies from the hip joint, pedicle bone grafting, and open reduction of posterior hip dislocations.

With the patient in the true lateral position or prone, a slightly curved 15-cm incision centered on the tip of the greater trochanter is made, superiorly in line with the fibers of the gluteus maximus and inferiorly in line with the femoral shaft. The deep fascia is incised in line with the skin incision to expose the vastus lateralis inferiorly and the gluteus maximus superiorly. Both the superior (branch of the internal iliac artery) and inferior gluteal arteries supply the gluteus maximus by branches that enter the deep surface of the muscle and branch throughout the muscle. These branches cross the muscle where it is to be split and need to be ligated.

The muscle fibers of the gluteus maximus are then split in line with the incision to expose the short external rotator muscles of the hip. The sciatic nerve is noted to lie posteriorly as it leaves the greater sciatic notch of the pelvis, exits distal to the piriformis, runs vertically down the back of the thigh, and finally crosses the obturator internus, the superior and inferior gemelli, and the quadratus femoris before running deep to the femoral attachment of the gluteus maximus. The trochanteric bursa can now be identified and partially resected. To expose the posterior hip capsule, the femur should be rotated internally and the short external rotator muscles should be detached from the femur beginning (from proximal to distal) with the piriformis, followed by the superior gemellus, obturator internus, inferior gemelli and commonly, part of the quadratus femoris. Significant bleeding can occur from the ascending branches of the medial femoral circumflex that are frequently located within the quadratus femoris. The tendinous insertion of the gluteus maximus at the femur can also be detached in order to improve mobility of the femoral shaft and to increase exposure of the acetabulum. After capsulotomy, the hip can then be dislocated by internal rotation and adduction.

The sciatic nerve may be damaged by excessive retraction during surgery, causing a compression neuropraxia, or by stretching during leg lengthening (conversion of a developmentally dysplastic hip to a total hip arthroplasty). The inferior gluteal artery (branch from the internal iliac artery) enters the buttocks inferior to the piriformis. Its branches to the gluteus maximus are frequently sacrificed when the gluteus maximus is split. The piriformis tendon insertion into the upper border of the greater trochanter is also a surgical landmark for the entry point for most femoral intramedullary rods. The piriformis is also an important landmark for neurovascular structures as they enter the buttock and lower extremity. Only the superior gluteal nerve and artery enter proximal to the piriformis. The inferior gluteal nerve and artery, pudendal nerve and internal pudendal artery, nerve to obturator internus, sciatic nerve, posterior femoral cutaneous nerve, and nerve to quadratus femoris enter distal to the piriformis.

The quadratus femoris has a vast blood supply consisting of cruciate anastomosis from the ascending branch of the first perforating artery, the descending branch of the inferior gluteal artery, and transverse branches of the medial and lateral femoral circumflex arteries. Because of this, the quadratus femoris has been used as a vascular muscle–bone pedicle to revascularize an avascular femoral head or neck or to aid in uniting a femoral neck nonunion.

Lateral Approach (Hardinge)

The direct lateral hip approach avoids trochanteric osteotomy, preserves the gluteus medius muscle, enables early mobilization of patients following surgery, and has been used for hemiarthroplasty and primary total hip arthroplasty. Since the approach does not provide as wide an exposure as the anterolateral approach with trochanteric osteotomy, it is generally not used for revision hip arthroplasty.

With the patient supine on the operating table, a 10-cm incision centered at the greater trochanter is made in line with the femur. This approach uses no internervous plane as the gluteus medius muscle (superior gluteal nerve), tendon, and fibers are split by the incision. Since the split occurs distal to the insertion of the superior gluteal nerve that supplies the muscle, it is not significantly denervated during the approach. The vastus lateralis muscle is also split during the approach. This muscle receives its innervation from the femoral nerve that enters more medially and anteriorly than the dissection. The deep fascia is incised in line with the skin incision to expose the tensor fasciae latae anteriorly and the gluteus maximus posteriorly. The gluteus medius and vastus lateralis are then incised, beginning at the apex of the trochanter. The incision is extended proximally in line with the fibers of the gluteus medius and distally onto the anterior surface of the femur by cutting through the vastus lateralis. The transverse branch of the lateral circumflex artery should be identified and ligated on the femur. The ligament of Bigelow and the anterior aspect of the gluteus minimus insertion onto the greater trochanter are then detached along with the insertion of the vastus lateralis on the

intertrochanteric line to expose the anterior capsule of the hip joint. After capsulotomy, the hip can then be dislocated by adduction and external rotation. Similar to the anterolateral approach, the structures within the femoral triangle are at risk from inappropriately placed retractors or excessive retraction.

Medial Approach (Ludloff)

The medial approach uses the intramuscular interval between the adductor longus and the gracilis. The medial approach is utilized for hip adductor releases, open reduction of developmental dislocation of the hip, biopsy and treatment of tumors near the lesser trochanter, psoas release, and obturator neurectomy. Patients should be positioned supine, with the affected hip flexed, abducted, and externally rotated. A longitudinal incision is made on the medial side of the thigh, starting at a point 3 cm below the pubic tubercle and extended distally over the adductor longus. The superficial dissection uses the intramuscular plane between the adductor longus and the gracilis, both innervated by the anterior division of the obturator nerve. Since both muscles receive their nerve supply proximal to the dissection, there is little risk of denervation.

The dissection is then carried more deeply between the adductor brevis (innervated by the anterior division of the obturator nerve) and the adductor magnus (innervated by both the posterior division of the obturator nerve and by the tibial division of the sciatic nerve). Care should be taken to protect the posterior division of the obturator nerve as it runs vertically down the thigh, superficial to the adductor magnus and deep to the adductor brevis. In cases of obturator neurectomy, the anterior division of the obturator nerve (innervates the adductor longus, the adductor brevis, and the gracilis) can be located on the medial side of the thigh between the adductor longus and the adductor brevis. The medial femoral circumflex artery is located on the medial side of the distal part of the psoas tendon and needs to be isolated, especially in children, before detaching the psoas tendon. The adductor compartment of the thigh consists of three muscle layers, with the two divisions of the obturator nerve in between each pair of layers. The superficial layer contains the adductor longus and the gracilis, the middle layer contains the adductor brevis, and the deep layer contains the adductor magnus.

THIGH

ANATOMY

The femur articulates with the pelvis at its upper aspect and with the patella (a sesamoid bone within a tendon) and tibia at its lower aspect. The proximal femur consists of a head, a neck, and greater and lesser trochanters. The angle of inclination between the femoral neck and shaft should average 126 degrees, with approximately 14 degrees of anteversion. The bony architecture of the proximal femur includes trabeculae that align along the stress-and-strain forces to which the femur is subjected. The spheroid femoral head is covered with articular cartilage except at the fovea capitis. The fovea is a depression located on the medial side of the femoral head to which the ligament of teres is attached. The femoral neck is smaller in diameter than the femoral head. The greater trochanter is located laterally and extends above the femoral neck. The lesser trochanter is located posteromedially just below the femoral neck. Both trochanters are important sites for the insertion of muscles that move the hip. The two trochanters are connected by the intertrochanteric crest; anteriorly, the intertrochanteric line is the attachment site of the hip capsule to the femur.

The femur is cylindrical below the trochanters until it flares out at the distal end to form the condyles. The pectineal line, which is a prominent ridge below the lesser trochanter, continues distally with prominent ridges both medially and laterally, known as the linea aspera. The distal end of the femur is formed by two rounded condyles, the medial condyle being larger. The medial and lateral epicondyles are located at the sides of the condyles, with the medial epicondyle containing a more prominent projection, the adductor tubercle.

The femur shaft begins to ossify in fetal week 7 or 8; the femoral head ossifies during postnatal year 1; the distal femoral epiphysis usually ossifies prior to birth. The greater trochanter epiphysis is ossified at 5 years, the lesser trochanter at 10 years, and the fusion of the head and the trochanters with the femoral shaft between years 16 and 18.

The sciatic nerve enters the thigh just distal to the piriformis muscle and runs posterior to the short external rotators to descend deep to the gluteus maximus tendon. The nerve then runs vertically between the semimembranosus and long head of the biceps posterior to the adductor magnus. Just prior to or at the apex of the popliteal fossae, it divides into the common peroneal nerve and tibial nerve (Fig. 19-2).

SURGICAL APPROACHES TO THE THIGH

There are four basic approaches to the thigh: lateral, posterolateral, anterolateral, and anteromedial. In each approach, the quadriceps muscle is penetrated.

Lateral Approach

The lateral approach can be used to expose almost the entire length of the femur. It is used for a variety of procedures, including open reduction and internal fixation of intertrochanteric fractures, closed or open reduction of femoral neck fractures, open reduction and internal fixation of femoral shaft fractures, slipped capital femoral epiphysis, subtrochanteric or intertrochanteric osteotomy, and supracondylar femur fractures. It is used also for the treatment of chronic osteomyelitis of the femur and for the biopsy and treatment of femoral bone tumors.

With the patient in either the supine or the lateral position, a longitudinal incision is made on the lateral side of the thigh in line with the femur. This approach has no internervous or intermuscular plane, since the vastus lateralis, which is innervated by the femoral nerve, is split. The muscle is not denervated because it receives its nerve supply high in the thigh. The fascia lata of the thigh is then incised in line with the skin incision in order to expose the vastus lateralis. The vastus lateralis is then split in the line of its fibers by blunt dissection, exposing several perforating branches of the profunda femoris artery that traverse the vastus lateralis and need to be ligated before they are avulsed. The femoral periosteum is incised, and the dissection is continued subperiosteally around the femoral shaft.

Posterolateral Approach

The posterolateral approach to the thigh can be used to expose the entire length of the femur by using the internervous plane between the vastus lateralis (innervated by the femoral nerve) and the hamstrings (sciatic nerve). It is useful for open reduction and internal fixation of femoral shaft fractures, open intramedullary rodding of femoral shaft fractures, treatment of femoral nonunions, femoral osteotomy, treatment of chronic or acute osteomyelitis, and biopsy and treatment of bone tumors.

With the patient in either the supine or the lateral position, a longitudinal incision is made on the posterolateral aspect of the thigh in line with the femur. The deep fascia of the thigh is incised in line with the skin incision to expose the vastus lateralis, which is then reflected anteriorly, dissecting between muscle and the lateral intermuscular septum. Several perforating branches of the profunda femoris artery cross this interval to supply the muscle and must be

ligated or coagulated. If these vessels are torn at the lateral intermuscular septum and not ligated, they may retract behind the lateral intermuscular septum and bleed. The dissection is continued posteriorly to the linea aspera of the femur, and the periosteum is incised in line with the femoral shaft.

Anterolateral Approach

As with the posterolateral approach, the anterolateral approach can also be used to expose the entire femoral shaft. The anterolateral approach is useful for open reduction and internal fixation of femoral shaft fractures, femoral nonunions, femoral osteotomy, treatment of chronic osteomyelitis, biopsy and treatment of bone tumors, and quadricepsplasty.

With the patient supine, a linear incision is made starting 5 cm below the anterior superior iliac spine and continuing toward the lateral border of the patella. This approach uses no true internervous plane, since the superficial dissection uses the interval between the rectus femoris and the vastus lateralis (both innervated by the femoral nerve). There is little risk of denervation because both muscles receive their nerve supply more proximally. The deep dissection splits the vastus intermedius muscle, also innervated proximally in the thigh and safe from denervation. The fascia lata is incised in line with the skin incision to expose the interval between the vastus lateralis and the rectus femoris. Numerous tributary vessels of the lateral femoral circumflex artery cross the intermuscular interval in the upper part of the incision and must be ligated. The nerve to the vastus lateralis (branch of the femoral nerve) must be identified and preserved as it enters the medial side of the muscle at the proximal portion of the femoral shaft. The vastus lateralis is then retracted laterally and the rectus femoris medially to expose the vastus intermedius. The fibers of the vastus intermedius are then split to expose the anterior femur. Next, the periosteum is incised longitudinally and the dissection continued subperiosteally.

Anteromedial Approach

The anteromedial approach is useful for exposure of the distal two-thirds of the femur and the knee joint. This approach can be used for open reduction and internal fixation of distal femur fractures (including intercondylar and supracondylar femur fractures), open reduction and internal fixation of femoral shaft fractures, treatment of chronic osteomyelitis, quadricepsplasty, and biopsy and treatment of bone tumors.

With the patient supine, a 10- to 15-cm longitudinal incision is made on the anteromedial aspect of the thigh; the incision can be extended to the medial part of the patella for a knee arthrotomy. The dissection uses an intramuscular interval between the vastus medialis and the rectus femoris (both innervated by the femoral nerve). The deep fascia of the thigh is incised in line with the skin incision, and the interval between the vastus medialis and the rectus femoris is developed. A knee arthrotomy can be performed, if necessary, by a medial parapatellar approach. The medial superior genicular artery must be ligated where it crosses the operative field just proximal to the knee. The dissection is then carried deep to reveal the vastus intermedius, which is split in line with its fibers to expose the femoral periosteum.

Posterior Approach

The posterior approach exposes the middle three-fifths of the femur and the sciatic nerve, but it is rarely applied. It is useful for treatment of chronic osteomyelitis, biopsy and treatment of bone tumors, and exploration of the sciatic nerve.

With the patient prone, a straight longitudinal incision is made in the midline of the posterior thigh. The internervous plane between the lateral intermuscular septum covering the vastus lateralis (femoral

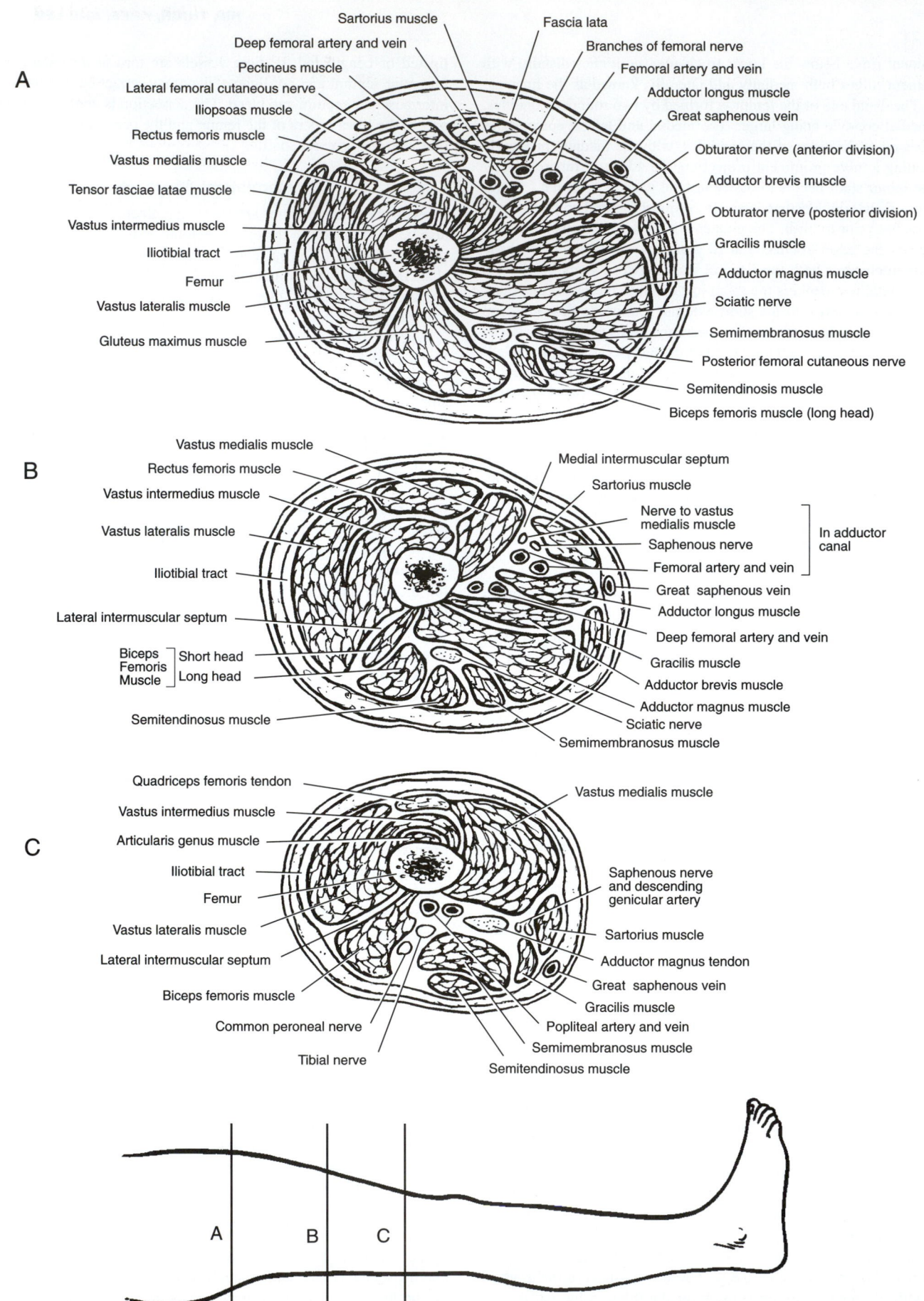

Figure 19-2

Serial cross sectional of the thigh. (Copyright 1989. Novartis. Reprinted with permission from the *Atlas of Human Anatomy*, illustrated by Frank H. Netter, M.D. All rights reserved.)

nerve) and the biceps femoris (sciatic nerve) is used. The deep fascia of the thigh is incised in line with the skin incision after care is taken to identify and protect the posterior femoral cutaneous nerve that lies in the groove between the biceps and the semitendinosus muscles. The interval between the biceps femoris and the vastus lateralis (covered by the lateral intermuscular septum) is then developed, with the long head of the biceps femoris retracted medially and the lateral intermuscular septum retracted laterally. The origin of the short head of the biceps is detached from the lateral lip of the linea aspera to expose the posterior femur. Distally, the long head of the biceps is retracted laterally to expose the sciatic nerve, which is also retracted laterally to expose the periosteum of the posterior femur.

KNEE

ANATOMY

The knee is a large synovial joint consisting of three intraarticular compartments: medial (articulation between the medial femoral condyle and the medial tibial plateau), lateral (articulation between the lateral femoral condyle and the lateral tibial plateau), and patellofemoral (articulation between the patella and the femoral intercondylar groove) (Fig. 19-3). Between the medial and lateral tib-

ial plateaus is the nonarticular intercondylar region that provides attachment sites for the anterior and posterior cruciate ligaments and the medial and lateral menisci. Both anterior and posterior cruciate ligaments are considered to be extraarticular, since they are enclosed by synovium. Within the intercondylar region are two intercondylar eminence or spines—medial (anterior) and lateral (posterior)—neither of which serve as attachment sites for the cruciate ligaments.

All the neurovascular structures of the leg are posterior to the knee joint and, as a result, the posterior approach is reserved for procedures involving those structures. The patella, which is the largest sesamoid bone, functions to protect the knee joint, to facilitate knee joint lubrication, and to increase the lever arm of the knee extensor mechanism. Deep to the patella tendon is the fat pad. The knee also contains the medial and lateral menisci, each attached to the tibia by the coronary ligament. The menisci increase joint stability (by increasing the joint concavity), act as shock absorbers to distribute forces across the knee more evenly, contribute to joint lubrication, and aid in knee rotation. The menisci structure is divided into an avascular "white zone" (peripheral one-third) and a vascular "red zone" (inner two-thirds).

The knee is stabilized by a complex array of ligaments, tendons, and soft tissues (Fig. 19-4). The ligaments on the medial side of the knee often merge with each other, making identification of each layer difficult. The medial side of the knee consists basically of three sep-

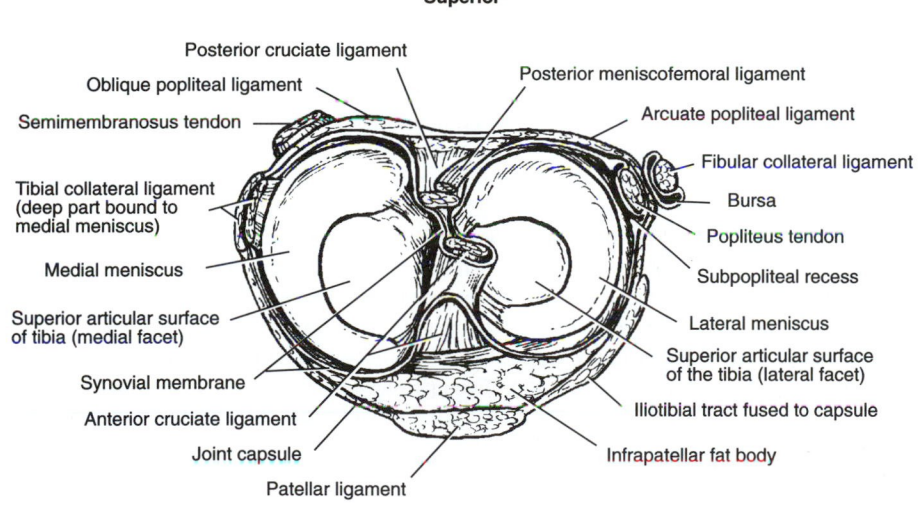

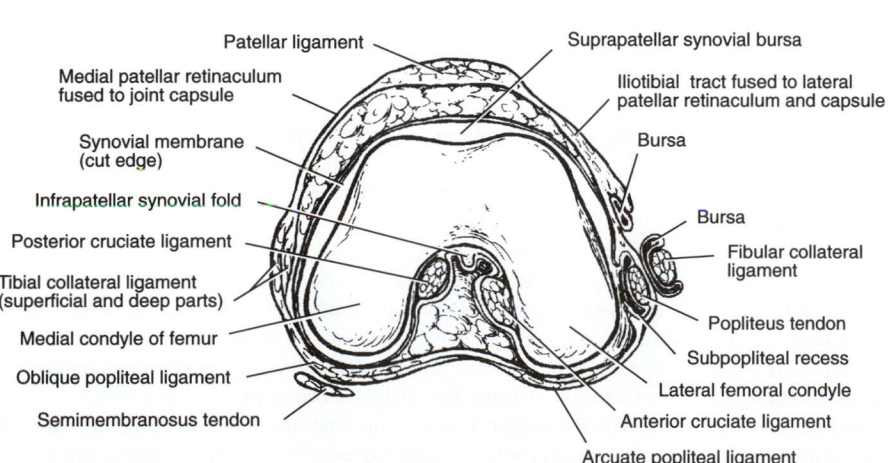

Figure 19-3

Intraarticular anatomy of the knee. (Copyright 1989. Novartis. Reprinted with permission from the *Atlas of Human Anatomy,* illustrated by Frank H. Netter, M.D. All rights reserved.)

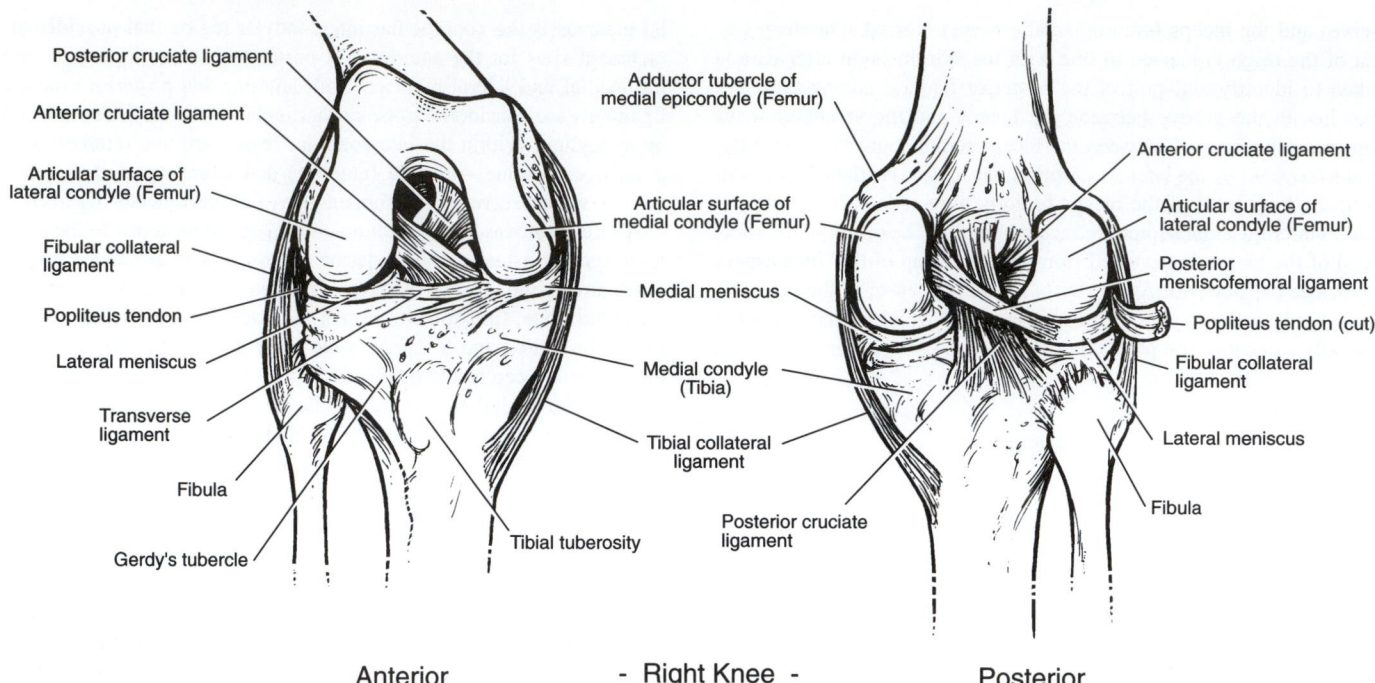

Figure 19-4
Bone, ligaments, tendons, and meniscal anatomy about the knee.

arate layers: outer, middle, and deep. The outer, or most superficial layer, is the deep fascia of the thigh whose fibers enclose the muscles and tendons of the pes anserinus before they insert into the tibia. The middle layer of the medial knee is the superficial medial collateral ligament that extends from just distal of the adductor tubercle to insert (as a quadrangular ligament) approximately 6 cm below the joint line into the subcutaneous border of the tibia. The superficial medial collateral ligament lies slightly posterior to the knee axis of rotation. Proximal and anterior to the insertion of the superficial medial ligament, a fibrous tissue band extends from the middle layer to the medial side of the patella as the medial patellofemoral ligament. The semimembranosus tendon continues posteriorly across the popliteal fossa and inserts into the posterior portion of the tibial medial condyle. The deep layer of the medial knee consists of the joint capsule, the deep medial collateral ligament (which extends from the medial epicondyle of the femur to the medial meniscus), and the coronary ligament (which anchors the medial meniscus to the tibia). Each of the three muscles that insert into the pes anserinus on the anteromedial tibia—the sartorius (femoral nerve), the semitendinosus (sciatic nerve), and the gracilis (obturator nerve)—has a different nerve supply. Since all three muscles originate from widely separated positions on the pelvis (the sartorius from the anterior superior iliac spine, the semitendinosus from the ischial tuberosity, and the gracilis from the inferior pubic ramus), they function powerfully to stabilize the pelvis on the leg, to flex the knee, and to rotate the tibia internally.

The lateral side of the knee also contains three layers: outer, middle, and deep. The outer layer consists of the deep fascia of the thigh, the iliotibial band (which inserts into the area of the lateral tibial condyle known as Gerdy's tubercle), the biceps femoris, and the lateral patellar retinaculum. The middle layer consists of the superficial lateral collateral ligament and the lateral inferior genicular vessels. The deep layer consists of the knee joint capsule, the popliteus muscle and tendon, and the deep lateral collateral ligament (which extends from the lateral femoral condyle to the fibular head).

The popliteal fossa is a diamond-shaped area that is formed inferiorly by the gap between the two heads of the gastrocnemius, by the

semimembranosus and semitendinosus medially, and by the biceps femoris laterally. Its inferior boundaries are the two heads of the gastrocnemius.

The tibial nerve (terminal branch of the sciatic nerve) runs lateral to the popliteal artery as it enters the popliteal fossa, crosses the artery at the midpoint to run medial to it, and then exits the fossa between the two heads of the gastrocnemius. The tibial nerve supplies motor branches to the plantaris, gastrocnemius, soleus, and popliteus muscles, and has a single sensory branch called the sural nerve. The common peroneal nerve diverges laterally to the medial side of the biceps tendon and enters the peroneus longus muscle prior to winding around the fibula. The common peroneal nerve divides into deep and superficial peroneal nerves within the peroneus longus muscle. The popliteal artery divides into its terminal branches—the posterior tibial, anterior tibial, and peroneal arteries—behind the gastrocnemius.

The popliteus, which is unusual in that its origin is distal to its insertion, functions to unlock the knee from its fully extended screw-home position by shifting the lateral femoral condyle behind the tibia and drawing the lateral meniscus posteriorly, preventing it from being trapped between the tibia and femur.

SURGICAL APPROACHES TO THE KNEE

Medial Parapatellar Approach

The medial parapatellar approach, which is the most commonly used approach to the knee, yields access to the suprapatellar pouch, the patella, and the medial aspect of the knee. The approach is used for synovectomy, medial meniscectomy, removal of loose bodies, ligamentous reconstructions, patellectomy, drainage of an infected knee, total knee or unicondylar arthroplasty, and open reduction and internal fixation of some intraarticular fractures.

With the patient supine, a midline incision is made on the anterior or just medial side from approximately 5 cm above the superior pole of the patella distally to the medial aspect of the patellar ligament and tibia tubercle. There is no internervous plane in this approach, since the quadriceps tendon is split between the vastus medialis and the rectus femoris (both innervated by the femoral nerve). Next, an incision is made in the medial aspect of the quadriceps tendon, making certain that a cuff of tissue medial to the patella and lateral to the quadriceps is present to facilitate wound closure. The patella is then dislocated laterally and inverted. Care should be take to avoiding the patella ligament from its insertion on the tibia tubercle. If the patella does not dislocate or invert, added mobility can be achieved by performing a quadriceps "snip" (a short transverse cut in the quadriceps tendon just proximal to the patella), by extending the quadriceps incision more proximally, or by performing a tibial tubercle osteotomy. The infrapatellar branch of the saphenous nerve is usually transected during this approach and may result in a postoperative neuroma. The area of sensation loss is usually not of clinical significance.

Anteromedial Approach

The anteromedial approach is very flexible. It can be performed using a variety of skin incisions or different positions for patients. The approach is useful for medial meniscectomy, partial meniscectomy, removal of loose or foreign bodies, and treatment of osteochondritis dissecans of the medial femoral condyle.

A skin incision is made at the inferomedial corner of the patella to 1 cm below the joint line. Care should be taken not to continue the incision more distally because that puts the infrapatellar branch of the saphenous nerve at risk. No internervous plane is used in this approach because the deep incision goes through the medial patellar retinaculum and joint capsule.

Medial Approach

The medial approach yields the widest exposure of the ligamentous structures (medial collateral ligament and capsule) on the medial side of the knee. This approach is used most often for repair of the medial collateral ligament and medial joint capsule. It is used rarely for medial meniscectomy in conjunction with ligamentous repair.

With the patient supine and the knee flexed at approximately 60 degrees, a curved incision beginning just proximal to the adductor tubercle is carried approximately 6 cm anterior and inferior to the tibia. There is no internervous plane in this approach, since the structures are subcutaneous and only the saphenous nerve and its tributaries are at risk. The saphenous nerve, which provides sensation for some of the nonweightbearing portions of the foot, exits the deep tissues between the gracilis and the sartorius muscles. The infrapatellar branch of the saphenous nerve is usually sacrificed because it is located perpendicular to the skin incision. The long saphenous vein, usually located in the posteromedial aspect of the wound, should be preserved.

The deep structures of the medial side of the knee form three layers. The deep incision should be planned to be either anterior or posterior to the superficial medial collateral ligament. Deep dissection carried anterior to the superficial medial collateral ligament is useful to expose the superficial medial collateral ligament, the anterior part of the medial meniscus, and the cruciate ligament. For this deep dissection, incise the fascia at the anterior border of the sartorius muscle and then retract the muscle posteriorly. This should uncover the semitendinosus and gracilis muscles, which should also be retracted posteriorly to expose the tibial insertions of the superficial medial collateral ligament (located deep and distal to the anterior edge of the sartorius). Deep dissection carried posterior to the superficial medial collateral ligament exposes the posterior horn of the medial meniscus and the posteromedial corner of the knee. Similar to the anterior approach, the fascia is incised along the anterior border of the sarto-

rius, and all three muscles are retracted posteriorly. The posteromedial corner of the knee is then exposed after separating the medial head of the gastrocnemius from the semimembranosus (both innervated by the tibial nerve well away from the plane of dissection) and then from the posterior knee capsule.

Arthrotomy posterior to the superficial medial collateral ligament can then be performed for either treatment of the collateral ligament, posteromedial corner, or posteromedial intraarticular or periarticular pathology. Care should be taken to identify and ligate, if necessary, the medial inferior genicular artery, because it may be disrupted during dissection of the medial belly of the gastrocnemius from the posterior knee capsule.

Lateral Approach

The lateral approach gives wide exposure to structures on the lateral side of the knee, and can be extended for intraarticular surgery. This approach is useful for assessment and treatment of ligamentous damage and, more rarely, for total knee arthroplasty with a valgus knee.

With the patient supine, a curved incision is made just lateral to the patella. The incision is extended distally to Gerdy's tubercle and proximally in line with the femur. The approach uses the internervous plane between the iliotibial band (superior gluteal nerve) and the biceps femoris (sciatic nerve). The fascia in between the iliotibial band and the biceps femoris should be incised. Care should be taken to identify and avoid the common peroneal nerve that is located on the posterior border of the biceps tendon. The iliotibial band is retracted anteriorly and the biceps tendon and the peroneal nerve retracted posteriorly to expose the superficial lateral collateral ligament (which extends from the femoral lateral epicondyle to the fibula head) and the posterolateral corner of the knee.

The knee joint may then be entered through an anterior or a posterior arthrotomy based on its location to the superficial lateral collateral ligament. The anterior arthrotomy is most useful for visualization of the lateral meniscus. The posterior arthrotomy is useful to visualize the posterior horn of the lateral meniscus. To complete the posterior arthrotomy, the lateral head of the gastrocnemius at its lateral femoral condyle origin must be dissected free from the posterolateral corner. The lateral superior genicular arteries must be ligated. Care must be taken when performing the posterior arthrotomy to avoid injury to the popliteus tendon that is located peripheral to the lateral meniscus. The common peroneal nerve, located on the posterior border of the biceps tendon, is at risk during the approach.

Posterior Approach

The posterior approach to the knee, which is reserved primarily for exposure of the neurovascular structures in the popliteal fossae, can be used for repair of these neurovascular structures, open reduction and internal fixation of avulsion fractures involving the posterior cruciate ligament attachment to the tibia, recession of gastrocnemius heads in cases of contracture, lengthening of hamstring tendons, excision of Baker's or other popliteal cysts, and access to the posterior knee capsule.

With the patient prone, an S-shaped incision is made beginning laterally over the biceps femoris, then continued obliquely across the popliteal fossa, and finally carried distally over the medial head of the gastrocnemius. This approach exposes the contents of the popliteal fossa by retracting three muscles from its margins, and therefore, does not use an internervous plane. After the skin flaps are raised, the small saphenous vein is identified as it runs proximally in the midline of the calf. The medial sural cutaneous nerve (a branch of the tibial nerve that innervates varying amounts of skin over the posterior calf), which is found on the lateral side of the saphenous vein, should also be identified. The fascia of the popliteal fossa, just medial to the small saphenous vein, is then incised, and the medial sural cutaneous nerve traced proximally to the tibial nerve. Once the tibial nerve is identified, it should be used as a guide to the apex of the popliteal fossa (formed on the medial side by the semimembranosus and on the lateral side by the biceps femoris). The common peroneal nerve is identified as it separates from the tibial nerve at the apex of the popliteal fossa. This nerve should be dissected from proximal to distal along the posterior border of the biceps femoris. Deep to the tibial nerve are the popliteal artery and vein (medial to the artery). Five main branches are given off the popliteal artery at the knee: two superior, two inferior, and one middle genicular artery, which may need to be ligated.

Approach for Lateral Meniscectomy

Various types of longitudinal, transverse, or oblique incisions can be used to expose the lateral meniscus. All incisions will expose the lateral compartment of the knee anterior to the superficial lateral ligament and can be used for lateral meniscectomy, removal of loose or foreign bodies, and treatment of osteochondritis of the lateral femoral condyle.

With the patient supine, a skin incision is made from the inferolateral corner of the patella and continued posterior and inferior for approximately 5 cm. There is no internervous plane in this approach, since the joint can be entered through the lateral patellar retinaculum and the joint capsule. The lateral inferior genicular artery is not at risk during the approach, but can be damaged during lateral meniscectomy because it lies next to the peripheral attachment of the lateral meniscus. The superficial lateral collateral ligament (fibular collateral ligament) extends from the head of the fibula to the lateral femoral condyle.

LEG

ANATOMY

The tibia and fibula, which differ in both structure and function, are of approximate equal length. The function of the tibia is to transmit the majority of the forces from the ankle to the knee. The fibula only transmits approximately 17 percent of the forces and is more important for ankle stability. The tibial shaft in cross section is triangular, with the apices anterior, medial, and posterolateral. The periosteum of the tibia supplies only 10 percent of the blood supply to the bone, with the rest coming from medullary vessels.

There are four muscular compartments in the leg: anterior, lateral, posterior (superficial and deep), and a deep flexor (Fig. 19-5). The anterior compartment consists primarily of the extensor muscles of the foot and ankle—all of which are innervated by the deep peroneal nerve and receive their blood supply from the anterior tibial artery. The lateral compartment consists of the foot evertors innervated by the superficial peroneal nerve. Since there is no artery in the lateral compartment, all the muscles receive their supply from peroneal artery branches. The posterior compartment (superficial and deep) contains the flexors of the foot and ankle. The flexors are innervated by the tibial nerve and receive their blood supply from either the posterior tibial artery or the peroneal artery. The muscles of the superficial posterior compartment are the gastrocnemius, the soleus, and the plantaris. Those of the deep posterior compartment include the flexor digitorum longus, the flexor hallucis longus, and the tibialis posterior.

The common peroneal nerve passes around the fibula neck and into the peroneus longus muscle, where it divides into deep and superficial branches. The deep peroneal nerve continues deep to the extensor digitorum longus to the anterior surface of the interosseous membrane and then runs vertically on the interosseous membrane between the tibialis anterior and the extensor hallucis longus to innervate all the muscles of the anterior compartment of the leg. The superficial peroneal nerve continues vertically down the peroneal compartment of the leg and supplies motor innervation to the peroneus longus and brevis as well as sensory innervation to the dorsum of the foot.

The popliteal artery enters the leg between the two heads of the gastrocnemius and divides into the anterior and posterior tibial arteries. The anterior tibial artery, which is the first branch of the popliteal artery, passes above the interosseous membrane to run with the deep peroneal nerve on the interosseous membrane and terminates in the foot as the dorsalis pedis artery. The posterior tibial artery continues deep in the posterior compartment of the leg, deep to the fibrous arch of the soleus. The peroneal artery is a main branch from the posterior tibial artery and is usually given off just distal to the popliteal fossa. The peroneal artery continues through the deep flexor compartment and terminates in calcaneal branches.

SURGICAL APPROACHES OF THE LEG

Anterior Approach to the Tibia

As the medial aspect of the tibia is subcutaneous, the anterior approach offers safe, easy exposure. It is useful for open reduction and internal fixation of tibial fractures, bone grafting for delayed or tibial nonunions, excision and biopsy of tumors, and tibial osteotomies. However, this approach should be avoided if there are soft tissue problems over this region of the tibia.

With the patient supine, a longitudinal incision is made just lateral to the tibia on the anterior surface of the leg. Since the dissection is from skin to subperiosteum, there is no internervous plane in this approach. Only the long saphenous vein located on the medial side of the calf is at risk during the development of skin flaps. A subperiosteal dissection is then used to reflect the tibialis anterior laterally to expose the tibia.

Posterolateral Approach to the Tibia

The posterolateral approach, which exposes the posterior middle two-thirds of the tibia and fibula, is used most often for bone grafting of tibial nonunions and occasionally for open reduction and internal fixation of fractures. With the patient in either the lateral or prone position, a longitudinal incision is made over the lateral border of the gastrocnemius. An internervous plane is developed between the gastrocnemius, soleus, and flexor hallucis longus muscles (innervated by the tibial nerve) and the peroneal muscles (innervated by the superficial peroneal nerve). Care is taken to identify and retract the short saphenous vein located on the posterolateral aspect of the leg. The fascia is incised in line with the skin incision, and the interval between the lateral head of the gastrocnemius and the soleus (posterior) and the peroneus brevis and longus (anterior) is developed. The peroneal artery often sends muscular branches that cross the intermuscular plane between the gastrocnemius and the peroneus brevis and must be ligated. Deep to this interval is the flexor hallucis longus (which originates from the posterior surface of the fibula) that must be detached along with the soleus origin from the fibula. As the dissection is carried deeper, the origin of the tibialis posterior must be dissected free from the interosseous membrane. The posterior tibial artery and nerve are safe during this exposure because they lie superficial to the muscle belly of the tibialis posterior and the flexor hallucis longus. The dissection then follows the interosseous membrane to the lateral border of the tibia, where it is continued subperiosteally.

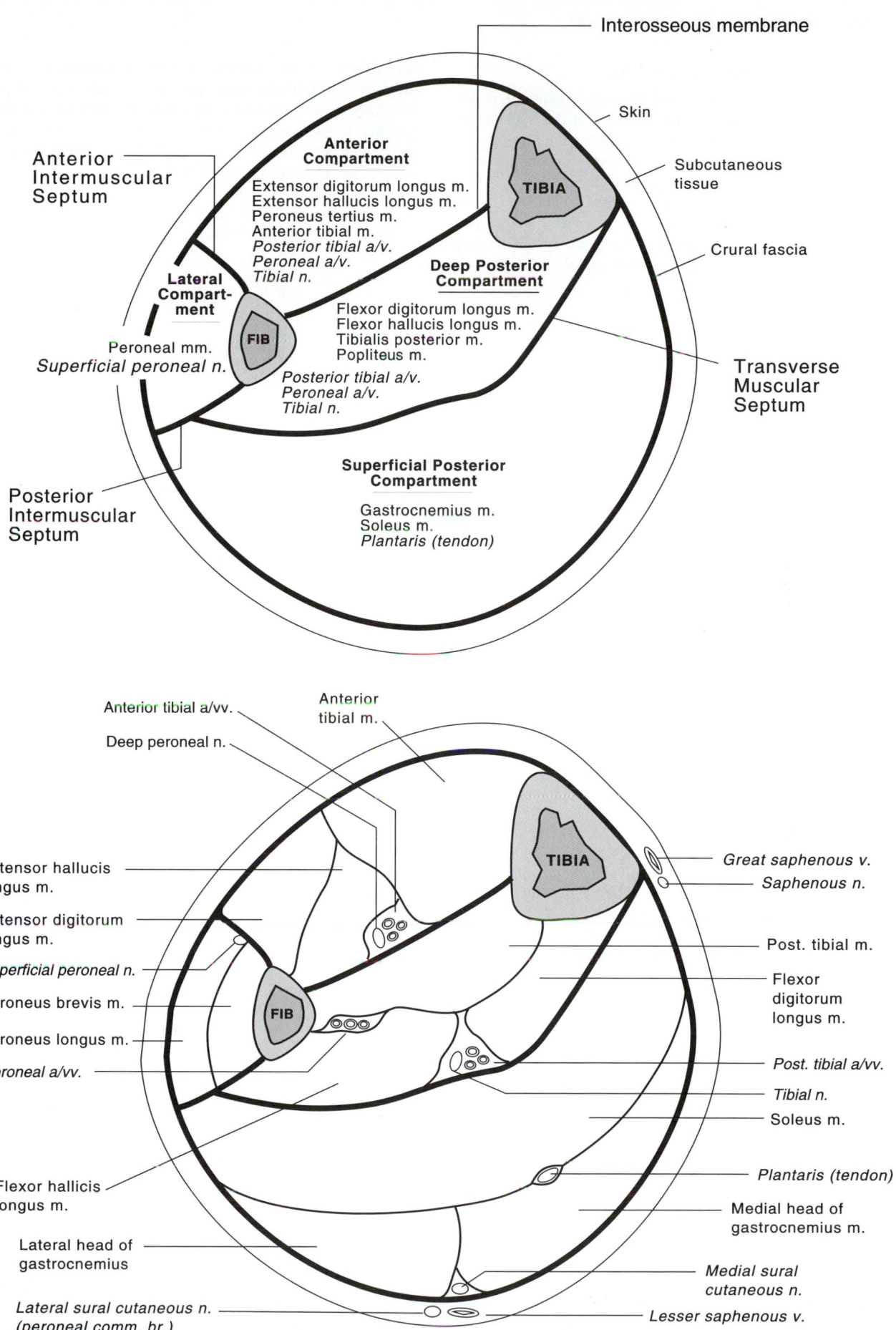

Figure 19-5
Cross sectional and compartmental anatomy of the mid-portion of the leg.

Approach to the Fibula

The approach, which enables the entire fibula to be exposed, is useful for fibula osteotomy or ostectomy, resection of the fibula to decompress all four compartments of the leg for a compartment syndrome, resection of tumors, treatment of osteomyelitis, and for open reduction and internal fixation of fibula fractures.

With the patient either supine or lateral, a vertical incision is made posterior to the fibula. Care should be take to avoid the common peroneal nerve because it is subcutaneous at the fibula neck. The deep fascia is incised in line with the skin incision, and the posterior border of the biceps femoris tendon and common peroneal nerve identified. A branch of the superficial peroneal nerve, which is located anteriorly at the distal and middle third of the fibula, can be injured, resulting in numbness on the dorsum of the foot. With the common peroneal nerve retracted anteriorly, an interval between the peroneal muscles and the soleus is developed. The deep dissection uses the internervous interval between the peroneal muscles (innervated by the superficial peroneal nerve) and the foot flexor muscles (innervated by the tibial nerve). The muscles are then dissected from the fibula by sharp dissection.

APPENDIX

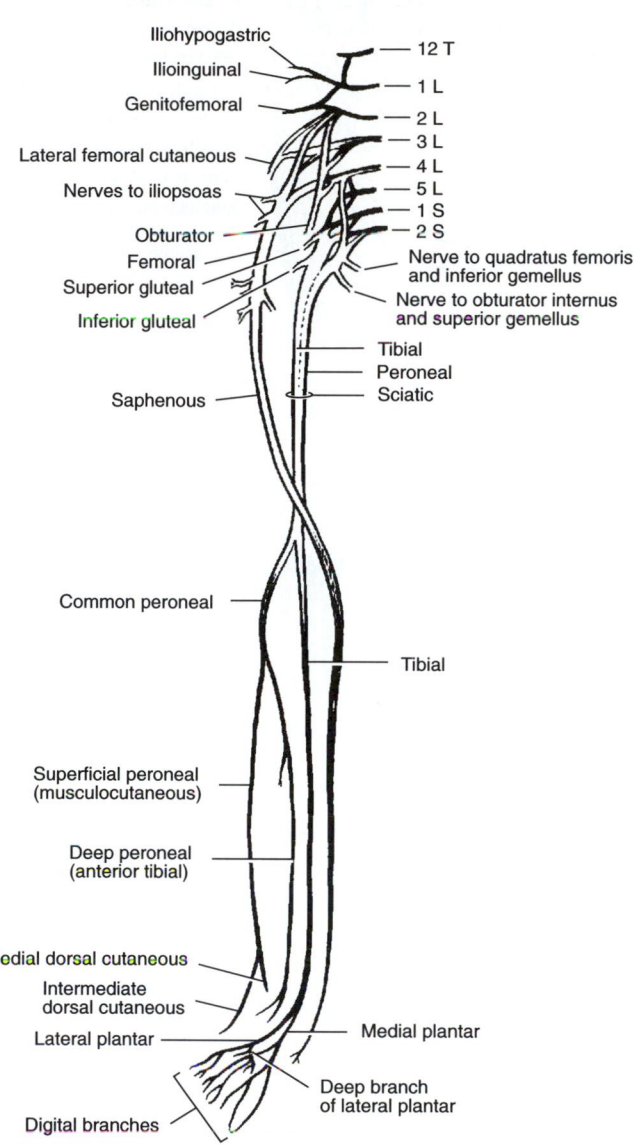

Figure 19-6
Nerves of the lower extremity. [Reproduced and modified with permission from Warfel JH: *The Extremities,* 4th ed. Philadelphia: Lea & Febiger (now Lippincott Williams & Wilkins); 1981:115.]

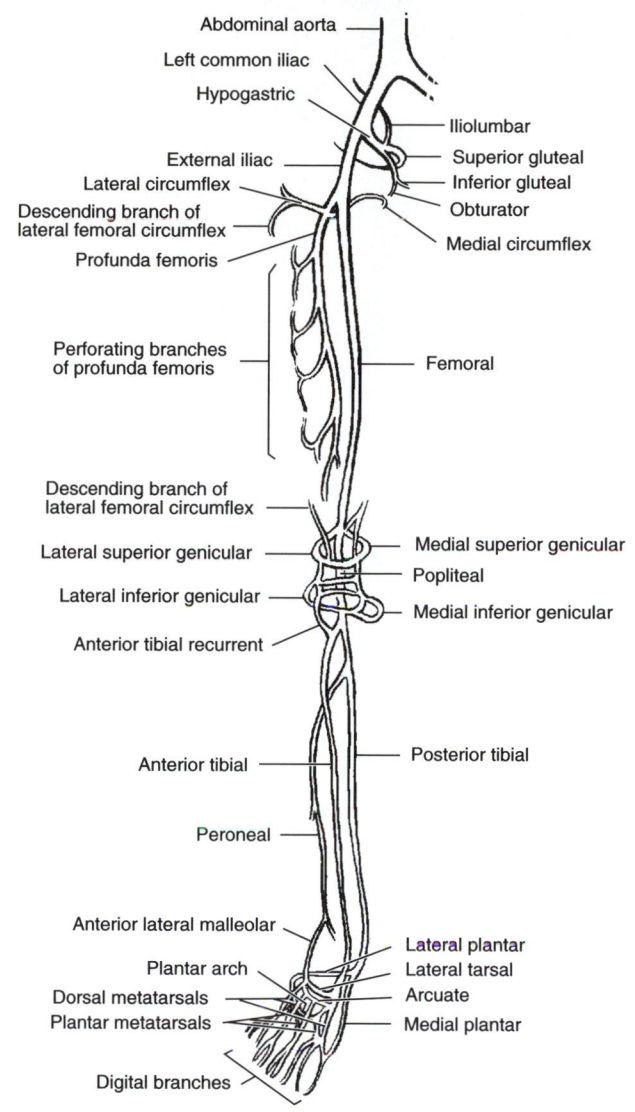

Figure 19-7
Arteries of the lower extremity. [Reproduced and modified with permission from Warfel JH: *The Extremities,* 4th ed. Philadelphia: Lea & Febiger (now Lippincott Williams & Wilkins); 1981:116.]

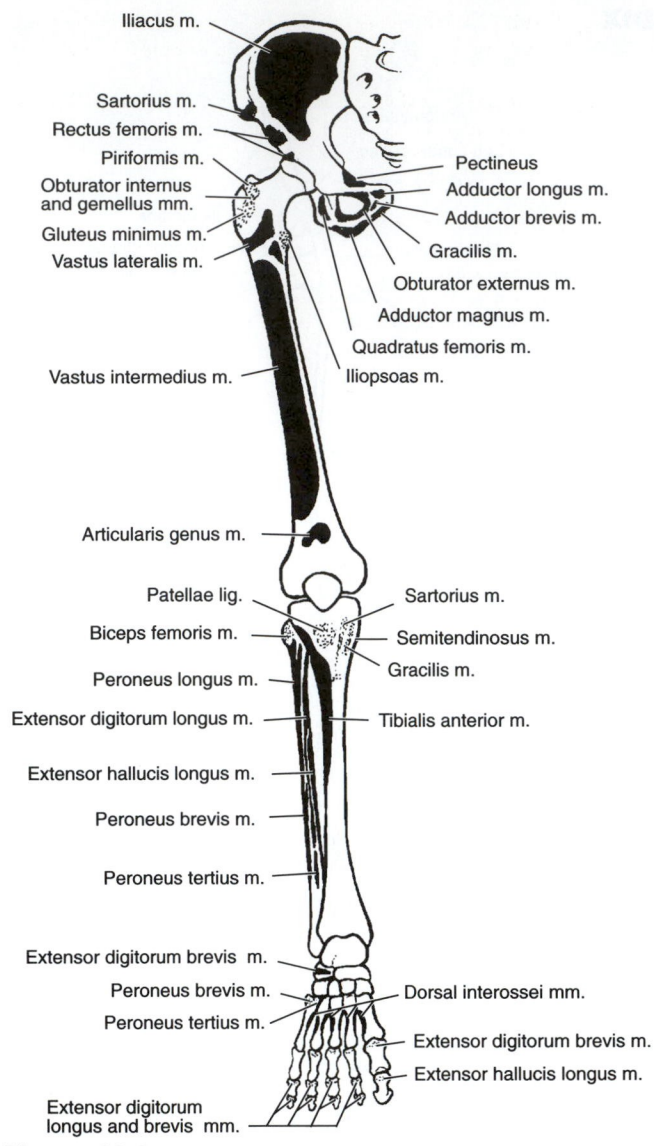

Figure 19-8

Muscles of the lower right extremity (anterior). (Muscle insertions, dotted; origins, solid.) [Reproduced and modified with permission from Warfel JH: *The Extremities,* 4th ed. Philadelphia: Lea & Febiger (now Lippincott Williams & Wilkins); 1981:119.]

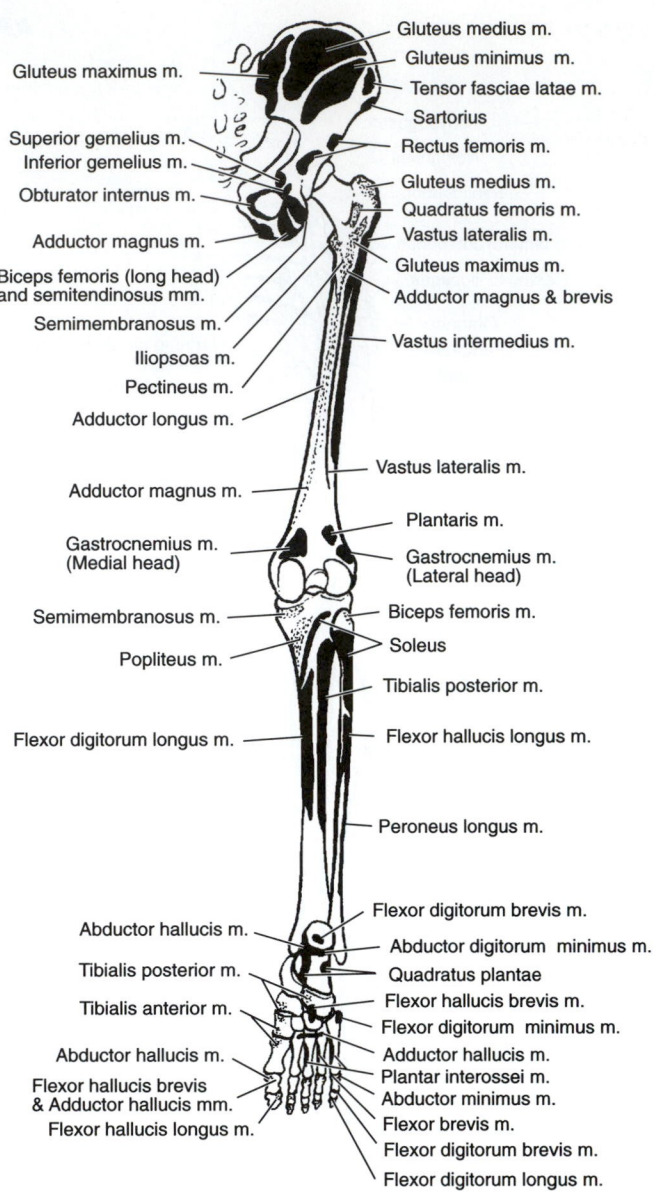

Figure 19-9

Muscles of the lower right extremity (posterior). (Muscle insertions, dotted; origins, solid.) [Reproduced and modified with permission from Warfel JH: *The Extremities,* 4th ed. Philadelphia: Lea & Febiger (now Lippincott Williams & Wilkins); 1981:120.]

SUGGESTED READINGS

Hoppenfeld S: *Surgical Exposures in Orthopaedics: The Anatomic Approach.* Philadelphia: JB Lippincott; 1994:303–511.

Netter FH: *Atlas of Human Anatomy.* Summit, NJ: CIBA-GEIGY; 1989.

O'Rahilly R (ed): The lower limb. In: *Gardner-Gray-O'Rahilly Anatomy: A Regional Study of Human Structure,* 5th ed. Philadelphia: WB Saunders; 1986:157.

Rosse C, Gaddum-Rosse P, Hollinshead WR (eds): *Hollinshead's Textbook of Anatomy,* 5th ed. Philadelphia: Lippincott-Raven; 1997.

Warfel JH: *The Extremities.* Philadelphia: Lea & Febiger; 1974.

Chapter 20

FOOT AND ANKLE: ANATOMY

Myles Rubin Samotin and Steven C. Sheskier

OSTEOLOGY

There are 26 foot bones (14 phalanges, 5 metatarsals, and 7 tarsal bones), not including the sesamoids and accessory bones.

TALUS

The talus is a bone of complex shape consisting of three parts: body, neck, and head. The surface is 60 percent cartilaginous. It forms the universal joint between the leg, hindfoot, and midfoot. There are no endogenous attachments to this bone. Hence, all of its motions are passive and occur through its linkage to surrounding bones. The blood supply is unique and prone to injury. The body is capped with a convex cartilaginous surface which subtends an arc of approximately 90 degrees. The talar dome articulates with the tibia and fibula in the ankle mortise. The anterior portion of the talar dome is wider than the posterior portion. Inferiorly, it is concave and articulates with the posterior and medial facets of the calcaneus. The body has medial and lateral processes. Posteriorly, there is a posterolateral process of variable length that may be nonunited and is called an *os trigonum.* This is present in 7 percent of the population and may be confused with a fracture. The posterior talofibular ligament attaches to this process.

The talar neck is devoid of cartilage and is the site of ligamentous, capsular, and vascular attachments. Its origin is medial to the center of the body and tends to deviate medially. Obliquely running on its under surface is a channel called the *tarsal canal.* A vascular leash, consisting of branches of the posterior tibial and peroneal artery, runs within the tarsal canal (Fig. 20-1).

The head of the talus is completely covered with cartilage and articulates with the navicular and anterior process of the calcaneus.

CALCANEUS

The talus is perched upon this complex bone via three articular surfaces: posterior, medial, and anterior facets, (convex, concave, and planar, respectively). It articulates with the cuboid anteriorly. The anteromedial aspect has a strong cortical surface, the sustentaculum tali, which overhangs horizontally and supports the middle articular facet of the talocalcaneal joint above it. Plantar vessels and nerves pass inferior to the sustentaculum tali.

MIDFOOT

The midfoot consists of five cancellous bones. The proximal bones, the cuboid and the navicular, articulate with the anterior portions of the calcaneus and talus, respectively. On the plantar lateral aspect of the cuboid lies a groove through which the peroneus longus tendon sweeps from the lateral aspect to the undersurface of the foot. The cuboid also articulates with the lateral cuneiform, as well as the fourth and fifth metatarsals. The navicular articulates with the medial, mid-

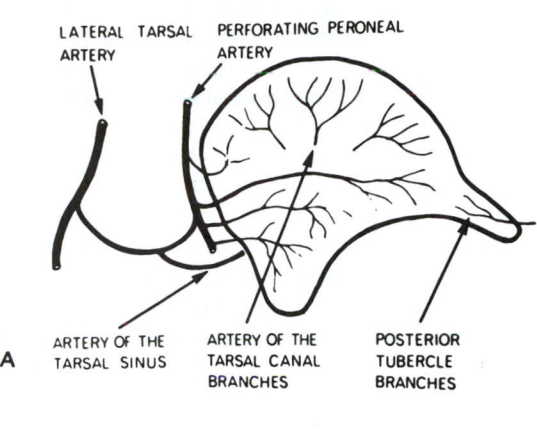

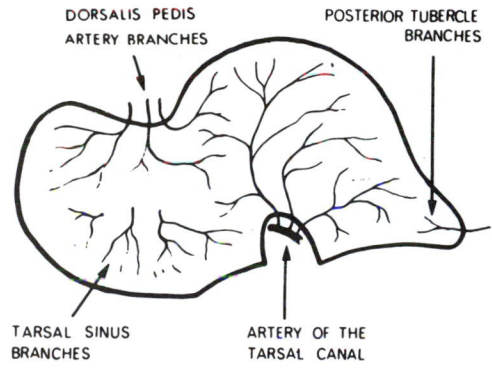

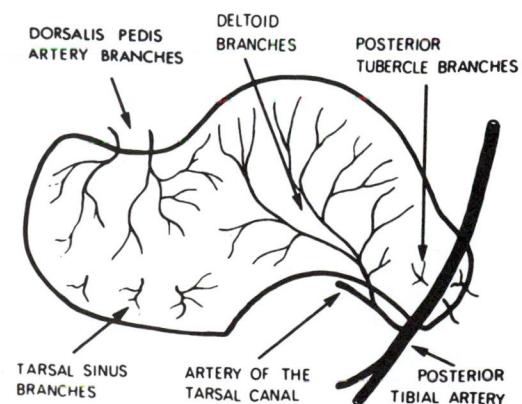

Figure 20-1

Blood supply to the talus in sagittal sections. (*A*) Lateral third of the talus. (*B*) The middle third of the talus. (*C*) Medial third of the talus. (Reproduced with permission from Sarrafian SK: Angiology. In *Anatomy of the Foot and Ankle: Descriptive, Topographic, Functional,* 2d ed. Philadelphia: Lippincott; 1993:334. Original source: Mulfinger GL, Trueta J: The blood supply of the talus. *J Bone Joint Surg [Br]* 1970; 52:160.)

dle, and lateral cuneiforms at its distal articulation. The three cuneiform bones lie anterior to the navicular and medial to the cuboid. They form the start of the transverse arch of the foot and provide the inset for the base of the second metatarsal, the keystone of the metatarsal arch.

FOREFOOT

The forefoot consists of five metatarsals and five sets of phalanges. The first metatarsal is distinguished by its increased width and cortical thickness, which is not surprising since it normally bears between 33 and 50 percent of body weight. Two sesamoids lie beneath the first metatarsal head, specifically within the substance of the flexor hallucis brevis tendon, separated by a crista. They are notorious for being bipartite or even tripartite, with the medial sesamoid being most commonly involved and usually larger than the uninvolved one. Other sesamoids are inconsistently present under the lesser metatarsal heads as well as the phalanges. The second metatarsal may be longer than the first metatarsal (Morton's foot) or equal in length. It also extends more proximally than the other metatarsals into the previously mentioned inset in the cuneiform bones. The fifth metatarsal is notable for its nonarticular posterior extension into which the peroneus brevis and lateral portion of the plantar fascia attach. The phalanges consist of three bones except for the first toe, which has two bones. The fifth toe commonly has a congenital fusion between the middle and distal phalanges.

JOINTS, ARTICULATIONS, AND LIGAMENTS

ANKLE

The distal tibia along with the distal fibula form the mortise that cups the articular surface of the talar dome. The ankle joint is known as a *ginglymus,* or hinge joint. The stability of the joint relies on its bony and ligamentous architecture. When weightbearing, the two malleoli help to prevent inversion and eversion of the ankle joint. Numerous ligamentous structures also help to prevent excess ankle inversion and eversion. Medially, the broad expanse of the deltoid ligament resists valgus forces. The deltoid ligament is divided into two portions: superficial and deep. The superficial portion of the deltoid ligament is comprised of three structures that all have as their origin the medial malleolus and insert respectively into the navicular tuberosity, sustentaculum tali, and the inner side of the talus. The deep portion of the deltoid ligament is the strongest portion of this ligament and is intraarticular. It has as its origin the medial malleolus and inserts into the medial surface of the talus.

On the lateral side of the ankle, three distinct ligaments are present. The anterior talofibular ligament has its origin at the lateral malleolus and extends forward transversely to insert onto the posterolateral portion of the talar neck. The anterior talofibular ligament is the weakest of the three lateral ankle ligaments and is therefore the most commonly injured ligament in lateral ankle sprains. The middle ligament, known as the calcaneofibular ligament, originates from the lateral malleolus as well and extends obliquely posteriorly to insert into the lateral wall of the calcaneus. The third lateral ankle ligament, known as the posterior talofibular ligament, originates at the lateral malleolus and extends transversely posteriorly to insert into the posterior aspect of the talus. The posterior talofibular ligament is the strongest of the three ankle ligaments and is only torn in the most severe lateral ankle sprains. The anterior talofibular ligament is most taut when the foot is in plantar flexion. The calcaneofibular ligament resists valgus forces when the foot is in neutral position. Anterior displacement of the talus on the tibia is resisted by the bony mechanical fit of the convex talus in the concavity of the distal tibial plafond

as well as by the combined efforts of both the deltoid and lateral ankle ligaments.

INFERIOR TIBIOFIBULAR JOINT

The inferior tibiofibular joint is formed by the medial aspect of the distal fibula, known as the *incisura fibularis,* and the lateral distal aspect of the tibia. There are four separate ligaments that bind this joint. The anterior inferior tibiofibular ligament binds the joint anteriorly while the posterior tibiofibular ligament, smaller in size than the anterior inferior tibiofibular ligament, binds the joint posteriorly. There is an additional posteriorly located ligament, known as the inferior transverse ligament, which lies just below the posterior tibiofibular ligament. An interosseous ligament serves as the fourth ligament to bind this joint.

SUBTALAR JOINT

The subtalar joint lies between the talus above and the calcaneus below and is responsible for heel inversion and eversion. This is not a pure motion and has been likened to a screw mechanism in which inversion has been associated with internal rotation in relation to the talus. *Chopart's joints,* the talonavicular and calcaneocuboid joints, work in conjunction with the subtalar joint by augmenting the amount of adduction and abduction associated with inversion and eversion respectively. When the heel is everted, Chopart's joints are loosely packed and allow motion through them. When the heel is inverted, Chopart's joints are tightly packed and lock into position. It is for this reason that, during subtalar fusion, it is best to place the subtalar joint in an everted or valgus position. This allows movement through Chopart's joints, also known as the transverse tarsal joints, to occur. The posterior tibial tendon, with its main insertion and six other accessory insertions across the midtarsal bones, acts as the dynamic controller of this locking mechanism across Chopart's or the transverse tarsal joint.

The talocalcaneal interosseous ligament, also known as the interosseous ligament as well as the cervical ligament, originates from the talus and inserts into the calcaneus and separates the posterior and medial facets of this joint. This ligament prevents excessive eversion of the talus on the calcaneus. The majority of the dorsal ligaments traversing Chopart's joints are thin and relatively inconsequential except for the dorsal extensions of the deltoid ligament. The spring ligament, also known as the plantar calcaneonavicular ligament, lies plantar medially, arises from the sustentaculum tali, and inserts into the navicular. It forms a hammock upon which the undersurface of the talar head rests. Lateral to the spring ligament lie the short and long plantar ligaments. The short plantar ligament, also known as the plantar calcaneocuboid ligament, extends from the calcaneus to the cuboid. This short plantar ligament is felt to be the main static strut of the longitudinal arch. The long plantar ligament, also known as the calcaneocuboid-metatarsal ligament, is of lesser importance in this regard and extends from the calcaneus to the cuboid and first through fifth metatarsals. On the lateral side of the foot lies the bifurcate ligament, also known as the calcaneocuboid/calcaneonavicular ligament, which originates on the anterior process of the calcaneus and divides into two strong bands that insert onto the cuboid and lateral portion of the navicular, respectively.

LISFRANC JOINTS

Lisfranc joints lie between the metatarsal and the midtarsal bones (the three cuneiform bones and the cuboid). Bony stability is achieved through the triangular configuration of the metatarsal bases forming a transverse arch, with the second metatarsal base forming the keystone of the arch, the latter being further stabilized by its inset into the cuneiforms. The strongest ligamentous structure stabilizing the configuration lies plantar to these joints and is the *Lisfranc ligament,* also known as the tarsometatarsal ligament. It originates on the plantar aspect of the medial cuneiform and extends to the base of the second metatarsal. This ligament is stronger in tension than the bone it inserts on. Hence, a Lisfranc fragment may be the only initial radiographic finding suggesting that a dislocation of this joint has occurred and spontaneously reduced. The lateral tarsometatarsal joints are the most mobile, with minimal motion at the second joint. While the lateral four metatarsal bases articulate with each other and are secured by ligaments to each other, the first metatarsal base does not. The first tarsometatarsal joint displays variable degrees of mobility from none to hypermobility and can be associated with pes planus and hallux valgus.

Metatarsophalangeal joints are similar in structure to their counterparts in the hand. They are stabilized by collateral ligaments as well as a volar plate plantarly. The first metatarsophalangeal sesamoid complex is more complex. The interphalangeal joints are supported mainly by their capsules (Fig. 20-2).

MUSCULOTENDINOUS ANATOMY

The majority of the motions of the foot and ankle are dependent on muscles that originate proximal to the ankle joint (Fig. 20-3). The in-

trinsic muscles of the foot play a moderating role on the extrinsic muscle action, especially evident in the toes. The action of these tendons on ankle, hindfoot, and forefoot motion is dependent upon their relationship to the various axes of motion to the joints in question. Though each tendon can be said to have a primary function, they can and do have secondary functions in both physiological and pathological conditions. For example, when there is a weakness of the anterior tibialis muscle, the extensor hallucis longus can act as a dorsiflexor of the ankle, but only after the great toe is maximally dorsiflexed. The majority of the extrinsic muscle functions are intuitively obvious, but some are not. The peroneus longus assists the brevis in eversion and plantar flexion of the ankle. However, due to its insertion on the plantar aspect of the first metatarsal, the peroneus longus is responsible for plantar flexion of the first metatarsal as well (Table 20-1). It is useful to divide muscles of the leg into their four compartments; anterior, lateral, posterior, and deep posterior, respectively. Muscles intrinsic to the foot are divided into four plantar layers as well.

NERVE ANATOMY

All nerves innervating structures of the foot and ankle originate from the sciatic nerve which branches into tibial and common peroneal branches.

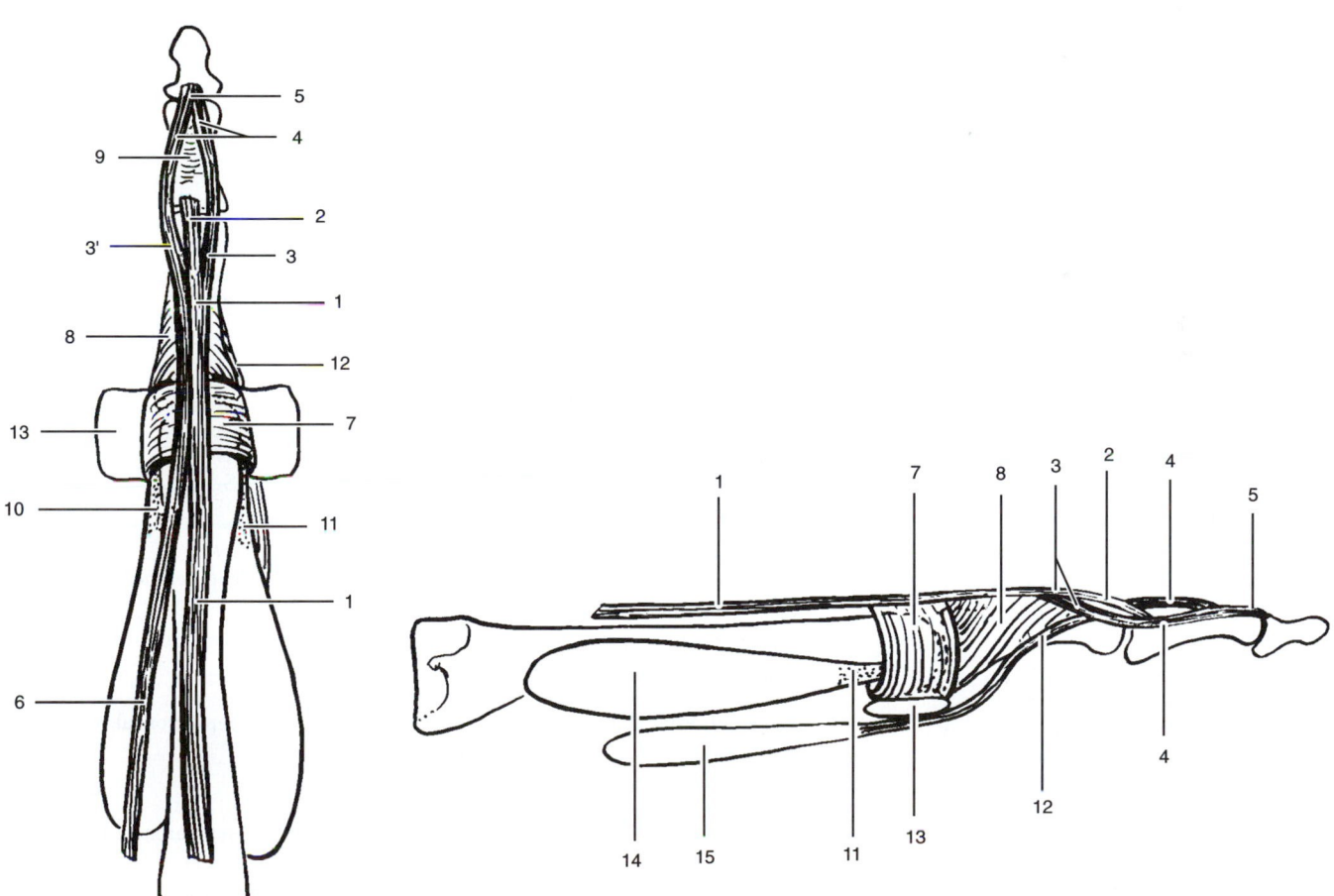

Figure 20-2
Extensor complex of a lesser toe: (1) extensor digitorum longus tendon, (2) middle slip of extensor tendon trifurcation, (3, 3') lateral slips of extensor tendon trifurcation, (4) lateral tendons of extensor tendon trifurcation, (5) terminal extensor tendon, (6) extensor digitorum brevis tendon, (7) transverse lamina of extensor aponeurosis or extensor sling, (8) oblique component of extensor aponeurosis forming the extensor hood or wing, (9) triangular ligament, (10, 11) interossei tendons, (12) lumbrical tendon, (13) deep transverse metatarsal ligament, (14) interosseous muscle, (15) lumbrical tendon. (Reproduced with permission from Sarrafian SK: Myology, In *Anatomy of the Foot and Ankle: Descriptive, Topographic, Functional,* 2d ed. Philadelphia: JB Lippincott; 1993:224.)

Table 20-1

Muscles of the Foot and Ankle

Muscle	Origin	Insertion	Action	Innervation
POSTERIOR COMPARTMENT				
1. Gastrocnemius	Posterior lateral and medial femoral condyles	Posterior calcaneus	1° Ankle plantarflexion 2° Foot inversion	Tibial nerve (S_1)
2. Soleus	Posterior fibula and tibia	Posterior calcaneus	1° Ankle plantarflexion 2° Foot inversion	Tibial nerve (S_1)
3. Plantaris	Lateral femoral condyle	Posterior calcaneus	Ankle plantarflexion	Tibial nerve (S_1)
DEEP POSTERIOR COMPARTMENT				
1. Flexor hallucis longus	Fibula	1st Toe, distal phalanx	1° 1st toe plantarflexion 2° Ankle plantarflexion 2° Foot inversion	Tibial nerve (S_1)
2. Flexor digitorum longus	Tibia	2d–5th Toes, distal phalanges	1° Lesser toe plantarflexion 2° Ankle plantarflexion 2° Foot inversion	Tibial nerve (S_1S_2)
3. Posterior tibial	Tibia, fibula, interosseous membrane	Tuberosity of navicular, inferior surface of medial cuneiform, middle cuneiform, lateral cuneiform, cuboid, bases of 2d, 3d, 4th, 5th metatarsals	1° Foot inversion 2° Ankle plantarflexion	Tibial nerve (L_4L_5)
LATERAL COMPARTMENT				
1. Peroneus longus	Proximal fibula	Plantar aspect of medial cuneiform Lateral tubercle of base of 1st metatarsal	1° Foot inversion 2° Ankle plantarflexion 1st metatarsal Plantarflexion Foot abduction	Superficial peroneal nerve (S_1)
2. Peroneus brevis	Distal fibula	Styloid apophysis of 5th metatarsal base	1° Foot eversion 2° Ankle plantarflexion	Superficial peroneal nerve (S_1)
ANTERIOR COMPARTMENT				
1. Anterior tibial	Lateral tibia	Medial aspect of medial cuneiform, inferior medial aspect of 1st metatarsal base	1° Ankle dorsiflexion 2° Foot inversion 2° Foot eversion	Deep peroneal nerve (L_4)
2. Extensor hallucis longus	Fibula	Dorsum of distal phalanx 1st Toe base	1° 1st Toe dorsiflexion 2° Ankle dorsiflexion 2° Foot eversion	Deep peroneal nerve (L_5)
3. Extensor digitorum longus	Tibia and fibula	Lesser toe Middle and distal phalanges	1° Lesser toe dorsiflexion 2° Ankle dorsiflexion 2° Foot eversion	Deep peroneal nerve (L_5)
4. Peroneus tertius	Fibula	Dorsum of 5th metatarsal base	2° Foot eversion 2° Ankle dorsiflexion	Deep peroneal nerve (S_1)

Table 20-1

Muscles of the Foot and Ankle *(Continued)*

Muscle	Origin	Insertion	Action	Innervation
INTRINSIC MUSCLES OF THE FOOT				
First Plantar Layer (Most Superficial)				
1. Abductor hallucis	Tuberosity of calcaneus	Base of 1st toe, proximal phalanx	1st Toe abduction 1st Toe MTP joint flexion	Medial plantar nerve
2. Flexor digitorum brevis	Posteromedial tuberosity of calcaneus	Inferior aspect of 2d–5th toes, middle phalanges	Flexion lesser toes	Medial plantar nerve
3. Abductor digiti minimi	Tuberosity of calcaneus	Plantar plate of 5th MTP joint, lateral aspect of 5th toe proximal phalanx	5th Toe abduction	Lateral plantar nerve
Second Plantar Layer				
1. Quadratus plantae	Lateral head: posterolateral calcaneal tuberosity Medial head: posteromedial aspect of calcaneal tuberosity	FDL tendon	2° Flexion distal phalanges Lesser toes, flexion MTP joints Extension IP joints	Lateral plantar nerve
2. Lumbricals (4)	FDL tendons	EDL tendons at extensor hood	Flexion MTP joints, extension IP joints	Medial and lateral plantar nerves
3. (FDL & FHL)[a]				
Third Plantar Layer				
1. Flexor hallucis brevis	Cuboid and lateral cuneiform	1st Toe, proximal phalanx	1st Toe, MTP joint flexion	Medial plantar nerve
2. Adductor hallucis	2 Heads: 1. 2d–4th Metatarsals 2. 3d, 4th, 5th MTP joints	Lateral aspect of proximal phalanx 1st toe Lateral sesamoid	Adduction 1st toe 1st Toe, MTP joint flexion	Lateral plantar nerve
3. Flexor digiti minimi brevis	Base of 5th metatarsal head, cuboid, plantar aponeurosis	Base of 5th toe, proximal phalanx; plantar plate of 5th toe MTP joint	5th Toe flexion	Lateral plantar nerve
Fourth Plantar Layer				
1. Dorsal interossei (4)	Lateral 1st, 2d, 3d, 4th metatarsal shafts	Medial and lateral aspect of 2d toe Lateral aspects of 3d, 4th toes	Flexion MTP joints Extension IP joints Abduction toes	Lateral plantar nerve
2. Plantar interossei (3)	Medial aspect of 3d, 4th, 5th metatarsal shafts	Medial aspect of 3d, 4th, 5th toes	Adduction toes Flexion MTP joints Extension IP joints	Lateral plantar nerve
3. (Peroneus longus and posterior tibial)[b]				
Dorsal Layer				
1. Extensor digitorum brevis	Anterolateral aspect of sinus tarsi	Lateral base of proximal phalanges of 1st, 2d, 3d, 4th toes [No slip of extensor brevis tendon to 5th toe]	Extension 1st, 2d, 3d, 4th toes	Deep peroneal nerve

[a]See above, under Deep Posterior Compartment.

[b]Peroneus longus, see under Lateral Compartment; Posterior tibial, see under Deep Posterior Compartment.

TIBIAL NERVE

The tibial nerve travels in the posterior aspect of the leg, coursing between the two heads of the gastrocnemius muscle. It then passes deep to the soleus muscle to arrive at the posterior aspect of the medial malleolus. The tibial nerve is the larger, medial, and terminal branch of the sciatic nerve. In the ankle region, the tibial nerve lies posterior to the flexor digitorum longus muscle and anterior to the flexor hallucis longus muscle. It curves anteroinferiorly behind the medial malleolus, between these two tendons, and deep within the flexor retinaculum. The tibial nerve gives off muscular, articular, calcaneal, medial, and lateral plantar, as well as osseous and vascular branches. The nerve terminates at the medial malleolar level by dividing into the medial and lateral plantar nerves. Muscular branches of the tibial nerve include those to the gastrocnemius, soleus, posterior tibial,

flexor digitorum longus, and flexor hallucis longus muscles. These branches are mostly given off in the upper third of the leg. Articular branches help to supply the ankle and superior and inferior tibiofibular joints. Under the flexor retinaculum, the tibial nerve splits into two branches. The *medial plantar nerve* is the larger of the two. It arises when the tibial nerve passes beneath the posterior part of the abductor hallucis muscle and then travels forward in the medial intermuscular septum between the abductor hallucis and flexor digitorum brevis muscles. Both the medial and lateral plantar nerves run in the second plantar foot layer. The medial plantar nerve supplies plantar sensation to the medial 3-1/2 digits and motor sensation to the flexor hallucis brevis, the abductor hallucis, the flexor digitorum brevis, and the first lumbrical (Fig. 20-4).

LATERAL PLANTAR NERVE

The lateral plantar nerve, which is smaller than the medial plantar nerve, runs obliquely under the quadratus plantae muscle. It provides innervation to the abductor digiti minimi and quadratus plantae muscles, the flexor digiti minimi brevis muscle, and sometimes the two interosseous muscles of the fourth interspace. It also supplies sensation to the lateral 1-1/2 digits of the foot. The usual bifurcation of the posterior tibial nerve into its medial and lateral plantar terminal branches occurs 1.3 cm proximal to the tip of the medial malellus. There is also a *cutaneous calcaneal branch of the posterior tibial nerve* that provides sensation to the skin of the medial malleolar area as well as the inner aspect of the heel. It should be noted that at the level of the tarsal tunnel the first branch coming off of the lateral plantar nerve is known as the *nerve to the abductor digiti quinti*. At the lower border of the abductor hallucis, this nerve turns and courses laterally in a transverse fashion passing immediately anterior to the medial calcaneal tuberosity. It is located between the quadratus plantae and the underlying flexor digitorum brevis-plantar aponeurosis complex. It then penetrates the abductor digiti quinti on its deep surface. A clinical association has been established between certain types of plantar heel pain and injury to this nerve.

COMMON PERONEAL NERVE

The common peroneal nerve is the smaller terminal division of the sciatic nerve. It winds around the fibular neck deep to the peroneus longus muscle and at this point divides into superficial and deep branches. The *superficial peroneal nerve* runs between the lateral and anterior compartments in the leg. It terminates in two cutaneous branches; the medial and the intermediate dorsal cutaneous nerves of the dorsum of the foot. The *intermediate dorsal cutaneous nerve* courses over the third intermetatarsal space to supply sensation to the dorsolateral aspect of the third toe and the dorsomedial aspect of the fourth toe. The *medial dorsal cutaneous nerve* is the largest branch of the superficial nerve and further divides into three branches: lateral, middle, and medial. These branches supply sensation to the dorsolateral portions of the second toe, the dorsomedial portion of the third toe, and the dorsomedial aspect of the first toe.

DEEP PERONEAL NERVE

The deep peroneal nerve, also known as the anterior tibial nerve, runs along the anterior portion of the interosseous membrane. Immediately above the ankle, the deep peroneal nerve is located between the ex-

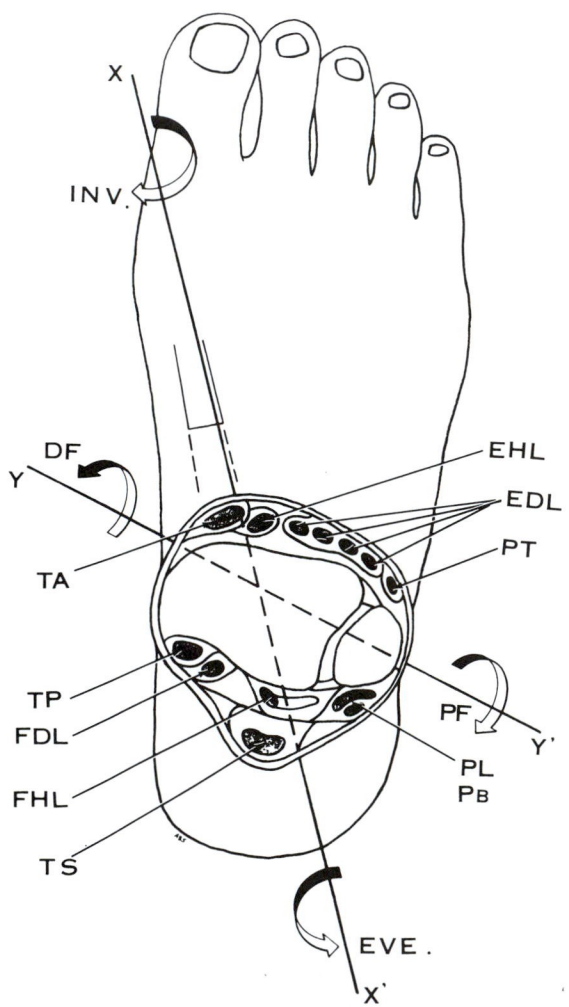

Figure 20-3

Motors of the ankle and hind foot. (XX', axis of motion of the talocalcaneonavicular joint; YY', axis of motion of the ankle joint; INV, inversion; EVE, eversion; DF, dorsiflexion; PL, plantar flexion). *Invertors:* TA, tibialis anterior; TP, tibialis posterior; FDL, flexor digitorium longus; FHL, flexor hallucis longus; TS, triceps surae. *Evertors:* PL, peroneus longus; PB, peroneus brevis; EHL, extensor hallucis longus; EDL, extensor digitorum longus; TA, tibialis anterior; PT, peroneous tertius. Plantar flexors: TP, FDL, FHL, TS, PL, PB. Dorsiflexors: TA, EHL, EDL, PT. (Reproduced with permission from Sarrafian SK: Functional anatomy of the foot and ankle. In *Anatomy of the Foot and Ankle: Descriptive, Topographic, Functional,* 2d ed. Philadelphia: JB Lippincott; 1993:551.)

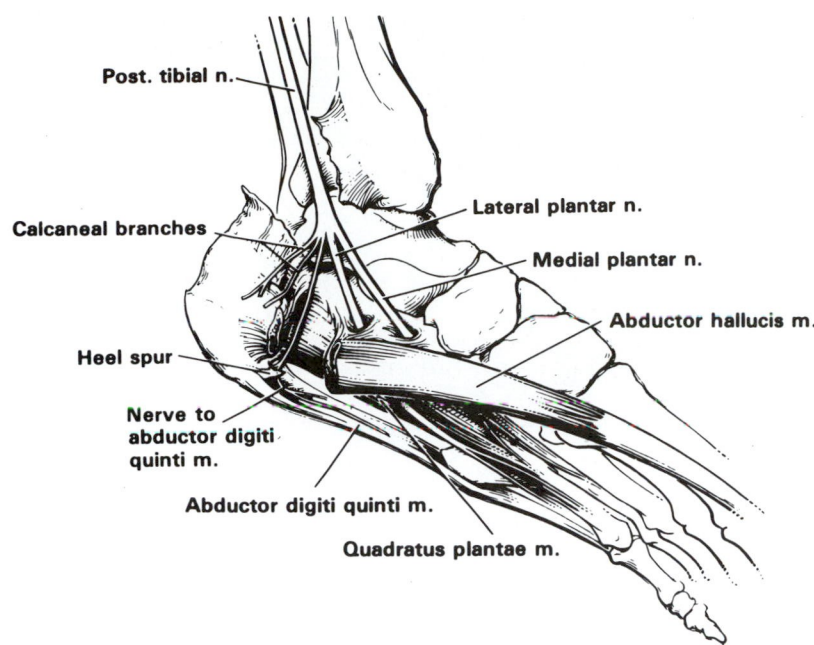

Post. tibial n.

Calcaneal branches

Heel spur

Nerve to
abductor digiti
quinti m.

Abductor digiti quinti m.

Quadratus plantae m.

Lateral plantar n.

Medial plantar n.

Abductor hallucis m.

Figure 20-4
Posterior tibial nerve and its terminal branches.
(Reproduced with permission from Baxter DE,
Thigpen CM: Heel pain–operative results. *Foot Ankle*
1984; 5:18.)

tensor hallucis longus and the extensor digitorum longus tendon, and is usually found lateral to the anterior tibial artery. Right above the ankle joint, it divides into medial and lateral terminal branches. The larger medial branch is located between the extensor hallucis longis tendon and the extensor hallucis brevis muscle. When it reaches the first intermetatarsal space, it pierces the dorsal aponeurosis of the foot and supplies sensation to the dorsolateral aspect of the first toe as well as the dorsomedial aspect of the second toe. The lateral branch of the deep peroneal nerve proceeds anterolaterally where it innervates the extensor digitorum brevis muscle.

SURAL NERVE

The sural nerve is formed by the union of branches of the tibial nerve with branches from the common peroneal nerve. The sural nerve then courses along the lateral aspect of the Achilles tendon. It passes around the posterior border of the lateral malleolus at a distance of approximately 1 to 1.5 cm from its tip. At the level of the fifth metatarsal tuberosity, it divides into lateral and medial terminal branches. The lateral branch provides sensory innervation to the dorsolateral aspect of the fifth toe. The medial branch provides sensory innervation to the dorsomedial aspect of the fifth toe and possibly the dorsolateral aspect of the fourth toe. Behind and slightly above the lateral malleolus, the sural nerve provides a lateral calcaneal branch that supplies sensation to the outer aspect of the heel.

SAPHENOUS NERVE

The saphenous nerve is the terminal branch of the femoral nerve, found on the medial aspect of the knee between the sartorius and gracilis muscles. It runs down the leg behind the medial border of the tibia, just posterior to the greater saphenous vein. Proximal to the ankle, it divides into two branches: the first branch terminates at the ankle level, and the second branch passes anterior to the medial malellus, providing sensation to the medial side of the foot.

VASCULAR ANATOMY

The *femoral artery* continues in the knee as the *popliteal artery,* which divides into anterior and posterior tibial arteries. The *anterior tibial artery* passes between the posterior tibial muscle and the interosseous membrane and runs distally on the anterior surface of the interosseous membrane between the anterior tibial muscle and extensor hallucis longus. It terminates as the *dorsalis pedis artery* which provides the blood supply to the dorsum of the foot. It divides into many branches with its largest branch, the *deep plantar artery,* running between the first and second metatarsals.

The *posterior tibial artery* runs down the leg in the deep posterior compartment. It passes behind the medial malleolus, coursing anteriorly and distally in the neurovascular bundle which is located between the flexor digitorum longus tendon and the flexor hallucis longus tendon. At the medial malleolar level, the posterior tibial artery terminates by dividing into *medial* and *lateral plantar arteries.* This occurs deep to the abductor hallucis muscle belly. The larger lateral plantar branch of the posterior tibial artery anastomoses with the deep plantar artery of the dorsalis pedis artery to form the arterial plantar arch, which is located in the fourth plantar layer of the foot.

SUGGESTED READINGS

Hoppenfeld S, deBoer P: The ankle and foot. In *Surgical Exposure in Orthopaedics: The Anatomic Approach,* 2d ed. Philadelphia: JB Lippincott Company; 1994:513.

Lutter LD, Mizel MS, Pfeffer GB (eds): *Orthopaedic Knowledge Update: Foot and Ankle,* Rosemont, IL: American Academy of Orthopaedic Surgeons; 1994.

Mann RA, Coughlin MJ: *Surgery of the Foot and Ankle,* 6th ed. St. Louis: Mosby; 1993.

Sarrafian SK: *Anatomy of the Foot and Ankle: Descriptive, Topographic, Functional,* 2d ed. Philadelphia: JB Lippincott Company; 1993.

Sarrafian SK: Topographical anatomy and surgical approaches to the ankle and foot. In Jahss MH (ed): *Disorders of the Foot and Ankle: Medical and Surgical Management,* vol 1, 2d ed. Philadelphia: WB Saunders; 1991:280.

Chapter 21

FOOT AND ANKLE: SURGICAL APPROACHES

Myles Rubin Samotin and Steven C. Sheskier

Surgical approaches to the structures of the foot and ankle are not generally complicated since most of the underlying bony structures are rather superficial. As a consequence of this, the soft tissue flap developed is frequently thin, and viability of this flap often remains a significant concern. For this reason it is important to evaluate the vascular and neurologic status of the foot and ankle prior to undertaking an operation. Ischemia or neuropathy presents ample reasons to avoid or delay surgery in this area.

SURGICAL APPROACHES TO THE ANKLE

ANTERIOR APPROACH

Indications for this approach include: drainage, debridement, synovectomy, excision of anterior osteophytes, internal fixation of fractures (anterior lip fractures and screw placement for posterior malleolus fractures), and ankle fusion. It provides wide exposure of the ankle joint, anteriorly, from medial malleolus to lateral malleolus. The incision can be extended both proximally to expose the distal subcutaneous tibia and distally to expose the talonavicular joint (Fig. 21-1).

With the patient in a supine position, a longitudinal incision is made midway between the inner border of the medial and lateral malleoli. One must be mindful of cutaneous branches of the peroneal nerve which lie immediately under the skin. If a tourniquet is used, the leg is exsanguinated by elevation, without using an Esmarch, in order to retain blood in the anterior tibial vessels. This facilitates identification of the deep peroneal nerve and maintenance of hemostasis. The proximal incision is continued down to the superior extensor retinaculum which is then incised between the anterior tibial and the extensor hallucis longus tendon (step cutting the retinaculum will facilitate its closure). Blunt dissection is performed down to the periosteum of the distal tibia, taking care to avoid the neurovascular structures that lie laterally. Any direct tributaries should be ligated with silk ties. A capsulotomy is made longitudinally and the joint capsule elevated sharply medially and laterally, allowing Homan retractors to be placed about the malleoli. Retraction, especially of the laterally placed Homan, should be relaxed whenever possible to avoid compression injury to the deep peroneal nerve.

ANTEROLATERAL APPROACH

This approach provides the easiest access to the anterior ankle joint since the ankle joint is almost subcutaneous in this area. The structure most at risk is the superficial peroneal nerve and its branches. The approach can be used for drainage and debridement, removal of loose bodies, treatment of anterolateral lesions of the talus, and exposure of the tibio-fibular syndesmosis. The incision can be developed distally to expose the contents of the sinus tarsi, the calcaneocuboid joint, and even portions of the talocalcaneal and talonavicular joints.

A bolster is placed under the supine patient in order to internally rotate the leg. A longitudinal incision is made between the anterior lateral malleolus and the lateral edge of the talus. Inverting the ankle may make the superficial peroneal nerve visible and therefore easier to avoid. During blunt dissection to approach the joint, the superficial peroneal nerve is moved to the side, medially. A few of the most superior fibers of the inferior extensor retinaculum may be incised. A capsulotomy is made from proximal to distal, taking care not to lacerate the anterior talofibular ligament. The amount of capsular detachment from the tibia is dependent upon the indication for the procedure.

In the superficial surgical dissection, the interval used is between the peroneus tertius laterally and the extensor digitorum longus medially, both of which receive their innervation from the deep peroneal nerve. In the deep surgical dissection, the extensor digitorum brevis is detached at its origin from the calcaneus in order to expose the dorsal portions of the calcaneocuboid and talonavicular joints.

MEDIAL APPROACH

The medial malleolus lies subcutaneously and is often accessed to provide exposure for open reduction of fractures. When utilized as part of an extensile anterior-medial approach for pilon fractures, the incision is placed anteriorly to the ankle joint and extended proximally along the anterior subcutaneous border of the distal tibia, while curving posteriorly at the distal extent. An osteotomy of the medial malleolus may be performed in order to gain exposure to the central and posterior talus. This is useful in exposing talar dome lesions, and also as an aid in the reduction of irreducible talar neck fractures where the body of the talus is trapped posteromedially (Fig. 21-2).

The placement of the incision is dependent upon the indication. A longitudinal incision is placed over the anterior third of the medial malleolus to facilitate anterior arthrotomy and to aid in visualization of articular reduction in fracture cases. A mid-malleolar incision is used if malleolar osteotomy is entertained. In all instances, the incision is carried down to the periosteum making certain to avoid laceration of the saphenous vein and to ligate all its tributaries. The superficial deltoid may be incised longitudinally for screw placement. However, care must be taken in doing so posteriorly, since the posterior tibial tendon is attached intimately to the posterior aspect of the medial malleolus and may be injured or lacerated accidentally.

If a medial malleolar osteotomy is performed, the dissection must be taken posteriorly, the anterior edge of the flexor retinaculum incised, and the posterior structures elevated and protected. The medial malleolus is scored longitudinally with an osteotome or cautery to

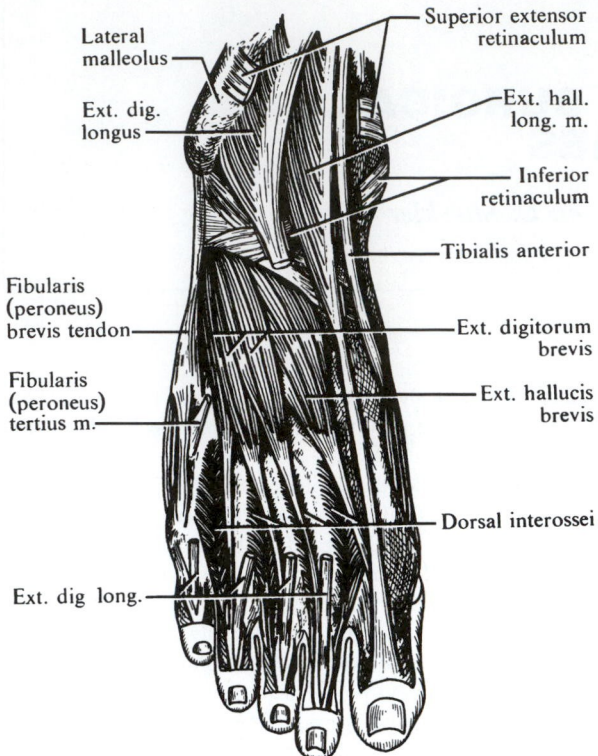

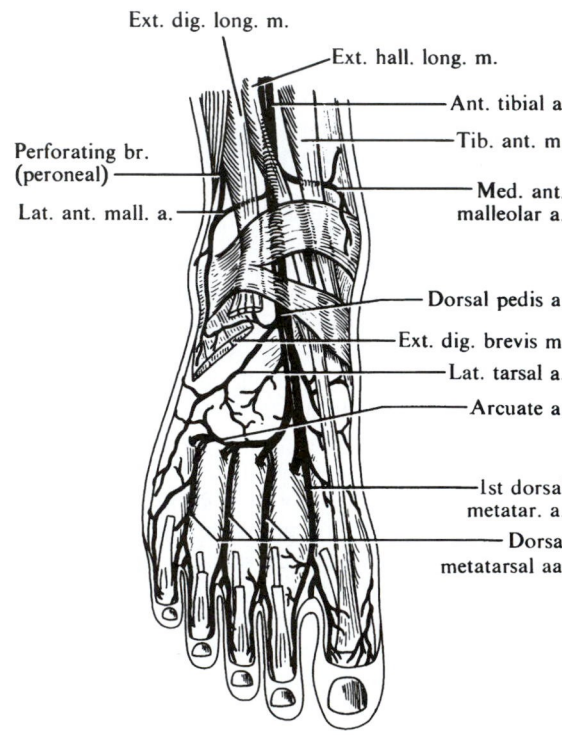

Figure 21-1
Anterior aspect of foot and ankle.

assure anatomic reduction. An arthrotomy is made anteriorly and posteriorly to guide the angle of the osteotomy, which is started proximal to the joint, entering it obliquely, to increase surface area. The osteotomy may be started with a saw, but it is recommended to be completed with an osteotome so that there is no bone or cartilage loss. The distal fragment should be predrilled and tapped for placement of a half-threaded cancellous screw when the osteotomy is replaced. One must watch for the saphenous nerve and the long saphenous vein, which course anteromedially across the medial malleolus. The posterior tibial tendon lies immediately posterior to the medial malleolus and must be retracted away.

LATERAL APPROACH

As in the medial approach, the lateral approach is most often utilized for fracture reduction. The lateral malleolar fragment can be turned down to aid in the exposure and reduction of posterior malleolar fractures as well. Lateral transmalleolar approaches have been used in a variety of ankle fusions as well. The sural nerve is in jeopardy as the incision proceeds distal to the tip of the malleolus. The superficial peroneal nerve is at risk as the dissection is developed proximally (Fig. 21-3).

With the patient in a supine position, a bolster is placed under the ipsilateral hip. This allows for greater internal rotation of the ankle,

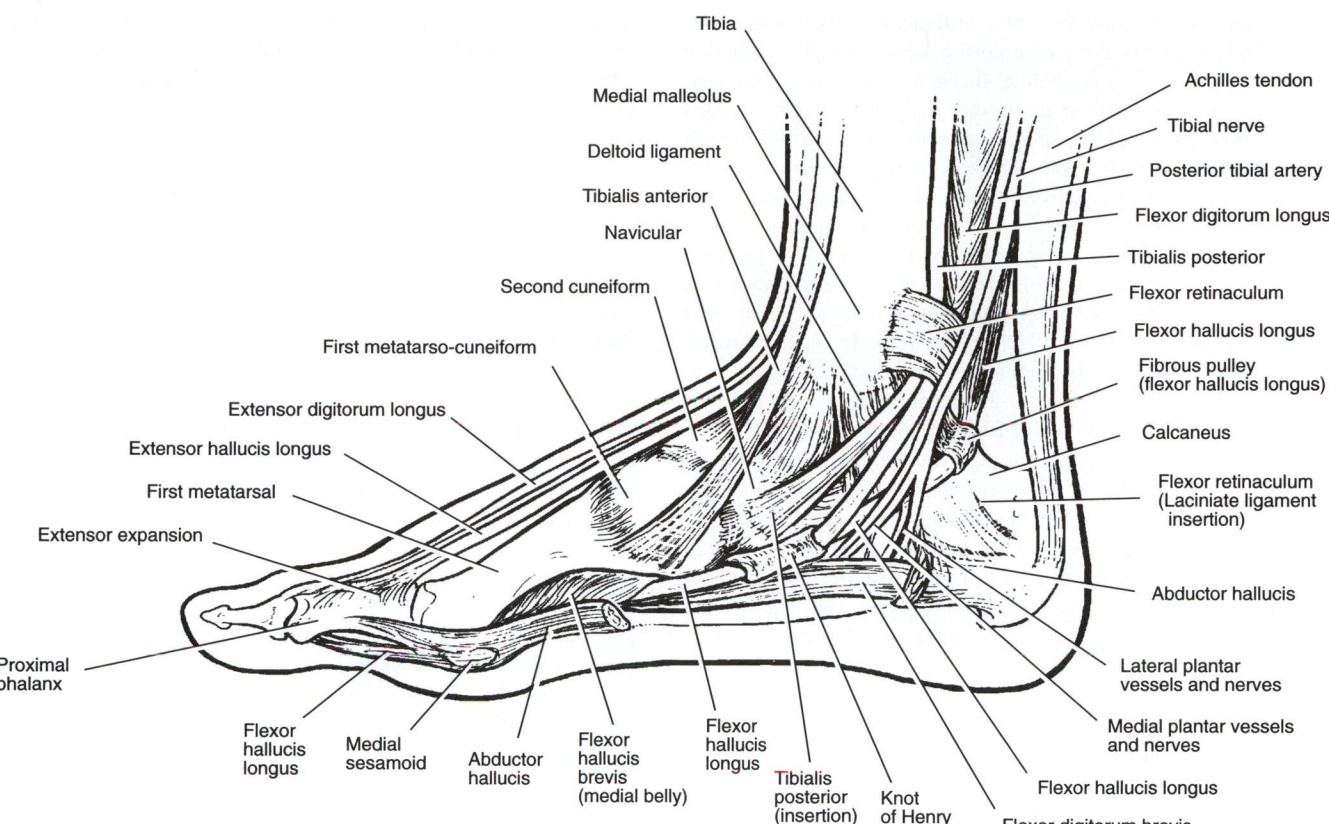

Figure 21-2
Medial aspect of foot and ankle.

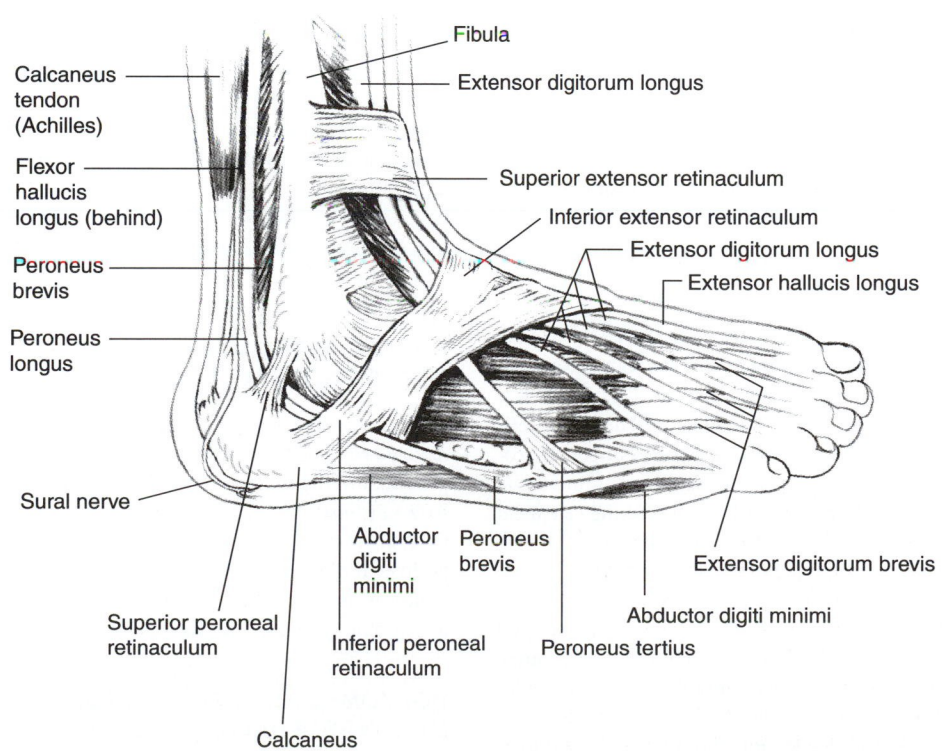

Figure 21-3
Lateral aspect of foot and ankle.

thus making the exposure possible. Sufficient internal rotation is needed to allow for the taking of a mortise view when post-reduction films will be needed. A longitudinal incision is made along the posterior aspect of the fibula to its tip. At this point, the incision is curved forward below the tip of the lateral malleolus. Dissection continues right down to subcutaneous bone. There is no true internervous plane. If the dissection is continued proximally, the plane is between the peroneus tertius which is innervated by the deep peroneal nerve and the peroneus brevis which is innervated by the superficial peroneal nerve. Structures to watch out for include the short saphenous vein which lies immediately posterior to the lateral malleolus. The sural nerve runs adjacent to the short saphenous vein. Terminal branches of the peroneal artery may be damaged if dissection is not kept subperiosteal on the medial surface of the distal fibula.

To expose a posterior malleolar fracture, the syndesmosis (which usually is disrupted) is released. The peroneal tendon sheath is opened with a step cut at the level of the retinaculum. Both anterior and posterior capsulotomies are performed, making sure to spare the anterior talofibular ligament. The lateral malleolus is then turned down, hinging on the lateral ligaments. This exposes the posterior portion of the distal tibia. The lateral malleolus is then reduced and held in place with appropriate lateral fixation and a syndesmotic screw.

POSTEROLATERAL APPROACH

A posterolateral approach midway between the Achilles tendon and the posterior edge of the lateral malleolus can allow one to gain access to the posterior ankle joint for os trigonum excision as well as procedures on the peroneal tendon sheath. For this approach, the patient must be prone or in a lateral position. The internervous plane lies between the peroneus brevis, which is innervated by the superficial peroneal nerve, and the flexor hallucis longus, which is innervated by the tibial nerve. As the skin flaps are mobilized, the short saphenous vein and sural nerve run in the anterior flap immediately behind the lateral malleolus. The peroneus brevis runs anterior to the peroneus longus at this level, and tends to be muscular while the peroneus longus is tendinous. This permits a fail-safe distinction between the two. Next, the peroneal retinaculum is incised in a step-cut fashion to allow exposure of these tendons, which should be retracted anteriorly. The flexor hallucis longus will then come into view, and when retracted posteriorly reveal the periosteum and joint capsule over the posterior aspect of the tibia (Fig. 21-4).

MISCELLANEOUS APPROACHES

An incision posterior to the medial malleolus can be used to expose the medial structures of the ankle (posterior tibial tendon, flexor digitorum longus tendon, and the posterior tibial nerve). This incision is made one finger breadth behind the medial malleolus. The flexor retinaculum is then encountered. The appropriate sheath is opened proceeding from proximal to distal, especially when entering the tarsal tunnel, since there may be many anomalous branches of the calcaneal nerve. If all of the above structures are retracted posteriorly, the posterior portion of the ankle joint may then be visualized. Once an ankle capsulotomy is performed, the ankle may be dorsiflexed to increase the amount of talar dome visualized. This may obviate the need to osteotomize the medial malleolus for visualization of this area.

A posterior approach to the ankle and subtalar joint may be developed by transecting the Achilles tendon (in a Z cut fashion). Extensile approaches to the Achilles tendon should be placed immediately posteromedial to the tendon at the level of the ankle joint. This incision should then be centralized if it is brought proximally. The incision can be extended transversely across the tendon at the

level of its insertion in order to gain better exposure distally. This medial incision avoids injury to the sural nerve distally. Care must be taken to avoid the sural nerve in the proximal portion of the incision as the sural nerve centralizes in the proximal calf region.

SURGICAL APPROACHES TO THE FOOT

Incisions on the foot must be made with caution and planning. In contrast to other areas of the body, because the foot is usually encased in a shoe, painful postoperative scars and pressure sensitive neuromas are a particular area of concern. Any surgical approach must therefore respect the abundant sensory nerves that course subcutaneously, especially on the dorsum of the foot, as well as avoid areas that are normally exposed to increased pressure. In the past, incisions on the plantar aspect of the foot were avoided for just this reason. However, if one avoids plantar pressure areas (e.g., directly under the metatarsal heads), painful scars can be avoided.

DORSAL APPROACH TO THE MIDFOOT

In a dorsal approach to the midfoot, a longitudinal incision is made directly over the area of concern. A dorsomedial incision can be used to expose the talonavicular joint, the navicular-medial cuneiform joint, and the first metatarsocuneiform joint, as well as the insertions of the posterior and anterior tibial tendons. A dorsolateral incision can be used to expose the calcaneocuboid joint, as well as the base of the fifth metatarsal. Longitudinal incisions centered directly over the Lisfranc joints (tarsometatarsal joints) may be used for open reduction and fixation of these joints in fracture dislocations, as well as for tarsometatarsal fusions. If a tourniquet is used, it is recommended that the foot be exsanguinated by elevation, rather than using an Esmarch bandage. This makes the deep peroneal nerve and its accompanying blood vessels easier to identify and thus protect. Longitudinal incisions are centered directly over the tarsometatarsal joints in question if an isolated ray is to be exposed. Otherwise, the incision can be centered midway between two to three metatarsal bases. Once through the skin, blunt dissection is used to avoid cutting the many branches of the superficial peroneal nerve. The inferior extensor retinaculum is then encountered and incised longitudinally. The muscle belly of the extensor digitorum brevis may be encountered as well. The first metatarsocuneiform joint can be approached medially being careful to avoid cutting the anterior tibial tendon (as it fans out plantar medially under the first metatarsal base) and the saphenous nerve branches in this area.

DORSAL APPROACH TO THE FIRST METATARSOPHALANGEAL JOINT

With the patient supine, a dorsal incision is made beginning immediately proximal to the interphalangeal joint and proceeding about 3 cm proximal to the metatarsophalangeal joint. The incision stays medial to the extensor hallucis tendon. This tendon is then retracted laterally to expose the joint capsule which is incised longitudinally. Subperiosteal dissection reveals the metatarsophalangeal joint. It is necessary to look for the dorsomedial cutaneous nerve to the great toe, a terminal branch of the saphenous nerve, during the dissection.

DORSOMEDIAL APPROACH TO THE FIRST METATARSOPHALANGEAL JOINT

This incision begins just proximal to the interphalangeal joint on the dorsomedial aspect of the first toe with the patient supine. The incision is brought dorsally over the joint itself and is continued medi-

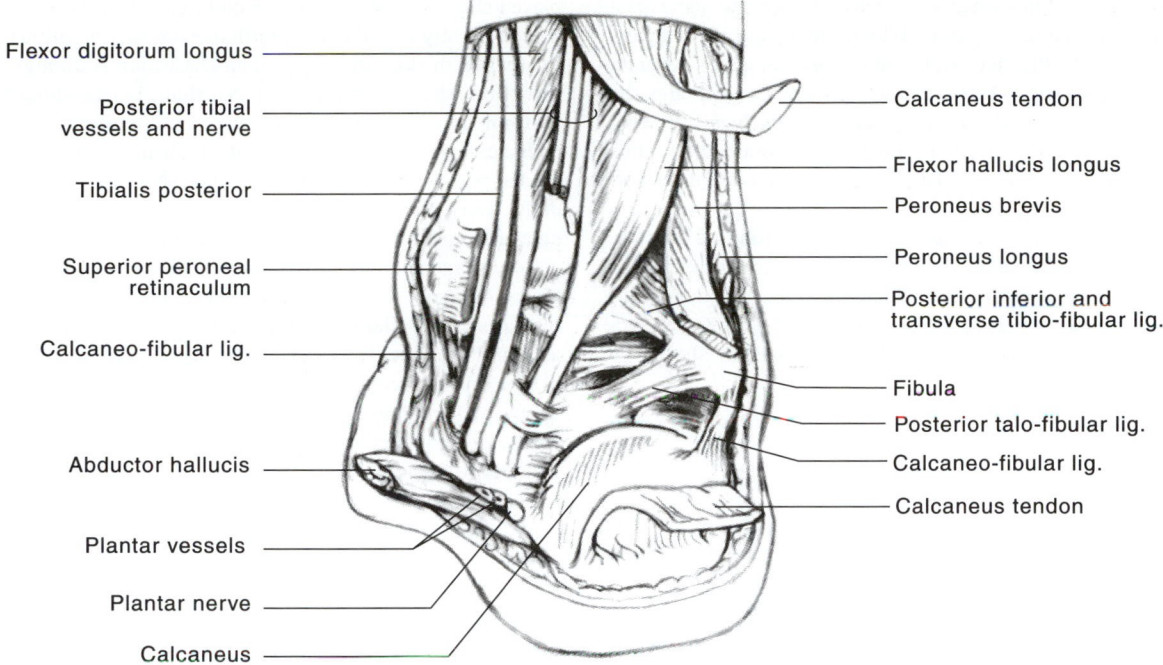

Flexor digitorum longus

Posterior tibial vessels and nerve

Tibialis posterior

Superior peroneal retinaculum

Calcaneo-fibular lig.

Abductor hallucis

Plantar vessels

Plantar nerve

Calcaneus

Calcaneus tendon

Flexor hallucis longus

Peroneus brevis

Peroneus longus

Posterior inferior and transverse tibio-fibular lig.

Fibula

Posterior talo-fibular lig.

Calcaneo-fibular lig.

Calcaneus tendon

Figure 21-4
Posterior aspect of foot and ankle.

ally to the extensor hallucis longus tendon. It then proceeds medially up the midshaft of the first metatarsal approximately 3 cm proximal to the joint. In this approach, it is important to watch out for the extensor hallucis longus tendon and retract it laterally. The dorsomedial cutaneous nerve is also seen during this approach and must be retracted anteriorly and laterally. The dorsal and dorsomedial approaches to the first metatarsophalangeal joint may be used to expose the joint for distal metatarsal osteotomy, hallux valgus correction, bunionectomy, metatarsophalangeal joint arthrodesis, and cheilectomy for hallux rigidus.

DORSAL APPROACH TO THE METATARSOPHALANGEAL JOINTS OF THE LESSER TOES

Indications for dorsal approach incisions include metatarsal head resection, distal metatarsal osteotomy, and capsulotomy. The lesser metatarsophalangeal joints can be exposed through hockey stick incisions over the joints (as in the hand). This helps to avoid extension contractures leading to cockup deformities at the metatarsophalangeal joints. Blunt dissection down to the level of the extensor tendon is performed. Care must be taken to ensure that the dorsal digital nerves are not cut during this exposure. The extensor tendons can be transected or Z-cut, depending upon the indication and procedure being performed. A dorsal capsulotomy can be performed by making a longitudinal incision between the extensor digitorum longus and brevis tendon without performing any tenotomy if this is desired. The joint can be dislocated plantarly by continuing the arthrotomy, proximally through the periosteum. The periosteum can then be stripped off of the metatarsal shaft. Similarly, the medial and lateral collateral ligaments can be detached, thus facilitating a good exposure to the joint.

APPROACH TO THE DORSAL WEB SPACES

In the second, third, or fourth web spaces, the following approach is most commonly used for excision of Morton's neuroma. It may also be used for draining a web space infection as well as gaining

access to the first web space, most commonly during a distal soft tissue procedure as part of hallux valgus correction. A longitudinal incision is used to approach the contents of the web spaces. The incision is placed directly between the metatarsal heads and is approximately 4 cm in length. Blunt dissection is used to navigate between the metatarsal heads, making sure to sweep the dorsal cutaneous nerves to the side. A bursa may be encountered between the metatarsal heads, and is sharply entered. At this point, a small laminar spreader can be inserted at the level of the metatarsal necks to gain better visualization. This will also result in a tensioning of the intermetatarsal ligament. Plantar pressure just distal to the metatarsal heads will force the web contents, including the neuroma, into view as well as delineate the distal edge of the intermetatarsal ligament. The ligament can be safely incised, after the underlying plantar digital nerve is freed from its undersurface and protected with a hemostat. Revision Morton neurectomies are commonly performed via a longitudinal plantar approach, making sure to avoid placing the incision directly under the metatarsal (weightbearing) head. Once through the skin and plantar fat, the distal edge of the plantar fascia is encountered and incised, allowing the plantar digital nerve or stump to be easily found. This is facilitated by extending the incision proximally into "virgin" territory.

APPROACH FOR RELEASE OF THE COMPARTMENTS OF THE FOOT

Recent work by Manoli and coworkers (1992) has shown there are nine compartments in the foot. These include the medial, lateral, superficial, calcaneal, four interosseous, and the adductor hallucis compartments. The medial, lateral, and superficial compartments run the entire length of the foot. The medial compartment contains the abductor hallucis and flexor hallucis brevis muscles. A lateral compartment contains the flexor digiti minimi brevis and the abductor digiti minimi muscles. The superficial compartment runs along the plantar aspect of the central portion of the foot and contains the flexor digitorum brevis muscle. In the forefoot, the interosseous muscles are found in individual compartments located between the metatarsal shafts. The adductor hallucis muscle is found in a separate compartment. In the hindfoot, the calcaneal compartment is also a separate compartment deep to the superficial compartment and contains the quadratus plantae muscle. The development of claw toes following foot compartment syndrome has been attributed to contracture of this muscle. Calcaneal fractures may also lead to involvement of the calcaneal compartment.

A complete release of the compartments of the foot includes releasing all of the above-mentioned nine compartments. There are two major techniques for compartment decompression. The dorsal approach is based on two longitudinal incisions which are over the second and fourth metatarsals, respectively. One incision should be

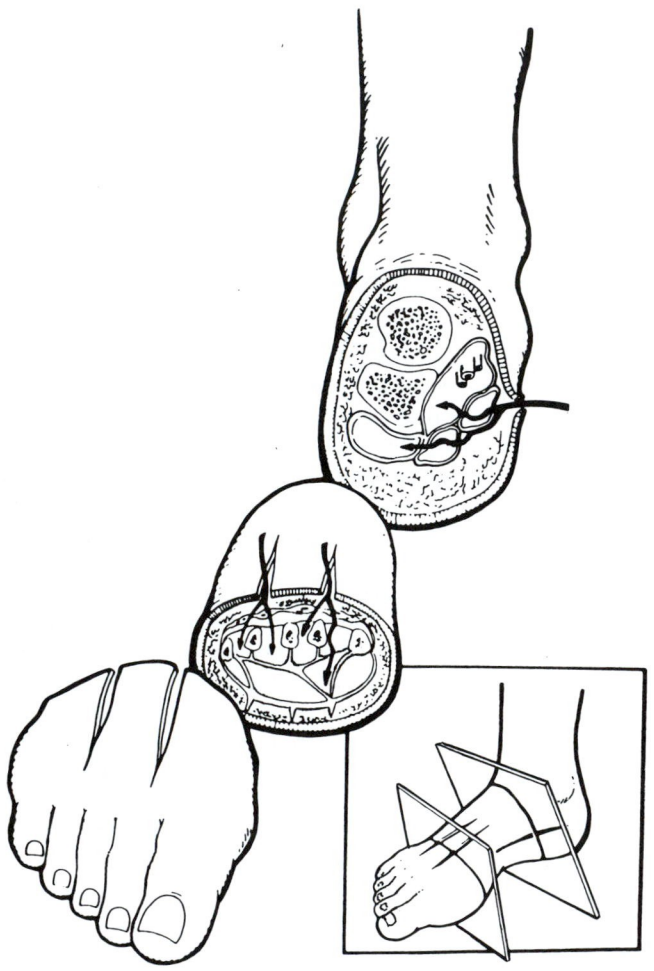

Figure 21-5
Approaches for release of nine foot compartments. (Reproduced with permission from Manoli A II, Fakhouri AJ, Weber TG: Compartmental catheterization and fasciotomy of the foot. *Operative Tech Orthop* 1992; 2:209.)

placed slightly medial to the second metatarsal with the other being placed slightly lateral to the fourth metatarsal, thus allowing the maximal width of skin bridge possible. Dissection is through the skin directly to both sides of the metatarsal shaft. Longitudinal dissection is performed in each interosseous space until a release is achieved. The adductor compartment is reached by stripping the muscles off the medial portion of the second metatarsal shaft and retracting them medially. Deep in the first interspace, the fascia overlying the adductor compartment is then seen and incised longitudinally.

For the medial approach, a 6-cm hindfoot incision is made. It begins 4 cm from the posterior aspect of the heel and 3 cm from the plantar surface. The incision extends distally, paralleling the plantar aspect of the foot. The fascia overlying the abductor hallucis muscle is seen and incised, thus releasing the medial compartment. The abductor hallucis muscle is then retracted superiorly, allowing visualization of the medial intermuscular septum, which is then opened longitudinally. This must be performed with great care since the lateral plantar neurovascular bundle lies just deep to the septum and can be easily injured. The quadratus plantae muscle is now seen, enabling a release of the calcaneal compartment. The medial plantar nerve must also be avoided as it lies just distal to the incision and at times is directly within the medial intermuscular septum or the calcaneal compartment. The dissection is continued inferior to the medial compartment, where the superficial compartment is encountered and opened on the plantar aspect of the foot, releasing the flexor digitorum brevis muscle. As this is done, the flexor digitorum brevis muscle is retracted plantarly, and the lateral compartment is seen. The compartment is opened longitudinally and released. Combining the two dorsal incisions with the medial hindfoot incision allows for a complete release of all nine foot compartments (Fig. 21-5).

SUGGESTED READINGS

Hoppenfeld S, deBoer P: The ankle and foot. In *Surgical Exposures in Orthopaedics: The Anatomic Approach*, 2d ed. Philadelphia: JB Lippincott; 1994:513.

Jahss MH: Surgical principles and the plantigrade foot. In Jahss MH (ed): *Disorders of the Foot and Ankle: Medical and Surgical Management*, vol 1, 2d ed. Philadelphia: WB Saunders; 1991.

Lutter LD, Mizel MS, Pfeffer GB (eds): *Orthopaedic Knowledge Update: Foot and Ankle.* Rosemont, IL: American Academy of Orthopaedic Surgeons; 1994.

Mann RA, Coughlin MJ (eds): *Surgery of the Foot and Ankle*, 6th ed. St. Louis: Mosby-Year Book; 1993.

Sarrafian SK: Cross sectional and topographic anatomy. In *Anatomy of the Foot and Ankle: Descriptive, Topographic, Functional*, 2d ed. Philadelphia: JB Lippincott; 1993:391.

Sarrafian SK: Functional anatomy of the foot and ankle. In *Anatomy of the Foot and Ankle: Descriptive, Topographic, Functional*, 2d ed. Philadelphia: JB Lippincott; 1993:474.

Sarrafian SK: Topographic anatomy and surgical approaches to the ankle and foot. In Jahss, MH (ed): *Disorders of the Foot and Ankle: Medical and Surgical Management*, vol 1, 2d ed. Philadelphia: WB Saunders; 1991: 280.

Chapter 22

SPINE

Paul M. Brisson

The physical examination of the spine should proceed in a systematic fashion similar to that of other body regions and should include inspection, palpation, and range of motion testing. Neurologic examination of the extremities is crucial for evaluation of spinal cord and nerve root function. In addition, specific provocative tests and maneuvers are described for the different regions of the spine.

INSPECTION

The examination should begin with both focal and global observations of the spine. On a focal level, skin lesions and irregularities may provide valuable insight to underlying pathology. However, it is equally important to make the necessary global observations regarding spinal contours and fluidity of movement.

Skin markings such as café-au-lait spots, hairy patches, birth marks, and lipomas often denote underlying neurologic or bone pathology. For example, a tuft of hair on the back may reflect a bony defect such as a spina bifida occulta or a diastematomyelia, a congenital bony or cartilagenous bar that separates the lateral halves of the spinal cord. Birth marks or unusually large port wine stains might also represent signs of underlying bony pathology. Lipomas (fatty masses) in the area of the low back may be a sign of spina bifida or, if dumbell-shaped, may extend into the cauda equina through a bony defect.

The normal contours of the spine in the sagittal plane include a lordosis (convexity anterior) in the cervical and lumbar region, and a kyphosis (convexity posterior) in the thoracic region. With patients standing fully erect, these sagittal contours should combine to allow the head to be positioned directly above the pelvis. Patients who remain with the head forward of the pelvis with their best attempt to stand erect are considered *decompensated* anteriorly.

A localized flattening of the cervical or lumbar lordosis with muscle spasm and decreased spinal mobility may suggest the possibility of a herniated intervertebral disc. An excessive lumbar curvature (hyperlordosis) may occur in order to compensate for the protuberant abdomen of marked obesity or pregnancy. Hyperlordosis may also be seen compensating for increased thoracic kyphosis or flexion contractures of the hips. A deep midline crease may sometimes be observed across the lumbar paravertebral muscles in this setting. An excessive thoracic kyphosis is common in the elderly, especially in women; however, when seen in adolescent patients, consider Scheuermann's Disease.

Look for any difference in the heights of the shoulders, the iliac crests, and the skin creases of the abdomen and below the buttocks. Unequal heights of the iliac crests (a pelvic tilt) may be due to unequal leg lengths. Such a tilt is abolished by placing supports under one foot. Clinical assessment of leg length is done using a tape to measure the distance between each anterior superior iliac spine (ASIS) and the ipsilateral medial malleolus. Scoliosis and adduction or abduction of the hip may also cause a pelvic tilt. Note whether an imaginary line dropped from the spinous process of T1 falls, as it should, through the gluteal cleft.

List is a lateral tilt of the spine. When a plumb line dropped from the spinous process of T1 falls to one side of the gluteal cleft, a list is present. A list should be measured in centimeters and recorded. Causes include a herniated disc and painful spasms of the paravertebral muscles. Scoliosis is inherent in a list but without compensation by a spinal deviation in the opposite direction. When a list is caused by a herniated disc in its typical location lateral to the nerve root, patients tend to list away from the side of the irritated nerve root, attempting to draw the nerve root away from the disc fragment. Herniation of the disc that is medial to the nerve root (in the nerve axilla) may instead produce a list toward the side of the irritated nerve root, as this position brings the nerve root away from the medial compression.

In scoliosis, the body generally compensates for the coronal curvature, and a plumb line from T1 drops through the gluteal cleft for most patients. When this does not happen, the patient is said to be *decompensated* in the coronal plane (measured in centimeters).

Structural scoliosis is typically associated with rotations of the vertebrae upon each other, and the rib cage is accordingly deformed. This deformity is seen best when the patient flexes forward. On the side of the thoracic convexity, the ribs bulge posteriorly and are widely separated. On the opposite side, they are displaced anteriorly and are close together. *Functional scoliosis* compensates for other abnormalities such as unequal leg lengths. It involves neither vertebral rotation nor thoracic deformity. The scoliosis disappears with forward flexion.

PALPATION

With the patient sitting, the spinous processes are palpable with the thumb. Begin with the fingers on the tops of the iliac crests and the thumbs on the midline at the same level, approximately the level of the L4/L5 disc space. Determine whether one spinous process seems unusually prominent in relation to the one above it. The presence of a "step-off" from the spinous process of L5 or possibly L4 may represent a spondylolisthesis, an anterior slip of a vertebral body.

Soft-tissue palpation surrounding the spinous processes is done to detect areas of localized tenderness and muscle spasm. The soft tissue of the lumbar spine has been classified into five clinical zones: midline raphe, iliac crest, posterior superior iliac spines, sciatic area, and the anterior abdominal wall/inguinal area.

Although made up of three distinct muscles (spinalis, longissimus, and iliocostalis), the midline sacrospinalis muscles must be palpated as a single unit. Having the patient place the head back during the examination helps relax the overlying fascia.

Inspect and palpate the paravertebral muscles for any atrophy, spasm, or tenderness. Due to their segmental innervation, the paraspinal muscles may be subject to local atrophy. A paravertebral muscle in spasm looks prominent, feels tight, and is usually tender. Palpate for tenderness in any other areas that are suggested by the patient's symptoms. Tenderness in the costovertebral angles may signify kidney infection rather than a musculoskeletal problem.

The iliac crest provides the site of origin for the gluteal muscles, where sometimes tender fibrofatty nodules can be the source of low back pain in some patients.

A skin dimple usually overlies the posterior superior iliac spine and guides you toward the sacroiliac area. Ankylosing spondylitis may produce sacroiliac tenderness. Additionally, the posterior superior iliac spines act as points of attachment for the sacrotuberous ligaments, which can be a source of pain for the patient.

The midpoint between the ischial tuberosity and the greater trochanter represents the location of the sciatic nerve as it exits through the sciatic notch. Nerve root compression can cause this spot to be tender to palpation. By positioning the patient such that the hip is flexed, one can most easily find the necessary bony landmarks.

As with the paraspinal muscles, the anterior abdominal wall has segmental innervation and thus can display local atrophy and weakness with nerve impingement. To best evaluate for these deficits, have the patient hold the position of a partial sit-up.

RANGE OF MOTION

To evaluate flexion, have the patient bend forward to touch the toes without bending the knees. The amount of flexion can be expressed as the number of degrees of the angle formed by the lumbar spine from vertical or measured in inches from the floor touching the toes. The latter method is more reproducible, but also includes hip, pelvic, and thoracic motion. Maximal neck flexion can also be expressed in degrees from the vertical or centimeters between the chin and chest. Note also the smoothness and symmetry of movement and the curve in the lumbar area. As flexion proceeds, the posterior cervical and lumbar concavities should flatten out. Paravertebral muscle spasm and ankylosing spondylitis may prevent this flattening, and lordosis may persist.

Extension, lateral bending, and rotation are also assessed. Normal ranges of motion for the cervical and lumbar regions are listed in Table 22-1.

NEUROLOGIC EXAMINATION

The neurologic examination of the spine places emphasis on patterns that emerge involving reflex, motor, and sensory deficits. Being familiar with the anatomy of a given reflex, the innervation of a muscle, and the sensory dermatomes allows one to better localize and perhaps isolate a disease process because of the spine's segmental nature (Fig. 22-1).

Recording the functional level of these modalities follows some standard guidelines. First, one side of the patient must always be compared with the other side, as asymmetrical findings are often the most significant. For example, symmetrical loss of reflexes in the elderly is not unusual, but inability to dorsiflex the big toe against resistance only on one side may require further investigation. Second, individual tests often represent multiple nerve root involvement. For example, the patellar reflex is a deep tendon reflex mediated through nerve roots from L2, L3, and L4, but predominantly from L4. When combined, however, the results of all three modalities often allow for the diagnosis of the nerve level most likely involved.

Reflexes are most commonly observed to be either increased, decreased, or normal. A hyperreflexia often suggests an upper motor neuron lesion, and thus loss of the regulatory control from the brain and its descending tracts. In contrast, an interruption in the basic reflex arc results in the loss of reflex, while pressure on the nerve itself may decrease its intensity and cause a hyporeflexia (Fig. 22-2).

Motor power is graded on a standardized scale from 0 to 5 (Table 22-2). Although discerning between grade 4 and 5 can be difficult at times, again asymmetry may provide a useful clue. Make note that a grade 3 (and above) muscle can move the joint through a full range of motion against gravity, while those below cannot.

Sensation of pain and temperature travels in the lateral spinothalamic tract, while sensation of vibration and light touch travels in the dorsal columns. Damage to the cord or nerve root results in loss of light touch first, and later on loss of sensation of pain. During the recovery phase, the opposite is true; sensation of pain returns before light touch. The test for sensation most often involves an examiner's light brushing with a finger tip over different dermatomal areas, as this will pick up the earliest deficits and latest recoveries. Descriptions of sensation include hyperesthetic (increased), hypesthetic (decreased), dysesthetic (abnormal), anesthetic (absent), or normal.

In addition, a complete neurologic survey includes testing of temperature sense (with test tubes filled with hot or cold water) and vibration (using a relatively low-pitch tuning fork tapped first on the heel of the examiner's hand and placed firmly over a distal interphalangeal joint of the patient's finger and of the big toe). Vibration sense is often the first sense to be lost in peripheral neuropathy, most commonly caused by diabetes or alcoholism. Vibration is also lost in posterior column disease, and testing sensation over the trunk area can often help delineate the level of the lesion. Some loss of vibration sense is expected with aging. Position sense is tested by holding the patient's big toe firmly and moving it up or down while the patient's eyes are closed, asking for confirmation of the correct position. Loss of position sense, like vibration, suggests either posterior column dysfunction or a peripheral nerve disease.

GAIT

Gait is observed by having the patient walk down the hall, turn, and come back. A gait that lacks coordination, with guarding and insta-

---

Table 22-1

Clinical Range of Motion of the Neck and Lower Back

	Flexion	Extension	Axial Rotation	Lateral Bend
Cervical	80 to 90°	70°	70 to 80°	20 to 45°
Lumbar	40 to 60°	20 to 35°	3 to 18°	15 to 20°

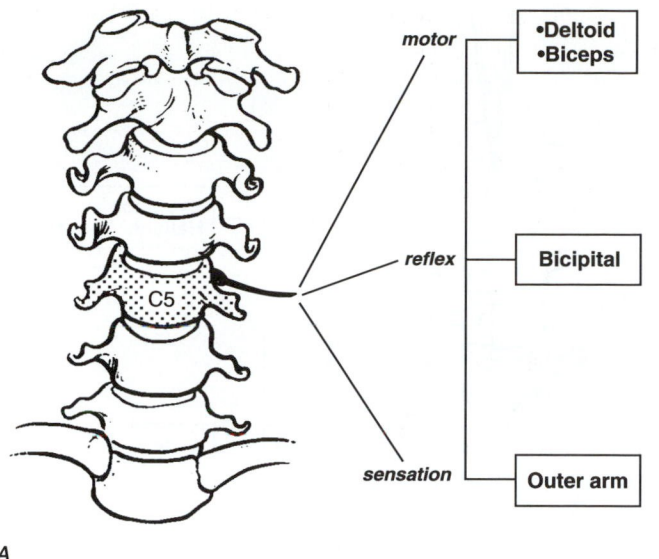

A

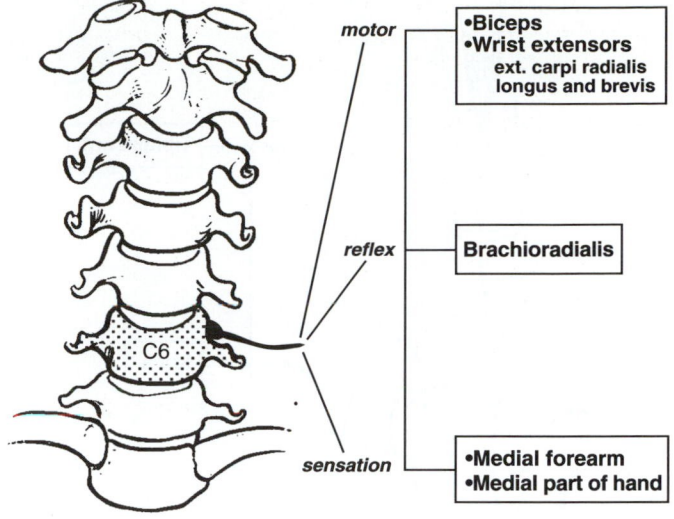

B

C

motor	•Wrist flexors •Finger extensors
reflex	Tricipital
sensation	Middle finger

D

motor	•Interossei Muscles •Finger flexors
reflex	None
sensation	Ulnar side of hand

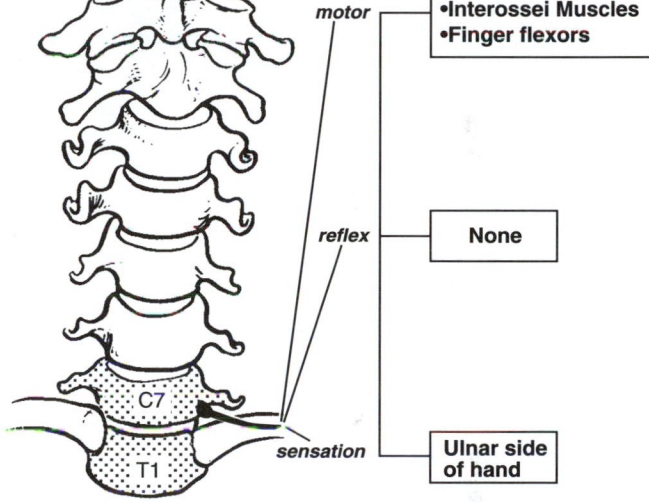

Figure 22-1
A. C5 root. *B.* C6 root. *C.* C7 root. *D.* C8 root. *E.* T1 root.

E

motor	Interossei Muscles
reflex	None
sensation	Inner arm

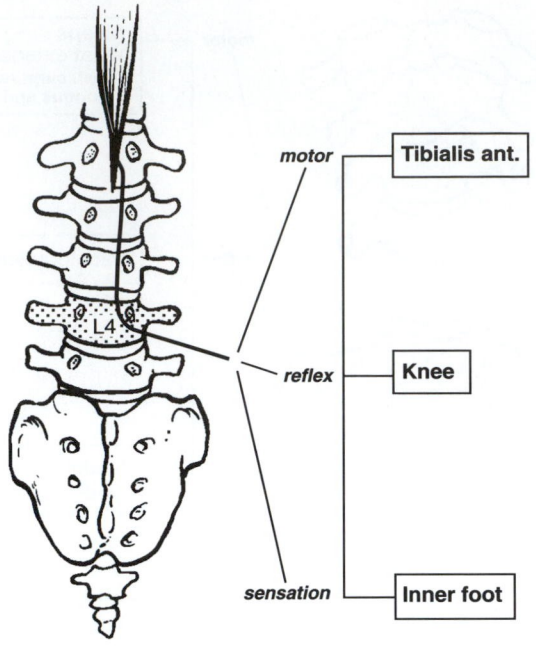

A

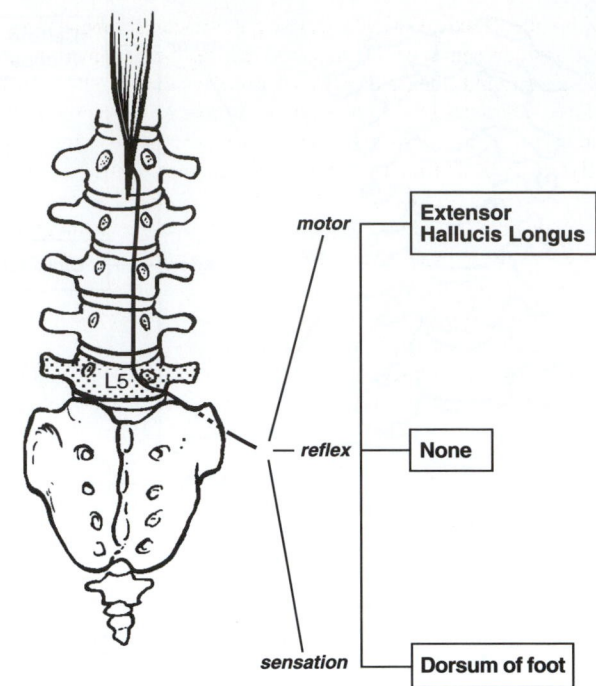

B

Figure 22-2
A. L4 root. *B.* L5 root. *C.* S1 root.

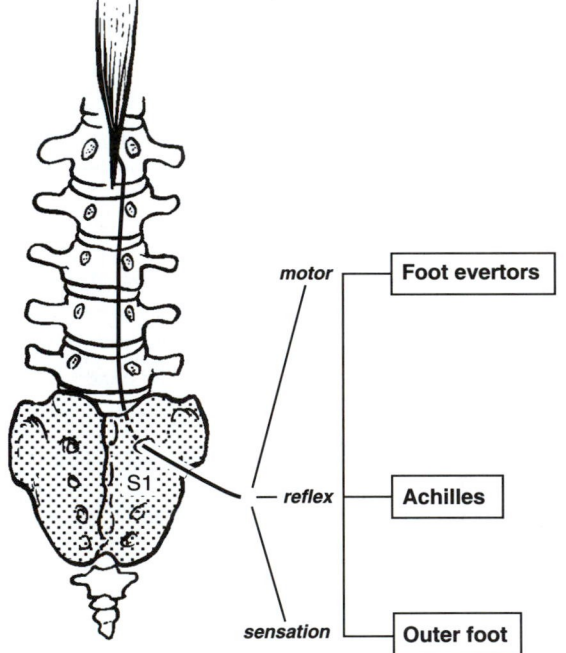

C

Table 22-2

Muscle Grading

Grade 5	Normal	Complete range of motion against gravity with full resistance
Grade 4	Good	Complete range of motion against gravity with some resistance
Grade 3	Fair	Complete range of motion only against gravity
Grade 2	Poor	Complete range of motion with gravity eliminated
Grade 1	Trace	Evidence of slight contractility. No joint motion.
Grade 0	Zero	No evidence of contractility

bility, is called ataxic. Causes of ataxic gait include cerebellar lesions, loss of position sense, or intoxication. Having the patient walk heel-to-toe in a straight line (tandem walking) may occasionally reveal an ataxia not otherwise observed. Walking on toes (S1), then heels (L4, L5) may reveal motor weakness secondary to radiculopathy not previously apparent. Difficulty bending on one knee suggests proximal muscle weakness (hip extensors), weakness of quadriceps (knee extensors), or both. In a home environment, this weakness may manifest itself as difficulty rising from a chair, stepping onto a stool, or going up or down steps.

The *Romberg test* helps to evaluate whether vision is in part compensating for a sensory loss, as in ataxia due to loss of position sense. The patient stands with feet together and open eyes; then, the patient closes his or her eyes for 20 to 30 s. If the patient loses balance, the test is positive. In cerebellar ataxia, the patient will lose balance regardless of whether the eyes are open or closed.

When the anterior tibial muscles are compromised secondary to lower motor neuron disease, a "foot drop" often prevails. All anterior tibial muscles function as dorsiflexors during walking, lifting the forefoot at toe-off and early swing phase, then dorsiflexing the foot as a whole so that the heel strikes the ground first and the forefoot does not rapidly follow and slap the ground. If these muscles are compromised, patients may either drag their foot or try to compensate by lifting them high with knees flexed ("high stepping" or steppage gait), thus appearing to climb stairs. As mentioned earlier, these patients are unable to walk on their heels.

PERIPHERAL CIRCULATION

No examination of the spine is complete without an evaluation of the peripheral pulses. This becomes extremely important in the lower limbs in order to help differentiate between vascular and neurogenic causes of extremity pain. Popliteal, posterior tibial, and dorsalis pedis pulses should be examined and documented. Also, the lower extremity skin should be examined for atrophic changes typical of vascular insufficiency disease.

SPECIAL MANEUVERS

Special diagnostic tests are best left toward the end of the examination because they are often used to confirm already suspected diagnosis.

Cutaneoabdominal reflexes are normally present. Gentle stroking of each of the four quadrans provokes a movement of the umbilicus

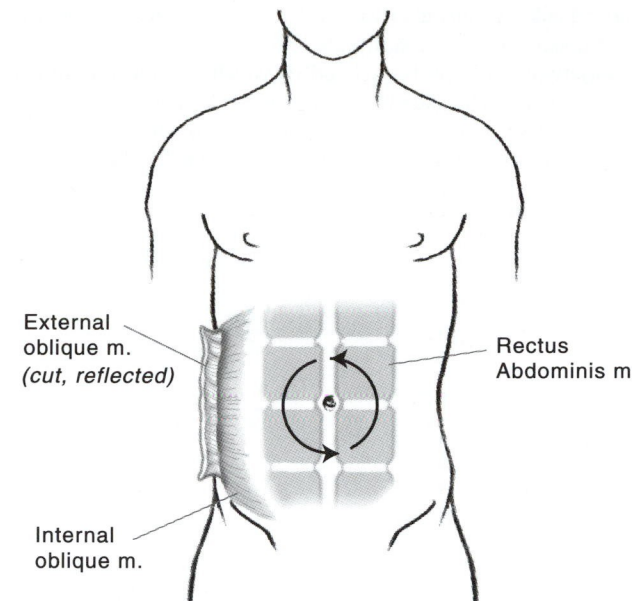

Figure 22-3
Cutaneoabdominal reflex.

secondary to a contraction of the oblique muscles (Fig. 22-3). Lack of response is abnormal. The suggestion is that an abnormal test in the case of scoliosis may indicate a neurogenic origin to the deformity.

Pathologic reflexes are tested for when spinal cord injury or compression is suspected. In the upper extremity, the *Hoffman sign* is elicited by quickly extending the middle finger while stabilizing the third metacarpal, examining for a reflex flexion response of the index finger and thumb. A positive test bilaterally may be normal in up to 10 percent of patients. The *pectoralis reflex,* always abnormal when present, is elicited by tapping the insertion of the pectoralis major and provoking a reflex contraction observed by humoral adduction and internal rotation

The *Babinski sign* is a pathologic lower extremity test indicative of an upper motor neuron lesion. It is done by stroking the lateral aspect of the foot with a key or handle of a neuro hammer and moving medially just before the toes. Normally, the toes should all be stimulated into flexion (Fig. 22-4A). A positive response manifests as dorsiflexion of the big toe and fanning of the other toes (Fig. 22-4B).

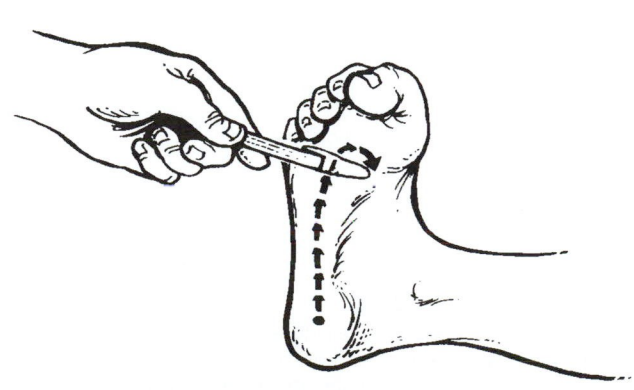

A

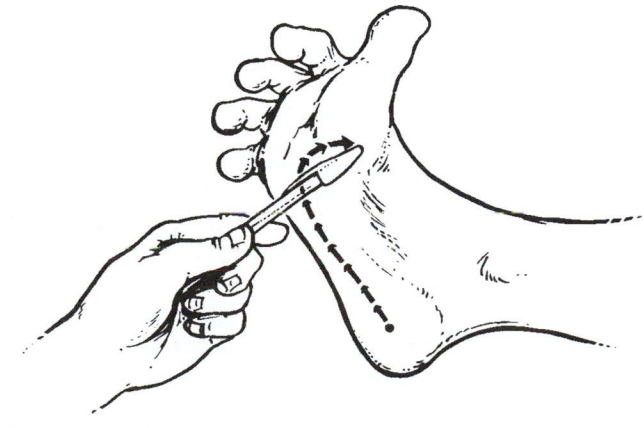

B

Figure 22-4
A. Negative Babinski. *B.* Positive Babinski.

Sustained ankle clonus after forced dorsiflexion is also an abnormal sign of upper motor neuron disease.

A variety of tests have been described which are indicative of lumbar nerve root tension due to compression. The *straight leg raising test,* also known as *Lasegue's test,* is performed with the patient in the supine position. The examiner then places one hand on the ilium to stabilize the pelvis and uses the other hand to slowly elevate one leg by the heel (Fig. 22-5A). The test is considered positive only if radiating leg pain is present, usually beyond the knee; back pain alone

is not sufficient. Often, the pain will abate with flexion of the knee. The *contralateral straight leg raise test* involves the same maneuvers, but on the leg that is not reported to be a source of pain. The test is considered positive if radiating pain is evoked in the leg that is not being raised, and is considered more specific for disc herniations medial to the nerve root in the axilla (Fig. 22-5B). The *bowstring test* is another tension root maneuver done with patient's ipsilateral knee in some flexion, and the examiner applying thumb pressure on the popliteal compartment. This action bowstrings the popliteal nerve. A

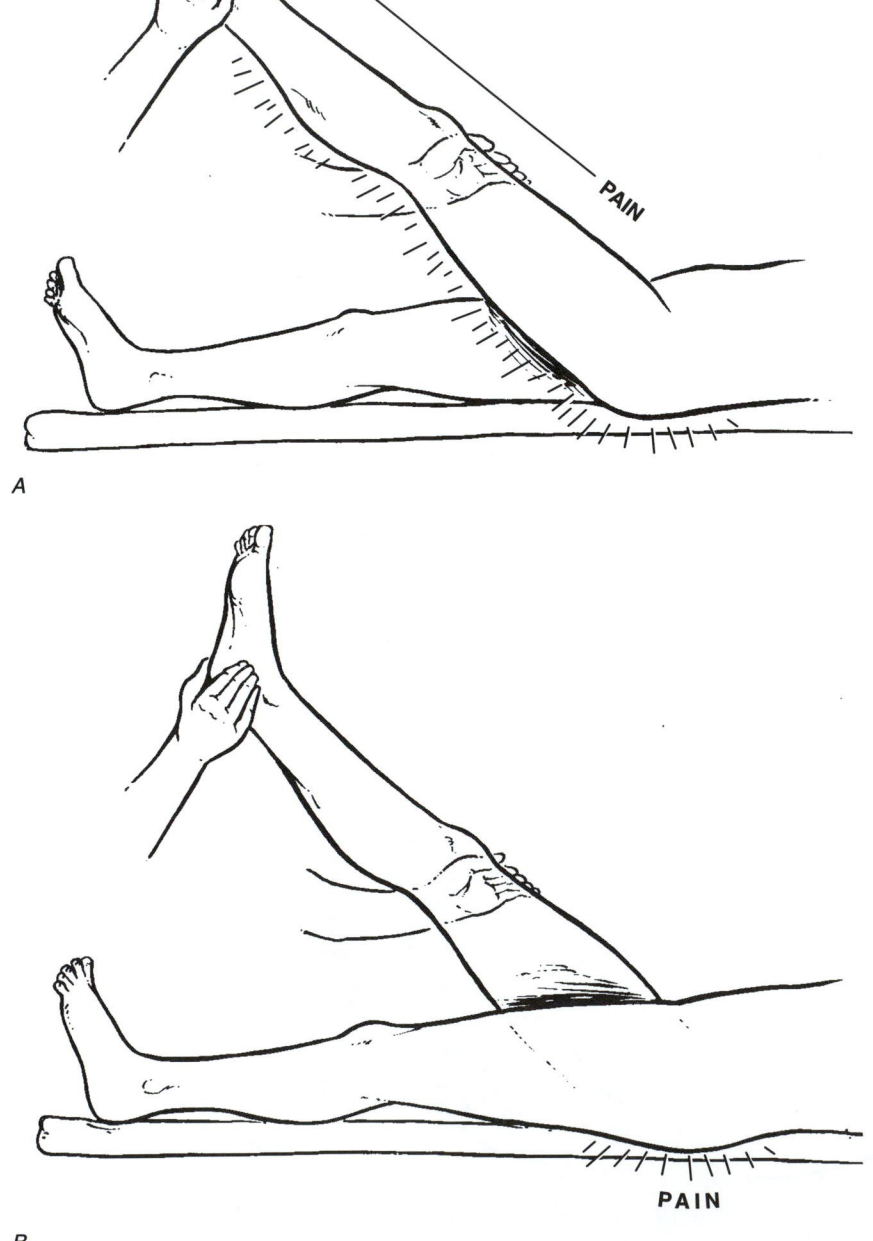

A

B

Figure 22-5
A. Straight leg raising test (positive if radiating pain is present, usually beyond knee). *B.* Contralateral straight leg raising test (positive if pain is evoked in leg not being raised).

positive test is one with pain reproduced in the buttock and hamstring. This test is viewed as an indicator of the acuity of the sciatica.

The *femoral stretch test*, also known as the *reverse strength straight leg raising test*, is done to assess for upper lumbar (L2-L4) radiculopathy. With the patient in the lateral position or prone, the affected leg is flexed at the knee and the hip is extended. This maneuver puts the femoral nerve on stretch, and relaxes the sciatic nerve.

SUGGESTED READINGS

Bates B, Bickley LS, Hockelman RA: *A Guide to Physical Examination and History Taking,* 6th ed. Philadelphia: JB Lippincott; 1995.

Hoppenfeld S: *Orthopaedic Neurology: A Diagnostic Guide to Neurologic Levels.* Philadelphia: JB Lippincott; 1977.

Hoppenfeld S: *Physical Examination of the Spine and Extremities.* Philadelphia: Appleton-Century-Crofts; 1976.

Neumann RD: Low back pain, lumbar disc disease, and spinal stenosis. In Brown D, Neumann RD (eds): *Orthopaedic Secrets.* Philadelphia: Hanley & Belfus; Mosby; 1995:185.

Stern JT: *Essentials of Gross Anatomy.* Philadelphia: FA Davis; 1988.

Chapter 23

SHOULDER

Frances Cuomo and Amaryllis J. Scott

Clinical evaluation of shoulder pathology requires an organized, logical approach in order to obtain an accurate diagnosis. A detailed history combined with a thorough physical examination and plain radiographs can often lead to the correct diagnosis, without requiring further diagnostic tests.

When obtaining the history, inquire about the patient's chief complaint. Is it pain, instability, loss of motion, or perhaps weakness? Identify the presence of a precipitating event, either traumatic or the result of a repetitive activity. If pain is present, characterize its quality and severity; note its location and whether it radiates. Assess the presence or absence of night pain and inquire about any aggravating or alleviating factors, as well as associated symptoms. Arm dominance, occupation and questions regarding repetitive activities also play a major role in determining an accurate diagnosis.

A thorough physical examination should include inspection and palpation of the shoulder, assessment of the range of motion and strength, and the performance of the appropriate provocative tests. In addition, a thorough examination of the cervical spine should be performed on all patients to rule out primary cervical pathology with referred pain to the shoulder. The neurological examination includes a complete motor and sensory evaluation, as well as testing of the reflex arcs. The duplication of the primary complaint of shoulder pain by range of motion of the neck or provocative testing is indicative of cervical spine pathology, rather than an intrinsic shoulder problem.

INSPECTION AND PALPATION

Inspection of the shoulder is both dynamic and static. Observation of patients as they enter the examination room and disrobe can provide valuable information regarding shoulder function. Look for fluidity of motion and symmetry of bony and soft tissue contour in comparison with the contralateral shoulder. Note any swelling or discoloration of the skin. Assess for muscular atrophy of the pectoralis, deltoid, supraspinatus, infraspinatus, teres minor, or trapezius. Check for scapular winging and symmetrical scapulohumeral synchrony.

Palpate along all bony contours and joints including the sternoclavicular and acromiclavicular joints, noting any areas of tenderness, deformity, or asymmetry. Palpate the greater tuberosity with the shoulder in extension and slight internal rotation, as this will bring the supraspinatus portion of the rotator cuff out from under the acromion. Palpation of the biceps is best performed with the arm in 10 degrees of internal rotation, evaluating for both tenderness or subluxation.

RANGE OF MOTION

Normal shoulder range of motion is divided into two components: glenohumeral and scapulothoracic. Although there is disagreement in the literature as to the exact contribution of each component, it is generally accepted that there is a 2:1 ratio, with a greater contribution from the glenohumeral component. The glenohumeral joint, therefore, provides 120 degrees of elevation, and the scapulothoracic articulation provides 60 degrees. Stabilization of the scapula as one assesses range of motion allows the examiner to determine the relative contribution of each component.

The American Shoulder and Elbow Surgeons society has recommended a standard protocol for testing the range of motion of the shoulder. The shoulder should be evaluated in the following planes of motion: forward elevation (active and passive), internal rotation (active or passive, as these are generally the same), and external rotation at the side and at 90 degrees of abduction (active and passive). Active range of motion is best assessed in the sitting or standing position. Passive range of motion is tested in the supine position for all planes of motion except internal rotation. Supine testing will eliminate any compensatory motion of the spine. The contralateral shoulder should always be examined for comparison.

Forward elevation is defined as flexion of the shoulder in the plane of the scapula with the angle formed between the arm and the posterior thorax. Assess for pain during forward elevation. A painful arc of motion within the 60 to 120 degree range may be indicative of rotator cuff pathology. External rotation is measured both with the arm at the side and the elbow flexed 90 degrees, as well as with the arm abducted 90 degrees. Internal rotation is assessed by having the patient reach behind his or her back and measuring the highest level reached by the outstretched thumb. This is recorded as buttock or greater trochanter, sacrum, iliac crest or L4, umbilicus or T12-L1, and inferior border of the scapula or T7. The exact level of the spinous process may also be counted directly.

MUSCLE TESTING

Strength of the shoulder is assessed using standard muscle grading (0 to 5) (see Table 22-2). The muscles tested include the shoulder flexors, extensors, abductors, adductors, and external and internal rotators, as well as the scapular muscles and the biceps.

The primary shoulder flexors include the anterior deltoid and the clavicular head of the pectoralis major. The secondary flexors include the coracobrachialis and the biceps. To test the shoulder flexors, have the patient forward-flex the shoulder against resistance, starting at 90 degrees of elevation. Isolated testing of the biceps brachii is performed by having the patient flex the elbow against resistance with the forearm held in supination.

The primary shoulder extensors are comprised of the latissimus dorsi, teres major, and the posterior deltoid. The teres minor and the long head of the triceps are the secondary extensors. These muscles are best evaluated with shoulder extension against resistance while maintaining the elbow at the side and flexed to 90 degrees.

The supraspinatus and the middle deltoid function as the primary shoulder abductors. The anterior and posterior deltoid and the serratus anterior (scapular stabilizer) act as secondary abductors. These muscles are best tested by gradually abducting the shoulder against resistance with the elbow slightly abducted from the side and flexed to 90 degrees. For isolated testing of the supraspinatus, the arm is abducted 90 degrees in the plane of the scapula, while pronating the forearm such that the thumb points toward the floor. With the arm maintained in this position, the arm is then abducted against resistance.

Adduction occurs mainly as a result of pectoralis major and latissimus dorsi function, and secondarily by teres major and anterior deltoid function. Adduction strength is measured by gradually adducting the shoulder against resistance with the elbow flexed 90 degrees and starting with the shoulder adducted 90 degrees.

External rotation is performed by the action of the infraspinatus and the teres minor. The posterior deltoid acts as a secondary external rotator. With the elbow in 90 degrees of flexion and neutral humeral rotation, stabilize the arm against the thorax and have the patient gently externally rotate against resistance to test these important rotator cuff muscles.

The subscapularis, pectoralis major, latissimus dorsi, and teres major function as primary shoulder internal rotators. The anterior deltoid acts as a secondary internal rotator. Strength testing involves flexing the elbow to 90 degrees in neutral humeral rotation and stabilizing the elbow against the thorax while the patient internally rotates against resistance.

Scapular motion occurs as a result of numerous muscular attachment actions. Scapular elevation is primarily a function of the trapezius and levator scapulae muscles, with the rhomboids secondarily assisting. To test the scapular elevators, stand behind the patient with hands placed on top of both shoulders while the patient shrugs his shoulders against resistance.

Scapular protraction is performed by the serratus anterior. Weakness in this muscle often presents with scapular winging and may be secondary to a long thoracic nerve injury. The integrity of the serratus anterior is best evaluated by the "push up" manuever, whereby the patient pushes against a wall with the arm forward flexed to 90 degrees. Observe for scapular winging indicating weakness of the serratus anterior.

In contrast, the rhomboids are the primary retractors of the scapula, aided secondarily by the trapezius. To evaluate scapular retraction strength, the shoulders are actively brought back against resistance applied by the examiner standing in front of the patient and holding the scapular spine and acromion forward.

PROVOCATIVE TESTS

Various provocative tests can be performed which will allow further assessment of shoulder function. Several tests in particular help evaluate for the presence of instability about the shoulder. The anterior apprehension test is performed in order to assess anterior instability. The patient is placed in the seated position with the arm abducted to 90 degrees while the shoulder is gradually externally rotated. The examiner's hand is placed over the humeral head and an anteriorly directed force is applied. Apprehension secondary to a sensation of impending dislocation as the humeral head translates anteriorly on the glenoid rim is considered a positive test. This may or may not be accompanied by pain (Fig. 23-1).

The *relocation test* is also suggestive of anterior instability. With the patient in the supine position and the involved shoulder off the edge

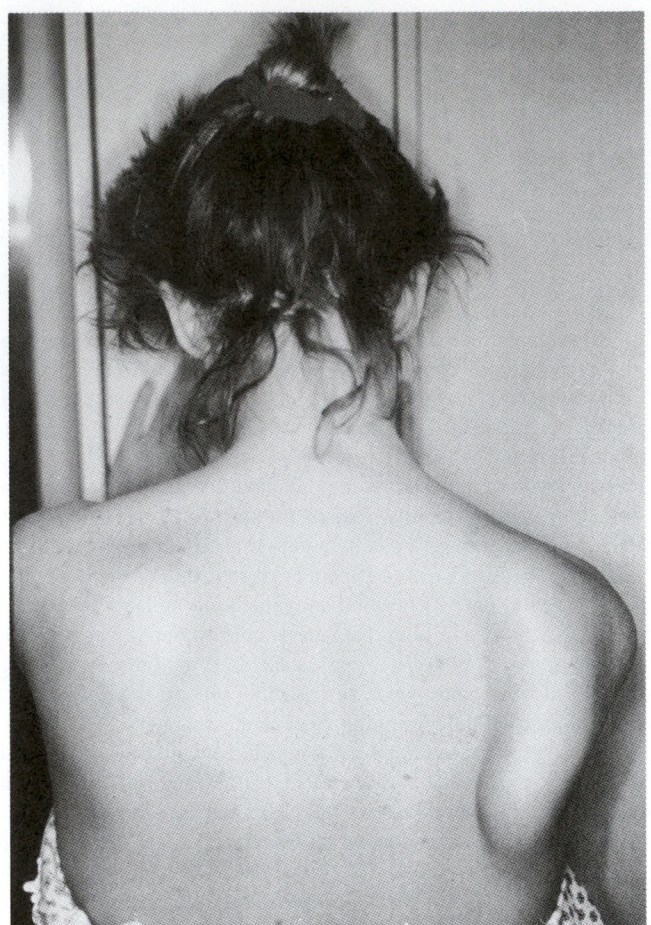

Figure 23-1
Scapular winging noted on right due to long thoracic nerve injury.

of the examination table, the arm is placed in a position of 90 degrees abduction and then maximally externally rotated. At the point where pain is noted, a posteriorly directed force on the humeral head is applied. Relief of pain is considered a positive test.

Posterior instability is evaluated by the use of the *posterior apprehension test*. With the patient in the seated position, the arm is placed in 90 degrees forward-flexion and slight adduction. The shoulder is then gently internally rotated while a posteriorly directed force is placed on the arm and humeral head. A sensation of apprehension secondary to impending dislocation or pain as the humeral head translates posteriorly on the glenoid rim is considered a positive test.

Dimpling of the skin adjacent to the acromion while direct inferior traction is applied to the arm is referred to as a *sulcus sign*. A positive sulcus sign is a common finding in patients with multidirectional instability and generalized ligamentous laxity. The presence of a sulcus sign signifies inferior capsular laxity but not necessarily instability (Fig. 23-2).

The *load and shift test* (also known as *anterior-posterior drawer* test) assesses the amount of humeral head translation in the affected shoulder. This test can help determine the presence of isolated increased anterior translation in patients with a questionable history of traumatic dislocation, as well as help identify those patients with multidirectional laxity. With the patient in the seated position, the humeral head is grasped between the examiner's thumb and forefingers. The

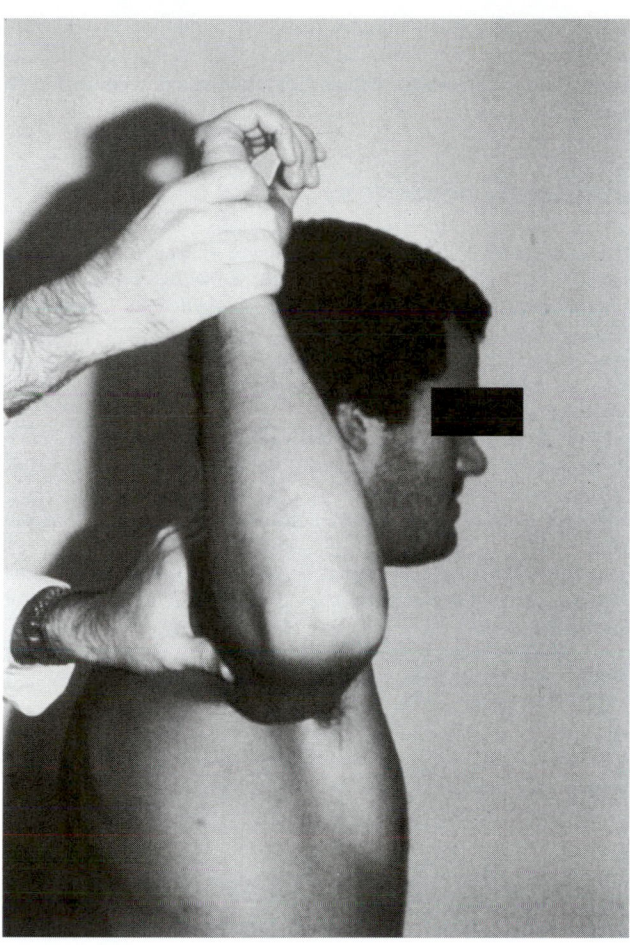

Figure 23-2
Anterior apprehension test to assess anterior instability. A positive test may or may not be accompanied by pain.

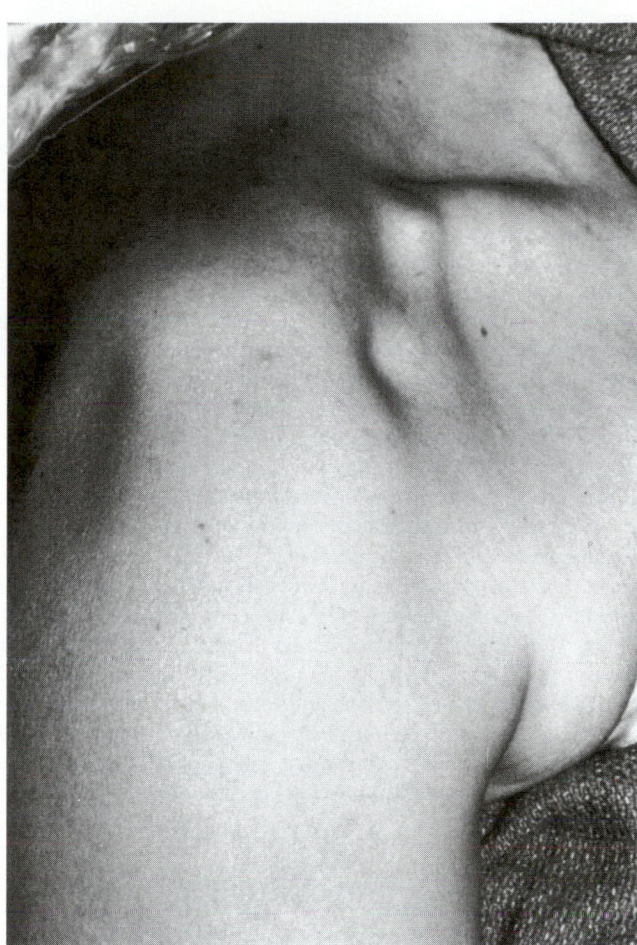

Figure 23-3
Dimpling adjacent to the acromion during direct inferior traction to the arm represents a positive sulcus sign.

examiner's opposite hand stabilizes the scapula. A gentle compressive "load" is then applied to reduce the humeral head against the glenoid. Once the head has been reduced, anterior and posterior forces are then applied. The amount of "shift" or translation is noted. The test should also be repeated in the supine position. The contralateral shoulder should always be examined for comparison.

Other provocative tests provide information regarding the presence of rotator cuff inflammation, bicipital tendonitis, or acromioclavicular arthrosis. Two classic impingement tests exist: the Neer test and the Hawkins test. Both tests evaluate the presence of rotator cuff tendonitis secondary to impingement. In addition, a lidocaine subacromial injection test can further elicit the diagnosis of impingement. Improvement of symptoms post-injection (a positive test) supports the diagnosis of rotator cuff pathology, while a negative test leads the physician to look elsewhere for the etiology of the patient's symptoms (Fig. 23-3).

The *Neer impingement test* is performed by forcibly forward-elevating the arm against a stabilized scapula. In a positive test, pain is elicited as the greater tuberosity impinges the inflamed supraspinatus tendon against the undersurface of the anterior acromion (Fig. 23-4).

The *Hawkins impingement test* is performed by first forward-flexing the arm to 90 degrees, followed by internal rotation. When positive, pain is elicited as the inflamed supraspinatus tendon is forced against the coracoacromial ligament and anterior acromion.

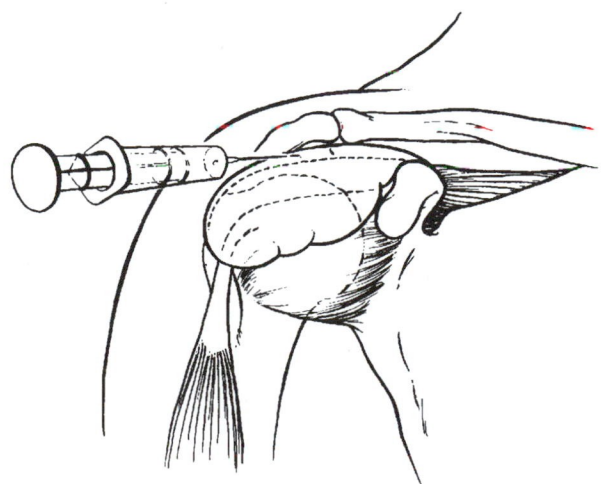

Figure 23-4
Subacromial lidocaine injection may facilitate confirmation of the diagnosis of impingement. [Reproduced by permission from Neer CS II: Cuff tears, biceps lesions, and impingement. In: *Shoulder Reconstruction*. Philadelphia: WB Saunders; 1990:80. Original source (with permission) Neer CS II: Impingement lesions. *Clin Orthop* 1983; 173:73.]

Specific provacative tests evaluate for bicipital tendonitis which is usually not an isolated finding, but occurs concomitantly with rotator cuff pathology. Two frequently used tests to assess for bicipital tendonitis are Speed's and Yergason's tests. In *Speed's test,* the arm is forward-elevated against resistance with the elbow extended and the forearm supinated. A positive test results in pain referred to the region of the bicipital groove, signifying pathology of the long head of the biceps.

Yergason's test is performed by supinating the forearm against resistance while maintaining 90 degrees of elbow flexion. A positive test will elicit pain in the region of the bicipital groove. In addition, the examiner should place his or her forefingers over the biceps tendon while performing this test to assess for any evidence of subluxation.

Subscapularis pathology can be evaluated with the *lift-off* test. With the arm internally rotated behind the lumbar spine, have the patient hold the arm off the back. Inability to perform this maneuver is indicative of subscapularis dysfunction or rupture. Pain without weakness may be an indicator of subscapularis inflammation.

Examination of the acromioclavicular joint includes a combination of direct palpation and the cross-arm adduction test. The test is performed by positioning the arm in 90 degrees of forward elevation and then passively adducting the arm across the chest. Pain elicited in the region of the acromioclavicular joint is considered a positive test. It should be noted that this test may also reproduce the pain of impingement. However, with impingement the pain is often not localized to the acromioclavicular joint, but rather anteriorly to the region of the rotator cuff. Similarily, the Hawkins test may elicit pain in patients with acromioclavicular arthrosis, but symptoms would not be referred directly to the acromioclavicular joint. A selective lidocaine injection into the acromioclavicular joint would aid in confirming the diagnosis in cases of ambiguity.

SUGGESTED READINGS

Cuomo F, Lonner JH, Spivak JM, et al: Clinical evaluation of the neck and shoulder. In Nordin M, Andersson GBJ, Pope MH (eds): *Musculoskeletal Disorders in the Workplace: Principles and Practice.* St. Louis: Mosby; 1996:359.

Flatow EL, Pollock RG: Shoulder: instability. In Kasser JR (ed): *Orthopedic Knowledge Update 5.* Rosemont, IL: American Academy of Orthopaedic Surgeons; 1996:223.

Hawkins RJ, Bokor DJ: Clinical evaluation of shoulder problems. In Rockwood CA Jr, Matsen FA III (eds): *The Shoulder,* vol 1. Philadelphia: WB Saunders; 1990:149.

Hawkins RJ, Hobeika P: Physical examination of the shoulder. *Orthopedics* 1983; 6:1270.

Hoppenfeld S: Physical examination of the shoulder. In *Physical Examination of the Spine and Extremities.* Norwalk, CT: Appleton-Century-Crofts;1976:1.

Jobe FW, VanderWilde RS: Chronic shoulder problems in athletes. In Griffin LY (ed): *Orthopedic Knowledge Update: Sports Medicine.* Rosemont, IL: American Academy of Orthopaedic Surgeons; 1994:153.

Neer CS II: Impingement lesions. *Clin Orthop* 1983; 170:70.

Post M: *Physical Examination of the Musculoskeletal System.* Chicago, IL: Mosby Year-Book Medical; 1987.

Chapter 24

ELBOW

Andrew S. Rokito

This chapter should provide the clinician with a clear, sequential method for examining the elbow that can be performed readily and is reproducible. When combined with an adequate record of the patient's medical history, a systematic examination of the elbow will lead to diagnostic success. Accurate examination of the elbow includes the history, inspection, palpation, range of motion testing, ligamentous stress testing, motor strength testing, and a neurovascular evaluation.

HISTORY

A careful documentation of the patient's medical history includes not only the chief complaint, but also a description of the pain in terms of its location and associated symptoms (e.g., swelling, radiation, locking, and/or paresthesias). The chronicity of the symptoms should also be ascertained, as well as the date of injury, when available. The history should also include the mode of onset of the symptoms (i.e., single event versus insidious) and any previous treatment that has been attempted.

When evaluating throwing athletes, particular attention should be paid to establishing when the symptoms occur with regard to the throwing motion. One should question whether the athlete's training program or biomechanics have been altered. A well-documented history gives the physician the necessary background to perform a comprehensive physical examination.

INSPECTION

Adequate examination of the elbow requires the patient to be appropriately attired such that both upper extremities can be completely evaluated simultaneously. The shoulder, wrists, and hands should always be generally inspected to exclude symptoms from a referred source.

The *carrying angle* should be examined first with the elbow extended, palm facing forward. Normally, the elbow has a valgus posture secondary to the obliquity of the trochlea. This angle is approximately 5 degrees in males and 10 to 15 degrees in females and can vary considerably, especially among athletes. It may be more clearly seen by placing a heavy object in the hand of the arm being examined.

Any increase in angulation (i.e., cubitus valgus) should be noted. This may have been caused by a childhood injury resulting in epiphyseal damage, such as following a lateral condyle fracture. A decrease in angulation (i.e., cubitus varus or "gunstock" deformity) should also be noted (Fig. 24-1). This is also a complication of childhood trauma, such as following a supracondylar humerus resulting in malunion or growth retardation of the distal humerus. The difference in degrees in the carrying angles between sides should be recorded.

The skin should be evaluated for such signs of trauma or infection as erythema, abrasions, or lacerations. The presence of an effusion must also be noted. It is important to determine whether the edema is localized, such as in olecranon bursitis, or diffuse, such as an intraarticular effusion in inflammatory arthritis.

RANGE-OF-MOTION TESTING

The elbow has been described as a hinge or ginglymoid joint; its planes of motion, however, have been found to be considerably more complex. While flexion and extension are the primary motions observed, pronation and supination are critical secondary components.

Flexion and extension take place at the ulnohumeral articulation and should be examined together in a single arc. Normal range of motion is from 0 (straight arm) to −5 degrees of extension to 150 degrees of flexion. The average person should be able to reach the ipsilateral shoulder with all of his or her fingers. Flexion may be limited by the presence of intraarticular loose bodies, articular surface defects, or muscle tightness (e.g., sprain). Extension is limited by the depth of the olecranon fossa and may be diminished secondary to posterior intraarticular loose bodies, overgrowth of the tip of the olecranon, or a scarred anterior capsule.

Pronation and supination should also be performed as one test because the two motions are described as a single arc. These motions should be tested with the patient's elbow flexed to 90 degrees and held by the examiner at waist level to prevent substitution with shoulder motion. The forearm should be rotated so that the palm faces upward (supination) and then downward (pronation). Average pronation and supination are 75 and 85 degrees, respectively. Range of motion should be tested both actively and passively. Range of motion can be limited by pathology at the shoulder, elbow, and/or wrist.

PALPATION

OSSEOUS STRUCTURES

Palpation of the elbow should begin with inspection of the bony prominences. The *olecranon process* is a good point of reference with which to begin palpating the elbow because it is easily felt with the elbow in 90 degrees of flexion as it moves out of the olecranon fossa. In this position, the olecranon and medial and lateral epicondyles form a triangle, such that the examiner's index finger on the tip of the olecranon is at the apex of the triangle.

The *olecranon fossa,* just proximal to the olecranon, may be difficult to palpate, because it is covered by the olecranon bursa and triceps tendon with its aponeurosis. It is more easily palpated with the elbow flexed 45 degrees, allowing the triceps tendon to slacken. The

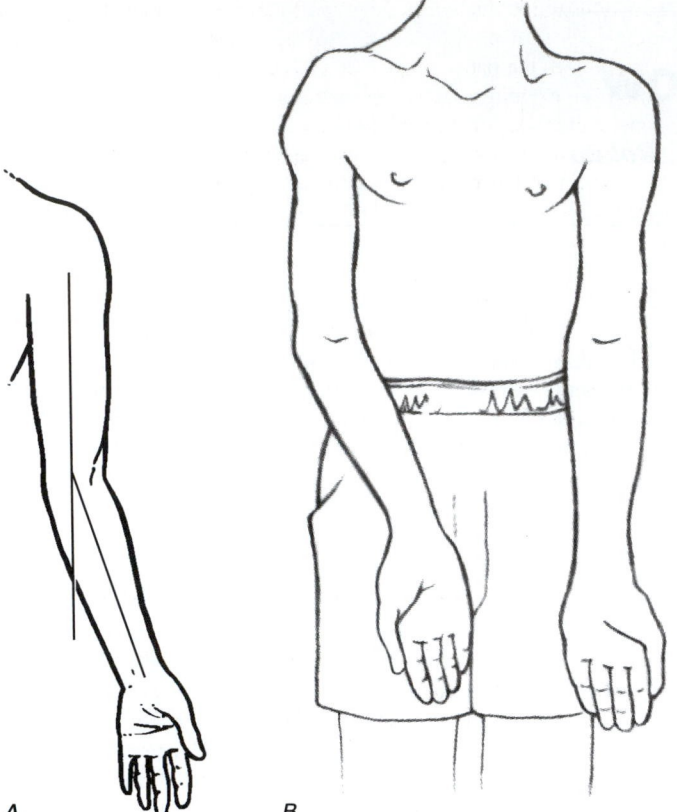

Figure 24-1
A. Normal carrying angle (cubitus valgus). *B.* Cubitus varus or "gun-stock" deformity (right elbow).

examiner should be able to distinguish between posteromedial and posterolateral tenderness.

The *medial epicondyle,* which is larger and more easily palpated than its lateral counterpart, should be gently palpated and assessed for tenderness and any abnormality in its contour. It is the most frequently fractured part of the elbow, especially in pediatric athletes, whose physes have not yet closed. The *medial supracondylar ridge* of the humerus can be assessed by palpating proximally in a linear fashion. Occasionally, osteophytes or ectopic calcifications are present that can impinge on the median or ulnar nerves. The *ulnar border* of the forearm can be palpated distally toward the ulnar styloid of the wrist.

The less prominent *lateral epicondyle* can then be palpated in a similar fashion. The *lateral supracondylar ridge* can be felt just proximal to the lateral epicondyle. The *radial head,* which is located deep within a depression in the skin distal to the lateral epicondyle and just medial and posterior to the wrist extensor group, can be more easily identified by instructing the patient to pronate and supinate the forearm. Pain in this region may be indicative of synovitis, fracture, degenerative joint disease, osteochondritis dissecans, dislocation, or subluxation.

SOFT TISSUE STRUCTURES

The *olecranon bursa* can be palpated overlying the olecranon process. When inflamed, this structure is tender and may feel boggy and thickened. Rheumatoid nodules may also be felt in this region and over the extensor surface of the forearm.

The wrist flexors originate as a common tendon from the medial epicondyle and then split into the individual muscles, which include the *pronator teres, flexor carpi radialis, palmaris longus,* and *flexor carpi ulnaris.* The order and course of these muscles can easily be remembered by placing one's hand over the medial border of the patient's forearm with the thenar eminence over the medial epicondyle (Fig. 24-2). In this way, the thumb corresponds to the patient's pronator teres, the index finger to the flexor carpi radialis, the middle finger to the palmaris longus, and the ring finger to the flexor carpi ulnaris. The wrist flexor muscles can be palpated as a unit and then individually, checking for localized tendinitis resulting from excessive forearm pronation, such as from playing golf or tennis, turning a screwdriver, or shaking hands.

As its name implies, the pronator teres functions to pronate the forearm. It is not directly palpable as it lies deep to the other muscles. The flexor carpi radialis acts to flex and radially deviate the wrist. The palmaris longus, which aids in wrist flexion, is a long, slender muscle that passes superficially across the wrist to end in the palmar aponeurosis. It is absent in one or both sides in approximately 12 percent of the population. The flexor carpi ulnaris lies on the ulnar side of the forearm and acts to flex and deviate the wrist in an ulnar direction.

The *wrist extensors,* which originate from the lateral epicondyle and supracondylar ridge, consist of the *brachioradialis, extensor carpi radialis longus,* and *extensor carpi radialis brevis.* Initially, these muscles can be palpated as a unit and then individually. They are most easily assessed with the patient's elbow flexed and the forearm in a neutral rotation. The brachioradialis can then be evaluated by asking the patient to flex the elbow against resistance. The entire length of the muscle can then be palpated, checking for tendinitis,

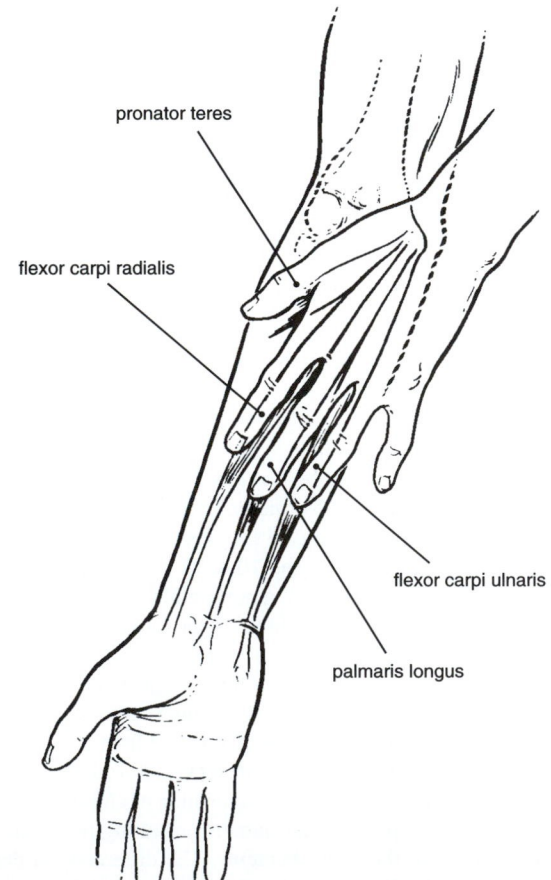

pronator teres

flexor carpi radialis

flexor carpi ulnaris

palmaris longus

Figure 24-2
The wrist flexors.

defects, hematomas, masses, etc. This muscle acts as an important elbow flexor and forearm supinator. The extensor carpi radialis longus and brevis are best evaluated with the examiner offering resistance to dorsiflexion of the wrist. Tenderness over the origin at the lateral epicondyle is indicative of lateral epicondylitis or *tennis elbow.* Pain or weakness associated with resistance of middle finger extension (i.e., *third digit sign*) is indicative of tendinitis or epicondylitis affecting the extensor carpi radialis brevis.

The *triceps surae* muscle spans two joints as the long head crosses both the shoulder and elbow. The three heads of the muscle can best be palpated with the elbow in extension in a weightbearing position, as with crutch walking or with having the patient support his or her weight on a table or desk. The long head is located posteromedially, the lateral head posterolaterally, and the medial head deep to the long head over the medial aspect of the distal humerus. The tendon is located proximal to the tip of the olecranon and should be palpated for areas of tenderness, calcifications, and defects.

The *cubital fossa* can be thought of as a triangle formed by the pronator teres medially, the brachioradialis laterally, and a line between the humeral epicondyles as the base. Within this triangle are two easily palpable structures: the *biceps brachii tendon* and the *brachial artery.* The tendon, with its expanse, the bicipital aponeurosis, is located lateral to the artery, and is more easily palpable with resistance to elbow flexion.

STRESS TESTING

The valgus stresses across the elbow associated with throwing lead to increased tensile forces over the *medial collateral ligament,* a fan-shaped structure that originates from the undersurface of the medial epicondyle and inserts onto the medial aspect of the coronoid process of the ulna, but is not directly palpable. It serves as a medial stabilizer of the ulnohumeral articulation and is best evaluated with the elbow in approximately 30 degrees of flexion so as to unlock the olecranon process from the fossa. A valgus force is then applied to the elbow to assess for tenderness over the ligament and increased laxity. Injury to this structure usually occurs secondary to a sudden valgus force or repetitive loading, as in baseball pitchers.

The *lateral collateral ligament,* which may also be injured by the repetitive forces of throwing or by direct trauma, is a ropelike structure that extends from the lateral epicondyle to the outer aspect of the annular ligament. The examiner should cup the patient's elbow with one hand and hold the wrist with the other while applying a varus stress across the joint in approximately 30 degrees of flexion. One should note whether the patient expresses pain, as well as the degree of laxity produced by this maneuver. In patients with recurrent subluxation due to a deficiency of the lateral collateral ligament, the results of a *pivot shift test* may be abnormal. This test is performed with the patient supine and the affected extremity held overhead. The examiner grasps the patient's wrist and elbow and applies a supination-valgus moment during flexion, which causes the elbow to subluxate, resulting in a typical apprehension response with reproduction of the patient's symptoms. Reproducing the actual subluxation and clunk with further flexion can usually be accomplished only with general anesthesia.

MOTOR STRENGTH TESTING

Manual muscle testing is used to evaluate further the integrity of the contractile structures about the elbow. Resistive maneuvers for elbow flexion–extension, forearm pronation–supination, and wrist flexion–extension are performed and can accurately assist in locating specific areas of pain and weakness.

NEUROVASCULAR STRUCTURES

These structures include the brachial artery, and the median, musculocutaneous, and ulnar nerves. As previously stated, the brachial artery is palpable just medial to the biceps tendon. The median nerve lies just medial to the brachial artery, exiting the elbow distally and piercing the pronator teres muscle. The musculocutaneous nerve located lateral to the biceps tendon, deep to the brachioradialis, approximately 1 to 2 inches above the joint line, is not directly palpable. It provides sensation to the lateral aspect of the forearm where it becomes the lateral antebrachial cutaneous nerve.

The *ulnar nerve* can be gently rolled under the examiner's fingers within the *ulnar groove* between the medial epicondyle and the olecranon process. It normally feels soft, round, and tubular, and any thickening, which is indicative of scarring, should be noted. Ease of displacement or subluxation should also be noted with elbow flexion and extension. The presence of a Tinel's sign over the groove or just superior to it may be indicative of ulnar neuritis.

SUGGESTED READING

Hoppenfeld S: Physical examination of the elbow. In *Physical Examination of the Spine and Extremities.* New York, Appleton-Century-Crofts, Division of Prentice-Hall, 1976:35.

Regan WD, Morrey BF: The physical examination of the elbow. In Morrey BF (ed): *The Elbow and Its Disorders,* 2d ed. Philadelphia: WB Saunders; 1993.

Chapter 25

HAND AND WRIST

Salvatore R. Lenzo

HISTORY

In any thorough assessment of a patient the history is critical. This is especially true in hand injuries where a diagnosis often can be made directly from the history. A variety of factors (e.g., dominant hand, sex, and occupation) are important in determining the prognosis and/or subsequent sequelae with regard to a particular hand injury. A simple illustration of this is seen in nerve injuries. Results of nerve grafting in a 60-year-old would be much less reliable than results in a 20-year-old person. In addition, understanding the functional demands of a patient's occupation is vital when determining the course of treatment. For example, a chronic laceration of the flexor digitorum profundus in a laborer would indicate that an arthrodesis of the distal interphalangeal joint is needed. However, in a concert violinist in which terminal active flexion is essential for performance, one might consider a staged tendon graft procedure.

After obtaining the above important data, the patient's chief complaint is the next information to address. With regard to complaints of pain it is important to assess whether there is rest pain, night pain, or perhaps morning pain. Does the patient have any complaints of deficits in sensation and/or motor function within the hand? Are there limitations with regard to activities of daily living or just in certain circumstances? Assessment of bilateral complaints is also important, and is especially true in peripheral neuropathies.

When managing hand injuries, the date of onset, type of injury, cause of injury, and prior treatment (e.g., a flexor tendon rupture, Leddy type I, one day old, or four weeks old) can dictate what type of treatment is indicated. Regarding cause for example, is the injury a burn secondary to hot water which tends to be superficial or is it a burn secondary to hot grease which tends to cause a very deep burn, as the oil retains heat? Regarding prior treatment, it may be critical to know if the patient received a tetanus shot at the time of the injury, or were antibiotics given?

Also important in the development of a good history is the mechanism of injury and the mode of onset. For example, was there a severe crush injury to a digit which may have compromised the vascularity of that finger? In this case, surgery for revascularization of the digit would be emergent.

Understanding the particular medical history is crucial to the treatment plan. Are there any systemic illnesses such as diabetes, inflammatory conditions, or prior hand injuries? The physician must also assess possibility for an immunocompromised state.

From the simple clinical examples above, one can see how a history can impact the initial overall assessment and plan of treatment in injuries of the hand and wrist.

EXAMINATION

EQUIPMENT NEEDED

Before performing a hand examination, several pieces of equipment are needed. These include a two point discriminator to assess sensory function, a goniometer to assess range of motion, a grip and pinch dynamometer to evaluate strength, a tape measure to assess length or width of a particular injured extremity, and finally, a Doppler flow meter to determine vascular function.

OBSERVATION

The initial evaluation of any injury and/or hand problem begins with observation. Is there gross atrophy of the thenar musculature as would be seen in advanced carpal tunnel syndrome? Does the finger lack good capillary fill after a crush injury indicative of vascular compromise? Is there abnormal pseudomotor function as would be seen in reflex sympathetic dystrophy? Is there gross swelling or ecchymosis within a finger, indicative of a possible phalangeal fracture? Is there an abnormal posture of a finger, such as could be seen with septic flexor tenosynovitis?

PALPATION

Assessing the temperature of a particular digit can provide significant information with regard to the viability of that finger following injury. In addition, palpation facilitates assessment of a possible vasospastic disorder which can be treated with a peripheral nerve block of the sympathetic system. Palpation is also critical in determining *areas of tenderness* and identifying underlying structures which have been injured.

For example, with regard to wrist injuries, careful palpation of the distal radius and distal radioulnar joint, as well as of the respective carpal bones should be performed. Even in the presence of a negative radiograph, an acute injury associated with tenderness within the radial snuff box should be considered suspicious for a scaphoid fracture, and treated as such. Palpation is also important in evaluating subcutaneous masses. Is there, for example, an associated clicking or locking phenomenon with a synovial cyst at the base of the flexor tendon sheath? Is there a tender nodule or cord, as with Dupuytren's contracture?

RANGE OF MOTION

Normal range of motion in the fingers is from 0 to 85 degrees of flexion at the metacarpophalangeal joint, and 0 to 65 degrees at the distal interphalangeal joint. The total of these respective joint motions is called TAM (total active motion). In assessing TAM, in addition to adding up the various ranges of flexion, any extension lag is subtracted from the total active flexion range (Table 25-1).

Other finger motions are abduction which is movement away from the middle finger and adduction which is movement towards the middle finger. *Thumb motions* include palmar abduction, opposition, retroposition, and radial abduction (Fig. 25-1). *Wrist motion* encompasses forearm pronation and supination with a normal value of 80 degrees in each direction, extension and flexion with a normal value

---
Table 25-1

Range of Motion for Fingers

Normal

1. MP joint: 0 to 85 degrees

2. PIP joint: 0 to 110 degrees

3. DIP joint: 0 to 65 degrees

---

of 75 to 80 degrees in each direction, and radial and ulnar deviation. Normal radial deviation is approximately 20 degrees and normal ulnar deviation is approximately 25 degrees.

NERVE TESTING

Sensory Evaluation

Each major nerve in the upper extremity has its own autogenous zone. The median nerve is best tested at the distal aspect of the index finger while the ulnar nerve should be tested at the distal aspect of the small finger. Radial nerve sensory examination is best tested in the first dorsal web space. When performing a thorough examination, however, it is also important to test the dorsum of the hand first in order to rule out the possibility of a high ulnar nerve compression (i.e., at the level of the cubital tunnel). In addition, sensation over the medial forearm is tested to help differentiate between a possible brachial plexus compression (i.e., compression of the medial antebrachial cutaneous nerve coming off the medial cord) versus compression of the ulnar nerve either at Guyon's canal or the cubital tunnel. With regard to evaluating median nerve function for possible compression at a more proximal site, it is important to assess the area innervated by the palmar cutaneous branch.

Peripheral nerve function can be assessed in an objective fashion. A tuning fork can be used in the initial stages of nerve damage to assess a decreased ability to perceive a stimulus. However, as compression continues, there is a decrease in innervation density. This results in abnormal findings on two-point discrimination. (Normal two-point discrimination is approximately 6 mm on the volar aspect of each finger and/or thumb.) Thus, abnormal two-point discrimination begins later in the sequence of damage to the nerve, and therefore gives some indication concerning the chronicity and/or severity of the nerve problem.

Additional objective testing for sensory function can be performed with the Ninhydrin test which documents the presence of sweat and its associated amino acids. An intact or regenerated nerve will have a positive Ninhydrin test. In addition, the wrinkle test can be used to assess sensory nerve function (i.e., a denervated finger when placed in water will not wrinkle).

Motor Function

Each of the three major nerves in the upper extremity innervates a defined group of muscles. In some instances, there is cross-over between innervations. The flexor pollicis brevis muscle, for example, is innervated by both the median and ulnar nerves (i.e., Riche-Cannieu communication). In the Martin-Gruber anastomosis, the median nerve supplies ulnar innervated muscle through a branch from the anterior interosseous nerve. Each nerve has its own major function. The ulnar nerve is important for the power grip as it innervates the intrinsic musculature and the flexor tendons on the ulnar aspect of the hand. The median nerve is important for precision grip, providing innervation to the index finger and thumb muscles. The radial nerve innervates the wrist extensors which are critical in stabilizing the wrist to prepare the hand to grip an object. The radial nerve bifurcates into a superficial branch, which continues to course underneath the muscle belly of the brachioradialis, and the posterior interosseous nerve, which courses through the supinator muscle at the level of the Arcade of Froshe. It is the posterior interosseous nerve which innervates the finger extensors including the extensor digitorum communis, extensor indices proprius, and extensor digiti minimi. It also innervates the extensor carpi ulnaris, extensor pollicis longus, extensor pollicis brevis, and the abductor pollicis longus tendons.

Further modes of testing the upper extremities include evaluation of reflexes. The biceps reflex tests nerve roots emanating from the C5-6 level. The brachioradialis reflex also tests the C5-6 nerve roots, while the triceps reflex tests the C7 nerve root.

Muscle strength is graded from 0 to 5. See Table 25-2.

Finally, there are specific findings associated with injuries to each of the three major nerves of the upper extremities. An example of a specific sign of injury to the ulnar nerve is Froment's sign: hyperflexion of the interphalangeal joint with key pinch. This is due to the intrinsic weakness of extending the interphalangeal joint of the thumb and flexing the metacarpophalangeal joint of the thumb. There is an over pull of the flexor pollicis longus causing flexed deformity of the interphalangeal joint.

The Bouvier test is important in the evaluation of ulnar intrinsic function, especially with a claw deformity resulting in an abnormal hyperextension deformity of the metacarpophalangeal joint. By blocking the metacarpophalangeal joint in flexion and asking the patient to extend the interphalangeal joints of the finger, the examiner can see if there is reasonably good intrinsic function within the proximal interphalangeal joint of the finger. This would be important in deter-

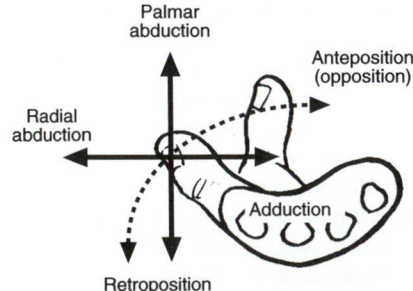

Figure 25-1
Motions of the thumb. [Redrawn with permission from the American Society for Surgery of the Hand (ASSH): The hand evaluation. In: *ASSH 1996 Regional Review Course Syllabus.* Englewood, CO: ASSH; 1996:4.]

Table 25-2

Grades for Muscle Strength

0	No contracture
1/5	Trace of contracture
2/5	Contraction without resistance
3/5	Fair resistance
4/5	Good resistance
5/5	Normal

mining what type of tendon transfer the surgeon would use to reconstruct a claw deformity of the hand secondary to ulnar nerve palsy.

The Phalen's test is used to evaluate compression of the median nerve at the level of the carpal tunnel. The patient is asked to hyperflex the wrist, and indicate to the examiner when he or she develops numbness in the median nerve distribution, the examiner noting the time at which this occurs (e.g., 5 s, 10 s). When evaluating for a proximal median nerve compression, (i.e., pronator syndrome) it is important to realize that there are three potential sites for compression. One can test for compression at the level of the lacertus fibrosis by asking the patient to resist the examiner while flexing the elbow. One can test for compression at the level of the pronator teres by asking the patient to actively pronate the forearm against resistance. Finally, the flexor digitorum sublimis arch can cause compression of the median nerve and this can be tested by asking the patient to flex his fingers about the examiner's hand at the level of the proximal interphalangeal joints of each finger. In each of these cases, the examiner assesses pain.

Specific findings when evaluating radial nerve function would include asking the patient to actively supinate against resistance. Symptoms elicited by this maneuver would indicate a possible compression at the level of the Arcade of Froshe.

TENDON TESTING

Flexor digitorum profundus test

The flexor digitorum profundi to the middle, ring, and small finger have a common muscle belly. The flexor digitorum profundus to the index finger has an individual muscle belly. It can be examined in each finger by blocking flexion of the proximal interphalangeal joint of the finger being tested and asking the patient to flex the distal interphalangeal joint of that finger.

The flexor superficialis test

The flexor digitorum profundus has a common muscle belly in the middle, ring, and small finger. By blocking the profundus muscle (i.e., flexion of the distal interphalangeal joint of the respective finger except for that finger being tested) one can assess flexor digitorum sublimis function (Fig. 25-2.)

Finger extensor tendon test

The extensor digitorum communis tendons have an integrated function due to their common muscle belly and the fact that they are attached further distally by the junctura tendinis.

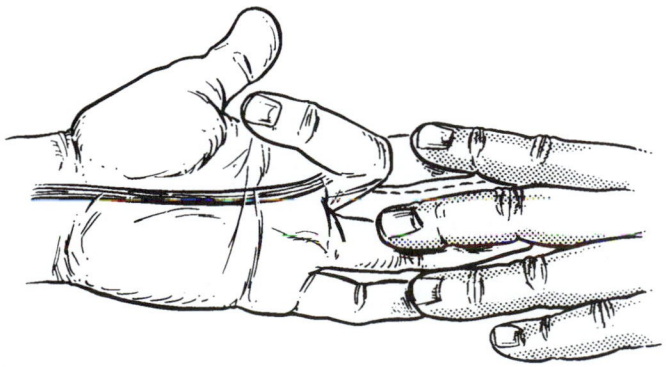

Figure 25-2
Testing flexor sublimis function to middle finger by taking advantage of common muscle belly of profundus. [Redrawn and modified with permission from the American Society for Surgery of the Hand (ASSH): The hand evaluation. In: *ASSH 1996 Regional Review Course Syllabus.* Englewood, CO: ASSH; 1996:7.]

By having the patient flex the middle two fingers (i.e., the middle and ring finger), one can test the extensor indicis proprius and the extensor digiti quinti. This is especially important if one is considering using these tendons for tendon transfers.

Assessing the tenodesis effect of tendons

In assessing the tenodesis effect of tendons with volar flexion of the wrist, the extrinsic tendons become taut, resulting in extension of the respective fingers. This is helpful to differentiate whether a laceration in the proximal forearm has resulted in injury to the posterior interosseous nerve or the muscle belly. Similarly, with extension of the wrist, the extrinsic flexors of the fingers also become taut and the patient exhibits flexion of the respective fingers and thumb. This tenodesis effect of wrist extension is lost with a flexor tendon laceration.

JOINT CAPSULAR TESTING

Restricted motion within a finger joint can be secondary to the following:

1. Inherent joint contracture
2. Intrinsic tightness
3. Extrinsic tightness

Capsular tightness

Capsular tightness is usually secondary to collateral ligament contracture or a volar plate contracture. It could also be due to contracture of the dorsal capsule and/or intraarticular adhesions and degenerative changes. Most commonly, this develops after improper splinting of a joint. Therefore, the metacarpophalangeal joint should be splinted in a position of 90 degrees and the interphalangeal joint should be splinted at 0 degrees, such that the collateral ligaments are at their longest length. The volar plate can often become contracted after splinting the interphalangeal joint in a flexed position, thus resulting in a "pseudoboutonniere-type" deformity.

Intrinsic tightness

Intrinsic tightness may have several causes. It can be seen in crush injuries to the hand, arthritic deformities as seen in rheumatoid patients, and spastic disorders as seen in patients with central nervous system injuries. Intrinsic tightness is determined by first flexing the metacarpophalangeal joint which relaxes the intrinsic muscles (as these course volar to the coronal axis to the metacarpophalangeal joint) and then assessing proximal interphalangeal joint flexion.

With intrinsic tightness, flexing the metacarpophalangeal joint allows the proximal interphalangeal joint to flex easily. However, with extension of the metacarpophalangeal joint which then puts the intrinsic muscles on stretch, the proximal interphalangeal joint does not flex easily. There is also an intrinsic tightness test which evaluates the ligament of Landsmeer. This ligament is volar to the coronal axis of the proximal interphalangeal joint. Thus, if there is a tightness within this ligament with extension of the proximal interphalangeal joint, there will be difficulty in passively flexing the distal interphalangeal joint.

Extrinsic tightness

Extrinsic tightness occurs when there are adhesions about the extrinsic extensor mechanism. With volar flexion of the wrist, and flexion of the metacarpophalangeal joints, the extrinsic tendons are put on stretch. If there are adhesions at these levels, there will be difficulty when passively flexing the proximal interphalangeal joints. Extending the wrist and metacarpophalangeal joints will release stretch on the adhesed tendon, and thus allow the examiner to readily passively flex the proximal interphalangeal joint.

The *quadriga* effect is seen in the flexor tendons to the fingers. This refers to the decreased active motion in an uninjured digit that has a common muscle origin with an adjacent injured digit with diminished tendon excursion. Finally, the examiner should be aware of the *lumbrical plus deformity* in a finger. This can be seen in the origin of the lumbrical muscle or in a tendon graft which has been sewn into the distal stump of the flexor digitorum profundus in a lax position. When a flexor tendon contracts, it puts tension on the origin of the lumbrical muscle, thus causing increased tightness in this muscle tendon unit. If the flexor cannot act distally, such as in a distal flexor profundus laceration or in a tendon graft that is sewn in loosely, the position of the finger will be contrary to what would be expected, i.e., instead of flexion of the proximal interphalangeal joint, there would be extension of this joint.

EVALUATION OF VASCULAR INJURIES

The vascular examination of hand and wrist injury includes assessment of color, pulses, pain, paresthesias, and possible paralysis. In addition, the examiner should also test for the temperature of the extremity. There are other tests done on physical examination to assess for vascular insufficiency or problems such as the Allen test at the level of the wrist, and/or individual finger. In the Allen test, the radial and ulnar arteries are occluded with pressure while the patient makes a sequential fist. The examiner then releases pressure on one of the arteries to determine which digit receives its blood supply from that artery. Special tests can also be used to assess vascular function, such as a Doppler exam, an arteriogram, and digital plethysmography.

It is important to remember that the arterial supply is volar to the nerve supply in the palm, while at the level of the digit, the nerve is volar to the artery. Thus, with volar laceration to a finger in which the patient reports that there was vigorous bleeding, the examiner can be assured that the digital nerve was also lacerated at the time of the injury. In addition, it should be noted that despite having lacerations of both the ulnar and radial digital arteries at the level of the proximal interphalangeal joint, capillary refill can be present in the nail bed after blanching. However, this would not preclude surgical intervention to repair the artery since there would be significant other deficits secondary to the dual laceration of the arteries, i.e. subsequent cold intolerance. The Allen test is especially important to perform when considering resection of a volar ganglion or when assessing trauma to the ulnar aspect of the wrist and/or possible ulnar neuropathy at the level of Guyon's canal. With either laceration of the radial or the ulnar artery at the level of the wrist, gross ischemia of the hand is not usually apparent; rather, a claudication of the intrinsic muscles is seen on stress. A traumatic thrombosis of the ulnar artery often causes more distal ischemic phenomenon secondary to distal vasospasm, i.e., subsequent to traumatic pseudoaneurysms at the level of the hook of the hamate. Finally, circulatory compromise of the hand can be seen in more proximal injuries such as at the level of the elbow or forearm (i.e., fractures). Often a gentle reduction of these fractures can release kinking of the artery and subsequent distal compromise of the circulation. Finally, the examiner should also always be aware of tight bandages and/or a cast which may cause circulatory embarrassment.

SUGGESTED READINGS

Beasley RW: *Hand Injuries*. Philadelphia: WB Saunders; 1981.

Overton DT, Uehara DT: Evaluation of the injured hand. *Emerg Med Clin North Am* 1993; 11(3):585.

Watson HK, Ashmead D 4th, Makhlouf MV: Examination of the scaphoid. *J Hand Surg [Am]* 1988; 13(5):657.

Chapter 26

HIP

Alan J. Dayan, Daniel W. Wilen, and Steven A. Stuchin

INSPECTION

Physical examination of the hip should begin with observation of the patient's gait. Any gait abnormality such as a limp, lurch, or an antalgic gait pattern should be noted and further assessment for primary hip pathology or other causes (e.g., neuromuscular) should be made. An antalgic gait is characterized by a rapid swing phase of the unaffected leg, thereby shortening the weightbearing, or stance phase, of the affected limb to counteract or lessen pain. A lurch is an alteration of a normal gait pattern typically used to offset muscle weakness about the hip. An abductor lurch results from a weak gluteus medius muscle; the direction of the lurch is lateral. This compensatory movement is performed to maintain hip abduction and prevent the pelvis from tilting toward the opposite side during midstance. The patient shifts his or her center of gravity over the involved hip by thrusting the thorax in that direction. An extensor lurch counteracts a weak gluteus maximus muscle, or weak hip extension. The direction of the extensor lurch is backward, and is the result of thrusting the thorax and center of gravity posteriorly to maintain hip extension during midstance (see Chap. 35).

The examination continues with the patient supine, and the hip joint appropriately exposed to examine the overlying skin. Abrasions, swellings, scars, draining sinuses, or areas of ecchymosis or erythema should be noted. The observed position of the leg can provide important clinical information, especially if the patient cannot ambulate. An underlying hip fracture may manifest as a shortened, externally rotated lower extremity. The positions of the anterior superior iliac spine (ASIS), iliac crest, and greater trochanter should be noted for any unusual configurations and/or lack of symmetry with respect to the contralateral side. If the bony anatomy is not symmetrical from side to side, pelvic obliquity may be present. Pelvic obliquity can have several causes including unilateral hip contracture, scoliosis, and limb-length inequality. The diagnosis of pelvic obliquity can be con-firmed by comparing the patient's true and apparent leg length discrepancy. True leg length is measured from the ASIS to the ipsilateral medial malleolus. Apparent leg length is assessed by measuring the distance from a non-fixed point, such as the umbilicus or the xiphisternal joint to the medial malleolus. A discrepancy between the true and the apparent leg length indicates a pelvic obliquity.

The degree of lumbar lordosis should also be observed and evaluated. The absence of normal lordosis may suggest paravertebral muscle spasm. Excessive lordosis, on the other hand, may indicate weak abdominal muscles or be secondary to a hip flexion contracture with a loss of normal hip extension. Increased lumbar lordosis allows the pelvis to rotate anteriorly and the thigh to fully rest on the examination table.

PALPATION

Pelvic and hip areas important to assess by palpation include the iliac crest, the greater trochanter, the femoral triangle, the posterior hip, the sciatic nerve, and the related musculature.

Palpation for pathology associated with the hips should begin with the patient in a supine position. Findings of tenderness, warmth, abnormal masses, and swelling are generally facilitated by examining both hips at the same time. Simultaneous assessment of both hips should start with the iliac crests and anterior superior iliac spines, continue posteriorly several centimeters to the iliac tubercles (the widest portion of the iliac crest), then proceed, distally and laterally, to the greater trochanters. The femur can be rotated to facilitate identification of the greater trochanter. Point tenderness over the greater trochanter or the trochanteric bursa may represent trochanteric bursitis. Finally, at the midline, the pubic tubercle can be palpated. This structure is located at the same level as the proximal aspect of the greater trochanter (Fig. 26-1).

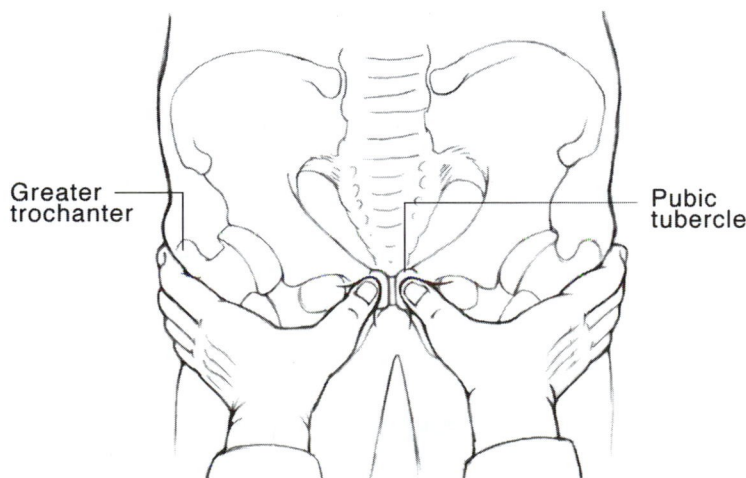

Greater trochanter

Pubic tubercle

Figure 26-1
Palpation of the pubic tubercles.

In order to best palpate the contents of the femoral triangle, the affected leg should be placed in a "figure of four" position by flexing, abducting, and externally rotating the hip (Fig. 26-2). The femoral triangle is bordered by the sartorius muscle laterally, the adductor longus muscle medially, and the inguinal ligament superiorly. Swelling or a "bulge" along the inguinal ligament may suggest the presence of an underlying hernia. The adductor longus muscle, which is often the source of a "groin pull," can be palpated from its origin at the pubic tubercle. The femoral *v*ein, *a*rtery, and *n*erve ("VAN") pass beneath the inguinal ligament from medial to lateral, respectively. The lymph nodes are situated at the most medial aspect of the triangle; enlargement of these nodes should suggest local or distal pathology such as infection or tumor.

The posterior aspect of the hip is examined with the patient lying on the contralateral side. The posterior portion of the iliac crest lies just below the subcutaneous tissue and is easily palpated. A small dimple can frequently be seen just distal to the posterior iliac crest and may serve as a guide to the posterior superior iliac spine (PSIS), which can be palpated deep to this surface landmark. By continuing further distally and laterally, the ischial tuberosity is palpated. The sciatic nerve can be palpated midway between the ischial tuberosity and the greater trochanter. Nerve trauma, muscle spasm, and disc herniation are among the possible causes of observed tenderness when palpating the sciatic nerve.

RANGE OF MOTION

Passive range of motion testing of the hip begins with the patient supine. The Thomas test is performed to evaluate for the presence of a hip flexion contracture. The contralateral hip is flexed to flatten the lumbar spine and stabilize the pelvis. If the involved leg does not completely extend with the contralateral hip fully flexed, then a hip contracture is likely. The extent of the hip flexion contracture can be

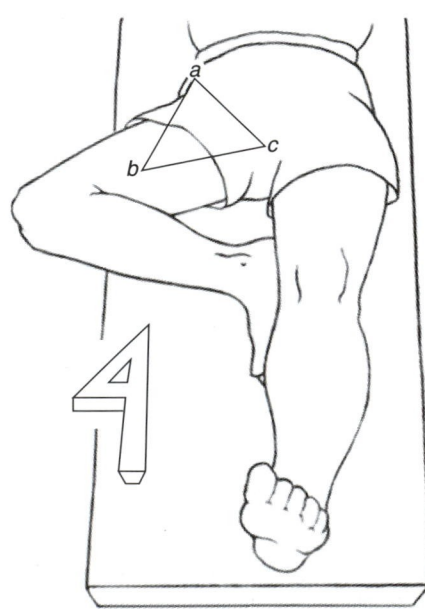

Figure 26-2
Femoral triangle (abc) with the leg in a figure-four position. Anterior iliac spine (a), pubic tubercle (c), inguinal ligament (ac), medial border of sartorius muscle (ab), medial border of adductor longus muscle (cb).

estimated by measuring the angle of the thigh (extended leg) relative to the examining table. Normal hip flexion is 120 to 130 degrees. This is assessed by flexing the hip maximally while also flexing the knee.

Abduction is assessed with the patient in a supine position. The pelvis should be stabilized with the examiner's forearm placed over the abdomen and the hand of the same arm positioned on the opposite anterior superior iliac spine; the leg (supported near the ankle by the examiner's other hand) should then be brought away from the midline and toward the examiner as far as comfortably possible. Normal abduction is approximately 45 degrees. The maximum distance obtained between the medial malleoli as both hips are abducted is an additional estimate of abduction and can be measured for comparison at subsequent visits.

To test *adduction*, the patient should be supine with the pelvis stabilized (see above); the leg should be supported near the ankle and then moved away from the examiner, or toward and across the midline of the body as far as comfortably possible. Normal hip adduction is approximately 20 to 30 degrees.

Assessment of *hip rotation* is performed with the patient prone. The examiner should be positioned at the patient's feet. Each hip is assessed individually. To test for extent of external hip rotation, the knee is first flexed 90 degrees. The examiner then grasps the ankle of the flexed leg and rotates the hip by moving the ankle toward the midline while stabilizing the pelvis with his other hand. Measurements can be made by observing the angle of displacement of the tibia from a neutral line (0 degrees). The normal range of external rotation is 45 degrees. Internal rotation is assessed by rotating the hip away from the body midline. The normal range of internal hip rotation during hip extension is 35 degrees.

An external rotation contracture is present if the extremity cannot be internally rotated to at least 0 degrees. Similarly, an internal rotation contracture is present if the extremity cannot be externally rotated to at least 0 degrees.

Femoral neck version (anteversion and retroversion) can be assessed by palpating the posterior edge of the greater trochanter as the hip is rotated. With the patient prone, the degree of internal rotation necessary to bring the flat posterior edge of the greater trochanter parallel with the floor is a measure of hip anteversion. Normal femoral neck anteversion is 15 degrees. Excessive anteversion can lead to in-toeing during gait. If external rotation of the hip is necessary to bring the flat portion of the greater trochanter parallel to the floor, the hip is retroverted. Femoral neck retroversion represents a decreased anterior angle, and may lead to an out-toeing during gait (Fig. 26-3).

Hip extension should be measured with the patient in a prone position and the pelvis stabilized by the examiner resting his forearm over the lower spine and the area of the posterior iliac crests. Since the rectus femoris muscle crosses both the hip and the knee joint, the knee should be extended to minimize the effect of any contracture in the quadriceps mechanism. With a contracture in the quadriceps mechanism, knee flexion will limit hip extension. Thus, with the knee extended, the examiner places a forearm to stabilize the pelvis, and with the other hand under the thigh, elevates the leg off the table, extending the hip. Extension is normally 20 to 30 degrees.

SPECIAL TESTS

The Ober test is used to evaluate a tight, contracted, or inflamed iliotibial band (ITB). The patient should be positioned on the noninvolved side on the examining table. The hip should be abducted as

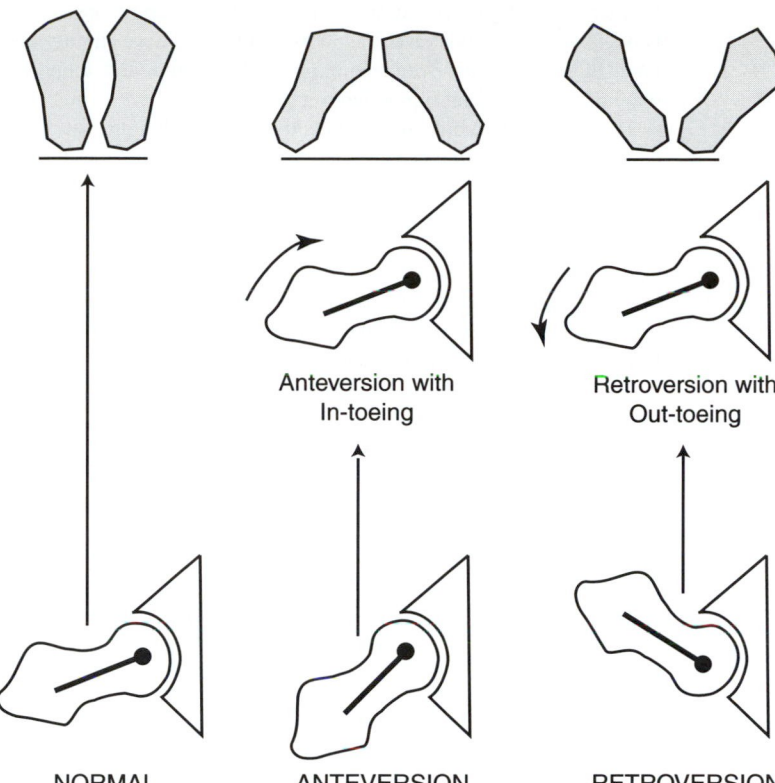

Anteversion with
In-toeing

Retroversion with
Out-toeing

NORMAL   ANTEVERSION   RETROVERSION

Figure 26-3
In-toeing associated with excessive femoral neck anteversion and out-toeing associated with femoral neck retroversion.

far as is comfortable for the patient, and the knee is then flexed 90 degrees while maintaining the hip in the abducted position. This maneuver will relax the ITB which inserts onto Gerdy's tubercle on the lateral side of the upper aspect of the tibia, at the knee. Next, the examiner releases the abducted leg, allowing the extremity to adduct. If the thigh remains abducted after the leg is released, the Ober test is positive, suggesting a possible contracture or other pathology of the ITB. Individuals with ITB friction syndrome frequently have a positive Ober test. These patients may have pain at the greater trochanter (the first bony prominence over which the ITB passes), over the ITB origin (the ASIS) or insertion (Gerdy's tubercle), or over the lateral femoral epicondyle (the second bony prominence over which the ITB passes).

A recently described provocative test may be used to evaluate for the presence of a labral detachment associated with hip dysplasia (acetabular rim syndrome). With the patient in a supine position, the hip is brought passively to a position of maximum flexion, adduction, and internal rotation. In patients with acetabular rim syndrome, this reproduces the symptoms by bringing the anterior portion of the femoral neck into contact with the torn labrum. Occasionally, possible hyperextension with external rotation may also reproduce this pain, thereby suggesting the presence of acetabular rim syndrome.

MOTOR EXAMINATION

Muscle strength is graded by manual muscle testing on a scale from 0 to 5 (see Table 22-2).

The primary hip flexors are the psoas major (flexion and external rotation of the thigh, flexion and lateral bending of the spine) and iliacus (flexion and external rotation of the thigh); because of the close association of these muscles, they are collectively termed the iliopsoas muscle. Innervation is mainly from the ventral rami of the L1 and L2 nerve roots. The iliacus is innervated mainly by the L2 nerve root and to a smaller extent by the L3 root (femoral nerve). To test *hip flexion*, the patient should be in a sitting position with knees flexed over the edge of the examination table. The examiner then places his or her hand on the distal thigh to resist flexion as the patient raises his thigh off of the table.

The primary hip extensor is the gluteus maximus muscle (extension and external rotation of the thigh). It is innervated by the inferior gluteal nerve which is derived from the L5, S1, and S2 roots. To test the gluteus maximus for *hip extension*, the patient should be in a prone position. The examiner then places one hand on the posterior thigh and offers resistance as the patient elevates his thigh off of the table.

The primary hip abductors are the gluteus medius and gluteus minimus muscles. They are both innervated by the superior gluteal nerve which is derived from the L4, L5, and S1 nerve roots. *Hip abduction* strength is tested with the patient lying on the contralateral hip: The examiner places a hand on the distal lateral thigh and offers resistance to abduction by the patient.

The Trendelenburg test is a gross motor test that also examines hip abduction strength, specifically strength or weakness of the gluteus medius muscle. The test is performed by having the patient stand on one leg and then flexing the contralateral knee and lifting the foot off the ground. If the patient maintains an erect posture during this single leg stance, the gluteus medius (on the supporting side) has adequately contracted. The pelvis on the unsupported side can be observed as slightly elevated. The Trendelenburg test in this case is considered negative (adequate hip abduction). If, however, the gluteus medius on the standing side is weak, hip abduction is abnormal, and the patient will begin to compensate; their posture will be un-

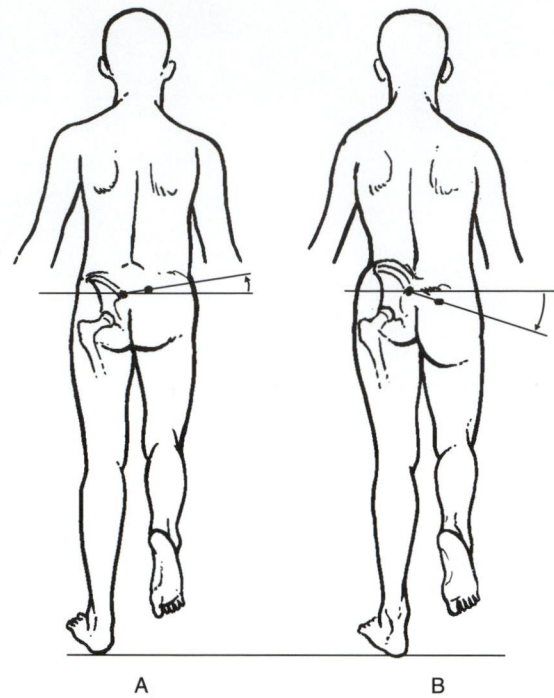

Figure 26-4
Trendelenburg test to examine hip abductor function. *A*, Negative; *B*, positive.

balanced, and the pelvis on the unsupported side can be observed to be level with the pelvis on the supported side or to have slightly lowered. In this case, the Trendelenburg test is positive and supports a diagnosis of abnormal hip abduction (Fig. 26-4).

The primary adductor of the hip is the adductor longus; secondary adductors are the adductor brevis, adductor magnus, and gracilis muscles. Innervation is by the obturator nerve (L2, L3, L4) with the exception of the pectineus muscle which is innervated predominantly by the femoral nerve with a minor contribution by the obturator nerve. To test the strength of the hip adductor muscles, the examiner places his or her hands on the medial aspect of each of the distal thighs which are slightly abducted; the patient then attempts to adduct, or bring together, his or her legs against the examiner's resistance.

SUGGESTED READINGS

Amstutz HC: *Hip Arthroplasty*. New York: Churchill Livingstone; 1991.

Anderson C: *Manual for the Examination of Bone*. Boca Raton, FL: CRC Press; 1982.

Hoppenfeld S: Physical examination of the hip and pelvis. In: *Physical Examination of the Spine and Extremities*. New York: Appleton-Century-Crofts; 1976.

Klaue K, Durnin CW, Ganz R: The acetabular rim syndrome. A clinical presentation of dysplasia of the hip. *J Bone Joint Surg [Br]* 1991; 73:423.

Netter FH: Lower limb: Hip and thigh. In: *Atlas of Human Anatomy*. Summit, NJ: Ciba-Geigy; 1989:457.

Nicholas JA, Hershman EB (eds): *The Lower Extremity and Spine in Sports Medicine*, 2d ed. St. Louis: Mosby-Year Book; 1995.

Chapter 27

KNEE

Andrew S. Rokito

Physical examination of the knee begins with documentation of the patient's complete medical history. The examiner should elicit information regarding the mechanism of injury, the nature of the onset of the symptoms (i.e., acute or gradual), the character and severity of the pain (i.e., dull ache, sharp, or intermittent), and the presence of swelling (at the time of the injury or subsequently), clicking, locking, catching, or giving way (i.e., does the knee feel unstable?). It is important to know whether there was a "pop" at the time of the injury. The patient should be asked whether any particular activities alleviate or exacerbate the symptoms.

INSPECTION

Patients should be observed getting on and off the examining table. Lower extremity alignment is noted with the patient standing, while the examiner looks for evidence of genu varum or valgum. Abnormalities in the gait pattern—such as patellar squinting, pronation of the feet, a Trendelenburg lurch, recurvatum thrust, or a varus moment of the knee—may provide insight to the underlying knee disorder.

With the patient supine, the examiner should inspect both knees for evidence of asymmetry. Muscular atrophy is detected by measuring thigh circumference at a fixed distance (i.e., 15 cm) from a fixed anatomic landmark (e.g., the medial joint line) and comparing it with the contralateral limb. The presence of a difference of greater than 0.5 cm may indicate underlying knee pathology. Inspect the knee for evidence of abrasion, ecchymosis, and erythema. Examine the knee for swelling. A small effusion can be identified by placing gentle thumb pressure over the lateral aspect of the patellofemoral joint and detecting a fluid wave with the index finger. In the ballottement test, one hand milks fluid from the suprapatellar pouch while the other hand presses down on the patella. The patella springing back indicates the presence of a larger effusion.

PALPATION

The bony and soft tissue anatomy of the knee is palpated systematically. With the knee extended, the patella can be gently displaced both medially and laterally to palpate its corresponding facets. The outer aspect of the patella and its prepatellar bursa can then be palpated and examined for evidence of swelling, fracture, or contusion. The quadriceps tendon and vastus medialis obliquus are also palpated and checked for continuity and areas of tenderness. Finally, the insertion site of the patellar tendon at the inferior pole of the patella should also be palpated.

Both the medial and the lateral joint lines are palpated for areas of tenderness, beginning anteriorly alongside the patellar tendon and proceeding posteriorly toward the popliteal fossa in a step-wise fashion. The superficial medial collateral ligament should be palpated at its mid-portion at the medial joint line and at its tibial and femoral attachment sites. The lateral collateral ligament can be identified and palpated more easily with the knee in the figure-of-four position. Palpate the patellar tendon, its tibial insertion site, and the tibial tubercle for tenderness. Check for tenderness over the pes tendons and its overlying bursa.

RANGE OF MOTION

A goniometer is used to assess active and passive ranges of motion with the patient supine. Range of motion is always compared with the contralateral side. The examiner should have the patient perform a straight leg raise and note the presence of any extensor lag. Loss of extension, however, can be better appreciated with the patient prone and by measuring the difference in heel height. Normal range of motion is approximately 0 to 35 degrees, but this should always be compared with the contralateral side to ascertain what is normal for that individual.

PATELLOFEMORAL JOINT

The evaluation of the patellofemoral joint begins with measurement of the Q angle, which is measured as the intersection of a line drawn from the anterior superior iliac spine to the center of the patella and the center line of the patellar tendon (Fig. 27–1). The normal Q angle is reported to range between 10 and 15 degrees with the knee in full extension. The apprehension test, which is used to assess patellofemoral malalignment or instability, involves attempted lateral displacement of the patella over the lateral femoral condyle while observing the patient for evidence of apprehension or discomfort during the maneuver.

More subtle tests of malalignment include the passive patellar glide and tilt tests performed with knee in full extension. The patella can be divided longitudinally into four quadrants. The examiner's thumb and index finger are used to displace the patella medially and laterally to determine the degree of parapatellar tightness. The ability to displace it laterally three quadrants is indicative of lax medial restraints, whereas four quadrants of lateral displacement defines a dislocatable patella. In the passive patellar tilt test, the examiner attempts to tilt the patella from its lateral side and compares the height of the medial to the lateral patellar border. The two borders should be level compared with the horizontal. Excessively tight lateral restraints will

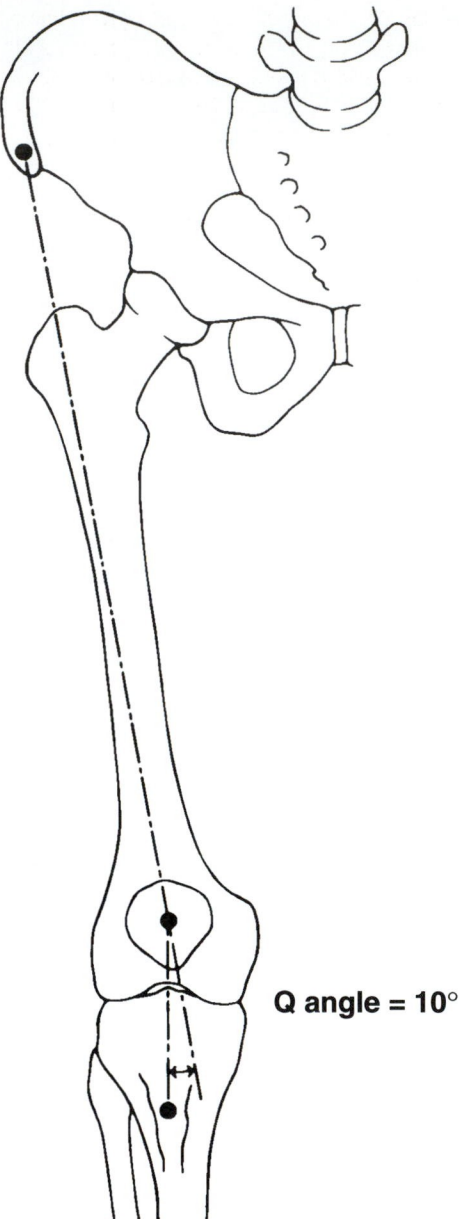

Q angle = 10°

Figure 27-1
The Q angle. (Reproduced by permission from McBeath AA: The patello-femoral joint. In Evarts CM (ed): *Surgery of the Musculoskeletal System*, 2d ed. New York: Churchill Livingstone; 1990; vol 4:3436.)

restrict the patella from reaching the neutral or horizontal position. The examiner should also observe for a "J" or jump sign. In cases of lateral patellar subluxation or dislocation, the patella will follow an inverted J-shaped course as the knee is extended from a 90 degree flexed position. Pain with patellofemoral compression is determined by having the patient perform a straight leg raise while restricting the patella. Although the presence of crepitus does not always correlate with the degree of disease, it should be felt for throughout the range of motion.

MENISCUS

The evaluation of meniscal injuries begins with joint line palpation. The patient should be observed for any evidence of specific joint line tenderness. One of the most reliable methods to assist in the diagno-

sis of meniscal tears is the McMurray test, which begins with the knee fully flexed and the examiner's fingers along the medial and lateral joint lines. The knee is then slowly extended to 90 degrees while valgus stress and external rotation, and then varus stress and internal rotation, are applied. A palpable "click" along the joint line with these maneuvers indicates the presence of a medial or a lateral meniscal tear, respectively.

LIGAMENT

Knee ligament integrity is assessed in each of the most common instability planes, beginning with the anterior cruciate ligament. The Lachman test, which is performed with the knee in 20 to 30 degrees of flexion, is the most accurate means for detecting anterior cruciate ligament insufficiency. The examiner stabilizes the femur and applies an anterior force to the tibia while assessing both the amount of anterior translation and the quality or proprioceptive nature of the endpoint. The latter can be graded as firm (normal), marginal, or soft. The opposite knee should always be examined for comparison. The anterior drawer test, which is not as sensitive or as reliable as the Lachman test, is performed with the patient supine and the knee flexed to 90 degrees. An anterior force is applied to the tibia while feeling for the degree of anterior translation.

Anterolateral rotatory instability also reflects anterior cruciate ligament insufficiency. The pivot shift test, which has been devised to assess anterolateral rotatory instability, is initiated with the examiner internally rotating the patient's foot while applying a valgus stress to the extended knee. The knee is then slowly flexed and, in the presence of anterior cruciate ligament disruption, the tibia subluxes anteriorly and rotates internally. As the knee flexes beyond 20 to 30 degrees, the iliotibial band tightens and becomes posterior to the axis of the knee, causing reduction of the tibial plateau. The reduction event is graded as 0 (absent), 1+ (glide), 2+ (moderate), or 3+ (severe). When this test is performed with the patient under anesthesia, the reduction may be striking, because it is no longer impeded by the pain and guarding that are frequently present in awake and acutely injured patients.

Posterior instability is much less common and can often be readily detected by the "sag" sign. In patients with an injury to the posterior cruciate ligament, the tibia sags posteriorly at 90 degrees of knee flexion, with loss of the normal anteromedial and anterolateral prominences of the plateau. As in the anterior drawer test, the posterior drawer test is performed with the knee in 90 degrees of flexion as the examiner attempts to translate the tibia posteriorly while assessing the degree of displacement. In the case of a posterior cruciate ligament disruption, it is important not to mistake the reduction of a posteriorly subluxed tibia for a positive anterior drawer. The quadriceps active drawer test is performed with the knee flexed between 70 and 90 degrees while the examiner supports the leg and thigh. The patient is then instructed to slide the foot down the examining table. Anterior tibial displacement resulting from quadriceps contraction confirms the presence of a posterior cruciate ligament injury.

Posterolateral rotatory instability is uncommon and may be quite subtle. The external rotation recurvatum test is performed by suspending the extremity by the great toe and looking for the presence of hyperextension–varus of the involved knee. In the posterolateral drawer test, a standard posterior drawer is performed with the tibia in neutral, internal, and external rotations. A positive posterior drawer in neutral or internal rotation suggests injury to the posterior cruciate ligament. In cases of posterolateral rotatory instability, the examiner will detect a posterior drawer sign that is more marked in external rotation. In the reverse pivot shift test, the examiner flexes the patient's knee to 70 to 80 degrees while externally rotating the tibia. In patients with posterolateral rotatory instability, this position will cause the lateral tibial plateau to sublux posteriorly. When the knee is extended, the examiner applies an axial and valgus load. As the knee approaches 20 degrees of flexion, the lateral tibial plateau reduces and a shift will be appreciated. It should be noted that in about 25 percent of asymptomatic individuals this test may be positive. A more simple method of detecting posterolateral rotatory instability is by noting the degree of tibial external rotation by measuring the thigh–foot angle at 30 and 90 degrees of knee flexion. Increased external rotation at 30 degrees is consistent with posterolateral rotatory instability. At 90 degrees, additional increased external rotation suggests posterior cruciate ligament damage as well.

Medial instability is detected by a valgus stress applied to the fully extended and 30 degree flexed knee. Placing the patient's leg in the axilla frees the examiner's hands to actually palpate the exact amount of joint line opening, which is graded as 0 (normal), I (1 to 4 mm), II (5 to 9 mm), or III (10 to 15 mm). Opening at 30 degrees implicates injury to the medial collateral ligament, whereas opening in extension reflects additional damage to the cruciate ligaments. On physical examination, grades I and II are found to have definite endpoints, whereas grade III tears have a soft or no endpoint.

Isolated straight lateral instability is rare, but can be detected by applying a varus stress to the fully extended and 30 degree flexed knee and noting the degree and end-point of joint line opening. The presence of varus laxity in 30 degrees of flexion, without any accompanying rotational instability, suggests the presence of isolated lateral collateral ligament injury. Opening in full extension, however, suggests additional significant lateral structure injury.

NEUROVASCULAR

As in any other examination, neurovascular assessment is critical, particularly in an acutely injured knee. The examiner must check for pulses and capillary refill, as well as sensory and motor function.

SUGGESTED READINGS

Daniel DM, Akeson WH, O'Connor JJ (eds): *Knee Ligaments: Structure, Function, Injury, and Repair.* New York: Raven; 1990.

DeLee JC, Drez D Jr, Stanitski CL (eds): The knee. In *Orthopaedic Sports Medicine: Principles and Practice,* vol 2. WB Saunders; 1994:1113–1549.

Hoppenfeld S: Physical examination of the knee. In: *Physical Examination of the Spine and Extremities.* New York: Appleton-Century-Crofts; 1976:171.

Chapter 28

FOOT AND ANKLE

Myles Rubin Samotin and Steven C. Sheskier

Examination of the foot and ankle entails visual inspection, palpation, range of motion (active and passive), neuromuscular evaluation, and testing joint stability. A complaint-related examination is guided by the patient's history, as well as having the patient point to the specific area of concern; for example, patients sometimes offer a detailed history of "ankle pain" only to point to the subtalar region.

Since all body weight is transmitted to the foot, it is subjected to much stress which results in many static deformities. The foot is protected from the external environment by shoewear which also serves to cause a myriad of other foot-related problems. Any foot-related examination must also closely evaluate the shoewear for appropriate size, length, width, and general fit, as well as protruding seams, foreign bodies within, or abnormal wear pattern (Table 28-1). The foot may also serve as a beacon to alert the clinician to any systemic conditions such as inflammatory arthritis or diabetic neuropathy.

SCREENING EXAM

Patients are asked to remove both shoes and stockings and elevate clothing above their knees, facing the examiner. Much can be learned by examining the foot and ankle during weightbearing since many conditions only appear at this time. The overall alignment of the lower extremities is noted, particularly genu varus/valgus. One can palpate both anterior superior iliac spines to rule out a gross leg length discrepancy. Formal measuring can be performed if there is any concern. Symmetry of the musculature and presence or absence of edema and skin pigmentation should be noted. Pes planus or cavus may be noted at this time. The patient is asked to turn away from the examiner. The alignment of the heel is determined by noting the angle that is formed by a line through the body of the calcaneus and a line down the midline of the ankle.

The ability to walk is the summation of most of the various components of the foot/ankle complex, and no exam is complete until it is observed. The patient is asked to walk so that any limp, limitation of motion, dynamic deformity, or paralysis may be noted. The examiner should be familiar with the different pathologic gait patterns, particularly foot drop with its high steppage and circumduction of the leg. The patient is then asked to walk on his or her toes, heels, and lateral and medial aspects of the foot. This screening provides an overall assessment of the patient's active range of motion, muscle strength, and balance. The patient should be requested at the outset of the exam to indicate if there is any discomfort and where, if provoked by the maneuvers, preferably at the time they occur.

INSPECTION

The patient is next asked to sit at the edge of the examination table with both feet dangling. Inspection begins with counting and assessing the attitudes of the toes. Are they straight, flat, disproportionately large or small, swollen, crooked, overlapping, or underlapping? Is there clawing, hammering, malleting, or deviation of the digits? The plantar aspect of the foot should be inspected for any lesions including abnormal callosities under pressure areas, scars, or warts.

Both feet are inspected for symmetry. Normally, the feet will rest in slight plantar flexion and inversion. The medial longitudinal arch, if nonexistent, indicates pes planus (Fig. 28-1) or, if too high, indicates pes cavus. Assessment is also made for excessive hindfoot valgus/varus or forefoot adductus.

BONY PALPATION

Palpation of the foot and ankle may be divided into bony and soft tissue components. Bony palpation can start at the first metatarsophalangeal (MTP) joint and the metatarsal head. Look for abnormalities indicative of arthritis (hallux rigidus) or gout. Proceed proximally up the first metatarsal shaft to the first metatarsocuneiform joint. Further proximally, the tubercle of the navicular may be found and its relative size, prominence, or any tenderness may be evaluated; tenderness may be associated with a painful accessory navicular or posterior tibial tendon insertion. Continuing proximally, the head of the talus may be palpated. Inversion and eversion of the forefoot helps in isolating the talonavicular joint. The talar head will be most prominent in pes planus.

The talonavicular joint can be examined by placing the thumb dorsal and index finger plantar to the talar neck. By adducting and abducting the navicular on the talar head, a midpoint position for head coverage can be ascertained. The foot is now said to be in its "neutral position." An appreciation of the forefoot's relationship to the hindfoot can be achieved by holding the navicular in this "neutral" position while dorsiflexing the forefoot.

Table 28-1

Foot Deformities with the Resulting Shoewear Pattern

Deformity	Pattern of Shoewear
Flat foot (pes planus)	Broken medial counter
Drop foot	Scuffing of toe box
Toe in	Excess wear on lateral sole
Hallux rigidus	Oblique creases in toe box
No toe off	No creases in toe box

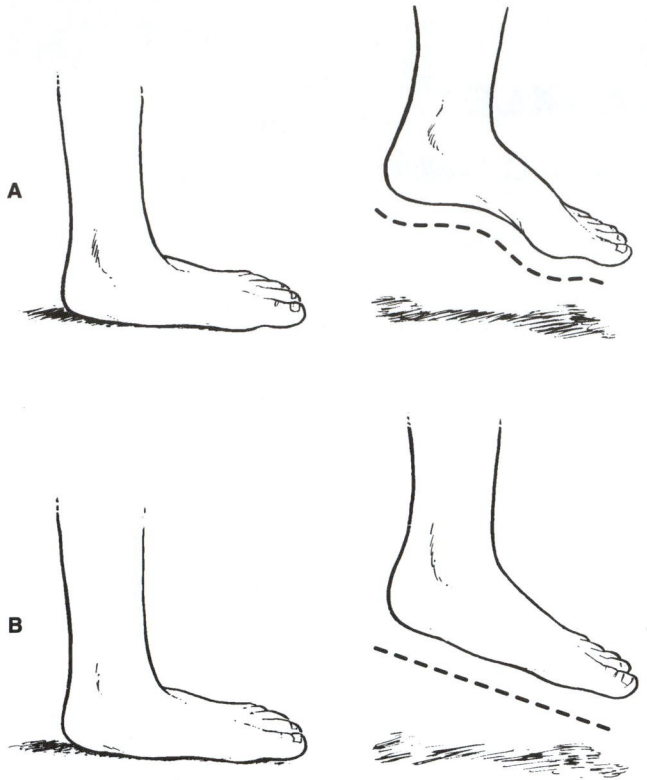

Figure 28-1
Supple (*A*) versus rigid (*B*) flat foot.

Proceeding proximally along the medial side of the foot, a prominent talar head may be palpated just proximal to the medial aspect of the navicular. This is most commonly seen in pes planus and is often secondary to posterior tibial tendon insufficiency, resulting in medial-plantar talar head displacement with loss of the medial longitudinal arch. This may also lead to a prominent callosity in this area.

Continuing proximally, the medial malleolus is palpated. About 1.5 cm plantar to the medial malleolus the sustentaculum tali can be found. This serves as an origin for the spring ligament and also supports the talus. Finally, the medial tubercle of the talus may be felt posterior to the medial malleolus.

On the lateral aspect of the foot, bony palpation proceeds as follows: Begin at the fifth MTP joint and palpate proximally along the shaft to reach the base, or the styloid process which is commonly fractured, as well as the insertion of the peroneus brevis. Just proximal to the styloid process is a groove on the anterior/inferior surface of the cuboid, through which the peroneus longus tendon passes as it travels from the lateral to the plantar surface of the foot. Proceeding again proximally, the lateral border of the calcaneus may be palpated. Fractures are often missed along the anterior process of the calcaneus.

Next, the lateral malleolus of the distal fibula is palpated. At the same time, place both index fingers on the tips of the medial and lateral malleoli to assess their relative lengths. The lateral malleolus is normally more posterior and extends distally to the medial malleolus. Distal to the tip of the lateral malleolus lies the small peroneal tubercle of the calcaneus which separates the peroneus brevis from the peroneus longus tendon.

The anterolateral talar dome is just anterior to the lateral malleolus and may be palpated with plantar and dorsiflexion of the ankle.

Anterior and distal to the tip of the lateral malleolus is a depression in which the sinus tarsi lies.

The inferior tibiofibular joint is palpated proximal to the talus. This is palpated anteriorly while compressing the tibia and fibula, assessing for signs of instability indicative of a syndesmotic injury. It is important, during the evaluation of ankle sprains, fractures, or syndesmotic injuries, to palpate the entire fibula in order to avoid missing a proximal fracture with resultant ankle diastasis or instability.

Both sides of the calcaneus are palpated immediately anterior to the Achilles tendon. This allows for assessment of the posterior one-third of the calcaneus. Diffuse tenderness on both sides may be due to a calcaneal stress fracture, while posterior heel tenderness in children may be due to calcaneal apophysitis. Tenderness over the weight-bearing medial tubercle of the calcaneus, which is located over the medial plantar aspect of the calcaneus, could indicate plantar fasciitis as this is the point of origin of the plantar fascia.

The tarsometatarsal or Lisfranc joints should be individually palpated while passively dorsi-and plantarflexing each joint. The lateral Lisfranc joints are the most mobile while the second, the "keystone" of the transverse arch, is the least mobile. Mobility of the first ray is variable. Exostoses may be palpable and may be associated with crepitus or a Tinel's sign, especially in the area of the second metatarsocuneiform joint, where the deep peroneal nerve is in close proximity.

Bony palpation of the plantar aspect of the foot is difficult due to the large amount of intervening soft tissue. It is important to palpate the medial and lateral sesamoids of the first MTP joint. These lie within the flexor hallux brevis tendon and each may bear one-sixth of the weight distributed to the forefoot. Tenderness may indicate sesamoiditis or sesamoid fracture. Each metatarsal head should be palpated, assessing for bony prominences (dropped metatarsal head) or tenderness (stress fracture, avascular necrosis).

The toes are then palpated assessing for abnormal attitude. A claw toe deformity consists of MTP joint hyperextension with proximal interphalangeal (PIP) and distal interphalangeal (DIP) joint flexion. Claw toes may be supple or rigid and generally involve all the toes. They are often associated with pes cavus deformity or systemic illness.

Hammer toe deformities consist of MTP and DIP joint hyperextension with PIP joint flexion, with typically isolated toe involvement. Mallet toes are characterized by flexion of the DIP joint.

SOFT TISSUE PALPATION

Soft tissue palpation can also begin at the first MTP joint. Assess first for the presence of a prominent medial eminence (associated with hallux valgus) and an associated bursitis in the soft tissues of this area. Soft tissue crepitations along with first MTP swelling may be indicative of gout.

There are many significant structures on the medial side of the ankle. The deltoid ligament can be palpated immediately below the medial malleolus. Tenderness may indicate a sprain or tear, especially when there is pain with hindfoot eversion. Just posterior to the medial malleolus lies the posterior tibial (*P*T) tendon, flexor digitorum longus (*F*DL) tendon, posterior tibial *a*rtery, tibial *n*erve, and flexor hallucis longus (*FH*L) tendon proceeding from anterior to posterior ("*T*om, *D*ick, *AN*d *H*arry"). The most sensitive test of PT tendon function is active resistance to inversion with the foot initially plantarflexed and everted. Tenderness may indicate synovitis or tear. Insufficiency or weakness may result in a planovalgus foot deformity while spasticity might manifest as a plantarflexed and inverted foot.

The FDL tendon may be palpated just posterior to the posterior tibial tendon by having the patient flex and extend the toes with the examiner attempting to appreciate the tendons' excursion.

The posterior tibial artery serves as the main blood supply to the foot and can be best appreciated with the ankle plantarflexed in order to relax the tendons.

The tibial nerve is just posterior to the artery. Although not easily palpable, percussing the length of this nerve, as well as its branches (calcaneal branch, medial plantar nerve, lateral plantar nerve, nerve to abductor digiti quinti) may result in a Tinel's sign, suggestive of tarsal tunnel syndrome or neuroma.

Finally, most posteriorly, lies the FHL tendon which actually courses along the posterior aspect of the ankle joint. Palpation is aided by flexing and extending the big toe. A sensitive test for FHL tenosynovitis is the Thomasen test which involves hyperextending the first MTP joint with the ankle, first, in plantarflexion, and then, in maximal dorsiflexion. FHL tenosynovitis or tightness will manifest itself as a decreased ability to hyperextend the toe with the ankle maximally dorsiflexed (Fig. 28-2).

On the dorsal aspect of the foot, from medial to lateral, lie the anterior tibialis (AT) tendon, extensor hallucis longus (EHL) tendon, dorsalis pedal artery, extensor digitorum longus (EDL) tendon, and the peroneus tertius tendon.

The AT tendon is the strongest foot inverter and ankle dorsiflexor and consequently can most easily be palpated with the foot inverted and the ankle dorsiflexed. It inserts into the base of the first metatarsal and medial cuneiform. Loss of AT function may result in foot drop.

The EHL tendon is best appreciated with first toe extension. It inserts onto the distal phalanx of the first toe.

Similarly, the EDL tendon is most readily palpated with extension of the lesser toes.

The dorsalis pedis pulse may be palpated between the EHL and the EDL. The dorsalis pedis artery is not the primary blood supply to the foot and may be absent in up to 15 percent of cases.

On the lateral side of the ankle, palpate the anterior talofibular ligament (ATFL), calcaneofibular ligament (CFL), and the posterior talofibular ligament (PTFL), all of which comprise the lateral collateral ligament complex of the ankle. The ATFL is the first and most commonly injured ligament in a lateral ankle sprain (inversion with plantarflexion) and may be palpated anterior to the lateral malleolus where it courses over the sinus tarsi to insert into the lateral talar neck (Fig. 28-3).

The calcaneofibular ligament is the next most commonly injured lateral ankle ligament. It courses plantarly from the distal tip of the lateral malleolus and inserts into the lateral calcaneal wall (Fig. 28-4).

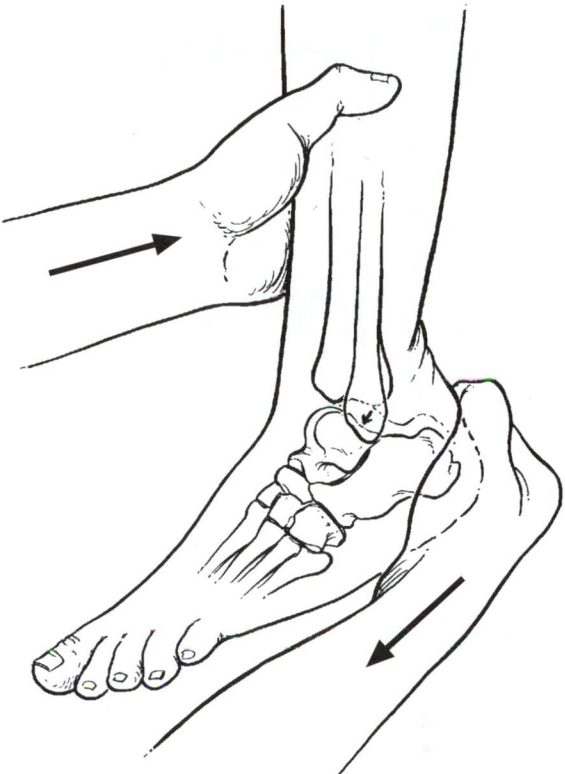

Figure 28-3
Anterior drawer sign.

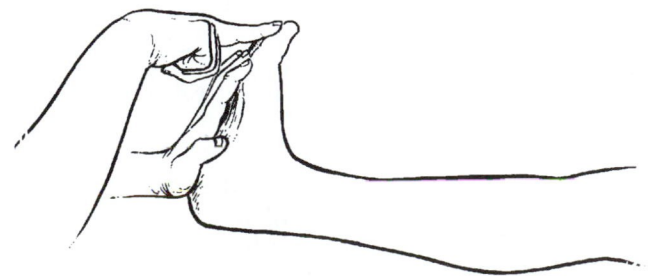

Figure 28-2
Test for functional hallux rigidus. (Redrawn with permission from Hamilton WG: Stenosing tenosynovitis of the flexor hallucis longus tendon and posterior impingement upon the os trigonum in ballet dancers. *Foot Ankle* 1982; 3:75.)

The posterior talofibular ligament is the strongest of the three lateral ligaments and is the last to be injured. It passes posteriorly from the posterior lateral malleolus to insert onto the lateral talar tubercle.

The peroneus brevis and longus tendons course posterior to the lateral malleolus with the brevis anterior to the longus. The peroneus brevis tendon can be palpated most easily with resisted foot eversion. The peroneus longus can be palpated with resisted foot eversion plus plantarflexion. Both tendons serve as primary evertors of the foot and secondary plantar flexors of the ankle. The examiner should palpate these tendons for thickening which is indicative of synovitis or dislocation. Acute peroneal tendon subluxation or dislocation typically presents with maximal tenderness at the posterior aspect of the fibula. Resisted foot eversion causes extreme discomfort. Chronic peroneal tendon subluxation or dislocation is best reproduced by having the patient move the inverted, plantarflexed foot into maximal eversion and dorsiflexion against resistance. This should reproduce the dislocation or cause apprehension suggestive of this problem. Deep tenderness over the sinus tarsi, a depression immediately anterior to the distal portion of the lateral malleolus, may indicate the presence of subtalar pathology (fracture or arthritis).

On the lateral side of the foot, there may be a prominent bursa over the fifth metatarsal head secondary to shoewear or associated with a bunionette deformity.

On the posterior aspect of the heel, palpate the interstitial or calcaneal bursa, the Achilles tendon, and the retrocalcaneal bursa proceeding from superficial to deep.

Thickening of either bursa might indicate a bursitis. The interstitial bursa, located immediately under the skin, superficial to the Achilles tendon, is usually inflamed secondary to tight or high heel

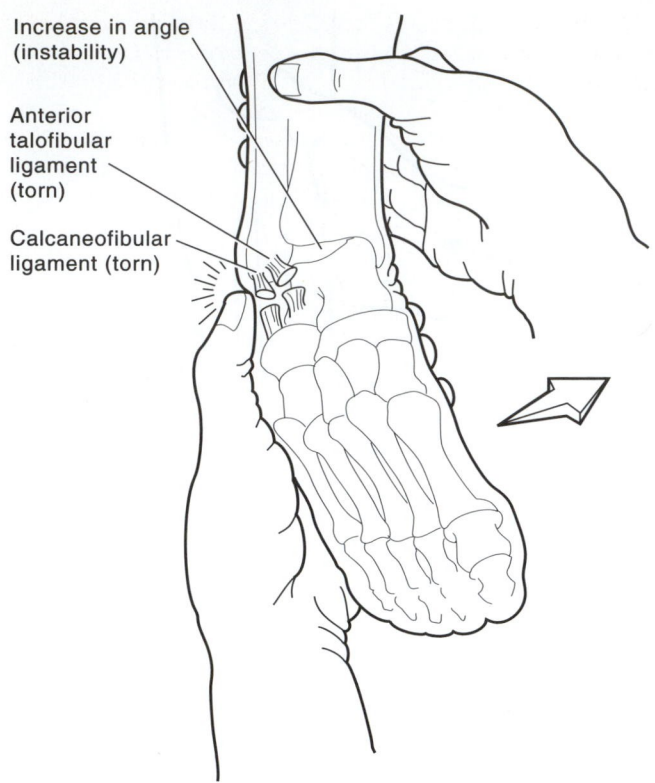

Increase in angle
(instability)

Anterior
talofibular
ligament
(torn)

Calcaneofibular
ligament (torn)

Figure 28-4
Talar tilt test.

counters (pump bumps). Thickening of the retrocalcaneal bursa may be secondary either to a prominent posterosuperior calcaneal tuberosity or to Achilles tendonitis.

The Achilles tendon may be palpated along its length. Thickening is indicative of tendonitis while a palpable gap is indicative of rupture. The Thompson test is a sensitive way of evaluating Achilles tendon rupture. With the patient prone and the foot hanging off the edge of the table, the calf is squeezed. Absent or decreased plantarflexion of the involved ankle may indicate rupture.

On the plantar surface of the foot, palpate the insertion of the plantar fascia on the medial tubercle of the calcaneus. Tenderness in this area may indicate proximal plantar fasciitis or heel pain syndrome. Palpate along the length of the plantar fascia as it fans out to insert near the metatarsal heads. Forced dorsiflexion of the ankle and the toes will help to accentuate the plantar fascia. Distal tenderness along the plantar fascia may indicate distal plantar fasciitis, a less common entity than proximal plantar fasciitis. Nodularities within the plantar fascia may represent plantar fibromatoses (Dupuytren's contractures). Callosities under the metatarsal heads may be diffuse or discrete, secondary to a localized (hammertoe or dropped metatarsal) or more diffuse (transfer metatarsalgia) problem. Plantar warts may be mistaken for a callosity; however, warts may be distinguished by the fact that they are most typically found on the nonweightbearing portion of the plantar forefoot.

Palpate the metatarsal heads for metatarsalgia and metatarsophalangeal synovitis. Palpate in between the metatarsal heads for interdigital (Morton's) neuroma; most commonly seen in the third web space followed by the second, first, and fourth interspaces, respectively (Fig. 28-5). Neuroma pain is best elicited by pushing the thumb up into the interspace while palpating dorsally with the index finger. The metatarsal heads are then compressed by the opposite hand and a sharp pain is experienced which at times is associated with a pal-

pable click (Mulder's) as the neuroma brushes against the metatarsal heads. The lesser MTP joints, especially the second, should be examined for instability, which may be displayed by a varus/valgus deformity or the presence of an increased drawer sign (Fig. 28-6). The drawer sign indicates that the volar plate is incompetent, thus allowing the proximal phalanx to sublux dorsally.

Soft corns are usually found between the toes secondary to maceration in an intertriginous area, whereas hard corns are located in areas of excessive bony pressure (i.e., osteophytes).

ACTIVE RANGE OF MOTION

Active range of motion of the ankle and subtalar joints can be assessed by asking the patient to move both extremities simultaneously and comparing their movements (Table 28-2). This is accomplished by asking the patient to pull their feet up (dorsiflex), point them down (plantarflex), turn them in (invert), and finally turn them out (evert). This will help to determine if there is any gross restriction in motion in the foot and ankle. Walking on toes, then heels, will help to test the ability to plantarflex and dorsiflex, respectively. Having patients walk on the lateral borders of their feet, then on the medial borders of their feet, will test the ability to invert and evert, respectively. This form of testing provides an overall gross assessment of active range of motion.

PASSIVE RANGE OF MOTION

Passive ankle range of motion may be tested with the patient sitting on the edge of the table with the legs hanging free. With the knee bent, the gastrocnemius is not under tension. The calcaneus is held with one hand to stabilize the subtalar joint and the forefoot is inverted to lock it into place with the hindfoot. The ankle is now maximally plantarflexed and dorsiflexed, eliminating all other joints as potential sources of motion. Ankle motion, particularly dorsiflexion, may be restricted as the result of an ankle fracture malunion. Since the talar dome that articulates within the mortise is widest in dorsi-

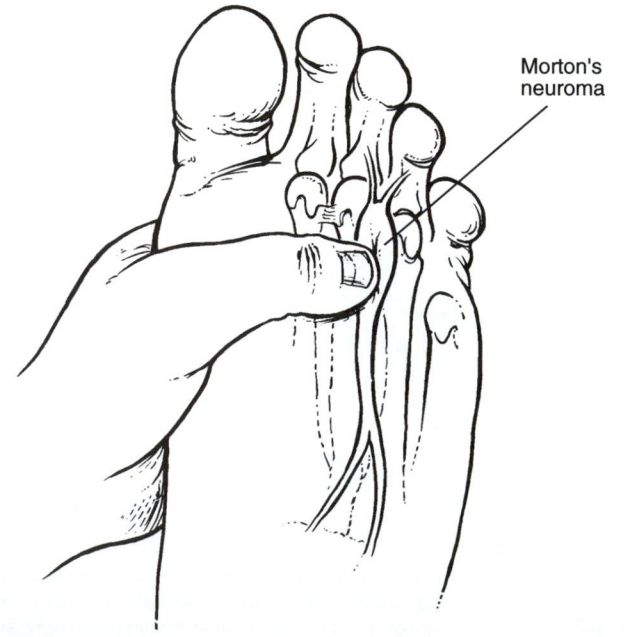

Morton's
neuroma

Figure 28-5
Morton's neuroma.

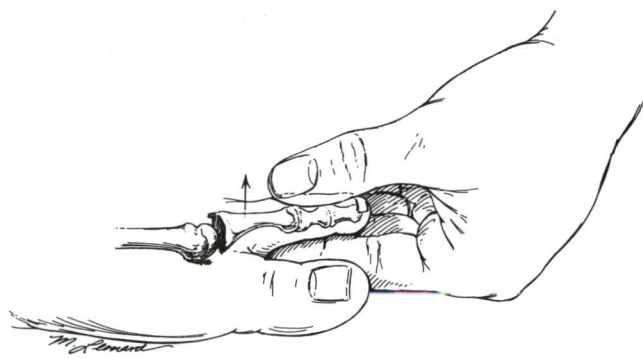

Figure 28-6
Positive drawer sign for MTP joint instability. (Reproduced with permission from Fortin PT, Myerson MS: Second metatarsophalangeal joint instability. *Foot Ankle Int* 1995; 16:308.)

flexion, dorsiflexion may be limited if the intermalleolar distance has been decreased secondary to an ankle fracture. Casting in equinus may also result in decreased ankle dorsiflexion. Ankle edema can also restrict ankle motion, as can any bony or soft tissue lesion causing impingement in the anterior aspect of the ankle joint.

Subtalar inversion and eversion may be tested by stabilizing the patient's lower tibia with one hand while grasping the calcaneus with the other hand. Try to maximally invert and evert the calcaneus to assess motion. This motion primarily takes place at three joints: the talocalcaneal, talonavicular, and calcaneocuboid joints. Subtalar motion is primarily used to help the foot to adapt to uneven surfaces such as climbing on rocks or walking on the beach. These activities may prove to be difficult if there is a limitation of subtalar motion which is often due to subtalar arthritis.

At the transverse tarsal joint, also known as the midtarsal joint, which consists of the talonavicular and calcaneocuboid joints, forefoot adduction and abduction take place. The calcaneus is stabilized in a neutral position directly under and in line with the tibia, using one hand, while the other hand is used to move the forefoot in a medial and lateral direction while motion is assessed. Subtalar inversion with forefoot adduction is known as supination. Subtalar eversion with forefoot abduction is known as pronation.

The first MTP joint may be tested by stabilizing the patient's first metatarsal with one hand while maximally flexing and extending the great toe through this joint. Limited range of motion, particularly in extension, may be an indication of hallux rigidus.

The first MTP joint may also be assessed. Palpating from distal to proximal along the dorsal aspect of the first metatarsal will lead to appreciation of a ridge. This is the location of the first metatarsocuneiform joint. With one hand grasping the medial cuneiform and the other hand grasping the metatarsal shaft, an attempt at dorsiflexion and plantarflexion, as well as translation about this joint, should result in minimal or no motion. With practice, an example of excess motion at this joint will be readily appreciated. This may develop in various conditions where there is ligamentous laxity as well as syndromes involving hypermobility of the first ray.

NEUROLOGIC EXAMINATION

The neurologic examination consists of sensory, manual muscle, and deep tendon reflex testing.

The sensory exam of the foot and ankle consists of testing for light touch, pain, vibratory, and position sense. The L_4, L_5, and S_1 dermatomes cover the foot and ankle. Both sides should be examined and compared (Figs. 28–7 to 28–10). Decreased light touch and pain sensation may be an indication of peripheral neuropathy. The superficial peripheral nerves may also be tested for sensation individually. These consist of the sural nerve, the superficial peroneal nerve, the

Table 28-2		
Normal Range of Motion of Joints of the Foot and Ankle		
Ankle	Dorsiflexion	20°
	Plantarflexion	50°
Subtalar	Inversion	50°
	Eversion	50°
Forefoot	Adduction	20°
	Abduction	10°
First metatarsophalangeal	Dorsiflexion	70–90°
	Plantarflexion	45°
Proximal interphalangeal joint of first toe	Extension	0°
	Flexion	90°

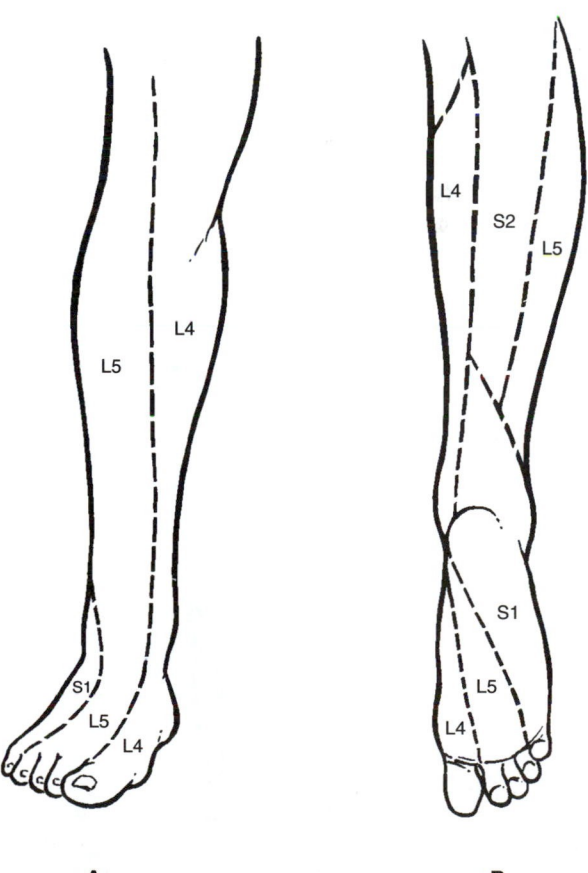

A   B

Figure 28-7
Segmental innervation of the lower extremity: (*A*) anterior, (*B*) posterior.

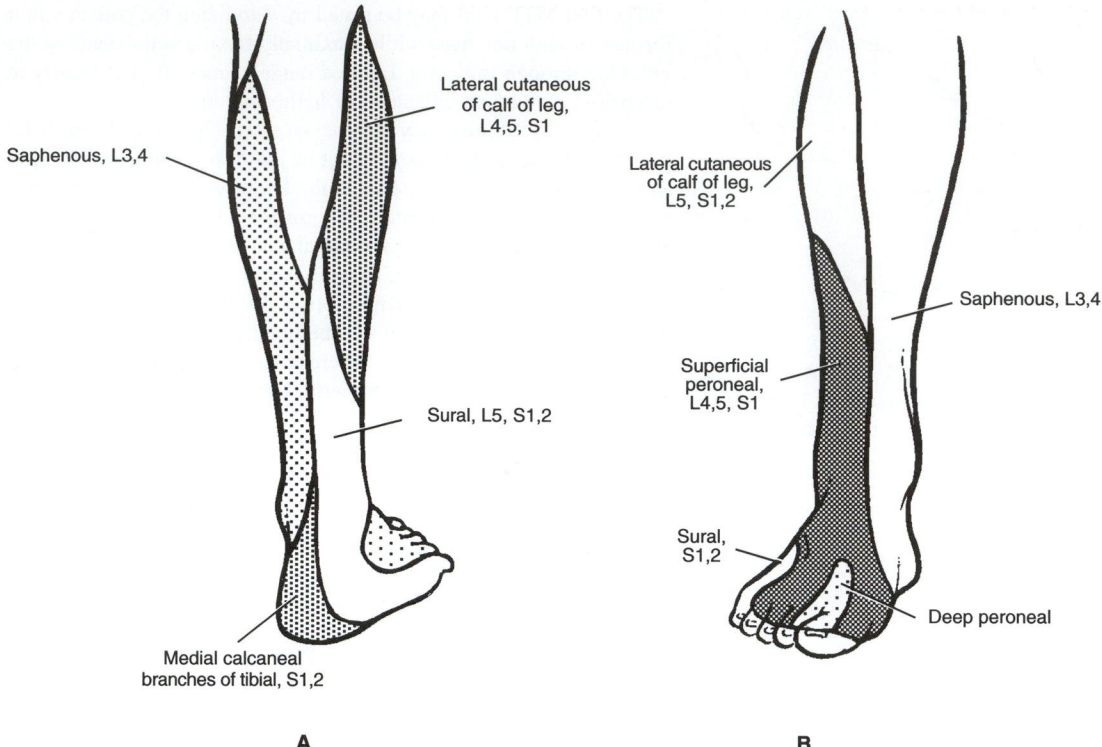

Figure 28-8
Cutaneous innervation of the lower extremity: (*A*) posterior, (*B*) anterior.

deep peroneal nerve, and the long saphenous nerve, as well as the posterior tibial nerve which divides into the medial plantar branch, the lateral plantar branch, the medial calcaneal branch, and the motor nerve to the abductor digiti quinti. Sensation to the lateral aspect of the foot is generally supplied by branches of the sural nerve. Branches of the superficial peroneal nerve usually supply sensation to the dorsum of the foot, as well as to the toes. The exception to this is the first web space, including the lateral aspect of the first toe as

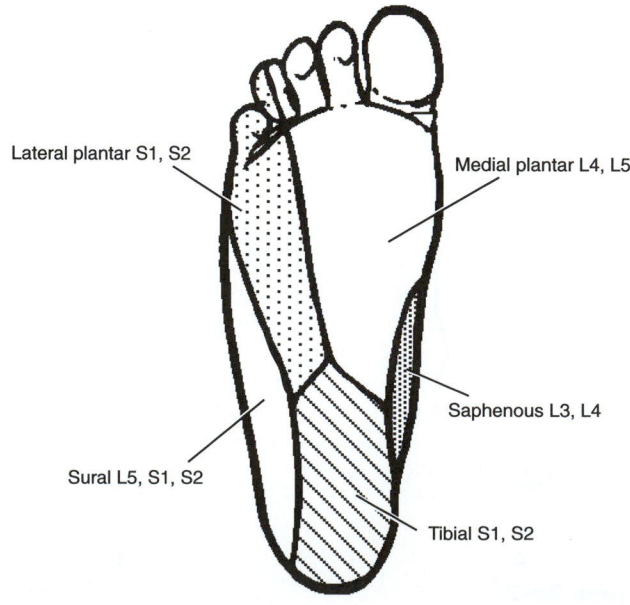

Figure 28-9
Distribution of the cutaneous nerves on the sole of the right foot.

well as the medial aspect of the second toe, which is supplied by branches of the deep peroneal nerve. The long saphenous nerve supplies sensation to the medial side of the foot. The posterior tibial nerve and its branches supply the plantar aspect of the foot. Familiarity with the distribution of the nerves is quite important. Since many of them are immediately subcutaneous in the foot, they are extremely prone to posttraumatic as well as postsurgical neuroma formation. These nerves should be lightly percussed along their length, assessing for a Tinel's sign. Vibratory sense, which may be diminished in the various peripheral neuropathies, may be tested by applying a tuning fork to the medial or lateral malleolus. The patient is then asked at which point vibration is no longer felt. At this point, the tuning fork is then applied to the styloid process of the distal radius. Vibratory sense should normally be equal in the upper and lower extremities. Any decrease in vibratory sense in the lower extremities should be noted. This same examination may be repeated comparing vibratory sense at the ankle level to the toe level.

The Achilles tendon reflex is the major deep tendon reflex that is tested in the foot and ankle. It is mediated through the gastrocnemius-soleus complex and is innervated largely by S1. With the leg dangling free, the foot is gently dorsiflexed to put the Achilles tendon under stretch. The tendon is then percussed using a reflex hammer. A normal reflex will result in plantarflexion of the ankle. This reflex may be more readily elicited by asking the patient to pull his or her clasped hands apart at the time of testing.

MANUAL MUSCLE TESTING

Ankle dorsiflexors include the anterior tibialis muscle, the extensor hallucis longus muscle, and the extensor digitorum longus and brevis muscles (Fig. 28-10). Since all four of these muscles are inner-

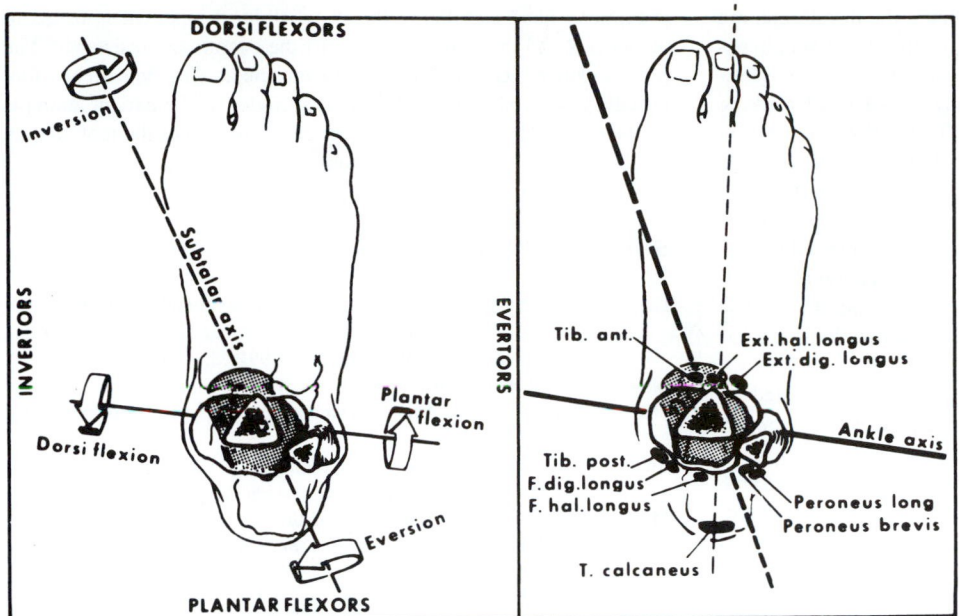

Figure 28-10
Musculature of the foot and ankle and their relationship to the axes of the ankle and subtalar joints. [Reproduced with permission from Mann RA: Overview of foot and ankle biomechanics. In Jahss MH (ed): *Disorders of the Foot and Ankle*, 2d ed. Philadelphia: WB Saunders; 1991:390. (Original source: American Academy of Orthopaedic Surgeons: *Atlas of Orthotics*, 2d ed. St Louis: CV Mosby; 1985.)

vated by the deep peroneal nerve, any injury to this nerve may result in a foot drop (Table 28-3).

The anterior tibialis muscle is the primary dorsiflexor of the ankle joint. Having the patient walk on heels with both feet inverted is a functional way of testing for this muscle. Manual testing of the anterior tibial muscle consists of stabilizing the distal tibia with one hand while placing the other hand on the dorsomedial border of the first ray. The patient is then instructed to push away the examiner's hand by simultaneously dorsiflexing and inverting his foot. The examiner, in turn, attempts to plantarflex and evert the patient's foot. The tendon of the anterior tibialis muscle may be clearly seen on the dorsomedial portion of the ankle and forefoot and can be readily palpated at this time.

Table 28-3

Muscles Crossing the Ankle Joint and Their Innervations

ANKLE DORSIFLEXORS

Extensor digitorum longus and brevis	L_5	Deep peroneal nerve
Extensor hallucis longus	L_5	Deep peroneal nerve
Anterior tibialis (primary ankle dorsiflexor)	L_4, L_5	Deep peroneal nerve

ANKLE PLANTARFLEXORS

Gastrocnemius and soleus (primary ankle plantarflexors)	S_1, S_2	Tibial nerve
Peroneus longus and brevis	S_1	Superficial peroneal nerve
Flexor hallucis longus	L_5	Tibial nerve
Flexor digitorum longus	L_5	Tibial nerve
Posterior tibialis	L_5	Tibial nerve

The extensor hallucis longus muscle may be manually tested with the foot dangling. The hindfoot is supported with one hand while the other hand is placed on the dorsum of the distal phalanx of the great toe. The patient attempts to actively dorsiflex the first toe while the examiner tries to push the distal phalanx into plantarflexion. The extensor hallucis longus tendon can be seen and palpated during this maneuver. If the examiner's hand is placed across or proximal to the IP joint of the first toe, the extensor hallucis brevis muscle is also being tested along with the extensor hallucis longus. The examiner's hand must be distal to the interphalangeal joint of the first toe in order to isolate the extensor hallucis longus muscle.

The extensor digitorum longus muscle may be tested functionally in the same way as the extensor hallucis longus muscle. The patient is asked to walk on his heel with his foot in a neutral attitude. The tendinous slips to the four lesser toes should be readily apparent. In order to manually test this muscle, the patient must sit on the edge of the examining table with legs dangling. The hindfoot is secured in a neutral position with one hand while the examiner's other hand is placed on the dorsum of the patient's lesser toes. The patient then tries to extend or dorsiflex the toes while the examiner tries to forcefully plantarflex them. The tendons of the extensor digitorum longus should be readily apparent and may be palpated at this time.

The muscle belly of the extensor digitorum brevis may be palpated in the sinus tarsi.

Plantarflexors of the ankle include the gastrocnemius/soleus complex, the peroneus longus and brevis, the flexor hallucis longus, the flexor digitorum longus, and the posterior tibialis. Some of these muscles also act as inverters and everters of the foot. The gastrocnemius/soleus complex are the strongest plantarflexors as well as the strongest muscles acting across the foot and ankle. The patient should walk on his or her toes to exhibit gross weakness of these muscles. Requesting the patient to jump up and down on the toes of one foot, with the other foot in the air, will help isolate weakness in this muscle complex.

The peroneus longus and brevis muscles serve as the major everters of the foot. They can be functionally tested by asking the patient to walk on the medial side of his foot. These muscles may be tested manually with the patient sitting on the edge of the examination table and the foot dangling. With one hand stabilizing the distal tibia, the patient should evert his foot. The examiner's other hand simultaneously provides resistance. This is primarily a test of the peroneus brevis muscle. The peroneus longus muscle may be isolated by asking the patient to attempt eversion while plantarflexing the foot. The examiner's hand should be attempting to dorsiflex and invert the patient's foot. Since the peroneus longus is the primary plantarflexor of the first ray complex, this is a rather sensitive test for this muscle.

The flexor hallucis longus muscle may be manually tested by stabilizing the patient's heel and resisting the patient's attempts at plantarflexion of the first toe; any weakness should be noted. The Thomasen test may be used to test for flexor hallucis longus tightness or tenosynovitis.

The flexor digitorum longus muscle may be manually tested by grasping the patient's calcaneus and asking the patient to plantarflex his toes. This motion is resisted by the examiner's other hand.

In addition to being a secondary plantarflexor of the ankle, the posterior tibialis is also the primary invertor of the foot. The flexor hallucis longus and the flexor digitorum longus are secondary invertors of the foot. The PT tendon is tested with the foot dangling. With the examiner's hand stabilizing the distal tibia, the patient is asked to plantarflex and invert the foot against the examiner's resistance. The most sensitive method of testing this muscle is with the patient's foot initially in a dorsiflexed and everted attitude. As the patient attempts to plantarflex and invert the foot, the examiner resists the motion; any weakness may be noted at this point.

SUGGESTED READINGS

Hoppenfeld S: Physical examination of the foot by complaint. In Jahss MH (ed): *Disorders of the Foot and Ankle: Medical and Surgical Management*, vol 1, 2d ed. Philadelphia: WB Saunders; 1991:52.

Jahss MH: Examination. In Jahss MH (ed): *Disorders of the Foot and Ankle: Medical and Surgical Management*, vol 1, 2d ed. Philadelphia: WB Saunders; 1991:35.

Lutter LD, Mizel MS, Pfeffer GB (eds): *Orthopaedic Knowledge Update: Foot and Ankle*. American Academy of Orthopaedic Surgeons; 1994.

Mann RA: Principles of examination of the foot and ankle. In Mann RA, Coughlin MJ (eds): *Surgery of the Foot and Ankle*, vol 1, 6th ed. St. Louis: Mosby; 1993:45.

Chapter 29

CONVENTIONAL RADIOGRAPHY AND TOMOGRAPHY

Steven Shankman

CONVENTIONAL RADIOGRAPHY

Conventional radiography is an essential tool in orthopaedic practice. Despite the newer imaging modalities that are readily available, the plain radiograph remains the first glance inward. Ideally, neither too few nor too many radiographs should be ordered in any given clinical situation. Standard examinations, therefore, have been developed for each bone and joint. Specific clinical concerns have led to the development of specialized techniques and projections.

HAND

Routine projections for the hand are the posterior-anterior (PA), lateral, and posterior oblique views.

PA Position—Forearm and hand on x-ray cassette with palmar surface down.
   Central ray: Perpendicular to the third metacarpophalangeal (MP) joint.
   Structures shown: A PA view of the carpals, metacarpals and phalanges (except the thumb), and the distal ends of the radius and ulna. This position yields an oblique view of the thumb. A true anterior posterior projection of the thumb is obtained by turning the hand into a position of extreme internal rotation and holding the extended fingers back with the opposite hand, with the dorsal surface of the thumb resting on the x-ray cassette.

Lateral Position—Forearm and hand on x-ray cassette, ulnar side down, with fingers superimposed.
   Central ray: Perpendicular to the MP joints.
   Structures shown: A lateral view of the bony and soft tissue structures. Anterior and posterior displacement of fracture fragments can be seen with this view.

Posterior Oblique Position—Forearm and hand on x-ray cassette, ulnar side down with the forearm pronated so that the fingers, which are slightly flexed, touch the cassette and the MP joints form an angle of approximately 45 degrees.
   Central ray: Perpendicular to the third MP joint.
   Structures shown: Oblique view of the bones and soft tissue of the hand. With slight adjustment of this position, a true lateral of the thumb can be obtained.
   In addition to these routine views, stress views of the first MP joint may be required for evaluation of ligamentous injuries. Specifically, abduction stress views of the injured and normal thumb may demonstrate widening of the ulnar aspect of the joint with radial subluxation of the proximal phalanx when the ulnar collateral ligament is disrupted, as with the "gamekeeper's thumb."

WRIST

Routine projections for the wrist are the PA, lateral, and posterior oblique views.

PA Position—Forearm and hand on x-ray cassette with palmar surface down; the hand is slightly arched (dorsiflexed), placing the wrist in close contact with the film.
   Central ray: Perpendicular to the midcarpus.
   Structures shown: PA projection of the carpus, the distal ends of the radius and ulna, and the proximal ends of the metacarpals.

Lateral Position—Elbow flexed 90 degrees, the forearm and arm on the x-ray cassette are ulnar side down.
   Central ray: Perpendicular to the carpus.
   Structures shown: Lateral view of the carpus, the proximal end of the metacarpals and the distal end of the radius and ulna.

Posterior Oblique Position—From the lateral position, the forearm is pronated until the wrist forms an angle of approximately 45 degrees with the plane of the film.
   Central ray: Perpendicular to the scaphoid.
   Structures shown: This position demonstrates the carpal bones on the lateral side of the wrist, in particular the scaphoid.
   An anterior oblique position or semi-supinated oblique view may be obtained for the evaluation of arthritis. From the lateral position, the forearm is supinated until the wrist forms an angle of approximately 45 degrees with the plane of the film. The pisiform-triquetral joint compartment is only seen with such a view. Early erosions that are associated with inflammatory arthritis, especially rheumatoid arthritis, may occur at this joint (Fig. 29-1). Stress views of the first carpal metacarpal joints can be obtained by pressing the tips of the thumbs together with the hands in a nearly lateral position. The central ray is directed perpendicular to the first carpal metacarpal joints. Radial subluxation of the first carpal metacarpal joint is most commonly seen in basal joint osteoarthritis.
   The carpal tunnel view is taken with the wrist hyperextended. The x-ray beam is angled along (parallel to) the volar aspect of the wrist, showing the bony anatomy of the carpal tunnel. This view will be helpful in detecting erosions in the carpal tunnel and may detect occult fractures of the hook of the hamate which may be difficult to see on routine radiographs.
   Motion series of the wrist may aid in the detection of ligamentous injuries that result in instability. This includes PA radial and ulnar deviation views and lateral volar and dorsiflexion views. Such static views may be normal in the setting of ligamentous injury and dynamic video fluoroscopy of the wrist may be required. The clenched fist anterior posterior (AP) view may demonstrate a scapholunate dissociation by driving the capitate proximally between the lunate and scaphoid. Specialized views of the scaphoid itself have been designed

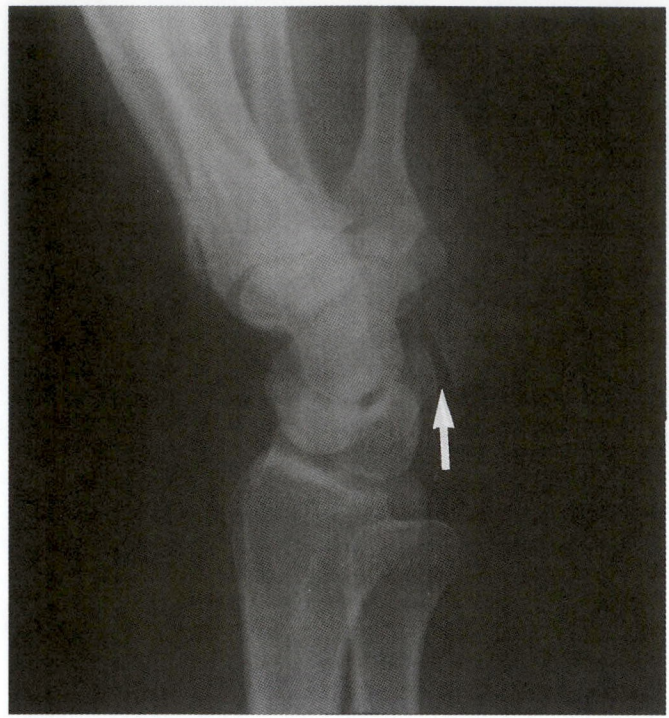

Figure 29-1
Semi-supinated oblique view of the wrist shows the pisiform-triquetral joint compartment (*arrow*).

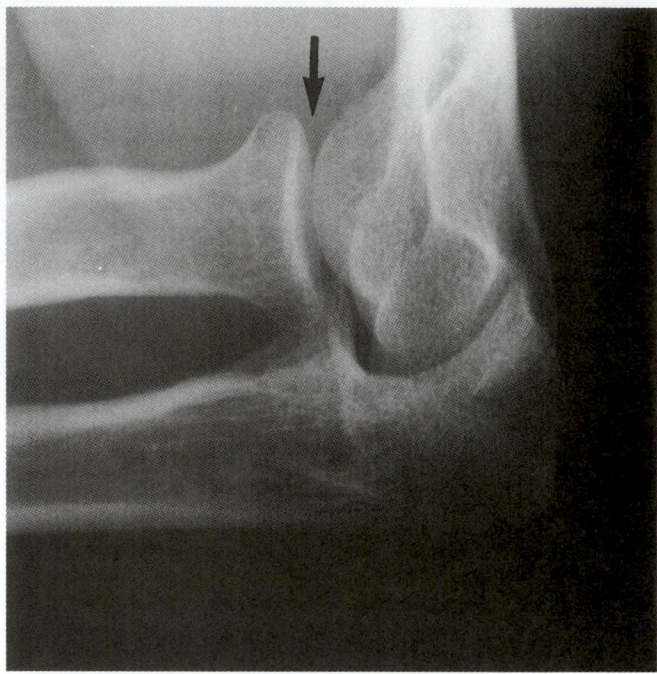

Figure 29-2
Radial-head-capitellum view projects the radial-head capitellum joint (*arrow*) cephalad to the ulna-trochlea articulation.

for the detection of occult fractures. In addition to the PA ulnar deviation view, the scaphoid may be elongated and projected free of other osseous structures when the central x-ray beam is angled 20 degrees proximally towards the elbow.

ELBOW

Routine projections for the elbow are the AP and lateral views.

AP Position—Elbow extended with the forearm supinated and patient leaning laterally until the anterior surface of the elbow is parallel with the plain x-ray cassette of the film.
   Central ray: Perpendicular to the elbow joint.
   Structures shown: An AP projection of the elbow joint, including the distal end of the humerus and the proximal end of the forearm.

Lateral Position—The elbow is flexed 90 degrees and the hand is in a lateral position.
   Central ray: Perpendicular to the elbow joint.
   Structures shown: A lateral view of the elbow joint, the distal arm and proximal forearm.

The radiocapitellar view is especially helpful in demonstrating radial head and capitellum fractures. On the lateral projection, angling the central beam cephalad projects the radiocapitellar joint free of the ulnar-trochlear articulation. These compartments are superimposed on the lateral view (Fig. 29-2). Views of the cubital tunnel are obtained with the elbow flexed approximately 45 degrees and the forearm supinated with its dorsal surface against the x-ray cassette. The central ray is angled approximately 20 degrees with respect to the olecranon process. This is particularly useful for looking at the bony aspect of the cubital tunnel where the ulnar nerve lies and can show osteophytes and loose bodies.

SHOULDER

Routine projections for the shoulder are the AP (internal and external rotation), axillary, and scapula "y" views.

AP Position—The patient is supine or erect, preferably erect, and slightly obliqued so the scapula is near parallel to the film. The forearm is supinated with slight abduction of the shoulder for external rotation and the elbow is slightly flexed. The back of the hand rests on the hip for internal rotation.
   Central ray: Perpendicular to the coracoid process.
   Structures shown: AP external rotation shows the anatomic position of the shoulder girdle with the greater tuberosity seen in profile, laterally. AP internal rotation shows a true lateral of the humerus and the lesser tuberosity seen in profile, medially.

Radiographic examination of the shoulder girdle may be tailored to the given clinical situation. A trauma series consists of an AP, axillary, and scapular lateral views. A true AP of the shoulder girdle is one in which the x-ray beam is perpendicular to the scapula. This requires obliquing the patient 45 degrees such that the scapula itself is parallel to the x-ray cassette. In this way, the glenohumeral joint is seen without overlap of the humeral head and glenoid fossa. The axillary view has many variations but essentially consists of the x-ray beam passing through the axilla from inferior to superior. The glenohumeral joint, coracoid process, and the acromion process are all seen. Numerous variations of the axillary view exist for the evaluation of shoulder instability. The West Point axillary view is obtained with the patient prone and with the tube angled 25 degrees cephalad and medial to the midline of the glenohumeral joint. This maximizes visualization of the anterior inferior glenoid rim, enhancing the detection of bony Bankart lesions. The Stryker notch view maximizes the visualization of the humeral head and Hill-Sach's lesion. This view is taken with the patient supine and the arm flexed (without abduction), and the cassette beneath the shoulder. The central ray is directed 10 degrees cephalad. One view that is helpful in the evaluation of impingement syndrome is the outlet view which centers the beam at the coracoacromial arch.

AC JOINTS

Routine projection for the acromioclavicular joints is the AP view.

AP Position—The patient erect with the arms hanging at the sides
Central ray: 15 degrees cephalad at the level of the coracoid process.
Structures shown: A bilateral frontal projection of the AC joints.
Stress views of the AC joints can be performed with 10- to 20-lb weights strapped to the patient's wrists to help differentiate incomplete from complete injuries. It is essential that the patient not hold these weights, in that muscle contraction may produce a false-negative examination.

STERNOCLAVICULAR JOINTS

Routine projection for the sternoclavicular joints is the PA view.

PA Position—Prone
Central ray: Perpendicular to the mid-point of the body at the level of the sternoclavicular joints.
Structures shown: A frontal view of the sternoclavicular joints and medial aspects of the clavicles.
Oblique views of the sternoclavicular joints can also be obtained by obliquing the patient or the central ray approximately 15 degrees. The serendipity view (patient is supine or erect, facing the tube) involves a 40-degree cephalic tilt and allows for evaluation of anterior and posterior dislocation.

SPINE

Cervical Spine

Routine projections for the cervical spine are the AP and lateral views.

AP Position—The patient is placed either supine or erect.
Central ray: 15 to 20 degrees cephalad at the most prominent point of the thyroid cartilage.
Structures shown: A frontal view of the lower five cervical bodies and the upper two or three thoracic bodies, the interpedicular spaces, the superimposed transverse and articular processes, and the intervertebral disc spaces.

Lateral Position—The patient is lateral to the x-ray cassette, either seated or standing.
Central ray: Perpendicular to the midneck.
Structures shown: A lateral view of the cervical bodies and their interspaces, the articular pillars, the lower five facets and the spinous processes. Depending on how well the shoulders can be depressed, the seven cervical vertebra and sometimes the upper one or two thoracic vertebra can be seen; all seven cervical vertebrae, particularly in trauma cases, must be seen.
Numerous other views aid in the evaluation of trauma and arthritis. Oblique views show the neural foramina clearly and osteoarthritic encroachment may be detected. The open-mouth odontoid view demonstrates the C1-2 articulation in the AP projection. Fractures of C1 and arthritic changes at the C1-2 facets may also be identified.

The Pillar view shows the pillars or lateral masses to advantage as the central beam is angulated parallel to their sloping course, caudad in the AP projection and cephalad in the PA projection. Occult fractures may be detected with this view. Flexion-extension views are particularly helpful in the evaluation of instability that may not be detected on routine neutral views.

Lumbar Spine

Routine projections for the lumbar spine are the PA or AP, and lateral views.

PA and AP Position—Either frontal projection is adequate and can be taken with the patient supine or erect. Patient comfort often dictates patient position. If the patient is supine, the knees and hips should be flexed.
Central ray: Perpendicular to L3
Structures shown: A frontal view of the lumbar vertebral bodies, their disc spaces, the interpedicular spaces, the lamina, and the spinous and transverse processes.

Lateral Position—Supine or erect. If supine, the left side is down with the hips and knees flexed to a comfortable position.
Central ray: Perpendicular to L3.
Structures shown: A lateral view of the lumbar vertebral bodies and their disc spaces, the spinous processes, the lumbosacral junction, and the sacrum and coccyx.
Oblique views of the lumbar spine not only show the neural foramina but also demonstrate the pars interarticularis to aid in the detection of spondylolysis. Flexion-extension views may enhance spondylolisthesis or retrolisthesis or demonstrate pivotal motion at a given disc. The Fergerson view is an AP view with cephalad angulation, which essentially compensates for the normal lordosis of the lumbosacral region and allows one to see this junction clearly. This is particularly helpful in the evaluation of postoperative cases when bone graft has been applied posteriorly between the transverse processes.

PELVIS

Routine projection for the pelvis is the AP view.

AP Position—Supine with the feet internally rotated approximately 15 degrees.
Central ray: Perpendicular to the midpoint of the pubic symphysis.
Structures shown: A frontal view of the pelvic girdle and proximal third of both femora.
Oblique views and inlet and outlet views may be obtained especially in the setting of trauma. The inlet view is obtained with the patient supine and the beam angled 10 degrees cephalad. The outlet view is obtained with the beam angled 15 degrees caudad. Both acetabular and pubic rami fractures are notorious for escaping detection or complete assessment and will be seen to advantage with these different views. The Judet oblique views of the pelvis involve rotating the injured side 45 degrees internally and externally. When the pelvis is rotated internally, an anterior oblique view or obturator oblique view is obtained. This view demonstrates the iliopubic (anterior) column and the posterior lip of the acetabulum. When the pelvis is rotated externally, a posterior oblique view or iliac oblique view is obtained. This view shows the ilioischial (posterior) column and the anterior acetabular rim.

HIPS

Routine projections for the hips are AP and lateral views.

AP Position—Supine with the feet internally rotated 15 degrees.

Central ray: Perpendicular to the midpoint of the film.

Structures shown: Frontal projection of the acetabulum and proximal femur

Lateral Position—The patient is turned to a near lateral position and toward the affected side with the hip and knee flexed. This is also termed a "frog-leg" lateral view.

Central ray: Perpendicular to a point midway between the anterior superior iliac spine and the pubic symphysis.

Structures shown: A lateral projection of the proximal femur with an oblique view of the acetabulum.

Cross table lateral filming is the best approximation of a true lateral film of the hip and is particularly useful in the setting of subtle subcapital fractures and the postoperative evaluation of hip arthroplasty. The patient is supine with the film cassette centered at the greater trochanter. The knee and hip of the unaffected side are flexed. The central ray is perpendicular to the long axis of the femoral neck and the film cassette.

SI JOINTS

Routine projection for the sacroiliac joints is the AP or PA view.

PA and AP Positions—The patient is either supine or prone with the lower extremities extended.

Central ray: Perpendicular to the level of the anterior superior iliac spine with the patient prone; 30 to 35 degrees cephalad with the patient supine.

Structures shown: Frontal view of the sacrum and SI joints and the lumbosacral junction.

Oblique views of the SI joints may also be obtained with the patient supine and the side of interest anteriorly obliqued approximately 20 degrees.

KNEES

Routine projections for the knee are AP and lateral views.

AP Position—Supine with the knee extended.

Central ray: 5 to 7 degrees cephalad to the knee joint.

Structures shown: Frontal view of the knee.

Lateral Position—Lateral with the affected side down and the knee flexed approximately 30 degrees.

Central ray: 5 degrees cephalad.

Structures shown: Lateral view of the distal end of the femur, the patella, the knee joint, and the proximal ends of the tibia and fibula.

Weightbearing views of the knees with and without flexion are particularly helpful in the evaluation of arthritis and the detection of joint space narrowing, which may not be as obvious with nonweightbearing or nonstanding views. Weightbearing with flexion is particularly helpful in the detection of osteoarthritis when focal cartilage loss can be seen posteriorly (Fig. 29-3).

Various views have been developed for the evaluation of the patellofemoral joints and their alignment. The merchant view is obtained with the patient supine and the knees flexed over the end of the x-ray cassette. The beam is directed toward the feet and the film cassette is held on the shins. The sunrise view is obtained with the patient prone and the knee flexed more than 90 degrees. The beam is angled perpendicular to the x-ray cassette.

ANKLES

Routine projections for the ankles are the AP, lateral, and mortise views.

AP Position—The patient supine with the foot vertical.

Central ray: Perpendicular to a point midway between the malleoli.

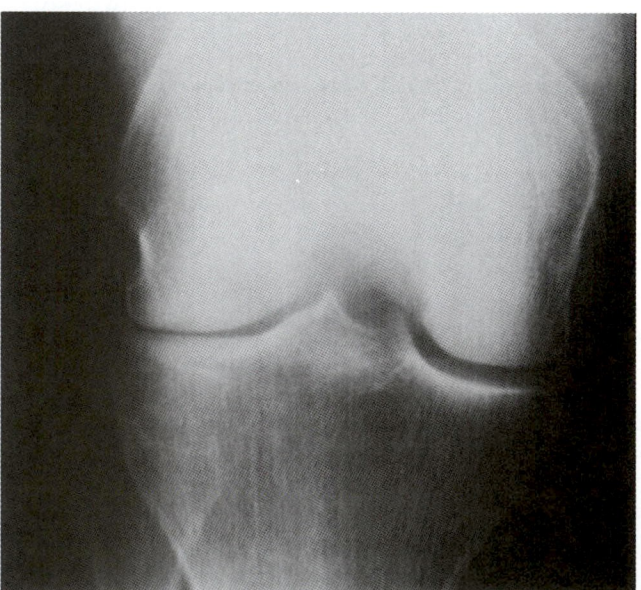

A   *B*

Figure 29-3

A. AP weightbearing view of the knee appears normal. *B.* AP weightbearing view of the knee in the same patient with 40 degrees of flexion shows narrowing at the lateral joint compartment.

Structures shown: Frontal projection of the ankle joint, the distal ends of the tibia and fibula, and the proximal portion of the talus. Neither the syndesmosis nor the inferior portion of the lateral malleolus is well demonstrated in this projection.

Lateral Position—Lateral side of the ankle down; the patient is supine and turned toward the affected side.

Central ray: Perpendicular to the lateral malleolus.

Structures shown: A lateral view of the distal third of the tibia and fibula, the ankle joint, and the hindfoot.

Mortise Position—Supine with the leg and the foot rotated internally approximately 15 degrees.

Central ray: Perpendicular to the ankle joint.

Structures shown: The syndesmosis is now well seen without overlap of the anterior process of the distal tibia. The distal aspect of the lateral malleolus is better visualized.

Stress views of the ankles are routinely utilized for assessment of instability and injury to the lateral collateral ligamentous structures. This is best performed with a calibrated standardized device needed to position and stress the ankle. Inversion stress produces increased talar tilt in injured patients (Fig. 29-4). Anterior drawer stress produces posterior joint space widening and may cause talar displacement in injured patients. Both the affected and normal side are examined for comparison. Complete tears of the deltoid ligament may be demonstrated with eversion stress.

FEET

Routine projections for the feet are the dorsiplantar, lateral, and medial oblique views.

Dorsiplantar Position—Supine, with the knee flexed and the sole of the foot resting on the x-ray cassette.

Central ray: Perpendicular to the base of the third metatarsal.

Structures shown: A frontal projection of the midfoot and forefoot

Lateral Position—Lateral side down with the patient supine.

Central ray: Perpendicular to the midfoot.

Structures shown: A true lateral projection of the foot, ankle joint, and distal leg.

Medial Oblique Position—Supine, with the knee flexed and the leg rotated medially until the sole of the foot forms an angle of 30 degrees to the plane of the film.

Central ray: Perpendicular to the midfoot.

Structures shown: The calcaneocuboid, cuboid- 4th and 5th metatarsal, cuboid cuneiform, and talonavicular articulations. The sinus tarsi is also well seen.

The Harris-Beath or axial view of the hindfoot best shows the posterior and medial subtalar joints (Fig. 29-5). Coalition at the medial facet can be detected with this view. Avulsion fractures at the medial or lateral aspects of the calcaneal tuberosity are also seen to advantage with this view.

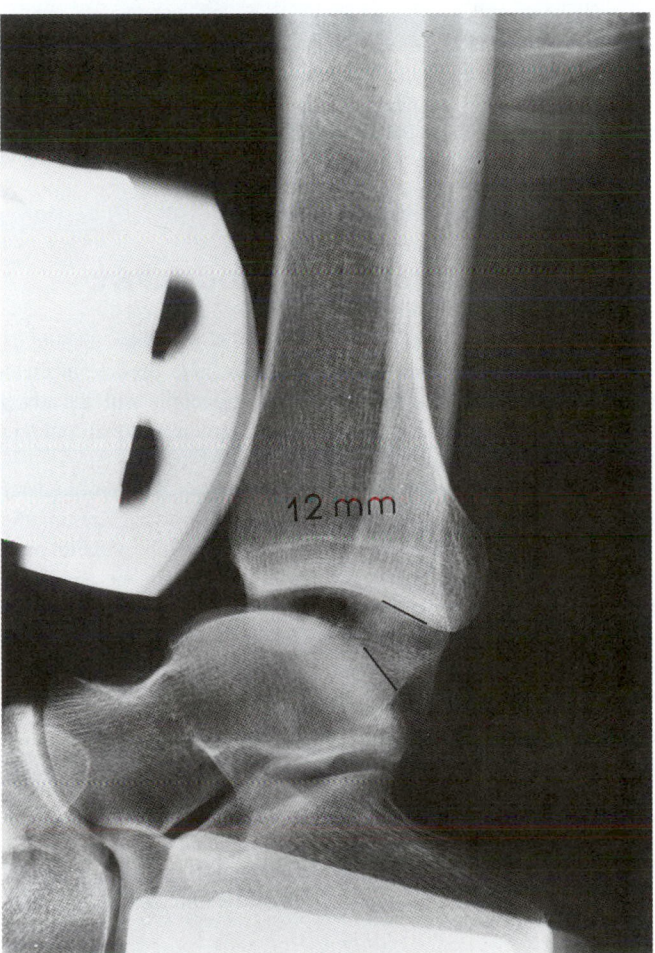

A

B

Figure 29-4

A. Inversion stress view of the ankle shows increased talar tilt. *B.* Anterior drawer stress view of the ankle reveals increased posterior joint space widening.

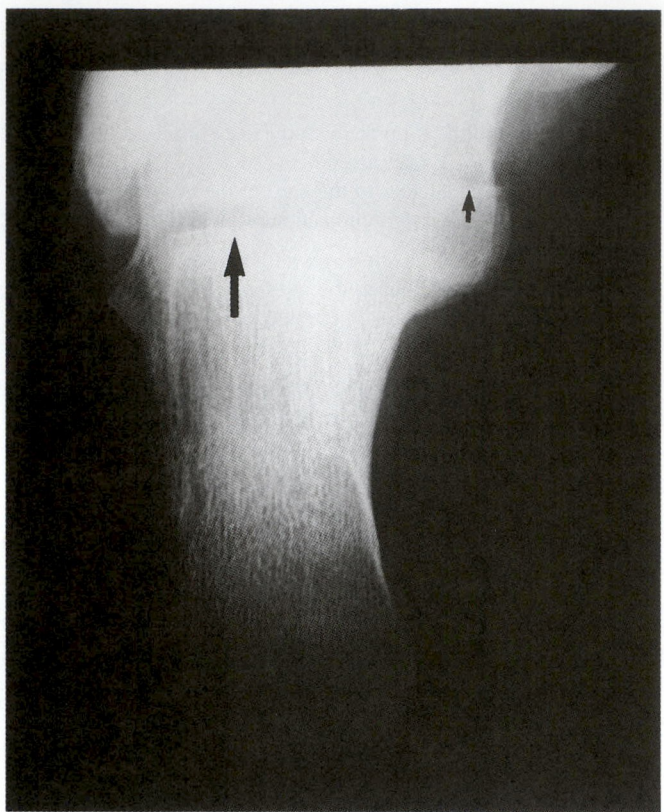

Figure 29-5
Harris-Beath view of the hindfoot shows the medial (*small arrow*) and posterior (*large arrow*) subtalar joints to advantage.

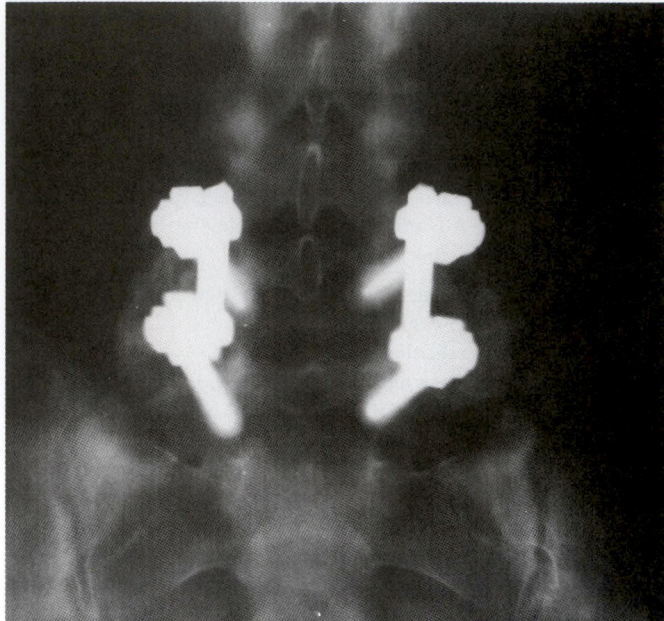

Figure 29-6
AP tomogram of the L-S spine shows the intertranverse process bone graft site. Osseous gap on the left proved to be pseudoarthrosis.

CONVENTIONAL TOMOGRAPHY

The utilization of conventional tomography has dramatically decreased as newer cross sectional modalities have become available and refined (i.e., MRI and CT). The latter, especially with the advent of spiral or helical CT, is virtually replacing conventional tomography in most institutions.

Conventional tomography shows structures in a given, predetermined plane of tissue, eliminating or blurring those structures in other planes. This is accomplished by motion. The x-ray tube and film move as the patient is stationary. Structures in the focal plane are always imaged whereas other planes are blurred. The basic principle of any tomographic system is that all parts of the object to be blurred that are perpendicular to the direction of the tube motion are maximally blurred, whereas those parts that are parallel to the direction of motion are not blurred, but merely elongated. The pattern of motion may be linear, circular, elliptical, spiral or hypocloidal, and pseudo-hypocloidal. Spiral motion provides for extremely thin tomographic sections, which is especially useful in the evaluation of small parts, such as the wrist. Narrow-angle tomography called zonography produces thicker sections useful for the evaluation of hip fracture. All cases, however, should be monitored by the radiologist.

The disadvantages of conventional tomography include the length of the exam and the radiation exposure. Certain joints, however, are well served by this modality. These include the sternoclavicular, temporomandibular, sacroiliac, costovertebral, apophyseal, atlantooccipital, atlantoaxial, subtalar, carpal, and tarsal joints.

Clinical situations commonly requiring tomographic imaging include the evaluation of wrist, hip, knee, and ankle trauma; spinal fusion; fracture healing; osteochondral lesions; and osteonecrosis. The detection of occult scaphoid, subcapital, and intertrochanteric fractures lends itself to conventional tomography. The degree of depression at a tibial plateau fracture is often assessed. The display of fracture fragmentation of pilon fractures is also shown. Fracture healing at any site may also be assessed. This is particularly useful at bone graft sites, especially fusion masses in the spine (Fig. 29-6). Small osteochondral lesions may be better defined when suspected on conventional radiographs. Likewise, subtle areas of articular collapse may be better seen in cases of osteonecrosis when the plain film is suggestive in the proper clinical setting.

SUGGESTED READINGS

Ballinger PW (ed): *Merrill's Atlas of Radiographic Positions and Radiologic Procedures,* 8th ed. St. Louis: Mosby Year-Book; 1995.

Resnick D: *Diagnosis of Bone and Joint Disorders,* vol 1, 3d ed. Philadelphia: WB Saunders; 1995.

Weissman B, Sledge CB: *Orthopaedic Radiology.* Philadelphia: WB Saunders; 1985.

Chapter 30

COMPUTED TOMOGRAPHY

Javier Beltran and Zehava Sadka Rosenberg

Before the introduction of magnetic resonance imaging (MRI), computed tomography (CT) was the technique of choice for the evaluation of lesions of the musculoskeletal system because of its improved soft tissue contrast resolution over x-ray techniques. Combined with the intraarticular injection of contrast material it has improved definition of lesions of articular surfaces, capsule, tendons, and other supporting structures of joints such as the shoulder, elbow, ankle, knee, and hip. Soft tissue masses are much better depicted with CT than with plain film radiography, especially when using intravenous injection of contrast material. Distinction between solid and fluid-containing lesions is possible, allowing more specific diagnoses to be made. Most of the indications for CT in the musculoskeletal system changed when MRI became available. There is still, however, a role for CT, as a complementary study, but also sometimes as the only study necessary to evaluate a lesion.

Recent technical developments have been introduced that allow very fast imaging time and almost immediate reconstruction in 2-D and 3-D modes. This has opened renewed interest in CT imaging of the musculoskeletal system.

TECHNIQUE

A CT scanner system consists of a scanning gantry which holds the x-ray tube and detectors (moving parts), a moving table or couch for the patient, an x-ray generator, computer processing unit, and a display console or work station (Fig. 30-1). Images are obtained in the

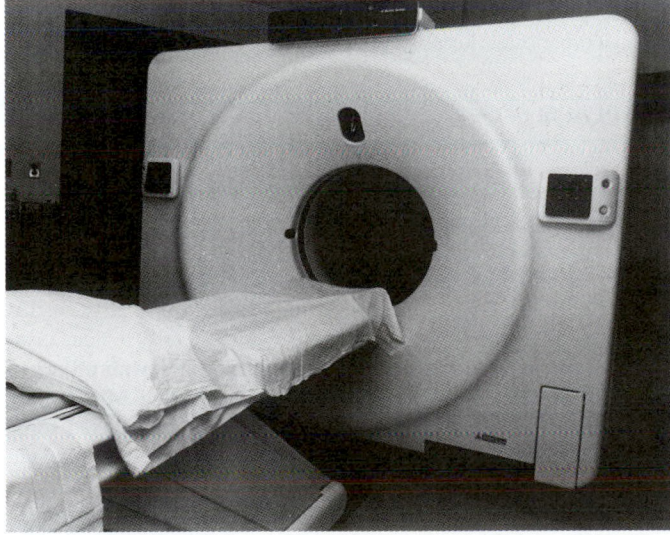

Figure 30-1
The scanning gantry (x-ray tube and detectors) and moving table of a computed tomography work station. The complete workstation also includes an x-ray generator, a computer processing unit, and a display console.

transverse (axial) plane of the patient's body by rotating the x-ray tube 360 degrees. The x-rays are absorbed in part by the patient's body. The amount of x-rays transmitted through the body is detected in the opposite side of the gantry by an array of detectors. The x-ray transmission through the body is determined by the combined attenuation properties of the tissues. For instance, calcium in bone will attenuate more x-ray photons than air in the lungs or fat in the subcutaneous tissues. The information obtained by the detector array is transferred to the computer system where the data is transformed and reconstructed to produce a diagnostic image.

The configuration of the array of detectors and motion of the tube has been modified through the years to optimize image quality and speed. In the newest generation of CT units, the x-ray tube is set in continuous motion and the array of detectors forms a complete stationary circumference. The table advances in a continuous motion while the tube rotates. Therefore sets of data are obtained in a spiral fashion, hence the term "spiral" or "helical" CT. Images are then reconstructed in the desired plane.

The CT image reflects the absorption coefficient values of the x-rays after traversing different tissues within the body. These attenuation values are expressed in Hounsfield units (HU) and are normalized to water. Hence, water measures 0 HU, bone (the highest absorption values) measures 1000 HU, and air (the lowest absorption values) measures −1000 HU. Adjusting the level and the width of the displayed range of HU (window) the operator can study different tissues optimally in the work station. Additionally, most display and operator consoles are equipped with postprocessing capabilities, including measurements of distances, volumes, and HU defined in regions of interest (ROI). Software improvements have been introduced through the years, allowing fast image reconstruction in any desired plane (2-D) or surface reconstruction (3-D). Surface reconstruction of the data can be displayed in different ways depending on the selection of tissues to be displayed. This operator selection function is used frequently in the spine and other complex areas of the musculoskeletal system to optimally depict fractures and other types of bone pathology.

IMAGE QUALITY

Image quality in CT imaging depends on a variety of factors which are mostly selected by the operator. Two parameters are used to define image quality of a given system: spatial resolution and contrast resolution. For improvement of spatial resolution (defined as the ability of the system to distinguish between two closely spaced objects) the operator should select a small matrix size (256 × 256), small field of view, and thin slices. Special reconstruction algorithms can also be chosen to improve spatial resolution. Other factors influencing spatial resolution, not controlled by the operator, are related to the patients themselves or to the configuration of the system. Contrast resolution is defined as the ability of a system to discriminate between two adjacent areas with different attenuation values. To improve contrast resolution the operator has several choices: appropriate selection of reconstruction algorithm, tube current [measured in milliamperes, (mA)], scanning time (measured in seconds), pixel size (matrix), and slice thickness. It is important to understand that increased tube current or scanning time will increase radiation dose. Another strategy to increase contrast resolution is to use contrast material, either intraarticular or intravenous.

Another important consideration is the scanning strategy. Although the axial plane is the most frequently used, other planes can also be imaged directly by changing the position of the patient within the gantry. These strategies are frequently used in musculoskeletal imaging. For instance, the wrist can be imaged in axial, sagittal, coronal, and oblique planes with the patient prone, the arm above the head, and changing the orientation of the wrist within the gantry. The same applies to the shoulder, ankle, foot, leg, and forearm.

CLINICAL APPLICATIONS

TRAUMA

CT has been applied extensively for the delineation of fractures and dislocations in areas with complex anatomy such as the pelvis, shoulder, and spine. The ability to depict intraarticular fragments of bone or cartilage or retro pulsed vertebral fragments are only two examples of the superiority of CT over plain film radiography. Adequate images of the traumatized spine can be obtained even in the presence of metallic hardware such as Harrington rods. In the spine, the transaxial nature of the images allows assessment of the size of the spinal canal and adjacent structures. CT has also been found to be superior to plain film radiography to display fractures involving the pedicle, lamina, or transverse processes. Complex fractures of the pelvis, hips, and sacrum are also better depicted with CT than with plain films using multiplanar and 3-D reconstruction techniques (Fig. 30-2). Important information about the condition of the acetabular roof, anterior and posterior columns, and quadrilateral plate can be obtained with CT.

In the shoulder, CT has helped to define comminuted fracture-dislocations of the proximal humerus and dislocations of the sternoclavicular joint. Coupled with the intraarticular injection of contrast and air (CT arthrography), this technique has been used extensively to investigate patients with glenohumeral joint instability. It has been used to assess the integrity of the labrum, capsule, and biceps tendon. CT arthrography with direct coronal or direct sagittal images also allows accurate depiction of small rotator cuff tears. In most practices, however, MRI has largely replaced CT arthrography, not only in the shoulder but also in the knee, ankle, wrist, elbow, and hip.

Occasionally, CT may be required to study complex fractures of the knee (tibial plateau fractures) and ankle (pilon fractures, triplane fractures; Fig. 30-3), for preoperative planning and also to assess surgical results following open reduction. Other potential indications of CT in trauma include suspected dislocation of the proximal tibio-fibular joint, distal radio-ulnar joint subluxation, and fractures of the hook of the hamate, scaphoid, lunate, or other carpal or tarsal bones. In many centers, CT has replaced conventional tomography in the evaluation of trauma for three reasons: better contrast resolution, decreased radiation, and many companies have stopped producing conventional tomography units.

INFECTION

The indications for CT for the diagnosis of musculoskeletal infection has been replaced by scintigraphy and MRI. CT can, however, be

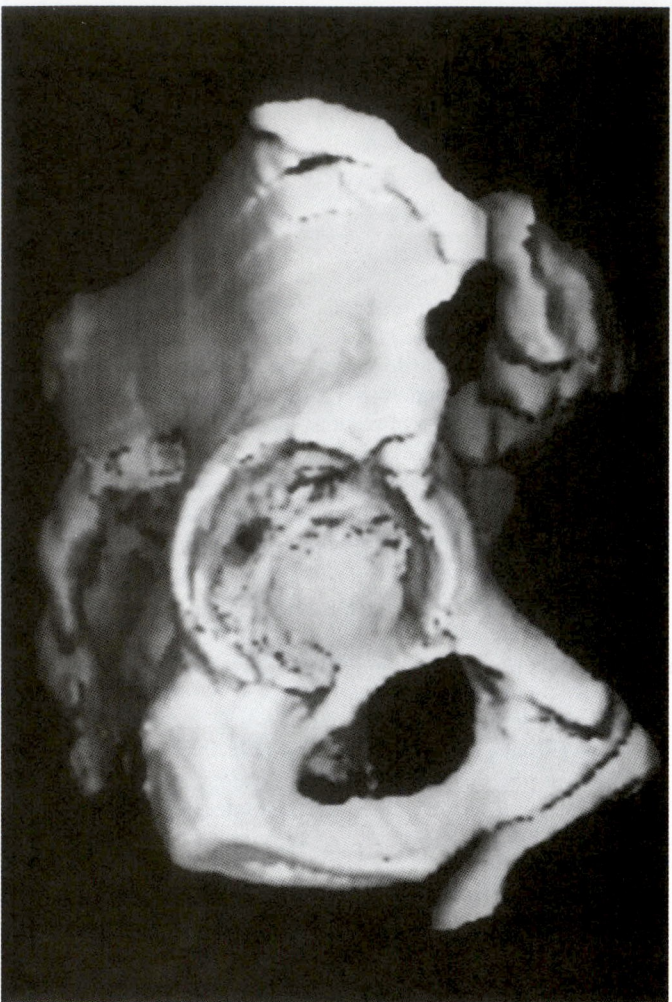

Figure 30-2
An acetabular fracture visualized on 3-D CT reconstruction.

used occasionally to depict bony detail such as sequestra, cortical defects, and periosteal reactions.

NEOPLASM

Although for many years CT was the best technique for detection of soft tissue tumors, at present, this is better accomplished with MRI. CT however, is still indicated in many cases of bone tumor because of its superior depiction of calcified tissue over MRI. Hence CT is used to determine cortical bone involvement (thinning, scalloping, expansion, destruction), the presence of sequestra or matrix calcifications (cartilaginous vs. osteoid matrix), or to identify a nidus in an osteoid osteoma. Periosteal reaction is well depicted with CT when the periosteum has become calcified. On the other hand, MRI can depict periosteal elevation before it calcifies. MRI is considered superior to CT to assess intramedullary tumor extension, soft tissue and articular extension and neurovascular involvement. While MRI is indicated for preoperative assessment in most cases of soft tissue tumors, CT and MRI have complementary roles in the preoperative staging of bone tumors.

ARTICULAR DISEASE

In most clinical situations, CT is not required for evaluation of articular disease. In some specific cases such as pigmented villonodu-

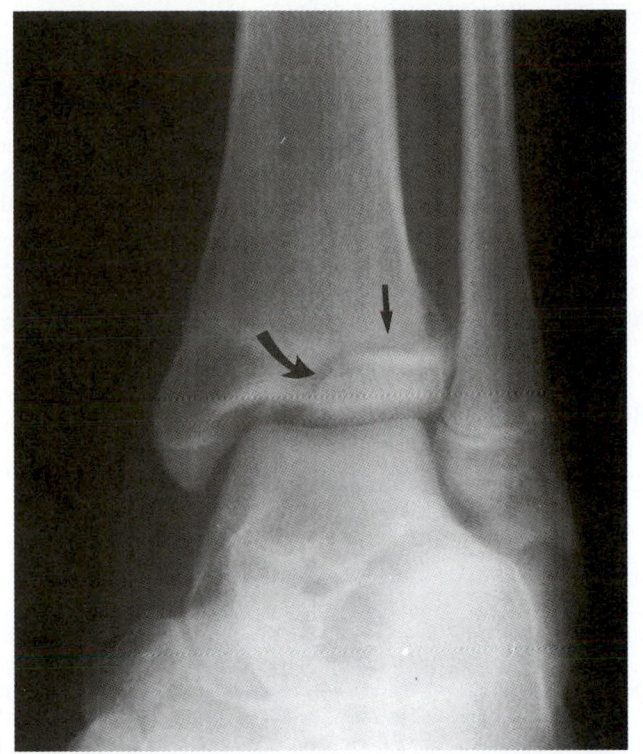

A

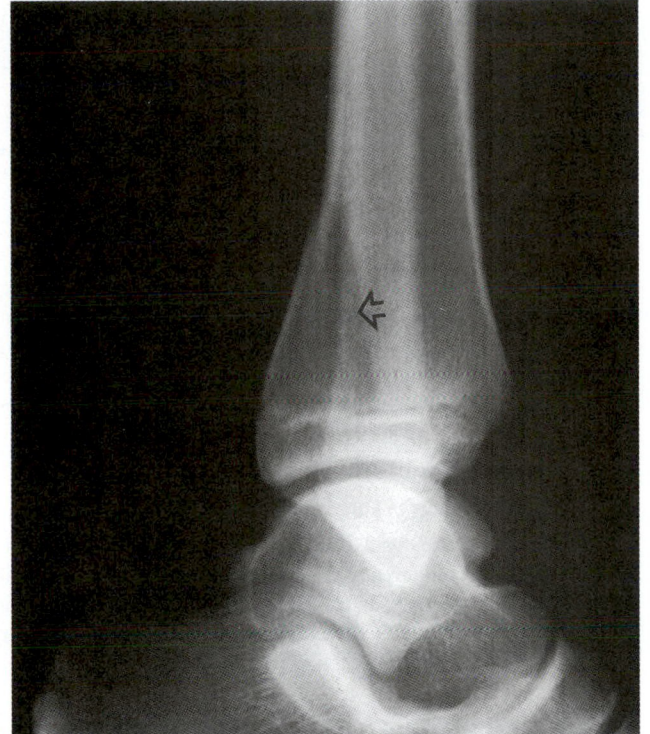

B

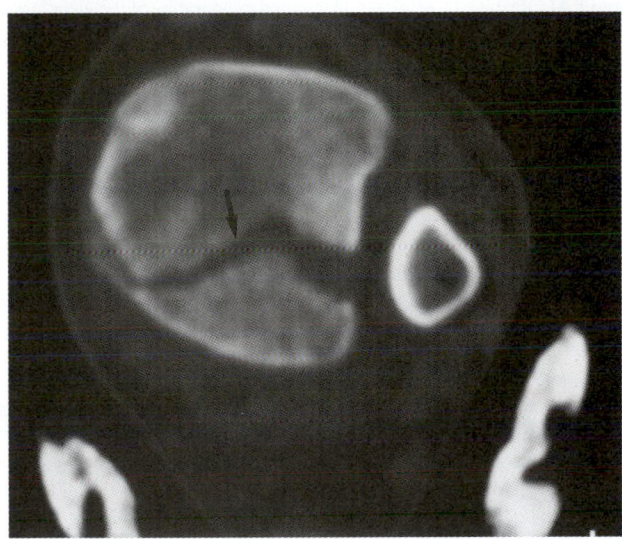

C

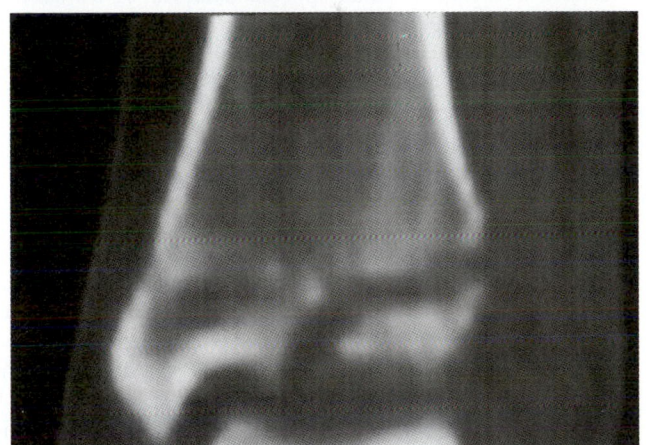

D

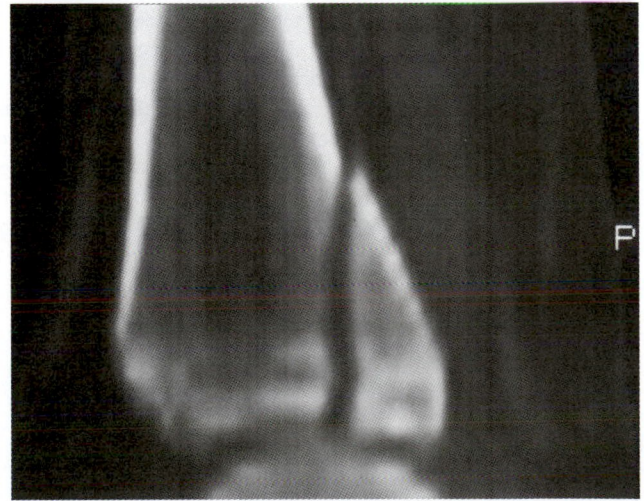

E

Figure 30-3

Triplane fracture in a 14-year-old. AP (*A*) and lateral (*B*) plain films demonstrate tibial epiphyseal fracture (*curved arrow*), growth plate fracture (*straight, closed arrow*), and metaphyseal fracture of distal tibia (*straight, open arrow*). Axial CT (*C*) demonstrates metaphyseal fracture (*arrow*). Coronal (*D*) and sagittal (*E*) 2-D reconstructions demonstrate the fracture lines to better effect.

lar synovitis, synovial chondromatosis, hemophilic arthropathy, or early inflammatory arthritis (i.e., sacroiliitis), CT was used in the past, but it has now been replaced by MRI because of its improved multiplanar capabilities and better soft tissue contrast resolution.

A potential indication of CT is for the 3-D surface display of articular diseases for subsequent creation of plastic models. It is also used to assess patellar tracking abnormalities.

VASCULAR DISEASE

MRI and scintigraphy are used for early diagnosis of avascular necrosis. CT may play a role in surgical planning for advanced disease involving the femoral head, to determine the involvement of the articular surface and degree of collapse, when osteotomy is contemplated instead of total joint replacement.

CONGENITAL AND DEVELOPMENTAL DISEASE

CT is used for the preoperative assessment of dysplastic deformities such as developmental dysplasia of the hip and tarsal coalition. Other applications in developmental disorders are based on the possibility of obtaining measurements in different planes. Hence, CT can be used to measure leg length discrepancy, anteversion angle of the femur or tibia, and degree of vertebral rotation in scoliosis.

OSTEOPOROSIS

Dedicated software and the use of a phantom with standardized values of different concentrations of calcium allow accurate measurements of bone mineral content of the lumbar spine in patients suspected of having osteoporosis. This technique has been used extensively in the last decade, but now it is being replaced by dual photon x-ray absorptiometry with dedicated equipment (DEXA scanners).

SPINE

The evaluation of patients with low back pain continues to be a controversial subject. Imaging techniques available include plain film radiography, scintigraphy, CT, CT post myelography, CT with intravenous injection of contrast, discography, CT post discography, and MRI. Although MRI has simplified the work up of these patients, CT with and without intrathecal contrast is still used as a complementary test for preoperative evaluation since it provides better evaluation of the bony structures of the spinal canal and neuroforamina than MRI. When MRI and CT myelography are combined, the overall accuracy of both techniques for disc disease is superior to the accuracy of each one of them when considered separately.

Discography followed by CT, although controversial, is still used in some centers to assess patients with multilevel lumbar disc disease, or in cases with discrepant results of MRI and CT-myelography. Supposedly, reproducibility of pain during intradiscal injection of contrast helps to identify the disc level responsible for the symptoms. CT following discography can depict radial and peripheral annular tears.

INTERVENTIONAL PROCEDURES

CT offers the ability to image a lesion and a biopsy needle or draining catheter. Careful measurements obtained prior to the introduction of the needle or catheter allow an accurate and safe approach. CT-guided biopsies have been used extensively in the musculoskeletal system for both superficial and deep lesions. This technique is especially valuable for lesions located near vital structures such as the aorta or pleura. Ultrasound is an alternative technique for needle or catheter guidance, but its use is limited when it comes to deeply located lesions or for lesions located in the spine or paraspinal area. Although some work has been performed with MRI-guided biopsies, CT continues to be the easiest and safest modality for this purpose.

SUGGESTED READINGS

Aitken AG, Flodmark O, Newman DE, et al: Leg length determination by CT digital radiography. *Am J Roentgenol* 1985; 144:613.

Burk DL Jr, Mears DC, Kennedy WH, et al: Three-dimensional computed tomography of acetabular fractures. *Radiology* 1985; 155:183.

Carrera GF, Foley WD, Kozin F, et al: CT of sacroilitis. *Am J Roentgenol* 1981; 136:41.

Cone RO 3d, Nguyen V, Flournoy JG, et al: Triplane fracture of the distal tibial epiphysis: Radiographic and CT studies. *Radiology* 1984; 153:763.

Destouet JM, Gilula LA, Murphy WA, et al: Computed tomography of the sternoclavicular joint and sternum. *Radiology* 1981; 138:123.

Deutsch AL, Resnick D, Campbell G: Computed tomography and bone scintigraphy in the evaluation of tarsal coalition. *Radiology* 1982; 144:137.

Deutsch AL, Resnick D, Mink JH: Computed tomography of the glenohumeral and sternoclavicular joints. *Orthop Clin North Am* 1985; 16:497.

Fishman EK, Magid D, Ney DR, et al: Three dimensional imaging. *Radiology* 1991; 181:321.

Guerra J Jr, Gafin Sr, Resnick D: Vertebral burst fractures. CT analysis of the retropulsed fragment. *Radiology* 1984; 153:769.

Handel SF, Lee YY: Computed tomography of spinal fractures. *Radiol Clin North Am* 1981; 19:69.

Kalender WA, Seissler W, Klotz E, et al: Spiral volumetric CT with single-breath-hold technique, continuous transport, and continuous scanner rotation. *Radiology* 1990; 176:181.

Lukens JA, McLeod RA, Sim FH: Computed tomographic evaluation of primary osseous malignant neoplasms. *Am J Roentgenol* 1982; 139:45.

Mack JA, Harley JD, Winquist RA: CT of acetabular fractures: Analysis of fracture patterns. *Am J Roentgenol* 1982; 138:407.

Martinez S, Korobkin M, Fondren FB, et al: Computed tomography of the normal patellofemoral joint. *Invest Radiol* 1983; 18:249.

Ney DR, Fishman EK, Kawashima A, et al: Comparison of helical and serial CT with regard to three-dimensional imaging of musculoskeletal anatomy. *Radiology* 1992; 185:865.

Norman A, Nelson J, Green S: Fractures of the hook of hamate: Radiographic signs. *Radiology* 1985; 154:49.

Rafii M, Firooznia H, Golimbu C, et al: Computed tomography of tibial plateau fractures. *Am J Roentgenol* 1984; 142:1181.

Rafii M, Firooznia H, Golimbu C, et al: CT arthrography of capsular structures of the shoulder. *Am J Roentgenol* 1986; 146:361.

Shirkhoda A, Brashear HR, Staab EV: Computed tomography of acetabular fractures. *Radiology* 1980; 134:683.

Weiner DS, Cook AJ, Hoyt WA Jr, et al: Computed tomography in the measurement of femoral anteversion. *Orthopedics* 1978; 1:299.

Chapter 31

INTERVENTIONAL RADIOLOGY AND ANGIOGRAPHY

Norman Y. Schoenberg

This chapter discusses the indications for contrast imaging of the joints, joint replacements, the spine, percutaneous needle biopsies, and angiography.

THE JOINTS

ARTHROGRAPHY

In recent years, the number of indications for conventional arthrography of the joints has diminished with the advent of magnetic resonance imaging (MRI). There are both *general* indications for arthrography and *specific* indications related to individual joints. The *primary general* indications for performing a conventional arthrogram are: (1) to confirm intracapsular positioning of a needle or catheter following a joint aspiration or prior to an anesthetic joint injection; (2) in place of an MR scan if it is not available, contraindicated, or if the patient is too obese for the gantry or is claustrophobic; and (3) for the diagnosis and treatment of adhesive capsulitis (brisement).

There are also *specific* indications related to the shoulder and wrist. Single- (iodine only) or double- (air and iodine) contrast shoulder arthrography is still a valid and simple test to perform in the diagnosis of partial and full-thickness rotator cuff tears. This test should be utilized as a second-line procedure should an MR scan of the shoulder be contraindicated or equivocal in a patient with a high index of clinical suspicion for a tear. A full-thickness rotator cuff tear is present when contrast crosses the rotator cuff space from the joint into the subacromial-subdeltoid bursa (Fig. 31-1). A tri-compartment wrist arthrogram is still the study of choice in the evaluation of interosseous ligament and triangular fibrocartilage tears. Due to the limited spatial resolution of MRI, small structures are difficult to visualize. Initially, 2 to 3 cc of iodinated contrast is injected into the radiocarpal joint under fluoroscopic control. Using careful monitoring, pre- and postexercise views of the wrist are performed to evaluate for a tear of the scapholunate or lunatotriquetral ligaments and the triangular fibrocartilage. Since a small percentage of patients can have a tear with unidirectional leakage, contrast injections are also performed in the intercarpal compartment and the distal radioulnar joint. An interosseous ligament tear is present if communication is identified between the radiocarpal and intercarpal compartments. A triangular fibrocartilage tear is noted when contrast leaks between the radiocarpal compartment and the distal radioulnar joint (Fig. 31-2).

CT ARTHROGRAPHY

CT arthrography has been the study of choice to evaluate the joint capsule, labrum, articular cartilage, joint space, and subchondral bone, that is, the joint contents. The spatial resolution is better than an MR scan. The disadvantages are x-ray exposure, an interventional procedure, and the small risk of an allergic reaction to the iodinated contrast agent. These studies are performed utilizing a small amount of contrast to coat the articular surfaces and capsule of a joint and a moderate to large amount of air to expand the surfaces so they can be visualized separately. The general indications for this study would include: evaluation of the articular surfaces for chondral defects, loose bodies, and synovial disorders. Specifically, in the shoulder, this test is primarily indicated in the evaluation of glenohumeral instability. Stripping of the anterior capsule from the scapula, anterior labral tears (Bankart lesions), and Hill-Sachs lesions are well seen (Fig. 31-3). Osteochondritis dissecans can occur in the elbow, hip, knee, or ankle. There are several stages to this disease. Treatment often is dependent upon whether the articular cartilage is intact. With an unstable lesion, contrast will insinuate between the fragment and subchondral bone (Fig. 31-4). The patellofemoral joint can also be evaluated for subluxation and chondromalacia. This study is performed from 0 to 40 degrees of flexion at 10-degree increments. Both patellae are evaluated for alignment and articular cartilage integrity.

Following open reduction for the correction of infantile hip dysplasia, an intraoperative hip arthrogram is performed, followed by a CT scan, to evaluate alignment (Fig. 31-5). In adult patients with hip clicking, a double-contrast CT arthrogram (as in the shoulder) can be performed to evaluate the size and configuration of the labrum.

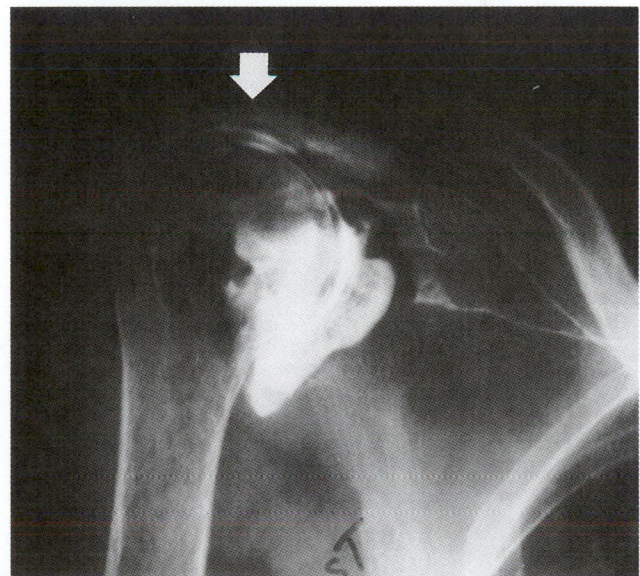

Figure 31-1
Rotator cuff tear. Following a double-contrast right shoulder arthrogram, an external rotation view of the right shoulder demonstrates contrast and air within the subacromial/subdeltoid bursa (*arrow*). This finding is compatible with a full-thickness rotator cuff tear.

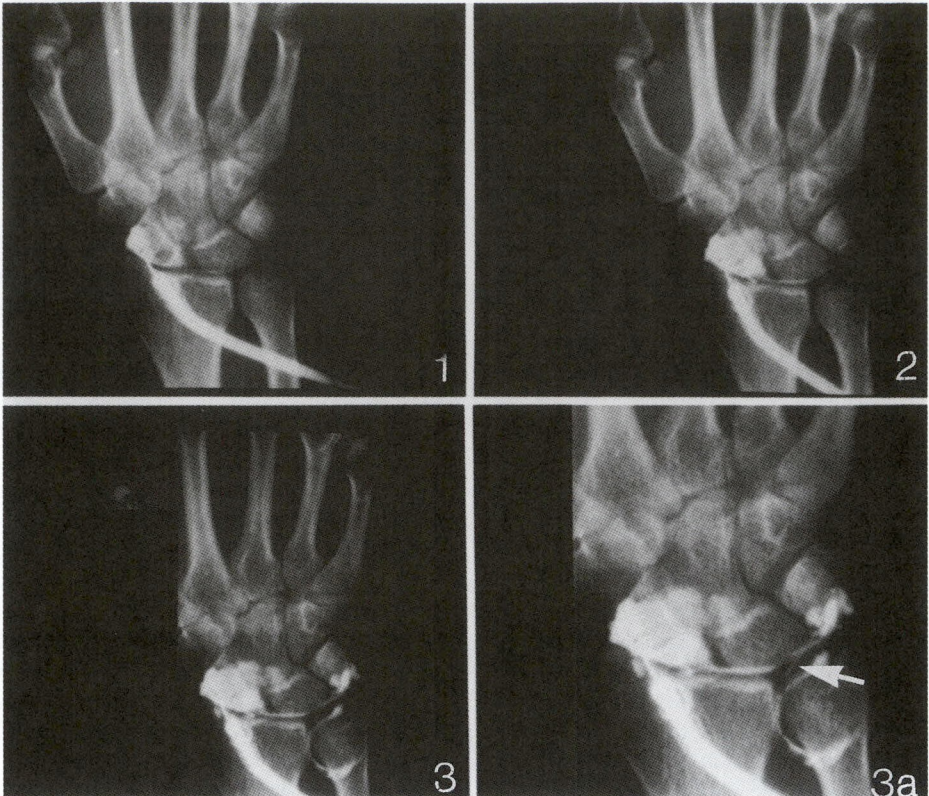

Figure 31-2
TFCC tear. Sequential filming of the right wrist in the PA projection, during a single-contrast injection in the radiocarpal compartment; demonstrates abnormal filling of the distal radioulnar joint. The arrow (3a) points to an obliquely oriented full thickness tear of the triangular fibrocartilage complex (TFCC).

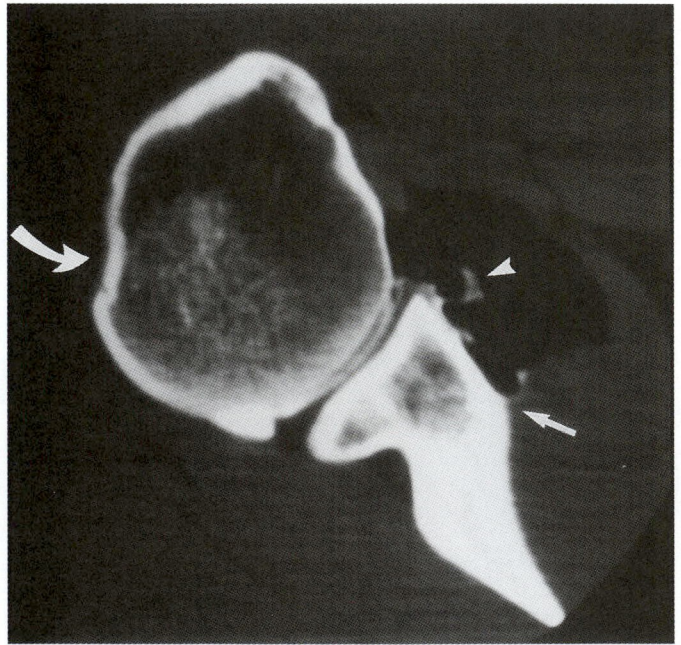

Figure 31-3
Glenohumeral instability. A double-contrast CT arthrogram of the right shoulder demonstrates several findings indicative of glenohumeral instability. The curved arrow is pointing to a Hill-Sachs lesion at the posterolateral aspect of the humeral head. The arrowhead demonstrates avulsion of the anterior labrum from the glenoid. The straight arrow points to anterior capsular stripping from the scapula.

MR ARTHROGRAPHY

MR arthrography is currently an investigative technique that should replace CT arthrography. This technique improves the accuracy in the diagnosis of partial and complete rotator cuff tears (Fig. 31-6) and may surpass the accuracy of CT arthrographic evaluation of glenohumeral instability (Fig. 31-7). In addition, superior labrum anterior posterior (SLAP) lesions are well visualized. There is a dramatic improvement in the ability to visualize and diagnose disruption of the interosseous ligaments of the wrist and triangular fibrocartilage of the wrist (Fig. 31-8).

Patients with recurrent knee pain following arthroscopy are difficult to evaluate with noncontrast MRI. The need to distinguish new and recurrent meniscal tears from chronic tears and postoperative changes have led some researchers to experiment with intraarticular contrast. In addition, infantile hip dysplasia, adult hip labral abnormalities, and osteochondritis dessicans can be assessed.

TOTAL JOINT REPLACEMENTS

Aspiration arthrography is often performed in the evaluation of loosening and/or infection of total joint replacements. Following needle placement into the joint space, an aspirate is obtained and sent for the usual cultures and cell count. If no fluid can be aspirated, saline is infused and reaspirated. The contrast injection merely confirms intraarticular positioning and can be photographed using conventional film or digital subtraction technique. Digital subtraction involves subtracting the scout view from the injected view, leaving only the con-

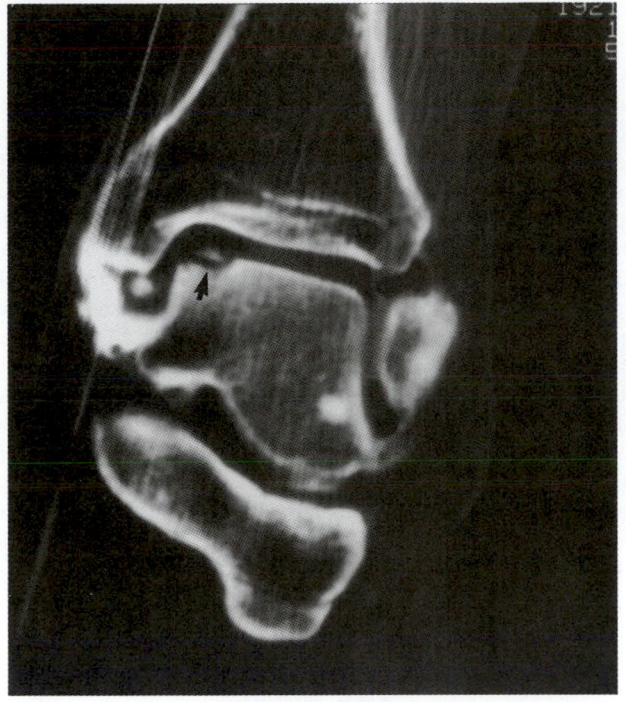

A

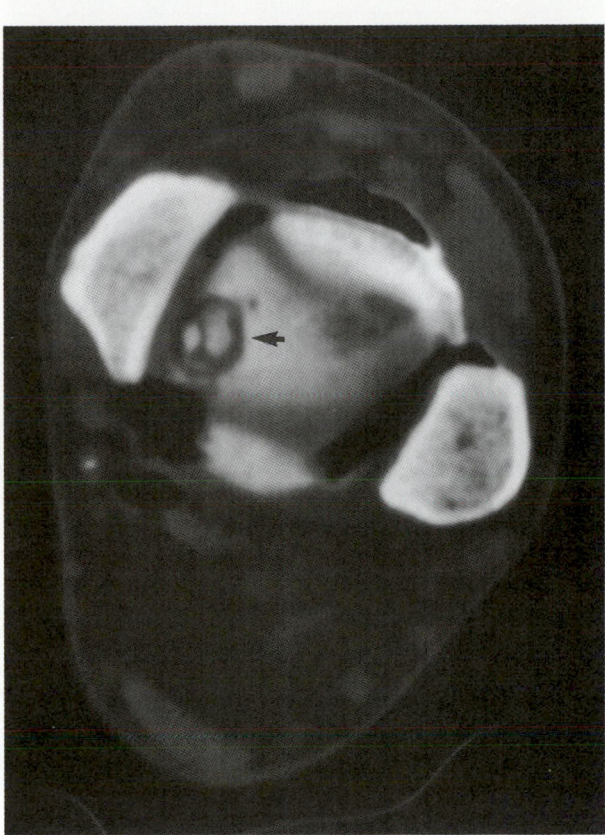

B

Figure 31-4

Osteochondritis dissecans in situ. Images *A* and *B* are taken from a double-contrast CT arthrogram of the right ankle performed in the coronal (*A*) and axial (*B*) planes using a bone window. The arrows point to osteochondritis dissecans in situ of the medial talar dome. Fragmentation is present. However, the lesion is stable since no contrast nor air has insinuated between the fragments and the talar bone.

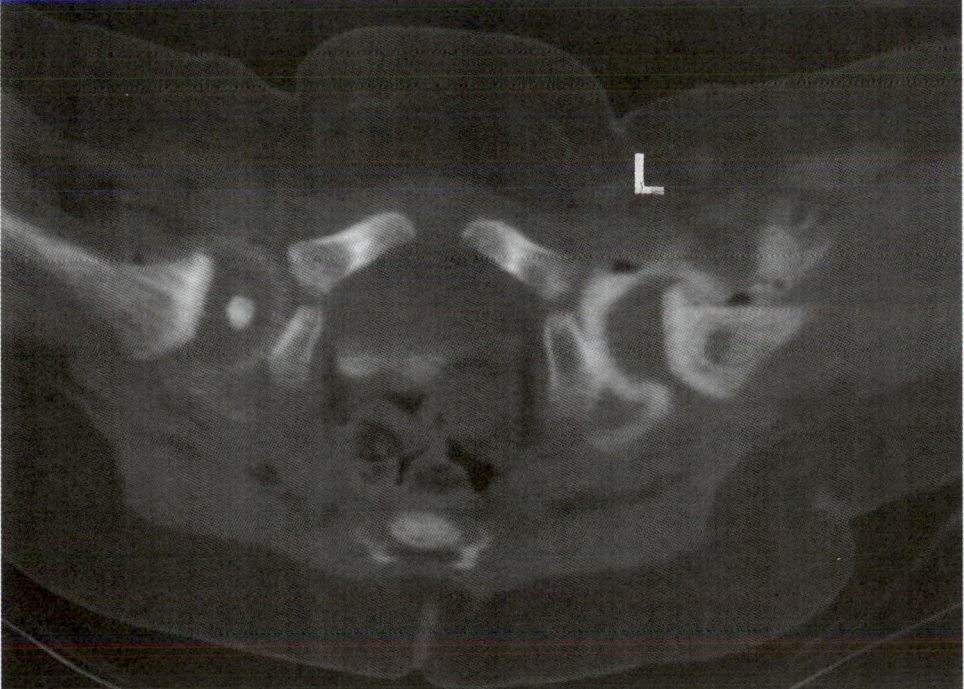

Figure 31-5

Infantile dysplasia of the hip. Following an intraoperative arthrogram of both hips and spica cast placement, a CT scan is performed to confirm intracapsular positioning. The left hip demonstrates delay in ossification of the proximal left femoral epiphysis and a flattened posterior acetabular column. Both findings are compatible with infantile hip dysplasia. The left hip has been restored to near anatomical alignment. The right hip is normal and available for comparison. L, left.

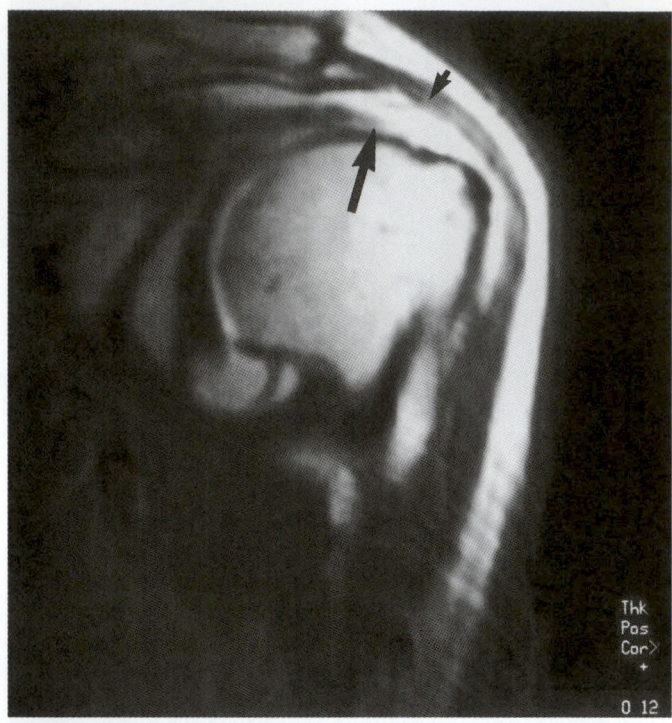

Figure 31-6
Full-thickness rotator cuff tear. A T1-weighted coronal image from an MR arthrogram of the left shoulder demonstrates retraction of the supraspinatus tendon [linear dark signal (*long arrow*)] and contrast filling of the left subacromial/subdeltoid bursa (*short arrow*).

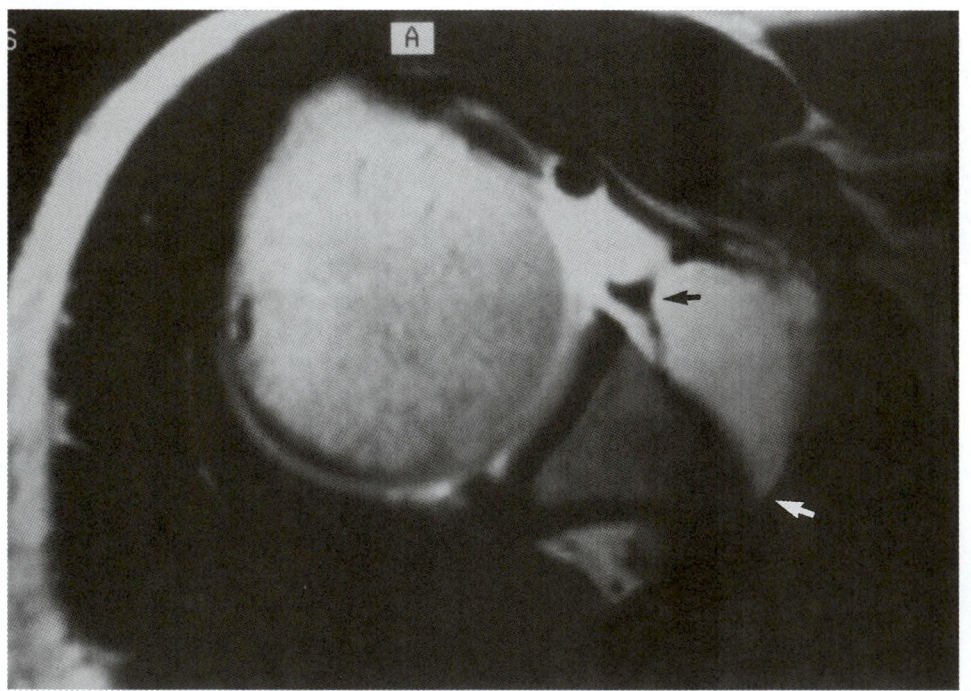

Figure 31-7
Glenohumeral instability. A T1-weighted axial image from an MR arthrogram of the right shoulder demonstrates evidence of glenohumeral instability. There is flattening of the posterolateral aspect of the right humeral head suggesting a subtle Hill-Sachs lesion (impaction fracture). The black arrow points to an avulsion of the anterior labrum and cortex from the glenoid consistent with a Bankart lesion. The white arrow points to anterior capsular stripping from the scapula compatible with redundant capsular insertion.

trast. The advantage of digital subtraction technique is that it allows the contrast medium to be differentiated from the radiopaque prosthesis and cement. Contrast tracking into the cement–bone or prosthesis–cement interfaces is compatible with loosening (Fig. 31-9). Pronounced widening of the cement–bone interface, endosteal scalloping, and periosteal reaction are aggressive features that are more compatible with infection of the prosthesis. Arthrographic findings suggesting infection would include an irregular contour to the joint capsule, filling of (non-bursal) cavities or an abscess, and sinus tract opacification (Fig. 31-10). Infected cavities are typically more irregular and "thick-walled" in appearance than a bursa, and tend to communicate with the capsule through a narrow neck. Complementary studies to this technique would include a three-phase technetium bone scan with a regional indium leukocyte scan. Aspiration following removal of an infected hip replacement is helpful prior to revision to ensure a sterile joint. The arthrogram is performed to demonstrate intracapsular positioning of the needle tip. Again, a technetium bone scan followed by an indium leukocyte scan would be complementary to this test.

THE SPINE

MYELOGRAPHY AND CT

MR scanning has become widely used in the evaluation of the spine after plain films. The causes for myelopathy, radiculopathy, low back pain, or sciatica can be evaluated. Disc degeneration and herniation, osteoarthritis of the facet joints, discitis, osteomyelitis, primary neoplasia, and metastatic disease can be identified. Unsuspected occult diseases can also be seen. An MR scan is not invasive and involves no radiation.

Myelography with CT scan is commonly used in patients where the MR scan is equivocal, unavailable, or contraindicated as in patients with pacemakers or intracranial aneurysm clips. Many surgeons also use myelography with CT scan as a procedure for preoperative planning. Myelography is still quite helpful in evaluating the degree of stenosis, spinal cord impingement, and nerve root impingement. Lumbar arachnoiditis is easily diagnosed on myelography. Another indication would include evaluation of traumatic nerve root avulsions, leaving an empty nerve root sleeve. An anterior impression on the thecal sac is usually secondary to a bulging disc. A large anterior or anterolateral defect suggests a herniation, whereas a posterolateral defect is more likely due to enlargement of the ligamentum flavum or hypertrophic osteoarthritis of a facet joint. Spinal stenosis typically shows an hourglass configuration resulting from both anterior and posterior impressions.

The postmyelogram CT scan provides better spatial resolution than that obtained with an MR scan. This study

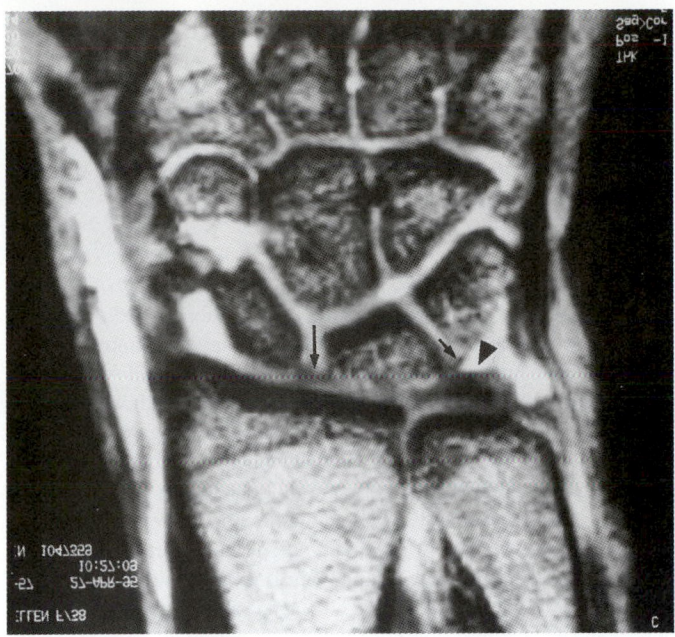

Figure 31-8

Normal MR arthrogram of the wrist. A three-dimensional gradient echo, coronal image from an MR arthrogram of the right wrist nicely demonstrates intact interosseous ligaments and the triangular fibrocartilage complex. Long arrow, scapholunate ligament; short arrow, lunotriquential ligament; arrowhead, triangular fibrocartilage complex.

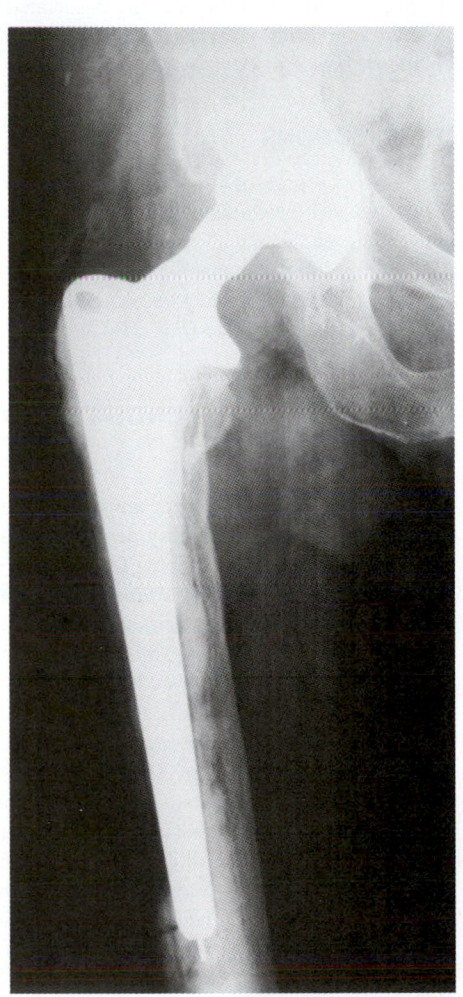

A

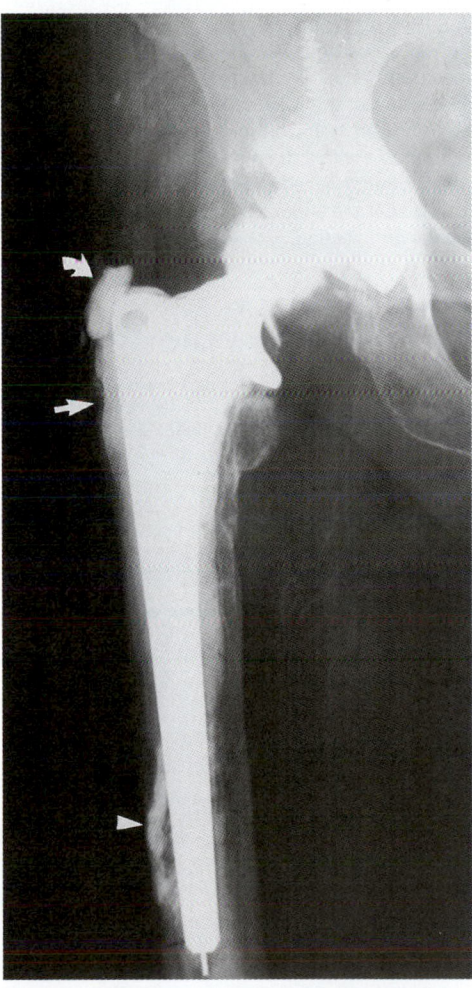

B

Figure 31-9

Prosthetic loosening. *A* represents an AP scout view of a hybrid right total hip replacement prior to arthrographic injection. Note there is an irregular lucency at the cement-bone interface of the femoral component suggesting loosening. *B* is the same anterior view, following single-contrast injection at the neck of the femoral component. There is a cuff of contrast surrounding the femoral neck compatible with the in-

tracapsular injection. The curved arrow shows filling of an incidental small bursa overlying the greater trochanter. The straight arrow demonstrates contrast leaking into the cement–bone interface of the femoral component compatible with loosening. The arrowhead demonstrates contrast leaking into a lateral cortical defect.

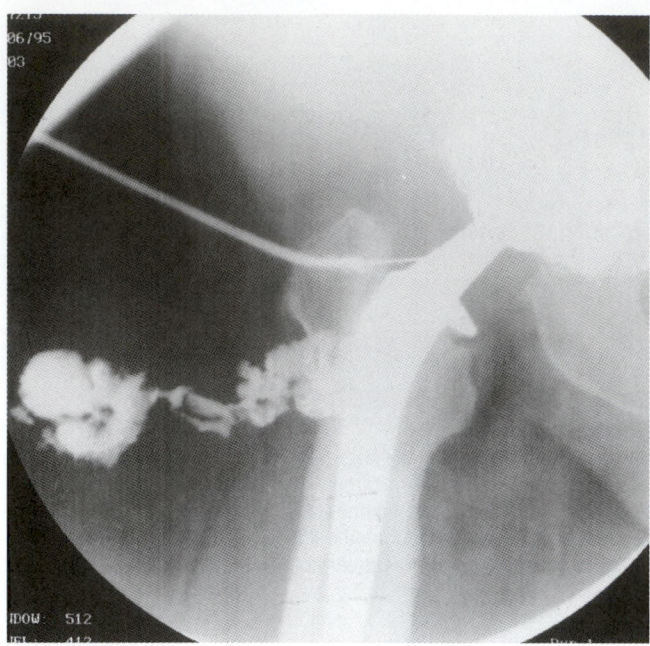

Figure 31-10
Prosthetic infection with sinus tract. An AP view of a noncemented right total hip replacement was obtained during arthographic injection. The needle tip is intracapsular, at the neck of the femoral component. The contrast immediately leaked from the joint space into a lateral sinus tract of the thigh compatible with a draining infection. Concurrent opacification of small- and moderate-sized infected cavities are present along the sinus tract. Also present are endosteal erosions at the cement–bone interface, compatible with infection.

is also excellent for measuring the size of a herniation or determining the degree of stenosis (Fig. 31-11). Ligamentum flavum enlargement and hypertrophic bone changes resulting in spinal cord or nerve root entrapment from stenosis of the spinal canal and lateral recesses are well visualized in this study.

DISCOGRAPHY

Discography is an uncommonly used examination in the evaluation of a patient with low back pain and/or radicular symptoms. The indications for a lumbar or cervical discogram are as follows: (1) severe or unremitting low back or neck pain with or without radicular symptoms in a patient with virtually negative imaging studies or degenerative disc disease; (2) for use in preoperative planning prior to spinal fusion to include only those painful disc levels; (3) in the evaluation of neural foraminal masses which may represent an extruded disc herniation or a nerve sheath tumor; (4) to determine accurate needle placement prior to chymopapain injection; and (5) persistent pain in the postoperative period. The test has a provocative pain component and an anatomic component. The discogram is considered positive at a disc level if it reproduces the patient's familiar (typical) pain that is moderate to severe in intensity associated with an abnormal disc, either demonstrating degeneration or a radial tear (the path for a herniation) (Fig. 31-12).

FACET INJECTIONS

Another elusive source of low back pain is facet joint arthropathy. The diagnosis and treatment of facet syndrome can be obtained by injecting the facet joints with an anesthetic agent and steroid preparation. Pain relief suggests that the facet joints are the primary source of pain. Any joint or nerve may be successfully blocked using a thin needle and imaging guidance (Fig. 31-13).

PERCUTANEOUS NEEDLE BIOPSY

There are three types of closed needle biopsy devices for soft tissue and bone lesions. The first and simplest type is an *aspiration* needle. Typically this is used to remove a small quantity of fluid or fluid mixed with clumps of cells. No histology is preserved. Most often this needle is used to evaluate for infection. The second type of needle is a *cutting* needle. This needle uses a cutting mechanism to provide a soft tissue specimen that is free of maceration. Soft tissue histology is preserved, so that the technique is very useful for primary soft tissue neoplasms, osteolytic lesions of the bone, and evaluation of the bone marrow. The last type of biopsy needle is a *trephine* needle. This needle provides a bone specimen. It is the largest of the three types of needles and also provides the largest specimen. This device is designed for osteoblastic masses (Fig. 31-14) that are deep in a bone, or tumors that incite a large area of surrounding reactive bone.

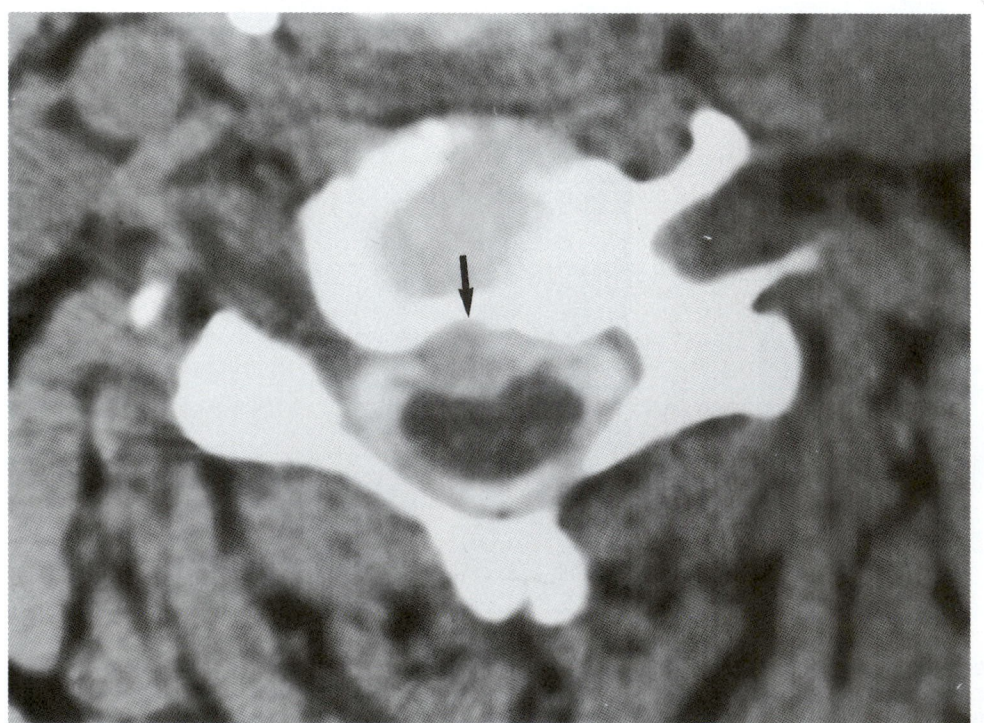

Figure 31-11
Disc herniation. Single axial CT image of the cervical spine at the C5-C6 level was obtained following a cervical myelogram and using a soft tissue window. The arrow points to a large central herniation at C5-C6 which is mildly impinging the spinal cord. No impingement of the exiting nerve root can be seen.

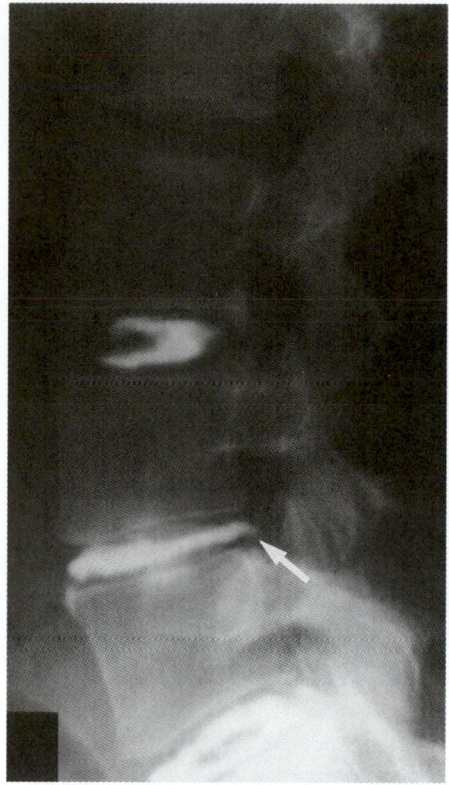
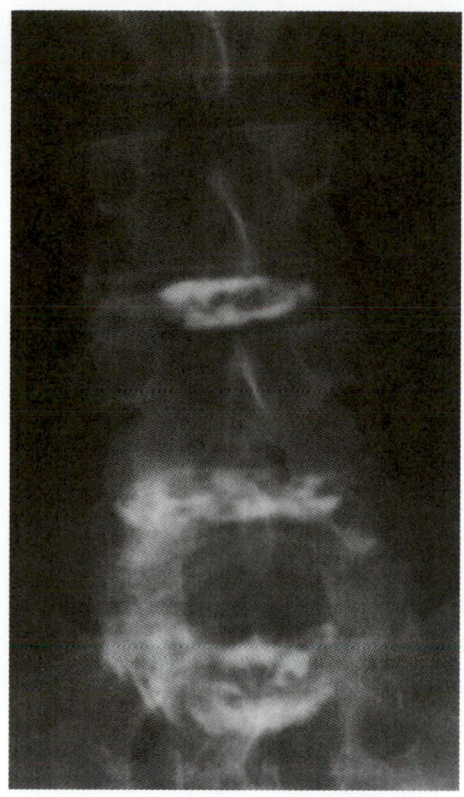

A   *B*

Figure 31-12

Lumbar discogram. *A.* Lateral lumbar spine. *B.* AP lumbar spine. Provocative injection reproduced familiar lower back pain at the L4-5 and L5-S1 levels. The L4-5 level demonstrates interspace narrowing and annular degeneration allowing contrast to extend to the disc margins. The arrow (*A*) points to a dorsal radial tear at L4-5 which has allowed a small contrast leak into the anterior epidural space. The L5-S1 level demonstrates a normal horizontal cleft but with contrast extension into the annular portion of the disc compatible with moderate degeneration. The L3-4 level demonstrates normal central pooling of the contrast associated with a normal horizontal lucent cleft. Mild opacification of the right posterolateral needle tract is incidentally noted.

The indications for a closed needle biopsy are as follows: (1) diagnosis of osteomyelitis, septic arthritis, or septic discitis; (2) neoplasm biopsy to confirm metastatic disease or recurrence; (3) multiple primary lesions; (4) debilitated patients who are not surgical candidates; (5) preoperative planning prior to definitive resection of primary bone or soft tissue tumors; and (6) synovial membrane biopsy to evaluate articular and inflammatory disorders. Multiple myeloma is excluded since it can be diagnosed using laboratory examination and an iliac crest marrow aspirate.

The advantages of a closed needle biopsy over an open needle biopsy are as follows: (1) a shorter period of time to acquire the specimen; (2) can be performed as an outpatient procedure without the need for general anesthesia; (3) imaging such as fluoroscopy, CT scanning, or ultrasound will confirm accurate needle placement; and (4) several specimens may be taken during the same session. The disadvantages of closed needle biopsies are as follows: (1) the specimens tend to be small and may be difficult to examine histologically and (2) there is a theoretical risk of dissemination of malignant tissue to neighboring or distant tissues. In one study an accurate diagnosis was made in up to 95 percent of patients with a primary neoplasm and 97 percent of patients with an inflammatory disorder. Disease was excluded in 80 percent of the patients.

The more common complications include mild pain and discomfort at the site of the biopsy, or a small hematoma, secondary to vascular injury, due to improper motion of the needle lacerating adjacent tissues. Rare complications include: significant hemorrhage from hypervascular tumors or arteriovenous malformations, vascular fistula, pneumothorax, sinus tract, or nerve root injury. There is a theoretical risk of malignant seeding along the needle tract. If there is a high index of suspicion for malignancy, then the course of the biopsy can be tailored such that the needle tract can be resected along with the neoplasm at the time of the definitive procedure.

ANGIOGRAPHY

There are several indications for musculoskeletal and peripheral angiography. Some of the diagnostic studies will be supplanted by MR angiography in the near future. The indications include: (1) as a diagnostic study, following possible vascular injury from trauma; (2) embolization of active bleeding sites not amenable to surgical control, such as within the pelvis; (3) evaluation of bone and soft tissue tumors [the findings will assess: the neovascularity of the lesion, the extent of the tumor, and invasion or impingement of major vessels (Fig. 31-15)]; (4) preoperative or palliative intraarterial embolization or chemotherapy; (5) diagnosis and treatment of AV malformations; (6) evaluation of the arterial anatomy prior to bone or soft tissue grafts; and (7) diagnosis of arteritis that is further complicating col-

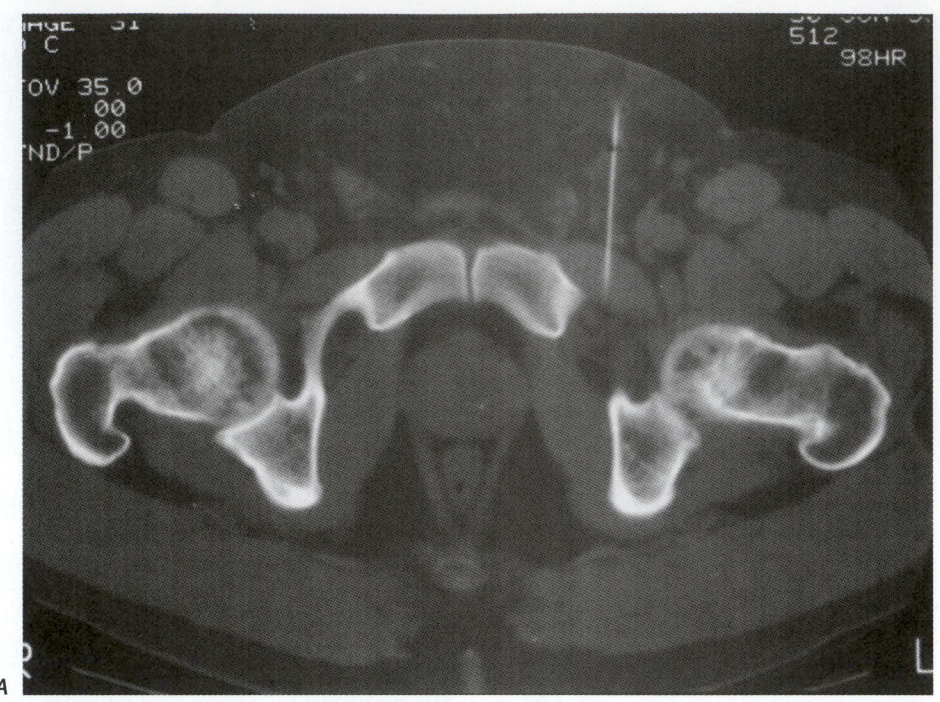

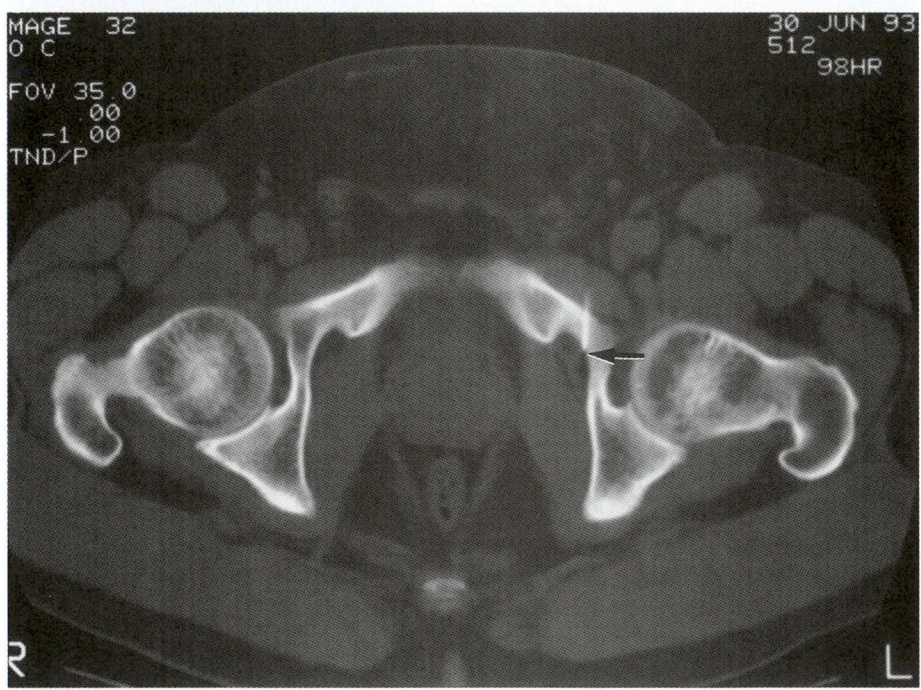

Figure 31-13

Left obturator nerve block. *A* and *B* are axial CT images, using a bone window, from a patient with chronic left pelvic pain suspected to originate from injury of the left obturator nerve. Using CT guidance, a thin needle was inserted from an anterior approach so that the tip (*arrow, B*) is present within the left obturator canal. A 3-cc mixture of 1% lidocaine and 40 mg of triamcinolone was injected to diagnose the origin of his pain and provide temporary therapeutic relief.

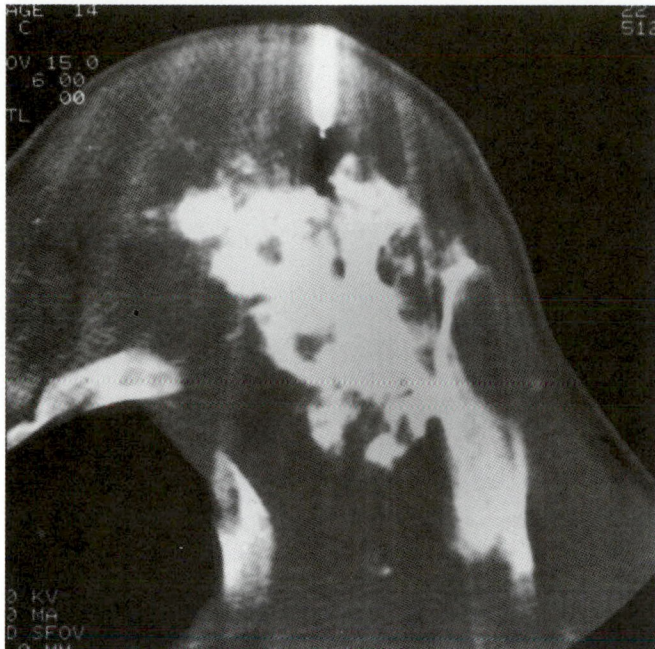

Figure 31-14
CT guided biopsy. This axial CT slice, using bone technique, was obtained to guide the biopsy of a large, possibly aggressive, and heavily centrally calcified soft tissue mass of the left scapula. Several core needle biopsy specimens were obtained to exclude malignant degeneration and assist in preoperative planning. The lesion proved to be a benign osteochondroma.

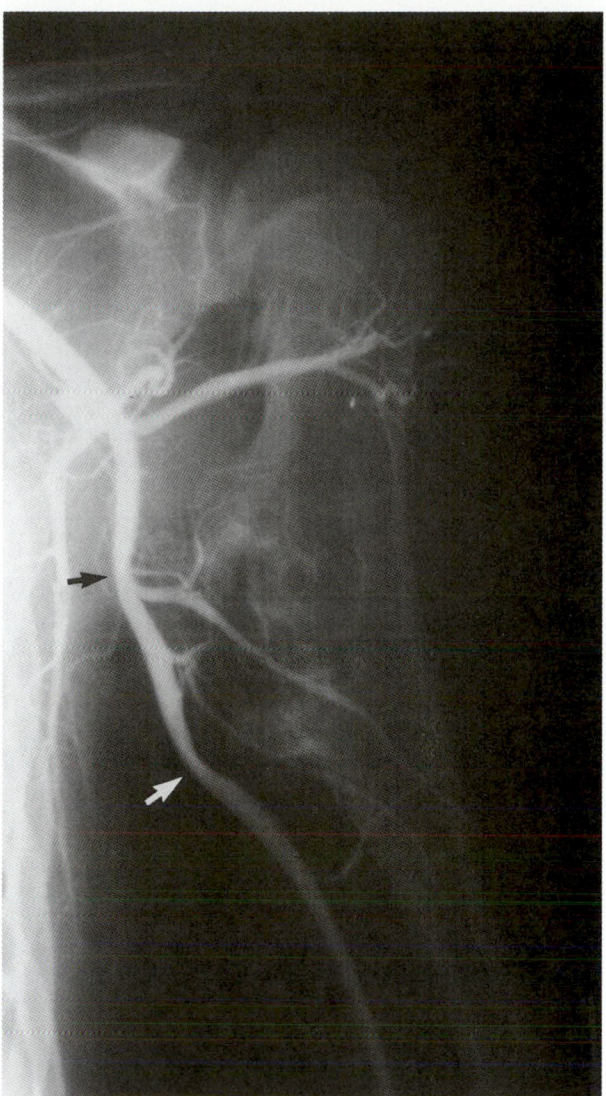

Figure 31-15
Brachial artery compression by tumor. Prior to resection of a broad-based and large osteochondroma of the proximal left humerus, the patient underwent a left upper extremity angiogram. The arrows indicate two areas of brachial artery compression from the cartilage cap of the tumor.

lagen vascular disease. Angiography can also be used as a second line study (after ultrasound and MRI) to differentiate vascular versus non-vascular masses such as occasionally occur behind the knee.

Venography, to evaluate deep venous thrombosis, has been largely supplanted by duplex sonography. Uncommonly, if the exam is equivocal due to obesity or prior phlebitis, a venogram may still be helpful.

SUGGESTED READINGS

Beige J: Musculoskeletal imaging takes interventional turn. *Diagn Imaging* 1995; 17:69.

Bookstein JJ: Angiography. In Resnick D (ed): *Diagnosis of Bone and Joint Disorders,* 3d ed. Philadelphia: WB Saunders; 1995:410.

Haughton V: Imaging techniques in intraspinal diseases, in Resnick D (ed): *Diagnosis of Bone and Joint Disorders,* 3d ed. Philadelphia: WB Saunders; 1995:237.

Rafii M: Shoulder. In Firooznia HF, Golimbu C, Rafii M, et al. (eds): *MRI and CT of the Musculoskeletal System.* St. Louis: Mosby-Year Book; 1992:chap 15.

Resnick D: Arthrography, tenography, and bursography. In Resnick D (ed): *Diagnosis of Bone and Joint Disorders,* 3d ed. Philadelphia: WB Saunders; 1995:277.

Resnick D: Needle biopsy of bone. In Resnick D (ed): *Diagnosis of Bone and Joint Disorders,* 3d ed. Philadelphia: WB Saunders; 1995:475.

Schoenberg NY, Beltran J: Contrast enhancement in musculoskeletal imaging: Current status. *Radiol Clin North Am* 1994; 32:337.

Weissman B: Imaging of joint replacements. In Resnick D (ed): *Diagnosis of Bone and Joint Disorders,* 3d ed. Philadelphia: WB Saunders; 1995:559.

Chapter 32

MAGNETIC RESONANCE IMAGING

Javier Beltran

BASIC PHYSICAL PRINCIPLES

Magnetic resonance imaging (MRI) is an imaging technique based on the use of magnetic fields, radio frequency (RF) waves, and complex image reconstruction techniques. Normally, the axes of protons in the body have a random orientation. However, if the body or part of the body is placed within a high magnetic field, protons will align themselves parallel with or perpendicular to the direction of the magnetic field. Protons also have a natural spinning motion at a specific frequency (Larmor frequency). When an RF pulse of the same frequency as that of the spinning protons within a magnetic field is applied, the protons will be deflected from their newly aligned axis by a specific angle. The degree of deflection is dependent on the strength of the applied RF wave pulse. The protons, now spinning synchronously or coherently at an angle with the magnetic field, induce a current in a nearby transmitter-receiver coil or antenna. This small nuclear signal is then recorded, amplified, measured, and localized (linked to the exact location in the body where the MRI signal is coming from), producing a high-contrast, clinically useful MR image.

Due to existing inhomogeneity within the magnetic field and interactions between adjacent protons, the signal starts to decay as soon as the RF pulse is discontinued and the protons begin to "relax" back to a state of equilibrium. The decaying of the signal is intimately related to two factors: the realignment of the protons within the magnetic field (longitudinal relaxation); and the loss of coherence or synchrony (dephasing) of the protons as they continue spinning at an angle to the magnetic field (transverse relaxation). These two phenomena, called relaxation times T1 and T2 respectively, are tissue-specific relaxation constants for different types of tissue and their molecular composition. T1 and T2 can be measured independently to create images that are dependent on different T1 values of the tissues (T1-weighted images, T1WI) or on different T2 values (T2-weighted images, T2WI). Images containing T1 and T2 information are called balanced images or proton density-weighted images (PDWI).

IMAGE CONTRAST AND IMAGE QUALITY

Contrast between tissues is dependent on the differences between T1, T2, and PD values on T1WI, T2WI, or PDWI. These different types of images can be obtained by changing imaging parameters such as the repetition time (TR), echo time (TE), or angle of deflection or flip angle (FA). By changing these parameters, one can control the rate of repetition of the RF pulses (TR), the time elapsed between an RF pulse and the production of a signal or echo (TE), and the intensity of the applied RF pulse which determines the FA. Images obtained using short TR and short TE will produce T1-weighted contrast. Images obtained with long TR and long TE will produce T2-weighted contrast, and images obtained with long TR and short TE will produce PD-weighted contrast. These are the main parameters governing a common pulse sequence design called spin echo (SE). There are other clinically useful pulse sequences that combine different TRs, TEs, and FAs to provide other types of information, such as blood flow. These are generically called gradient echo pulse sequences (GRE). To enhance contrast between water-rich tissues and fat, other sequences are applied using the parameter of inversion time (TI) to create images where the signal intensity from fat is suppressed (short tau inversion recovery or STIR).

When evaluating image contrast and image quality, other parameters to take into consideration are the strength of the magnetic field and the use of surface coils. Low field magnets (0.2 Tesla) and medium field magnets (0.5 Tesla) produce less signal than the high field magnets (1.0 to 1.5 Tesla). Image quality is superior at high field strengths. Surface coils are used very frequently in musculoskeletal imaging because they produce significant improvement of the signal-to-noise ratio when imaging small areas such as the joints. Most manufacturers of MRI devices include a variety of surface coils designed for specific joints.

CLINICAL APPLICATIONS

JOINTS

Shoulder

Rotator cuff pathology, glenohumeral joint instability, and shoulder pain of unknown etiology are the main indications for MRI of the shoulder. Images are obtained in the axial, oblique coronal, and oblique sagittal planes, following the orientation with the coronal plane of the scapula and the supraspinatus tendon. The use of intraarticular contrast (gadolinium) MR arthrography (MRA) may improve the delineation of the inner aspect of the capsule, glenohumeral ligaments, intracapsular portion of the long head of the biceps tendon and glenoid labrum. Thickening and increased signal intensity (SI) are signs of tendinitis or intrasubstance degeneration of the supraspinatus tendon. Bursal or articular surface defects indicate partial thickness rotator cuff tears. Complete discontinuity of the tendon indicates a full-thickness rotator cuff tear. Tendon retraction, muscle atrophy, a fatty degeneration, the condition of the biceps tendon, and osseous lesions can also be evaluated with MRI. MRA can provide good depiction of labral and capsulo-ligamentous lesions, as well as tears at the insertion of the biceps tendon (SLAP lesions, superior lebrum anterior posterior) (Fig. 32-1).

MRI has also been used to assess miscellaneous painful lesions of the shoulder including: osteonecrosis, compressive neuropathies, and inflammatory conditions. MRI evaluation of compressive neuropathies of the suprascapular nerve or the axillary nerve may disclose nerve enlargement or a mass lesion compressing the nerve, such as a ganglion cyst (Fig. 32-2). The denervated muscle can show increased SI on T2WI during the early stages, followed by atrophy.

Elbow

MRI has been applied to the elbow joint to study mass lesions, tendon and ligamentous lesions, osteochondral lesions, pediatric elbow

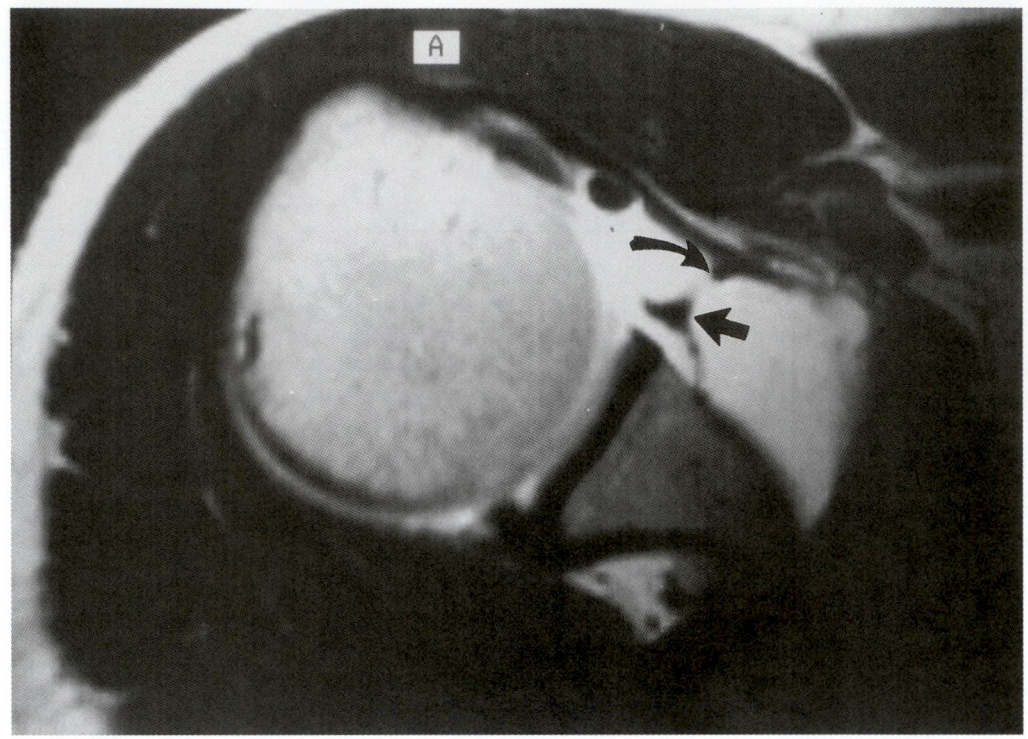

Figure 32-1
MR-arthrogram of the shoulder. Axial T1-weighted image obtained following intraarticular injection of gadolinium. There is an anterior labral tear. A fragment of the anterior labrum (*arrow*) is separated from the glenoid margin, but it remains attached to the superior glenohumeral ligament (*curved arrow*). Note that the injected gadolinium is hyperintense on T1-weighted images.

fractures, compressive neuropathies, and miscellaneous conditions. Most tumors will demonstrate low SI on T1WI and high SI on T2WI. Injuries of the tendons and ligaments may appear as focal areas of increased SI on T2WI, or discontinuity of the fibers with complete tears. This has been useful in assessing lateral epicondylitis (tennis elbow), collateral ligament disruption, and biceps and triceps tendon tears. MRI has been helpful in the assessment of osteochondral lesions (osteochondritis dissecans, OCD). It has been used to determine the size of the lesion, viability of the fragment, congruity of the articular surface (depression, elevation) and stability of the fragment. In general, however, CT is considered superior to MRI in evaluating intraarticular loose bodies.

Pediatric elbow fractures are sometimes difficult to assess with plain film radiography. MRI can depict the extension of fracture lines through a nonossified epiphyses. In compressive or entrapment neuropathies, MRI can also demonstrate the presence of a mass lesion, the location of the compression, changes in SI, or size of the nerve (Fig. 32-3).

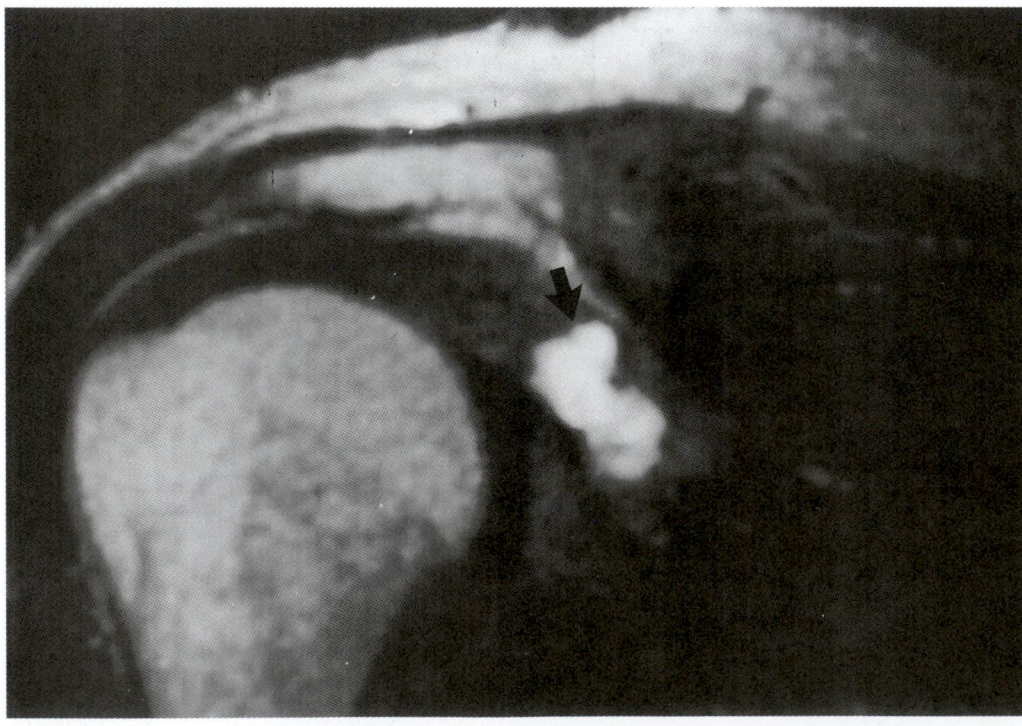

Figure 32-2
Ganglion cyst. Coronal T2-weighted image shows a hyperintense mass (*arrow*) located in the region of the suprascapular notch, producing compressive neuropathy of the suprascapular nerve.

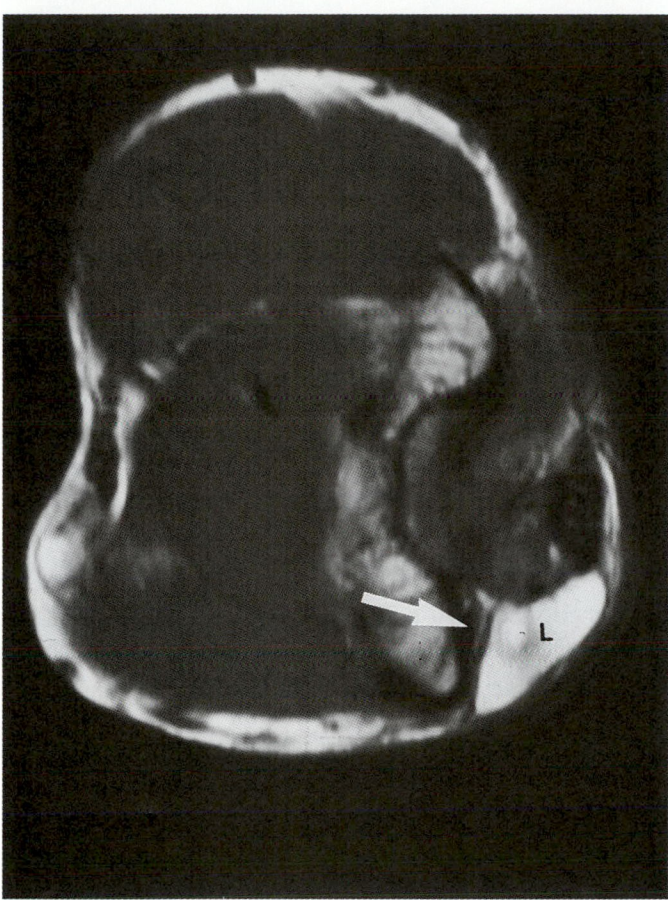

Figure 32-3
Lipoma of the elbow. Axial T1-weighted image demonstrates a soft tissue mass (L) located in the posterior aspect of the elbow, adjacent to the medial epicondyle. The ulnar nerve (*arrow*) is compressed between the tumor and the bone, producing a cubital tunnel syndrome. Note the hyper-intense signal of the tumor, similar to that of the subcutaneous fat.

Hand and Wrist

The most frequent indications for MRI of the hand and wrist include: the evaluation of palpable mass lesions, ligamentous tears, triangular fibrocartilage complex (TFCC) tears, posttraumatic avascular necrosis (AVN) of the scaphoid, Kienböck's disease, tendon tears, and compressive neuropathies. The most frequent palpable mass lesions around the wrist are ganglion cysts. The nature, location, and relationship of a ganglion cyst to adjacent structures are demonstrated well by MRI. Solid, soft tissue tumors are relatively infrequent in the region of the hand and wrist. Giant cell tumors of the tendon sheaths, sarcomas, fibromas, fibrolipomas, and neuromas are among some of the histologic varieties. MRI characteristics are nonspecific, perhaps with the exception of fibrolipomatous hamartoma, which can show a characteristic striated pattern, most often in the distribution of the median nerve.

Ligamentous and TFCC lesions can be demonstrated on MRI with an accuracy ranging between 50 and 90 percent, depending on the ligament involved. TFCC injuries are more easily demonstrated than scapholunate or lunotriquetral ligament lesions. MR arthrography may be more accurate than plain MRI for the diagnosis of ligamentous lesions. Ulnar collateral ligament tears of the first metacarpophalangeal joint ("gamekeepers' thumb" or "skier's thumb"), and

its relationship with the aponeurosis of the adductor policis (Stener lesions), can also be depicted with MRI.

AVN of the scaphoid or lunate appears as a loss of the normal SI of the fatty marrow on T1- and T2-weighted pulse sequences. Intravenous injection of gadolinium may help to determine tissue viability. Tendon tears are diagnosed clinically, but MRI can provide information regarding the site and extent of the tear. Compressive neuropathies (median nerve, carpal tunnel syndrome; ulnar nerve, Guyon's canal syndrome) are also diagnosed clinically, and with electromyography, but MRI may demonstrate the location and etiology of the compression.

Hip

MRI is most commonly used in the hip is to evaluate for the presence of AVN of the femoral head. The most significant advantage of MRI in the evaluation of AVN of the femoral head is its high sensitivity, and the possibility for accurately assessing the size of the lesion. The MRI signs of AVN include areas of abnormal SI in the anterior half of the femoral head, surrounded by an irregular line or band of decreased SI, known as the reactive interface. Occasionally, a second band of higher SI on T2 WI can be found adjacent to the first band (the double line sign). Its appearance is considered diagnostic for AVN.

Transient osteoporosis of the hip is another relatively frequent condition that can be diagnosed with MRI. This is by virtue of the edema-like pattern of SI involving the femoral head and neck that is seen without the focality of AVN. In some instances, patients with an MRI pattern consistent with transient osteoporosis develop MRI changes consistent with AVN. Osteochondral lesions, tumors, synovial chondromatosis, and pigmented villonodular synovitis (PVNS) are other indications for MRI evaluation of the hip.

The Knee

The knee is one of the areas of the musculoskeletal system most commonly imaged by MRI. Meniscal and ligamentous injuries can be diagnosed with an accuracy of almost 95 percent. Meniscal tears appear on MRI as an abnormally high SI area, extending to the articular surface (Fig. 32-4). Peripheral tears and small radial tears may be difficult to detect with MRI. Ligamentous tears can be seen as areas of swelling, with partial or complete disruption of the fibers. Similar findings apply to tendon injuries. Partial or complete tears of the patellar tendon, quadriceps tendon, popliteal tendon, and semimembranosus tendon can be diagnosed with MRI.

Cartilaginous lesions can be demonstrated with MRI using only conventional pulse sequences when the lesion is advanced or large (type 3, 4), or in cases of osteochondritis dissecans (OCD). Small cartilaginous lesions (type 1 or 2) can be diagnosed only when using specific pulse sequences designed for cartilage. Most of these sequences involve 3-D data acquisition, fat suppression and very thin-slice reconstructions. Recently, magnetization transfer sequences have been used successfully to depict very small cartilaginous lesions of the knee.

Bone marrow abnormalities detected with MRI include: contusions (bone bruise), occult fractures, osteonecrosis, tumors, and infection. Inflammatory or tumoral synovial lesions can also be shown with MRI. The use of intravenous gadolinium has helped to differentiate between joint effusion and inflamed synovium.

Ankle and Foot

The most common indications for MRI of the ankle include: tendon lesions, OCD, chronic ankle instability, and pain of unknown etiology. The MRI signs described for ligamentous and tendon lesions of

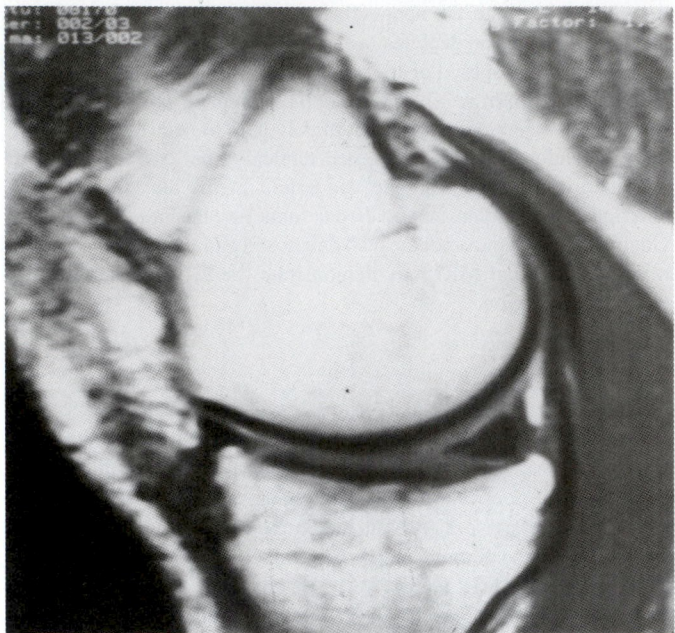

Figure 32-4
Meniscal tear. Sagittal proton density-weighted image demonstrates a tear of the posterior horn of the medial meniscus extending to the articular surface.

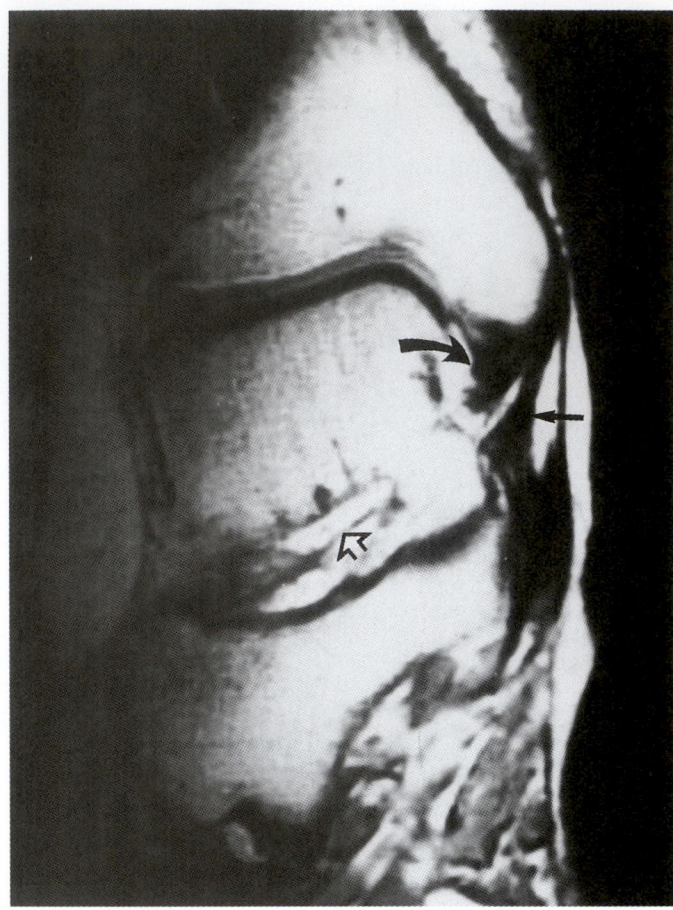

Figure 32-5
Normal deltoid ligament of the ankle. Coronal T1-weighted image demonstrating the tibia talar (*curved arrow*) and tibia calcaneal (*arrow*) components of the deltoid ligament. Observe the normal interosseous ligament in the region of the sinus tarsi (*open arrow*).

the knee also apply to other joints, including the ankle and foot (Fig. 32-5). Lateral and deltoid ligament tears can be diagnosed with an accuracy of 75 to 80 percent, increasing to about 95 percent with the use of intraarticular injection of gadolinium. The most frequent tendons studied with MRI are the Achilles tendon (Fig. 32-6) and the tibialis posterior tendon. Tendinitis, degeneration, and tears are frequent in these locations. MRI may help to confirm the diagnosis, as well as determine the location and size of the tear (Fig. 32-7). MRI can be used to assess OCD lesions involving the talar dome. The size, location, viability, stability, and congruency of the lesion can be determined by MRI.

A number of syndromes involving the ankle and foot can be studied with MRI. These include: sinus tarsi syndrome, tarsal tunnel syndrome, heel pain syndrome (plantar fasciitis), metatarsalgia, and Morton's neuroma, among others.

BONE MARROW

Normal hematopoietic marrow is found in the adult skull, ribs, sternum, spine, pelvis, proximal humeri, and proximal femora. The remaining skeletal marrow space consists of yellow or fatty marrow. Normal red marrow appears as intermediate or low SI on all pulse sequences, whereas yellow marrow demonstrates signal intensity similar to fat. Different processes may affect the bone marrow and produce SI changes on MR images. Reconversion of yellow marrow to red marrow occurs in anemic states (chronic anemia, sickle cell anemia). MRI will demonstrate the presence of red marrow in the expected location of yellow marrow. Bone marrow edema can be seen on MRI in cases of trauma, tumors, infection, osteonecrosis, transient osteoporosis, or transient bone marrow edema. MRI findings of bone marrow edema include low SI on T1WI and high SI on T2WI. Bone marrow replacement by cellular infiltrates (tumor, lymphoma, leukemia, myeloma, infection) presents as areas of decreased SI on T1WI and increased SI on T2WI; this is similar to edema, but within a more focal region. Fatty infiltration of the spine can occur in se-

vere osteoporosis, and also in regions of the skeleton that have been irradiated for therapeutic purposes.

MRI allows an early diagnosis of osteonecrosis with characteristic changes, including areas of abnormal SI surrounded by bands of low SI. It has also been shown to be useful for determining the size of the infarct to plan for appropriate therapy in cases of AVN of the femoral head (Fig. 32-8). It has been found to be especially helpful in diagnosing pre-clinical and pre-radiographic cases of AVN of the femoral head (i.e., contralateral hip).

BONE AND SOFT TISSUE TUMORS

The value of MRI in evaluating bone tumors is that it allows an accurate determination of the location and size of the tumor. In general, SI characteristics of most bone tumors are nonspecific. In fact, some benign tumors, such as osteoid osteomas, chondroblastomas, and eosinophilic granulomas, may display areas of bone and soft tissue edema that simulate the appearance of malignant lesions. Soft tissue tumors can be more accurately detected with MRI than with CT. In addition, the multi-planar capabilities of MRI allow for better staging. As in bone tumors, the SI characteristics of most soft tissue tumors are nonspecific. Occasionally, tumors with hemosiderin deposition (PVNS, hemorrhage) or with a fibrous component (fibromas), may demonstrate areas of low SI on all pulse sequences.

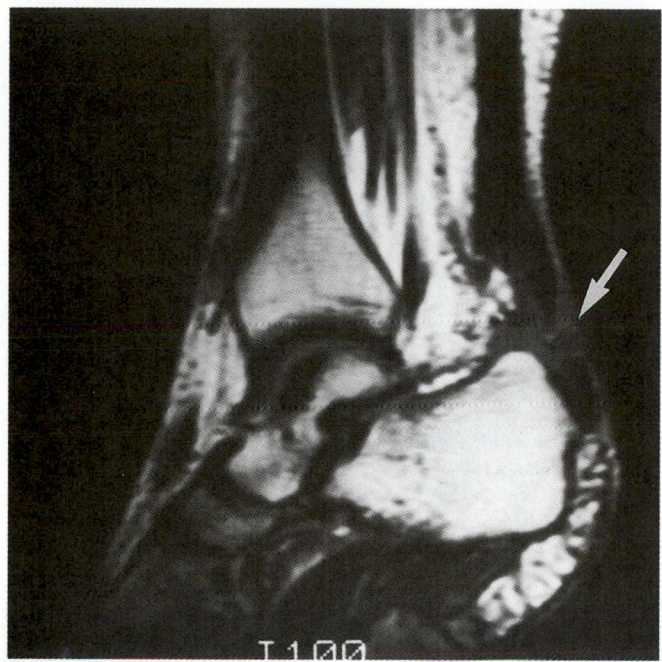

Figure 32-6

Achilles tendon tear. Sagittal T1-weighted image shows thickening and discontinuity of the fibers of the distal Achilles tendon (*arrow*), with about 1 cm separation. This image was obtained with the foot in plantar flexion, to assess the space between the ends of the ruptured tendon after casting.

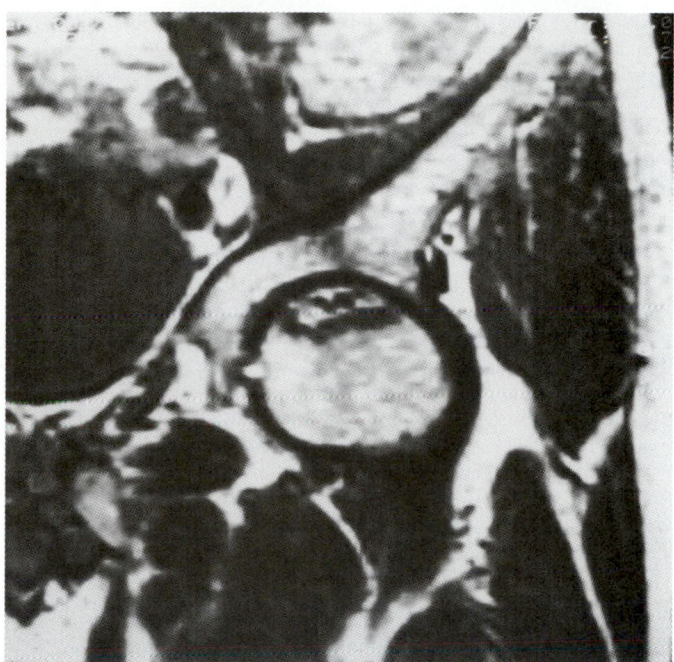

Figure 32-8

Avascular necrosis (AVN) of the femoral head. Coronal T1-weighted image demonstrates large areas of AVN of the femoral head surrounded by a band of decreased signal intensity, representing the reactive interface.

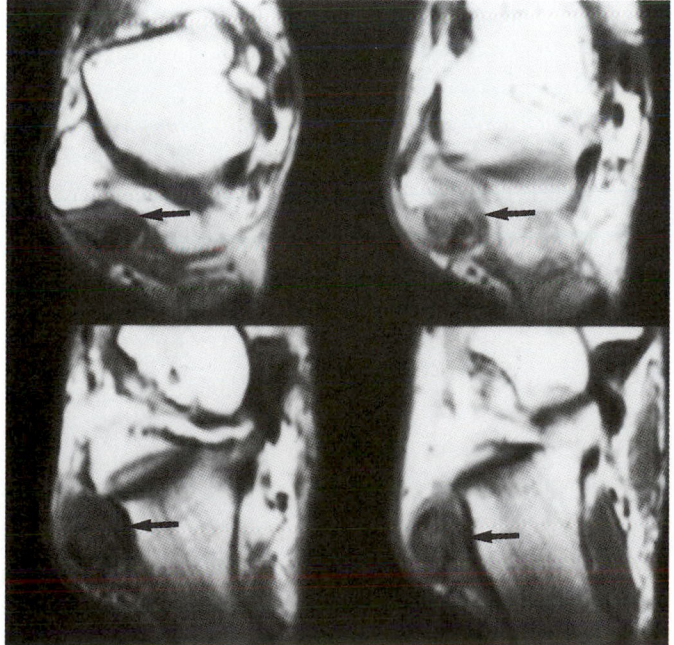

Figure 32-7

Tear of the peroneal tendons. Axial proton density-weighted images obtained at four different levels, from the region of the lateral malleolus to the calcaneus. Observe the irregularity and discontinuity of the fibers of the peroneus brevis and longus tendons (*arrows*), indicating a complete tear of both tendons.

SPINE

MRI has become the screening technique of choice for the evaluation of patients with suspected disc herniation, spinal stenosis, cord tumors, and traumatic, degenerative, and congenital disorders. The combination of multi-planar capabilities and high contrast resolution are ideal for spine imaging. Detection of annular bulges, disc protrusions, extrusions, and sequestrations with MRI can be accomplished with an accuracy rate in the range of 90 percent. MRI is also ideal for the evaluation of patients with recurrent symptoms following discectomy. In these cases, contrast-enhanced MRI can help in distinguishing between recurrent disc herniation and scar tissue. Recurrent disc herniation will appear as an area of intermediate SI, similar to the adjacent disc, surrounded by a rim of enhanced granulomatous tissue. Scar tissue, on the other hand, demonstrates a more diffuse enhancement pattern. MRI is also the technique of choice for detection and staging of demyelinating disorders involving the spine (multiple sclerosis) and syringomyelia.

SUGGESTED READINGS

Beltran J, Munchow AM, Khabiri H, et al: Ligaments of the lateral aspect of the ankle and sinus tarsi: An MR imaging study. *Radiology* 1990;177:455.

Cartland JP, Crues JV 3d, Stauffer A, et al: MR imaging in the evaluation of SLAP injuries of the shoulder: Findings in 10 patients. *Am J Roentgenol* 1992;159:787.

Chandnani V, Ho C, Gerharter J, et al: MR findings in asymptomatic shoulders: A blind analysis using symptomatic shoulders as controls. *Clin Imaging* 1992;16:25.

Chandnani VP, Yeager TD, DeBerardino T: Glenoid labral tears: Prospective evaluation with MR imaging. MR arthrography and CT arthrography. *Am J Roentgenol* 1993;161:1229.

Erickson SJ, Rosengarten JL: MR imaging of the forefoot: Normal anatomic findings. *Am J Roentgenol* 1993;160:565.

Farley TE, Neumann CH, Steinbach LS, et al: Full-thickness tears of the rotator cuff of the shoulder: Diagnosis with MR imaging. *Am J Roentgenol* 1992;158:347.

Goldman AB, Schneider R, Pavlov H: Osteoid osteomas of the femoral neck: Report of four cases evaluated with isotopic bone scanning, CT and MR imaging. *Radiology* 1993;186:227.

Hodler J, Haghighi P, Trudell D, et al: The cruciate ligaments of the knee: Correlation between MR appearance and gross and histologic findings in cadaveric specimens. *Am J Roentgenol* 1992;159:357.

Kier R, Dietz MJ, McCarthy SM, et al: MR imaging of the normal ligaments and tendons of the ankle. *J Comput Assist Tomogr* 1991;15:477.

Kier R, McCarthy S, Dietz MJ, et al: MR appearance of painful conditions of the ankle. *Radiographics* 1991;11:401.

Klein MA, Spreitzer AM: MR imaging of the tarsal sinus and canal: Normal anatomy, pathologic findings, and features of the sinus tarsi syndrome. *Radiology* 1993;186:233.

Kornick J, Trefelner E, McCarthy S, et al: Meniscal abnormalities in the asymptomatic population at MR imaging. *Radiology* 1990;177:463.

Metz VM, Schratter M, Dock WI, et al: Age-associated changes of the triangular fibrocartilage of the wrist: Evaluation of the diagnostic performance of MR imaging. *Radiology* 1992;184:217.

Mink JH, Deutsch AL: Occult cartilage and bone injuries of the knee: Detection, classification, and assessment with MR imaging. *Radiology* 1989;170:823.

Morrison WB, Schweitzer ME, Bock GW, et al: Diagnosis of osteomyelitis: Utility of fat-suppressed contrast-enhanced MR imaging. *Radiology* 1993;189:251.

Palmer WE, Brown JH, Rosenthal DI: Labral-ligamentous complex of the shoulder: Evaluation with MR arthography. *Radiology* 1994;190:645.

Recht MP, Kramer J, Marcelis S, et al: Abnormalities of articular cartilage in the knee: Analysis of available MR techniques. *Radiology.* 1993;187:473.

Ruwe PA, Wright J. Randall RL, et al: Can MR imaging effectively replace diagnostic arthroscopy? *Radiology* 1992;183:335.

Smith DK, Snearly WN: Lunotriquetral interosseous ligament of the wrist: MR appearances in asymptomatic volunteers and arthrographically normal wrists. *Radiology* 1994;191:199.

Stoller DW, Martin C, Crues JV 3d, et al: Meniscal tears: Pathologic correlation with MR imaging. *Radiology* 1987; 163:731.

Chapter 33

ULTRASONOGRAPHY

Stephane Grijseels and Javier Beltran

Ultrasonography has been extensively used in the musculoskeletal system to diagnose pathologic conditions that are located superficially enough to be detected by the transducer. The technique is very operator dependent, perhaps more than any other imaging modality. The images obtained do not display the anatomic detail identified with other techniques requiring more time to get familiar with this imaging modality. Technical considerations are also important, because it is necessary to operate with high-resolution transducers to obtain images with sufficient diagnostic information. Despite its disadvantages, ultrasonography has its obvious advantages. In most facilities, it is a readily available technique, enabling a fast diagnosis. It is less expensive than most other imaging modalities (with the exception of plain films), does not involve ionizing radiation, and is noninvasive. It allows real-time imaging, a feature that is very useful for some conditions, such as snapping tendon syndrome or developmental dysplastic hip, where dynamic imaging provides additional information. With real-time imaging, anatomic structures are visualized on the monitor as they move, because the reconstruction of each image frame is instantaneous.

The following discussion includes the basic physical principles of ultrasonography and its most frequent clinical applications, including imaging joints, muscle, tendons, subcutaneous soft tissues, foreign bodies, and the performance of ultrasonographically guided procedures.

TECHNIQUE

A diagnostic ultrasound system is composed of a set of transducers, a power system, and computer unit with a display screen. The transducer, which is the device that sends and receives the ultrasound waves, is composed of an array of quartz crystals that generate these waves. Each transducer is designed to operate at a specific frequency, in the range of 2 to 12 MHz.

As ultrasound waves are transmitted through the body, they are reflected at tissue interfaces. The reflectivity of the wave is influenced by two factors: the *acoustic impedance* of the two tissues composing the interface and the *angle of incidence* of the sound beam. Acoustic impedance is the product of the density of the material and the speed of sound transmission within that substance. The reflectivity is greatest at the interfaces between tissues of dissimilar acoustic impedance. When the angle of incidence of the sound beam is 90 degrees or perpendicular to the tissue interface, the reflectivity is highest and decreases with decreasing angle. At highly reflective interfaces, almost all of the energy of the sound beam is reflected, producing a sound void area beneath the interface. This occurs between soft tissues and air or calcium. The sound beam appears enhanced when it passes through tissues such as water or other fluids that do not absorb ultrasound, therefore showing as sound void areas.

Occasionally, one can observe an artifact called *comet tail* because of its characteristic bands of increased echogenicity deep to the object. This phenomenon is observed within metal or glass objects, and is an artifact that can be used to help localize a foriegn body. Another artifact occurs when the sound beam hits objects not perpendicular; the sound is bent, resulting in an image that depicts structures as less echogenic than they actually are. To prevent this distortion artifact, the sound should be directed perpendicular to the tissues under examination. Another artifact, called *reverberation,* occurs at highly reflective interfaces. The beam is reflected back and forth within the body, resulting in phantom structures. This occurs more frequently in the pelvis and around the diaphragm.

CLINICAL APPLICATIONS

THE SHOULDER

Although preliminary results of ultrasonography of the shoulder region were disappointing, recent technological developments (high-resolution software and high-frequency transducers) have produced impressive results comparable to those of magnetic resonance imaging (MRI) for the diagnosis of rotator cuff tears. The sensitivity and specificity of ultrasonography have been reported in the range of 97 to 100 percent, respectively, for full-thickness tears, and 94 and 94 percent, respectively, for partial tears. Depending on the orientation of the transducer, the rotator cuff tendons demonstrate some degree of *echogenicity,* which can be defined as the amount of echosignal generated by a tissue. Tears, on the other hand, show different degrees of echogenicity. One of the advantages of ultrasonography is its capability of identifying small amounts of fluid, enabling the diagnosis of small rotator cuff tears, biceps tendon tears, joint effusion, and synovitis. Biceps tendon subluxation or dislocation can also be diagnosed with ultrasonography, using its real-time features.

The disadvantages of ultrasonography of the shoulder include the difficulty of assessing tissues located beneath the acromion, as well as deeply located structures such as the labrum and articular cartilage.

The proper role of ultrasonography in the shoulder is actually difficult to assess due to its significant dependence on operator expertise. In some institutions ultrasonography is being used only to screen patients for massive rotator cuff tears, whereas in other hospitals its use has been expanded to such a degree that MRI is reserved for special circumstances.

THE ELBOW

As in other joints, the evaluation of superficially located soft tissue lesions is a common indication for ultrasonography. Tendinitis involving

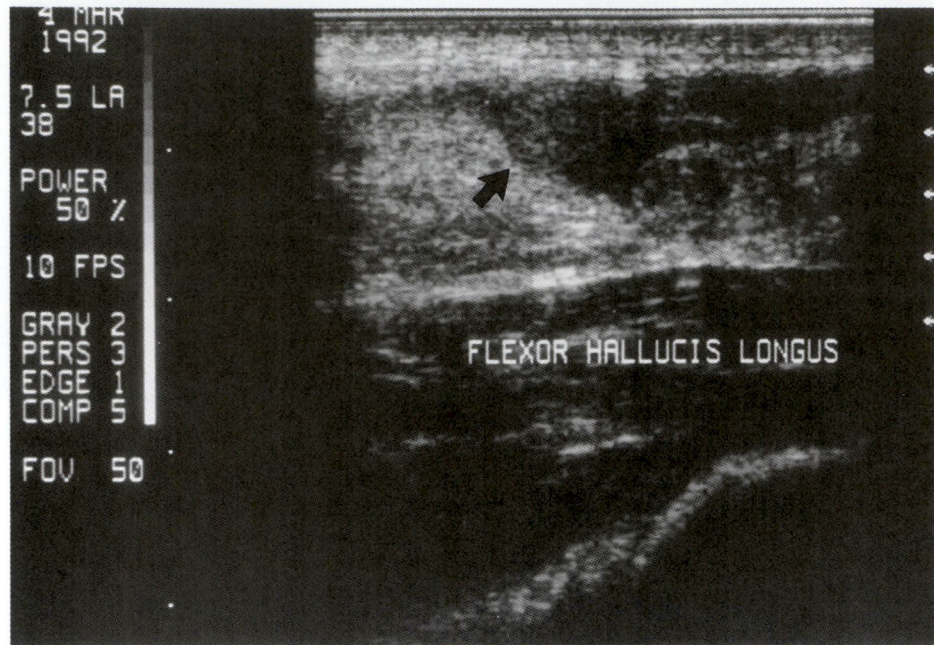

4 MAR
1992

7.5 LA
38

POWER
50 %

10 FPS

GRAY 2
PERS 3
EDGE 1
COMP 5

FOV 50

FLEXOR HALLUCIS LONGUS

Figure 33-1
Achilles tendon rupture: longitudinal ultrasound study. Note the interruption of the Achilles tendon (*arrow*) and the presence of hypoechoic area representing the hematoma.

the extensor tendons (lateral epicondylitis) appears as a hypoechoic area. It is important to compare the involved side with the uninvolved side in the same location and transducer position. Other indications for ultrasonography of the elbow include avulsion of the ossification centers in the immature skeleton, tears of the ulnar collateral ligament, joint effusion, loose bodies, and tendon tears (biceps and triceps).

THE HAND AND WRIST

The suspected presence of tendinitis and tenosynovitis in patients with carpal tunnel syndrome is a common indication for ultrasonography of the hand and wrist. Scar tissue and thickening of the flexor retinaculum in cases of recurrent carpal tunnel syndrome can also be assessed with ultrasonography. Other indications include tendon tears, soft tissue masses such as ganglion cysts and tumors, and synovial proliferation in inflammatory arthritis.

THE HIP

Utrasonography plays a major role in the evaluation of infants suspected of having developmental dysplastic hip. With this modality, it is possible to determine not only the presence of dislocation or subluxation of the nonossified femoral head, but also the degree of acetabular dysplasia, femoral head coverage, and morphology of the adjacent soft tissues, such as the labrum, ligamentium teres, psoas tendon, and pulvinar.

Joint effusion, bursitis, loose bodies, and the so-called snapping psoas tendon syndrome are other potential indications for ultrasonography of the hip. The use of real-time imaging enables dynamic evaluation of the hip joint in developmental dysplastic hip as well as in the snapping tendon syndrome. Ultrasound-guided aspiration of the hip joint may be indicated in cases of suspected hip infection, soft tissue abscess, and bursitis.

THE KNEE

Indications for ultrasonography of the knee include evaluation of fluid collections (e.g., a joint effusion, prepatellar and infrapatellar bursi-

tis, popliteal cyst, and popliteal artery aneurysm) and detection of tendon and ligamentous pathology (e.g., patellar tendinitis, quadriceps tendon ruptures, and collateral ligament tears). Although some preliminary work has been performed in ultrasound evaluation of anterior cruciate ligament and meniscal tears, its role for this type of pathology has not yet been defined.

THE ANKLE AND FOOT

Tendinitis, tenosynovitis, tendon rupture (partial or complete), and ligament rupture are among the most common indications for ultrasonography of the ankle and foot. Typically, Achilles tendon pathology, including tears and inflammation, has been studied with ultrasonography with a reported high accuracy rate (Fig. 33-1). Joint effusion and other fluid collections can also be easily evaluated with this technique.

MUSCLE PATHOLOGY

Muscle tears can be identified with ultrasonography, and their healing assessed with follow-up examinations. This technique may be helpful to determine the timing of rehabilitation and to prevent scar formation in athletes. The more common site of application of ultrasound to assess muscle injuries is in the region of the thigh, where tears of the rectus femoris muscle often occur.

MISCELLANEOUS INDICATIONS

Ultrasonography has been used extensively for guiding needle aspiration of solid masses or fluid collections located in the superficial soft tissues. Real-time imaging allows continued monitoring of the needle position to the desired depth. Foreign body localization is another practical indication for ultrasound. Although metallic and glass fragments are easily seen on plain radiographs, wood splinters are more difficult to visualize. Ultrasonography has been found to be accurate for precise detection of most types of foreign bodies, as long as they are within reach of the transducer.

SUGGESTED READINGS

Burk DL Jr, Karasick D, Kurtz AB, et al: Rotator cuff tears: Prospective comparison of MR imaging with arthrography, sonography, and surgery. *Am J Roentgenol* 1989; 153:87.

Charboneau JW, Reading CC, Welch TJ: CT and sonographically guided needle biopsy: Current techniques and new innovations. *Am J Roentgenol* 1990; 154:1.

Downey DJ, Simkin PA, Mack LA, et al: Tibialis posterior tendon rupture: A cause of rheumatoid flat foot. *Arthritis Rheum* 1988; 31:441.

Gevers G, Dequeker J, van Holsbeeck M, et al: A high dose (up to 200 mg) tolerance and efficacy study of intra-articular rimexolone (Org 6216) in rheumatoid synovitis of the knee. *Clin Rheumatol* 1994; 13:103.

Koski JM, Anttila PJ, Isomaki HA: Ultrasonography of the adult hip joint. *Scand J Rheumatol* 1989; 18:113.

Koski JM: Ultrasonographic evidence of hip synovitis in patients with rheumatoid arthritis. *Scand J Rheumatol* 1989; 18:127.

Koski JM: Ultrasonography in detection of effusion in the radiocarpal and midcarpal joints. *Scand J Rheumatol* 1992; 21:79.

Marcelis S, Daenen B, Ferrara MA, et al: *Peripheral Musculoskeletal Ultrasound Atlas.* Stuttgart, New York: Georg Thieme Verlag, 1996.

Middleton WD, Edelstein G, Reinus WR, et al: Sonographic detection of rotator cuff tears. *Am J Roentgenol* 1985; 144:349.

Miller CL, Karasick D, Kurtz AB, et al: Limited sensitivity of ultrasound for the detection of rotator cuff tears. *Skeletal Radiol* 1989; 18:179.

Terjesen T: Ultrasonography for diagnosis of slipped capita femoral epiphysis. *Acta Orthop Scand* 1992; 63:653.

Tikkakoski T, Paivansalo M, Siniluoto T, et al: Percutaneous ultrasound-guided biopsy: Fine needle biopsy, cutting needle biopsy, or both? *Acta Radiol* 1993; 34:30.

Van Holsbeeck MT, Eyler WR, Sherman LS, et al: Detection of infection in loosened hip prosthesis: Efficacy of sonography. *Am J Roentgenol* 1994; 163:381.

Van Holsbeeck MT, Introcaso JH: *Musculoskeletal Ultrasound.* St. Louis, CV Mosby, 1991.

Wiener SN, Seitz WH: Sonography of the shoulder in patients with tears of the rotator cuff: Accuracy and value for selecting surgical options. *Am J Roentgenol* 1993; 160:103.

Chapter 34

MUSCULOSKELETAL SCINTIGRAPHY

Jo Ellen Finkel

RADIOPHARMACEUTICALS

BONE AGENTS

Technetium-labeled diphosphonate derivatives including methylene diphosphonate (MDP) and methylene hydroxydiphosphonate (HDP) are currently the bone agents of choice. Both agents have rapid blood clearance. Approximately 50 percent of the radionuclide is cleared by the kidneys and excreted in the urine.

Physiologic determinants of uptake of these agents are: (1) metabolic activity: bony turnover is the most important determinant of uptake of radiopharmaceuticals (this accounts for increased uptake seen at growth plates and osteoblastic lesions); (2) blood flow: flow must be present for delivery of radiopharmaceutical, if not, there will be a cold defect; (3) sympathetic tone: loss of sympathetic tone causes local increased blood flow which results in increased tracer accumulation.

BONE MARROW AGENTS

^{99m}Tc sulfur colloid is used to image the bone marrow. It may be used to diagnose osteonecrosis and is also useful to demonstrate altered bone marrow or replacement of bone marrow by infection when combined with an indium 111–labeled WBC study.

INFLAMMATION AND INFECTION AGENTS

A. Indium 111–labeled leukocyte scan. The patient's WBCs are separated out and labeled in vitro with indium-111 oxine. A dose of 500 mCi(18.5 Mbq) of the indium 111–labeled leukocytes is injected intravenously. Images are obtained 18 to 24 h later.
B. Gallium-67 Citrate scan. A dose of 5 to 10 mCi(185 to 370 Mbq) of gallium-67 citrate is injected intravenously, and images of specified areas of interest or the whole body are obtained at 24 to 72 h. Bowel cleansing and additional 96h delayed scintiphotos may be needed to evaluate abdominal activity.
C. Technetium-99m hexamethylpropylene amine oxime (HMPAO) labeled leukocytes have been studied as an alternative for indium-labeled leukocytes. Images are obtained at 4 h postinjection. Initial studies have yielded results similar to indium-111 oxine in patients with chronic osteomyelitis and orthopaedic implants.
D. Newer agents are being studied which avoid handling of blood and blood products. These agents include: human polyclonal (nonspecific) immunoglobulin G (IgG) (labeled to indium-111 or technetium-99m) and technetium 99m–labeled monoclonal antigranulocyte antibody.

TECHNIQUES

BONE SCAN

Patient preparation is not required other than good hydration. The adult patient is injected with 15-20 mCi(555-740 Mbq) of technetium-labeled diphosphonate intravenously, and imaging is performed with a gamma camera 2 to 4 h later. Whole body or spot views, patient positioning, and the number of views employed depend on the indication for the examination.

THREE-PHASE BONE SCAN

The three-phase bone scan consists of the following image phases:

1. Flow study. The injection is the same as for a routine bone scan, but imaging is begun immediately after the injection. Sequential images are obtained every 2 to 3 s for 60 s.
2. Blood pool. Immediately following the flow study, a blood pool image is obtained over the area of interest. This image serves as a marker of extravascular tissue activity.
3. Delayed static images. After a minimum of 2 h, images are obtained over the area of interest. These images demonstrate radioisotope uptake in the osseous structures. The four-phase bone scan involves acquisition of a 24-h delayed image. Selected clinical applications of the three-phase bone scan include: evaluation of stress fractures, differentiation between osteomyelitis and cellulitis, and evaluation of reflex sympathetic dystrophy syndrome. In patients with diabetes mellitus and/or peripheral vascular disease and suspected osteomyelitis, the overall accuracy is improved by the addition of a 24-h image. The scan is positive for osteomyelitis if images show progressively increasing lesion to background activity ratios over time.

PINHOLE COLLIMATED IMAGING

Pinhole collimated images are useful in pediatric patients and to magnify small structures.

SPECT SCAN

Single photon emission computed tomography (SPECT) scanning improves both detection and localization of the scintigraphic abnormality by permitting spatial separation of bony structures that overlap on standard planar images. After acquisition of the study, the computer is used to reconstruct images in the axial, sagittal and coronal planes. The SPECT study requires extra time to image and process.

To date, bone SPECT has been found to be of particular clinical value in studies of the vertebral column. In patients with chronic low back pain, SPECT scintigraphy has been shown to be more sensitive than plain film radiology, with the majority of SPECT lesions corresponding to identifiable disease on CT. Only one-third of the SPECT abnormalities are visible on planar images. SPECT scanning enables abnormalities to be localized to the vertebral body or to the posterior elements. This is useful in the evaluation of facet syndrome. Not only is it a sensitive technique, but it can help predict which patients are more likely to benefit from local facet joint injections.

SPECT scanning is a highly sensitive means of detecting spondylolysis, a fracture of the pars interarticularis. It is also useful in various clinical settings. If there is low back pain and the radiographs are normal, then the bone scan with a SPECT study can be performed to evaluate for a possible occult pars injury which is not yet evident radiographically. If on the other hand, the spondylolysis is noted on radiographs, in a patient with low back pain, an abnormal bone scan indicates a metabolically active or acute stress injury of the pars (Fig. 34-1). A normal bone scan in this setting, indicates that the injury is old and has healed by fibrous union, and the defect is not the cause of the low back pain.

SPECT scanning is useful to evaluate symptomatic patients following spinal fusion. It is more sensitive than planar imaging and radiography in detecting pseudarthrosis. Another clinical use of SPECT is the diagnosis of avascular necrosis of the hips. A comparison study of planar and SPECT imaging found that planar had a sensitivity of 55 percent, compared to 85 percent for SPECT.

CLINICAL APPLICATIONS

NEOPLASM

Metastatic Disease

The bone scan is significantly more sensitive than radiographs for the detection of metastases. Of patients with positive bone scans, 30 to 50 percent will have negative radiographs. Tumors most likely to metastasize to bone include: breast, lung, prostate, lymphoma, thyroid, renal, and neuroblastoma. The most common pattern of metastatic disease is multiple asymmetric areas of increased uptake predominantly involving the axial skeleton. In a patient known to have a primary malignancy, the likelihood that a solitary abnormality on a bone scan represents metastatic disease varies depending on the location. Only 10 percent of solitary rib lesions are due to metastatic disease, whereas 60 to 70 percent of axial and 40 to 50 percent of appendicular lesions are due to metastatic disease.

Two other patterns may be seen in metastatic disease. One is the super-scan in which there is uniformly increased activity throughout the skeleton. This is associated with almost total absence of soft tissue activity. This pattern is most commonly caused by metastatic prostate cancer. Other tumor metastases which may cause this appearance are: breast, lung, bladder, and lymphoma. Non-tumor causes of a super-scan include: hyperparathyroidism, osteomalacia, Paget's disease, and fibrous dysplasia. The other pattern is the flare phenomenon which occurs when there is worsening of the bone scan, as noted by an increasing intensity of lesions or even new lesions, despite clinical response to new treatment. A repeat bone scan will show improvement after 4 to 6 months.

Approximately 5 percent of patients with metastatic diagnosis will have negative bone scans and positive radiographs. Tumors which may cause false negative bone scans include: multiple myeloma, thyroid cancer, and some anaplastic tumors and purely lytic lesions.

Benign Bone Tumors

Benign bone lesions that have mild to moderate uptake on bone scan include bone islands (greater in size than 3 cm or actively growing), nonossifying fibromas and fibrous cortical defects, bone cysts, enchondromas, and stable osteochondromas. Increased uptake of radioisotope is seen with giant cell tumors, bone cysts with pathologic fracture, osteochondroma that is actively growing, fibrous dysplasia, and Paget's disease. Bone infarcts and eosinophilic granulomas show variable uptake.

The bone scan has excellent sensitivity for the diagnosis of osteoid osteoma. A negative scan virtually rules it out. A typical appearance on the third phase of the bone scan is the double density sign. The nidus appears as an intense focus of uptake within an area of less intense uptake representing reactive sclerosis. When the nidus is in an area that is difficult to identify surgically, intraoperative scanning with a gamma camera or Geiger counter can aid in localization.

INFECTION

Osteomyelitis

Sensitivity of the three-phase bone scan in the detection of osteomyelitis in adults has been reported as 90 to 100 percent and specificity as 73 to 89 percent. The sensitivity may be lower in the neonatal and elderly patient. The scan is usually positive within 24 h of symptoms whereas plain films may be normal for the first 10 to 14 days. The scintigraphic appearance of osteomyelitis is: (1) increased activity on the flow study, (2) increased activity in the area of interest on the blood pool phase, and (3) increased activity on the delayed images. The bone/soft tissue ratio at the site increases up to 24 h (four-phase bone scan), and the activity is usually more focal than in cellulitis.

Cold defects may be seen early in osteomyelitis. This can be attributed to (1) increased pressure reducing blood flow, (2) stripping of the periosteum by pus, or (3) interruption of blood supply by sludging and thrombosis.

The specificity of the three-phase bone scan decreases when osteomyelitis occurs as a complication of a disease process that causes increased bone turnover such as fracture, osteotomy, active arthritis,

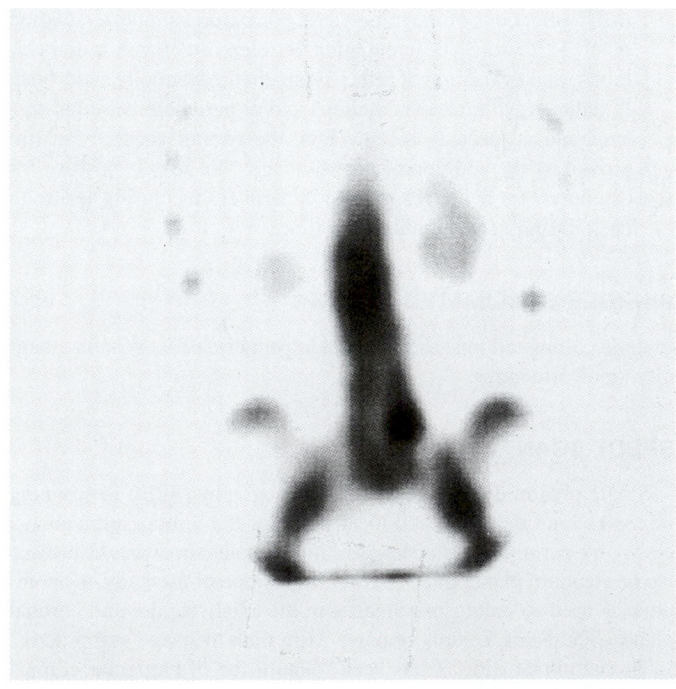

Figure 34-1
The coronal SPECT image shows a focal area of increased uptake in L5 on the left side representing a stress injury of the pars interarticularis.

or neuropathic changes. Each of these will also cause hyperemia on all three phases. In such cases or when the bone scan is negative yet a high clinical suspicion exists, gallium-67 citrate or indium-111 leukocyte imaging may be used as an adjunct to technetium imaging. There are advantages, limitations, and potential pitfalls of each. The diagnostic sensitivity is equally high for ^{67}Ga and ^{111}In WBCs, but ^{111}In WBC studies achieve higher specificity for a wide variety of clinical conditions, ranging from abscess to osteomyelitis to infected prosthesis. The summed results of numerous studies yield a mean sensitivity of 88 percent and a specificity of 85 percent for indium 111–labeled WBCs versus a sensitivity of 81 percent and a specificity of 69 percent for gallium. Several studies have suggested a higher accuracy of the gallium scan in detecting a response or lack of response of the infection to antibiotic treatment.

Gallium is an easier and less costly agent to use. It is the preferred isotope for imaging young children given the higher incidence of false negative bone scans, and that children are unlikely to have underlying bony abnormalities to complicate the interpretation. Gallium images are obtained at 24 and 48 h after injection of an adult dose of 5 mCi. Imaging is delayed to allow for clearance of high background activity. Proposed mechanisms for ^{67}Ga concentration at inflammatory sites include: hyperemia, increased capillary membrane permeability, protein binding mediated by iron-chelating siderophores, and direct leukocyte incorporation. For combined bone and gallium scans, several patterns have been described, but it is only the pattern in which the abnormal gallium uptake that exceeds the abnormal bone scan uptake that indicates active bone infection reliably.

In treated osteomyelitis, the bone scan remains hot during the healing phase. Gallium activity tends to fade with successful therapy. Because gallium is a weak bone agent, interpretation is difficult in patients who have had orthopaedic surgery. Labeled leukocytes, on the other hand, do not normally accumulate at these sites.

In-WBC labeling is a time consuming in vitro process. The adult dose should not exceed 0.5 mCi because of the relatively high absorbed dose to the spleen. The migration to and localization of the labeled cells in infectious foci depends on factors such as the site (it is less sensitive for vertebral osteomyelitis), duration of the infection, the host response, and possibly concomitant drug therapy. Imaging is routinely performed at 24 h following infusion of the labeled cells. Limitations for use include patients with leukopenia, impaired chemotaxis, or abnormal WBCs.

Cellulitis

The scintigraphic appearance of cellulitis on the bone scan is: (1) increased activity on the flow study, (2) increased activity or normal activity on the blood pool phase, and (3) mild, diffuse increased activity or normal activity on the static images. The bone/soft tissue ratio falls on delayed images. Gallium will localize in the soft tissues with cellulitis.

Septic Arthritis

The bone scan shows increased flow and blood pool activity around the joint. On the third phase, there is diffusely increased juxtaarticular uptake. Reflex sympathetic dystrophy will have a similar appearance. Gallium uptake is localized to the soft tissues of the joint more than the bones, and therefore may be helpful in differentiating osteomyelitis from septic arthritis.

PROSTHESIS EVALUATION

The normal bone scan will show no increased flow or blood pool activity. The appearance of a total hip arthroplasty (THA) on the delayed images depends on whether the prosthesis is cemented or noncemented. Increased activity in the greater trochanter is common with

a noncemented femoral component and persistent activity after 24 months may still be normal. Increasing uptake with time, however, is suspicious for infection. The presence of increased acetabular uptake in these patients is ubiquitous and has little significance. Any increase in uptake on serial scans is again suspicious for infection. Uptake at the distal tip segment is also common and its presence does not predict either loosening or infection. The trend for distal tip activity on serial scans is to remain stable or decrease. Lateral tip segment activity, although less common, demonstrates a similar overall trend on serial scanning. More prostheses, however, may show increased activity with time in this region, which does not necessarily imply an infection. Medial segment activity, on the other hand, is much less common and any increased uptake after the first few months postoperatively should be viewed with suspicion.

The uncomplicated cemented THA shows increased activity around the prosthesis for 9 to 12 months, which then tends to diminish, especially at the tip.

The bone scan findings are not specific enough to reliably make the distinction between loosening and infection. Classically, with loosening, the bone scan shows normal flow and blood pool images, with increased uptake around the prosthesis on the delayed images, usually at the tip. Infection will also show increased activity, which may be quite diffuse. The blood flow and blood pool images, however, show increased activity. The best combination of sensitivity and specificity for detecting an infected prosthesis is with indium 111–labeled WBCs (Fig. 34-2). Increased uptake at the tip of the femoral component on the Indium scan can be seen normally after surgery and will sometimes persist for years. The intensity, however, is low grade and decreases over time. Any increase or change in the distribution suggests infection. Indium activity may be diffusely increased in the femur distal to the tip. This represents marrow packing due to the surgery. A bone marrow scan using ^{99m}Tc sulfur colloid can differentiate compressed marrow from infection. No infection is present if the In–111 leukocyte study shows an uptake pattern identical to that seen on the marrow scan.

TRAUMA

Fractures

Traumatic fractures are almost always diagnosed by clinical examination and standard radiographs. There are instances in which the bone scan may be helpful. This is especially true with covert fractures in which the initial radiographs are negative or indeterminate. Two common examples are injuries of the scaphoid bone and nondisplaced fractures of the hip and pelvis. Since radiographic changes may not be seen for seven to ten days following the injury, the earlier diagnosis with bone scan is quite helpful. Scanning can be done even if the limb is in a cast.

Acute Fractures

In general, fracture sites tend to show increased accumulation of tracer within hours after injury. The minimum time for the bone scan to show positive findings after the fracture occurs appears to be age dependent. For patients under 65 years of age, 95 percent of fractures will be positive on bone scan by 24 h, and 100 percent will be positive by 3 days after the injury. For older patients, the respective percentages are 80 and 95 percent.

Three scintigraphic phases of fracture healing have been described. In the acute phase, lasting three to four weeks, all three phases of the bone scan are positive. On the delayed images, the fracture site shows intense activity, the margins of which often appear blurred. In the subacute phase, which occurs for the next 8 to 12 weeks, the angiographic phase becomes normal, and the activity on the delayed images, al-

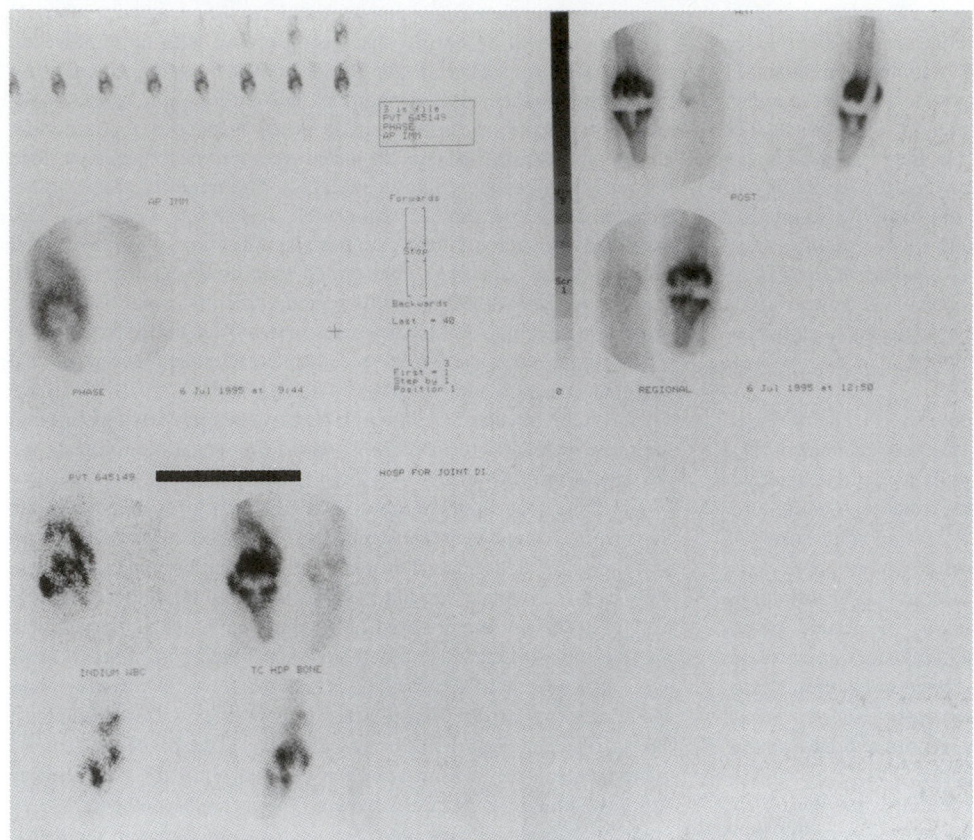

Figure 34-2
Infected right total knee arthroplasty. There is intense arterial phase hyperemia (*upper left*) and abnormally increased blood pool activity in this patient who is status post right TKA. Delayed static images demonstrate abnormal activity adjacent to the arthroplasty (*upper right*). The combined Indium–111 WBC images and 24-h delayed ^{99m}Tc bone scan images (*lower left*) show diffuse abnormal WBC localization consistent with an infected prosthesis.

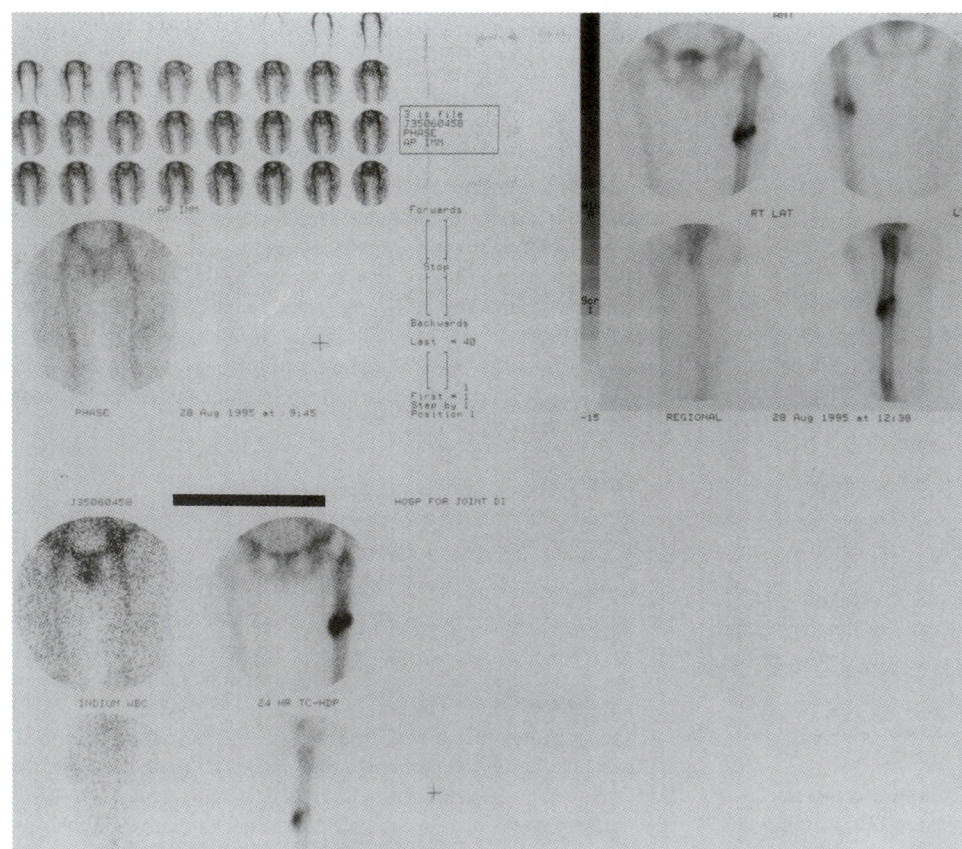

Figure 34-3
Left femoral fracture non-union. The three-phase bone scan demonstrates normal flow, minimally increased activity on the blood pool image (*upper left*) and intense uptake at the fracture site on the delayed images (*upper right*). The combined ^{111}In WBC and the ^{99m}Tc bone scan (*lower left*), shows no abnormal WBC localization, indicating that this is an aseptic nonunion.

though still very intense becomes more focal. The blood pool image will stay positive for 6 to 8 weeks. In the chronic stage corresponding to the end stages of healing and remodeling, the angiographic and blood pool activity returns to normal. The amount of tracer uptake on the third phase of the bone scan gradually diminishes and reaches normal levels after a variable period. In weightbearing bones, mechanical stresses can maintain slightly increased levels of tracer uptake at fracture sites for many years, particularly if the bone fragments were malaligned. Comminuted fractures, fractures that are openly reduced, and fractures requiring internal fixation, usually remain positive for a considerably longer period. Also, as a general rule, bone scans return to normal in uncomplicated healed fractures earlier in younger patients than in older patients. By two years after injury, approximately 90 percent of fractures return to normal on bone scan and by three years, the percentage approaches 100 percent.

A bone scan is not useful in distinguishing delayed union from hypertrophic nonunion, because both demonstrate focal uptake at the fracture site (Fig. 34-3). Atrophic nonunion will demonstrate a focal defect at the site.

While a bone scan may be useful in suspected child abuse cases to detect fractures, there are some limitations: old, healed fractures will not be detected, it is difficult to diagnose metaphyseal corner fractures adjacent to the normally intense epiphyseal uptake, and skull fractures may be missed.

In an attempt to distinguish a fracture from metastatic disease in the patient with a known primary malignancy elsewhere, there are certain useful clues to look for, particularly with regard to rib lesions. Discrete focal lesions aligned longitudinally almost always represent fractures (Fig. 34-4). Linear or fusiform activity is highly suggestive of tumor or Paget's disease and randomly scattered multifocal lesions favor the diagnosis of neoplasm.

The three-phase bone scan is useful to predict successful clinical outcome in patients with vascularized fibular or iliac bone grafts. The presence of increased perfusion and blood pool activity at the graft site at 1 to 2 weeks post-surgery indicates graft viability.

Stress Injuries

Stress fractures occur in the normal bones of healthy individuals in response to the unaccustomed stress of repetitive activities. The chief value of scintigraphy is in early diagnosis, since radiographic changes

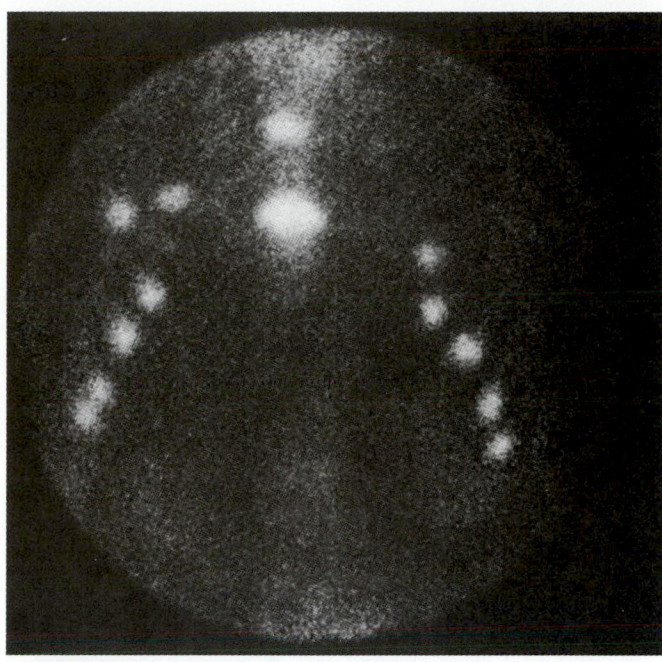

Figure 34-4
Rib fractures as a result of a motor vehicle accident. Note the linear arrangement of focal activity. These fractures were not seen on radiograph because they occurred at the costochondral junction. A fracture through the body of the sternum is also noted.

are often not apparent for 10 to 12 days after the injury is established. A stress fracture appears as a focal fusiform area of radionuclide activity on the delayed images. If a three-phase scan is performed, the radionuclide angiogram will show increased perfusion for three to four weeks after the onset of pain. Increased blood pool activity is noted for 6 to 8 weeks. The third phase of the bone scan, which remains positive during the entire healing process, may show increased activity for as many as 16 to 20 weeks or longer (Fig. 34-5).

Shin splints, also known as tibial stress syndrome, are another form of skeletal injury caused by stress. Plain films are negative, and as with stress fractures, bone scintigraphy is the diagnostic test of choice. The characteristic appearance is a linear area of increased activity

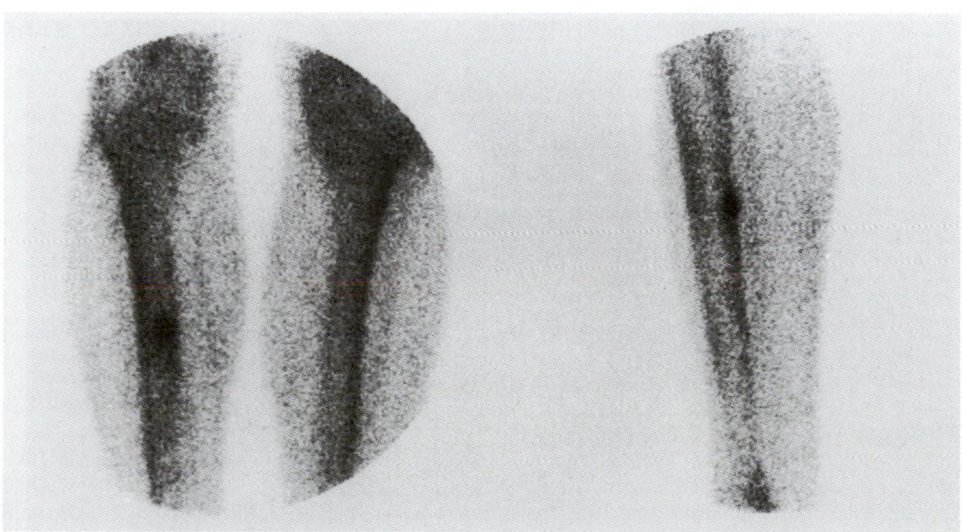

Figure 34-5
Stress fracture. The bone scan in this runner with leg pain and normal radiographs shows a focal area of increased uptake at the posteromedial cortex of the right tibia consistent with a stress fracture.

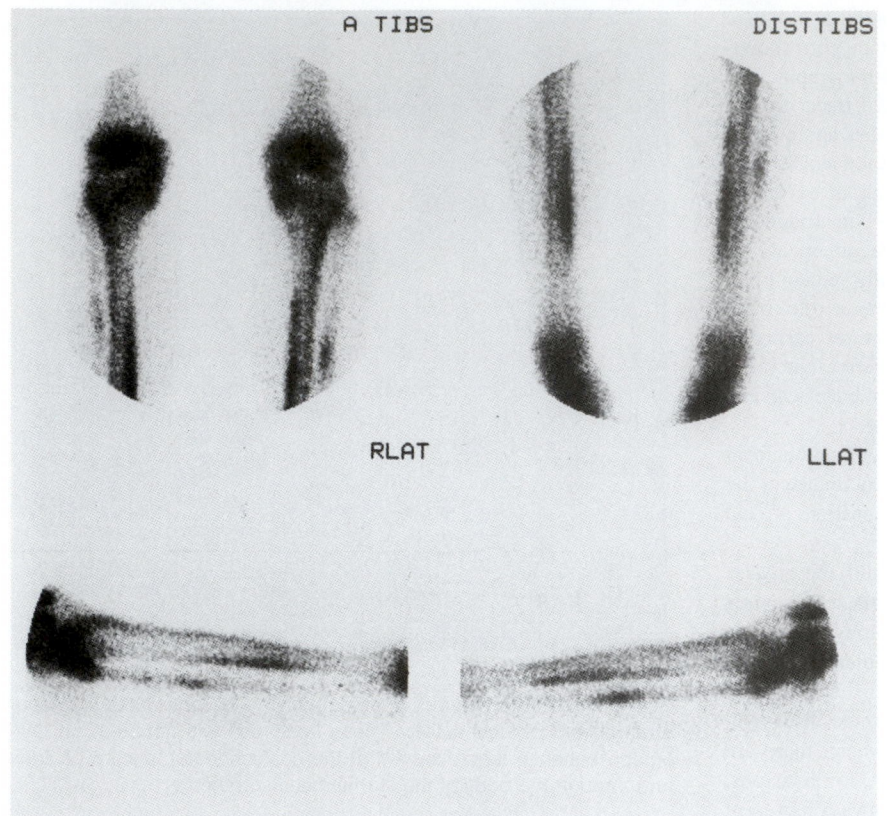

Figure 34-6
Typical appearance of bilateral tibial shin splints. AP and lateral views show linear activity along the posteromedial tibial cortices. The patient also has a nonspecific "stress reaction" of both fibulae.

present along the cortex (usually posterior) of the tibia. The abnormal activity is best visualized on the lateral view (Fig. 34-6). In contrast to the acute stress fracture, the arterial and blood pool phases are normal.

Insufficiency fractures result from normal or physiologic stress placed on bone with deficient elastic resistance. The common sacral insufficiency fracture in the elderly osteoporotic patient often has a characteristic H or butterfly appearance. The central area of uptake represents a horizontal sacral fracture. This is joined by adjacent vertically oriented uptake representing bilateral alar fractures (Fig. 34-7).

SUGGESTED READINGS

Abreu S, Van Nostrand D, Ziessman HA: *Selected Atlases of Bone Scintigraphy.* New York: Springer-Verlag; 1992.

Alazraki N: Radionuclide techniques. In Resnick D, Niwayama G (eds): *Diagnosis of Bone and Joint Disorders.* Philadelphia: WB Saunders; 1995:460.

Collier BD, Fogelman I, Rosenthall L: *Skeletal Nuclear Medicine.* St. Louis: Mosby-Year Book; 1996.

Datz FL: *Handbook of Nuclear Medicine.* St. Louis: Mosby-Year Book; 1993:61.

Finkel J: Scintigraphy of musculoskeletal trauma. In Taveras J, Ferrucci J (eds): *Radiology-Diagnosis-Imaging-Intervention.* Philadelphia: JB Lippincott; 1995:chap 109:1.

Fogelman I (ed): *Bone Scanning in Clinical Practice.* New York: Springer-Verlag; 1987.

Thrall JH, Ziessman HA: *Nuclear Medicine—The Requisites.* St. Louis: Mosby-Year Book; 1995.

Vande Streek PR, Caretta RF, Weiland FL: Nuclear medicine approaches to musculoskeletal disease. *Radiol Clin North Am* 1994; 32:227.

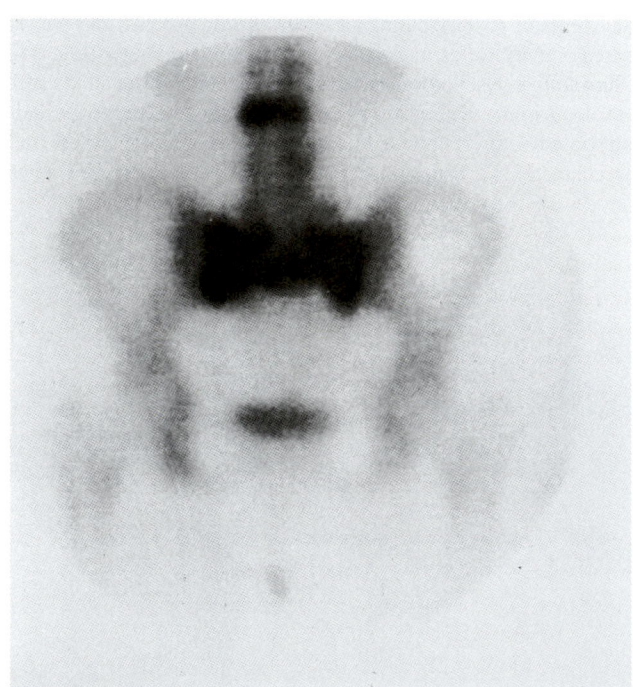

Figure 34-7
Sacral insufficiency fracture. There is a typical H-shaped appearance of radionuclide uptake in both sacral ala and the body of the sacrum characteristic of an insufficiency fracture. The patient also has a compression fracture of L2.

Chapter 35

GAIT ANALYSIS

Ann E. Barr

Clinical gait analysis encompasses techniques ranging from visual observation to measurement with highly technological instruments. This chapter will provide an overview of clinical gait analysis methods, definitions of the components of normal gait, and a discussion of illustrative pathologic gait patterns and the usefulness of gait analysis in directing and assessing their treatment.

TYPES OF GAIT ANALYSIS METHODS

The major strengths and limitations of the following six gait analysis methods are summarized in Table 35-1. *Observational gait analysis* consists of the observation of an individual's gait by the trained eye of a clinician and the notation and classification of certain over-

---

Table 35-1

Strengths and Limitations of Gait Analysis Methods

Gait Analysis Method	Strengths	Limitations
Observational Analysis	1. Widely available 2. Can be enhanced by simple video taping 3. Allows classification of gross gait patterns 4. Inexpensive	1. Subjective 2. Not able to measure more subtle phenomena
Stride Analysis	1. Provides quantitative information regarding time-distance parameters 2. Easy and fast 3. Low space requirements 4. Relatively inexpensive	1. Does not permit angular kinematic and kinetic analysis 2. Requires that patients have distinct swing phase in which floor contact is broken
Angular Kinematic Analysis	1. Permits precise measurement of joint angular excursions 2. Objective and quantitative	1. Requires technically trained personnel for measurement and interpretation of results 2. High space requirements 3. Limited portability 4. Costly
Force Plate and Pressure Plate Analyses	1. Permits precise measurement of external loads 2. Permits inverse dynamics analyses 3. Provides information regarding load patterns and distributions on stance limb	1. Limited usefulness in isolation 2. May require permanent installation in "gait lab" 3. Requires technically trained personnel for measurement and interpretation of results 4. Costly
Electromyographic Analysis	1. Provides measurement of motor performance and functional role of musculature 2. Enhances interpretation of kinematic and kinetic parameters	1. Requires technical expertise for measurement and interpretation 2. Subject to interference and artifact during sampling 3. Invasiveness of intramuscular technique poses risk to patients 4. Costly

all movement behaviors. *Stride analysis* involves the temporal quantification of stance and swing. *Joint angular kinematics* during gait are most frequently measured by electrogoniometry, accelerometry, or optoelectronic techniques. Electrogoniometers and accelerometers are attached directly to the body segments on either side of the joint or joints of interest. Optoelectronic techniques involve the use of video cameras to capture images of an individual walking followed by the digitization of pertinent anatomic landmarks in order to reconstruct time histories of segmental movement trajectories. *Force plates* measure the resultant ground reaction force and its point of application beneath the foot. *Pressure plates* or *insoles* additionally measure the load distribution beneath the foot. *Electromyography* (EMG) involves the recording of muscle activation and helps to explain the motor performance that underlies gait.

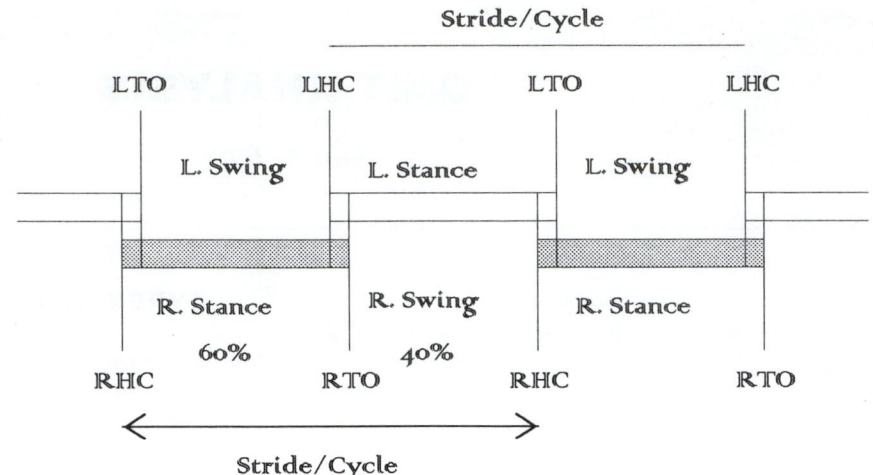

Figure 35-1
Schematic diagram of the temporal sequence of the gait cycle showing complete right (shaded bars) and left strides. HC, heel contact; TO, toe off; R, right; and L, left. The areas of overlap between HC and TO represent periods of double limb support, which coincide with the occurrence of preswing on the trailing limb and foot flat on the leading limb. In the case of the right stride, initial double limb support (lasting ~ 10 percent of the gait cycle) occurs from RHC to LTO, and terminal double limb support (lasting ~ 10 percent of the gait cycle) occurs from LHC to RTO.

THE COMPONENTS OF NORMAL GAIT

SIX DETERMINANTS OF GAIT

Saunders (1953) first proposed that excursions of the body's center of mass (COM) during gait could be minimized through the optimization of six determinants. *Pelvic rotation* reduces total hip flexion-extension and attenuates vertical oscillations of the COM. *Pelvic tilt* attenuates the vertical COM displacement and facilitates the hip abductor mechanism during single limb support. *Knee flexion* in stance phase smoothes directional changes in vertical displacements of the COM. The *ankle mechanism* lengthens the lower extremity at heel contact, owing to the posterior projection of the heel with respect to the ankle joint axis, then shortens the lower extremity through midstance, thereby mediating controlled downward vertical acceleration of the COM. The *foot mechanism* lengthens the lower extremity during terminal stance, owing to the anterior projection of the mid- and forefoot with respect to the ankle joint axis, thereby facilitating upward vertical acceleration of the COM. *Lateral displacement* of the COM is reduced through the narrowness of the base of support and slight valgus inclination at the knee joints.

THE GAIT CYCLE

Bipedal locomotion is cyclic and symmetrical and consists of stance and swing phases. A full *gait cycle* is defined by the occurrence of sequential stance and swing phases by one limb, or a *stride* (Figs. 35-1 and 35-2). *Stance phase* occupies 60 percent of the gait cycle and consists of two periods of *double limb support* (initial and terminal), when the contralateral foot is in contact with the ground, and an intermediate period of *single limb support,* when the contralateral limb is engaged in swing phase. Stance consists of six events or periods: *heel contact,* when the foot makes contact with the floor; *foot flat,* during which the sole of the foot comes into contact with the floor and which coincides with the end of initial dou-

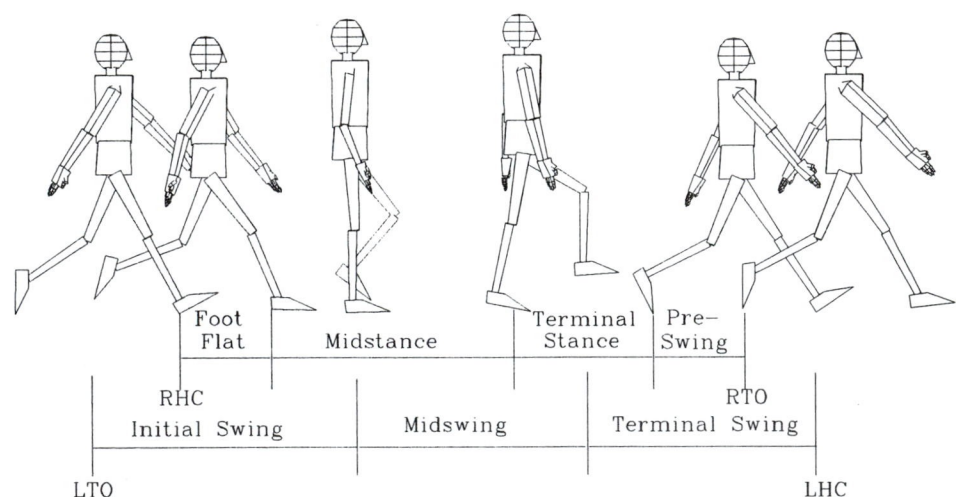

Figure 35-2
Schematic diagram of the spatial sequence of the gait cycle showing stance phase on the right and swing phase on the left. HC, heel contact; TO, toe off; R, right; and L, left. Stance phase is demarcated by two events, HC and TO, and broken into four periods, foot flat (from ~ 0 to 10 percent of gait cycle), midstance (from ~ 10 to 30 percent of gait cycle), terminal stance (from ~ 30 to 50 percent of gait cycle), and preswing (from ~ 50 to 60 percent of gait cycle). Swing phase is demarcated by two events, TO and HC, and broken into three periods, initial swing (from ~ 60 to 70 percent of gait cycle), midswing (from ~ 70 to 85 percent of gait cycle), and terminal swing (from ~ 85 to 100 percent of gait cycle).

ble limb support; *midstance,* during which the tibia rotates over the stationary foot and the beginning of which coincides with single limb support; *terminal stance,* during which the body weight is transferred from the hind and midfoot onto the forefoot and which coincides with the beginning of terminal double limb support; *preswing,* during which weight is transferred onto the contralateral limb and which coincides with terminal double limb support; and *toe off,* when the foot breaks contact with the floor. *Swing phase* occupies 40 percent of the gait cycle and consists of three periods: *initial swing,* which comprises about one-third of swing phase from toe-off until the swinging foot is opposite the stance foot; *midswing,* which ends when the tibia of the swinging limb is vertically oriented; and *terminal swing,* which ends at heel contact.

TIME-DISTANCE PARAMETERS

Time-distance parameters are derived from the temporal and spatial occurrence of stance and swing phases. Normal values of these quantities are provided in Table 35-2. *Stride,* which is synonymous with *gait cycle,* is defined as the occurrence of an event on one foot until the next occurrence of that same event on the same foot and is usually delineated by sequential ipsilateral heel contact. *Stride time* is the time it takes to perform a single stride. *Stride length* is the distance covered by a stride in the direction of locomotion. *Step* is defined as the occurrence of an event on one foot until the next occurrence of that same event on the opposite foot and is usually delineated by sequential contralateral heel contact. *Step length* is the distance covered by a step in the direction of locomotion. *Step width* is the distance covered by a step perpendicular to the direction of locomotion. Two sequential steps comprise a stride. *Cadence* is the number of steps taken per unit time. *Velocity* is the distance covered in the direction of locomotion per unit time.

Table 35-2

Ranges of Normal Values for Time-Distance Parameters of Adult Gait at Free Walking Velocity

Stride or cycle time	1.0 to 1.2 m/sec[a]
Stride or cycle length	1.2 to 1.9 m[b]
Step length	0.65 to 1.1 m[a]
Step width	7.7 to 9.6 cm[a]
Cadence	90 to 140 steps/minute[b]
Velocity	0.9 to 1.8 m/sec[b]

[a]Values adapted from multiple sources as summarized in Craik and Oatis, 1995.
[b]Values adapted from Whittle, 1991.

ANGULAR KINEMATIC PARAMETERS

Kinematics most frequently refers to the analysis of *joint angular displacements,* which are depicted in Fig. 35-3 for flexion-extension of the lower limb joints. *Ankle motion* is bimodal with peak stance phase dorsiflexion (i.e., flexion) occurring late in midstance and peak swing phase dorsiflexion occurring in terminal swing. *Knee motion* is bimodal with peak stance phase flexion occurring early in midstance, and peak swing phase flexion occurring at midswing. *Hip motion* is unimodal with peak flexion occurring during terminal swing. *Pelvic motion* reaches maximum anterior rotation of 5 degrees at heel

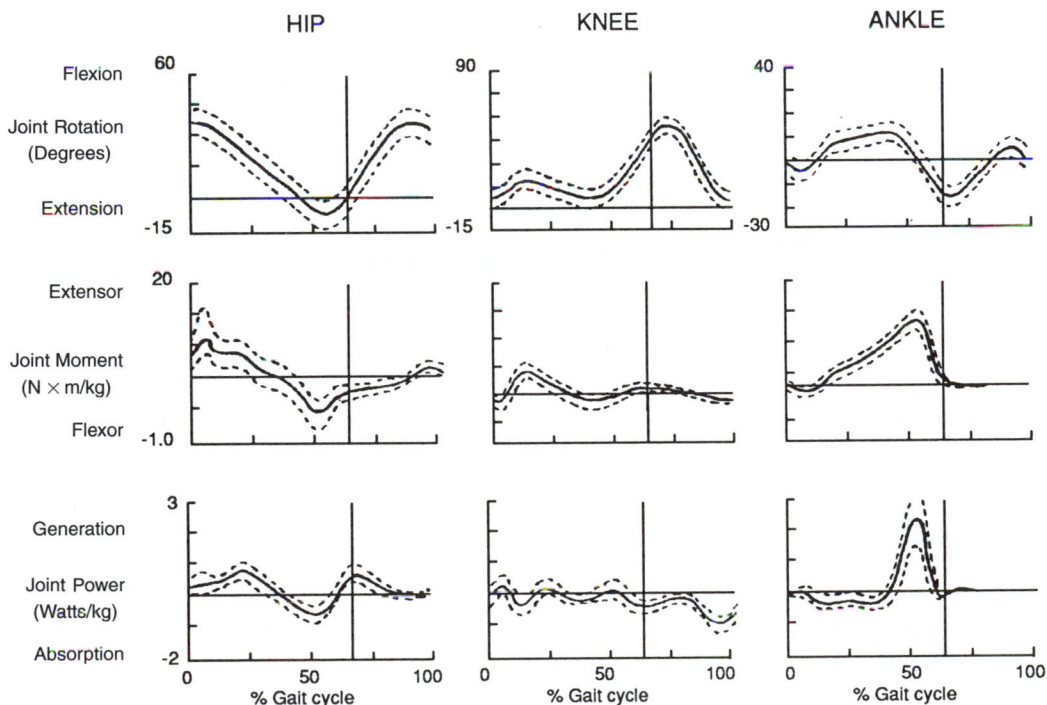

Figure 35-3
Graphic representation of the time histories of angular kinematics, internal joint moments, and joint powers about the sagittal plane (i.e., flexion-extension motion axes) of the hip, knee, and ankle joints during the normal gait cycle as determined by combined angular kinematic and force plate analyses. Vertical lines indicate stance (from 0 to 60 percent of the gait cycle) and swing (from 60 to 100 percent of the gait cycle) phases. (Reproduced with permission from Gage JR: *Gait Analysis in Cerebral Palsy.* London:Mac Keith Press; 1991:31.)

contact, maximum upward tilt of 5 degrees during foot flat, and a maximum anterior tilt of approximately 7 degrees during stance phase. *Trunk motion* during gait is opposite to the rotational and tilting motions of the pelvis. The body's *center of mass* is anterior to the sacrum throughout the gait cycle, and it undergoes sinusoidal displacements of approximately 3 cm vertically, 4 cm laterally, and 2 cm in the fore-aft direction.

LINK-SEGMENT KINETIC PARAMETERS

Joint moments and *joint power* are the most frequently reported *kinetic* parameters of gait.

A *moment* is defined as the cross-product of a force vector and the perpendicular distance from the joint center to the line of action of that force vector. Moments cause a tendency for joint rotation. In this discussion, the term moment refers to the *internal moment* generated about the joint in question. A *knee extensor moment,* for example, is the internal moment of force that tends to rotate the knee joint in the direction of extension and occurs when the line of action of the tibiofemoral reaction force vector passes posteriorly to the axis of knee flexion-extension (i.e., when the *external moment* tends to cause knee flexion). Activation by the knee extensors is required to counterbalance the tendency for knee flexion. Internal moments, assumed to result from the muscles, soft tissues, and contact forces acting on the joint, are an expression of the *net* effect of internal active and passive structures and are strictly accurate when a muscle group is unopposed by antagonist activation. The internal moments occurring about the lower extremity joints are depicted in Fig. 35-3.

Joint power is defined as the product of joint angular velocity and the internal moment at a given point in time. Joint power indicates the generation or absorption of mechanical energy by muscle groups. Profiles for normal joint power are depicted in Fig. 35-3. Positive joint power values indicate concentric, power generating muscle contractions, whereas negative joint power values indicate eccentric, power absorbing muscle contractions. For example, during preswing, a high magnitude power generation peak by the concentrically contracting plantarflexors represents about two-thirds of the total energy generated during walking and is believed to contribute significantly to propulsion in gait. Alternatively, from heel contact to foot flat, power absorption by the eccentrically contracting quadriceps controls knee flexion as weight is accepted by the stance limb.

MUSCULAR ACTIVITY

Muscle activation patterns also are cyclic during gait (Fig. 35-4). Muscle contraction type varies between the eccentric control of joint angular accelerations, such as in hamstrings activation during terminal swing, and the concentric initiation of movement, such as in tibialis anterior activation in preswing. In normal individuals, agonist-antagonist coactivation is of relatively short duration and occurs during periods of kinematic transition.

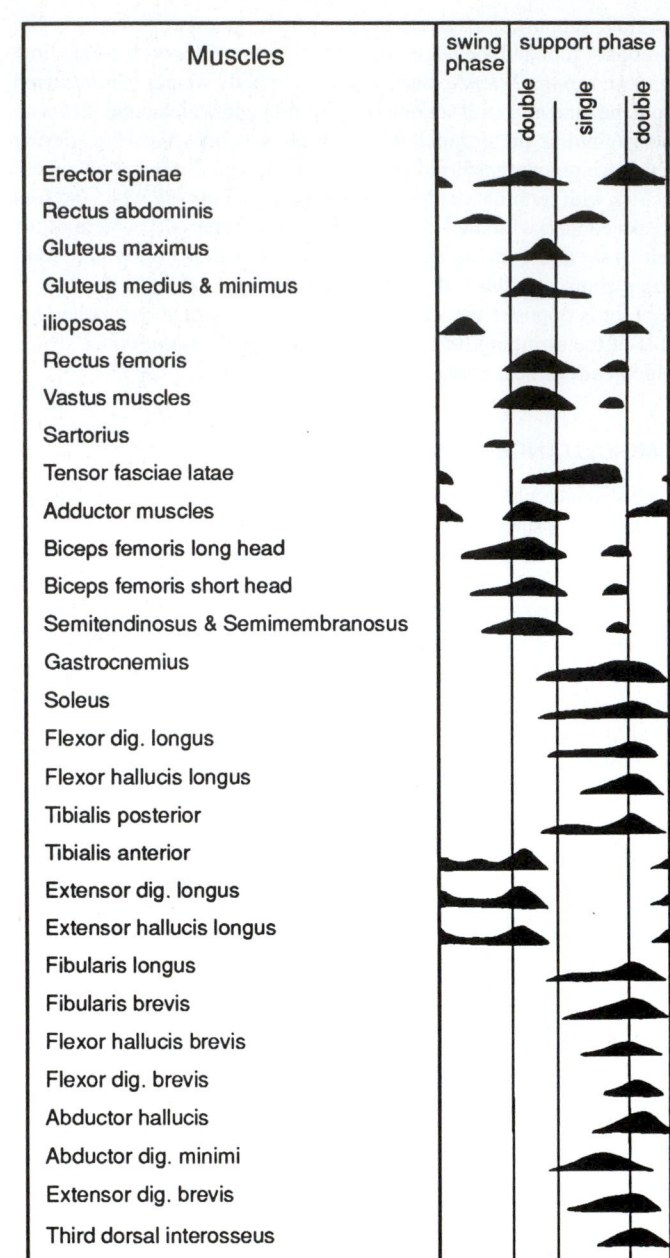

Figure 35-4

Schematic representation of muscle activation patterns during the normal gait cycle as determined by electromyographic analysis. Both onset and amplitude of activation are indicated. (Reproduced with permission from Carlsöö S: *How Man Moves: Kinesiological Studies and Methods.* London:Heinemann; 1972, p 117.)

CLINICAL APPLICATIONS OF GAIT ANALYSIS

Clinical gait analysis assesses the impact of clinical practice on an important functional activity. This section will highlight some of the disorders and conditions for which gait analysis has been particularly useful. Tables 35-3 to 35-5 summarize gait abnormalities associated with additional disorders.

ANTERIOR CRUCIATE LIGAMENT DEFICIENCY

Some individuals with anterior cruciate ligament (ACL) deficiency demonstrate a quadriceps avoidance gait pattern associated with reduction of the stance phase knee extensor moment by as much as 140 percent. This adaptation probably prevents unrestrained anterior translation of the tibia by the patellar tendon through reduction in quadriceps activation, and may prevent degenerative changes associated with chronic ACL deficiency.

Table 35-3

Gait Abnormalities in Arthritic Disease and Associated Conditions and Treatment Examples

	GAIT ABNORMALITIES				
Disorder	Observational	Time-Distance	Angular	Kinetic and EMG	Treatment
Osteoarthritis of the hip, unilateral involvement	Lateral lurch gait pattern	1. ↑ Stance time, uninvolved side 2. ↑ Double limb support 3. ↑ Step time, involved side 4. ↓ Step length, involved side 5. ↓ Velocity	↓ Hip flexion-extension excursion, involved side	↓ Hip abductor moment	1. Cane or crutches 2. THA
Rheumatoid arthritis with hindfoot pain and deformity	1. Antalgic gait pattern 2. Flat foot gait pattern	1. ↓ Velocity 2. ↓ Single limb support, involved side 3. ↓ Cadence 4. ↓ Stride length 5. Delayed heel rise	1. ↑ Knee flexion during stance 2. ↑ Dorsiflexion during stance 3. ↓ Plantarflexion during terminal stance 4. ↑ Subtalar eversion during terminal stance	↑ Tibialis anterior activation during terminal stance and preswing	1. Cane 2. Rigid AFO or hindfoot orthosis 3. Rocker bottom shoes 4. TAA
Total knee arthroplasty, unilateral		1. ↓ Single limb support, involved side 2. ↓ Stride length	↓ Knee flexion during stance	↓ Knee extensor moment	N/A

NOTE: THA, total hip arthroplasty; AFO, ankle foot orthosis; TAA, total ankle arthroplasty.

TOTAL JOINT ARTHROPLASTY

Gait analysis can be used to evaluate and improve surgical techniques and component design for lower extremity total joint arthroplasty (TJA). Table 35-3 summarizes gait abnormalities associated with total knee arthroplasty and of arthritic conditions for which TJA is frequently indicated.

During stair climbing, posterior cruciate ligament-retaining total knee arthroplasty designs are associated with normal angular kinematics. Total condylar and posterior stabilized total condylar designs (i.e., cruciate-sacrificing) are associated with decreased peak knee flexion and forward lean of the body, both of which contribute to a reduced knee extensor moment, and with increased EMG activity of the soleus during stair climbing, which indicates control of knee flexion through the restraint of forward tibial rotation. These compensations are probably in response to reduced femoral rollback with knee flexion, which would reduce the effective length of the knee extensor moment arm, thereby increasing the requirements for knee stabilization by the quadriceps.

Varus alignment of the femoral stem in cemented total hip arthroplasty (THA) is more geometrically similar to an intact femur, but it results in decreased hip flexion-extension motion, increased hip extensor moment during the first half of stance, decreased hip flexor moment during the latter half of stance, and decreased stride length. These compensations probably reduce symptoms associated with component instability and, ultimately, loosening. THA with valgus alignment, on the other hand, results in normal postoperative gait.

CEREBRAL PALSY

Five major parameters have been identified as crucial in restoring normal gait function in children with cerebral palsy (CP): (1) stance phase stability; (2) swing phase clearance; (3) foot preposition in terminal swing; (4) adequate step length; and (5) energy conservation. Gait analysis can help to identify the *primary* causes of these gait disturbances.

Rectus femoris transfer, usually performed in combination with hamstring lengthening, is indicated for "stiff-knee" or "crouched" gait. If kinematic and EMG analysis show these gait abnormalities in conjunction with prolonged activation of the rectus femoris (RF) during swing plus normal stance phase activation of the other heads of

---

Table 35-4

Gait Abnormalities Associated with Muscle Weakness and Treatment Examples

	GAIT ABNORMALITIES				
Disorder	Observational	Time-Distance	Angular	Kinetic and EMG	Treatment
Dorsiflexor paresis or paralysis	1. Steppage gait pattern 2. Foot slap gait pattern	1. ↓ Time to foot flat 2. ↓ Step length, uninvolved side	1. Ankle plantarflexion during swing 2. ↑ Hip and knee flexion during swing	↓ Dorsiflexor moment	AFO
Hip abductor weakness	1. Trendelenberg gait pattern 2. Lateral lurch gait pattern	1. ↑ Double limb support 2. ↓ Step length, uninvolved side 3. ↓ Velocity	1. ↑ Hip adduction during midstance, with Trendelenberg 2. ↑ Lateral trunk tilt with lateral lurch 3. ↓ Pelvic tilt during swing, involved side, with Trendelenberg	↓ Hip abductor moment during stance with lateral lurch	1. Cane 2. Crutches
Plantarflexor paresis or paralysis	No pattern discernible	1. Prolonged midstance 2. ↓ Step length, uninvolved side 3. ↓ Single limb support, involved side	1. ↑ Stance phase knee flexion 2. ↑ Stance phase dorsiflexion	1. ↓ Plantarflexor power during late stance 2. Prolonged stance phase quadriceps activation	AFO

NOTE: AFO, ankle foot orthosis.

the quadriceps femoris, the RF can be transferred to act as a knee flexor during swing without compromising knee stability during stance, particularly if preoperative knee ROM during gait is less than 80 percent normal. *RF release* is more effective in alleviating "stiff-knee" gait when preoperative knee ROM during gait is greater then 80 percent normal. *Selective dorsal rhizotomy* (SDR) is indicated in individuals with significant spasticity in the presence of good or slightly impaired selective motor control. SDR results in improved hip, knee, and ankle flexion-extension; velocity and stride length; and phasic muscle activation patterns. A negative outcome of SDR is increased anterior pelvic tilt, which may be indicative of inadequate control of hip extension by the hamstrings. *Equinovarus deformity* in CP results in "toe-walking" during stance phase and "toe-dragging" during swing phase. Combined foot switch and EMG analysis permits the identification of the muscle(s) contributing to this abnormal foot posturing, thereby indicating the need for either an ankle foot orthosis (AFO) or tendon lengthening or transfer.

PAIN IN THE LOWER LIMB

Pain in the lower limb results in an *antalgic gait pattern,* which is detectable by observational gait analysis and is characterized by decreased single limb support time on the involved side, or a limp. Walking aides, such as a cane or crutches, usually correct this ab-

normality by enabling patients to share loading of the painful lower extremity with the upper extremity. A cane should be held in the hand *opposite* the painful limb to maximize the base of support and facilitate normal rotational excursions of the trunk and upper extremities.

VARUS GONARTHROSIS

Candidates for *high tibial osteotomy* to correct varus gonarthrosis, who demonstrate low abductor moments (i.e., less than 4 percent body weight × height) about the knee joint during stance phase, have been shown to have a better long-term surgical result, even when preoperative knee scores and varus deformities were indistinguishable from candidates with high preoperative knee abductor moments. The compensation used by the low abductor moment group is out-toeing with decreased stride length, which suggests that patients with high abductor moments might benefit from training in conjunction with corrective surgery.

MUSCLE WEAKNESS

Lower limb paresis or paralysis during gait leads to either insufficient control of accelerating body segments or inability to initiate and sustain properly timed movements. The resulting gait patterns are often detectable by observational gait analysis. Common gait patterns associated with weakness are shown in Table 35-4.

Table 35-5

Gait Abnormalities Associated with Neurologic Disorders and Treatment Examples

Disorder	GAIT ABNORMALITIES				Treatment
	Observational	Time-Distance	Angular	Kinetic and EMG	
Ataxia	"Ataxic" gait pattern	Variable stride to stride	Variable stride to stride	Variable stride to stride	1. Orthotic stabilization to control movement variability 2. Walking aids (e.g., crutches, walker)
Hemiplegia from stroke	1. "Stiff-legged" gait pattern 2. Equinus or equinovarus gait pattern 3. Circumduction	1. ↑ Double limb support 2. ↓ Step length, involved side 3. Delayed heel rise 4. ↓ Velocity 5. ↓ Stride length 6. ↓ Cadence 7. Absent heel contact 8. Toe-drag during swing	1. ↑ Plantarflexion during swing 2. ↓ Knee flexion during stance and swing	1. ↑ Knee flexor moment during stance 2. ↓ Amplitude of joint powers 3. Abnormal timing of muscle activation (i.e., mass synergy patterns)	1. AFO 2. Rectus femoris release 3. Tendo-achilles lengthening 4. Tendon transfer, foot and ankle 5. FES
Parkinson's disease	1. "Shuffling" gait pattern 2. "Frozen" gait pattern	1. ↓ Stride length 2. ↓ Step length 3. ↓ Step width 4. ↑ Cadence 5. ↓ Velocity	↓ Angular excursions throughout	Agonist-antagonist coactivation with "frozen" pattern	Pharmaceutical/medical management

NOTE: AFO, ankle foot orthosis; FES, functional electrical stimulation.

PROSTHETIC AND ORTHOTIC EVALUATION

Gait analysis can be used to evaluate how well prosthetic and orthotic designs achieve their intended purpose. For example, energy storing prosthetic feet have been shown to store and return mechanical energy with a higher efficiency than non-energy storing devices during level walking and running.

NEUROLOGIC DISORDERS

Functional ambulation in paraplegia is an important area of clinical research and there are several ambulation orthoses now available, including those employing functional electrical stimulation (FES). Gait analysis will continue to prove valuable in assessing these devices. Many neurologic disorders, both upper and lower motoneuron in origin, cause a variety of gait abnormalities ranging from weakness patterns to spasticity and other indicators of compromised motor control. In addition to examples already touched upon, gait abnormalities in other common neurologic disorders are summarized in Table 35-5.

SUMMARY

Clinical gait analysis continues to progress as sophisticated technology becomes more accessible, and as clinical researchers apply its methods to the investigation of ever-increasing numbers of pathologic conditions. The wealth of clinical and scientific gait analysis literature spanning the last several decades reflects these advances and, in many disease populations, the emergence of consensus regarding the interpretation of gait analysis results. The inclusion of quantitative detail contained in such a large volume of literature in these few paragraphs is not feasible. The intent here is to present the basic terminology and concepts underlying gait analysis with an emphasis on the clinical applicability of the information it provides. The disorders and conditions highlighted were chosen to illustrate the unique contributions clinical gait analysis can make to treatment planning and outcome assessment. As such, this introduction to gait analysis is a mere glimpse into the original works on which it is based.

SUGGESTED READINGS

Allard P, Stokes IAF, Blanchi J: *Three-Dimensional Analysis of Human Movement.* Champaign, IL: Human Kinetics; 1995.

Andriacchi TP: Dynamics of knee malalignment. *Orthop Clin North Am* 1994; 25:395.

Barr AE, Siegel KL, Danoff JV, et al: Biomechanical comparison of the energy-storing capabilities of SACH and Carbon Copy II prosthetic feet during stance phase of gait in a person with below-knee amputation. *Phys Ther* 1992; 72:344.

Colborne GR, Wright V, Naumann S: Feedback on triceps surae EMG in gait of children with cerebral palsy: A controlled study. *Arch Phys Med Rehabil* 1994; 75:40.

Craik RL, Oatis CA: Gait analysis, in: *Theory and Application.* St. Louis:Mosby-Yearbook, Inc; 1995.

Dorr LD, Ochsner JL, Gronley J, Perry J: Functional comparison of posterior cruciate-retained versus cruciate-sacrificed total knee arthroplasty. *Clin Orthop* 1988; 236:36.

Gage JR: *Gait Analysis in Cerebral Palsy.* London:Mac Keith Press; 1991.

Gundersen LA, Valle DR, Barr AE, et al: Bilateral analysis of the knee and ankle during gait: An examination of the relationship between lateral dominance and symmetry. *Phys Ther* 1990; 69:640.

Hodge WA, Andriacchi TP, Galante JO: A relationship between stem orientation and function following total hip arthroplasty. *J Arthroplasty* 1991; 6:229.

Hurwitz DE, Andriacchi TP, Guyton J, et al: How surgical approach influences walking and stair climbing in patients with cementless total hip re-placements. *Proc Am Soc Mech Eng (ASME) Biomech Symp (Applied Mech Div)* 1991; 120:313.

Lafortune MA, Cavanagh PR, Sommer HJ 3d, et al: Three-dimensional kinematics of the human knee during walking. *J Biomech* 1992; 25:347.

Lehmann JF: Push-off and propulsion of the body in normal and abnormal gait: Correction by ankle foot orthoses. *Clin Orthop* 1993; 288:97.

Malezic M, Hesse S, Schewe H, et al: Restoration of standing, weight-shift and gait by multichannel electrical stimulation in hemiparetic patients. *Int J Rehabil Res* 1994; 17:169.

Perry J: *Gait Analysis: Normal and Pathological Function.* Thorofare, NJ: SLACK; 1992.

Prodromos CC, Andriacchi TP, Galante JO: A relationship between gait and clinical changes following high tibial osteotomy. *J Bone Joint Surg [Am]* 1985; 67:1188.

Rose J, Gamble JG: *Human Walking,* 2d ed. Baltimore:Williams & Wilkins; 1994.

Saunders JBDM, Inman VT, Eberhart HD: The major determinants in normal and pathological gait. *J Bone Joint Surg [Am]* 1953; 35:543.

Sutherland DH, Olshen RA, Biden EN, et al: *The Development of Mature Walking.* London:Mac Keith Press; 1988.

Ueno E, Yanagisawa N, Takami M: Gait disorders in Parkinsonism: A study with floor reaction forces and EMG. *Adv Neurol* 1993; 60:414.

Winter DA: *Biomechanics and Motor Control of Human Gait: Normal, Elderly and Pathological.* Waterloo:University of Waterloo Press, 1991.

Chapter 36

BASIC ELECTROPHYSIOLOGY

John T. Hughes

Neurophysiologic techniques are powerful diagnostic tools employed to study the central and peripheral nervous system and neuromuscular functions. Nervous system disease and dysfunction are manifested by a relatively narrow clinical spectrum of symptoms and signs. Orthopedic injuries are frequently associated with neurologic complications involving the peripheral nervous system. The narrow clinical expression of peripheral nerve dysfunction may present as atrophy, muscle weakness, paresthesia, dysesthesia, sensory loss, and pain. The complexities of neurologic anatomy are responsible for the varied, although stereotypical, clinical presentations of peripheral nervous system dysfunction. Nerve conduction studies, electromyography, and somatosensory evoked potentials (SEPs) are sensitive modalities used to probe the effects of various diseases on the peripheral and central nervous system.

The initial clinical impression is based on the history and clinical examination. Electrodiagnostic testing is an objective method to assess for neurogenic lesions and is an extension of the physical examination. The clinical history and physical examination must be considered and relied upon when planning the electrodiagnostic evaluation. The information obtained from both the clinical and electrodiagnostic examinations serves as the basis for the diagnosis. The physical examination is often limited and sometimes misleading due to the uncertainties introduced by the presence of fractures, immobilization, fixation devices, pain, or disuse. Subjective complaints and uncertainties can largely be discerned by electrodiagnostic testing. The goal of electrodiagnostic testing is first to identify and ultimately localize the neurogenic lesion. This can be accomplished to a high degree of certainty and accuracy with currently available electrodiagnostic techniques.

MOTOR AND SENSORY CONDUCTION STUDIES

Electrical stimulation of nerves results in a compound muscle action potential (CMAP) and a sensory nerve action potential (SNAP) which can be recorded using surface electrodes. The transcutaneous measurement of evoked potential parameters such as *distal latency, amplitude of evoked responses,* and *conduction velocity* offers important information about peripheral nervous system integrity and the ability of motor and sensory nerves to conduct electrical impulses. Standardization of parameter measurements has made nerve conduction study (NCS) a reliable and reproducible method for neurogenic lesion localization. Demyelination and axonal loss are two major categories of peripheral nerve disorders. Based on conduction studies, characteristic abnormalities such as demyelination or axonal loss can be assessed.

Conduction velocity is a measure of the speed of impulse propagation over an axon and it is based on latency measurements along a nerve. *Latency* is measured using the onset of an evoked response

and therefore conduction velocity is a measure of the fastest and largest fiber conduction. *Amplitude of the evoked response* is a reflection of the number and synchrony of the conducting fibers in a peripheral nerve. Diminished amplitudes may be an indicator of axonal loss provided there is normal synchrony of axonal impulses. A 50 percent decrement in amplitude when comparing sides is considered clinically significant and usually indicates axonal loss (Fig. 36-1). *Temporal dispersion* of an evoked motor or sensory response is seen when there are large conduction velocity differences between the fastest and slowest fibers in a nerve. Temporal dispersion will alter the evoked potential response curve and will result in a diminished amplitude with a longer duration response. Although the evoked potential amplitude is decreased, the overall area of the response remains unchanged with temporal dispersion. This loss of amplitude of the evoked response seen in association with excessive temporal dispersion is not an indicator, therefore, of axonal loss. This is an indicator of abnormal conduction (myelin problem). A more accurate measurement of peripheral nerve axon density is the *response curve area* and not absolute amplitude. A significant drop in amplitude with proximal nerve stimulation, provided significant temporal dispersion

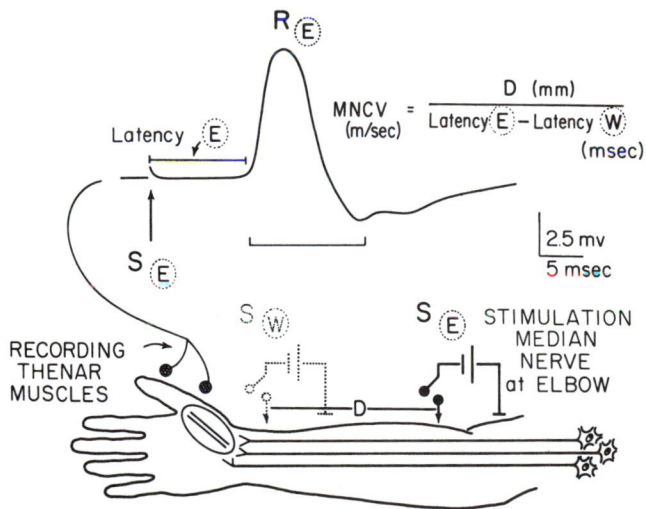

Figure 36-1
Compound muscle action potential recorded from the thenar eminence after stimulation of the median nerve at the elbow. The nerve conduction time from the elbow at the wrist equals the latency difference between the two responses elicited by the distal and proximal stimulation. The motor nerve conduction velocity (MNCV), calculated by dividing the surface distance between the stimulus points by the subtracted times, concerns the fastest fibers. (Reproduced by permission from Kimura J: Principles of nerve conduction studies. In *Electrodiagnosis in Diseases of Nerve and Muscle: Principles and Practice,* 2d ed. Philadelphia: FA Davis, 1989:84.)

is absent, would indicate the presence of a conduction block due to mechanical or immunological factors.

There are three degrees of nerve injury. *Neurapraxia* involves local myelin injury which manifests as conduction block. *Axonotmesis* is defined as axonal disruption with intact endoneurium. *Neurotmesis* is a severe injury with total disruption of axons and supporting connective tissue. In neurapraxia full recovery is usual and typically takes several days to weeks. The prognosis for regeneration in axonotmesis is usually good. Effective antegrade reinnervation occurs via intact endoneurial pathways provided the lesion in not too proximal. Recovery periods are variable and will be directly related to injury severity and the distance the regenerating nerve must travel. This time is usually measured in months. In neurotmesis, surgical anastomosis or autogenous nerve graft is necessary to effect recovery.

Conduction failure is seen with stimulation proximal to the lesion in all three forms of nerve injury. The degenerative changes seen in a nerve after a crush or section are commonly referred to as wallerian degeneration. The axons and myelin sheaths distal to the injury site will break down. Wallerian degeneration will occur in axonotmesis and neurotmesis and this typically occurs 4 to 6 days after nerve injury (Fig. 36-2). An evoked response is present with distal stimulation acutely in all three forms of injury. Once wallerian degeneration has occurred, intact distal conduction occurs only in neurapraxia due to continuity of axons at and beyond the lesion site. The clinical as well as electrophysiologic distinction between axonotmesis and neurotmesis is important and can be difficult. The presence of partial sensory or motor function or partial evoked response after nerve stimulation may serve to differentiate between them. SEPs may also be helpful. Complete absence of a SEP usually indicates neurotmesis, although this can not fully exclude axonotmesis with partial conduction block at the lesion site.

Standard nerve conduction techniques test the distal one-third of the peripheral nervous system (PNS) and provide little information regarding the more proximal nerve segment or root. F waves are motor responses elicited with supramaximal antidromic activation of motor fibers and subsequently anterior horn cells. This is an indirect probe of the more proximal parts of PNS. The F wave may be helpful in segmental localization but it is not useful in lesion localization along the reflex arc. The H reflex is a motor response produced by submaximal stimulation of the Ia afferent fibers of a monosynaptic reflex arc. The Ia afferent nerve fibers originate in muscle, enter the dorsal horn of the spinal cord, and synapse with the alpha motor neurons. Stimulation of the afferent arch results in anterior horn cell discharge and subsequent motor response. H reflexes are limited to the calf muscles and the flexor carpi radialis at rest. H-reflex latency is a measure of nerve conduction along the entire afferent and efferent arc. A delay or absence of the H reflex or F wave may be an indication of polyneuropathy as well as radiculopathy (i.e., S_1 nerve root).

The peripheral sensory neuron has unique anatomical features which offer an electrodiagnostic advantage over motor nerves. A lesion anywhere along a segmental motor nerve, including motor neuron degeneration seen in motor neuron diseases, may result in nonlocalizing denervative features on NCS and EMG studies. The sensory neuron is a unipolar neuron. The cell body is situated in the dorsal root ganglion (DRG), in the neural foramen between the sensory root and distal peripheral nerve. There is a single axon which bifurcates into two major processes. One projects distally as the peripheral nerve and the other centrally as the sensory root and dorsal column (Fig. 36-3). Lesions disrupting axons proximal to the DRG (i.e., root lesions) will cause wallerian degeneration proximal to the dorsal root ganglion and fibers distal to the DRG (peripheral nerve) remain intact. In this situation, the patient has hypesthesia or anesthesia with a normal SNAP. Disruption of sensory fibers distal to the DRG will cause wallerian degeneration of fibers within the peripheral nerve and this will be reflected in a diminished or absent SNAP. Central projections proximal to the DRG remain unaffected. NCS can be very useful in localizing lesions distal to the DRG such as in the plexopathy or peripheral nerve lesions. Active denervation within a peripheral myotome and paraspinal muscles in association with a normal SNAP is a typical signature found in radiculopathy.

ELECTROMYOGRAPHY

Electromyography (EMG) is helpful in identifying patients with neurogenic as well as myopathic conditions. Both types of patients frequently seek orthopaedic attention. The usefulness, diagnostic power, and accuracy of EMG are realized only when the exam is planned and interpreted in light of the patient's history and physical examination. The EMG examination parameters which will serve as the ba-

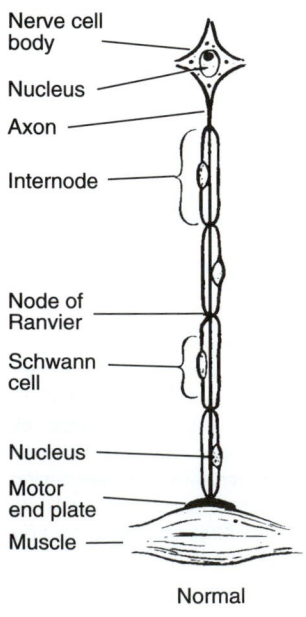
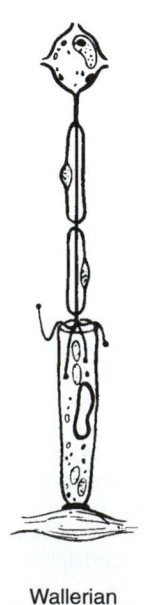
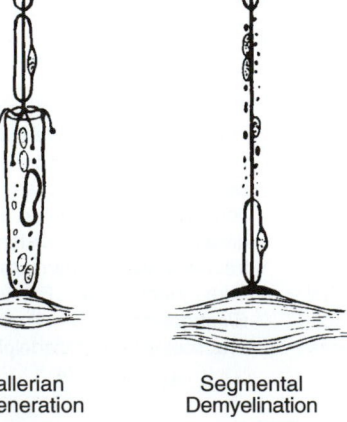
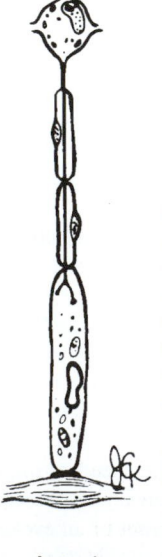

Normal   Wallerian Degeneration   Segmental Demyelination   Axonal Degeneration

Figure 36-2
(*Left*) Normal nerve axon and myelin sheath. (*Right*) Types of degeneration: wallerian degeneration (following transection of the fiber), segmented demyelination, and axonal degeneration (secondary to disorders of the nerve cell). (Reproduced by permission from Asbury AK, Johnson PC: Basic pathologic mechanisms. In: *Pathology of Peripheral Nerve. Major Problems in Pathology,* vol 9. Philadelphia: WB Saunders; 1978:51.)

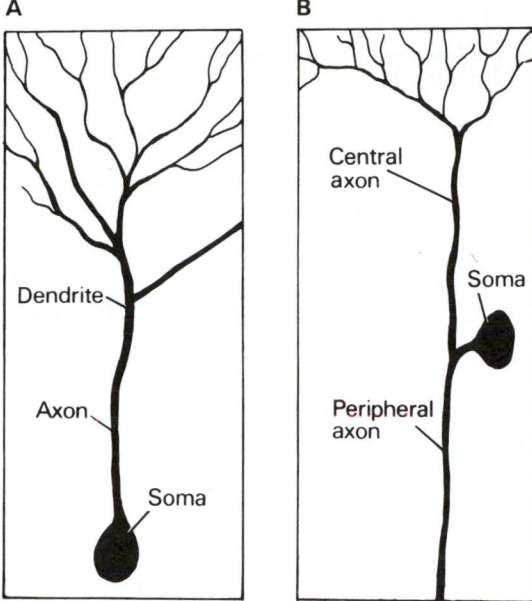

Figure 36-3
Unipolar cells. *A.* Invertebrate neuron. *B.* Dorsal root ganglion cell. Unique structure of large fiber somatic afferent neuron. (Reproduced by permission from Kandel ER: Nerve cells and behavior. In Kandel ER, Schwartz JH: *Principles of Neural Science,* 2d ed. New York: Elsevier; 1985:16.)

sis for diagnosis include: (1) insertional activity, (2) spontaneous activity, (3) motor unit morphology, (4) interference pattern.

Insertional activity (IA) is the brief burst of electrical activity which accompanies the insertion of the needle electrode into the muscle. This reflects an "injury potential" which results when the needle elec-

trode stimulates the muscle membrane. Analysis of such a response is dependent upon the speed and forcefulness of needle penetration; however, a semiquantitative analysis is possible. Decreased IA is typically seen in fibrotic muscle and is associated with progressive neurogenic or myogenic conditions. Increased IA indicating hyperexcitability can be seen in denervated muscle and in myopathic diseases such as myopathies, myositis, and myotonic disorders. Further characterization of the pathologic process will depend on other EMG parameters such as motor unit potentials (MUP) morphology and recruitment patterns.

Spontaneous EMG activity includes fibrillation potentials, positive sharp waves, fasciculations, complex repetitive discharges, and myokymic discharges. Fibrillations and positive sharp waves are seen in denervated muscle and in a number of myogenic diseases (Figs. 36-4 and 36-5). Denervated muscle fibers develop as much as a 100-fold increase in sensitivity to circulating acetylcholine (Ach) molecules. This increase in sensitivity to Ach in combination with lowered resting membrane potentials and increased sodium conductance contributes to the generation of spontaneous discharges. Fibrillation and positive sharp waves are typically observed two weeks after denervation occurs. Fibrillations and positive sharp waves are single muscle fiber potentials which are not observable on the clinical examination. Fasciculations are isolated spontaneous discharges of the motor unit (Fig. 36-6). These are observed on physical examination as individual muscle twitches. Fasciculations are most commonly associated with anterior horn cell diseases such as amyotrophic lateral sclerosis; however, they may be associated with radiculopathy, nerve entrapments, and cervical spondylitic myelopathy. Metabolic disorders such as tetany, thyrotoxicosis, and anticholinesterase intoxication can cause fasciculations. Myokymia are grouped complex repetitive discharges which typically occur in brain stem lesions in association with multiple sclerosis, gliomas, and chronic peripheral nerve disorders such as Guillain-Barré syndrome, radiation plexopathies, and

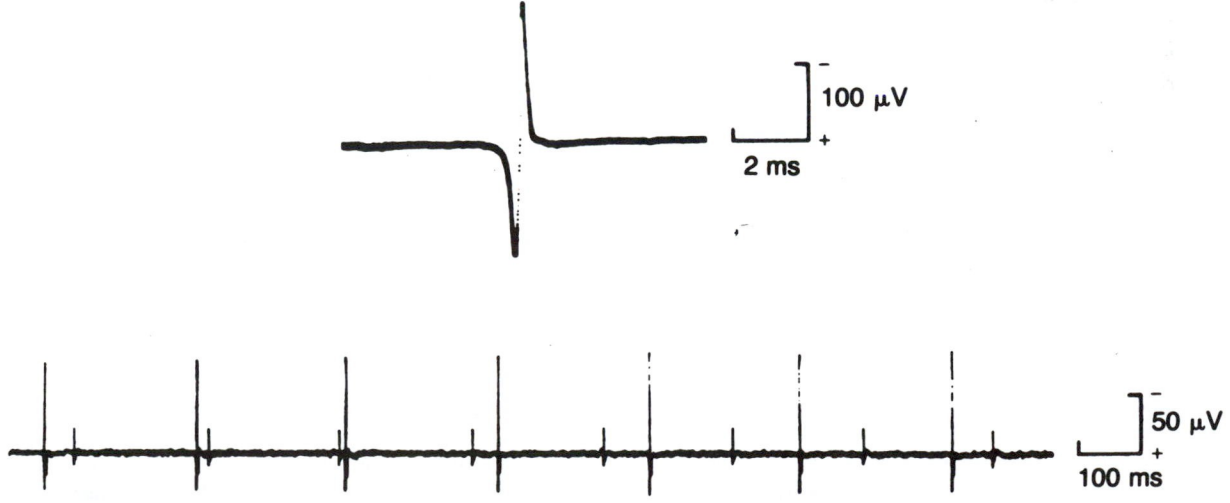

Figure 35-4
Fibrillation potential. The top trace shows a single *fibrillation potential* waveform. The bottom trace shows the pattern of discharge of two other *fibrillation potentials* which differ with respect to amplitude and discharge frequency. A fibrillation potential is the electric activity associated with a spontaneously contracting (fibrillating) muscle fiber. It is the action potential of a single muscle fiber. The action potentials may occur spontaneously or after movement of the needle electrode. The potentials usually fire at a constant rate, although a small proportion fire irregularly. Classically, the potentials are biphasic spikes of short duration (usually less than 5 ms) with an initial positive phase and a peak-to-peak amplitude of less than 1 mV. When recorded with concentric

or monopolar needle electrode, the firing rate has a wide range (1 to 50 Hz) and often decreases just before cessation of an individual discharge. A high-pitched regular sound is associated with the discharge of fibrillation potentials and has been described in the old literature as "rain on a tin roof." In addition to this classic form of fibrillation potentials, *positive sharp waves* may also be recorded from fibrillating muscle fibers when the potential arises from an area immediately adjacent to the needle electrode. (Reproduced by permission from Dumitru D: AAEM glossary of terms. In: *Electrodiagnostic Medicine.* Philadelphia: Hanley & Belfus; 1995:1194.)

POSITIVE SHARP WAVE

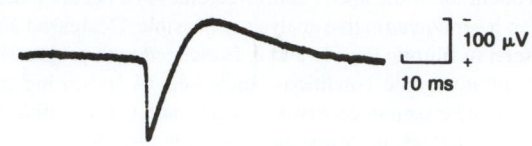

TRAIN OF POSITIVE SHARP WAVES

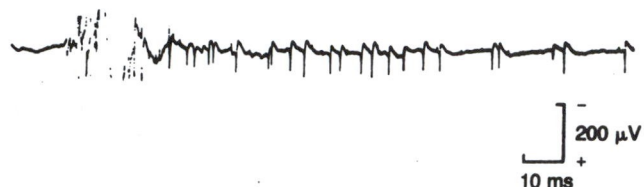

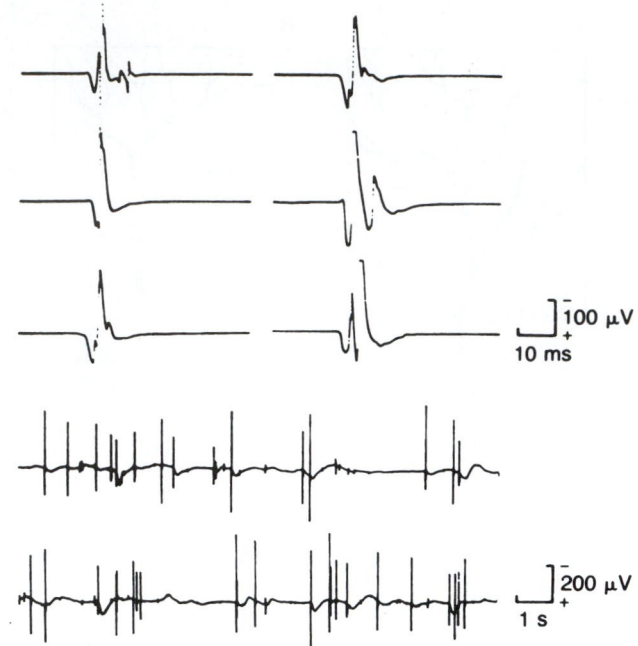

Figure 36-5

The top trace shows a single *positive sharp wave.* The bottom trace shows the pattern of initial discharge of a number of different *positive sharp waves* after movement of the recording needle electrode in detonated muscle. A *positive sharp wave* is a biphasic, positive-negative *action potential* initiated by needle movement and recurring in a uniform, regular pattern at a rate of 1 to 50 Hz; the discharge frequency may decrease slightly just before cessation of discharge. The initial positive deflection is rapid (1 ms), its duration is usually less than 5 ms, and the amplitude is up to 1 mV. The negative phase is of low amplitude, with a duration of 10 to 100 ms. A sequence of positive sharp waves is commonly referred to as a *train of positive sharp waves.* Positive sharp waves can be recorded from the damaged area of fibrillating muscle fibers. Its configuration may result from the position of the needle electrode which is felt to be adjacent to the depolarized segment of a muscle fiber injured by the electrode. Note that the positive sharp waveform is not specific for muscle fiber damage. *Motor unit action potentials* and potentials in *myotonic discharges* may have the configuration of positive sharp waves. (Reproduced by permission from Dumitru D: AAEM glossary of terms. In: *Electrodiagnostic Medicine.* Philadelphia: Hanley & Belfus; 1995:1195.)

Figure 36-6

Fasciculation potential. Six different *fasciculation potentials* are displayed in the top traces with a time scale to permit characterization of the individual waveforms. The bottom two traces display *fasciculation potentials* with a time scale to demonstrate the random discharge pattern. A *fasciculation potential* is the electric potential often associated with a visible *fasciculation,* which has the configuration of a *motor unit action potential* but which occurs spontaneously. Most commonly these potentials occur sporadically and are termed "single fasciculation potentials." Occasionally, the potentials occur as a grouped discharge and are termed a "brief repetitive discharge." The occurrence of repetitive firing of adjacent fasciculation potentials, when numerous, may produce an undulating movement of muscle (see *myokymia*). Use of the terms *benign fasciculation* and *malignant fasciculation* is discouraged. Instead, the configuration of the potentials, peak-to-peak amplitude, duration, number of phases, and stability of configuration, in addition to frequency of occurrence, should be specified. (Reproduced by permission from Kimura J: Appendices: AAEE Glossary of terms in clinical electromyography. In: *Electrodiagnosis in Diseases of Nerve and Muscle: Principles and Practice,* 2d ed. Philadelphia: FA Davis; 1989:659.)

motor neuron diseases (Fig. 36-7). Complex repetitive discharges are a sign of irritation and are actually a group of muscle fibers which fire in repetitive bursts. The bursts start abruptly, are regular, and end abruptly. Complex repetitive discharges are associated with muscular dystrophies, myositis, and chronic denervating entities such as motor neuron diseases, radiculopathies, and polyneuropathies (Fig. 36-8).

Motor unit potential (MUP) morphologies are helpful in discerning between myopathic and neurogenic processes. Amplitude, duration, and number of phases are key quantifiable EMG parameters. Amplitude is an indicator of muscle fiber density per axon near the tip of the needle electrode. Duration is an indicator of motor unit territory. Both amplitude and duration are increased in neurogenic lesions as denervated fibers are incorporated into surrounding motor units. In myopathic conditions muscle fibers are lost and amplitude and duration of MUPs are both diminished.

Motor unit phases are MUP waveform positive and negative deflections from the baseline. Most of the MUPs observed during an EMG examination have four or less phases. Polyphasia is a semiquantitative assessment of the number of MUPs with excessive phase reversals. In normal muscle, up to 15 to 20 percent of the MUP

potentials may have five or more phases (increased polyphasia). Degenerating or regenerating distal nerve fibers conduct poorly. These fibers may be immature, very thin, poorly myelinated, and myoneural junction transmission efficiency may be markedly diminished. These factors cause an increase in temporal dispersion in terminal nerve and muscle fiber membrane conduction. This desynchronization of nerve fiber conduction and muscle fiber discharges results in increased polyphasia which can be assessed with EMG. Polyphasia will increase in myopathy and neurogenic lesions such as radiculopathy, nerve entrapments, polyneuropathy, and anterior horn cell disease. Increased polyphasia is usually seen in subacute lesions and therefore can be helpful in dating neurogenic lesions.

Recruitment patterns are determined by motor unit discharge rate and the total number of motor units firing. Normally, greater muscle tension requires recruitment of previously inactive motor units as well as a higher firing frequency of recruited motor units. A normal recruitment pattern is defined as an appropriate number of motor units with a firing rate commensurate with the contractile force. In order to compensate for neurogenic or myogenic induced weakness,

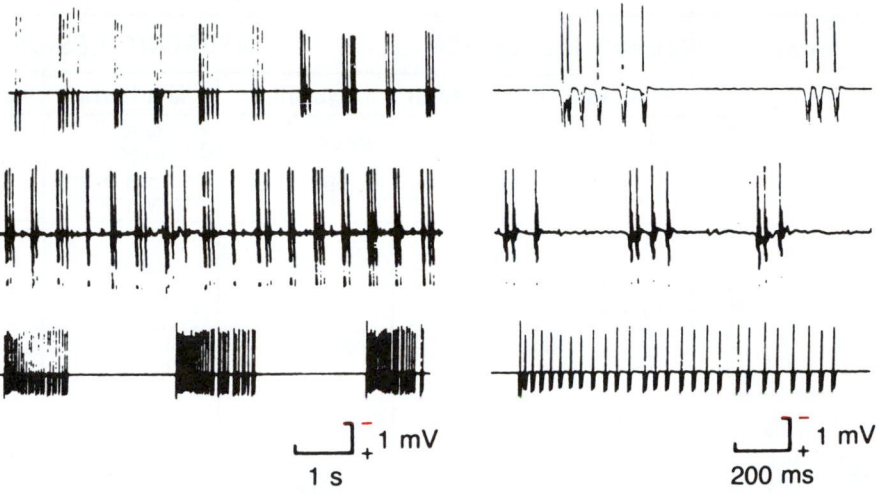

Figure 36-7

Myokymic discharge. Tracings of three different *myokymic discharges* displayed with a time scale (*left*) to illustrate the firing pattern and with a different time scale (*right*) to illustrate that the individual potentials have the configuration of a *motor unit action potential*. A *myokymic discharge* is a group of *motor unit action potentials* that fire repetitively and may be associated with clinical myokymia. Two firing patterns have been described. Commonly, the discharge is a brief, repetitive firing of single units for a short period (up to a few seconds) at a uniform rate (2 to 60 Hz) followed by a short period (up to a few seconds) of silence, with repetition of the same sequence for a particular potential. Less commonly, the potential recurs continually at a fairly uniform firing rate (1 to 5 Hz). Myokymic discharges are a subclass of *grouped discharges* and *repetitive discharges*. (Reproduced by permission from Kimura J: Appendices: AAEE Glossary of terms in clinical electromyography. In: *Electrodiagnosis in Diseases of Nerve and Muscle: Principles and Practice*, 2d ed. Philadelphia: FA Davis; 1989:660.)

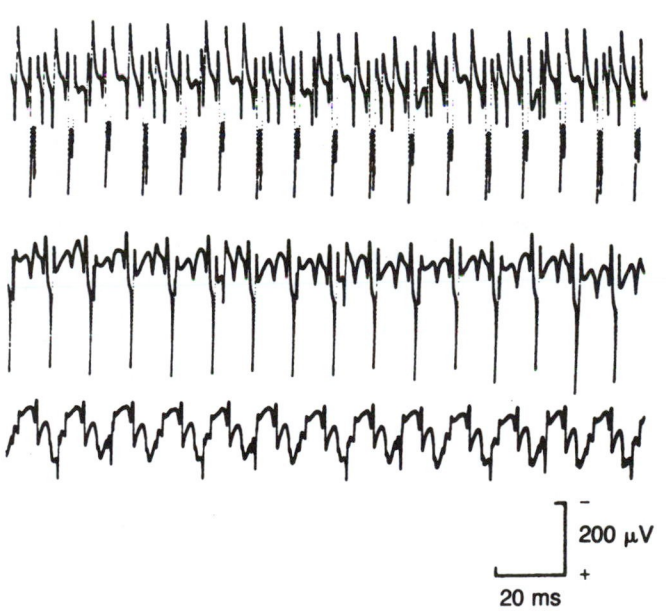

Figure 36-8

Complex repetitive discharge. This is a polyphasic or serrated potential that may begin spontaneously or after a needle movement. They have a uniform frequency, shape, and amplitude, with abrupt onset, cessation, or change in configuration. Amplitude ranges from 100 μV to 1 mV and frequency of discharge from 5 to 100 Hz. This term is preferred to *bizarre high frequency discharge, bizarre repetitive discharge, bizarre repetitive potential, near constant frequency trains, pseudomyotonic discharge,* and *synchronized fibrillation*. (Reproduced by permission from Dumitru D: AAEM glossary of terms. In: *Electrodiagnostic Medicine*. Philadelphia: Hanley & Belfus; 1995:1196.)

changes occur in the numbers of motor units recruited for a given muscle tension and firing frequency. These EMG quantitated changes can be characterized as neurogenic or myogenic. Neurogenic disorders such as motor neuron disease, peripheral nerve lesions, and polyneuropathy are associated with motor axon loss. Fewer, high amplitude, long duration MUPs are observed which fire at higher than normal frequency rate. This results in overall diminished interference and recruitment patterns. In myogenic disorders, muscle contraction is inefficient. The MUPs are low amplitude and short duration. In myopathic muscle, more diseased muscle fibers must be recruited for a desired muscle tension. The EMG will show disproportionately large numbers of "myopathic MUPs" (low amplitude, short duration MUPs). A full recruitment pattern is observed with less than a full contraction indicating an early or increased recruitment (Fig. 36-9).

SOMATOSENSORY EVOKED POTENTIALS

SEPs are elicited by stimulation of mixed peripheral nerves or dermatomal sensory cutaneous nerves. Computer-enhanced signal-averaging and special filtering techniques have made it possible to record time locked spinal and cortical SEP responses. Signal-averaging "cancels" random background EEG activity, muscle EMG artifact, and other extraneous artifacts. Through repetitive stimulation characteristic waveforms with constant latencies can be recognized and recorded at various sites along peripheral or central sensory pathways. Routine evaluation includes right and left unilateral nerve stimulation and comparison of spinal as well as contralateral hemispheric short latency peaks.

The SEP response is mediated by the Ia sensory fibers in peripheral nerve-dorsal column-medial lemniscus-cortical radiation sensory

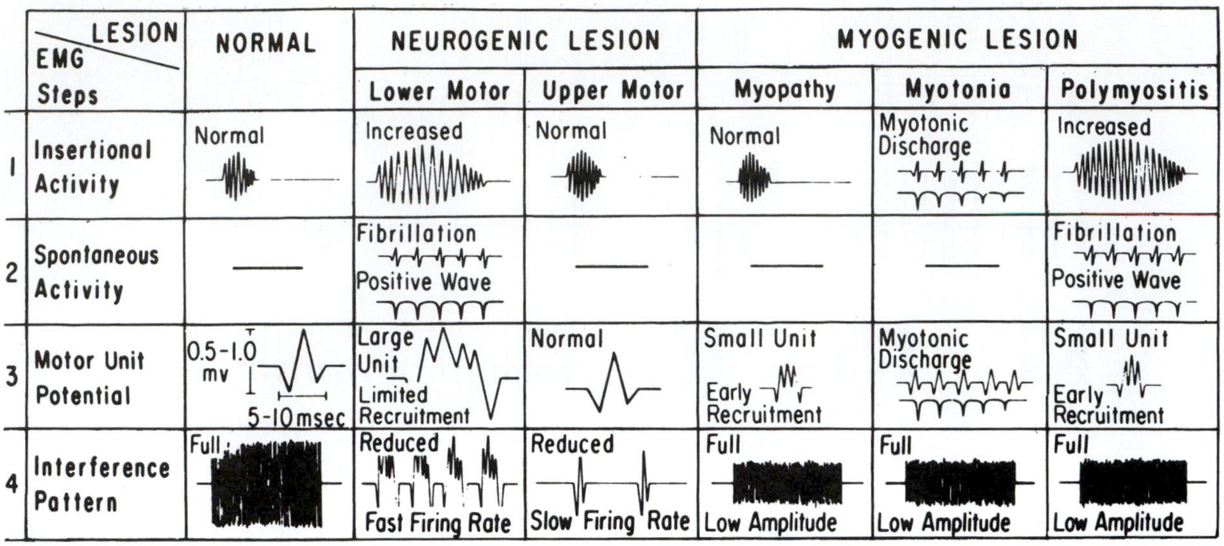

LESION EMG Steps	NORMAL	NEUROGENIC LESION		MYOGENIC LESION		
		Lower Motor	Upper Motor	Myopathy	Myotonia	Polymyositis
1 Insertional Activity	Normal	Increased	Normal	Normal	Myotonic Discharge	Increased
2 Spontaneous Activity	—	Fibrillation Positive Wave	—	—	—	Fibrillation Positive Wave
3 Motor Unit Potential	0.5-1.0 mv 5-10 msec	Large Unit Limited Recruitment	Normal	Small Unit Early Recruitment	Myotonic Discharge	Small Unit Early Recruitment
4 Interference Pattern	Full	Reduced Fast Firing Rate	Reduced Slow Firing Rate	Full Low Amplitude	Full Low Amplitude	Full Low Amplitude

Figure 36-9

The EMG changes which can be expected with various neurogenic or myogenic lesions are summarized. (Reproduced by permission from Kimura J: Types of abnormality. In: *Electrodiagnosis in Diseases of Nerve and Muscle: Principles and Practice,* 2d ed. Philadelphia: FA Davis; 1989:252.)

pathway. SEPs assess the entire length of the afferent sensory pathway and a lesion anywhere along the pathway may cause an abnormal SEP response. The common sites of stimulation include the tibial nerve at the ankle, peroneal nerve at the knee, and the median and ulnar nerves at the wrist. Neural generators for SEP responses for the upper extremity nerves are at Erb's point (brachial plexus), cervical spine, and contralateral sensory cortex. The lower extremity generators include the lower lumbosacral spine (roots), conus, and midline somatosensory cortex.

A single, abnormal SEP response by itself may not be helpful in localizing lesions in the peripheral or central nervous system. Present peripheral responses (i.e., Erb's point and cervical spine responses) with absent cortical responses obviously indicate a central nervous system lesion. However, often both peripheral and central responses are present, making localization difficult. The lesion site may be deduced from the pattern of abnormal responses observed when comparison is made to contralateral as well as other peripheral nerve SEP responses. For example, symmetric prolongation of all SEP responses from the lower or upper extremities is suggestive of dorsal column dysfunction frequently associated with myelopathy. The pattern of delayed tibial nerve cortical SEP latency with distal stimulation (ankle) and normal peroneal nerve latency with proximal stimulation (knee) suggests a polyneuropathy. Polyneuropathy causes disproportionate conduction slowing in the longest fibers, therefore the tibial responses are prolonged while the peroneal latencies are within the normal range. Patchy, asymmetric abnormalities of tibial, peroneal, and saphenous nerve SEP responses would strongly suggest the presence of multilevel lumbosacral radiculopathies, often seen in patients with spinal stenosis. Stimulation of a nerve above and below a suspected nerve lesion can also identify and confirm the lesion site. This can be very useful in evaluating sciatic, peroneal, lateral femoral cutaneous, and saphenous nerve lesions, especially in patients with superimposed conditions such as radiculopathy and polyneuropathy.

Routine NCS is used in evaluating the distal segments of the peripheral nervous system. SEPs complement peripheral nerve conduction studies. Evaluation of the inter-peak latencies between spinal and cortical generators allows differentiation between central and pe-

ripheral dysfunction. SEP techniques have a definite advantage in evaluating proximal neuropathies such as patients with Guillain-Barré syndrome, chronic inflammatory demyelinating polyneuropathy (CIDP), and brachial and lumbosacral plexopathies. SEP studies can be also helpful in evaluating proximal sciatic nerve lesions, thoracic outlet syndrome, and cervical spondylitic myelopathy. The diagnostic yield in lumbosacral radiculopathies is more variable; however SEPs can be particularly useful in showing patterns which are characteristic for spinal stenosis.

The phenomenon of central synaptic amplification makes it possible to record cortical SEPs when the peripheral nerve response is either too small or temporally dispersed for subcortical SEP responses or SNAPs to be detectable. Central amplification of peripheral responses is a unique feature seen with SEPs and makes SEPs a very sensitive probe for investigating nerve lesions, nerve regeneration, and the success of surgical repair of nerve lesions. Peripheral conduction studies are often insensitive and show absent responses with incomplete nerve lesions after trauma and with early nerve regeneration. It is possible to confirm with SEPs whether some sensory fibers remain in continuity or if effective regeneration is taking place after partial traumatic nerve section or crush injury. The presence of a cortical SEP response indicates that a traumatic nerve lesion is incomplete. SEP techniques have potential value in assessing regeneration of surgically repaired peripheral nerves. SEPs may be the first indication of successful nerve regeneration and can track progress of nerve regeneration.

SUGGESTED READINGS

Brown W, Bolton C: *Clinical Electromyography,* 2d ed. Boston: Butterworth-Heinemann; 1993.

Dumitru D: *Electrodiagnostic Medicine.* Philadelphia: Hanley & Belfus; 1995.

Jones S: Somatosensory evoked potentials II: Clinical observations and applications. In Halliday AM (ed): *Evoked Potentials in Clinical Testing,* 2d ed. London: Churchill Livingstone; 1992:421.

Kandel ER, Schwartz JH: *Principles of Neural Science,* 3d ed. New York: Elsevier Science; 1991.

Kimura J: *Electrodiagnosis in Diseases of Nerve and Muscle: Principles and Practice,* 2d ed. Philadelphia: FA Davis; 1989.

Kimura J: Nerve conduction studies and electromyography. In Dyck P, Thomas P, Griffin J, et al (eds.) *Peripheral Neuropathy,* 3d ed. Philadelphia: W.B. Saunders; 1993: 598.

Mumenthaler M, Schliack H: Principles of the operative treatment of peripheral nerve lesions. In Mumenthaler M, Schliack H (eds.): *Peripheral Nerve Lesions,* 6th ed. Stuttgart: Georg-Thieme-Verlag (New York: Thieme Medical Publishers); 1991:95.

Seddon HJ: A classification of nerve injuries. *Br Med J* 1942; 2:237.

Seddon HJ: *Surgical Disorders of the Peripheral Nerves,* 2d ed. Edinburgh: Churchill Livingstone; 1975.

Seddon HJ: Three types of nerve injury. *Brain* 1943; 66:237.

Chapter 37

CLINICAL NEUROPHYSIOLOGY

Aleksandar Berić

NERVE DISORDERS

RADICULOPATHY

Needle electromyography (EMG) is the most sensitive and valuable clinical neurophysiological test to diagnose radiculopathy. Characteristic motor-unit changes and the presence of denervation can confirm radiculopathy in a particular spinal segment as well as determine the acute, subacute, or chronic nature of the lesion. Acute radiculopathy (<6 weeks) is characterized by active denervation and loss of motor units, with the remaining motor units having normal features (Fig. 37-1A). A subacute lesion is characterized by active denervation together with some reinnervation. Polyphasic and prolonged duration motor units are suggestive of a subacute process which occurs at least 6 weeks after the onset of dysfunction (Fig. 37-1B). Chronic lesions, at least six months after the initial root injury, are characterized by active denervation together with consolidated collateral reinnervation, which is seen as large amplitude, rounded motor units (Fig. 37-1C). Residual radiculopathy is characterized by a slight loss of motor units with the presence of large, rounded amplitude motor units without polyphasics, longer duration motor units, or active denervation. This represents an inactive process which indicates that at least 6 months ago there was root injury followed by collateral (within muscle) reinnervation, in which there is an attempt to repair the loss of axons. Axonal lesions at the root level (alpha motor neuron) do not have the capacity to regenerate and regrow to muscles.

Localizing the root injury is complex because most muscles in the body are innervated by multiple spinal or root segments. For this reason, several different muscles must be examined by EMG to find out which ones are abnormal. In addition, the degree of abnormality in each of the various muscles helps to determine the root most likely damaged. The electromyographic guidelines for root innervation of muscles are the same as for the clinical assessment. Some muscles, however, are easily accessible to EMG and can be readily activated by the patient, while other muscles usually used for the clinical diagnosis of root lesions are less suitable for EMG.

The degree of root lesion can also be estimated by neurophysiologic testing. Needle EMG is sensitive to even minor axon loss. Even a 5 to 10 percent loss can be detected by EMG. With a minor loss, the patient may have pain without obvious weakness, but due to the sensitivity of the needle EMG, this test may be abnormal and confirm the presence of root damage. In contrast, a nerve conduction study looks at the compound muscle action potential (CMAP) represented by the entire population of axons innervating the muscle under the recording electrode. Since the CMAP represents the spared portion of nerve fibers, it can be used to semi-quantitatively measure the amount of fiber loss. For example, complete loss of CMAP would represent total or near-total loss of fibers innervating that particular muscle. An 80 or 90 percent reduction in amplitude would represent an 80 or 90 percent loss of fibers. Nerve conduction studies tend to correlate better with muscle weakness than do EMGs. Weakness appears when there is a loss of approximately 50 percent of the fibers.

Sensory nerve action potentials (SNAPs) are useful in radiculopathy only when it is necessary to exclude the presence of a peripheral nerve lesion or polyneuropathy. SNAPs should be normal and preserved in root lesions. As the root lesion is proximal to the sensory ganglion, the continuity of the peripheral axon at the point of stimulation within the ganglion ensures viability of the axon and normal parameters of the SNAPs, including sensory nerve conduction velocity. Sensory dysfunction in root lesions can be assessed with spinal and cortical somatosensory evoked potentials (SEPs). The SEP responses are generated by stimulation of the peripheral nerve below the root lesion with recordings above the root lesion at the cervical cord or the primary sensory cortex. By stimulating small cutaneous nerves in appropriate dermatomes, the dermatomal SEPs can be obtained in addition to large trunk sensory and mixed nerve stimulation.

In conclusion, needle EMG is a very sensitive test for any loss of motor fibers and can readily be used to diagnose radiculopathy. It is not particularly suitable for quantification and therefore not appropriate for quantitative follow-up. However, it is useful for staging reinnervation by assessing changes of features of the motor units. The overall percentage loss of motor fibers can be determined by the amplitude decrease of a CMAP in a motor nerve conduction study. The loss of sensory fibers is estimated by the amplitude decrease in the cortical SEP. SNAPs should be normal in root lesions. The presence of any abnormality of the SNAP does not necessarily rule out the presence of a root lesion; however, it does suggest an additional peripheral nerve lesion, plexus lesion, or polyneuropathy that should be further investigated and documented.

PLEXOPATHY

Nerve plexus lesions are frequently caused by injury. There is also a significant number of compressive plexopathies due to tumors, as well as idiopathic forms which are now being considered to be autoimmune. The diagnosis of plexopathy depends on the distribution of the abnormality which can be tested by appropriate motor and sensory nerve conduction studies, as well as needle electromyography. Detailed knowledge of the brachial plexus, as well as the lumbar and lumbosacral plexuses, is absolutely necessary for diagnosis. Needle EMG may be more sensitive than the clinical examination in finding more widespread abnormalities than clinically obvious weakness of one or more muscles. Needle EMG can also be used for staging of nerve regeneration and recovery of the lesion. The appearance of true reinnervation can be followed in cases of complete or severe injuries by the appearance of nascent motor units, usually long before there is any clinical improvement. CMAP amplitude can also be used to assess the degree of regeneration, as it correlates with reinnervation and the return of muscle power. In plexopathy, the lesion consists of a severing of the connection between the peripheral portion of the nerve and the ganglion. Therefore, the SNAPs are abnormal. The distribution of the degree of loss of amplitude of different nerve SNAPs is very useful in assessing plexopathy.

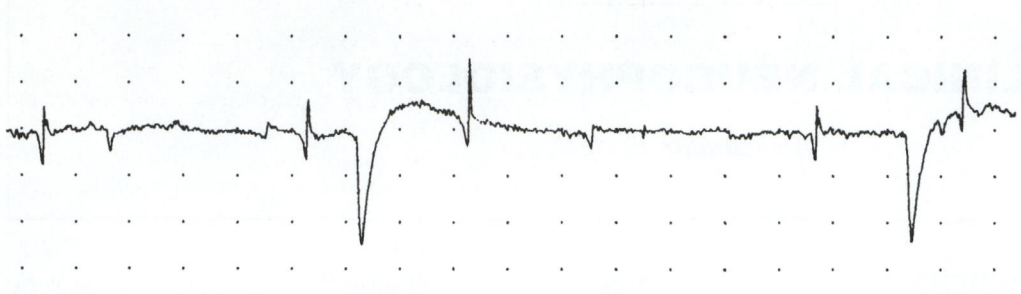

A

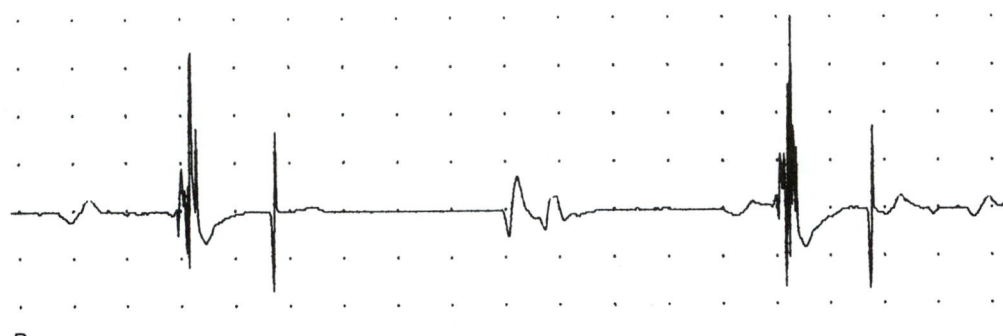

B

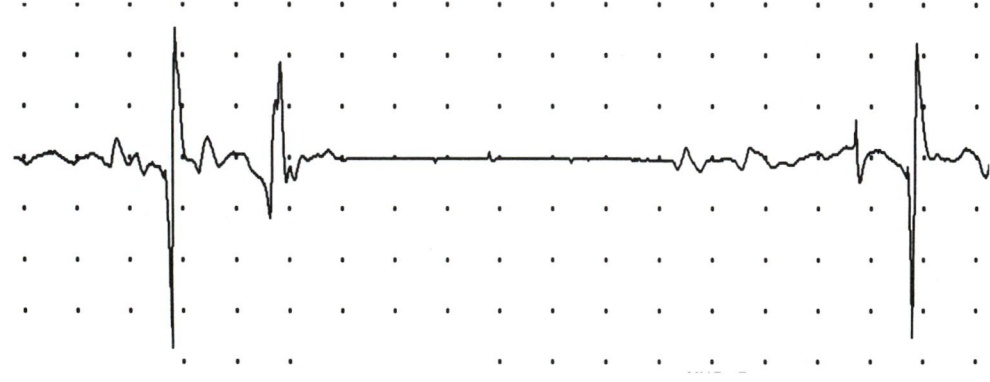

C

Figure 37-1

A. Fibrillations and positive sharp waves—sign of an active denervation usually seen in an acute lesion. Horizontal calibration is 10 ms/division in the entire figure, vertical calibration is 50 µV/division. *B.* Polyphasic potentials with a large number of turns—sign of an early reinnervation in a subacute lesion. Vertical calibration is 200 µV/division. *C.* Large amplitude motor unit—sign of a completed reinnervation in a chronic or residual lesion. Vertical calibration is 1000 µV/division.

One particular diagnostic problem is the differentiation of severe traumatic brachial plexopathy with and without concomitant cervical root avulsion. The absence of sensory perception in the appropriate distribution of the upper extremity with preservation of the SNAP is indicative of a root avulsion. Loss of SNAP amplitude is suggestive of a brachial plexus lesion, but cannot exclude the presence of an additional root avulsion. Additionally, cortical SEPs after peripheral nerve stimulation may be absent while the amplitude of the SNAPs may only be somewhat reduced. This would suggest an additional root avulsion together with a brachial plexus injury.

PERIPHERAL NEUROPATHY

Peripheral neuropathy is a relatively common clinical disorder, especially in the elderly population. There are two main types of peripheral neuropathies. The more common one is axonal, which primarily affects the axons of the longest nerves. It is usually of a "dying back" type in which the peripheral ends of the neurons degenerate first. For this reason, the axonal polyneuropathies start distal in the extremities, usually in the feet, with proximal progression toward the knees. When the neuropathy affects the lower leg to the level of the knees, the upper extremities are usually involved from the fingers, proximally. The most frequent causes of axonal polyneuropathies are diabetes, vitamin deficiencies (B_{12}), and toxic exposures to agents such as alcohol, heavy metals, and some antineoplastic medications such as cis-platinum. It is worth noting that diabetic neuropathy can present in several different forms where symmetrical distal polyneuropathy is one of the most frequent. It may present as multifocal mononeuropathy where several different peripheral nerves are involved in the upper and lower extremities in any combination. Diabetic neuropathy can also present as diabetic amyotrophy which usually involves the thigh muscles. This is a form of combined lumbar plexus and lumbar root lesions. It can also present as a small fiber neuropathy involving only small myelinated and unmyelinated fibers. Clinical symptoms include pain in the feet, in which case a nerve conduction and EMG may be totally normal as they assess only large nerve fiber function.

The other form of peripheral neuropathy is demyelinating, in which case the myelin is attacked as part of an autoimmune process. Initially, the axons are intact and only the conduction velocity is slowed together with a presence of a conduction block as the insulation is broken and conduction in normal saltatory mode cannot be maintained. The acute form of demyelinating neuropathy is called Guillain-Barré syndrome which usually starts as a weakness in the lower extremities and sometimes spreads proximally to involve respiratory muscles. This is a neurologic emergency and one of the rare electromyographic emergencies apart from myasthenia gravis and botulinum intoxication. The chronic form of demyelinating neuropathy is called chronic inflammatory demyelinating polyneuropathy (CIDP), which is usually associated with remissions and relapses and involves the upper extremities more often than the lower extremities.

There is a separate group of inherited polyneuropathies which can be either axonal or demyelinating. In some of these there is a specific gene defect, such as in Charcot-Marie-Tooth (CMT) neuropathy. CMT usually progresses very slowly and if it is mild, can be recognized in adults but may not appear in childhood or adolescence.

In general, treatment of axonal polyneuropathies is etiologic. Demyelinating neuropathies are usually considered autoimmune and can be treated with plasmapheresis, IV gamma-globulins, or sometimes corticosteroids.

ENTRAPMENT NEUROPATHY

The usual entrapment sites of nerves are at the wrist (carpal tunnel syndrome), the elbow (ulnar nerve palsy), and at the fibular head (peroneal nerve palsy). Rare and disputed entrapment sites are the thoracic outlet and the tarsal tunnel. The hallmark of entrapment is compression with local demyelination and conduction block that can be detected by prolonged latency due to slowed conduction across the compression site. These entrapment neuropathies usually have a good prognosis. When the compression is removed, remyelination occurs and full conduction is regained. If the compression is for a prolonged period of time and more severe, there will be some damage to the axons which may require a longer recovery time. Sometimes the compressions are neglected for a very long time and complete atrophy of the muscles and sensory fibers distal to the compression site can be found. In this case, recovery is poor and can be very painful during sensory nerve regeneration. Special sensory and motor nerve conduction studies are used to diagnose these localized compression neuropathies. For example, a transcarpal orthodromic nerve conduction study, inching technique for carpal tunnel, and a three-point ulnar and peroneal nerve stimulation study for ulnar and peroneal nerves can be used. It is important to note that peripheral entrapment neuropathy can be present together with cervical radiculopathy, as in the "double crush syndrome."

Neurophysiologic diagnostic studies have a high specificity and sensitivity for diagnosing entrapment syndromes.

MOTOR NEURON DISEASE

The two major subgroups of motor neuron disease are spinal muscular atrophy and amyotrophic lateral sclerosis (ALS). Spinal muscular atrophies are hereditary and involve a loss of spinal motor neurons. This results in lower motor neuron weakness of the lower and sometimes upper extremities. Typical EMG findings of giant motor units and histological findings of muscle atrophy and fiber type grouping are consistent with collateral reinnervation. ALS, or Lou Gehrig's disease, is found primarily in adults. There is a relatively rapid and progressive loss of alpha motor neurons within the spinal cord. It usually starts with atrophy of the distal upper extremities with progression to the respiratory muscles, ultimately resulting in death. There are now some recognized, treatable forms of motor neuron diseases which resemble ALS. The best known form is a multifocal motor neuropathy. This form has a relatively benign prognosis, especially when treated with IV gamma-globulins. Neurodiagnostic tests, together with the presence of the anti-GM-1 and anti-MAG antibodies, are crucial in differentiating this entity from ALS.

NEUROMUSCULAR JUNCTION DISORDERS

The neuromuscular junction (NMJ) consists of a presynaptic nerve terminal where the transmitter, acetylcholine (ACh), is stored in vesicles. When the nerve ending is depolarized, calcium is released and the vesicles are emptied into the synaptic cleft. The ACh diffuses, binds with the ACh receptors on the muscle, and generates the depolarization potential. After the potential reaches the threshold, a muscle action potential is elicited which depolarizes the muscle membrane. The NMJ is a highly specialized structure and any abnormality in the pre- or postsynaptic aspect can result in intermittent neuromuscular transmission, variability in transmission, or complete cessation of transmission resulting in either intermittent, partial, or total muscle weakness. There are a large number of hereditary and congenital abnormalities which require highly sophisticated in vitro neurophysiologic measurements and electromicroscopic assessments of muscle biopsy. The most common forms are acquired. Myasthenia gravis is an autoimmune disease that results from the presence of antibodies to ACh receptors. EMG and nerve conductions are usually normal in myasthenia gravis; however, repetitive nerve stimulations will show an abnormal decrement, and single fiber electromyography will show an increased neuromuscular jitter with fiber blocking. These are the signs of variable and intermittently interrupted neuromuscular transmission. Botulinum intoxication impairs neuromuscular transmission and can be fatal if not diagnosed promptly. Lambert-Eaton myasthenic syndrome (LAMS) can be idiopathic as well as paraneoplastic, associated with carcinoma of the lung. LAMS is caused by a pre-synaptic abnormality which can be improved by brief exercise. LAMS can sometimes precede cancer or can be the first objective sign of the cancer. Therefore, unexplained weakness in the adult and elderly population should be carefully investigated.

MUSCLE DISORDERS

Myopathies can be divided into hereditary-congenital and acquired types. It is important to note that hereditary myopathies can appear in different forms at any age in life. These forms are infantile, juvenile, and adult. This variability in the onset of the disease makes the diagnosis of hereditary myopathy rather difficult. Genetic markers, such as dystrophin levels in Duchenne's muscular dystrophy and multiple copies of some genes, as in myotonic dystrophy, can help in diagnosis.

Acquired myopathies are usually more diagnostically complex. They can be seen as side effects of treatment, such as with steroids. Both hypo- and hyperthyroidism can also cause myopathy. A separate subgroup of myopathies is inflammatory. This usually affects more women than men in the fourth and fifth decade of life. These myopathies start insidiously with some proximal joint pains and muscle sensitivity to pressure. If not treated, this can also lead to severe weakness of the axial muscles. Steroids and immunosuppressants are used for treatment of this condition. There are typical electromyographic features which can distinguish inflammatory myopathies from other types of myopathies. Diagnosis is usually confirmed by monocytic infiltration seen in muscle biopsy.

INTRAOPERATIVE MONITORING

During surgery, many neural structures can be at risk for damage, due to either vascular or compressive causes. As the patient is under anesthesia, no continuous feedback is possible. During spine surgery, there is a relatively high risk of overcorrection for scoliosis or placement of screws very close to or within the root. In cervical spine surgeries, there is a possibility of vascular compromises with changes in blood pressure as well as vascular spasms. Somatosensory evoked potentials with recordings from below and above the surgical site may detect any abnormalities in the functions of the posterior portion of the spinal cord. In addition, anterior spinal cord stimulation or transcranial motor stimulation above the surgical site, at the brain level, with recording below the surgical site can assess the function of the fast descending motor tracts. This can prevent lesions of the anterior portion of the spinal cord. There have been a number of false positive and false negative cases for both somatosensory and motor recordings reported. However, a combination of monitoring both systems will yield almost no false negatives. False positivity depends on the experience of the monitoring personnel and technical conditions of the recording as well as proper monitoring of anesthesia and interaction with the anesthesiologist. Dysfunctions from circulatory or compressive causes and pressure palsies due to inadequate positioning can be avoided by using intraoperative spinal monitoring.

SUGGESTED READINGS

Aminoff MJ. *Electrodiagnosis in Clinical Neurology,* 3d ed. New York: Churchill Livingstone; 1992.

Brown WF, Bolton CF. *Clinical Electromyography,* 2d ed. Newton, MA: Butterworth-Heinemann; 1993.

Chiappa KH. *Evoked Potentials in Clinical Medicine,* 2d ed. New York: Raven Press; 1990.

Dumitru D. *Electrodiagnostic Medicine.* Philadelphia: Hanley & Belfus Medical Publishers; 1995.

Liveson JA. *Peripheral Neurology: Case Studies in Electrodiagnosis,* 2d ed. Philadelphia: FA Davis; 1991.

Kimura J. *Electrodiagnosis in Disease of Nerve and Muscle: Principles and Practice,* 2d ed. Philadelphia: FA Davis; 1989.

Mumenthaler M, Schliack H. *Peripheral Nerve Lesions: Diagnosis and Therapy.* Stuttgart: Georg Thieme Verlag; 1991.

Oh SJ. *Clinical Electromyography: Nerve Conduction Studies,* 2d ed. Baltimore: Williams & Wilkins; 1993.

Chapter 38

GENERAL PRINCIPLES

Jess H. Lonner and Samuel Kenan

Primary tumors of the musculoskeletal system account for less than 1 percent of all tumors diagnosed in the United States each year (approximately 4000 cases annually). Since many patients with benign bone tumors are asymptomatic, the exact incidence of bone tumors is uncertain. Despite their relative paucity, these tumors represent a diverse group of pathologic entities, exhibiting a broad spectrum of clinical behavior and aggressiveness. Consequently, the diagnosis and treatment of these lesions are equally complex and varied.

Strategies exist to simplify the evaluation of these tumors and ultimately ensure appropriate treatment. These strategies include such methods as establishing consistency in nomenclature, understanding the site- and age-specific predilections of particular tumors, and characterizing the radiographic and histologic characteristics of each tumor. The following discussion specifically considers the diagnosis and treatment of common primary and secondary benign and malignant tumors affecting the musculoskeletal system.

CLINICAL EVALUATION

The definitive diagnosis of bone tumors requires a combined effort and collaboration among the clinician, radiologist, and pathologist. The most important criteria to be taken into consideration are the patient's medical history, age, location, radiographic features, and pathologic findings.

MEDICAL HISTORY

It is important to establish the clinical presentation. The first question is what made the patient seek medical attention? Was it an incidental finding during a routine check-up? Is there a history of trauma; post-traumatic ossifying hematoma may resemble a malignant tumor. Information about the patient's occupation is as important as the type and level of sport activity the patient may participate in; long-distance runners may present with a stress fracture that could mimic an osteogenic sarcoma. The pain pattern (intensity and duration) are also important factors. Pain at rest during day and night and nocturnal pain suggest osteoid osteoma; pain at rest that is also associated with activity suggests multiple stress fractures. Rapid onset of pain over a short period of time suggests an aggressive process such as osteomyelitis, eosinophilic granuloma, or Ewing's sarcoma. Any history of metabolic conditions such as Paget's disease, Gaucher's disease, or hyperparathyroidism should also be taken into consideration in forming the differential diagnosis.

AGE DISTRIBUTION

Benign bone tumors are far more commonly seen in young patients; metastatic tumors are seen almost exclusively in adult patients. Bone tumors in a 1-year-old infant suggests a metastatic neuroblastoma. The age of detection for a simple bone cyst, aneurysmal bone cyst, and eosinophilic granuloma is during the first decade of life. Through the second decade, *with the adolescent years,* chondroblastoma, Ewing's sarcoma, and osteosarcoma are more commonly seen. In the third decade of life, giant cell tumor is a more visible disorder. The age of detection for chondrosarcoma and malignant fibrous histiocytoma is seen in the adult patient, above the fourth decade of life. In old patients, myeloma is the most common primary bone tumor.

LOCATION

Certain tumors favor a specific anatomic site (Table 38-1). Most primary bone tumors tend to develop in areas of rapid bone growth; particularly in the distal end of the femur, proximal tibia, and proximal femurs. Metastatic tumors are more commonly seen in persistent, active hematopoietic red marrow bones such as the axial skeleton and the proximal end of the extremities. Round cell tumors such as Ewing's sarcoma are more often seen in the diaphysis metaphyseal region of the long tubular bone. A frequent site of adamantinoma is the mid shaft of the tibia. Non-ossifying fibroma are more often found eccentrically along the metaphyseal diaphysial region of the long tubular bone. Chondroblastomas are exclusively epiphysial. Giant cell tumors are almost invariably extended up to the end of the long tubular bone, just adjacent to the subchondral bone. A parosteal osteosarcoma is more commonly seen over the posterior aspect of the distal femur.

Most primary bone tumors are solitary. Multiple bone lesions in young patients may be seen in conditions such as fibrous dysplasia, osteochondromatosis, or enchondromatosis. Multiple bony lesions in adult patients suggest a metastatic tumor.

RADIOGRAPHIC FEATURES

A plain radiograph is the most important initial study for evaluation. In select conditions, a plain radiograph is sufficient to establish the correct diagnosis. Plain radiographs also provide information about the biological activity and aggressiveness of the lesion. The pattern of bone destruction and marginal characteristics as seen in radiographs are an index of the biological activity and growth rate. The most important radiographic features to be identified and evaluated are the pattern of bone destruction, marginal characteristics, type of permeation, tumor matrix, and type of periosteal reaction. The pattern of bone destruction is reflected by the tumor cells and factors that may stimulate osteoclastic proliferation and bone resorption. Cancellous bone is destroyed more rapidly than cortical bone. However, a cancellous bone destruction is less noticeable on plain roentgenogram. Destruction of cortical bone occurs at a lower rate, but it is more easily noticeable on plain radiographs.

Geographic patterns of bone destruction demonstrate a large cavity with a narrow zone of a transition. Geographic latent (Stage 1) lesion demonstrates a well delineated and well demarcated lesion which is surrounded by a sclerotic margin. Such lesions are seen in nonossifying fibroma (Fig. 38-1), simple bone cyst, fibrous dysplasia, chondromyxoid fibroma (Fig. 38-2), and rarely, giant cell tumor

Table 38-1

Bone Location/Site Predilection

Epiphyseal	Eosinophilic granuloma	Eosinophilic granuloma	Chondromyxoid
Chondroblastoma	Osteoid osteoma	Pelvis	fibroma
Giant cell tumor	Adamantinoma	Chondrosarcoma	Parosteal
Clear cell chondrosarcoma	Lymphoma	Metastatic disease	Myositis
Brodie's abscess osteochondritis	Fibrous dysplasia	Multiple myeloma	Osteosarcoma
		Aneurysmal bone cyst	Chondrosarcoma
Metaphyseal	Axial skeleton	Paget's disease	Chondroma
Simple cyst	Osteoblastoma	Ewing's sarcoma	
Fibrous dysplasia	Aneurysmal bone cysts		Multiple lesions
Osteoblastoma	Multiple myeloma	Proximal humerus	Metastasis
Chondromyxoid fibroma	Plasmacytoma	Chondroid lesions	Myeloma
Osteosarcoma	Metastatic lesions		Hemangioma
Aneurysmal bone cyst	Chordoma	Fibula	Fibrous dysplasia
Non-ossifying fibroma	Giant cell tumor	Ewing's sarcoma	Osteochondromas
	Paget's disease		Enchondromas
Diaphyseal	Hemangioma	Tibia	Histiocytosis X
Ewing's sarcoma		Adamantinoma	

(Fig. 38-3). These lesions may be observed or be treated by a simple curetting procedure. Following such procedures, local recurrence is negligible.

Geographic active (Stage 2) lesion has a well-defined but nonpermeated margin. There is no sclerotic interface. The host bone tumoral interface is sharply delineated as could be seen in giant cell tumor (Fig. 38-4). Simple curettage may leave behind traces of tumor which will be associated with a local recurrence rate up to 38 percent. Those lesions should be treated by aggressive curettage.

Geographic aggressive (Stage 3) lesions have ill-defined permeated margins as is demonstrated in some aggressive giant cell tumors where breakthrough of the outer cortex, and joint invasion has been noted (Fig. 38-5). Such a pattern of aggressive processes has been described in malignant tumors. Because of the high risk of local recurrence, those lesions should be treated by wide surgical margins.

Moth-eaten destruction represents an intermittent growth rate with no clear margination (Fig. 38-6). The lesion typically demonstrates multiple, ill-defined processes such as those seen in malignant lymphoma.

Permeative bone destruction represents a high-grade malignant tumor with rapid growth, the bone permeates before apparent bone destruction as can be seen in Ewing's sarcoma and osteosarcoma (Fig. 38-7).

The above radiographic classification has proven to demonstrate good correlation between the radiographic grade and the local recurrence rate, and also provides a useful guideline for treatment.

Periosteal Reaction

The periosteal reaction seen on radiographs reflects the intensity and aggressiveness of the lesion and the stage of maturation. The extent of periosteal reaction is also related to the patient's age. Since young children have a thick, active periosteum, any inciting process would cause extensive periosteal reaction. Adult patients have thin, nonactive periosteum; a large metastatic tumor may not be accompanied by a noticeable periosteal reaction.

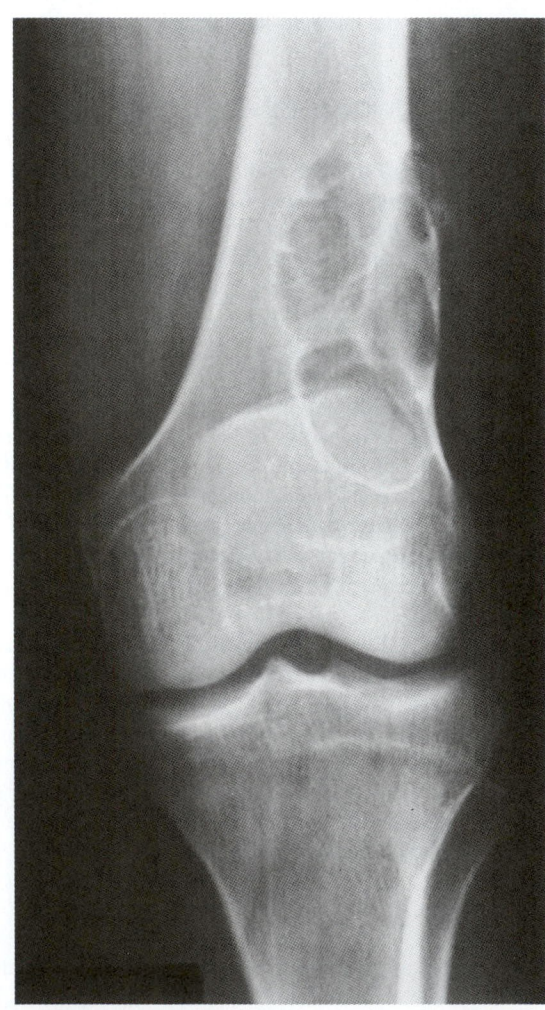

Figure 38-1

Geographic stage 1 latent lesion. Nonossifying fibroma of the distal femur. The lesion is well circumscribed by sclerotic margins.

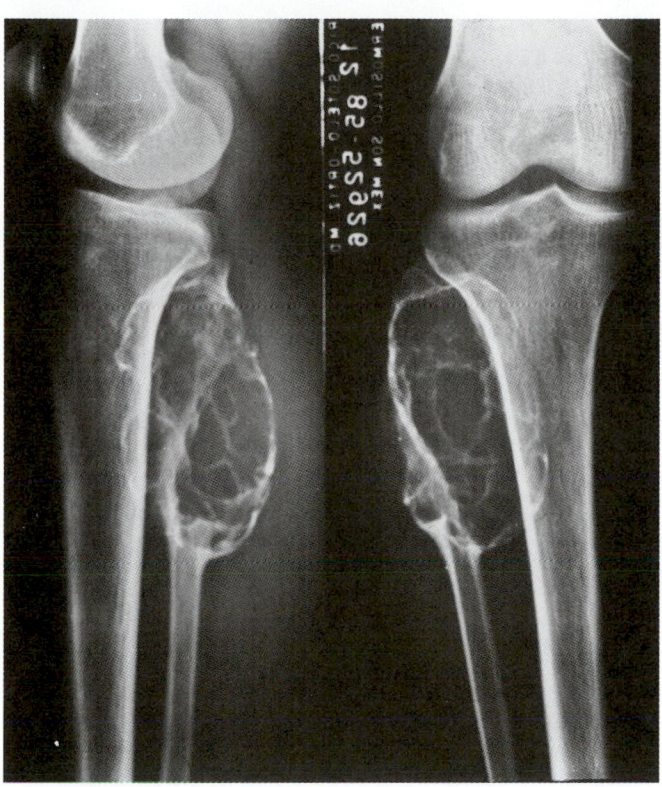

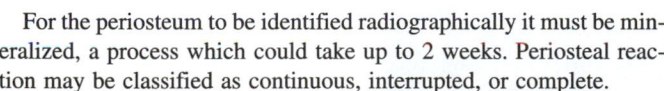

A

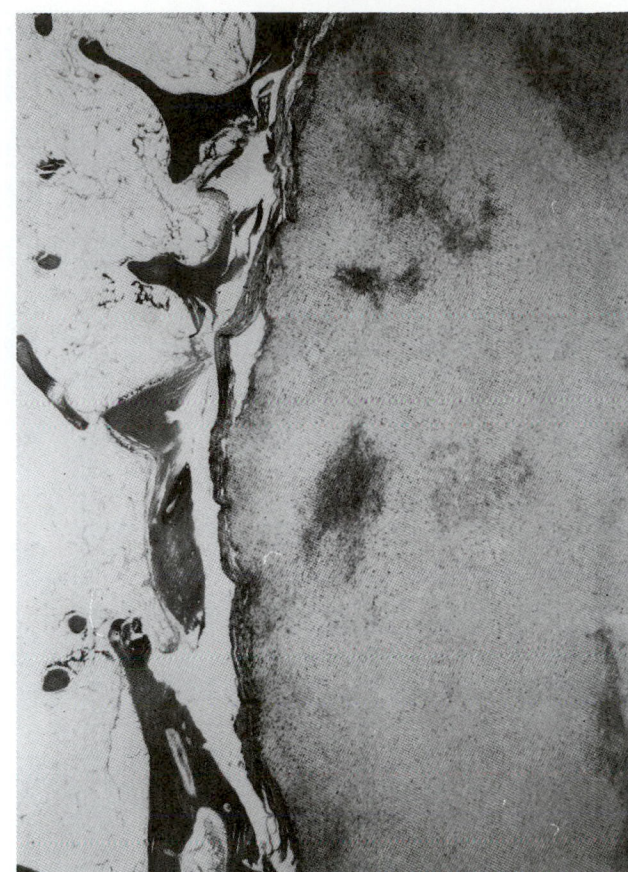

B

Figure 38-2

Geographic stage 1 latent lesion chondromyxoma fibroma of the proximal fibula demonstrating a radiolucent expansile lesion, surrounded by fine sclerotic margins (*A, left,* lateral view; *A, right,* AP view).

Histologically, a cleft space separating the lesional tissue from the sclerotic margin (*B*).

For the periosteum to be identified radiographically it must be mineralized, a process which could take up to 2 weeks. Periosteal reaction may be classified as continuous, interrupted, or complete.

Single uninterrupted lamellar reaction is seen in a biologically nonactive process such as a subperiosteal hematoma or subperiosteal abscess (Fig. 38-8). Uninterrupted multilamellar reaction is seen in biologically active processes such as eosinophilic granuloma or osteomyelitis (Fig. 38-9).

Interrupted multilamellar reaction is seen in biologically aggressive processes such as Ewing's sarcoma or osteosarcoma.

Speculated reaction (sun-burst) indicates a rapid growth of the tumor with breakthrough of the cortex into the subperiosteal space. This elevates the periosteum and stretches the perpendicular-oriented Sharpy's fibers, as can be seen in osteosarcoma and Ewing's sarcoma (Fig. 38-10).

Solid periosteal reaction represents a chronic, slow-growing biologically active process such as seen in osteoidosteoma and periosteal chondroma (Fig. 38-11). The linear radiolucent spaces between the layers are filled with dense new bone formation giving the impression of solid, thick cortical hyperostosis.

A periosteal shell and a rigess are seen in slowly growing processes where bone resorption is slower as compared to new bone formation. Widening of the cortical outline with expansion of the bone and preservation of the cortical thickness signifies a process where the endosteal bone resorption is balanced by periosteal new bone formation. Such conditions are seen in simple bone cysts and chondromyxoid fibroma (Fig. 38-2). However, the thinning of the cortical outline with expansion of the bone signifies a more aggressive process where the endosteal bone resorption exceeds periosteal new bone formation, as is seen in both aneurysmal bone cyst and giant cell tumor.

TUMOR MATRIX

Many tumors are named according to the tumor matrix that they produce. The matrix is the extracellular substance that is produced by mesenchymal cells. It may be fibrous as in fibrous dysplasia (Fig. 38-12), cartilaginous as with enchondroma (Fig. 38-13), or osteoid as in osteoid osteoma and osteosarcoma (Fig. 38-14). It should be emphasized that nonmineralized matrix is not visible on radiographs. Mineralized cartilaginous matrix can be identified by calcification.

BIOPSY

The final and definitive diagnosis is confirmed by biopsy. The biopsy is done only after a complete radiographic work-up and consideration of the definitive treatment. The biopsy site should be planned very carefully. The incision should be small, longitudinal, and re-

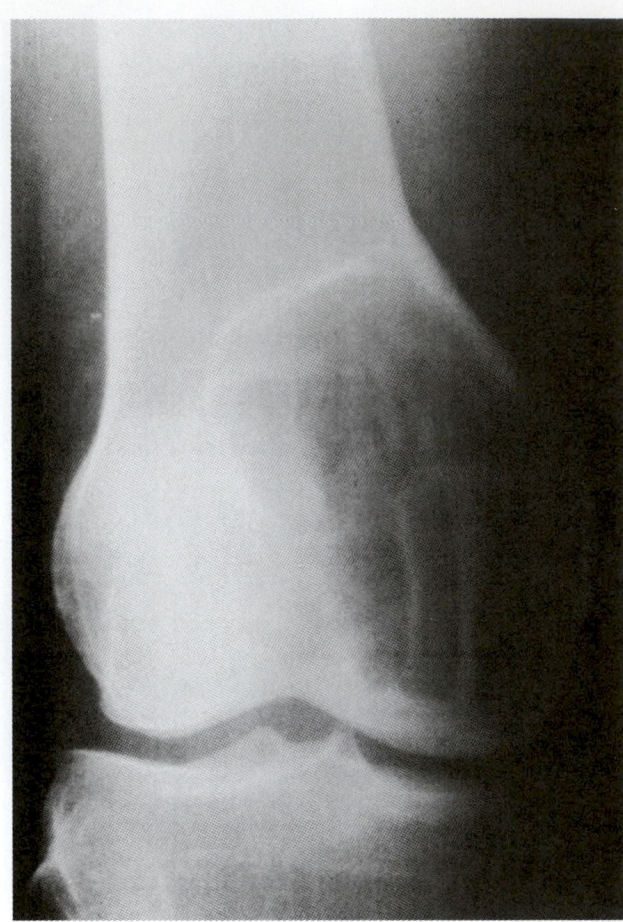

A

Figure 38-3
Geographic stage 1 lesion. 55-year-old female with a giant cell tumor
of the distal femur which is circumscribed by a fine sclerotic margin.
Such radiographic presentation is relatively rare for giant cell tumor.
(*A*) AP view. (*B*) CT.

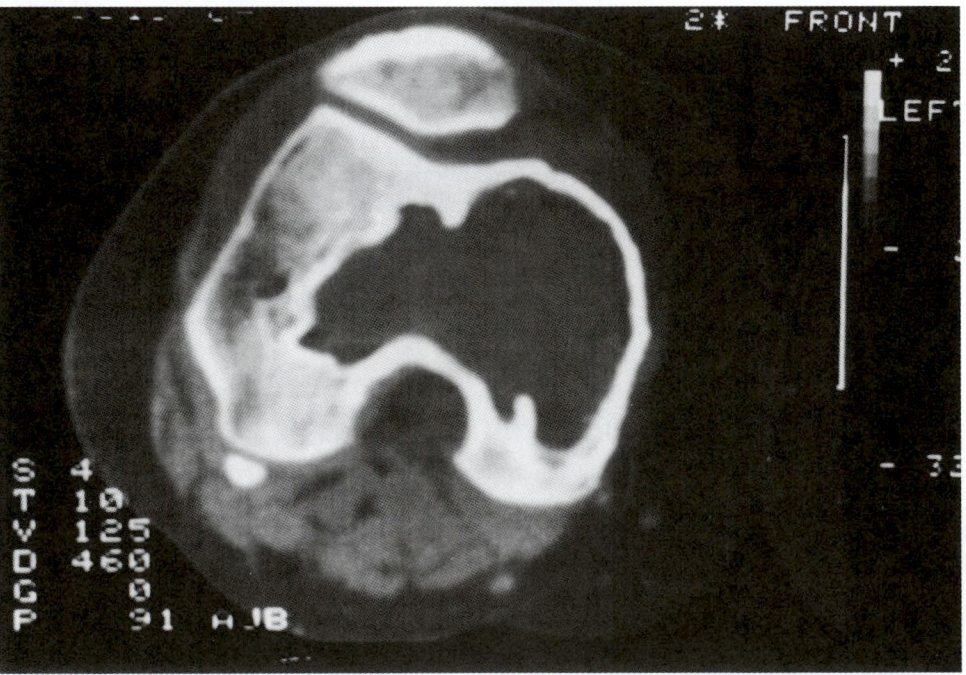

B

sectable without contamination of the surrounding tissue. Tissue samples should reflect the nature of the tumor and should be representative. A large irreversible surgical procedure based solely on the frozen section is often not recommended.

Preoperatively, the surgeon should discuss with the pathologist the medical history, and review the radiographic features. This allows the pathologist to be prepared for the frozen section and to handle the tissue in the best manner. The choice of open biopsy versus needle

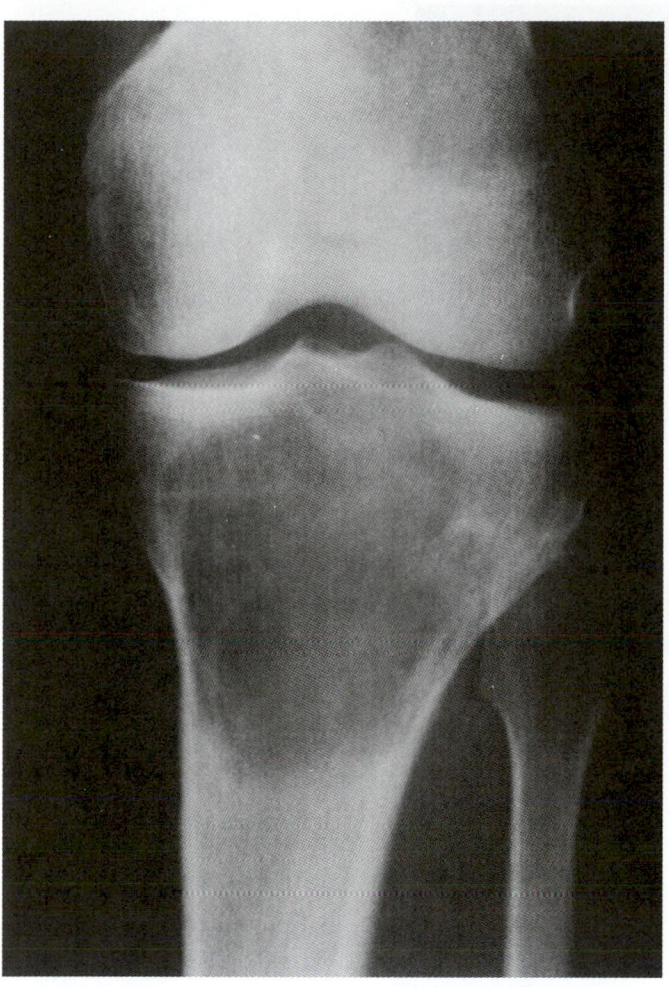

A

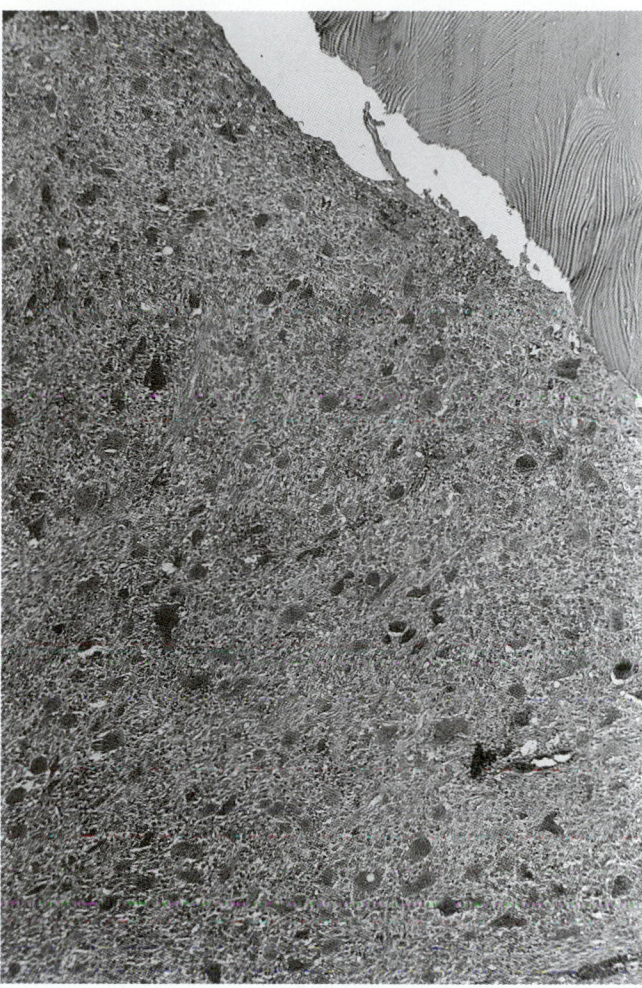

B

Figure 38-4

Geographic stage 2 active lesion. *A.* 45-year-old female with giant cell tumor of proximal tibia manifested radiographically as a radiolucent lesion with a sharp margin. *B.* Histologically, the host bone tumor interphase is sharply delineated.

biopsy depends upon the individual situation as well as the particular preference of the surgeon and pathologist.

IMAGING OF MUSCULOSKELETAL TUMORS

A variety of imaging methods are available to assist in determining or predicting the biologic activity of a tumor. If the lesion is well-circumscribed, it is generally considered lower grade or less aggressive. Alternatively, a tumor that exhibits tremendous heterogeneity, edema, and invades tissue planes is generally biologically aggressive.

RADIOGRAPHS

Several radiographic features may be seen that help predict the biologic activity and behavior of a particular lesion. Enneking has devised a system of four questions, which should be systematically addressed when characterizing a tumor based on radiographs (Table 38-2). These questions include: What is the anatomic location involved? What effect does the lesion have on the surrouding bone? What, if any, is the response of the bone to the lesion? And, what are the unique characteristics of the tumor? A lesion is referred to as geographic when bone destruction is slow. This geographic appearance may be well-defined, with an encasing rim of reactive bone, a so-called stage 1 lesion (Fig. 38-1). An example is a nonossifying fibroma. When there is a well-defined geographic appearance, but no rim of reactive bone, the lesion is referred to as a stage 2 lesion (Fig. 38-4). This radiographic appearance is indicative of ongoing bone destruction, as in a slow-growing chondroblastoma. In a stage 3 lesion, the appearance is still geographic, but the margins are even more ill-defined, as in a giant cell tumor (Fig. 38-5).

A moth-eaten appearance represents intermediate growth rate, with no clear margination of the bony lesion (Fig. 38-6). Finally, a permeative pattern of bone destruction, representative of an aggressive, high-grade lesion, occurs when lesional growth is so rapid that it invades host bone before the bone is resorbed. In these cases, the boundaries of the tumor are usually far beyond those that can be seen on radiographs. A classic example of this pattern is seen in Ewing's sarcoma and osteosarcoma.

Periosteal response also gives a clue as to the aggressiveness of the tumor. In general, absent periosteal reaction depicts a non-aggressive tumor, whereas more aggressive tumors will frequently cause

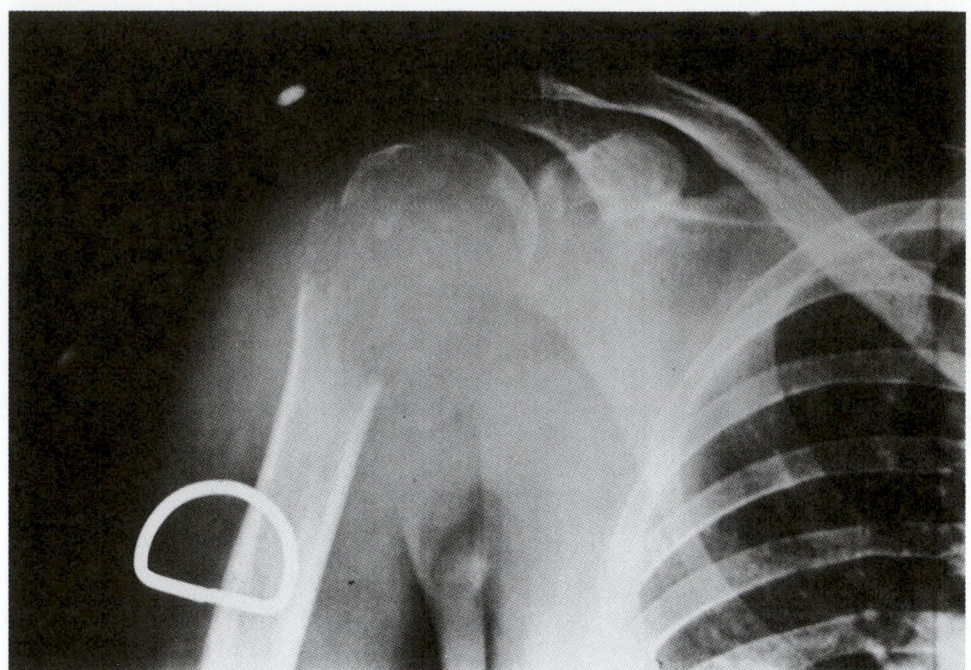

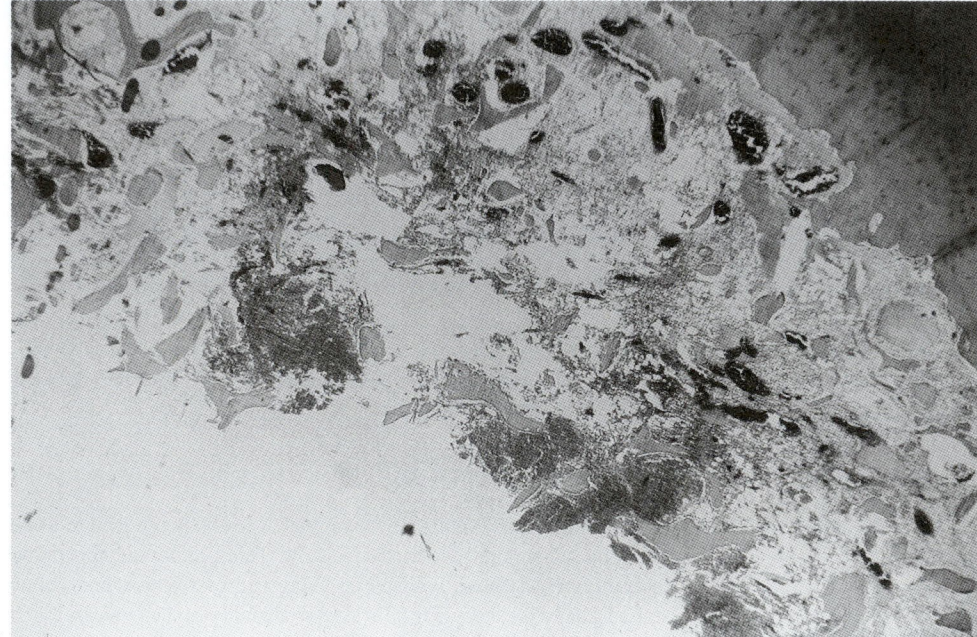

Figure 38-5
Geographic stage 3 aggressive lesion. *A.* 25-year-old male with aggressive giant cell tumor with cortical destruction and extraneous extension with pathologic fracture. *B.* Histologically, the margins are ill-defined and infiltrated with hyperemic vascular reaction.

periosteal elevation with a resultant onionskin appearance or a Codman's triangle that represent deposition of subperiosteal bone. Interrupted Codman's triangles or lamellation, or a speculated sunburst appearance (as is classically seen with osteosarcoma) is associated with a greater rate of bone destruction and aggressiveness (Fig. 38-10).

Particular tumors have specific radiographic characteristics that will be addressed later.

COMPUTED TOMOGRAPHY

Computed tomography (CT) scans are useful for demonstrating the extent of the tumor within bone and the cortical integrity. CT scans are not very effective for visualizing the soft-tissue components of the tumor, although differences in tissue densities may be evident.

TECHNETIUM 99 PYROPHOSPHATE BONE SCANS

Technetium-labeled nuclear scans are valuable for localizing tumors in bone, with the early phase of three-phase scans sometimes helping to establish the vascularity of the tumor. The bone scan is the most effective scan for identifying skeletal metastases. Certain tumors stimulate little reaction, resulting in so-called "cold" scans. These include myeloma, lymphoma, eosinophilic granuloma, and thyroid, renal, and neuroblastoma metastases.

Table 38-2

Enneking Staging System for Benign and Malignant Musculoskeletal Tumors

Stage	Characteristics		
Benign			
1 (latent)	G0	T0	M0
2 (active)	G0	T1	M0
3 (aggressive)	G0	T2	M0-M1
Malignant			
1A	G1	T1	M0
1B	G1	T2	M0
2A	G2	T1	M0
2B	G2	T2	M0
3A	G1/2	T1	M1
3B	G1/2	T1	M1

NOTE: G, Grade; G0, benign; G1, low grade malignant; G2, high grade malignant; T, site; T0, intracapsular; T1, extracapsular, intracompartmental; T2, extracapsular, extracompartmental; M, metastases; M0, none; M1, regional or distant.

MAGNETIC RESONANCE IMAGING

MRI is the most effective technique for determining the true anatomic extent of tumors, particularly in the soft tissues. Unless high in fat content, musculoskeletal neoplasms tend to be darker on T1-weighted images, because relaxation times tend to be prolonged. In T2-weighted images, tumors tend to have a higher signal intensity and appear lighter. Malignant neoplasms will often appear heterogeneous, indicative of hemorrhage and cell necrosis. Contrast enhancement (with gadolinium or other agents) will help to distinguish tumor from scar and reactive or edematous zones.

LABORATORY STUDIES

Laboratory tests may be of some value in the evaluation of musculoskeletal tumors. Erythrocyte sedimentation rate is frequently elevated in a number of neoplastic conditions but lacks the sensitivity to be considered a valuable tool. Alkaline phosphatase may be elevated in such disease states as Paget's disease and osteosarcoma. Urinary hydroxyproline levels are helpful in diagnosing Paget's disease and following the therapeutic response. Serum electrophoresis, and serum and urine immunoelectrophoresis are routine tests in diagnosing and following the course of multiple myeloma. Urinary Bence-Jones proteins are pathognomonic for myeloma. Quantitative paraprotein levels in the SPEP can be used to follow the disease.

DIAGNOSIS AND EVALUATION

ENNEKING SYSTEM

The staging system currently used by the Musculoskeletal Tumor Society for musculoskeletal lesions was developed by William Enneking. The system is based on the biologic characteristics of the neoplasm, taking into account three factors: the histologic grade of the tumor (G), its anatomic location as defined by compartmentalization (T), and the presence or absence of metastases (M) (Table 38-2). Its purpose is to promote guidelines for surgical planning and

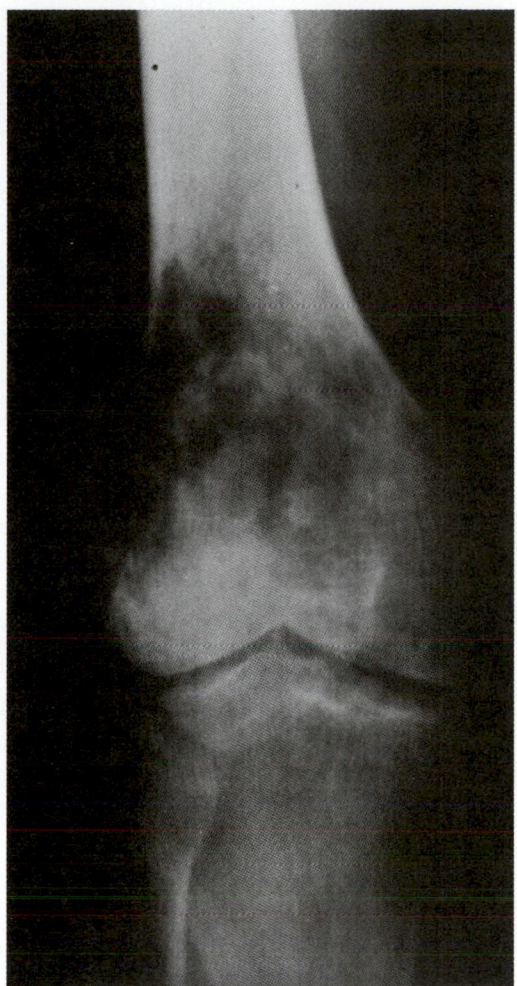

Figure 38-6
Malignant lymphoma radiographically showing "moth-eaten" destructive process.

chemotherapy, to predict prognosis, and to facilitate interdisciplinary communication.

The most important prognostic criteria is the histologic grade. All benign tumors, no matter how aggressive they may be, are classified as G0. Malignant tumors are classified as G1 for low-grade malignancies (such as parosteal osteosarcoma) or G2 for high-grade lesions (such as conventional osteosarcoma). G1 malignant tumors are classified as stage 1 lesions; G2 tumors are stage 2 lesions. G1 malignant tumor has a low rate of metastasis, less than 10 percent. G2 has a high rate of metastasis, over 50 percent.

Compartments are bounded by fascial structures or bone which act as barriers towards the spread of actively growing lesions. A combination of imaging studies, such as plain radiographs, nuclear studies, CT scan, and magnetic resonance imaging studies, are key tools in establishing the extent of anatomic involvement. Examples of compartmental barriers include the bony cortex, articular cartilage, periosteum, joint capsule, skin and subcutaneous tissue, and fascia. A T0 lesion remains intracompartmental and within its capsule. T1 lesions display extracapsular extension, but both the tumor and its surrounding reactive zone remain within the compartment of origin. T2 lesions have extracompartmental extension, either by direct tumor growth, trauma, or surgical seeding. Tumors that involve major neurovascular bundles are generally classified as T2. Malignant lesions that remain intra-

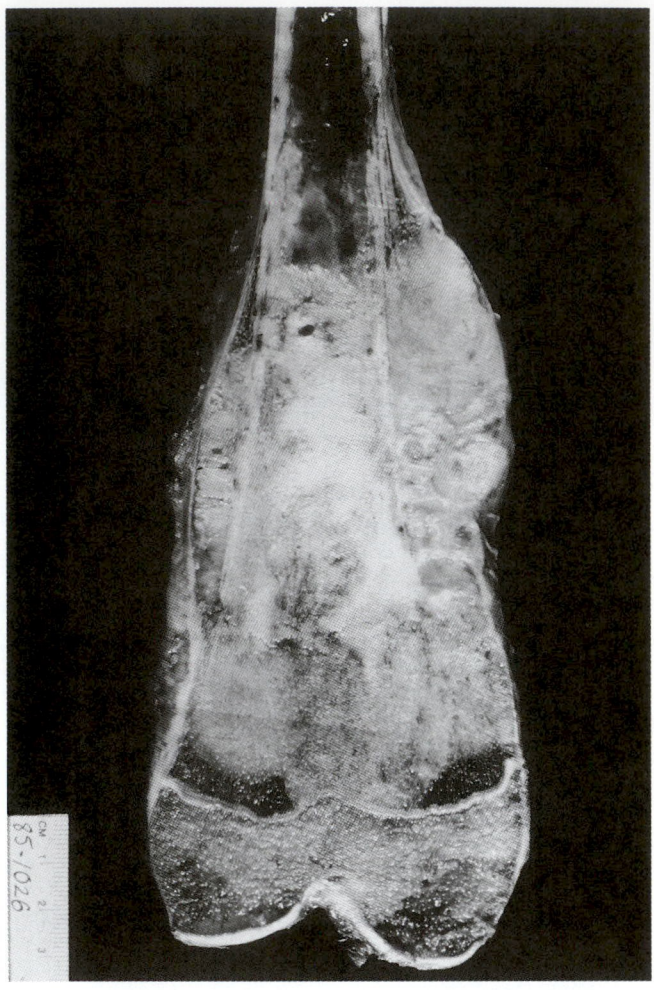

A

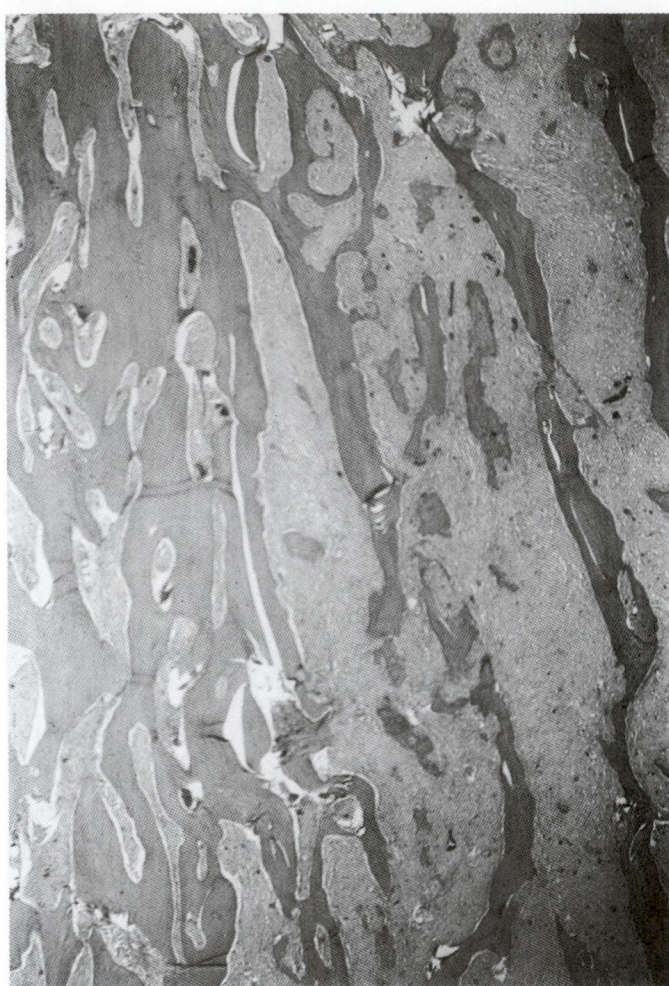

B

Figure 38-7
Osteosarcoma. The tumor permeates the cortex with extraneous extension. Specimen (*A*). Histology (*B*).

compartmental are classified as stage I-A for low-grade sarcomas and stage II-A for high-grade lesions. If they are extracompartmental, the stages are I-B or II-B for G1 and G-2 tumors, respectively.

The absence of metastases is classified as M0; regional or distant metastases qualify the lesion as M1. When patients present with metastases, they are automatically classified with Stage III disease, regardless of the histologic grading or the compartmental involvement.

The system for benign lesions characterizes tumors as latent, active, or aggressive. Stage 1 (latent) lesions are intracapsular, with a course that is considered unchanging or self-limiting (Figs. 38-1 and 38-2). They are usually diagnosed incidentally or because of a structural problem like a pathologic fracture. An example is a simple cyst in the proximal humerus. Stage 2 (active) lesions undergo slow growth and activity within the confines of the capsule. An example is a giant cell tumor that has not invaded the cortex of the distal femoral condyle (Fig. 38-4). These lesions have a 5 to 10 percent local recurrence rate after curettage. Stage 3 (aggressive) lesions undergo extracapsular penetration and may remain intracompartmental or extend extracompartmentally (Fig. 38-5). These lesions mimic low-grade malignancies in their locally aggressive behavior. An example is an aggressive giant cell tumor that has broken through the cortex, extending into the soft tissues or the joint. They are destructive processes

and recurrence rates from 10 to 20 percent after intralesional or marginal excision. Chondroblastomas and giant cell tumors have the capacity to metastasize to the lungs. In such cases, however, they are still classified as benign Stage 3 lesions.

PRINCIPLES OF INTRALESIONAL BIOPSIES

Biopsy should be considered only after a complete radiographic workup and thorough evaluation of the patient. The biopsy must be carefully planned so as not to compromise the definitive surgical procedure, if necessary. An ill-planned biopsy can jeopardize the potential for limb salvage and the overall course of the disease. Generally, the most active portion of the tumor is located peripherally; necrotic regions are centrally located. In order to best establish the type and biologic behavior of the tumor, biopsies should be representative and preferentially be taken from the periphery of the lesions, including the capsule or pseudocapsule.

Needle biopsies may be adequate for lesions that are easily diagnosed with small samples. Needle biopsy tracts must be excised at the time of definitive surgery. Open biopsies, however, are more reliable and less likely to yield inaccurate diagnoses. With the latter technique, larger amounts of tissue can be analyzed, special stains

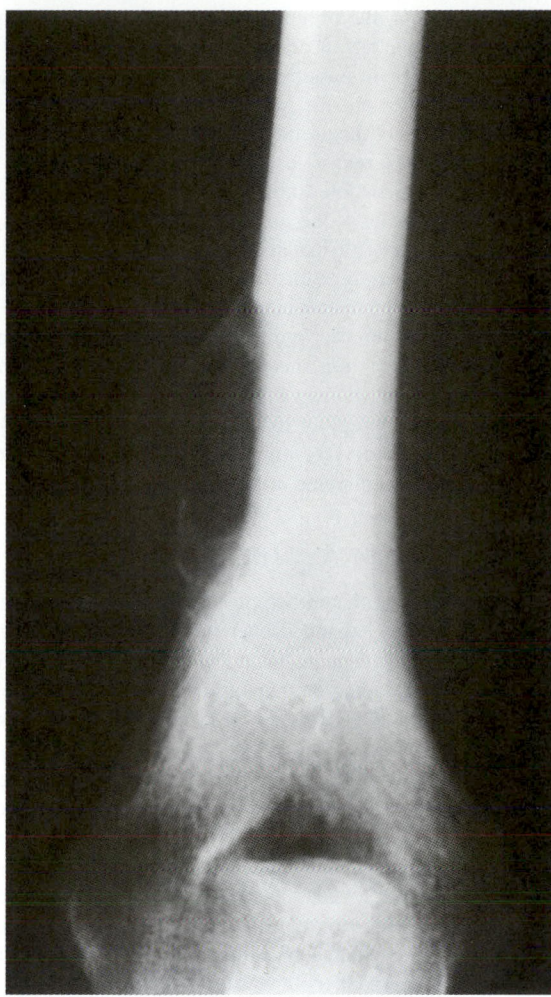

Figure 38-8
Subperiosteal hematoma of the distal humerus, surrounded by mineralized periosteal reaction.

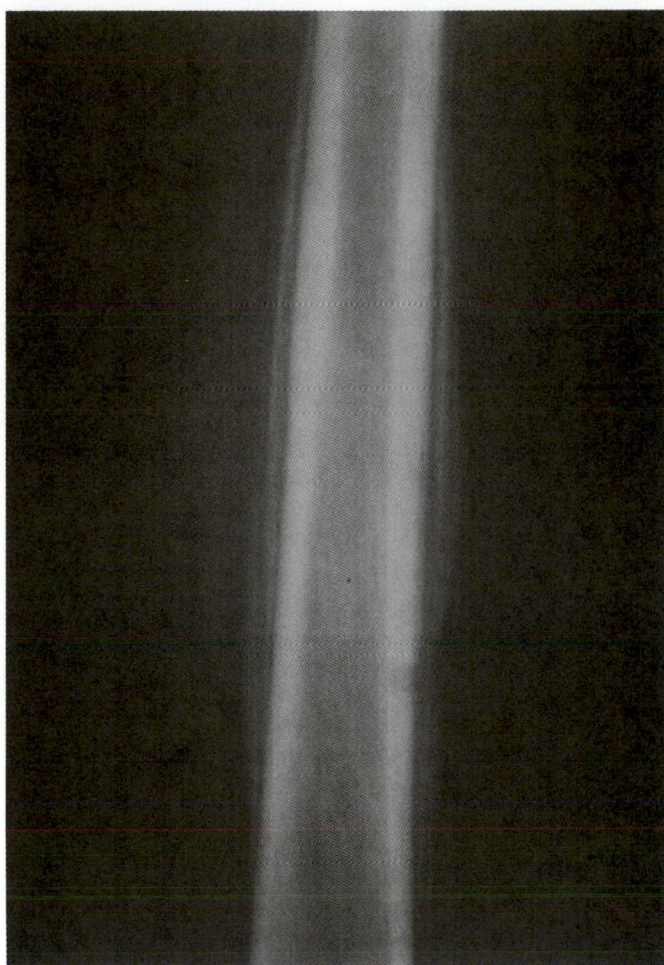

Figure 38-9
Osteomyelitis of midshaft region of femur, manifested by uninterrupted multilamellar periosteal reaction.

performed, and a more accurate assessment of biologic activity made. Frozen section analysis should be performed routinely. It serves to confirm sampling of lesional tissue and may establish an early working diagnosis. The overall accuracy of noninvasive staging studies in differentiating between benign and malignant lesions is approximately 90 percent; this increases to 97 and 99 percent for frozen and permanent section analysis, respectively. Irreversible procedures based soley on frozen section are not recommended.

Several key surgical principles must be followed when considering the biopsy of tumors. Lesions that are obviously benign and small can be excisionally biopsied; aggressive lesions, or those with uncertain diagnoses, are better suited to incisional biopsies. Open biopsies should be oriented longitudinally; the entire biopsy tract must later be excised if the lesion is malignant and definitive surgery performed. Biopsies are performed through muscle-splitting approaches without using traditional internervous planes. All biopsy samples should be sent for bacteriologic analysis. Finally, biopsy of aggressive or malignant lesions should be done at the institution where the definitive surgery is to be performed. Otherwise, surgical margins are more likely to be compromised, there will be a higher incidence of amputations of extremities that are amenable to limb salvage procedures, and misdiagnosis by nonmusculoskeletal pathologists will be higher.

TREATMENT

PRINCIPLES OF SURGICAL TREATMENT

The appropriate treatment of any musculoskeletal tumor is determined by location and Enneking stage. Regarding benign tumors, latent lesions can generally be observed, unless actual or impending pathologic fracture has occurred or neurovascular compromise by the mass developed. Active and aggressive benign bone tumors can usually be adequately treated by intralesional curettage and reconstruction with autograft, allograft, or polymethylmethacrylate. Prophylactic stabilization may be used as necessary.

The goal of treatment of musculoskeletal sarcomas is to resect the lesion and minimize the risk of local recurrence. Limb salvage, while an attractive option, should only be considered if local tumor control is at least equal to that after amputation and if the salvaged limb is functional. A variety of surgical resections exist, with variable margins, each appropriate for different tumors with different stages. There are four types of oncologic surgical procedures. (1) An *intralesional margin* is one in which tumor is removed by curettage or in a piecemeal fashion. Gross disease is frequently left in situ; therefore, this technique is generally reserved for benign lesions. (2) A *marginal zone of resection* passes through the pseudocapsule or reactive zone

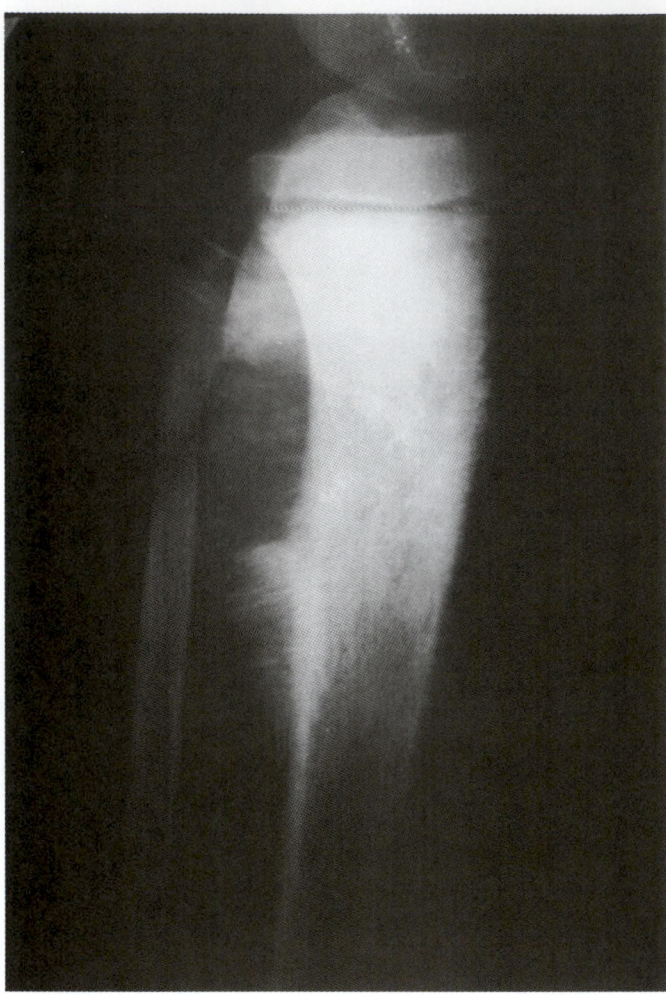

Figure 38-10
Osteosarcoma proximal tibia. Radiographically demonstrates aggressive sunburst and spiculated periosteal reaction.

of the tumor. Residual microscopic disease in the form of skip and satellite lesions may be left, accounting for a local recurrence of 25 to 50 percent in malignant tumors treated by this method. (3) A *wide surgical resection* takes out the tumor with a cuff of normal tissue beyond the boundaries of the pseudocapsule. Skip lesions may be left, but the local recurrence rate is less than 10 percent. Stages 1A and 1B tumors are most amenable to this form of treatment. (4) A *radical surgical margin* includes the tumor and the entire involved compartment, including the full extent of muscle, ligaments, and connective tissues. This margin results in complete removal of the tumor and any possible intracompartmental skip lesions. Functional limb salvage is rarely possible after radical resection. Stages 2A and 2B lesions are best treated by this method, although wide excision may be appropriate for certain tumors that have shown adequate response to neoadjuvant chemotherapy or irradiation. Stages 3A and 3B have metastases with 5-year survivorship approaching zero. Treatment of these patients should be directed at palliation.

PRINCIPLES OF ADJUVANT THERAPY

The role of multi-agent chemotherapy for the treatment of musculoskeletal sarcomas has expanded over the last decade. The appropriate utilization of these agents has allowed smaller margins of tumor resection while reducing the rate of local tumor recurrence. This in turn has improved the prospects of limb salvage and disease-free survival. Preoperative (so-called "neoadjuvant") multi-agent chemotherapy are now commonly utilized, with proven efficacy, for high-grade osteosarcoma, rhabdomyosarcoma, and Ewing's sarcoma. Most chondrosarcomas are not responsive to these agents or to irradiation. Most contemporary protocols consist of neoadjuvant chemotherapy for 8 to 12 weeks, followed by postoperative maintenance chemotherapy for up to one year. The adjunctive use of chemotherapy has improved survival in stages 2A and 2B disease to as high as 40 to 60 percent (compared to 20 percent without adjuvant therapy). In the presence of metastatic disease, chemotherapy has been shown to prolong survival times but not increase the rate of survival.

Radiation therapy has a role in the treatment of all soft tissue sarcomas, Ewing's sarcoma, myeloma, lymphoma, and metastatic disease. The radiation-induced fibrous ring that forms around soft tissue sarcomas makes this an effective adjunct to surgery for these malignancies. Local beam irradiation has limited systemic effects; however, postirradiation sarcoma (in the form of osteosarcoma, malignant fibrous histiocytoma, or fibrosarcoma) and pathologic stress fractures remain potential complications.

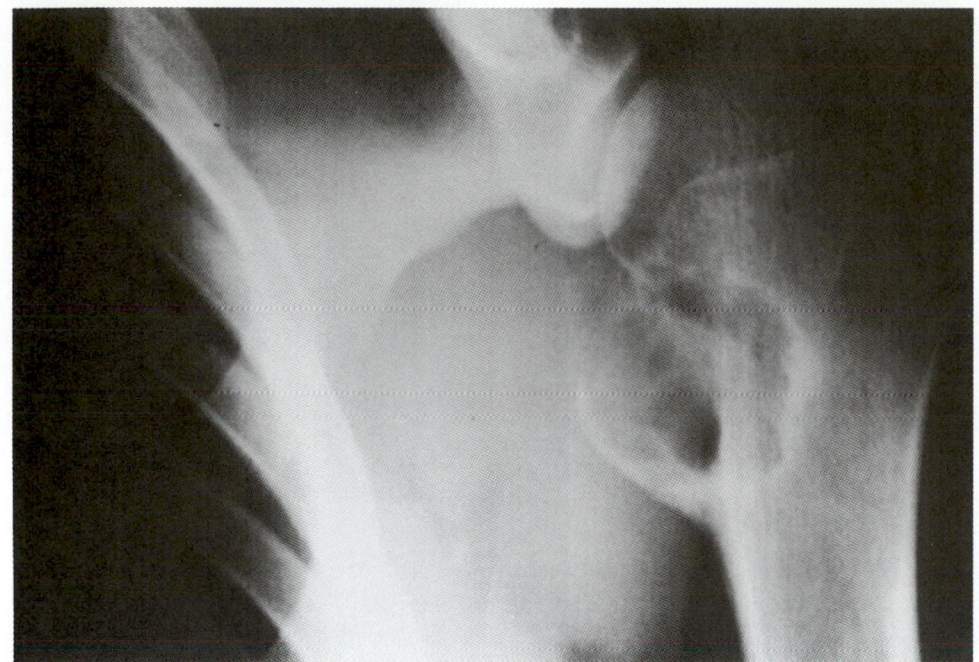

A

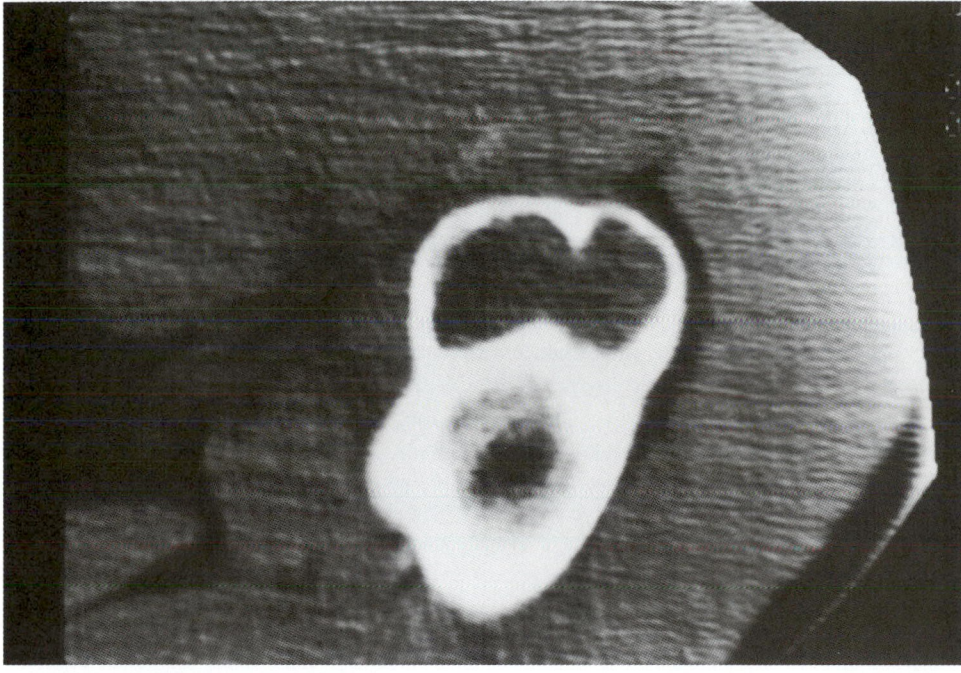

B

Figure 38-11
Periosteal chondroma. The lesion is surrounded by a buttress of solid bone formation, indicating a slow growing tumor. *A.* AP view. *B.* CT.

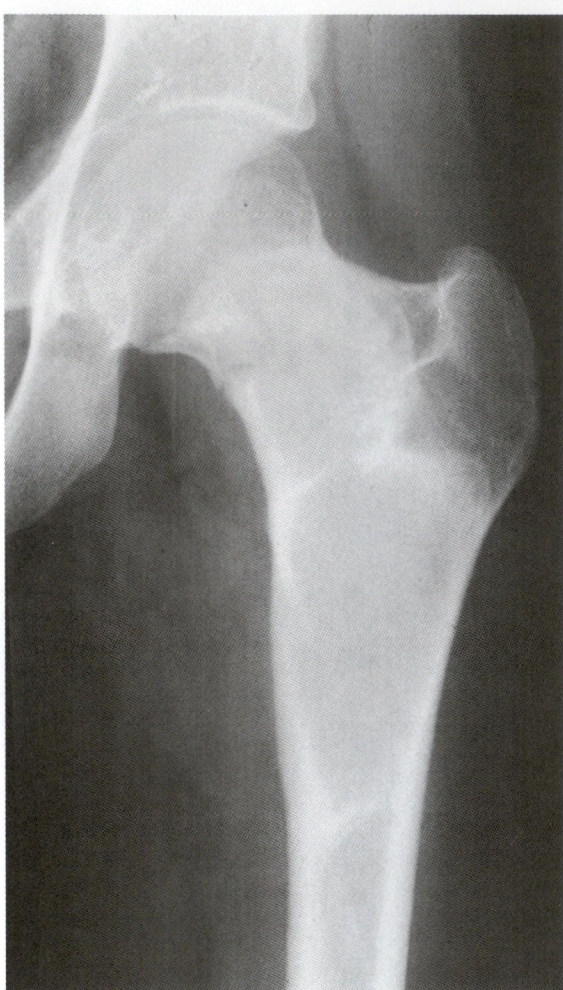

Figure 38-12
Fibrous dysplasia of proximal femur. Radiographically, the matrix demonstrates a "ground glass" appearance.

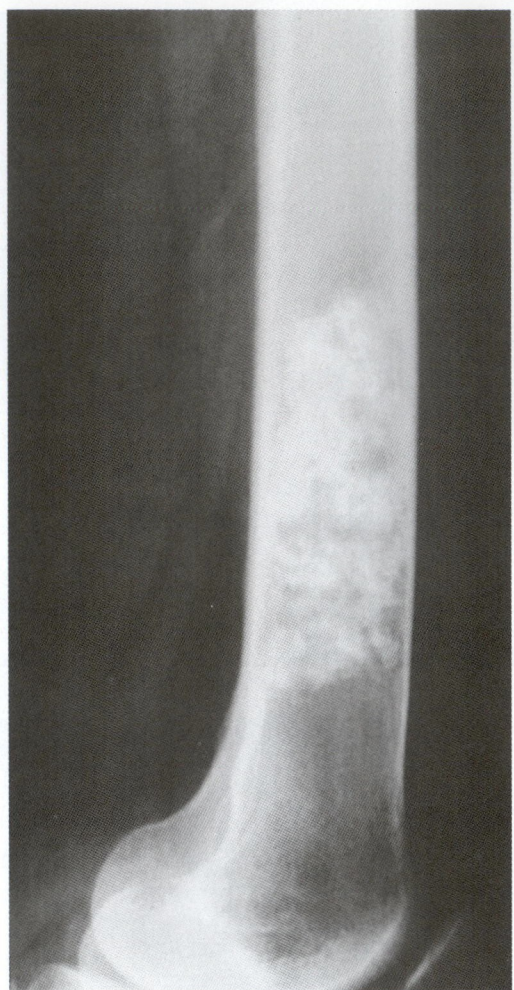

Figure 38-13
Enchondroma of distal femur. Radiographically, the matrix demonstrates popcorn calcification.

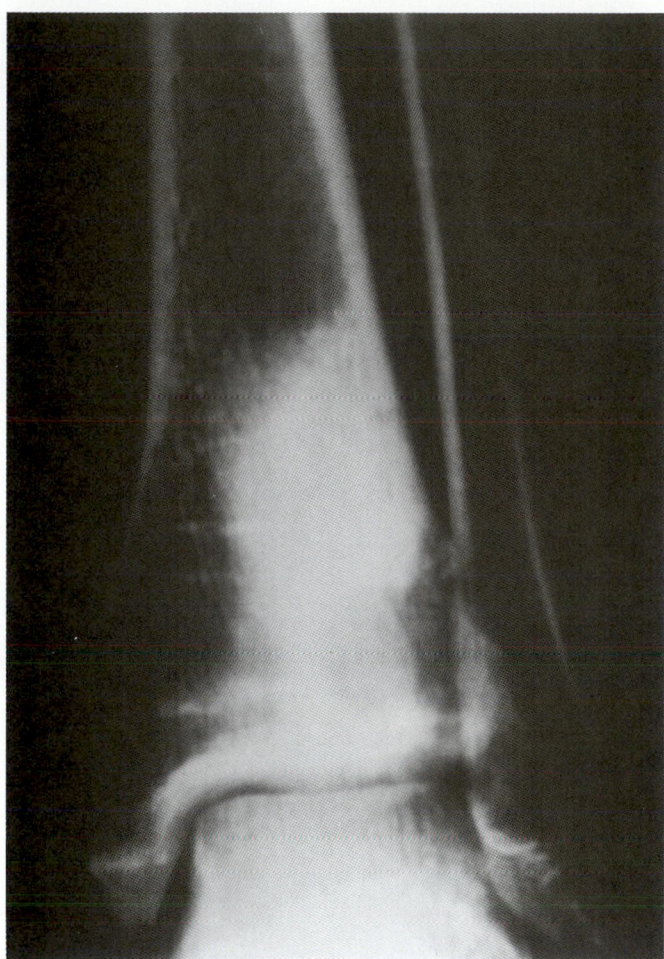

Figure 38-14
Osteosarcoma of distal tibia. The matrix demonstrates blastic neoplastic new bone formation.

SUGGESTED READINGS

Dorfman HD, Czerniak B: *Bone Tumors*. St. Louis: Mosby; 1998.

Enneking WF, Dunham W, Gebhardt MC, et al: A system for the functional evaluation of reconstructive procedures after surgical treatment of tumors of the musculoskeletal system. *Clin Orthop* 1993; 286:241.

Enneking WF, Spanier SS, Goodman MA: A system for the surgical staging of musculoskeletal sarcoma. *Clin Orthop* 1980; 153:106.

Fechner RE, Mills SE: Tumors of the bones and joints. In: *Atlas of Tumor Pathology*. Washington, DC: Armed Forces Institute of Pathology; 1993.

Holland JF, Bast RC Jr, Morton DL, et al. (eds): Principles of chemotherapy. In: *Cancer Medicine,* vol 2, 4th ed. Baltimore: Williams & Wilkins; 1997:chaps. 52–59.

Holland JF, Bast RC Jr, Morton DL, et al. (eds): Chemotherapeutic agents. In: *Cancer Medicine,* vol 2, 4th ed. Baltimore: Williams & Wilkins; 1997:chaps. 60–68.

Madewell JE, Ragsdale BD, Sweet DE: Radiologic and pathologic analysis of solitary bone lesions. Part I: Internal margins. *Radiol Clin North Am* 1981; 19:715.

Mankin HJ, Mankin CJ, Simon MA: The hazards of the biopsy, revisited. *J Bone Joint Surg [Am]* 1996; 78:656.

McDonald DJ, Capanna R, Gherlinzoni F, et al: Influence of chemotherapy on perioperative complications in limb salvage surgery for bone tumors. *Cancer* 1990; 65:1509.

Mirra JH: *Bone Tumors: Clinical, Radiographic, and Pathologic Correlations.* Philadelphia: Lea & Febiger; 1989.

Postma A, Kingma A, De Ruiter JH, et al: Quality of life in bone tumor patients comparing limb salvage and amputation of the lower extremity. *J Surg Oncol* 1992; 51:47.

Ragsdale BD, Madewell JE, Sweet DE: Radiologic and pathologic analysis of solitary bone lesions. Part II: Periosteal reactions. *Radiol Clin North Am* 1981; 19:749.

Schajowicz F: *Tumors and Tumorlike Lesions of Bone: Pathology, Radiology, and Treatment,* 2d ed. New York: Springer-Verlag; 1994.

Sim FH: *Diagnosis and Management of Metastatic Bone Disease: A Team Multidisciplinary Approach.* New York: Raven Press; 1988.

Sweet DE, Madewell JE, Ragsdale BD: Radiologic and pathologic analysis of solitary bone lesions. Part III: Matrix patterns. *Radiol Clin North Am* 1981; 19:785.

Unni KK: *Dahlin's Bone Tumors: General Aspects and Data on 11,087 Cases,* 5th ed. Philadelphia: Lippincott-Raven; 1996.

Wold LE, McLeod RA, Sim FH, et al: *Atlas of Orthopaedic Pathology.* Philadelphia: WB Saunders; 1990.

Yasko AW, Land JM: Chemotherapy for bone and soft tissue sarcomas of the extremities. *J Bone Joint Surg [Am]* 1991; 73:1263.

Chapter 39

BONE FORMING TUMORS

Jess H. Lonner, German C. Steiner, and Samuel Kenan

BENIGN TUMORS

OSTEOID OSTEOMA

This tumor is a small circumscribed osteoblastic lesion that presents most frequently in males in their second decade. The proximal femur (particularly, the femoral neck) is affected nearly 30 percent of the time, followed by the tibia, other long bones, phalanges, and spine, although any bone may be involved.

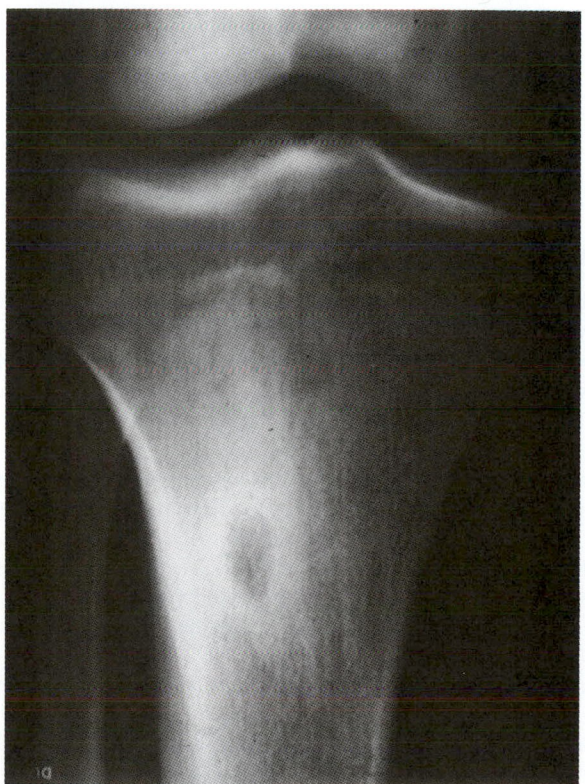

Figure 39-1
Osteoid osteoma of the proximal tibia in a 25-year-old male who complained of knee pain for 3 years. Radiograph shows a small, ill-defined lucency with peripheral sclerosis.

Symptoms are classic, with dull pain that is worse at night, relieved with salicylates in most cases. If the lesion is in a vertebrae, the patient may present with painful scoliosis; if in the appendicular skeleton, subcutaneous swelling and a limp may be noted.

Radiographically, a lucent "nidus" surrounded by dense reactive bone is characteristic. The lesion is generally less than 1 cm in diameter. At times, a central ossified lesion may be present. (Figs. 39-1 and 39-2)

Grossly the nidus is red in color, with a granular texture. The nidus may be difficult to see, but in some cases, preoperative labeling with oral tetracycline shows fluorescence of the nidus under ultraviolet light. Histologically, haphazardly arranged, thin osteoid trabeculae with varying degrees of mineralization comprise the nidus. The trabeculae are lined by uniform osteoblasts and surrounded by fibrovascular connective tissue with scattered multinucleated giant cells (Fig. 39-3). The nidus is clearly delineated from the surrounding reactive bone.

Surgical resection is the recommended treatment. CT localization, intraoperative radiographs, and tetracycline labeling are helpful aids for ensuring removal of the tumor.

OSTEOBLASTOMA

This tumor occurs most commonly in males in their second decade. It is less frequent and larger in size than osteoid osteoma. The posterior spinal elements are most frequently involved, but sporadic long bone involvement is often seen. Long-standing pain, localized to the affected area, is the typical presenting symptom. A painful scoliosis may be present in the setting of spinal involvement.

The radiographic appearance of osteoblastomas may be quite variable and nonspecific. They often look like large osteoid osteomas, more than 2 centimeters in diameter; 50 percent of tumors are radiodense. Posterior spinal elements may be expanded by the tumor (Fig. 39-4).

Grossly, the tissue is hemorrhagic, reddish, and granular, with well-defined reactive rims. Histologically, the lesion is characterized by irregularly arranged trabeculae of osteoid and woven bone, similar to the nidus of osteoid osteoma. However, in osteoblastoma, the trabeculae are less organized and mineralized than osteoid osteoma and the tumor is more cellular and more vascular (Fig. 39-5).

Treatment generally includes curettage and grafting. Care must obviously be taken in treating lesions of the spine to preserve nerve roots and maintain stability.

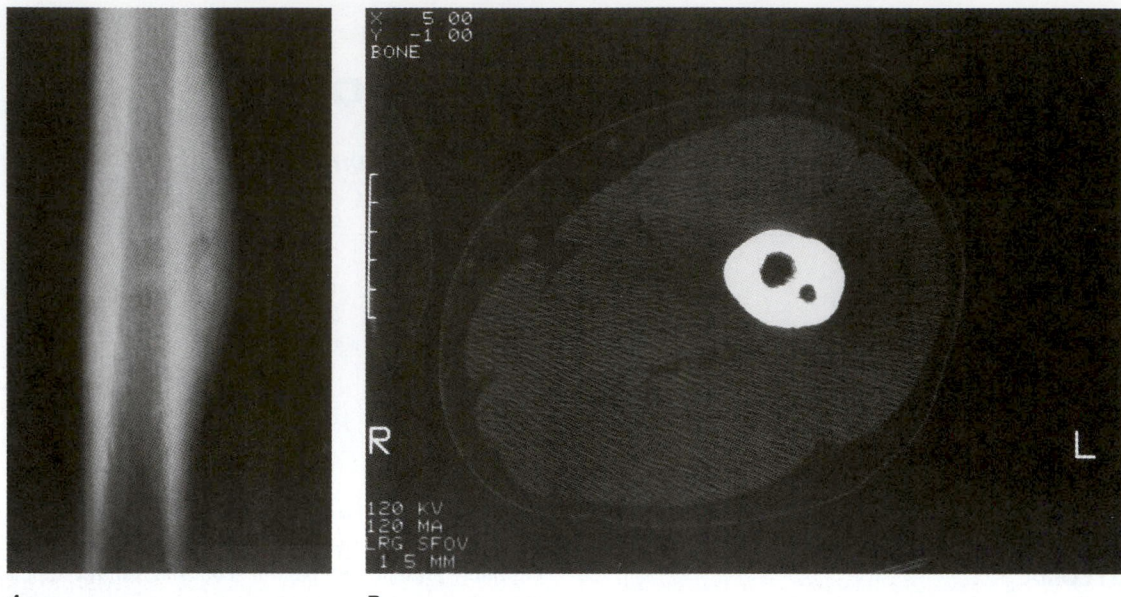

Figure 39-2

Osteoid osteoma of the shaft of the femur. Radiograph (*A*) reveals an area of cortical thickening with a small radiolucent center. The intra-cortical nidus is well demonstrated in the CAT scan (*B*).

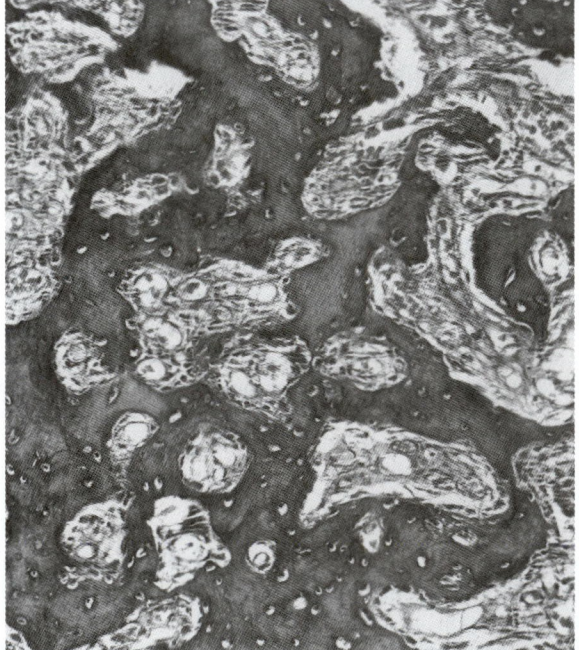

Figure 39-3

Osteoid osteoma. It consists of a rather organized pattern of trabeculae of woven bone separated by a fibrovascular stroma. The trabeculae are lined by osteoblasts.

MALIGNANT TUMORS

OSTEOSARCOMA (CONVENTIONAL)

Excluding multiple myeloma, osteosarcoma is the most common primary malignant bone tumor. It is most frequent in children and adolescents, usually afflicting those in the second decade of life. Males are slightly more affected than females, in a ratio of approximately 1.4:1. The distal femur and proximal tibia are the most common sites, followed by proximal humerus.

Pain and swelling of short duration are the most frequent presenting symptoms. On examination a tender mass may be obvious due to soft tissue tumor extension. Characteristically, these lesions have a predilection for the long bone metaphyses. The radiographic appearance of this tumor is diagnostic in the majority of the cases. It is usually a metaphyseal medullary lesion that often extends to the soft tissues. The tumor shows frequent mineralization including the soft tissue component. Trabecular and cortical bone destruction is common, the tumor frequently poorly circumscribed, and periosteal elevation on a bed of new bone takes on a characteristic appearance, known as the *Codman's triangle* (Figs. 39-6 and 39-7). Rarely, osteosarcomas can be multicentric.

Grossly, the tumor occupies the medullary cavity, but usually has violated the bony cortex and a soft tissue mass is present. It has a gritty consistency, owing to its osseous components; areas of necrosis and hemorrhage account for softer areas. Skip lesions occur in a very small percentage of cases. Histologically, the main feature of

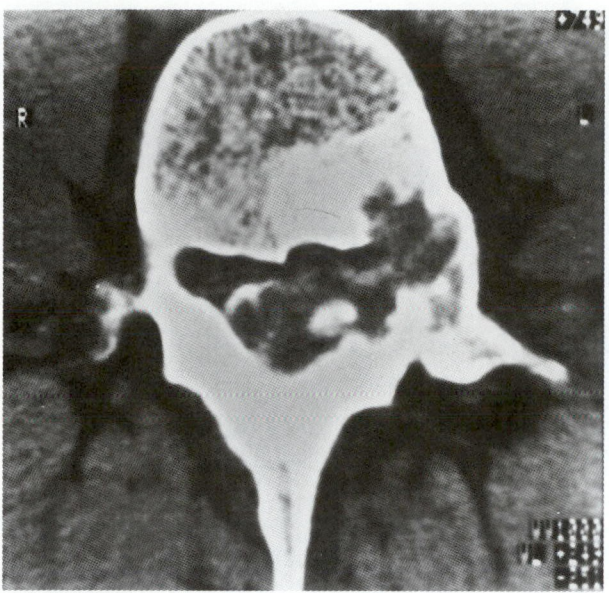

Figure 39-4
Osteoblastoma of the 4th lumbar vertebra in a 24-year-old male who complained of back pain for 3 years. CAT scan reveals a focally calcified tumor involving the spinal canal and destroying part of the vertebral body and posterior elements, with reactive sclerosis.

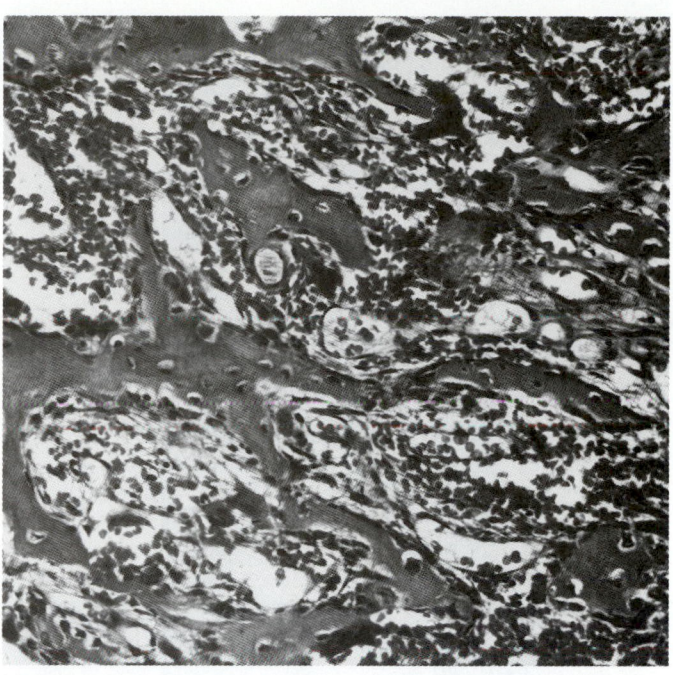

Figure 39-5
Osteoblastoma. It consists of trabeculae of woven bone that are loosely arranged in a cellular fibrovascular stroma. There is focal mineralization of the bone and prominent osteoblastic and osteoclastic activity.

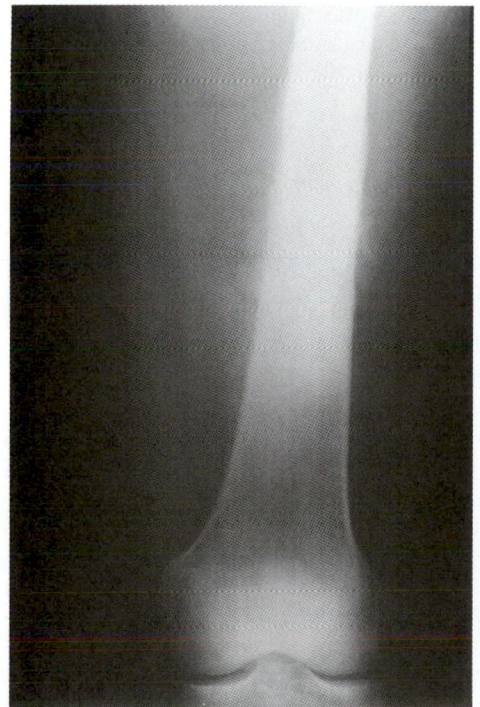

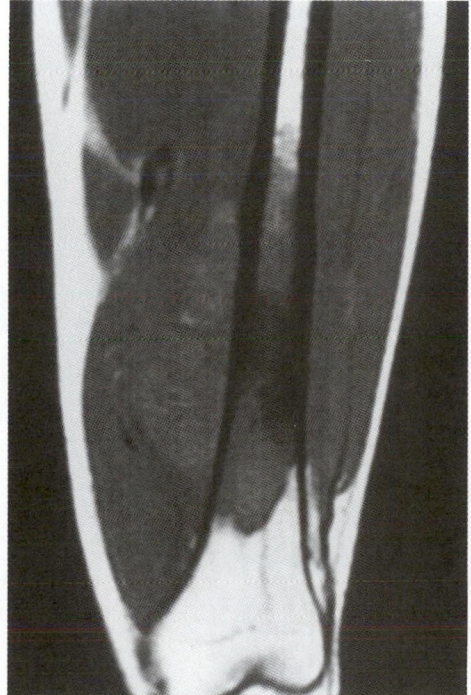

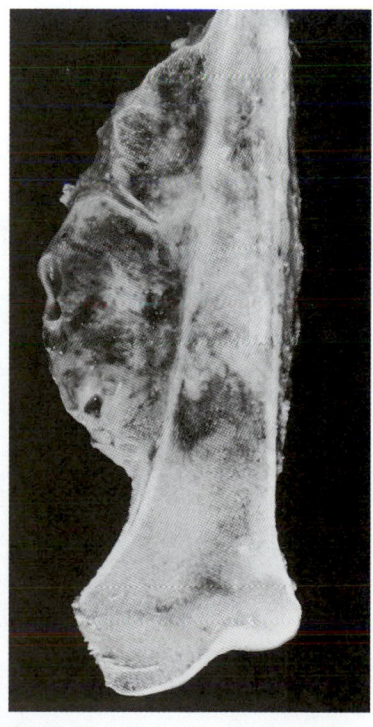

A   *B*   *C*

Figure 39-6
Osteosarcoma of the distal shaft of the femur in an 18-year-old male. Pretreatment radiograph (*A*) shows increased density in the medullary cavity of the femur, associated with a radiodense soft tissue mass, periosteal reaction, and a Codman triangle. *B*. MRI demonstrates the extent of medullary and soft tissue involvement. *C*. Photograph of resected specimen obtained after chemotherapy treatment. Although the tumor showed no apparent decrease in size, there was good chemotherapy response with more than 90 percent of tumor necrosis.

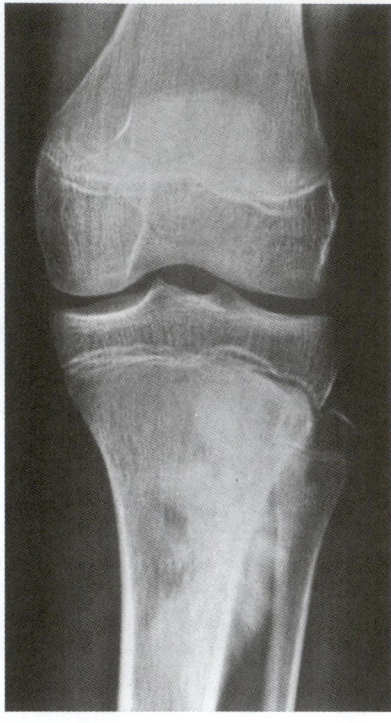

Figure 39-7
Radiograph of osteosarcoma of proximal tibia. The tumor shows increase medullary density with extension into the soft tissues.

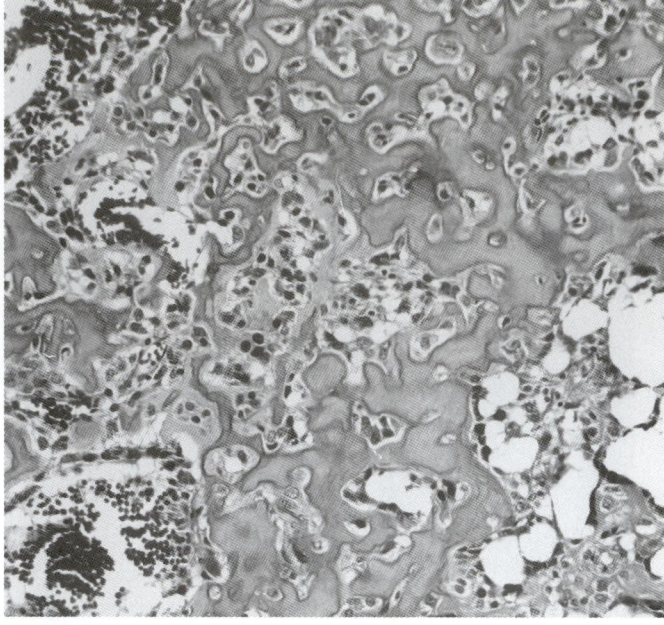

Figure 39-8
Photomicrograph of osteosarcoma. It consists of tumor osteoid and bone in a lacelike pattern around tumor cells.

osteosarcoma is the presence of malignant osteoid and woven bone. The tumor cells are ovoid to spindle-shaped, with marked pleomorphism, hyperchromatic nuclei, and mitotic figures. The tumor is generally hypercellular (Figs. 39-8 and 39-9). In areas containing neoplastic bone, the tumor cells in the bone are small with minimal pleomorphism. Besides the osteoblastic component, chondroblastic and fibroblastic components may be present (Fig. 39-10).

On rare occasions, medullary osteosarcoma consists of small round cells mimicking Ewing's sarcoma, and is designated as small cell osteosarcoma.

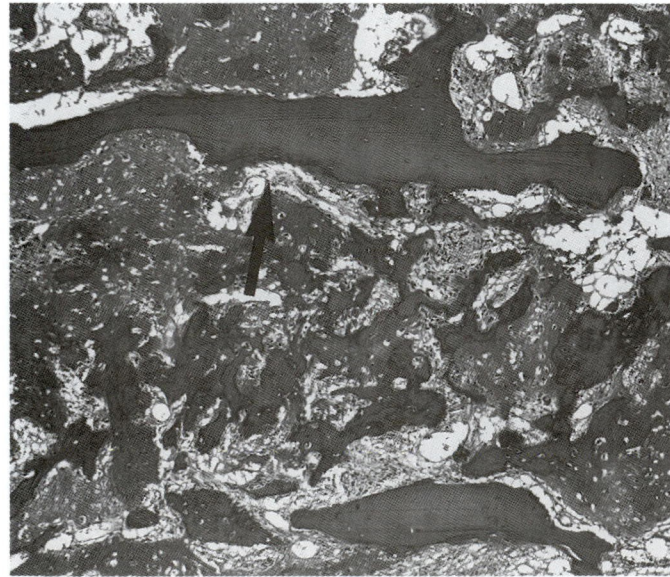

Figure 39-9
The tumor is infiltrating into the marrow spaces between preexisting cancellous bone (*arrow*).

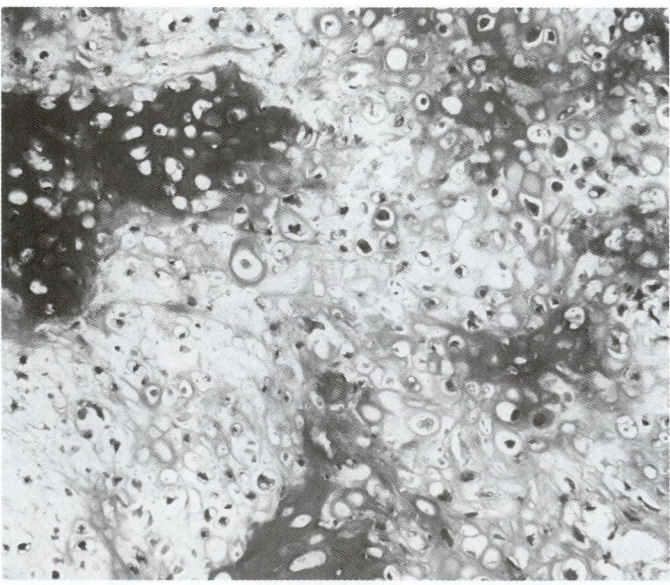

Figure 39-10
Chondroblastic component of osteosarcoma. Other areas of the tumor contained malignant bone formation.

Preoperative chemotherapy and tumor ablation by radical resection in the form of amputation or limb-salvage with wide margins are the recommended treatment options. In the event that limb salvage is a feasible option, limb reconstruction with a custom joint prosthesis, osteochondral allograft, or resection arthrodesis may be considered depending on the remaining bone stock and patient needs. Limb salvage is not an option in the setting of neurovascular involvement, pathologic fractures, infection, or extensive soft tissue involvement. Preoperative chemotherapy may cause up to 100 percent tumor necrosis as demonstrated by histologic examination of the resected specimen, enhancing survival and improving the outcome after limb-sparing surgery. The 5-year survival rate is more than 50 percent, particularly in patients who have at least 90 percent of histologic evidence of tumor necrosis. Unfortunately, even in the most responsive tumors, recurrence after limb salvage is approximately 6 percent.

Osteosarcoma can occur secondary to pre-existing bone disorders such as Paget's disease, bone infarct, and irradiated bone. The patients are usually older than 50 years and the prognosis in general is worse than primary osteosarcoma. For further comments on this subject, see Chap. 47.

TELANGIECTATIC OSTEOSARCOMA

It is a rare variant of osteosarcoma, accounting for less than 5 percent of all osteosarcomas. This tumor has a similar age and site predilection as the conventional osteosarcoma, and often presents in a similar fashion. Unlike the former, this tumor is purely lytic, with considerable medullary and cortical bone destruction and ill-defined margins (Fig. 39-11). Lesional tissue is hemorrhagic with extensive blood clot. Histologically, osteoid production is limited and focal. Blood-filled sinuses and multinucleated giant cells give this an appearance that may be confused with an aneurysmal bone cyst; however, malignant pleomorphic cells are seen within the cellular septa and cystic walls. Treatment is like that for conventional osteosarcomas. The use of preoperative chemotherapy has substantially improved the prognosis of this tumor, which now is similar to conventional osteosarcoma.

LOW-GRADE CENTRAL OSTEOSARCOMA

This rare tumor has been identified in recent years and accounts for 1 to 2 percent of all osteosarcomas. Unlike the above-mentioned osteosarcomas, this tumor typically is not associated with swelling or focal signs other than pain. Radiographically and histologically, it is frequently difficult to determine whether the tumor is benign or malignant. These are medullary lesions, tend to be large and sclerotic, and often extend to the bone ends (Fig. 39-12).

While the tumor is usually confined to the intramedullary cavity, focal areas of cortical disruption may be seen without local soft tissue invasion. Grossly, these lesions tend to be gritty. Histologically, these tumors are often indistinguishable from parosteal osteosarcoma, as the bone trabecula are well organized and the spindle cells show little pleomorphism, mitotic activity, or anaplasia (Fig. 39-13). Other cases resemble fibrous dysplasia.

Treatment should include wide surgical resection. Adequate surgical margin is associated with a less than 10 percent recurrence rate. Because it is difficult to distinguish from fibrous dysplasia, these tumors are frequently treated inadequately, accounting for multiple recurrences and biopsies. Following recurrence, some of these tumors may transform into high-grade osteosarcoma.

SURFACE BONE FORMING TUMORS

Parosteal Osteosarcoma

This tumor arises from the external surface of a bone, occurs most commonly in the third decade of life, and involves the distal posterior femur in approximately 70 percent of cases. It usually presents as a painless mass behind the knee and is frequently present for several years. Radiographically, these are lobulated radiodense lesions with broad-based origins off the metaphyseal cortex and have no continuity with the medullary cavity (Fig. 39-14). Larger tumors may encircle the bone.

Microscopically, it is a low-grade malignant tumor. Osteoid and woven trabeculae are separated by intervening fibroblastic stroma with minimal cytologic atypia. The bony trabeculae may undergo lamellar transformation and appear like normal bone (Fig. 39-15). A cartilaginous cap may be present, giving it the appearance of an osteochondroma.

Wide surgical resection provides good local control. The prognosis is excellent, with a 5-year survival rate of more than 80 percent, and metastases are rare. Neither adjuvant chemotherapy or radiotherapy are necessary for the typical lesions; however, for the more rare aggressive variant, the so-called dedifferentiated parosteal osteosarcoma, multi-agent adjuvant chemotherapy is an important component of treatment.

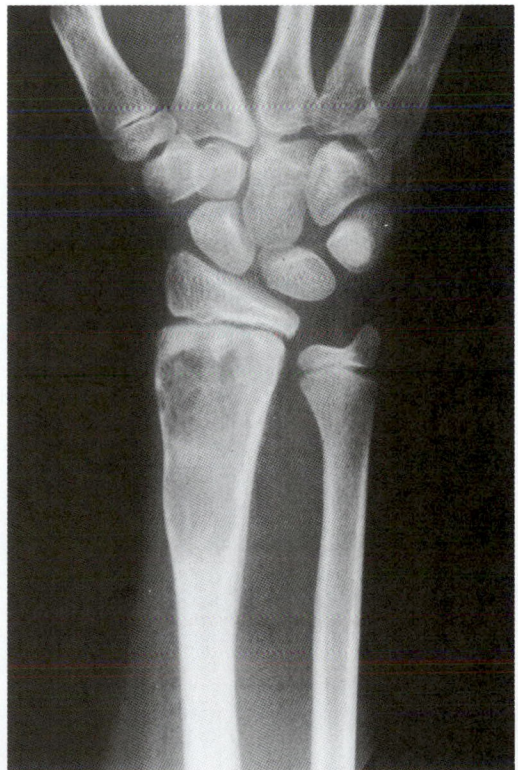

Figure 39-11
Telangiectatic osteosarcoma of the distal radius in a 10-year-old girl, with pain in the forearm of short duration. At the time of surgery, a cavity was found containing blood and scanty amount of tissue. This tumor can be mistaken for an aneurysmal bone cyst.

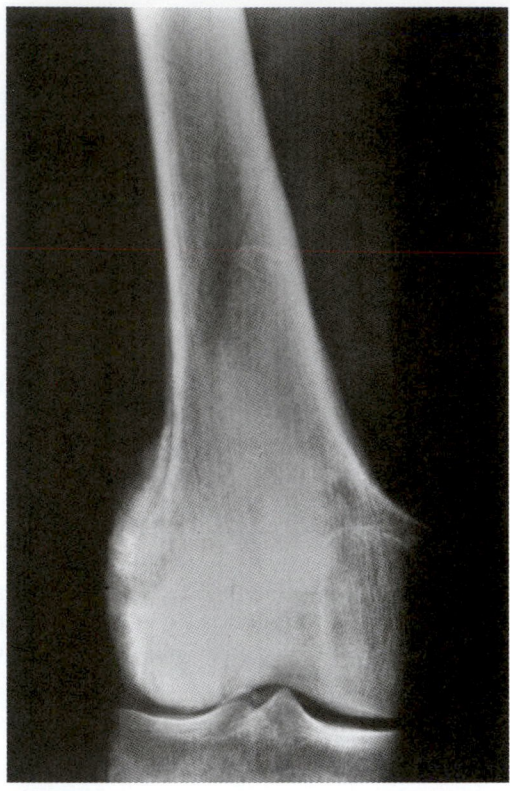

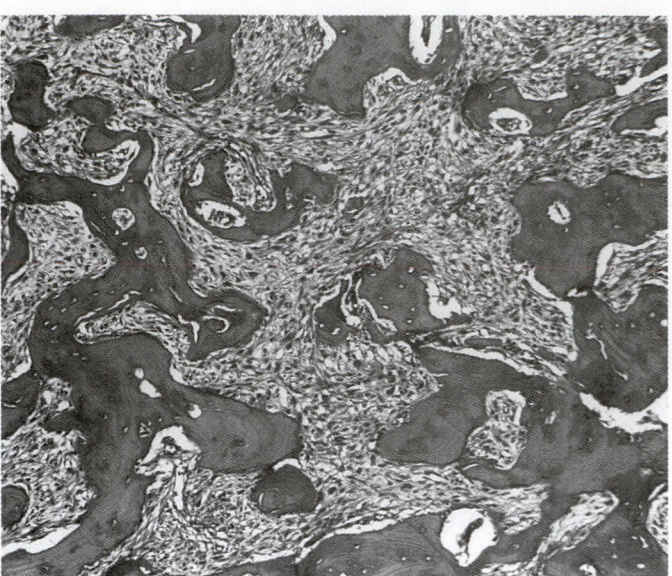

Figure 39-13
Photomicrograph showing well-organized, mostly lamellar trabecular bone, separated by a spindle stroma with little pleomorphism. This lesion can be misinterpreted for fibrous dysplasia.

Figure 39-12
Low-grade surface osteosarcoma in a 26-year-old male who complained of right knee pain for 10 months. Radiograph shows an ill-defined intramedullary density in the distal femur, associated with cortical destruction and periosteal reaction.

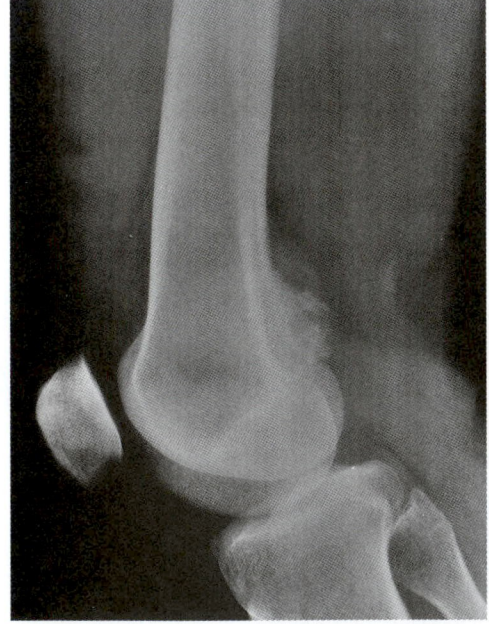

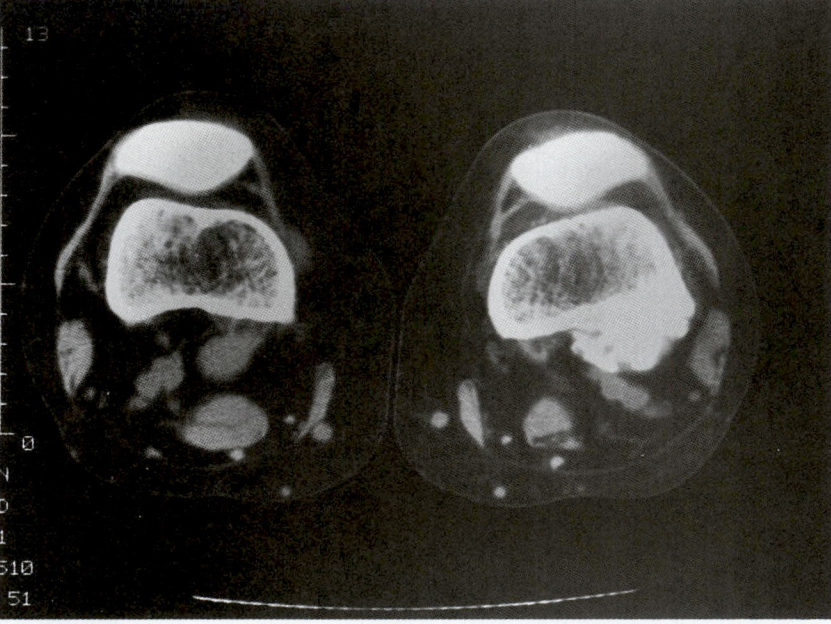

A   *B*

Figure 39-14
A. Radiograph of parosteal osteosarcoma in a 35-year-old female. A radiodense mass is seen in the distal femur, attached to the posterior cortex. *B.* CAT scan shows the cortical origin of the tumor.

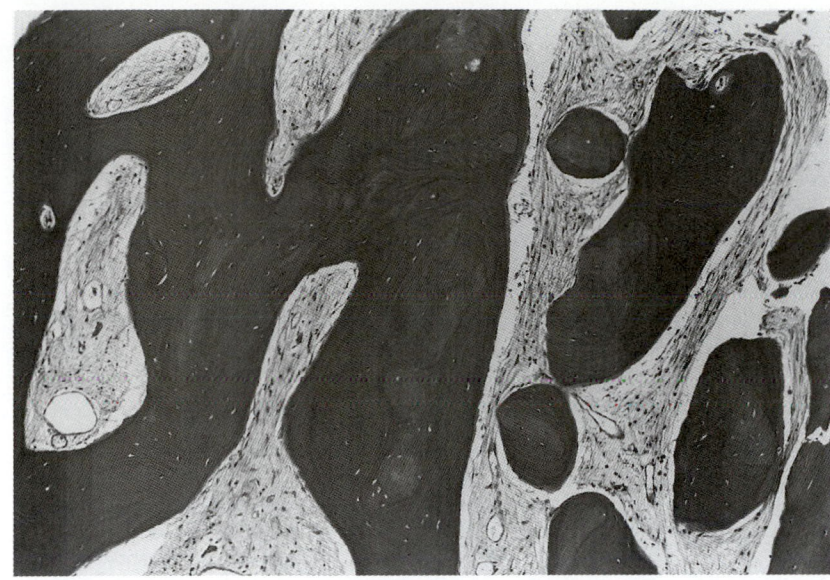

Figure 39-15
Parosteal osteosarcoma. Photomicrograph shows well-organized trabecular bone separated by a stroma composed of small fibroblasts. There is mild cell pleomorphism and atypia.

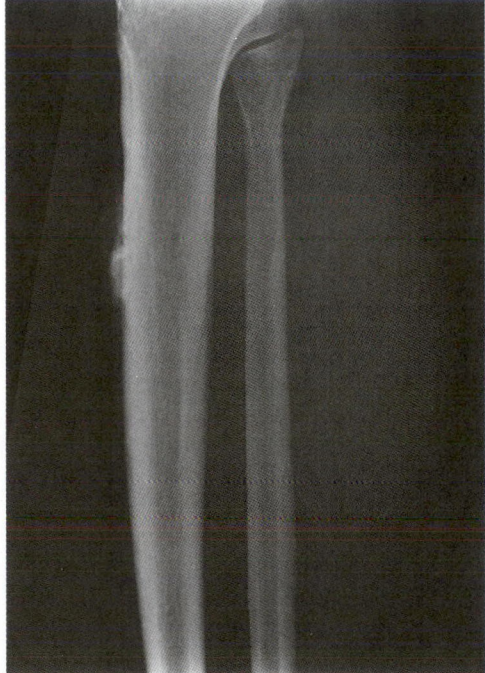

Figure 39-16
Periosteal osteosarcoma. Twenty-nine-year-old female with a painful mass in the tibia of 6 months' duration. Radiograph demonstrates a lesion in the anterior cortex of the tibia, with irregular mineralization.

Periosteal Osteosarcoma

This neoplasm has a peak incidence in the second decade, occurring most commonly on the diaphysis of the tibia and femur. It generally presents as a painful mass. Radiographically, it is characterized as an ill-defined diaphyseal surface lesion with variable matrix mineralization, with a "scooped-out" appearance. Perpendicular spicules of bone may be seen (creating a characteristic "sunburst" appearance), as well as periosteal reaction and a Codman's triangle. Usually, no marrow involvement is present (Fig. 39-16).

Histologically, these tumors show a predominant cartilaginous component with neoplastic osteoid production. The tumor is lobulated, with peripheral condensations of spindle cells that gives it a well-circumscribed appearance. The malignant chondroid and osteoid cells show a moderate degree of differentiation (Fig. 39-17). Treatment involves wide surgical resection, with neoadjuvant chemotherapy.

Of the surface tumors, periosteal osteosarcoma shows intermediate degree of malignancy between the low-grade malignant parosteal osteosarcoma and high-grade surface osteosarcoma.

High-Grade Surface Osteosarcoma

This rare tumor seems to peak in the second decade. It generally presents as a painful mass; the skin may be warm and erythematous. It is highly aggressive. Radiographically, it is marked by a poorly defined surface origin on long bones (usually the femur), cortical destruction, and reactive bone formation. There is no significant intramedullary involvement (Fig. 39-18). Histologically, it looks like conventional osteosarcoma, with marked cellular and nuclear pleomorphism and anaplasia with brisk mitotic activity. Lacelike osteoid and neoplastic production is identifiable, with varying degrees of chondroid and spindle cell formation. Treatment is similar to conventional osteosarcoma, with wide surgical resection or amputation and adjuvant chemotherapy.

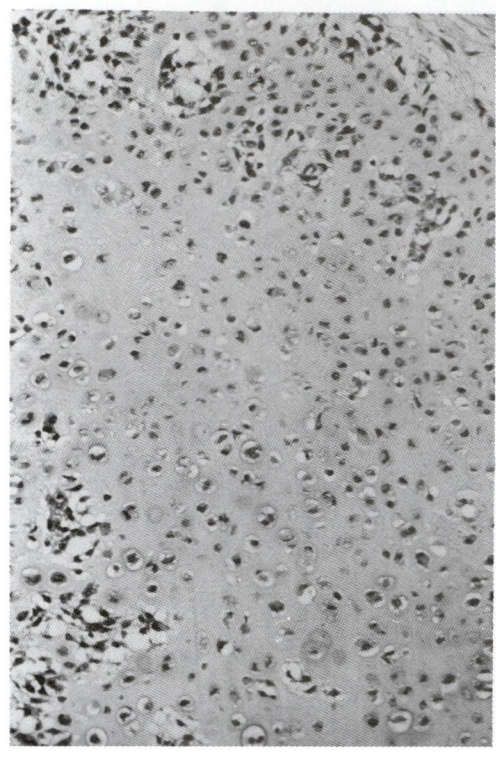

A

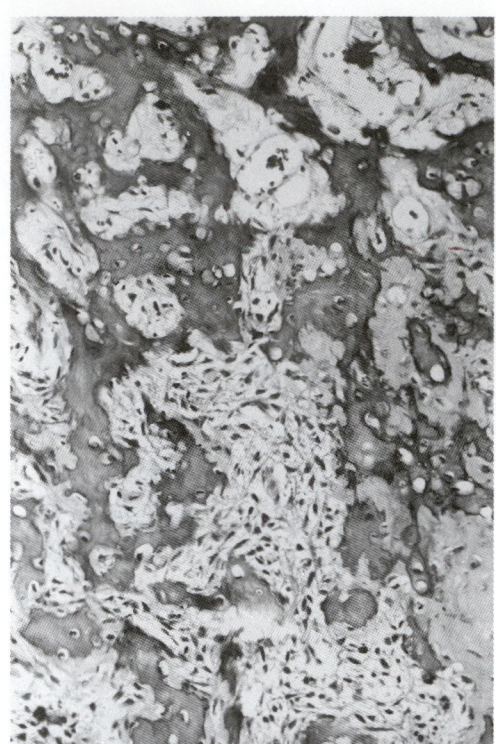

B

Figure 39-17
Periosteal osteosarcoma. *A.* A photomicrograph showing the chondroblastic component of the tumor with high degree of cellularity and moderate pleomorphism. The cartilage is frequently the major component of the lesion. *B.* Another area of the tumor showing malignant bone-forming tissue.

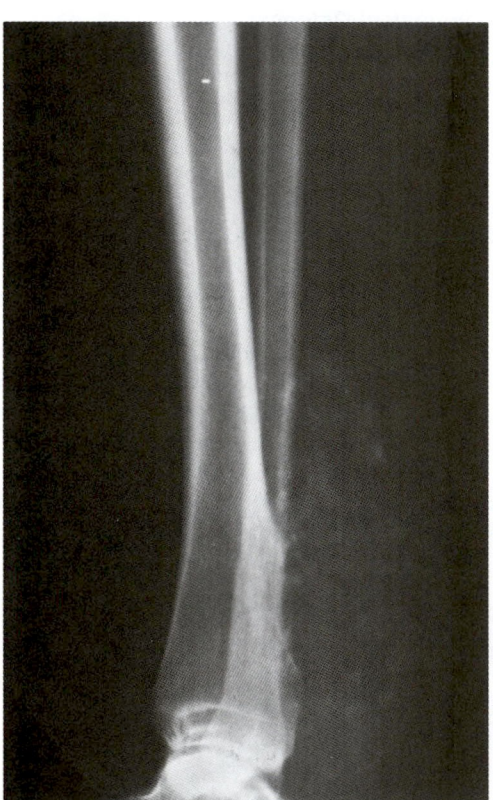

Figure 39-18
High-grade surface osteosarcoma. Radiograph shows a large tumor mass in the soft tissue with cortical destruction of the tibia. Patchy mineralization is seen within the tumor. Histologically, the tumor was a conventional osteosarcoma with telangiectatic areas, destroying the cortical bone without medullary extension.

SUGGESTED READINGS

Fechner RE, Mills SE: Tumors of the bones and joints. In: *Atlas of Tumor Pathology.* Washington, DC: Armed Forces Institute of Pathology; 1993:3d series, fascicle 8.

Gitelis S, Wilkins R, Conrad EU 2d: Benign bone tumors. *Instr Course Lect* 1966; 45:425.

Huvos AG: *Bone Tumors. Diagnosis, Treatment, and Prognosis,* 2d ed. Philadelphia: WB Saunders; 1991.

Mirra JH: *Bone Tumors: Clinical, Radiographic, and Pathologic Correlations.* Philadelphia: Lea & Febiger; 1989.

Schajowicz F: Bone-forming tumors. In: *Tumors and Tumorlike Lesions of Bone: Pathology, Radiology, and Treatment,* 2d ed. New York: Springer-Verlag; 1994:29.

Unni KK, Dahlin DC: *Dahlin's Bone Tumors: General Aspects and Data on 11,087 Cases,* 5th ed. Philadelphia: Lippincott-Raven; 1996.

Wold LE, McLeod RA, Sim FH, et al: *Atlas of Orthopaedic Pathology.* Philadelphia: WB Saunders; 1990.

Chapter 40

CARTILAGE-FORMING TUMORS

Jess H. Lonner, German C. Steiner, and Samuel Kenan

BENIGN CARTILAGE-FORMING TUMORS

OSTEOCHONDROMA

This represents the most common benign bone tumor, and accounts for approximately 35 to 50 percent of all benign bone neoplasms. It occurs most frequently in the second decade, and most lesions are located in the distal femur, proximal tibia, and proximal humerus. These lesions result from disordered enchondral bone growth, probably from displaced epiphyseal cartilage. They arise from the metaphyseal surface of bone, adjacent to the physis. They may be sessile or pedunculated and often grow away from the epiphysis. These tumors may rarely arise in bone that was previously irradiated during childhood.

Osteochondroma usually presrent as a painless mass unless the tumor has fractured, which rarely occurs. The overlying structures may be compressed, and sometimes a painful bursa develops over the tumor. Tumor growth is seen during childhood and usually ceases after skeletal maturity.

The radiographic feature of an osteochondroma is the presence of a bony projection arising from the metaphyseal surface of the cortex in which there is continuity between the cortex and medullary bone of the lesion and that of the affected bone (Fig. 40-1).

Grossly, the lesion, either pedunculated or sessile, consists of trabecular bone beneath a cartilage cap. There is continuity between it and the underlying trabecular bone. A bursa often covers the lesion. Histologically, the cap consists of hyaline cartilage covered by thin fibrous periosteum. At the junction with the underlying bone, the cartilage cap often resembles an epiphyseal growth plate with active endochondral ossification. The chondrocytes are arranged in a columnar fashion and have small, darkly stained nuclei that lack cytologic atypia (Fig. 40-2).

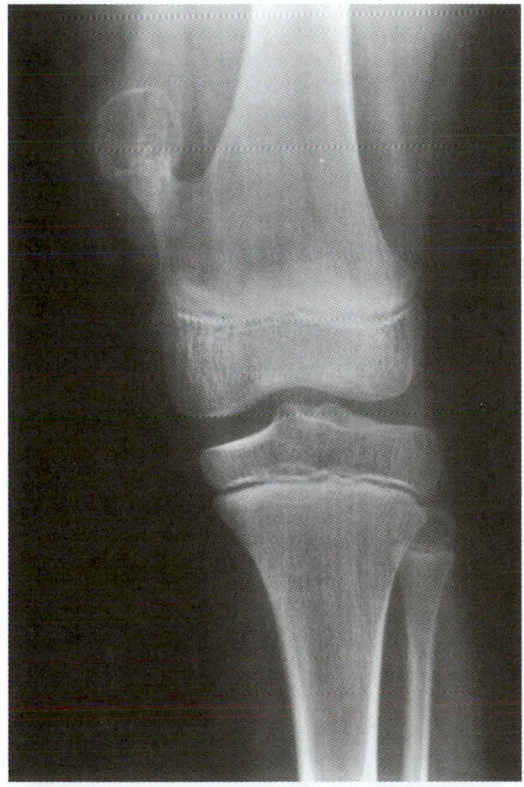

Figure 40–1
Osteochondroma of the distal femur in an 8-year-old boy. The lesion is pedunculated, arises from the distal metaphysis and there is continuity with the cortex and medullary bone.

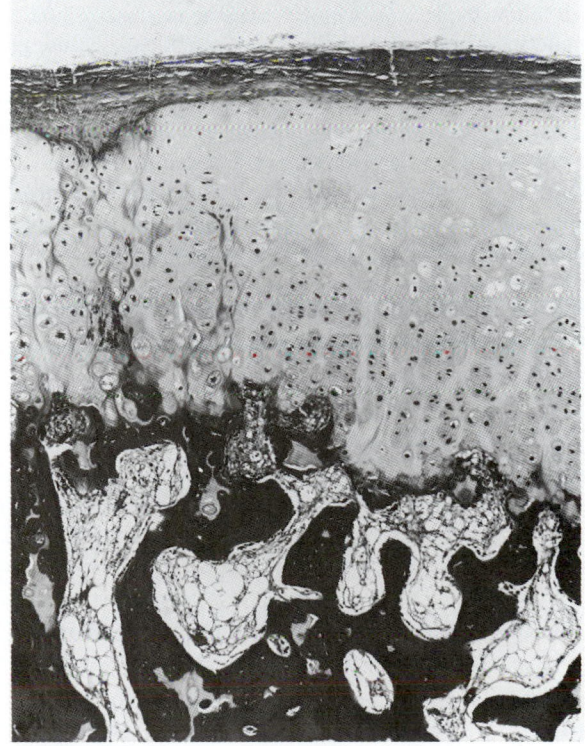

Figure 40–2
Photomicrograph of osteochondroma. The cartilage cap is covered with periosteum and the chondrocytes tend to be oriented in a columnar fashion in the deeper layer. Endochondral ossification is present at the cartilage-bone junction.

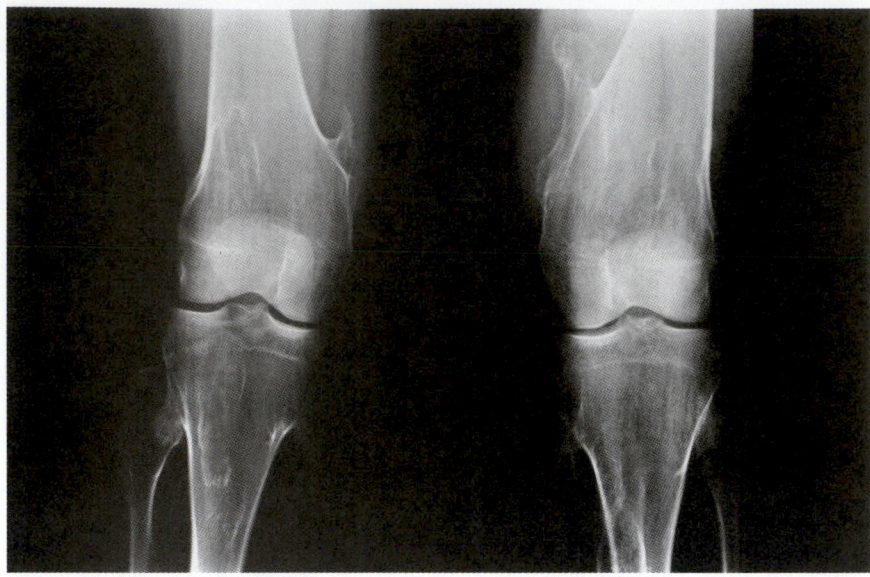

Figure 40-3
Osteochondromatosis. Radiograph shows multiple osteochondromas involving the distal femur and proximal tibia, bilateral.

There is a risk of malignant transformation to chondrosarcoma. This risk is less than 1 percent in solitary lesions. The risk of transformation seems to be related to the thickness of the cartilage cap. The cartilage cap is usually less than 1 cm thick; a thicker bosselated cap, particularly one over 2 cm should be worked up for malignancy. CT scanning is useful for the evaluation of the cartilage cap and the degree of mineralization. (see Chap. 47).

Most osteochondromas are asymptomatic and therefore no treatment is necessary. Annual examination and radiography should be used to follow the lesions, with CT scans to evaluate painful or enlarging lesions. Lesions about the elbow or ankle may cause growth disturbance or interfere with motion at those joints. In such cases excision may be indicated. Excision of an osteochondroma must be done at the base of the stalk and include the cap and periosteum. Care should be taken to avoid disrupting the cap and periosteum.

Osteochondromatosis (multiple hereditary exostosis) is an autosomal dominant disorder in which the patients have multiple tumors involving several bones (Fig. 40-3). The disorder is often marked by a mild decrease in stature, leg length discrepancy, and angular deformities of the knee, elbow, and ankle. The risk of malignant transformation to chondrosarcoma is probably less than 5 percent.

Subungual Exostosis

Subungual exostosis is a bony projection arising from the subungual region of the distal phalanx, usually from the great toe. The lesion is composed of trabecular bone covered with fibrocartilage and hyaline cartilage. Subungual exostosis is a reactive process probably related to trauma or infection, and is apparently unrelated to osteochondroma.

Bizarre Parosteal Osteochondromatous Proliferation of the Hands and Feet (BPOP)

Bizarre parosteal osteochondromatous proliferation of the hands and feet (BPOP) is a benign lesion arising from the cortical surface of short tubular bones and is composed of cartilage, bone, and fibrous tissue. It is different from osteochondroma and is probably posttraumatic. It has also been described in the long bones.

ENCHONDROMA

This is a relatively common benign tumor of mature hyaline cartilage, originating within the medullary cavities of long bones, possibly from remnants of the epiphyseal plate. It accounts for approximately 10 percent of the benign bone tumors. Endochondromas occur most commonly in the second, third, and fourth decades of life, but are seen in all age groups. They are most typically found in the short tubular bones of the hands and feet, but are frequently seen in the femur and humerus as well.

Most enchondromas are painless and are diagnosed incidentally on radiographs. Pain should raise the question of a pathologic fracture or malignancy if the lesion is in a long bone. Radiographically these tumors display the characteristic punctate calcifications common to

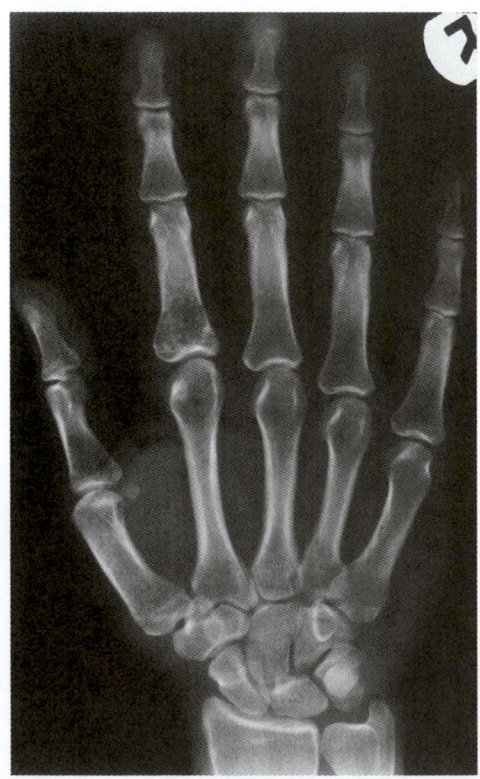

Figure 40-4
Enchondroma of the proximal phalanx of the index finger in a 34-year-old female. Radiograph shows stippled calcification with focal expansion of the bone and cortical thinning.

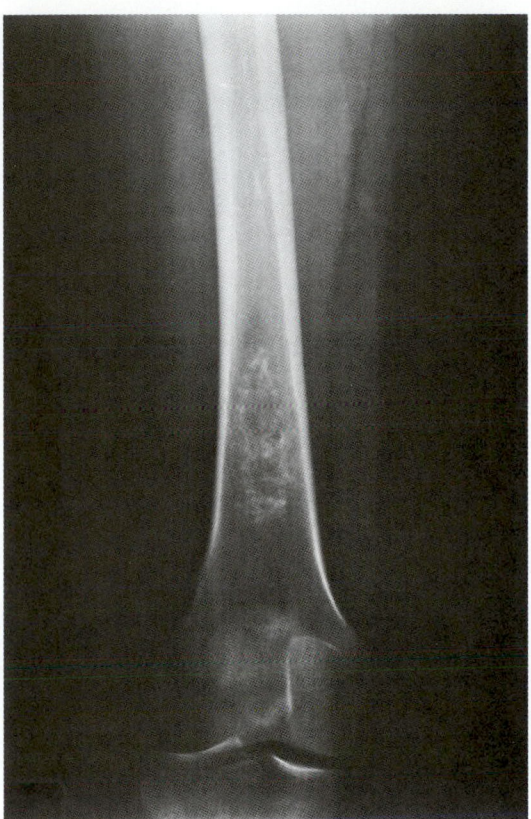

Figure 40-5
Radiograph of enchondroma of the distal femur, showing patchy medullary calcification. This lesion can be confused radiologically with bone infarct.

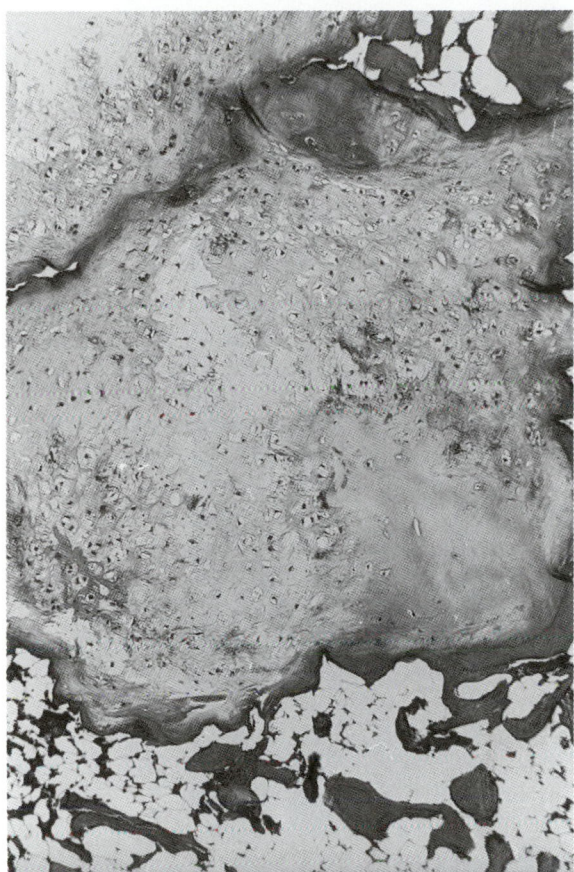

Figure 40-6
Enchondroma. The lesion is lobulated with peripheral ossification. It is hypocellular and the chondrocytes are small, have uniform appearance and show no atypical features.

cartilage-forming tumors. The tumors are usually well-defined with clear demarcation between them and the surrounding normal bone. In the phalanges, they tend to expand the bone and thin the cortex (Fig. 40–4). The matrix may be focally calcified. Enchondromas of long bones may sometimes be difficult to distinguish radiographically from a bone infarct or low-grade chondrosarcoma (Fig. 40-5).

Grossly the tumor is translucent and blue-gray in color. Histologically, it is lobulated and usually hypocellular, with a typical cartilaginous matrix containing normal-appearing chondrocytes located within lacunae. The cells have small uniform nuclei lacking atypia (Fig. 40-6). The matrix may be focally calcified. Enchondromas of the hands and feet are often more cellular than those of the long bones.

Asymptomatic lesions can simply be observed and followed longitudinally. Symptomatic lesions should be biopsied to confirm the benignity of the lesion, and at the same time should be curetted and bone grafted.

Ollier's disease is the eponym for multiple enchondromatosis (Fig. 40-7). It is usually unilateral and has an incidence of malignant transformation to chondrosarcoma that is reported to be 10 to 30 percent. Maffucci's syndrome is characterized by multiple enchondromas with soft tissue angiomas. The incidence of malignant transformation in this condition is probably higher than in enchondromatosis.

PERIOSTEAL CHONDROMA

This uncommon lesion arises from the outer cortex of long and short tubular bones, beneath the periosteum. It is most commonly seen in patients in their second to third decades of life. The proximal humerus and proximal and distal femur and phalanges are common locations. The tumor may present as a palpable mass with local tenderness.

Radiographically, these tumors are well-defined, small metaphyseal surface lesions with erosion of the outer cortex and reactive periosteal bone formation (Fig. 40-8). One-third are calcified. Histologically, they exhibit lobulated hyaline cartilage, but they are usually more cellular with greater pleomorphism and cell binucleation than enchondromas.

The recommended treatment is en bloc resection.

CHONDROBLASTOMA

Fifty to 65 percent of these benign tumors occur in the second decade of life and are most commonly found in the proximal humerus, distal femur, or proximal tibia. The lesion is characteristically centered in the epiphysis, but it may be in an apophysis or the triradiate cartilage of the pelvis.

Pain localized to the region of the tumor is the most common presenting symptom. Physical findings are often subtle, and may include tenderness, a limp, or pain on motion of the affected joint. Radiographically, the lesion is radiolucent, with well-defined sclerotic borders that clearly define its limits from the surrounding epiphyseal trabecular bone. The amount of mineralization within the bone is variable, occurring in at least 25 percent of cases. The tumor may cross an open physis and expand the surrounding bone (Fig. 40-9).

Grossly, the lesional tissue is grayish-pink in color, measuring between 1 to 7 cm (usually less than 3 cm). Calcific foci may be ap-

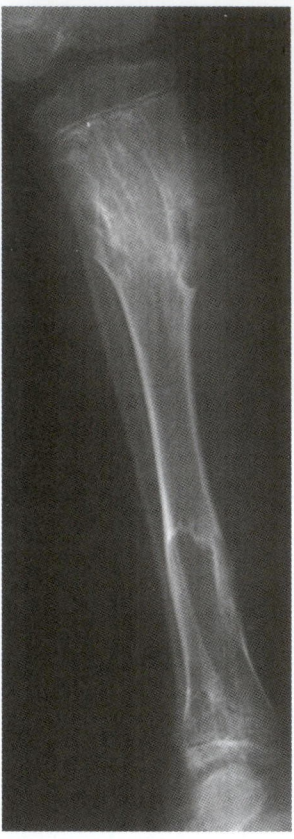

Figure 40-7
Enchondromatosis of the tibia involving the proximal and distal metaphysis. Areas of linear lucencies and densities are seen proximally in the tibia.

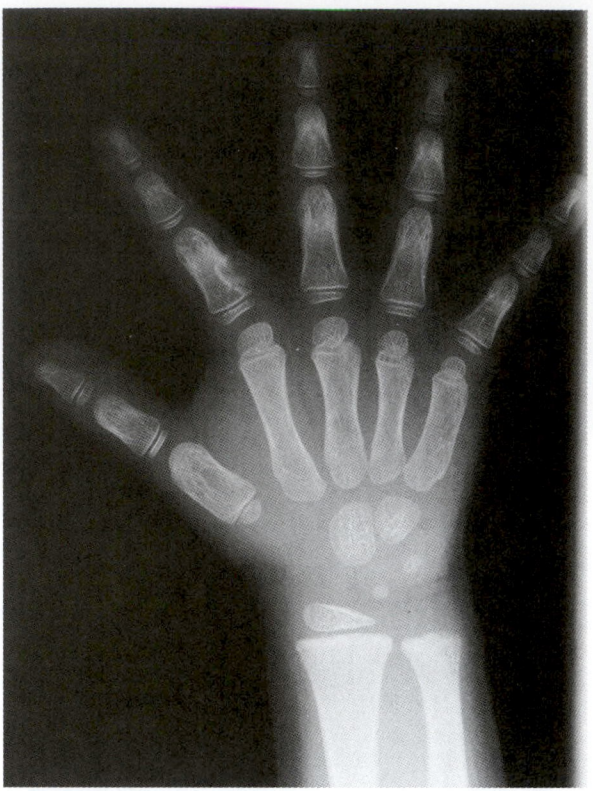

Figure 40-8
Periosteal chondroma in a 3-year-old girl, with pain and swelling of the right index finger for 3 months. Radiograph shows cortical scalloping of the proximal phalanx with a soft tissue mass.

parent in the tissue. Since a secondary aneurysmal bone cyst component may be present, hemorrhagic tissue may be prominent.

Microscopically, the predominant cells are round to polyhedral with well-defined cell borders containing often-indented nuclei. Varying degrees of chondroid differentiation are seen (Fig. 40-10*A*). Matrix calcification may take on a characteristic "chicken wire" appearance around the individual cells (Fig. 40-10*B*). Multinucleated giant cells may be present—scattered and sometimes in large numbers. Cystic spaces resembling aneurysmal bone cyst are seen in approximately 20 percent of the cases. Immunohistochemical studies have shown that the chondroblastoma cells react positively to S-100 protein. Because of its epiphyseal location and the presence of giant cells, chondroblastoma may be confused with giant cell tumor.

Most chondroblastomas can be successfully treated with curettage and bone grafting with an approximate 90 percent cure rate. Rarely, chondroblastomas can be locally aggressive or can metastasize to the lungs. There are rare documented cases of malignant transformation.

CHONDROMYXOID FIBROMA

This rare benign cartilage tumor occurs most commonly in the second and third decades, with two-thirds occurring in long bones and approximately 25 percent localized to the proximal tibia. While some of these are picked up as incidental findings, the majority are painful. In some cases, local swelling and a palpable mass are noted. Physical exam is usually unremarkable, other than occasional tenderness.

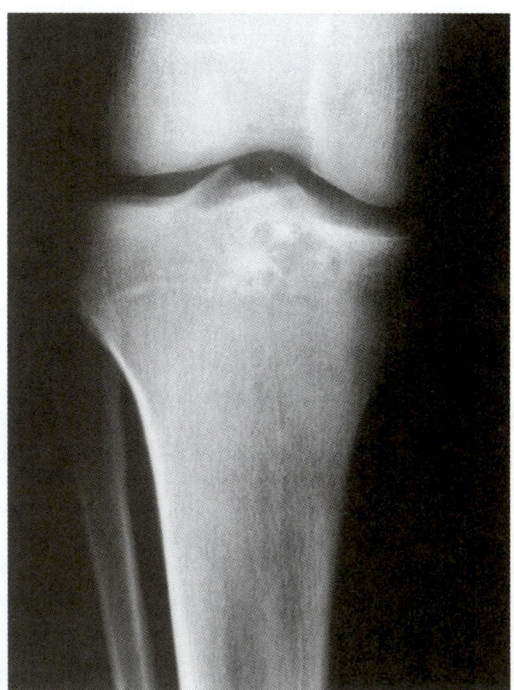

Figure 40-9
Chondroblastoma of the proximal epiphysis of the tibia in an 18-year-old male. An ill-defined lesion is seen with focal calcification.

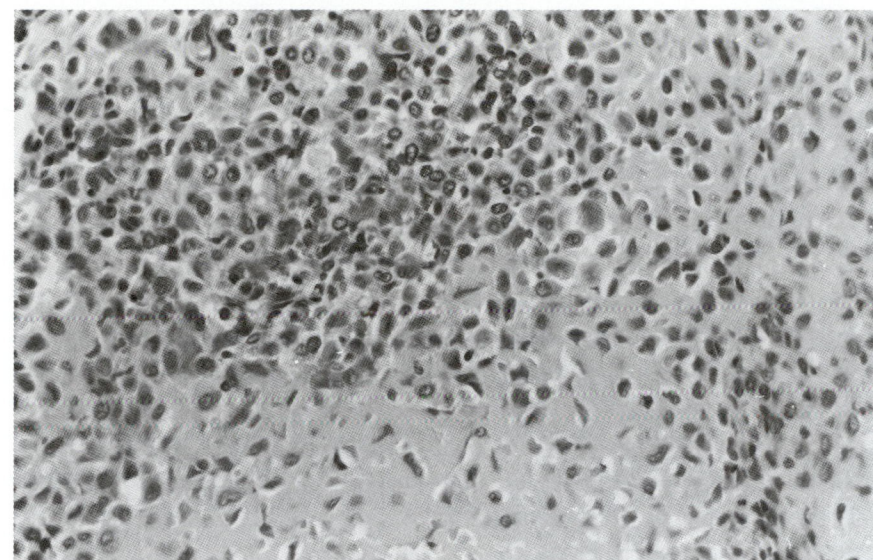

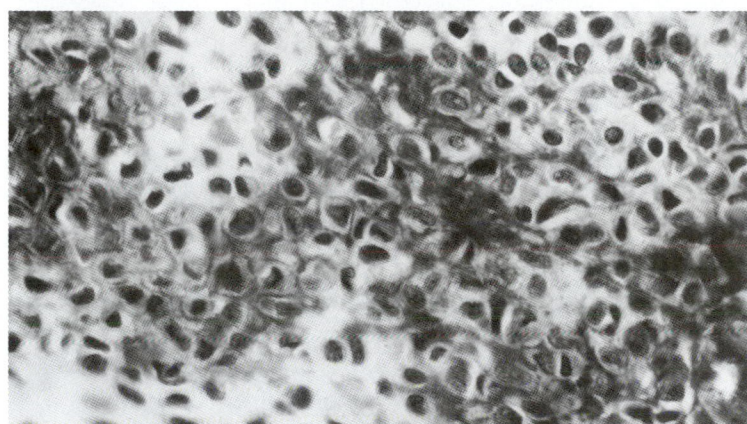

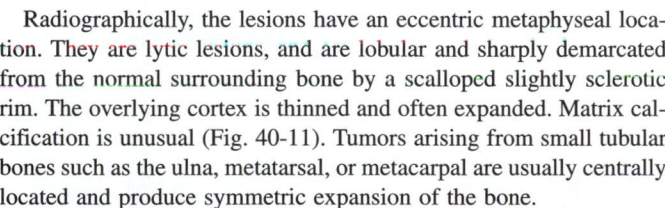

A

B

Figure 40-10

A. Chondroblastoma. The tissue consists of polygonal cells with indented nuclei, disposed in dense aggregates with focal areas of chondroid matrix. *B.* High-power photomicrograph shows calcification around individual cells in a "chicken wire" pattern.

Radiographically, the lesions have an eccentric metaphyseal location. They are lytic lesions, and are lobular and sharply demarcated from the normal surrounding bone by a scalloped slightly sclerotic rim. The overlying cortex is thinned and often expanded. Matrix calcification is unusual (Fig. 40-11). Tumors arising from small tubular bones such as the ulna, metatarsal, or metacarpal are usually centrally located and produce symmetric expansion of the bone.

Grossly, the tumor may take on a well-circumscribed, lobulated appearance, with translucent bluish-gray color that resembles cartilage. Microscopically, the tumor is poorly lobulated and contains spindled and stellate cells with an abundant myxoid matrix. Peripheral hypercellularity of the lobules is common; multinucleated giant cells are often found in the fibrous tissue between the lobules, and round cells resembling chondroblasts may be seen in these areas. Well-developed hyaline cartilage is unusual in these tumors. Cellular atypism with hyperchromatism may be found, but mitoses are rare (Fig. 40-12).

Treatment usually involves intralesional curettage and bone grafting. Recurrence rate is approximately 10 to 15 percent. In some cases, the tumors are locally aggressive and extend into soft tissues, requiring wider local resection. Malignant transformation to chondrosarcomas is exceptional.

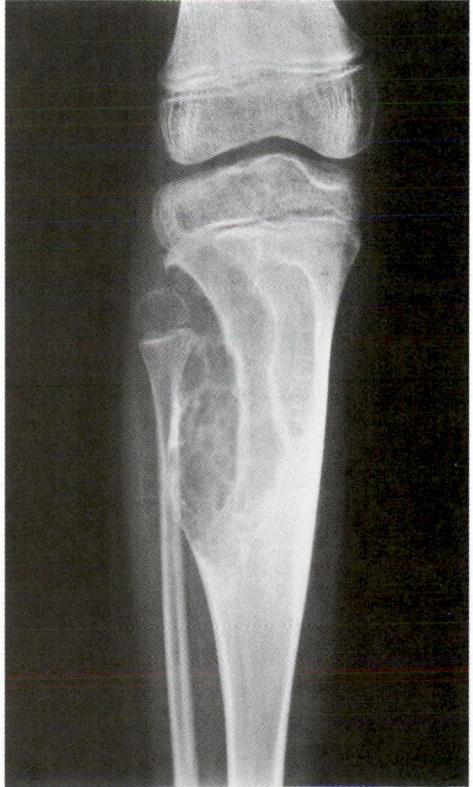

Figure 40-11

Chondromyxoid fibroma of the tibia in an 8-year-old girl with 6 months history of pain in the right knee. A large lytic lesion is seen in the proximal metaphysis and shaft of the tibia, with sclerotic margins, bone expansion, and cortical thinning.

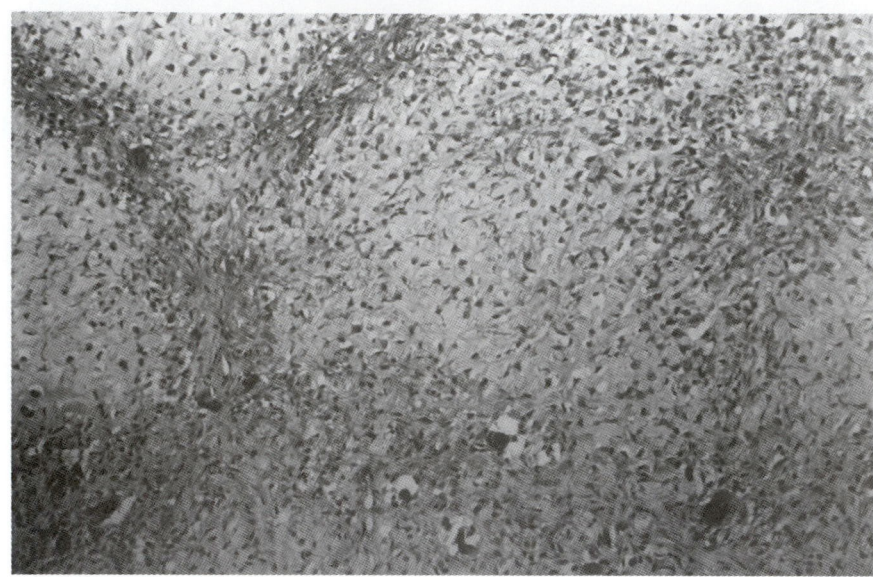

Figure 40-12
Chondromyxoid fibroma. It consists of poorly lobulated myxoid tissue with stellate cells with increased cellularity at the periphery. Giant cells are present between the lobules.

MALIGNANT CARTILAGE-FORMING TUMORS

CHONDROSARCOMA (CONVENTIONAL, CENTRAL)

This represents a common malignant neoplasm of cartilage cells that is seen predominantly in adults between 40 and 70 years of age, rarely in patients younger than 20. If multiple myeloma is excluded, chondrosarcoma is the second most common primary malignant tumor of bone after osteosarcoma. Most lesions occur in the pelvis or proximal femur, followed by the scapula and proximal humerus. The most common presenting symptom is localized pain of relatively long duration, anywhere from several months to more than 10 years. Physical findings are often subtle and may include pain on examination of the adjacent joint, mild muscular atrophy, tenderness, a palpable mass, and an antalgic gait.

Radiographic features are characteristic, often diagnostic. Central chondrosarcomas of long bones occur primarily in the metaphysis or diaphysis. There is cortical thickening, endosteal scalloping, and often fusiform expansion of the bone. Matrix calcification in a stippled or ring-like pattern is frequently seen, particularly in low-grade malignant tumors. Soft tissue extension may be seen with larger tumors and is associated with cortical destruction (Fig. 40-13). Involvement of the medullary cavity by tumor may be extensive. Pain, in association with endosteal scalloping and cortical thickening, is important diagnostic clues in distinguishing low grade chondrosarcoma from the benign enchondroma.

Grossly chondrosarcomas tend to be lobulated, with a blue-gray translucent cartilaginous appearance, interspersed with white areas of calcification. Areas of myxoid degeneration, necrosis, and liquefaction help distinguish this malignant tumor from the benign cartilage-forming lesions. Histologically, the tumors vary greatly in their degree of cellularity and matrix composition. In well-differentiated chondrosarcomas (grade 1), the tissue is lobulated and contains chondrocytes lying within lacunae separated by abundant hyaline matrix. The cells show mild to moderate nuclear pleomorphism and are often binucleated. The tumor is moderately cellular and no mitosis are seen. Although some grade 1 chondrosarcomas can be indistinguishable histologically from enchondroma, the presence of tumor infiltration of the marrow spaces and the aggressive radiographic

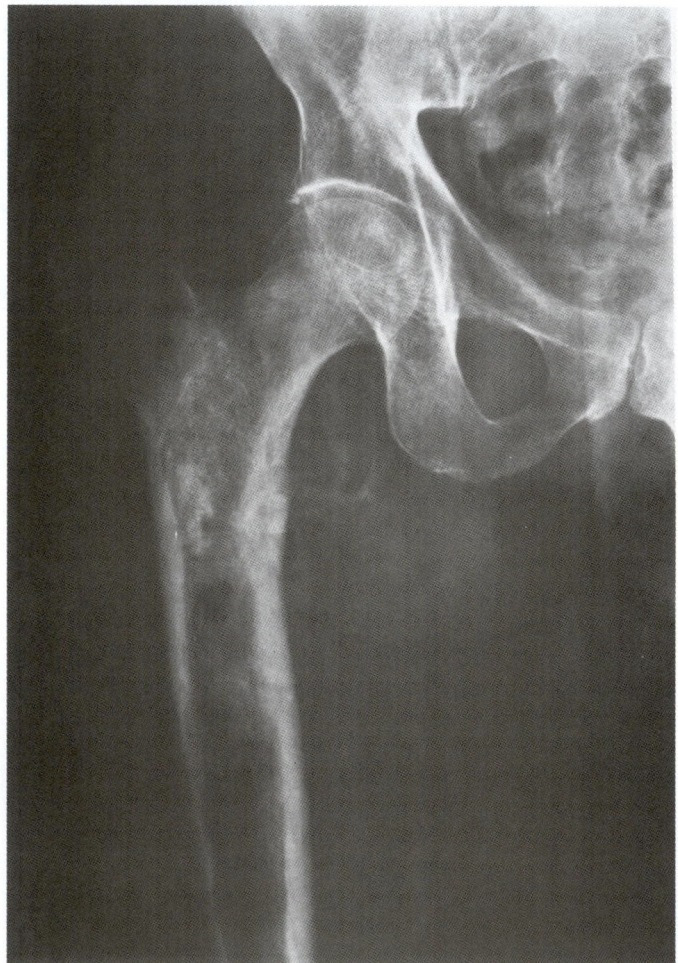

Figure 40-13
Conventional chondrosarcoma of the femur in a 79-year-old male, with right leg pain for 1 year. Radiograph shows an extensive lytic medullary lesion in the femur, with focal calcification. There is cortical thickening and endosteal scalloping. The area of calcification (see arrow) medial to the femur represents tumor extension in the soft tissue.

appearance favor malignancy (Fig. 40-14). In grade 2 chondrosarcomas, there is an increase in cellularity and nuclear atypia as well as the presence of multinucleated tumor cells, and occasional mitoses. Myxoid changes are common. The grade 3 chondrosarcomas show highly malignant cells and less evidence of cartilaginous differentiation.

Secondary chondrosarcomas, as opposed to primary central chondrosarcomas, arise at the site of preexistent benign cartilage tumors such as endochondromatosis, osteochondromatosis, and solitary osteochondroma, and rarely in solitary enchondroma. They are usually well-differentiated (grade 1).

Treatment of this malignancy is predominantly surgical, consisting of wide surgical resection with adequate margins. Amputation may be necessary, but reconstruction can be considered depending on the location. These tumors are not considered responsive to routine chemotherapy or irradiation. The most important prog-nostic factors appear to be the size of the tumor, anatomic location, and the histologic grade. The overall 5-year survival rate is approximately 50 to 60 percent.

DEDIFFERENTIATED CHONDROSARCOMA

This represents the most malignant cartilage tumor; dedifferentiation complicates approximately 10 percent of all chondrosarcomas. It has a peak incidence in the fifth to seventh decades of life, with a similar site predilection as the conventional chondrosarcomas. Pain is typical, often varying with the rate of tumor growth. The presence of an intraosseous tumor that radiographically resembles enchondroma or chondrosarcoma, but showing cortical destruction and soft tissue invasion without mineralization, strongly suggests dedifferentiated chondrosarcoma (Fig. 40-15).

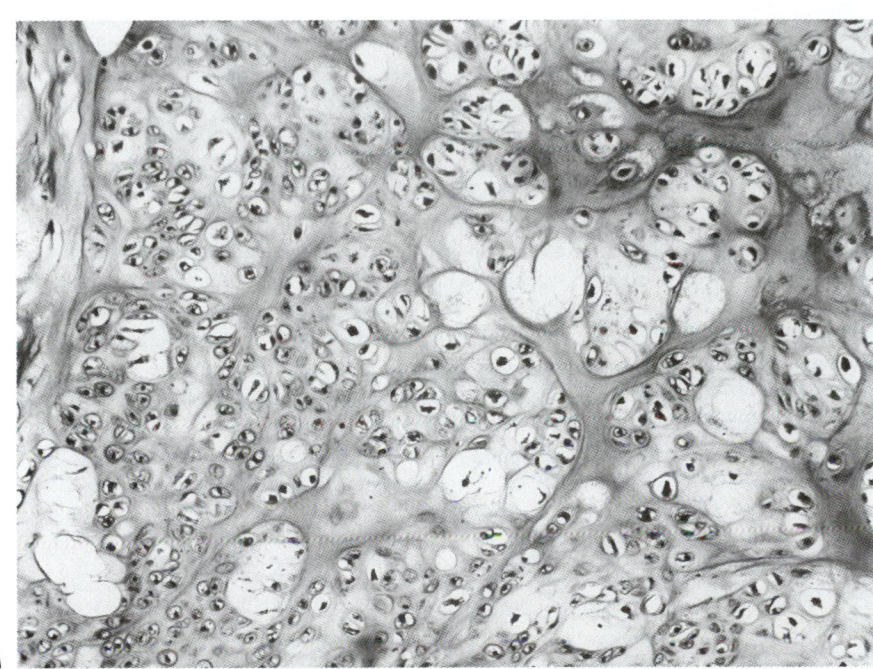

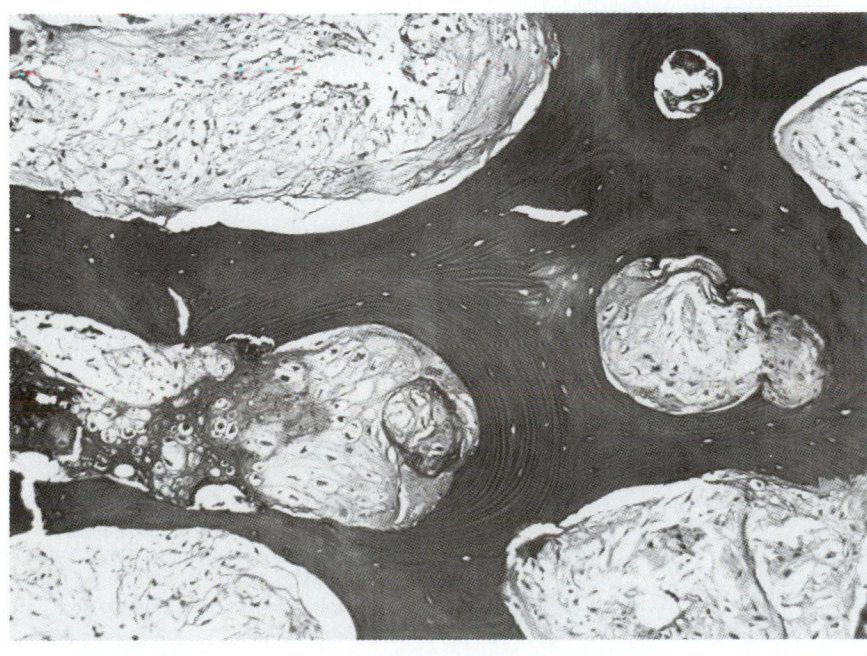

Figure 40-14
A. Photomicrograph of well-differentiated chondrosarcoma (grade I). The lesion is moderately cellular with mild to moderate atypia. B. There is tumor infiltration into the marrow spaces between the pre-existing bone. This finding is diagnostic of malignancy.

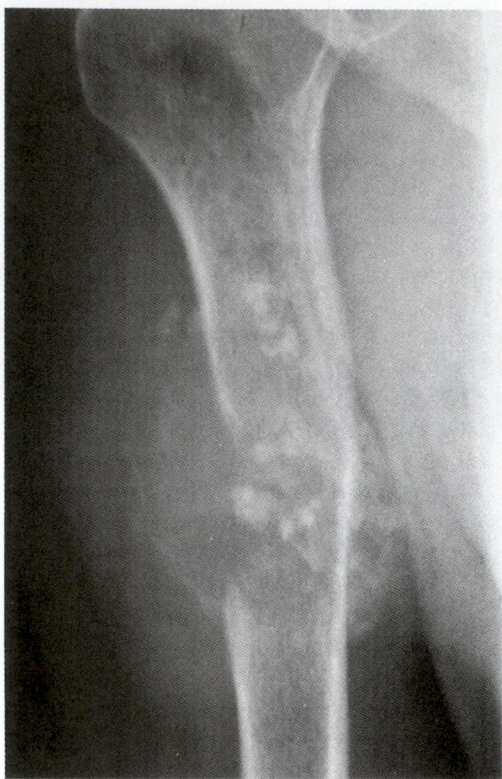

Figure 40-15
Dedifferentiated chondrosarcoma. Eighty-one-year old male who fell 5 weeks before and sustained a pathologic fracture of the right humerus. Radiograph reveals multiple foci of intramedullary calcification in the humerus, with a fracture, cortical destruction, and a soft tissue mass.

Histologically, the tumor consists of a cartilaginous tumor of low-grade malignancy and a noncartilaginous high-grade malignant component. There is sharp transition between the two tissue elements. The low-grade cartilage component has features similar to ordinary chondrosarcoma (usually grade 1); the high-grade component may be malignant fibrous histiocytoma, fibrosarcoma, or osteosarcoma (Fig. 40-16). This latter component is the most aggressive of the tumor and extends into the soft tissue.

Long-term survival is less than 10 percent. Metastatic sites demonstrate the high-grade noncartilaginous component. Amputation is usually necessary unless wide margins can be achieved. Multiagent adjuvant chemotherapy is important for addressing the spindle cell component.

MESENCHYMAL CHONDROSARCOMA

This rare tumor has a peak incidence in the third decade of life, but is spread over a wide age range. Approximately one-third of the patients have had pain for more than 1 year prior to diagnosis. One-third of cases occur in the soft tissues; osseous predilection is in the pelvis, ribs, proximal femur, and jaw.

There are no characteristic radiographic features that help to differentiate this tumor from ordinary chondrosarcoma. In the bone, the lesion is lytic and stippled with calcifications, cortical destruction, and soft tissue extension (Fig. 40-17). Histologically, it consists of a bimorphic pattern with well-differentiated chondrosarcoma intimately associated with hypercellular noncartilaginous tumor consisting of round, oval, or spindle cells. This latter component has a conspicuous vascular proliferation with a hemangiopericytomatous pattern of growth. The histologic appearance of the areas containing round cells is reminiscent of Ewing's sarcoma (Fig. 40-18). Areas of cartilage may be quite small, and reactive osteoid may be present. Mitoses are sparse.

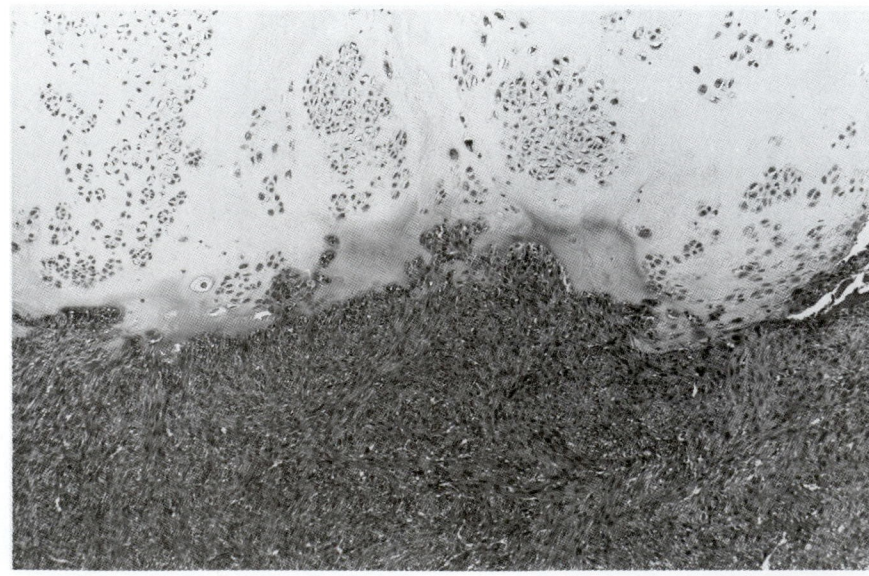

Figure 40-16
Dedifferentiated chondrosarcoma. The tumor consists of two different components: a well-differentiated cartilaginous tissue at the upper part of the illustration and a noncartilaginous tumor tissue consistent with malignant fibrous histiocytoma at the lower part. Notice the sharp transition between the two components.

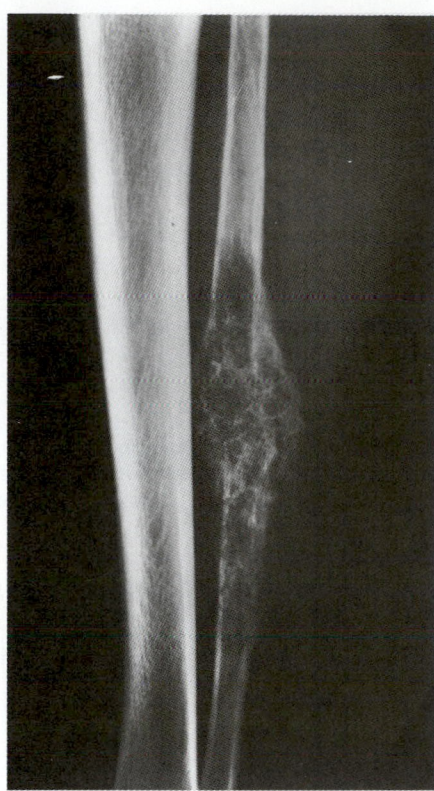

Figure 40-17
Mesenchymal chondrosarcoma. Thirty-one-year old male with discomfort in the lower leg for 5 months. A lesion was palpable in the mid-leg. Radiograph shows a large lesion in the fibula containing lucent and dense areas, at the site of an old fracture.

Treatment is surgical, requiring surgical resection with wide margins. Adjuvant radiation and chemotherapy offer no proven benefit. Long-term prognosis is poor.

CLEAR CELL CHONDROSARCOMA

This rare, low-grade malignant neoplasm afflicts patients from the second to ninth decades, with a peak incidence in the third and fourth decades. Patients, usually male, often have pain and other subtle symptoms for several years prior to diagnosis. Approximately 50 percent of cases affect the femoral head; the proximal humeral epiphysis, the distal femur, and proximal tibia are the next most frequently involved sites.

Radiographically, in its early stages, the tumor may look benign, with sharp margins; focal calcification may be present. Larger, more advanced lesions are poorly circumscribed, with marked cortical destruction (Fig. 40-19).

Grossly a bluish-gray matrix may be difficult to see; hemorrhagic cystic spaces may be present. Histologically, the tumor cells have abundant clear cytoplasm, bland nuclear features, and the chondroid matrix is sparse and distributed between the clear cells and is focally calcified. Scattered bone trabeculae, as well as multinucleated giant cells, are frequent components of this tumor (Fig. 40-20). Because of its epiphyseal location, clear cell chondrosarcoma should be distinguished from chondroblastoma, both radiologically and histologically.

Wide surgical resection without adjuvant therapy is the recommended treatment.

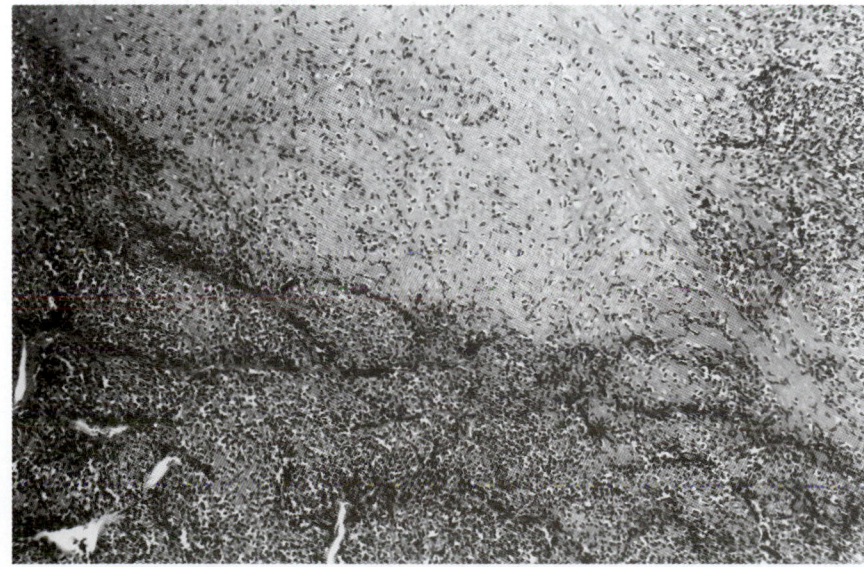

Figure 40-18
Mesenchymal chondrosarcoma. The tumor consists of a well-differentiated cartilaginous tissue (*upper part*) merging into a small round cell undifferentiated tumor (*lower part*). The vascular spaces seen in the left lower corner are part of the hemangiopericytomatous pattern of the tumor.

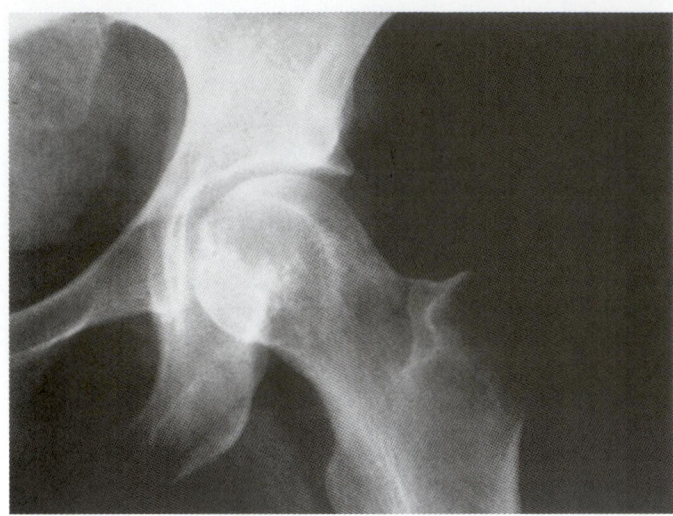

Figure 40-19
Clear cell chondrosarcoma of the femoral head in a 40-year-old female. A circumscribed lytic lesion is seen with marginal sclerosis and focal central calcification. The lesion resembles a chondroblastoma.

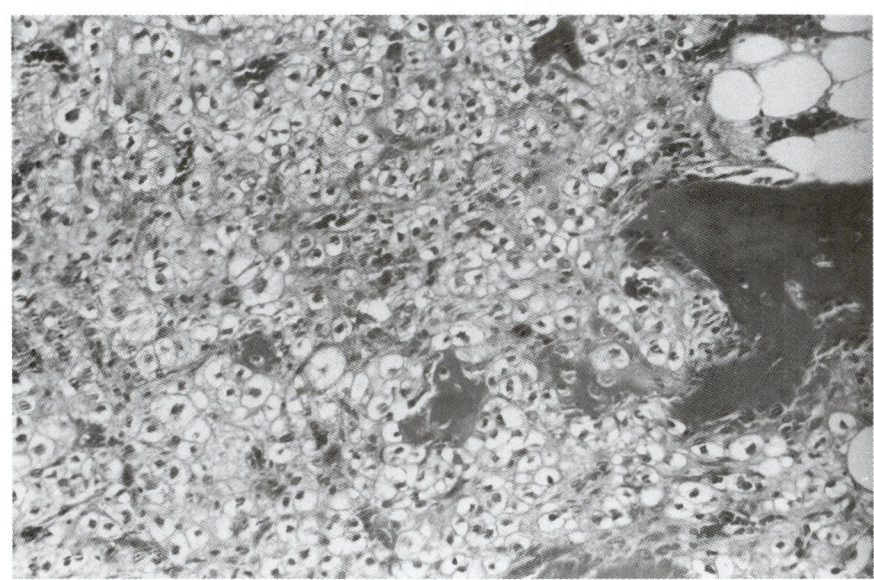

Figure 40-20
Clear cell chondrosarcoma. The tumor consists of cells with clear cytoplasm disposed in dense aggregates with sparse matrix. Focal ossification and multinucleated giant cells are seen.

SUGGESTED READINGS

Dorfman HD, Czerniak B: *Bone Tumors*. St. Louis: Mosby, 1998.

Fechner RE, Mills SE: Tumors of the bones and joints. In: *Atlas of Tumor Pathology*. Washington, DC: Armed Forces Institute of Pathology; 1993:3d series, fascicle 8.

Huvos AG: *Bone Tumors. Diagnosis, Treatment, and Prognosis*, 2d ed. Philadelphia: WB Saunders; 1991.

Mirra JH: *Bone Tumors: Clinical, Radiographic, and Pathologic Correlations*. Philadelphia: Lea & Febiger; 1989.

Schajowicz F: Cartilage-forming tumors. In: *Tumors and Tumorlike Lesions of Bone: Pathology, Radiology, and Treatment*, 2d ed. New York: Springer-Verlag; 1994:141.

Springfield DS, Gebhardt MC, McGuire MH: Chondrosarcoma: A review. In: Pritchard DJ (ed): *Instructional Course Lectures*. Rosemont, Ill: American Academy of Orthopaedic Surgeons; 1996; 45:417.

Unni KK: *Dahlin's Bone Tumors: General Aspects and Data on 11,087 Cases*, 5th ed. Philadelphia: Lippincott-Raven; 1996.

Wold LE, McLeod RA, Sim FH, et al: *Atlas of Orthopaedic Pathology*. Philadelphia: WB Saunders; 1990.

Chapter 41

FIBROUS AND FIBROHISTIOCYTIC TUMORS

Brian C. Toolan, German C. Steiner, and Samuel Kenan

BENIGN TUMORS

BENIGN FIBROUS HISTIOCYTOMA

Benign fibrous histiocytoma is a rare lesion that is microscopically indistinguishable from a nonossifying fibroma. It occurs exclusively in adults, often older than 25 years of age. The pelvis and the ribs are the most common sites for a benign fibrous histiocytoma. The tumor may also be found in the long bones, but tends to appear in the epiphysis or diaphysis. The epiphyseal lesions may be indistinguishable histologically from giant cell tumor. Regardless of their location, these lesions are always painful, a characteristic that clearly distinguishes the tumor from a nonossifying fibroma which is usually painless. Controversy exists as to whether benign fibrous histiocytoma is a distinct entity or a reactive lesion associated with a preexisting condition. The prognosis of benign fibrous histiocytoma is similar to other benign fibrous tumors and treatment with curettage and bone grafting has been demonstrated to prevent recurrence.

DESMOPLASTIC FIBROMA

Desmoplastic fibromas are rare, benign aggressive fibrous lesions seen in adolescence and young adulthood. They occur in the metadiaphyseal region of long bones such as the femur, tibia, and humerus, as well as the pelvis and jaws. On radiograph they are lytic lesions with cortical thinning, and the margins may be sharp or ill-defined. A trabecular pattern may be present within the lesion (Fig. 41-1). Histologically, the tumor consists of abundant collagen fibers and small benign-appearing fibroblasts, and resembles fibromatosis (Fig. 41-2). Microscopic extensions into adjacent reactive bone are present and may account for the recurrence in reported cases treated with curettage and bone grafting. Intralesional curettage is the treatment of choice. Differentiation between desmoplastic fibroma and low-grade fibrosarcoma may be difficult and sometimes both lesions overlap.

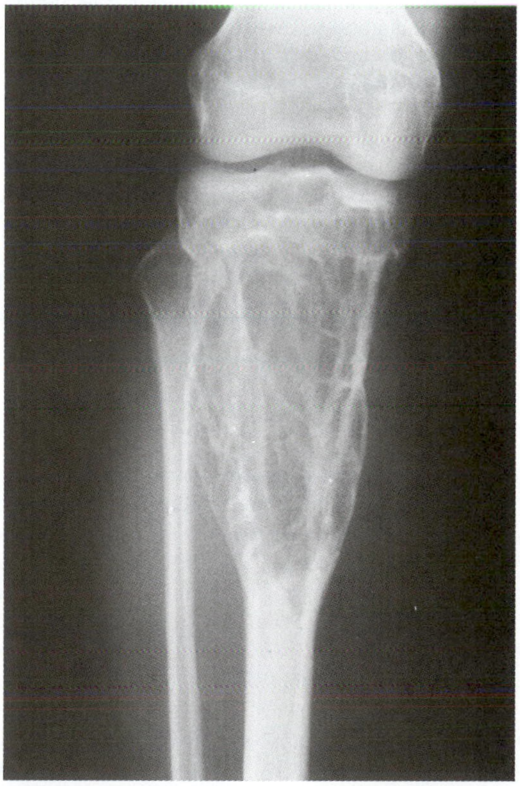

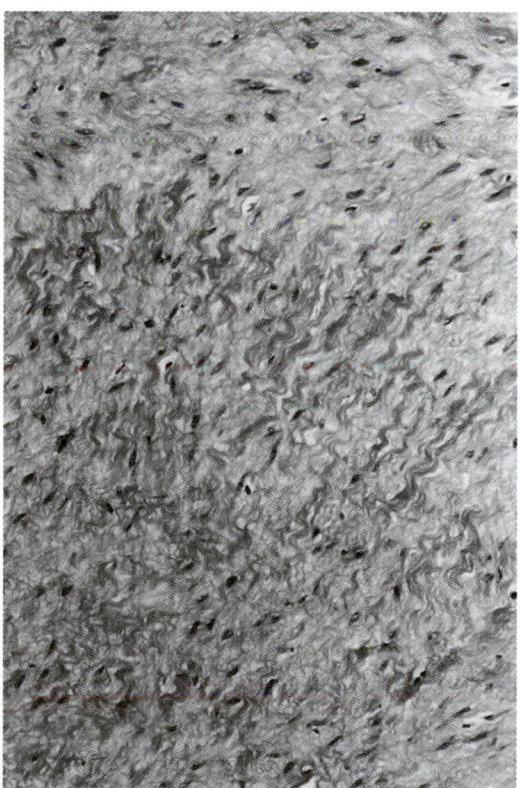

Figure 41-1
Desmoplastic fibroma. Twenty-eight-year old female with an expansile, large lytic lesion of the proximal tibia. It contains coarsely trabeculated bone.

Figure 41-2
Desmoplastic fibroma. There is a sparse population of small fibroblasts separated by abundant collagen bundles. The lesion resembles fibromatosis.

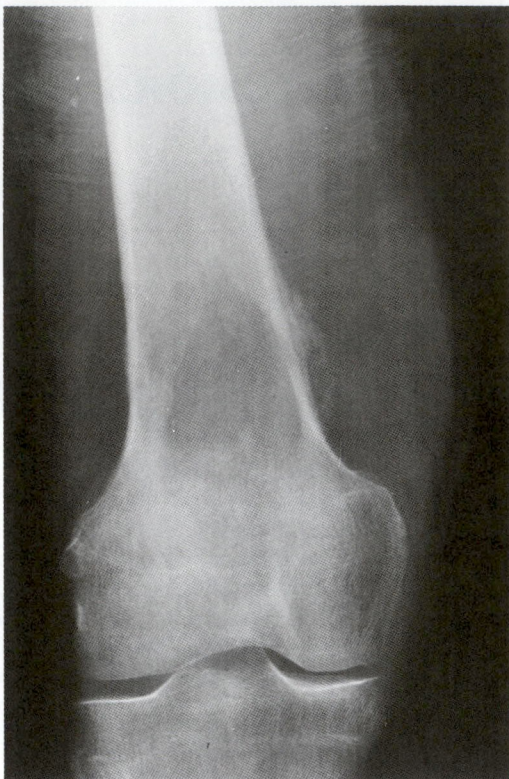

Figure 41-3
Malignant fibrous histiocytoma of the distal femur in a 67-year-old male. There is an ill-defined lytic lesion in the metaphyseal region. The periosteal reaction is due to cortical destruction by the tumor with soft tissue extension.

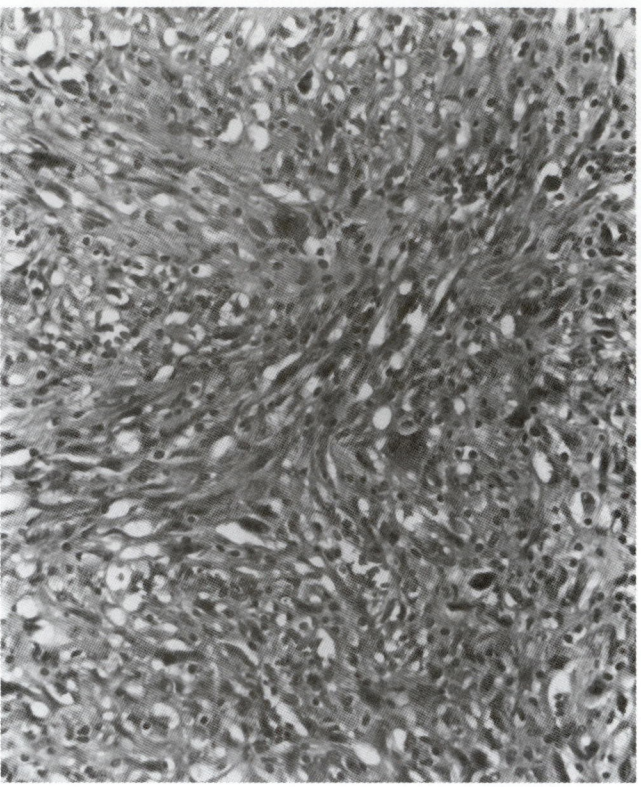

Figure 41-4
Malignant fibrous histiocytoma. The tumor shows intersecting fascicles of atypical fibroblasts with a storiform pattern. There are also large atypical cells present in the tissue. [Reproduced with permission by Steinberg GC: Tumors and tumor-like conditions. In Johannessen JV (ed): *Electron Microscopy in Human Medicine*, vol 4. New York: McGraw-Hill; 1998:112.]

MALIGNANT TUMORS

MALIGNANT FIBROUS HISTIOCYTOMA

Malignant fibrous histiocytoma of bone was described in 1972 as a neoplasm composed of spindle cells, histiocytic-type cells, and giant cells, with spindle-cells disposed in a fascicular arrangement that is called storiform pattern. Recent studies suggest that this tumor derives from fibroblasts rather than histiocytes.

It frequently arises in the metadiaphyseal region of long bones of adults, most often the distal femur. The symptoms of pain and swelling associated with a tender mass, usually present for at least 6 months, are the most common presenting complaints. The lesions appear lytic on radiograph; however, they can also appear mixed with sclerosis on occasion. There is cortical destruction with minimal periosteal reaction, and a soft tissue mass can be seen on the plain film (Fig. 41-3). Histologically, the lesional tissue features spindle cells and histiocytoid cells, as well as scattered multinucleated giant cells and lipid-laden histiocytes. The spindle cells are often arranged in a storiform or cartwheel pattern, where they form fascicles that intersect in a central hypocellular area. The cells show a varying degree of cell pleomorphism (Fig. 41-4). Many cases that were originally diagnosed as fibrosarcoma are now reclassified as malignant fibrous histiocytoma. Osteosarcomas and leiomyosarcomas have areas that resemble malignant fibrous histiocytoma, but proper tissue sampling and immunohistochemical studies are helpful in the differential diagnosis. The surgical treatment involves a wide resection. The bene-

fits of chemotherapy are inconclusive. Five-year survival rate is approximately 50 percent. Malignant fibrous histiocytoma may result from malignant transformation of bone involved with Paget's disease, bone infarct, or previous radiation therapy for an unrelated tumor. Patients with this secondary malignant fibrous histiocytoma have a poor prognosis.

FIBROSARCOMA

Fibrosarcoma is a primary malignant tumor that arises from fibroconnective tissue of the marrow cavity. Secondary fibrosarcoma can arise from a precursor lesion such as a bone infarct or Paget's disease, or from previously irradiated bone. The tumor may occur at any location; however, it has a strong predilection for the metaphyseal region of the femur and tibia. Patients with primary fibrosarcoma of the bone present in the middle decades of life and may have long-standing complaints of pain and swelling prior to seeking medical attention. The lesion has an aggressive nonspecific appearance on radiograph. They are usually large, eccentrically based lytic lesions that are poorly marginated and often lack a rim of reactive sclerosis. Cortical destruction with erosion into the soft tissues may occur. Microscopically, the tumor is comprised of spindle cells arranged in a "herringbone" pattern. The spindle cells from low-grade lesions demonstrate little cellular atypia and few mitotic figures, while the high-grade tumors have marked pleomorphism and significant mitotic activity.

Fibrosarcoma should be differentiated histologically from fibroblastic osteosarcoma and malignant fibrous histiocytoma, but this distinction is often difficult. It is possible that many fibrosarcomas are examples of malignant fibrous histiocytoma. Fibrosarcoma is treated with a wide resection. Radiation therapy may be of use for surgically inaccessible lesions. The overall prognosis for fibrosarcoma of bone is less than 50 percent reported survival rate at 5 years.

SUGGESTED READINGS

Dorfman HD, Czerniak B: *Bone Tumors*. St. Louis: Mosby, 1998.

Fechner RE, Mills SE: Tumors of the bones and joints. In: *Atlas of Tumor Pathology*. Washington, DC: Armed Forces Institute of Pathology; 1993:3d series, fascicle 8.

Huvos AG: *Bone Tumors. Diagnosis, Treatment, and Prognosis*, 2d ed. Philadelphia: WB Saunders; 1991.

Mirra JH: *Bone Tumors: Clinical, Radiographic, and Pathologic Correlations*. Philadelphia: Lea & Febiger; 1989.

Schajowicz F: Other connective tissue tumors. In: *Tumors and Tumorlike Lesions of Bone: Pathology, Radiology, and Treatment*, 2d ed. New York: Springer-Verlag; 1994:403.

Unni KK: *Dahlin's Bone Tumors: General Aspects and Data on 11,087 Cases*, 5th ed. Philadelphia: Lippincott-Raven; 1996.

Wold LE, McLeod RA, Sim FH, et al: *Atlas of Orthopaedic Pathology*. Philadelphia: WB Saunders; 1990.

Chapter 42

ROUND CELL TUMOR

Brian C. Toolan, German C. Steiner, and Samuel Kenan

Ewing's Sarcoma

Ewing's sarcoma is a small round cell tumor of bone and is the fourth most common malignant bone neoplasm after myeloma, osteosarcoma, and chondrosarcoma. The tumor can appear anywhere in the skeleton, but the majority are found in the pelvis and long tubular bones, particularly the femur. Ewing's sarcoma occurs during adolescence with pain and swelling at the tumor site. The patient may present with an associated fever, tender mass, an elevated white cell count, and anemia that may confuse the clinical picture with infection. Radiographs reveal a poorly marginated, permeative lytic lesion of the medullary cavity. There is periosteal new bone formation with an "onion-skin" pattern; this is a consistent radiographic finding, but is not pathognomonic for Ewing's sarcoma. It results from the reactive bone production secondary to the tumor violating the periosteum (Fig. 42-1). The soft tissue mass that usually is present may be seen on plain films; however, its extent of tumor involvement is better defined with an MRI or CT scan (Fig. 42-2). A Ewing's sarcoma has a semi-solid, liquefied gray-white gross appearance with areas of hemorrhagic necrosis. In keeping with its mimicking an infection, the lesional tissue can be mistaken for pus. Microscopically, the lesion is very cellular with minimal matrix production. It demonstrates small, rounded, closely packed cells with round uniform nuclei and indistinct cell membranes. The cells have scant cytoplasm and are two to three times the size of normal lymphocytes. They are arranged in dense sheets or nests separated by thin fibrous septa (Fig. 42-3). Areas of necrosis may be extensive, and viable cells can be identified around the capillary vessels. In some cases, rosette-like structures are noted in which the center contains necrotic cells. Periodic acid-Schiff (PAS) stain with diastase digestion identifies glycogen in the cytoplasm of Ewing's sarcoma cells in approximately 70 to 75 percent of the cases. The presence of glycogen is an important finding, but is not specific for Ewing's sarcoma cells. Immunohistochemical stains help to differentiate Ewing's sarcoma from other round cell tumors of bone. The Ewing's sarcoma cells are positive for Vimentin, which is a mesenchymal marker, and are negative for leukocyte common antigen (LCA), a marker for lymphoid cells. The cells react positively to the HBA-71 and 013 antibodies, which localize a glycoprotein produced by the gene *MIC2*. This latter finding and the presence of reciprocal translocation of chromosomes 11:22 (q24; q12) indicate that Ewing's sarcoma belongs to the group of neuroectodermal tumors.

Ewing's sarcoma is best treated with chemotherapy. Radiation therapy may be combined with chemotherapy to treat visceral and lymphatic metastases. Surgical resection is recommended after chemotherapy in locations where complete removal is possible. Radiotherapy is indicated in inoperable cases such as in the spine, and in cases with contaminated margins following surgery. The poor prognosis of Ewing's sarcoma relates to its fulminant clinical course and propensity for widespread metastases. The initial dismal 5-year survival rate for Ewing's sarcoma has improved with modern treatment protocols to over 40 percent.

Neuroectodermal tumor of bone (PNET) is a malignant neoplasm that has been recently described. It is basically indistinguishable from Ewing's sarcoma on clinical, radiologic, and histologic grounds. Both tumors share the same abnormal chromosomal translocation and the gene *MIC2*. However, neuroectodermal tumor demonstrates more ev-

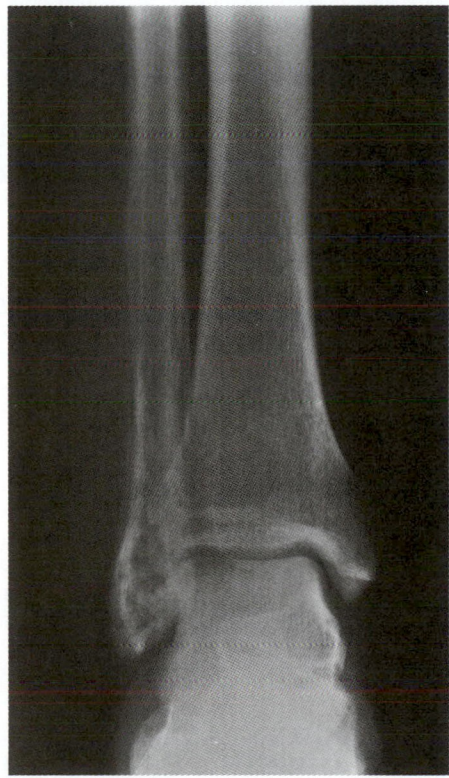

Figure 42-1

Ewing's sarcoma. A 24-year-old male with pain and swelling of the ankle for 8 months. Radiograph reveals irregular demineralization of the distal fibula with periosteal reaction.

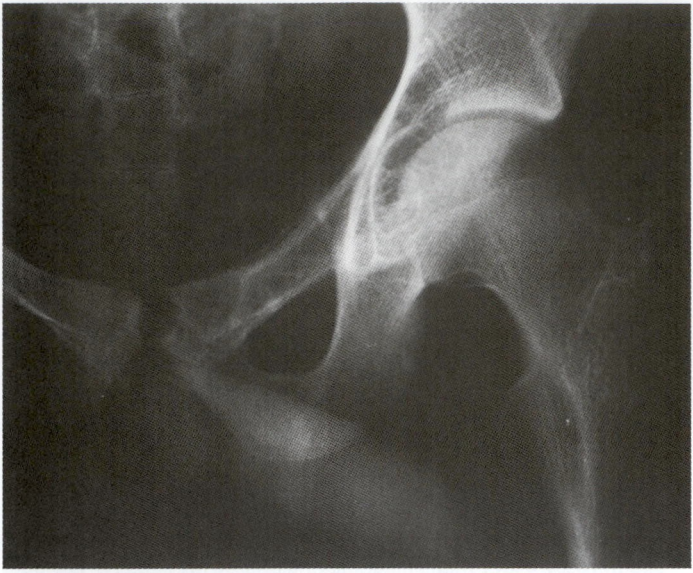

A

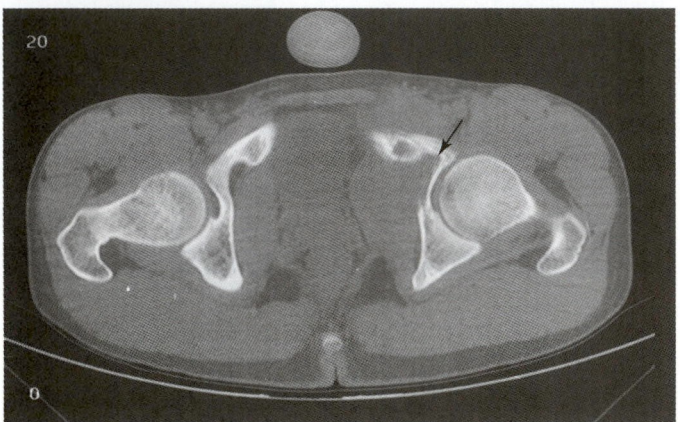

B

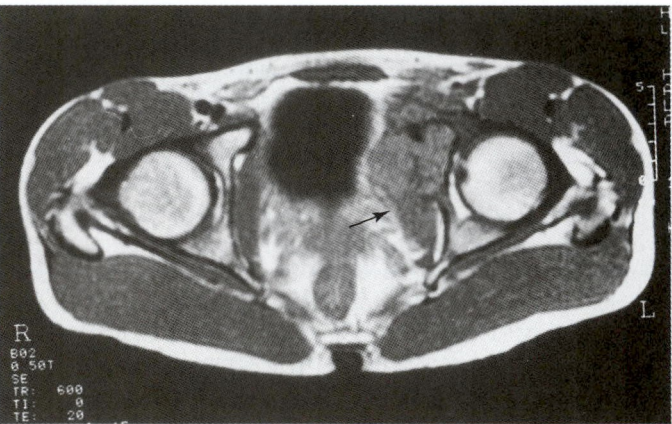

C

Figure 42-2
Ewing's sarcoma of the left pelvis in a 20-year-old male. (*A*) Radiograph shows a lytic lesion in the left pubic bone with periosteal reaction. (*B*) CT scan demonstrates bone destruction (*arrow*) in the left pubic ramus and the acetabular region. (*C*) MRI confirms the presence of a tumor in that area with soft tissue invasion (arrow).

idence of neural differentiation than Ewing's sarcoma. Some authors do not distinguish between these tumors and refer to them as Ewing's sarcoma/PNET. It is possible that they represent the same neoplasm in different stages of differentiation.

MALIGNANT LYMPHOMA (NON-HODGKIN'S LYMPHOMA)

Primary malignant lymphoma of bone is defined as a tumor arising within the bone and remaining localized at the original site without extraosseous involvement for at least 6 months. It is a rare tumor with an indolent clinical presentation during adulthood, particularly the

third decade. The patients complain of pain and swelling in a localized bone. These symptoms are often long-standing and the patients do not have constitutional complaints. The patients can present with soft tissue masses if the lesion penetrates the cortex and can have neurologic complaints due to compression of the spinal cord or nerve roots by tumor. The knee is the most common location of this tumor with the distal femur and proximal tibia involved in nearly half of the cases. Malignant lymphoma of bone appears as a poorly marginated, destructive permeative lesion in the diaphysis of long bones. The "moth eaten" bone may appear lytic or sclerotic or a mixture of both. There may be periosteal reaction, and the cortex may be thickened (Fig. 42-4). Grossly, the tumor appears whitish-gray and the residual bone trabeculae of this permeative lesion give it a gritty consistency.

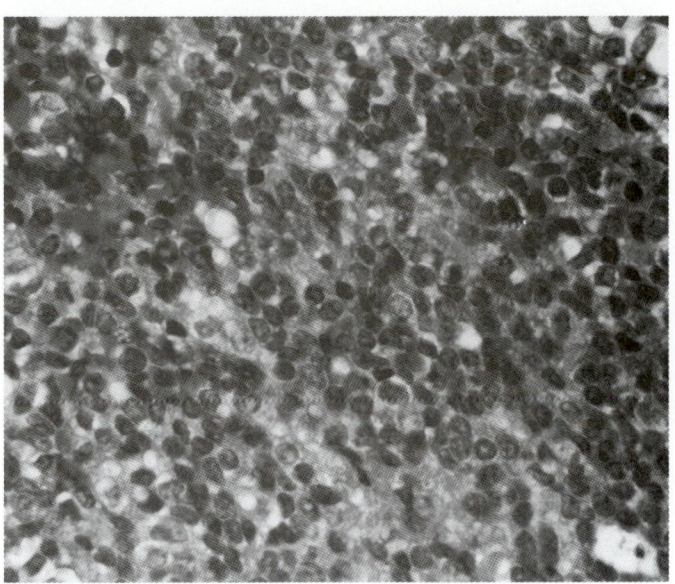

Figure 42-3
Photomicrograph of Ewing's sarcoma. It consists of a uniform population of round cells with indistinct cell borders. The nuclei are also rounded and uniform in size and the cytoplasm is sparse.

Histologically, a diffuse infiltration of round lymphoid cells is seen, varying from small lymphocytes to large cells, which often have grooved nuclei and conspicuous nucleoli (Fig. 42-5). Areas of spindle cell proliferation with fibrosis are focally seen. The majority of primary lymphomas are classified as diffuse large B-cell type. The tumor cells react immunohistochemically with (LCA) and B-cell markers (L-26). The considerable variation in size and shape of the lymphoma cells help to distinguish morphologically this tumor from Ewing's sarcoma, in which the cells are uniformly rounded. Adequate biopsy material and the application of immunomarkers help to distinguish malignant lymphoma from chronic osteomyelitis. Radiation therapy and chemotherapy are the primary modes of treatment. The prognosis depends on whether the lesion remains localized in the bone or disseminates to other organs. The 5-year survival rate varies from 20 to more than 50 percent.

Primary bone lymphoma should be distinguished clinically from secondary bone involvement by lymphoma arising in the lymph nodes or other extraosseous sites.

Hodgkin's disease involving bone as a primary clinical manifesta-

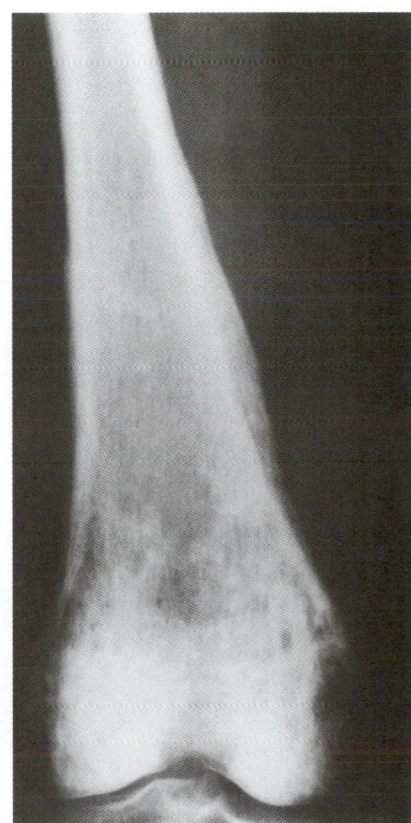

Figure 42-4
Malignant lymphoma of the distal femur in a 21-year-old female who complained of pain for 2 years. There is a large mottled lesion with areas of sclerosis and lucencies, as well as a smooth periosteal reaction on the right.

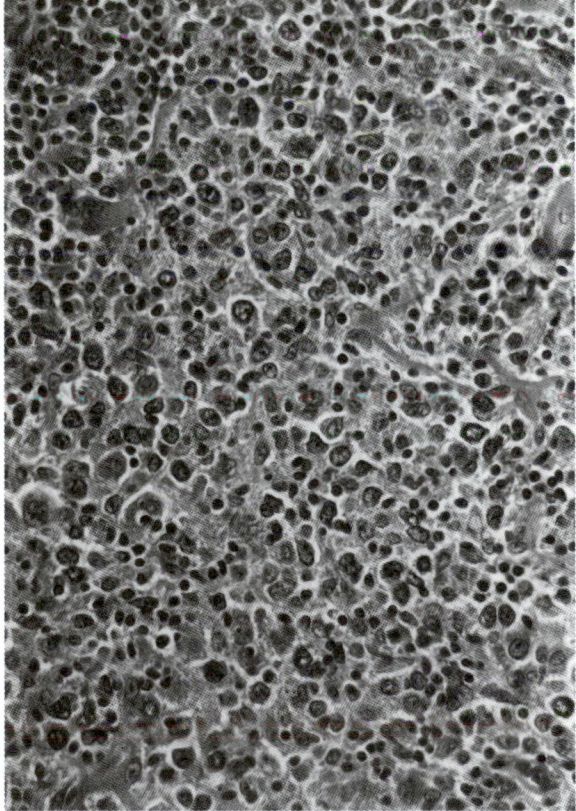

Figure 42-5
Malignant lymphoma. There is a dense, mixed population of large cells and small lymphocytes. The large cells have irregular nuclei and conspicuous nucleoli. Most primary bone lymphomas are of B-cell phenotype.

tion is rare. Most of the patients have detectable extraosseous lesions following staging studies.

Myeloma

Myeloma is a malignant plasma cell neoplasm originating from the marrow that usually presents with multiple osseous lesions (multiple myeloma). It is the most common primary malignant bone tumor. This condition affects males twice as often as females, most commonly in the sixth decade of life. The patient usually has bone pain, is anemic, and has elevated serum calcium proteinuria and plasmacytosis in bone marrow (>30%). Serum electrophoresis reveals a globulin spike, and immunoelectrophoresis usually demonstrates high levels of monoclonal immunoglobulins (M component) in the serum and a monoclonal light chain in the urine (Bence Jones proteinuria). Solitary myeloma is less frequent than multiple myeloma and presents as a single bone lesion. The majority of these tumors eventually become disseminated.

In very rare cases, myeloma presents at an extramedullary site with nasopharyngeal tumors or with neurologic findings due to vertebral compression fractures.

On radiographs, the tumors appear as multiple small, well-circumscribed "punched-out" lytic lesions at one or many sites such as the vertebrae, ribs, or pelvis. There is little or no reaction by the sur-

rounding host bone, but endosteal scalloping and medullary expansion may be appreciated. When the tumor involves a long bone and penetrates the periosteum it creates a soft tissue mass and may result in a pathologic fracture (Fig. 42-6). The above radiographic and laboratory findings and a marrow biopsy establish the diagnosis of myeloma. On gross examination, the tissue appears as a reddish gray homogeneous soft mass. The lesion consists of tightly packed plasma cells with an eccentrically located nucleus, abundant pink cytoplasm, and a pale-stained juxtanuclear halo that represents the Golgi apparatus. There is no background stroma with this tumor, and in some cases it can be mistaken for a lymphoma (Fig. 42-7). There may be amyloid deposits in the tumor, either as nodular foci or broad areas within the lesion. Intracytoplasmic inclusions (Russell bodies) are frequently seen at the light microscope and an increased amount of rough endoplasmic reticulum is noted in the myeloma cells with the electron microscope. The clinical course and prognosis are apparently related to the clinical stage of the disease and, less important, to the histologic degree of differentiation of the tumor. Well-differentiated solitary lesions have a longer median survival than poorly differentiated disseminated disease. Chemotherapy is the recommended treatment for myeloma, however radiation is effective for solitary lesions. Patients with impending pathologic fractures in the long bones require internal fixation. Vertebral lesions associated with myelopathy should be treated with decompressive laminectomy and may need instrumentation if the spine is unstable. The role of wide excision for solitary lesions is controversial.

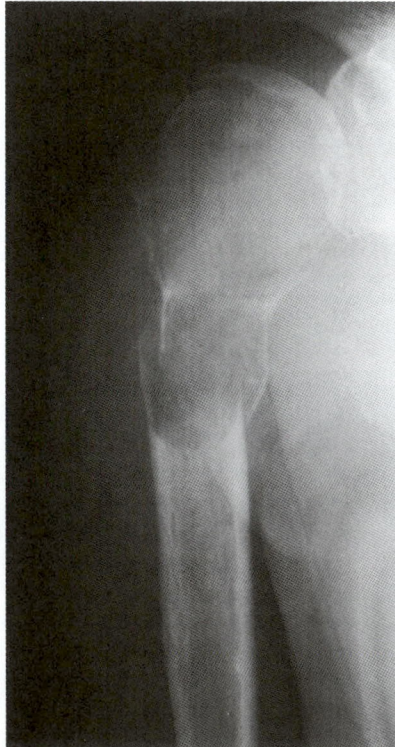

Figure 42-6
Radiograph of myeloma, showing a large lytic lesion involving the proximal humerus, associated with a pathologic fracture.

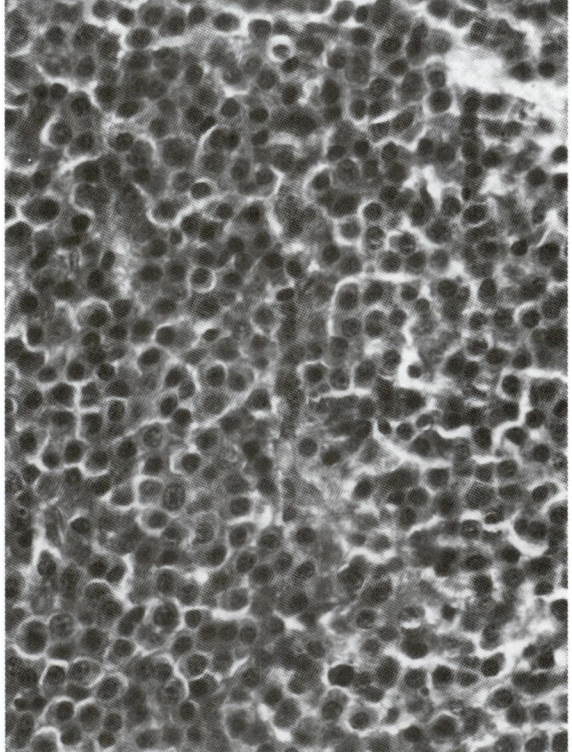

Figure 42-7
Myeloma. Photomicrograph showing densely packed well-differentiated plasma cells with round eccentric nuclei and clear cell borders.

SUGGESTED READINGS

Dorfman HD, Czerniak B: *Bone Tumors*. St. Louis: Mosby; 1998.

Fechner RE, Mills SE: Tumors of the bones and joints. In: *Atlas of Tumor Pathology*. Washington, DC: Armed Forces Institute of Pathology; 1993:3d series, fascicle 8.

Huvos AG: *Bone Tumors. Diagnosis, Treatment, and Prognosis*, 2d ed. Philadelphia: WB Saunders; 1991.

Mirra JH: *Bone Tumors: Clinical, Radiographic, and Pathologic Correlations*. Philadelphia: Lea & Febiger; 1989.

Schajowicz F: Marrow tumors (round cell tumors). In: *Tumors and Tumorlike Lesions of Bone: Pathology, Radiology, and Treatment*, 2d ed. New York: Springer-Verlag; 1994:301.

Unni KK: *Dahlin's Bone Tumors: General Aspects and Data on 11,087 Cases*, 5th ed. Philadelphia: Lippincott-Raven; 1996.

Wold LE, McLeod RA, Sim FH, et al: *Atlas of Orthopaedic Pathology*. Philadelphia: WB Saunders; 1990.

Chapter 43

GIANT CELL TUMOR

Brian C. Toolan, German C. Steiner, and Samuel Kenan

Giant cell tumor of bone derives from cellular elements of the bone marrow. Both the mononuclear and giant cells of the tumor show evidence of histiocytic differentiation. The giant cells apparently originate by fusion of the mononuclear cells. The mononuclear cells are the principal cells of this lesion. Multinucleated giant cells are present in many tumors, thus their presence in lesional tissue does not confirm the diagnosis of giant cell tumor.

The incidence of giant cell tumor peaks during the third decade of life and rarely presents before the age of 20 years. There is a slight female predominance.

Giant cell tumors are epiphyseal lesions that extend to the articular surface. The distal femur and proximal tibia are the most common locations of giant cell tumors followed by the distal radius and proximal humerus. These are painful lesions that may be accompanied by a mass or swelling, or may be associated with limitation of motion of the joint adjacent to the tumor and, on rare occasion, a pathologic fracture. The primary radiographic features of giant cell tumors relate to their eccentric, well-delineated epiphyseal location with metaphyseal extension, and the lack of reaction by the host bone. It is the lack of a sclerotic margin and the presence of soft tissue infiltration that can give giant cell tumors a rapidly destructive appearance and lead to mistaking them for malignant processes (Figs. 43-1 and 43-2). The tissue has a hemorrhagic, gray-brown appearance and may have liquefied cystic and necrotic areas. The surrounding cortical bone is thinned and there may be extension of the tumor into the adjacent soft tissues. The lesion may extend to the articular cartilage which is rarely

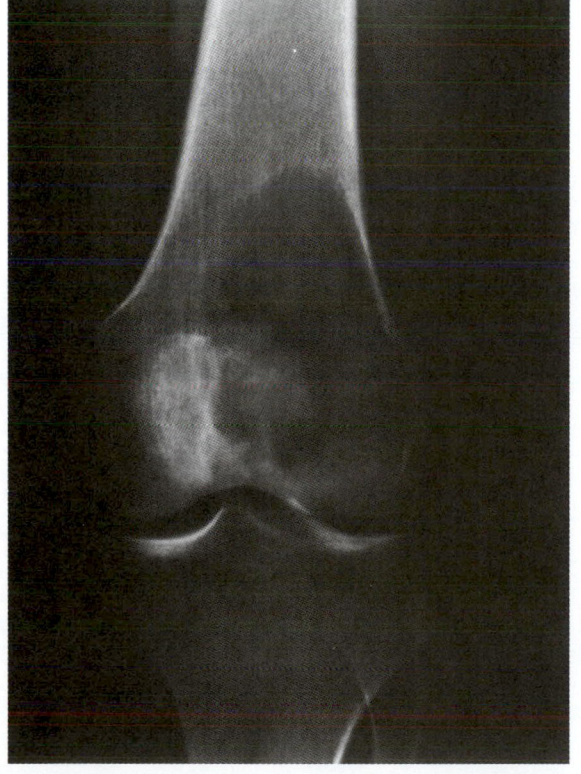

A

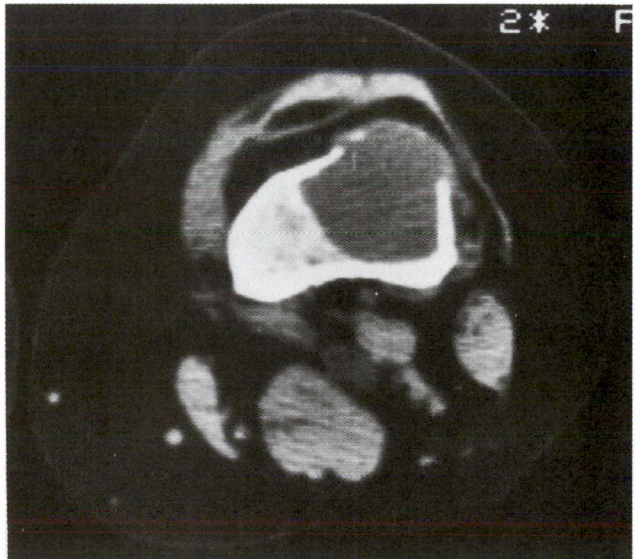

B

Figure 43-1
Giant cell tumor of distal femur. A 26-year-old female with pain in the knee for 5 months. Radiograph (*A*) reveals a large circumscribed lytic lesion with ill-defined margins, that reaches the articular end of the femur. CAT scan (*B*) shows anterior expansion of the femur with cortical destruction.

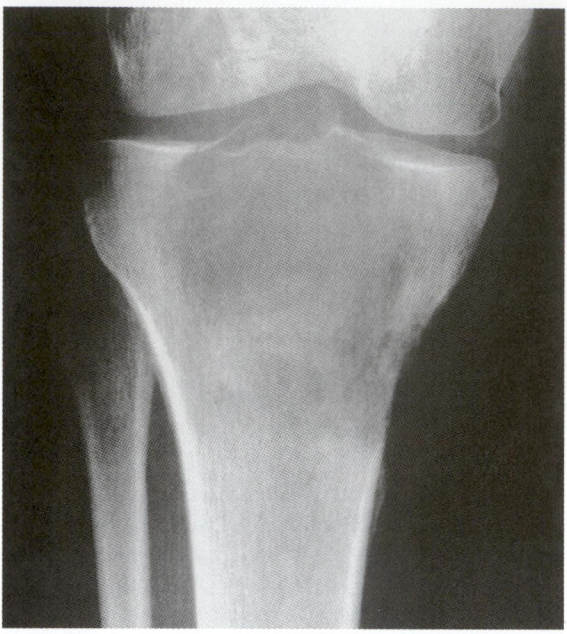

A

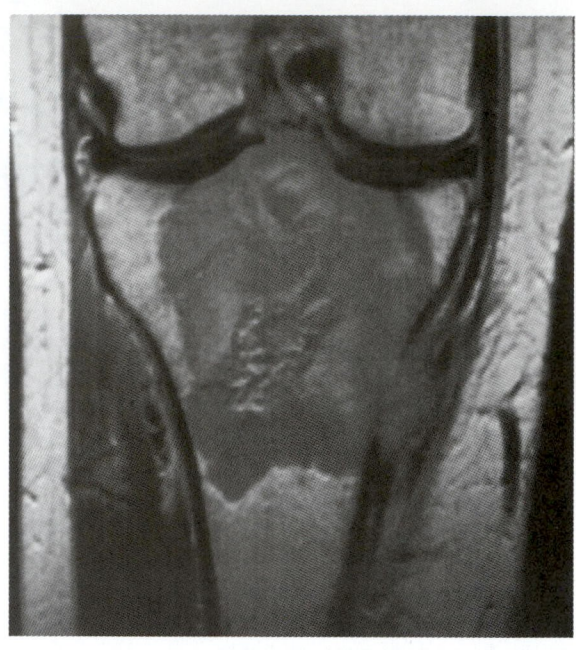

B

Figure 43-2
Recurrent giant cell tumor of the proximal tibia in a 23-year-old female, who had a previous curettage 4 months ago. Radiograph (*A*) shows a large central lucency with ill-defined margins and focal cortical de- struction on the medial cortex of the tibia. MRI (*B*) demonstrates the medullary involvement of the lesion which extends to the articular end, and the focal invasion of the soft tissues medially.

perforated. Under the light microscope the tissue is composed of nu- merous multinucleated giant cells that are uniformly distributed and separated by spindle and oval shaped mononuclear cells. Both types of cells have a rather uniform appearance and mitotic figures are pres- ent in the mononuclear cells (Fig. 43-3). The histologic appearance of the tumor may be altered when regressive or "healing changes" take place or when a pathologic fracture has occurred. The tumor typically lacks matrix production, but not infrequently, reactive new bone for- mation may be found. The majority of giant cell tumors are benign and the degree of local recurrence following curettage is not related to the histologic grading of the tumor (grade 1 or 2). Therefore, the grading has no practical value. Rarely, these lesions can metastasize to the lungs. Malignant giant cell tumor (grade 3) without previous radiation is extremely rare. Giant cell tumor should be differentiated from other benign lesions with giant cells, such as nonossifying fi- broma, aneurysmal bone cyst, giant cell reparative granuloma, and Brown tumor of hyperparathyroidism. The age of the patient, labora- tory data, tumor location, and radiograph, as well as the histologic ap- pearances of the lesions are important distinguishing features.

The treatment and prognosis of the tumor depends upon its clini- cal and radiographic presentation. Patients with radiographic stage 1 and 2 lesions (Enneking) may be treated with curettage and bone grafting or methylmethacrylate packing. Stage 3 lesions which show marked cortical destruction and prominent soft tissue infiltration are best suited to en bloc resection. Cryosurgery and chemical ablation have been utilized as adjuvants to local resection. Unresectable tu- mors may be treated with radiation; however concerns regarding the potential for malignant degeneration of irradiated giant cell tumors limits the efficacy of this treatment option. Aggressive local soft tis- sue and joint involvement may necessitate either amputation or ex- tensive joint reconstruction. Recurrence rate following curettage only

has been reported in the past to be as high as 40 percent. Recently, thorough curettage with cement packing has decreased recurrence to less than 25 percent.

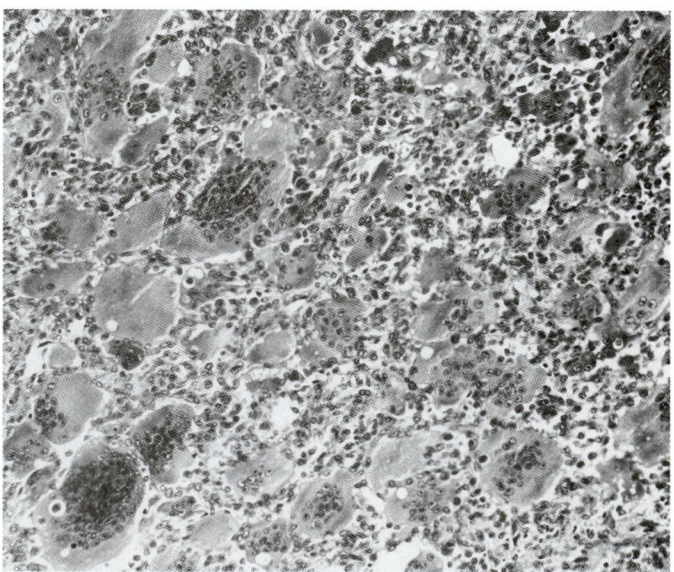

Figure 43-3
Photomicrograph of typical areas of giant cell tumor. It consists of mul- tinucleated giant cells which are uniformly distributed in the tissue, and are separated by round to ovoid mononuclear stromal cells.

SUGGESTED READINGS

Dorfman HD, Czerniak B: *Bone Tumors*. St. Louis: Mosby; 1998.

Fechner RE, Mills SE: Tumors of the bones and joints. In *Atlas of Tumor Pathology*. Washington, DC: Armed Forces Institute of Pathology; 1993:3d series, fascicle 8.

Huvos AG: *Bone Tumors. Diagnosis, Treatment, and Prognosis*, 2d ed. Philadelphia: WB Saunders; 1991.

Mirra JH: *Bone Tumors: Clinical, Radiographic, and Pathologic Correlations*. Philadelphia: Lea & Febiger; 1989.

Schajowicz F: Giant cell tumor (osteoclastoma). In *Tumors and Tumorlike Lesions of Bone: Pathology, Radiology, and Treatment*, 2d ed. New York: Springer-Verlag; 1994:257.

Unni KK: *Dahlin's Bone Tumors: General Aspects and Data on 11,087 Cases*, 5th ed. Philadelphia: Lippincott-Raven; 1996.

Wold LE, McLeod RA, Sim FH, et al: *Atlas of Orthopaedic Pathology*. Philadelphia: WB Saunders; 1990.

Chapter 44

VASCULAR TUMORS

Brian C. Toolan, German C. Steiner, and Samuel Kenan

BENIGN VASCULAR TUMORS

HEMANGIOMA

Hemangioma is a benign tumor of blood vessels of adulthood that infrequently involves the bone. Its common osseous sites are the skull, vertebrae, ribs, and long bones. Symptomatic lesions are rare and the patient usually presents with an incidental finding on radiography. Skull or rib lesions may manifest a sunburst pattern on x-ray due to radiating bone spicules in the tumor. Radiographs of the spine demonstrate prominent thickening of the vertical bony trabeculae of the vertebral body, or a "honeycombed" pattern. Vertebral body hemangiomas may weaken the bone and allow a compression fracture to occur (Fig. 44-1). Histologically, most of these hemangiomas are of the cavernous type. Large, blood-filled channels lined with endothelial cells are seen. The endothelial cells are inconspicuous and be-

nign appearing which helps to distinguish these lesions from hemangioendothelioma and angiosarcoma (Fig. 44-2). The primary treatment is observation for asymptomatic lesions. Radiation may ablate painful vertebral lesions and laminectomy may be required if cord compression is present. Care must be taken during surgery as these lesions may bleed extensively.

Massive osteolysis is a rare condition, also known as Gorham's disease, that is characterized by slow and progressive destruction of multiple contiguous bones. It predilects areas such as the shoulder and pelvis. Most patients are children and young adults. The bones are replaced by delicate endothelial lined channels which are indistinguishable from hemangioma.

GLOMUS TUMOR

Glomus tumor is a rare tumor composed of round, uniform cells resembling smooth muscle cells, associated with vascular spaces. The most common location is the subungual region of the finger. Secondary erosion of the distal phalanx may occur. They are always associated with pain. Glomus tumors arising from within the bone are extremely rare.

INTERMEDIATE VASCULAR TUMORS

HEMANGIOENDOTHELIOMA

It is a vascular tumor of intermediate degree of malignancy characterized by the presence of vascular structures lined by plump endothelial cells. It usually affects young adults. The tumor involves mostly the bones of the axial skeleton such as the pelvis and vertebrae, as well as the bones of the lower extremities including the foot. The lesion can be multifocal in several bones within the same area, such as the foot. Radiologically, they are osteolytic and are often well outlined and have sclerotic margins (Fig. 44-3). Histologically, there are anastomosing vascular spaces and the endothelial lining cells are round to polygonal and prominent, often with pink cytoplasm (Fig. 44-4). The degree of vascular differentiation is variable, and mitotic activity is also variable. Inflammatory infiltration with eosinophils is often present. In epithelioid hemangioendothelioma, the endothelial cells resemble epithelial cells by their appearance.

Distinction between epithelioid hemangioendothelioma and hemangioma may be difficult, particularly in hemangiomas that have prominent epithelioid features. Hemangioendothelioma should be differentiated from metastatic adenocarcinoma and angiosarcoma. The treatment is curettage for low-grade lesions, and the prognosis is good. Metastasis occur only in high-grade tumors. There is apparently no difference in prognosis between solitary and multifocal lesions.

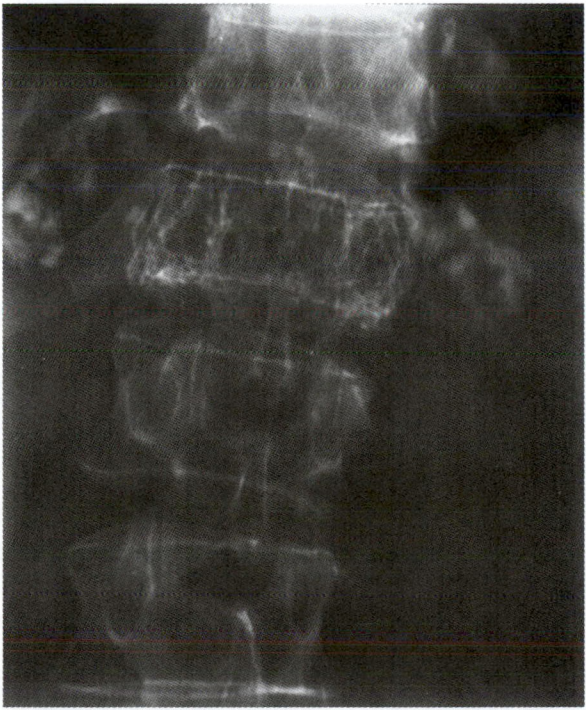

Figure 44-1
Hemangioma of the 12th thoracic vertebra in a 73-year-old female who complained of low back pain for several weeks, radiating to both legs. Radiograph shows a partial collapse of the 12th vertebra with coarse trabeculation with "honeycomb" appearance.

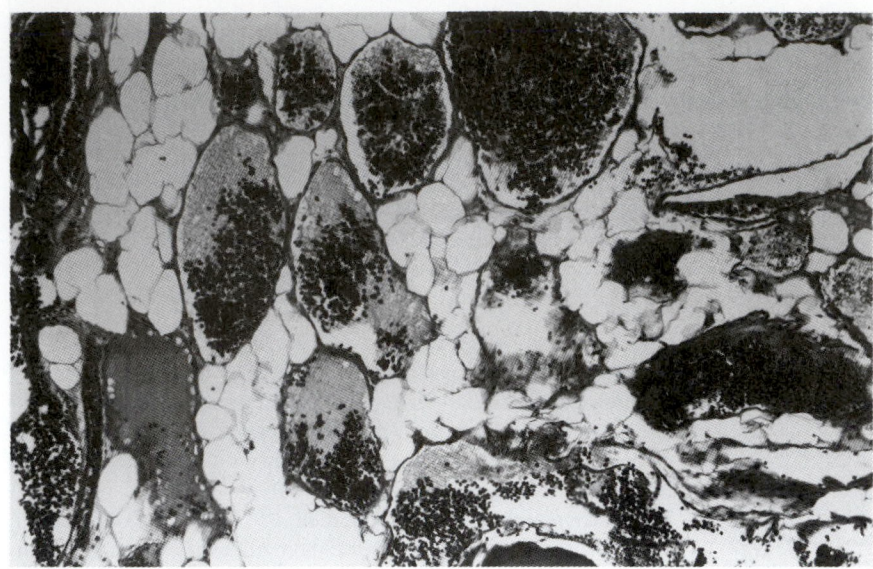

Figure 44-2
Photomicrograph of vertebral hemangioma. The lesion consists of large, thin-walled vascular spaces separated by adipose tissue. The vessel wall is lined by flat endothelial cells.

MALIGNANT VASCULAR TUMORS

ANGIOSARCOMA

Angiosarcoma is a rare vascular tumor, even less frequent than hemangioendothelioma. It has been reported at skeletal sites such as the femur, tibia, and humerus. The lesions may involve multiple bones or multiple locations in a single bone. Pain is the usual presenting

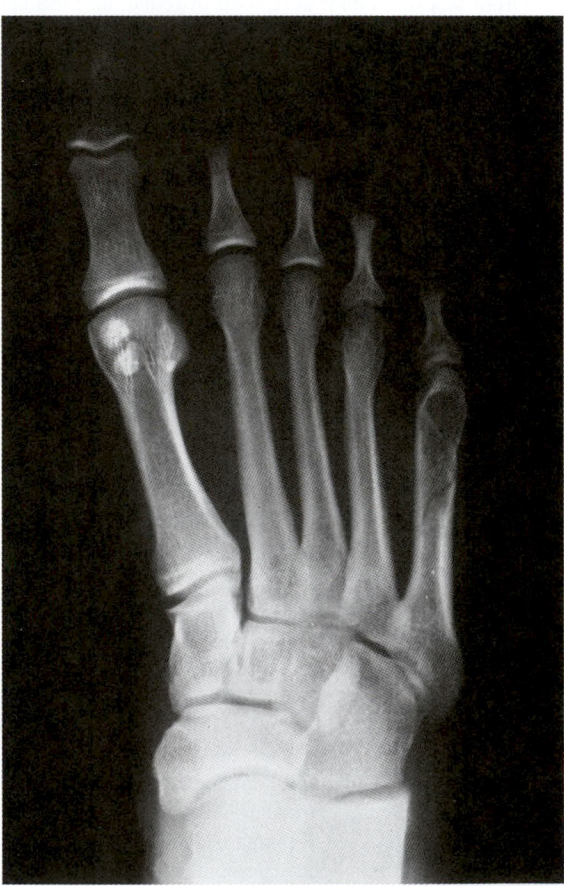

Figure 44-3
Hemangioendothelioma in a 19-year-old male who presented with a pathologic fracture in the right fifth metatarsal bone. A lytic lesion with bone expansion and cortical thinning is seen in the metatarsal bone in addition to the fracture.

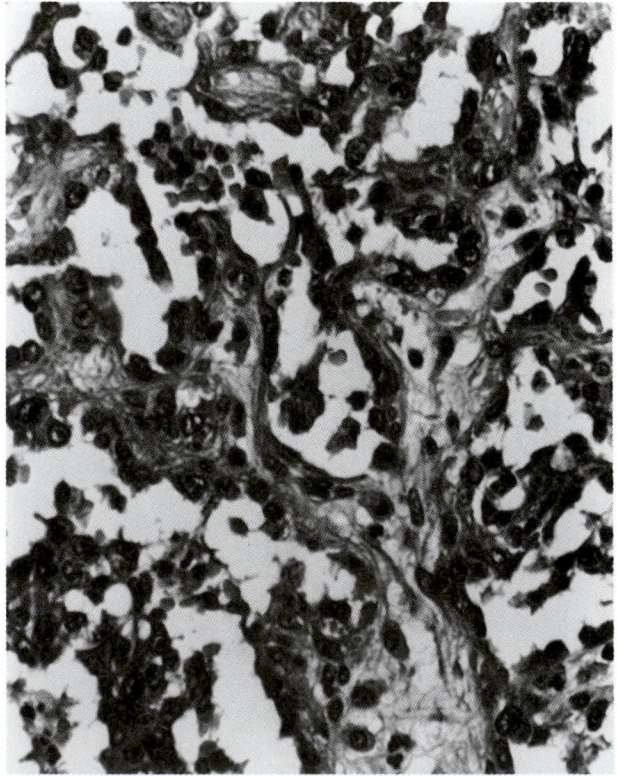

Figure 44-4
Hemangioendothelioma. The tumor consists of anastomosing vascular spaces which are lined by a prominent layer of large, round to polygonal endothelial cells.

complaint. Radiographs are nonspecific and demonstrate destructive lytic lesions with cortical destruction and soft tissue extension. Histologic examination reveals highly atypical endothelial proliferation. The neoplastic cells are usually poorly differentiated, and vascular formation is minimal. The lesions are treated by a wide margin resection or amputation. Radiation and chemotherapy are also indicated. Angiosarcomas metastasize widely to the viscera and lymphatics and carry a dismal prognosis for this reason.

HEMANGIOPERICYTOMA

Hemangiopericytoma is an extremely rare malignant vascular tumor consisting of abnormal proliferation of capillary channels and pericytes. The lesions occur in the adult pelvis and present as a tender mass. It has a nonspecific radiographic appearance, but is most often lytic. Occasionally, a honeycombed appearance may be seen. Hemangiopericytomas can occur as multiple lesions in a single bone or in adjacent bones. Microscopically, this hypercellular tumor has many thin-walled vessels branching throughout, with prominent perivascular proliferation of oval to elongated pericytic cells. Cellular atypia is present as well as mitotic figures, however the degree of

these findings is highly variable. The treatment ranges from radiotherapy to chemotherapy or surgical ablation depending on the location and grade of the tumor.

SUGGESTED READINGS

Dorfman HD, Czerniak B: *Bone Tumors*. St. Louis: Mosby; 1998.

Fechner RE, Mills SE: Tumors of the bones and joints. In *Atlas of Tumor Pathology*. Washington, DC: Armed Forces Institute of Pathology; 1993:3d series, fascicle 8.

Huvos AG: *Bone Tumors. Diagnosis, Treatment, and Prognosis*, 2d ed. Philadelphia: WB Saunders; 1991.

Mirra JH: *Bone Tumors: Clinical, Radiographic, and Pathologic Correlations*. Philadelphia: Lea & Febiger; 1989.

Schajowicz F: Vascular tumors. In *Tumors and Tumorlike Lesions of Bone: Pathology, Radiology, and Treatment*, 2d ed. New York: Springer-Verlag; 1994:369.

Unni KK: *Dahlin's Bone Tumors: General Aspects and Data on 11,087 Cases*, 5th ed. Philadelphia: Lippincott-Raven; 1996.

Wold LE, McLeod RA, Sim FH, et al: *Atlas of Orthopaedic Pathology*. Philadelphia: WB Saunders; 1990.

Chapter 45

TUMOR-LIKE LESIONS

Brian C. Toolan, German C. Steiner, and Samuel Kenan

SIMPLE BONE CYST

Simple (unicameral or solitary) bone cysts are solitary, fluid-filled cystic lesions located in the metaphysis of long bones near the epiphyseal plate of children and adolescents. These lesions predominantly occur in the proximal humerus and the proximal femur, although they have been reported in the bones of the forearm, leg, and foot. A solitary bone cyst is often asymptomatic. It commonly presents as a radiographic finding in a child with a fracture associated with minimal trauma. The pathogenesis of this lesion is unclear. It may result from resorption and cystic changes at the site of a post-traumatic hematoma or arise from a local disturbance of bone growth with the formation of fibrous tissue and the accumulation of fluid within the bone. Radiographically, it appears as a radiolucent, trabeculated lesion with well-defined borders (Fig. 45-1). The cyst contains straw-colored or blood-tinged fluid with thin, bony ridges that give the lesion its multiloculated appearance on x-ray. The cyst is lined with a loose connective tissue membrane containing small numbers of fibroblasts, giant cells, and hemosiderin-laden macrophages (Fig. 45-2). The treatment of a simple bone cyst varies with its location and the age of the patient. Up to 15 percent of cysts may heal after fracture with observation alone. A nonsurgical approach of aspiration and multiple steroid injections has proven to be effective in the healing of cysts. A surgical approach of curettage and bone grafting improves the healing rate and provides mechanical support. A higher rate of recurrence is associated with large lesions (involving more than one-eighth of the overall length of the bone), proximal humeral cysts, and cysts occurring in young (<10 years of age) males.

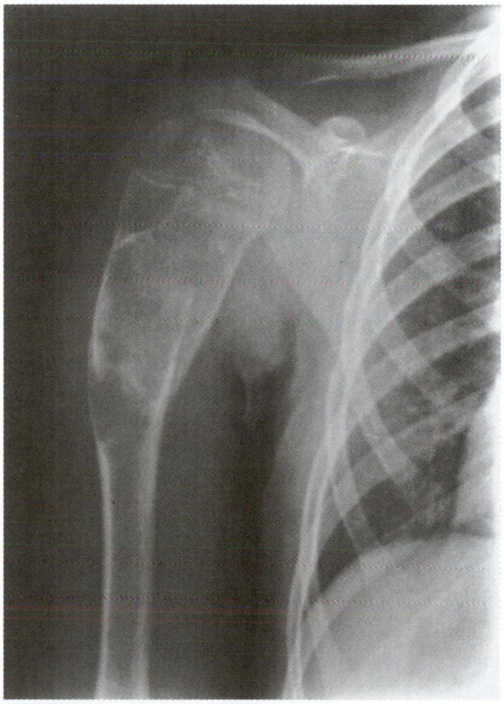

ANEURYSMAL BONE CYST

An aneurysmal bone cyst is a solitary expansile lesion located in the metaphysis of long bones, flat bones, and vertebrae. It presents in the second decade of life and, unlike a simple bone cyst, pain is the presenting complaint along with tenderness and swelling at the site of the lesion. There may be an associated limitation of motion of nearby

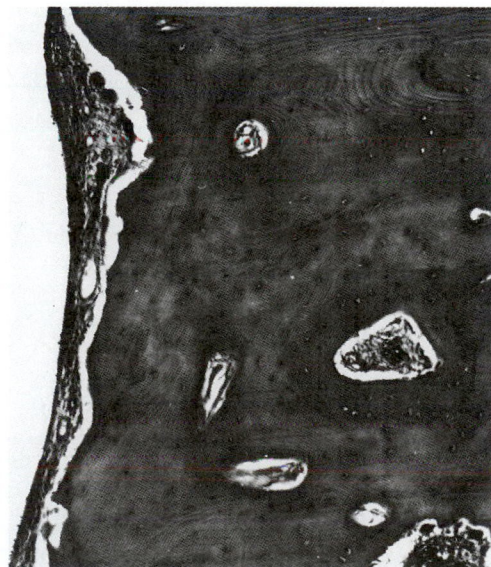

Figure 45-1
Simple bone cyst: 13-year-old female with a lytic lesion in the proximal metaphyseal region of the humerus. She developed a pathologic fracture 3 months prior to treatment.

Figure 45-2
Simple bone cyst: A thin, fibrous membrane containing few cells is seen lining the inner surface of the cortex on the left.

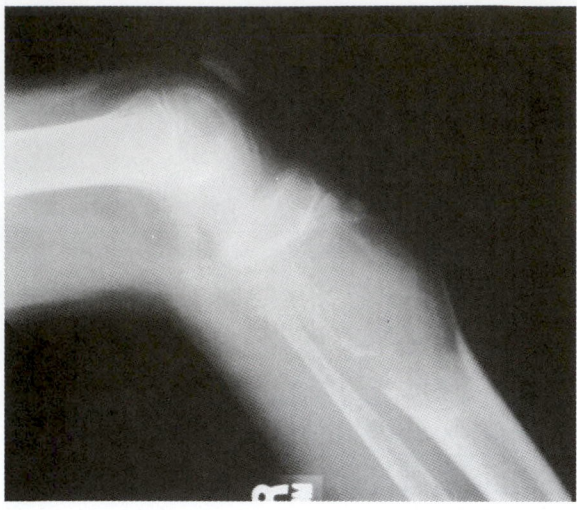

A

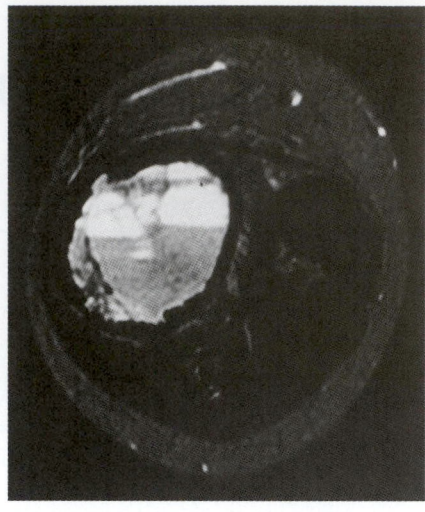

B

Figure 45-3
Aneurysmal bone cyst. *A.* A 10-year-old boy with an expansile lytic lesion of the proximal tibia with cortical thinning. *B.* MRI revealed typical fluid-fluid level within the lesion which is consistent with a blood-filled cystic cavity.

joints. Vertebral lesions can present with the signs and symptoms of cord or root compression due to bony expansion of the posterior elements. Radiographs demonstrate an expansile eccentric lesion surrounded by a thinned cortex with periosteal new bone formation and a characteristic "fluid-fluid" level within the cavity may be seen on CT scan or MRI (Fig. 45-3). The etiology of this lesion is unknown. A vascular disturbance in bone such as arteriovenous communication or an alteration of a preexisting fibro-osseous lesion has been offered as possible causes for aneurysmal bone cysts. Gross inspection of these lesions reveals a honeycombed appearance of bony trabeculae or fibrous tissue bands enclosing cystic spaces of various sizes filled with unclotted blood. Microscopically, the blood spaces are separated by cellular septa lacking an endothelial cell lining and containing a variety of cells such as fibroblasts, multinucleated giant cells, and histiocytes with hemosiderin deposits, as well as metaplastic bone

(Fig. 45-4). Large, solid cellular areas may also be seen. Aneurysmal bone cysts can be treated by excision, curettage, and bone grafting. A wide margin resection may be performed when the lesion is located in areas of nonessential bone. Cryosurgery and chemical cautery have also been employed successfully in the treatment of these lesions.

INTRAOSSEOUS GANGLION

It is a benign cystic lesion located in the subchondral region adjacent to the joint. It occurs in adults and has a predilection for the bones of the knee, ankle, hip, wrist, and carpal joints. The lesion may be incidentally found, but most often pain near the joint is a common presentation. Radiographs demonstrate a well-outlined lytic defect in the subchondral bone, usually measuring 1 to 2 cm in the greatest dimension. The lesion extends to the articular cartilage and has sclerotic margins. The affected joint shows minimal or no evidence of osteoarthritis (Fig. 45-5). Grossly, it consists of fibromembranous tissue with mucinous material. Histologically, the cyst wall contains fibrous tissue and may have myxoid areas (Fig. 45-6).

The pathogenesis of this lesion is unknown and probably is a reactive process. The cyst usually does not communicate with the joint. Intraosseous ganglion should not be confused with subchondral cysts of osteoarthritis. If pain persists treatment is by curettage and bone grafting.

FIBROUS DYSPLASIA

Fibrous dysplasia is a dysplasic disorder of bone characterized by the presence of trabeculae of immature bone presenting at one or many skeletal sites. It may represent disordered bone maturation, and often results in progressive bony deformity that may be associated with pathologic fracture. It often presents during the second or third decade of life with local pain and swelling. This condition can be monostotic or polyostotic. A rare polyostotic variant associated with precocious puberty and café-au-lait spots predominantly seen in young girls is known as Albright's syndrome. On x-ray, the lesion has a "ground glass" appearance and is sharply marginated with a rim of sclerotic bone. There is expansion, endosteal scalloping, and deformity of the affected bone (Figs. 45-7 and 45-8). The classic "shepherd's crook" deformity of the proximal femur arises from bowing of the bone and multiple pathologic fractures. The lesion may contain numerous cysts

Figure 45-4
Aneurysmal bone cyst. Photomicrograph showing vascular spaces separated by cellular septa containing numerous multinucleated giant cells and fibroblasts. The spaces are not lined by endothelial cells.

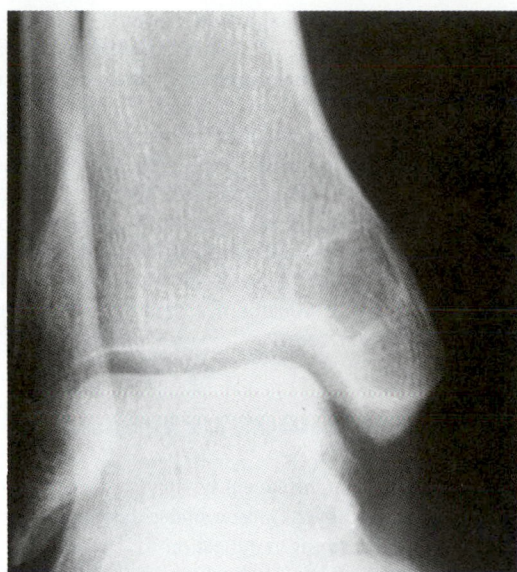

Figure 45-5
Intraosseous ganglion of the distal tibia. There is a subchondral lytic lesion in the tibial malleolus, with mild peripheral sclerosis. The ankle joint is normal.

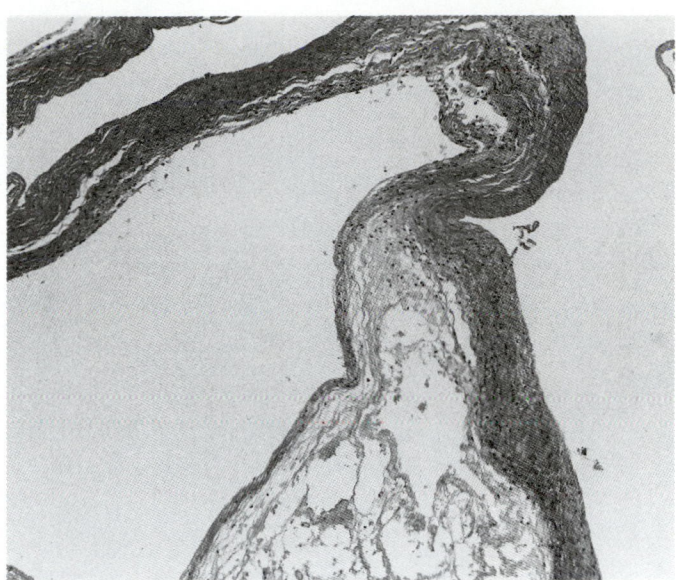

Figure 45-6
Intraosseous ganglion: It shows a thin, fibrous membrane containing few cells and areas of myxoid degeneration.

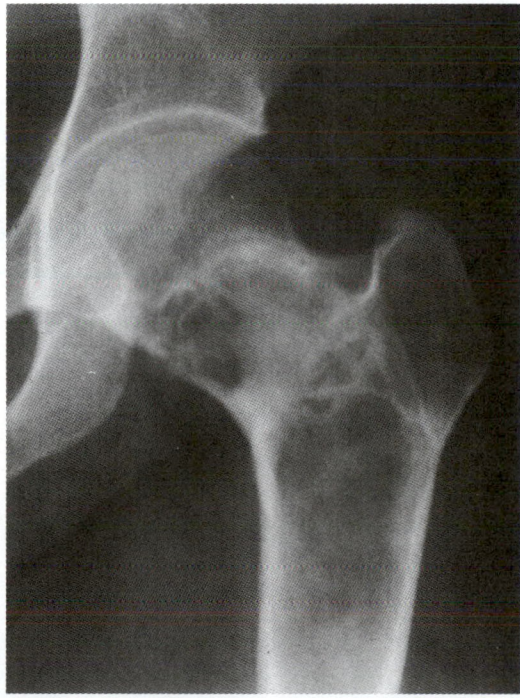

Figure 45-7
Fibrous dysplasia, monostotic. An intraosseous process is seen in the proximal femur, showing areas of lysis and sclerosis and the typical "ground glass" appearance. A pathologic fracture is also noted in the femoral neck.

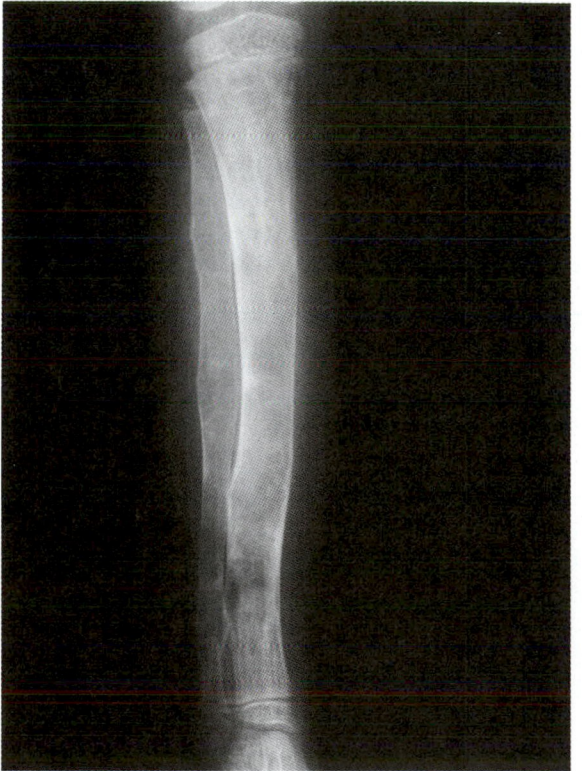

Figure 45-8
Fibrous dysplasia, polyostotic: There is extensive medullary involvement of the tibia and fibula with a "ground glass" appearance, expansion, and cortical thinning.

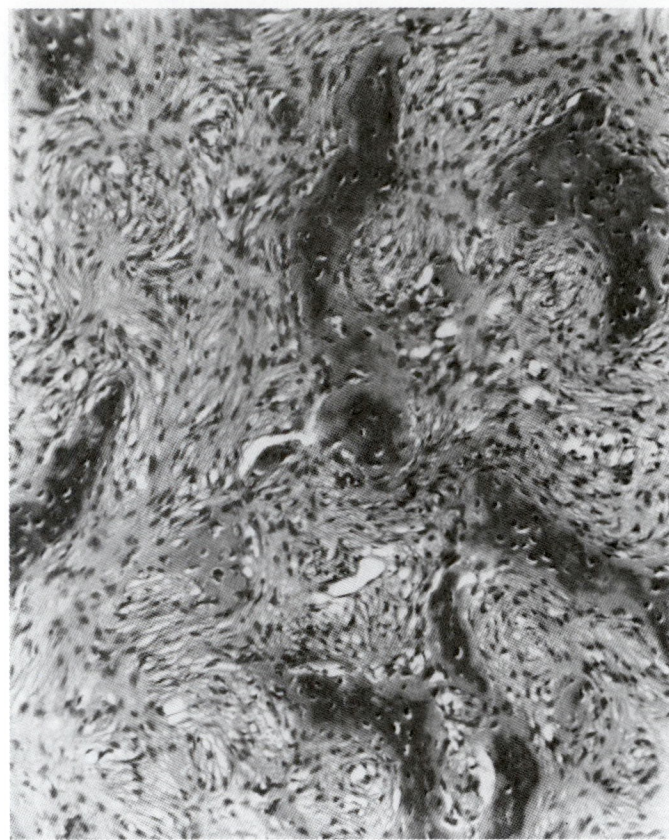

Figure 45-9
Fibrous dysplasia. It consists of irregular trabeculae of woven bone separated by a fibroblastic stroma. Occasional flat osteoblasts are seen rimming the bone trabeculae.

surrounded by a dense fibrous tissue with a gritty consistency. Histologically, a collagenous matrix containing proliferating fibroblasts surrounds irregularly shaped trabeculae of immature bone arranged in haphazard pattern classically described as "Chinese letters." The paucity of osteoblasts rimming the bony trabeculae distinguishes this lesion from osteofibrous dysplasia (Fig. 45-9). Cartilaginous tissue may occasionally be present in this condition. Monostotic fibrous dysplasia in the non-weightbearing skeleton can be treated with observation while bone grafting and internal fixation is often necessary for proximal femoral lesions. The prognosis of fibrous dysplasia is good, although sarcomatous transformation has been reported on very rare occasion in the polyostotic form.

OSTEOFIBROUS DYSPLASIA

Osteofibrous dysplasia is an infrequent benign fibro-osseous lesion of bone, originally described by Kempson under the name ossifying fibroma. This lesion has a strong predilection for the tibia and occurs in the first two decades of life. Radiographs reveal lytic defects involving the anterior cortex of the tibial shaft. There is usually associated sclerosis surrounding the lesions and anterior bowing deformity is not uncommon (Fig. 45-10). Histologically, there is a fibroblastic stroma associated with trabecular bone resembling fibrous dysplasia. The trabeculae, however, are lined by prominent osteoblasts (Fig. 45-11). This and the cortical location in the tibia distinguish osteofibrous dysplasia from fibrous dysplasia, which is a disorder of the medullary bone. There is strong evidence in the literature to suggest a relationship between osteofibrous dysplasia and adamantinoma. Both lesions involve the anterior cortex of the tibia, and it is known that adamantinoma may have areas that resemble osteofibrous dysplasia. In addition, osteofibrous dysplasia often shows keratin-positive cells in the fibrous stroma. The relationship between these two disorders is still unclear. The treatment of osteofibrous dysplasia is curettage, particu-

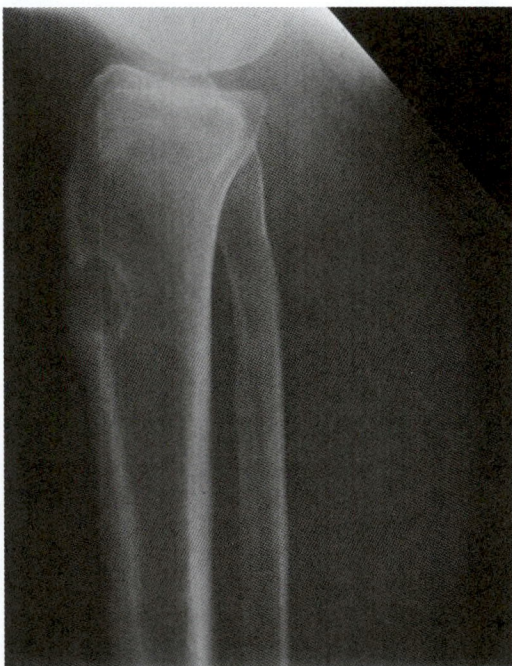

Figure 45-10
Osteofibrous dysplasia. A 20-year-old female who noticed a bump in the anterior aspect of the tibia. A circumscribed lytic lesion in the anterior cortex of the tibia is seen with medullary extension and sclerotic margins.

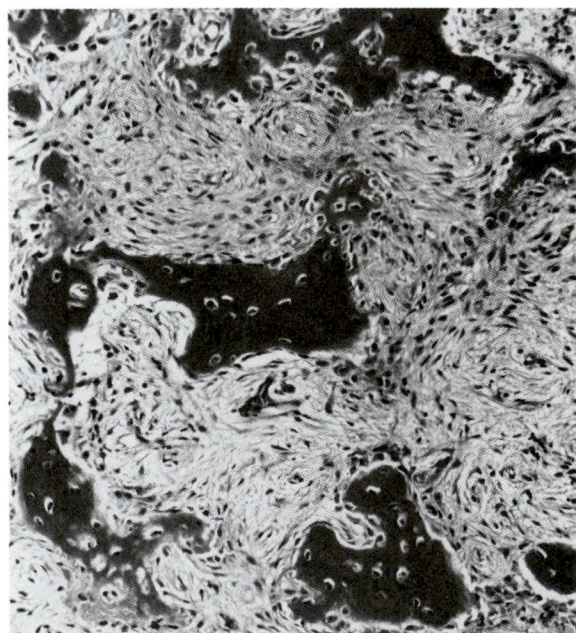

Figure 45-11
Osteofibrous dysplasia. Photomicrograph showing irregular bone trabeculae lined by a conspicuous layer of osteoblasts. The stroma consists of a moderately cellular fibroblastic proliferation

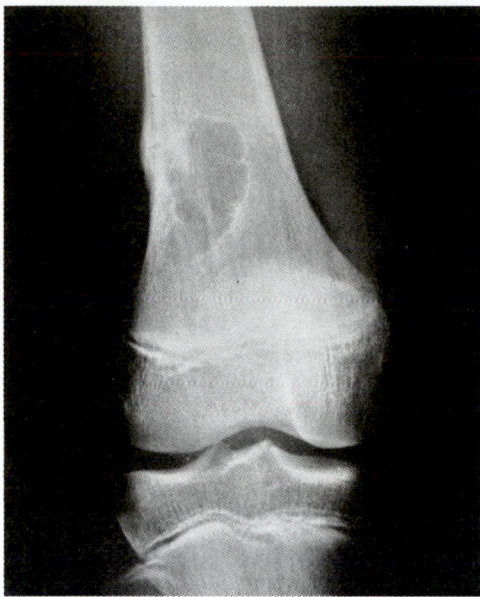

Figure 45-12
Nonossifying fibroma of the right distal femur in a 15-year-old male. He complained of right thigh pain for 4 weeks following a minor injury. There is a well-outlined eccentric lesion with marginal sclerosis. The periosteal reaction is secondary to a cortical fracture.

larly in enlarging lesions during the second decade of life. Recurrence may occur.

NONOSSIFYING FIBROMA

A nonossifying fibroma is a well-defined, eccentric metaphyseal fibrous lesion of long bones, particularly around the knee. It is distinguished from a fibrous cortical defect, which is characterized as a localized area involving the cortex. Most authors consider nonossifying

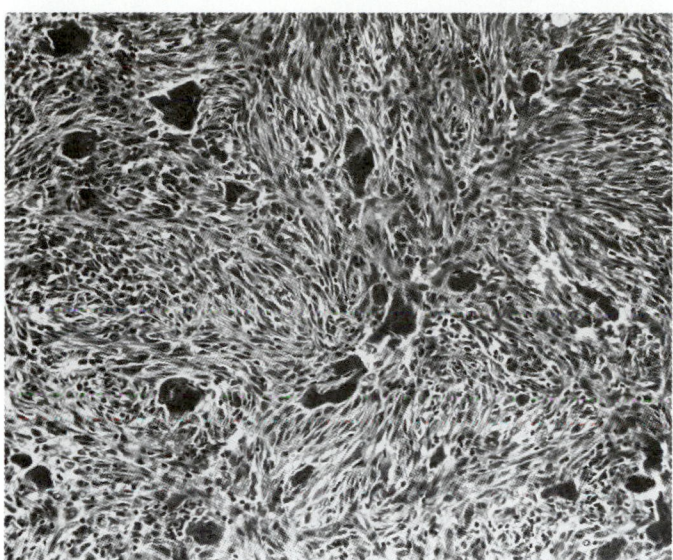

Figure 45-13
Photomicrograph of a typical nonossifying fibroma, showing scattered multinucleated giant cells separated by a fibroblastic stroma with a storiform pattern.

fibromas as advanced forms of fibrous cortical defects because they are no longer confined to the cortex but extend into the medullary canal. These lesions appear to arise as a result of some nonspecific developmental aberration of the tissue or as a consequence of an intraosseous hemorrhage. Fibrous cortical defects are usually asymptomatic and present on radiographs taken for unrelated conditions in the distal femur and proximal tibia of children. They may also be seen in the distal radius. Nonossifying fibromas may be painful and can present with pathologic fracture. They appear as clearly demarcated, eccentric, multilocular expansile lesions with scalloped, sclerotic margins (Fig. 45-12). Multiple and bilateral cortical defects are common. The cortex may be attenuated in areas adjacent to the lesion but remains intact unless pathologic fracture has occurred. Histologic examination reveals spindle cells arranged in a storiform pat-

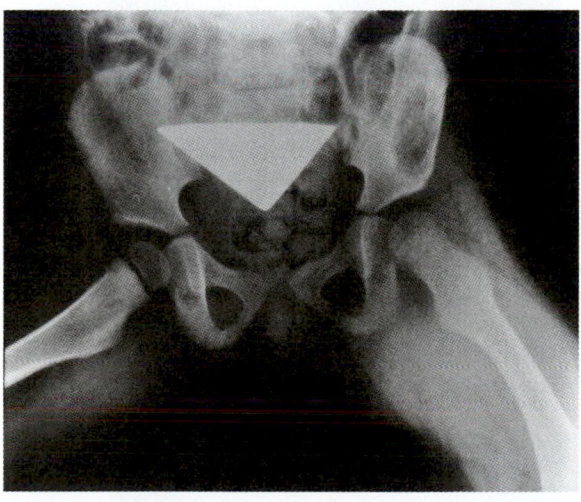

A   B

Figure 45-14
Eosinophilic granuloma of the left ilium in a 20-month-old girl who presented with a limp. The radiograph depicts a large lytic lesion with mildly sclerotic margins (A). MRI (B) shows expansion of the left ilium and a soft tissue mass.

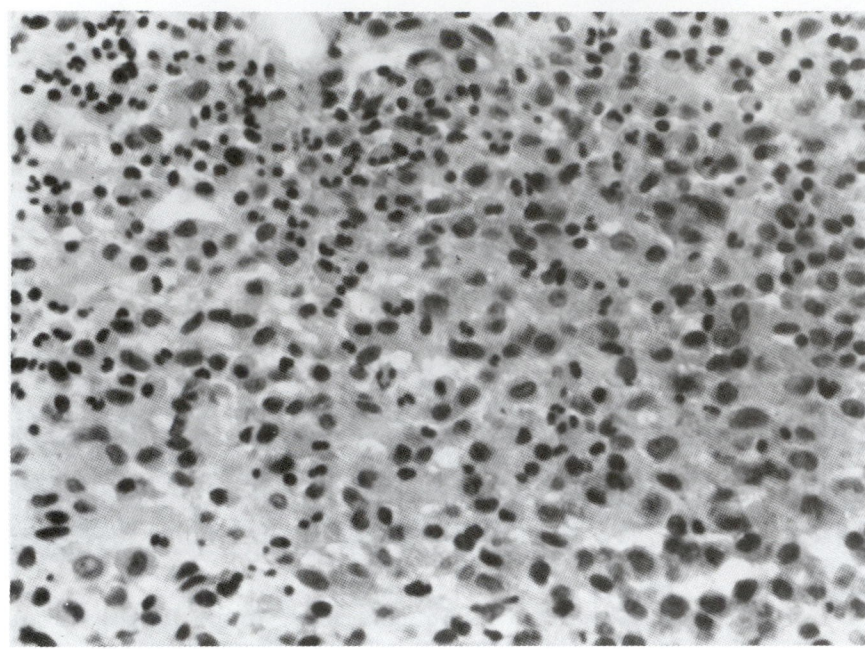

Figure 45-15
Eosinophilic granuloma. There are numerous Langerhans cells, some of which have indented nuclei. Small cells with bilobed nuclei typical of eosinophils are also seen scattered in the tissue.

tern. These whorls of connective tissue are often interspersed with multinucleated giant cells and lipid-laden macrophages (foam cells) (Fig. 45-13). The giant cells tend to be widely scattered, unlike the more uniform distribution seen with a giant cell tumor. Nonossifying fibromas and fibrous cortical defects are self-limited lesions that eventually ossify by the third decade of life and therefore may be managed with observation. Large lesions that encompass more than half of the bone diameter may require curettage and bone grafting to prevent pathologic fracture.

LANGERHANS CELL GRANULOMATOSIS

It is a nonneoplastic proliferation of Langerhans cells associated with eosinophils, and other chronic inflammatory cells. Eosinophilic granulomas present as solitary lesions in the long bones, pelvis, ribs, and vertebrae of young children, most commonly between the ages of 5 to 10 years. Histiocytosis X was a term used in the past for this condition that comprises eosinophilic granuloma, Hand-Schüller-Christian disease, and Letterer-Siwe disease. They often manifest with local symptoms of pain and swelling. When the lesions appear in long bones, they are found in the metaphysis or diaphysis and may show end osteal scalloping, and there may be a periosteal reaction if there is local cortical destruction (Fig. 45-14). These lesions may be more sharply defined when they present in the cranial or mandibular bones. Spinal lesions may manifest with vertebra plana due to compression of the vertebral body. Grossly, the tissue is soft with a loose consistency and is yellow in color. Histologically, it consists of Langerhans cells containing a vesicular, indented nucleus with a small, centrally placed nucleolus and abundant pale, granular eosinophilic cytoplasm. These cells are arrayed in sheets or clusters, and they are surrounded by eosinophils, various chronic inflammatory cells, and macrophages (Fig. 45-15). Small areas of necrosis may be seen. Electron microscopy of the Langerhans cells reveals the characteristic "Birbeck granules": racquet-shaped cytoplasmic structures. The Langerhans cells react immunohistochemically with S-100 protein. The surgical

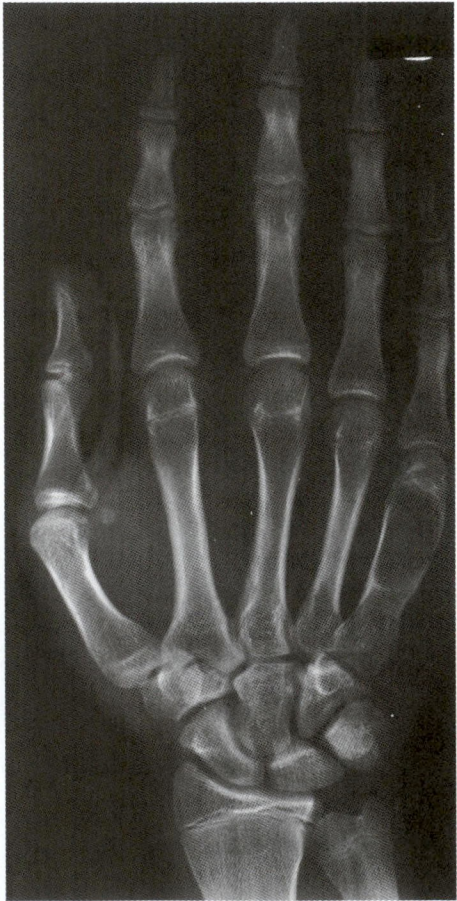

Figure 45-16
Giant cell reparative granuloma. A 14-year-old boy who had trauma in the hand 5 months before. There is a circumscribed lytic lesion in the fifth metacarpal bone, with expansion and cortical thinning.

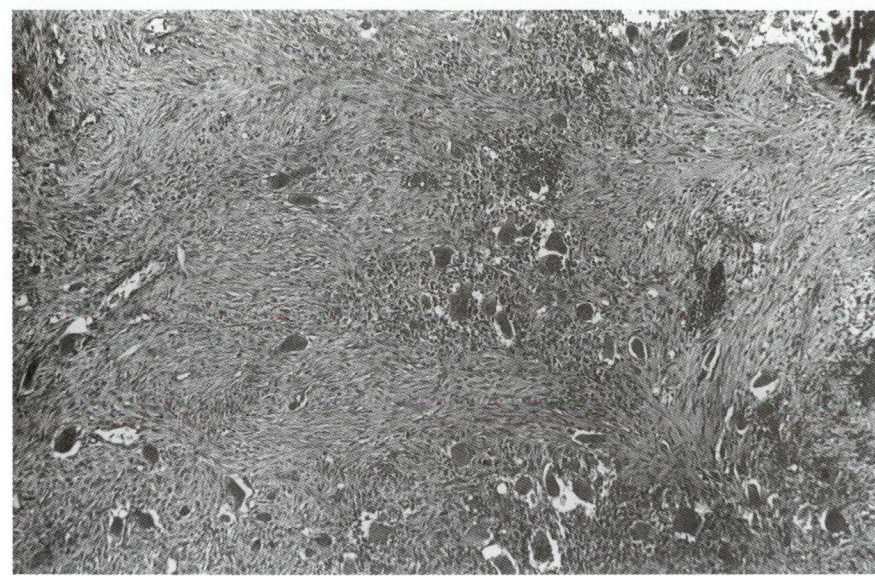

Figure 45-17
Giant cell reparative granuloma. Photomicrograph showing patchy aggregates of multinucleated giant cells, separated by abundant fibroblastic stroma with focal hemorrhage.

treatment of esinophilic granuloma includes simple intraosseous curettage and bone grafting. In other cases, a conservative approach by intralesional injection of steroids has proved to be effective.

Other clinical manifestations of Langerhans cell granulomatosis include Hand-Schüller-Christian and Letterer-Siwe disease. Hand-Schüller-Christian disease is a systemic process involving multiple bones, particularly the skull, as well as the liver, lungs, spleen, and skin. Letterer-Siwe disease demonstrates fewer skeletal lesions but has an aggressive clinical course due to widespread involvment of the skin, viscera, and lymphatics. The histologic features of these two conditions are similar to eosinophilic granuloma.

GIANT CELL REPARATIVE GRANULOMA

It is a benign process that was originally described in the jaw but was found also to occur in the short tubular bones of the hands and feet. A few cases have been recently described in long bones. It is more common in children and young adults but has a wide age distribution. Radiographs show a lytic intramedullary lesion in the phalanges, metacarpals, or metatarsals, sometimes associated with bone expansion and thinning of the cortex (Fig. 45-16). Histologically, there is fibroblastic proliferation associated with scattered aggregates of giant cells, stromal hemorrhage, and bone reaction (Fig. 45-17).

Giant cell reparative granuloma is a reactive nonneoplastic process. It usually can be distinguished histologically from giant cell tumor, where the giant cells are distributed uniformly in the tissue. The lesion has histologic similarities with aneurysmal bone cyst, particularly the solid areas, and probably the two processes are closely related. It is indistinguishable from brown tumor of hyperparathyroidism, but the patients have normal serum calcium and phosphate levels. As far as distinction from nonossifying fibroma, it is exceedingly rare in the bones of the hands and feet. Curettage is the recommended treatment. Recurrence is not uncommon.

SUGGESTED READINGS

Fechner RE, Mills SE: Tumors of the bones and joints. In: *Atlas of Tumor Pathology*. Washington, DC: Armed Forces Institute of Pathology; 1993:3d series, fascicle 8.

Huvos AG: *Bone Tumors. Diagnosis, Treatment, and Prognosis*, 2d ed. Philadelphia: WB Saunders; 1991.

Lieberman PH, Steinman RM, Erlandson RA, et al: Langerhans cell (eosinophilic) granulomatosis: A clinical study encompassing 50 years. *Am J Surg Pathol* 1996; 20:519.

Mirra JH: *Bone Tumors: Clinical, Radiographic, and Pathologic Correlations*. Philadelphia: Lea & Febiger; 1989.

Schajowicz F: Tumorlike lesions. In: *Tumors and Tumorlike Lesions of Bone: Pathology, Radiology, and Treatment*, 2d ed. New York: Springer-Verlag; 1994:505.

Unni KK: *Dahlin's Bone Tumors: General Aspects and Data on 11,087 Cases*, 5th ed. Philadelphia: Lippincott-Raven; 1996.

Wold LE, McLeod RA, Sim FH, et al: *Atlas of Orthopaedic Pathology*. Philadelphia: WB Saunders; 1990.

Chapter 46

MISCELLANEOUS TUMORS

Brian C. Toolan, German C. Steiner, and Samuel Kenan

ADAMANTINOMA

Adamantinoma is an uncommon primary bone neoplasm with a strong predilection for the tibia. Recent studies have confirmed the epithelial nature of this tumor. Adamantinomas present most frequently during early adulthood as painful leg masses with variable symptom duration, ranging from a few months to a few years. These tumors appear in the tibial diaphysis as a well-circumscribed, eccentric, lytic, sometimes multicystic lesion with surrounding sclerosis. The long bone is often expanded and the cortex may or may not be intact, but there is no periosteal reaction (Fig. 46-1). The lesional tissue is grossly graywhite in color and rubbery-firm in consistency, and cystic regions containing blood or straw-colored fluid may be present. Adamantinomas

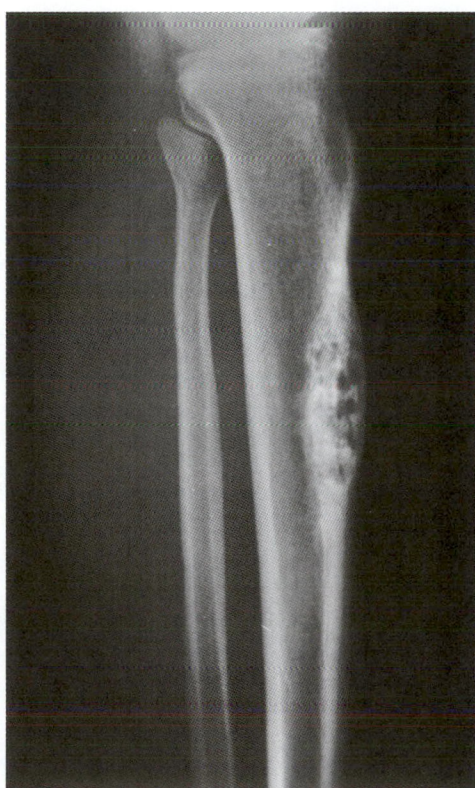

Figure 46-1
Adamantinoma of the tibia in a 54-year-old male. Radiograph shows an intracortical lesion in the tibia with lucent and dense areas, with expansion of the cortex.

have a wide variety of histologic appearances. Most frequently, the tumor has a basaloid pattern, composed of groups of cells which peripherally have palisading epithelial cells (Fig. 46-2). Other histologic patterns are tubular, spindle, and squamoid. Between these islands of epithelial cells is a hypocellular, poorly organized, fibrous connective tissue, which often contains areas resembling osteofibrous dysplasia. The tubular pattern may be confused histologically with a vascular tumor. Immunohistochemical studies of adamantinoma demonstrate the presence of cytokeratin in the tumor cells, and absence of endothelial markers. At the electron microscope level, the cells show epithelial features. The treatment of adamantinoma is en bloc excision with amputation reserved for large, unresectable, or recurrent lesions. This tumor has been reported to metastasize to the lungs in approximately 20 to 25 percent of costs.

There is recent evidence in the literature that there is a new type of adamantinoma called osteofibrous dysplasia-like or "differentiated" adamantinoma. It is more common among younger patients, contains a prominent osteofibrous dysplasia-like tissue, and has a good prognosis following curettage alone.

CHORDOMA

A chordoma is a rare tumor arising from remnants of the primitive notochord. It is a solitary lesion found in the midline at either end of the spine, most commonly first at the sacrococcygeal region (50 to 60 percent) and second at the sphenooccipital region. Other sites of the spine are less frequently involved. Chordomas have a predilection for middle-aged males and present with pain of gradual onset and of long duration. There may be a large presacral rectal mass that is palpable on rectal examination, and the patient may present with bowel or bladder dysfunction from compression of the sacral roots. Chordomas of the sphenoid or cervical spine may present with a cranial nerve palsy or nasopharyngeal mass. Radiographically, the tumor is destructive and associated with an expansile soft tissue mass (Fig. 46-3). MRI or CT scan may help to delineate the extent of the tumor. On gross inspection the tumor appears gray, lobulated, gelatinous, and encased in a pseudocapsule. Histologically, the cells are polyhedral in shape and often have eosinophilic cytoplasm and numerous vacuoles which displace the nucleus (physaliphorous cells). The tissue has a lobular architecture and the cells are disposed in cords, trabeculae, or sheets, which are separated by abundant mucoid and myxoid matrix (Fig. 46-4). Immunohistochemically, chordoma cells show positive reaction to S-100 protein, cytokeratin, and epithelial membrane antigen. These studies help to distinguish chor-

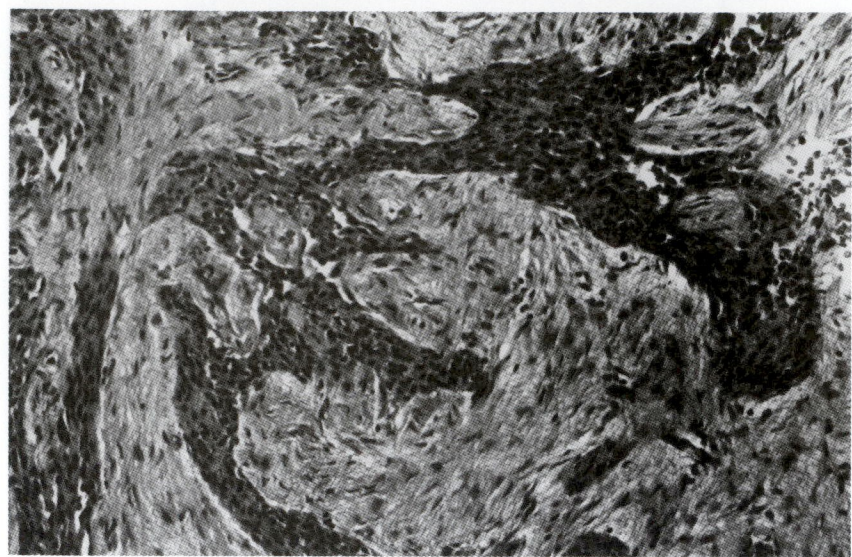

Figure 46-2
Adamantinoma. Photomicrograph showing large, solid areas and cords of epithelial cells separated by a fibroblastic stroma. The tumor cells are cytokeratin positive.

doma from other malignant tumors such as myxoid chondrosarcomas and metastatic adenocarcinomas.

Wide local resection is the recommended treatment; however, because the patients often present late in the clinical course and because of its close proximity to neurologic structures, the tumor is usually not resectable. Radiation is indicated. These tumors have a very high rate of recurrence even with surgical treatment. Metastases develop rather frequently to the lungs, liver, and other tissues.

A small percentage of chordomas of the sphenooccipital region have a prominent chondroid component and are designated as chondroid chordomas. They apparently have a better prognosis than conventional chordomas. Rarely, chordomas may have a high-grade sarcomatous component adjacent to it, usually resembling malignant fibrous histiocytoma. These tumors are called dedifferentiated chordomas and have a bad prognosis.

LIPOMA

Lipomas primary in bone are rare. They occur in adults and predilect the femur, fibula, tibia, and calcaneous. Radiographs demonstrate a lytic lesion with well-defined margins. Central areas of radiodensity

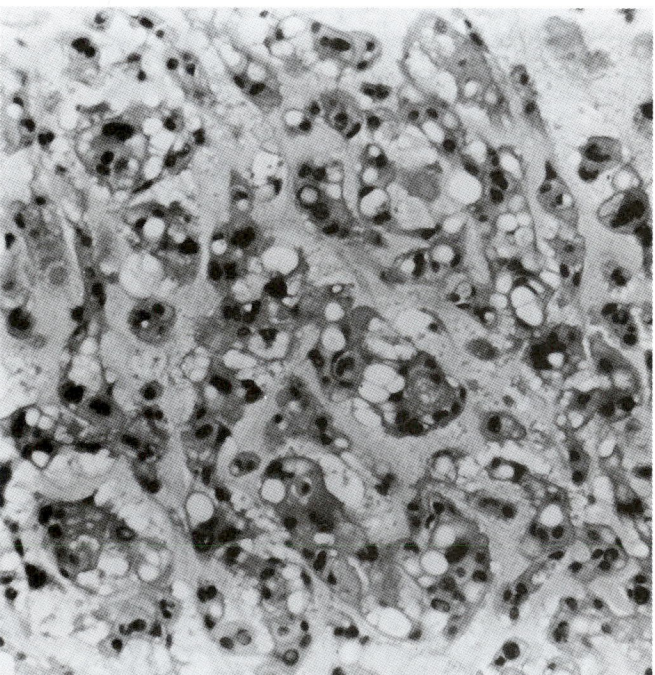

Figure 46-4
Photomicrograph of chordoma. The tumor consists of multivacuolated cells (physaliphorous cells) which are arranged in cords or trabeculae, separated by a loose mucoid matrix. [Reproduced with permission from Steiner GC: Tumors and tumor-like conditions. In Johannessen JV (ed): *Electron Microscopy in Human Medicine*, vol 4. New York: McGraw-Hill; 1998:115.]

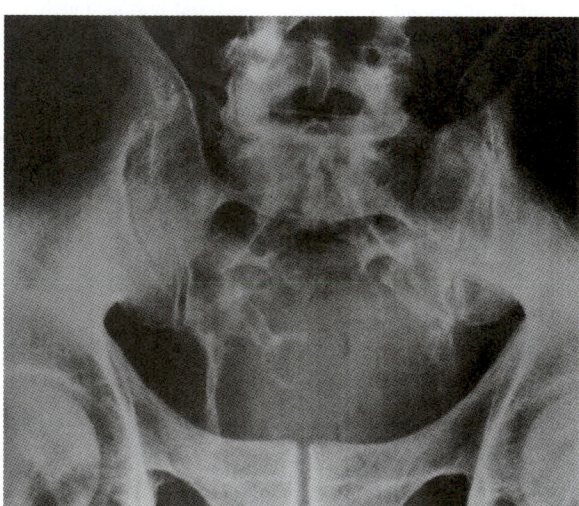

Figure 46-3
Radiograph of chordoma showing a large lytic and destructive lesion of the sacrum.

may be seen. MRI is helpful in the diagnosis of lipoma, showing high signal intensity in both T1- and T2-weighted images. Histologically, there is mature adipose tissue with atrophic bone trabeculae. Fat necrosis and calcification also may be seen. Treatment is by curettage. Liposarcoma is exceedingly rare.

LEIOMYOSARCOMA

Leiomyosarcoma is a rare tumor affecting adults and most commonly predilecting the femur and tibia. Radiographs show nonspecific lytic changes of a malignant nature. Histologically, there are spindle cells with acidophilic cytoplasm, and the nuclei show varying degrees of atypia and mitotic activity. There is a dense fascicular pattern. Immunohistochemical reactivity to muscle markers are important findings in order to differentiate this tumor from malignant fibrous histiocytoma and fibrosarcoma. En bloc resection or amputation is recommended. At least 50 percent of patients die of metastases. Primary leiomyosarcoma of bone should be distinguished clinically from metastatic leiomyosarcoma to bone, particularly from the uterus.

SCHWANNOMA

Intraosseous schwannomas are rare and arise from the sacrum, mandible, and other bones. Radiographically, they are lytic lesions, and microscopically, they show the typical features of Antoni A and B tissue as seen in the soft tissue counterparts. In most cases of neurofibroma with bone involvement, the tumors are located in the soft tissue with secondary extension into bone.

SUGGESTED READINGS

Dorfman HD, Czerniak B: *Bone Tumors*. St. Louis: Mosby; 1998.

Fechner RE, Mills SE: Tumors of the bones and joints. In: *Atlas of Tumor Pathology*. Washington, DC: Armed Forces Institute of Pathology; 1993:3d series, fascicle 8.

Huvos AG: *Bone Tumors. Diagnosis, Treatment, and Prognosis*, 2d ed. Philadelphia: WB Saunders; 1991.

Mirra JH: *Bone Tumors: Clinical, Radiographic, and Pathologic Correlations*. Philadelphia: Lea & Febiger; 1989.

Schajowicz F: Other tumors. In: *Tumors and Tumorlike Lesions of Bone: Pathology, Radiology, and Treatment*, 2d ed. New York: Springer-Verlag; 1994:453.

Unni KK: *Dahlin's Bone Tumors: General Aspects and Data on 11,087 Cases*, 5th ed. Philadelphia: Lippincott-Raven; 1996.

Wold LE, McLeod RA, Sim FH, et al: *Atlas of Orthopaedic Pathology*. Philadelphia: WB Saunders; 1990.

MALIGNANT TUMORS ARISING IN PREEXISTING CONDITIONS OF BONE

Samuel Kenan and German C. Steiner

The majority of primary malignant bone tumors originate in normal-appearing bone. Malignant tumors arising in benign preexisting lesions of bone are rare. The association of certain conditions with sarcomatous transformation has been well documented.

Malignant transformation describes a process whereby the cells have lost their histologic differentiation, resulting in increased anaplasia and increased mitotic rate to become a malignant tumor. Such malignant processes have been noted in bone, Paget's disease, infarct, radiation osteitis, osteochondromatosis, enchondromatosis, and less frequently in chronic osteomyelitis, fibrous dysplasia, synovial chondromatosis, osteoblastoma, giant cell tumor, and chondroblastoma. In a long-standing indolent process such as bone infarct, the primary lesion is surrounded by a reparative process and it is possible that malignant transformation occurs in these areas of reparative activity.

Malignant transformation is seen in adult patients who have a long-standing history of preexisting conditions. Adult patients who have one of the above underlying conditions and who present with a change in the clinical course with a rapid onset of pain, swelling, and constant change in the appearance of the radiographic features should be suspected of having malignant transformation. Early recognition and treatment are of vital importance.

SARCOMATOUS TRANSFORMATION

BONE INFARCT

Sarcomas arising in bone infarcts are extremely rare. Such events are seen in middle-aged patients in whom the bone infarct has been present for many years. Such cases have been reported in patients with idiopathic bone infarct, sickle cell disease, and in caisson workers. Histologically, the sarcomatous process in most of the cases is malignant fibrous histiocytoma followed by osteosarcoma and fibrosarcoma (Fig. 47-1).

PAGET'S DISEASE

The most serious and devastating complication of Paget's disease is the development of sarcomatous transformation. The incidence of sarcomatous change varies in different reports. It is estimated to be under 1 percent. Osteosarcoma is the most common histological type. Paget's sarcoma is very rare in patients under the age of 50 years. The majority of the patients are in their sixth and seventh decades. Males are affected more often than females. Sarcomatous change is more commonly seen in patients with polyostotic Paget's disease. The most common anatomical sites are the femur, humerus, pelvis, and cranium. Radiographically, the sarcomatous change could be lytic, blastic, or mixed type (Fig. 47-2). The average duration of symptoms before diagnosis is about 6 months. The presenting symptoms are pain and swelling. The overall prognosis of Paget's sarcoma is poor with a short life expectancy. In most cases, surgical extirpation is only palliative, and radiotherapy and chemotherapy do not change the clinical course.

RADIATION INDUCED SARCOMA

Radiation is associated with a variety of skeletal complications. The most devastating complication is radiation-induced sarcoma. Malignant fibrous histiocytoma is the most common histologic type. The criteria for radiation-induced sarcoma are: (1) the involved bone should be included in the radiation field; (2) there should be a latent period of several years, at least 3 to 4 years; and (3) histologic verification of sarcoma (Fig. 47-3).

The mean latent period until sarcomatous change in adults is about 16 years. A shorter mean latent period of 9.6 has been reported in children. Postradiation sarcomas are very aggressive with high rates of metastases and shorter life expectancy.

CHRONIC OSTEOMYELITIS

Squamous cell carcinoma is known to occur in chronic draining sinuses of osteomyelitis. This complication is reported to occur in less than 0.5 percent of cases of chronic osteomyelitis. Pain and swelling with progressive radiographic changes should alert the clinician to the possibility of malignant change.

OSTEOCHONDROMA AND OSTEOCHONDROMATOSIS

It appears that the risk of malignant change in osteochondroma has been grossly overestimated. The wide range of incidence reported is probably related to the different age group distribution and different histologic criteria. A realistic incidence of malignant change for solitary osteochondroma is less than 1 percent and for multiple osteochondromatosis is less than 5 percent. The risk of malignant change increases with larger lesions and with lesions which are localized closer to the axial skeleton such as the pelvis and spine. The average age of sarcomatous change is usually beyond the third decade of life. Malignant change should be suspected whenever one of the follow-

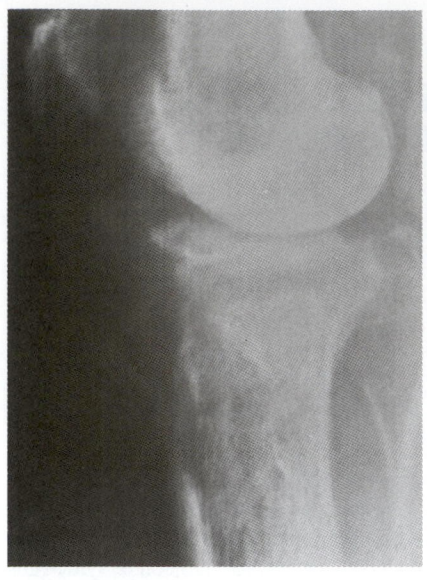 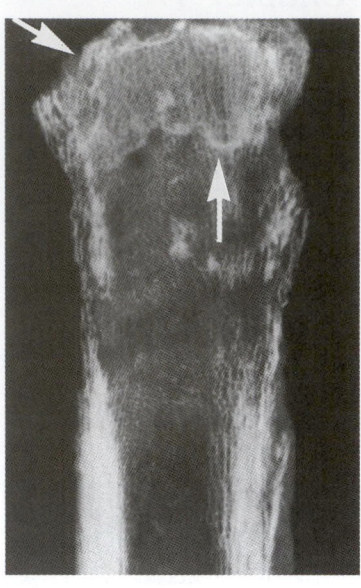 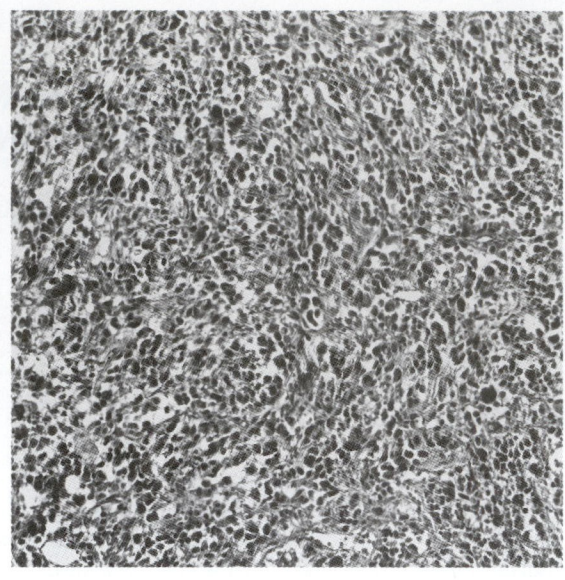

A   *B*   *C*

Figure 47-1

A. Sarcoma arising in bone infarct. A 46-year-old male with knee pain for 2 months. Radiographs shows a destructive tumor involving the proximal tibia with soft tissue extension. *B.* Radiograph of the amputated specimen demonstrates destruction of the medullary and cortical bone. The preexistent bone infarct is seen in the proximal tibia (*arrows*) with peripheral calcification. *C.* Photomicrograph of pleomorphic malignant fibrous histiocytoma arising in the bone infarct in the proximal tibia.

ing criteria is present: (1) osteochondroma that continues to grow after the second decade of life; (2) large cartilage cap over 2 cm in patients beyond the second decade of life; (3) scattered peripheral calcification embedded within the cartilaginous cap; and (4) permeation of the adjacent bone (Fig. 47-4). Histologically, most chondrosarcomas arising in osteochondromas are low-grade malignancy and have a favorable prognosis and low metastatic rates.

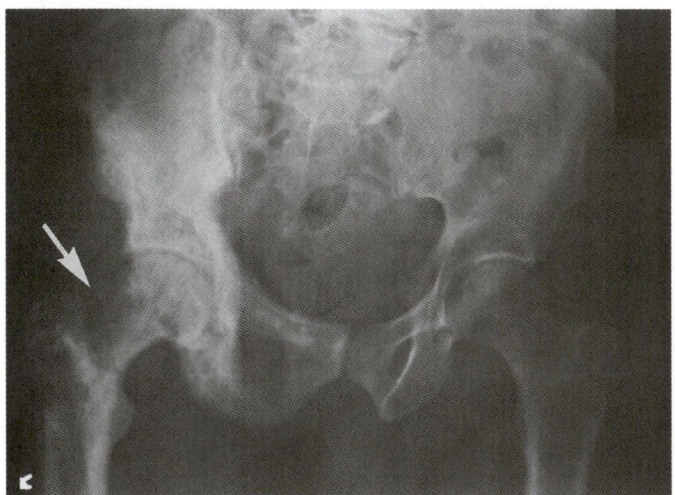

Figure 47-2

Paget's sarcoma. A 62-year-old male with Paget's disease of the right pelvis and right femur. He fell and developed pain in the right hip. Radiograph shows a destructive process in the proximal femur at the site of Paget's disease (*arrow*), with a pathologic fracture. A biopsy demonstrated a malignant fibrous histiocytoma.

ENCHONDROMA AND ENCHONDROMATOSIS

The rate of transformation of enchondroma to chondrosarcoma varies from center to center. Unni from the Mayo Clinic is very skeptical about such a possibility of sarcomatous change. Huvos maintained that occasionally a chondrosarcoma may arise in a preexisting enchondroma. Mirra speculated that about half of all central chondrosarcomas originated from preexisting enchondroma. In our experience the rate of malignant transformation is very low.

The distinction between cellular enchondroma and low-grade chondrosarcoma presents a significant diagnostic problem to the bone pathologist. Clinically, insidious pain with progressive radiographic change such as endosteal scalloping raises the possibility of malignant transformation. Histologically, permeation of tumor into the marrow spaces and preexisting bone is the most important criterion to establish the diagnosis for chondrosarcoma.

The incidence of chondrosarcoma arising in enchondromatosis (Ollier's disease) is much higher and is estimated to be 10 to 30 percent during a lifetime (Fig. 47-5). The average age of these patients is 40 years. In most cases, the chondrosarcoma is of low-grade malignancy. The prognosis for chondrosarcoma is directly related to the histologic grade; low grade tumors have a good prognosis.

FIBROUS DYSPLASIA

Sarcoma arising in fibrous dysplasia is extremely rare. So far, over 100 cases have been reported. Approximately, one-third of these patients received radiation therapy prior to the development of the sarcoma. The diagnosis of low-grade central osteosarcoma always should be ruled out before making the diagnosis of sarcomatous transformation.

The histologic type in most cases is osteosarcoma followed by fibrosarcoma. The prognosis is poor.

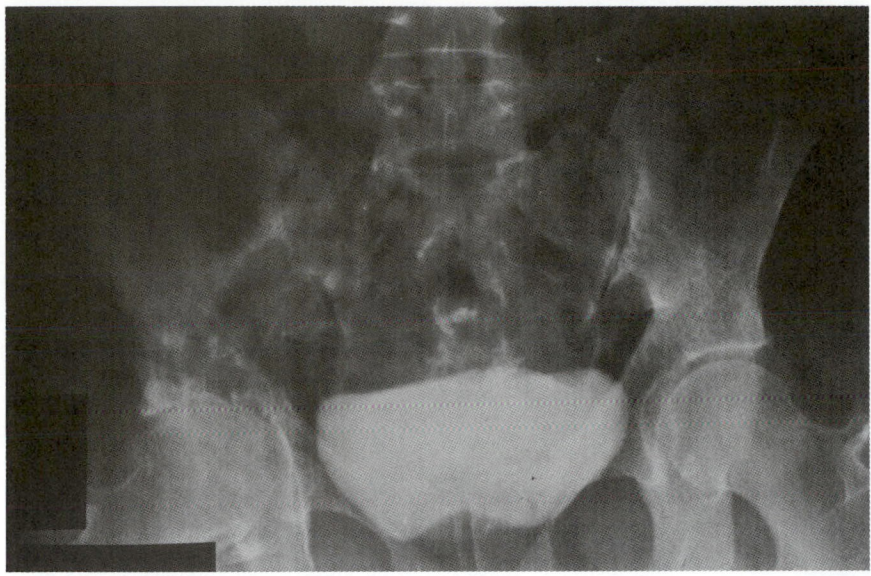

Figure 47-3
Radiation-induced sarcoma in a 68-year-old female, who complained of bilateral hip pain, particularly the right, associated with weakness. She had history of uterine cancer 16 years ago, treated with surgery and radiotherapy including radium implants. Radiograph shows a large destruction of the right ilium and acetabulum. A biopsy showed a malignant fibrous histiocytoma.

SYNOVIAL CHONDROMATOSIS

Chondrosarcoma arising in synovial chondromatosis is extremely rare. So far, only 20 cases have been reported. Most patients had a prolonged history of synovial chondromatosis with an interval of at least 10 years and multiple surgical procedures. In both conditions (synovial chondromatosis and chondrosarcoma arising in synovial chondromatosis) the clinical presentation is similar, namely pain, swelling, loss of range of motion, and multiple previous surgical procedures. The diagnosis should be based on the histologic findings. Histologically, chondrosarcoma arising in synovial chondromatolosis should demonstrate chondrocytes which have lost their clustering pattern, myxoid changes of the matrix, necrosis, and spindling of the cells.

GIANT CELL TUMOR

Lung metastases in histologically benign giant cell tumor is seen in less than 2 percent of the cases. Those metastatic lesions should not

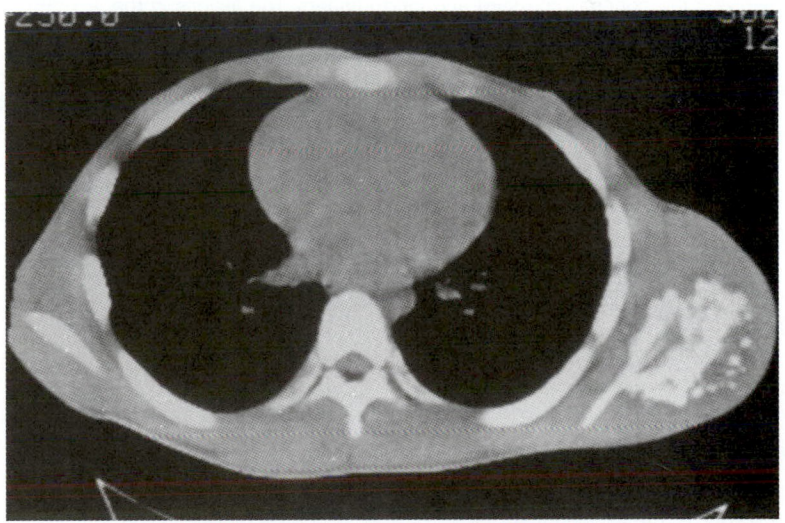

A   *B*

Figure 47-4
Chondrosarcoma arising in a solitary osteochondroma. A 17-year-old male who noticed a mass in the left scapula from approximately 2 years. *A.* Plain x-ray showed a sessile exostotic lesion in the left scapula. Irregular foci of calcification are seen far from the tumor in the soft tissue (*arrow*). *B.* CT scan demonstrates a broad-based osteochondroma of the left scapula with abnormal stippled calcifications in the cap, suspicious of malignant transformation. Biopsy revealed a grade I chondrosarcoma.

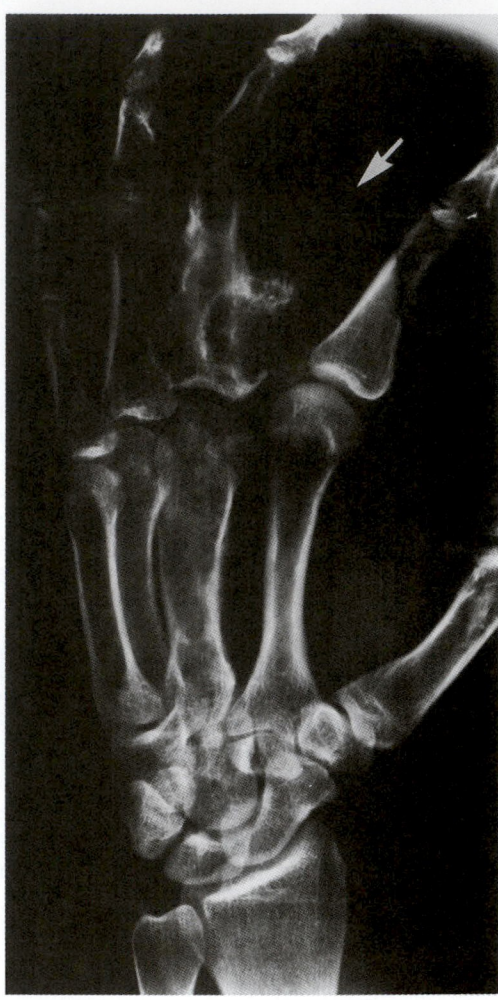

Figure 47-5
Chondrosarcoma arising in enchondromatosis. A 38-year-old male with progressive swelling of the right middle finger for the last 10 years. Radiograph of the right hand showing multiple intramedullary lesions involving the bones of the third and fourth fingers. The lesions in the proximal phalanx of the third finger is destroying the cortex producing a large soft tissue mass with focal calcification (*arrow*). [Reproduced with permission from Steiner GC: Benign cartilage tumors. In Taveras JM, Ferrucci JT (eds): *Radiology.* Philadelphia: JB Lippincott; 1986:chap 78:12.]

be confused with malignancy and should be described as deposits of benign tumor cells in the lung. They are self-limited in their growth potential and in most cases remain static and may even regress spontaneously. Malignant giant cell tumor without an antecedent history of radiation is extremely rare. The tumor can be malignant at the initial presentation, or malignancy may occur at the side of a previously documented benign giant cell tumor.

CHONDROBLASTOMA

Sarcoma arising in chondroblastoma is extremely rare. Only rare cases have been reported without previous irradiation. Lung metastases have been reported in histologically benign chondroblastoma. Those should not be confused with malignancy. They are self-limited in growth and carry an excellent prognosis.

OSTEOBLASTOMA

Osteoblastoma is a rare, benign bone-forming tumor. It is estimated that local recurrence following intralesional curettage occurs in 10 percent of the cases. Cases of aggressive osteoblastoma have been reported. Aggressive osteoblastoma histologically demonstrates increased cellularity with large epithelioid osteoblasts, but the presence of these cells does not necessarily indicate aggressive behavior. The distinction between aggressive osteoblastoma and osteoblastoma-like osteosarcoma is very difficult even for an experienced bone pathologist. There are a few well-documented cases of osteoblastoma that after multiple local recurrences transformed to osteosarcoma.

SUGGESTED READINGS

Dorfman HD, Czerniak B: *Bone Tumors.* St. Louis: Mosby; 1998.

Fechner RE, Mills SE: Tumors of the Bones and Joints. In: *Atlas of Tumor Pathology.* Washington, DC: Armed Forces Institute of Pathology; 1993:3d series, fascicle 8.

Huvos AG: *Bone Tumors. Diagnosis, Treatment, and Prognosis,* 2d ed. Philadelphia: WB Saunders; 1991.

Mirra JH: *Bone Tumors: Clinical, Radiographic, and Pathologic Correlations.* Philadelphia: Lea & Febiger; 1989.

Schajowicz F: Tumors arising at site of preexisting bone tumors. In: *Tumors and Tumorlike Lesions of Bone: Pathology, Radiology, and Treatment,* 2d ed. New York: Springer-Verlag; 1994:485.

Unni KK: *Dahlin's Bone Tumors: General Aspects and Data on 11,087 Cases,* 5th ed. Philadelphia: Lippincott-Raven; 1996.

Wold LE, McLeod RA, Sim FH, et al: *Atlas of Orthopaedic Pathology.* Philadelphia: WB Saunders; 1990.

Chapter 48

METASTATIC BONE DISEASE

Brian C. Toolan and Samuel Kenan

Metastatic bone disease is the most common malignancy of bone. Factors contributing to an observed increase in the overall incidence of bone metastases over the past 25 years include: an increase in life span of the general population with an attendant increase in the number of persons contracting cancer and an increase in the long-term survival of patients with malignant disease. The vast majority of skeletal malignant tumors are of metastatic origin rather than a primary bone tumor. Virtually every cancer has the potential to metastasize to bone. Skeletal metastasis represents the major orthopaedic complication of failed cancer treatment. Public health projections estimate over 3 million individuals are living with skeletal metastases in the United States. Following metastasis to the lymph node, lung, and liver, the skeleton is the fourth most common site. Metastatic tumors arise most frequently from breast carcinoma followed by lung, kidney, prostate, gastrointestinal, thyroid, and other miscellaneous sites. Patients who present with skeletal metastases of unknown origin have a poor prognosis with a short life expectancy. At autopsy it has been reported between 30 to 85 percent of the patients who die from cancer show occult skeletal metastases. Many of those lesions are too small to be detected radiographically.

Metastatic lesions that result in net loss of bone are described as osteolytic. Such conditions are seen in disorders such as myeloma, metastatic renal cell carcinoma, and thyroid carcinoma (Figs. 48-1 and 48-2). When the process involves bone formation with a net increase in bone, these lesions are described as blastic processes, as can be seen in metastatic prostate carcinoma (Fig. 48-3). Other metastatic processes may demonstrate a mixed type of lesion with lytic and blastic areas such as seen in some breast carcinoma (Fig. 48-4).

The mechanisms of bone reabsorption are primarily osteoclastic mediated. Hypercalcemia associated with skeletal metastasis is a common metabolic complication and a life-threatening disorder. The clinical symptoms associated with hypercalcemia are weakness, nausea, vomiting, dehydration, polyuria, anorexia, lethargy, confusion, stupor, and eventually coma. Hypercalcemia is most commonly associated with myeloma and carcinoma of the breast. Hypercalcemia is related to the secretion of hypercalcemic factors by the tumor cells. The two major mechanisms of cancer-related hypercalcemia are secretion of local osteolytic factors and systemic factors. The local factors are related to osteoclastic mediated bone resorption and bone destruction. The systemic factors are associated with the production of circulating hypercalcemic factors, the tumor being the secretory gland and the target organ being the osteoclast in the skeleton. A systemic parathyroid hormone-like mediated hypercalcemia is seen in squamous cell carcinoma and renal, bladder, and other carcinoma.

METASTATIC SITES AND SPREAD

All bones of the skeleton have been reported to be involved with metastases. The most common sites are the vertebrae, pelvis, ribs, skull, and proximal femur. The thoracolumbar vertebral bodies are the most common site for skeletal metastasis, not only because of the presence of red marrow but also because of the special paravertebral venous-plexus system which was described by Batson. Batson's vertebral plexus is a low intraluminal pressure network of thin-walled veins that connects the pelvic venous circulation to the spinal column,

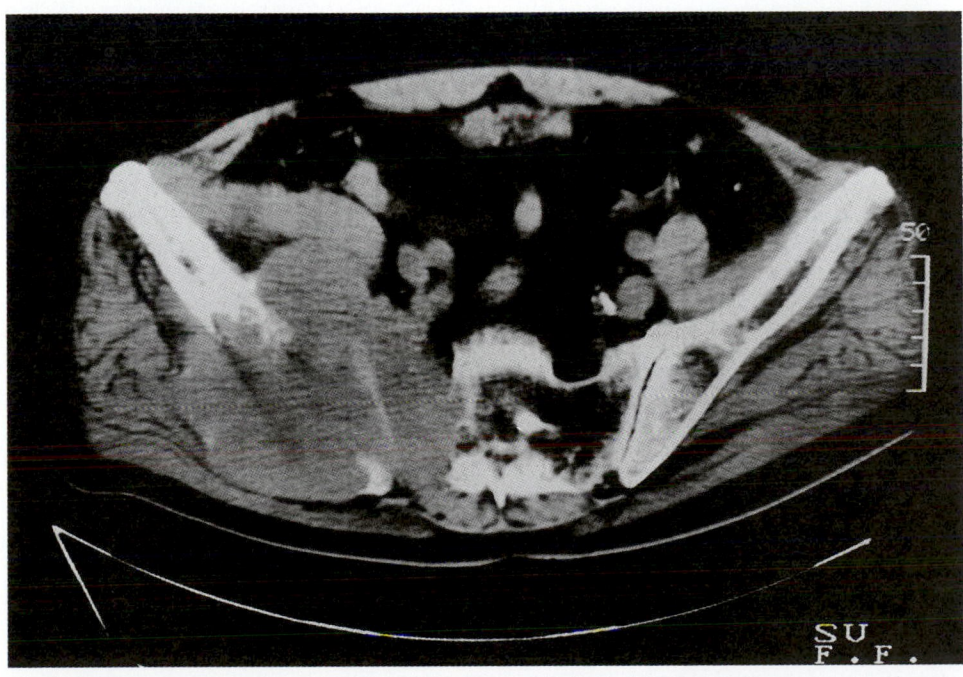

Figure 48-1
Metastatic thyroid carcinoma. Large lytic process involving the posterior right iliac crest and associated with a large soft tissue mass.

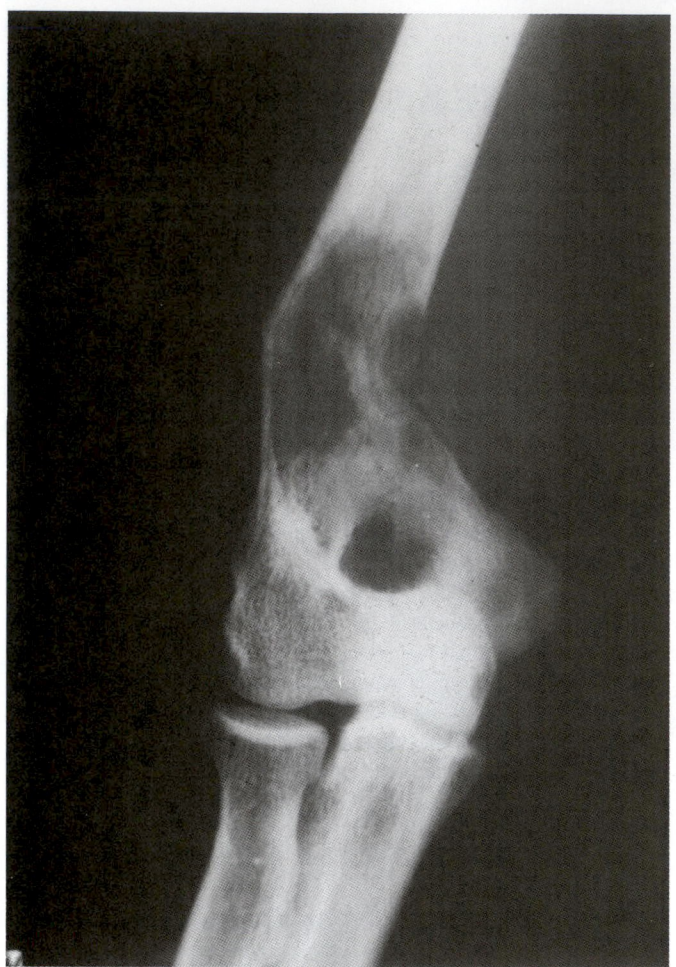

A

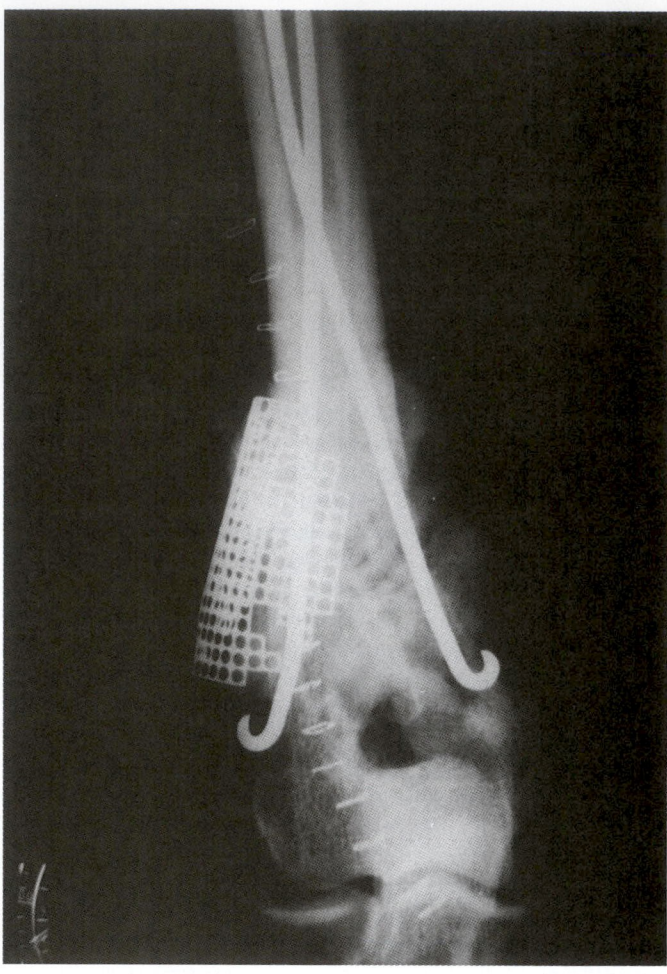

B

Figure 48-2
Metastatic hypernephroma. Lytic lesion of distal humerus with a pathological fracture (*A*). Treated by curettage and internal fixation with cement packing (*B*).

trunk, head, and neck independent of the vena cava. Because of the rarity of vascular marrow distal to the knee and elbow, metastases are relatively rare at these sites. The proximal femur was found to be the site of metastases in 11 percent of all patients with metastatic tumor. However, because of the high stress distribution at this location, they are often likely to fracture (Fig. 48-4). Highly anaplastic and rapidly growing vascular lesions are associated with a higher risk of fracture.

Although vascular dissemination of tumor cells predominately occurs through the venous system, metastases can occur by arterial or lymphatic means. In addition to the circulation theory to explain the distribution of tumor cells, the soil hypothesis states that local factors present in the tissues either facilitate or hinder the development of metastatic lesions. The pH, oxygen tension, presence of nutrients or hormones, or other local environmental factors may affect the viability of tumor cells once transported to a distant site. Finally, the spread of cancer may also depend on the ability of the tumor cells to secrete factors that foster the establishment of a metastatic focus.

PATHOGENESIS

Metastatic lesions destroy bone through a combination of direct replacement of host bone with tumor and its subsequent extension into

the adjacent tissues and indirectly through the production of cell-mediating factors by the tumor that stimulate osteoclasts to resorb bone. Osteoclasts are the primary cells involved in early bone destruction. They form a resorption front in bone that precedes the invading tumor cells. The tumor cells secrete osteoclast-activating factor, parathyroid hormone, prostaglandins, and other factors which control osteoclast-dependent osteolysis. Only in the latter stage of bone destruction, once the cancer completely encircles the bone, does direct tumor cell-mediated osteolysis occur. Some have postulated that direct pressure from the tumor mass or bone ischemia and necrosis induces bone resorption by this mechanism.

New bone formation occurs with most osseous metastases, with round cell tumors the predominant exception. Bone forms in these lesions by two mechanisms. Fibroblasts located in the stroma surrounding tumor foci are stimulated by osteoinductive factors to differentiate into osteoprogenitor cells and ossify their fibrous matrix. Bone also forms in direct response to bone destruction. Changes in stress distribution and the normal physiologic coupling between osteoblasts and osteoclasts induce bone formation adjacent to sites of bone resorption. The lytic or blastic appearance of a metastatic lesion on x-ray depends on the relative rates of osteoclast and osteoblast activity and the degree of coupled bone turnover at that site.

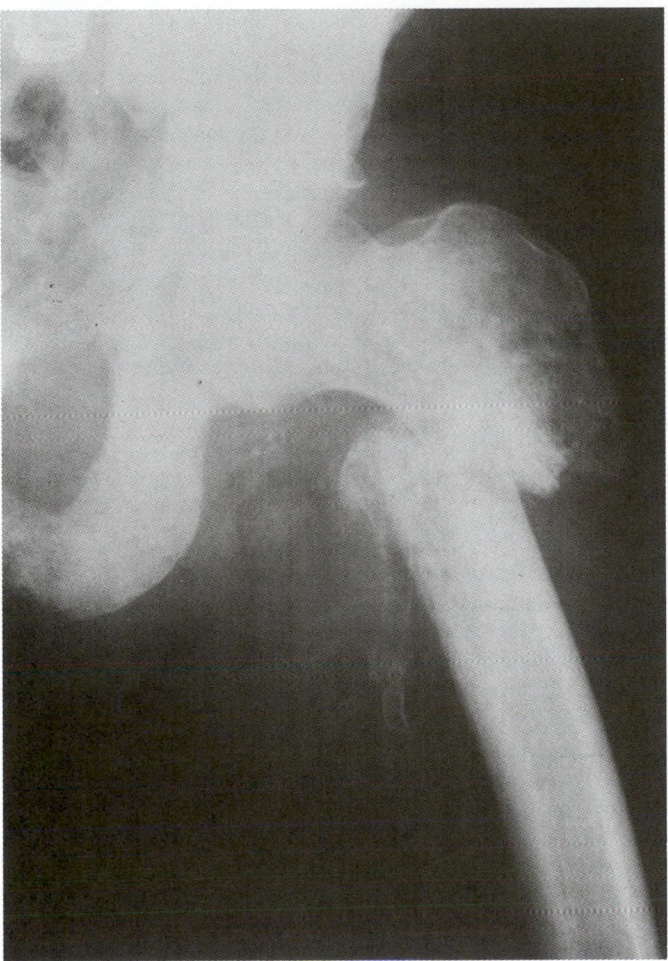

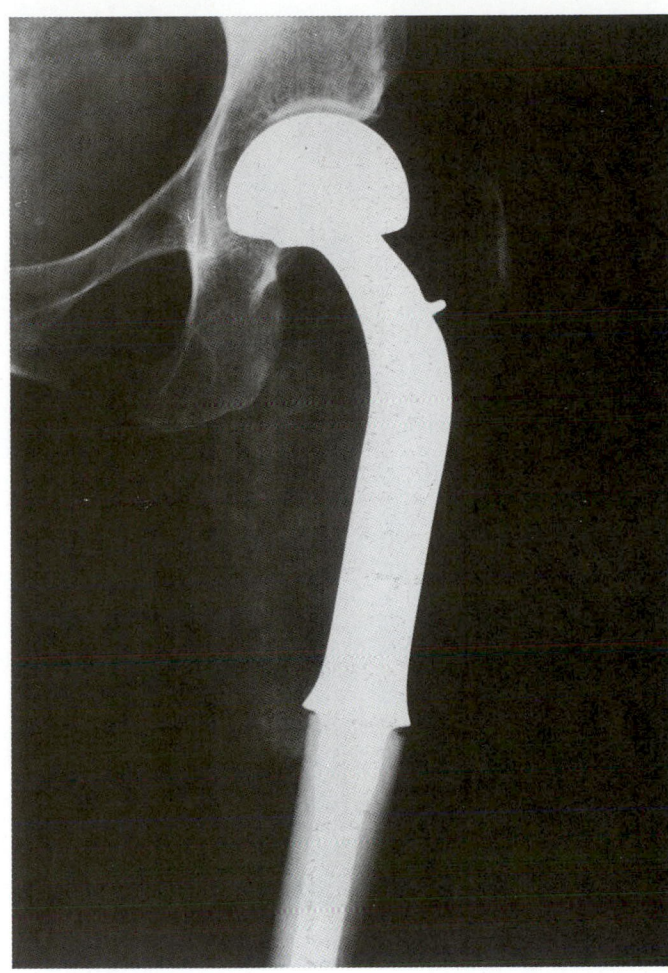

A   *B*

Figure 48-3
Metastatic prostate. Blastic lesion with pathologic fracture of the proximal femur. Treated by proximal femoral resection (*A*) and replacement by proximal femoral prosthesis (*B*).

DIAGNOSIS AND RADIOGRAPHIC EVALUATION

Metastatic bone disease is not difficult to diagnose. Pain is the most frequent symptom associated with skeletal metastases. It has an insidious onset, becoming gradually more severe over the course of weeks to months. The patient may describe an ache, commonly worse at night or with rest after activity. Metastases to the spine often present in this manner. Long-bone lesions manifest with mechanical symptoms and pain with activity that is relieved with rest. Although the patient perceives pain, the underlying lesion may not be evident on plain films. The clinician should be suspicious of osseous metastases when a patient with a known malignancy complains of pain. Despite pain commonly associated with metastatic bone disease, most lesions are asymptomatic. For this reason, the clinician must initiate a diagnostic radiographic workup. Concurrent with these efforts, a comprehensive history and physical exam must be performed to determine the overall state of the patient and to detect the presence of associated conditions that may require treatment. Anorexia, dehydration, anemia, and hypercalcemia are the most common nutritional and metabolic dysfunctions associated with metastatic disease. In rare instances, metastatic bone disease will present as an incidental radiographic abnormality. In this case, the workup is directed towards identifying the primary lesion and the general health of the patient.

The evaluation of metastatic bone disease begins with diagnostic bone imaging. Plain radiographs may not demonstrate an early metastatic lesion because bone loss must exceed 50 percent before the lesion becomes visible. Therefore, small occult metastatic lesions, which may not be painful, may also not be detected radiographically. When cortical bone is destroyed, a lesser degree of destruction is needed for radiographic detection.

A total body bone scan is the initial modality to screen for osseous metastases. It is the most sensitive method for detecting skeletal lesions except multiple myeloma. It locates suspicious sites for further inspection with plain radiographs, CT scans, and MRI. In patients with a primary malignancy known to metastasize to bone, a bone scan can serve as a surveillance tool to detect occult metastases. A CT scan can determine the extent of intra- and extramedullary involvement of the tumor through imaging in the transverse plane. It can guide a biopsy or surgical approach to the lesion and help to determine the fields for radiation therapy. Computed tomography (CT) is also helpful in detecting lesions of the spine and pelvis.

MRI is less sensitive in displaying bone destruction and more sensitive in demonstrating marrow infiltrates. An MRI can provide additional information through imaging in the sagittal and coronal planes. It is more sensitive than CT scan in demonstrating the presence and extent of marrow involvement or an associated soft tissue mass and in the evaluation of bone and soft tissue for recurrent tumor. An

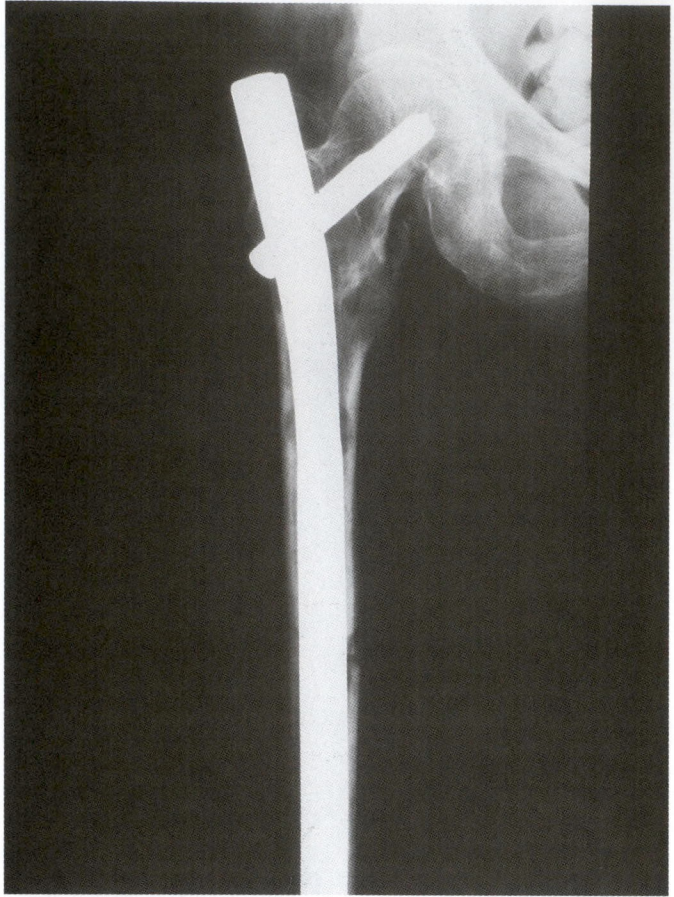

Figure 48-4
Metastatic breast carcinoma. Multifocal lytic and blastic lesions along the proximal femur; treated by intramedullary nailing.

MRI is useful for spine lesions in order to rule out potential spinal cord compression due to tumor in the spinal canal. Finally, the importance of obtaining a chest film to rule out metastases to the pulmonary parenchyma must never be overlooked during the workup of metastatic bone disease.

Three radiographic patterns have been described for a metastatic lesion to bone. A *geographic* lesion consists of well-circumscribed lytic areas more than 1 cm in diameter. There is often a rim of sclerotic bone surrounding the lesion. This delineates a narrow transition zone between normal and involved bone and indicates a slow-growing lesion, a feature more common to benign than malignant tumors. It is an unlikely presentation of skeletal metastases. A lesion with a "*moth-eaten*" appearance consists several small lytic lesions, less than 1 cm in size, in close proximity with ill-defined margins. This radiographic pattern signifies extensive cortical bone destruction and indicates a more aggressive tumor. A *permeative* lesion demonstrates a highly aggressive tumor. Multiple, small, destructive tumor foci, approximately 1 mm in size are interspersed throughout normal bone. This signifies a rapidly growing tumor that has extensively infiltrated the bone. This is the more common appearance of metastatic bone disease. Metastatic lesions may present with a "moth-eaten" pattern alone or in combination with a permeative appearance. Although more common to primary bone tumors, metastatic lesions may demonstrate a periosteal reaction, especially those tumors that tend to be osteoblastic such as prostate, bladder, and GI carcinomas. Skeletal metastases may display a lytic, blastic, or mixed appearance on plain radiograph (Table 48-1). Many tumors possess a mixed appearance with predominately lytic or blastic features with osteolytic lesions the more common presentation. It is difficult to identify the origin of a skeletal metastasis based solely on its radiographic appearance; however purely lytic lesions are typical of bronchial carcinoma.

Biopsy establishes an accurate tissue diagnosis of an osseous lesion. In patients with skeletal metastasis the biopsy site should be selected carefully. Frozen sections should be obtained to confirm that adequate tissue was obtained. In selected patients with impending fracture, if frozen section is diagnostic for metastatic disease, prophylactic internal fixation can be carried out immediately. In any case, the purpose of the biopsy is to provide an adequate and representative tissue sample for histopathologic analysis without adversely affecting the prognosis or treatment of the patient. This process requires a clear line of communication between the surgeon and pathologist before, during, and after the procedure to achieve this objective.

TREATMENT

Treatment of patients with skeletal metastasis should involve a multi-disciplinary team approach including the oncologist, radiotherapist, and orthopaedic surgeon, as good judgment and considerable experience are necessary in the selection of a patient's full range of therapy. The main goals of treatment are to relieve pain, to ease nursing care, and to allow early mobilization in order to return the patients as soon as possible to their previous environment and level of activity. Advances in surgical techniques and internal fixation devices have resulted in a great improvement in controlling pain. The criteria for internal fixation are: (1) patients with a lytic lesion involving greater than 2.5 cm of the cortex; (2) medullary lesions that are greater than 50 percent of the cross-section of the bone; and (3) progressive painful lesions that do not respond to radiotherapy. An avulsion fracture of the lesser trochanter and pain in weightbearing bones containing a metastatic lesion despite radiation therapy are also indications for surgery.

The approach to treatment of metastatic bone disease considers the nature and location of the lesion and the health of the patient. Lesions that do not present with impending fracture can be treated successfully by radiotherapy alone to relieve pain. Radiation therapy can diminish bone pain, maintain functional status, and prevent pathologic fractures. It is especially useful for patients with widely disseminated metastases. Radiation therapy is indicated for the treatment of radiculopathy and myelopathy secondary to compression by spinal metastases. Radiation therapy can also play a curative role when combined with surgical extirpation for a solitary lesion. The most common metastatic carcinomas are radiosensitive, and palliative effects are seen in 80 percent of these patients for up to 1 year. There are several complications of radiation therapy with orthopaedic implications. A 5 percent incidence of osteonecrosis is associated with prophylactic or postoperative radiation of femoral head and neck lesions. The devascularization of irradiated bone may induce osteitis or result in fracture. For this reason, stabilization of hip and long-bone lesions is recommended prior to the initiation of radiation therapy. Radiation-induced sarcoma was a critical issue prior to the development of current techniques. However, its long latency period continues to make it a prevalent concern.

Metastatic lesions to the femoral neck are best treated by bipolar prosthesis replacement. Larger trochanteric lesions with pathologic fracture may be treated by proximal femoral replacement using other medullary prostheses (Fig. 48-3). Femoral mid-shaft lesions should be treated by intramedullary nailing; if necessary, to be augmented by cement fixation (Fig. 48-4). Metastatic lesions to the femoral condyles can be treated by intralesional curettage and cement packing followed by radiation. Other lesions with larger processes may be treated with a distal femoral replacement. The same principles should be used in other sites of the extremities (Fig. 48-5). Lesions of the acetabulum with large lytic processes could be treated by curettage and cement packing followed by radiation therapy.

Table 48-1

Radiographic Appearance of Primary Tumors

Primary Tumor	Radiographic Appearance
Lung	Lytic; blastic esp. adenocarcinoma (25–33%)
Breast	Lytic; occ. blastic or mixed
Prostate	Blastic; older pts. more likely lytic
GI tract	Lytic; stomach and pancreas can be blastic
Bladder	Lytic; occ mixed, transitional cell blastic
Kidney	Lytic
Thyroid	Lytic; medullary cell can be blastic
Ovary (rare skeletal metastases)	Lytic; occ blastic
Cervix	Lytic or mixed
Skin (melanoma) (rare skeletal metastases)	Lytic
Neuroblastoma	Lytic; rarely blastic
Rhabdomyosarcoma	Lytic
Retinoblastoma	Lytic or blastic
Intracranial (rare skeletal metastases)	Lytic, blastic, or mixed

---

Most vertebral lesions initially are occult and painless. Metabolic lesions that do not compromise stability may remain asymptomatic. Pain occurs when a significant amount of bone destruction has occurred. Pathologic fractures of the vertebral body are of a compressive type and usually are stable. Radiosensitive lesions may be treated by irradiation alone. Surgical decompression may be indicated in those patients who do not respond to radiation and develop instability and progressive neurologic deterioration. The result of anterior decompression with vertebral body resection and reconstruction by cement spaces and bracing has proved to be very effective in stabilizing the spine and preventing further neurologic deterioration.

Chemotherapy directed towards the primary disease also must be included in the treatment plan. This includes cytotoxic agents, hormonal therapy, and radionuclide treatments. Breast and prostate cancers respond well to hormonal manipulations, and thyroid cancer can be treated with radioactive iodine. The efficacy of chemotherapy directly relates to tumor size. It is most successful as an adjuvant following surgical or irradiative debulking of the tumor. The use of brachytherapy to deliver high concentrations of chemotherapeutic agents intraarterially to a lesion after surgical debulking may prove amenable to the treatment of metastatic bone disease.

The patient must be treated for the metabolic imbalances that accompany metastatic disease such as hypercalcemia of malignancy, anorexia, and dehydration. Hypercalcemia may be present in as many as 30 percent of patients with metastatic bone disease. Severe acute cases require vigorous intravenous hydration accompanied with diuretics. Chronic hypercalcemia of malignancy is currently treated with oral bisphosphonates or calcitonin. A nutritional assessment identifies patients with protein-calorie malnutrition from inadequate nutrient intake. Serum albumin concentration below 3.5 g/dl and total iron-binding capacity less than 240 mg/dl are simple laboratory screening tests to detect nutritional deficiency.

PATHOLOGIC FRACTURE

Lesions that present with impending pathologic fracture can be treated by a closed intramedullary nailing followed by local irradiation. Lesions with a large area of bone loss and a risk of telescoping and migration of the bone fragments, could be stabilized by intramedullary nailing augmented by methyl methacrylate. Each anatomic site may require a specific attention and treatment approach. Overall, pathologic fracture occurs in approximately 10 percent of skeletal metastases. Advances in treatment have prolonged the survival of cancer patients and have increased their risk of sustaining a pathologic fracture. Over 60 percent of all pathologic fractures secondary to metastatic disease occur in patients with carcinoma of the breast because they have the longest survival after the onset of skeletal metastases. With their primary malignancy successfully managed, a pathologic fracture looms as the greatest threat to the quality of life for a cancer patient.

The goals of orthopaedic management are to alleviate pain, ease nursing care, and restore functional activity. Achieving these objectives depends on stabilization of the fracture to permit early mobilization of the patient. The recovery of independent ambulation improves the pyschosocial well-being of the patient and enhances the overall care of the patient. For these reasons, survival expectancy should not be the sole determinant for surgical intervention. These predictions are often inaccurate. Instead, the potential benefits of surgery must be weighed against the patient's overall condition and survivability. The opportunity of 4 to 6 weeks of improved quality of life after surgery is a strong indication to operate. The timing of the procedure must be coordinated with all the other aspects of the patient's care to maximize the surgical benefit. The surgical approach, technique, and choice of implant should be individualized for each patient and be flexible, should intraoperative findings require changing the initial plan. This preoperative assessment should take into ac-

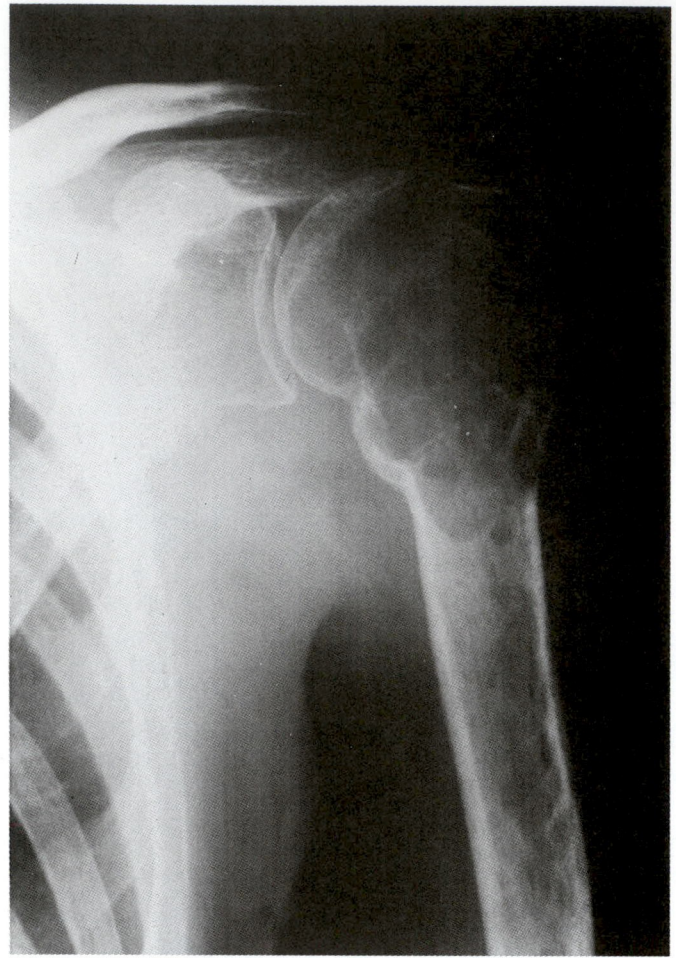

A

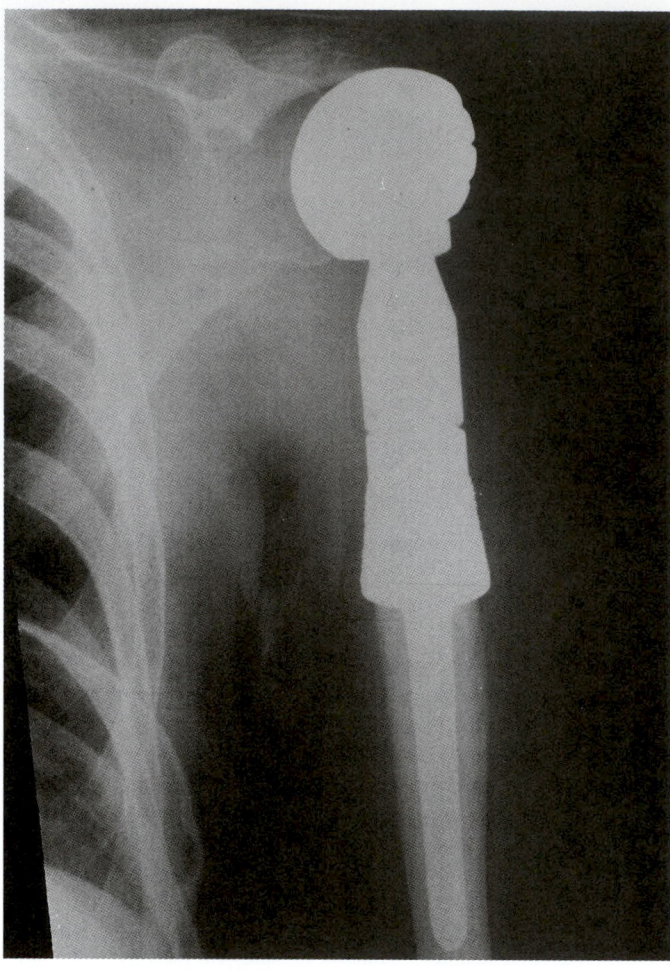

B

Figure 48-5
Metastatic breast carcinoma. Lytic lesion involving the proximal humerus treated by resection (*A*) and proximal humerus replacement (*B*).

count the location of the lesion, the quality of adjacent bone, and the presence of other lesions requiring fixation.

Several studies have demonstrated superior clinical results when polymethylmethacrylate (PMMA) augments internal fixation or accompanies prosthetic replacement of impending or actual pathologic fractures secondary to metastatic bone disease. The use of PMMA enhanced pain relief and functional ambulation and increased the 1-year survival rate of patients when compared to those patients who were stabilized without PMMA. There was also a decreased clinical incidence of implant failure and loss of fixation that corroborated biomechanical studies demonstrating a higher load to failure for constructs augmented with PMMA. Stable fixation is imperative in light of the low rate of union with pathologic fracture. The results of several studies suggest less than one-third of fractures unite, even after effective internal fixation. This result may reflect the discrepancy between the time necessary for complete consolidation and the patient's survival rather than the potential for fracture healing. Preoperative radiation and chemotherapy, the cell type of the tumor, the presence of viable tumor at the fracture, and interposition of PMMA between the fracture fragments have all been identified as factors contributing to nonunion. Bone grafting is ineffective at promoting union unless 6 months has elapsed since radiation therapy. Metastatic bone disease of the spine may result in destabilization and cord or root compression from vertebral collapse. This situation may necessitate decompression and stabilization with spinal instrumentation.

SUGGESTED READINGS

Dorfman HD, Czerniak B: *Bone Tumors.* St. Louis: Mosby; 1998.

Fechner RE, Mills SE: Tumors of the bones and joints. In: *Atlas of Tumor Pathology.* Washington, DC: Armed Forces Institute of Pathology; 1993:3d series, fascicle 8.

Holland JF, Bast RC Jr, Morton DL, et al (eds): Principles of chemotherapy. In: *Cancer Medicine*, vol 2, 4th ed. Baltimore: Williams & Wilkins; 1997: chaps 52–59.

Holland JF, Bast RC Jr, Morton DL, et al (eds): Chemotherapeutic agents. In: *Cancer Medicine*, vol 2, 4th ed. Baltimore: Williams & Wilkins; 1997: chaps 60–68.

Huvos AG: *Bone Tumors. Diagnosis, Treatment, and Prognosis*, 2d ed. Philadelphia: WB Saunders; 1991.

Mirra JH: *Bone Tumors: Clinical, Radiographic, and Pathologic Correlations.* Philadelphia: Lea & Febiger; 1989.

Rougraff BT, Kneisel JS, Simon MA: Skeletal metastases of unkown origin: A prospective study of diagnostic strategy. *J Bone Joint Surg [Am]* 1993; 75:1276.

Schajowicz F: *Tumors and Tumorlike Lesions of Bone: Pathology, Radiology, and Treatment*, 2d ed. New York: Springer-Verlag; 1994.

Unni KK: *Dahlin's Bone Tumors: General Aspects and Data on 11,087 Cases*, 5th ed. Philadelphia: Lippincott-Raven; 1996.

Wold LE, McLeod RA, Sim FH, et al: *Atlas of Orthopaedic Pathology.* Philadelphia: WB Saunders; 1990.

Chapter 49

HIP

Patrick A. Meere, Paul E. Di Cesare, and Alan J. Dayan

Arthritis, which is the most common disorder of the hip, can be classified into two broad categories based on whether its etiology is degenerative or inflammatory. Regardless of etiology, the morbidity associated with hip arthritis leads to progressive pain and loss of function that, if left untreated, can ultimately result in chronic pain, crippling joint ankylosis, and eventual loss of the ability to ambulate. Over the last three decades, considerable advances have occurred in both the surgical and medical management of arthritis. Clinical results from surgical management have been impressive, and many believe that total hip arthroplasty (THA) is the most effective surgical procedure for the restoration of function and normal daily living. There has also been great progress in understanding the various disease processes that lead to hip pain; the result has been improved early diagnosis and better medical management.

This chapter is divided into two sections: *primary hip reconstruction* for previously untreated hip conditions, and *revision hip reconstruction* for the evaluation and management of failed hip reconstructions previously treated by arthroplasty.

PRIMARY HIP RECONSTRUCTION

The source of acute or chronic hip pain can be intrinsic (within the articular joint) or extrinsic (outside the joint). Intrinsic hip pain, whether caused by degenerative or inflammatory arthritides, signals articular cartilage degeneration and varying reactive periarticular bone changes leading to loss of congruency and decreased joint function. There may be significant overlap between the broad classes of arthritis, as mechanical degenerative changes often superimpose on preexisting disease. Extrinsic causes of hip pain include referred pain from other areas, inflammatory process related to tendons crossing the hip joint, and unrelated general surgical causes.

Degenerative (mechanical) arthritis—osteoarthritis—can be either primary (idiopathic) or secondary, that is, resulting from preexisting pathologic conditions such as pediatric sequelae, osteonecrosis, previous septic joint, or trauma. Among the inflammatory processes, rheumatoid arthritis is the most common, followed by systemic lupus erythematosus and the seronegative arthritides.

EVALUATION

A careful documentation of the patient's medical history, a physical examination, and radiographs are the cornerstones of the evaluation of hip pain. The specific hip-related assessment must be viewed as a complement to a comprehensive medical examination. Evaluation of the history should consider the possibility of an inflammatory disease and define the nature of the pain, its location, any pertinent radiation,

whether it occurs at night, and worsening or alleviating factors. If previous treatment has been initiated, results should be documented. A standard assessment of functional level is paramount, and several functional scoring systems have been used in an attempt to standardize documented outcomes. Most such systems take into account performance of activities of daily living, pain, and physical and radiologic findings; more elaborate systems integrate a social questionnaire.

The physical examination effectively begins with the observation of the patient standing up from a sitting position in the waiting area. The relative difficulty with which patients perform this task in addition to their gait pattern and the use of walking aids should be noted. While recording the history, the general status of the patient is observed, and any stigmata of chronic disease or generalized inflammatory arthritis must be noted for later examination. The comprehensive exam of the hip should start with an assessment of leg length inequality (true versus apparent) and the presence of a positive Trendelenburg's sign or lurch. A full active and passive range-of-motion exam of both hips is then performed, including a Thomas test to see whether there are hip flexion contractures. The exam is completed by a thorough distal neurovasculature exam and examination of the adjacent joints: the sacroiliac, the lumbosacral, and the ipsilateral knee. Among the various arthritides, there is no major difference in the physical deficit of the hip joint. Leg length inequality and abductor weakness may be more pronounced in mechanical arthritides by virtue of the proximal femoral migration. Rotational range of motion is the first and hip flexion is usually the last to be affected in the degenerative hip.

Serologic evaluation of hip arthritis aims at ruling out an inflammatory or infectious process. Specific tests are performed on clinical suspicion that are not part of the systematic evaluation. The baseline infectious work-up consists of a differential white cell (WBC) count, an erythrocyte sedimentation rate (ESR), and a C-reactive protein (CRP) level. A positive value may lead to further testing, such as hip aspiration or radionucleotide scans. The basic inflammatory work-up, in addition to the elements of the infectious work-up, include rheumatoid factor, ANA factor, complement levels, and Lyme titers.

Basic radiologic studies include standard anteroposterior (AP) films of the pelvis and AP and lateral films of the involved hip. Specific tests include Judet (internal and external oblique) views, computed tomography (CT) and magnetic resonance imaging (MRI) of the pelvis. The difference between various types of arthritis is most pronounced on evaluation of roentgenographic changes. Inflammatory changes typically consist of concentric joint space narrowing, diffuse periarticular osteopenia, relative paucity of peripheral osteophytes, paucity of subchondral cysts, and absence of subchondral sclerosis. Osteoarthritic joints show nonconcentric or asymmetric joint space narrowing with superolateral erosion of the acetabulum and complementary medial wall osteophytic deposition, subchondral sclerosis, multiple subchondral erosion cysts, and varying degrees of peripheral osteophytic bone formation. Degenerative arthritides secondary to preexisting hip pathology present certain particular features. A degenerative dysplastic hip (DDH) arthritis is characterized by a high-riding proximal femur with coxa valga, excessive anteversion of the femoral neck, and a stenotic canal. Acetabular changes vary depending on the final outcome of the DDH. Untreated cases that result in complete hip dislocation have an osteopenic virginal dysplastic acetabular fossa and a degenerative pseudoacetabulum, which may lie at a variable distance on the proximal external ilium. Cases resulting from chronic subluxation in DDH display more typical erosive segmental destruction of the superolateral acetabular wall. Degenerative arthritis after slipped capital femoral epiphysis (SCFE) demonstrates poor congruence, with the femoral head tilted posteromedially. Usually, the remnant of the cortical neck is visible posteriorly, with a concomitant absence of head anterolaterally (positive Klein line). Arthritis that develops after Legg-Calvé-Perthes (LCP) disease reveals a large femoral head (coxa magna), flattening of the head (coxa plana), and possibly a shortened neck (coxa breva). An abduction hinge and underdeveloped greater trochanter are often seen. Adult avascular necrosis (AVN) routinely presents in the later stages (e.g., stage V), at which point the acetabular side has been involved. The specific changes are femoral head collapse and severe sclerosis with cystic erosions. Earlier stages of AVN of the femoral head should be investigated by MRI to determine the location and percentage of femoral head involvement and the stage of the destructive process. Posttraumatic arthritis may show a malunion and sclerosis of an acetabular fracture or fracture-dislocation, which is best visualized on the Judet (internal and external oblique) views or the CT scan of the pelvis. There may be superimposed AVN of the femoral head with collapse. Postinfectious arthritis is less pathognomonic. Joint destruction is more concentric, but the femoral head shows patchy sclerosis with cystic erosions. The diagnosis of an active or residual infection is confirmed by radionucleotide scan (technetium, gallium, and/or indium scans) or by MRI (T2 phase will show greater femoral head uptake).

TREATMENT

Nonsurgical Treatment

The natural history for most intrinsic hip pain is a slow progression of increased pain and decreased function. Although medications, therapy, rest, and/or orthotics can provide symptomatic relief and improve function, they do not arrest the degenerative process. The clinical response to these treatment modalities is extremely variable because they do not address the underlying pathology. Initial management of osteoarthritis is combined medical treatment, physiotherapy, ambulatory aids, and weight control. The primary line of medication is nonsteroidal anti-inflammatory drugs (NSAIDs). The inflammatory arthritides are customarily treated and followed by the rheumatologist. Three lines of pharmacologic agents can be used and tailored to the specific patient. The first level consists of NSAIDs. The second-line and third-line drugs modulate the underlying disease processes and can have severe side effects. Second-line drugs, termed *remittive agents,* include penicillamine, gold, and the antimalarials. Third-line drugs such as systemic corticosteroids and cytotoxic agents are immunosuppressive and potentially highly toxic. The clinical success of surgical treatment in the last decades has been such that it may now be considered as an adjunct to the comprehensive rheumatologic treatment armamentarium rather than a traditional salvage procedure. The term *conservative management* for this initial phase of

arthritis treatment is a misnomer; it should rather be referred to as *nonsurgical management.*

Surgical Treatment

Debridement   Arthroscopic joint debridement is indicated in select patients to decrease symptoms and improve function. Conditions such as synovial chondromatosis or loose bodies within the hip joint may be improved by removal of these bodies.

Resection arthroplasty (Girdlestone)   Resection arthroplasty is often considered to be an end-stage solution for hip pain in nonambulatory patients, in cases with chronic infection with osteomyelitis, and in debilitated patients (usually with severe immunosuppression, such as in steroid dependency, end-stage rheumatoid arthritis, and AIDS). Finally, it is also an option in cases where reconstruction is thwarted by major bone loss on both the femoral and the acetabular sides. The problems associated with resection arthroplasty include pain, instability, limb shortening, and abductor weakness. Ambulatory patients with a resection arthroplasty will require ambulatory aids as well as a shoe lift.

Osteotomy   Femoral or pelvic osteotomies are usually indicated for the early, symptomatic mechanical types of arthritis secondary to pediatric hip malformation. The goal of the osteotomy is to provide pain relief and to improve joint mechanics and contact area. This procedure, however, should not be done if it will compromise structural alignment such that it complicates or precludes subsequent salvage by arthroplasty. The effectiveness of hip osteotomies for arthritis is moderate. The selection should favor younger age, lean habitus, and a focal lesion with enough surrounding intact hyaline cartilage to ensure successful load redistribution. Best results should be obtained with an incongruent hip joint that is realigned by osteotomy. Osteotomy of the femur and/or pelvis should be planned to address the presenting patient deformity.

Acetabular Osteotomies   The periacetabular redirectional pelvic osteotomies used in the adult are the Salter, Steel, Dial, and Ganz procedures (Fig. 49-1). The goal of these procedures is to correct acetabular dysplasia by realignment of the hyaline cartilage of the acetabulum over the lateral and anterior aspects of the femoral head. Acetabular augmenting osteotomies for incongruent joint space, such as the Chiari, can achieve lateral femoral head coverage by metaplasia of the joint capsule into fibrocartilage. Patient selection for these osteotomies must be careful and the surgical execution precise in order to obtain satisfactory results.

Femoral Osteotomies   The femoral redirectional osteotomies can also be technically challenging. The preoperative assessment must include adduction-abduction and rotation films to assess optimal coverage of the femoral head and calculate the biplanar intertrochanteric closed wedge resection (modified Southwick). Intertrochanteric osteotomy (varus, valgus, or displacement) has been indicated for the treatment of osteoarthritis in younger adults if congruity can be improved. Pain relief following osteotomy has been noted to deteriorate with time, with only about 25 percent of patients maintaining a good result after 10 years.

In patients with AVN, Sugioka (1992) has reported good results with a transtrochanteric "rotational" osteotomy. The size of the lesion should be less than 50 percent of the femoral head surface, however, and a favorable outcome beyond 10 years should not be expected.

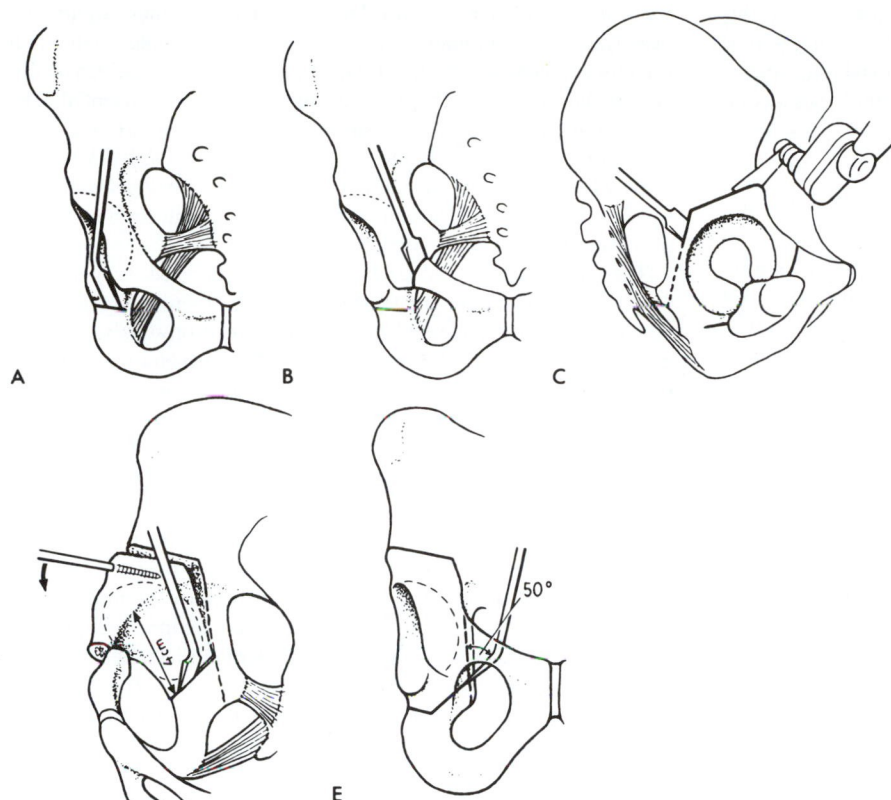

Figure 49-1

Bernese acetabular osteotomy. *A.* The angled chisel is introduced into the space between the psoas tendon and capsule and the ischium is notched 5 to 10 mm deep at the infracotyloid groove. *B.* Osteotomy of the pubis immediately adjacent to the acetabulum. *C.* Roof-shaped osteotomy viewed from the outside. The anterior leg of the osteotomy is made with an oscillating saw starting proximal to the anteroinferior iliac spine. The anterior portion of the posterior leg is osteotomized from inside and outside at an angle of 120 degrees using the chisel. The remainder of that osteotomy will break spontaneously toward the ischial spine (dotted line). *D.* Introduction of a Schanz screw into the supra-acetabular bone tilts the fragment laterally. Osteotomy of the ischium from the quadrilateral surface is done with the angled chisel 4 cm below the well-visualized pelvic brim. The dorsal pillar and sacropelvic connections remain intact. *E.* Using a distance of 4 cm from the pelvic rim, a 50-degree angle between the blade of the chisel and the quadrilateral surface will result in an osteotomy posterior to the acetabulum. (Reproduced with permission from Ganz R, Klaue K, Vinh TS, et al: A new periacetabular osteotomy for the treatment of hip dysplasias. Technique and preliminary results. *Clin Orthop* 1998; 232:29.)

Arthrodesis The relative success of the functional outcome of arthroplasties has made the treatment option of arthrodesis (in selected cases) difficult for many patients and surgeons to accept. Indications are (1) mechanical arthritis in a young active male (e.g., a heavy laborer) with unilateral disease and a nonarthritic lumbosacral spine and ipsilateral knee, (2) previous pyogenic or tuberculous joint sepsis, and (3) salvage of a failed arthroplasty or osteotomy. Strict contraindications include (1) bilateral disease and (2) polyarticular connective tissue disease. Relative contraindications are (1) female, (2) AVN or inflammatory arthritides by virtue of potential bilateral diseases, and (3) a sedentary life style or limited life span.

The currently favored technique of arthrodesis is with plate (i.e., cobra) fixation. Great care must be taken to protect the abductor mechanism in anticipation of eventual conversion to an arthroplasty. The final position of the femoral shaft should be in 30 degrees of flexion, 5 degrees of adduction, and 5 to 10 degrees of external rotation. Once union has been achieved, the anticipated level of function is quite good. Pain relief should be excellent and gait minimally perturbed. A circumduction gait is typical of excessive abduction. Complications of arthrodesis are classified into early and late. Early complications include sciatic nerve (peroneal branch) palsy, shortening greater than 2 cm (especially with the cobra plate technique), nonunion, and pseudarthrosis. Implant failure is possible with delayed union or nonunion. Fatigue failure distal to the plate is also reported, but can be successfully treated (98 percent union rate) with open reduction, internal fixation using a compression plate, and autograft. Late complications include the development of lumbosacral, ipsilateral knee, and/or contralateral hip degenerative changes and arthritic pain due to the increased load transmission to these joints from the maximally constrained arthrodesed hip. These changes are accelerated with improper position or malunion of the arthrodesis. Anticipated results with the use of a cobra plate for hip arthrodesis include an approximate incidence of 8 percent pseudoarthrosis and 16 percent malposition. Long-term follow-up of more than 20 years has shown 80 percent patient satisfaction; however, approximately one-third of women and one-quarter of men report moderate impairment of sexual function.

Joint Replacement: Partial Approaches *Hemiarthroplasty* With either a bipolar or unipolar prosthesis hemiarthroplasty is rarely indicated in the treatment of symptomatic arthritis (both sides of the joint are usually involved). This alternative is usually reserved for the treatment of displaced femoral neck fractures in the elderly. The presence of preexisting acetabular arthritis in displaced femoral neck fractures, however, is preferentially treated by THA. In cases of symptomatic femoral head AVN with a radiologically intact acetabulum, the selection of a hemiarthroplasty replacement is ill-advised, because retrieval studies have shown significant abnormalities of the acetabular cartilage. The 5-year clinical outcome of such cases has been shown to be fair to poor.

Surface Replacement This procedure was developed to maintain bone stock in anticipation of subsequent revision; only the articulating cartilage surface and subchondral bone of the femoral head are replaced. The failure rate of this implant was reported to be 12.3 percent in a series of 584 hips. Other series, however, have found a revision rate of up to 26 percent in the short-term to midterm interval.

The role of fixation appears to be particularly important with this implant. Encouraging results have been seen with the new porous cementless fixation systems. Although the functional outcome is comparable to that with THA, the surface replacement is not recommended for younger, more active patients.

Total Hip Arthroplasty *Indications* Since the 1980s the indications for THA have expanded due to the clinical success of the operation. Indications can now be considered as incapacitating pain refractory to nonsurgical treatment and not being a candidate for osteotomy. The pain should be persistent and there should be significant limitation of function causing a severe impact on quality of life. Not uncommonly, patients less than 50 years of age require secondary arthroplasty reconstruction, as in complex cases of degenerative arthritis secondary to pediatric conditions, osteonecrosis, or trauma. Accordingly, the minimum acceptable age requirement for primary arthroplasty is being increasingly challenged as clinical series report good to excellent results.

Contraindications can be systemic or specific to the hip joint. Systemic contraindications include a preexisting severe medical condition, limited life expectancy, nonambulatory status, and skeletal immaturity. Absolute specific contraindications are the presence of active infection, functional loss of the abductor muscle, a progressive neurologic disease, and advanced bone destruction. Relative specific contraindications include a prior history of joint sepsis, a neurotrophic hip joint, young age, and limited rehabilitation potential.

Implant Designs and Principles of Fixation Once the patient has been clinically indicated, the next step is the selection of the implant and mode of fixation. A THA can conceptually be divided into five segments: the acetabular-bone interface, the acetabular component, the hip joint (acetabular-femoral head interface), the femoral component, and the femoral-bone interface. The principles of implant fixation evidently apply to the first and last of these segments. Implant design theories concern the middle three segments. Since the advent of modularity, further subdivision has occurred to include the interface between the acetabular liner and shell, as well as that between the femoral neck and the head and/or between the femoral stem and any modular attachments. Design variables for each component include geometry and material properties. These, in turn, determine mechanical stability and rate of wear with articulating components. The overall stiffness of a component depends both on its geometry (especially diameter) and on the material elasticity.

The original acetabular design was made of full-thickness polyethylene. The quality of the material used now has been standardized to ultra-high-molecular-weight polyethylene (UHMWPE). The rate of wear caused by friction of the femoral head occurs by two modes: penetrating (point) and volumetric wear. The type of wear that predominates depends mostly on the femoral head diameter. Smaller head sizes (e.g., 22 mm) cause deeper focal penetration into the polyethylene liner, whereas greater head sizes (e.g., 32 mm) result in more superficial but overall greater volumetric wear. The all-polyethylene design was modified in the 1980s in an attempt to minimize aseptic loosening at the acetabular-bone interface. The rationale was to dampen the load transmission by using a metal acetabular shell while simultaneously eliminating cement fixation, as particulate polymethylmethacrylate (PMMA) debris was thought to be the primary cause of osteolysis (previously known as cement disease). The clinical success of this design theory has been mixed. Osteolysis was still found, now originating from UHMWPE particles, which are produced at a greater rate because of the stronger reactive force onto the hip joint from the stiff metal shell. Another new problem was backside

wear at the modular interface between shell and liner. Significant osteolysis has been found directly adjacent to screw holes in the shell used for supplemental acetabular fixation. Acetabular wear rate is linear for the first 10 to 15 years and then becomes exponential. The linear rate after the first year is approximately 0.1 mm/year. Catastrophic acetabular failure has also been seen with flawed designs with incongruent matching of liner to shell and/or insufficient rim or wall thickness. Current recommendations call for a minimum of 8 mm of polyethylene wall thickness.

The ideal femoral head size has been long debated. Larger heads (e.g., 32 mm) may offer greater stability at the expense of greater volumetric wear and decreased range of motion. Conversely, smaller-diameter heads (e.g., 22 mm) have more focal penetration and relatively less stability but a greater range of motion. Current practice is to use 26- to 28-mm-diameter femoral heads as long as the minimal acetabular thickness criteria are met. When a small acetabular component is employed, it is advisable to use a 22-mm femoral head to maximize the thickness of the UHMWPE liner.

Some newer acetabular designs vary in material properties. Ceramic heads have excellent stiffness and wear properties, but have been associated with catastrophic failure because of their highly brittle nature. Metal-on-metal and ceramic-on-ceramic articulations have also attracted renewed interest as modern production techniques allow precise joint congruency and minimal friction. Both of these alternatives may eventually obviate the need for UHMWPE and minimize production of particulate debris that leads to osteolysis and premature implant failure.

The role of the rigidity of the implant has particular importance for the femoral component. The ideal goal is isoelasticity with the proximal femur. Design variables influencing elasticity are the type of metal used and the diameter of the implant. The latter is more influential because it varies with the fourth power of the radius. For smaller implants, however, metallurgical strength is critical. Catastrophic failures (stem fractures) are now rare with the superalloys routinely used: chrome-cobalt (Cr-Co) and titanium (Ti), the former being significantly stiffer. Stiffness can also be increased through the production process of forging (machining the implant from a block of metal) instead of casting (pouring liquid metal into a mold). The rigidity of large noncemented stems, particularly of the distal fit design, often exceeds that of the native surrounding bone and results in load bypass through the stem to the hip. This, in turn, results in proximal femoral bone (calcar) resorption. The clinical significance of this phenomenon remains controversial. Periprosthetic femoral fracture comprises another danger with excessively stiff implants. The initiation point of the fracture, in the absence of underlying osteolysis and subsidence, usually corresponds to an abrupt stress transition zone. To address this problem, some larger-caliber implant designs have a thinner waist, as well as such other stiffness-reducing features as distal fluting or clothespin features. Cement fixation has a protective role, since its stiffness lies between that of bone and the superalloys and thus reduces the net stiffness of the construct and acts as a dampening device.

The role of the calcar collar on the femoral stem is controversial. Suggested functions are to prevent subsidence of cemented stems, transfer mechanical load to the calcar to prevent bone resorption, and to serve as a shield to prevent the passage of UHMWPE particles into the femur-bone cement or implant-bone interface. To prevent the latter, many femoral stem designs have incorporated a full-circumference surface coating at the proximal stem level. Corrosion fretting between metallic modular parts of the femoral implant has been identified as another source of particulate debris that leads to osteolytic destruction. More precise fitting and avoidance of metallurgical mismatch may partially correct the problem.

Fixation principles for hip arthroplasty differ for cemented and noncemented fixation. In cemented hip arthroplasty, which was developed first, both the acetabular and femoral components are fully coated with a mantle of PMMA cement that serves as a complete interface between implant and host bone. The cement has no particular chemical bonding property; rather, it acts as a grout with macrodigital penetration into the irregular contour of the recipient bone surfaces. First-generation cementing technique involved insertion of the PMMA cement by digital application and packing. This was later modified by the introduction of a cement restrictor into the femoral canal and mechanical cleansing of the femoral canal followed by retrograde filling using a long-nozzle cement gun (on the femoral side) and pressurization. Third-generation cementing technique focused on porosity reduction of the PMMA cement by vacuum mixing or centrifugation prior to insertion. Such treatment in the liquid phase of the monomer is intended to minimize the number and size of trapped air vacuoles that could weaken the structural strength of the compound and potentially play a role in microfracture propagation. This was considered necessary because of evidence of premature mechanical failure with valgus position yielding less than 2 mm of distal cement mantle. Fourth-generation cementing technique introduced coated or textured component surfaces in order to increase the bonding area. Recent results using fourth-generation techniques have not been all that favorable, and most surgeons currently use the third-generation cementing technique.

In response to evidence of osteolysis (originally called "cement disease") and of shorter-term failure of total hip implants in younger patients, efforts were made to achieve implant fixation without cement, and total joint components of varying designs emerged. Two classes of acetabular component gained popularity: the hemispherical press-fit fixation and the threaded-ring fixation. The former evolved with dual-radius geometry, surface coating to enhance bone ingrowth, and allowance for supplemental screw fixation. The latter design, though still popular in Europe, has largely been abandoned in North America. It relies on rim fixation and is often bottomless. A large wingspan and pitch have been associated with superior implant performance. The surgical technique is exacting and unforgiving.

Cementless femoral stem fixation is achieved by a stable osseous ingrowth or ongrowth at the bone-implant interface. Design strategies may be classified into two major groups, based on the anatomic site of purchase: metaphyseal locking ("proximal fit") or diaphyseal locking ("distal fill") prosthesis. The former attempts a proximal, anatomically contoured metaphyseal fit, whereas the latter opts for a tight interference-like fill of the midsegments and distal segments of the stem. Thigh pain, which has not been a problem with cemented femoral stems, has been associated with the use of noncemented femoral stems and an apparent greater incidence with the use of larger, stiffer implants.

The primary determinant of mechanical stability in noncemented implants remains the immediate fit. A minimum of three-point cortical contact is required to that effect. The degree of osseous ongrowth or ingrowth of the implant-host interface is later critical for the long-term survival of the arthroplasty. This can be achieved by microinterlocking of cancellous bone within an applied latticework or by chemical bonding. Various surface-coating designs exist, the most popular being sintered beads (porous coating) and adfixed wire mesh. Hydroxyapatite coating is the major application of chemical bonding. The extent of surface coating is also variable. Most proximal fitting designs coat the metaphyseal area, whereas distal filling designs extend the coated surface further down the diaphysis.

Cemented arthroplasties are the treatment of choice for elderly (older than age 75) and sedentary patients. For young and active patients, noncemented implant fixation is favored. Several studies have

now established the long-term clinical success of the newer-generation cemented arthroplasty techniques. One of these, the hybrid hip arthroplasty, consisting of a cementless acetabulum and a cemented femoral component, is considered the standard of care for patients older than age 55 (Fig. 49-2). A high-demand patient (usually male) with sufficient femoral bone stock will be best treated with a cementless reconstruction; a more sedentary patient would be best treated with a hybrid. The issues of physiologic age and anticipated load are thus paramount in the selection of the implant.

Once the implant type has been selected, a careful preoperative analysis of the radiograph will determine the exact position, model, and size of the implant. Preoperative templating starts with a verification of the leg length discrepancy by measuring the relative height of the lesser trochanters on the AP pelvis film. Next, the original contour of the acetabulum is delineated, that is, medial wall (teardrop),

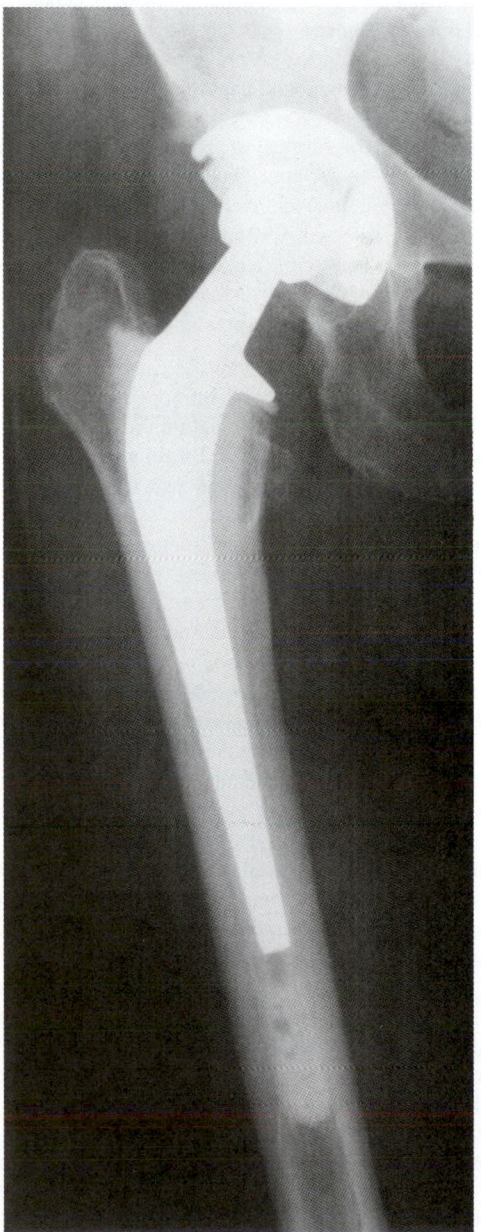

Figure 49-2
AP radiograph demonstrating satisfactory radiologic outcome of a primary total hip reconstruction for osteoarthritis. Note the acetabular vertical inclination, anteversion, and rim fit. The femoral component shows satisfactory cement technique, position, and distal column length.

inferomedial, and superolateral margins. A proper template fit is obtained and the center marked. A preliminary sizing of the better-preserved contralateral acetabulum is often required. The femoral templating is more complex, with outcome variables of size and length of the component, length and degree of offset of the neck, height of the neck cut based from the lesser trochanter, and the size of the head. Cemented implants require a minimum of 1 to 2 cm of cement distal to the femoral stem and a circumferential cement mantle of 2 mm.

Surgical Approach   The most common surgical approaches utilized in primary hip arthroplasty are the posterior approach with posterior dislocation and the anterolateral approach with anterior hip dislocation. The posterior approach has been significantly associated with postoperative posterior dislocation, this complication being less common with other approaches. Anterior and anterolateral approaches, however, are often associated with a persistent abductor limp. The transtrochanteric approach is seldom used for primary hip arthroplasty because, although it provides excellent exposure, the associated morbidity is high, with a trochanteric nonunion rate of up to 10 percent.

The selection of the surgical approach is usually a matter of the surgeon's personal choice and experience. Specific indications include acetabular columnar deficiencies, where a corresponding approach should be selected. Contraindications for the posterior approach are cases of spasticity (e.g., Parkinson's disease), so as to decrease the chance of posterior dislocation, and in recumbent patients with fecal incontinence, so as to preclude wound contamination.

Complications   The complications associated with hip arthroplasty can be classified chronologically. Intraoperative complications include: hemodynamic insufficiency and failure secondary to excessive blood loss or predisposing associated medical conditions, complications associated with polymethacrylate use, fractures, and neurologic injuries. Cementing poses a specific risk as extravasation in the liquid phase can reach neurovascular structures and cause thermal injuries. Pressurization of the monomer is associated with pulmonary embolization, which may trigger cardiopulmonary compromise. Mechanical complications include acetabular and femoral fractures. Excessive leg lengthening may cause a neuropraxia stretch injury to the peroneal branch of the sciatic nerve. Although most of these injuries are incomplete, the potential for full nerve recovery is usually guarded. Electromyographic documentation should be obtained at 6 weeks postoperatively. The generally accepted limit for lengthening is 2 to 4 cm or 6 to 8 percent of the femoral length. The femoral nerve may also incur damage, usually the result of forceful anterior retraction. The prognosis is similar to that of sciatic injuries.

Immediate postoperative complications include: infection, deep venous thrombosis (DVT), pulmonary embolus, and dislocation. The incidence of DVT may be as high as 10 percent (range, 5 to 20 percent). Of these, up to 10 percent may embolize to cause symptomatic pulmonary emboli. Only 30 percent of patients who have a fatal pulmonary embolism are clinically diagnosed with either a DVT or pulmonary embolism. Most patients, therefore, lack the typical clinical profile of shortness of breath, chest pain, leg pain, and swelling that can lead to the diagnosis of DVT and pulmonary embolism. Following THA, patients are at increased risk for thromboembolic disease because of the triad of stasis, activation of the clotting cascade, and damage to venous endothelium during surgery. The inciting factors for thromboembolic disease originate at the time of surgery, with detectable thrombi in the thigh beginning at 24 to 48 h after surgery, peaking at days 5 to 7, and dropping in incidence after day 10. The probability of embolization increases with proximal extension of the thrombus. For this reason, anticoagulation prophylaxis is a standard component of postoperative arthroplasty protocols. Prevention of

DVT consists of early mobilization and rehabilitation, lower extremity exercises, elastic stockings, external pneumatic compression devices, and medications. Currently recommended medications for DVT prophylaxis are either low-molecular-weight subcutaneous heparin injections or oral warfarin therapy. The clinical diagnosis of DVT should be entertained from a high clinical suspicion, since most patients do not present with such classic symptoms as a positive Homans' sign, edema, pain, or thrombosis. It is reported that the accuracy of clinical diagnosis alone shows only a 33 percent sensitivity and a 50 percent specificity. If DVT is suspected, then the diagnosis should be confirmed by duplex scanning (93 percent sensitive and 98 percent specific in the diagnosis of thigh thrombosis) or venography. If pulmonary embolus is clinically suspected, the diagnosis should be confirmed by immediate ventilation-perfusion scan and chest radiographs with supportive measures initiated. In cases where the diagnosis is still in doubt, pulmonary angiography may be necessary to confirm the diagnosis. Once the diagnosis has been confirmed, treatment should consist of systemic intravenous heparin anticoagulation followed by 3 to 6 months of oral Coumadin (warfarin) anticoagulation therapy. In selected cases where systemic anticoagulation is contraindicated, an inferior vena caval filter should be placed.

Dislocation is the most common immediate postoperative complication, with an incidence of 1 to 3 percent. The causes of dislocation are varied and include component malposition, inadequate soft tissue tension, insufficient neck length or offset, infection, impingement of the femoral component on bone or acetabular components, and traumatic dislocation (Fig. 49-3). Posterior dislocation is the most common type (from a posterior approach) and can be the result of insufficient anteversion of the acetabular component (relative retroversion) and/or insufficient anteversion of the femoral component. Though usually implicated when present, the role played by an excessively vertically tilted acetabular component remains unclear. Inadequate restoration of the soft tissue envelope tension is usually preventable and generally stems from improper vertical or horizontal offset restoration, but may also be the result of excessive dissection or ab-

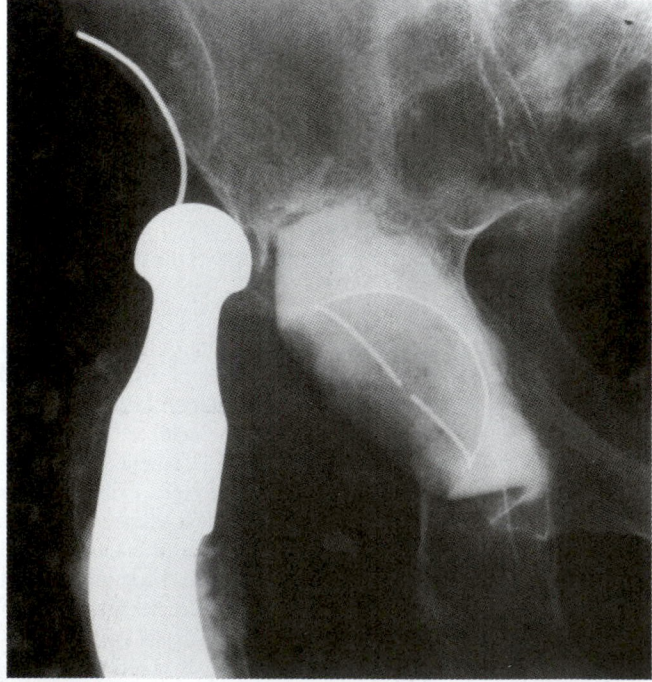

Figure 49-3
AP radiograph of the right hip demonstrating chronic dislocation and broken trochanteric fixation wire.

ductor muscle injury. The corrective measure is to lengthen the leg within acceptable limits and/or perform a trochanteric advancement. Infection may occasionally play a role by dilation and inhibition of the capsule and local musculature, leading to dislocation. The treatment of postoperative dislocations must address the cause. Careful radiographic analysis must rule out component malposition. In traumatic or idiopathic cases, the first line of treatment consists of closed reduction followed by restriction of hip range of motion by either stricter hip precautions or by an abductor brace. Six weeks of treatment is generally sufficient. Recurrent dislocations and identified component malposition are indications for either surgical revision or trochanteric advancement.

Late postoperative complications include heterotopic ossification, septic and aseptic loosening, and periprosthetic fractures (Fig. 49-4). Formal discussion of the latter three is presented in the following section on "Revision Hip Reconstruction." Heterotopic ossification, which has an incidence as high as 53 percent of patients, is most often classified according to the Brooker system into four levels of severity: class I consists of islands of bone occurring in the soft tissues about the hip, class II is noted by the appearance of bone spurs extending from either the pelvis or proximal femur, class III occurs when the space between the bone spurs is less than 1 cm, and class IV is defined by bony ankylosis at the hip. The majority of patients suffer little functional disability. Associated factors include male gender, young age, previous history of heterotopic ossification, traumatic arthritis, ankylosing spondylitis, and diffuse idiopathic skeletal hyperostosis syndrome. Heterotopic bone formation in patients at risk is prevented by administration of either postoperative radiation (600

to 800 rad in one or two doses) given before postoperative day 4 or indomethacin (75 mg/day for 3 weeks). The probability of subsequent radiation-induced sarcoma is small. If surgical removal of the heterotopic bone is indicated, this should be delayed until at least 6 months after the index operation, and prophylactic radiation therapy should be used.

OSTEONECROSIS

Osteonecrosis of the femoral head represents a collection of pathologic conditions of various etiologies leading to a common pathway of cellular death and architectural collapse, which in turn yields to incongruency of the hip joint and eventual secondary degenerative arthritis. There are numerous risk factors for the development of non-traumatic osteonecrosis of the femoral head (Table 49-1). Of these, alcohol abuse and corticosteroid use are the most frequently associated factors. Primary idiopathic osteonecrosis is the most common. The quantity of alcohol required to be a causative agent is very high: 400 ml/week. The danger associated with the use of corticosteroids involves mostly sudden high-systemic regimens. A particularly strong association with systemic lupus erythematosus is noted. To date, there is no significant evidence of association with local intraarticular or trigger-point injections. Traumatic osteonecrosis may develop after femoral neck fractures (20 percent) or hip dislocations (10 percent).

Four pathomechanical pathways have been described: (1) intraosseous venous hypertension with secondary compartment syndrome, (2) extraosseous flow disruption (e.g., trauma), (3) extrinsic vessel pressure from fat cells (Gaucher's disease and corticosteroids), and (4) internal vessel thromboembolic injury (e.g., sickle cell disease).

The several classification systems for AVN of the femoral head have been modified with advances in diagnostic radiology, most notably scintigraphy, MRI, and, more recently, single photon emission computed tomography (SPECT). MRI has a high specificity for the early diagnosis of osteonecrosis of the femoral head. The Association Internationale de Recherche sur le Circulation Osseuse (ARCO) has

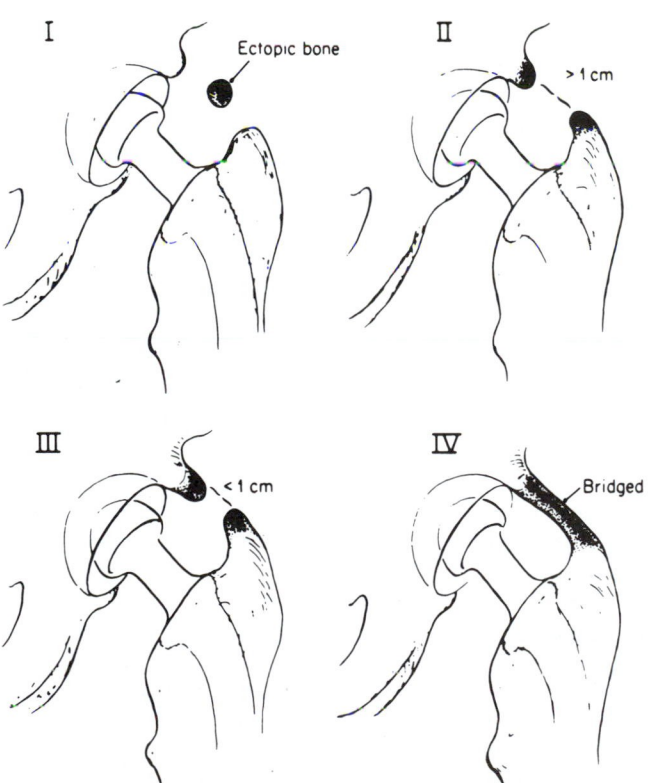

Figure 49-4
Brooker classification system. Class I, islands of bone; Class II, ectopic bone, leaving a space of more than 1 cm between the opposing surfaces; Class III, bone spurs that reduce the space between the opposing surfaces to less than 1 cm; Class IV, bony bridging or apparent roentgenographic "ankylosis." [Reproduced with permission from Thomas BJ: Heterotopic bone formation. In Amstutz HC (ed): *Hip Arthroplasty.* New York: Churchill Livingstone; 1991:407.]

Table 49-1

Clinical Events and Conditions Associated with Osteonecrosis

Alcoholism
Anticoagulant deficiencies
Brain/spinal surgery
Chemotherapy
Diabetes mellitus
Dysbaric phenomena—decompression sickness
Hemoglobinopathies
Hypercortisonism
Hyperlipemia
Inflammatory bowel disease
Nephrotic syndrome
Pancreatitis
Serum sickness
Sickle-cell crisis
Storage diseases—Gaucher's disease
Systemic lupus erythematosus
Toxic shock
Vascular disorders—arteriosclerosis

now suggested a uniform staging system for osteonecrosis with a five-stage system: stage 0, histology only; stage 1, with a positive diagnostic test; stage 2, with a positive x-ray with no radiographic collapse; stage 3, with positive radiograph with collapse; and stage 4, with a positive radiograph with osteoarthritis. Each stage can be subclassified according to the percent of head involvement or surface collapse: subclass A, minimal with less than 15 percent femoral head involvement or with less than 2 mm of surface collapse; subclass B, moderate with 15 to 30 percent head involvement or with 2 to 4 mm of surface collapse; and subclass C, extensive with more than 30 percent femoral head involvement or with more than 4 mm of surface collapse. One entity that is not uncommonly encountered, however, is transient osteoporosis of the proximal femur. This condition is usually self-limiting and need not be treated by surgical decompression. The zone of marrow signal changes is more diffuse than in osteonecrosis. Some authors nevertheless warn that it may represent a possible early stage of AVN, and that careful observation is mandatory. The critical stage of all classifications is the development of the crescent sign representing a chondral lucency, a harbinger of subchondral collapse. Once this is present, the therapeutic value of decompressive surgery plummets. The last stage in most classifications indicates acetabular degeneration, and usually implicates the need for reconstructive surgery.

Prior to the development of the crescent sign on x-ray, treatment options include observation, restriction of weightbearing, electrical stimulation, surgical core decompression with or without strut grafting (with either avascular or vascularized fibular graft), and proximal femoral osteotomies. Restricted weightbearing has consistently proven inefficient at halting the progression of the osteonecrosis (70 to 90 percent probability of progression). Electrical stimulation (pulsed electromagnetic fields), although pending approval by the Food and Drug Administration, offers an optimistic treatment alternative. In stages I and II (Ficat, 1983), it has been shown to be comparable to core decompression, whereas it was slightly superior with stage III.

Core decompression, which remains controversial, consists of a decompressive tunnel created through the femoral neck from the lateral cortical margin. Its success rate beyond Ficat stage III is poor. There is also a strong correlation with the size of involvement of the femoral head, with significantly better results with smaller lesions and sparing of the lateral column. When considered as a unified group, the probability of progression to end stage (requiring arthroplasty) has been found to vary between 20 and 60 percent. As a supplement to the decompression, several authors have recommended structural bone grafting. In this procedure, the decompression tunnel is filled with a nonvascular (Bonfiglio) or vascular fibular strut graft. The results with recognized section collapse are no better than with core decompression alone (20 percent conversion rate to arthroplasty). Recent results with vascularized fibular strut graft have been encouraging in short-term follow-up.

Osteotomies for osteonecrosis are of two types: angulation and rotational. In both applications, the failure rate increases with the size of the femoral head defect. Beyond 50 percent involvement, the procedure is contraindicated by virtue of poor outcome (over 70 percent conversion to THA at 10 years). Angulation osteotomy should be of the varus type for central or medial head involvement, whereas valgus osteotomy is reserved for superolateral head defects. Rotational intertrochanteric osteotomies, such as popularized by Sugioka (1992), are highly technical, and clinical success has been variable.

Once subchondral collapse has taken place, there is no longer any significant role for the aforementioned treatment modalities. Assuming no medical contraindications, these young and active patients are generally best treated by total joint arthroplasty. Because of the high incidence of bilaterality in nontraumatic osteonecrosis (up to 80 percent, depending on etiology), arthrodesis is a limited option. Hemiarthroplasty may appear attractive in the presence of radiologic sparing of the acetabulum, but anatomic studies have demonstrated advanced degenerative changes, rendering the long-term outcome of this procedure fair to poor. It should be emphasized that, although THA is the best option for this stage, it does not present an ideal long-term solution, because the failure and complication rates of osteonecrosis as a class are significantly higher than for comparable groups with osteoarthritis. More specific reasons for this may include an underlying continuing condition such as sickle cell disease or the age and activity level of these patients.

REVISION HIP RECONSTRUCTION

The popularity of arthroplasty in the treatment of degenerative and inflammatory hip diseases has increased continuously over the last three decades, which has led to a high prevalence of implants with intrinsic (limited) mechanical longevity. Understandably, the incidence of acute and progressive implant failures has risen accordingly. Although the exact mode of failure varies and is often complex, the similarity in the evaluation and treatment of failed hip arthroplasties warrants a focused discussion.

Arthroplasties can fail for many reasons at different time intervals. In the short term (i.e., the first 3 months), the most common cause of failure is infection or recurrent dislocation due to component malposition. The midterm failures (within 1 year of surgery) usually are due to infection, either from a latent microorganism from the original operation or a new acute hematogenous process. The long-term failures (after 1 year of implantation) are due to either mechanical (aseptic) or septic loosening process. A third failure scenario, independent of postoperative stage, is that of acute mechanical failure from a periprosthetic fracture.

Independent of osteolytic weakening effect, the reconstruction may fail because of bad design, metallurgy factors (fatigue fracture), or individual implant-to-bone mismatch. Certain acetabular metal-backed designs have insufficient UHMWPE at the rim of the liner, leading to premature catastrophic liner failure. In other cases, smaller (usually less than 9 mm diameter) femoral stems fracture from excessive fatigue. More commonly, poor choice of implant selection or technical errors during implantation are responsible. Technical errors on the acetabular side include insufficient superolateral coverage, excessive coronal tilt (vertical), insufficient medialization, and femoral-head-to-liner-thickness mismatch. Technical errors on the femoral side include varus placement of the stem, inadequate anteversion, intraoperative fracture or perforation, inadequate canal filling for biologic fixation, and unsatisfactory cement technique for cemented implants.

EVALUATION

In addition to the medical history leading to the initial diagnosis and previous treatment for hip arthritis, a comprehensive assessment of the postoperative course is essential. This includes a detailed account of the postoperative pain relief and functional recovery to date, noting postoperative complications and their management, and any subsequent trauma or infection.

The physical evaluation of the failed arthroplasty hip includes most elements of the primary hip examination. In addition, however, a detailed examination for signs of infection, mechanical failure, or trauma is required. Of particular importance, one may note a painful hip with the leg held in flexion and external rotation (sepsis), painful grinding of components (polyethylene fracture), or shortening and malrotation (periprosthetic fracture). The previous surgical approach should be also noted.

Laboratory evaluation is of critical importance to distinguish septic from aseptic loosening, since management of these two conditions is significantly different. An acute infection typically gives rise to an elevated WBC count with a left shift on the differential count. The ESR and CRP level are sensitive but nonspecific indicators of a chronic process. Chronically immunosuppressed anergic patients may not be capable of mounting a defensive hematologic response to infection, and the absence of such a response must be evaluated with caution in such cases.

The standard roentgenographic evaluation consists of AP and lateral films of the hip and an AP view of the pelvis. These films are analyzed for any radiologic evidence of loosening. A set of well-defined criteria are then used to quantify the degree of erosive changes as probable or definite radiologic loosening in cases of aseptic failure. Moreover, the acetabular and femoral areas have been divided in zones for analytical purposes. Zone distributions based on the works

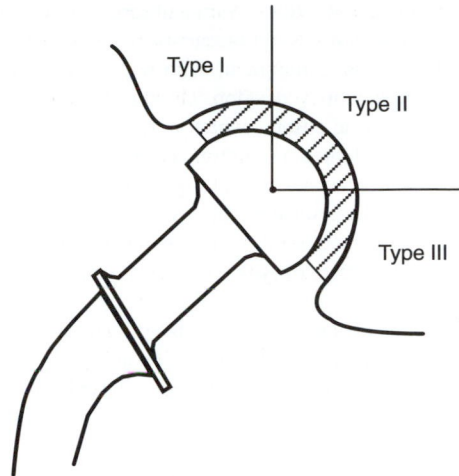

Figure 49-6
DeLee and Charnley Zones. Division of circumference of acetabular bone-cement interface in zones type I, type II, and type III. (Reproduced with permission from DeLee JG, Charnley J: Radiological demarcation of cemented sockets in total hip replacement. *Clin Orthop* 1976; 121:22.)

of DeLee and Charnley for the acetabulum and Gruen for the proximal femur are generally used (Figs. 49-5 and 49-6).

On the acetabular side, signs of wear may be seen as an asymmetric position of the femoral head within the acetabular liner (eccentric wear) (Fig. 49-7); in turn, there may be radiolucent lines at the implant-bone or cement-bone interface. These become cause for

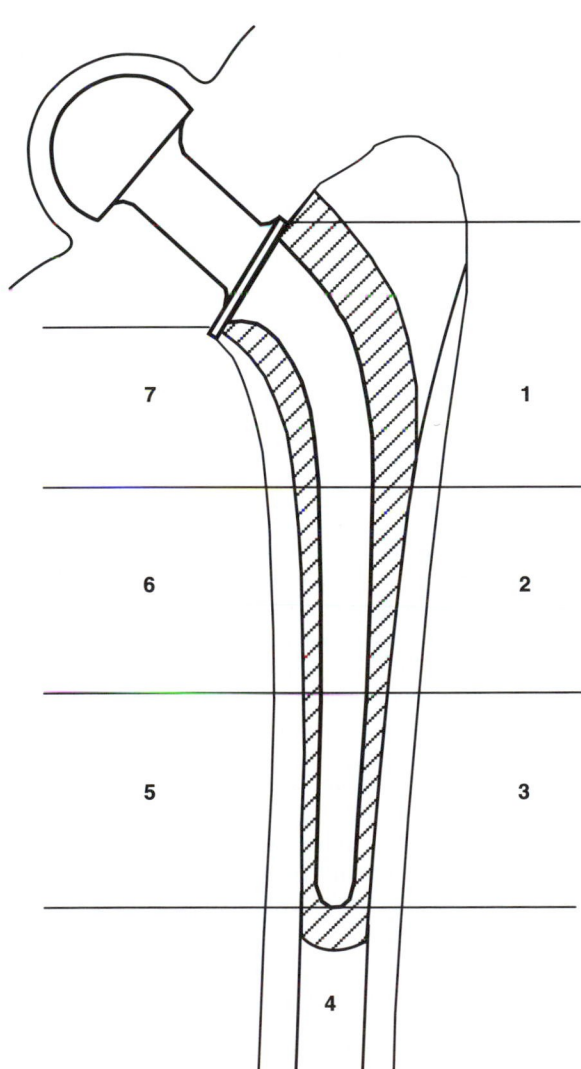

Figure 49-5
Gruen Zones. Seven delineated sections around the femoral component for zonal evaluation of looseness and progressive loosening. (Reproduced with permission from Gruen TA, McNeice GM, Amstutz HC: "Modes of failure" of cemented stem-type femoral components. A radiographic analysis of loosening. *Clin Orthop* 1979; 141:18.)

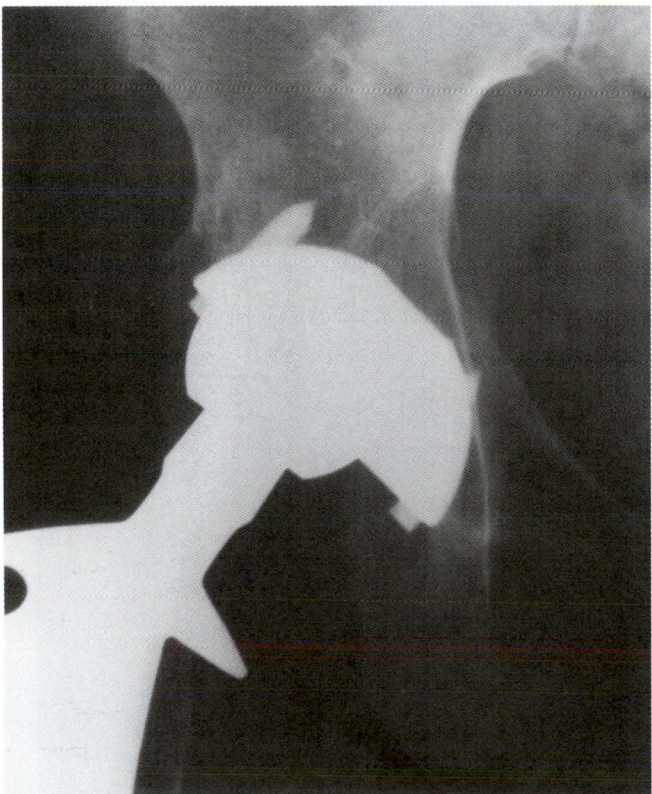

Figure 49-7
AP radiograph of the right hip demonstrating catastrophic polyethylene failure. Note the eccentric position of the femoral head in the acetabulum.

concern if they are greater than 2 mm and progressive or continuous over more than one zone. Radiolucencies in acetabular zone III are associated with a loose component. With worsening osteolysis, cystic or cavitary defects may develop. Once loosening has reached a critical stage, migration ensues, which may result in tilting or shifting of the implant. Central migration results in gradual protrusion, whereas shear erosion causes typical superolateral segmental defects. If the destruction is so extensive as likely to require supplementation, a more precise visualization of the acetabular defect can be obtained through a CT scan and possibly three-dimensional CT reconstruction imaging.

Radiologic signs of femoral osteolysis will vary according to type of fixation (cemented or noncemented). The aging cemented implant (usually first-generation cement technique) will typically demonstrate fusiform ballooning with thin wall expansion of reactive bone about a sheath of osteolytic debris within the loosened cement-bone interface (Fig. 49-8). Varus migration and distal cortical penetration or periprosthetic fracture are not uncommon findings. Aseptic loosening of noncemented implants is suggested by the appearance of femoral diaphyseal radiolucent lines, adaptive cortical changes, endosteal lysis, formation of distal osseous intramedullary pedestal, or

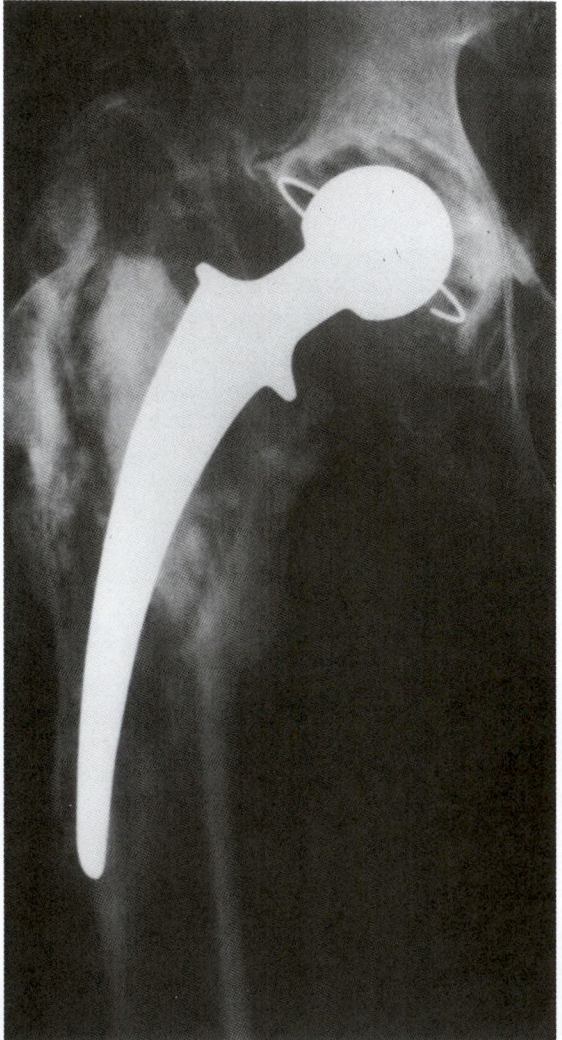

Figure 49-8
AP radiograph of the right hip demonstrating advanced aseptic loosening of a cemental femoral component with subsidence and varus migration.

implant subsidence. It is of paramount importance to note the progression of radiographic change as an indication of whether the component is loose.

If the diagnosis of possible periprosthetic infection is still in question, special tests before revision hip surgery can be helpful. Plain radiographs alone cannot be used definitively to diagnose infection. Abnormal blood values of the WBC count, ESR, and CRP level may suggest an infection, but are not diagnostic. The role of preoperative hip aspiration arthrogram remains controversial, because some authors report poor accuracy (40 percent false-negative rate) due to infectious loculations, the potential morbidity of an iatrogenic infection, and possible false-positive results from skin contaminants. Nonetheless, it is of value if the cultured organism is of high virulence, since the subsequent management is significantly altered by this finding. Technetium-99m bone scans can reveal areas of increased bone activity about loose implants, but do not enable one to distinguish between septic and aseptic loosening. Indium-111-labeled leukocyte scans have a high false-positive rate, with only approximately 55 percent of cases with a positive scan being a septic failure. A positive technetium scan with a negative indium scan, however, is about 95 percent predictive of aseptic loosening. Technetium-gallium imaging has also been used, but has a reported accuracy of only approximately 60 percent for identifying the presence of an infected implant. In a prospective study performed at the authors' institution, results from frozen sections of the periprosthetic tissue obtained intraoperatively showed that more than 10 polymorphonuclear leukocytes per high-power field had a sensitivity of 84 percent and a specificity of 99 percent for predicting infection at revision surgery. Research being conducted on the use of the polymerase chain reaction to detect bacterial RNA shows promise.

ASEPTIC LOOSENING

Aseptic loosening, which is the predominant mode of fixation failure of cemented and noncemented implants, can be attributed to various biologic, mechanical, and material factors as well as implant designs. Osteolysis results from a biologic reaction to foreign particles, including those of PMMA and metal; however, polyethylene is the main contributor. Osteolysis and aseptic loosening contribute greatly to the bone deficiencies seen at revision surgery, with each revision increasingly more demanding to reconstruct.

A four-mode classification system of failure has been devised for cemented stems: *Pistoning* occurs when the stem and/or cement mantle are loose. *Medial midstem pivot* is characterized by proximal medial and distal lateral motion. *Calcar pivot* occurs when the stem is fixed proximally and the distal stem rotates about this axis in windshield-wiper fashion. *Cantilever failure* occurs when a distally well-fixed stem is loose proximally and the stem itself fractures. This last category of failure has become increasingly rare with the use of superalloys. Stress shielding can also contribute to bone loss and is typically more significant in diaphyseal locking press-fit noncemented stems, especially if the porous-coated stem diameter is greater than 13.5 mm.

As the proximal femoral bone deficiency increases, so does the need for distal fixation of the revision construct. Femoral defects can be classified as type I, intact metaphysis and diaphysis; type II, nonsupportive metaphysis but intact diaphysis; or type III, nonsupportive metaphysis and diaphysis with distal diaphyseal support usually remaining.

Several extended trochanteric osteotomies have been described that can aid in femoral implant and/or cement extraction. In addition to the various osteotomes, drills, and slap hammers, ultrasound-driven instruments are available to assist in cement removal from the canal.

Perforation of the femoral cortex during extraction is a frequent complication. When present, fixation of the revision stem should bypass the perforation by two bone diameters.

Once the implant is removed, multiple methods exist to reconstruct the femur. If a cemented technique is chosen, a long-stem component is required; proximal bone loss will result in inadequate cement fixation, and distal purchase is needed to improve the results of revision surgery. Similarly, if a porous-coated stem is used, an extensively coated implant for diaphyseal purchase is needed. Impaction grafting technique, which seems promising for reconstructing cavitary defects of the proximal femur, uses morselized cancellous allograft compressed in the proximal femur and a polished collarless stem cemented into the graft bed.

Several additional options are available to manage femoral bone deficiencies. Cortical strut allografts can be used to enhance the strength of a femoral construct and to restore cortical bone loss. Segmental bone loss of the proximal femur may require a proximal femoral allograft for reconstruction. A long stem that bypasses the host-allograft junction by at least two bone diameters is cemented into the allograft and either press-fitted or cemented into the host bone. Alternatively, a custom proximal femoral-replacing prosthesis, as used in tumor surgery, can be implanted.

Acetabular defects are broadly categorized as contained or non-contained. Contained defects are pockets, with an intact, supportive rim in and around the acetabulum, whereas noncontained defects do not have a supportive rim. Cemented acetabular revisions have high, early loosening rates. More successful fixation is achieved with a porous-coated press-fitted prosthesis. A contained defect can be filled with morselized allograft. Noncontained acetabular defects can be reconstructed using either femoral head, distal femur, or occasionally whole acetabular structural allografts. With massive acetabular defects, antiprotrusion cages fixed to the ilium and ischium can be used to suspend a prosthetic socket in difficult reconstruction cases.

SEPTIC LOOSENING

Sepsis following THA occurs in stages. Stage I infections are acute, fulminate postoperative infections that generally occur within the first 3 months. Stage II infections are the delayed or indolent infections that occur between 6 and 24 months postoperatively, with no pain-free period. Stage III infections occur more than 24 months after surgery, have a pain-free period, and are seeded hematogenously from a distant site. The incidence of stage I infections has declined to 0.05 percent since the advent of THA. The incidence of stage III infections appears to increase with the life of, and wear on, a THA device and accounts for half of the infected cases.

Although a recent report suggests that the administration of rifampin and oxacillin together for 6 months may eradicate *Staphylococcus aureus* infection in 70 percent of infected total joint arthroplasties, the follow-up was short and the individuals may have had only a suppressed infection. In general, antibiotic suppression therapy should be reserved for older patients with a securely fixed prosthesis and medical contraindications to surgery. There are also patients who require a resection arthroplasty to eradicate the infection, but are not candidates for reimplantation and are left with a resection arthroplasty as a definitive procedure.

The vast majority of patients with an infected THA will require staged reconstruction. It is essential to identify the infecting organism and its drug sensitivities with preoperative and/or intraoperative cultures. If the organism causing the infection is of low virulence (e.g., *Staphylococcus epidermidis,* methicillin-sensitive *Staphylococcus aureus,* β-hemolytic *Streptococcus*) and gross purulence is not seen at surgery, some authors recommend a one-stage exchange: the

infected total hip components are removed, the wound is thoroughly debrided, and a new THA is cemented using antibiotic-impregnated acrylic cement. The patient is then treated with organism-specific parental antibiotics for 2 weeks, followed by oral antibiotics for 4 weeks.

Most surgeons will treat an infected THA with a two-stage exchange. Certainly, if gross purulence is found at surgery and/or the organism cultured is virulent (e.g., *Pseudomonas aeruginosa,* group D *Streptococcus,* or methicillin-resistant *S. aureus*), then a two-stage procedure should be performed consisting of a resection arthroplasty followed by a delayed reconstruction. Antibiotic-impregnated acrylic cement spacers are used to maintain the space to be used in the reconstruction and to deliver a high local concentration of antibiotics. Parenteral antibiotics are given for 4 to 6 weeks after the resection arthroplasty. Reconstruction can be performed as early as 3 months after the resection for low-virulence organisms, but should be delayed 1 year for high-virulence organisms. The second-stage reconstruction procedure is performed with a cemented or noncemented implant. If a cemented arthroplasty is chosen, antibiotic-impregnated cement is often used.

Finally, a three-stage reconstruction can be considered in infected patients with significant bone destruction. The first stage includes resection arthroplasty, antibiotic-impregnated cement spacers, and parenteral antibiotics for 4 to 6 weeks. As a second stage, 3 to 6 months later, bone graft reconstruction of the acetabulum and/or femur is performed. Then, 9 to 12 months after the second stage, prosthetic components are reimplanted. Failure to remove all of the acrylic cement when performing the resection arthroplasty greatly increases the likelihood of reinfection after the delayed reconstruction. Following these guidelines, successful reconstruction of an infected THA can be accomplished in approximately 75 to 95 percent of cases.

PERIPROSTHETIC FRACTURES

Periprosthetic fractures are a distinct class of arthroplasty failure that can be thought of as acute mechanical failure (Fig. 49-9). One must nonetheless always consider the possibility that underlying septic or aseptic loosening might have predisposed the patient to an acute event. It is useful to reconstruct the fragments on paper to obtain an immediate prefracture image, which might reveal the cause for the fracture, such as lateral diaphyseal osteolysis and migration (ballooning). A sequential analysis of recent films will often reveal an undetected fracture line that led to full propagation. The incidence of periprosthetic hip fractures is 1 to 3 percent, with the vast majority occurring on the femoral side.

Periacetabular fractures, which are rare and usually occur intraoperatively or with significant trauma, are classified by the same descriptive system as acetabular fractures without implants, and are combined with a classification of the acetabular aseptic loosening, if present. The management of periacetabular fracture can be operative or nonoperative. The latter treatment is reserved for simple nondisplaced fractures in debilitated patients where the morbidity of a surgical intervention poses a significant risk. The principle of operative treatment is aimed at the restoration of the structural integrity of the acetabular rim and a stable bone-implant interface that can be achieved in either one or two stages. In the latter option, a first procedure provides osteosynthesis and converts a noncontained defect into a contained one. The second stage then reconstructs the cavitary defect by using the same principles as for the treatment of aseptic loosening. A one-stage operation combines osteosynthesis and reconstruction into one session. This is favored whenever the intermediate immobilization jeopardizes a patient's overall condition.

Femoral periprosthetic fractures have been classified according to

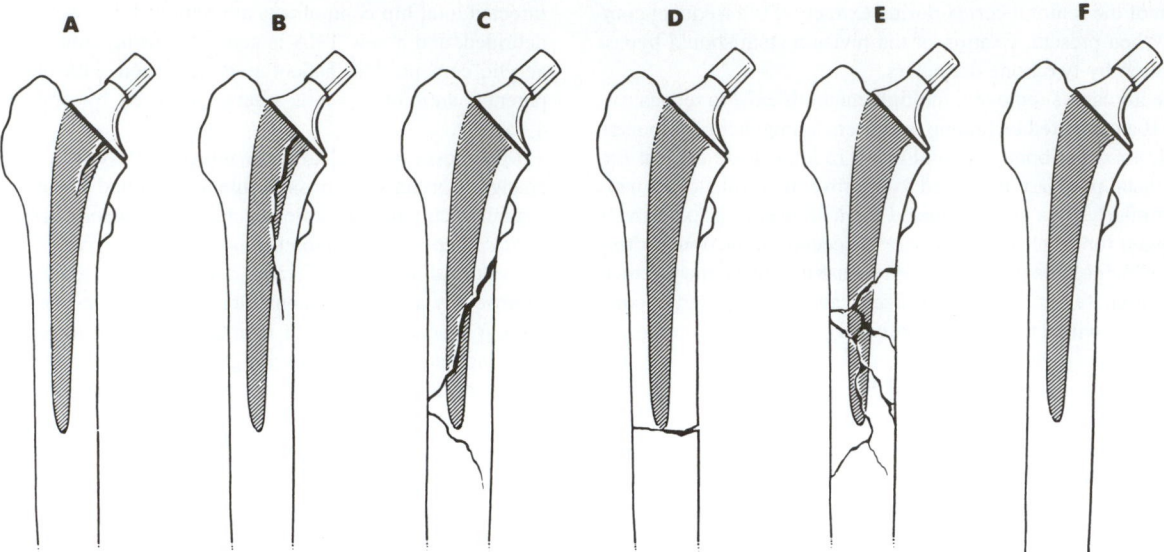

Figure 49-9

Classification (AAOS) of femoral fractures associated with total hip arthroplasty based on location and pattern of fracture. Type I (*not shown*), located proximal to intertrochanteric line, commonly occurs preoperatively and does not alter the treatment of total hip arthroplasty. *A.* Type II is vertical or spiral fracture (split) that does not pass the lower margin of the lesser trochanter. *B.* Type III is vertical split or spiral fracture that extends to or beyond the lower margin of the lesser trochanter but does not pass the junction of middle and lower third of femoral stem. *C.* Type IV includes area of femoral stem tip; IVA is spiral, and IVB is transverse (*D*). *E.* Type V extends distal to stem with comminution. *F.* Type VI fracture line is located distal to prosthesis. (Reproduced with permission from Eftekhar NS: Associated femoral fractures. In: *Total Hip Arthroplasty.* St. Louis: Mosby; 1993:1613.)

fracture location with respect to the prosthesis. Postoperative femoral fractures have been reported to occur in as high as 4 percent of revision and in 0.1 percent of primary hip arthroplasty cases. The Johansson (1981) classification is widely used: type I is a fracture at the distal tip of the implant, type II is a fracture that is proximal to the distal tip of the femoral stem with the stem dislodged from the distal fragment, and type III fractures are those that occur entirely distal to the femoral component. Nonoperative treatment on the femoral side should be restricted to simple, noncomminuted fractures in debilitated patients. There should be distal internal splinting by a radiologically stable implant over a distance of at least two shaft diameters. The operative treatment for periprosthetic femur fracture is generally performed in one stage and is dependent on the fixation of the femoral component. If the femoral stem is loose, then revision surgery with a long-stem cemented or noncemented implant is the treatment of choice, with or without bone grafting. Revision of the femoral implant is often facilitated by the open fracture site. If the femoral stem is well fixed, then open reduction with internal fixation of the fracture is indicated (without revision of the femoral stem) using either cerclage cables alone, plates with cerclage cables and screws, or onlay cortical strut allografts with cerclage fixation. The goal is the restoration of axial structural integrity, as well as circumferential integrity of the femur.

SUGGESTED READINGS

Ahnfelt L, Herberts P, Malchau H, et al: Prognosis of total hip replacement: A Swedish multicenter study of 4,664 revisions. *Acta Orthop Scand* 1990; 238(suppl):1.

Amstutz HC, Campbell P, Kossovsky N, et al: Mechanism and clinical significance of wear debris-induced osteolysis. *Clin Orthop* 1992; 276:7.

Callaghan JJ, Dennis DA, Paprosky WG, et al. (eds): *Orthopaedic Knowledge Update: Hip and Knee Reconstruction.* Rosemont, IL: American Academy of Orthopaedic Surgeons; 1995.

Charnley J: *Low Friction Arthroplasty of the Hip: Theory and Practice.* Berlin, Springer-Verlag; 1979.

Ficat RP: Treatment of avascular necrosis of the femoral head. *HIP* 1983: 279.

Fitzgerald RH: Infected total hip arthroplasty: Diagnosis and treatment. *J Am Acad Orthop Surg* 1995; 3:249.

Fitzgerald RH, Hanssen AD: Postoperative deep wound infection. In Morrey BF (ed): *Joint Replacement Arthroplasty.* New York: Churchill Livingstone; 1991:8350.

Galante JO, Lemons J, Spector M, et al: The biologic effects of implant materials. *J Orthop Res* 1991; 9:760.

Gie GA, Linder L, Ling RS, et al: Contained morselized allograft in revision total hip arthroplasty: Surgical technique. *Orthop Clin North Am* 1993; 24:717.

Johansson JE, McBroom R, Barrington TW, et al: Fracture of the ipsilateral femur in patients with total hip replacement. *J Bone Joint Surg [Am]* 1981; 63:1435.

Johnston RC, Fitzgerald RH Jr, Harris WH, et al: Clinical and radiographic evaluation of total hip replacement: A standard system of terminology for reporting results. *J Bone Joint Surg [Am]* 1990; 72:161 [Erratum, *J Bone Joint Surg [Am]* 1990; 73:948].

Kasser JR (ed): *Orthopaedic Knowledge Update 5: Hip and Pelvis: Reconstruction.* Rosemont, IL: American Academy of Orthopaedic Surgeons; 1996:389.

Laupacis A, Bourne R, Rorabeck C, et al: The effect of elective total hip replacement on health-related quality of life. *J Bone Joint Surg [Am]* 1993; 75:1619.

Livermore J, Ilstrup D, Morrey B: Effect of femoral head size on wear of the polyethylene acetabular component. *J Bone Joint Surg [Am]* 1990; 72:518.

Lonner JH, Desai P, Di Cesare PE, et al: The reliability of analysis of intra-operative frozen sections for identifying active infection during revision hip or knee arthroplasty. *J Bone Joint Surg [Am]* 1996; 78:1553.

McDonald DJ, Fitzgerald RH, Ilstrup DM: Two-stage reconstruction of a total hip arthroplasty because of infection. *J Bone Joint Surg [Am]* 1989; 71:828.

Merkel KD, Brown ML, Dewanjee MK, et al: Comparison of indium labeled leukocyte imaging with sequential technetium-gallium scanning in the diagnosis of low grade musculoskeletal sepsis. *J Bone Joint Surg [Am]* 1985; 67:465.

Mulroy RD Jr, Harris WH: The effect of improved cementing techniques on component loosening in total hip replacement: An 11-year radiographic review. *J Bone Joint Surg [Br]* 1990; 72:757.

Paproski WG, Magnus RE: Principles of bone grafting in revision total hip arthroplasty. *Clin Orthop* 1994; 298:147.

Schulte KR, Callaghan JJ, Kelley SS, et al: The outcome of Charnley total hip arthroplasty with cement after a minimum twenty-year follow-up: The results of one surgeon. *J Bone Joint Surg [Am]* 1993; 75:961 [Erratum, *J Bone Joint Surg [Am]* 1993; 75:1418].

Sofue M, Kono S, Kawaji W, et al: Long-term results of arthrodesis for severe osteoarthritis of the hip in young adults. *Int Orthop* 1989; 13:129.

Spector M, Shortkroff S, Sledge CB, et al: Advances in our understanding of the implant-bone interface: Factors affecting formation and degeneration. In Tullos HS (ed): *Instructional Course Lectures.* Park Ridge, IL: American Academy of Orthopaedic Surgeons, 1991; 50:101.

Sugioka Y, Hotokebuchi T, Tsutsui H: Transtrochanteric anterior rotational osteotomy for idiopathic and steroid-induced necrosis of the femoral head. Indications and long-term results. *Clin Orthop* 1992; 277:111.

Zimlich RH, Fulbright BM, Friedman RJ: Current status of anticoagulation therapy after total hip and total knee arthroplasty. *J Am Acad Orthop Surg* 1996; 4:54.

Chapter 50

KNEE

Paul E. Di Cesare

SYNOVECTOMY

Synovectomy is indicated for selected patients with rheumatoid arthritis, pigmented villonodular synovitis, synovial chondromatosis, and hemophilia synovitis. The clinical outcome of synovectomy is often only temporary, because the decreased pain and stiffness from the synovitis frequently recur, with approximately half of the synovectomized patients later requiring another surgical procedure within 4 years. Only patients with at least 6 months of clinical symptoms of pain, effusion, stiffness, and synovitis despite medical management and those classified as a functional class I or II by the American Rheumatological Association's criteria for rheumatoid arthritis, with minimal radiographic changes, and quiescent systemic disease activity should be indicated for synovectomy. Arthroscopic synovectomy offers many advantages over open synovectomy, such as lower morbidity, lower risk of infection, performance as an outpatient procedure, and minimal loss of knee motion. Expected results are decreased pain and swelling in approximately 80 percent of patients after 2 years; by 4 years after synovectomy, however, approximately 50 percent of the patients with rheumatoid arthritis will have recurrent persistent pain and 25 percent will have recurrent synovitis. Arthroscopic synovectomy is usually performed using full-radius shavers through anterolateral, anteromedial, and posterior (needed to remove synovium from the posterior knee joint) portals. Care must be taken to preserve the menisci and cruciate ligaments and not to damage the articular cartilage. Chemical and radiation synovectomy have also been advocated as alternatives to either open or arthroscopic synovectomy. Chemical synovectomy performed with intraarticular alkylating agents or osmic acid has mostly been abandoned because of the risk of articular cartilage damage. Radiation synovectomy with gold or yttrium has been shown to decrease symptoms for up to 3 years in approximately 50 percent of properly indicated patients. Potential risk of using these isotopes is diffusion to other organ systems due to their long half-lives (2 to 3 days). More recently, dysprosium 165 linked to ferric hydroxide macroaggregates has been used for radiation synovectomy with comparable clinical results and fewer potential side effects due to its shorter half-life (2 h) and larger molecular mass of the composite.

DEBRIDEMENT PROCEDURES

Arthroscopic surgery with both joint debridement and lavage has been performed on osteoarthritic knees in the hope of postponing total knee arthroplasty; however, the success of this has not been proven. The patients who may benefit best from this procedure are those who have recent onset of mechanical symptoms with minimal radiographic changes and also have evidence of intraarticular crystal deposition. Controversy still exists as to whether articular lavage alone is as effective as arthroscopic debridement with lavage. Advocates of this procedure note the low morbidity and mortality and suggest that removal of cartilage debris, crystals, and inflammatory factors will result in decreased pain and stiffness. Clinical trials, however, have resulted in only short-term benefits, with a failure rate of over 50 percent by 2 years. This procedure should be contraindicated in patients with longstanding arthritis, severe articular cartilage loss, and/or joint deformity.

Drilling of subchondral bone or abrasion chondroplasty has not been shown to produce an adequate cartilaginous repair in osteoarthritic knees and usually exacerbates symptoms of pain and stiffness. These procedures should be avoided because they appear to accelerate the degenerative process and do not treat the underlying disease processes.

OSTEOTOMY

Since all joint replacements have the common long-term problem of aseptic loosening, osteotomy and realignment procedures can provide pain relief for patients who are young, perform heavy labor, and/or have unicompartmental degenerative arthritis, with only one joint involved. This procedure is only palliative since the majority of patients will require total knee arthroplasty by 15 years after osteotomy, and most will have decreased symptoms for approximately 7 to 10 years. Later conversion to total knee arthroplasty is usually more technically difficult after high tibial osteotomy, but, if well performed, one can achieve results as good as with a primary knee arthroplasty. Osteotomy is most commonly performed for medial compartment disease on the tibial side.

The rationale for osteotomy and realignment is to decrease the joint reactive forces to the arthritic compartment of the knee and redistribute those forces to the less-involved compartment. Normally the knee experiences forces that are two to four times the body weight, with 60 percent of those forces across the medial tibiofemoral compartment. With joint degeneration in one compartment along with malalignment, the mechanical axis of the limb [passes from the center of the femoral head to the center of the ankle plafond (Fig. 50-1)] shifts the joint reactive forces from the center of the intercondylar region of the tibial plateau to the affected compartment. The anatomic axis of the femur is that formed from the center of the femoral canal to the long axis of the tibia. The normal angle between the mechanical and anatomic axes is approximately 5 degrees in men and 7 degrees in women. Knee malalignment is a direct result of a combination of either the anatomic axis, the net loss of cartilage and bone in one compartment, or widening of the other compartment due to the attenuated and stretched ligamentous and soft tissue from the tension of the mechanical axis in the contralateral compartment. As a general rule, each degree of angulation is the result of each millimeter of joint space narrowing or separation.

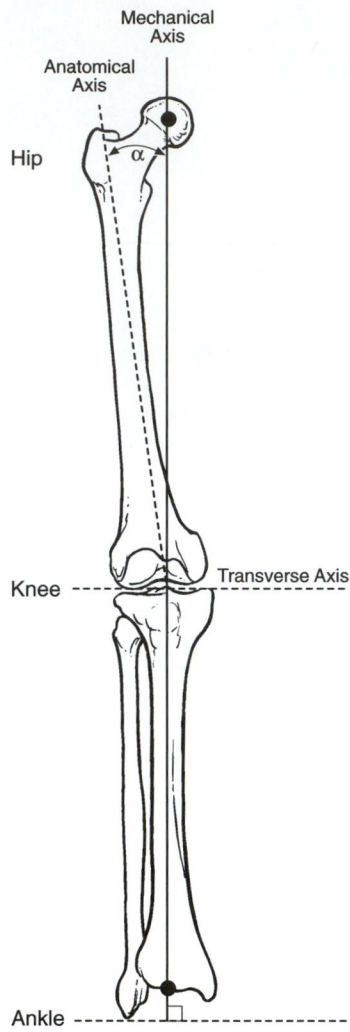

Figure 50-1
Anatomic and mechanical axis of the femur. The normal angle (α) formed is approximately 5 degrees in men and 7 degrees in women.

HIGH (PROXIMAL) TIBIA VALGUS OSTEOTOMY

The high tibial valgus osteotomy is indicated for pain relief and functional improvement in patients younger than age 60 who have medial compartment disease and a functional arc of motion of at least 90 degrees. Absolute contraindications include a flexion contracture greater than 15 degrees, inflammatory arthritis, severe tricompartmental disease, subluxation of the tibia on the femur of more than 1 cm, significant ligamentous instability resulting from more than 1 cm of cartilage and bone loss, joint incongruity, and varus malalignment of greater than 15 degrees. Relative contraindications include mild degenerative changes in the lateral compartment, age older than 70, peripheral vascular disease, and severe patellofemoral arthritis.

Full-length, weightbearing radiographs are essential for preoperative planning of the amount of correction (Fig. 50-2). Although many techniques have been advocated, a lateral closing wedge osteotomy with internal fixation combined with either a fibular osteotomy or division of the proximal tibiofibular joint is most often used. The best long-term clinical outcomes with osteotomy have been with young heavy patients (younger than age 60) in whom a slight overcorrection of the mechanical axis by 2 to 3 degrees has been achieved (final angle between the mechanical and anatomic axis of 8 to 10 de-

grees of valgus). Long-term clinical studies of patients with high tibial osteotomy for varus deformity have demonstrated satisfactory results in 60 to 80 percent of patients at a 10-year follow-up, and no further surgery in 80 percent of patients at 6 years, which decreases to 60 percent by 7 years. Most recently, it has emerged that the dynamic adduction forces across the knee during gait, as a result of the upper body position relative to the knee and the walking speed, may be more important than static angular deformity on standing radiographs in determining the success with osteotomy.

The surgical technique for high tibial osteotomy involves either a closing wedge or dome osteotomy approximately 2 cm distal to the knee joint with fluoroscopic guidance. Potential intraoperative complications include a too proximal osteotomy with the resultant thin proximal fragment that can either fracture or progress to avascular necrosis; a too distal osteotomy that disrupts the tibial tubercle and knee extensor mechanism; or malrotation due to a poorly planned osteotomy and fixation. Because of the higher infection rate with external fixation and the probability of conversion to total knee arthroplasty, it is recommended to use either casting with no internal fixation or internal fixation of either staples and casting or plates and screws with early knee range of motion.

The most common complication, which occurs in approximately 20 percent of cases, is inadequate correction at the time of osteotomy. Since varus deformity recurs in as many as one-third of osteotomy patients, under-correction is associated with increased need for reop-

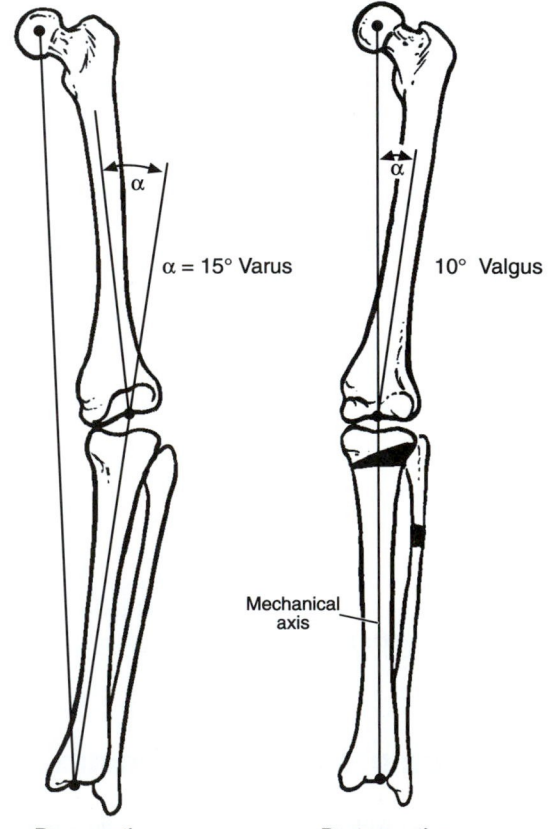

Figure 50-2
High tibial osteotomy to correct medial compartmental degenerative disease with 15 degrees of varus to 10 degrees of valgus. [Redrawn and modified with permission from Goldberg VM, Kettelkamp DB, Colyer RA: Osteoarthritis of the knee. In Moskowitz RW, Howell DS, Goldberg VM (eds): *Osteoarthritis: Diagnosis and Medical Surgical Management*, 2d ed. Philadelphia: Saunders; 1992:607.]

eration and an earlier recurrence of clinical symptoms. Neurologic injuries (peroneal nerve palsy) have been reported in up to 10 percent of patients, occurring most frequently with the use of external fixation, fibular head or neck osteotomy, or in cases of more than 15 degrees of correction. Osteonecrosis of the proximal fragment or nonunion can occur if the proximal fragment is too thin. Delayed union or nonunion has been reported in only 0 to 3 percent of patients. Postoperative infections occur relatively infrequently except in the cases where external fixation is used (infection rate, 1 to 8 percent). Compartment syndrome, although quite rare, has also been reported, so either prophylactic anterior compartment release and/or drains should be used postoperatively.

Since high tibial osteotomy usually results in only temporary symptomatic relief, many patients will require total knee arthroplasty. Approximately 25 percent of patients will undergo total knee arthroplasty 9 years after high tibial osteotomy.

Total knee arthroplasty after high tibial osteotomy is technically more demanding than primary total knee arthroplasty and in some series had worse clinical results than primary total knee arthroplasty (result equivalent to revision knee arthroplasty). Many cases include patella infera, so more attention needs be directed toward proper patella tracking. Patients who had a high tibial osteotomy followed by total knee replacement are at increased risk of needing a lateral retinacular release and quadriceps turndown for exposure to prevent patella tendon avulsion, and have an increased incidence of infection (4.4 percent).

DISTAL FEMORAL VARUS OSTEOTOMY

Valgus malalignment with degenerative knee disease occurs less frequently than varus malalignment and can be the end result of trauma, inflammatory arthritis, renal osteodystrophy, rickets, or infantile poliomyelitis. As a result of the increased valgus deformity, the medial collateral ligament may become stretched, leading to further joint instability. Correction of valgus malalignment must be addressed to the femoral side and, when properly performed, yields results similar to those attained by high tibial valgus osteotomy. The alignment of the distal femur to the shaft is normally in valgus, and therefore any correction done on the tibial side will result in the knee joint line being oblique and angled superolaterally. An oblique joint line will cause marked shear forces across the knee during gait and eventually result in lateral tibial subluxation as the distal femur slides off the medial tibial plateau.

Distal femoral osteotomy is indicated in those instances where the angle between the anatomic and mechanical axis is greater than 15 degrees of valgus or when the joint line is greater than 10 degrees from being parallel to the floor (Fig. 50-3). The osteotomy should slightly overcorrect the angle between the anatomic axis of the femur and the mechanical axis of the tibia to 0 to 2 degrees of valgus in order to decrease the joint reactive forces in the lateral tibiofemoral compartment and to prevent recurrence. Expected clinical results at 4 years postoperatively for properly performed distal femoral osteotomies are good to excellent in approximately 80 to 90 percent of properly selected patients. Reported complications are similar for high tibial valgus osteotomy, with femoral nonunion being the most prevalent.

Distal femoral varus osteotomy is usually performed through a medial approach to the distal femur or can be performed through a midline approach, since many patients will eventually require knee replacement. Varus correction is most often achieved by a medial closing wedge osteotomy in the distal supracondylar femur fixed with a blade plate or equivalent device. Medial displacement of the distal

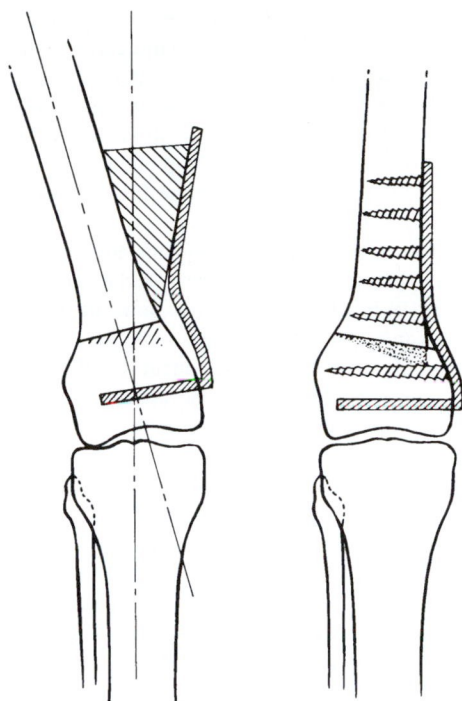

Figure 50-3
Supracondylar femoral osteotomy fixed with a blade plate for valgus malalignment with lateral compartment degenerative disease. A distal medial wedge of bone is removed to correct the limb so the mechanical axis will fall in the midline to medial compartment of the knee.

fragment is also desired because it will restore the mechanical axis to the center of the knee joint.

Patient selection is the same for high tibial valgus osteotomy, with the goal of pain relief and functional improvement in patients who are younger than age 60 with lateral compartment disease and a functional arc of motion of at least 90 degrees and a flexion contracture no greater than 15 degrees. The procedure is contraindicated in patients with inflammatory arthritis, severe tricompartmental disease, subluxation of the tibia on the femur of more than 1 cm, significant ligamentous instability, or joint incongruity.

ARTHRODESIS

Knee arthrodesis is rarely indicated as a primary treatment for the arthritic knee except in young patients, who are heavy laborers, with marked knee ligamentous instability. The recommended position of the knee fusion is 10 to 15 degrees of flexion, 0 to 7 degrees of valgus, and slight external rotation. Arthrodesis is more often indicated as the definitive treatment for patients with recurrent or persistent septic knee arthritis or those who have had a failed knee replacement and are poor candidates for reimplantation because of the lack of an extensor mechanism or sepsis. Some controversy still exists regarding treatment of patients with neuropathic knee joint disease, but these patients have been adequately treated by arthrodesis. The primary indication for knee arthrodesis is pain relief. Patients with a successfully fused limb will have some functional limitations. If the fused limb is made long, patients will have difficulty clearing the fused limb during gait and must circumduct the leg. Patients with a fused limb that is much shorter than the contralateral limb will have a short leg gait unless a shoe lift is used. Patients will also have difficulty getting in and out of automobiles and using public transportation, and must alter their sitting posture so that the fused limb does not project at 90 degrees from the chair.

Fusion rates after failed knee replacements differ based on both the previous knee implant and the arthrodesis technique. Key principles to achieve a successful fusion are to maximize the bone contact areas, to stabilize and compress the bones to be fused, and to preserve the vascularity of the bone and surrounding soft tissues. After a through irrigation and debridement and appropriate antibiotic therapy, knee fusion can be performed even in the presence of active infection by certain bacteria. Fusion rates are much higher for failed resurfacing-type total knee implants (approximately 80 percent fusion rate of failed condylar components) as compared with failed hinged-type total knee implants (approximately 55 percent fusion rate for failed hinged implants) as a result of less initial bone resection. Fusion can be achieved by either internal or external fixation. All internal fixation techniques require a closed wound that has been adequately treated for infection. Of all the internal fixation techniques, intramedullary nail fixation for arthrodesis has had the highest reported fusion rates of up to 85 percent (Fig. 50-4). The advantages

of this method include early ambulation and weight bearing. Disadvantages compared with other methods are longer surgical times; more technically demanding, significant blood loss; and risk of fat embolism. With the use of an intramedullar device, the knee is fused in full extension; this is not a problem, however, because of the limb shortening that occurs and, as a result, circumduction of the limb during gait is avoided. Internal fixation with either a tension-band plate or dual plates can also be used to achieve fusion of the previously infected knee replacement. External fixation can achieve knee fusion in approximately 75 percent of patients. The advantage of this method is that it can be used in patients without a closed wound. Disadvantages include a higher incidence of postoperative complications primarily related to the pin tracts, an increase risk of peroneal nerve palsy, patient dissatisfaction with a bulky external devise, and loss of compression due to pin loosening. With all techniques, knee fusion should occur in 4 to 6 months.

ARTHROPLASTY

UNICOMPARTMENTAL KNEE ARTHROPLASTY

Arthroplasty can be performed to replace only the medial compartment or the lateral compartment (unicompartmental) of the knee in unicompartmental disease. Advantages over total knee arthroplasty are preservation of a greater postoperative knee range of motion, more normal knee kinematics due to retention of the both cruciate ligaments, fewer postoperative complications, possible preservation of tibial bone stock for revision, and a shorter rehabilitation time. Patients indicated for unicompartmental knee arthroplasty should have single-compartment disease and not be candidates for realignment osteotomy; they should be older than age 60, relatively inactive, and thin [weigh less than 80 kg (180 lb)], have a preoperative knee range of motion of at least from 5 to 90 degrees, and have a maximum angle between the anatomic and mechanical axis of no more than 15 degrees of valgus or 10 degrees of varus, both of which can be passively correctable to neutral. The procedure is contraindicated in patients with multicompartmental joint degeneration, fixed deformities, inflammatory arthritis, ligamentous instability, or a flexion arc of less than 90 degrees; and who are young, active, obese, or perform heavy labor. In properly indicated patients, unicompartmental knee arthroplasties have a reported survivorship of 90 percent at 9 years, 85 percent at 10 years, and 82 percent at 11 years, with reported good to excellent results in approximately 90 percent of patients (Fig. 50-5).

Potential complications after unicompartmental knee arthroplasty include infection, implant loosening, and tibial component subsidence. Unicompartmental replacements are also at risk for further joint degenerative in the nonreplaced knee compartments and for patella impingement on the femoral component.

Since the most common complication of unicompartmental arthroplasty is aseptic loosening, meticulous technique with regard to the alignment of the tibial component is essential. The tibial component should be inserted perpendicular to the mechanical axis of the tibia, with the postoperative mechanical axis passing through the center or just medial to the center of the knee. Over-correction of the deformity should be avoided, because this generates greater loosening forces about the implant. Although some centers are still experimenting with uncemented components, cemented femoral and metal-backed polyethylene tibial components have yielded the best clinical results. The use of unicompartmental replacement remains controversial, as many surgeons believe results with total knee components have a more predictable result and a longer survivorship.

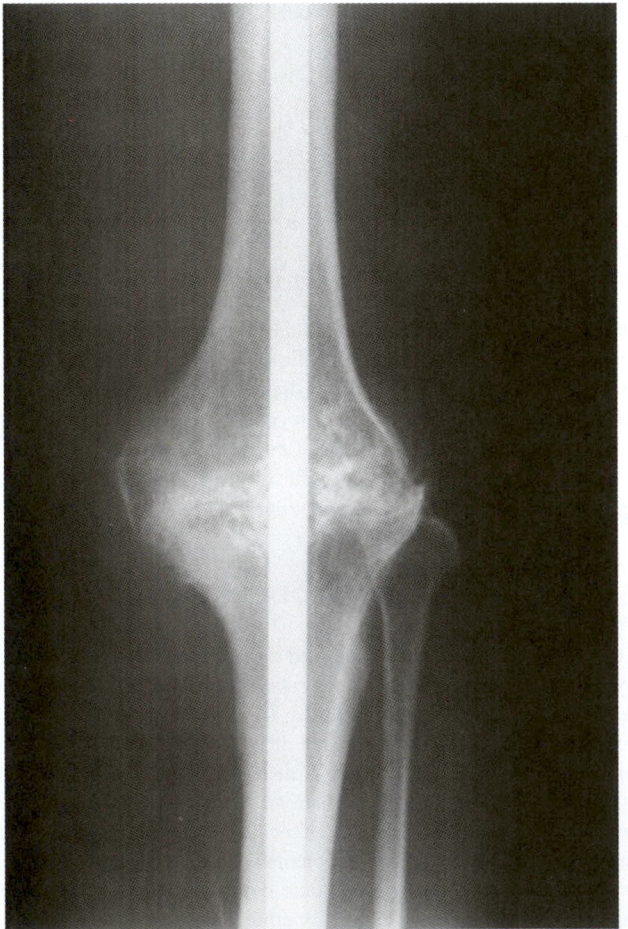

Figure 50-4
Arthrodesis after an infected total knee arthroplasty with loss of extensor mechanism with an intramedullary nail.

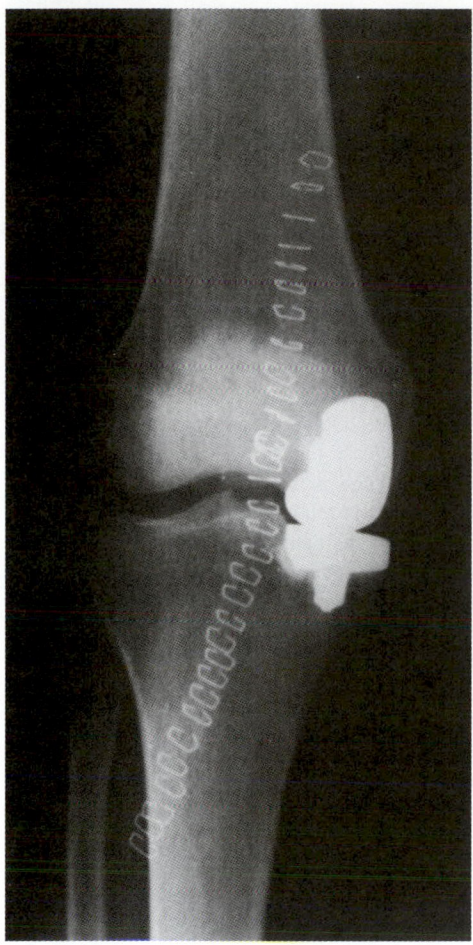

A

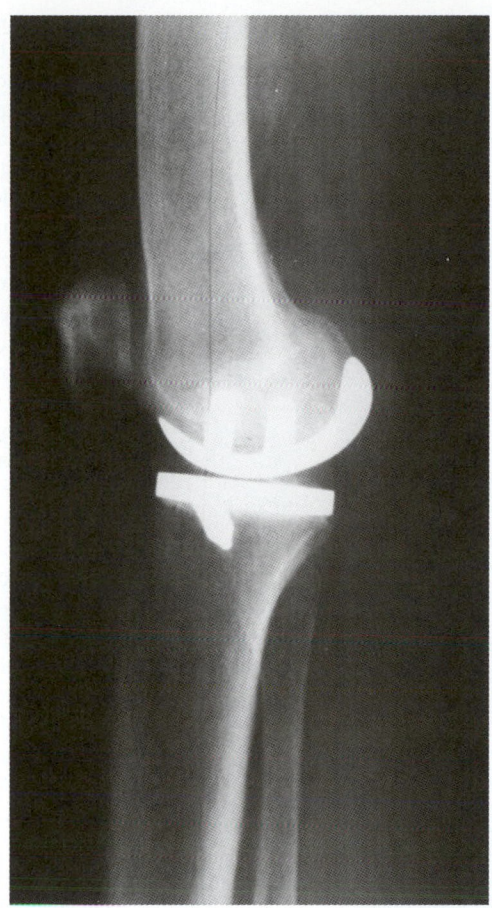

B

Figure 50-5
Unicompartmental arthroplasty radiographs for the treatment of unicompartmental degenerative disease secondary to avascular necrosis: *A,* anteroposterior; *B,* lateral.

TOTAL KNEE ARTHROPLASTY

Total knee arthroplasty is indicated for patients who have disabling knee pain, a functional impairment from knee joint degeneration and radiographs consistent with significant joint degeneration. Patients indicated for knee replacement should have failed a trial of nonoperative treatment and not be more appropriately treated by another surgical procedure, such as realignment osteotomy. The procedure is contraindicated in patients without a functioning extensor mechanism, without neuromuscular control, in those with active sepsis, a well-functioning knee arthrodesis, or a neuropathic joint (controversial). Relative contraindications include patients with significant peripheral vascular disease, those with a history of prior knee sepsis or osteomyelitis, and the nonambulatory. Patients with previous tuberculosis arthritis can undergo a successful total knee implantation if the infection is not active and the patients are administered both preoperative and postoperative chemotherapy. Implant selection to more or less constrained implants should be appropriately chosen based on the patients' deformity and ligamentous stability. Whenever possible, the least-constrained implants should be used, because they should have the best longevity due to the decreased loosening forces.

OPERATIVE CONSIDERATIONS

More complications are related to the surgical wound when knee arthroplasty is performed in patients who have had previous surgery.

The blood supply to the skin in the anterior knee is more tenuous because of the lack of an underlying muscular pedicle. As a result, the surgical incision used to perform knee replacement should incorporate previous incisions and, if possible, the new incision should intersect the prior incision at a 90-degree angle. In cases where a parallel incision is used, a skin bridge of at least 7 cm should be present. For the knees that have not been previously operated on, an anterior midline skin incision is used, followed by an anteromedial capsulotomy and a longitudinal incision in the quadriceps tendon. Some surgeons prefer the subvastus or Southern approach (the vastus medialis is reflected laterally) because this preserves the entire extensor mechanism, allowing for a faster rehabilitation program, and preserves the supreme geniculate arterial blood supply to the patella. Alternatively, an anterolateral capsulotomy also can be used in cases with marked valgus deformity.

The alignment of the implants in the coronal, sagittal, and transverse planes is critical for a long-term successful clinical outcome after knee replacement (Fig. 50-6). Malalignment of the implants with the mechanical axis not passing through the midline of the proximal tibia after arthroplasty has an increased incidence of component loosening. Most surgeons recommend cutting the proximal tibia in 0 to 3 degrees of varus in relation to its longitudinal axis and cutting the distal femur in approximately 7 degrees of valgus in relation to the anatomic axis of the femur for the proper coronal alignment. When properly performed, the mechanical axis should be approximately 0 degrees. Either the distal femur or proximal tibial cuts can be made

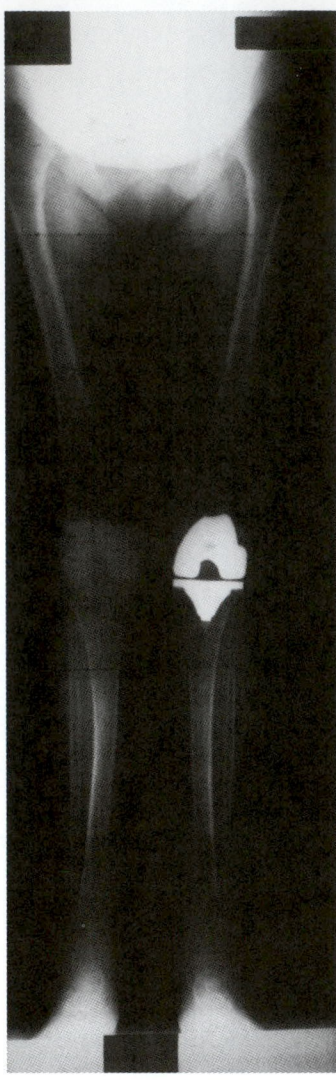

Figure 50-6
Leg length film showing proper alignment after total knee arthroplasty.

with the aid of either extramedullary and intramedullary guides. For the femur, the intramedullary alignment guide is more accurate than the extramedullary alignment guides. The intramedullary alignment guide usually results in a cut to within 1 to 2 degrees of varus or valgus. An extramedullary alignment system may have to be used when the femoral canal is occluded or malaligned. Both intramedullary and extramedullary alignment guides are accurate for aligning the proximal tibial cut. Preoperative full-length tibial radiographs should be obtained prior to use of an intramedullary guide, because marked variations in the tibial bow can result in malalignment.

The posterior slope of the tibial implant and the flexion–extension of the femoral component determines the sagittal (lateral view) alignment. The tibial component should be placed within 3 to 7 degrees of posterior slope. Since the normal tibia has a posterior slope, the sagittal alignment of the tibial component should be perpendicular to the proximal tibia trabeculae and avoid removing excessive anterior tibia, which results in a weaker tibial support. If the femoral component is placed in excessive extension, the anterior femur may be notched. Notching the distal femur has been associated with a greater incidence of late postoperative supracondylar femur fractures. If the

femoral component is placed in excessive flexion, the knee range of motion can be altered with the greatest decrease in knee extension.

The rotational alignment of the tibial and femoral components represents the axial alignment, which is most critical for patella tracking. The tibial component should be slightly externally rotated so that the midpoint of the implant is aligned with the medial third of the tibial tubercle. If the tibial component is internally rotated, the Q angle will be increased from the lateral displacement of the tibial tubercle and will increase patellar instability. The femoral component should be externally rotated 3 to 4 degrees relative to the posterior border of the femoral condyles for best patella tracking and to equalize collateral ligament tension. Like the tibial component, if the femoral component is placed in excessive internal rotation, problems with patella tracking are increased.

The postoperative joint line should be the same as the preoperative joint line in order to decrease loosening forces to the implants and promote patella tracking. This is more important in cases where the posterior cruciate ligament is retained, because a change in the joint line will adversely affect the balance of the posterior cruciate ligament and may impede knee range of motion (Fig. 50-7).

Ligamentous balancing is necessary for proper knee stability. Both medial and lateral collateral ligaments should have equal tension throughout the entire range of knee motion. To achieve collateral ligament balancing, after the bony cuts are made, trial total knee components in place or trial blocks should be used to ensure that the flexion and extension gaps are equal (Fig. 50-8). If the knee is not balanced, then ligamentous release on the narrower or tighter side needs to be performed. When the posterior cruciate ligament is retained, this must be balanced as well. To balance the flexion–extension gap during surgery, further bony resections may be needed. A knee has an increased flexion gap if it is loose in flexion and lacks full extension. An increased flexion gap is easily corrected by removing more distal femur. A knee has an increased extension gap if it is loose in extension and lacks flexion. An increased extension gap is rarer but can be corrected most often by increasing the posterior slope of the tibial resection or by shifting the femoral component more anteriorly, thereby removing more of the posterior femoral condyle. If the knee is tight in both flexion and extension then the tibial bone cut has usually not been sufficient and can be corrected by removing more proximal tibia. In general, approximately 10 mm of proximal tibia and 6 to 8 mm of distal femur are removed, depending on the components used.

The patella should also be resurfaced by either recessed or resurfacing components. The patella thickness should be restored with the patella component. Most patella components are 10 mm thick and therefore require the same amount of patella bone resection. If the patella is too thin (i.e., resection leaving less than 10 mm of patella bone), then either the patella should not be resurfaced or less bone resected, because of the increased risk of spontaneous patella fracture. Metal-backed patella components are rarely used, because they have been associated with wear through the polyethylene and metal-on-metal abrasive wear. The patella should track in the femoral trochlear groove without subluxation. If the patella does not track well, then a lateral retinacular release, usually performed from inside the knee joint, needs to be performed. If a lateral transecting retinacular release is performed, an attempt should be made to avoid the superolateral geniculate artery. If a tourniquet is used, it should be released prior to closure to ensure that, if the vessel is transected, it is ligated; if ignored, a large postoperative hemarthrosis can occur.

There are many different designs of total knee components. Implants can be classified based on the amount of constraint and

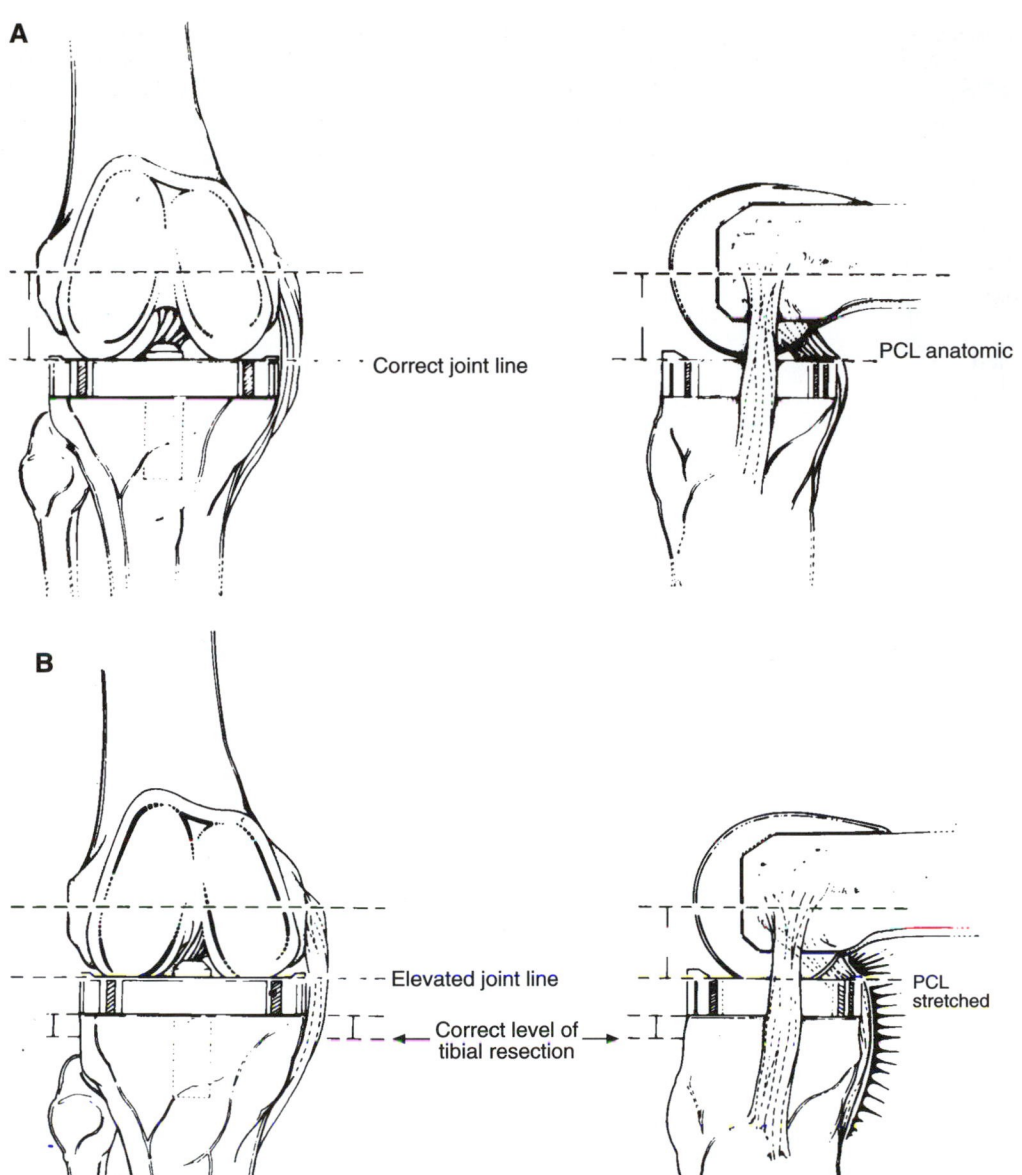

A

Correct joint line

PCL anatomic

B

Elevated joint line

Correct level of tibial resection

PCL stretched

Figure 50-7
The correct tibial cut should be made to maintain an anatomic joint line (*A*). In cases where the joint line is elevated (*B*) and the posterior cruciate ligament is retained, a poor clinical result may occur as a result of stiffness and pain. (Reproduced by permission from Dorr LD, Boiardo RA: Technical considerations in total knee arthroplasty. *Clin Orthop* 1986; 205:9.)

whether the posterior cruciate ligament is retained or sacrificed and whether the posterior cruciate ligament is substituted (Fig. 50-9). Conforming total knee components are most often used. Hinge or linked implants are the most constrained and should be used only in patients with gross ligamentous instability. Fully constrained implants have been associated with high rates of tibial loosening, increased wear, and high infection rates. Some implant designs, which are rarely used, retain both cruciate ligaments, but they are more technically difficult to insert and to achieve ligamentous balance. Conforming total knee components typically have a condylar femoral component made of cobalt–chrome alloy and either all-polyethylene or metal-backed tibial components. These implants all sacrifice the anterior cruciate ligament. In some designs, the implants also sacrifice the posterior cruciate ligament. If the posterior cruciate ligament is sacrificed, some designs substitute for that ligament and are referred to as posterior stabilized.

Cemented total knees, including the femoral, tibial, and patellar components, have yielded the best long-term clinical results. Implant longevity with cemented components depends on final limb alignment, maximal coverage of the cut surface of the proximal tibia, and implant design. Survivorship analysis of cemented total condylar design total knee arthroplasty (all-polyethylene tibial component) has revealed a 15-year survival rate of over 90 percent. Another survivorship study on varied cemented component designs revealed a 5-year survival rate of 98 percent and a 10-year survival rate of 91 percent. Cementless components for total knee were introduced for the theoretical advantages of avoiding cement as a potential source of particulate debris, for use in younger patients where biologic fixation could increase longevity, and for avoiding the heat-induced bone necrosis that occurs with cement. Clinical trials with cementless total knee components, however, have failed to show any improvements over cemented total knee components. Clinical trials have revealed

Flexion gap

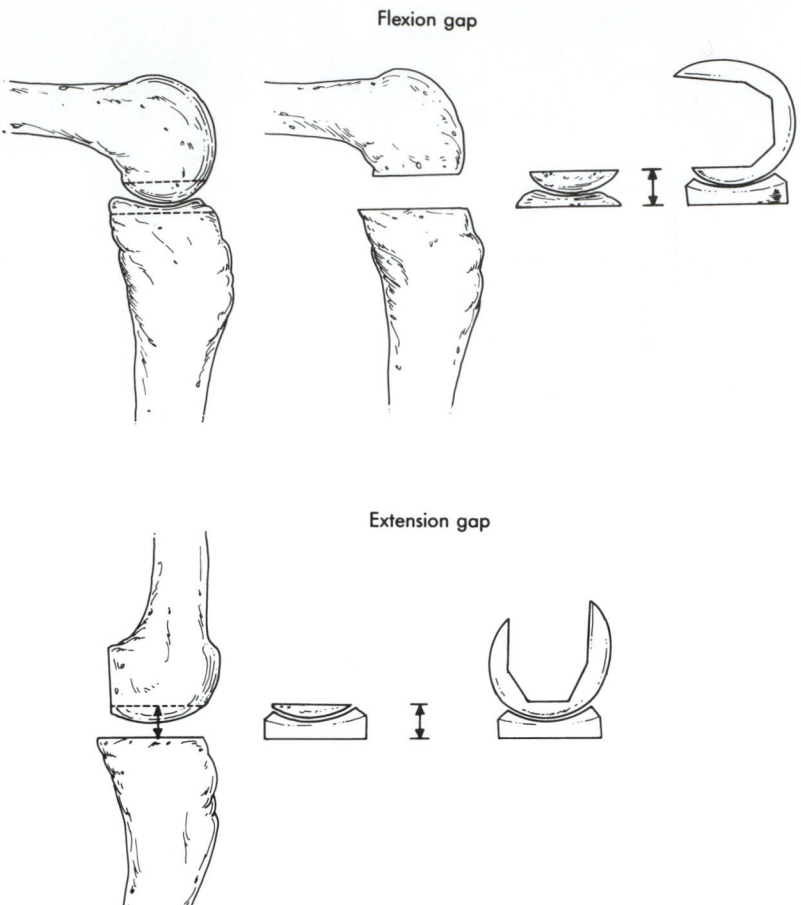

Extension gap

Figure 50-8
Bony resection should be made so that the resultant flexion and extension gaps are equal and, when resurfaced, restore the joint line to the anatomic position. (Reproduced by permission from Krackow RA: Intraoperative alignment and instrumentation, in: *The Technique of Total Knee Arthroplasty*. St. Louis: CV Mosby; 1990:141.)

decreased longevity of the implants, poorer clinical outcomes, increased frequency of metal fatigue, increased problems with the patella component, implant migration and subsidence, and inadequate biologic fixation (primarily on the tibia). As a result of these poorer results, most surgeons use total knee designs with cement because of superior clinical results and decreased cost. Proponents of cementless fixation are still experimenting with alternate designs that may limit micromotion in order to improve biologic fixation and to avoid stress shielding the proximal tibia that can occur with ingrowth stems, keel, or pegs. Various designs using either a keel, 6.5-mm cancellous screws, stems, or the addition of bone paste to improve the immediate fixation of the tibial component and enable biologic fixation are currently under investigation. Hybrid total knee arthroplasty (cemented tibial component and cementless femoral component) has been advocated to avoid problems of the cementless tibial components. The results of clinical trials have been reported to be good or excellent in over 90 percent of patients at up to 7 years postoperatively. No long-term data are available on hybrid total knees, but current concerns over the increased cost of uncemented implants without documented proof of improved clinical outcomes may limit their use.

The theoretical advantages of retaining the posterior cruciate ligament are more normal knee kinematics (with axial tibial rotation and roll-back of the femur on the tibia) and retention of the ligament's proprioception. Disadvantages of retaining the posterior cruciate ligament include more intraoperative difficulty in balancing the knee ligaments and the necessity to reproduce the preoperative joint line. If the joint line is raised, then the posterior cruciate ligament will function to increase joint reactive forces, and alter the knee kinematics, and may result in increased polyethylene wear and poorer knee motion. Knee replacement designs that sacrifice and substitute for the posterior cruciate ligament typically have a central polyethylene post (which may be supported by an intrapost metallic peg) on the tibial component. The post then fits centrally within a femoral component in which a central box has been created. The post within the box functions as a cam during knee movements. Total knee arthroplasty after previous patellectomy should have a posterior stabilized prosthesis because it aids in anterior–posterior knee stability and patients have more predictable pain relief and improved function than those in which the posterior cruciate ligament is retained.

Clinical results of well-performed total knee replacements using either posterior cruciate ligament-sacrificing implants (with or without substitution) or posterior cruciate ligament-retained implants have only shown a difference in gait. Gait analysis has demonstrated that patients with total knee replacement without a posterior cruciate ligament will shift their weight farther forward during stair climbing as a result of the lack of femoral roll-back. There has not been shown to be any difference in patients with either type of implants during

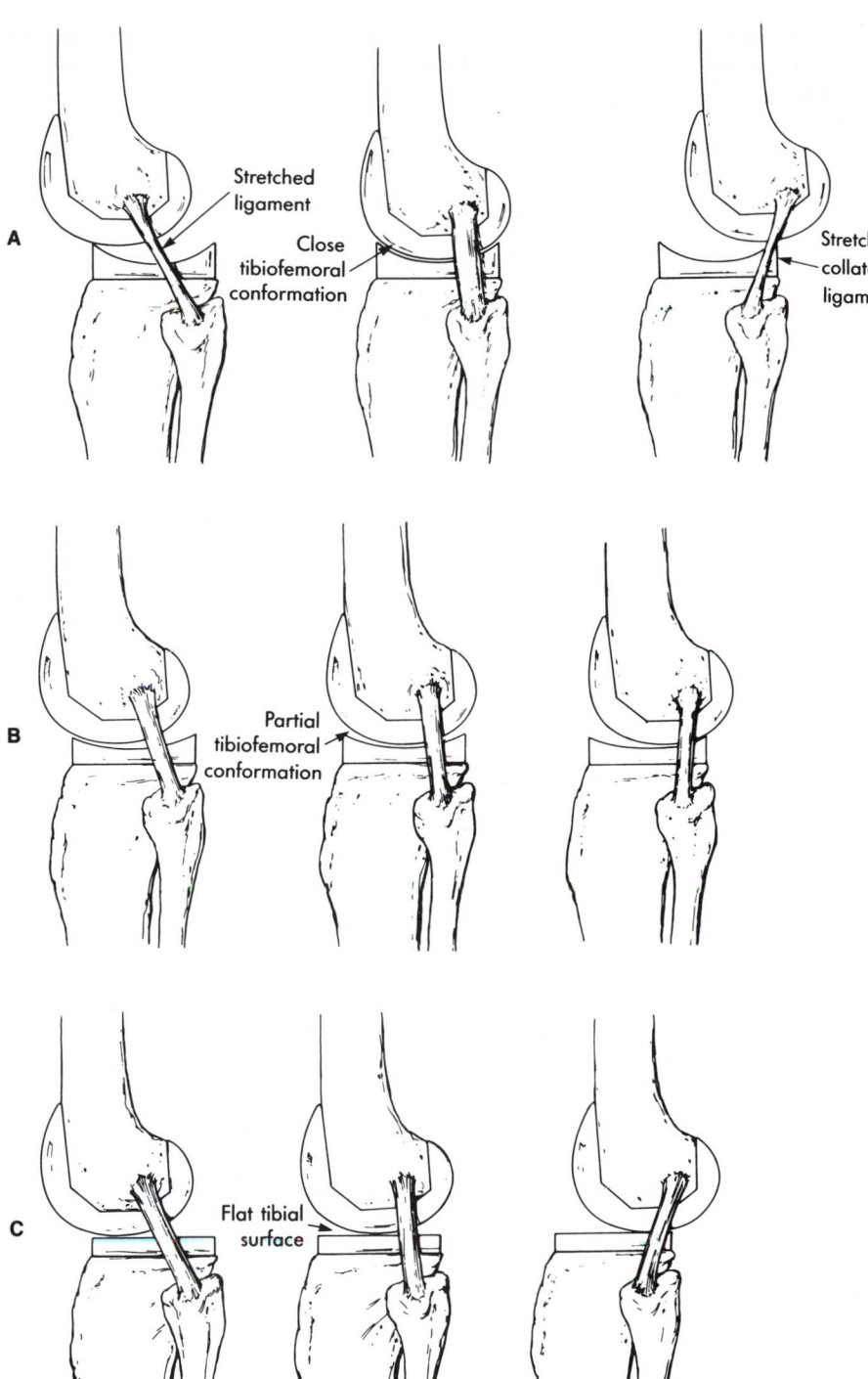

Stretched ligament

Close tibiofemoral conformation

Stretched collateral ligament

A

Partial tibiofemoral conformation

B

Flat tibial surface

C

Figure 50-9
Representation of various tibial tray conformations: complete tibiofemoral conformation (*A*), partial tibiofemoral conformation *(B)*, and a flat tibial surface (*C*). Most implant designs that retain the posterior cruciate ligament have a flat tibial surface to enable axial tibial rotation and femoral rollback. (Reproduced by permission from Krackow RA: Prosthesis selection, in: *The Technique of Total Knee Arthroplasty*. St. Louis: CV Mosby; 1990:59.)

gait on level surfaces. All types of implants that retain, sacrifice, or substitute the posterior cruciate ligament have been reported to achieve excellent results. Clinical results of posterior cruciate ligament-sacrificing total condylar arthroplasty (all-polyethylene tibial components) have been reported to be 88 percent good to excellent after 10 to 12 years, but more than 50 percent of cases had radiolucent lines at the tibial bone–cement interface. As a result, the material of the tibial components was changed to use a metal-backed tibial component. When a posterior cruciate ligament–sacrificing total condylar arthroplasty with a metal-backed tibial component was used, survivorship increased to 96 percent at 11 years after surgery. Clinical series of patients with posterior cruciate ligament-substituting implants also report good to excellent results in 83 percent of patients at up to 8 years postoperatively. Clinical series with posterior cruciate-preserving implants have reported 88 percent good to excellent clinical results with a 3 percent revision rate after 5 to 9 years.

Total knee implants have also shown catastrophic wear of the polyethylene inserts. Catastrophic wear has most often resulted from component malalignment, component design flaws, thin polyethylene, and the material properties of the polyethylene. In the case of malaligned components, increased point loading on the margins of the polyethylene can result in asymmetric wear. Flat or unconstrained tibial polyethylene trays have decreased areas of femoral–tibial component contact and therefore have higher point loading to the components.

Metal backing of the tibial component was introduced for many reasons. These components allowed for the introduction of uncemented tibial designs, increased ease at ligament balancing intraoperatively, decreased polyethylene deformation and wear, and the more even distribution of forces at both the implant–cement and the implant–bone interfaces. Metal-backed tibial components have been shown to have improved survivorship as compared with all-polyethylene tibial components. The main disadvantage of metal-backed tibial components is that they often use a thinner polyethylene insert. Based on finite element analysis, only in cases where the polyethylene was less that 6 mm did the contact stresses on the insert exceed the yield strength of the polyethylene. The potential concern of backside wear (wear between the polyethylene and the metal backing) is a complication that has been more of a concern in modular metal-backed acetabular components. Although of great interest, newer fabrication processes to improve the wear characteristics of the polyethylene have failed to demonstrate improved clinical outcomes. Neither heat pressing nor carbon fiber reinforcement of polyethylene has done well clinically, and both have been shown to have increased wear.

Many factors influence the final range of knee motion after total knee arthroplasty. Most patients should achieve approximately 0 to 110 degree final range of motion independent of the total knee design. Most patients will regain their preoperative motion arc, albeit in an improved functional arc. Long-term studies have shown that postoperative flexion contracture of up to 30 degrees will correct by 2 years with physical therapy. The results of the use of continuous passive motion (CPM) on outcomes after total knee arthroplasty continue to be conflicting. Advocates of CPM report improved early range of motion, decreased incidence of deep vein thrombosis, pulmonary embolus, faster pain relief, and briefer hospitalization. There have also been reports, however, of an increased incidence of wound complications and no long-term benefit to the use of CPM. The use of CPM may decrease, given the current trend toward a shortened hospital stay after surgery and cost containment. If CPM is used, it is recommended that a rate of 1 cycle/min with 40 degree maximum flexion be used for the first 3 days to avoid wound problems. Poor knee flexion of less than 90 degrees for up to 6 weeks afterward may be improved by operative manipulation.

No long-term results of total knee arthroplasty performed on young patients have been reported. One would predict that, like patients with total hip arthroplasty, these young patients are at increased risk of early arthroplasty failure. Studies on total knee replacement in young rheumatoid arthritis patients have reported clinical results that are relatively similar to those in older osteoarthritic patients in midterm follow-up. One report comparing cemented total knee arthroplasty in osteoarthritic patients younger than age 55 with patients with rheumatoid arthritis and older osteoarthritic patients has shown similar radiographic and clinical outcomes at 6-year follow-up.

Patients weighing more than 150 percent of ideal body weight are considered obese and thus are at increased risk for complications during total knee arthroplasty, although 2- to 6-year follow-up shows similar clinical results. Obese patients have a higher incidence of patella complications, most likely caused by increased joint reactive forces at the patellofemoral articulation. Obese patients do not have a higher rate of other postoperative complications such as deep vein thrombosis, knee hematoma, prolonged rehabilitation, or delayed wound healing. The long-term results of total knee arthroplasty in obese patients have not been reported, but concerns exist because of the increased incidence of radiolucent lines at the bone–cement interface under the tibial component.

Patients with diabetes mellitus have an increased incidence of wound problems, an increased rate of infection (up to 7 percent), an increased revision rate, and an increased mortality rate. Rates of deep vein thrombosis are similar for diabetic and nondiabetic patients.

Paget's disease of the tibia or femur can present with tibial or femoral deformity, thereby predisposing the knee to joint degeneration. Despite the radiographic changes consistent with knee arthritis, the etiology of the symptoms should be confirmed by either pain relief after an intraarticular local anesthetic injection or pain relief after systemic pharmacologic therapy. At 7-year follow-up, patients with Paget's disease who are treated with cemented total knee arthroplasties had clinical and radiographic results similar to those of total knee arthroplasties in patients without Paget's disease. During total knee arthroplasty, surgeons may need to use extramedullary cutting guides if technical difficulties arise due to bowing of either the tibia or the femur because of the underlying bone disease.

Because of recurrent hemarthrosis, hemophilic patients have an increased risk of knee joint degeneration and, when undergoing total knee replacement, are at increased risk for complications. Complication rates of over 50 percent have been reported primarily because of an increased risk of nerve palsies, postoperative bleeding, and infection. To reduce complications, the intraoperative factor VIII level should be maintained at 100 percent instead of the previously recommended 80 percent and then slowly tapered postoperatively. To decrease the risk of future bleeding, a complete synovectomy should also be performed at knee replacement. Clinical follow-up has reported good clinical results at a mean of 5 years; however, there are bone–cement radiolucent lines at the tibial component in approximately 75 percent of patients, thereby raising concerns about long-term clinical outcomes.

Complications of total knee arthroplasty can have devastating clinical outcomes. Approximately 1 percent of cases become infected. Patients with rheumatoid arthritis, ipsilateral skin ulcers, or prior knee surgery are all at increased risk for infection. Although they appear to be associated with joint infections, obesity, urinary tract infections, and oral steroids have not been proven to increase the infection risk. Preoperative antibiotics and either room or surgeon air-flow systems have been demonstrated to decrease the infection rate significantly. Preoperative intravenous antibiotics should be administered 5 min before the tourniquet is inflated. Controversy still exists regarding the use of antibiotic-impregnated cement. Some studies have shown a reduced infection rate in both primary and revision knee arthroplasties with the use of antibiotic cement. Long-term concerns, however, persist because gentamicin released from the antibiotic-impregnated cement may affect the local bone metabolism, increasing the rate of implant loosening, and long-term low-dose exposure may predispose the patient to antibiotic-resistant bacterial strains.

An infected total knee arthroplasty should be suspected in any postoperative patient with persistent knee pain and effusion. This is more readily diagnosed if there is early implant loosening, joint inflammation, drainage, and sepsis.

Patients often will present with an elevated serum white blood cell count, a positive C-reactive protein, and/or an elevated sedimentation rate. However, the high false-negative rates of the results of these tests make a negative test result inconclusive. White blood cells labeled with indium followed by nucleotide scanning have been reported to predict infection about total joint implants in approximately 80 percent of infected cases. However, more recent studies demonstrate indium scans to have a lower positive predictive value and sensitivity, thereby making the scan alone unreliable for predicting infection. Although aspiration and culture is still the "gold standard" in predicting infection about total knee implants, the aspiration and culture will be negative in approximately 25 percent of infected cases, so it is still paramount to obtain operative cultures.

Treatment options for an infected total knee prosthesis are antibiotic suppression, irrigation and debridement with retention of the implants, irrigation and debridement with removal of the implants and cement and possible placement of antibiotic spacer, or above-knee amputation. Antibiotic suppression is indicated for patients who are not medically cleared for another surgical procedure, have well-fixed components, and are infected with a bacteria of low virulence that is sensitive to oral antibiotics. Antibiotic suppression with oral antibiotics must be continued indefinitely and will not cure the infection. For acute total joint infections that have been present for less than 4 weeks in otherwise healthy patients without a sinus track, debridement and retention of well-fixed components can be performed in cases with antibiotic-sensitive gram-positive organisms. Surgical debridement must be thorough, with removal of the modular polyethylene tibial tray and a complete synovectomy prior to replacement of a new polyethylene tray. If, after multiple debridements, the operative cultures are still positive, then all of the components and cement need to be removed. The best method for curing an infected knee remains irrigation and debridement, and removal of the components and cement, with a 4- to 6-week course of intravenous antibiotics (bactericidal titer of 1:8). Multiple debridements may needed, and the surgical wound should be closed over silicone-based suction drains.

To facilitate future reimplantation of a total knee arthroplasty and to increase the local level of antibiotics, an antibiotic-impregnated methylmethacrylate spacer block can be used. Typically, because of its thermal stability, lack of allergic response, and wide bacterial coverage, tobramycin is mixed in powder form with Palicos-brand methylmethacrylate. Second-stage treatments after the infection has been considered adequately treated include resection arthroplasty, reimplantation, or arthrodesis. Resection arthroplasty is rarely indicated, because it is reserved for debilitated patients with limited rehabilitation potential who will probably not become ambulators. Functional results after resection arthroplasty are generally poor, and most patients will require a cast or a brace about the knee for stability. Second-stage reimplantation of a total knee is the treatment of choice for most patients who are in good health and have an antibiotic-sensitive infecting organism (either gram-positive or gram-negative), a healed wound, and an intact extensor mechanism. The previous infection must be cured prior to reimplantation. During reimplantation, surgical technical difficulties encountered include difficulties in exposure, bone defects, and ligament instability. The length of antibiotic treatment after second-stage reimplantation has varied, but if the operative cultures are negative, then the antibiotics can be discontinued.

When properly performed, the two-stage reimplantation treatment of an infected total knee will be successful in up to 95 percent of patients. These patients, however, have a poorer clinical result, with only approximately 65 percent having good to excellent clinical results at a mean follow-up of 4 years. For cases of continued sepsis about an infected total knee despite other measures to cure the infection, in nonambulatory patients and in those patients who are medically ill and cannot undergo further attempts at reconstruction, above-knee amputation is the salvage treatment of choice.

Deep venous thrombosis after total knee arthroplasty has been reported to occur in more than 50 percent of patients, mostly in the calf of the operative leg. Deep venous thrombosis in the contralateral leg is less common, occurring in approximately 3 percent of patients. Most deep venous thromboses are asymptomatic and are not treated with anticoagulation therapy. Pulmonary embolism is also common and asymptomatic in approximately 15 percent of patients. Symptomatic pulmonary embolism occurs in approximately 0.5 to 3 percent of patients and is fatal in 3 per 1000 patients. Prophylactic measures (mechanical or pharmacologic) should be used in all patients to decrease the rate of these complications. Mechanical measures for prophylaxes include intermittent pneumatic compression devices, compressive thigh-high stockings, and CPM. The use of an operative tourniquet has not been shown to increase the incidence of deep venous thrombosis. Prophylactic pharmacologic drugs commonly used include warfarin, low-dose heparin, aspirin, dextran, low molecular weight heparin, and antithrombin III. The combination of mechanical (sequential pneumatic compression devices) and pharmacologic (warfarin or low molecular weight heparin) prophylactic measures may be the most effective.

Vascular injury is rare (fewer than 5 cases per 10,000) during total knee arthroplasty. Arterial injuries include thrombosis, traumatic aneurysm, and transection of either the femoral or the popliteal arteries. If an arterial injury occurs, but is not recognized and treated immediately, subsequent limb ischemia can result in the need for limb amputation. Arterial injuries can be caused by the tourniquet on atherosclerotic vessels and therefore should not be used in patients with either documented atherosclerotic disease, radiographic arterial calcification, or absent pedal pulses.

Nerve injury occurs in fewer than 3 cases per 100. Most frequently, the peroneal nerve is injured in patients who have a combination of a flexion and valgus deformity. Most often, the nerve is injured by traction or compression either intraoperatively or postoperatively caused by the dressing or a hematoma. If a peroneal nerve palsy occurs, the patient's knee should be immediately flexed and all compressive dressings removed. Most patients with a peroneal nerve palsy will have at least a partial return of function, and slightly more than half will have complete return. Probability of recovery is also related to the degree of the nerve palsy. Approximately 80 percent of patients with only a partial nerve palsy recover completely, whereas approximately 35 percent of patients with a complete nerve palsy recover complete nerve function.

Most patients will lose approximately 2 units of blood (between 1000 and 1500 ml) from total knee arthroplasty surgery. Plugging the femoral canal after the use of an intramedullary guide significantly decreases the post-operative blood loss. The use of either cement fixation, CPM, a tourniquet, or intraoperative hemostasis prior to closure has not been statistically shown to decrease total blood loss.

Periprosthetic fractures after total knee arthroplasty (usually in the femur) occur in approximately 1 case in 100. Most patients have a factor predisposing to fracture, such as anterior femoral notching, osteoporosis, or distal femoral bone loss and, as a result, fractures occur with minimal trauma. The goals in treating these fractures are to unite the fracture and to maintain limb alignment and knee motion. Revision knee arthroplasty with long-stem components at the time of fracture treatment should be performed only in cases where the components are loose. Fractures can be treated by either closed or open reduction with either locked femoral or supracondylar nails, plates (condylar, blade, or dynamic condylar), and/or cerclage cables. In some cases, fractures can be managed closed in a cast or brace, but this is often accompanied by loss of knee motion and malalignment.

Fat embolism occurs in approximately 3 cases in 100 during or after total knee replacement surgery. The intraoperative use of either components with intramedullary stems or intramedullary alignment guides increases the risk for fat embolism. Bilateral one-stage total knee arthroplasty also increases the risk of fat embolism. Patients with fat embolism will have either pulmonary or neurologic symptoms and, when diagnosed, are treated by respiratory support.

Problems with wound healing after total knee arthroplasty are increased in patients with a poor nutritional status [low white blood cell count (less than 1500 cells/mm^3) and low albumin level (less than 3.5 g/dL)], previous knee surgery, rheumatoid arthritis, or diabetes mellitus. Postoperative wound hematoma or persistent wound drainage also increases the risk of infection. Controversy still remains regarding the routine use of drains. In prospective randomized studies, no significant differences were noted between those cases that were or were not drained during single-stage bilateral total knee arthroplasty. Drains left in place for more than 48 h are associated with an increased the risk of infection. If drains are used, they should always be removed before 48 h, irrespective of the drain output. If an area of skin necrosis occurs, immediate irrigation and debridement should be followed by a local soft-tissue flap (usually the medial or the lateral head of the gastrocnemius) and skin grafting to achieve a closed wound.

The most common complications following total knee arthroplasty are related to the patella. Patella problems occur in up to 10 percent of cases and account for approximately 50 percent of all complications following total knee arthroplasty. Patella complications include problems with the actual component, the patellofemoral joint, and patella tracking. Component problems include the failure of metal-backed implants and implant loosening. Patellofemoral problems include patella instability, patella fracture, osteonecrosis of the patella, and disruption of the knee extensor mechanism.

Because of the high incidence of patella problems, some surgeons continue to not resurface the patella. Problems with the unresurfaced patella have been reported to occur in as many as 25 percent of patients. Most surgeons would agree that the patella should be resurfaced in all patients with inflammatory arthritis or in any patient with marked degenerative disease in the patella. If the patella is to be resurfaced, it should be done with an all-polyethylene component. High failure rates of the metal-backed patellar components have been reported for most of this type of design, due to either wear through the polyethylene, dissociation of the polyethylene from the metal, material failure at the metal peg–plate junction, or a lack of biologic fixation into the porous surface. Patients with a failed metal-backed patella usually have anterior knee pain, swelling, knee effusion, and crepitus. Radiographs with patella (sunrise or merchant) views will often confirm the implant failure by showing either contact between the metal-backing of the patella component with the femoral component, metallic debris about the knee, or dissociation of the polyethylene with migration to the suprapatellar pouch. If radiographs are not confirmatory, either knee aspiration demonstrating metallic debris or arthroscopic examination of the knee demonstrating fragmented, delaminated, or dissociated polyethylene can confirm the diagnosis. The appropriate treatment of the failed metal-backed patella implant is for revision to an all-polyethylene component, synovectomy, and possible revision of the femoral component if significant metal burnishing or scratching has occurred.

The design of cemented all-polyethylene patella components is important for proper patella function. Most designs differ with regard to polyethylene thickness and conformity within the patellofemoral joint. All polyethylene patella components can be either dome shaped or asymmetric in design and can either be used to resurface or be inset within the patella. The corresponding trochlear groove on the femur can be either flat (unconstrained) or deep (constrained) and can be either symmetric or asymmetric. Unconstrained patella–femoral articulations have significantly lower forces and therefore less poly-

ethylene wear than more constrained articulations. Also, more constrained patellofemoral articulations may also inhibit patellar rotation and may predispose the implant to loosening. At 4-year follow-up, inset patella components appear to be function better than those that have been resurfaced.

Later problems with the patellofemoral joint can often be avoided by proper surgical technique and implant positioning. Preoperative valgus deformity is more often associated with patellofemoral tracking problems due to contracted lateral retinacular structures that need to be balanced by lateral retinacular release. Both the femoral and the tibial components should be placed at neutral to slight external rotation to facilitate patella tracking. The femoral component should also be placed as far lateral as possible to facilitate patella tracking. The resultant thickness of the patella implant and host bone should match the preoperative patella thickness. Minimal patella thickness prior to insertion of the patella component should be no thinner than 12 mm, because this predisposes the patella to fracture. Prior to surgical closure, proper patellar tracking must be evaluated and adjusted intraoperatively. Generally, either removal of patellar osteophytes, lateral retinacular release, and/or medial retinacular reefing will result in proper patella tracking as long as the femoral and tibial components are not malrotated. During lateral retinacular release, care should be taken to try to preserve the lateral geniculate vessels, because this may decrease the risk of patella osteonecrosis. In cases with patellar instability, treatment should be directed at its cause. If the femoral or tibial components are malrotated or malaligned, then they may also need to be revised. If the femoral and tibial components are correctly aligned, then a lateral retinacular release combined with medial retinacular reefing may be sufficient to correct the instability. In rarer cases, a distal realignment osteotomy of the tibial tubercle with medial translation may be needed.

Treatments for the failed patella component are either revision, removal of the implant rather than resurfacing, or patellectomy. In most cases, as long as adequate host bone is present, the treatment of choice will be revision. If insufficient host bone is present or the patella cannot be resurfaced for other reasons, then the patella should be left unresurfaced after removal of all polyethylene and cement. Patellectomy should rarely be performed, but can be considered if a posterior stabilized total knee implant is in place. In all cases, proper patella tracking should be present. If the patella is not resurfaced or if patellectomy is performed, then weakness of the knee extensor mechanism and a possible extensor lag can be anticipated.

Arthroscopic treatment of the symptomatic total knee arthroplasty is most commonly performed for patella clunk or tethered patella syndrome (Fig. 50-10), a condition that develops when a fibrous nodule forms at the junction between the posterior aspect of the quadriceps tendon and the proximal pole of the patella. With the knee in flexion, the nodule becomes impinged below the anterior flange of the femoral component in the intercondylar notch and, as the knee is extended, the nodule becomes entrapped and is finally released at about 30 to 45 degrees of full extension, causing the nodule to clunk out of the intercondylar notch. Several other complications after total knee arthroplasty can be successfully treated by arthroscopy. Patients with persistent synovitis can be treated by arthroscopic synovectomy. Other indications for arthroscopy of total knee replacements include removal of loose bodies, resection of a symptomatic pseudomeniscus, resection of scar tissue in patients with arthrofibrosis, lateral retinacular release for patella maltracting, and for the diagnosis of symptomatic arthroplasties with an unknown etiology.

Treatment of periprosthetic patellar fracture depends on the amount of displacement of the fragments and whether the patella component has been loosened. Fractures that are nondisplaced or minimally displaced with a patellar component that is not loose can be treated with

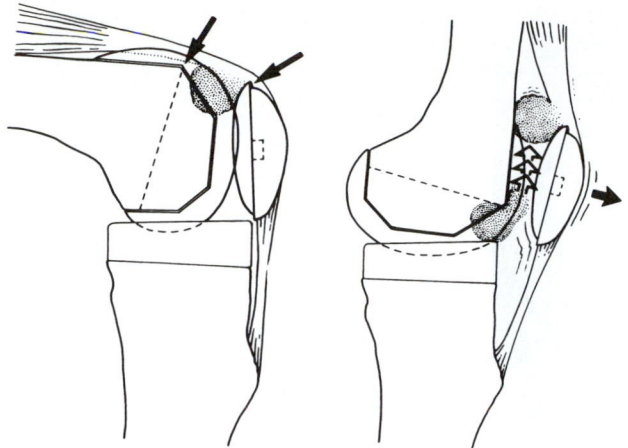

Figure 50-10
Patella "clunk" syndrome occurs when the patella catches during knee extension and tracks roughly. Patients usually have an excellent amount of flexion, and a posterior stabilized implant femoral design. This can be effectively managed with arthroscopic debridement of the scar tissue. (Reproduced by permission from Hozack WJ, Rothman RH, Booth RE Jr, et al: Patellar clunk syndrome. *Clin Orthop* 1989; 241:206–207.)

cast or knee immobilization for approximately 6 weeks. Patella fracture fragments that are significantly displaced with a marked extensor lag in which the patella component is still well fixed can be treated by a combination of open reduction and internal fixation of the patella with repair of the knee retinaculum. Following repair, controlled range of motion and immobilization during ambulation should be performed for approximately 6 weeks or until fracture union has occurred. If the patella component has become loose after the patella fractures, then the patella implant and cement often must be removed. In rare cases of marked comminution, a partial or total patellectomy with repair of the extensor mechanism can be performed.

Avulsion of the patellar tendon can occur either intraoperatively or postoperatively. During surgery, the insertion of the patella tendon may be partially or completely avulsed during knee flexion and must always be guarded against. Patients who have had previous knee surgery or a high tibial osteotomy or are having revision surgery are at increased risk for patella tendon avulsion. In cases where the insertion of the patella tendon is under high stress and at risk of avulsion, intraoperative measures such as a more complete soft tissue release from the proximal tibia, a V–Y quadricepsplasty, or a tibial tubercle osteotomy should be performed to improve exposure and prevent avulsion. Recommended treatment of a patellar tendon avulsion is primary repair with protection of the repair by a cerclage wire from the tibial tubercle to the patella. In cases of primary repair failure, reconstruction of the extensor mechanism with allograft (tibial tubercle–patella tendon–patella–quadriceps tendon) has been used successfully as a salvage in some cases. In extreme cases in which the extensor mechanism cannot be repaired, knee fusion may be the last resort. Rupture of the quadriceps tendon and loss of knee extension occurs much more rarely. Quadriceps tendon rupture is more easily treated by healthy viable soft tissue repair after the scarred tissue has been resected.

REVISION TOTAL KNEE ARTHROPLASTY

The basic principals in revision total knee arthroplasty are the same as for primary knee arthroplasty. However, many more technical prob-

lems are encountered, such as removal of components and then reconstruction, with either severe osseous or soft tissue deficiencies. Before performing revision knee arthroplasty, preoperative planning is essential to choose implants properly and to restore the knee joint line to its proper position. A thorough physical examination is needed to assess the knee ligaments and preoperative planning of the surgical incision is needed, based on the location of previous incisions. Infection workup should be performed prior to surgery, and intraoperative cultures and possible frozen-section analysis performed prior to receiving perioperative antibiotics. Because of scar tissue and contractures from previous surgery, the operative exposure may be more difficult. More extensive medial and posterior tibial soft tissue dissections often are necessary, and either a V–Y quadriceps tendon incision or a tibial tubercle osteotomy occasionally may be necessary to improve exposure and so as not to avulse the patella tendon. Revision total knee systems often can increase constraint to compensate for soft tissue imbalance and can have either wedges or blocks with or without intramedullary stems to compensate for bony defects. In cases of severe ligamentous instability, hinged total knee design components can be used. Because of the marked constraint of hinged total knee components, they have a higher loosening rate and infection rate (approximately 5 percent or higher) than primary knee arthroplasty. Results of revision knee arthroplasty are not as good as with primary knee arthroplasty, because of the increased risk of infection, difficulties in compensating for soft tissue and bony deficiencies, increased rate of wound complications, higher incidence of deep venous thrombosis, increased problems with patella tracking, and increased rate of pulmonary embolism. Most studies comparing the short-term to midterm clinical results of primary to revision knee arthroplasties report approximately 10 to 20 percent more good or excellent results in the primary group. Revised total knees also had a higher reoperation rate and an increased incidence of radiolucent lines at the bone–cement and implant–cement interfaces.

The management of bony defects during either primary or revision total knee surgery depends on the location, depth, and containment of the defect by host bone (Fig. 50-11). Typically, patients with a varus deformity will have an uncontained bony defect on the posteromedial proximal tibia. Patients with a valgus deformity often have a contained defect in the posterolateral proximal tibia and bone loss of the distal lateral femoral condyle. Central contained defects in either the femur or the tibia are usually encountered after removal of primary knee components or are the end result of component subsidence. Because it is difficult to determine the exact extent of these bony defects, surgeons should be prepared to address each one during surgery. The goal of the final result will be to have the joint line restored and the components aligned properly, and to reestablish the proper mechanical axis. Bone defects can be managed by resection of more bone to eliminate the defect or fill the defect. More bone can be resected to eliminate a bony defect if the defect is small and not more than 10 mm of proximal tibia needs to be resected. In cases of small peripheral defects, smaller components can be placed away from the defect. Defects can be filled with either cement alone, cement with screw support, bone graft (autograft or allograft), modular metal wedges or blocks, or custom implants. When a defect is filled, it is generally accompanied by intramedullary stems. Cement filling (with or without screw support) of defects is the least technically demanding procedure and can be used for all defects of less than 10 mm. Cement filling for defects larger than 10 mm is mechanically weaker than other methods. Autograft bone during primary knee replacement can be fixed to peripheral host bone defects by screws or pins, or wedge fit into contained defects without internal fixation. When autograft is used, care must be taken to avoid interposition of cement into the host–graft interface, because this will block autograft

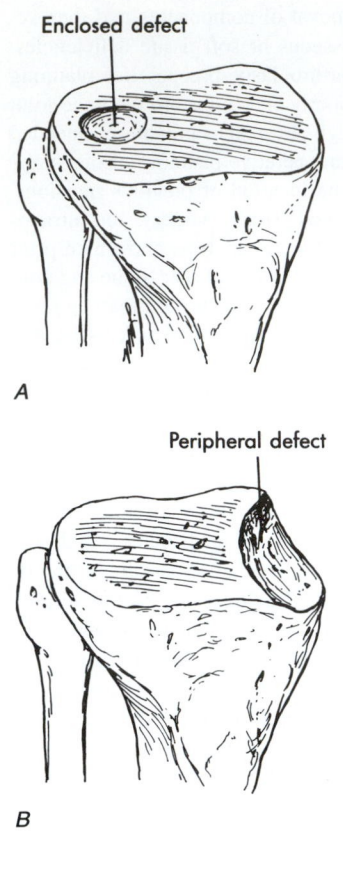

Enclosed defect

A

Peripheral defect

B

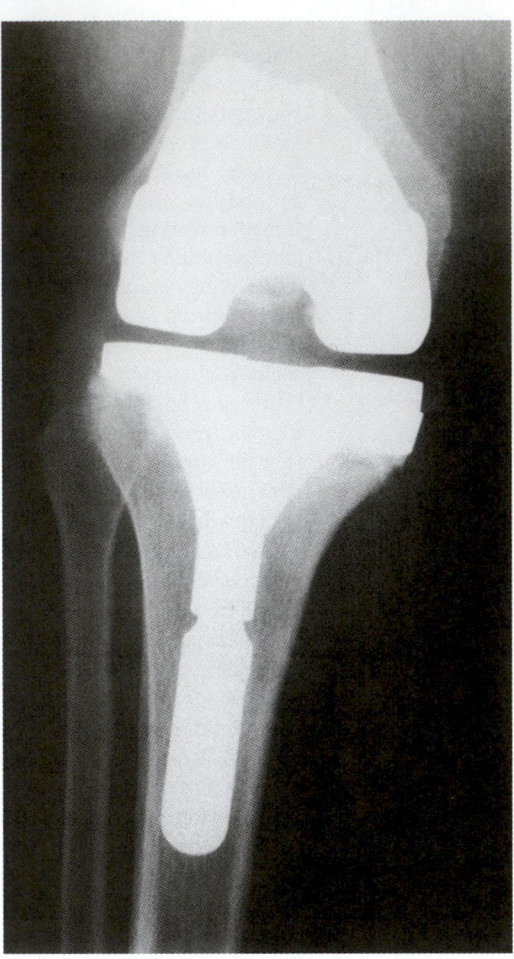

C

Figure 50-11
Enclosed or contained (*A*) and peripheral defect (*B*) present after the proper tibial bone cut is made. *C*, Peripheral defect can be effectively managed by metal wedges (radiograph). (Reproduced by permission from Krackow RA: Management of bone defects, in: *The Technique of Total Knee Arthroplasty*. St. Louis: CV Mosby; 1990:238.)

union to the host. Studies on the clinical results of autogenous bone graft for tibial bone defects have reported radiographic graft–host bone union in more than 65 percent of cases. Better results have be obtained with autografts used to fill contained defects as compared with those used for uncontained defects. Uncontained autografts have been reported to fail in approximately 15 percent of cases at short-term to midterm follow-up. In revision cases, sufficient autograft is usually not available, and therefore bulk and morselized allograft bone can be used in a similar fashion as the autograft bone. Although the long-term results for allograft bone are not yet known, short-term follow-up shows radiographic union or incorporation in more than 90 percent of cases. Modular metal wedges have been shown both in biomechanical testing and in short-term clinical reports to be more advantageous when compared with the use of bone graft or cement for bone defects. Some clinical concerns exist with the use of modular metal wedges and include debonding of the metal wedge from the metal component or the generation of metal debris from that interface. In all cases of managing bony defects, minimal further resection of host bone should be performed. In cases where bone loss exceeds that for metallic wedges or blocks, custom-made implants should be used, but are very expensive and require precise preoperative planning.

When managing bone defects, the addition of an intramedullary stem to the component is advantageous, because it transfers up to 30 percent of the forces from the bone subjacent to the implant to regions further away from the joint surface. Controversy still exists regarding fixation of the intramedullary stems. Generally, press-fit intramedullary stems should be used because, if infection does occur, they would be easier to remove. In some cases, however, it may not be possible to press-fit the stem or, if shorter stems are used, it may be advantageous to use cement.

SUGGESTED READINGS

Callaghan JJ, Dennis DA, Paprosky WG, et al (eds): *Orthopaedic Knowledge Update: Hip and Knee Reconstruction.* Rosemont, IL: American Academy of Orthopaedic Surgeons; 1995.

Chmell MJ, Moran MC, Scott RD: Periarticular fractures after total knee arthroplasty: Principles of management. *J Am Acad Orthop Surg* 1996; 4:109.

Grelsamer RP: Unicompartmental osteoarthrosis of the knee. *J Bone Joint Surg [Am]* 1995; 77:278.

Jacobs JJ, Shanbhag A, Glant TT, et al: Wear debris in total joint replacements. *J Am Acad Orthop Surg* 1994; 2:212.

Krackow KA: *The Technique of Total Knee Arthroplasty.* St. Louis: CV Mosby; 1990.

Scuderi GR, Insall JN, Scott N: Patellofemoral pain after total knee arthroplasty. *J Am Acad Orthop Surg* 1994; 2:239.

Windsor RE, Bono JV: Infected total knee replacements. *J Am Acad Orthop Surg* 1994; 2:44.

Chapter 51

SHOULDER

Howard J. Luks and Frances Cuomo

HISTORY

In the 1800s, surgery for severe afflictions of the shoulder included arthrodesis, resection arthroplasty, or amputation. One of the first attempts to replace any joint prosthetically was made by Pean, in France, in 1893, who placed a platinum and rubber total shoulder into a patient suffering from tuberculous arthropathy (see Lugli, 1978). The prosthesis had to be removed 2 years later because of overwhelming sepsis, and little else was mentioned of total shoulder arthroplasty (TSA) until Neer (1953, 1955) published his pioneering work in the 1950s. Neer had used a Vitallium (cobalt–chromium alloy) prosthesis to replace the humeral portion of the joint in patients with degenerative, traumatic, and inflammatory conditions affecting the shoulder. Kenmore (1973, 1974) was the first to propose and design a polyethylene glenoid liner for use with the Neer prosthesis. Many different design changes, especially with regard to the glenoid component, have taken place over the years, but the Neer (1974) prosthesis remains widely used today.

SURGICAL INDICATIONS

The general indications for prosthetic replacement of the glenohumeral joint are severe shoulder pain with significantly restricted motion that compromises activities of daily living. Radiographs should show advanced glenohumeral arthritis. Patients should have undergone a program of nonsurgical management that proved unsuccessful prior to being considered for TSA. Appropriate nonoperative modalities include rest, nonsteroidal anti-inflammatories, and a well-structured physical therapy program. In selected patients with mild involvement due to inflammatory arthritides (hemophilic arthropathy or rheumatoid arthritis), an arthroscopic or open synovectomy may provide significant pain relief and may be considered as a temporizing measure.

DISEASE CHARACTERISTICS

OSTEOARTHRITIS

Patients with advanced osteoarthritis (OA) generally tend to be older and are more commonly male. It may present as a monoarticular problem, although it is not uncommon to have more than one joint involved. The rotator cuff is much less frequently involved in these patients than in those with rheumatoid arthritis (RA). Only 5 percent of patients with OA of the shoulder will have a full-thickness rotator cuff tear at the time of surgery. Anterior capsular contraction, resulting in severe loss of external rotation, is common. Radiographic ex-

amination of patients with glenohumeral OA will show dense, sclerotic bone and extensive osteophyte formation (Fig. 51-1). Humeral abnormalities include osteophytes at the articular margin, usually at the anterior and inferior portions of the humerus. Glenoid abnormalities include marginal osteophyte formation, mainly along the inferior two-thirds, and central and posterior erosion. Bone loss, in general, is not a problem in patients with OA. Osteophyte formation, however, will make it necessary to identify the bony anatomy carefully at the time of TSA.

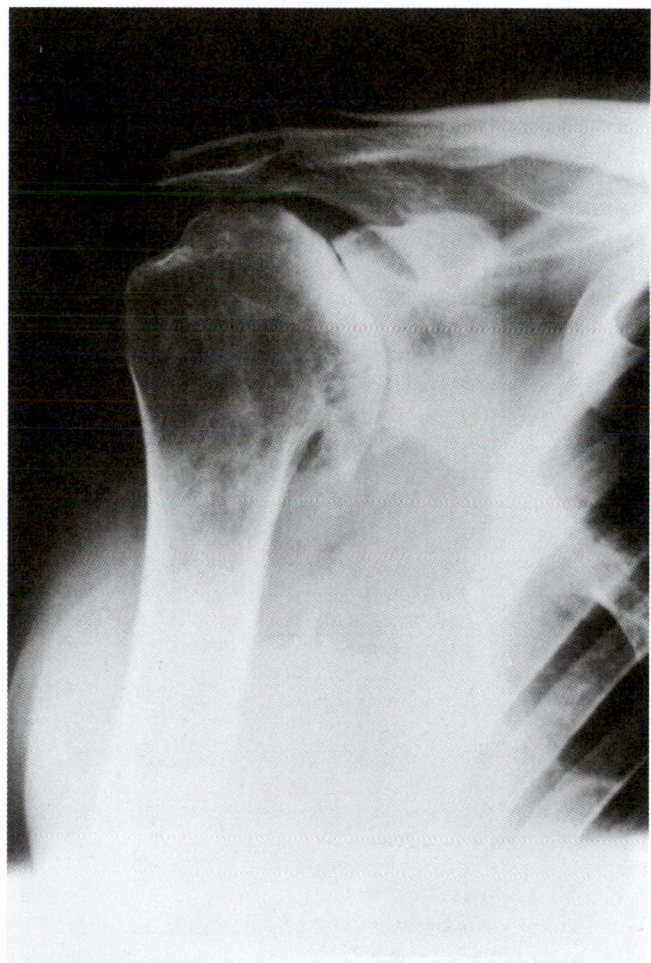

Figure 51-1
Dense sclerotic bone and marginal osteophyte formation associated with glenohumeral osteoarthritis.

RHEUMATOID ARTHRITIS

Patients with advanced RA of the glenohumeral joint are typically younger and tend to be female, reflecting the epidemiologic aspects of the disease. These patients typically have multiple joint involvement, including both the upper and lower extremities. Recognizing this is a key aspect of the surgical timing for TSA. Patients with RA may have systemic manifestations of their disease that require medical evaluation preoperatively, and instability of the cervical spine must be evaluated prior to induction of a general anesthetic.

Surgical considerations in the rheumatoid patient are numerous since many different shoulder structures can be involved. The glenohumeral joint, subacromial bursa, rotator cuff, and acromioclavicular joint may all be involved. Upward of 75 percent of patients with RA have marked abnormalities of the rotator cuff and 30 percent will have a full-thickness rotator cuff tear at the time of surgery. Marked soft tissue contracture is commonly encountered, as is extensive erosion of the humeral head and the glenoid. Early in the disease, the bone about the shoulder may be normal or show only osteopenia. With continuing synovial disease, marginal erosions develop. Initially, bone resorption on the humeral side is minimal. Erosion of the glenoid can range from minimal posterior bone loss to very significant medial glenoid bone loss resulting in medialization of the glenohumeral joint (Fig. 51-2).

Several rare complications or associations with RA in the glenohumeral joint have been reported. These include pseudothrombosis,

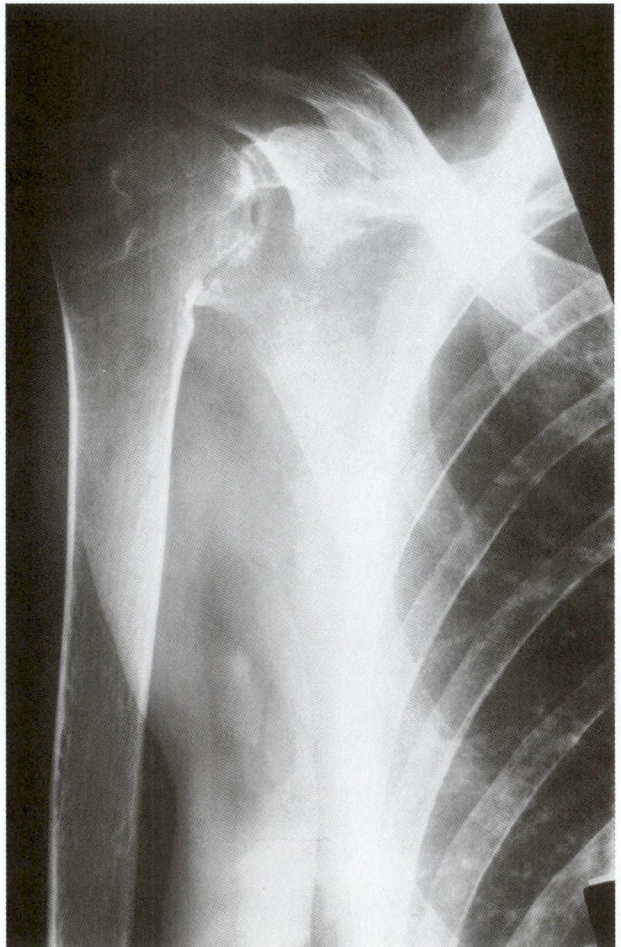

Figure 51-2
Medialization of the glenohumeral joint as a consequence of severe bone loss from rheumatoid arthritis with concentric joint space narrowing.

serratus anterior disruption, superimposed septic arthritis, and neuropathic arthropathy secondary to cervical spine disease.

POSTTRAUMATIC ARTHRITIS

There is no clear male or female predominance noted in this population, and the patients may be young or old. Radiographically, it is common to find malunion of the tuberosities or the articular segment. Malalignment of the shaft with respect to the proximal humerus may also be present. The bone is usually sclerotic, and collapse of small segments or of the entire humeral head is indicative of coexistent osteonecrosis. Due to the humeral asymmetry, irregular glenoid wear with posterior erosion is frequently encountered.

Chronic, missed or fixed dislocations of the proximal humerus pose a significant reconstructive problem. An axillary radiographic view is essential to confirm the diagnosis of shoulder dislocation. A computed tomographic (CT) scan can also aid in the diagnosis by defining the glenohumeral articulation and size of the articular defect (Fig. 51-3). Significant distortion of the anatomy, retraction of the tuberosities, loss of humeral height, and scarring of the rotator cuff tend to make identification of anatomic structures and soft tissue mobilization difficult. There also may be associated nerve injuries involving the axillary nerve, the suprascapular nerve, or the brachial plexus, which should be evaluated prior to considering surgical intervention. In the elderly population, magnetic resonance imaging may demonstrate the presence of a massive rotator cuff avulsion in association with a dislocation. In this circumstance, if the rotator cuff is irreparable, controversy exists as to whether TSA or humeral head replacement alone is the better treatment, as the uneven glenoid pressure distribution that is present may increase the rate of loosening.

In general, a hemiarthroplasty is recommended for dislocations that are more than 6 months old or if the humeral head defect involves more than 45 percent of the articular surface. If the glenoid surface is markedly abnormal, a TSA may be performed. A careful physical exam is necessary in this patient population to identify the presence of cuff pathology or a concomitant neurologic deficit. The complication rate for TSA and proximal humeral hemiarthroplasty performed for chronic dislocations is significantly higher than that for TSA performed for other conditions.

CUFF TEAR ARTHROPATHY

The end stage of rotator cuff disease, cuff tear arthropathy, is an uncommon entity that is usually encountered in the elderly of either sex. Many of these patients will have had prior rotator cuff surgery.

On examination, there is often a significant amount of swelling about the shoulder and extensive atrophy of the rotator cuff musculature. Fluid within the subacromial bursa is seen on physical exam as the classic "fluid sign." It is not uncommon for all four rotator cuff tendons to be torn, resulting in loss of joint integrity, with resultant upward migration of the humeral head. Subsequent secondary erosive changes on the undersurface of the acromion and the acromioclavicular joint are noted (Fig. 51-4). Complete absence of the rotator cuff results in marked shoulder instability, and the humeral head is frequently subluxated anteriorly and superiorly. Replacement in this setting is very challenging, and the goals need to be realistically portrayed to the patient. While relief from pain can be accomplished, significant gains in motion postoperatively are unlikely.

OSTEONECROSIS

Osteonecrosis is generally encountered in younger patients with underlying medical problems. Predisposing conditions include exogenous steroids, systemic lupus erythematosus, alcohol abuse, and

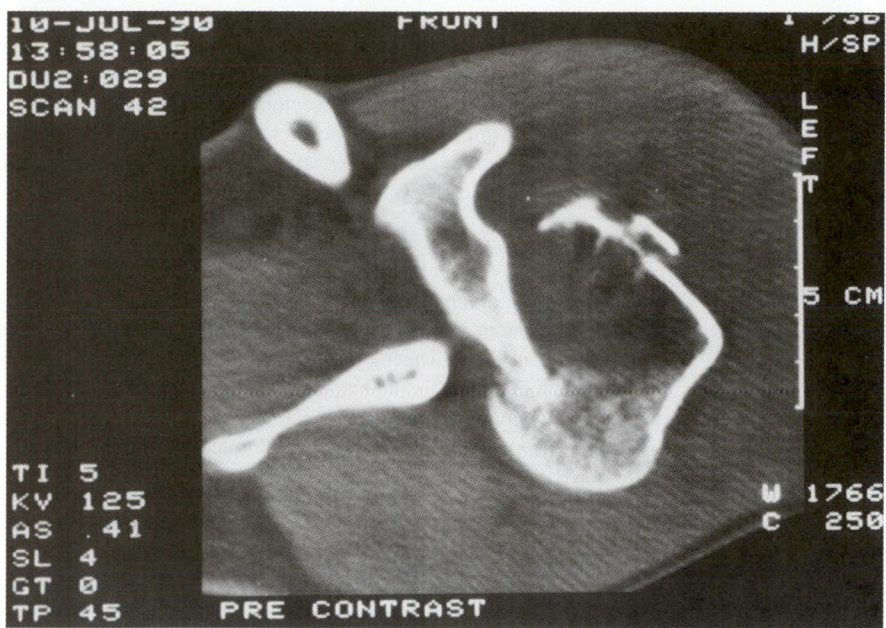

Figure 51-3
CT scan demonstrating posterior dislocation and articular surface defect.

sickle cell anemia. Osteonecrosis differs from the other conditions discussed in that significant relief from pain can be accomplished by nonsurgical means, especially in mild forms. This is because research has demonstrated that symptom progression is rare in patients with mild disease, and the vast majority of patients can be managed successfully without surgery. When these nonoperative modalities fail to

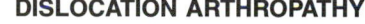

relieve pain adequately, surgical intervention, consisting of proximal humeral replacement or TSA, may be necessary.

Early in the process, the soft tissues about the shoulder are relatively spared. If the disease progresses and the humeral head deforms, joint incongruity results in secondary erosive changes of the glenoid and significant soft tissue contracture from chronically restricted motion.

DISLOCATION ARTHROPATHY

Arthritis of dislocations is more commonly encountered in the younger, male population. The vast majority of these patients have undergone previous surgery for recurrent instability of the gleno-humeral joint. The resultant degeneration may be due to malposition of the hardware used during prior surgical intervention or it may be secondary to overtightening of the soft tissues on one side of the joint which led to fixed subluxation on the opposite side and eventual degenerative arthritis. The most common scenario is seen in patients with multidirectional instability who were misdiagnosed as having unidirectional instability. The surgery then resulted in overtightening of the anterior capsule, and a fixed posterior subluxation may be present. When TSA is indicated, a number of factors need to be considered. The anatomy may be distorted, particularly if the coracoid was transferred. In addition, neurovascular structures may be displaced. The axillary nerve is at particular risk for injury during surgery due to its proximity to the inferior aspect of the joint capsule. The integrity of the soft tissues is one of the most important operative considerations in this patient population. Soft tissue balancing, in order to achieve a stable prosthetic reconstruction, will usually require an anterior capsule release and subscapularis lengthening. Occasionally, a posterior capsulorraphy will need to be performed to maintain the appropriate soft tissue tension. In addition, the surgeon may need to adjust the version of the components to enhance stability.

CRYSTALLINE ARTHROPATHY

Crystalline arthropathy may present as gout, pseudogout, or hydroxy-apatite disease. In general, this is an uncommon cause of arthropathy that is found in older individuals, with a slight male predominance.

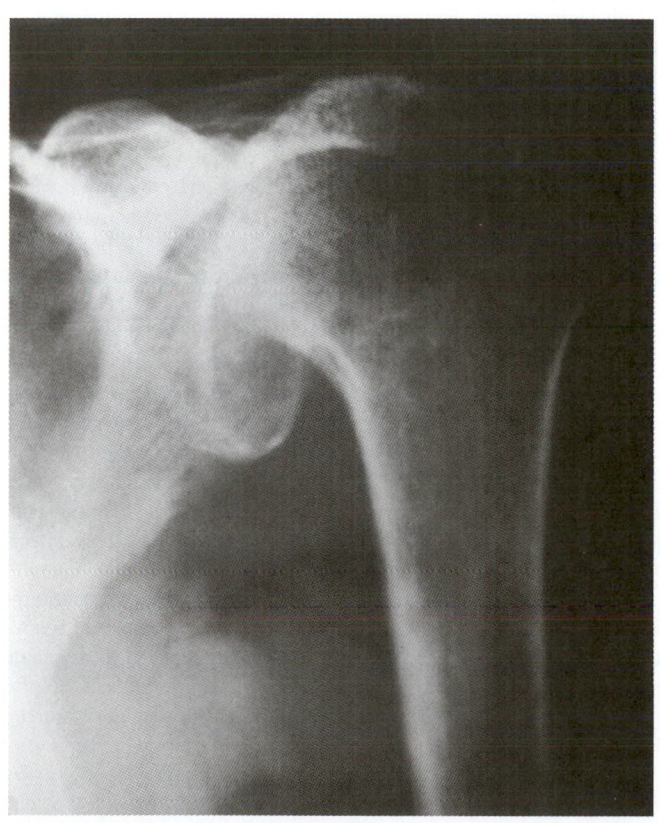

Figure 51-4
Cuff tear arthropathy representing the end stage of rotator cuff disease. Note resultant upward migration of the humeral head.

The clinical picture is quite variable and ranges from the appearance of mild inflammatory arthritis to one of extensive soft tissue and bony erosion.

HEMOPHILIC ARTHROPATHY

Hemophilic arthropathy is generally encountered in patients with either factor VIII and factor IX deficiencies, or von Willebrand's disease. Because of the sex-linked nature of the disease, it is more common in males. The clinical picture is similar to that of any other inflammatory arthritides. The arthropathy is due to synovial hypertrophy, and the disease is characterized by progressive bony erosion and soft tissue compromise. Before significant bony changes have occurred, arthroscopic synovectomy may be a reasonable option. This procedure results in fewer joint bleeds, and relief of pain, but it has not been shown otherwise to alter the course or progression of the disease. When significant erosion and joint destruction have occurred, these patients are candidates for TSA.

CLINICAL EVALUATION

Evaluation of patients with glenohumeral arthritis includes a careful history, physical exam, and radiographic evaluation. Pain and functional deficit are usually the presenting complaints. A standard trauma radiographic series is obtained and includes an anteroposterior view in internal and external rotation, an axillary view, and a scapular Y view. In patients with posttraumatic arthritis, a CT scan may be necessary to delineate the tuberosity anatomy. A preoperative electromyogram may be warranted in posttraumatic or postsurgical patients to rule out any preexisting neurologic dysfunction.

Patients with OA may demonstrate fullness posteriorly due to a posteriorly subluxed humeral head. Patients with full-thickness cuff tears may demonstrate fluid in the acromioclavicular joint and subacromial bursa. Rheumatoid patients may show flattening of the lateral aspect of the shoulder due to extensive glenoid erosion and resultant medial subluxation of the humeral head. Due to its prognostic significance, atrophy and weakness of the rotator cuff musculature must be assessed meticulously, and its etiology defined, prior to surgery. Screening for coexistent conditions in the cervical spine, ipsilateral upper extremity, and bilateral lower extremities must be performed since this can impact on the timing of TSA and the use of a general anesthetic.

If the glenohumeral arthritis is unusually severe, bony fragmentation is present, the bones are resorbing, or the shoulder is unstable, a neuropathic component to the arthritis should be considered and a careful neurologic evaluation undertaken. This is especially true in the rheumatoid patient who may have C-spine instability or neural compression.

SURGICAL TREATMENTS

Numerous surgical treatments have been proposed for patients with glenohumeral arthritis. Proximal humeral replacement or TSA has superseded nearly all other treatment alternatives, but each of the following treatments may play a role in selected patients.

SYNOVECTOMY

RA and hemophilic arthropathy are diseases where synovial hypertrophy is responsible for the symptoms attendant to the condition. Many surgeons feel that there remains a limited role for shoulder synovectomy. In rheumatoid patients, with at least 50 percent of the thickness of the articular cartilage remaining and an intact rotator cuff, synovectomy has been proven to decrease the pain associated with marked synovial hyperplasia. Synovectomy, however, has not been shown to protect the rotator cuff nor delay the need for TSA in the future. Similar results have been obtained in hemophiliacs with significant shoulder pain and limitation of activities of daily living.

DEBRIDEMENT

An isolated debridement remains a viable alternative in young patients with moderate OA who are not clinically and psychologically ready for replacement. During a debridement, the offending osteophytes, bursal hypertrophy, and reactive synovitis are excised. These patients will generally obtain pain relief and an increase in motion as long as the disease is not far progressed. Patients must be informed, however, that this remains a temporizing measure and that replacement may be required in the future.

RESECTION ARTHROPLASTY

Although once a commonly performed procedure during the preprosthetic era, resection arthroplasty is generally reserved for patients with uncontrolled septic arthritis of the glenohumeral joint. It may also be employed in situations where marked bone loss has resulted from a previous attempt at TSA. Pain relief has been reported as moderate, and stability is surprisingly adequate, but range of motion remains severely affected following resection of the glenohumeral joint.

ARTHRODESIS

There remain very few indications for arthrodesis of the shoulder. Most shoulder fusions performed today are done for paralysis of the deltoid and rotator cuff, uncontrollable infection, or failed reconstructive procedures. Recommended position of fusion includes 40 degrees of flexion, 20 degrees of abduction, and 20 degrees of internal rotation. External rotation must be avoided.

PROSTHETIC ARTHROPLASTY

Several important factors must be recognized and carefully considered in planning a TSA. Radiographs of the involved shoulder provide the basis for an evaluation of the bony anatomy. The bony structures must be evaluated for quality, quantity, and deformity. Quantity refers to the degree of bone loss (both to the glenoid and to the humeral head) that may be present as a result of inflammatory, degenerative, or traumatic processes. Quality refers to the structure of the available bone stock. Severe osteopenia and sclerosis can be very problematic if not accounted for prior to the onset of surgical intervention. Bone deformity is especially important in posttraumatic situations where the tuberosities or the shaft may be malunited. This can lead to difficulty in soft tissue mobilization, in obtaining adequate stability, and in the ability to place the stem of the humeral component properly.

A complete radiographic assessment, including scapular anteroposterior views in internal and external rotation, axillary, and scapular lateral views, can be supplemented with a CT scan to delineate the bony anatomy adequately. CT scans may be particularly helpful in localizing the tuberosities, assessing the degree of bone loss, and determining the version of the glenoid and proximal humerus.

The condition of the soft tissues about the shoulder is an equally important preoperative consideration. The range of motion that can be obtained postoperatively and hence the degree of improvement of shoulder function depend in large measure on intact, functioning soft tissues. The deltoid and the rotator cuff are the most important components to be addressed. The deltoid may be scarred from previous trauma or surgery. Detachment of the anterior deltoid, due to prior shoulder surgery, is a particularly difficult problem to overcome. Assessment of the integrity of the rotator cuff preoperatively will aid in determining the expected surgical result, because of the positive correlation that exists between a well-functioning rotator cuff and a good clinical outcome.

The question frequently arises regarding whether to replace the glenoid in performing a shoulder arthroplasty. In general, humeral head replacement alone is indicated when the glenoid is either uninvolved or does not possess adequate bone quantity or quality to obtain secure prosthetic fixation. Replacement of the glenoid is also controversial in patients with a severely deficient rotator cuff where glenoid replacement would prohibit adequate rotator cuff closure.

In select patients with OA, osteonecrosis, posttraumatic arthritis, and cuff tear arthropathy, a humeral hemiarthroplasty is well tolerated and can yield good clinical results. In general, a prerequisite for considering a hemiarthroplasty versus a TSA is a relatively spared glenoid. Patients with RA, and glenoid bone stock that will accept a prosthesis, should receive a TSA. RA will always continue to progress in the presence of articular cartilage, and thus a hemiarthroplasty is of limited use except in patients with severe joint medialization as a result of profound glenoid bone loss. In patients with massive, functionally deficient rotator cuff tears, a humeral component alone can provide good pain relief and function well in the limited goals category.

If patients are to be considered good candidates for a TSA, they must possess enough glenoid bone stock to seat the prosthetic component properly. Most patients with severe arthritis of the glenohumeral joint will fit into this category, but one must always be cognizant of the relative prerequisites for a TSA and be prepared to alter the surgical plan as necessary.

As discussed previously, soft tissue or bony abnormalities that exist need to be addressed intraoperatively. In patients with limited external rotation, with or without posterior subluxation, an anterior release and subscapularis lengthening will need to be performed. This is a critical consideration, because this will determine how the subscapularis will be cut during the initial approach to the glenohumeral joint. Once the joint is exposed, the version of the humeral component will need to be determined. For this, the arm is placed at the side and externally rotated 30 to 40 degrees. This ensures that the proximal humeral cut is in 30 to 40 degrees of retroversion. Only the articular portion of the humeral head is to be removed. Removal of an excess amount of humerus will result in prominence of the greater tuberosity and impingement on the acromion. The glenoid is then assessed for any bony deficiency. A burr is used to cut out the portion of the glenoid where the keel of the glenoid component is to be seated. The surface of the glenoid is then burred free of any remaining articular cartilage, being careful not to remove any of the bone stock, and the component is cemented in place. The humeral trial component is then seated, and an assessment of the stability is made. It is imperative that the humeral component be seated in its correct version. Aligning the fin of the prosthesis just posterior to the bicipital groove will often place the component in 30 to 40 degrees of retroversion. With the arm at the side and the elbow flexed to 90 degrees and in neutral rotation, the humeral component should face the glenoid cavity. The humeral head should be cephalad to the greater tuberosity to ensure the maintenance of humeral height and the avoidance of postoperative impingement. Many of the newer modular total shoulder systems allow for easy exchange of humeral head components in order to adjust the soft tissue tension appropriately (Fig. 51-5).

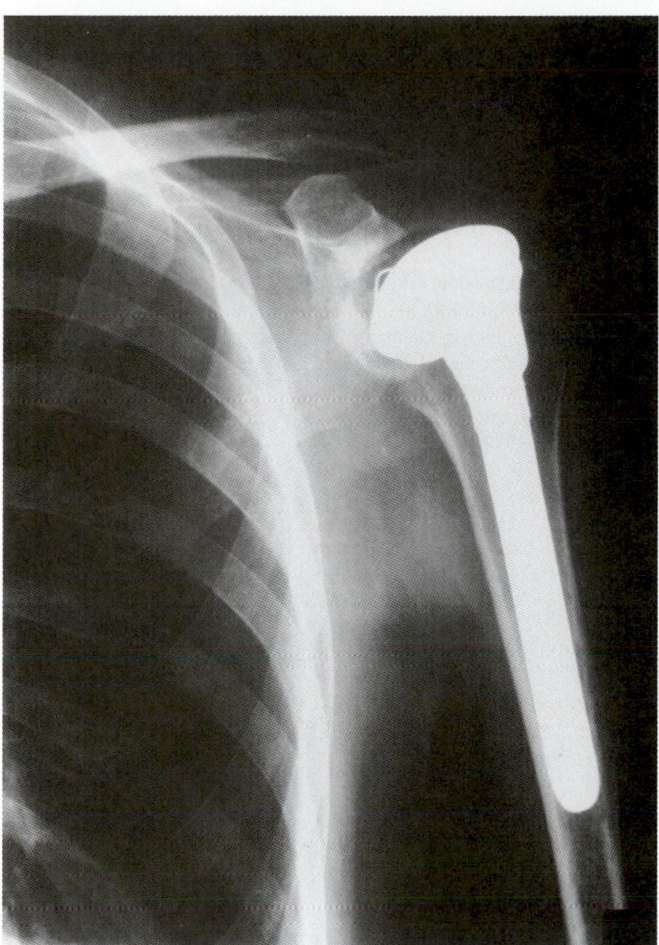

Figure 51-5
Total shoulder arthroplasty employing modular system with uncemented humeral component and cemented glenoid.

Associated degenerative problems of the upper extremity must also be carefully considered. In patients with polyarticular inflammatory arthritis, ipsilateral involvement of the elbow, wrist, and hand may be present and require careful staging of the surgical procedures. It may be optimal initially to complete hand and wrist reconstructions prior to proceeding with TSA. Associated degenerative problems of the lower extremity must also be considered carefully. A patient in need of a TSA as well as a total hip or knee replacement must completely recover from the lower extremity procedure prior to having the TSA. The need to use assistive walking devices can adversely affect the outcome of TSA in the first 6 to 9 months following the procedure.

Complications relating to TSA include, but are not limited to, infection (0.51 percent), fracture (1.4 percent), nerve injury (0.68 percent), instability (2 percent), ectopic calcification (0.17 percent), and rotator cuff tear or tuberosity malunion (3.4 percent). In the acute setting, the most common complication is instability of the TSA components. This is especially true in the setting of a TSA performed for a fixed anterior or posterior dislocation. In patients with fixed posterior dislocations, the humeral component should be placed in a relatively anteverted position or only slight retroversion, whereas in patients with a fixed anterior dislocation, retroversion of the humeral component to 45 to 60 degrees may be necessary to prevent postoperative instability.

The most common late complication of TSA involves loosening of the glenoid component (2.6 percent at 5 to 10 years). In patients with a proximal humeral replacement for fracture of the proximal humerus, the most common complication relates to the improper seating of the humeral component with failure to restore the height of the greater tuberosity and myofascial tension within the system, leading to instability of the components postoperatively.

SUGGESTED READINGS

Cofield RH: Total shoulder arthroplasty with the Neer prosthesis. *J Bone Joint Surg [Am]* 1984; 66:899.

Figgie HE III, Inglis AE, Goldberg VM, et al: An analysis of factors affecting the long-term results of total shoulder arthroplasty in inflammatory arthritis. *J Arthroplasty* 1988; 3:123.

Kenmore PI: A simple shoulder replacement. Clemson University Biomaterials Symposium, 1973.

Kenmore PI, MacCartee C, Vitek B: A simple shoulder replacement. *J Biomed Mater Res* 1974; 8:329.

Lugli T: Artificial shoulder joint by Péan (1893). The facts of an exceptional intervention and the prosthetic method. *Clin Orthop* 1978; 133:215.

Neer CS II: Articular replacement for the humeral head. *J Bone Joint Surg [Am]* 1955; 37:215.

Neer CS II: Replacement arthroplasty for glenohumeral osteoarthritis. *J Bone Joint Surg [Am]* 1974; 56:1.

Neer CS II, Brown TH Jr, McLaughlin HL: Fracture of the neck of the humerus with dislocation of the head fragment. *Am J Surg* 1953; 85:252.

Neer CS II, Watson KC, Stanton FJ: Recent experience in total shoulder replacement. *J Bone Joint Surg [Am]* 1982; 64:319.

Zuckerman JD, Cuomo F: Glenohumeral arthroplasty: A critical review of indications and preoperative considerations. *Bull Hosp Joint Dis* 1993; 52:21.

Chapter 52

ELBOW

Neal L. Hochwald and Joseph D. Zuckerman

RHEUMATOID ARTHRITIS

Elbow involvement, primarily the ulnohumeral articulation, is present in 20 to 50 percent of patients with rheumatoid arthritis (RA). The initial presentation of the inflammatory process is movement-limiting pain that frequently leads to soft tissue contracture. The main causes of pain are elbow capsule distention and synovitis. If unresolved, hyaline cartilage erosion occurs with joint space narrowing, subchondral cyst and osteophyte formation, and subchondral bone loss ensuing. In addition, destruction to the annular and anteromedial ligaments leads to joint instability and specifically, the potential for subluxation. Continued progression of the synovitis can result in intraosseous synovial cyst formation and subsequent ulnar or radial nerve compression. Rheumatoid disease can also cause enlargement of the olecranon bursa and formation of rheumatoid nodules on the extensor surface of the ulna, both being prone to irritation and in-fection. Elbow involvement in juvenile idiopathic arthritis (JIA), formerly termed juvenile rheumatoid arthritis (JRA), may cause anky-losis or severe growth disturbances because the disease process most often occurs when the epiphyseal plates are still open. Synovitis in JIA may cause either premature closure or overgrowth of the epiphyses, resulting in misshaping of the distal humeraus and prox-imal ulna and occasionally dislocation of the radial head.

Physical examination of the rheumatoid elbow includes assessment of radial and ulnar nerve function, inspection for bursa or nodules, go-niometric measurements of range of motion, and evaluation of the pa-tient's ability to perform activities of daily living. Early radiographs in these patients may show joint space narrowing and marginal erosions along the ulnohumeral joint and changes at the radiocapitellar joint (Fig. 52-1). The initial treatment is nonoperative, and may include sal-icylates, non-steroidal anti-inflammatory drugs (NSAIDs), remittive agents, immunosuppressive agents, and corticosteroids. Physical ther-apy and occupational therapy may be used to maintain range of mo-tion. Splinting can be helpful for initial pain relief and prevention of contractures. Static splints can be worn at night to protect the elbow, or when the patient is using the elbow for specific activities. A hinged splint may be useful to protect the elbow from varus and valgus stresses if instability is present. Periodic intraarticular injections of cortico-steroids may be of benefit to minimize painful synovitis.

Operative intervention should be considered for progressive elbow pain and dysfunction which prove refractory to nonoperative treat-

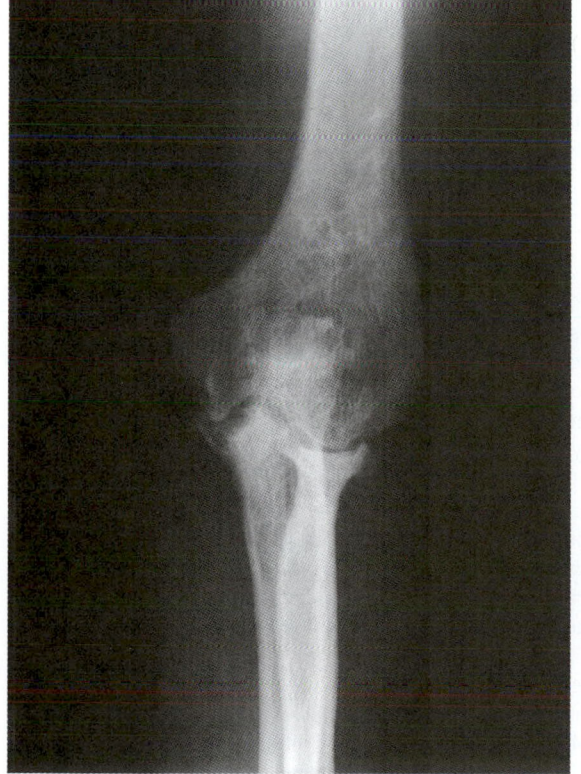

A

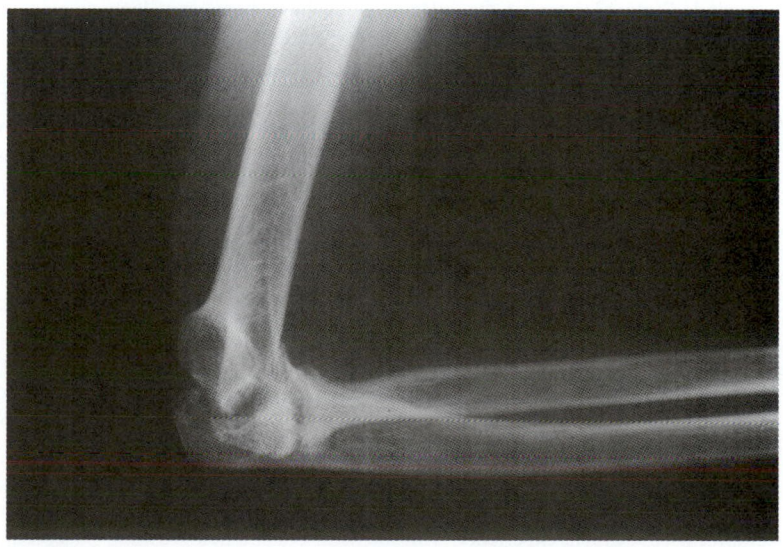

B

Figure 52-1
Severe rheumatoid involvement of the elbow showing marked collapse and deformity. *A.* AP view.
B. Lateral view.

ment. The hand, wrist, and shoulder should also be examined to determine the extent of involvement. If multiple joints of the upper extremity are painful and a source of significant disability, the hand and wrist should be corrected first, followed by either the elbow or shoulder, whichever is more symptomatic.

Elbow synovectomy and debridement with or without radial head excision should be considered for the painful elbow with uncontrolled synovitis. Younger patients with more extensive joint destruction may benefit most from this procedure since treatment options for this group are limited. Contraindications to elbow synovectomy include gross instability and severe stiffness. The technique involves a complete synovectomy, capsular release, and usually a radial head excision through a posterolateral (Kocher) approach to the elbow joint. Arthroscopic synovectomy affords rapid return of motion, but it is technically demanding and associated with a significant risk to the neurovascular structures lying just anterior to the joint capsule. Therefore, open synovectomy is the procedure of choice for most orthopaedic surgeons. Satisfactory pain relief is reported in approximately 70 to 90 percent of patients, but increased joint motion is much less predictable. Better results are obtained when the procedure is performed at earlier stages of the disease.

Another operative option for the younger patient with painful synovitis, joint instability, ankylosis, or advanced joint destruction is interposition arthroplasty with fascia lata or cutis. Through an extensive posterolateral approach, the elbow joint is debrided and the remaining articular surfaces are reshaped and covered with the interposition substance. If extensive capsular releases are performed and the joint is extremely unstable, a hinged external fixation device that holds the joint in a distracted and stable position should be utilized since it allows early motion in the first few weeks following interpositional arthroplasty. Resection arthroplasty or arthrodesis of the elbow, although used previously, are no longer recommended treatment options. These surgical treatments are rarely used because of poor functional outcomes reported and the availability of improved procedures.

Total elbow arthroplasty is the procedure of choice for older patients with advanced levels of joint destruction, severe pain, and poor elbow function that restricts the ability to perform activities of daily living. Pain relief and restoration of motion and function can be expected. Survival rates of the arthroplasties have been excellent and the indications are expanding to younger patients. An absolute contraindication to elbow replacement is the presence of an active infection.

The two primary elbow prostheses used today are the minimally constrained and semi-constrained designs. The minimally constrained prosthesis functions as a surface replacement, has no coupling between components, and receives little inherent stability from its articulation, thus relying on surrounding soft-tissue constraints for stability. The main problem reported or identified in series of patients with this type of replacement has been instability with rates of up to 20 percent. Loosening rates have been low with long-term follow-up. The semi-constrained design is characterized by a coupling between the ulnar and humeral components which affords stability and prevents dislocation (Fig. 52-2). It also provides sufficient laxity to transfer loads across the elbow from the cement-bone interface to the soft tissues. Due to its inherent stability, the semi-constrained prosthesis may be better suited for elbow joints with significant bone loss or soft tissue compromise. Clinical experience with the semi-constrained prosthesis has demonstrated low loosening rates and a less demanding insertion technique; it is the design most commonly utilized.

The most common complications requiring revision are infection, instability, loosening, component failure, and polyethylene wear. Other complications frequently encountered that can usually be treated nonoperatively are delayed wound healing and ulna nerve neuropraxia.

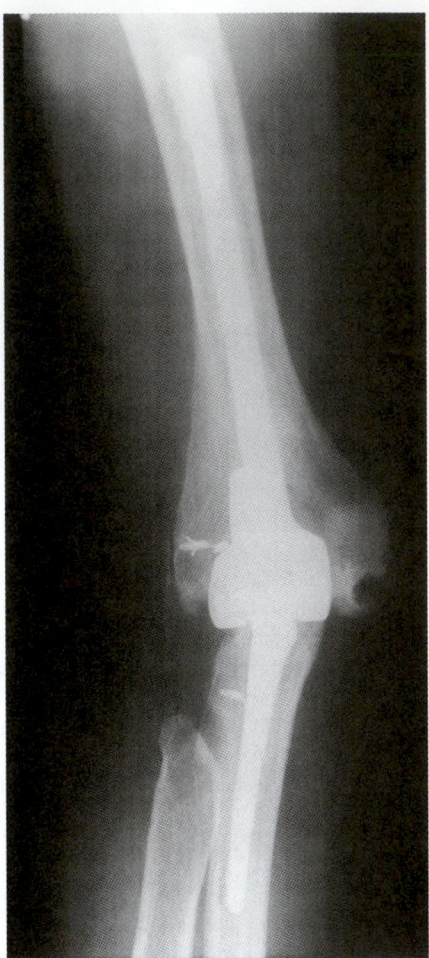

Figure 52-2
Postoperative radiograph of a cemented semi-constrained total elbow arthroplasty.

OSTEOARTHRITIS

Primary osteoarthritis of the elbow comprises only 1 to 2 percent of all arthritic elbows. It affects males almost exclusively, and the usual presentation is 50 years of age. The most common precipitating factor is repetitive use, and overwhelmingly involves the dominant extremity. Typical complaints are mild to moderate pain at the extreme ranges of flexion and extension, loss of full extension, and stiffness. Excessive osteophyte formation may produce ulnar nerve irritation. Radiographs are often diagnostic, with routine anteroposterior and lateral views revealing osteophyte formation on the anterior coronoid and posterior olecranon processes, and within the olecranon and coronoid fossae. MRI may be useful to detect loose bodies and to evaluate the size and extent of osteophytes.

The nonoperative management of elbow osteoarthritis begins with symptomatic treatment of avoiding painful activities, application of heat or cold, and splinting. Range of motion exercises should be encouraged to maintain mobility and muscle strengthening exercises (avoiding excessive joint loading) should be performed regularly. Operative management is indicated if nonoperative treatment is ineffective. Arthroscopy is minimally invasive and can be used to remove osteophytes and loose bodies.

A more extensive open debridement of the joint may be performed in the patient with painful terminal extension. This procedure, the

Outerbridge-Kashiwagi or ulnohumeral arthroplasty, exposes the elbow from the posterior aspect allowing osteophyte removal from the olecranon and the olecranon fossa. The fossa is then penetrated anteriorly and widened with a burr to facilitate exposure of the anterior aspect of the joint for excision of coronoid osteophytes (Fig. 52-3). Aggressive therapy and splinting are used postoperatively to maintain any gains in range of motion. Results with this procedure show that 80 to 90 percent of patients will have pain relief and increased range of motion. However, with several years of follow-up, recurrence of pain and decreased motion may develop. Interpositional arthroplasty has proven more favorable in the osteoarthritic than the rheumatoid elbow because of better bone stock and stability. Finally, as in rheumatoid patients, older patients with osteoarthritis and severe elbow dysfunction may be managed with total elbow arthroplasty.

CRYSTALLINE-INDUCED ARTHROPATHIES

Acute gouty arthritis is an inflammatory reaction to the formation of monosodium urate crystals within synovial spaces. These crystals are deposited on and within the articular cartilage, synovium, and bur-

sae, initiating the process of phagocytosis. Gout may initially present in the elbow as acute olecranon bursitis with tophi formation. Calcium pyrophosphate dehydrate crystals (pseudogout) can also affect the elbow, causing synovitis. The patient often presents with an acutely painful elbow and flexion contracture. Radiographs may show a linear calcification in the joint space. Joint aspirates will show negative birefringent crystals with gout and positive birefringent crystals with pseudogout. Treatment with other NSAIDs, colchicines, or intra-articular injection of corticosteroids should be used in conjunction with rest and splinting. When the acute, painful crisis subsides, range of motion exercises should be initiated. Synovectomy is rarely beneficial in these patients.

SEPTIC ARTHRITIS

Infection of the elbow joint in adults is very uncommon and usually occurs in patients with predisposing risk factors. These include rheumatoid arthritis, immunodeficiency, prior elbow surgery, and direct inoculation of bacteria from trauma. Ages at risk include children and the elderly. Symptoms of pain, swelling, and limited motion are most common. Passive motion of the elbow is extremely

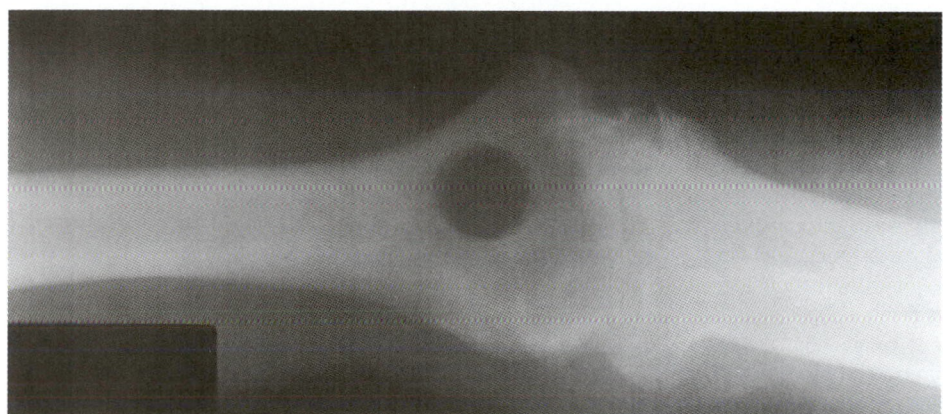

A

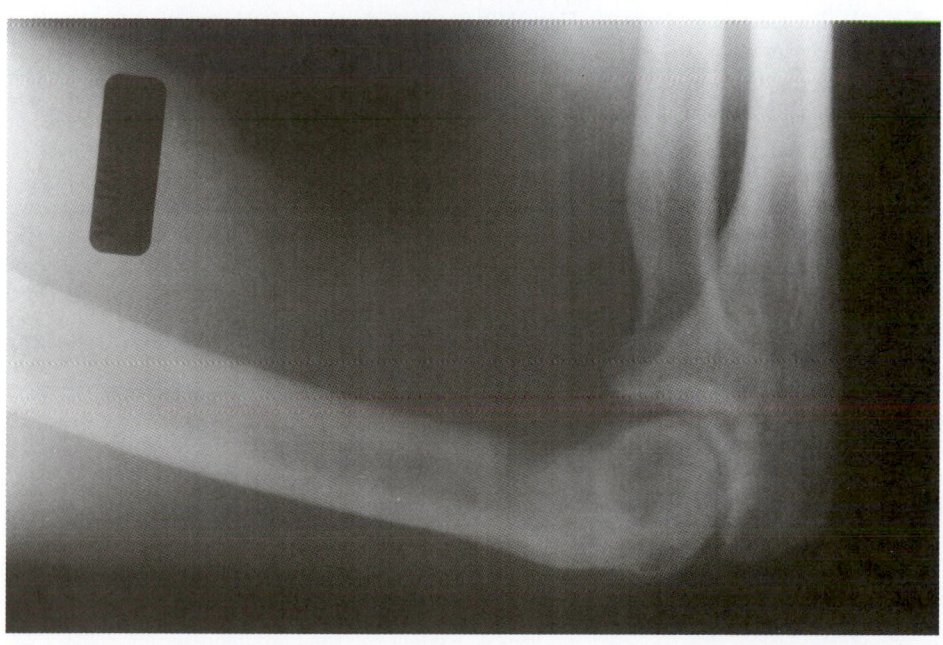

B

Figure 52-3
A. Postoperative anteroposterior radiograph of an ulnohumeral arthroplasty performed in a patient with early osteoarthrtis. B. Lateral view of the same elbow.

painful. An elevated serum white blood cell count, erythrocyte sedimentation rate (ESR), and C-reactive protein are frequently seen. Initial radiographs may show a posterior fat pad sign due to increased synovial fluid. Long-standing joint infections lead to osteopenia, bone erosion, loss of articular cartilage, and destruction of subchondral bone.

Differential diagnosis in adults includes rheumatoid arthritis with secondary infection, gout, or pseudogout. In children, juvenile idiopathic arthritis, osteomyelitis, trauma, acute rheumatic fever, and transient synovitis should all be considered as alternative diagnoses. Osteomyelitis should be distinguished by the location of tenderness and the level of tolerance to passive range of motion.

Aspiration of the elbow between the radial head, lateral epicondyle, and olecranon will confirm the diagnosis. Bacterial cultures are most commonly positive for *Staphylococcus aureus* in adults. In children, *Haemophilus influenzae* should be a suspected pathogen. Coliform and gram-positive organisms are common in the infant. Treatment consists of administration of intravenous antibiotics and surgical irrigation and debridement to remove cellular debris and harmful enzymes. Arthroscopy or open arthrotomy may be utilized. Results are most favorable with early diagnosis and treatment, and initiation of a physical therapy program to regain motion.

HEMATOLOGIC ARTHRITIS

Hemophilia and sickle cell disease can both affect the elbow. Hemophilia is due to a deficiency in plasma coagulation factors and may cause elbow arthropathy due to recurrent hemarthroses. An acute hemarthrosis is often spontaneous and presents with pain and stiffness, progressing to a warm and swollen joint. The elbow is held in a flexed position with a painful and restricted arc of motion. Recurrent hemarthroses can lead to a chronic arthropathy. The elbow synovium hypertrophies with pannus formation, hemosiderin staining, and fibrillation of cartilage. Progression to complete joint destruction and fibrotic, contracted periarticular structures may result.

Treatment for the initial acute hemarthrosis is coagulation factor replacement therapy and splinting. Joint aspiration is usually not needed, but physical therapy with early mobilization is important to retain motion as soon as the acute bleeding has stopped. Surgical synovectomy can be considered for recurrent hemarthroses which effectively reduces bleeding episodes and may decrease pain. For the patient with a chronic arthropathy and symptoms of severe pain and limitation of motion, total elbow arthroplasty may be performed.

Patients with sickle cell disease may have vasoocclusive crises which can affect the elbows. Acute onset of pain, swelling, warmth, and limited motion is the usual presentation. Osteomyelitis, particularly due to salmonella, must be ruled out in these patients. Radiographs may show evidence of prior bone infarction or periostitis, but degenerative changes are unusual. Treatment includes fluid replacement, pain management, and physical therapy to maintain joint motion. Surgery is rarely needed.

POSTTRAUMATIC ARTHRITIS

Nonoperative management of posttraumatic arthritis is the same as for osteoarthritis: avoidance of painful activities, range of motion exercises, and splinting. Early stages of posttraumatic arthritis consist-

ing of flap tears or chondral injuries to the articular surface may be treated by arthroscopic or open debridement. Interposition arthroplasty may be used in the younger patient with more advanced arthritic changes.

Patients with large bony defects around the elbow may be managed with resection arthroplasty. However, this procedure is more predictable of relatively pain-free motion with stability if the columns of the distal humerus, olecranon, and coronoid remain in place. Another option is osteochondral allograft replacement of the deficient arthritic segment of the elbow. Osteochondral replacement may restore bone stock; however, complications of bony nonunion, fracture, infection, and cartilage degeneration are common and the procedure remains investigational.

In addition, comminuted intraarticular distal humerus fractures and malunions and nonunions of the distal humerus in the elderly have recently been managed with total elbow arthroplasty. This procedure has the potential to rapidly return these patients to their former lifestyle by minimizing the number of subsequent surgical procedures. The experience, however, has been quite limited and preliminary and this approach is considered to be under investigation. It should be noted that the outcome in patients who undergo total elbow arthroplasty for the traumatic indications mentioned above are not as successful as for those in whom osteoarthritis or rheumatoid arthritis is the primary indication.

SUGGESTED READINGS

Butters KP, Morrey BF: Septic arthritis. In Morrey BF (ed): *The Elbow and Its Disorders.* 2d ed. Philadelphia: WB Saunders; 1993:784.

Cooney WP: Elbow arthroplasty: Indications and implant selection. In Morrey BF (ed): *The Elbow and Its Disorders,* 2d ed. Philadelphia: WB Saunders; 1993:629.

Ewald FC, Simmons ED Jr, Sullivan JA, et al: Capitallocondylar total elbow replacement in rheumatoid arthritis. Long-term results. *J Bone Joint Surg [Am]* 1993; 75:498.

Gilchrist GS, Bolander M: Hematologic arthritis. In Morrey BF (ed): *The Elbow and Its Disorders,* 2d ed. Philadelphia: WB Saunders; 1993:794.

Goldberg VM, Figgie HE 3d, Inglis AE, et al: Total elbow arthroplasty. *J Bone Joint Surg [Am]* 1988; 70:778.

Inglis AE, Figgie MP: Rheumatoid arthritis. In Morrey BF (ed): *The Elbow and Its Disorders,* 2d ed. Philadelphia: WB Saunders; 1993:751.

Lonner JH, Stuchin SA: Synovectomy, radial head excision, and anterior capsular release in stage III inflammatory arthritis of the elbow. *J Hand Surg [Am]* 1997; 22:279.

Morrey BF: Primary degenerative arthritis of the elbow: Treatment by ulnohumeral arthroplasty. *J Bone Joint Surg [Br]* 1992; 74:409.

Morrey BF: Primary degenerative arthritis of the elbow: Ulnohumeral arthoplasty. In Morrey BF (ed): *The Elbow and Its Disorders,* 2d ed. Philadelphia: WB Saunders; 1993:774.

Morrey BF, Adams RA: Semiconstrained arthoplasty for the treatment of rheumatoid arthritis of the elbow. *J Bone Joint Surg [Am]* 1992; 74:479.

O'Driscoll SW: Elbow arthritis. Treatment options. *J Am Acad Orthop Surg* 1993; 1:106.

Tompkins RB: Nonheumatoid inflammatory arthritis. In Morrey BF (ed): *The Elbow and Its Disorders,* 2d ed. Philadelphia: WB Saunders; 1993:767.

Tulp NJ, Winia WP: Synovectomy of the elbow in rheumatoid arthritis: Long-term results. *J Bone Joint Surg [Br]* 1989; 71:664.

Chapter 53

NEUROPATHIC ARTHROPATHY

Joseph D. Zuckerman

Neuropathic arthropathy is a chronic, progressive, and degenerative disorder most commonly associated with diabetes, syphilis (tabes dorsalis), and syringomyelia, and less so with other neurologic conditions such as leprosy and myelomeningocele. It occurs in joints that develop abnormal sensory innervation with diminished proprioceptive sensation and are simultaneously unprotected from the effects of minor trauma—a devastating, aggressive combination of neurologic and local injury that leads to rapid and total joint destruction in undiagnosed or neglected cases. Clinical presentation includes joint swelling and instability in one or more peripheral and/or vertebral articulations, usually accompanied by only mild pain. Today, the terms Charcot's joints, neurotrophic joints, neuropathic osteoarthropathy, tabetic arthropathy, and neuropathic arthritis are used interchangeably to describe an arthritis that is associated with sensory neural deficit.

PATHOGENESIS

The pathogenesis of neuropathic arthropathy has remained controversial since Charcot's era. Various patterns of joint degeneration and tissue injury have been described, depending on the associated disorder. The most widely accepted "neurotraumatic" theory postulates that initial injury to the nociceptors of the joint and to the periarticular tissues by chronic infection (syphilis), metabolic disease (diabetes), or mechanical trauma leads to abnormal sensation, diminished proprioception, and joint instability.

Neuropathic joints also have increased blood flow, which has been reported to be up to five times the normal rate in diabetic neuropathy. A second hypothesis, the "neurovascular" theory, suggests the underlying disease produces a hypervascularized area within subchondral bone, possibly mediated by direct nerve damage or sympathetic disjunction. The region becomes characterized by increased osteoclastic resorption and osteoporosis. These neurovascular changes result in pathologic microfractures, eventual subchondral collapse, and joint destruction. However, the observation of active resorption of subchondral trabeculae by osteoclasts in vascular connective tissue reticulum characterized by dilated channels has been an inconsistent finding in histologic studies.

Affected joints progress through three discrete phases: destructive, reparative, and quiescent. The destructive or atrophic phase is typified by joint swelling, hyperemia, and active osteoclastic bone resorption. The hypertrophic reparative sclerotic phase begins when the joint is placed "at rest"—protected from further injury. During repair, a dense fibrous tissue forms within the joint, and dense sclerotic bone is deposited at the joint line and within the surrounding tissue. The reparative or hypertrophic phase may actually provide improved joint stability from the combined effect of osteophyte production, myositis ossificans, and the accumulation and fusion of dense, sclerotic bone. The quiescent phase is distinguished by a decrease in vascularity, a stabilizing of the periarticular reaction and associated tissues, and significant osseous sclerosis.

HISTOLOGY

Distinguishing histologic features include (Fig. 53-1) the appearance of osseous and cartilaginous debris deep within the synovium (most reliable finding), normal metachromatic staining of neuropathic cartilage, frequent appearance of hemosiderin from intraarticular hemorrhage, and metaplastic tissue characteristics (requires specialized staining).

IMAGING

Early radiographic findings may resemble the beginning of osteoarthritic disease. Two imaging patterns reflect the atrophic and

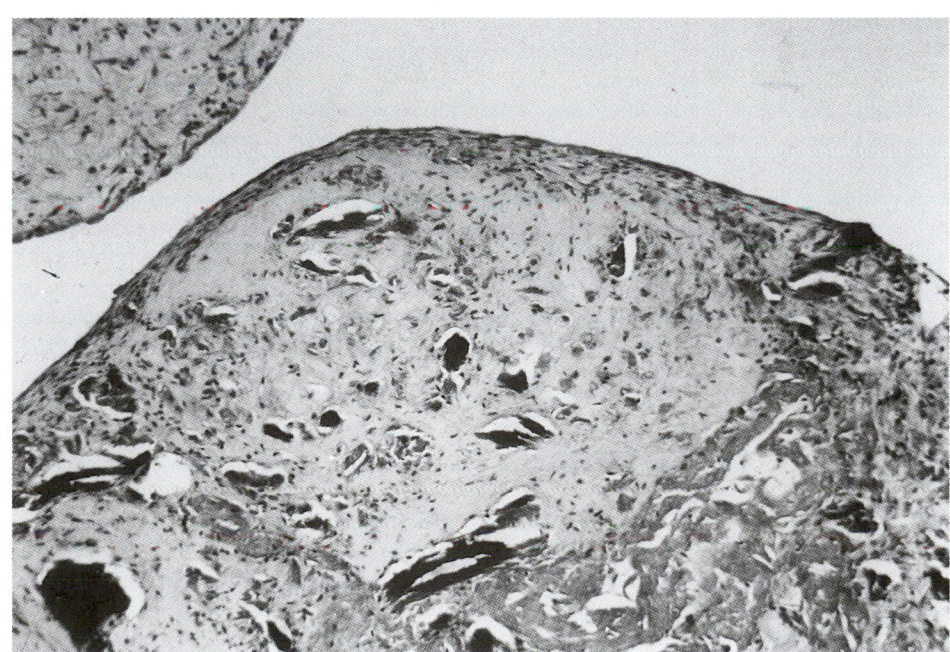

Figure 53-1
Photomicrograph of synovial tissue containing embedded fragments of bone debris consistent with neuropathic joint (×110).

hypertrophic phases described. The atrophic pattern is characterized by massive bone resorption and rapid disintegration of the joint, a pattern encountered most commonly in the hip, shoulder, and foot. The hypertrophic pattern is characterized by severe joint destruction, periarticular new bone formation (speckled calcification), osteophytes, fractures, and osseous debris. Migration of bony fragments along tissue planes has also been described. Hypertrophic patterns are commonly seen in the knee, elbow, and ankle.

CLINICAL PRESENTATION

The typical presentation is that of a diffusely swollen, warm, erythematous joint. Although neuropathic joints have occasionally been described as "painless," patients usually do have some degree of pain which is much less than would be expected based on the degree of changes present. Most patients provide a nonspecific history of trauma. One-third reportedly do not demonstrate a neurologic deficit. During the early course, a large joint effusion is generally present. In later stages, swelling may subside. Swelling is often associated with mild erythema that raises the suspicion of septic arthritis. As the disease progresses, joint instability is more evident. If significant fragmentation has occurred, palpation of soft tissues surrounding superficial joints may reveal the presence of osseous debris. In advanced cases, joints may feel similar to a "bag of bones."

Neuropathic arthropathy occurs in fewer than 1 percent of patients with diabetes mellitus (most common cause) and in 5 percent of those with peripheral neuropathy. Commonly affected joints include the tarsal, midtarsal, tarsometatarsal, metatarsophalangeal, and interphalangeal.

Neuropathic arthropathy secondary to syphilis occurs in 5 to 10 percent of patients (usually >60 years of age) with tabes dorsalis. Joints commonly involved are the hip, knee, or spine. Upper-extremity involvement is less common.

Neuropathic joints occur in 20 to 40 percent of patients with syringomyelia (most common cause of upper extremity neuroarthropathy). The majority have a monarticular presentation of the shoulder, and less commonly the elbow, and 20 percent of cases present with involvement of multiple, upper-extremity joints.

Additional peripheral neuropathies associated with neuropathic joint include leprosy, amyloidosis, Charcot-Marie-Tooth disease, multiple sclerosis, chronic demyelinating polyradiculopathy, gigantism, and alcoholism. Multiple intraarticular steroid injections have also been described as producing a type of neuropathic arthropathy. Subclinical inherited neuropathy is a term recently described in the literature to account for primary disease of idiopathic origin. Neuropathic joints in the pediatric population are usually associated with congenital insensitivity to pain, spinal dysraphism, or the Riley-Day syndrome.

MANAGEMENT

Management varies from protection and bracing to arthrodesis. Treatment of the underlying neurologic disorder (if treatable) associated with systemic disorders is the essential first step in management. Patient education, joint protection strategies, and early detection of fractures are general management principles. Protective measures include limb immobilization, restricted weightbearing, and functional bracing. Surgery, which is reserved for cases of advanced joint destruction with marked disability, is performed during quiescent rather than active stages of the disease, to decrease the risk of failure.

THE SPINE

Neuropathic spine has been historically associated with syphilis. Recently, syringomyelia, diabetes, congenital insensitivity to pain, spinal cord injury, and old age have also been identified as etiologic. The thoracolumbar junction and lumbar spine are most frequently involved; cervical spine involvement occurs in syringomyelia. Patients usually exhibit a painless, progressive spinal deformity, varying from significant hypermobility to ankylosis. Nerve root compression or bowel/bladder dysfunction can be present in long-standing cases.

Radiographically, massive new bone formation is characteristic. Destruction of facets occurs in conjunction with the development of marginal osteophytes secondary to instability ("parrot's beak"). Disc space narrowing and retrolisthesis can occur with frank dislocation in severe cases. The differential diagnosis includes severe osteoarthritis, osteomyelitis, Paget's disease, and skeletal metastases.

Traditionally, long-term cast or brace immobilization is used to stabilize the hypermobile segment(s). A higher-risk, combined anterior and posterior fusion technique with instrumentation and bone grafting has recently been advocated to prevent disastrous neurologic sequelae that may accompany instability and marked deformity.

THE UPPER EXTREMITY

Neuropathic joints of the upper extremity typically exhibit less symptomatology and more joint destruction and instability than the weight-bearing lower extremities and may be underreported. The affected shoulder is usually associated with syringomyelia, but has been noted in syphilis, diabetes, Arnold-Chiari malformation, cervical spondylosis, adhesive arachnoiditis, tuberculous arachnoiditis, and post-traumatic syringomyelia. Painless swelling and limited active motion with passive motion maintained are typical clinical features. Aspiration yields a straw-colored fluid with particulate debris. Cultures are taken to rule out infection. Radiographic findings are characterized by osteolysis and osseous fragmentation and destruction that may culminate in subluxation or frank dislocation (Fig. 53-2).

Initial treatment includes restricted activity and immobilization with a sling. Arthrodesis can be considered when marked instability is present. Chronic erosion/resorption presents difficulties for arthrodesis in glenohumeral disease and for joints in the acute inflammatory stage. Prosthetic arthroplasty is an unacceptable choice, because of inadequate glenoid bone stock, prosthetic loosening, and instability secondary to soft tissue compromise.

Neuropathic elbows usually occur in association with syringomyelia, syphilis, and congenital insensitivity to pain, and less commonly with diabetes, Charcot-Marie-Tooth, and a rare idiopathic form. Significant swelling may be present. Late radiographic findings include marked joint destruction and subluxation of radiohumeral and ulna-humeral articulations (Fig. 53-3). Sclerosis, osteophytes, periarticular swelling, and calcification may also be evident.

Functional bracing should provide functional flexion and extension while neutralizing varus and valgus stresses. Arthrodesis can be considered; however, long periods of immobilization are required for successful fusion, and the nonunion rate is high.

Neuropathic arthropathy of the wrist and hand may occur with diabetes, leprosy, congenital indifference to pain, syringomyelia, and syphilis. In the absence of significant pain or history of trauma, patients usually present with swelling and deformity of the wrist. Radiographic findings include narrowed intercarpal spaces, disorganized carpal alignment and resorbed carpal bones, subchondral sclerosis, diffuse periostitis, cysts, and joint debris.

Management focuses on protection using immobilization and functional bracing. Arthrodesis may be appropriate when marked instability is present. Total wrist arthroplasty and arthroplasty of the small joints of the hand are contraindicated.

Rare sternoclavicular joint involvement is associated with syringomyelia. There is massive, progressive swelling of the medial portion of the clavicle. Osteomyelitis and tumor should be part of the differential diagnosis. If a neuropathic etiology is confirmed, supportive, symptomatic treatment is applied unless vital structures posterior to the sternum are at risk of being compromised.

THE LOWER EXTREMITY

Neuropathic arthropathy of the hip is most commonly associated with syphilis. Two patterns have been described: femoral head or neck fracture produced by minimal trauma, and an "arthritic" type characterized by progressive wear and fragmentation of the femoral head and acetabulum, leading to extensive joint destruction. Patients usually present with a progressive, painless limp. Range of motion is maintained. Crepitus may be present. Radiographic findings include extensive resorption of the femoral head and neck, and periarticular new bone deposits and fragmentation.

Management focuses on symptomatic relief. Some patients will only require a cane even with extensive radiographic changes. Debridement and synovectomy with loose body removal can provide limited pain relief in selected patients; periarticular bone and scar tissue should not be disturbed, because they provide some degree of joint stability.

When an acute femoral neck fracture occurs, treatments include closed reduction and internal fixation, or primary resection arthroplasty. The nonunion rate with internal fixation is extremely high; prolonged postoperative protection with traction or a spica cast is recommended. Prosthetic replacement also has a high complication rate and has only been infrequently utilized. Arthrodesis is rarely successful.

The neuropathic knee joint is especially susceptible to instability and progressive destruction from the effects of weightbearing activity. Affected joints occur more frequently with syphilis and diabetes. Clinical findings include swelling, instability, pain, and crepitus; spontaneous dislocation has been reported. Progressive bony destruction, fragmentation, hypertrophic new bone formation, and subluxation are radiographic findings (Fig. 53-4).

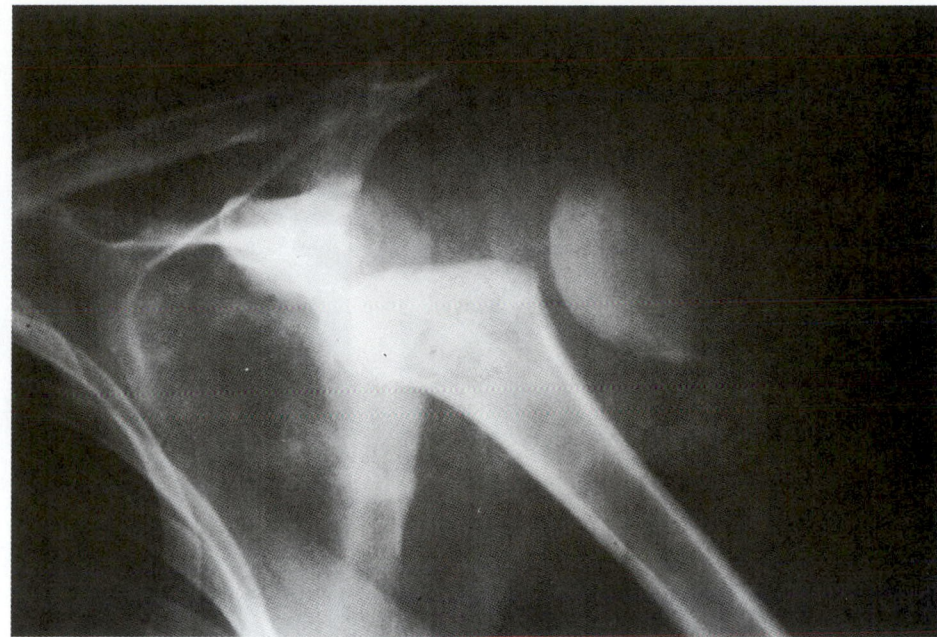

Figure 53-2
Anteroposterior radiograph of a neuropathic shoulder with fragmentation and dissolution of the proximal humerus.

Management includes protective bracing to enhance stability and to reduce shear stresses. Arthrodesis has enjoyed reasonable success and is an option if bracing fails to provide adequate stability and functional improvement. Local swelling and warmth should be controlled with casting or bracing prior to arthrodesis; successful union requires operating during the quiescent disease phase. Total knee arthroplasty is controversial and cannot be recommended.

Since weightbearing force-transmission biomechanically links the ankle with all of the joints of the foot, any disturbance will induce

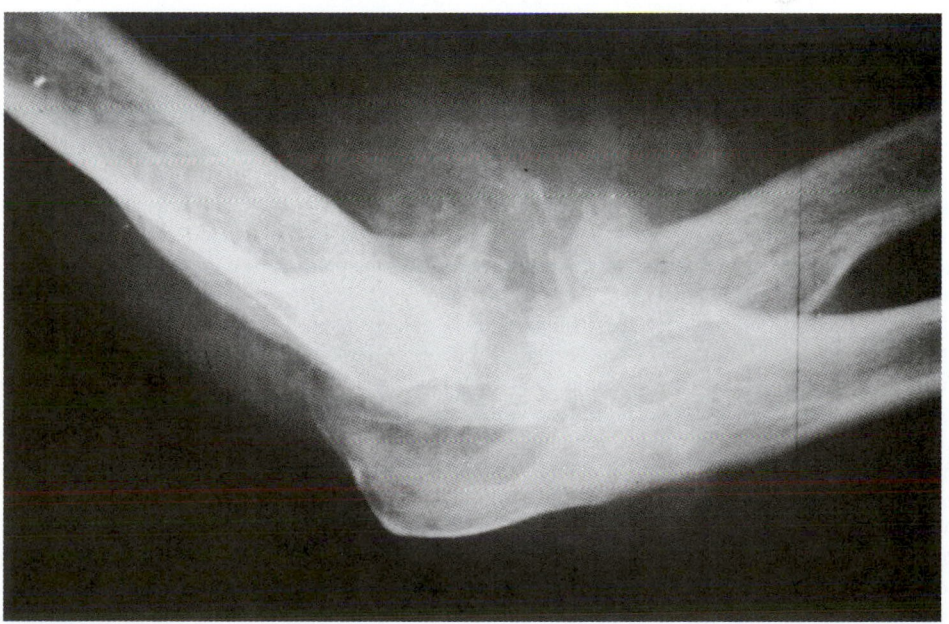

Figure 53-3
Lateral radiograph of the elbow in a patient with syringomyelia. There is destruction of the ulnohumeral and radiohumeral joints. Note the periarticular calcification and osteophyte formation.

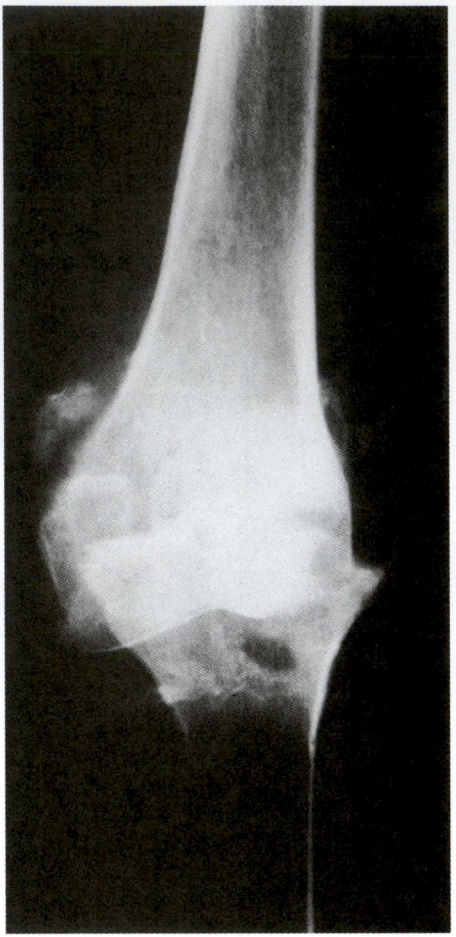
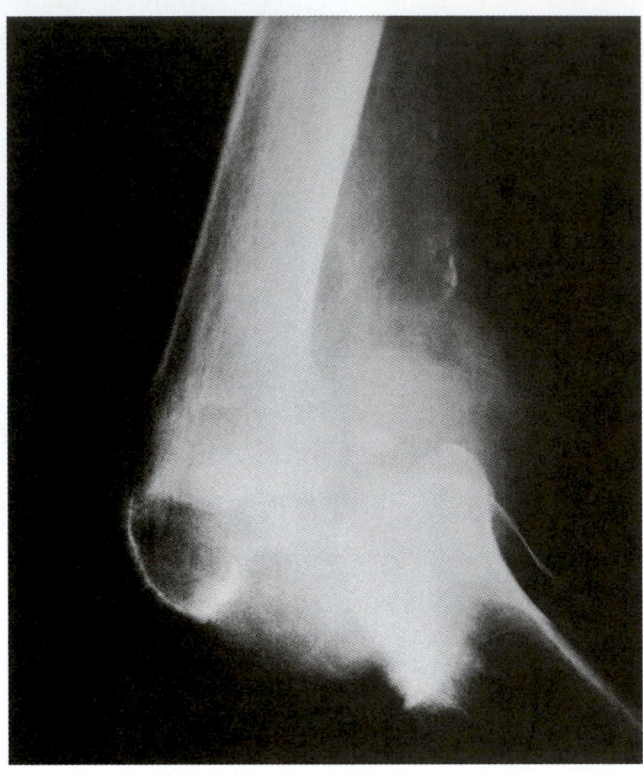

A   B

Figure 53-4
Anteroposterior and lateral radiographs of the knee in a patient with tabes dorsalis. There is gross
subluxation of the tibiofemoral joint as well as joint space obliteration and periarticular calcification.

changes in other joints, a complex linkage that may explain the progression to the severe destructive changes encountered in neuropathic arthropathy.

A common cause of neuropathic arthropathy in the foot and ankle is long-standing diabetic peripheral neuropathy. Patients are typically older (50 to 60 years) and present with diminished vibratory sense, anhidrosis, loss of ankle reflexes, and often exhibit unilateral involvement. Bilateral involvement occurs in up to 25 percent of patients and does not appear to be related to disease severity or the presence of retinopathy and nephropathy.

Clinical presentation includes the insidious onset of a painless, warm, swollen, and erythematous foot or ankle. Patients often complain that their shoes no longer fit. Examination may show fixed varus or valgus deformities of the ankle, a shortened/thickened foot, rocker-bottom deformity from collapse of the longitudinal arch, or ulcers and painful callosities from hammer-toes and thinning of the fat pad beneath the metatarsal heads.

Radiographs may demonstrate fractures or peritalar dislocations, and loose bodies, subchondral sclerosis, tibiofibular dissociation, osteophytes, and vascular calcification are frequently seen (Fig. 53-5). Valgus or varus deformity is often present. The talus may show osteonecrosis with collapse leading to disintegration. Generally, changes are hypertrophic with differing patterns and stages of fragmentation, resorption, sclerosis, periarticular calcification, and new bone formation (Fig. 53-6). Bony prominences leading to plantar ulceration may

develop from collapse of arches. Less often, navicular dislocations, Lisfranc's fracture-dislocations, calcaneal tuberosity avulsions, and cuneiform destruction can occur.

Metatarsophalangeal joint involvement can result in dorsal dislocation of the proximal phalanx. Plantar callosities and ulcerations are frequent. Dissolution of the metatarsal neck and shaft, from infection or a hypervascular state, results in a "pencil-in-cup" deformity. Similar pathology in the proximal phalanges can produce an hourglass-shaped deformity.

The differential diagnosis includes psoriatic arthritis, rheumatoid arthritis, gout, neoplasm, tuberculosis, and osteomyelitis. Differentiating osteomyelitis from neuropathic arthropathy can be problematic because of the potential to occur together. It is essential to distinguish between these two conditions because the management differs significantly. The "gold standard" for diagnosis appears to be histologic study of synovium and bone biopsy. Less successful approaches include three-phase bone scans (uptake in all three phases for both disorders), gallium scans (nonspecific), magnetic resonance imaging (nonspecific), white blood cell scan with indium labeling (possible false positives), and dynamic bone scanning (three-phase bone scan plus a computerized blood flow study; reported success, experience limited).

Treatment of the neuropathic ankle and foot starts with patient education and management of the underlying disease. Daily inspection and meticulous foot care are cornerstones of therapy and should be effective if instituted prior to development of arthropathy. Supplements of vitamin B_{12}, thiamine, and pyridoxine have been efficacious in patients with leprosy.

A protective well-padded cast or polypropylene splint should be used for 6 to 12 weeks to reduce swelling and associated inflammatory changes. Patients should be kept nonweightbearing until there is radiographic evidence of bony consolidation. Casting may continue for as long as 6 months. Custom-molded, extradepth shoes are recommended for further protection after weightbearing is permitted. Double upright patella tendon-bearing orthoses have also been recommended to decrease weightbearing across the foot and ankle. The orthosis may be continued for up to 1 year or until osteopenia has resolved.

Occasionally, nonoperative measures are not effective in controlling plantar ulceration and progressive instability. In these cases, the option of aggressive surgical debridement of ulcers and

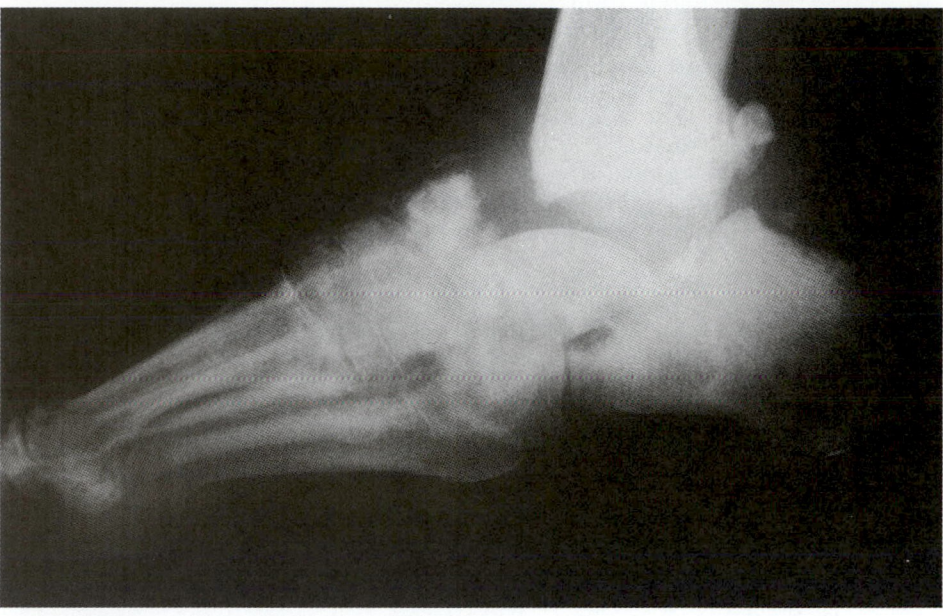

Figure 53-5
Lateral radiograph of the foot in a patient with insulin-dependent diabetes mellitus. There is extensive destruction of the talus extending into the midfoot.

exostectomy of bony prominences should be considered. Arthrodesis can be successful with the goals to reestablish normal weightbearing axes, restore the plantigrade foot, and remove the need for long-term bracing. Prolonged immobilization is necessary to increase the probability of a successful outcome. Surgery should be undertaken during the quiescent phase of the disease. Both internal and external fixation have been used. Early weightbearing, even in the presence of abundant callus formation, can result in resorption at the fusion site and subsequent nonunion. Long-term bracing may be necessary to obtain successful arthrodesis. Joint replacement has not been reported in neuropathic disease of the foot or ankle. Uncontrollable infection or severe, disabling instability may ultimately require amputation.

Neuropathic arthropathy is an uncommon, potentially devastating joint disease. Early diagnosis and management of the underlying neurologic disorder and the neuropathic joint represents the optimal treatment plan to prevent the progressive destruction that is inevitable in the neglected case.

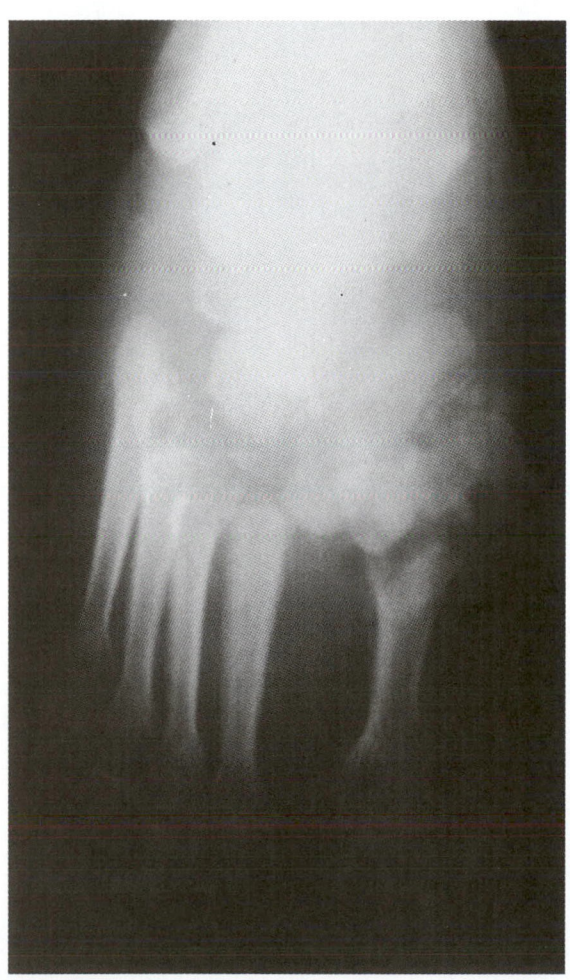

Figure 53-6
Anteroposterior radiograph of the foot of a patient with diabetes. Note the massive destruction of the tarsometatarsal articulation (Lisfranc's joint).

SUGGESTED READINGS

Bhaskaran R, Suresh K, Iyer GV: Charcot's elbow. *J Postgraduate Med* 1981; 27:194.

Bono JV, Roger DJ, Jacobs RL: Surgical arthrodesis of the neuropathic foot: A salvage procedure. *Clin Orthop* 1993; 296:14.

Brower AC, Allman RM: Pathogenesis of the neurotrophic joint: Neurotraumatic vs. neurovascular. *Radiology* 1981; 139:349.

Clohisy DR, Thompson RC Jr: Fractures associated with neuropathic arthropathy in adults who have juvenile-onset diabetes. *J Bone Joint Surg [Am]* 1988; 70:1192.

Devlin VJ, Ogilvie JW, Transfeldt EE, et al: Surgical treatment of neuropathic spinal arthropathy. *J Spinal Dis* 1991; 4:319.

Drennan DB, Fahey JJ, Maylahn DJ: Important factors in achieving arthrodesis of the Charcot knee. *J Bone Joint Surg [Am]* 1971; 53:1180.

Eloesser L: On the nature of neuropathic affections of the joints. *Ann Surg* 1917; 66:201.

Fitzgerald JA, Manning CW: Neuropathic arthropathy secondary to atypical congenital indifference to pain. *Proc Royal Soc Med* 1968; 61:663.

Harrelson JM: Management of the diabetic foot. *Orthop Clin North Am* 1989; 20:605.

Harrison MJ, Sacher M, Rosenblum BR, et al: Spinal Charcot arthropathy. *Neurosurg* 1991; 28:273.

Hoppenfeld S, Gross M, Giangarra C: Nonoperative treatment of neuropathic spinal arthropathy. *Spine* 1990; 15:54.

Johnson JT: Neuropathic fractures and joint injuries: Pathogenesis and rationale of prevention and treatment. *J Bone Joint Surg [Am]* 1967; 49:1.

Jordan WR: Neuritic manifestations in diabetes mellitus. *Arch Intern Med* 1936; 57:307.

Norman A, Robbins H, Milgram JE: The acute neuropathic arthropathy—a rapid, severely disorganizing form of arthritis. *Radiol* 1968; 90:1159.

Papa J, Myerson M, Girard P: Salvage, with arthrodesis, in intractable diabetic neuropathic arthropathy of the foot and ankle. *J Bone Joint Surg [Am]* 1993; 75:1056.

Robb JE, Rymaszewski LA, Reeves BF, Lacey CJN: Total hip replacement in a charcot joint: brief report. *J Bone Joint Surg [Br]* 1988; 70:489.

Sinha S, Munichoodappa CS, Kozak GP: Neuro-arthropathy (Charcot joints) in diabetes mellitus (clinical study 101 cases). *Medicine* 1972; 51:191.

Soudry M, Binazzi R, Johanson NA, et al: Total knee arthroplasty in Charcot and Charcot-like joints. *Clin Orthop* 1986; 208:199.

Stuart MJ, Morrey BF: Arthrodesis of the diabetic neuropathic ankle joint. *Clin Orthop* 1990; 253:209.

Williams B: Orthopaedic features in the presentation of syringomyelia. *J Bone Joint Surg [Br]* 1979; 61:314.

Chapter 54

DEGENERATIVE DISORDERS: CERVICAL

Nissim Ohana and Jeffrey M. Spivak

The mobile cervical spine is prone to degeneration, which often proceeds asymptomatically but may be the source of pain. *Cervical spondylosis* refers to degenerative disease of the cervical motion segments, with the associated vertebral body osteophytes and facet arthropathy. *Cervical disc herniation* may occur in an otherwise healthy appearing disc or in the setting of more advanced spondylosis.

The cervical spine is commonly divided into the upper cervical spine, from the occiput to C2, and the lower cervical spine, from C2 to T1. Degenerative disease of the cervical spine commonly affects only the lower cervical spine. With the exception of a brief review of arthritis of the atlantoaxial joint, this chapter discussion is limited to diseases of the lower cervical spine.

ANATOMY

There are seven cervical vertebrae and eight cervical nerves. The cervical spinal nerves exit above the named pedicle (above the lateral mass and lamina for C1) except for the C8 nerve, which exits between the C7 and T1 pedicles. The cervical nerve roots form and exit almost directly laterally, with little caudal excursion as in the lumbar spine; in fact, the upper cervical nerves pass somewhat cephalad to their exit foramina. Therefore, a disc herniation in the cervical spine causes compression of the forming and exiting nerve (C5 nerve at the C4-5 disc level, for example), unlike the lumbar spine where the forming or traversing root is affected from a typical posterolateral disc herniation (L5 nerve at the L4-5 disc level). However, as the roots exit above the named pedicle in the cervical spine and below the named pedicle in the lumbar spine, the typical posterolateral disc herniation in either location affects the root named by the vertebral level cephalad to the disc (as in the above examples).

The cervical *neural foramen* is oriented to allow for anterior passage of the cervical nerves within the foramen. It is located more laterally than the lumbar neural foramen, lateral to the vertebral body. Its borders are the pedicles superiorly and inferiorly, the uncovertebral joint anteromedially, and the facet joint posterolaterally. The cervical spinal nerves pass anteriorly and laterally through the foramen, posterior to the vertebral artery and vein, traveling longitudinally within the foramen transversarium of the transverse process.

The *uncovertebral joints*, also known as neurocentral joints or the joints of Lushka, are synovial joints located at the posterolateral corners of the cervical vertebrae which develop from the disc space during the childhood years. Cervical disc degeneration commonly leads to degeneration of the uncovertebral joints with osteophyte formation.

The cervical *facet joints* are located posterolaterally with respect to the vertebral bodies. The articular processes form the superior and inferior surfaces of the *lateral masses*, cylindrical columns of bone connected to the vertebral bodies by the cervical pedicles and connected left and right by the cervical laminae. Arthritic enlargement of the cervical facet joints commonly narrows the neural foramen, but, unlike the lumbar spine, generally does not directly affect the more medial spinal canal.

PATHOPHYSIOLOGY

Spondylosis can occur throughout the spine but is more common in the midcervical and the lower lumbar regions, due at least in part to the large amount of motion in these areas. Primary anatomic factors include disturbances in blood supply and bony architecture. The initial lesion is the deterioration of the intervertebral disc, usually insidious and most often asymptomatic. Reactive hyperostosis and osteophyte formation occur, which increase the diameter of the vertebral body at the level of the disc space. Posterior vertebral and posterolateral uncovertebral osteophytes may significantly reduce the cross sectional area of the spinal canal and neural foramen, respectively, at the spondylotic level (Fig. 54-1).

As the process continues, the progressive encroachment on the spinal canal and neuroforamina leads to compression of the spinal cord and nerve roots. Chronic spinal cord compression results in intrinsic changes including degeneration of the posterior and lateral white matter tracts and destruction of neurons by phagocytosis (neuronophagia) and gliosis in the anterior and posterior horns of the gray

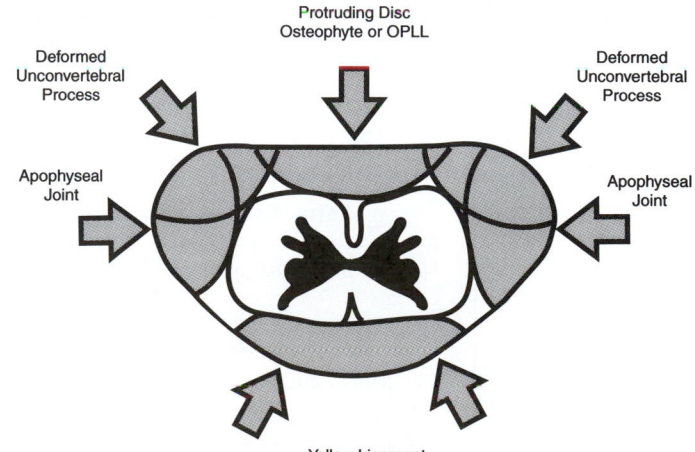

Figure 54-1

Anatomic structures which may encroach along the circumference of the spinal canal. (Reproduced with permission from Bernhardt M, Hynes RA, Blume HW, et al: Current concepts review. Cervical spondylotic myelopathy. *J Bone Joint [Am]* 1993; 75:120.)

matter. Atrophy of the dorsal nerve root fibers may occur, and to a lesser degree, the ventral nerve roots fibers. Experimentally, it has been shown that a number of pathophysiologic changes occur in the spinal cord before gross demyelinization and destruction of the white matter, including blockage of axoplasmic flow and stretching of the intrinsic transverse terminations of the anterior spinal artery.

In the early stage of cervical spondylosis, the disc becomes dehydrated and eventually collapses. At this stage, complete posterior annular tears may allow the disc to herniate as a soft fragment without concomitant chondroosseous spurs. In time, spurs commonly form along the posterior and the posterolateral margins in response to the altered anatomy and biomechanics of the motion segment. The most common location of a soft disc herniation is posterolaterally; however, herniation may occur anteriorly or posteriorly (a central herniation) through the posterior longitudinal ligament (PLL). Anterior herniation with concomitant osteophyte formation can occasionally cause extrinsic compression of the esophagus and dysphagia; the vast majority remain asymptomatic.

The typical age of clinical presentation for cervical spondylosis is 40 to 50 years old; cervical disc herniations present at a somewhat younger age. Men are affected more commonly than women. Risk factors include frequent lifting and excessive driving and smoking. The most commonly affected level is C5-6, followed by C6-7 and C4-5.

CLINICAL PRESENTATION

Degenerative disease of the cervical spine may present with one or a combination of four sets of clinical symptoms and signs: headache, neck pain, radiculopathy, and myelopathy.

Generalized occipital headaches are common in patients with cervical spondylosis as well as neck pain and stiffness. Headache is also common in both acute and chronic cervical strain injuries. The etiology of the headache is unclear in this latter setting. Headache alone without neck pain and stiffness is uncommon, and not likely to be related to any cervical spine disease. Unilateral occipital headache may be related to unilateral arthritis of the C1-2 facet joint with irritation of the ipsilateral C2 (greater occipital) nerve.

Neck pain is the most common presenting symptom for both osseous and soft tissue disorders of the cervical spine. The actual source of the pain is commonly unclear, but the pain may be related to the discs, ligaments, musculature, and/or neural elements. Posterior neck pain with stiffness is common in cervical spondylosis, muscular strain syndromes, and instability due to trauma, degenerative disease, and inflammatory disease. Neck pain related to these disorders may also be unilateral, with radiation to the scapula, shoulder, or anterior chest wall. Typical patterns of referral of sclerotomal pain, elicited by facet joint injection, have been described. Acute central disc herniations, with elevation and stretch of the PLL, may also present as acute neck pain. Posterolateral disc herniations of the upper cervical spine, with pain along the C3 or C4 roots, typically present as unilateral neck pain only, representing the dermatomal distribution of these root levels.

Radiculopathy refers to radiating pain from the neck into one or both upper extremities, due to irritation and/or compression of one or more cervical spinal nerves. Most commonly only one extremity is involved, and the pain radiates along a typical dermatomal distribution (Fig. 54-1). Radicular pain is typically accompanied by complaints of sensory disturbance (e.g., numbness, tingling, burning) and muscular weakness. The most common causes of cervical radiculopathy are acute cervical disc herniations and compression due to progressive cervical spondylosis. The differential diagnosis of radicular pain and neurologic dysfunction is listed in Table 54-1.

Myelopathy is the term used to describe the clinical signs and symptoms of spinal cord dysfunction. This can be caused by a compression of the spinal cord within the spinal canal (compressive myelopathy) or medical processes affecting the spinal cord and spinal cord function (medical myelopathy). The differential diagnosis of myelopathy is listed in Table 54-2. Myelopathy due to cervical spondylosis is the most common type of spinal cord dysfunction in patients who are greater than 55 years of age. Cervical spondylotic myelopathy can be divided into five distinct syndromes on the basis of clinical presentation: lateral, medial, combined, vascular, and anterior. Table 54-3 summarizes the differences among the five clinical patterns.

PHYSICAL EXAM

The physical exam begins by inspection of the patient's gait, the head and neck position, and the presence or absence of muscle atrophy of the extremities. Gait abnormalities in cervical myelopathy include spasticity and poor balance with unsteadiness. *Dysdiadochokinesia,* defined as difficulty with tandem gait, is an early sign of myelopathy. A generalized weakness of the lower extremities may also be found, but is uncommon.

Table 54-1

The Differential Diagnosis of Cervical Radiculopathy

Tumors: intraspinal and extraspinal

Entrapment syndromes of the upper extremity
  Median nerve: pronator syndrome, anterior interosseous syndrome, carpal tunnel syndrome, palmar cutaneous nerve syndrome
  Ulnar nerve: cubital tunnel syndrome, Guyon's canal entrapment
  Radial nerve: radial tunnel syndrome (PIN syndrome)

Thoracic outlet syndrome

Brachial plexus disorder
  Idiopathic branchial neuritis
  Brachial plexopathy

Table 54-2

The Differential Diagnosis of Myelopathy

Compressive myelopathy
  Cervical spondylosis with stenosis
  Cervical disc herniation
  Fracture
  Spondylolisthesis
  Tumor
    Vertebral column primary tumor
    Metastatic tumor
  Infection
    Epidural abscess
    Discitis or osteomyelitis with epidural extension
  Epidural hematoma
  Syringomyelia

Medical myelopathy
  Idiopathic acute or subacute transverse myelitis
  Postinfectious and postvaccination myelitis
  Multiple sclerosis
  Amyotrophic lateral sclerosis
  Infectious myelitis: viral, bacterial, fungal, parasitic
  Arachnoiditis
  Vascular disease of the pinal cord
    Atherosclerosis
    Epidural arteriovenous malformation
  Connective tissue disease
  Paraneoplastic myelopathy
  Metabolic and nutritional disease of the spinal cord
    Vitamin B_{12} deficiency
    Chronic liver disease
  Toxins
  Decompression illness (Caisson's Disease)
  Electrical injury
  Radiation injury (postradiation therapy)
  Necrotic myelopathy of unknown cause

Palpation of the neck is done to assess for possible tenderness, abnormal bony contours, and paraspinal muscle spasm. Limitations in neck range of motion are noted.

A thorough neurologic exam is necessary to evaluate for focal neurologic defects (common in radiculopathy) and for upper motor neuron signs (common in myelopathy). Compression of a cervical nerve root may cause sensory disturbances (e.g., hypesthesia, numbness), reflex diminution or loss, and motor weakness in a specific dermatomal pattern (Table 54-4).

Hyperactive or abnormal reflexes in the upper and lower extremities may indicate an upper motor neuron lesion due to cervical myelopathy. The *Hoffmann reflex* is present if the ipsilateral interphalangeal joints of the thumb and index finger flex when the volar surface of the terminal phalanx of the long finger is rapidly extended. Extension of the patient's neck may increase the appearance of a positive reflex. One must remember that a Hoffmann reflex is found bilaterally in 10 to 15 percent of the normal population, but a unilateral Hoffman reflex is always considered pathologic. Another abnormal finding is the *inverted radial response*, characterized by spontaneous flexion of the digits when the examiner attempts to elicit the brachioradialis reflex. Examination for a *jaw jerk reflex* is done in patients with signs of myelopathy. A positive response is a reflex jaw contraction following a hammer tap opening the jaw. The jaw jerk should be negative in cervical myelopathy. If positive, this implies that the source of the spinal cord dysfunction is above the foramen magnum.

Patients may describe an electric shock–like sensation while doing neck flexion and extension (most commonly during flexion); this is known as a positive *Lhermitte's sign*. The *Babinski sign* is an abnormal plantar response (extensor or splaying) of the toes with stimulation of the plantar foot surface. It commonly does not appear until the myelopathy becomes severe. *Clonus* of the lower extremities, seen as sustained rapid ankle plantarflexion in response to forced dorsiflexion, is also a sign of profound upper motor neuron dysfunction.

Diffuse nondermatomal sensory changes commonly occur in cervical myelopathy, including abnormal sensation of pain, temperature, or light touch stimulus. A more specific sensory finding is a loss of position and vibratory sensation. Subtle deficits in fine motor control are commonly found early in cervical myelopathy.

Two specific nerve root tension tests have been described in the upper extremity which are part of the standard exam for cervical

---

Table 54-3

Characteristics of the Different Syndromes of Cervical Spondylotic Myelopathy

Syndrome	Pain	Gait Abnormality	Involvement of Extremities	Laterality
Lateral (radicular)	Yes	Sometimes	Upper	Often unilateral
Medial (myelopathic)	No	Yes	Lower	Usually bilateral
Combined	Sometimes	Yes	Upper and lower	Unilateral in upper extremities, bilateral in lower extremities
Vascular	No	Yes	Upper and lower	Bilateral
Anterior (painless weakness of the upper extremity)	No	No	Upper	Often unilateral

Table 54-4

Neurologic Testing of Upper Extremity Nerve Root Function

Nerve Root	Reflex	Sensation	Muscle
C4	None	Posterolateral neck	None
C5	Biceps	Lateral arm	Deltoid, biceps
C6	Brachioradialis	Lateral forearm and thumb	Wridst extensors Biceps
C7	Triceps	Middle finger	Triceps, wrist flexors Finger extensors
C8	None	Ring, little fingers	Finger flexors, intrinsics
T1	None	Medial arm and forearm	Intrinsics

radiculopathy. *Spurling's test* is performed by having the patient extend the neck and rotate and laterally bend the head toward the affected side; an axial compressive force is then applied by the examiner to the top of the patient's head. The test is considered positive when the maneuver elicits the patient's typical radicular arm pain. The *shoulder abduction relief sign* is tested for in patients with active radicular arm pain. The palm of the hand of the patient's affected arm is placed on the top of the patient's head. The sign is present if the maneuver results in the patient experiencing relief of the radicular pain, due to shortening of the nerve path length with resultant relaxation of the stretch along the brachial plexus. Some patients may even report during the intake history that pain is relieved with placing the affected arm overhead, and some may even maintain the arm in this position while being examined.

In order to quantify the severity of myelopathy and its impact on daily activities and function, different scales have been developed. The two most popular are Nurick's classification and the assessment scale of the Japanese Orthopaedic Association (JOA). *Nurick's classification* of clinical disability in cervical spondylotic myelopathy is mainly on the basis of gait, with five grades as follows:

Grade 0:   Only root signs and symptoms, no cord involvement
Grade I: Clinical signs of cord involvement, normal gait
Grade II: Mild gait abnormality, able to be employed
Grade III: Gait abnormality preventing employment
Grade IV: Can ambulate only with assistance
Grade V: Unable to ambulate (chairbound or bedridden)

The *JOA assessment scale* for cervical myelopathy is a more elaborate quantitative scoring system involving four categories: motor dysfunction of the upper extremity, motor dysfunction of the lower extremity, sensory deficit, and sphincter dysfunction. Within each category, scores can range from 0 (severe disability) to 3 or 4 (no disability), with a maximal score of 17 for patients with no clinical dysfunction.

The shoulder joint is often a potential source for some or all of the patient's pain and complaints. A thorough shoulder evaluation is important when indicated by the patient's pain. This includes shoulder range of motion testing, examining for signs of impingement and rotator cuff pathology, and examination of the acromioclavicular joint.

In some cases, a lidocaine injection of the subacromial space may be helpful in differentiating the source of a patient's pain.

RADIOLOGIC EVALUATION

Plain radiographs of the cervical spine are used as a basic radiologic screening exam for patients with neck pain, radiculopathy, and clinical myelopathy. Plain radiographs are indicated in patients with neck pain greater than 4 to 6 weeks in duration; patients with a history of trauma; constitutional symptoms (fever, chills, fatigue, weight loss); previous tumors; and in patients over age 60.

Anterior-posterior (AP) and lateral views allow for evaluation of the overall vertebral column contour and the presence or absence of significant spondylotic changes (vertebral body and uncovertebral joint spurs, disc space narrowing), subluxations, and fractures.

Oblique views visualize the neuroforamina, including their anteromedial and posterolateral borders, the uncovertebral and facet joints, respectively. Dynamic flexion-extension lateral radiographs are useful in the evaluation of cervical segmental instability.

The AP diameter of the spinal canal can be estimated on the lateral radiograph. The posterior canal border is the spinolaminar line and the anterior border is the posterior aspect of the vertebral bodies. Most authors agree that the normal AP diameter of the spinal canal is approximately 17 to 18 mm from C3 to C7 with only slight variation between males and females. An AP diameter of less than 11 mm, with magnification taken into account, correlates with a high risk of cervical spondylotic myelopathy. The *Pavlov ratio* is the AP distance of the canal divided by the AP diameter of the vertebral body at its midportion, measured at each vertebral level on the lateral radiograph. As the measurement is expressed as a ratio, it is not affected by differences in radiographic magnification. A ratio of 1.0 or greater is considered normal; a ratio of less than 0.8 is indicative of a narrow spinal canal.

Advanced imaging studies, including CT scanning, MRI, and CT-myelography, provide additional anatomic detail of the spinal canal and neural elements. An advanced imaging study should be obtained whenever a profound focal neurologic deficit or signs of myelopathy are found on physical examination.

High-field-strength MRI provides optimal visualization of the soft tissue structures, including the intervertebral discs and spinal cord. Increased signal intensity within the spinal cord on T2-weighted images may represent scarring or myelomalacia. Dynamic MRI studies can be obtained with the neck in maximum flexion and extension to document the presence of dynamic spinal cord compression.

CT scanning provides better detail of the bony elements, and allows for more clear identification of ossification of the PLL. CT scans also provide the clearest evaluation of the neuroforamina and potential stenosis from uncovertebral and facet hypertrophy. Myelography with post-myelogram CT scanning can best visualize the neural and bony elements and can best differentiate between the hard (osteophyte) and soft tissue (disc, ligamentum flavum) aspects of spinal cord compression.

The *compressive ratio* can be calculated from the axial MRI or the post-myelography CT scan images. This is the ratio of the smallest AP diameter of the spinal cord to the broadest transverse diameter at a given spinal level. This ratio has been shown to have prognostic value; a ratio of less than 0.4 following decompression portends a guarded prognosis for recovery, while an increased ratio of more than 0.4 correlates with significant clinical recovery.

ELECTROPHYSIOLOGIC STUDIES

Electrophysiologic studies which may be useful in the evaluation of neurologic involvement in cervical disc disease include: electromyogram (EMG), nerve conduction velocity (NCV), and somatosensory evoked potentials (SSEP). EMG studies are very sensitive for cervical root irritation but are nonspecific. Overall, electrophysiologic studies are not used routinely; however, they may be helpful in establishing the diagnosis in questionable cases. They are particularly useful in differentiating between cervical radiculopathy, peripheral nerve entrapment syndrome, and peripheral neuropathy. They may also be useful in pinpointing the level of a cervical radiculopathy in cases without hard neurologic deficits and multilevel foraminal stenosis.

NATURAL HISTORY

Acute cervical radiculopathy, due either to an acute disc herniation or spondylotic spurs, is generally expected to resolve in 90 percent or more of cases within 6 to 12 weeks. The presence of hard neurologic deficits does not alter the expected recovery rate, but significant functional motor deficits may prompt a more rapid workup and surgical management.

The natural history of cervical myelopathy is variable. The disease course is prolonged, with long periods of nonprogressive disability common; however, some patients present with a progressively deteriorating course. Therefore, the spectrum of disease varies from a minor degree of dysfunction with few neurologic deficits over a long period of time to acute and catastrophic deterioration over a relatively short period of time. Unfortunately, it is currently impossible to predict which patients will have a rapid deteriorating course and to what degree patients can expect improvement after operative treatment. The prevention of further deterioration is a reasonable indication for surgery, but the best overall patient outcome may come from early operative intervention before major irreversible functional neurologic loss has occurred.

TREATMENT

NONOPERATIVE TREATMENT

All patients with neck pain and radiculopathy without major motor weakness and clinical myelopathy should be given an initial period of nonoperative treatment. The different treatments currently in use include immobilization, medications, and physical therapy including therapeutic modalities and exercises.

An initial short period of immobilization may be useful to rest the neck and reduce the inflammatory response to local soft-tissue injury. A soft foam cervical collar is most commonly used, and maintains the neck in neutral or slight flexion. Use of the collar should not exceed 2 weeks, and generally only a few days of collar use is appropriate before beginning mobilizing neck exercises. Prolonged use can lead to a dependency of the collar, both psychologically and by disuse weakening of the paracervical musculature.

Nonsteroidal anti-inflammatory drugs (NSAIDs) are the most commonly used medications for acute neck and radicular arm pain. It is believed that inflammatory reaction around the nerve root is an important factor in the generation of radicular pain, not only mechanical compression. Currently, there is a vast spectrum of NSAIDs in use; no single NSAID has been proven superior to the others.

Another group of medications commonly prescribed are muscle relaxants, which may improve pain by reduction of muscle spasm in acute neck pain. Their efficacy remains unproved. Severe pain may warrant the use of narcotic analgesics in the acute phase of radicular pain.

Steroid medications given orally in a high-dose, rapidly tapering schedule are also commonly used for severe acute radicular pain with or without focal neurologic findings. Cervical epidural steroid injections may also be helpful in pain reduction by diminishing the edema and local inflammatory response surrounding the nerve root. However, this procedure is invasive and without clearly proven efficacy.

Therapeutic modalities, including heat, cold, electrical stimulation, ultrasound, traction, trigger point injections, and manipulation, may help to improve muscle spasm and achieve some temporary pain relief, but their efficacy in the treatment of acute neck and radicular arm pain is unproved. Therapeutic exercises, including neck stretching, strengthening, and general fitness exercises may be of benefit. A patient education component to the therapy program is also considered by many to be useful.

OPERATIVE TREATMENT

The indications for surgery in cervical degenerative disease are based on the patient's complaints and clinical findings in correlation with the pathoanatomy seen on diagnostic testing. In general, pathoanatomic conditions amenable to surgery include segmental instability and compression of the neural elements from a disc herniation, advanced spondylosis, or vertebral subluxation. Surgery for degenerative disc disease without neurologic compression or instability remains controversial, as its efficacy compared to the natural history of the degenerative process is unclear.

Surgery for cervical degenerative disease is generally reserved for persistent symptoms despite adequate nonoperative treatment. More urgent surgical treatment is indicated for significant myelopathy and spinal cord compression and progressive nerve root dysfunction due to compression.

Factors to be considered in choosing the type of surgical treatment for cervical radiculopathy or myelopathy include the location and extent (number of levels) of the compression, the tissues causing the compression, the neural elements being compressed, and the overall sagittal alignment of the compressed portion of the cervical spine. Both anterior and posterior techniques can be used.

Anterior techniques include single or multilevel anterior cervical discectomy and *corpectomy* (vertebral body resection). The anterior cervical spine is approached through a transverse skin incision, dissecting between the sternocleidomastoid muscle laterally and the strap muscles medially, then between the carotid sheath laterally and the trachea and esophagus medially (see Chap. 13). One or more discs can be removed from anterior to posterior, and the midline portion of the intervening vertebral body can be removed using a high-speed burr.

Fusion of the interbody (disc) space is always recommended following anterior discectomy; multiple anterior iliac crest graft geometries have been described (Fig. 54-2). Following corpectomy, reconstruction can be achieved using tricortical anterior iliac crest graft, fibula strut graft, titanium mesh cylinders, and others. Bone cement and metallic pin reconstruction should be reserved for reconstruction following tumor resection, not for degenerative disease with a longer postoperative life expectancy. Anterior plate fixation of the cervical spine is becoming more common following multilevel discectomy and corpectomy, and may obviate the need for rigid postoperative external immobilization.

Posterior procedures can also accomplish both decompression and fusion of the cervical spine. *Keyhole foraminotomy*, which can be done at one or multiple sites, involves a small laminotomy at the root take-off with lateral extension to remove the medial one-third to one-half of the facet joint. This decompresses the posterolateral border of the nerve root foramen. Removal of the epidural venous cuff covering the root origin and exploration of the anterior epidural space for soft disc material or uncovertebral osteophytes using a microangled dissector may not be necessary to afford adequate nerve root decompression. Benefits of posterior foraminotomy include the lack of need for fusion, lack of risks of the anterior approach, and a more rapid patient recovery. Foraminotomy does not address any component of axial neck pain which may be due to spondylosis. It also cannot be used to decompress the spinal canal and spinal cord from central compression.

Posterior *cervical laminectomy* is historically the most common surgical procedure for multilevel cervical spondylotic myelopathy. Central posterior decompression of the spinal canal is achieved, and the laminectomy can be combined with foraminotomy for root decompression as well. One common technique for laminectomy includes bilateral troughs created with a burr at the lamina-facet joint junction, followed by completion of the troughs with a 1- or 2-mm Kerrison rongeur and direct posterior removal of the involved lamina. This technique avoids the use of any undercutting instruments in the central region where the spinal cord is being compressed. The most commonly reported complication of cervical laminectomy is postoperative instability and the development of spondylolisthesis and kyphosis. For this reason, laminectomy should only be performed in cervical spines with normal lordosis and preferably some spondylotic stiffening. In fact, laminectomy is ineffective in relieving anterior compression and therefore contraindicated for decompression of cervical stenosis in patients with a rigid kyphotic deformity.

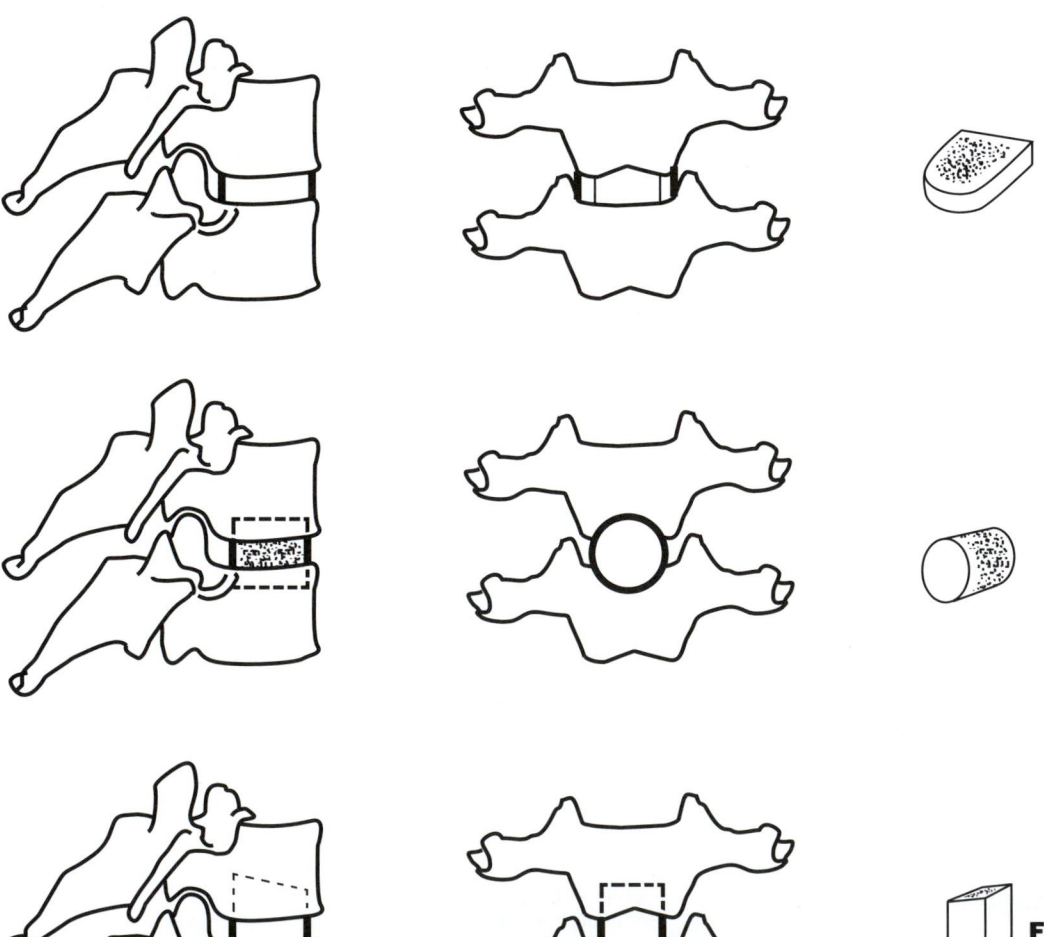

Figure 54-2
Types of anterior cervical interbody bone grafts. Upper, Smith-Robinson type tricortical graft; middle, Cloward-type bicortical graft; lower, Simmons-type keystone graft.

Cervical laminoplasty is an excellent alternative to laminectomy for multilevel posterior central decompression of the spinal canal, with improvement in postoperative spinal stability as compared to laminectomy. In laminoplasty, the position of the posterior lamina is shifted, not removed, to effect an increase in the cross-sectional area of the spinal canal. Multiple techniques have been described, including a single opening door, z-shaped osteotomies of the laminae, and a central-opening french-door configuration. Although they maintain increased stability, laminoplasty procedures also stiffen the cervical spine somewhat as compared to laminectomy. Like laminectomy, laminoplasty is contraindicated in patients with kyphosis or loss of the normal cervical lordosis.

Spinal fusion can also be accomplished posteriorly. Internal fixation techniques with intact midline posterior elements include spinous process wiring, sublaminar wiring, and hook/rod constructs, and lateral mass plate fixation. Following laminectomy, lateral mass plate fixation provides optimal stability when fusion is indicated (such as in segmental instability or a reducible multilevel kyphosis). Screw fixation through the plates pass into the medially directed pedicles at C2, C7, and T1, and laterally into the lateral masses at C3-C6.

Depending on the clinical scenario and pathoanatomy, anterior and/or posterior procedures may represent reasonable surgical options. Spinal fusion for neck pain and degenerative disc disease is commonly performed anteriorly. In cases of neck pain and segmental instability, both anterior fusion and posterior fusion with internal fixation are reasonable surgical options.

Radiculopathy due to an acute posterolateral soft disc herniation can be approached anteriorly with discectomy and fusion or posteriorly with foraminotomy and disc fragment excision. Foraminotomy should not be done if the disc herniation crosses the midline or causes central spinal cord compression. In patients with preexisting spondylosis and significant axial neck pain preexisting the radiculopathy, the anterior approach is generally chosen; interbody fusion is done to treat the spondylotic axial neck pain. In patients with radiculopathy due to uncovertebral or facet joint osteophytes, either anterior or posterior decompression can be performed.

In patients with myelopathy and cord compression due to anterior pathology at one or two levels, anterior decompression and fusion is generally recommended. With three or more levels of compression, posterior laminectomy or laminoplasty may be less morbid than three or more anterior discectomies or multilevel corpectomy, but is only an option for decompression in the nonkyphotic cervical spine.

OSSIFICATION OF THE POSTERIOR LONGITUDINAL LIGAMENT

Ossification of the posterior longitudinal ligament (OPLL) is seen most commonly in people of Asian descent; however, it is being reported with increasing frequency and similar clinical and radiographic manifestations in non-Asian populations. Of the patients who have OPLL 50 percent also have diffuse idiopathic skeletal hyperostosis (DISH). The pathogenesis in OPLL is an idiopathic ossification of the PLL causing an anterior compression of the spinal cord. Most commonly the disease involves the ligament at multiple levels, the segmental type. It may be segmented, continuous, localized, or mixed (Fig. 54-3).

The average age of onset is about 50. Almost all patients with OPLL have only mild subjective complaints such as neck pain or numbness in the hand, and do not have disturbances in the activity of daily living. About 10 to 15 percent of patients will have a spastic gait or clumsiness of the fingers. An acute aggravation of tetraparesis after a minor trauma such as a simple fall has been reported in about 20

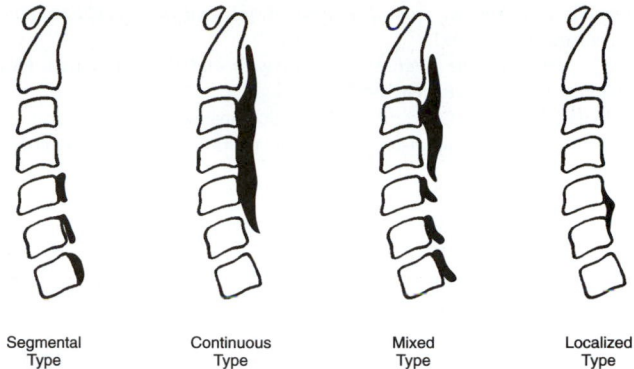

| Segmental Type | Continuous Type | Mixed Type | Localized Type |

Figure 54-3

Patterns of OPLL. Reproduced with permission from Satomi K, Hirabayashi K: Ossification of the posterior longitudinal ligament, in Rothman RH, Simeone FA (eds): *The Spine.* Philadelphia: WB Saunders; 1992; chap 21:641.

percent of the patients undergoing surgical treatment. A useful way to describe the clinical severity of the myelopathy in OPLL is the JOA score, described previously.

The continuous and mixed types of OPLL can be easily diagnosed on plain lateral radiographs; localized and segmental types may be overlooked. CT scanning with sagittal reconstructions is the most useful imaging test in determining the configuration of the ossification. Plain sagittal tomography can be useful for demonstration of small foci of ossification. MRI is much less effective in diagnosing and evaluating the anatomy of the ossification, but it is extremely useful in visualizing intraparenchymal pathology of the spinal cord.

In general, surgical intervention is indicated in patients who score 6 to 12 points on the JOA score. The final decision is made based upon the patient's age. The preferable surgical treatment is a posterior decompression through cervical laminoplasty. With anterior decompression, serious and potentially fatal complications can occur due to persistent cerebrospinal fluid leak with fistula formation and infection, as the dura may be absent or adherent to the ossified PLL.

UNILATERAL C1-2 FACET ARTHROSIS

An uncommon cause of unilateral upper neck pain and suboccipital headaches is from unilateral arthritis of the C1-2 facet joint. The suboccipital headache occurs from compression or irritation of the greater occipital nerve, the major branch of the posterior primary ramus C2, which exits between C1 and C2 adjacent to the facet joint.

Initial radiographs of patients with neck pain and unilateral suboccipital headaches should include an AP open-mouth view, where the C1-2 joints can be assessed. Unilateral facet arthrosis can be confirmed with CT scan coronal reconstructions or coronal tomograms. A fluoroscopic-guided lidocaine/steroid injection can be used as both a diagnostic test and treatment option. Persistent symptoms despite adequate nonoperative treatment can be successfully treated with a posterior spinal fusion of C1-2.

SUGGESTED READINGS

Bernhardt M, Hynes RA, Blume HW, et al: Current concepts review. Cervical spondylotic myelopathy. *J Bone Joint Surg [Am]* 1993; 75:119.

Boden SD, McCowin PR, Davis DO, et al: Abnormal magnetic-resonance scans of the cervical spine in asymptomatic subjects. A prospective investigation. *J Bone Joint Surg [Am]* 1990; 72:1178.

Bridwell KH, DeWard RL (eds): *The Textbook of Spinal Surgery*. Philadelphia: Lippincott-Raven; 1991.

Frymoyer JW (ed): *The Adult Spine. Principles and Practice*, 2d ed. Philadelphia: Lippincott-Raven; 1997.

Herkowitz HN, Kurz LT, Overholt DP: Surgical management of cervical soft disc herniation. A comparison between the anterior and posterior approach. *Spine* 1990; 15:1026.

Herkowitz HN: A comparison of anterior cervical fusion, cervical laminectomy, and cervical laminoplasty for the surgical management of multiple level spondylitic radiculopathy. *Spine* 1988; 13:774.

Lee F, Aldren Turner JW: Natural history and prognosis of cervical spondylosis. *Br Med J* 1963; 2:1607.

Rothman RH, Simeone FA (eds): *The Spine*, 4th ed. Philadelphia: WB Saunders; 1998.

Chapter 55

DEGENERATIVE DISORDERS: LUMBAR

Jeffrey M. Spivak and Nissim Ohana

Most degenerative lumbar spine disorders are related either to aging or to altered biomechanical stresses within the lumbar spine, resulting from trauma or deformity. Kikaldy-Willis and Farfan emphasized the importance of the three-joint complex of the motion segment (also known as the "functional spinal unit"), defined as two adjacent vertebrae and the connecting intervertebral disc, facet joints, and ligaments. Injury or degenerative involvement of any of the three joints, which form a functional tripod, causes abnormal biomechanical stresses that can affect the other joints and cause pain, instability, and deformity, with resulting disability and morbidity.

HERNIATED LUMBAR DISC

ANATOMY

The intervertebral disc is composed of the central nucleus pulposus and the outer annulus fibrosus. In the lumbar spine, the anterior annulus is considerably thicker and stronger than the posterior annulus. The posterior annulus is covered posteriorly by the posterior longitudinal ligament (PLL), a central longitudinal band with segmental expanses at each disc level. A disc is named by the vertebrae (or first sacral segment) surrounding it.

The *conus medullaris* is the sacral end of the spinal cord, typically at the L1-2 disc space. Below this, the lumbar and sacral nerve roots extend caudally as the *cauda equina* within the thecal sac. At each vertebral level, the left and right spinal nerves exit below their named vertebral pedicle (the L4 spinal nerve inferior to the L4 pedicle for example). These nerves typically form and separate from the thecal sac at the disc space above the pedicle. The lateral border of the forming spinal nerve is known as the *shoulder* of the nerve. The region of the acute angle between the formed spinal nerve and the continuing thecal sac is known as the nerve *axilla*. At times, two nerve roots may form from a single stalk off the thecal sac, and only later divide. This normal variant is known as a *conjoined nerve root*, and if compressed by a disc herniation, may present with symptoms of dysfunction of two segmental nerve levels.

CLASSIFICATION

Lumbar disc herniations are commonly described by the relationship of the herniated material to the posterior annulus fibrosus and posterior longitudinal ligament (PLL) and the continuity of the herniated material with the remainder of the disc. These descriptive terms are often confusing (Fig. 55-1). All types of true disc herniations must be differentiated from a *disc bulge*, a diffuse outpouching of the annulus fibrosus due to early disc degeneration and disc space collapse. A true *disc herniation* is a more focal anatomic derangement limited to a specific circumferential region of the annulus. Sometimes, this seemingly simple difference between a bulge and a herniation is not so clear, as some herniations may be quite broad based and appear as more diffuse bulges. True disc herniations can be *contained*, covered by an intact veil of posterior annulus and PLL, or *noncontained*, with the herniated fragment directly in contact with the anterior epidural space through a complete defect in the posterior annulus and PLL. Contained disc herniations are also known as *protrusions*, where herniated disc material is covered by some amount of intact posterior annulus and PLL. Noncontained disc herniations include *extrusions*, where the herniated material is in continuity with the disc space but extending completely into the epidural space, and *sequestrations*, where the herniated disc material has broken continuity with the disc space and is a free fragment of material in the epidural space. Generally speaking, when disc material extends from the disc space posterior to the vertebral body, it is noncontained. If it is covered by a remaining PLL, it is sometimes called a *subligamentous* extrusion.

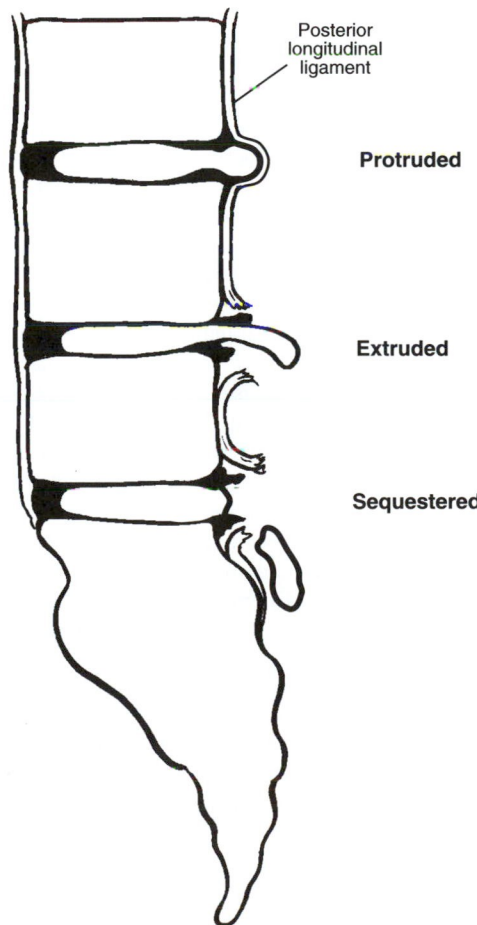

Figure 55-1
Types of disc herniations.

Lumbar disc herniations are also described by their anatomic location along the circumference of the annulus fibrosus. Anterior herniations (through the thicker anterior annulus) cause no neural element compression, and are not clinically significant for this reason. Herniations along the posterior annulus can be *central* (midline), *posterolateral* (most common, along the weaker lateral expansion of the PLL), *foraminal* (or *lateral*), or *extraforaminal* (or *far lateral*, lateral to the neural foramen). Broad herniations can easily extend into two or more of these zones. Central disc herniations may affect the spinal canal as a whole, causing stenosis, or can narrow one or both lateral recesses, affecting the forming nerve root at that level (L5 roots at the L4-5 disc space for example). Posterolateral herniations affect the forming nerve root at the level of the herniation. Foraminal and extraforaminal herniations affect the exiting nerve root at the level of the herniation (the L4 root at the L4-5 level for example).

Another descriptive term sometimes used is an *axillary disc herniation*. Most commonly, a typical posterolateral disc herniation compresses along the lateral border (the shoulder) of the forming spinal nerve. A noncontained disc herniation may extend superiorly into the axilla of the nerve root exiting above (an L4-5 herniation extending superiorly into the L4 root axilla for example). When a herniation causes this type of medial compression on the forming nerve, it is considered *axillary* in position. Axillary disc herniations may also arise from inferior migration of the disc material to affect the axilla of the forming nerve root at that level (an L4-5 herniation extending inferiorly to compress medially in the axilla of the L5 root).

PATHOPHYSIOLOGY

The intervertebral disc degenerates naturally through a series of events, including dehydration, intradiscal fissure, and fragmentation. This is followed by progressive annular disruption from the inner annular layers progressing more superficially, ultimately resulting in a complete annular tear and herniation of disc material into the spinal canal. Patients commonly experience episodes of back pain, often with radiation to the posterior thigh, during the time when fissuring and fragmentation take place and the annular layers are disrupting. Once disc material herniates into the canal, the pressure on the annulus by the fragment and the intradiscal pressure is relieved. Typically this is when sciatic lower extremity pain replaces the back pain. There are two basic mechanisms believed to be responsible for the lower extremity pain seen in disc herniations. The first one is a *tension mechanism*, common in young patients, and is the result of the spinal nerve stretching over the herniated disc material. The second is a *compressive mechanism*, more common in older patients, which occurs when the spinal nerve is compressed between the herniated disc material and a rigid portion of the spinal canal, including the lamina and ligamentum posteriorly and the medial border of the pedicle laterally. In both mechanisms, pain is generated by the pressure, which initiates an inflammatory response.

The two most common levels of disc herniation are L4-5 and L5-S1. Together, herniations at these levels comprise 90 percent of all symptomatic lumbar disc herniations. The L3-4 level is the next most common. A symptomatic disc herniation occurs during the lifetime of about 2 percent of the population. The peak age of occurrence is 30 to 50 years old.

CLINICAL PRESENTATION

Patients typically complain of severe radiating lower extremity pain (*radiculopathy*). Pain from typical low lumbar nerve dysfunction travels posterior in the thigh and leg, radiating in a dermatomal pattern to the sole and lateral foot (S1) or the dorsal aspect of the ankle and foot (L5). Upper lumbar nerve pain radiates to the anterior thigh (L2, L3) and anterior knee and medial leg (L4). The pain is usually abrupt in onset rather than insidious, and may or may not be related to a specific injury or activity. Often there is a months-to-years history of more central back pain, which may improve or abate totally with the onset of the lower extremity pain. The leg pain is commonly described as sharp or stabbing. It is more commonly constant but may vary in intensity with position or activity. Patients are usually more comfortable standing rather than sitting, and some describe the pain as intensified when supine.

Patients may list to one side, more commonly away from the side of the pain in order to bring the compressed nerve root away from the more typical posterolateral disc herniation with lateral root pressure. Leaning toward the side of the leg pain may indicate medial root compression from an axillary disc herniation (Fig. 55-2).

An uncommon clinical presentation of a lumbar disc herniation is the *cauda equina syndrome*, a clinical syndrome due to excessive compression of the entire cauda equina in the lumbar spine. When due to disc herniation, it is most commonly a large central disc herniation at L4-5 or L3-4. Clinically, patients present with low back pain, bilateral lower extremity pain, saddle anesthesia or dysesthesia, and motor weakness in the lower extremities. Bowel and bladder incontinence may occur, and signifies severe global lumbosacral root dysfunction. Dysfunction may also be in the form of urinary frequency or retention and bowel constipation.

The presence of a cauda equina syndrome clinically represents an indication for emergent imaging of the spinal canal via MRI or CT-myelography and emergent surgical decompression. Unfortunately, studies have shown that an acute onset of symptoms correlates with a poor prognosis whereas patients with an insidious onset have a better chance for overall recovery.

PHYSICAL EXAMINATION

The gait and stance of the patient with a painful lumbar disc herniation are characteristic: the gait is antalgic, with the painful leg held flexed and the patient reluctant to place the foot flat on the floor. In the acute phase, paravertebral muscle spasm may be noted with a loss of the normal lumbar lordosis. Patients commonly stand and walk with a 'sciatic scoliosis' or list. Lumbar motion is commonly severely limited.

On palpating the back, pain may be elicited along the midline or the paravertebral region at the involved disc level. When spasm is present, palpation will reveal remarkable firmness in the contracted muscle mass. Palpation should also be done along the course of the sciatic nerve, from the sciatic notch distally. Tender motor points represent the main neuromuscular junction in the involved muscle groups. Patients with true radiculopathy commonly have tender motor points in the myotome corresponding to the probable segmental level of nerve root involvement. The main application of the motor points examination is prognostic, as it correlates directly with disability. In the absence of radiculopathy, back pain patients with tender motor points remain disabled nearly three times as long as those without tenderness. The presence of back pain, in addition to radiculopathy, increases the chance for disability for nearly four times as long.

Neurologic evaluation for the patient with a suspected nerve root irritation should include a careful motor and sensory examination. Compression of the motor fibers of the nerve root results in weakness or paralysis of the muscle group in its distribution. With long-standing compression, atrophy of the muscle belly may be seen. The pattern of sensory involvement usually follows the dermatome of the affected root, although sensory exam is the most nonspecific portion of the neurologic exam. Table 55-1 summarizes the specific sensory,

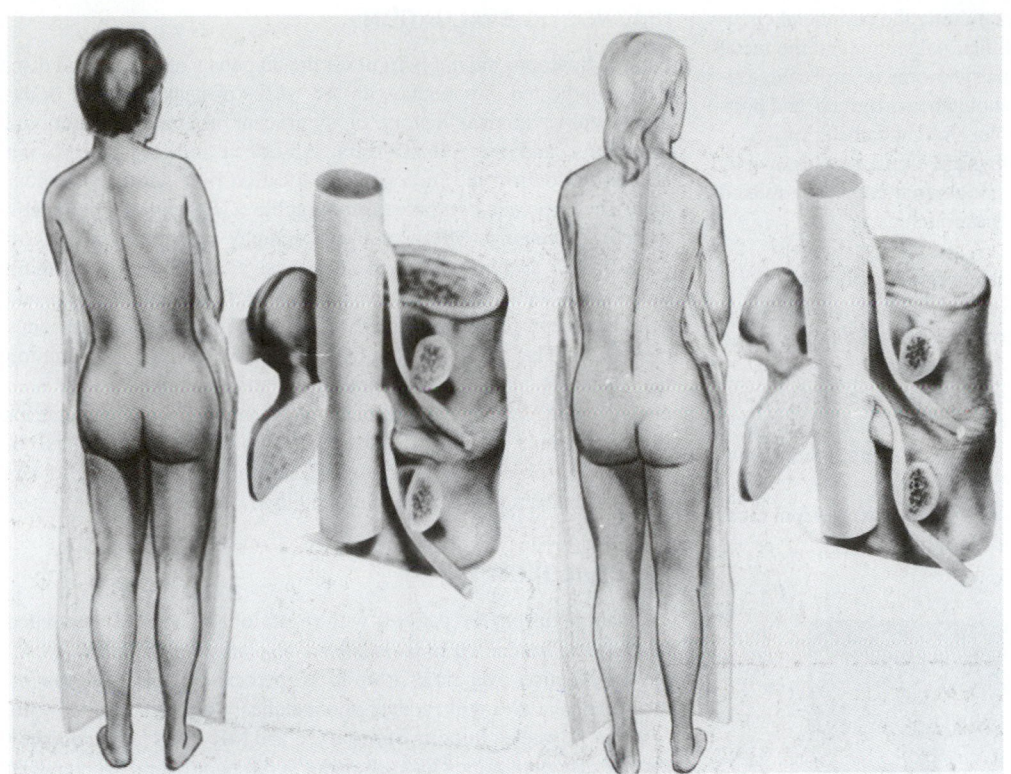

Figure 55-2
Sciatic listing. (*Left*) Listing is away from the side of pain for the common posterolateral disc herniation with lateral nerve root compression. (*Right*) Listing is toward the side of pain in the case of an axillary disc herniation with medial nerve root compression. [Reproduced with permission from Wisneski RJ, Garfin ST, Rothman RH: Lumbar disc disease. In Rothman RH, Simeone RA (eds): *The Spine*, 3d ed. Philadelphia: WB Saunders; 1992:690.]

motor, and reflex patterns of common lumbosacral root involvement.

In addition to the focal neurologic exam, testing is also done for specific nerve root *tension signs*. The overall excursion of the L5 and S1 spinal nerves is 2 to 6 mm at the level of the foramen. The L4 root moves a lesser distance, and the more proximal lumbar roots show little motion with lower extremity motion. The *straight leg raising* (SLR) test, also known as the *Lasègue sign*, is performed when the examiner slowly elevates the affected lower extremity by the heel with the knee fully extended. Only reproduction or worsening of radiating pain below the knee makes this a truly positive test. Buttock, back, and posterior thigh pain may be provoked, but may not be due to nerve root tension. A positive SLR is seen in nearly all patients ≤30 years old with a symptomatic disc herniation. The absence of a positive SLR in a patient ≤30 makes a herniated disc unlikely; after age 30, however, the SLR test may be negative in the presence of a true symptomatic low lumbar disc herniation. The *bowstring sign* is another variation of the SLR test: the leg is elevated as usual until pain

is provoked and the knee flexed to reduce pain. Finger pressure is then applied to the popliteal fossa and recurrence of the pain is considered to be a positive test.

The *crossed straight leg raising test* is when pain is elicited in the painful leg while elevating the other leg; a positive crossed-SLR is felt to be more specific of a disc herniation, especially one in the axillary position. The *seated-SLR* (or "flip-test") is performed with the patient seated over the side of the examination table. Pain is elicited or the patient is forced to lie backwards with elevation of the leg extending the knee. A negative seated SLR and a grossly positive supine SLR may indicate malingering.

The *reverse SLR (femoral stretch test)* is used to examine for nerve root tension of the upper lumbar nerves, L2-L4. It is performed with the patient prone or on his or her side, and the examiner extends the affected leg at the hip and then flexes the knee. This maneuver stretches the femoral nerve, and is positive with the reproduction of anterior thigh pain.

Table 55-1

Neurologic Testing of the Lower Extremity

Nerve	Reflex	Sensation	Muscles
L4	Patellar	Posterolateral thigh, anterior knee, anteromedial leg	Quadriceps
L5	None (or posterior tibial)	Posterior thigh, anterolateral leg, dorsal foot to great toe	Extensor hallucis longus (EHL)
S1	Achilles	Posterior thigh, posterior leg, lateral foot and sole	Gastrocsoleus, flexor hallucis longus (FHL)

The physical exam is completed by examining the peripheral circulation, hip and knee joint motion, abdominal palpation, and the rectal tone and sensation. Also, if a cauda equina syndrome is suspected, testing of perianal sensation and rectal tone should be performed, and postvoid residual urine should be measured via straight catheterization.

Waddell described a group of five physical signs, now known as *Waddell signs,* which are indicative of nonorganic pathology related to a patient's complaint of back pain. These include:

1. *Tenderness* to light touch or in a nonanatomic distribution
2. Pain with *simulation* of lumbar movement, including axial loading of the skull or passive simultaneous rotation of the pelvis and shoulders
3. Loss of a positive physical finding (such as a positive SLR) by *distracting* the patient
4. *Regional disturbances* of sensation or motor strength (in a nonanatomic distribution)
5. *Overreaction*, in the form of verbalization, facial expression, muscle tension and tremor, collapsing, or sweating

DIAGNOSTIC EVALUATION

Plain radiographs are not helpful for the diagnosis of a herniated disc, but are indicated in patients with >6 weeks of back pain and in patients with a clinical history of significant trauma, constitutional symptoms, and previous cancers. Advanced imaging studies are needed to confirm the presence and location of a herniated lumbar disc. These include computed tomographic (CT) scanning, magnetic resonance imaging (MRI), and myelography with post-myelogram CT scan. CT scanning is the least expensive, and is best at imaging the osseous elements. MRI provides the best imaging of the discs and neural elements, and can examine the entire lumbar canal to the conus medullaris (Fig. 55-3). Sagittal MR images are useful for examining the neural foramen, but far-lateral disc herniations may best be seen on CT scans. Intrathecal contrast (myelography) provides superior detail compared to plain CT scans, and is indicated if MRI is not available or for patients in whom MRI is contraindicated (due to cardiac pacemakers and brain aneurysm clips).

NATURAL HISTORY

The natural history for patients with radiculopathy and a documented lumbar disc herniation is spontaneous resolution of symptoms without intervention over time in up to 90 percent of cases. In general, most patients who will recover spontaneously will do so within the first 6 to 12 weeks. Reports of serial CT and MR scans in documented lumbar disc herniations have shown a significant overall decrease in size of the herniated material over time, presumably due to dehydration of the disc fragments and possibly due to resolution of the herniation by a vascular inflammatory response. This process has been documented in histologic studies in animals. Some studies have sug-

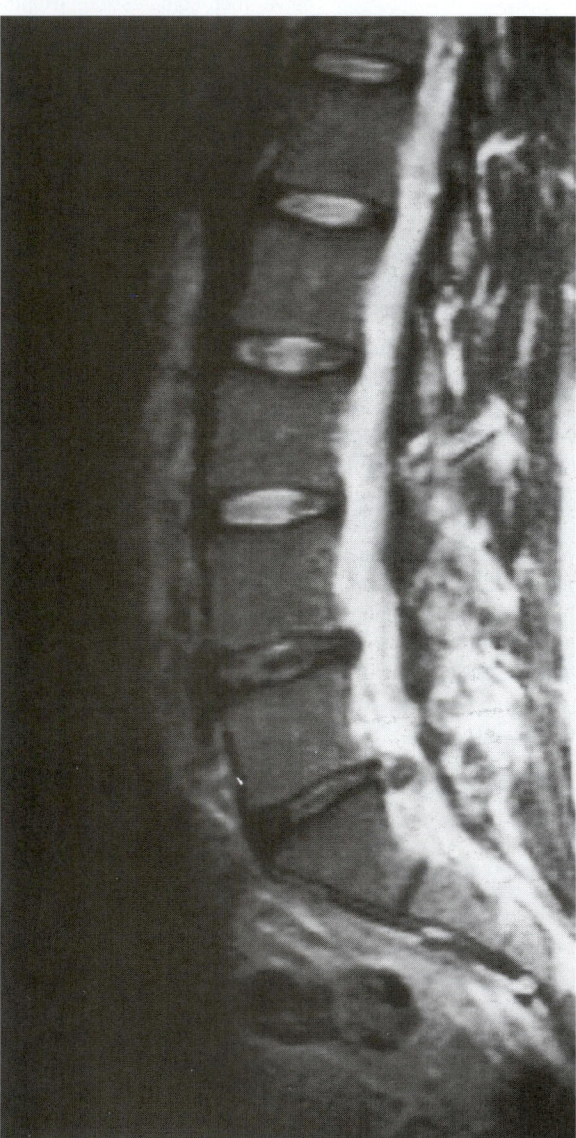

A

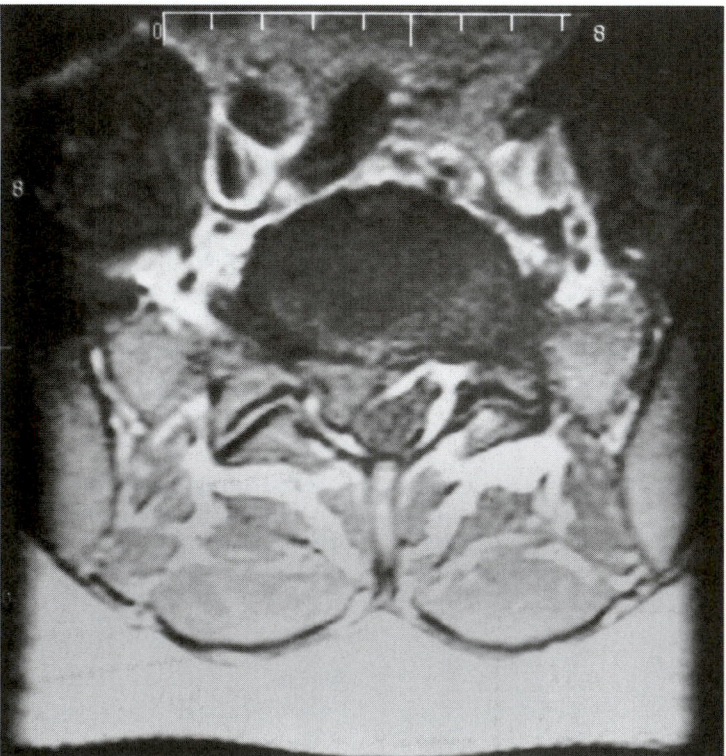

B

Figure 55-3
Lumbar disc herniation seen on MRI. *A.* Sagittal image. *B.* Axial image.

gested that older patients with a negative SLR may have less favorable prognosis overall for spontaneous resolution.

Based on Weber's prospective study, surgery for the patients with persistent radiculopathy has significantly superior results to nonoperative treatment after 1 year of follow-up. Results remained better in the surgical group of patients but were not statistically significant after 2 to 4 years of follow-up.

NONOPERATIVE TREATMENT

Cauda equina syndrome and a progressive motor weakness are the only definite indications for immediate operative decompression in lumbar disc herniations. In most cases, a nonoperative approach is utilized. In the acute setting, an initial period of 3 to 5 days of bedrest may be appropriate. Longer periods of bedrest are actually detrimental to overall recovery. Useful medications include aspirin and nonsteroidal anti-inflammatory pain relievers. An initial course of high dose-rapid taper steroid medication has been shown to be effective in improving the symptoms and signs associated with an acute disc herniation. Narcotic medications can also be used judiciously for short periods if the pain is severe. Muscle relaxants and prolonged narcotic usage have no place in the treatment of radiculopathy from an acute disc herniation.

After the initial period of rest, progressive return of daily activities is recommended. A formal program of physical therapy may be useful, but a simple set of home exercises and aerobic fitness training is often adequate. Epidural steroid injections may be helpful in improving symptoms, although the effects may be temporary.

OPERATIVE TREATMENT

The primary goal of the surgical treatment is to decompress the nerve root with the minimum damage to the surrounding structures. It is essential that the nerve root be completely visualized and explored and be free of all external pressure and tension. Surgery is most commonly done via a limited-open approach, through a 1-in. midline incision and a small ipsilateral laminotomy at the operative level, with improved visualization through the use of surgical loupes or an operative microscope. For most patients, this approach can be done on an outpatient basis or with an overnight hospital stay.

Microdiscectomy through an off-midline muscle-splitting approach has also been described. This procedure offers somewhat less complete visualization than the limited open approach and has a significant learning curve. However, it offers the potential benefits of a more rapid postoperative recovery and return to activities due to less muscle stripping during the approach.

ALTERNATIVE FORMS OF DISC EXCISION

Chemonucleolysis refers to the chemical degeneration of the nuclear portion of the intervertebral disc via an infectable agent. *Chymopapain*, the most commonly utilized chemical agent, is a proteolytic enzyme extracted from the tropical fruit papaya. It is the most specific enzyme in its activity on nucleus pulposus and the least antigenic. Chymopapain hydrolyzes the proteoglycans that are the dominant part of the nucleus, and thus interferes with its ability to hold water. This hydrolysis deflates the nuclear bulge and may reduce pressure on the nerve root. Problems reported with chymopapain injection include severe postinjection low back pain and potential complications including anaphylaxis, arachnoiditis, and delayed transverse myelitis. Overall, the results of chymopapain injection are significantly inferior to limited open discectomy.

Minimally invasive disc excision refers to a group of procedures including *automated percutaneous lumbar discectomy* (APLD), *per-*

cutaneous discectomy, *laser discectomy*, and *arthroscopic discectomy*. Of these, only arthroscopic discectomy affords the visualization needed to excise focally herniated disc material. The other procedures attempt to decompress the disc using various manual means, effecting an indirect decompression similar to chemonucleolysis. The results of these procedures have been less favorable than limited open discectomy, and the argument that the procedures are minimally invasive is a poor one. Complications of nerve root injury can cause irreversible nerve dysfunction and pain. Although the learning curve is long and steep, arthroscopic-assisted percutaneous disc excision can be used to safely remove many contained disc herniations. This procedure may also be particularly useful for foraminal and extraforaminal disc herniations. Its use for noncontained disc herniations should be reserved for only the most experienced hands. Again, the benefits of this technique over standard limited open discectomy are unproved.

LUMBAR SPINAL STENOSIS

ANATOMY

The spinal canal is bounded anteriorly by the disc, the posterior longitudinal ligament, and the vertebral body. The posterior border is formed by the ligamentum flavum and lamina. The lateral border is formed by the pedicles, the medial border of the facet joints, and lateral expanse of ligamentum flavum. Those structures create a spinal canal which, in cross section, has three basic forms: round, ovoid, and the less common trefoil "delta" shape (more often seen with congenital stenosis). The normal A-P diameter of the spinal canal is 12 mm or more, with a critical size of 75 ± 13 mm cross-sectional area.

The *lateral recess* zone is that region of the spinal canal between the lateral border of the dural sac and a line connecting the medial borers of the pedicles. The anterior border is formed by the vertebral body and disc and the posterior border is formed by the anterior surface of the superior articular process of the facet joint and the lateral expanse of the ligamentum flavum. The lumbar nerve root forms in the lateral recess zone, generally at the level of the disc space, and travels caudally along the medial border of the pedicle until it enters the neural foramen.

The *neural foramen* is the space between adjacent pedicles, through which the spinal nerves pass segmentally. The cephalad half of the anterior border is made by the vertebral body and the caudal half is formed by the intervertebral disc. The posterior border is the facet joint, mainly the superior articular process of the more caudal vertebra.

The overall length of the nerve root path has also been described in terms of four zones: the entrance zone, the middle zone, the exit zone, and the far lateral zone (Fig. 55-4).

CLASSIFICATION

Lumbar spinal stenosis can be defined as a narrowing of the spinal canal resulting in compression of the neural elements before their exit from the neural foramen. The stenosis may be limited to a single motion segment or it may extend over two or more motion segments. Etiologic and anatomic classifications of lumbar spinal stenosis have been described. The etiologic classification, originally described by Arnoldi, separates congenital and developmental stenosis from acquired or degenerative spinal stenosis (Table 55-2). The congenital and developmental type is the result of either an idiopathic narrowing of the spinal canal or from narrowing secondary to a bone dysplasia such as achondroplasia. Acquired lumbar stenosis is most com-

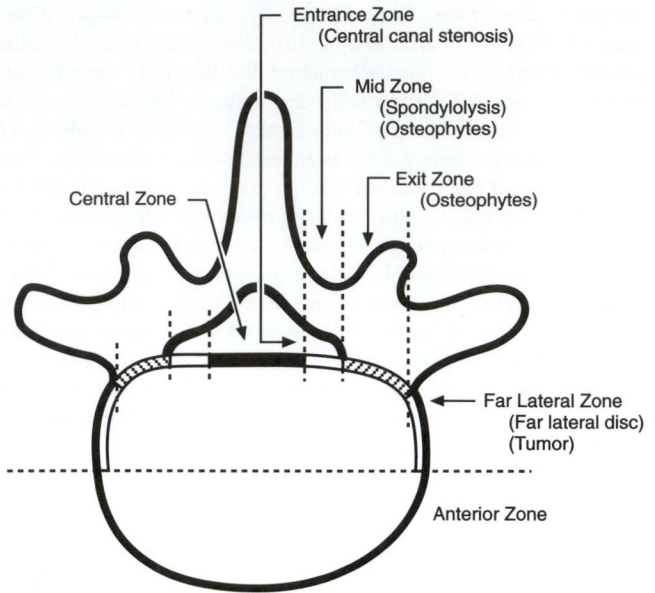

Figure 55-4
The four nerve root zones of the lumbar spine with potential causes of regional stenosis in each zone.

monly degenerative in origin, but it may also occur due to an underlying metabolic disorder (such as Paget's disease), tumor, infection, posttraumatic arthritic changes, and instability with listhesis resulting from previous operative intervention (iatrogenic).

The anatomic classification of lumbar spinal stenosis includes central, lateral recess, and foraminal stenosis. *Central stenosis* includes a narrowing of the entire spinal canal, with central compression of the thecal sac and cauda equina. By necessity, central stenosis on a degenerative basis also implies compression of the lateral recess as well. It is most commonly due to a combination of disc bulging or herniation and/or facet joint hypertrophy, with central encroachment of the inferior articular processes. *Lateral recess stenosis* refers to entrapment of a nerve root in its lateral recess, as or after it forms and separates from the thecal sac but before it enters the neural foramen. It also occurs most commonly due to facet hypertrophy, with posterior compression from an enlarged superior articular process. *Foraminal stenosis* refers to narrowing and compression of the nerve root in the nerve foramen, between the pedicles, which can be due to disc bulging or herniation, facet hypertrophy, and/or vertebral body osteophytes.

Table 55-2

Etiologic Classification of Lumbar Spinal Stenosis

Congenital-developmental
   Idiopathic
   Achondroplastic
Acquired
   Degenerative
   Spondylolisthetic/spondylolytic
   Iatrogenic (postlaminectomy)
   Posttraumatic
   Miscellaneous (Paget's disease, fluorosis, tumor, infection)

PATHOPHYSIOLOGY

The degenerative process which results in lumbar spinal stenosis usually begins with degeneration of the intervertebral disc. Disc degeneration is most commonly seen at the L4-5 and L5-S1 levels, as these are the most mobile segments in the lumbar spine. By the age of 40, 80 percent of male and 65 percent of female discs are moderately degenerated.

As the disc space collapses, there is concomitant settling of the facet joints, which come under increased load. Normally, the lumbar facet joints transmit about 15 percent of total axial load. Initially, the facet cartilage is intact and has a well-contoured gliding surface. Under increased and abnormal stresses, the joint surfaces become irregular and osteophytes develop. Facet joint hypertrophy, redundancy and possible hypertrophy of the ligamentum flavum, and bulging of the posterior annulus of the disc act to narrow the lateral recess and/or central spinal canal.

Disc space narrowing and bulging also cause decreased cross-sectional area in the neuroforamen and some degree of compromise of the spinal nerve root as it exits the canal. In addition, retrolisthesis and osteophytes develop along both the posterior vertebral body and the anterior aspect of the facet joint and increase the stenosis and pressure on the nerve roots in the region of the dorsal ganglia.

Studies on the effect of cauda equina constriction on neurologic deficits in a dog model found that 50 percent or greater acute constriction of the cross-sectional area of the cauda equina elicited motor and sensory deficits. Constant mechanical compression of the thecal sac cannot explain the intermittent nature of the typical pain in spinal stenosis. Another explanation of pain in the lumbar spinal stenosis relates to the arterial and nutritional support systems of the cauda equina. Arterial dilatation occurs with exercise, and oxygen use increases with stimulation of the nerve. Along the spinal nerve roots and cauda equina, an area of relative hypovascularity is noted where the central and radicular systems approach each other. Spinal stenosis with constriction of the neural elements and their blood supply can thus diminish oxygen supply, especially during physical activity when oxygen demand is higher, and can cause ischemia. When this occurs the dorsal root ganglion, which has a very rich and extensive microvascular network, may be stimulated by diffusion of the toxic metabolic substances from the stenotic segment.

CLINICAL PRESENTATION

Typically, patients with degenerative spinal stenosis are females (3:1 to 5:1 female-to-male ratio) in their late fifties or older. Back pain is the most common complaint. The pain is more often insidious in its onset rather than acute; patients rarely have a sciatic list or significant back spasm as seen in disc herniation. The quality of the pain is more an ache with stiffness, often worse in inclement weather, and mechanical in nature. Radiation of the pain to the buttocks and coccyx is typical.

Most of the patients with symptomatic spinal stenosis seek medical attention because of lower extremity pain. Two types of pain have been described. Type I, seen more in lateral stenosis, is more like typical sciatica with aching or sharp pain following a specific dermatomal distribution. Type II is the more classic neurologic claudication pain associated with spinal stenosis. The patient commonly describes the symptoms as pain, numbness, tingling, weakness, cramping, or burning in one or both legs. Typically, the pain begins in the low back or buttocks, radiating diffusely into the legs without a specific dermatomal distribution. Classically, walking or standing worsen the symptoms, whereas sitting and leaning forward or lying down alleviate the discomfort.

Vascular claudication is the primary differential diagnosis to the type II pain of spinal stenosis. The pain in peripheral vascular disease

(PVD) is more commonly a cramping or tightness in the calves. The symptoms usually start distally and progress proximally and are relieved by simply standing still. The PVD patient usually experiences the pain after walking a certain distance while in lumbar stenosis a variable distance is commonly described before symptoms occur. The pain due to PVD does not occur while standing still, unlike neurogenic claudication. In addition, the pain in PVD worsens when walking uphill (increased energy utilization) and improves when walking downhill (lessened energy requirement). The opposite is true of neurogenic claudication due to the flexed position going uphill and the extended position going downhill. Finally, the pain due to PVD worsens with riding a stationary bike, which will have less of an effect in lumbar spinal stenosis due to the maintenance of a flexed position.

Another medical condition that may be confused with lumbar spinal stenosis is peripheral neuropathy. Patients with peripheral neuropathy, most commonly due to diabetes, complain of burning or hypersensitivity beginning in the feet and progressing proximally. The pain has no correlation to activity and is worse at night. A "stocking glove" distribution of discomfort below the knees, unrelated to activity, is the hallmark of neuropathy.

Urinary dysfunction due to spinal stenosis is uncommon. It occurs in 3 to 4 percent of the patients and the chief complaint is urinary frequency or incontinence.

PHYSICAL EXAMINATION

Pain is commonly reproduced with extension of the lumbar spine, and may also be elicited by palpation of the sciatic notch. Flexion is generally full and painless, except in cases with associated unstable spondylolisthesis. The straight leg raising test and other nerve root tension signs are usually negative in spinal stenosis unless there is an associated disc herniation. Neurologic evaluation commonly shows no focal neurologic deficits, but may reveal a mild weakness of the extensor halucis longus or tibialis anterior muscles. Reflex testing is unreliable since reflex loss is common in the elderly. Sensory deficits are uncommon; whenever a diffuse sensory deficit occurs, peripheral neuropathy should be considered.

Since spinal stenosis is related to activity, during a static examination the neurologic evaluation may be normal. If the diagnosis of lumbar stenosis is suspected, symptoms and focal neurologic findings may be produced by asking the patient to walk down the hallway and then repeating the examination.

DIAGNOSTIC EVALUATION

Standing AP and lateral radiographs form the initial evaluation. When isthmic spondylolisthesis is suspected, Ferguson oblique views (with the beam tilted to better view the low lumbar laminae due to lordosis) should be added. Plain radiograph abnormalities may include disc space narrowing, facet osteoarthritis, spondylosis, degenerative scoliosis, spondylolisthesis, settling of the spinous processes and narrowing of the interpedicular distance as seen in cases of congenital spinal stenosis.

Plain radiographic abnormalities can only be suggestive of stenosis. Confirmation of the diagnosis can only be made by an advanced imaging study. Magnetic resonance imaging (MRI) or computed tomographic (CT) scanning can be used. MRI is noninvasive, and supplies more information about the soft tissue components of the spine including the disc, ligamentum flavum, and neural elements (Fig. 55-5). CT scanning gives better detail about the bony component of the stenosis, and is better at evaluating facet arthrosis.

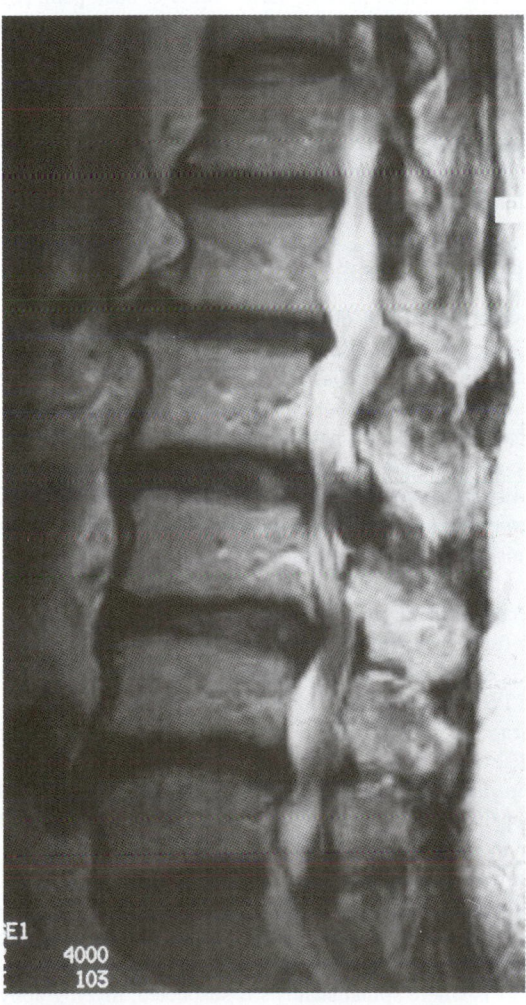

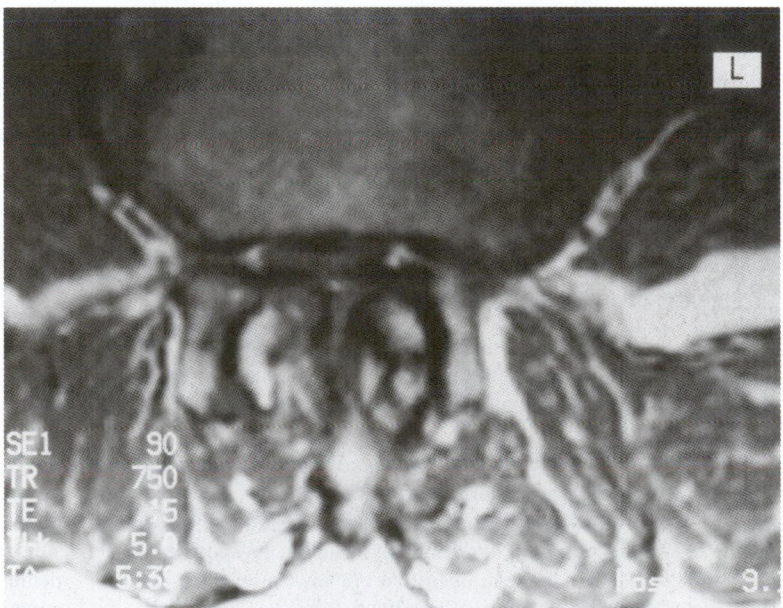

A

B

Figure 55-5
Lumbar spinal stenosis seen on MRI. *A.* Sagittal T2-weighted image. *B.* Axial T1-weighted image at the L2-3 level.

CT-myelography, although invasive, gives excellent information about the bony elements and the extent of the stenosis. Flexion-extension lateral myelographic images can demonstrate a dynamic component of the stenosis. Because it is invasive, CT-myelography is usually reserved as a preoperative study when more anatomic detail than provided in the other diagnostic studies is needed. It is not used routinely simply to make the diagnosis of stenosis.

The surgical correlation of CT-myelography and MRI are almost equal, reported to be 83 percent and 82.6 percent, respectively.

Electrophysiologic studies, including electromyography (EMG), nerve conduction velocity, and somatosensory evoked potentials (SSEP), are not considered part of the routine evaluation of lumbar spinal stenosis. In patients with diabetes and lumbar stenosis, however, EMG and SSEP evaluation can be useful in differentiating between radiculopathy from nerve compression and diabetic neuropathy affecting the peripheral motor and sensory nerves. EMG can also be useful in differentiating active denervation from chronic inactive changes in peripheral nerves. Normal electrophysiologic studies do not rule out the presence of symptomatic lumbar stenosis; however, the more typical pattern found in symptomatic patients is that of a polyradiculopathy, with multiple root level radiculopathies which are often bilateral. Also, SSEP evaluation performed both before and after physical exercise may help determine the more involved nerve roots in a patient with lumbar spinal stenosis.

TREATMENT

Nonsurgical management consists of a physical therapy regimen including flexion exercises, abdominal strengthening, and gentle aerobic fitness exercises. Use of nonsteroidal anti-inflammatory medications and epidural steroid injections may be helpful.

Indications for surgical intervention include persistent functional impairment, persistent neurologic deficit, and intractable pain with concomitant impairment of life-style. Urgent operative decompression is indicated only in cases with a progressive neurologic deficit or the presentation of a cauda equina syndrome.

The mainstay of surgical treatment usually consists of an adequate decompression of the neural elements of the involved segment. The standard decompressive laminectomy includes midline decompression and undercutting lateral decompression with partial medial facetectomy, preserving the pars interarticularis and the majority of each facet joint. Concomitant spinal fusion is not recommended routinely. It is reserved for cases of preoperative instability (as in degenerative spondylolisthesis and degenerative scoliosis) and iatrogenic instability from excessive facet joint resection (generally less than one facet in total remaining).

DEGENERATIVE SPONDYLOLISTHESIS

Degenerative spondylolisthesis is one of the common causes of lumbar spinal stenosis. It most commonly affects the L4-L5 segment, is more common in females, and increases in prevalence with increasing age.

The most common anatomic predisposition for degenerative spondylolisthesis is relative immobility of the lumbar segment below the lesion. The immobility is most commonly due to relative sacralization of L5, but can also result from long-standing degenerative disc disease of the L5-S1 segment, or from a previous surgical fusion. A higher incidence of degenerative spondylolisthesis has been reported in diabetics and in woman who have undergone oophorectomy; the reasons for these findings are not known.

Biomechanically, the body weight transmitted through the spinal column tends to displace the cephalad lumbar vertebra of each motion segment anteriorly. This force is normally resisted by soft tissue and the posterior articulation. Normally, the plane of the inferior articular facet is at a right angle to the pedicles and the superior facet prevents its anterior slippage. The early dysfunction that starts the listhetic process is unknown; a more sagittal orientation of the facet joints and disc degeneration likely play a significant role.

As the process continues, there are repetitive erosions and tropism of the inferior articular process of the cephalad vertebra (usually L4), allowing gradual displacement of L4 anteriorly to the point where the L4 isthmus and inferior articular process impinge on the superior articular facet and posterosuperior aspect of the L5 vertebral body. Unless there is a concomitant isthmic lesion (pars defect, see Chap. 64) of L4, the slippage will never progress more than 30 percent of the vertebral body.

Up to 82 percent of patients with degenerative spondylolisthesis present with signs and symptoms of lumbar spinal stenosis. Back pain, tight hamstring muscle tightness, and a clinically palpable spinous process step-off are more prominent findings in these patients as compared to those with degenerative lumbar spinal stenosis without spondylolisthesis.

Surgical treatment should be considered when the disease becomes functionally incapacitating, similar to lumbar spinal stenosis without spondylolisthesis. Surgical stabilization of the listhetic level by spinal fusion is generally recommended. Spinal instrumentation may improve the fusion rate and may provide earlier relief of back pain, and is recommended by many. Instability, documented as >3 to 4 mm translational motion on preoperative flexion-extension radiographs, strengthens the indication for instrumented spinal fusion. In older patients without clinically significant back pain, despite the spondylolisthesis, a narrowed disc space and bridging osteophytes may provide enough stability to obviate the need for instrumentation or for spinal fusion altogether.

DEGENERATIVE SCOLIOSIS

Coronal plane deformity with Cobb angle > 10 degrees may arise in adulthood due to degenerative disc disease. It is associated with other manifestations of degenerative disease of the spine, including disc degeneration and facet joint arthrosis. This deformity is related primarily to mechanical insufficiency of the spine.

Degenerative scoliosis generally presents with back pain with or without lower-extremity symptoms (claudication or radiculopathy). Patients may experience nonspecific symptoms like low back and leg pain and diminished sensory perception along the lateral aspect of the thigh. Intermittent claudication can be the main complaint whenever there is a concomitant spinal stenosis.

Risk factors for curve progression include a Cobb angle greater than 30 degrees, significant apical rotation, an intercrestal line that passes through L5, and vertebral translation >6 mm.

Plain radiographs can demonstrate the different characteristics of degenerative disc disease, with asymmetric disc narrowing, osteophyte formation, facet arthrosis, and listhesis. In one series of 200 patients with degenerative scoliosis, 55 percent of cases demonstrated a significant spondylolisthesis and 78 percent had a lateral listhesis. Decreased lumbar lordosis was found in 85 percent of patients. Significant differences in the vertebral alignment and Cobb measurement between standing and supine lumbar radiographs may help demonstrate a significant "collapsing" instability. In the cases of degenerative scoliosis where spinal stenosis is suspected, myelography and post-myelogram CT scanning provide superior anatomic detail as compared to MRI. Stenosis at the apex is common, and nerve entrapment may produce more symptoms in the lower extremity on the side of the concavity of the curve.

The management of patients with back and leg pain due to degenerative scoliosis begins with the usual nonoperative measures, including anti-inflammatory pain medications and activity modifications including physical therapy. Application of a lumbar orthosis may provide some temporary relief in patients with significant deformity and instability. In female patients, attention should be given to the treatment of osteopenia.

Indications for surgery include failed nonoperative treatment with persistent back pain or, more commonly, lower extremity symptoms due to the spinal stenosis. The surgical procedure is done primarily for decompression of the neural elements. Currently, the addition of a spinal fusion of the curve with posterior segmental instrumentation and curve balancing is recommended in most cases. An extremely limited decompression may not require fusion in certain select cases.

DIFFUSE IDIOPATHIC SPINAL HYPEROSTOSIS

Diffuse idiopathic spinal hyperostosis (DISH), also known as *Forestier's disease*, is a syndrome that affects 5 to 10 percent of men >65 years old. It is characterized by calcification and ossification of the anterolateral aspects of at least three contiguous vertebral bodies. There is an extraspinous extension of DISH, usually to the extremities, which is commonly manifested as elbow and heel spurs. DISH is more common in diabetic patients (40 percent) and in patients with gout.

Although the most common area of the spine to be affected by DISH is the right side of the lower thoracic region, the process can involve the thoracolumbar spine as well. Thoracolumbar DISH is almost always asymptomatic, and although some patients can complain of stiffness, the range of motion is usually normal.

The typical radiographic manifestation of DISH is the bridging bony spurs that cross the disc space from one vertebra to another. Bone spur formation can also be seen in osteoarthritis, segmental instability, and ankylosing spondylitis or other spondyloarthropathies. Each of these has characteristic features (Fig. 55-6).

Osteophytes, usually formed at the anterolateral surface of the vertebral body, represent pathologic new bone formation at the attachment of the ALL or the intervertebral disc. They have a typical horizontal orientation associated with disc space narrowing.

Traction (Macnab) spurs arise secondary to instability at the site of ligamentous attachment. They are also horizontally oriented and originate 2 mm away from the distal border of the anterolateral margin of the vertebral body.

Marginal syndesmophytes are seen in ankylosing spondylitis and characterized by thin, vertically oriented ossification across the lateral margin of the disc space.

Nonmarginal syndesmophytes have the same orientation as marginal syndesmophytes; however, they are broader and coarser and arise along the waist or midportion of the vertebral body.

DISCOGENIC BACK PAIN

Discogenic pain can be defined as incapacitating back pain without a radicular component and with no evidence of neural compression or segmental instability. The concept of discogenic pain as a clinical and treatable entity remains controversial.

The posterior structures of the spine are highly enervated. Afferent nerve fibers supply the PLL, vertebral periosteum, facet capsule, interspinous ligament, and the ligamentum flavum. This overlapping and rich nerve network makes the localization of a single painful focus difficult. The disc itself has no nerve supply; however, studies have shown that a pressurized disc can produce back pain through stimulation of the nociceptors in the PLL.

The diagnosis of discogenic pain is one of exclusion, considered only after other anatomic causes of back pain are ruled out. The patient usually has a long history of mechanical back pain, localized mainly in the midline lower back and often with radiation to the posterior thigh, waist, and buttocks on one or both sides. On physical examination, paraspinal muscle spasm may be present, with decreased range of lumbar motion. Nerve root tension signs are generally negative, and neurologic examination is nonfocal.

Routine radiographs may be normal or may demonstrate a variety of degenerative changes, including decreased disc height (anteriorly or uniformly with a loss of lumbar lordosis), anterolateral or lateral subluxation, vertebral sclerosis, osteophytes, apophyseal joint malalignment, facet hypertrophy, narrowing of the interlaminar space, and gas within the disc (the so-called vacuum phenomenon). Plain radiographs are usually accompanied by dynamic flexion-extension views to rule out lumbar instability as the cause of the pain.

MRI is commonly used to make the diagnosis of degenerative disc disease. A loss of signal intensity on the T2-weighted sagittal image ("black disc disease") is considered by many as equivalent to degenerative disc disease, but may only represent a very small, clinically insignificant decrease in disc hydration. Annular tears, with fluid seen within the posterior annulus, may be more indicative of a painful disc. This so-called high intensity zone, seen on T2-weighted images, has

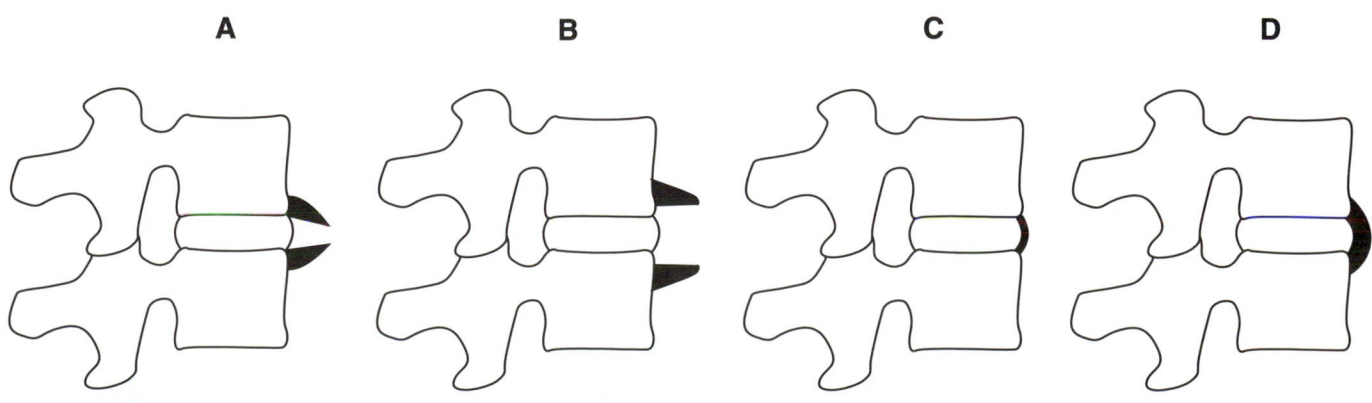

Figure 55-6
Types of lumbar bone spurs. *A.* Osteophytes. *B.* Traction spurs. *C.* Marginal syndesmophytes. *D.* Nonmarginal syndesmophytes.

been shown to correlate with positive pain provocation on discography (see below).

Changes of disc degeneration are certainly not diagnostic of a discogenic source for the back pain. Almost one-third of healthy asymptomatic volunteers have similar changes on MRI in one or more discs; clinical correlation must be made with care.

Discography can be used to attempt to correlate the degenerative changes with the patients pain. In this test, fine needles are placed in a sterile fashion under fluoroscopic guidance into the lumbar discs to be tested and contrast is injected under pressure. The anatomic portion of the test (including the post-discogram CT scan) adds little more information than a good quality MRI. However, the provocative component of the test may provide additional information with regard to the disc as a source of the patient's typical pain. Provocation of pain which is not familiar to the patient is considered a negative response. A positive discogram is considered a provocative familiar pain response in one or more discs, each with some type of anatomic abnormality. A positive test should also include a normal level as a reference.

The treatment protocol for patients with discogenic low back pain is primarily based on nonoperative measures. Patients may benefit from a course of physical therapy stressing an aggressive exercise approach with minimal use of modalities. Nonsteroidal anti-inflammatory medications are commonly used for pain relief. Orthotic devices, although widely used, are of no proven benefit. Surgery is considered only in compliant patients who fail extensive nonoperative treatment. Surgery consists of segmental spinal fusion, which may be done posterolaterally, interbody, or circumferentially. The use of segmental spinal instrumentation and interbody fusion cages are becoming more common.

THORACIC DISC HERNIATION

The incidence of symptomatic herniation of a thoracic disc has been reported to be 1:1,000,000 per year. Overall, thoracic disc herniations account for only 0.25 to 0.75 percent of all symptomatic disc herniations. Patients are most commonly in the third to fifth decade of life (80 percent), with a peak incidence in the fourth decade (33 percent). The T11-12 level is most commonly affected (28 percent), with 75 percent of all symptomatic thoracic disc herniations occurring below T8. The majority of herniations are central or posterolateral.

Thoracic disc herniations may present clinically in a variety of ways. Presenting symptoms include anterior band-like chest pain, paresthesia and weakness in the lower extremities, interscapular or lower thoracic pain, and epigastric pain. Coughing and sneezing may aggravate the pain. An upper thoracic disc herniation may mimic cervical radiculopathy and may present with a Horner's syndrome. Midthoracic disc herniations can present similar to cardiac or abdominal disease. Lower thoracic herniations may produce pain radi-

ating to the groin, similar to ureteral calculi or renal disease; the pain may also radiate to the lower extremity, similar to a lumbar disc herniation. Multisegmental sensory or motor dysfunction, sphincter dysfunction, gait abnormality, and clinical signs of myelopathy from thoracic spinal cord compression (isolated hyperreflexia of the lower extremities, clonus, and a positive Babinski sign) should raise suspicion for a thoracic disc herniation.

The course of the disease can be extremely variable, but is generally considered benign in patients not presenting with signs of spinal cord compression. It is unknown whether or not neurologic signs or symptoms would ever have developed in patients operated on for pain only. In many patients with local or radicular pain, the pain improves spontaneously, similar to lumbar and cervical disc herniations. Progressive neurologic involvement is uncommon but can occur.

Nonoperative treatment includes nonsteroidal anti-inflammatory pain medications and physical therapy. Steroids are indicated for clinical evidence of spinal cord compression prior to early surgical intervention. Surgical treatment is also indicated for patients with persistent pain despite nonoperative treatment. Posterior decompression via laminectomy and discectomy is contraindicated because of the risk of neurologic deterioration.

Posterolateral decompression via costotransversectomy is one surgical option and is especially useful for posterolateral herniations with foraminal root compression. Anterior discectomy via open thoracotomy or thoracoscopy is the most common, reliable, and safe surgical method for treatment of thoracic disc herniations. Concomitant fusion may help prevent postoperative back pain and progressive degenerative disease, but is usually not indicated on the basis of instability due to the stabilizing effect of the thoracic cage.

SUGGESTED READINGS

Boden SD, McCowin PR, Davis DO, et al: Abnormal magnetic-resonance scans of the lumbar spine in asymptomatic subjects. A prospective investigation. *J Bone Joint Surg [Am]* 1990; 72:403.

Bridwell KH, DeWard RL (eds): *The Textbook of Spinal Surgery,* 2d ed. Philadelphia: Lippincott-Raven, 1996.

Brown CW, Deffer PA Jr, et al: The natural history of thoracic disc herniation. *Spine* 1992; 17(suppl 6):S97.

Frymoyer JW (ed): *The Adult Spine. Principles and Practice,* 2d ed. Philadelphia: Lippincott-Raven; 1997.

Herkowitz HN, Kurz LT: Degenerative lumbar spondylolisthesis with spinal stenosis. *J Bone Joint Surg [Am]* 1991; 73:802.

Johnsson K-E, Rosén I, Udén A: The natural course of lumbar spinal stenosis. *Clin Orthop* 1992; 279:82.

Stillerman CB, Weiss MH: Managment of thoracic disc disease. *Clin Neurosurg* 1992; 38:325.

Waddell G, McCulloch JA, Kummel ED, et al: Nonorganic physical signs in low-back pain. *Spine* 1980; 5:117.

Weber H: Lumbar disc herniation. A controlled, prospective study with ten years of observation. *Spine* 1983; 8:131.

Chapter 56

DEFORMITY

Lynn J. Letko and Paul L. Kuflik

ANKYLOSING SPONDYLITIS

Ankylosing spondylitis (Marie Strumpell's disease) is an HLA-B27-positive, seronegative inflammatory arthritis that involves the axial skeleton. In the United States, the incidence is 0.2 to 0.3 percent. Males are more frequently affected than are females. The incidence, however, may be higher in females than was previously thought, with females being less severely afflicted.

Two types of ankylosing spondylitis have been described: juvenile onset and adult onset. Juvenile onset begins before age 16, whereas adult onset begins after age 16. The adult onset typically starts with bilateral sacroiliac (SI) joint involvement, low back pain, and stiffness that progresses in a cephalad manner. Progressive ossification with SI joint fusion and decreased motion of the hips, spine, and chest wall occurs. This disease process frequently becomes quiescent by the fourth or fifth decades.

The main orthopaedic spinal manifestations of ankylosing spondylitis relate to fixed spinal deformity, most commonly kyphosis. The kyphosis often develops from microfractures through the disc spaces, which heal in a flexed position. Hip flexion contractures may aggravate the deformity. Progressive deformity may result in an inability to see ahead of oneself, ribs may compress on the abdominal viscera, and diaphragmatic respiration may be diminished. The result is functional impairment.

Assessment of patients with ankylosing spondylitis includes several measurements. The chin-brow to vertical angle is the measurement of the angle formed by a line from the brow to the chin and a vertical line perpendicular to the floor (Fig. 56-1). Chest expansion should be measured at the nipple line. The normal chest excursion in a male is at least 5 cm. Hips should be evaluated for hip flexion contractures. Consideration should be given to total hip replacement if significant contractures exist. The Schober test is done by measuring 10 cm above and 5 cm below the lumbosacral junction. On maximal forward flexion, the distance between the two marks should increase greater or equal to 5 cm.

Radiographic assessment of patients with ankylosing spondylitis should include full-length erect anteroposterior and lateral radiographs, as well as localized films of the area of deformity and flexion-extension views. C-spine flexion-extension views should be obtained to rule out C1-2 instability. Tomograms or a bone scan may be useful to diagnose fractures of the fused spine. Typical early radiographic findings seen in ankylosing spondylitis include squaring of the anterior corners of the vertebral bodies and syndesmophyte formation. Late findings include the bamboo spine and the trolley-track appearance of the spine secondary to ossification of the facet joint capsules, ligamentum flavum, interspinous, and supraspinous ligaments (Fig. 56-2).

Problems associated with ankylosing spondylitis include temporomandibular joint involvement, the presence of aortic stenosis, decreased pulmonary function, postoperative ileus, gastric ulceration, and superior mesenteric artery syndrome. Two other spinal surgical considerations in these patients include vertebral osteopenia and adherence of or thinning of the dura.

Kyphotic deformity is more frequently seen in the lumbar spine than in the thoracic or cervical spine in these patients. Operative treatment for significant deformity in the lumbar spine consists of sagittal

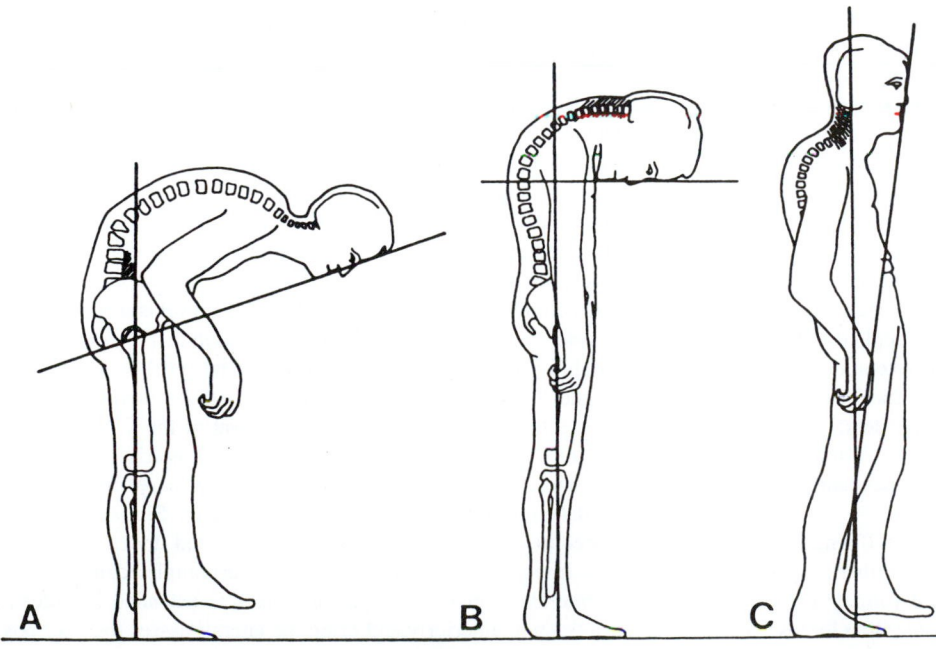

Figure 56-1
Chin-brow to vertical angle. *A.* Increased secondary to thoracolumbar kyphosis. *B.* Increased secondary to cervicothoracic kyphosis. *C.* Correction of cervicothoracic deformity by lower cervical osteotomy. [Reproduced with permission from Simmons ED Jr, Simmons EH: Ankylosing spondylitis. In Farcy JP (ed): *Spine: State of the Art Reviews—Complex Spinal Deformity*, vol 8. Philadelphia: Hanley & Belfus; 1994:593.]

A   B   C

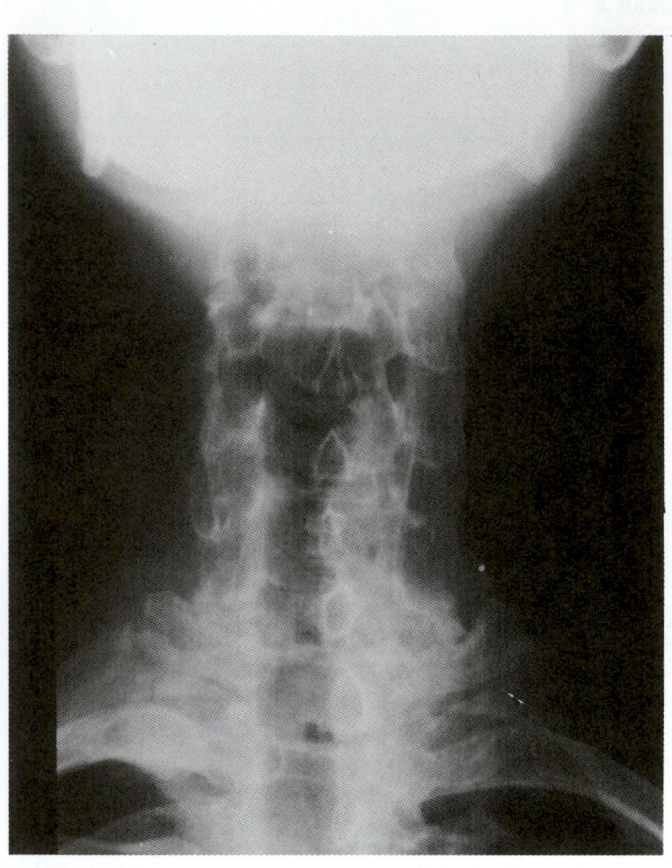

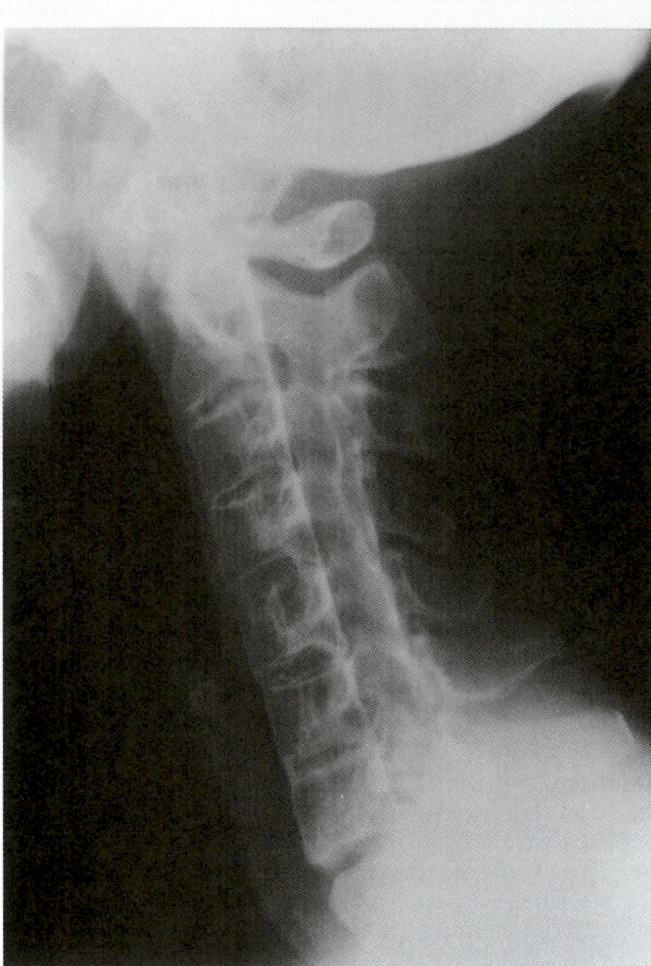

A

B

Figure 56-2
C-spine radiographs of a patient with ankylosing spondylitis. *A.* Anteroposterior. *B.* Lateral.

correction to restore the chin-brow to vertical angle to as close to normal as possible. The amount of correction needed is calculated from the chin-brow to vertical angle, and the appropriate amount of bone is removed through one or more V-shaped osteotomies in order to shift the weightbearing line posterior. Simmons (1977) has advocated a single-level osteotomy done below the level of termination of the spinal cord. Others advocate multiple-level osteotomies to obtain harmonious correction and reduce the incidence of neurologic complications. Undercutting of the laminae with or without that of the pedicles is necessary to avoid impingement of the neural elements on extension. Anterior osteoclasis is accomplished through hyperextension of the hips and pelvis. A posterior force is applied to the upper chest while an anterior force is applied to the osteotomy site to result in a greenstick fracture. Coexistent scoliosis may be corrected by taking unequal amounts of bone at the osteotomy site(s). Internal fixation may be used with or without cast or orthosis immobilization. Cast or orthosis immobilization may be used independently for up to six months (Fig. 56-3).

Kyphosis is rarely corrected at the thoracic level. If a mild to moderate thoracic kyphosis and a rigid or flattened lumbar region exist, a lumbar osteotomy can be used to correct the deformity. A more severe thoracic kyphosis with normal cervical and lumbar lordoses may occur. If incomplete ossification of the thoracic spine or an extensive

area of destructive spondylodiscitis exists, treatment consists of preliminary correction in halo traction followed by multiple posterior thoracic osteotomies with instrumentation and bone graft. For a rigid thoracic kyphosis with complete anterior ossification, an anterior release and grafting through a transthoracic approach followed by halo traction and then by a posterior approach with multiple V osteotomies and instrumentation has been advocated. However, high rates of significant neurologic injuries have been reported with this approach.

Deformity of the cervical spine frequently occurs at the cervicothoracic junction. For significant deformity, correction is obtained by an osteotomy at the C7-T1 level. The C7-T1 level is recommended for the osteotomy site because the spinal canal in this region is wider, less disability results from C8 nerve root damage than with higher levels, and the vertebral artery is not likely to be damaged at this level. Osteotomy is accomplished by removal of the C7, as well as portions of C6 and T1, spinous processes and posterior arches. The laminae above and below are undercut. The C8 nerve root is completely decompressed. As originally described by Simmons (1972), the procedure is done with the patient sitting and under local anesthesia with sedation. After the laminectomy is completed, a short-acting barbiturate is given. The patient's neck is extended in order to create a fracture anteriorly and bring the lateral masses together posteriorly. Internal fixation is used or the patient is immobilized in a

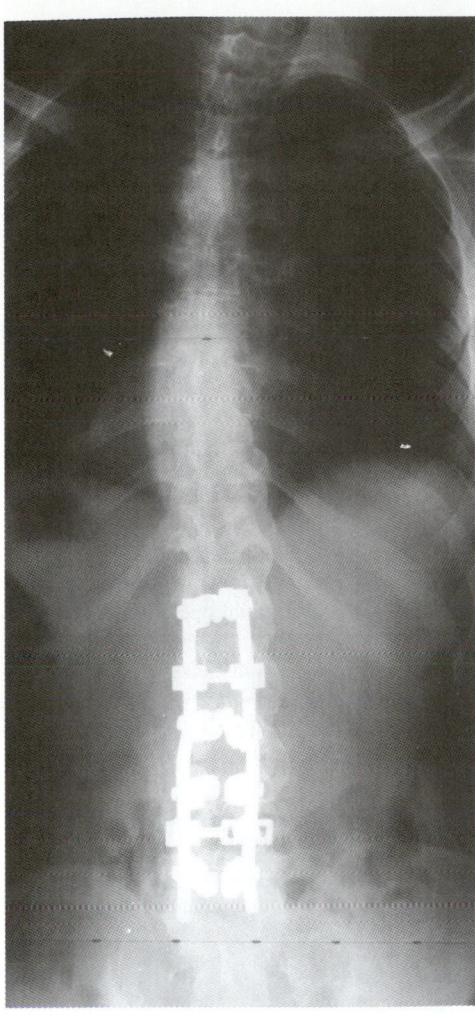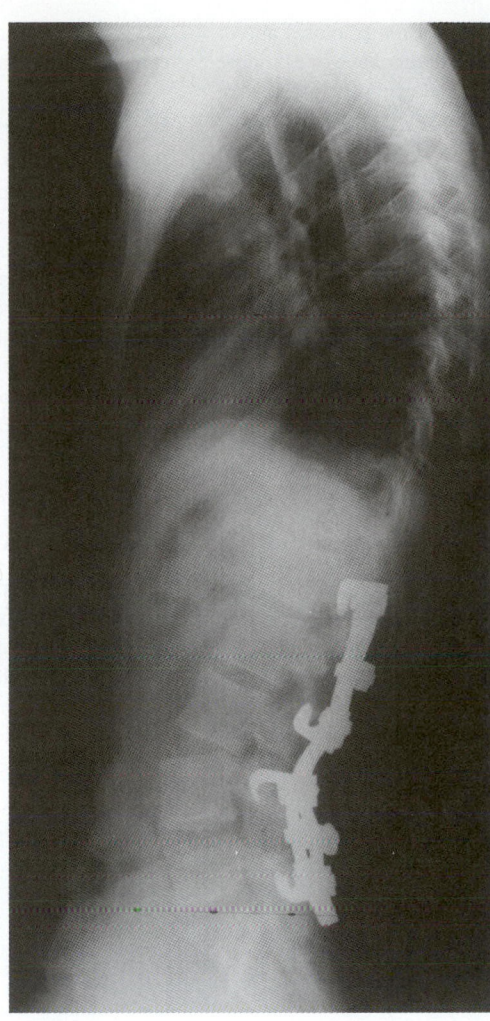

A   B

Figure 56-3
Postoperative radiographs after lumbar osteotomy for ankylosing spondylitis. *A.* Anteroposterior. *B.* Lateral.

halo body cast for 4 months, followed by SOMI (skull occiput mandibular immobilization) for 2 months. The corrected position should enable the patient to look down at a desk as well as straight ahead.

Spondylodiscitis, in ankylosing spondylitis, is thought to be either due to a posttraumatic pseudarthrosis or result from the inflammatory process. It is most commonly found at the thoracolumbar junction. Pain from spondylodiscitis may respond to nonsteroidal anti-inflammatory pain medications and bracing. Persistent pain may be an indication for debridement and bone grafting. Deformity may occur through an area of spondylodiscitis if translation or anterior collapse occurs in that region. Simmons (1977) recommends an extension osteotomy in the thoracolumbar region in an attempt to decrease the stress and increase the compression across the area of the spondylodiscitis to enhance the likelihood of spontaneous healing.

With trauma, the ankylosed spine fractures like a long bone. Fractures occur through the disc space or in the adjacent bone. The lack of normal soft tissue supports makes these injuries highly unstable. Fractures may occur after a seemingly minimal injury and are initially not diagnosed in many cases. Most fractures in ankylosing spondylitis occur in the cervical region. Patients complain of pain with or without neurologic injury. Significant translation at the fracture site may result in complete paralysis. Correction of a previously existing spinal deformity through a fracture site in patients with anky-

losing spondylitis is dangerous. It should not be done. Instead, the patient must be immobilized and stabilized in the deformed prefracture position. Neurologic compromise in these fractures may also result from hematoma. Any progressive neurologic deficits must be evaluated by magnetic resonance imaging or computed tomography/myelography because urgent decompression may be indicated. Cervical fractures may be treated by halo traction followed by a halo vest for 3 to 6 months. Surgical treatment consists of a posterior approach and open reduction with internal fixation. C1-2 subluxation/dislocation has been described as the result of posterior erosive fractures. Treatment consists of halo traction followed by posterior stabilization of the occiput to C2 with or without excision of the arch of C1. Fixed C1-2 subluxation with anterior spinal cord compression may require transoral decompression with or without reduction and posterior stabilization.

ADULT KYPHOSIS

SENILE KYPHOSIS

Senile kyphosis is described as an increasing kyphosis with decreased lumbar lordosis that occurs with aging. It is believed to be due to a loss of posterior muscle and ligamentous tone or to the loss of anterior support secondary to osteoporotic compression fractures and/or degenerated discs. Among white women, 40 percent have one or more compression fractures by the age of 80, and 5 percent of white women over the age of 80 have one or more osteoporotic burst fractures.

On presentation, the deformity may be flexible unless there is associated spondylosis. Patients may have mechanical pain and cervical hyperlordosis as well as fatigue pain with lumbar hypolordosis.

Nonoperative treatment in the form of nonsteroidal anti-inflammatory drugs (NSAIDs), analgesics, orthoses, and treatment of the underlying metabolic disease is the cornerstone of management in these patients. Indications for surgery are rare as a high complication rate is associated with surgical management of these patients. Indications for surgery include:

1. Debilitating pain unresponsive to medical management
2. Progressive kyphosis
3. Neurologic compromise

Full correction of the deformity is not the priority. Relief of pain and/or neural compression are the main goals of any surgical treatment. Various surgical approaches have been described, including posterior spinal fusion with instrumentation, anterior decompression and fusion for senile burst fractures with neurologic compromise and acute local kyphosis, and transpedicular decompression with posterior spinal fusion and instrumentation in situ followed by immobi-

lization in a thoracolumbosacral orthosis for 6 months for those who cannot tolerate anterior surgery (Fig. 56-4).

POSTLAMINECTOMY KYPHOSIS

Postlaminectomy kyphosis, which is seen more commonly in children than in adults, is most likely secondary to imbalance of the bone and ligamentous structures. Three cases have been reported after decompression for spinal stenosis in patients with unrecognized compression fractures. Adult postlaminectomy kyphosis most frequently involves the cervical spine, but less commonly can also involve the thoracic and lumbar spine. These cases are followed and managed nonoperatively. Indications for surgical intervention include progressive deformity and neurologic impairment. Neurologic compromise generally occurs anteriorly, necessitating anterior decompression. Stabilization and fusion may be done anteriorly, posteriorly, or by a combined approach.

POSTTRAUMATIC KYPHOSIS

Posttraumatic kyphosis, which is generally localized and acute, most commonly results from a failure of the initial operative or nonoperative fracture treatment to restore spinal stability and sagittal balance. As with any kyphotic deformity, progression causes the sagittal vertical axis to move further anterior, increasing the bending moment at the apex of the deformity and increasing the tendency toward wors-

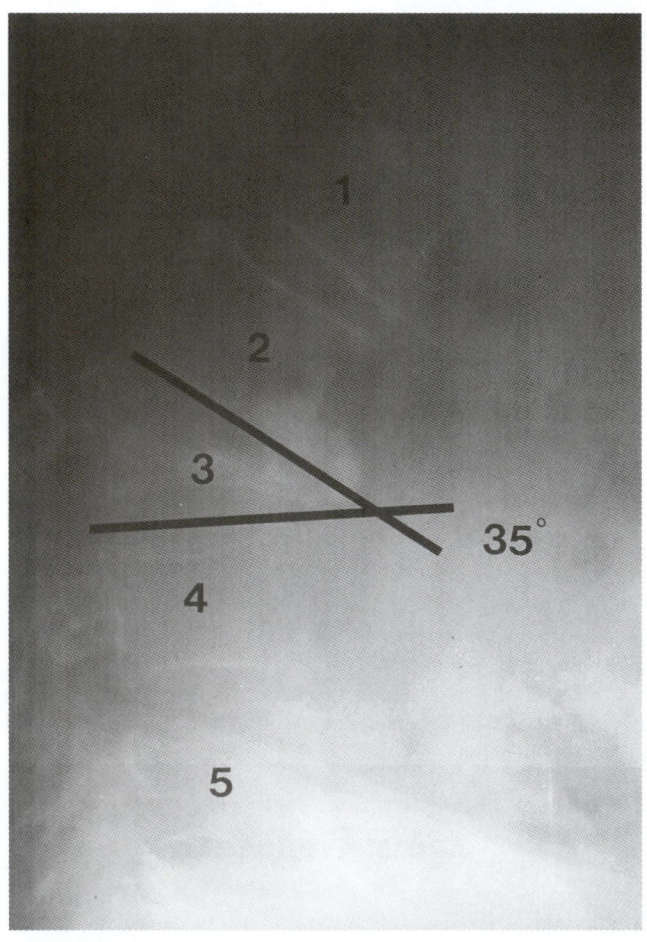

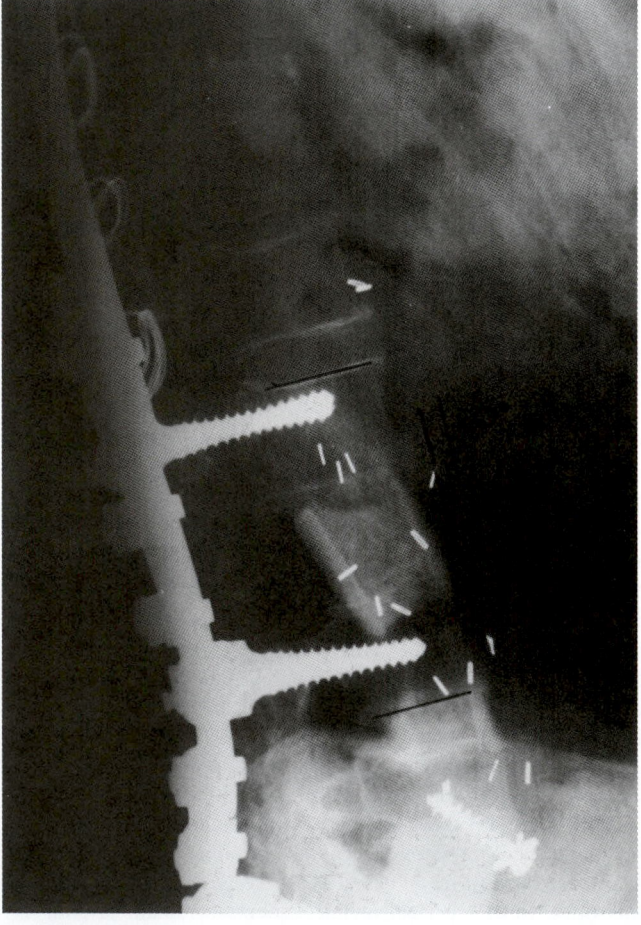

A   *B*

Figure 56-4
A. Localized 35-degree L3 kyphotic deformity secondary to senile burst fracture. *B.* Correction of this with a localized senile muscular thoracic kyphosis by a combined approach.

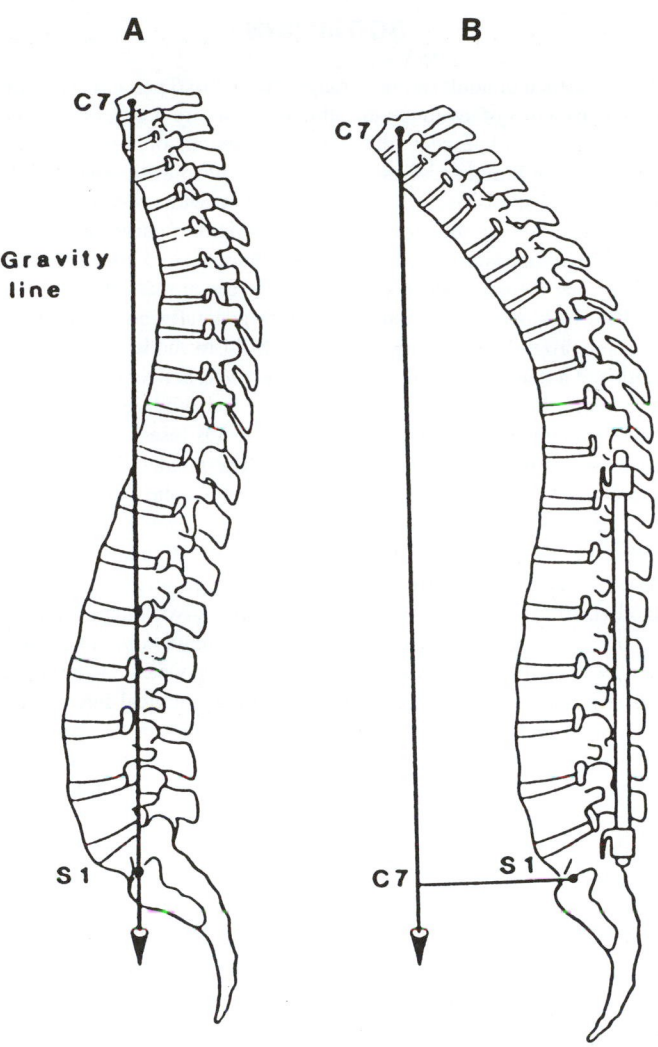

Figure 56-5
Measurement of the sagittal vertical axis. *A.* Normal sagittal contours. *B.* Anterior decompensation secondary to iatrogenic flat back. (Source with permission, from LaGrone MO: Loss of lumbar lordosis: A complication of spinal fusion for scoliosis. *Orthop Clin North Am* 1988; 19:386.)

ening of the deformity. This is the length of a perpendicular drawn from the sagittal vertical axis to the sacral promontory. Normally, this distance is 2 cm anterior to 2 cm posterior to the sacral promontory (Fig. 56-5). The worst prognosis for the development of postlaminectomy kyphosis is after an unstable fracture that is treated with a laminectomy.

Certain factors that predispose the spine to the development of a worsening posttraumatic kyphosis include the presence of greater than 30 degrees of local kyphosis, loss of greater than 30 percent of anterior vertebral body height especially at the thoracolumbar junction, compression fractures at two or more adjacent vertebral levels, and an unstable fracture treated with a laminectomy.

Indications for surgical intervention include painful deformity, progressive deformity, persistent instability, and persistent or progressive neurologic compromise. When treating this deformity, the compromised columns need to be realigned or reconstructed. Posterior instrumentation and fusion are generally not enough unless the kyphosis is reducible on an extension radiograph, and the height of the middle column of the spine is preserved. The posterior graft is under tension, which results in an increased pseudarthrosis rate. With 30 to 40 degrees of local kyphosis and a stable posterior column, patients

may be treated with anterior surgery alone. Anterior decompression is needed in the presence of incomplete or increasing neurologic deficit as well as in the presence of significant canal compromise. Local kyphosis of greater than 30 to 40 degrees with instability, previous laminectomy, or multilevel anterior column deficit generally requires anterior and posterior surgeries. Posterior compression instrumentation using hooks and/or screws provides the most stable construct. With restoration of the normal sagittal alignment, the likelihood of fusion increases and the stress on the instrumentation decreases.

FLAT-BACK SYNDROME

Flat-back syndrome was first recognized in the late 1970s with the use of distraction instrumentation in the lumbar spine to correct scoliosis. In addition to the coronal plane correction, the posterior distraction also resulted in increased kyphosis of the thoracic spine and in decreased lordosis of the lumbar spine. This became particularly evident if fusion was stopped at the apex of the kyphosis. Biomechanically, the decrease in upper lumbar lordosis results in a compensatory hyperlordosis and in increased stress at L4-5 and L5-S1, which hastens the development of degenerative changes. In time, the ability of the lower lumbar segments to compensate through hyperlordosis decreases. As a result, patients become more anteriorly decompensated. This loss of lumbar lordosis with distraction instrumentation is proportional to the number of levels fused. The worst results occur with fusion to the sacrum, where the anteriorly displaced sagittal vertical axis is fixed.

Patients with flat-back syndrome present with long-standing back discomfort. They complain of fatigue and anterior thigh pain secondary to prolonged knee flexion. Posture is stooped with flexion of the knees and extension of the upper spine in an attempt to attain upright posture. Impairment of functional activities is common. SI joint pathology should be ruled out.

The type of pain with which the patient presents may vary. Four pain patterns have been described:

1. Low back pain (frequently associated with a lumbar region pseudarthrosis)
2. Upper and midthoracic pain (tends to be worse at the end of the day and is secondary to increased muscle stress or fatigue; lying and sitting provide relief)
3. Cervical muscle strain (caused by attempts to hold the head maximally extended to allow for visualization; lessened by lying down)
4. Knee pain (caused by knee flexion in an attempt to compensate for the loss of lordosis; may be associated with patellofemoral symptoms)

Radiographic evaluation should consist of long-plate erect lateral radiographs with the knees fully extended. The sacral inclination provides information regarding the ability of the hips and pelvis to compensate. The sagittal vertical distance should be measured.

Flat-back syndrome is best prevented by preserving the normal lumbar lordosis. This is facilitated by positioning of the patient with the hips in full extension at the time of surgery and by the use of posterior segmental compression correction forces across the convexities of lumbar deformities.

Nonoperative treatment of a painful iatrogenic flat back consists of NSAIDs and therapeutic exercise. Pain symptoms may be significantly improved, although the underlying deformity will usually require surgical correction as degeneration and decompensation tend to progress. Orthotic treatment is rarely indicated except for temporary stabilization of a pseudarthrosis. Orthotic treatment for a painful flat back due to causes other than pseudarthrosis fails to control the problem and results in trunk and abdominal muscle weakness and worsening of the overall problem.

Indications for surgical intervention in flat-back syndrome include repair of pseudarthrosis, cephalad extension of the fusion to treat the development of a junctional kyphosis or progression of a cephalad kyphosis, caudal extension of the fusion to treat the juxtafusion degenerative disease with or without stenosis, and realignment of the fused spine. Posterior closing wedge osteotomies alone may be used to correct the alignment when mild to moderate iatrogenic-loss lumbar lordosis exists in the absence of significant thoracic kyphosis. The best results have been reported with combined anterior and posterior procedures with internal fixation (Fig. 56-6).

Correction of flat-back syndrome is not without potential complications and may be incomplete secondary to failure of fusion or collapse. Pseudarthrosis may develop at the osteotomy site. Neurologic compromise may occur as the result of foraminal encroachment from lateral impingement or centrally as the result of impingement from the closing wedge osteotomy, secondary to inadequate undercutting at the osteotomy site. Decompensation, loss of fixation, and dural complications are additional reported complications that occur with surgical correction of flat-back syndrome.

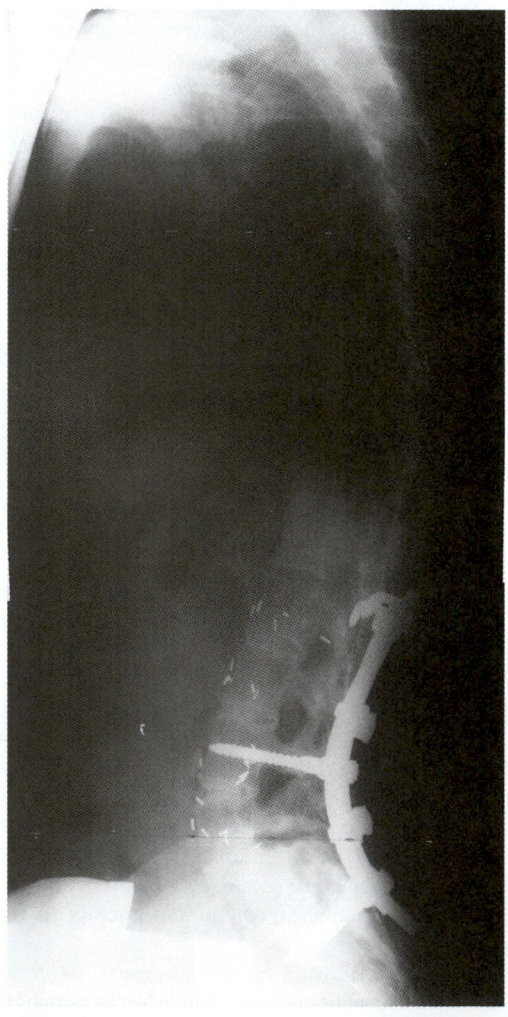

Figure 56-6
Correction by osteotomy of flat back after scoliosis surgery.

SCOLIOSIS

The incidence of adult scoliosis ranges from 4 to 6 percent. The most common causes of symptomatic adult scoliosis are progression or degeneration of adolescent idiopathic, congenital, or neuromuscular curves. Adult lumbar scoliosis may arise *de novo* as the result of degenerative disc disease, often in combination with osteoporosis, osteomalacia, or compression fractures. Adolescent curves at greatest risk for progression in adulthood are thoracic and thoracolumbar curves that measure between 50 to 75 degrees at maturity.

Mild to moderate scoliotic curves are generally not at increased risk for progression during pregnancy. Mild to moderate curves do not have a deleterious effect on pregnancy and delivery.

The development of degenerative changes in operatively treated scoliosis patients is related to the lowest level that is fused. The incidence increases as more distal levels are fused. The incidence increases as more distal levels are fused. Twenty percent of scoliosis patients who undergo spinal fusion that includes L2 develop degenerative changes. When L3 is included, the percentage increases to 30 percent. With L4 fused, 60 percent of patients demonstrate changes, and when L5 is included, 80 percent of patients develop degenerative changes. The development of kyphosis and spinal stenosis is more common in adult scoliotics with degenerative changes. These secondary changes may result in back pain that may require additional surgical intervention.

History and physical examination are important in the evaluation of adult scoliosis. Worsening of pain and functional disability need particular attention because these are important factors for surgical consideration in patients with adult scoliosis. Change in height, fit of clothes, rib prominence, and waistline should be documented. Patients may find that they are leaning more forward or to one side (evidence of decompensation) with time. Serial full-length erect anteroposterior and lateral radiographs are necessary for documentation of progression. With significant deformity, computed tomography/myelography may be more helpful than magnetic resonance imaging in the evaluation of concomitant spinal stenosis. Discography and/or facet blocks have been used to determine whether specific degenerative changes are the source of pain.

When considering the treatment of adult scoliosis, the patient's symptoms are more important than the degree of deformity. Nonoperative treatment consisting of NSAIDs, physical therapy, and the use of orthoses is generally tried first. Operative indications include pain not responsive to nonoperative treatment, curve progression documented by history or radiographs, structural imbalance with excessive rotation and/or decompensation, iatrogenic flat back, and neurologic compromise.

Anterior correction of adult scoliosis is less useful in the presence of true kyphosis, which may be worsened by this approach. Combined anterior and posterior approaches are advocated for kyphoscoliosis in the lumbar spine in patients older than age 50. An isolated anterior approach may be used in mobile curves in the absence of osteoporosis or spinal stenosis. Fusion to the sacrum is indicated only when the last motion segment has been determined to be a source of pain. When indicated, fusion to the sacrum should be done both anteriorly and posteriorly.

Thoracoplasty can significantly improve cosmesis in thoracic curves with rotation even without significant improvement of the scoliotic curve. Severe rigid curves of 75 to 180 degrees require anterior releases with or without anterior and/or posterior osteotomies. Degenerative lumbar scoliosis with spinal stenosis is best treated by fusion with instrumentation in addition to decompression. Indirect decompression by correction of the deformity is an alternative surgical strategy.

Potential complications of operative management of adult scoliosis include instrumentation failure with pseudarthrosis and/or loss of correction. Medical complications are common, especially with combined anterior and posterior procedures. Most complications are minor. Overall complication rates are lower in simultaneous combined procedures, especially in patients with significant medical problems.

SUGGESTED READINGS

ANKYLOSING SPONDYLITIS

Hammerberg KW: Ankylosing spondylitis. In Bridwell K, Dewald R (eds): *Textbook of Spinal Surgery*, vol 1, 2d ed: Philadelphia; JB Lippincott, 1997:1109.

Hehne HJ, Zielke K, Bohm H: Polysegmental lumbar osteotomies and transpedicled fixation for correction of long-curved kyphotic deformities in ankylosing spondylitis: Report on 177 cases. *Clin Orthop* 1990; 258:49.

Kostuik JP: Ankylosing spondylitis: Surgical treatment. In Frymoyer JW (ed): *The Adult Spine: Principles and Practice*, vol 1, 2d ed. New York: Lippincott-Raven, 1997:845.

Simmons EH: The surgical correction of flexion deformity of the cervical spine in ankylosing spondylitis. *Clin Orthop* 1972; 86:132.

Simmons EH: Kyphotic deformity of the spine in ankylosing spondylitis. *Clin Orthop* 1977; 128:65.

Simmons EH, Duncan CP: Fracture of the cervical spine in ankylosing spondylitis: An analysis of its influence in severe deformity presenting for spinal osteotomy [abstr]. *Clin Orthop* 1978; 133:277.

Simmons EH, Simmons ED Jr: Ankylosing spondylitis. In Khan MA (ed): *State of the Art Reviews: Spine*. Philadelphia: Hanley & Belfus, 1990; 4:598.

Smith-Petersen MN, Larson CB, Aufranc OE: Osteotomy of the spine for correction of flexion deformity on rheumatoid arthritis. *J Bone Joint Surg [Am]* 1945; 25:1.

KYPHOSIS

Abitol JJ, Garfin SR: Complications associated with posterior instrumentation of the spine. In Rothman RH, Simeone FA (eds): *The Spine,* 3d ed. Philadelphia, WB Saunders, 1992; 2:1846.

Cummings SR: Epidemiology of osteoporotic fractures. In Genant HK (ed): *Osteoporosis Update 1987*. San Francisco: Radiology Research and Education Foundation; 1987:7.

Denis F: Iatrogenic loss of lumbar lordosis. In Farcy JP (ed): *State of the Art Reviews: Spine*. Philadelphia: Hanley & Belfus 1994; 8:659.

Farcy JP: Iatrogenic thoracolumbar spine deformity. In Farcy JP (ed): *State of the Art Reviews: Spine*. Philadelphia: Hanley & Belfus, 1994; 8:673.

Hammerberg KW: Kyphosis. In Bridwell KH, Dewald RL (eds): *Textbook of Spinal Surgery*. Philadelphia, JB Lippincott, 1991:501.

Sutherland CJ, Miller F, Wang GJ: Early progressive kyphosis following compression fractures: Two case reports from a series of "stable" thoracolumbar compression fractures. *Clin Orthop* 1983; 173:216.

Tupper JW, Gunn DR: Factors influencing stability of spine fractures. *Orthop Trans* 1977; 1:132.

ADULT SCOLIOSIS

Aaro S, Ohlen G: The effect of Harrington instrumentation on the sagittal configuration and mobility of the spine in scoliosis. *Spine* 1983; 8:570.

Bradford DS: Adult scoliosis: Current concepts of treatment. *Clin Orthop* 1988; 229:70.

Kostuik JP: Adult scoliosis. In Bridwell KH, Dewald RL (eds): *Textbook of Spinal Surgery*, vol 1, 2d ed. Philadelphia: JB Lippincott, 1997:733.

Weinstein SL, Ponseti IV: Curve progression in idiopathic scoliosis. *J Bone Joint Surg [Am]* 1983; 65:447.

Winter RB, Lonstein JE, Denis F: Pain patterns in adult scoliosis. *Orthop Clin North Am* 1988; 19:339.

Chapter 57

INFLAMMATORY ARTHRITIS OF THE CERVICAL SPINE

Ronald Moskovich

Rheumatoid arthritis is the archetypal inflammatory arthritis affecting the cervical spine. Seronegative spondyloarthropathies often behave in a fashion similar to rheumatoid arthritis and can only be distinguished by serologic testing. It is rare to see cervical involvement due to Reiter's syndrome or the spondyloarthritis associated with inflammatory bowel disease. Psoriatic spondyloarthritis affecting the cervical spine usually manifests as premature degenerative disc disease, and is rarely associated with instability. Systemic lupus erythematosus may also affect the vertebral column. Other inflammatory arthritides such as ankylosing spondylitis are covered elsewhere. Rheumatoid arthritis affects the synovial joints of the neck similarly to other joints in the body. Instability at the atlantoaxial junction or subaxially may become evident when the patient with long-standing rheumatoid arthritis presents with pain or decreased function. Occipital neuralgia is a common symptom of atlantoaxial subluxation.

The incidence of rheumatoid atlantoaxial subluxation varies with the population studied. Although an incidence of 3.2 percent has been reported in patients with rheumatoid arthritis, 6.4 percent of those with clinical disease had subluxation. In rheumatoid patients who are admitted to hospital, the incidence of subluxation has been reported as 19 to 37 percent of patients. The incidence of atlantoaxial subluxation does appear to increase with time from the onset of arthritis, although it is present in 12 percent within 2 years of onset of the arthritis. Craniocervical complications arise in 30 to 50 percent of patients who have had rheumatoid arthritis for more than 7 years, and atlantoaxial subluxation with myelopathy develops in 2.5 percent of those with rheumatoid arthritis for more than 14 years. Subaxial instability may also develop in addition to the cephalad pathology or may occur independently.

EVALUATION

Evaluation of patients with long-standing rheumatoid arthritis is complicated and often limited by the presence of chronic polyarthritis and deformity. Joint contractures and multiple large and small joint arthroplasties are common in patients with chronic disease. Muscle atrophy commonly occurs, and root symptoms are common due to the multilevel subaxial arthritis. Peripheral entrapment neuropathies and polyneuropathies may also be present. Classical neurologic examination is thus often difficult in patients who have suffered from rheumatoid arthritis for many years. It may be impossible, for example, to assess whether the plantar responses are up- or downgoing, due to forefoot arthritis or arthroplasty. Neuraxial compression may result in little more than increased upper extremity reflexes and the presence of pectoralis reflexes. Other methods of assessment such as the Health Assessment Questionnaire may act as a gauge of declining function. The American Rheumatological Association or Steinbrocker classification of function (Table 57-1) and the Ranawat index (Table 57-2) are useful indices of arthritis and neurologic function, respectively. Neurologic complications occurred at a mean of 19 to 20 years after the onset of arthritis in the author's series and occur in approximately 2.5 percent of patients with long-standing disease. The prognosis is poor after signs of spinal cord compression develop, with 50 percent of patients dying within 1 year of diagnosis.

PATHOANATOMY

The facet joints, as well as the synovial joints around the dens, may be affected by rheumatoid arthritis. Rheumatoid synovitis may result in subluxation and, later, destruction of these joints. Clinical instability may be identified on lateral flexion and extension radiographs. Clinical destruction of the dens may also occur, resulting in additional apparent instability or fracture of the dens with instability (Fig. 57-1). Upward migration of the C2 body and dens towards the foramen magnum is known as vertical subluxation of the axis or, more descriptively, cranial settling (Table 57-3).

Table 57-1

Steinbrocker Functional Classification of Rheumatoid Arthritis

Class I	Complete ability to carry on all usual duties without handicaps
Class II	Adequate for normal activities despite handicap of discomfort or limited motion at one or more joints
Class III	Limited to little or none of the duties of usual occupation or self-care
Class IV	Incapacitated, largely or wholly bedridden or confined to wheelchair, little or no self-care

Table 57-2

Ranawat Classification of Neurologic Function

Class 1	No neurologic deficit
Class 2	Subjective weakness with hyperreflexia and dysesthesia
Class 3	Objective findings of weakness and long-tract signs 3A Ambulatory 3B Quadriparetic and nonambulatory

RADIOLOGY

Vertical dislocation may be diagnosed when the tip of the dens lies significantly above McGregor's palato-occipital line, or when it is situated above the level of the foramen magnum. It is sometimes difficult to assess the position of the apex of the dens on conventional radiography, because of overlying structures, poor technique, or destruction of the dens. The distance between McGregor's line and the lower end-plate of the C2 vertebra can usually be measured easily, which obviates the confusion that may arise from use of the other methods (see Fig. 60-3C). A distance of less than 34 mm in men and 29 mm in women between the center of the lower end-plate of the C2 vertebra and the palato-occipital line is defined as vertical subluxation. With increasing vertical subluxation, the atlanto-dens interval tends to decrease. This is related to the morphology of the axis vertebra, which is somewhat of an inverted cone. As the atlas settles on the axis, and even though the anterior ring of C1 may approach the C2 body, the space available for the cord progressively decreases (Fig. 57-2). In patients with developing or established myelopathy due to atlantoaxial anterior subluxation, the treatment modalities will be predicated on the degree of reducibility of the subluxation. Pannus around the dens may be a major cause of cord compression and contribute to mortality.

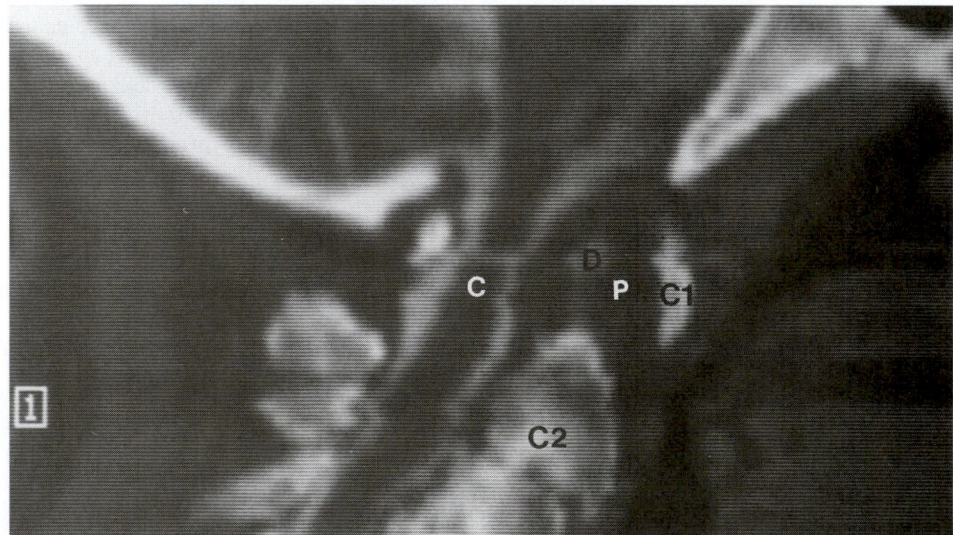

A

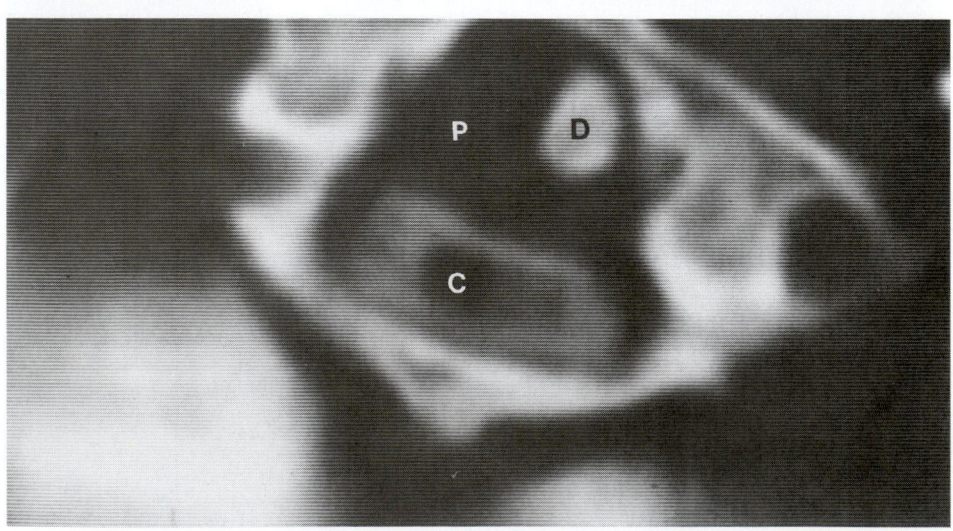

B

Figure 57-1
Computed tomographic reconstruction following myelography (CT-myelography) demonstrates marked erosion of the dens with a large soft tissue component (rheumatoid pannus) which is compressing the cervicomedullary junction. _A._ Sagittal CT- myelography. _B._ Axial CT-myelography. (C, cord; D, dens; P, pannus.)

Table 57-3

Rheumatoid Instability

Subluxation	Pathology
Anterior atlantoaxial	Ligamentous
Vertical atlantoaxial	Osseous
Lateral/Posterior atlantoaxial	Combination
Stepwise subaxial	Diskogenic

The upper cervical spine and cranial junction, as well as the subaxial spine, may be visualized using either magnetic resonance imaging (MRI) or contrast-enhanced computed tomography (CT-myelogram). Additional information about the neuraxis is obtained with the use of flexion and extension views (Fig. 57-3). These views are easier to obtain using CT rather than MRI because of the current technical limitations of MRI hardware, although the MRI units are rapidly improving. The radiologic abnormalities of rheumatoid arthritis are shown in Figs. 57-4 and 57-5.

MANAGEMENT

Education of rheumatoid patients is an important component of their care. The physician should counsel the patient regarding the potential risks associated with the disease. Rheumatoid patients should try to keep their hands free while walking to improve their balance and to be able to break a trip or fall. Use of a headrest and seat belts while driving are imperative. The correct position of the headrest should be emphasized: it should be adjusted so that the mid-part of the headrest aligns with the back of the occiput, and not the neck. An isometric exercise program is an excellent aid to general well-being and to greater flexibility and improved balance. Regular medical and radiologic evaluations by the physician are also important. Progressive subluxation or neurologic involvement is an indication for surgery to decompress the neuraxis and stabilize the cranioverte-bral column. The onset of myelopathy is a serious complication of the disease which generally may be prevented by active medical and/or surgical management.

The results of treating myelopathic rheumatoid patients have been studied. Nonambulatory patients (Ranawat class 3b) differed significantly in the degree of weakness, spasticity, and the presence of bladder and bowel control. Radiologically, they were characterized by a smaller cross-sectional spinal cord area and a greater degree of vertical translocation of the odontoid peg through the foramen magnum. Moreover, surgical intervention for rheumatoid atlantoaxial subluxation in bed-bound myelopathic patients was associated with a significantly higher postoperative complication rate, longer hospital stay, poorer neurologic and functional outcome, and ultimately decreased survival. The mortality in those without neurologic involvement (Ranawat class 1) was 1 percent.

Agarwal and coworkers (1992) reported on 110 patients who had undergone surgery for rheumatoid atlantoaxial subluxation. Of patients who had a C1-2 fusion 5.5 percent required additional surgery for subaxial problems a mean of 9 years after the index procedure. In contrast, 36 percent of those who had occipitocervical fusion required addition surgery after a mean of 2.6 years. They also found that no patients who had undergone atlantoaxial fusion developed vertical subluxation of the dens. These findings have been confirmed and supported by other researchers. Earlier surgery for patients with atlantoaxial subluxation will reliably prevent the development of vertical subluxation of the dens, decrease the necessity for subsequent surgery, and likely prevent those patients from requiring more major salvage procedures, such as resection of the dens.

The indications for surgical treatment of rheumatoid subluxation used to be limited to the development of cord compression. Severe neck symptoms or marked subluxation were relative indications. A combination of two of the following parameters is now an indication

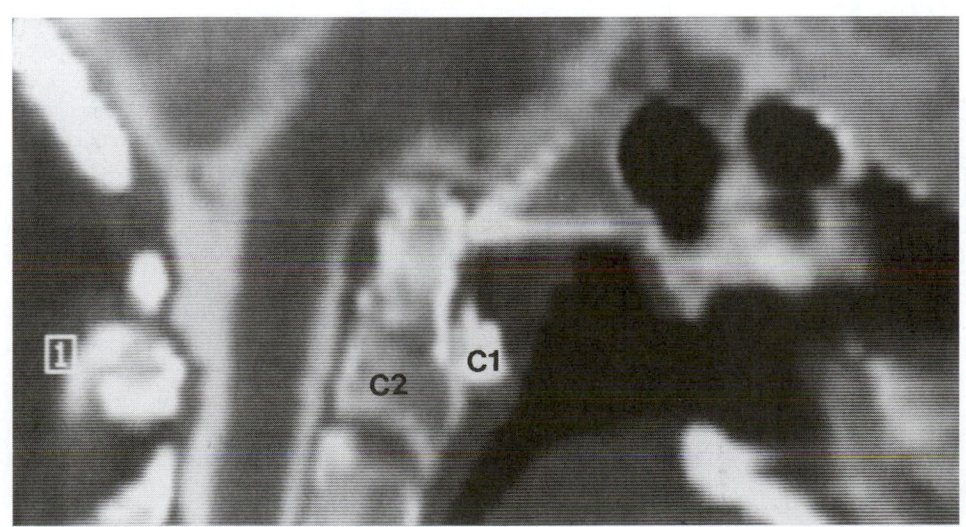

Figure 57-2

Sagittal CT-myelography of a rheumatoid patient with myelopathy. Marked vertical translocation of the dens is evident. The dens protrudes through the foramen magnum and impinges on the medulla oblongata. Note that the atlantodens interval is minimal in this situation.

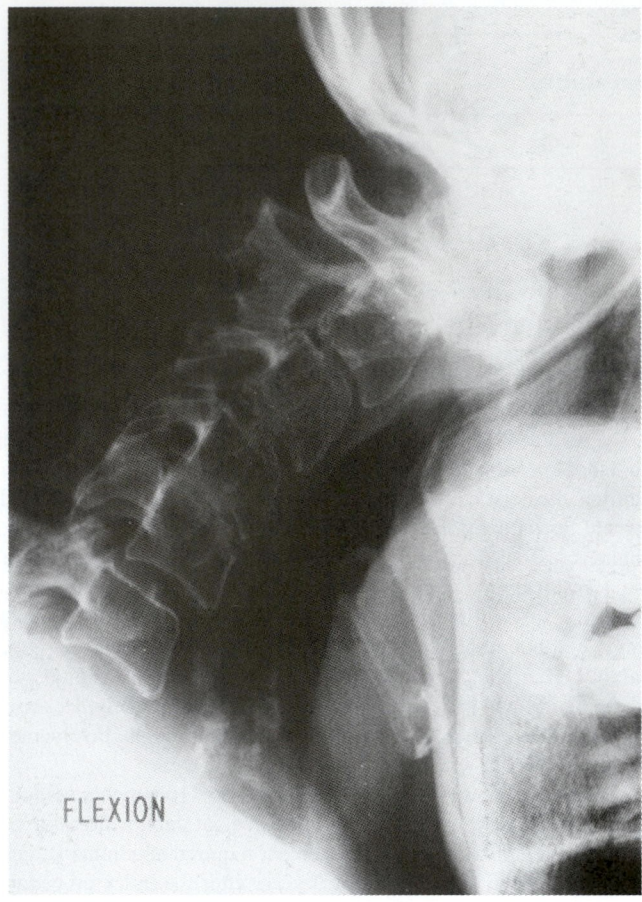

FLEXION

A

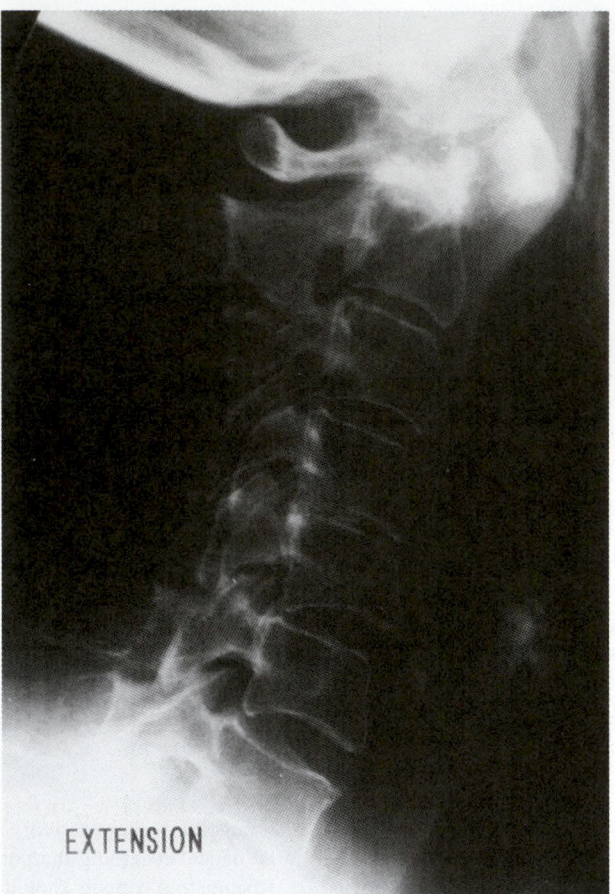

EXTENSION

B

Figure 57-3
Lateral cervical spine radiographs demonstrate vertical and anterior atlantoaxial subluxation in a patient with long-standing rheumatoid arthritis. The patient was referred for treatment after her neurologic function deteriorated. The anterior subluxation is largely fixed, and does not reduce with neck extension. Also note moderate subaxial arthritic changes. *A*. Flexion radiograph. *B*. Extension radiograph.

Atlantoaxial subluxation

Erosion of dens

Loss of disk height

Multiple subluxations

End-plate erosions

Facet joint erosions

Facet joint attenuation

Figure 57-4
The radiologic changes that may occur in rheumatoid arthritis.

for surgical intervention: Myelopathy, delayed central motor latency, reduction in spinal cord anteroposterior diameter to 6 mm or less or the spinal canal to 10 mm or less, inflammatory tissue behind the dens greater than 10 mm in thickness, and an increasing atlantodens interval or interval greater than 10 mm, or Redlund-Johnell measurement less than 34 mm in males or 29 mm in females. Surgical stabilization for atlantoaxial subluxation greater than 6 mm has been recommended in rheumatoid patients who are otherwise well. The natural history of rheumatoid atlantoaxial subluxation is bleak following development of spinal cord compression, as noted above.

Posterior atlantoaxial fusion should be performed if adequate reduction is possible. A solid fusion usually results in a reduction of pannus. In the face of a severe neurologic deficit, or if satisfactory reduction cannot be obtained, then the value of a posterior C1-2 fusion alone is questionable. It is undoubtedly true that stabilization may prevent some of the repetitive cord concussion that occurs with normal motion, but the anterior cord or medullary compression may persist, with suboptimal results. When a patient has basilar invagination associated with the Chiari malformation, we elect to perform an anterior decompression as a first stage, because surgical activity may impact the upper cervical cord/medulla onto the translocated odontoid peg, resulting in severe neurologic morbidity. The same situation pertains in the patient with a loss of joint-position sensation caused by compression of the cord by the posterior arch of C1. The passage

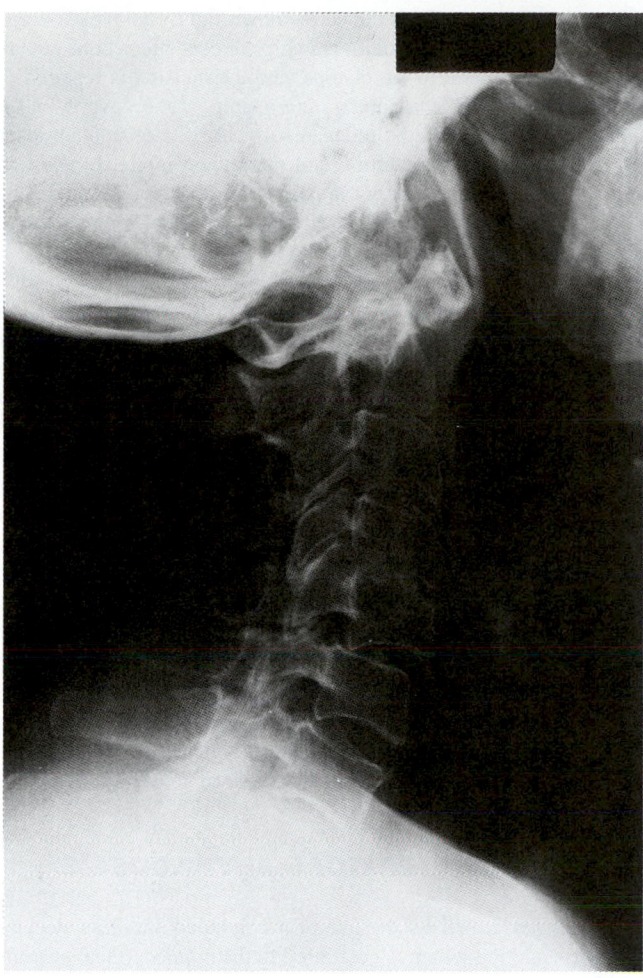

Figure 57-5
Lateral radiograph. Note marked vertical and anterior atlantoaxial sub-luxation. Spontaneous subaxial ankylosis has occurred at C4-5 and the C5-6 level has subluxed. The patient presented with severe occipital neuralgia and decreasing function, and was clinically myelopathic.

of instruments and wires beneath the lamina may result in significant neurologic morbidity, so an anterior decompression with or without stabilization should be the initial surgical approach.

Because of the relatively high rate of nonunion in rheumatoid patients who undergo posterior arthrodesis alone, other techniques to increase the fusion rate or at least to ensure initial stability of the arthrodesis have been used. The application of polymethylmethacry-late (PMMA) bone cement to the posterior elements has been advocated, and used successfully by some groups. PMMA used posteriorly to augment spinal arthrodeses is not without risk, however, and should be used with great caution as there is little evidence of long-term maintenance of fusion. Several anecdotal reports suggest that implantable bone growth stimulators increase the rate of solid fusion.

The problems and risks of bone harvesting are compounded in the rheumatoid patient who may have poorer quality skin, more depressed immunity, and greater postoperative immobility than average patients. Autograft is generally recommended when performing posterior arthrodesis with rigid fixation, or for anterior interbody arthrodesis for subaxial disease. Another surgical option is to omit bone grafting for occipitocervical arthrodesis when using a contoured modified Luque rectangle (the Hartshill-Ransford loop by Surgicraft. Redditch, Worcestershire, United Kingdom) and sublaminar wire fixation. The

long-term results (2 to 12 years) of this procedure have been equivalent to those using bone autograft while avoiding any of the complications of bone harvest. Patients with rheumatoid craniocervical and upper cervical instability generally will not have the same level of demand on the skeleton as active, age-matched individuals, and less rigorous application of the traditional role of bone grafting to achieve permanent stability has proved satisfactory.

Meijers and coworkers (1974) found that initial traction, posterior arthrodesis, and then traction for a further 3 to 6 months in a circo-electric bed for craniocervical instability in 14 patients resulted in the deaths of four patients of neurologic complications, and 10 of the 14 were dead within 1 to 8 years. One patient deteriorated suddenly after being on daily intermittent cervical traction for 1 year. A subsequent report on that series 10 years later (Meijers et al., 1984) warned of the high rate of deep venous thrombosis and pulmonary embolism in rheumatoid patients managed with recumbency. Other reports have also detailed the failure of this form of treatment to achieve consistent bony healing and patient survival. The inability of halo-vest fixation to ensure union was also demonstrated more recently by Papadopoulos, who reported that of 17 atlantoaxial (C1-2 only) stabilization procedures in patients with rheumatoid arthritis, only 76 percent fused and one patient died postoperatively despite the universal use of the halo-vest.

It is a widely held misconception that brainstem dysfunction and cranial nerve palsies in patients with rheumatoid arthritis are common and related to the vertical translocation of the odontoid process. In our database of 235 patients with seropositive rheumatoid arthritis and craniocervical junction involvement, we have found a very low incidence of such problems. The larynx, particularly the cricoarytenoid joint, is said to be commonly involved in rheumatoid arthritis. The symptoms and signs related to cricoarytenoid arthritis, such as hoarseness, dysphagia, and nocturnal stridor, may be incorrectly attributed to bulbar nerve dysfunction. Long tract signs were common, but loss of proprioception (joint position sensation) as the sole neurologic deficit was rare. Nystagmus was found to be associated with the tonsillar herniation of a Chiari 1 malformation and loss of joint position sensation with severe compression of the posterior aspect of the spinal cord at the craniocervical junction.

The surgical implications of these neurologic findings are obvious, but nonetheless extremely important. A patient with a Chiari 1 malformation, in whom there is herniation of the cerebellar tonsils into the upper cervical canal, will be particularly at risk during a posterior fixation procedure in which there is passage of wires around the foramen magnum and posterior arch of the atlas. The manipulation may lead to quadriparesis, respiratory arrest, or cardiac standstill and may account for some of the early postoperative deaths published.

Anterior approaches to the upper cervical spine and base of the skull may be performed via the retropharyngeal route or transorally. The retropharyngeal exposure is complex, requires extensive surgical dissection, and crosses major nerve planes. The transoral approach provides a direct exposure to the upper cervical spine extending from the clivus to the base of C3. Dissatisfaction with the complications and hazards of prolonged bed rest, skeletal traction, staged surgery, and halo-vest use in these rheumatoid patients resulted in the development of a one-stage transoral decompression with posterior fusion for instability and compression at the craniocervical junction. This approach avoids the problems of recumbency associated with a staged procedure. The transoral approach also has the advantage of providing a midline approach to the vertebrae, direct exposure of unstable vertebrae, and also reduces the risk of lateral approaches to the vertebral arteries and laterally placed neurovascular structures in the upper neck.

Enthusiasm for the transoral approach has been tempered by reports of complications such as failure of wound healing, cerebrospinal fluid fistula, hydrocephalus and meningitis, and respiratory arrest and tetraplegia. Rejection of transoral bone grafts have also been reported, but by and large these have not proved to be a major problem. The approach has been described in detail by Bonney, Menezes, and Crockard. The surgical techniques described by Crockard have reduced operative time for both the transoral decompression and the posterior fusion to the benefit of the patient and the surgeon alike.

TRANSORAL DECOMPRESSION

Surgery may be performed with the patient in the lateral position, or supine if an appropriate rotating table is used. After fiberoptic nasotracheal intubation has been performed, the patient is anesthetized and spinal cord monitoring is initiated. Tracheostomy is rarely required. Its use may cause complications because of the shortened necks of these patients and is an additional source of wound complications.

The skull is fixed in the Mayfield skull vise and the oral retractor is inserted. The tubercle of C1 is palpated to identify the midline and a vertical incision performed to expose the C1 arch and the body of C2. The anterior arch C1 is burred down and the pannus resected with diathermy or laser. The odontoid is thinned with a burr and separated from the corpus of C2, enabling the surgeon to pull down the dens and cut the alar and apical ligaments and remove the dens. It is then possible to observe the dural pulsations before closing the pharyngeal wall in two layers.

Postoperative care should consist of frequent oral cleansing, in addition to the use of prophylactic antibiotics (metronidazole and a third-generation cephalosporin). Elevation of the head reduces the swelling, and airway control is ensured by elective intubation for 48 h postoperatively.

ATLANTOAXIAL ARTHRODESIS

Anesthetic induction, endotracheal intubation, and positioning of the patient with cervical instability should be performed carefully to avoid iatrogenic neurologic injury. "Awake intubation" and subsequent repositioning of the patient into the prone position, followed by induction of general anesthesia, permits neurologic assessment to ensure that no further compromise has occurred.

Following surgical exposure of the atlas and axis, a variety of posterior fixation techniques are available. The traditional Gallie or Brooks-Jenkins posterior wire fixation techniques are sometimes compromised in patients with rheumatoid arthritis who have osteopenia and thinning of the posterior elements, which may not provide adequate support for wire tightening. Another technique utilizes interlaminar clamps. With this fixation it is not required to remove the ligamentum flavum or posterior atlantooccipital membrane.

Interlaminar (Halifax) clamps of correct size are selected so that when they are locked tightly, C1 and C2 are in the appropriate position, that is, not too closely approximated which would make the motion segment hyperlordotic. Two triangular cross-section wedges of bone are then harvested from the posterior iliac crest using osteotomes or a microoscillating saw. The wedges should be larger than the cross-sectional dimensions of the C1 posterior ring, measuring about 1.5 by 1.2 to 1.5 cm on the posterior cortical surface and 1 to 1.2 cm deep. It is advisable to harvest the grafts slightly larger than required as they may need contouring to lie precisely in the C1-2 interspace, on the C1 arch and C2 lamina. The graft bed (adjacent laminar surfaces of C1 and C2) is meticulously cleared of soft tissue before the graft is applied and punctate bleeding should be provoked with a burr. The clamps are then applied and tightened with the right-angled screwdriver. Final tightening should provide a solid construct, locking the C1 arch, bone graft, and C2 lamina into one unit (Fig. 57-6).

Care must be taken to lock the screw down tightly to avoid the risk of the screw backing out. Additional chips of cancellous bone are laid posteriorly and lateral to the clamps, and the incision is repaired.

The major advantage of interlaminar clamp fixation over wire fixation at a single level is the reduced surgical risks of implant insertion, including dural penetration and neurologic injury. In addition, rigid external fixation does not appear to be critical. A Philadelphia or foam collar worn for 3 months should adequately protect the construct while fusing.

None of the techniques of arthrodesis guarantee solid fusion. Both rotation and anteroposterior C1-2 motion should ideally be restricted to provide optimum conditions for fusion to occur and to reduce the risk of postoperative displacement. A combination of transarticular screw fixation and posterior arthrodesis may provide the optimum conditions. The trade-off, however, is the increased risk of screw insertion.

Transarticular C1-2 fusion is performed with the patient's head and neck positioned as straight as possible, to reduce the natural lordosis. Only the posterior elements of C1 and C2 need be exposed as the instrumentation may be applied percutaneously. The entrance for the screw lies on the dorsal, caudal edge of the facet of the axis, about halfway between the median line and the bony lateral boundary. The guide hole is drilled 0 to 10 degrees medial to the sagittal plane. Too lateral a hole may injure the vertebral artery. Lateral fluoroscopic control is essential to monitor the drill position. The hole is then depth-gauged and a 3.5- to 4.5-mm cortical screw inserted (Fig. 57-7). This is performed bilaterally. It is also recommended that a posterior interlaminar fusion be performed using one of the techniques described above (see Fig. 60-4).

OCCIPITOCERVICAL ARTHRODESIS

Fixation is performed by the use of a contoured stainless steel occipitocervical loop which is contoured to the craniocervical anatomy and affixed using sublaminar wires. The basiocciput and the laminae are exposed as far laterally as the facet joints. The junctional spinous processes and ligaments are preserved but the ligamentum flavum is excised at each level to be instrumented. Paired burr holes are made in the occiput and wires passed through those to fix the occipital part of the metal loop. Attempting to use one burr hole and passing the wires around the foramen magnum increases the risk of neurologic complications. Careful sublaminar wire passage at each cervical level is necessary, achieving a minimum six point fixation of the rod. The minimum configuration is occiput-C1-2 but additional laminae may be included if either the C1 ring is weak and fixation cannot be obtained or a staircase phenomenon is present with subaxial subluxations, which may be included in the fixation (Fig. 57-8). Instrumentation may also be extended to levels which are ankylosed, thereby providing improved fixation.

Sublaminar wiring in this population makes use of the strongest elements of the axial skeleton for fixation, and obviates the potential problems of cancellous purchase of other devices such as lateral mass screws in rheumatoid bone. The loop itself is precontoured for ease of use, and the current version incorporates a flare in the limbs of the device which act, in concert with C2 sublaminar wiring, as a simple method to maintain occipitocervical (occiput-C2) distraction without using external traction, halo-devices, or PMMA bone cement to maintain the reduction. It provides low-profile segmental fixation.

If transoral or other anterior surgery is performed, posterior stabilization should be performed under the same anesthetic. This will permit early mobilization of the patient and reduce the need for restrictive external support. In general, the surgeon should attempt to limit postoperative external support to either a standard Philadelphia collar or a soft cervical collar if the patient cannot tolerate the firmer support, and avoid the use of a halo-vest.

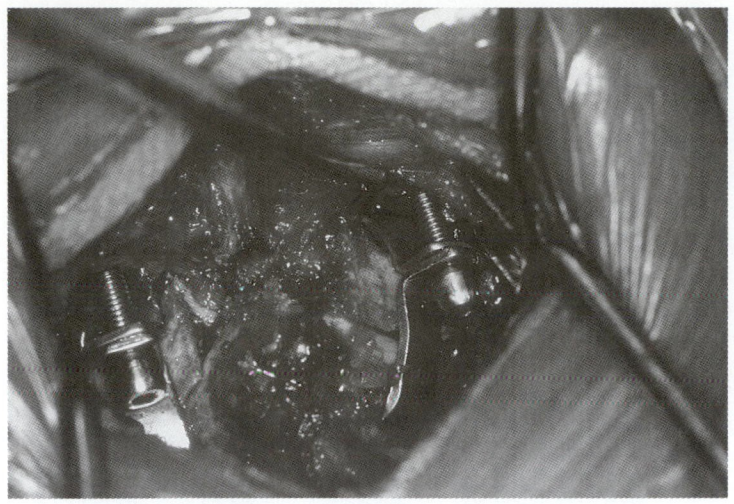

A

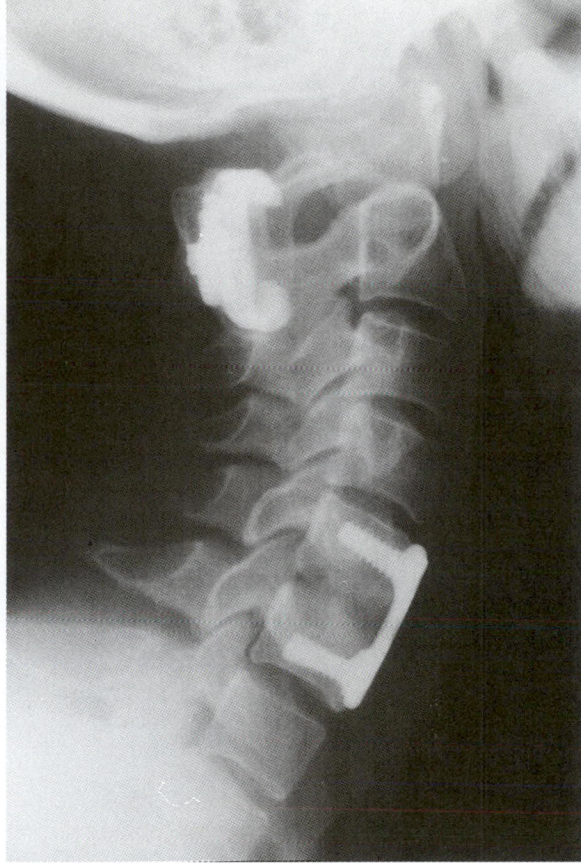

C

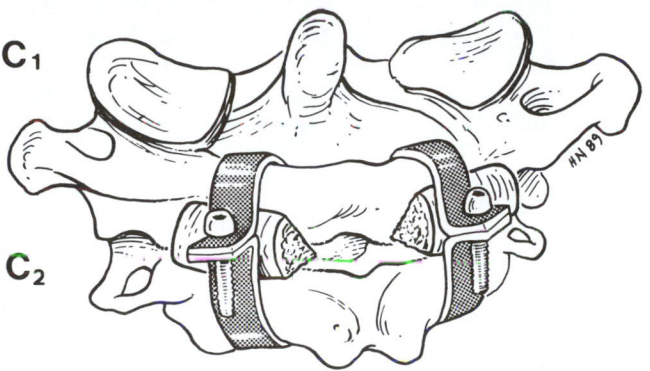

B

Figure 57-6

A and *B*. Halifax clamp fixation of the atlantoaxial complex provides initial stabilization. It is important to completely tighten the clamps over the laminae and interposed bone graft to avoid subsequent clamp loosening. *C*. A 40-year-old patient with long-standing rheumatoid arthritis developed myelopathy due to atlantoaxial subluxation. Treatment was by resection of the den and pannus and posterior atlantoaxial arthrodesis using Halifax clamps. Her symptoms resolved after surgery and a mature, solid fusion can be seen 3 years later. She subsequently suffered a C5-6 disc herniation which was treated by anterior cervical discectomy and interbody arthrodesis. The procedure was augmented by internal fixation because of the increased risks of nonunion in rheumatoid arthritis. [Panel *A* reprinted with permssion from Moskovich R: Cervical instability (rheumatoid, dwarfism, degenerative, others). In Bridwell KH, DeWald RL (eds): *The Textbook of Spinal Surgery,* 2d ed. Philadelphia: Lippincott-Raven; 1997:980. Panel *B* reprinted with permission from Moskovich R, Crockard HA: Atlantoaxial arthrodesis using interlaminar clamps: An improved technique. *Spine* 1992; 17:264.]

ANTERIOR SUBAXIAL ARTHRODESIS

In the presence of localized subaxial spondylolisthesis, anterior interbody arthrodesis may be necessary. Posterior fixation alone is adequate only in the absence of any neurologic deficit. Sometimes additional internal fixation or posterior arthrodesis may also be required to provide adequate stability (Fig. 57-6*C*). Approaches to the subaxial cervical spine were originally described in detail by Robinson and Smith and Cloward and are now well known. Structural interbody

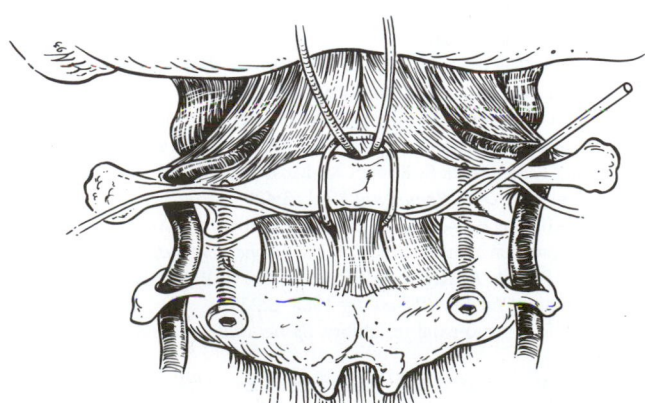

Figure 57-7

The position of transarticular screws used for atlantoaxial arthrodesis. While they eliminate translation, posterior wire fixation and bone grafting are necessary to eliminate flexion and extension. [Reprinted with permssion from Moskovich R: Cervical instability (rheumatoid, dwarfism, degenerative, others). In Bridwell KH, DeWald RL (eds): *The Textbook of Spinal Surgery,* 2d ed. Philadelphia: Lippincott-Raven; 1997:996.]

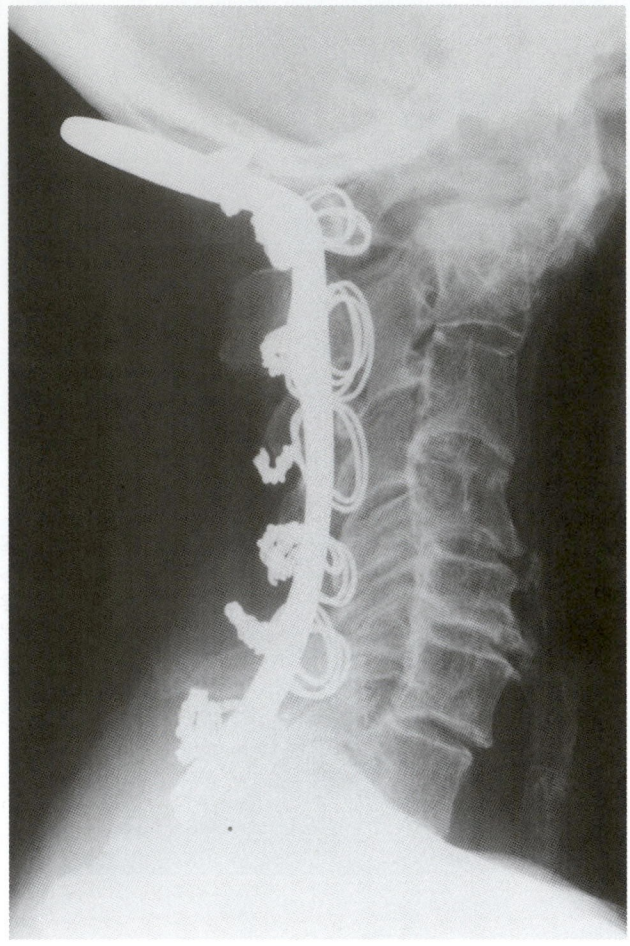

A

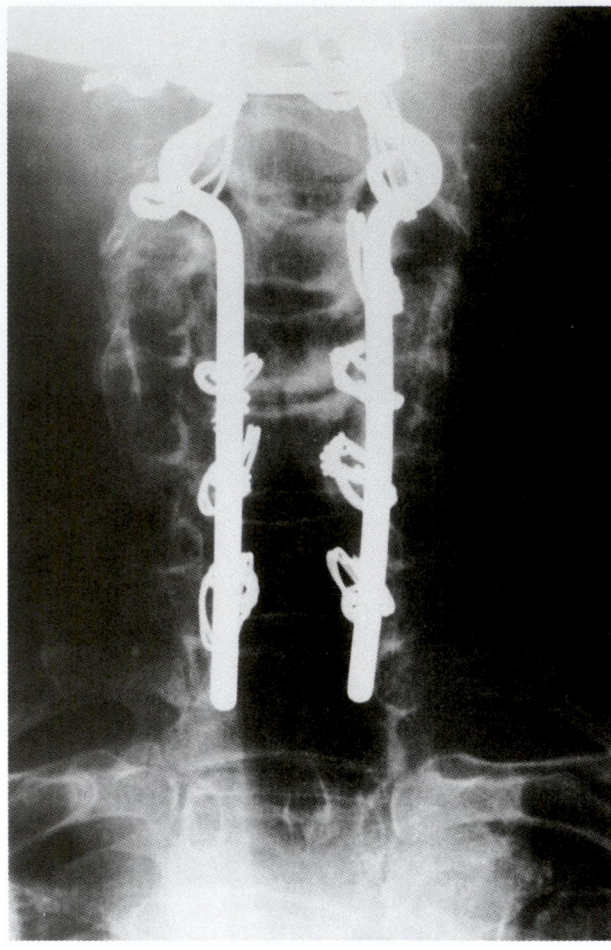

B

Figure 57-8

A and *B*. Occipitocervical stabilization without bone grafting was performed in a 68-year-old male who had long-standing rheumatoid arthritis and developed myelopathy. A transoral resection of the dens was performed because of a fixed atlantoaxial subluxation associated with marked neuraxial compression. Fixation was extended to include all the unstable subaxial levels which demonstrated a "staircase" phenomenon. No bone graft was used; nevertheless, ankylosis and complete stability of the subaxial spine developed.

grafting is usually performed to obtain adequate stability. Discectomy without interbody grafting is contraindicated.

CONCLUSION

The therapeutic regimen for rheumatoid cervical disease is one of compromise. An understanding of the natural history of the disease process, in combination with considerable technical advances, allows spinal surgeons to better manage these complex problems. These patients are also subject to an increased risk of cancer, which appears related to immune dysfunction, and a reduced life expectancy. Despite any surgical treatment, inevitably the basic pathology remains.

Our surgical objectives are to decompress the neuraxis, stabilize and correct deformity, relieve pain, anticipate further deterioration, and prevent overloading adjacent joints. It must be emphasized that when comparing treatment regimens and assessing morbidity and mortality (M&M), one should be cognizant of the total management M&M, not just the operative M&M. The rate of deep venous thrombosis and pulmonary embolism is significantly increased with recumbency. Constant clinical audit is essential to improve patient management proficiency. The incidence of complications may be reduced by a team approach, addressing all aspects of patient management. Rheumatoid patients are often fragile and all medical and nursing procedures require constant vigilance.

Active management of the rheumatoid patient is usually rewarding. The appropriate surgery is often well tolerated and patients experience an improved quality of life.

SUGGESTED READINGS

Agarwal AK, Peppelman WC, Kraus DR, et al: Arthritis following previous fusion: Can disease progression be prevented by early surgery? *J Rheumatol* 1992; 19:1364.

Casey AT, Crockard HA, Bland JM, et al: Surgery on the rheumatoid cervical spine for the non-ambulant myelopathic patient—too much, too late? *Lancet* 1996; 347:1004.

Crockard HA: The transoral approach to the base of the brain and upper cervical cord. *Ann Royal Coll Surg Engl* 1985; 67:321.

Helewa A, Goldsmith CH, Smythe HA: Independent measurement of functional capacity in rheumatoid arthritis. *J Rheumatol* 1982; 9:794.

Konttinen YT, Santavirta S, Kauppi M, Moskovich R: The rheumatoid cervical spine. *Curr Opin Rheumatol* 1991; 3:429.

Meijers KAE, Van Beusekom G, et al: Dislocation of the cervical spine with cord compression in rheumatoid arthritis. *J Bone Joint Surg [Br]* 1974; 65:668.

Meijers KAE, Cats A, Kremer HPH, et al: Cervical myelopathy in rheumatoid arthritis. *Clin Exp Rheumatol* 1984; 2:239

Moskovich R: Atlanto-axial instability. *Spine: State of the Art Reviews* 1994; 8:531.

Moskovich R, Crockard HA: Atlantoaxial arthrodesis using interlaminar clamps. An improved technique. *Spine* 1992; 17:261.

Chapter 58

INFECTIONS

Lynn J. Letko and Michael G. Neuwirth

Infections of the adult spine include pyogenic vertebral osteomyelitis, granulomatous vertebral osteomyelitis, postoperative disc space infections, and epidural abscesses. Spinal infections have been known since antiquity. Tuberculous spondylitis was first reported in Hippocratic texts. Lannelonge recorded the first pyogenic spine infection in 1897.

PYOGENIC VERTEBRAL OSTEOMYELITIS

Pyogenic vertebral osteomyelitis occurs through hematogenous spread, contiguous spread, or direct contamination. Trauma is not believed to play an etiologic role. Risk factors for pyogenic vertebral osteomyelitis include diabetes, extremes of age, intravenous drug use, and immunocompromised status. *Staphylococcus aureus* is the most common causative organism. *Escherichia coli, Proteus,* and *Pseudomonas* are the most common gram-negative organisms. *Pseudomonas* is seen with higher frequency in intravenous drug abusers. *Staphylococcus epidermidis* and other low-virulence organisms may result in a prolonged indolent course. These low-virulence organisms should not be regarded as contaminants when cultured.

Infection is most likely spread through the end arteriole anastomoses within the metaphyseal region of the vertebral body. Other proposed theories include spread of infection by back pressure through Batson's venous plexus. In pyogenic infections, the infection spreads from the body to the disc. This differs from tuberculous osteomyelitis, in which the disc is spared until relatively late in the disease process. The lumbar spine is most frequently involved, followed by the thoracic, cervical, thoracolumbar, and lumbosacral regions.

Diagnosis of pyogenic infection is frequently delayed. Of cases of pyogenic vertebral infections, 50 percent present in the chronic stage with a longer than 3-month history of symptoms: Only 20 percent present acutely (fewer than 3 weeks of symptoms), whereas the remaining 30 percent present subacutely (3 to 12 weeks of symptoms). The most common symptom of acute pyogenic vertebral osteomyelitis is neck or back pain. Fever is only present in approximately 50 percent of patients. Muscle spasm may limit spinal motion. In subacute and chronic cases, pain is frequently present. Other symptoms are usually vague and atypical. The magnitude of the presenting complaints and signs is affected by both the virulence of the organism and host resistance. The differential diagnosis includes tuberculosis and granulomatous conditions, fungal infections, metastatic disease, round cell tumors, trauma, degenerative disease, and epidural abscess.

Initial laboratory studies should include erythrocyte sedimentation rate (ESR), C-reactive protein (CRP), and white blood cell count (WBC). CRP and ESR are consistently elevated in these patients, while WBC elevation may be seen in approximately 42 percent.

Radiographic changes often lag behind clinical findings by up to 2 months. Radiographic changes are usually not seen for the first 2 to 4 weeks of the disease process. Disc space narrowing is commonly the first radiographic finding, followed by end-plate osteopenia. At 3 to 6 weeks, lysis of the vertebral body may be noted. Reactive bone and sclerosis with or without bony destruction and collapse are noted with healing. Computed tomographic (CT) scans may show the early erosive bony changes well. However, magnetic resonance imaging (MRI) is the imaging modality of choice: it is 96 percent sensitive, 93 percent specific and, overall, 94 percent accurate in diagnosing vertebral osteomyelitis. Changes are seen as early with MRI as they are with nuclear medicine scans, but the MRI changes are more specific. On T1-weighted images, decreased signal intensity is noted in the involved vertebral bodies and discs. The signal is increased on T2 images. Gadolinium enhancement of T1-weighted images results in increased signal intensity in vascular lesions such as tumor and infection. With vertebral osteomyelitis, this increased signal is seen in the vertebral body, whereas in disc space infections it is noted in the vertebral endplates.

Nuclear medicine studies demonstrate changes prior to those seen radiographically. Technetium-99 and gallium-67 citrate together have a 94 percent accuracy. Technetium-99 remains hot during the healing stages. Gallium-67 citrate becomes normal during healing and can be used to follow resolution of the infection. Indium 111 has poor sensitivity in the spinal infections. Its use is not indicated.

In septic patients, blood cultures may be positive. Typically, however, closed needle or open biopsy is needed to obtain tissue for culture and sensitivity. Closed needle biopsy is definitive in 68 to 86 percent of patients. All nonseptic patients should have a positive biopsy result prior to beginning antibiotics. More than one biopsy attempt may be needed. Multiple negative biopsies may be an indication for empiric antibiotic treatment without definitive identification of the causative organism. Definitive medical treatment is with intravenous antibiotics for a minimum of 6 weeks.

Patients are routinely treated with intravenous antibiotics for a minimum of 2 weeks once the CRP is negative. Oral antibiotics are used after intravenous antibiotics to ensure a total of 3 months of antibiotic coverage. The ESR should decrease by one-half to one-third by completion of successful antibiotic therapy.

Short-term bed rest, followed by mobilization in an orthosis for 3 to 4 months, is used in conjunction with antibiotic treatment. Surgery is indicated when closed techniques fail to provide a positive culture or to drain significant abscesses, in cases unresponsive to medical treatment, and to correct significant associated deformity. Surgery is urgently indicated in patients with spinal cord compression. Anterior debridement is best in almost all cases because it addresses and treats the pathology. Posterior stabilization may also be indicated.

Most patients do well if treated for 4 or more weeks with IV antibiotics. Many will develop a painless fibrous ankylosis rather than a solid fusion. The mortality rate in treated cases is less than 5 percent.

GRANULOMATOUS VERTEBRAL OSTEOMYELITIS

Granulomatous vertebral osteomyelitis is an uncommon entity most frequently seen in immunocompromised individuals. Etiologic organisms include bacteria such as tuberculosis, brucellosis, and nocardia; fungi such as candida and cryptococcus; and spirochetes such as syphilis. Tuberculosis is the most common of these etiologic agents. Bone and joint involvement is seen in 10 percent of all tuberculosis cases; tuberculous spondylitis, or Pott's disease, is seen in 5 percent. Tuberculous spondylitis is the most common cause of atraumatic paraplegia, with 10 to 47 percent of cases developing some degree of neurologic compromise.

Tuberculous spondylitis may result from hematogenous spread from other foci or may be secondary to direct extension from involved viscera. Paraspinal abscesses are more commonly seen with tuberculosis than in pyogenic vertebral osteomyelitis (Fig. 58-1). Four types of spinal involvement have been described:

1. Peridiscal, 33 percent: Starts in metaphysis. Extends under the anterior longitudinal ligament (ALL).

2. Central, 11.6 percent: Starts and stays in one body. Frequently with collapse and deformity.

3. Anterior, 52.8 percent: Spreads beneath the ALL over several segments.

4. Atypical: (*a*) neural arch, 2 to 10 percent; and (*b*) in the spinal canal, without bony involvement

The clinical presentation of tuberculous spondylitis is variable. Classically, the presentation consists of pain, weight loss, malaise, intermittent fever, local tenderness, muscle spasm, and limited motion. The thoracic spine is most frequently involved, followed by lumbar, cervical, and sacral involvement. ESR and CRP are elevated with a positive purified protein derivative (PPD). Biopsy specimen is needed to confirm the diagnosis.

Radiographic findings vary with the stage and location of the disease. Early, rarefaction is seen. Changes may appear advanced when compared to those of pyogenic infections. Less sclerosis and reactive bone is seen with healing. More deformity tends to occur than in cases of pyogenic vertebral osteomyelitis (Fig. 58-2). MRI is the imaging modality of choice in tuberculous spondylitis. Bone and gallium scans have false negative rates of 35 percent and 70 percent of cases, respectively.

The mainstay of treatment of tuberculous spondylitis is chemotherapy. Pharmacologic agents include isonicotinoylhydrazine (INH), rifampin, streptomycin, ethambutol, and pyrazinamide. Multiple drugs are used because of the development of resistance to single agents.

Indications for surgery in tuberculous spondylitis include:

1. Biopsy
2. Management of myelopathy, abscess, or sinus tracts
3. Failure to respond to 3 to 6 months of chemotherapy
4. Instability after healing
5. Recurrence of the disease
6. Unacceptable spinal deformity

When surgery is indicated, the Hong Kong operation (radical debridement and fusion) allows for earlier fusion, a higher fusion rate,

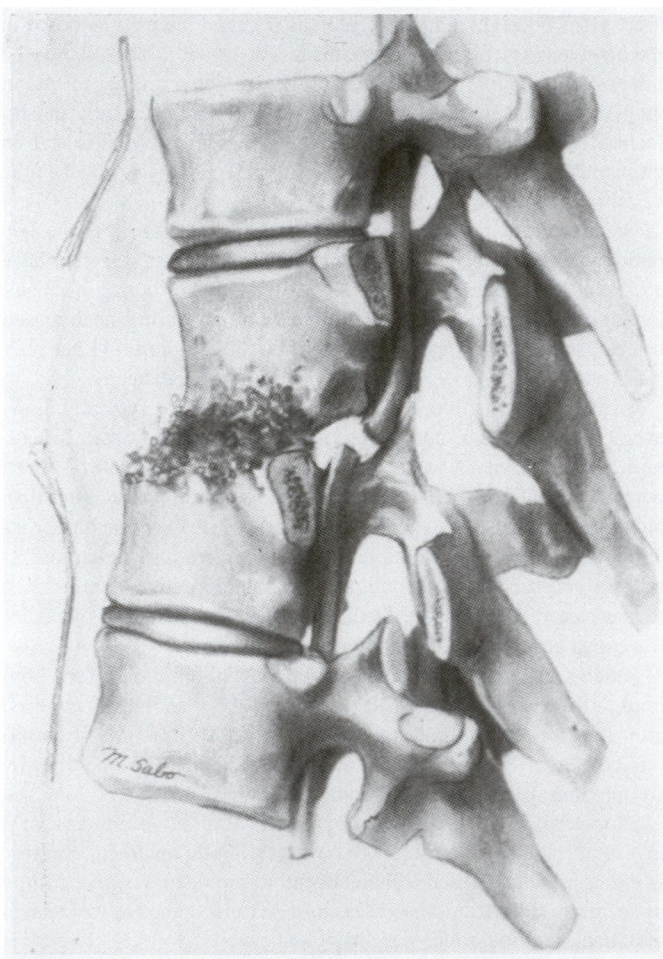

Figure 58-1
Collapse of the interspace with associated paraspinal abscess secondary to disc space infection with associated vertebral osteomyelitis. [Reproduced by permission from HH Bohlman, Department of Orthopaedics, University Hospitals of Cleveland, Ohio. Source is Currier BL, Eismont FJ: Infections of the spine. In Rothman RH, Simeone FA (eds): *The Spine,* 3d ed. Philadelphia: WB Saunders, 1992:1328.]

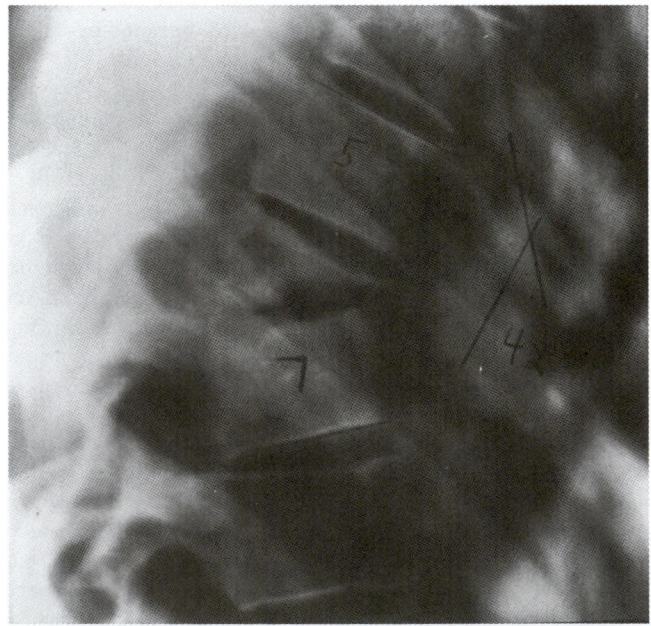

Figure 58-2
Kyphotic deformity and collapse secondary to tuberculosis spondylitis of T6.

less kyphotic deformity, and less back pain when compared to debridement with no fusion or with solely medical management. Anterior decompression and fusion with strut grafting also improves neurologic recovery when compared to nonoperative treatment. Costotransversectomy can be used to drain thoracic spine paravertebral abscesses. A retroperitoneal approach is advocated for drainage of psoas abscesses. Laminectomy is indicated only for atypical tuberculosis involving the posterior elements and for rare posterior epidural granulomas that exist without neurologic involvement.

Prognosis in patients with tuberculous spondylitis depends on patient factors such as age, health, and neurologic status. Resistance of the organism, duration, and severity of the disease also play a role. The mortality rate should be less than 5 percent if tuberculous spondylitis is diagnosed early and if patients are compliant with treatment. In patients with neurologic deficit secondary to tuberculous spondylitis, the prognosis improves with early surgery. Even those patients with long-standing paraplegia do better with aggressive surgical treatment.

POSTOPERATIVE DISC SPACE INFECTIONS

Postoperative disc space infections present in a typical manner. Patients return weeks or months after discectomy with increasingly severe back pain, occasional leg pain, and a benign surgical wound. Differential diagnosis includes recurrent herniated nucleus pulposus (HNP), HNP at another level, and mechanical low back pain. CRP and ESR are consistently elevated. The WBC is usually normal.

Plain films may show decreased disc height as the only finding. Later, blurring of the end plates is seen, followed by end-plate erosion. Reactive bone formation of the adjacent metaphysis may be observed. Advanced cases may show vertebral body collapse, indicating bony extension. With healing, obliteration of the disc space and bridging trabeculae are noted.

Technetium-99 bone scans alone are not helpful in the postoperative period, because they show increased uptake. Sequential ^{99}Tc and ^{67}Ga citrate scans are 94 percent accurate in such cases. Indium-111 scans have mixed results. MRI is the imaging modality of choice, with 94 percent accuracy. T1-weighted images show decreased signal intensity in the disc and adjacent marrow. T2-weighted images show increased signal intensity in the disc space. Changes are seen early within 3 to 5 days after the onset of the infection. MRI also allows for examination of epidural abscess or recurrent HNP.

Bed rest, immobilization, and intravenous antibiotics for 4 to 6 weeks are the mainstay of treatment for postoperative disc space infections. Indications for surgery include sepsis, cauda equina syndrome, advanced neurologic deficit with epidural abscess, failure of nonoperative treatment, and severe or intractable pain. Early, a posterior surgical approach can be used to incise and drain the disc space. In chronic cases, an anterior approach with incision and drainage followed by grafting is appropriate treatment. The prognosis for treated postoperative disc space infections is favorable.

EPIDURAL ABSCESS

Most cases of epidural abscess occur in adults. The incidence is reported to be 0.2 to 1.2/10,000 hospital admissions per year. An increased incidence is seen in persons with a history of intravenous drug use, diabetes mellitus, pregnancy, and back trauma, and 10 percent occur secondary to direct inoculation at the time of surgery or a spine procedure. *Staphylococcus aureus* is the most common causative organism, with an increased incidence of gram-negative or-

ganisms noted in patients with a history of intravenous drug use. Differential diagnosis should include epidural metastases and subdural abscess.

The clinical presentation of epidural abscesses is variable. Approximately 50 percent are initially misdiagnosed. Patients who present in the acute phase tend to have better-defined symptoms—including fever, chills, back pain, and spinal tenderness—than those who present in the chronic phase. CRP, ESR, and WBC are elevated. Blood cultures are positive in approximately 60 percent of cases. Cerebrospinal fluid cultures are positive in approximately 17 percent.

Radiographs are generally normal unless there is an associated osteomyelitis or disc space infection. The results of nuclear medicine studies are nonspecific. MRI is the study of choice (Fig. 58-3). CT myelogram should be done if MRI is negative in patients suspected of having an epidural abscess. Most epidural abscesses are located dorsally in the thoracic and lumbar spines. Ventral location may occur with abscesses resulting from spread of vertebral body or disc space infections. Four stages of progression without treatment are described: local spine pain, radicular pain, weakness, and paralysis that may occur unpredictably suddenly or after months of symptoms.

An epidural abscess should be treated as a medical and surgical emergency. Prognosis is directly related to the duration and severity of neurologic symptoms. Untreated, epidural abscesses progress relentlessly to paralysis. Patients with paralysis of less than 36 h duration

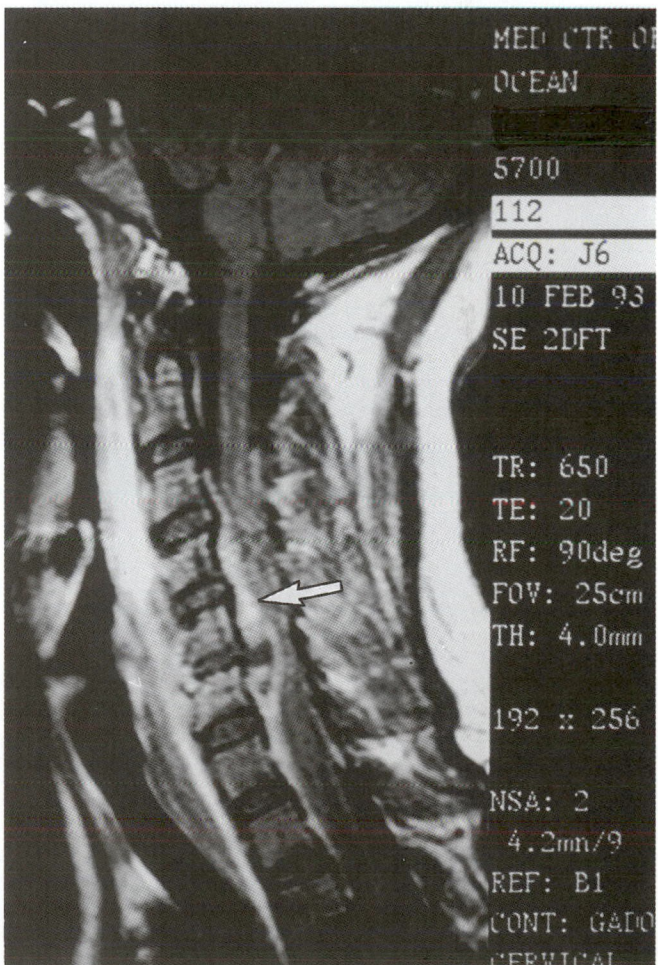

Figure 58-3
T1-weighted magnetic resonance image showing an epidural abscess (*arrow*) extending from a disc space infection at C5-6. Operative treatment using an anterior approach via C5-6 discectomy was performed.

tend to recover. Acute progression of complete paralysis within 12 h and complete sensory loss are poor prognostic indicators. Treatment consists of intravenous antibiotics in all cases and surgical decompression in cases with associated compressive neurologic symptoms. The surgical approach, anterior via discectomy or posterior via laminectomy, depends on the location of the abscess. Intravenous antibiotics are used for a minimum of 2 to 4 weeks, and up to 6 to 8 weeks in cases with coexisting vertebral osteomyelitis.

SUGGESTED READINGS

Currier BL, Eismont FJ: Infections of the spine. In Rothman RH, Simeone FA (eds): *The Spine,* vol 2, 3d ed. Philadelphia: WB Saunders; 1992:1319–1380.

Eismont FJ, Bohlman HH, Soni PL, et al: Pyogenic and fungal vertebral osteomyelitis with paralysis. *J Bone Joint Surg [Am]* 1983; 65:19–29.

Medical Research Council Working Party on Tuberculosis of the Spine: A 10 year assessment of controlled trials of inpatient and outpatient treatment and of plaster-of-Paris jackets for tuberculosis of the spine in children on standard chemotherapy. Studies in Masan and Pusan, Korea. *J Bone Joint Surg [Br]* 1985; 67:103–110.

Meyers SP, Wiener SN: Diagnosis of hematogenous pyogenic vertebral osteomyelitis by magnetic resonance imaging. *Arch Intern Med* 1991; 151:683–687.

Sapico FL, Montgomerie JZ: Pyogenic vertebral osteomyelitis: Report of nine cases and review of the literature. *Rev Infect Dis* 1979; 1:754–776.

Sapico FL, Montgomerie JZ: Vertebral osteomyelitis in intravenous drug abusers: Report of three cases and review of the literature. *Rev Infect Dis* 1980; 2:196–206.

Stauffer RN: Pyogenic vertebral osteomyelitis. *Orthop Clin North Am* 1975; 6:1015–1027.

Szyprt EP, Hardy JG, Hinton CE, et al: A comparison between magnetic resonance imaging and scintigraphic bone imaging in the diagnosis of disc space infection in an animal model. *Spine* 1988; 13:1042–1048.

Tuli SM: Results of treatment of spinal tuberculosis by "middle-path regime." *J Bone Joint Surg [Br]* 1975; 57:13–23.

Upadhyay SS, Sell P, Saji MJ, et al: Surgical management of spinal tuberculosis in adults. Hong Kong operation compared with debridement surgery for short and long-term outcome of deformity. *Clin Orthop Related Res* 1994; 302:173–182.

Upadhyay SS, Saji MJ, Sell P, et al: Longitudinal changes in spinal deformity after anterior spinal surgery for tuberculosis of the spine in adults: A comparative analysis between radical and debridement surgery. *Spine* 1994; 19:542–549.

Wiley AM, Trueta J: The vascular anatomy of the spine and its relationship to pyogenic vertebral osteomyelitis. *J Bone Joint Surg [Br]* 1959; 41:796–809.

Chapter 59

TUMORS

John A. Bendo and Michael G. Neuwirth

Tumors of the vertebral column, both primary and metastatic, have been well described in the literature. Appropriate preoperative work-up, staging, systemic therapy, and aggressive surgical treatment have improved both the short- and long-term outcomes. This chapter will outline the general principles of management, as well as specify details for extradural lesions with a predilection for the spine.

PRIMARY TUMORS

Primary tumors of the spine are a rare entity, with metastatic carcinoma being 40 times more prevalent. It is estimated that up to 70 percent of patients with primary carcinoma will develop skeletal metastases before death. The most common primary benign tumors of the spine are osteochondroma, osteoid osteoma, osteoblastoma, giant cell, hemangioma, and eosinophilic granuloma. Primary malignant tumors of the spine include osteosarcoma, chondrosarcoma, chordoma, Ewing's sarcoma, multiple myeloma, plasmacytoma, and lymphoma.

Symptoms secondary to a spinal tumor develop when one or more of the following occurs: (1) expansion or erosion of the cortex of the vertebral body by tumor mass leading to fracture and invasion of paravertebral soft tissues; (2) compression of nerve roots; (3) compression of the spinal cord; and (4) spinal instability secondary to bone and ligament destruction. Rapid progression of pain and neurologic compromise generally imply an aggressive lesion with a more guarded prognosis.

The age of the patient and location of the tumor within the vertebrae are also important prognostic factors. Most spinal tumors in patients younger than 21 are benign. In patients older than 21, the vast majority of spinal tumors are malignant. In addition, most tumors involving the posterior elements tend to be benign, whereas those in the anterior elements or body are more commonly malignant.

Pain is the most common symptom associated with spinal tumors. It can present as localized back pain or less frequently as radicular pain. Pain tends to be constant and progressive and very often worsens during rest or at night. Neurologic deficits are also common. Up to 70 percent of patients have weakness at the time of presentation. Bowel and bladder dysfunction can also occur. Spinal deformity may coincide with the onset of pain, secondary to paraspinal muscle spasm or vertebral body relapse. Up to 20 percent of cases may present with a palpable mass. Up to 5 percent of cases are asymptomatic at the time of diagnosis.

Imaging studies used to evaluate spinal neoplasms consist of plain radiographs, bone scan, computed tomography (CT) scan, magnetic resonance imaging (MRI), and myelogram. Anteroposterior (AP) and lateral radiographs should be obtained on every patient in which a neoplasm is suspected. Radiographic patterns of bony destruction include geographic, moth-eaten, and permeative, ordered from least to most aggressive. Radiographic evidence of trabecular bone destruction is usually not evident until 30 to 40 percent of the trabeculae

have been destroyed. Additional radiographic signs on the AP view include "the winking owl sign" (absence of pedicle), vertebral collapse, and soft tissue calcification. Radiographs obtained in the sagittal plane may reveal vertebral body collapse with disc space sparing commonly seen in spinal tumors. Osteolytic metastatic lesions are most commonly derived from breast, thyroid, and lung tumors, whereas osteoblastic lesions often are commonly from prostate, bladder, and gastrointestinal tumors.

Technetium-99 bone scanning remains a very sensitive test for the detection of spinal tumors larger than 2 mm, multiple lesions, and skip lesions. An aggressive osteolytic lesion with little reactive bone formation, such as multiple myeloma, may yield a false negative finding.

CT scanning provides excellent bony detail, can detect small irregularities not visible on plain radiographs, and can be used to evaluate for soft tissue extension of bony lesions. CT may be indicated for evaluation of vertebral compression fractures if a pathologic fracture is suspected.

MRI has become the gold standard for the evaluation of spinal tumors. It is particularly useful for evaluating epidural metastases and spinal cord compression. It is noninvasive and offers excellent soft tissue contrast with multiplanar images. Malignant tumors will have increased density on T2 and decreased density on T1. Gadolinium enhanced images also help to differentiate tumor versus a fluid filled cyst.

Myelography followed by CT can also provide an accurate assessment of spinal cord compression and epidural metastases. The possibility of acute neurologic deterioration following myelography in cases with a high grade block makes MRI the study of choice. Together, MRI and plain CT scan provide a complete anatomic evaluation of most spinal tumors.

BENIGN PRIMARY TUMORS

Osteochondromas (sessile, pedunculated) are slow growing benign cartilaginous lesions commonly arising from the posterior elements. They present in adolescence and may become painful. Neurologic compromise is exceedingly rare. Treatment involves simple excision if symptomatic or if sarcomatous changes are suspected.

Vertebral osteoid osteomas are usually found in the pedicles, transverse processes, or facet joints in teenagers and young adults. They show active uptake on bone scan and can often be seen on plain radiographs, tomograms, and CT scans. The classic presentation of a spinal osteoid osteoma is back pain worse at night, relieved by antiinflammatory medication, or it can present as a painful scoliosis. When associated with scoliosis, the tumor is usually located at the apex within the concavity of the curve. Treatment is surgical resection (curettage). The scoliosis will often resolve if the tumor is excised early and the child is young. Osteoblastomas share most of the same characteristics although they tend to be larger (>2 cm) and are often associated with a large soft tissue component. Spinal canal invasion results in a higher incidence of neurologic compromise. Pretreatment with tetracycline and the use of a Wood's lamp on the lesion will help to assess if the nidus has been removed.

Aneurysmal bone cysts typically present in the second decade of life and represent a dilatation of bony architecture by vascular channels within the neural arch. Rarely, they may arise in the anterior elements as well. Radiographs show the cortical expansion and a "soap bubble" appearance. They are quite vascular, making preoperative embolization beneficial to minimize surgical blood loss. Recommended treatments include total excision if possible, curettage, and low-dose radiotherapy. Recurrence rates of up to 25 percent have been reported following subtotal excision.

Hemangiomas are usually found incidentally on plain radiographs, MRI, or CT scan. Plain films reveal thick sclerotic bands of bony trabeculae resembling "jailhouse striations" within normal-sized vertebral bodies (expanded in Paget's disease). Axial CT images reveal "speckled spikes of bone." MRI shows increased signal intensity on both T1 and T2 images. They most commonly occur in the thoracic spine and in some instances may become expansile, painful masses that progress and cause collapse of the vertebral body and paraparesis. Treatment is observation, and radiation if conservative care fails. Anterior resection and fusion following embolization is rarely indicated, being reserved for resistant cases or cases with neurologic compromise and pathologic collapse.

Eosinophilic granuloma (Langerhans cell granulomatosis) is usually seen in the juvenile/adolescent age group and is commonly located in the vertebral body. It often presents radiographically as vertebrae plana. The disorder can occur as a solitary lesion or as a more systemic process. These lesions are usually self-limiting and vertebral body height is often reconstituted. Bracing may prevent kyphosis in the interim. Low-dose radiation or an incomplete curettage are alternate forms of treatment that are occasionally employed.

Giant cell tumors can involve all three columns of the vertebral body in young adults and remain one of the more common types of tumors in the sacrum. Treatment is usually surgical excision and bone grafting although the reported local recurrence rate remains quite high.

MALIGNANT SPINAL TUMORS

Solitary plasmacytoma and *multiple myeloma* present in older age groups as osteolytic osteopenic lesions, most commonly in the pedicle and vertebral body. Abnormal laboratory values include hypercalcemia, anemia, high globulin count in serum and urine electrophoresis, and Bence-Jones protein in the urine. These tumors are very radiosensitive, making radiotherapy the main form of tumor treatment. Chemotherapy is reserved for systemic disease. Larger lesions with compromised spinal stability are best treated by a combination of surgical debridement, reconstruction, and radiotherapy (3000 to 4000 centigrays). Postoperative radiation should be delayed an average of 2 to 3 weeks to diminish the incidence of wound dehiscence and allow for early bone graft vascularization.

Chordomas are slow-growing lesions most commonly involving the sacrum, base of the skull, and cervical spine. They have a predilection for anterior elements. They may present with abdominal pain or a presacral mass palpable on rectal exam. The treatment of choice is aggressive surgical resection and radiation therapy. Up to half the sacral roots (unilateral) may be resected with minimal sequelae. The local recurrence rate is high.

Ewing's sarcoma, osteosarcoma, and *chondrosarcoma* are uncommon lesions of the spine. They may be primary or metastatic and often involve all three columns of the spine. They are usually associated with a poor prognosis. An aggressive surgical debridement along with radiation is the mainstay of treatment. Unlike the extremities, wide margins of resection are usually not feasible in the spine. Neural structures should be preserved in most cases.

Lymphoma usually presents in the fifth or sixth decade, often in one or more vertebral bodies. It usually occurs in the lumbar and thoracic spine and can present as "ivory" vertebral bodies. Lymphomas are often very radiosensitive and may be treated with radiotherapy and chemotherapy if there is evidence of systemic disease.

METASTATIC DISEASE

The spine is the most common location for *skeletal metastases*. Breast, prostate, lung, and renal tumors are among the most common neoplasms that disseminate to the skeletal system. There are four potential pathways of metastasis to the spine: arterial, venous, direct extension, and lymphatic. The venous route via Batson's plexus has been considered the most common pathway of metastatic embolization to the vertebral column, mainly effecting the lumbar spine. Asdourian and colleagues have outlined the stages of spinal deformity associated with typical metastatic disease (Fig. 59–1). Their classification system is the first attempt to describe the successive stages of vertebral deformity secondary to tumor invasion.

The treatment options available for metastatic spinal disease include radiation therapy, hormonal manipulation, chemotherapy, surgical intervention, and most commonly, a combination of two or more of these treatment modalities.

GENERAL TREATMENT PRINCIPLES

The goals of treatment of spinal tumors include the following: (1) obtain a definitive diagnosis by imaging studies or biopsy, (2) institute appropriate medical/surgical care, (3) preserve (or restore) neurologic function, (4) maintain spinal stability, and (5) relieve pain.

Biopsies should be performed under control of the treating physician. They may be percutaneous (fluoroscopy, CT guided) or open (excisional versus incisional). The specimen should be taken from the margin of the soft tissue mass and meticulous hemostasis must be maintained.

Radiation therapy is appropriate for the treatment of symptomatic spinal metastases and primary tumors when: (1) the patient has a radiosensitive tumor, (2) the neurologic deficit is mild and the spinal canal compromise is a result of soft tissue impingement, (3) multiple myelographic blocks are present, (4) there is no evidence of spinal instability, (5) the condition of the patient precludes surgical treatment, and (6) the prognosis for long term survival is poor.

Prior to surgical intervention, the patient's immunologic, nutritional, and pulmonary status should be evaluated, and the life expectancy taken into consideration. Well-accepted surgical indications include: (1) intractable pain unresponsive to nonoperative measures such as bracing and radiotherapy, (2) progressive neurologic changes, (3) the presence of a radioresistant tumor, (4) decompression of the neural elements with tumor debulking, and (5) spinal instability or major destruction of vertebral architecture. The patient must be immunocompetent. This requires an absolute PMN count of greater than 1000.

The location of the neoplasm within the vertebrae or spinal canal determines the signs and symptoms produced, and dictates the surgical approach required for treatment. The vertebral body can be divided into anatomic zones which allows for objective preoperative

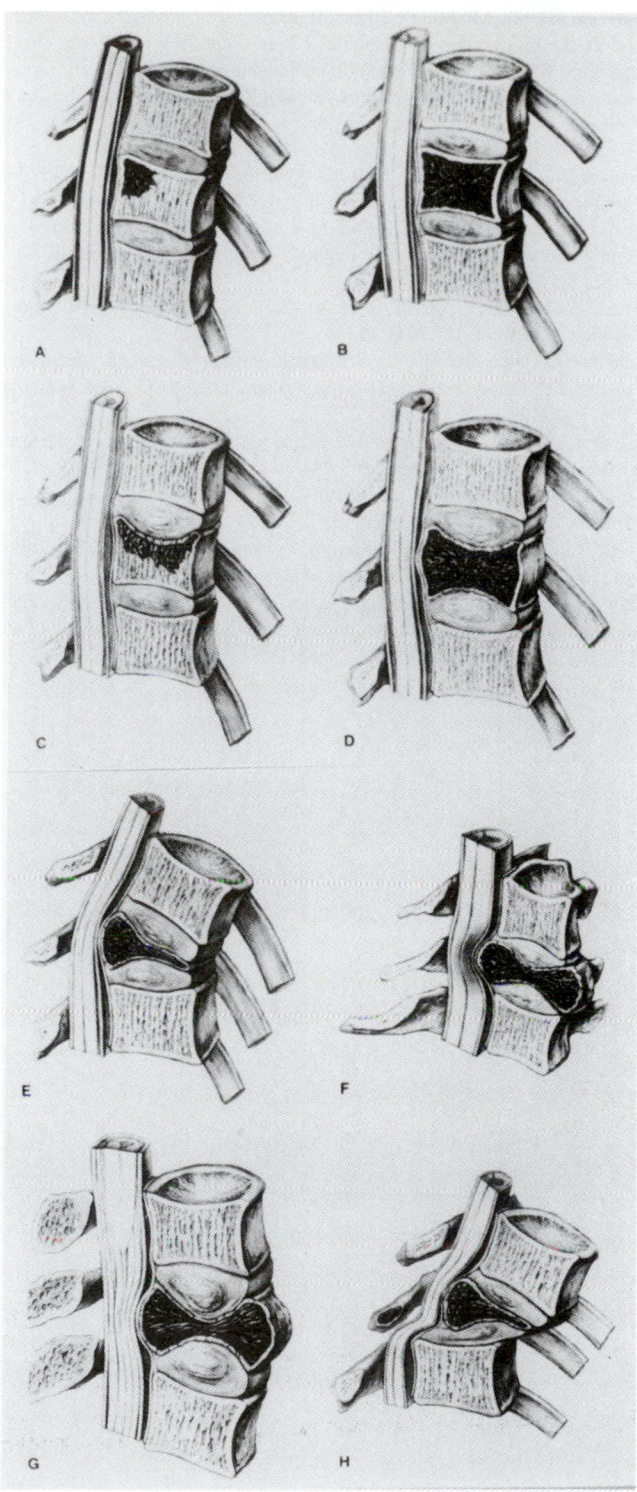

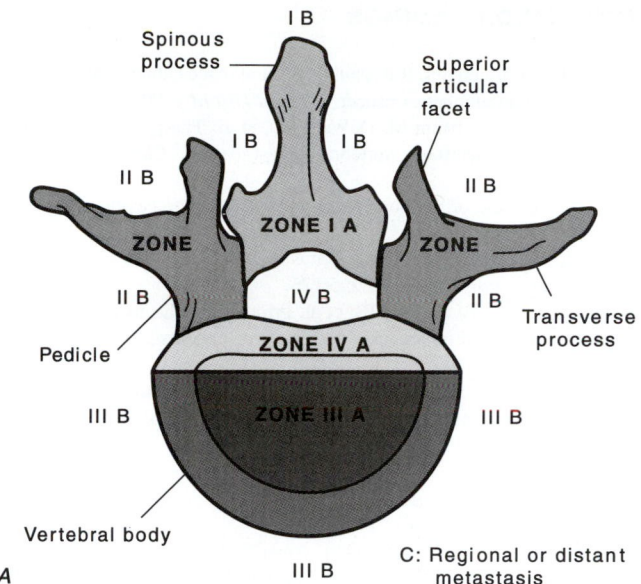

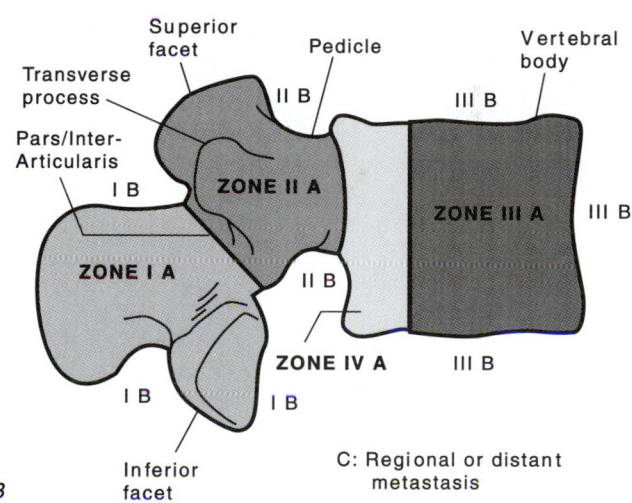

Figure 59–2
Anatomic extent of spinal tumor by zone. *A.* Axial cut through L1 (Zone I-IVA). *B.* Lateral through L1. [Reproduced with permission from Weinstein JN, McLain RF: The spine. In: Rothman RH, Simeone FA (eds): *The Spine*, vol I. Philadelphia: WB Saunders; 1992:1305.]

Figure 59-1
Diagrammatic representation of progressive vertebral metastatic involvement. *A.* An early metastatic deposit within vertebral body. *B.* Complete marrow replacement. *C.* Asymmetric involvement vertebral body resulting in fracture adjacent endplates. *D.* Early collapse with fracture of both endplates. *E.* End-stage collapse thoracic vertebrae. *F.* End-stage collapse cervical vertebrae. *G.* End-stage collapse lumbar vertebrae. *H.* Vertebral body deformity with associated translation of spine. [Reproduced with permission from Asdourian PL: Metastatic disease of the spine. In: Bridwell KH, DeWald RL (eds): *The Textbook of Spinal Surgery.* Philadelphia: JB Lippincott; 1991: 1192,1193.]

planning (Fig. 59–2). The surgical approaches for spinal decompression are divided into those that provide anterior access (vertebral body resection), posterior access (laminectomy), or lateral access (costotransversectomy or posterolateral).

Spinal reconstruction and stabilization should be considered when more than 50 percent of the vertebral body is involved or collapsed, when tumor involves both pedicles, when involvement of the posterior elements is complete, or with multilevel disease. The use of bone autograft or allograft to encourage biologic healing is preferred with a prolonged life expectancy; otherwise, methylmethacrylate is often useful for structural support. Segmental posterior instrumentation fixed in compression is commonly employed for immediate stabilization. Anterior instrumentation may obviate the need for adjunctive posterior instrumentation, depending on the tumor location and quality of bone. Adequate preoperative planning is mandatory for these patients and care must be coordinated with the radiation oncologist and the medical oncologist.

SUGGESTED READINGS

Asdourian PL, Mardjetko S, Rauschning W, et al: An evaluation of spinal deformity in metastatic breast cancer. *J Spinal Disord* 1990; 3:119.

Asdourian PL, Weidenbaum M, DeWald RL, et al: The pattern of vertebral involvement in metastatic vertebral breast cancer. *Clin Orthop* 1990; 250:164.

Batson OV: The role of vertebral veins in metastatic processes. *Ann Intern Med* 1942; 16:38.

Black P: Spinal metastasis: Current status and recommended guidelines for management. *Neurosurgery* 1979; 5:726.

Bohlman HH, Sachs BL, Carter JR, et al: Primary neoplasms of the cervical spine. Diagnosis and treatment of twenty-three patients. *J Bone Joint Surg [Am]* 1986; 68:483.

DeWald RL, Bridwell KH, Prodromas C, et al: Reconstructive spinal surgery as palliation for metastatic malignancies of the spine. *Spine* 1985; 10:21.

Enneking WF, Spanier S, Goodman MA: A system for surgical staging of musculoskeletal sarcoma. *Clin Orthop* 1980; 153:106.

Fidler MW: Anterior decompression and stabilisation of metastatic spinal fractures. *J Bone Joint Surg [Br]* 1986; 68:83.

Fielding JW, Pyle RN Jr, Fietti VG Jr: Anterior cervical vertebral body resection and bone grafting for benign and malignant tumors. A survey under the auspices of the Cervical Spine Research Society. *J. Bone Joint Surg [Am]* 1979; 61:251.

Gertzbein SD, MacMichael D, Tile M: Harrington Instrumentation as a method of fixation in fractures of the spine. *J Bone Joint Surg [Br]* 1982; 64:526.

Harrington KD: The use of methylmethacrylate for vertebral-body replacement and anterior stabilization of pathological fracture-dislocations of the spine due to metastatic malignant disease. *J Bone Joint Surg [Am]* 1981; 63:36.

Johnson JR, Leatherman KD, Holt RT: Anterior decompression of the spinal cord for neurologic deficit. *Spine* 1983; 8:396.

Kostuik JP: Anterior spinal cord decompression for lesions of the thoracic and lumbar spine, techniques, new methods of internal fixation results. *Spine* 1983; 8:512.

Manabe S, Tateishi A, Abe M, et al: Surgical treatment of metastatic tumors of the spine. *Spine* 1989; 14:41.

Mankin HJ, Lange TA, Spanier SS: The hazards of biopsy in patients with malignant primary bone and soft-tissue tumors. *J Bone Joint Surg [Am]* 1982; 64:1121.

Pettine KA, Klassen RA: Osteoid-Osteoma and Osteoblastoma of the spine. *J Bone Joint Surg [Am]* 1986; 68:354.

Siegal T, Siegal T: Current considerations in the management of neoplastic spinal cord compression. *Spine* 1989; 14:223.

Stener B, Johnsen OE: Complete removal of three vertebrae for giant cell tumor. *J Bone Joint Surg [Br]* 1971; 53:278.

Weinstein JN, McLain RF: Primary tumors of the spine. *Spine* 1987; 12:843.

Weinstein JN: Surgical approach to spine tumors. *Orthopedics* 1989; 12:897.

Chapter 60

CERVICAL SPINE

Nissim Ohana and Ronald Moskovich

The anatomic characteristics of the cervical spine of the infant and the child differ significantly from those of the adults. Until about 3 to 5 months of age, the average child is incapable of adequately supporting the head and is therefore vulnerable to the stresses that may be applied to the neck during delivery, parental shaking, or trauma. The characteristics of the immature cervical spine are: hypermobility, incomplete ossification, presence of epiphyses, synchondroses, unique vertebral configuration, and hyperlaxity of ligamentous and capsular structures. Some congenital cervical spine problems present clinically during infancy or early childhood while others may remain obscure until late childhood. The approach to the pediatric patient with a cervical spine problem should be based on the fact that while cervical spine conditions and diseases in adults are almost uniformly painful, the infant or young child usually presents with deformity rather than pain as the primary symptom.

TORTICOLLIS

Torticollis is a combined deformity that includes head tilt and rotation of the cervical spine. It usually indicates the existence of a C1–2 problem since 50 percent of cervical spine rotation occurs at this joint. Many different approaches to the pediatric patient with torticollis have been proposed. Table 60-1 indicates the large differential diagnosis of torticollis. In broad terms they can be divided to soft tissue versus osseous causes.

CONGENITAL TORTICOLLIS (WRYNECK)

Congenital torticollis is the most common cause of torticollis in infancy. The deformity is caused by contracture of the sternocleidomastoid muscle which creates tilting of the head toward the involved side, while the chin is rotated to the opposite side. The exact etiology is unknown. Theories of local soft tissue compression with a histologic picture similar to compartment syndrome, or in utero crowding have been proposed.

The problem is often diagnosed during the first 6 to 8 weeks of life by the typical combination of head tilt and chin rotation. Sometimes a mass can be palpated in the muscle on the involved side—the "sternocleidomastoid tumor." A coexistent congenital hip dysplasia or dislocation can be found in as many as 20 percent of the patients. Cranial and facial asymmetry (plagiocephaly) can develop within the first year of life if the deformity is progressive. Cervical spine radiographs should be always obtained to ensure the torticollis is purely muscular, and to exclude congenital lesions of the bony elements.

Table 60-1

Causes of Torticollis

Soft tissue

Congenital wryneck
Acquired torticollis
   Atlantoaxial rotary subluxation
   Sandifer's syndrome
   Infections and inflammatory
      Juvenile idiopathic arthritis
      Intervertebral disc calcification
      Cervical adenitis, retropharyngeal abscess, Grisel's syndrome
   Neurogenic
      Spinal cord tumors, posterior fossa tumors, syringomyelia, Arnold-Chiari malformation, ocular dysfunction, bulbar palsies

Osseous

Occipitocervical anomalies
   Basilar impression, atlanto-occipital anomalies, asymmetry of the occipital condyles, unilateral absence of C1 facet, odontoid anomalies, Klippel-Feil syndrome and familial cervical dysplasia
Tumors
   Osteoid osteoma, aneurysmal bone cyst

Treatment is mainly nonoperative. Good results can be expected with stretching exercises in up to 90 percent of the cases. Other treatments include modifying the child's toys and crib so that the neck will be stretched when the infant is reaching for or looking at objects of interest.

Surgery is indicated if the deformity persists after 1 year of age since continued stretching is usually unsuccessful. Bipolar release combined with Z-plasty of the sternal head of the sternocleidomastoid is the recommended surgical option. Simple transection of the sternal head may provide an unsatisfactory cosmetic result. The postoperative protocol is based on a short period of immobilization followed by stretching exercises.

ACQUIRED TORTICOLLIS

Acute onset of torticollis in the previously healthy child should be carefully investigated. The patient should be evaluated for injury, febrile disease, and upper respiratory illness, as well as for associated medical problems.

ATLANTOAXIAL ROTARY SUBLUXATION

Atlantoaxial rotary subluxation is the most common cause of childhood torticollis. The onset may occur spontaneously following minor or major trauma, an upper respiratory infection (Grisel's syndrome) or following head and neck surgery.

In the typical "cock robin" deformity, the head is tilted to one side, resisting any attempt at correction, while sternocleidomastoid spasm is noted on the opposite side (unlike congenital torticollis). There is usually pain associated with this type of torticollis, which tends to subside if the deformity becomes fixed. In long-standing cases, plagiocephaly and facial flattening may develop.

On true lateral cervical spine radiography the posterior arches of C1 fail to superimpose because of the head tilt, resulting in an oblique view of the atlas. There is also anteriorization of the C1 lateral mass relative to C2. On the open mouth (dens) view there is medial offset of one lateral mass (the mass looks wider and closer to the midline), while the other lateral mass exhibits a lateral offset (narrower mass, away from the midline). This radiographic finding can sometimes be obscured by the malalignment of the skull or the x-ray beam. It may be difficult to distinguish between a rotary subluxation and a normal child whose head is rotated. In that case, a dynamic CT scan in which the head is rotated maximally to both sides, should be taken. A fixed relationship of C1 to C2 is diagnostic (Fig. 60-1).

Rotary dislocation can be divided into four types (Fig. 60-2): (1) no anterior shift; (2) up to 5 mm of anterior shift; (3) more than 5 mm of anterior shift (reflecting progressively severe ligamentous injury); and (4) a subluxation with posterior atlantoaxial subluxation.

In most patients the atlantoaxial rotary subluxation resolves spontaneously, but occasionally the pathology becomes fixed. The duration of symptoms and degree of deformity should be taken into account when planning therapy.

Early deformity can be treated with a soft collar only, along with mandatory close follow-up. The patient should be admitted for halter traction if reduction fails to occur. If reduction occurs and no anterior displacement is noted (clinically and with CT), cervical support is needed until symptoms have subsided. In the case of proven anterior displacement, the patient should continue immobilization for at least 6 weeks. Indications for surgery are: failure of reduction, neurologic involvement, or presence of deformity for more than 3 months. Posterior arthrodesis should be performed. A further attempt at re-duction of the deformity should be made intraoperatively so that fusion occurs in the most neutral position possible. These maneuvers increase the neurological risks and should be only undertaken by a surgeon who is experienced in complex cervical surgery.

SANDIFER'S SYNDROME

Sandifer's syndrome consists of gastroesophageal reflux and torticollis. It is commonly seen in infancy or in children with cerebral palsy. The etiology is unclear. However, it is believed that the torticollis is reactive to the esophagitis caused by the reflux.

Upon examination of these infants, one can eliminate the possibility of congenital torticollis since none of its manifestations exist. The diagnosis of Sandifer's syndrome should be made after excluding other possible causes of torticollis and by demonstrating the reflux (upper GI study and pH monitoring).

Once the diagnosis has been made, therapy should be aimed towards the basic problem either medically or surgically. Surgical management of the reflux by fundoplication results in the disappearance of the torticollis.

NEUROGENIC TORTICOLLIS

Central nervous system-related causes for torticollis are relatively rare. The most common among them are tumors of the posterior fossa and spinal cord, syringomyelia, Arnold-Chiari malformation, ocular dysfunction, and paroxysmal torticollis of infancy.

Posterior fossa and cervical cord tumors, although rare, can present with torticollis. In contrast to cervical cord tumors, those of the posterior fossa present with torticollis in the late stage of the disease.

Cervical cord tumors can mimic congenital torticollis, obstetrical birth palsy, muscular dystrophy, and cerebral palsy.

The type I Arnold-Chiari syndrome consists of tonsillar elongation that projects into the upper cervical canal along with the medial part of the inferior lobe of the cerebellum. Chiari type I malformation occurs more commonly in children with at least half of the cases presenting with torticollis. In the type II Arnold-Chiari syndrome there is also elongation of the fourth ventricle into the spinal canal, a medullary kink, and hydrocephalus.

The infantile presentation of the malformation in its most severe form is usually associated with spina bifida and myelomeningocele.

The torticollis in ocular dysfunction is very unusual, since this is a positional deformity. In attempts to maintain a central gaze, the patient can turn his face about a vertical axis, or tilt his head toward one shoulder in order to keep the face in the frontal plane. No muscle spasm or other manifestations of structural torticollis are present and this deformity can be passively reduced without difficulty.

Paroxysmal torticollis is a very rare disease that presents as an episodic attack of torticollis, lasting minutes to days and recovering spontaneously. This syndrome is more common in girls, can be associated with lateral trunk curvature, eye movements, and alternating side torticollis. It has been suggested that paroxysmal torticollis is a migraine headache equivalent since there is a positive family history of migraine in 29 percent of cases.

INFLAMMATORY CAUSES OF TORTICOLLIS

Inflammatory conditions can involve the cervical spine and be expressed as torticollis.

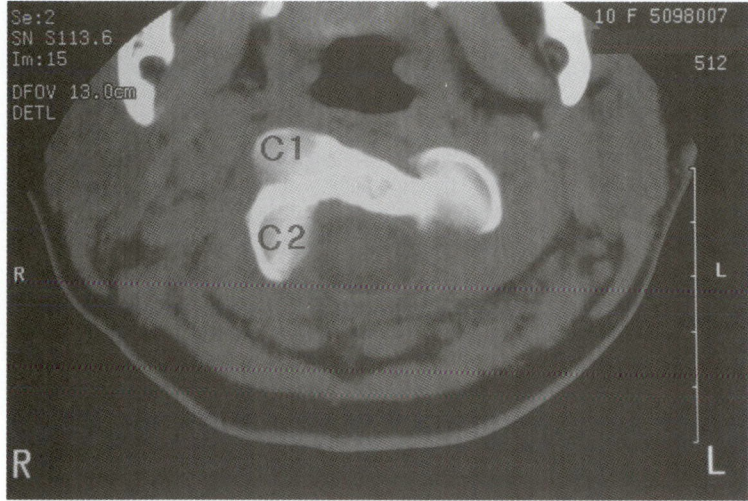

A

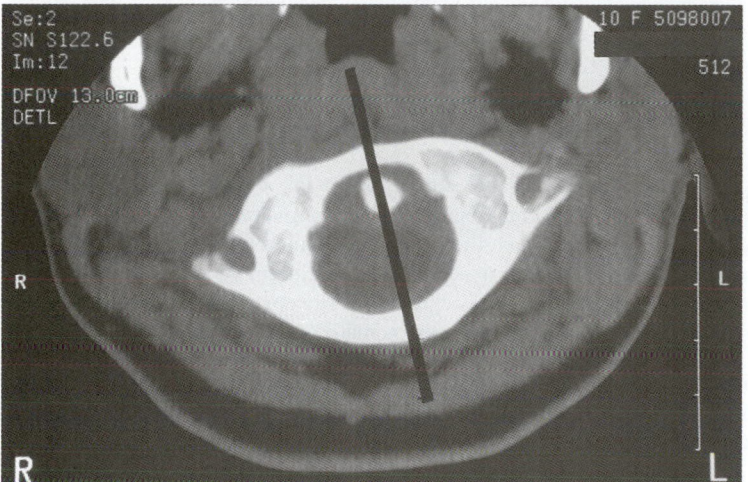

B

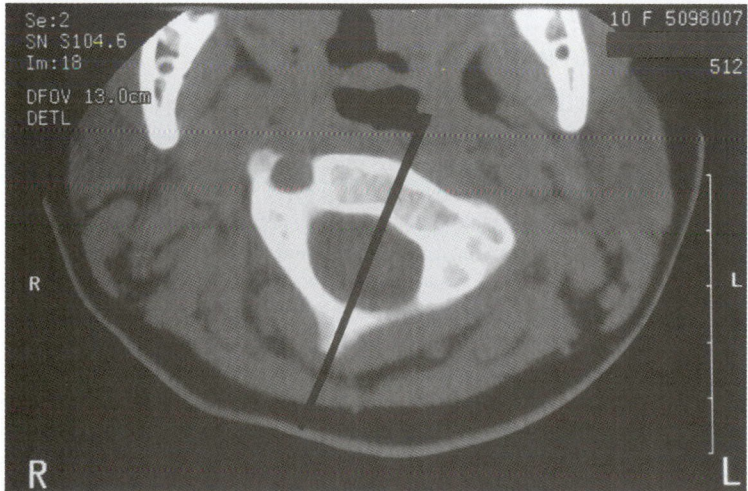

C

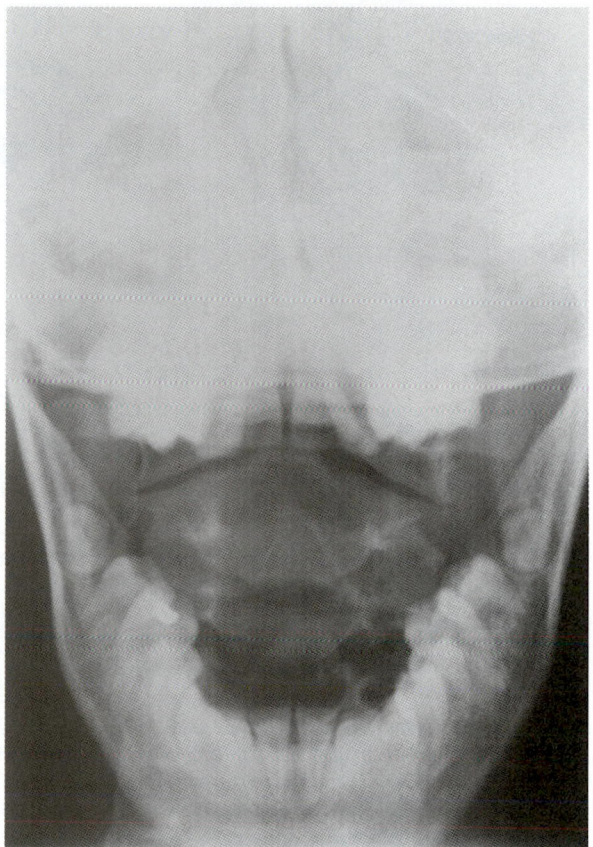

D

Figure 60-1

A. Computed tomographic axial view of the atlantoaxial junction in a 10-year-old patient with a 3-month history of neck pain and torticollis. The onset was a day following dance practice, with no specific trauma. Early active manipulation exacerbated her deformity. The CT shows a type I atlantoaxial rotary subluxation, with C1 and C2 seen malaligned on the axial scan. *B.* C1 is rotated +12 degrees relative to the sagittal plane. *C.* C2 is rotated −20 degrees relative to the same plane, resulting in a fixed 32-degree relative rotatory subluxation. The ADI is not increased. *D.* Halter and subsequent skeletal fraction failed to reduce the subluxation. Transoral open reduction of the "jumped" facets was performed, and the reduced position was maintained in a halo-vest for three months. She remained stable with a return to normal atlantoaxial relationships and a normal range of cervical motion. The open mouth view demonstrates symmetry of the lateral masses relative to the dens.

Juvenile Idiopathic Arthritis

Juvenile idiopathic arthritis (JIA) is a chronic inflammatory synovitis that can affect the apophyseal joints of the cervical spine as part of the generalized disease. This condition has traditionally been known as juvenile rheumatoid arthritis (JRA) or juvenile chronic arthritis (JCA). Although five types have been described, only the polyarticular and systemic onset types usually involve the cervical spine. The pauciarticular type affects it only rarely, when it progresses to a juvenile ankylosing spondylitis. Cervical spine involvement occurs most commonly during the first 2 years after onset of the arthritis. Clinically, patients present with stiffness and pain. Torticollis is rare and when this occurs other causes such as fractures, infection, or tumor should be suspected.

The radiographic appearance of JIA may include: anterior erosion of the dens, anterior-posterior erosion of the dens ("apple core" odontoid), C1–2 subluxation, soft tissue calcification, apophyseal joints

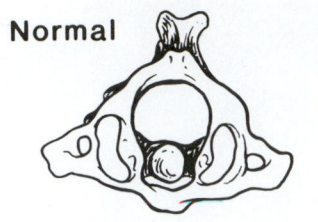

Normal

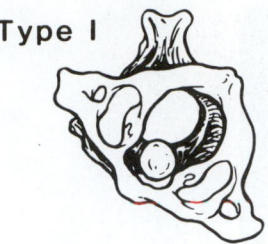

Type I

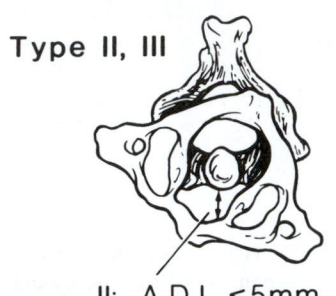

Type II, III

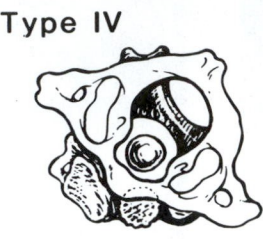

Type IV

II: A.D.I. <5mm

III: A.D.I. >5mm

Figure 60-2
Classification of atlantoaxial rotary subluxation: ADI, atlantodens interval. [Reprinted with permission from Moskovich R: Cervical instability (rheumatoid, dwarfism, degenerative, others). In Bridwell KH, DeWald RL (eds): *The Textbook of Spinal Surgery*, 2d ed. Philadelphia: Lippincott-Raven; 1997:972.]

ankylosis, vertebral growth abnormalities, and subaxial subluxation. As in the adult type of rheumatoid arthritis, complications such as C1–2 instability may occur, but cervical myelopathy and craniocervical subluxation are uncommon.

Treatment of JIA patients with cervical spine involvement is mainly symptomatic with rheumatologic care. Surgical intervention should be reserved only for patients with documented instability and progressive neurologic involvement.

Intervertebral Disc Calcification

Intervertebral disc calcification is uncommon, affecting boys more than girls with an average age at presentation of 8 years. Clinically, patients present with an abrupt onset of neck pain (50 percent), torticollis (25 percent), and fever (23 percent). Decreased range of motion and spinal tenderness are common.

Radiculopathy and myelopathy are seen only rarely. Nucleus pulposus calcification is visible radiographically, while advanced imaging studies, such as MRI reveals detectable protrusion of the disc in 38 percent of the cases.

The disease is generally self-limiting; two-thirds of the patients will recover within 3 weeks and 95 percent by 6 months. Regression of the deposits on radiographs occur in 90 percent of the cases. Symptoms should be managed with analgesics and rest in a soft collar; traction may be helpful for more severe cases.

Grisel's Syndrome

Grisel's syndrome, described in 1930, refers to the atlanto-axial rotary subluxation that occurs in the absence of trauma and is caused by chronic and acute inflammatory diseases of the neck and throat. Torticollis in those cases may be secondary to severe muscle spasm that holds the neck in flexion and aggravates the usual forward displacement of atlas on axis.

There is no relation between the severity, or intensity, of the inflammatory process and the torticollis. The etiology is a primary infection in the throat, or a remote focus draining into the cervical lymph nodes.

The clinical presentation seemingly evolves following resolution of the original infection, and the pain varies from mild to agonizing. The deformity heals spontaneously, usually following reduction and immobilization, even if the causative inflammation persists.

NEOPLASM

The most common neoplasm causing torticollis is osteoid osteoma. The lesion is most commonly located in the lamina but it also found in the pedicle and body. The intense inflammatory nature of the lesion and its proximity to the neural elements cause nerve root irritation, painful muscle spasm, and torticollis.

Osteoid osteomas do not undergo malignant transformation. However, if significant deformity results, surgical resection should be considered. Untreated osteoid osteoma tends to "burn out" as the patient matures.

OCCIPITOCERVICAL ANOMALIES

Occipitocervical synostosis, basilar impression, and dens anomalies are the most common developmental malformations in the occipitocervical region (1.4 to 2.5 per 100 children). The cause is faulty development of the neocranium and adjacent vertebral skeleton during embryonic life. Although these are congenital malformations, they often do not become symptomatic until adolescence or adulthood.

Clinically, these patients have an appearance similar to that of those with Klippel-Feil syndrome: a short broad neck, low hair line, high scapula, and torticollis. Sometimes the skull is deformed and shaped like a "tower skull," and patients may have associated anomalies such as dwarfism, funnel chest, jaw anomalies, cleft palate, congenital ear deformities, genitourinary defects, and syndactyly.

BASILAR IMPRESSION

In basilar impression, the tip of the dens is more cephalad and sometimes protrudes into the opening of the foramen magnum. There are two main types of impression: primary and secondary. Primary basilar impression, the most common type, is a congenital anomaly, often associated with other vertebral defects such as Klippel-Feil, odontoid abnormalities, atlantooccipital fusion and C1 hypoplasia, Arnold-Chiari malformation, and syringomyelia. Secondary basilar impression is a developmental condition attributed to softening of the osseous structures at the base of the skull. It can be secondary to metabolic bone diseases, Paget's disease, renal osteodystrophy, rickets and osteomalacia, osteogenesis imperfecta, achondroplasia, neurofibromatosis, and rheumatoid arthritis.

Clinically, patients present with a short neck, painful range of motion, and asymmetry of the skull or the face. Neurologic signs and symptoms are often present and can range from pyramidal syndromes to cerebellar involvement (when the impression is associated with an Arnold-Chiari malformation) and cranial nerve involvement. Osteogenesis imperfecta sometimes presents radiographically with invagination of the skull base settled down over the spine like an Irish cloth hat or "Tam O'Shanter." A variety of radiographic criteria to diagnose basilar impression have been proposed. Chamberlain, McRae, and McGregor, based their recommendations on the position of the tip of the dens in relation to various skull-base lines. The Redlund-Johnell measurement relates the base of C2 to the palatooccipital line of McGregor which avoids the confusion caused by overlapping bony

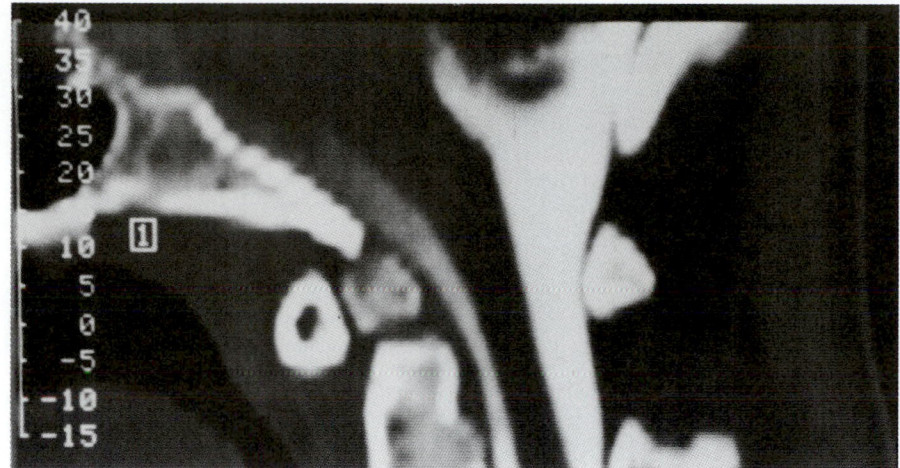

Figure 60-3
Sagittal CT reconstruction, following myelography, of a patient with an os odontoideum. The patient presented with acute myelopathy after hitting the top of his head on the underside of a diving board. He had considerable multidirectional instability. Treatment was by posterior atlantoaxial arthrodesis.

shadows of C1, the dens, and the mastoid air cells (Fig. 60-1). When it is difficult to assess the exact relation between the dens and the foramen magnum, an MRI or sagittally reconstructed CT scan can show the anatomic relationships and impingement of the neuraxis.

Treatment of basilar impression is primarily surgical. It is difficult and usually requires a multidisciplinary approach involving orthopedic surgery, neurosurgery, and neuroradiology.

CONGENITAL ANOMALIES OF THE ODONTOID

Three variations of odontoid anomalies have been described: aplasia, hypoplasia, and, the most common, os odontoideum. Aplasia is extremely rare and is associated with complete absence of the base of the odontoid. Hypoplasia has been described as a short, stubby projection just above the C1–2 articulation. Os odontoideum is a congenital or most likely acquired nonunion of the dens. It appears as a round ossicle of variable size, located at the position of the normal odontoid tip, and separated from the axis by a radiolucent line (Fig. 60-3).

The real frequency of dens anomalies is unknown since most of them are found incidentally, following trauma or after the spontaneous onset of symptoms sufficient to require radiologic investigation. In certain congenital disorders, these anomalies are recognized more frequently (Table 60-2).

UNILATERAL ABSENCE OF C1

Hemiatlas is often associated with other anomalies that are commonly associated with congenital spine deformities such as tracheoesophageal fistula. About 65 percent of the cases present at birth with painless torticollis and without the usual manifestation of wryneck, although plagiocephaly can develop. There is a decreased range of motion of the cervical spine. Neurologic signs such as headaches, vertigo, and myelopathy can be found in one-quarter of the patients.

The diagnosis is rarely made on routine radiographic studies, but plain tomography or CT suffice. Three types of hemiatlas have been described: type I is an isolated hemiatlas; type II is hemiatlas with

Table 60-2

Heritable Disorders in Which Atlantoaxial Instability and/or Odontoid Aplasia/Hypoplasia Is a Feature

Disorder	Atlantoaxial instability	Odontoid hypoplasia/aplasia
Chondroplasia punctata (Conradi-Hunermann type)	+	+
Diastrophic dysplasia	+	+
Dyggve-Melchior-Clausen	+	+
Hypochondrogenesis	+	—
Klippel-Feil	+	+
Lichtenstein	+	—
Marfan	+	—
Metaphyseal chondrodysplasia (McKusick type)	+	+
Metatropic dysplasia	+	+
Neurofibromatosis	+	—
Spondylo-epi-metaphyseal dysplasia (Strudwick disease)	—	+
Spondyloepiphyseal dysplasia	+	+
Kniest dysplasia	—	(?)
Morquio	—	+

SOURCE: The authors would like to acknowledge the assistance of E. Moran, M.S., Growth Center, Hospital for Joint Diseases Orthopaedic Institute. Reprinted and modified with permission from Scott CI, Jr. Pectoral girdle, spine, ribs, and pelvic spine. In Stevenson RE, Hall JG, Goodman RM: *Human Malformations and Related Anomalies.* New York: Oxford University Press; 1993; vol 2:668, 670.

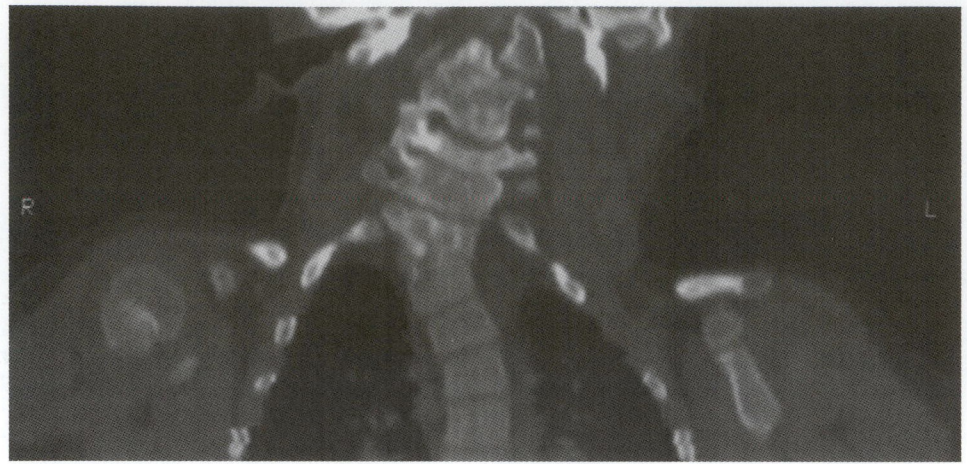

Figure 60-4
Klippel-Feil syndrome. Coronal reconstruction of a 6-year-old patient with multiple block vertebrae and cervicothoracic hemivertebrae. The patient has a short webbed neck. She is neurologically completely intact and participates in normal activities.

other anomalies of the cervical spine such as C3–4 fusion or congenital bar of the lower cervical spine; and type III is associated with partial or complete atlantooccipital fusion, sometimes with anomalies of the dens or the lower cervical spine.

Treatment in these cases is usually surgical. Surgery is recommended between the ages of 5 and 8. Angiography, MRI, and sometimes myelography may be necessary to complete the workup. Preoperative halo traction is used for gradual correction over 6 to 8 days. After a period of traction an occiput to C2 or C3 posterior

fusion is performed. Decompression should be performed only if there is coexistent spinal stenosis.

FAMILIAL CERVICAL DYSPLASIA

This autosomal dominant atlas deformity was described only recently. It includes a variety of occipitocervical anomalies such as: partial absence of the C1 posterior ring, hypoplastic facet of C2, occiput-C1 instability, and C1–2 instability.

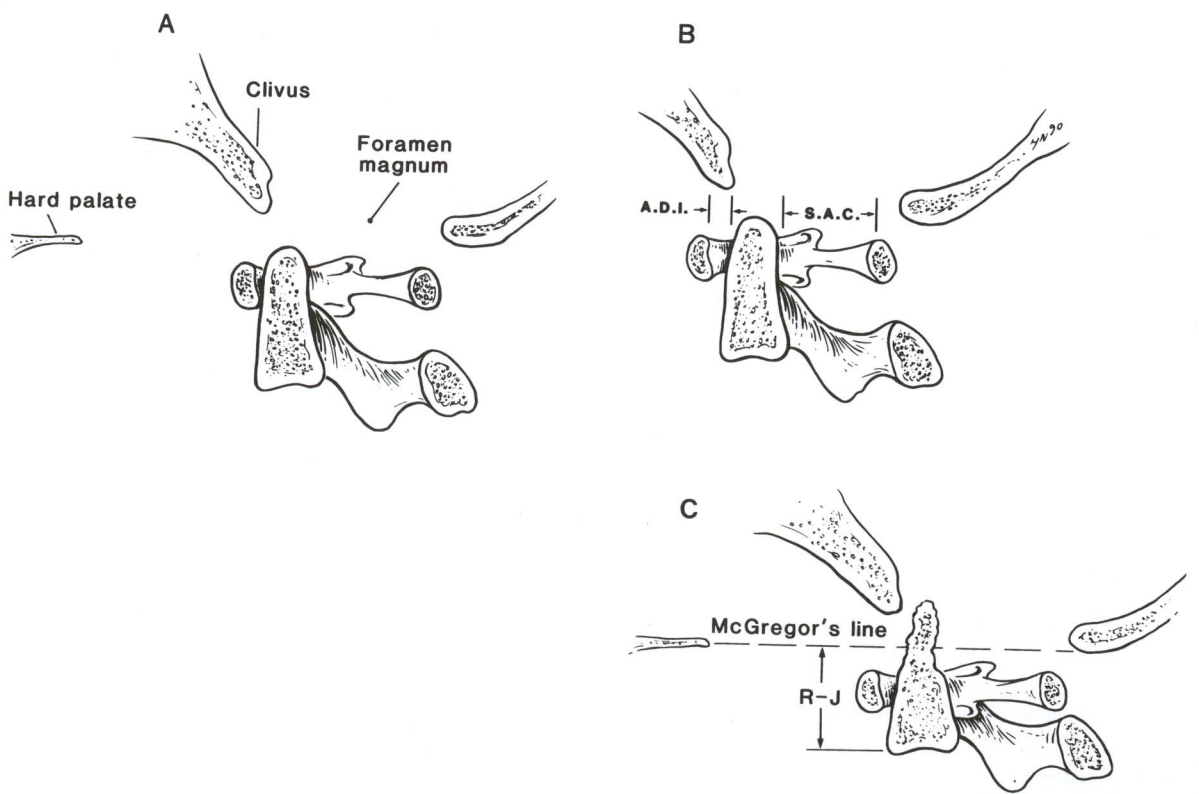

Figure 60-5
A. Normal craniocervical relationships, as would be seen on lateral radiography or sagittal computerized scans. B. Atlantodens interval (ADI) is the space between the anterior margin of the dens and posterior border of the anterior ring of the atlas. The space available for the cord (SAC) is the distance from the posterior aspect of the odontoid to the nearest posterior structure, either the foramen magnum or the posterior ring of the atlas. C. Vertical atlantoaxial subluxation, according to the method of Redlund-Johnell, is measured from the lower endplate of C2 to McGregor's palatooccipital line. [Reprinted with permssion from Moskovich R: Cervical instability (rheumatoid, dwarfism, degenerative, others). In Bridwell KH, DeWald RL (eds): *The Textbook of Spinal Surgery,* 2d ed. Philadelphia: Lippincott-Raven; 1997:970.]

Patients should be observed closely. Any evidence of neurologic compromise should be evaluated with dynamic MRI. Documented compression at the occipitocervical junction is an indication for surgery.

KLIPPEL-FEIL ANOMALY

Klippel-Feil syndrome (Fig. 60-4) is a triad of failure of segmentation of two or more cervical vertebrae, a short neck with limitation of head movement, and a low hairline. Most of the patients have normal intelligence.

Since its original description by Klippel and Feil in 1912, the syndrome was found to affect systems other than the cervical spine. Besides the classic stigmata of low hairline and short, wide neck, there can also be webs of soft tissue which tent the skin between the mastoid process of the skull and the acromion of the shoulder, or even Sprengel's anomaly. Other associated anomalies are: scoliosis; cervical ribs; spina bifida occulta; cleft vertebrae; hemivertebrae and occipitalization of the atlas; cleft palate; ocular anomalies and neurologic abnormalities such as facial nerve palsy, meningocele, encephalocele, Arnold-Chiari malformation, syringomyelia, and hydrocephalus; renal agenesis; and genital anomalies (hypospadias and cryptorchidism in males and absent vagina, uterus, and Fallopian tubes in females).

Congenital fusion of cervical segments may predispose to instability at remaining mobile segments. Occipitalization of the atlas combined with congenital fusion of C2–3 is the Klippel-Feil bony anomaly which most commonly predisposes the atlantoaxial joint to subluxation.

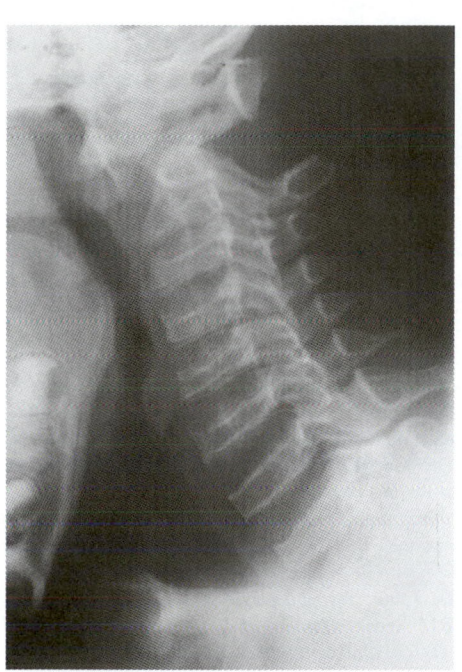

A

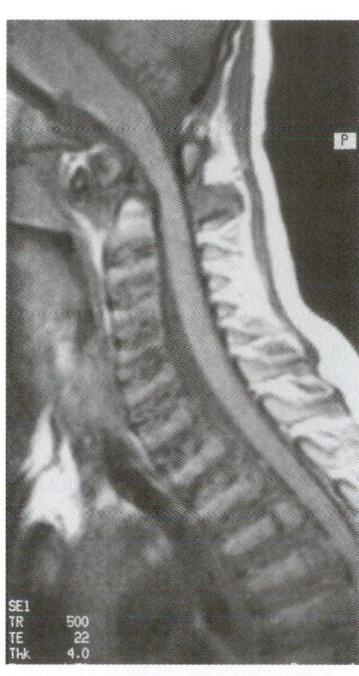

B

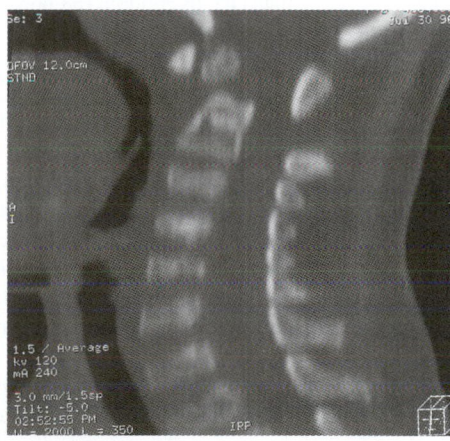

C

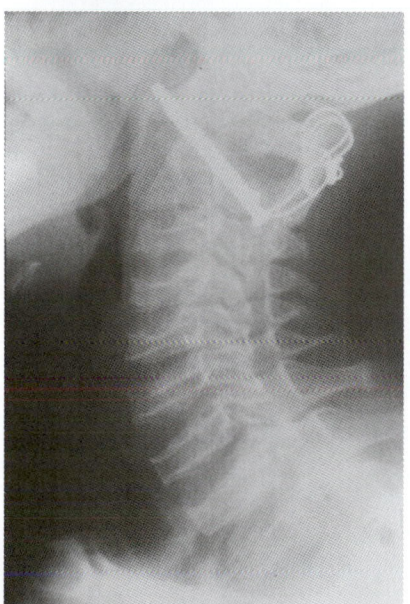

D

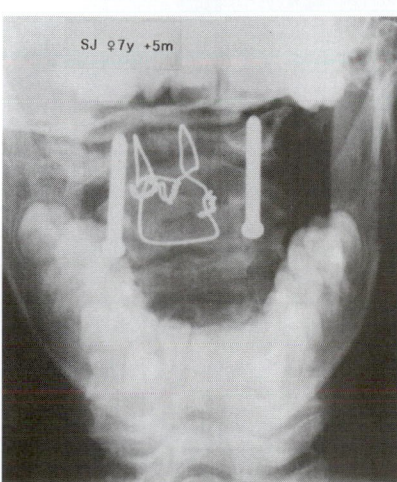

E

Figure 60-6

Seven-year-old patient with metatropic dysplasia and progressive C1-2 instability. *A.* Lateral cervical radiograph showing 10-mm atlantoaxial subluxation. Note the subaxial platyspondyly which occurs in this condition. *B.* Sagittal MRI demonstrates the neuraxial compression and the presence of an os odontoideum. *C.* CT of the same, clearly showing the separate, subluxed os odontoideum. *D.* Lateral and (*E*) anteroposterior radiographs demonstrate solid atlantoaxial fusion. Transarticular transfacet screw fixation augmented by posterior bone and wire arthrodesis was stable enough to permit early mobilization without external support.

ATLANTOAXIAL INSTABILITY

The C1-2 articulation is the most rotationally mobile segment of the vertebral column. Because there is no intervertebral disc, the odontoid process acts as a bony buttress to prevent hyperextension, while the transverse ligament forms the posterior wall of the "socket" for the dens and prevents the anterior atlantoaxial subluxation. The normal range of motion is maintained and depends on the integrity of the surrounding ligaments and capsular structures.

The atlantooccipital joint normally allows a few degrees of flexion-extension; in rotation the atlas and head turn as a unit. The C2-3 articulation permits flexion-extension but is restricted in rotation. Thus, the occiput-C3 complex has the extremely mobile and structurally weak atlantoaxial joint between these two relatively fixed points. Motion of the atlantoaxial articulation is usually accentuated in patient with bony anomalies above (atlantooccipital fusion) or below (C2-3 synostosis) that level.

RADIOLOGIC CRITERIA FOR C1-2 INSTABILITY

The basic study to evaluate atlantoaxial instability is the lateral cervical spine or lateral skull radiograph (Fig. 60-5). Dynamic studies, taken in flexion and extension, enhance our ability to detect abnormal intersegmental motion. The space between the anterior aspect of the dens and posterior border of the anterior ring of the atlas, is the atlas-dens interval (ADI). In children the normal ADI, particularly in flexion, may measure up to 4.0 mm. The normal ADI in adults is less than 3 mm and is a valuable index in assessing acute neck injury. An ADI of more than 5 mm in an acute injury indicates rupture of the transverse ligament. However, in chronic atlantoaxial instability, that measurement is of limited value. Under these conditions the dens can be hypermobile with increased ADI, particularly in flexion, but may be clinically insignificant. For such cases, attention should be directed to the amount of the space available for the cord (SAC). The SAC is determined by measuring the distance from the posterior aspect of the odontoid to the nearest posterior structure, either the foramen magnum or the posterior ring of atlas. It is generally accepted that a reduction to 13 mm or less may be associated with neurologic problems. Spinal cord impingement can be either posterior (from the C1 ring) or anterior (from the body of C2). Carefully supervised motion

studies (flexion-extension), are often necessary to demonstrate cervical spine instability. MRI can provide further information regarding the relationship of the brain stem and spinal cord to the surrounding structures.

Steel divided the anterior-posterior diameter of the spinal canal at the C1 level into thirds: one-third for the spinal cord, one-third for the odontoid, and one-third "empty space"—Steel's rule of thirds. The "space" is the safe zone in which displacement can occur without neurologic impingement, roughly it is equivalent to the transverse diameter of the odontoid (about 1 cm). Up to that point, the alar ligament functions as a second line of defence after a failure of the transverse ligament. Displacement beyond 1 cm implies rupture of even the alar ligament, and loss of ligamentous protection, with possible cord impingement and neurologic compromise.

Several congenital syndromes such as trisomy 21 and many of the skeletal dysplasias (Table 60-2) are predisposed to instability of C1–2. These patients should be followed clinically and radiographically to detect significant or progressive instability. If such instability is detected, surgical stabilization is indicated (Fig. 60-6).

SUGGESTED READINGS

Bland J: Cervical spine in infancy and childhood. In JH Bland (ed): *Disorders of the Cervical Spine*. Philadelphia: WB Saunders; 1994:405.

Hensinger RN: Congenital anomalies of the cervical spine. In Rothman RH, Simeone FA (eds): *The Spine*, 3d ed. Philadelphia: WB Saunders; 1992:261.

Kahn ML, Davidson R, Drummond DS: Acquired torticollis in children. *Orthop Rev* 1991; 20:667.

Loder R, Hensinger R: Developmental abnormalities of the cervical spine. In Weinstein SL (ed): *The Pediatric Spine: Principles and Practice*. New York: Raven Press; 1994:397.

Moskovich R: Cervical instability (rheumatoid, dwarfism, degenerative, others). In Bridwell KH, DeWald RL (eds): *The Textbook of Spinal Surgery*. Philadelphia: Lippincott-Raven; 1997:969.

Raynor R: Congenital malformations. In Sherk HH (chrmn), Cervical Spine Society. Editorial Committee: *The Cervical Spine*, 2d ed. Philadelphia: JB Lippincott; 1989.

Scott IC Jr: Pectoral girdle, spine, ribs, and pelvic gridle. In Stevenson RE, Hall JG, Goodman RM (eds): *Human Malformations and Related Anomalies*. New York: Oxford University Press; 1993:655.

Chapter 61

CONGENITAL SPINAL DEFORMITY

John A. Bendo, Jeffrey M. Spivak, Donald J. Cally, and Lynn J. Letko

EMBRYOLOGY OF THE SPINE

During week 3 of embryonic life, invagination of the midline ectoderm creates the notochordal process. Notochordal cells then separate, forming a solid notochord. The neural tube is created by the proliferation and then infolding of the ectoderm. The remaining ectoderm and neural tube separate from each other. The neural tube then closes, initially in the middle and then extending cranially and caudally. The process of the neural tube forming and then closing is called neurulation.

Further formation of the neural tube includes development of the somites, which are mesodermal cells that develop into paired segments. The somites further proliferate and differentiate and develop as distinct entities. The outer cell mass of the somite closest to the ectoderm develops into the dermatome, which gives rise to the skin. The cells medial to the dermatome evolve into the myotome and into the sclerotome. The myotome ultimately becomes skeletal muscle. Sclerotomal cells further differentiate and ultimately surround the notochord; they undergo segmentation at approximately 5 to 6 weeks of development. Each somite is related to a spinal nerve. Pre-chordal disc cells lie opposite the developing spinal nerve. The sclerotome development goes on to form the vertebral body. The neural arches, which migrate dorsally to surround the neural tube, develop from the lateral cells. The arches, which go on to form the lamina, unite initially in the lumbar area and then progress cranially and caudally from there.

Development of the vertebral bodies and neural arches is influenced differently, and thus congenital spine abnormalities may affect the posterior elements independently or the vertebral body independently or may affect both. If only one-half of the somite were to develop, this would cause the development of a hemi-vertebra. If the intervertebral sclerotome cells fail to develop, a fused vertebra would result (two fused vertebral bodies). If this failure of separation (segmentation) were to occur unilaterally, the result could be a unilateral bar. Each sclerotome contributes the cranial half of the vertebral body below, the disc, and the caudal half of the vertebral body above. The cranial and caudal halves of the sclerotome are divided by the sclerotomic fissure. At the time of birth, a typical vertebra consists of a centrum, in the center of the vertebral body, which is ossified and two arches that are ossified as well. The area between the ossified arch and centrum is a cartilaginous area known as the central synchondrosis. There is a cartilaginous end plate that is formed at the caudal and cranial ends of the vertebral body. These end plates are the sites of growth for each of the vertebrae, and are sites of en-

dochondral ossification. Secondary sites of ossification develop at the ring apophyses and at the junction of the end plate and the disc.

The primary growth center of the vertebrae, the physis, contributes to both the circumferential as well as the longitudinal growth of each vertebra. Individual vertebra do not contribute equally to growth of the spine. Greater contributions are obtained from the lumbar vertebrae than from the thoracic vertebrae. The growth of each thoracic segment from birth to skeletal maturity is 1.1 cm versus 1.6 cm in the lumbar spine. As there are 12 thoracic vertebrae and only five lumbar vertebrae, the total contribution to growth is still greater for the thoracic spine than for the lumbar spine.

During fetal development, the spinal cord ascends within the vertebral canal. By the age of 2 months, the caudal aspect of the cord normally reaches the L1-2 disc space, which is the level at which it remains throughout life. The presence of the end of the conus below the L2 vertebral body is abnormal.

As the neural tube and the vertebral bodies develop at the same time during embryonic development, it is not uncommon for abnormalities of the vertebral bodies and the neural elements to both be present. Other organ systems developing at the same time, especially the genitourinary and cerebrovascular systems, may also have congenital abnormalities.

CONGENITAL SPINAL DEFECTS

Congenital scoliosis can be defined as a lateral curvature of the spine as a result of abnormal vertebral development. Vertebral abnormalities that are present at birth cause deformity during growth. All forms of congenital scoliosis can be divided into either failures of formation and/or failures of segmentation as part of a single deformity. (Fig. 61-1) (Table 61-1). There can be combinations of failures of formation or failures of segmentation as part of a single deformity. Failures of formation typically include a hemivertebra or wedged vertebra. Failures of segmentation are generally unsegmented bars or a block vertebra. An unsegmented bar can also be present with a contralateral hemivertebra. As mentioned above, longitudinal growth of the spine occurs from the end plates. If there is an imbalance in the number of endplates or their rate of growth on one side of the spine versus the other, a lateral curvature will develop, resulting in scoliosis. If this imbalance is in the sagittal plane, a sagittal plane deformity occurs such as kyphosis or lordosis. The degree of deformity will depend on the severity of the imbalance. The natural history of any par-

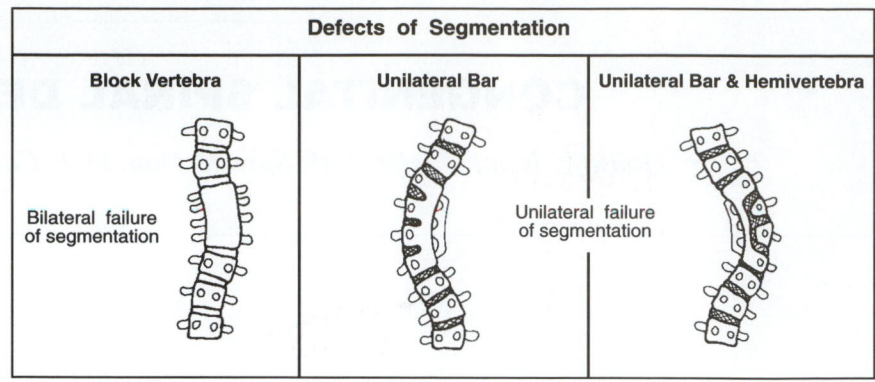

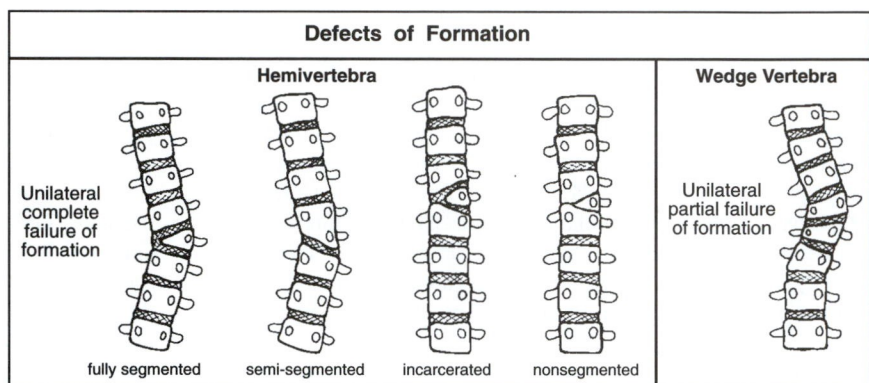

Figure 61-1
Anatomic defects in congenital scoliosis. [Reproduced with permission from McMaster MJ: Congenital scoliosis. In Weinstein SL (ed): *The Pediatric Spine: Principles and Practice.* New York: Raven Press (Lippincott Williams & Wilkins); 1994:229.]

ticular curve can be estimated by an understanding of the pathologic anatomy and its propensity to progress or not.

A segmentation defect may occur either unilaterally or bilaterally. The typical unilateral failure of segmentation is an unsegmented bar. On one side of the spine, two vertebrae are fused together, resulting in the loss of a growth segment. The growth on this side of the spine will be less than on the opposite side. Fusions of the ribs on the same side are frequently present and may be a tip-off as to the presence

---

Table 61-1

Types of Developmental Vertebral Anomalies Causing Congenital Scoliosis

DEFECTS OF SEGMENTATION

Unilateral
  Unsegmented bar
  Unsegmented bar with contralateral hemivertebrae
Bilateral
  Block vertebra

DEFECTS OF FORMATION

Complete unilateral
  Hemivertebra: Fully segmented, semisegmented, nonsegmented, incarcerated
Partial unilateral
  Wedge vertebra

MIXED OR UNCLASSIFIABLE ANOMALIES

SOURCE: Reproduced with permission by McMaster MJ: Congenital scoliosis. In Weinstein SL (ed): *The Pediatric Spine: Principles and Practice.* New York: Raven Press (Lippincott Williams & Wilkins); 1994:228.

---

of congenital scoliosis. When combined with a contralateral hemivertebra the risk of progression is extremely high. Complete failure of segmentation between two adjacent vertebrae will result in a block vertebra; this generally does not result in any deformity, as the loss of growth is circumferential and balanced.

A failure of formation may be relatively mild, with only anterior wedging of a vertebral body or a complete loss of one-half of the vertebral body, resulting in a hemivertebra (Fig. 61-2). Hemivertebrae may be classified as being segmented, semi-segmented, or unsegmented. If they have growth plates above and below the hemivertebrae, they are fully *segmented*. This type is most common. If they are fused either above or below they are *semi-segmented*, and if there are no growth plates both above and below they are *unsegmented*. An *incarcerated* hemivertebra is one that tends to fit into the contour of the spine such that the vertebra above it and the vertebra below it have changed shape to accommodate the hemivertebra. *Nonincarcerated* hemivertebra are frequently fully segmented and create more deformity. A line drawn through the pedicles will generally intersect the pedicle of an incarcerated hemivertebra, whereas that same line will lie medial to a nonincarcerated hemivertebra. The prognosis for nonincarcerated hemivertebra is much worse, as an incarcerated hemivertebra will rarely cause a scoliosis that exceeds 20 degrees and generally does not require treatment. Hemivertebrae may exist on opposite sides of the spine and thereby balance each other. This phenomenon is known as a *hemimetameric shift*. The severity of the deformity depends on the relative location of the hemivertebrae.

ASSOCIATED ABNORMALITIES

Associated intraspinal anomalies most commonly include diastematomyelia, tethering of the spinal cord, and syringomyelia. Diastematomyelia is a sagittal split in the spinal canal, resulting in either a split of the spinal cord or cauda equina. This split may be the result of either a bony or a cartilaginous spur that projects into

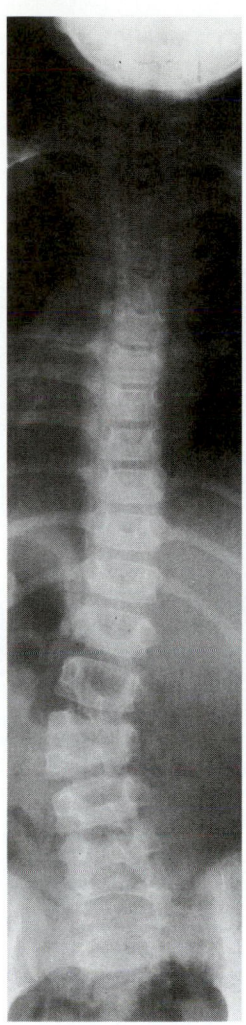

Figure 61-2
AP radiographic view of semisegmented nonincarcerated hemivertebrae in a 5-year-old male. The lumbar deformity stabilized at 32 degrees at skeletal maturity. He remained balanced in the coronal and sagittal planes, and required no active treatment.

the spinal canal from the back of one or more vertebral bodies. Diastematomyelia is present in 5 to 20 percent of patients with congenital scoliosis. Associated with diastematomyelia are other congenital neural abnormalities such as intrathecal lipomas, teratomas, and epidermoid or dermoid cysts. Tethering of the spinal cord to the sacrum is the result of a thickened filum terminale or fibrous bands. This results in a block to the normal ascension of the spinal cord with the conus medullaris remaining below the L2 vertebral body. These abnormalities, which can result in abnormal spinal cord function and clinical symptoms and signs, can generally be diagnosed using magnetic resonance imaging (MRI) or myelography. MRI is generally the preferred modality for evaluation of the spinal canal. Myelography may at times be necessary for satisfactory evaluation of the entire canal, especially in the presence of a significant deformity. It is widely accepted that an intraspinal anomaly that tethers the spinal cord should be surgically released if there is progressive neurologic deficit or before attempting to correct a spinal deformity.

In congenital scoliosis, there is also a high association of other congenital abnormalities outside of the spinal column. Approximately 25 percent of patients with congenital scoliosis have genito-urinary abnormalities such as unilateral kidney, duplication of the kidney, or pelvic kidney. All patients with congenital scoliosis should have a renal ultrasound performed. Klippel-Feil syndrome can be found in 25

percent of patients and congenital heart disease in 10 percent of patients with congenital scoliosis. Sprengle's deformity (elevation of the scapula) is also associated with congenital scoliosis.

CLINICAL EVALUATION

Evaluation of patients with congenital scoliosis begins with a complete medical history, which should include a history of the mother's pregnancy, including the possible use of a teratogenic drug and whether the deformity was noted at birth or thereafter. Any other associated congenital abnormalities should be investigated. Examiners should ask about the development of normal milestones, in particular ambulation and bladder and bowel control. The physical examination of children with congenital scoliosis is essentially the same as that of other children with scoliosis. In particular, any nevi or hairy patches overlying the spine should be documented. Superficial abdominal reflexes should also be assessed. Routine anteroposterior and lateral radiographs are generally sufficient to diagnose the presence and type of congenital scoliosis. In addition to looking at the spine, the examiner should evaluate the rib cage as well as the hip joints for the presence of abnormalities. Further imaging studies should be performed in any patient for whom surgical treatment is being contemplated. In the past, myelography has been the study of choice, but this has more recently been replaced by MRI (Fig. 61-3). Anteroposterior tomography may be of help to define better the anatomy and the type of vertebral anomaly. MRI or computed tomograph with coronal and sagittal plane views may similarly be helpful in determining the bony anomaly and the presence of growth plates. Curves are measured by the routine Cobb angle technique.

NATURAL HISTORY

McMaster and Ohtsuka (1982) have reviewed the natural history of congenital scoliosis. Only 11 percent of the curves did not progress, whereas 75 percent of the curves progressed significantly. The rate of progression depends on the type of congenital abnormality and the location within the spine. The worst prognosis was for a unilateral unsegmented bar with a contralateral hemivertebra. Diminishing risk of progression was observed for a unilateral unsegmented bar, a double convex hemivertebra, a single free convex hemivertebra, and a block vertebra (least risk of progressive deformity).

The location within the spine of the congenital abnormality contributes significantly to the prognosis. Abnormalities at the thoracic and thoracolumbar junctions are generally more significant than those in the upper thoracic spine or in the lumbar spine. The age of the patient at the time of diagnosis also contributes to the prognosis. The younger the patient, the worse the prognosis.

The true incidences and prevalence of this disorder is unknown because many anomalies produce minimal deformity and go unrecognized. Wynne-Davies (1975) found an increased risk to siblings of parents with multiple congenital vertebral anomalies. However, an isolated single anomaly is usually sporadic which poses no increased risk to siblings. The etiology of congenital scoliosis is more likely multifactorial with genetic and environmental components.

MANAGEMENT

Congenital scoliosis can at times be managed by simple observation. Curves with a relatively benign natural history can be followed. Such examples would be an incarcerated hemivertebra, which rarely causes a curve in excess of 20 degrees. Balanced contralateral hemivertebrae

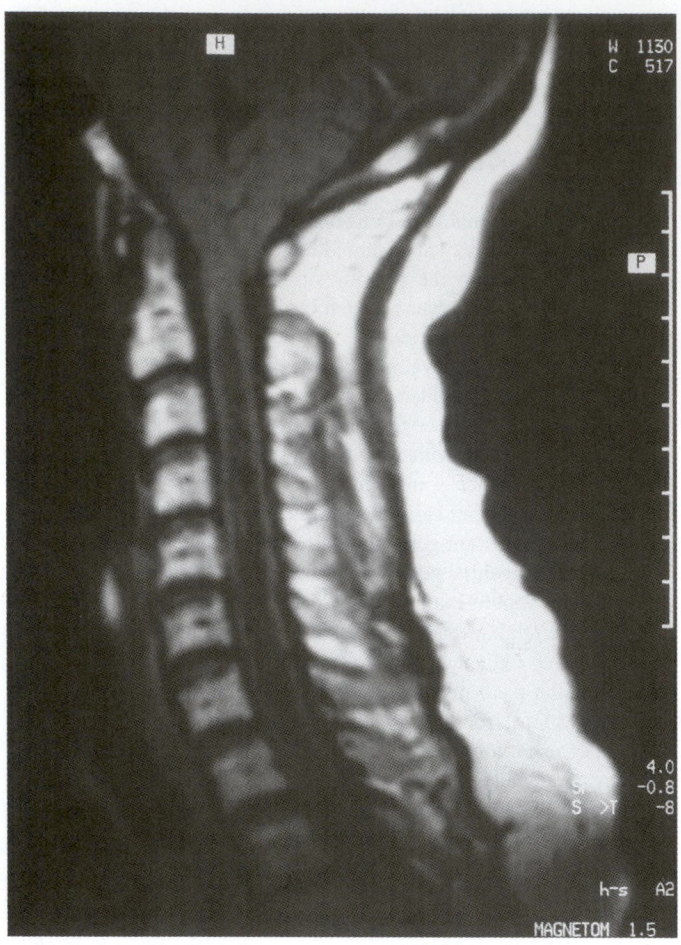

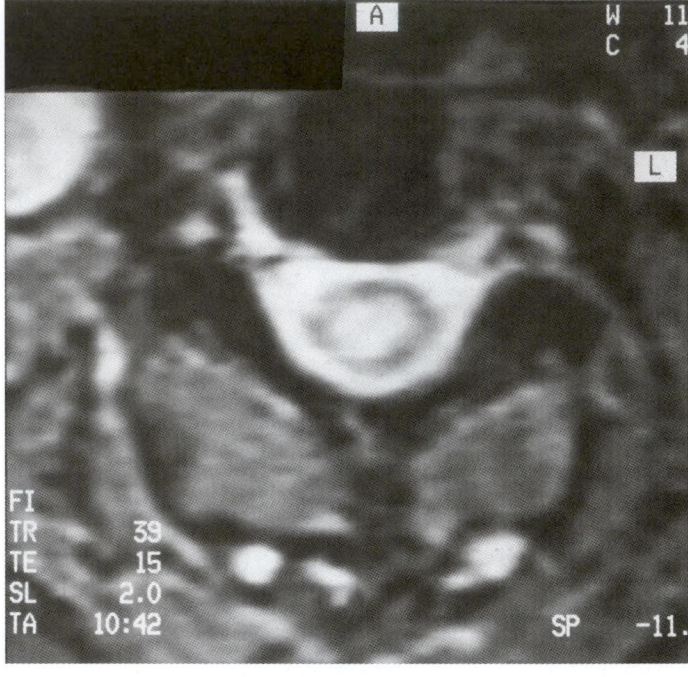

A

B

Figure 61-3
Sixteen-year-old female with left thoracic congenital scoliosis. Preoperative MRI survey of the entire
spine revealed a syrinx within the cervical spinal cord. The syrinx appears as a low-intensity signal
on the T1-weighted image (*A*) and a high-intensity signal on the T2-weighted image (*B*).

similarly rarely cause a curve of sufficient magnitude to require surgical intervention.

Bracing is rarely appropriate for the management of congenital scoliosis. There may occasionally be a patient who could benefit from
bracing to delay an anticipated surgical procedure. In general, the use
of a rigid orthosis or cast in young patients with congenital scoliosis
is contraindicated because of the adverse effect it has on the developing respiratory system. The forces of growth imbalance will overcome an orthotic device. Idiopathic-type curves in association with
congenital scoliosis are amenable to bracing, as are flexible compensatory curves.

Surgical management of congenital scoliosis is frequently the
treatment of choice, can be performed at any age, and may even be
indicated during infancy. The natural history of a curve can be determined by the nature of the vertebral anomaly. Decision making can
be instituted at an early age. Curves with a poor prognosis, such as
a segmented hemivertebra with contralateral bar, should be fused early
to prevent significant deformity that may require more extensive procedures if performed later. Two ipsilateral hemivertebrae have the
next worst prognosis and should also be fused early.

The mainstay of surgical management remains posterior fusion in
situ. The purpose of the fusion in situ is to create a solid posterior
fusion mass that will prevent progression of the deformity. Some correction can occasionally be obtained by postoperative casting. This
does not address significant compensatory curves above or below. If

a significant number of normal vertebrae are included within the
curve, or large compensatory curves exist, continued bracing may be
necessary postoperatively. In cases of severe imbalance, or with very
immature patients (< 10 years, Risser O), the continued anterior
growth may cause further progression of the scoliosis (crankshaft phenomenon), and circumferential fusion should be considered in such
situations. A large deformity in patients with an unsegmented bar and
contralateral hemivertebra may best be treated by circumferential fusion and postoperative casting. In general, for young children, it is
best to try to avoid instrumentation. If instrumentation is used, it is
generally to stabilize the spine and not to impart corrective forces.
Posterior fusion may at times be appropriate to slow the progression
of a curve in young patients to allow for further growth of the spine
before performing a longer fusion when the children are older. This
may be combined with the use of subcutaneous rods as well. In children who are older and have severe deformity, instrumentation and
correction of the spine may be indicated. It is mandatory that all patients for whom correction of the anomaly is being contemplated undergo preoperative myelography or MRI of the entire spine. An intraspinal lesion such as a tethered cord or diastematomyelia should
be corrected prior to any instrumentation of the spine. Management
can be accomplished either as a single stage or as a staged procedure,
depending on the complexity of the anomaly and the surgical time
expected. The mere presence of a diastematomyelia or thickened
filum or other intraspinal lesion does not necessitate surgical inter-

vention. That decision is based on the presence of neurologic findings and on whether manipulation of the spine is being contemplated. Occasionally, the presenting symptom in such patients may be the loss of bladder function. Instrumentation for posterior spinal fusions may also lower the pseudoarthrosis rate.

Hemiarthrodesis/hemiepiphysiodesis is a procedure performed on the convex side of the curve to prevent further growth of the spine on that side. The posterior elements and disc space on the convex side of the curve are fused. This necessitates two surgical procedures (anterior and posterior) that are generally performed during the same anesthetic. The indication for hemiarthrodesis/hemiepiphysiodesis is a curve usually of less than 60 degrees, involving six or fewer vertebrae in a child 6 years of age or younger. In this setting, the procedure allows for full growth of the spine on its concave side, resulting in some degree of correction of the curve with time. Even if correction does not occur, further progression of the curve is prevented. Care is taken not to dissect the concave side of the curve subperiosteally and, when the disc excisions are being performed, not to involve the concave side of the vertebral bodies. In young children, an allograft is generally used with satisfactory results. As much bone as can be used should be placed adjacent to the spine. This is true in all fusions for congenital scoliosis. Only those vertebrae that one plans to fuse should be exposed, because of the high fusion rate associated with the subperiosteal stripping of the muscles off the posterior elements.

Hemivertebra excision is occasionally indicated for congenital scoliosis arising from a hemivertebra. It is a challenging procedure that enables the deformity to be corrected by essentially performing a closing-wedge osteotomy (Fig.61-4). There is considerable risk of injury to the spinal cord and/or neural elements. The procedure is performed in two stages, removing the anterior and the posterior portions during each stage. Because of possible injury to the blood flow to the spinal cord, it is occasionally advocated that the hemivertebra excisions be staged. Although the excision could theoretically be performed for hemivertebrae at any level, the best indication is a lumbosacral hemivertebra that often causes severe imbalance and pelvic obliquity.

Osteotomy of the spine, which is a salvage procedure that is rarely indicated, is used in mature patients with severe deformity. It is best performed with the patient lying on his or her side, with simultaneous exposure of the spine anteriorly and posteriorly. Significant correction can be obtained. The indication needs to be weighed against the risk of severe neurologic injury from either direct spinal cord injury or ischemia to the cord. There is also the risk of significant blood loss from either the epidural vein or direct great vessel injury. The osteotomies can also be staged by initially performing the anterior osteotomies or vertebral excisions, followed by posterior osteotomy and instrumentation.

Since the natural history of congenital scoliosis is largely predictable, the thrust of treatment should be directed at early intervention to avoid the development of significant deformity requiring more difficult surgical procedures with more limited expected improvement.

CONGENITAL KYPHOSIS

Congenital deformity in the sagittal plane, similar to that in the coronal plane, is the result of a failure of formation, a failure of segmentation, or both. Congenital kyphosis is thus classified into type 1, fail-

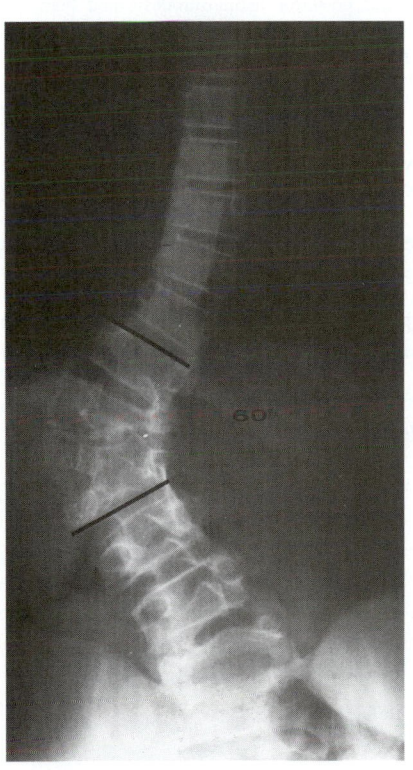
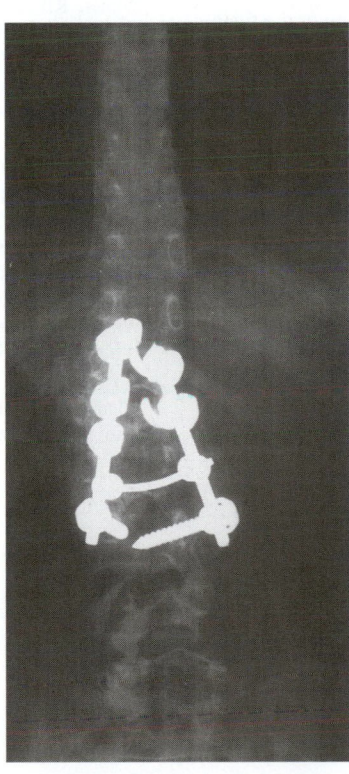
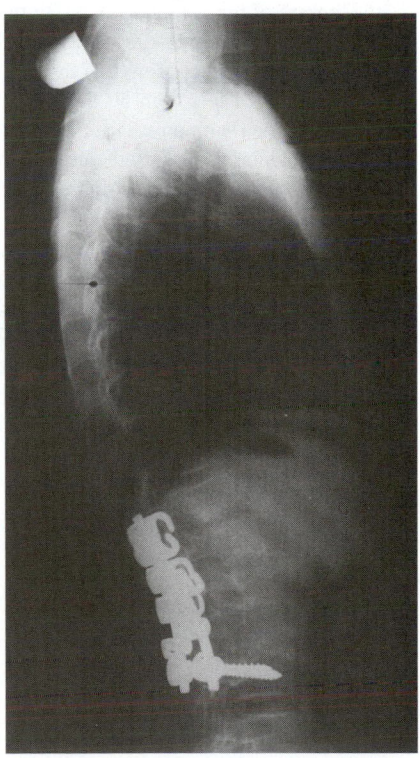

A   B   C

Figure 61-4

Twelve-year-old male who underwent posterior in situ fusion at age 2 years for a progressive congenital scoliosis secondary to a hemivertebrae with contralateral bar. The deformity continued to progress (crankshaft) during the adolescent growth spurt. He then underwent a vertebrectomy and fusion via an anterior/posterior approach with subsequent correction and stabilization of the deformity. Preoperative AP radiograph (A). Postoperative AP radiograph (B). Postoperative lateral radiograph (C).

ure of formation; type 2, failure of segmentation; and type 3, mixed. Type 1 deformities generally go on to form the most severe kyphosis. These deformities are rarely in the sagittal plane alone; the kyphosis is frequently combined with a scoliosis. Occasionally, however, a pure kyphotic deformity may occur. As in congenital scoliosis, these deformities may be associated with other vertebral anomalies, nervous system anomalies or other organ system abnormalities. Winter reported on the natural history of congenital kyphosis showing rapid progression of untreated curves with a significant incidence of paraplegia. All patients with paraplegia had type 1 lesions.

Patients with congenital kyphotic deformity should have an MRI of their entire spine performed for evaluation of the spinal canal. In those patients with an associated scoliosis, a myelogram may provide better visualization because of the coronal plane deformity. Patients with severe kyphosis ($\geq$100 degrees) in the thoracic region are at risk for development of respiratory problems. However, the most severe respiratory abnormalities are seen in patients with lordosis and/or lordoscoliosis, which causes marked diminution of the pleural cavity.

There is essentially no role for nonsurgical management of congenital kyphosis. Bracing is not an effective form of treatment. Because of the rapid progression of the curve causing significant deformity and the high incidence of paraplegia, surgical treatment is generally advised at a young age for those patients with progressive deformity or with high risk for progression. All patients undergoing surgical treatment for sagittal plane deformity need to have an extensive preoperative evaluation. It should include cardiopulmonary assessment, evaluation of the urogenital system, and careful examination for any neurologic deficit. A detailed physical examination should be performed, particularly with attention to the above. All patients should undergo ultrasound of the kidneys as well as an MRI or myelogram of the complete spine. In the young patient the fusions should be performed over short segments of the spine whenever possible to allow for further growth of the remainder of the spine. In general, a kyphosis of less than 50 degrees in patients under 5 years of age can be treated with a posterior in situ fusion. Patients with larger curves may benefit from both anterior and posterior arthrodeses. Patients who present with neurologic abnormalities secondary to their deformity should be decompressed at the time of their surgery. The spinal cord is usually draped over the kyphotic deformity. Surgical intervention often entails an anterior decompression with removal of the posterior portion of the vertebral bodies at the apex of the curve. Anterior strut grafting immediately follows the decompression. Positioning of the anterior strut grafts more than 4.0 cm from the spinal cord is associated with a high incidence of fracture. Vascularized rib grafting is an alternative technique that can lead to graft hypertrophy, thereby providing significant structural support. Instrumentation may be used to aid in the correction of the kyphotic deformity. However, its role is limited in the very young, immature patient. Posterior distraction over the kyphotic deformity is contraindicated due to the high incidence of paraplegia. Preoperative traction is also contraindicated in patients with congenital kyphosis secondary to the possibility of further spinal cord compromise. If traction is used, patients need to be monitored carefully for the development of any neurologic change.

SELECTED READINGS

Bradford DS, Boachie-Adjei O: One stage anterior and posterior hemi-vertebra resection arthrodesis. *J Bone Joint Surg [Am]* 1990; 72:536.

Dubousset J: Congenital kyphosis and lordosis. In Weinsten JL (ed): *The Pediatric Spine: Principles and Practice.* New York: Lippincott-Raven; 1994.

Hall JE, Herndon WA, Levine CR: Surgical treatment of congenital scoliosis with and without Harrington instrumentation. *J Bone Joint Surg [Am]* 1981; 63:608.

King JD, Lowry GL: Results of lumbar hemivertebral excision for congenital scoliosis. *Spine* 1991; 16:778.

McMaster MJ: Occult intraspinal anomalies and congenital scoliosis. *J Bone Joint Surg [Am]* 1984; 66:588.

McMaster MJ, Ohtsuka K: The natural history of congenital scoliosis: A study of two hundred and fifty-one patients. *J Bone Joint Surg [Am]* 1982;64:1128.

Ogden JA, Ganey TM, Sasse J, et al: Development and maturation of the axial skeleton. In Weinstein S (ed): *The Pediatric Spine Principles and Practice.* New York, Lippincott-Raven, 1994.

Winter, RB: Convex anterior and posterior hemiarthrodesis and hemiepiphysiodesis in young children with progressive congenital scoliosis. *J Pediatr Orthop* 1981; 1:361.

Winter, RB, Moh JH, Eilers VE: Part 1: Natural History. Congenital scoliosis: A study of 234 patients treated and untreated. *J Bone Joint Surg [Am]* 1968; 50:15.

Winter RB, Moe JH, Eilers VE: Part II: Treatment Congenital scoliosis. A study of 234 patients treated and untreated. *J Bone Joint Surg [Am]* 1968; 50:1.

Winter RB, Lonstein JE, Bouchie-Adjei O: Congenital scoliosis. In Pritchard DJ (ed): *Instructional Course Lectures.* Rosemont, IL: American Academy of Orthopaedic Surgeons; 1996; 45:117.

Winter RB, Moe JH, Wang JF: Congenital kyphosis. Its natural history and treatment as observed in a study of 130 patients. *J Bone Joint Surg [Am]* 1973; 55:223.

Wynne-Davies R: Congenital vertebral anomalies: Etiology and relationship to spina bifida cystica. *J Med Gen* 1975; 12:280.

Chapter 62

IDIOPATHIC SCOLIOSIS AND KYPHOSIS

Lynn J. Letko

Idiopathic scoliosis refers to scoliosis that is structural in nature without known etiology. Three categories of idiopathic scoliosis have been described based on the age of onset: infantile, juvenile, and adolescent. Infantile idiopathic scoliosis has an onset from birth to three years. Juvenile idiopathic scoliosis occurs between the ages of 4 and 10 years. Adolescent idiopathic scoliosis has an onset after the age of 10 years. Differentiation between the three types is important in treatment and prognosis. The diagnosis of idiopathic scoliosis is one of exclusion of other causes of scoliosis.

Increased thoracic kyphosis (round back) is a common problem responsible for adolescent visits to the orthopeadic surgeon. It is frequently the parents who bring the child in for evaluation because they are unhappy about the patient's posture. There may or may not be associated pain. Pain may be over the apex of the curve, above or below. There are essentially three causes of increased thoracic kyphosis in the adolescent patient: postural kyphosis, Scheuermann's disease, or less commonly congenital kyphosis.

INFANTILE IDIOPATHIC SCOLIOSIS

INCIDENCE AND ETIOLOGY

The incidence of infantile idiopathic scoliosis is variable. A higher incidence is reported in Europe than in North America. Two theories have been suggested regarding the etiology of infantile idiopathic scoliosis: intrauterine molding and the postnatal pressure as the result of the infant being placed in the supine or slightly decubitus position. The intrauterine molding hypothesis has fallen out of favor as infantile idiopathic scoliosis is frequently not present for some time after birth. The standard in positioning of babies in Europe is in the supine or slightly decubitus position. In North America, it is the prone position. Placing the baby in the supine or slightly decubitus position is thought to result in molding of the immature spine and hence infantile idiopathic scoliosis. The incidence of infantile idiopathic scoliosis is also noted to be greater in hypotonic babies.

In contrast with adolescent idiopathic scoliosis, 75 percent of the curves in patients with infantile idiopathic scoliosis are observed to be left thoracic and males are affected more frequently than females. The overall incidence of infantile idiopathic scoliosis has been reported to be declining in recent years.

Two types of idiopathic infantile curves are reported: a resolving type (approximately 85 percent) and a progressive type (approximately 15 percent). Recognition and appropriate treatment of infantile idiopathic curves is important because curves that result in significant thoracic deformity prior to the age of 5 years may result in subsequent cardiopulmonary compromise, with the development of restrictive lung disease and ultimately pulmonary arterial hypertension.

WORKUP AND RADIOGRAPHIC FINDINGS

Neurologic disorders, congenital hypotonia, and congenital scoliosis must be ruled out as the cause of the patient's scoliosis as idiopathic infantile scoliosis is a diagnosis of exclusion. This is accomplished by physical exam and radiographic evaluation. Radiographs should be examined for congenital vertebral abnormalities. Also, lordosis is generally noted at the apex of infantile idiopathic scoliotic curves. If indicated, MRI and/or myelography are ordered to rule out intrathecal abnormality.

PROGNOSIS

Age of onset of the curve, curve magnitude, curve rigidity, rib-vertebral angle difference of Mehta (RVAD), the presence of secondary curves and association with other developmental anomalies are important prognostic indicators. Curves that develop after one year of age, curves of greater magnitude, more rigid curves, curves associated with developmental anomalies and secondary curves, and curves with a rib-vertebral angle difference of greater than 20 degrees have a poorer prognosis. Mehta's RVAD is measured on an AP radiograph. The apical vertebra is utilized. The angle created by the neck of the rib and the vertical axis is measured on each side of the spine. The difference between these two angles is calculated. Curves with an RVAD of greater than 20 degrees have a high incidence of progression. The RVAD should be measured on serial radiographs as it is at times difficult to measure (Fig. 62-1).

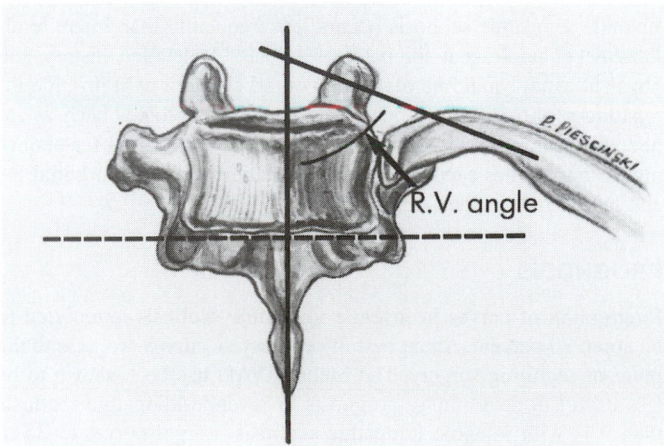

Figure 62-1
Method of measurement of Mehta's rib vertebral angle (RVA). First, draw a perpendicular line to the end-plate of the apical vertebra. Second, draw lines bisecting the head and neck of the ribs on each side of the apical vertebra. The angle formed by the intersection of these two lines is the RVA. (Reproduced with permission from Tachdjian MO: Scoliosis. In: *Pediatric Orthopaedics,* vol 3, 2d ed. Philadelphia: Saunders; 1990:2288.)

TREATMENT

The mainstay of management of infantile idiopathic scoliosis remains nonsurgical. Patients with resolving infantile idiopathic scoliosis are followed with physical examinations and radiographs every 3 to 6 months. The prone sleeping position is advocated. Most curves resolve in 1 to 2 years with vertebral rotation resolving last.

With progressive curves, serial casting or bracing is the initial treatment of choice. Posterior fusion alone should be avoided as it may worsen the thoracic lordosis. Serial casts or braces are used in an attempt to correct the deformity by the application of pressure over the prominence on the convex side of the curve. Curves that are not successfully managed in this manner by the age of 4 or 5 may require surgical consideration. Anterior discectomy and fusion may be followed by posterior instrumentation with fusion or by subcutaneous rod placement to allow for incremental distraction with posterior growth.

JUVENILE IDIOPATHIC SCOLIOSIS

INCIDENCE AND ETIOLOGY

Juvenile idiopathic scoliosis occurs between the ages of 3 and 10 years. It accounts for 12 to 21 percent of all cases of idiopathic scoliosis. The presentation may resemble either infantile idiopathic or adolescent idiopathic scoliosis. In the younger age of onset of juvenile idiopathic scoliosis, the male to female incidence is similar. The incidence of females to males in the older age of onset is 8 to 10:1. This is similar to that seen in adolescent idiopathic scoliosis. The types of curve patterns seen in juvenile idiopathic scoliosis are thoracic > double thoracic > thoracolumbar > lumbar.

Two periods of rapid growth of the spine occur. The first is between the ages of 0 to 4 years. The second occurs during the adolescent growth spurt. From the ages of 3 to 10 years, spine growth is relatively constant. Despite this relative plateau, children with juvenile scoliosis tend to progress during this time rather than during the adolescent growth spurt.

WORK UP AND RADIOGRAPHIC FINDINGS

Juvenile idiopathic scoliosis occurs less frequently than infantile idiopathic or adolescent idiopathic scoliosis. A detailed history and physical exam should be performed on all children with juvenile idiopathic scoliosis to rule out other potential etiologies such as intraspinal abnormalities. There should be a low threshold for obtaining further studies such as MRI in this patient population. Initial PA and lateral radiographs are obtained.

PROGNOSIS

Progression of curves in juvenile idiopathic scoliosis is reported to be about 70 percent. About half of progressive curves progress to the point of requiring surgery. The Mehta RVAD has been shown to be less useful in determining prognosis in juvenile idiopathic scoliosis than it is with infantile idiopathic scoliosis. Larger curves (>35 to 45 degrees) with less than 20 degrees of thoracic kyphosis on the initial radiographs have an increased likelihood of progression.

TREATMENT

The mainstay of management for juvenile idiopathic scoliosis is bracing. The parameters for bracing are generally more liberal than are those for adolescent idiopathic scoliosis. Children with curves in excess of 25 degrees should generally be braced. Initially, bracing is instituted on a full-time basis. Radiographs are done every 4 to 6 months. Part time use may be indicated after a year of full-time bracing if stabilization of the curve occurs. An RVAD of greater than 10 degrees has been associated with the need for full-time bracing. When curves continue to progress despite bracing, bracing may still be continued to allow for further spinal growth prior to fusion. Orthotic treatment of a juvenile idiopathic curve may be continued until the curve measures 50 to 60 degrees in an attempt to allow for further spinal growth. This may allow for enough growth such that posterior spinal fusion alone may be all that is needed.

When surgery is indicated several options exist, including posterior fusion with instrumentation or combined anterior and posterior fusions with instrumentation. With posterior surgery alone, the crankshaft phenomenon may develop. The crankshaft phenomenon describes the progressive bending of the posterior fusion mass as the result of continued anterior spinal growth at the previously fused posterior levels. The younger the child, the greater amount of remaining growth and the greater the magnitude of the curve, the greater the likelihood that anterior surgery will be necessary to prevent the crankshaft phenomenon. If the child is younger and less correction can be obtained posteriorly, the effect of the crankshaft phenomenon will be greater with an unacceptable end result. In contrast, an older child undergoing an isolated posterior procedure, may develop crankshaft and only 5 to 10 degrees of progression and a satisfactory end result. An open triradiate cartilage is associated with an increased incidence of crankshaft. Combined anterior and posterior procedures reduce the incidence of crankshaft phenomenon and are indicated in patients who are at high risk for crankshaft. Insertion of subcutaneous posterior rods with or without an apical posterior fusion has been indicated in this patient population. This is performed using Harrington rod instrumentation. The rod is distracted or exchanged for a longer rod periodically as mandated by the patient's growth until such time as definitive spinal fusion is required. Electrical stimulation has not been found to be of value in the treatment of juvenile idiopathic scoliosis.

ADOLESCENT IDIOPATHIC SCOLIOSIS

INCIDENCE AND ETIOLOGY

The prevalence of adolescent idiopathic scoliosis is reported to be 2 to 3 percent. To be diagnosed as idiopathic scoliosis, there must be at least 10 degrees of curvature along with rotation and lateral deviation on a standing radiograph (<10 degrees is considered normal). The incidence of adolescent idiopathic scoliosis among males and females is equal with progression of curve magnitude noted more frequently in females. The etiology of adolescent idiopathic scoliosis is not known. Proprioceptive disorders have been proposed but not proven. There does appear to be a familial tendency in adolescent idiopathic scoliosis and patients and their families should be appropriately informed. Adolescent idiopathic scoliosis is not a physically painful condition. Should the patient have a painful scoliosis, other etiologies such as osteoid osteoma should be sought.

Scoliotic curves are named by the location of the curve apex on radiograph:

Cervical: C1-C6
Cervicothoracic: C7-T1
Thoracic: T2-T11
Thoracolumbar: T12-L1
Lumbar: L2-L4
Lumbosacral: L5-S1

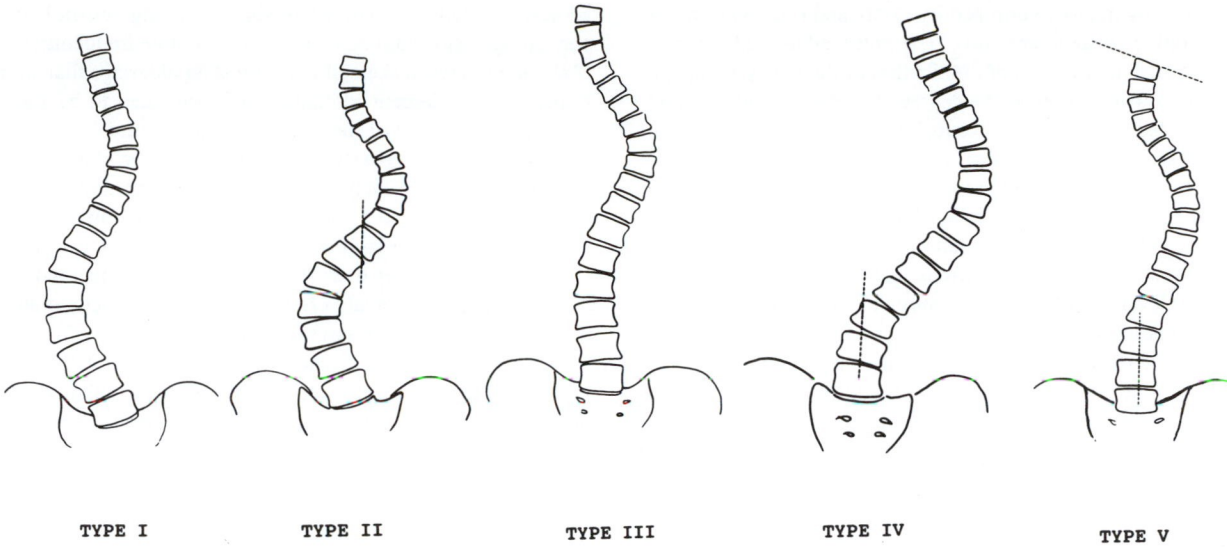

TYPE I   TYPE II   TYPE III   TYPE IV   TYPE V

Figure 62-2

Five types of scoliotic curves. [Reproduced with permission from King HA, Moe JH, Bradford DS, et al: The selection of fusion levels in thoracic idiopathic scoliosis. *J Bone Joint Surg [Am]* 1983: 65:1302. (Photo source; Miller MD: Pediatric orthopaedics. In: *Review of Orthopaedics.* Philadelphia: Saunders; 1992:15.]

Curves may be further described as being major or minor. A major curve refers to a fixed deformity with little flexibility. A minor curve is frequently referred to as being compensatory. This type of curve retains its flexibility longer. The most common curve types seen in adolescent idiopathic scoliosis are right thoracic followed by double major (right thoracic left lumbar), left lumbar, and right lumbar. Left thoracic curves of magnitude of greater than 20 degrees are rare. These curves have a high incidence of associated intraspinal anomalies. MRI is recommended for evaluation of the spine when a left thoracic curve is present.

King has further classified thoracic curves into five types (Fig. 62-2):

Type I: primary lumbar, secondary thoracic
Type II: primary thoracic, secondary lumbar
Type III: thoracic without structural lumbar
Type IV: long thoracic curve extending to L4
Type V: double thoracic curve with T1 tilting into the upper curve

These classifications allow for treatment recommendations based on prognosis for the different curve types. It is unclear if King's recommendations are applicable to current segmental fixation instrumentation systems.

WORKUP AND RADIOGRAPHIC FINDINGS

Workup for adolescent idiopathic scoliosis includes a complete history including inquiry about age of onset of menarche and family history of scoliosis. Physical exam includes height and weight at each visit, examination for level shoulders and pelvis, plumb line measurement for decompensation, Adam's forward-bend test with use of a scoliometer and measurement of rib and/or lumbar prominence, leg length measurement, flexibility assessment, and sagittal plane balance assessment. In addition, a complete assessment of deep tendon reflexes, plantar reflexes, clonus, and abdominal reflexes should be made. Abnormalities in abdominal reflexes may indicate intraspinal pathology such as syringomyelia.

Radiographic workup includes initial PA and lateral full-length erect radiographs for those patients with a scoliometer reading of

greater or equal to 5 to 7 degrees. PA rather than AP radiographs are used to decrease the amount of radiation to the breast tissue. Use of the 5- to 7-degree scoliometer reading as a guide to obtaining radiographs should prevent missing curves of 20 degrees or greater.

Scoliotic curves are measured on radiographs by the Cobb method to determine the degree of curvature. This measurement is made by drawing a perpendicular to a line drawn across the superior endplate of the upper end (most tilted) vertebra and the inferior endplate of the lower end vertebra. The angle formed by the intersection of the two perpendicular lines is the Cobb angle, a measure of the magnitude of the curve (Fig. 62-3).

A) Cobb Angle

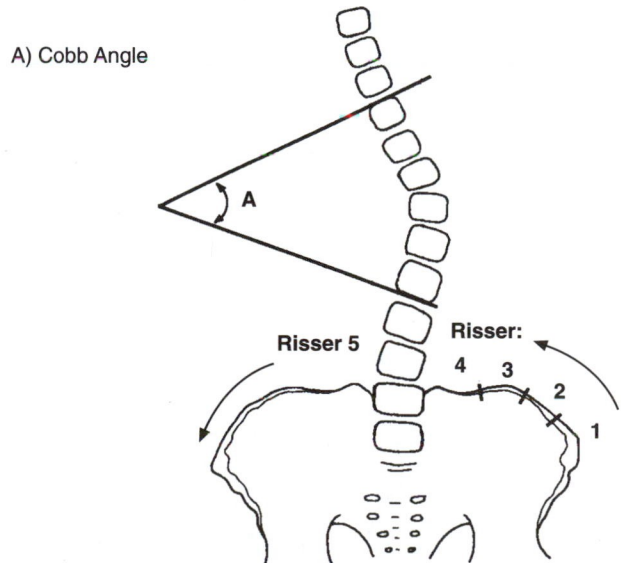

Figure 62-3

Illustration of measurements in idiopathic scoliosis. Cobb Angle, (A) and Risser staging. (Reproduced and modified with permission from Miller MD: Pediatric Orthopaedics. In: *Review of Orthopaedics.* Philadelphia: Saunders; 1992:14.)

Degree of wedging, as determined by Cobb, and rotation using the Nash-Moe rating system are also frequently addressed on radiographs. Risser sign or degree of ossification of the iliac crest apophysis is also assessed to appraise the degree of skeletal maturity. Risser staging is divided into six degrees of fusing and capping the iliac crest apophysis. Risser zero indicates no apophysis and skeletal immaturity while Risser 1 to 4 indicate progressive apophysis and Risser 5 indicates fusion. Each iliac crest apophysis fuses from lateral to medial and then caps from medial to lateral (Fig. 62-4).

Additional radiographic observations that have been used to help determine the levels to be fused when surgical intervention is deemed appropriate. These include the stable zone of Harrington, the stable vertebra, and the neutral vertebra as described by Moe.

The stable zone of Harrington includes those vertebrae that fall within the area of two vertical parallel lines drawn up from the S1 pedicles. The stable vertebra is the vertebra bisected by the central sacral line which is drawn through the midpoint of the sacrum perpendicular to the pelvis. The neutral vertebra is described as the vertebra having no rotation and symmetric pedicles on the RA radiograph. On the lateral radiograph, sagittal plane alignment is assessed as is incidental spondylolisthesis. The presence of thoracic lordosis or hypokyphosis may preclude brace treatment.

The presence of spondylolisthesis may influence the vertebra selected as the lowest level of the fusion.

PROGNOSIS

Only approximately 10 percent of adolescent idiopathic curves that are greater than 10 degrees in magnitude will require active treatment. Several risk factors for curve progression have been determined. These include younger age at the time of initial diagnosis, the female patient being premenarcheal at the time of diagnosis, having a lower Risser sign at the time of diagnosis, and having a curve of greater magnitude at the time of initial diagnosis. Although the incidence of

adolescent idiopathic curves is similar among females and males, curve progression has been noted to occur more frequently in females. Males tend to reach skeletal maturity at an older age than do females. Males with adolescent idiopathic scoliosis need to be followed for curve progression until they are skeletally mature.

Several risk factors exist for risk of progression of idiopathic curves in adulthood. These include thoracic and thoracolumbar curves that are greater than 50 to 55 degrees at skeletal maturity. These curves have been reported to increase at the rate of 1 degree per year. Lumbar curves that are greater than 30 degrees in magnitude and have more than 33 degrees of apical vertebral rotation at skeletal maturity have a greater tendency to progress in adulthood.

When scoliotic curves reach a magnitude of greater than 90 degrees, cardiopulmonary function may become impaired. These patients are at increased risk for cardiopulmonary complications such as cor pulmonale and restrictive lung disease. Thoracic lordosis and hypokyphosis have been implicated in loss of pulmonary function.

Prior to undertaking operative intervention for large curves and in patients with thoracic hypokyphosis or lordosis, pulmonary function tests should be obtained to evaluate the degree of pulmonary impairment.

In patients with curves that are not of the above magnitude, mortality rate and incidence of low back pain are not reported to vary significantly from the general population. Cosmesis is a primary reason for many adolescent idiopathic scoliotics to seek treatment. The risk of curve progression with pregnancy is somewhat controversial. We recommend that patients follow up and have radiographic evaluation after delivery so that the curve may be assessed for progression.

TREATMENT

The treatment of choice for adolescent idiopathic scoliosis depends on the magnitude of the curve and the patient's degree of skeletal maturity. Curves of 0 to 25 degrees in a skeletally immature patient are followed with serial observations and radiographs. Should the curve progress 5 degrees or more and the patient continue to be skeletally immature, then bracing is recommended. Skeletally immature patients may be braced for curves up to 40 to 45 degrees after which, bracing is no longer effective and surgery should be considered. In skeletally mature patients, surgery is considered in patients with curves of 50 degrees or greater because of the increased risk for progression. Electrical stimulation has no role in the treatment of adolescent idiopathic scoliosis. Exercises have not been proven effective in halting curve progression. They may be of benefit in improving or maintaining general conditioning during the treatment period.

Orthotic treatment of adolescent idiopathic scoliosis is used in attempt to prevent curve progression rather than to achieve any final curve correction. Orthotic treatment is indicated in skeletally immature patients. This includes those patients who are Risser 0, 1, or 2 and are premenarcheal or less than one year postmenarcheal and have curves between 30 to 40 degrees or between 20 to 30 degrees with documented progression of 5 degrees. Recently, brace treatment has also been advocated for 25 to 30 degree curves in patients with Risser scores of 0 and 1 in the absence of documented progression. The orthotic is used until the patient reaches skeletal maturity or the curve progresses to the point where surgical intervention is indicated. Attainment of skeletal maturity is defined as being more than 2 years postmenarcheal, at least a Risser 4, and having closed vertebral epiphyses. At this time orthotic use is weaned as the patient continues to be followed for curve progression.

Three types of orthoses are used in the treatment of adolescent idiopathic scoliosis: the Milwaukee brace; underarm TLSOs such as the Boston, Wilmington, or Miami brace; and the Charleston night-

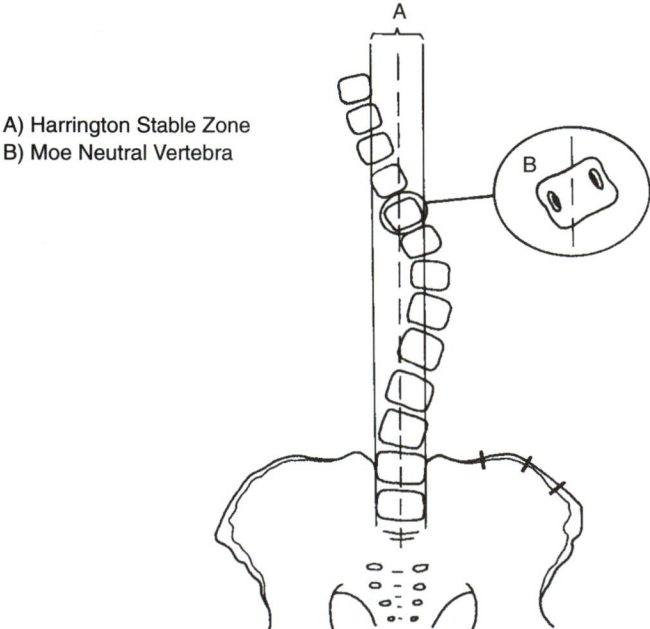

A) Harrington Stable Zone
B) Moe Neutral Vertebra

Figure 62-4

Illustration of measurements in idiopathic scoliosis. Harrington's stable zone (A) and stable (neutral) vertebra (B). (Reproduced and modified with permission from Miller MD: Pediatric orthopaedics. In *Review of Orthopaedics*. Philadelphia: Saunders; 1992:14.)

time bending brace. The Milwaukee brace, which has been proven to be effective in the treatment of adolescent idiopathic scoliosis, is used less frequently today because of less acceptance of its cosmetic appearance. The underarm TLSOs are generally better accepted cosmetically and are worn 23 h per day during the years of remaining skeletal growth. There have been reports of part-time (16 h) bracing showing comparable results to full-time use. The Charleston nighttime bending brace holds the patient in an acutely bent position opposite of the scoliotic curve. It is worn only at night for at least 8 h. Insufficient data is available at this time to prove its efficacy.

Surgical treatment of adolescent idiopathic scoliosis is indicated in cases of curve magnitude ≥45 degrees, and in curves of 30 to 45 degrees with documented progression despite proper brace treatment. Surgical goals include halting progression of the deformity, achieving some correction of the deformity, and achieving or maintaining both coronal and sagittal spinal balance. Prior to surgical intervention, supine lateral bending radiographs are obtained to determine the flexibility of the curves. The surgical goals can be accomplished through posterior fusion with segmental instrumentation, anterior release with fusion and instrumentation, or a combined approach. Many instrumentation systems are available. The surgical approach is determined by the curve magnitude, skeletal maturity of the patient at the time of surgery, and the type of curve. Determination of the levels to be fused is made based on the curve characteristics. In most cases when posterior instrumentation is used, fusion extends from the stable end vertebra to stable end vertebra. The use of anterior correction and rigid rod instrumentation in lumbar and thoracolumbar curves has become more common. Fusion levels are determined by locating the apex of the curve. If it is at a disc, the discs above and below are included in the fusion. If the apex is at a vertebra, the vertebra above and below are included. Usually the vertebrae that are most tilted into the curve on the standing radiograph are instrumented. Combined approaches may be indicated when there is concern about crankshaft, in very large curves where anterior release may provide some correction of the curve, and in adult patients with adolescent idiopathic scoliosis where the fusion rate may be improved with combined surgery.

Thoracoplasty either from a posterior or anterior approach, can be performed in large curves with significant rib prominence to improve cosmetic results. Patients with poor pulmonary function are not good candidates for thoracoplasty as this procedure, at best temporarily, diminishes vital capacity.

Potential complications of surgery include neurologic injury; this is minimized by the use of somatosensory evoked potential intraoperative monitoring and a Stagnara wake-up test (for motor function) as needed. The incidence of infection and pseudarthrosis is generally low in this patient population (1 to 2 percent). The need for homologous blood transfusions is minimized by the use of hypotensive anesthesia, hemodilution, intraoperative cell saver, and autologous blood donation. Painful hardware may be removed after the spine is fused. Use of lower profile systems may be helpful in preventing this problem. Other potential complications include flatback (lumbar hypolordosis) and degeneration below the level of fusion. The incidence of these problems is minimized by careful attention to the sagittal plane balance during surgery and fusing only those vertebrae necessary.

POSTURAL KYPHOSIS

The patient with postural kyphosis, or postural roundback, is more often than not brought in by a parent who complains about the adolescent's posture. Pain is rarely associated with the complaint of de-

formity. Frequently the parent is more disturbed by the deformity than the patient. As always, a detailed history should be obtained and a complete physical examination performed. There is generally nothing in the history of concern. At times, the adolescent has undergone the growth spurt at a younger age than typical. In females, the kyphotic posture is sometimes maintained by the child to hide the development of breasts. In males, it may be an attempt to draw attention away from being tall.

On physical examination a gentle rounded increased kyphosis is apparent over the entire thoracic spine with a compensatory increased lumbar and cervical lordosis. On the Adam's forward bend test, the kyphotic deformity is apparent without localized marked angular deformity. The spine is generally non-tender. The most important finding in postural kyphosis is the marked flexibility of the curve and the ability to correct the kyphotic deformity with the erect posture or extension of the spine. If the patients are allowed to sit for a period of time, they will return to the postural kyphotic slouching that brought them to the physician in the first place. Radiographs of the patient with a postural kyphosis will reveal a gentle kyphotic deformity of the entire thoracic spine. The generally accepted upper limit of normal thoracic kyphosis is 45 degrees. The child with postural kyphosis will have a measurement greater than 45 degrees but typically less than 60, though this is not always the case. There will be an absence of structural changes noted on the radiograph, that is, no wedging of the vertebrae, no wedging of the discs, absence of Schmorl's nodes or irregularities of the end plate. The neurologic examination of the patient with postural kyphosis is normal although occasionally there will be mild hamstring tightness.

Treatment includes reassurance that no significant deformity exists and encouragement to maintain a more upright posture. Extension exercises, abdominal and scapulothoracic strengthening exercises may be beneficial to strengthen the posterior musculature and assist the child in maintaining a more upright posture. In more extreme cases, particularly when the curve is less flexible, bracing may be appropriate. Postural kyphosis can become structural in time. Follow up examinations should be performed in 4 to 6 months. Progression of the deformity may require bracing, though this is unusual.

SCHEUERMANN'S KYPHOSIS

Scheuermann's disease was first described in 1921 by Holger Scheuermann. The etiology of Scheuermann's disease remains unknown. There is a defect of endochondral ossification. There is weakening of the cartilaginous endplate with decreased growth anteriorly and resultant kyphosis. The further compression of the anterior vertebral endplates further retards growth in this area resulting in worsening of the deformity. This is consistent with the Heuter-Volkman law of excessive physeal pressure resulting in decreased growth. Others have suggested that Scheuermann's kyphosis is a form of osteochondrosis. An autosomal dominant inheritance pattern with a variable degree of penetrance and expressivity has also been suggested. The incidence of Scheuermann's kyphosis has been reported to be between 0.4 and 8 percent. Male to female ratio varies greatly from study to study with an apparent equal incidence in both sexes. There are no reported cases of Scheuermann's disease in a child under 10 years of age. The presenting complaint of the adolescent with Scheuermann's kyphosis is either pain and/or concern over the deformity. The pain tends to be an annoyance. It is rarely severe and complaints of severe pain should warrant further investigations. It is frequently the cosmetic deformity that bothers the teenager the most. Pain associated with Scheuermann's kyphosis is generally centered over the apex, but it may also be diffuse over the entire thoracic spine.

There may also be pain in the lower back as a result of the compensatory hyperlordosis or in the neck from the compensatory cervical lordosis. There is an increased incidence of spondylolisthesis in patient's with Scheuermann's kyphosis and this may also be a contributing factor to the pain.

Physical examination of the patient with Scheuermann's kyphosis will immediately reveal the kyphotic deformity. In contrast to postural kyphosis, the deformity is more angular. It usually occurs near the apex of the normal thoracic kyphosis (T7-8), but it can also be present at the thoracolumbar junction. As the normal sagittal contour of the thoracolumbar junction is essentially neutral, a kyphotic deformity at this area is particularly apparent. The kyphosis becomes more prominent on the forward bending Adam's test. The kyphosis is generally fairly rigid with only mild to moderate correction noted on hyperextension of the spine. A mild scoliotic deformity is typically noted as well in the patient with Scheuermann's disease. Hamstring tightness is frequently noted. A detailed neurologic examination should be performed. Although typically normal, neurologically, there have been reports of paralysis associated with Scheuermann's kyphosis and any abnormality upon neurologic testing should be followed up with an MRI study of the entire spine.

Standard erect full length AP and lateral scoliosis radiographs should be obtained. In addition a hyperextension lateral should be obtained, performed with the patient in the supine position, and a wedge placed under or just caudal to the apex of the deformity. The classic description of Scheuermann's kyphosis includes irregularity of the vertebral endplates, anterior wedging of three or more vertebrae of 5 degrees or more and kyphosis in excess of 45 degrees. There may be considerable variability in the presentation with some patients having one or two of the above findings and others having all. Previous recommendations suggesting that three adjacent vertebrae all needed to have wedging may be too stringent; some consider a single wedged vertebra as acceptable for this diagnosis. In lumbar Scheuermann's disease, irregularity of the vertebral endplates and Schmorl's nodes may be the only radiographic finding. Clinically, patients with lumbar Scheuermann's do not have any deformity, although they may present with complaints of pain. Rarely the lumbar spine is frankly kyphotic (Fig. 62-5).

An increased incidence of lumbar isthmic spondylolysis has been reported in Scheuermann's kyphosis. An extensive follow-up of patients with Scheuermann's kyphosis was reported on by Murray et al. Although a greater incidence of back pain was reported in the group with Scheuermann's kyphosis this difference was not great. There was no significant statistical difference noted between pain that interfered with everyday life, fatigue, self esteem, psychological disturbances, type of employment or time lost from work as a result of back pain or sciatica. This suggests that the natural history of Scheuermann's kyphosis is relatively benign and patients and parents can be reassured of that fact. The chief presenting complaint of these patients is often cosmesis; the treatment needs to address this issue on an individual basis. Families can be reassured that cardiac or respiratory difficulties are not a concern. Only very large kyphotic deformities (>100) have been associated with decreased respiratory function.

TREATMENT OF SCHEUERMANN'S DISEASE

Those patients presenting with relatively small amounts of hyperkyphosis, less than 55 degrees, may be treated by observation and physical therapy. Physical therapy should be directed at strengthening of the spinal and abdominal musculature and encouraging extension type of exercises and activities. In the skeletally immature patient with a significant kyphosis, that is either painful or troublesome

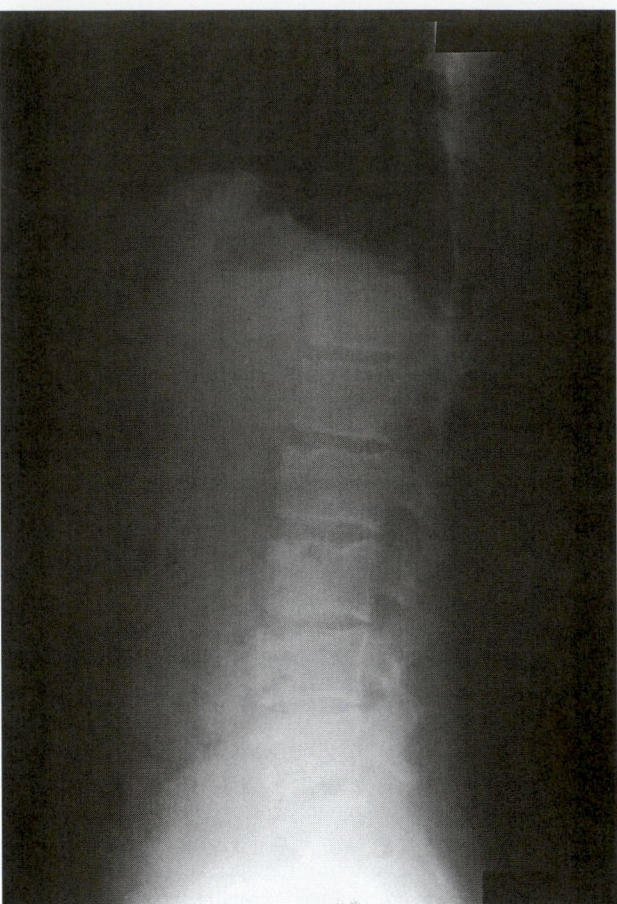

Figure 62-5
Lateral radiograph of lumbar Scheurmann's disease.

because of cosmesis, brace treatment may be indicated. The standard brace used is the Milwaukee brace. If the apex of the curve is below T7, an underarm TLSO with outriggers to apply posterior pressure on the shoulders may be used. Bracing needs to be continued until skeletal maturity. One can see reversal of the radiographic changes in many patients who are braced. Bracing can provide lasting correction of the curve in contrast to scoliosis bracing, where the goal of bracing is only to halt progression. By unloading the anterior column, increased growth anteriorly may result in correction of the deformity. If bracing is stopped too early, loss of correction may occur. Patients with kyphotic deformities that are greater than 75 degrees may be candidates for surgery. The most reliable treatment is an anterior release followed by posterior instrumentation. The fusion needs to be carried distally to the first lordotic segment, usually being the L1-2 or L2-3 interspace. The occasional patient with very flexible deformity that corrects to 55 degrees or less on extension can be treated with posterior surgery alone. Using segmental spinal instrumentation one should attempt to get three pedicle-transverse process claws proximal to the apex of the deformity. The correction is obtained by gentle three-point pressure on the apex of the deformity and by posterior compressive forces.

Lumbar Scheuermann's disease can be treated with a Boston type underarm brace for immobilization in those patients who are sufficiently symptomatic. Surgery is rarely required, but may be indicated for significant thoracolumbar junctional kyphosis.

SUGGESTED READINGS

Browne D: Congenital postural scoliosis. *Proc R Soc Med* 1956; 49:395.

Davies G, Reid L: Effect of scoliosis on growth of alveoli and pulmonary arteries and on the right ventricle. *Arch Dis Child* 1971; 46:623

McMaster MJ, MacNicol MF: The management of progressive infantile idiopathic scoliosis. *J Bone Joint Surg [Br]* 1979; 61:36.

Mehta MH: The rib-vertebra angle in the early diagnosis between resolving and progressive infantile scoliosis. *J Bone Joint Surg [Br]* 1972; 54:230.

Wynne-Davies R: Infantile idiopathic scoliosis. Causative factors, particularly in the first six months of life. *J Bone Joint Surg [Br]* 1975; 57:138.

JUVENILE IDIOPATHIC SCOLIOSIS

Dubousset J, Herring JA, Shufflebarger H: The crankshaft phenomenon. *J Pediatr Orthop* 1989; 9:541.

Lonstein JE, Carlson JM: The prediction of curve progression in untreated idiopathic scoliosis during growth. *J Bone Joint Surg [Am]* 1984; 66:1061.

Mannherz RE, Betz RR, Clancy M, et al: Juvenile idiopathic scoliosis followed to skeletal maturity. *Spine* 1988; 13:1087.

ADOLESCENT IDIOPATHIC SCOLIOSIS

Federico DJ, Renshaw TS: Results of treatment of idiopathic scoliosis with the Charleston bending orthosis. *Spine* 1990; 15:886.

King HA, Moe JH, Bradford DS, et al: The selection of fusion levels in thoracic idiopathic scoliosis. *J Bone Joint Surg [Am]* 1983; 65:1302.

Lonstein JE, Winter RB: The Milwaukee brace for the treatment of adolescent idiopathic scoliosis. A review of one thousand and twenty patients. *J Bone Joint Surg [Am]* 1994; 76:1207.

Moskowitz A, Moe JH, Winter RB, et al: Long-term follow-up of scoliosis fusion. *J Bone Joint Surg [Am]* 1980; 62:364.

Nash CL, Moe JH: A study of vertebral rotation. *J Bone Joint Surg [Am]* 1969; 51:223.

Schwend RM, Hennrikus W, Hall JE, et al: Childhood scoliosis: clinical indications for magnetic resonance imaging. *J Bone Joint Surg [Am]* 1995; 77:46.

Weinstein SL, Ponseti IV: Curve progression in idiopathic scoliosis. *J Bone Joint Surg [Am]* 1983; 65:447.

KYPHOSIS

Bradford DS, Ahmed KB, Moe JH, et al: The surgical management of patients with Scheuermann's disease: A review of twenty-four cases managed by combined anterior and posterior spine fusion. *J Bone Joint Surg [Am]* 1980; 62:705.

Lonstein JE, Winter RB, Moe JH, et al: Neurologic deficits secondary to spinal deformity. A review of the literature and reports of 43 cases. *Spine* 1980; 5:331.

Lowe TG. Scheuermann's disease. *J Bone Joint Surg [Am]* 1990; 72:940.

Murray PM, Weinstein SL, Spratt KF. The natural history and long-term follow-up of Scheuermann's kyphosis. *J Bone Joint Surg [Am]* 1993; 75:236.

Ogilvie JW, Sherman J: Spondylolysis in Scheuermann's disease. *Spine* 1987; 12:251.

Scheuermann HW. Kyfosis dorsalis juvenilis. *Ugeskr Laeger* 1920; 82:385.

Tolo VT: Postural kyphosis and Scheuermann's disease. *Semin Spine Surg* 1992; 4:216.

Chapter 63

NEUROMUSCULAR SCOLIOSIS

David S. Feldman

Neuromuscular scoliosis is a curvature of the spine in patients who have a disorder of the neuromuscular system. The disease states are quite diverse but can be divided into neuropathic and myopathic. Neuropathic diseases can affect primarily the upper or lower motor neurons or be a combined problem. These diseases may include cerebral palsy (upper), spinal cord trauma (upper), poliomyelitis (lower), or spina bifida (mixed). Myopathic diseases include muscular dystrophy as well as arthrogryposis. Children with neuromuscular disorders have an increased risk of scoliosis. The specific disorder will dictate the type of curve encountered and its risk of progression. In general, scoliosis associated with neuromuscular disease is longer (more segments involved) than idiopathic scoliosis and often includes the pelvis in the major curve, causing a pelvic obliquity. In addition, unlike idiopathic curves, neuromuscular scoliosis may progress rapidly and well after skeletal maturity.

A severely deformed spine in neuromuscular patients will have an adverse effect on their sitting ability and subsequently on pulmonary function. Children with neuromuscular scoliosis will often have pre-existing pulmonary dysfunction, particularly with clearing secretions. They often suffer from several other medical disorders. If the scoliosis becomes severe, sitting becomes impossible, necessitating an increasingly reclining position and decreased pulmonary clearance and consequent recurrent pneumonia.

GENERAL PRINCIPLES

EVALUATION

The evaluation of neuromuscular scoliosis is often multidisciplinary due to the multisystem dysfunction in children with this disorder. Children need to be evaluated based on their level of function. If a child who previously sat upright and performed activities with his hands is now leaning and supporting himself, then this behavior may represent a significant deterioration of his ability to be independent—therefore impacting his quality of life. The nutritional status of these children is essential if surgery is to be contemplated (see further discussion).

IMAGING STUDIES

The standardization of scoliosis radiographs is difficult but essential in order to determine a treatment plan. Little physical support should be given to the child. If the child can stand, then a long plate standing film is ideal; however, if the child cannot stand then a non-supported sitting film should be obtained. If the child is too young or cannot sit with minimal support, then a supine film is performed. In patients with a presumed neuromuscular disorder and a rapid progression of the scoliosis, the clinician should be certain there are no intramedullary causes for the scoliosis, such as syringomyelia or tethered cord. An MRI is indicated if there is a concern of an underlying spinal cord pathology contributing to the scoliosis. This is particularly true of children with spina bifida.

MANAGEMENT

The nonoperative management of neuromuscular scoliosis is often ineffective over the long term; however, it is essential in the overall management of the child during his or her growing years. While bracing a neuromuscular curve may be ineffective in halting its overall progression, it may be quite useful in delaying the need for surgery in a very young patient, allowing additional spinal growth prior to fusion. After puberty, bracing is ineffective and there is probably no reason to delay surgery any further. The clinician must be wary of decubitus ulcers in the insensate or spastic child with a brace.

The operative treatment of neuromuscular scoliosis requires a different approach than that of an idiopathic curve. While the principle of fusing a balanced spine over the sacrum is the same, the means of achieving this end are different. Often the patient is osteopenic and small and therefore will require segmental fixation, such as sublaminar wires. The pelvis is often incorporated into the fusion in order to balance the spine. Anterior fusion is frequently required due to the absence of posterior elements such as with spina bifida or due to the severity or rigidity of the curve.

Allograft is often used to achieve fusion due to the deformed pelvis and the frequent need to perform Galveston fixation (extension of rod fixation to the posterior ileum). Significantly more blood loss is expected in neuromuscular scoliosis surgery due to the osteopenia, the poor paraspinal musculature (particularly in Duchenne's muscular dystrophy), and the multiple laminotomies performed in order to achieve fixation.

Postoperative care is more difficult due to the poor pulmonary function and nutritional status in many of these patients. The patients are mobilized from bed early with aggressive pulmonary toilet. Both pre- and postoperative nutritional supplementation should be considered. The need for postoperative bracing depends on the fixation achieved with the instrumentation. It is most often not necessary.

SPECIFIC NEUROMUSCULAR DISORDERS

CEREBRAL PALSY

Scoliosis is a common finding in children with cerebral palsy (CP). Although it may be found in all types of cerebral palsy, it is most prevalent in patients with total body involvement. The etiology of the scoliosis is probably not secondary to the muscle imbalance as much as to the central proprioception dysfunction. The more severe the CP the more likely the child is to develop scoliosis. The curve is most commonly a long C-shaped curve into the pelvis; however, it may have an idiopathic configuration (Fig. 63-1). The idiopathic configuration is usually found in children with spastic diplegia who are ambulators.

The child must be evaluated initially for cognitive level of function, level of sitting and ambulatory function, any recent deterioration of physical function, Tanner stage, and pulmonary and general medical condition. The importance of a complete history and functional evaluation cannot be stressed enough as this will often influence the treatment to be administered.

Treatment depends on the age of the patient, the severity of the curve, and, most importantly, on evidence of deterioration of function. The curve should be evaluated for its configuration as well as for the extent of the structural component. Scoliosis due to poor trunk control may be positional but over time can become structural. In curves less than 45 degrees and in very young patients, orthotic use with a brace or custom wheelchair inserts are helpful. In patients with curves in excess of 50 degrees, posterior spinal fusion with segmental instrumentation is indicated. In children with severe CP and a fixed pelvic obliquity, fusion to the sacrum is necessary. Any child with a long C-shaped curve undergoing surgery should have fusion from the upper thoracic spine (T2) to the sacrum. Ending the fusion short of the sacrum will inevitably lead to a progressive pelvic obliquity and decompensation. If the fusion starts in the mid thoracic or thoracolumbar region, there is a risk that the patient will decompensate above with a junctional kyphosis or increasing scoliosis.

In very rigid curves or curves greater than 70 to 80 degrees, ante-rior release and fusion is required prior to undergoing the posterior fusion with instrumentation. Often this surgery can be performed in one day. The need for anterior and posterior surgery is to balance the spine as well as to prevent hardware failure posteriorly.

There are two issues that differ in the child with CP with regard to postoperative care. First, the child may not have a cough reflex; this requires extensive pulmonary toilet as well as a possible delay in extubation. Second, the child may have secondary hip and knee contractures which make positioning difficult. If the child has had a fusion to the pelvis via the Galveston technique, postoperatively the hips should not be forcibly extended. The child should be maintained in the normal resting position. If hip or knee releases are needed, they may be performed at a later date.

MUSCULAR DYSTROPHY

Although all forms of muscular dystrophy are associated with scoliosis, Duchenne's muscular dystrophy has the most rapidly progressive curve and requires aggressive and timely intervention. Children with Duchenne's will ordinarily be diagnosed in the second or third year of life. They show a steady decline in both girdle and axial strength. The patient will often become wheelchair-bound by the age of thirteen. It is at that time the patient develops scoliosis (Fig. 63-2).

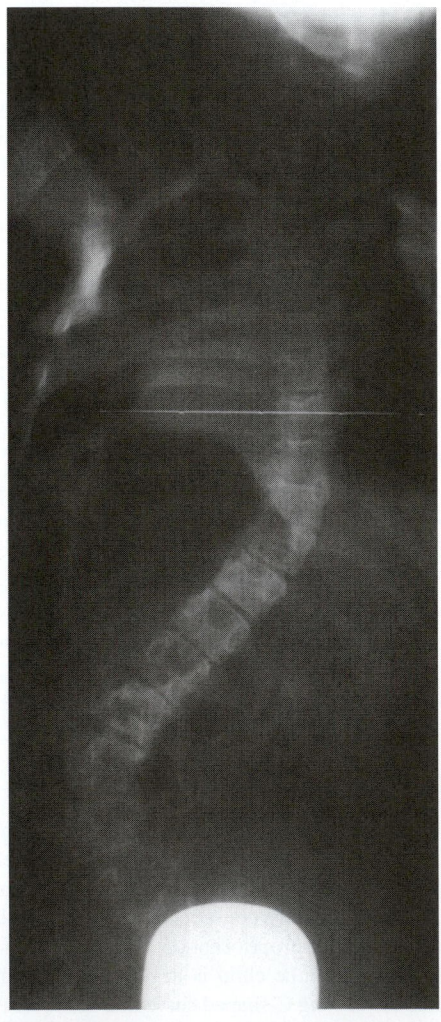
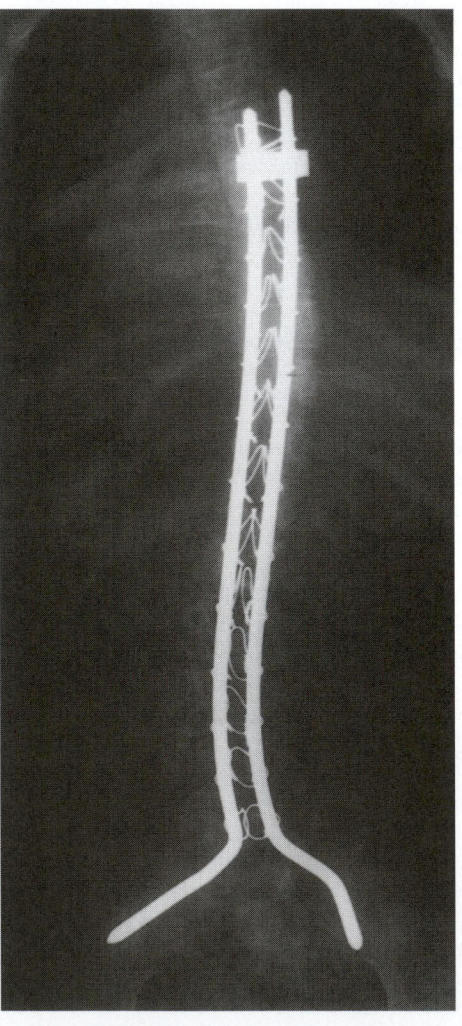

A *B*

Figure 63-1
A 13-year-old female with spastic quadriplegia and 70-degree scoliosis (*A*). Postoperative Luque instrumentation with a well-compensated spine (*B*).

Up to 95 percent of children with Duchenne's muscular dystrophy will develop progressive scoliosis. The goal of management is to maintain the patient as a stable sitter. As soon as the child is wheelchair-bound and scoliosis is evident and approaching twenty to twenty-five degrees, surgery should be performed. The child with Duchenne's will often have a rapid progression and the larger the curve, the greater the loss of vital capacity and the younger the age of death. The scoliosis progresses an average of 10 degrees per year, but some may progress 40 degrees during the first year the patient becomes wheelchair-bound.

The loss of vital capacity is a significant problem in determining if the patient can undergo surgery. It remains controversial whether surgery slows the inevitable decline in vital capacity, but certainly a vital capacity below 40 percent of predicted is a risk for the need for permanent ventilatory support postsurgery. A child with a vital capacity of less than 30 percent should not be operated on due to the probable permanent need for ventilatory support.

Standard surgery in this clinical situation consists of posterior spinal fusion from T2 to the pelvis. The instrumentation most frequently used is segmental sublaminar wire fixation to long rods extending into the pelvis ("Galveston technique"). In an attempt to minimize postoperative pseudoarthrosis and pain, a number of surgeons have attempted to leave the pelvis unfused in patients with minimal or no fixed pelvic obliquity. This has been met with varied success, although, if there is no fixed pelvic obliquity, fusion to L5 can be performed. Any patient with a pelvic obliquity above ten degrees should be fused to the pelvis. Anterior spinal surgery in children with Duchenne's is not performed due to the poor pulmonary capacity in these patients. Surgical blood loss is a consistent problem in these children due to the lack of contractile paraspinal musculature as well as osteoporosis.

Postoperative management includes ventilator support and hemodynamic stabilization. Children are mobilized to the sitting position in a body jacket as soon as possible, and if preoperatively the vital capacity is above 40 percent of predicted, the patient should not require prolonged ventilatory support.

There are other forms of muscular dystrophy. Becker's, which is phenotypically a milder form of Duchenne's, is commonly associated with scoliosis; however, it occurs at a later age and may not be inevitably progressive. Fascioscapular muscular dystrophy ordinarily presents after growth has ceased and therefore, is not associated with scoliosis. There is a less common, more severe form of the disease which presents in infancy and is often associated with scoliosis. Treatment depends on the age and severity of the curve. Bracing is often utilized early on in order to allow for spinal growth prior to surgery. Limb-girdle muscular dystrophy and myotonic dystrophy are not associated with scoliosis.

ARTHROGRYPOSIS

Arthrogryposis is a varied group of disorders associated with severe joint contractures at birth. The clinical presentation involves a varying degree of muscle weakness and contracture. Scoliosis occurs in about one-quarter of all patients with arthrogryposis. It is most often a long C-shaped curve; however, it may resemble an idiopathic curve. Curves measuring greater than 45 degrees in a growing child should be fused. Bracing is useful only in a very small child in order to delay surgery until more spinal growth has occurred (Fig. 63-3).

SPINA BIFIDA

Scoliosis associated with myelomeningocele is quite common and often very difficult to treat. The child with spina bifida may have the scoliosis secondary to the posterior element deficiency, may have a congenital scoliosis with hemivertabrae and unilateral bars, or they may have an idiopathic-like curve above the deficiency (Fig. 63-4). Patients must be evaluated carefully for neurologic function as a deterioration of function associated with scoliosis often means there is an underlying cause. Progressive scoliosis in a child with spina bifida warrants a work-up including an MRI to rule out a tethered cord, syringomyelia, or decompensated hydrocephalus. Scoliosis is nearly universal in thoracic level patients and becomes less common in the lower lumbar level patients. Sagittal plane deformity, particularly kyphosis, is common in high lumbar and thoracic level patients.

The treatment of the scoliosis in spina bifida depends on the age of the patient, progression and magnitude of the curve, and the ambulatory ability of the child. A number of difficulties arise in treating spina bifida patients with scoliosis. First, the patients are ordinarily insensate, which makes brace wear very difficult and fraught with a risk of skin breakdown and chest wall deformity. Second, the lack of posterior elements makes fusion and instrumentation in the lumbar spine difficult to achieve. Third, in ambulatory patients with spina bifida, if the fusion extends to the pelvis, this will hamper and diminish their ambulatory ability. Also, the patients with scoliosis are often young and small. The scoliosis can present as young as two years of age. The issue of spinal growth arises.

Therefore, the management of scoliosis with spina bifida is complex. Brace wear is ordinarily not advised, although a well-molded thoracic-lumbar-sacral orthosis (TLSO) can be utilized to allow ad-

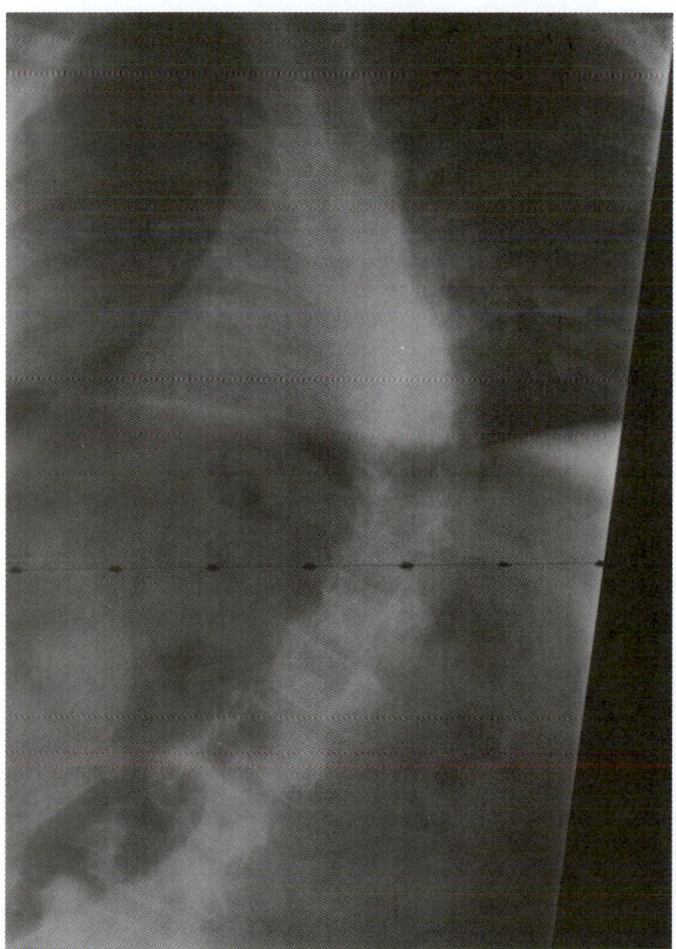

Figure 63-2
Long C-shaped curve in a 12-year-old child with muscular dystrophy.

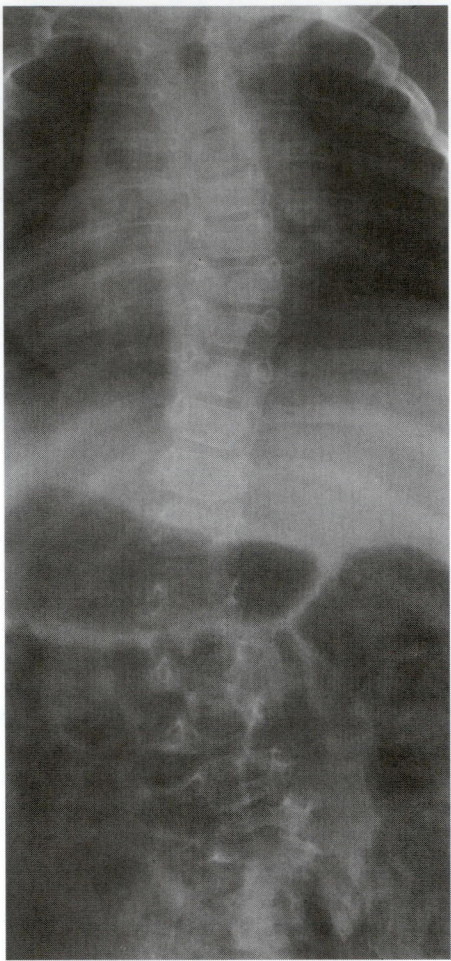

Figure 63-3
A 9-year-old boy with arthrogryposis and idiopathic type curve.

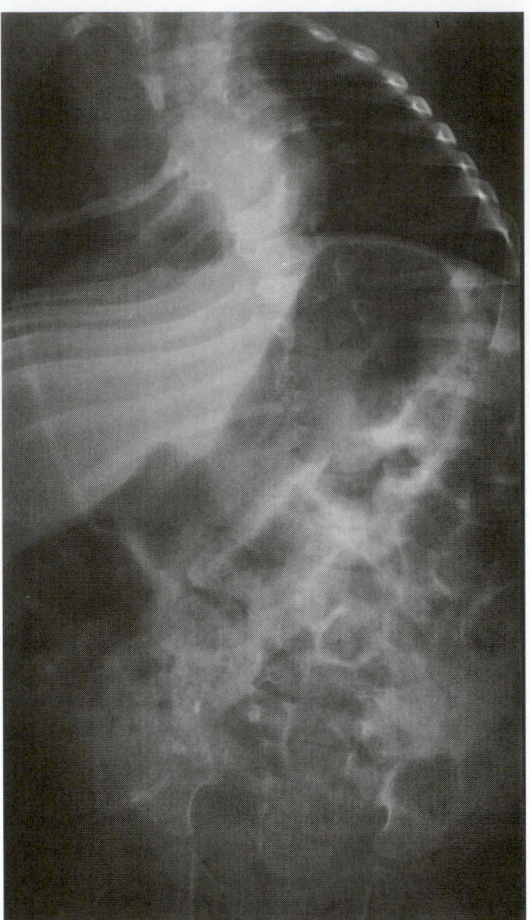

Figure 63-4
Scoliosis in 2-year-old child with thoracic myelomeningocele.

ditional spinal growth. Posterior fusion and instrumentation can be achieved with a combination of sublaminar wires and pedicle screws. This is recommended for a progressive scoliosis above 40 degrees in a growing child. Fusion to the pelvis should be performed if a pelvic obliquity of over 15 degrees exists or if the patient has a high lumbar or thoracic level. In children with large curves and no posterior elements in the lumbar spine, anterior fusion and instrumentation with a posterior fusion and instrumentation is the management of choice. In very young children, segmental posterior instrumentation without fusion is advised. This will often require fusion and re-instrumentation when the child reaches maturity.

Kyphosis in a child with spina bifida presents a unique problem. The kyphosis has an apex at the level of the defect, ordinarily, in the mid- to upper lumbar spine. The kyphosis is often rapidly progressive and may develop a fixed lordosis above. Correction of the kyphosis can be treated in infancy with resection and wiring; however, most often the child is treated in early adolescence. Indications to resect the kyphosis include skin breakdown with osteomyelitis of the kyphus, and inability of the children to use their hands due to the need to support themselves on their thighs. Surgery includes apical resection with segmental fixation and rods curved over the S1 foramen in order to maintain correction. Skin coverage posteriorly is often a problem, and tissue expanders and cross muscle flaps are helpful in achieving coverage of the orsthumentation.

FRIEDREICH'S ATAXIA

Patients with Friedreich's ataxia ordinarily present in early adolescence and often suffer from significant scoliosis. The curve pattern is most often similar to idiopathic scoliosis and can be treated in a similar fashion. Fusion to the pelvis is rarely necessary.

RILEY DAY SYNDROME (FAMILIAL DYSAUTONOMIA)

Riley Day syndrome is a rare autosomal recessive disorder effecting Jewish children of eastern European descent. The syndrome is associated with severe autonomic dysfunction, pain insensitivity, and progressive kyphoscoliosis. Progression may be rapid, and surgery has a high complication rate of infection and hardware failure. The mortality rate from all causes 1 year after surgery approaches 40 percent.

SPINAL CORD INJURY

Children and adolescents with thoracic-level paraplegia will often develop scoliosis. The risk of significant scoliosis is related to the age of the development of the paraplegia. Children who are age 9 and below will universally develop scoliosis. Once again, bracing has little effect on the natural history, and surgical fusion is most often needed.

SPINAL MUSCULAR ATROPHY

Spinal muscular atrophy (SMA) is a group of autosomal recessive disorders that cause a loss of anterior horn cells in the spinal cord and result in a progressive weakness, particularly in the trunk and proximal musculature. The severity of the disease is variable with onset from infancy to early adolescence.

Scoliosis is almost universal in children who survive with spinal muscular atrophy. The onset and severity of the scoliosis depends on the severity of the illness. Children with SMA who walk for a period of time have less progressive and less severe scoliosis than those children with infantile onset and non-ambulators. The curves are most often long C-shaped into the pelvis with a pelvic obliquity.

Treatment of the scoliosis depends on the age of the child, the magnitude of the curve, and the pulmonary function of the patient. A long C-shaped curve that approaches 50 degrees should undergo posterior spinal fusion from T2 to the sacrum with Luque segmental sublaminar instrumentation and Galveston fixation to the pelvis. The use of anterior surgery in children with SMA is reserved for those patients with rigid curves above 80 degrees. Anterior surgery is not well tolerated by these patients and should be undertaken with caution.

Postoperative complications may occur in up to half of the patients with SMA undergoing spinal surgery. Hardware failure due to ostepenia, pneumonia and atalectasis, severe ileus, wound infection, deterioration of function, and severe blood loss are not uncommon. The child should be mobilized early postoperatively and have extensive pulmonary support.

POLIOMYELITIS

Although poliomyelitis has been nearly eradicated in the United States, it continues to be a major health concern in countries without widespread vaccination programs. Moreover, the sequelae of polio is still felt from patients who suffered from the disease decades ago.

Scoliosis, as a sequelae of poliomyelitis, is estimated to occur in up to one-third of patients. It is thought to be caused by an imbalance of the paraspinal and other chest and abdominal musculature. The curve is most commonly a double major curve with a pelvic obliquity. Severe pelvic obliquity occurs in up to one-half of the patients with scoliosis. Other curve types include long C-shaped, lumbar, and thoracic curves in descending order of frequency. Most postpolio curves are not progressive, and simply require close observation.

Treatment of scoliosis depends on the age of the patient as well as the magnitude and type of the curve. Bracing is useful only to delay the inevitable need for surgery in children. Curves greater than 40 degrees should be considered for posterior spinal fusion. Segmental fixation is the instrumentation of choice due to the presence of osteoporosis. Patients who ambulate utilizing pelvic motion to achieve swing may have great difficulty in ambulation after fusion to the pelvis.

RETT SYNDROME

Rett syndrome is a neurologic disorder that affects females. It is progressive and of unknown etiology. Children are born normal and continue to meet normal milestones for up to the first 18 months of life. The children then undergo a rapid deterioration of mental and physical function. These children develop a progressive encephalopathy which leads to hyptonicity and eventual spasticity.

Scoliosis occurs in the vast majority of children with Rett syndrome. A long C-shaped curve is the most common deformity. Treatment depends on the magnitude of the curve. Once again, bracing may be utilized as a temporizing measure in young children with curves between 25 and 40 degrees. Curves above 40 degrees should be treated with posterior spinal fusion and segmental instrumentation with fusion to the pelvis if a pelvic obliquity exists. These neuromuscular curves can be very rapidly progressive and become very rigid. Therefore, surgery should be performed in most children with Rett syndrome when the curve reaches 40 degrees.

SUGGESTED READINGS

Boachie-Adjei O, Lonstein JE, Winter RB, et al: Management of neuromuscular spinal deformities with Luque segmental instrumentation. *J Bone Joint Surg [Am]* 1989; 71:548.

Galasko CS, Delancy C, Morris P: Spinal stabilization in Duchenne muscular dystrophy. *J Bone Joint Surg [Br]* 1992; 74:210.

Lonstein JE, Akbarnia A: Operative treatment of spinal deformities in patients with cerebral palsy or mental retardation. An analysis of one hundred and seven cases. *J Bone Joint Surg [Am]* 1983; 65:43.

Piggott H: The natural history of scoliosis in myelodysplasia. *J Bone Joint Surg [Br]* 1980; 62:54.

Rubery PT, Spielman JH, Hester P, et al: Scoliosis in familial dysautonomia. *J Bone Joint Surg [Am]* 1995; 77:1362.

Chapter 64

BACK PAIN IN CHILDREN

David S. Feldman

Children with spinal pathology present with various symptoms, such as back pain, scoliosis, weakness, paraparesis, and foot deformity. Some studies have indicated that back pain in children is an uncommon complaint and between 66 to 85 percent of these children will have a demonstrable and often treatable cause. Therefore, children with back pain frequently undergo extensive investigation due to the belief that organic pathology will be found in the majority of instances. However, epidemiologic studies have reported that 11 to 33 percent of school-age children complain of significant low back pain. This suggests that back pain in childhood may be a common and possibly benign complaint. Thus, many children with back pain may undergo expensive and unnecessary investigations. Back pain in young athletes has received more recent attention, with an emphasis on correct training techniques, proper equipment, and sound fitness as a means of preventing back injuries.

EVALUATION

Children presenting with back pain require careful evaluation. The history and physical examination are essential. The duration of the pain, its nature, and its constancy are detailed, and alleviating and aggravating factors for the pain should be carefully documented. Traumatic events and recreational activities that the child participates in are important in understanding causative factors for the pain. The patient needs to be asked about radiating pain and leg pain, as well as bladder, bowel, and (age-appropriate) sexual dysfunction.

Various disease states have quite specific presentations and symptoms. For instance, low back pain that is activity-related in an avid young female gymnast is likely to be a spondylolysis. A 13-year-old boy with night back pain that awakens him from sleep and that is alleviated with nonsteroidal anti-inflammatory medication or aspirin may have an osteoid osteoma.

Physical evaluation includes a thorough neurologic examination including reflexes (also abdominal reflexes) as well as motor and sensation ability. Range of motion of the spine and motion that incites the pain are important as well. The presence of a positive straight leg raise, loss of the normal sagittal or coronal contours of the spine, or hamstring tightness should be noted.

Laboratory evaluation is important in evaluating a young child with back pain and constitutional symptoms; a complete blood count (CBC) and erythrocyte sedimentation rate (ESR) are useful in the initial evaluation. Further studies such as rheumatoid factor, ANA, ASO, HLA B27 and Lyme titer are important if an inflammatory process is considered. A CBC is particularly important in young children below the age of 8 due to the possibility of leukemia.

Imaging studies performed depend on the age of the child and the location and nature of the pain, as well as concomitant physical findings. Not every child or teenager necessarily requires a bone scan. Plain films should be obtained. Further studies should be performed depending on the level of suspicion for a specific entity. Magnetic resonance imaging (MRI) is useful if the neuraxis is to be evaluated. In children with painful scoliosis, as well as abnormal neurologic findings, this becomes particularly important. Bone scan, or more specifically, single proton emission computed tomography (SPECT) is best utilized in evaluating or diagnosing spondylolysis. CT scan may be utilized to analyze the bony margins of an osseous tumor or with myelography if an MRI cannot be obtained.

TUMOR

The greatest concern of the physician treating children with back pain is delay in diagnosis of a malignant neoplasm. There are a number of factors that are of concern in a child. If the child is very young (i.e., below the age of 10), complains of constant pain and/or night pain or if a neurologic deficit is found on physical examination, then an evaluation for a possible tumor should be performed. A bone scan is insufficient to rule out spinal neoplasm as the tumor may be extraosseous. MRI is the best study to confirm or rule out a tumor.

Tumors of the spine may be benign or malignant and intraosseous or extraosseous. While no tumor with the exception of a benign intraosseous hemangioma is common, certain tumors have a propensity for involving the spinal elements. These tumors include osteoid osteoma, osteoblastoma, aneurysmal bone cyst, and eosinophilic granuloma (Fig. 64–1).

Malignant tumors such as neuroblastoma may present with spinal involvement, although children more commonly present with an inability to walk rather than back pain. Primary bone tumors such as Ewing sarcoma or osteogenic sarcoma may present in the spine, although rarely as the primary site of involvement. Up to 6 percent of children with acute lymphocytic leukemia will present with back pain, but usually the diagnosis is made by the pediatrician due to concomitant constitutional symptoms such as fatigue and easy bruisability.

DISC DISORDERS

Herniated nucleus pulposus is observed in children and adolescents. Patients often present with back pain and lower extremity radiation. Plain radiographs may demonstrate a scoliosis; however, the test of choice is MRI. Neurologic deficits are uncommon in the pediatric population. Treatment is the same as in adults, with nonoperative treatment consisting of rest and anti-inflammatory medications for up to 3 months prior to considering surgical intervention. Surgical treatment generally consists of discectomy without fusion. Although the children complain of back pain, fusion is usually not necessary as discectomy alone often relieves all of the symptoms. Congenital spinal stenosis may be a concomitant finding in children with a symptomatic herniated disc and can be diagnosed on CT scan or MRI. Degenerative disc disease has been seen in normal children with no back pain and is probably not the etiology for back pain in children in most instances.

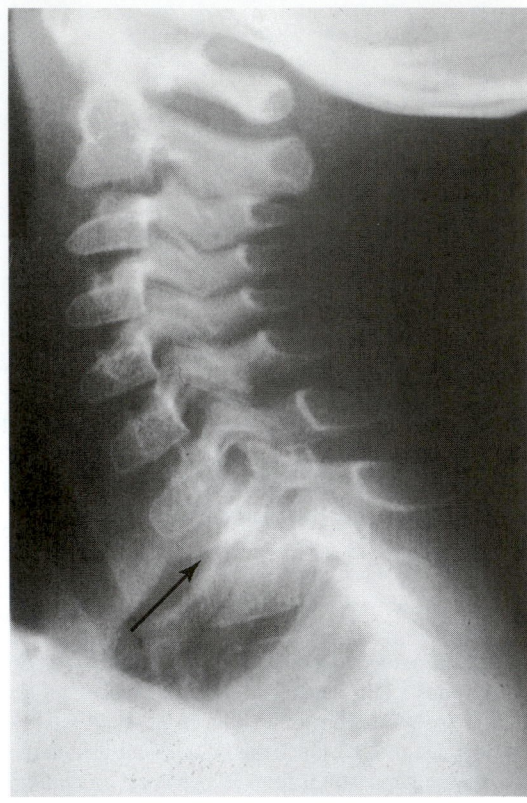

Figure 64-1
5-year-old boy with upper thoracic back pain secondary to eosinophilic granuloma (*arrow*).

During evaluation one should be certain there is not a slipped vertebral apophysis. This can be seen as a bony fleck within the spinal canal on plain radiographs or be diagnosed with MRI or CT scan, if suspected. CT scan is preferred as the bone fragment may not be well visualized on MRI. This most often occurs in adolescents as an acute event, such as lifting a heavy weight. It can occur from L3 to the sacrum, but is most commonly the inferior rim of L4. Treatment is surgical with excision of the bone fragment.

There are numerous other etiologies of back pain that will be discussed in various other chapters. Infection, such as discitis and osteomyelitis, must be considered (Fig. 64-2). Spondylolysis, spondylolisthesis, and Scheuermann's kyphosis may cause pain as well. Juvenile idiopathic arthritis (formerly termed juvenile rheumatoid arthritis) and ankylosing spondylitis may similarly cause pain, but usually have additional findings, such as large joint involvement and stiffness.

In summary, children with back pain need to be carefully evaluated. Appropriate laboratory and imaging studies should be ordered depending on the results of the plain radiographs and the level of suspicion. Young children with constant or night pain with a short duration of symptoms should be most closely evaluated.

SUGGESTED READINGS

Harvey J, Tanner S: Low back pain in young athletes. A practical approach. *Sports Med* 1991; 12:394.

Ramirez N, Johnston CE, Browne RH: The prevalence of back pain in children who have idiopathic scoliosis. *J Bone Joint Surg [Am]* 1997; 79:364.

Ransford AO, Pozo JL, Hutton PAN, et al: The behaviour pattern of the scoliosis associated with osteoid osteoma or osteoblastoma of the spine. *J Bone Joint Surg [Br]* 1984; 66:16.

Salminen JJ, Pentti J, Terho P: Low back pain and disability in 14-year-old school children. *Acta Paediatr Scand* 1992; 81:1035.

Taylor LJ: Painful scoliosis: A need for further investigation. *Br Med J* 1986; 292:120.

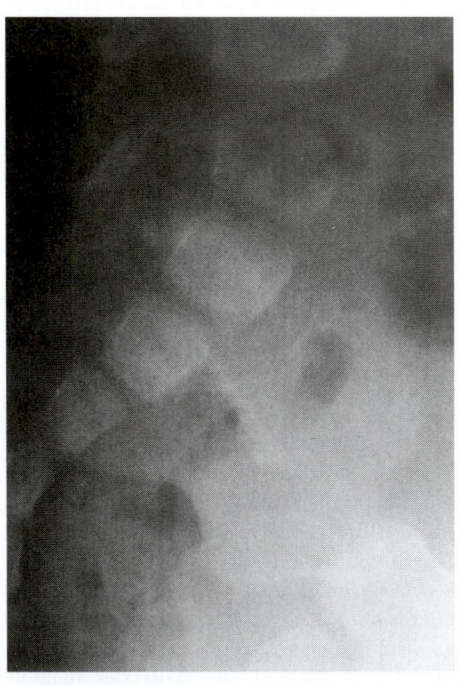
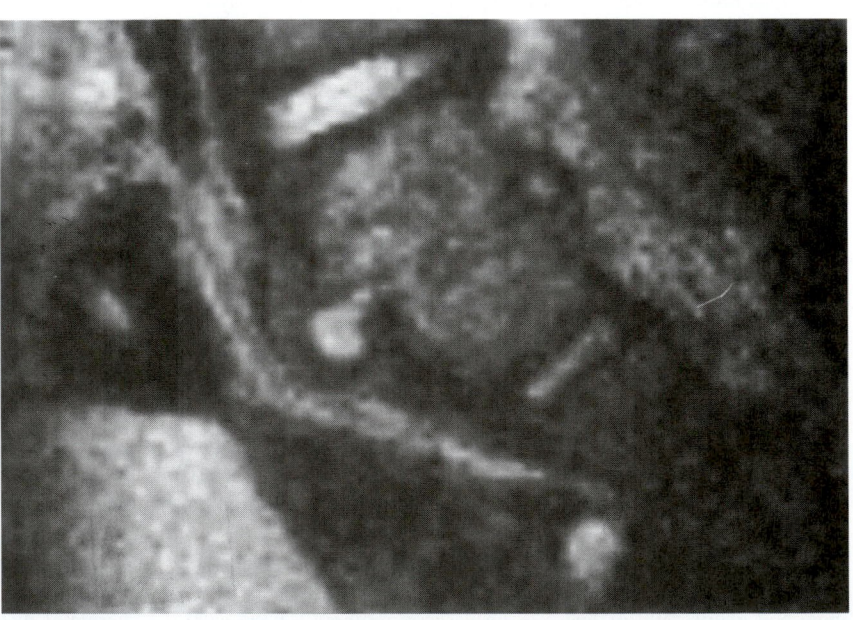

A   *B*

Figure 64-2
A. Normal radiograph in 2-year-old boy with back pain. *B.* MRI demonstrates disc space infection.

Chapter 65

SPONDYLOLISTHESIS

Gerard J. Girasole, Paul L. Kuflik, and Jeffrey M. Spivak

DEFINITIONS

A unilateral or bilateral defect in the pars interarticularis (aspect of the posterior arch of a vertebra that lies between the inferior and superior facets) without displacement of the vertebra is known as spondylolysis. This is the most common anatomically visible cause of low back pain in childhood or adolescence. The pars defect generally develops in childhood between the ages of 5 and 8, but is more common at the age of 7 or 8. The incidence increases until age 20 and thereafter remains constant. Spondylolisthesis is defined as a slipping forward of one vertebra onto another. The origin of the word is from the Greek "spondylos" meaning vertebra and "olisthesis," meaning to slip.

ETIOLOGY/DEMOGRAPHICS

For the majority of spondylolysis and spondylolisthesis associated with pars defects, the etiology remains unknown. The most accepted concept is that there is a congenital predisposition, often in association with acute or repetitive traumatic stress on the pars interarticularis. A defect of the pars has not been identified at birth. It is believed that lumbar lordosis is accentuated by the normal flexion contractures of the hip in childhood, and that this posture increases the force of weightbearing on the pars interarticularis. Anatomic studies have suggested that when the lumbar spine is extended there is greater shear stress on the pars. Physiologic loads during cyclic flexion–extension motion of the lumbar spine can cause a fatigue fracture of the pars interarticularis. These stresses may be further accentuated by lateral flexion movements on the extended spine, as is seen in gymnastics.

The overall incidence of spondylolysis is 5 to 6 percent. There is an increased prevalence (up to 12 percent) in adolescents with Scheuermann's disease, weight lifters, athletes such as football linemen, and gymnasts, versus the expected range of 4 to 8 percent in the general population. In Scheuermann's disease, the increased thoracic kyphosis causes a compensatory increase in lumbar lordosis. These developmental factors, repetitive activities, and postural changes may lead to stress fractures of the pars interarticularis. To date there are no cases of spondylolysis or spondylolisthesis that have been described in patients who were nonambulators.

Several studies have suggested a congenital predisposition for spondylolysis. The prevalence among family members of affected individuals is between 27 and 69 percent. Spondylolisthesis is associated with an increased incidence of sacral spina bifida (28 to 42 percent) and congenital deficiency of the sacrum and superior sacral facets. These posterior defects of the lumbosacral junction are found in 94 percent of patients who have dysplastic spondylolysis and in 32 percent of isthmic cases. This lack of integrity of the posterior structures may predispose individuals to spondylolisthesis.

The vast majority of pars defects occur in L5, with the remainder at L4 and much less commonly cephalad to L4. In 25 percent of the patients with L4 isthmic defects, a partial or complete sacralization of the fifth lumbar vertebra is present. This is more common in males, and becomes symptomatic more commonly in young adults than in children or adolescents. Pain and functional impairment are greater when the spondylosis is at the fourth vertebra, and the incidence of neurologic signs and spinal stenosis is also increased. There is commonly progression to a grade I spondylolisthesis, but severe slipping is unusual.

CLASSIFICATION

The most widely used classification of spondylolysis and spondylolisthesis has been derived by Wiltse and his associates (1976):

Type I. Congenital or dysplastic spondylolisthesis. This subtype is characterized by a dysplasia of the upper sacrum and L5-S1 facet joints. Because of this dysplasia, there is insufficient strength to resist shear stress, and forward slippage occurs. The pars interarticularis usually remains intact. With increasing anterior shear stress, the pars can become thinned out and elongated. Eventually, a pars stress fracture may occur. The pars defect in this case is a result rather than a cause of the slippage. The pars remains intact and causes compression of the cauda equina early on. Two subtypes are based on the congenital abnormality:

Subtype A. The articular processes are axially oriented.

Subtype B. The articular processes are sagittally oriented.

The first sacral vertebra or lowest lumbar vertebra has congenital changes that render the joint incapable of withstanding the forward thrust of the body weight. Other congenital defects such as a deficient sacral lamina an L5 spina bifida occulta are also common. This type is likely to go on to a high-grade slip.

Type II. Isthmic spondylolisthesis. The lesion here is a defect in the pars interarticularis. There are three subtypes:

Subtype A. A true bony defect in the pars interarticularis due to repetitive stress with eventual fracture and nonunion.

Subtype B. In this type, the pars becomes elongated secondary to repeated fracture and healing of the pars.

Subtype C. There is an acute fracture of the pars secondary to significant trauma. This type is usually associated with spondylolysis but not olisthesis and is quite uncommon.

Type III. Degenerative. This type, which is due to long-standing segmental instability, is more common in females and is most common at the L4-5 level. Slipping generally does not exceed 30 percent, because the intact posterior elements eventually abut the vertebral body below, blocking further slippage. The predisposing factor is believed to be a stable lumbosacral joint that puts increased stress on the adjacent L4-5 level. This leads to decompensation of the ligaments and increased mobility of the articular processes.

Type IV. Traumatic. This type is secondary to an acute injury that fractures some part of the bony hook other than the pars interarticularis. This is usually associated with major trauma.

Type V. Pathologic. There is generalized or localized bone disease to the pedicle, pars interarticularis, or articulating process.

Risk factors for progression in spondylolisthesis are age at onset, sex, type of slip, degree of deformity, and radiologic evidence of instability. Spondylolisthesis progresses primarily during the adolescent growth spurts (10 to 15 years of age). The earlier the onset, the greater is the risk of slipping. The overall incidence of spondylolysis and spondylolisthesis is lower in girls, but they are more prone to severe displacement, earlier increase of deformity, and more clinical symptoms than boys. More girls require surgical stabilization than do boys. Recurrent episodes of back pain caused by spondylolisthesis are associated with increased incidence of progression. Dysplastic spondylolisthesis is more likely to progress and have persistent symptoms than the isthmic type. Degree and angle of the slip are associated with progression. When the degree of the slip is equal to or greater than 50 percent, there is an increased likelihood for progression. An increasing slip angle accurately reflects the increased risk for continued progression, deformity, and pain. Radiographically, those children with a dome-shaped or vertical sacrum, a trapezoidal fifth lumbar vertebral body (teeter-totter appearance), and lack of sclerotic changes at L5-S1 are also more likely to have progression.

CLINICAL FINDINGS

The presenting symptoms of spondylolysis or spondylolisthesis differ in children and adolescents from those in adults. Symptoms are relatively uncommon in children, and the onset of complaints, if any, is usually during the adolescent growth spurt. Rarely are the symptoms severe enough to cause patients to seek medical attention. A study by Lafond (1962) found that only 23 percent of patients with spondylolysis or spondylolisthesis experienced the onset of complaints before age 20. Of this 23 percent, only 9 percent sought medical attention during childhood or adolescence.

In adults, pain is the predominant complaint, but many children do not have pain and are evaluated medically because of a postural deformity or an abnormal gait resulting from tight hamstring muscles. When children do complain of pain, it is usually one of two types. The first type is generally localized in the low back and occasionally radiates to the posterior aspect of the buttocks and thighs. Pain is usually initiated by strenuous activity or participation in competitive sports. The symptoms are decreased by rest or restriction of activities. The second type is minimal low back pain with a significant radicular component to the lower extremity. Adolescents rarely have pain distal to the knee or in the foot. Disc herniation is uncommon and, unlike adults, children seldom have objective signs of nerve-root compression, such as motor weakness, reflex changes, or sensory deficits. Physical findings may correlate with the degree of slippage. In a child with spondylolysis or a mild (grade I to II) spondylolisthesis, the findings on physical examination may be normal. With more significant slippage, there may be postural or gait abnormalities. A visible and palpable step-off at the lumbosacral junction will be apparent. Hamstring tightness as noted by restricted hip flexion causes the peculiar gait in these patients. It is believed that this tight-

ness is due to nerve-root irritation, but there is no evidence to support this. The excessively tight hamstring muscles cause the pelvis to tilt posteriorly (external) and limit hip flexion. Patients develop subsequently a bizarre gait pattern, the Phalen-Dixon sign, which is a stiff-legged and short-strided gait that is called the pelvic waddle. There may be splinting as well as guarding and restrictive side-to-side motion of the lower back.

Paraspinal muscle spasm with trunk deviation on forward bending is common. As the slip progresses, compensating mechanisms produce significant deformity. Distortion of the pelvis and trunk begin to become apparent in late grade II and grade III spondylolisthesis. As the L5 vertebra begins to slip further, the body's center of gravity is displaced anteriorly. To compensate for this, the lumbar spine above the lesion hyperextends, and the upper part of the trunk is displaced backward, which creates a lordosis that extends into the upper thoracic spine. With increasing slippage, the lumbosacral kyphosis increases, which causes the pelvis to become more retroverted, so that the sacrum becomes vertical. To maintain an upright posture, patients must stand with the knees partially flexed and the thoracic and upper lumbar spine in a hyperlordotic posture. When viewed from the back, the ilia appear flared and the buttocks are heart shaped. As the slippage becomes even greater, the trunk is shortened, with an absence of the waistline. When viewed from the front, the lower part of the abdomen appears to be thrust forward, forming a transverse abdominal crease at the level of the umbilicus.

Scoliosis may be associated with spondylolisthesis: It has been found in 23 to 48 percent of the patients with symptomatic spondylolisthesis, but in only 13 percent of the patients with spondylolysis. It is often not a structural curve and is related to lumbar muscle spasm. The scoliosis usually resolves with recumbency, the relief of symptoms, or both. The presence of scoliosis is more common in patients with dysplastic spondylolisthesis (59 percent) than in those with the isthmic type (42 percent). It is more common in girls and patients with severe slips.

The term for lumbar curves caused by muscle spasm is sciatic scoliosis, which is usually not structural and resolves with recumbency and rest. A torsional lumbar curve with asymmetric displacement and rotation that begins at the spondylolytic defect is called olisthetic scoliosis. Approximately two-thirds of the lumbar and olisthetic curves resolve after surgical stabilization of the spondylolisthesis. Those curves that do not improve seldom progress. Finally, patients who have idiopathic scoliosis have a slightly higher prevalence (6.2 percent) of spondylolysis or spondylolisthesis than the general population.

RADIOGRAPHIC FINDINGS

The standard radiographic evaluation of the lumbosacral spine in children suspected of having spondylolysis or spondylolisthesis, includes anteroposterior, lateral, and oblique radiographs (Fig. 65-1). The gold standard for visualizing spondylolisthesis is a standing lateral film. Marked changes in the position of the lumbar vertebra have been found in children and adolescents when they move from the supine to the standing position or from flexion to extension of the spine. Oblique radiographs are best for visualizing spondylolysis. A Ferguson oblique radiograph, with sagittal angling of the beam to be more perpendicular to the L4 and L5 lamina, is preferred. The Scotty dog sign of Lachapèle (1939) is seen on the oblique view as a defect in the "collar" around the dog's neck. In patients with an acute injury the gap is narrow with irregular edges, whereas in those with a long-standing defect the gap is wider with smooth and rounded edges. Unilateral defects occur in 20 percent of cases, making the diagno-

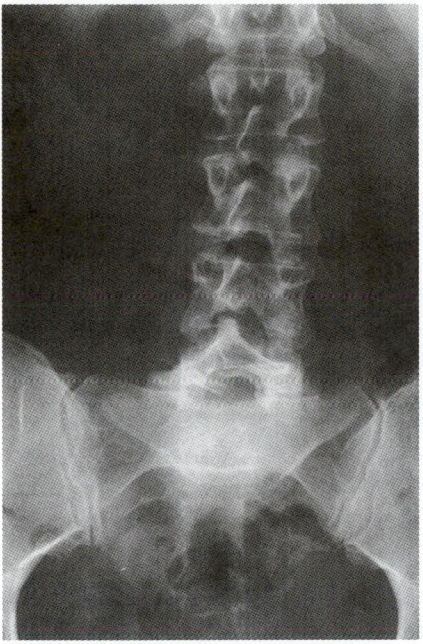
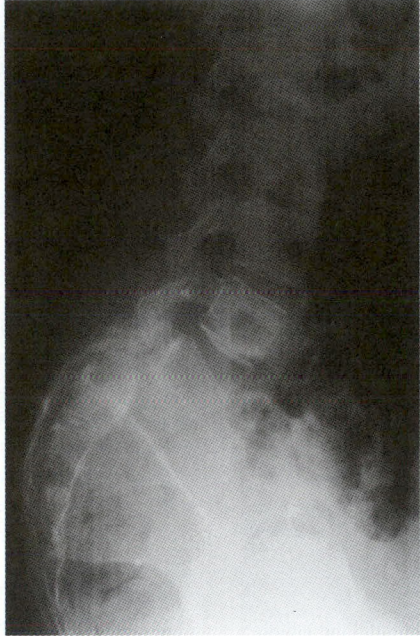
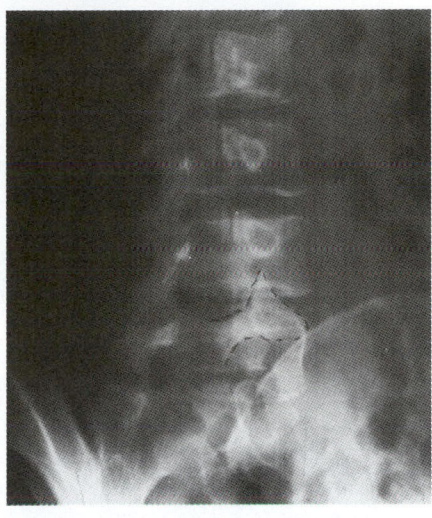

A   B   C

Figure 65-1

Radiographic evaluation of spondylolisthesis. (*A*) AP standing film, showing the "reverse Napoleon hat" sign of L5; (*B*) lateral radiograph; (*C*) oblique view of a spondylytic defect (the "collar" on the "Scotty-dog").

sis difficult without proper radiographs. Spondylolysis should be suspected if there is asymmetry of the neural arch and unilateral wedging of the vertebral bodies.

Computed tomography is helpful in diagnosing those patients suspected of having spondylolysis that cannot be confirmed by plain radiographs (Fig. 65-2). Technetium-99m bone scanning is also helpful in defining the pathologic defect in those patients who have acute diffuse lumbar pain, but is not recommended for patients who have had symptoms for more than 1 year or for those who are asymptomatic. Bone scans are helpful in distinguishing between patients with a nonunion from those who are still healing and may benefit from immobilization.

MRI, although not routinely needed, is beneficial in those cases with neurologic involvement. It is helpful in detecting cauda equina compression or disc herniation. In patients with significant leg pain or neurologic deficit, or who will undergo open reduction, MRI is recommended as a preoperative study. Nerve-root compression by granulation tissue in the area of the pars defect can also be visualized.

The most widely accepted grading system for spondylolithesis was originally described by Meyerding (1932) and is based on the percentage of anterior translation: grade 1 is a slippage of 0 to 25 percent, grade 2 is slippage of 25 to 50 percent, grade 3 is slippage of 50 to 75 percent, and grade 4 is slippage of 75 to 100 percent. Slippage of greater than 100 percent, also known as spondyloptosis, is considered grade 5, which is usually accompanied by some amount of inferior migration of L5 links to the pelvis.

There are several techniques of measuring translational or tangential displacement from a standing lateral radiograph. The most important are percentage of slippage, the slip angle, and sacral inclination (Fig. 65-3).

The percentage of slippage is calculated by a line drawn along the posterior border of the first sacral vertebra as a reference point for all measurements. The width of the sacrum is calculated at its widest dimension to give the denominator. In cases with any remodeling of the anterior sacral border, the anterior–posterior dimension of the inferior border of L5 is used as the denominator. A perpendicular line is drawn from the posterior inferior cortex of L5. The amount of displacement as compared with the width of the sacrum gives the percentage of slippage.

The slip angle is calculated by first drawing a line perpendicular to the reference line of the sacrum and then a second line that is parallel to the upper end plate of the L5 vertebral body. The superior end plate is used. The lower end plate can be distorted and difficult to visualize, because the L5 vertebra remodels and becomes more trapezoidal. The normal slip angle should be 0 degrees or less.

Sacral inclination is calculated by a line drawn perpendicular to the floor and the angle formed from this line to the reference line along the posterior aspect of the sacrum. The normal value for this should be greater than 30 degrees.

NATURAL HISTORY

Several long-term studies have examined the natural history of spondylolisthesis. In cases followed into adulthood, a high incidence of neurologic deficits (18 percent), lower back pain (91 percent), and sciatica (55 percent) has been reported. Slippage greater than 25 percent, a low lumbar index at L5, spondylolysis at L4, and early disc degeneration were associated with an increased risk for lower back symptoms. Among the cases followed for an average of 18 years, 36 percent of the patients stated that the back problem had influenced their choice of occupation, 45 percent avoided strenuous lifting, and many limited their recreational activity. MRI has shown disc degeneration to occur at the level below the defect, which would be

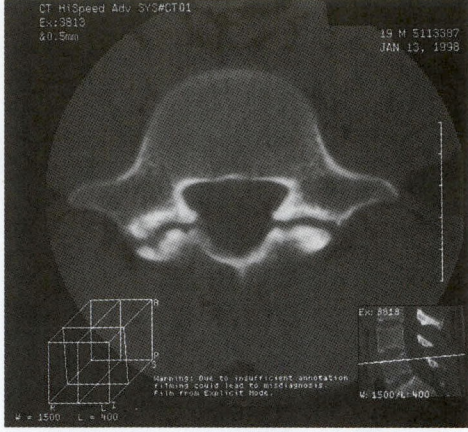

A

B

Figure 65-2
A. Axial CT image showing bilateral lytic pars defects, which can be confused with nearby facet joints. *B.* Sagittal reconstruction clearly showing lytic defect (*arrow*) separate from surrounding L4-5 and L5-S1 facet joints.

uncommon in patients younger than age 25. The incidence of disc herniation of the disc below the level of the defect rises significantly in the older population. The disc above, however, is no more likely to show degeneration than it is among the general population.

TREATMENT OF SPONDYLOLYSIS

NONOPERATIVE TREATMENT

Adolescents and children with spondylolysis are rarely symptomatic. For those who do become symptomatic, treatment may include limited initial bed rest, restriction of activities, and brace immobilization. Activities are permitted progressively as symptoms improve. If patients remain asymptomatic, then there is no need to restrict activities. Acute pars fractures due to a traumatic episode or repetitive trauma can be treated with a cast or brace. Not all defects heal after treatment with immobilization. Even though the defect remains, the patient's symptoms may improve. A bone scan or computed tomography may be helpful in assessing the age of the defect and its healing. Hamstring tightness is an excellent clinical guide for determining the level of healing and the success or failure of treatment. Recurrent symptoms despite all attempts at nonoperative treatment would be an indication for surgery.

OPERATIVE TREATMENT

As just mentioned, repeated failure of nonoperative treatment is an indication for surgical management. The types of procedures available are lateral fusion *in situ* and pars interarticularis repair. Lateral fusion consists of a midline or bilateral skin incision, muscle-splitting approach as described by Wiltse and Jackson (1976). Instrumentation is not required, and most authors recommend postoperative immobilization in either a brace or cast with a thigh cuff. In adult patients, transpedicular internal fixation may increase the fusion rate.

Repair of the defect in spondylolysis can be considered for L1 to L4 defects, for patients younger than age 25, and for a symptomatic defect without slippage. A variety of techniques have been described, all of which include bone grafting of the pars defect and fixation across the defect with wire and/or screws.

Figure 65-3
Radiographic measurements in spondylolisthesis. *A.* Percent slip. *B.* Slip angle. *C.* Sacral inclination. [Reproduced and modified with permission from Bradford DS: Spondylolysis and Spondylolisthesis. In Lonstein JE, Winter RB, Bradford DS, et al (eds): *Moe's Textbook of Scoliosis and Other Spinal Deformities*, 3d ed. Philadelphia: WB Saunders; 1978:406.]

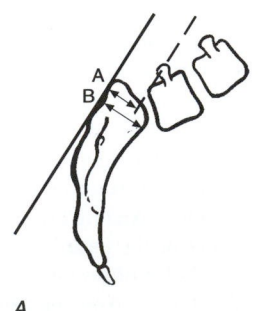
A

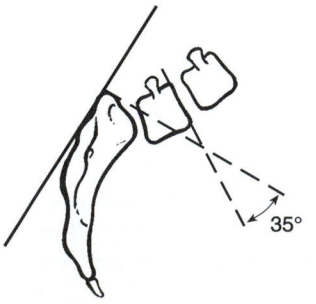
B

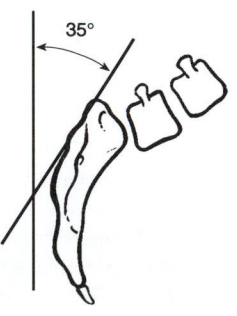
C

TREATMENT OF SPONDYLOLISTHESIS

NONOPERATIVE TREATMENT

The treatment of spondylolisthesis is based on the age of the patient, the degree of slippage, and the severity of symptoms. In children with slippage of less than 30 percent and in all adults, treatment consists of restricted activities and temporary use of a lumbosacral corset or plastic orthotic. Patients may resume activities once symptoms subside. Wiltse and Jackson (1976) proposed that activities need not be restricted if a slip is less that 25 percent. They recommended that, for slips greater than 25 percent, contact sports and activities that are associated with a high risk of back injury should be avoided.

OPERATIVE TREATMENT

The indications for surgical intervention are persistent back and sciatic pain despite nonoperative treatment, skeletally immature patients with high-grade slips (more than 30 to 50 percent) or documented progression even in the absence of symptoms, and patients with neurologic deficits along with nerve tension signs.

The procedure of choice is bilateral lateral arthrodesis with or without decompressive laminectomy. In grade I or II spondylolisthesis, arthrodesis of the transverse process of the fifth lumbar vertebra to the sacral alar is sufficient. In higher-grade slips (III or IV), the fusion should be extended to the transverse process of the fourth lumbar vertebra. Laminectomy (the Gill procedure) alone is contraindicated. Complete removal of the posterior elements can lead to worsening instability and is associated with an increased incidence of further progression of the slip and a significant increase in pseudarthrosis. Decompression is rarely indicated, due to the low incidence of associated herniated disc or nerve-root impingement in children with spondylolisthesis. Posterolateral arthrodesis is performed through a midline or bilateral skin incision with a paraspinal muscle-splitting approach (Wiltse and Jackson, 1976). Fusion is extended from the transverse process of the fifth or fourth vertebra to the sacral alar by using autologous iliac bone for grafting.

Postoperative brace or casting is recommended, especially for high-grade slips, and should include one or both thighs. In patients with less than 50 percent slips and in whom laminectomy has not been performed, ambulation is begun soon after surgery. Some feel that patients with high-grade slips should remain supine for 3 to 4 months in a body cast or brace with one hip in hyperextension. Patients are not permitted to engage in vigorous activities or contact sports during the first postoperative year, but may do so later if there is radiographic evidence of a solid arthrodesis. In patients with a slippage of greater than 50 percent and a slip angle greater than 55 degrees, progression of the deformity may continue even in the presence of a solid fusion. Some authors believe that the fusion biomechanically is under tension, so it may progress. This is an argument for reduction.

The pseudarthrosis rate ranges from 0 to 25 percent. Relief of symptoms does not always correlate with a successful fusion. Postoperative cauda equina syndrome has been reported in 6 percent of cases following in situ arthrodesis. Treatment of this complication consists of immediate decompression.

Anterior fusion in situ, either through a transperitoneal or retroperitoneal approach, has been described to treat spondylolisthesis. In addition, good results have been reported with interbody fusion through a posterior approach using an interbody dowel technique. These procedures are best for high-grade slips where posterolateral fusion alone is not likely to succeed.

REDUCTION

The first reduction for spondylolisthesis was performed in 1936 by Jenkins, and the efficacy of the technique is still debated. Because of the technical difficulties in reducing the slip, and the risk of neurologic impairment (mainly L5 nerve injury and postoperative foot drop), most surgeons remain discouraged. In patients with high-grade (III and IV) slips, progression has been reported in as many as 10 to 45 percent following posterolateral fusion. In addition, the loss of sagittal alignment may be cosmetically unacceptable to these patients and there is still a risk of cauda equina associated with in situ fusion. This has led surgeons in the last decade to devise techniques for safer reductions. Most agree that improvement in the sagittal deformity is more important than complete translational reduction.

Reduction can be performed either by a closed-cast method, open posterior instrumentation, or a combined anterior–posterior approach. The current suggested benefits of reduction are:

1. Restore alignment in high-grade slips
2. Prevent progression especially when decompression is necessary
3. Improve the fusion rate

The closed-cast technique can be used in skeletally immature patients with high-grade slips where further progression is likely if fusion in situ is done alone. The lumbosacral kyphosis should be partially correctable as demonstrated on flexion and extension films. In high-grade slips, L4 and the L5 vertebral bodies are kyphotic in reference to the sacrum. The goal of the reduction is to restore the lordotic position of L4 to the sacrum, which is accomplished by placing L4 parallel in relation to the sacrum, which is known as the stable or anatomic zone. This position of lordosis places the fusion mass under compressive forces to facilitate union. Halo iliac pin traction can be used to facilitate reduction in the cast.

Posterior instrumental reduction is done by gradual distraction and posterior translation, using transpedicular screw fixation. After reduction with or without discectomy and interbody bone grafting, compression is applied to restore lordosis and stability. This offers the most stability biomechanically, and the greatest ability for correction. The use of pure distraction implants should be avoided because of the loss of lumbar lordosis associated with these devices. This technique actually aggravates the sagittal alignment. Decompressive laminectomy is generally necessary prior to any posterior reduction.

COMBINED APPROACHES

Combined anterior and posterior techniques provide the greatest stability, the widest release of the constraints of the deformity, and the highest rate of fusion.

The resection of the L5 vertebral body [Gaines (1985) procedure] is an alternative to reduction in cases of spondyloptosis, but carries a very high rate of complications. In one study of eight vertebrectomies performed for spondyloptosis, four of the eight patients experienced postoperative neuropraxias. Two of these patients partially recovered, but only one recovered completely.

Surgical reduction should be performed only by experienced surgeons. Anatomic reduction is not necessary and fusion in situ is still the most acceptable procedure for spondylolisthesis. The complications associated with these methods of treatment include pseudarthrosis, neurologic deficits, progression of the grade or slip, and retrograde ejaculation in males after an anterior procedure. A review of the literature indicates an approximately 1 percent incidence of retrograde ejaculation in males following anterior lumbar surgery. In one series, pseudarthrosis was found in four (18 percent) of 22 patients who were managed with combined anterior–posterior reduction and stabilization, and three (14 percent) had neurologic complications. Similar results have been reported by other authors. There is a need for larger long-term studies to determine whether the increased risks of reduction justify the benefits.

SUGGESTED READINGS

Abdu WA, Wilber RG, Emery SE: Pedicular transvertebral screw fixation of the lumbosacral spine in spondylolisthesis. *Spine* 1994;19:710.

Ani N, Keppler L, Biscup RS, et al: Reduction of high-grade slips (grades III–V) with VSP instrumentation: Report of a series of 41 cases. *Spine* 1991; 16(suppl):S302.

Boos N, Marchesi D, Zuber K, et al: Treatment of severe spondylolisthesis by reduction and pedicular fixation. *Spine* 1993; 18:1655.

Bradford DS: Spondylolysis and spondylolisthesis. In Lonstein JE, Bradford DS, Winter RB, et al (eds): *Moe's Textbook of Scoliosis and Other Spinal Deformities*, 3d ed. Philadelphia: WB Saunders; 1995:399.

Bradford DS, Boachie-Adjei O: Treatment of severe spondylolithesis by anterior and posterior reduction and stabilization: A long term follow-up study. *J Bone Joint Surg [Am]* 1990; 72:1060.

Bradford DS, Iza J: Repair of the defect in spondylolysis or minimal degrees of spondylolithesis by segmental wire fixation and bone grafting. *Spine* 1985; 10:673.

Dewald RL, Faut M, Taddonio R, Neuwirth M: Severe lumbosacral spondylolithesis in adolescents and children. *J Bone Joint Surg [Am]* 1981; 63:619.

Esses S, Natout N, Kip P: Posterior interbody arthrodesis with a fibular strut graft in spondylolisthesis. *J Bone Joint Surg [Am]* 1995; 77:172.

Gaines RW, Nichols WK: Treatment of spondyloptosis by two stage L5 vertebrectomy and reduction of L4 onto S1. *Spine* 1985; 10:680.

Hensinger RN: Spondylolysis and spondylolisthesis in children and adolescents. *J Bone Joint Surg [Am]* 1989; 71:1098.

Jenkins SA: Spondylolisthesis. *Br J Surg* 1936; 24:80.

Lachapèle HP: Un simple moyen pour faciliter la lecture des radiographies vertébraies obliquies de la région lombo-sacrée, Bull. et mém. Soc. élect.-radiol. med. franç. 1939; 27:175.

Lafond G: Surgical treatment of spondylolisthesis. *Clin Orthop* 1962; 22:175.

Meyerding HW: Spondylolisthesis. *Surg Gynecol Obstet* 1932; 54:371.

Schoenecker P, Cole H, Herring J, et al: Cauda equina syndrome after *in situ* arthrodesis for severe spondylolisthesis at the lumbosacral junction. *J Bone Joint Surg [Am]* 1990; 72:369.

Whitecloud TS III, Butler JC: Anterior lumbar fusion utilizing transvertebral fibular graft. *Spine* 1988; 13:370.

Wiltse LL, Jackson D: Treatment of spondylolisthesis and spondylolysis in children. *Clin Orthop* 1976; 117:92.

Wiltse LL, Winter R: Terminology and measurement of spondylolisthesis. *J Bone Joint Surg [Am]* 1983; 65:768.

Wiltse LL, Newman PH, Macnab I: Classification of spondylolysis and spondylolisthesis. *Clin Orthop* 1976; 117:23.

Chapter 66

INFECTIONS

David S. Feldman

Spinal infections in children are uncommon, but they are often a diagnostic dilemma and may require prompt treatment. Children are more susceptible to osteomyelitis than adults. Similarly, infections of the spine are more common in children. Discitis and osteomyelitis are now thought to be a spectrum of the same disease. Initially, the disc space is involved, particularly at the level of the endplates. Eventually, if untreated, the vertebral body becomes involved with subsequent destruction of the body and possible abscess formation.

Osteomyelitis and discitis are most commonly bacterial (*Staphylococcus aureus*); however, tuberculosis and atypical fungal infections must be ruled out.

PYOGENIC INFECTIONS

PATHOGENESIS

The disc spaces have traversing vascular channels that connect the endplates. With the colonization of an endplate after a transient bacteremia, the infection develops in the disc space involving both endplates. If untreated the infection may further spread to the vertebral body, causing destruction and possibly abscess formation (Fig. 66-1).

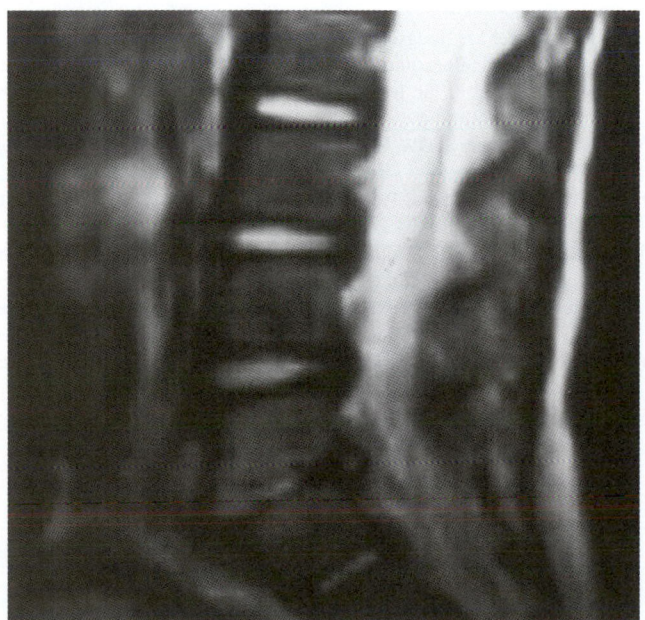

Figure 66-1
MRI demonstrating disc space infection in a 2-year-old child.

PRESENTATION

Children may present at any age with discitis although young children between the ages of 1 and 5 years are most commonly affected. The symptoms include fever, inability to ambulate, back pain, or abdominal pain. The varied presentation often makes the diagnosis difficult. The child may have back stiffness, loss of the lumbar lordosis, a positive straight leg raise, and hamstring tightness. Focal neurologic deficit is very unusual in the early stages of the disease. White blood cell count (WBC), erythrocyte sedimentation rate (ESR), and C-reactive protein (CRP) are often elevated. However, a normal WBC, ESR, and CRP do not preclude the diagnosis. Blood cultures may be positive, although this is more commonly seen in infections of the appendicular skeleton.

RADIOGRAPHIC EVALUATION

Although plain radiographs are negative early in the disease, they are essential to obtain in order to rule out other disorders that may cause back pain. Later in the disease process radiographs may demonstrate disc space narrowing or variable degrees of vertebral collapse. Bone scan is a useful tool in diagnosing discitis; however, false negatives are possible. Where MRI is readily available, it is the diagnostic tool of choice, and should include the sacroiliac joints. MRI is useful in assessing both the infection and the presence or absence of an epidural abscess.

DIFFERENTIAL DIAGNOSIS

Discitis may be confused with various other diseases due to the presenting symptoms. If abdominal pain is the main complaint, an intra-abdominal process should be considered. If the clinician is aware of the varied presentation as well as the imaging studies appropriate to evaluate for discitis, there should be little difficulty confirming the diagnosis. Neoplasms such as histiocytosis X and osteoblastoma may mimic discitis; however, an MRI will demonstrate that the tumor primarily involves the vertebral body and spares the disc space. Other forms of spinal infection such as tuberculosis must be considered, particularly if more than one vertebral segment is involved.

CLINICAL MANAGEMENT

The initial management of the early stages of discitis is intravenous antibiotics covering *S. aureus*. The patient should respond clinically within 4 to 5 days of initiating therapy. Ambulation, although tentative, should resume and the WBC and ESR should decrease. Bed rest and bracing are not mandatory unless there has been significant vertebral collapse. Bracing, however, may be useful in the early treatment period to provide support and diminish pain. If the patient does not respond clinically, that is, if they continue with significant pain, fever, and elevated WBC, then needle aspiration, biopsy, and possible debridement are indicated. Surgical debridement is restricted to patients with poor or incomplete response to antibiotics and an abscess.

TUBERCULOSIS

Although tuberculosis (TB) was at its nadir during the mid-1980s, there has been a resurgence of this disease, particularly in children and in developing countries. Children have a more fulminant course of the disease and bone involvement is relatively common. Children, unlike adults, are rarely paralyzed from TB, even though abscess formation is the rule as opposed to the exception.

CLINICAL PRESENTATION

Bone involvement from TB is related to the duration of the illness. TB is usually present for about 2 years before bone and joint involvement becomes evident. In cases of osseous involvement, the anterior spine is most commonly affected. Osseous involvement is always secondary to the primary organ involved, most often the lung.

The most common presenting symptom is back pain over the involved area. The thoracolumbar junction is the most frequently affected region of the spine. In children the high thoracic and lower cervical vertebrae are also commonly affected, and these cases may present with tracheal compression or symptoms of asthma from a paravertebral abscess. Children will often have flulike symptoms, such as fever, malaise, fatigue, and anorexia. The child may also demonstrate a gait abnormality from psoas irritation or signs of meningitis with actual neurologic deficit. This can be due to compression from a paravertebral abscess into the spinal canal or to actual involvement of the meninges with the TB.

INITIAL EVALUATION

Evaluation of the child with spinal TB depends on the stage of the disease. In patients presenting early with active disease, plain radiographs will help demonstrate the region of the disease as well as the portion of the vertebral body that is involved; i.e., anterior, central, or posterior. Other neoplasms of the spine can be confused with spinal TB. There is often more than one level involved and there is a variable amount of vertebral collapse. The disc space is often obliterated, and soft tissue abscess may or may not be evident on the plain radiograph. The abscess in TB may be calcified.

An MRI will demonstrate soft tissue involvement, including paraspinal abscesses. It will also demonstrate any spinal compression, if present.

The evaluation of the patient with chronic TB includes assessment of the degree of kyphosis, the presence of any neurologic compro-

mise, and the extent of previous medical management. Severe kyphosis secondary to TB is a common entity and is associated with an anterior soft tissue mass. This scar and granulation tissue may be adherent to the viscera anteriorly and to the dura posteriorly.

MANAGEMENT

TB is a disease that is primarily managed through prolonged chemotherapy with streptomycin, isoniazid, and rifampin. Due to the increasing incidence of drug-resistant TB, ethambutol and pyrazinamide may have to be added if there is a poor clinical response. Drug therapy should begin at least 1 week prior to surgical intervention.

The role of surgery for spinal TB is to prevent progression of the kyphosis and thereby prevent the possibility of the late sequelae, particularly progressive paraparesis. In the presence of active disease most authors advocate medical management followed by debridement, resection of the lesion, and autogenous strut grafting in order to prevent kyphosis. If there is significant bony destruction on multiple levels, then stabilization posteriorly may also be indicated. Posterior decompression is almost never indicated with the sole and rare exception of spinal TB involving the posterior elements.

Treatment of the late sequelae of TB is quite difficult. While surgical management of the acute disease has had favorable results, surgical treatment of either late onset paraplegia or severe kyphosis has a very high complication rate. Anterior release and decompression at the level of the kyphosis with strut grafting is required. In very severe cases with spontaneous fusion posteriorly, an anterior osteotomy and debridement are followed by a posterior osteotomy and then halopelvic traction followed by a circumferential fusion. This procedure is fraught with serious complications including death and should be reserved for cases where there are no other alternatives; children should be referred to centers capable of managing and monitoring pediatric patients in prolonged spinal traction.

SUGGESTED READINGS

Bailey HL, Gabriel M, Hodgson AR, et al: Tuberculosis of the spine in children. Operative findings and results in one hundred consecutive patients treated by removal of the lesion and anterior grafting. *J Bone Joint Surg [Am]* 1972; 54:1633.

Crawford AH, Kucharzyk DW, Ruda R, et al: Diskitis in children. *Clin Orthop* 1991; 266:70.

Du Lac P, Panuel M, Devred P, et al: MRI of disc space infection in infants and children. Report of 12 cases. *Pediatr Radiol* 1990; 20:175.

Medical Research Council Working Party on Tuberculosis of the Spine: A ten-year assessment of a controlled trial comparing debridement and anterior spinal fusion in the management of tuberculosis of the spine in patients on standard chemotherapy in Hong Kong. *J Bone Joint Surg [Br]* 1982; 64:393.

Wenger DR, Bobenchko WP, Gilday DL: The spectrum of intervertebral disc-space infection in children. *J Bone Joint Surg [Am]* 1978; 60:100.

Chapter 67

GENERAL CONSIDERATIONS

David S. Feldman

GENERAL

While certain general principles may be applied to children from adult orthopaedics, pediatric orthopaedic surgery is not to be thought of as performing orthopaedic surgery on "little people." Due to the differences between pediatric and adult bone, joints, and growth/remodeling potential, children's injuries should be treated as a unique discipline. This is particularly true in discussing pediatric orthopaedic trauma. At times, growth will be of value in remodeling fractures that would be unacceptable in an adult, such as in a child with a 45-degree angulation of a proximal humerus fracture; at other times, continued growth may cause a problem, such as in a supination adduction injury to the ankle with closure of the distal medial tibial physis and subsequent progressive varus deformity. The purpose of this chapter will be to review the principles of fracture treatment in children, stressing those fractures and situations that require special attention.

ANATOMY

Pediatric bone has a higher water content and lower mineral content per unit volume than adult bone. Therefore, pediatric bone has a lower modulus of elasticity (less brittle) and a higher ultimate strain-to-failure ratio than adult bone.

The physis (growth plate) is a unique cartilaginous structure that varies in thickness, depending on patient age and location of the physis. It is frequently weaker than bone in torsion, shear, and bending, predisposing the child to injury through this delicate area.

The periosteum in a child is a thick fibrous structure (up to several millimeters) that encompasses the entire bone except the articular ends. The periosteum thickens and becomes continuous with the physis at the perichondral ring, offering additional resistance to shear force.

As a general rule, ligaments in children are functionally stronger than bone. Thus, a high proportion of injuries that produce sprains in adults result in fractures in children.

The blood supply to the growing bone includes a rich metaphyseal circulation with fine capillary loops, ending at the physis (in the neonate, small vessels may traverse the physis, ending in the epiphysis). This differs from adult bone.

MECHANISM OF INJURY

Because of structural differences, pediatric fractures tend to occur at lower energies than adult fractures. The majority are a result of compression, torsion, or bending moments.

Compression fractures are found most commonly at the metaphyseal-diaphyseal junction and are referred to as "buckle fractures" or "torus fractures." Torus fractures rarely result in physeal injury; instead they generally result in acute angular deformity. Because torus fractures are impacted, they are stable and rarely require manipulative reduction. If manipulated, they usually regain the original fracture deformity as swelling subsides.

Torsional injuries result in two distinct patterns of fracture depending on the maturity of the physis. In the very young child with a thick periosteum, the diaphyseal bone fails before the physis, resulting in a long spiral fracture. In the older child, a similar torsional injury results in a physeal fracture.

Bending moments in the young child cause "greenstick fractures." These are fractures in which the compression side of the bone is incompletely fractured and is plastically deformed, while the tension side of the bone has fractured. In the older child, bending moments result in transverse or short oblique fractures. Occasionally, a small butterfly fragment may be seen; however, as pediatric bone fails more easily in compression, there may only be a buckle of the cortex.

CLINICAL EVALUATION

Children are not good historians; therefore, keen diagnostic skills are required for even the simplest problems. Parents are not usually present at the time of injury and cannot always provide an accurate history. It is important to evaluate the entire extremity, because young children cannot always localize the injury.

As a general rule, children will tolerate more pain than adults, especially if they understand what you are about to do and trust you. It is therefore important to explain everything to children, listen to their suggestions whenever possible, and stop when they ask you to do so.

RADIOGRAPHIC EVALUATION

Radiographs should always include the joint proximal and distal to the suspected area of injury. Should there be uncertainty as to the location of a suspected injury, the entire extremity may be placed on the radiographic plate. Comparison views of the opposite extremity may aid in localizing a minimally displaced fracture. Soft signs such as the posterior fat pad sign in the elbow should be closely evaluated. CT scans and tomograms are useful in evaluating complicated intraarticular fractures in the older child. MRI can be invaluable in the preoperative evaluation of a complicated fracture in a young child and may also help evaluate a fracture not clearly identifiable on plain films. Arthrograms may be essential to the intraoperative evaluation of intraarticular fractures.

CLASSIFICATION

SALTER-HARRIS/OGDEN

Pediatric physeal fractures have traditionally been described by the five-part Salter-Harris classification. The Ogden classification has extended the Salter-Harris classification to include periphyseal fractures, which do not radiographically appear to involve the physis but which may interfere with the physeal blood supply and result in growth disturbance (Fig. 67-1).

Salter-Harris Types I to V

Type I: Transphyseal fracture involving the hypertrophic and calcified zones. Prognosis is usually excellent, although complete or partial growth arrest may occur in displaced fractures.

Type II: Transphyseal fracture that exits the metaphysis. The metaphyseal fragment is known as the Thurston-Holland fragment; the periosteal hinge is intact on the side with the metaphyseal fragment. The prognosis is excellent, although complete or partial growth arrest may occur in displaced fractures.

Type III: Transphyseal fracture that exits the epiphysis, causing intraarticular disruption. Anatomic reduction and fixation without violating the physis is essential; prognosis is guarded, as partial growth arrest and resultant angular deformity are common problems.

Type IV: Fracture that runs from the articular surface, across the physis, and out the metaphysis. Anatomic reduction and fixation without violating the physis is essential; prognosis is guarded, as partial growth arrest and resultant angular deformity are common problems.

Type V: Crush injury to the physis. Diagnosis is generally made retrospectively; prognosis is poor, as growth arrest and partial physeal closure are common problems.

Ogden Types VI to IX

Type VI: Injury to the perichondral ring at the periphery of the physis, usually the result of an open injury. Close follow-up may allow early identification of a peripheral bar that is amenable to excision; prognosis is guarded, as peripheral physeal bridges are common.

Type VII: Fracture involving the epiphysis only. It includes osteochondral fractures and epiphyseal avulsions. Prognosis is variable and depends on the location of the fracture and the amount of displacement.

Type VIII: Metaphyseal fracture. Primary circulation to the remodeling region of the cartilage cell columns is disrupted; hypervascularity may cause angular overgrowth.

Type IX: Diaphyseal fracture. It interrupts the mechanism for appositional growth (the periosteum). Prognosis is generally good if reduction is maintained; cross-union between the tibia and fibula and between the radius and ulna may occur if there is intermingling of the respective periostea.

Peterson (1994) has added a primarily transverse metaphyseal fracture with an extension to the physis as an additional type of physeal injury, as well as describing the injury in which a portion of the physis is amputated or missing, such as after a lawn mower accident.

TREATMENT

The difference between management of a fracture in a child versus an adult is based on the presence of a thick periosteum in the case of a diaphyseal fracture or open physis in metaphyseal fractures.

An initial neurovascular status evaluation is mandatory. Pulses are important, but more important is the evaluation of the extremity, as cold or warm. A grossly ischemic limb, cold and pulseless, is a dire emergency while a warm hand with good capillary refill even with absent pulses may be acceptable. Periodic evaluation for compartment syndrome should be performed. When the femur is fractured, intracompartmental blood loss can be a serious problem in a young child.

Prereduction planning is mandatory, as is a review of the neurovascular anatomy. The thick periosteum can be an aid to reduction for those who understand the anatomy or, to the frustration of many, it can prevent an adequate reduction. The periosteum on the concave side of the deformity is usually intact and can be made to serve as a hinge, preventing overreduction. Longitudinal traction will not reliably unlock the fragments when the periosteum is intact. Controlled re-creation and exaggeration of the fracture deformity is an effective means of disengaging the fragments to obtain reduction. A careful neurovascular examination should be performed and documented before and after fracture manipulation.

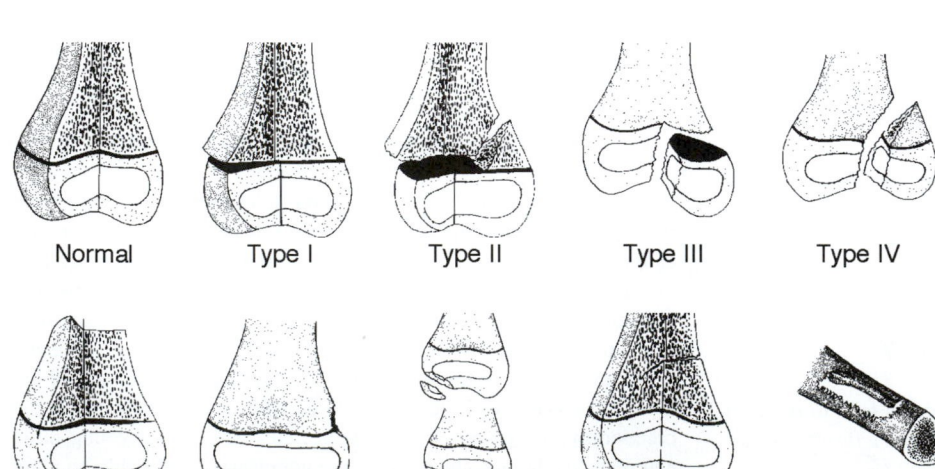

Figure 67-1
Salter-Harris (I–V) and Ogden (I–IX) classifications of physeal injuries in children. (Reproduced by permission from JA Ogden: *Pocket Guide to Pediatric Fractures.* Baltimore: Williams & Wilkins; 1987:25-42.)

Normal   Type I   Type II   Type III   Type IV

Type V   Type VI   Type VII   Type VIII   Type IX

Despite these measures, certain fractures may not be reducible by closed means. Nerves, particularly at the elbow and tendons, frequently become entrapped in the fracture site, preventing reduction. In difficult situations, the fracture should be splinted and the child prepared for general anesthesia, which allows complete relaxation and image intensification to be utilized.

Unlike the adult, considerable fracture deformity may be permitted, as the remodeling potential of the child is great. As a rule of thumb, the closer the fracture is to the joint (physis), the more deformity is permissible; such as at the shoulder or radial neck where 45 to 60 degrees of angulation in a young child may be permissible, while the midshaft fracture of the radius or tibia should be brought to within 10 degrees of normal alignment. Rotational deformity does not spontaneously correct, even in the young child, and should be avoided.

Intraarticular fractures, Salter-Harris type III and IV, require anatomic reduction (<1 to 2 mm of displacement both vertically and horizontally) to restore normal joint congruity and minimize physeal bar formation. Severely comminuted fractures (i.e., femur fracture) may require skin or skeletal traction. Traction pins should be placed proximal to the nearest distal physis, however, care should be taken not to place them through the physis.

Once the fracture has been reduced, either a splint or bivalved cast should be applied. Ideally, if the fracture is stable after reduction, the extremity should be immobilized in the neutral position. Univalving, particularly with a synthetic cast, does not provide adequate flexibility to accommodate swelling of the extremity.

Immobilization, such as with a short or long leg cast, depends on the inherent stability of the fracture. In as little as 2 days after cast application, children will run on short leg casts or climb monkey bars in short arm casts. All fractures should be elevated to the level of the heart, iced, and frequently monitored by responsible individuals. It is too easy to pass off the continued crying of a child as fracture pain when, in fact, a compartment syndrome is developing. In cases when the reliability of the guardian is in question, for any reason, hospital admission is warranted.

Operative indications include

- Open fractures
- Intraarticular fractures (Salter-Harris type III or IV)
- Fractures with vascular injury
- Fractures with an associated compartment syndrome
- Unstable fractures which require abnormal positioning to maintain closed reduction

COMPLICATIONS

Complications unique to pediatric fractures include the following:

- Complete growth arrest
- Progressive limb length inequalities, with the fractured limb being either too short or too long

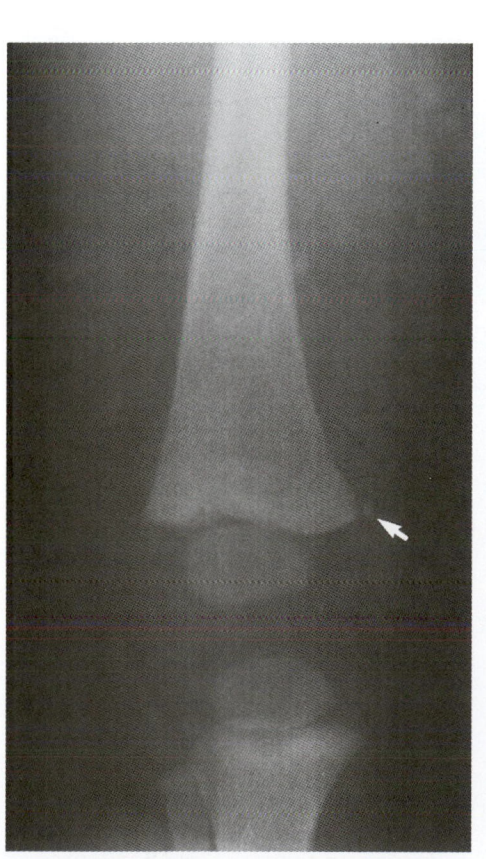
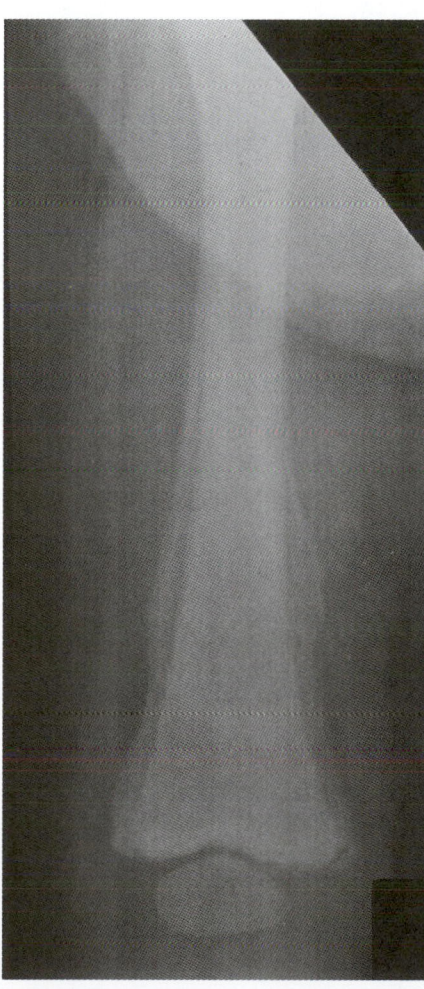

A

B

Figure 67-2
"Corner" metaphyseal fracture associated with child abuse (*A*). Three weeks after injury demonstrating extent of periosteal injury (*B*).

- Progressive angular deformities
- Other unusual joint deformities due to osteonecrosis of the epiphysis and partial physeal closure

CHILD ABUSE

Child abuse is a concern for physicians treating children with any injury, particularly those that are musculoskeletal. Child abuse must be suspected under the following circumstances:

- Fractures of the long bones in a nonambulating child; while spiral fractures may be due to twisting, all fracture patterns may be seen in abuse
- A history (mechanism of injury) that does not seem to fit the fracture pattern
- An unwitnessed injury that results in fracture
- Multiple fractures in various stages of healing
- Skin bruising suggestive of abuse
- Specific fracture patterns, such as a "corner" fracture (avulsion fracture from the metaphyseal side of the physis). (Fig. 67-2)

It is the obligation of the physician to ensure that the child is in a safe environment. If there is any question as to abuse, the child should be admitted to the hospital and social services notified.

The radiographic evaluation of child abuse should include a skeletal survey: anteroposterior and lateral views of the skull, anteroposterior view of the thoracolumbar spine, and an anteroposterior view of the extremities and chest in one view, if possible.

Not all children with multiple or suspicious fractures have been abused. The differential diagnosis for multiple fractures or multiple bones with periosteal elevation is extensive, and includes osteogenesis imperfecta, congenital syphilis, vitamin C or D deficiency, hypophosphatemic ricket, and leukemia. A thorough history, examination, and lab work are indicated to rule out other causes of the osseous and clinical appearance of the child.

SUGGESTED READINGS

Aponte JE Jr, Ghiateas A: Acute plastic bowing deformity: A review of the literature. *J Emerg Med* 1989; 7:181.

Loder RT, Bookout C: Fracture patterns in battered children. *J Orthop Trauma* 1991; 5:428.

Moseley CF: General features of fractures in children. In Eilert RE (ed): *Instructional Course Lectures*. Park Ridge, IL: American Academy of Orthopaedic Surgeons; 1992; 41:337.

Peterson HA: Physeal fractures: Part 3. Classification. *J Pediatr Orthop* 1994; 14:439.

Salter RB, Harris WR: Injuries involving the epiphyseal plate. *J Bone Joint Surg [Am]* 1963; 45:587.

Chapter 68

SPINAL TRAUMA

David S. Feldman

FRACTURES OF THE THORACIC AND LUMBAR SPINE

Injuries to the spine are quite rare in children. Although children most frequently injure their cervical spine, injuries to the thoracic and lumbar spines may also occur in childhood. Most children sustain injuries, however, secondary to motor vehicle accidents; injuries may also occur due to falls from a height. Adolescent children may injure their spine through sporting activities. Injuries of the spine in children are quite different than those in adults. The presence of the cartilaginous vertebral body as well as the larger disc space creates a hyperelastic spine.

ANATOMY

The centrum vertebral body appears quite small in infants. This is due to an increased cartilage/bone ratio. As a child ages and the vertebral body grows and ossifies, the mature disc space becomes apparent. The vertebral apophyses represent the secondary centers of ossification. They occur at the superior and inferior end plates of the vertebral body. These apophyses are larger at the periphery than they are in the center and are called ring apophyses. Each apophysis has a growth plate, the physis, attached to the vertebral body. These vertebral apophyses may be mistaken for a fracture or avulsion on plain radiographs.

The spinal segments in a child are quite elastic. This elasticity will account for the occurrence of a spinal cord injury without radiographic abnormality (SCIWORA). The spinal cord may be injured even without fracture; this is unique to the young child.

CLASSIFICATION

Fractures are defined by their mechanism of injury. Compression in a child may cause slipping of the vertebral apophyses. The child can have three types of slipped apophyses. Type I apophyseal separation is a separation of the posterior rim of the vertebrae. Type II is a large bony avulsion fracture, and type III represents a small portion of the avulsion fracture as opposed to a large segment as in type II. These fractures can occur from a simple compression force (Fig. 68-1).

A child can sustain a pure flexion injury. During compression of the spine, a child's vertebral disc is less likely to herniate than the vertebral body is to fracture. This is due to the hyperelasticity of the discs and the relative weakness of the bones (Fig. 68-2). Children may sustain multiple level fractures during a pure flexion injury. Other types of injuries such as a Chance fracture or distraction shear fracture may occur with seat belt injuries. These are similar to those seen in adults. Visceral injury in children is not uncommon with these types of injuries (Fig. 68-3).

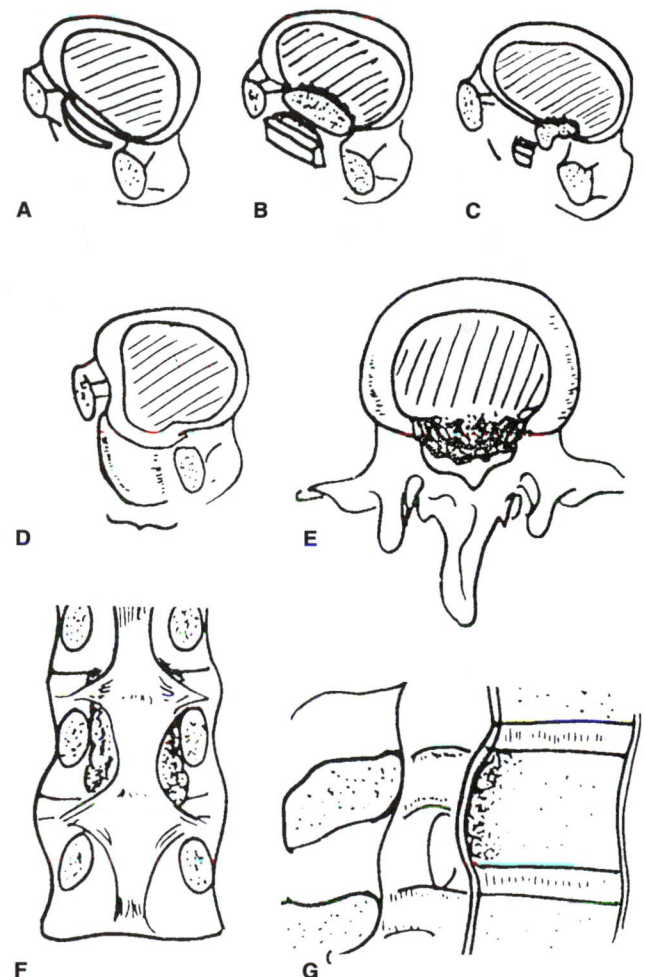

Figure 68-1

Schematic diagram of fractures to the vertebral limbus. *A.* Type I: simple separation of the entire posterior vertebral margin. *B.* Type II: avulsion of fracture of some of the substance of the vertebral body, including the margin. *C.* Type III: more localized lateral fracture of the posterior margin of the vertebral body. *D* to *G.* Type IV: fracture that extends both beyond the margins of the disc and for the full length of the vertebral body between the end plates. The type IV fracture effectively displaces the end plates. The type IV fracture effectively displaces bone in the posterior direction, filling the floor of the spinal canal with a combination of reconstituted cortical and cancellous bone accompanied in part by scar formation. (Reproduced with permission from Epstein NE, Epstein JA, Mauri T: Treatment of fractures of the vertebral limbus and spinal stenosis in five adolescents and five adults. *Neurosurgery* 1989; 24:596.)

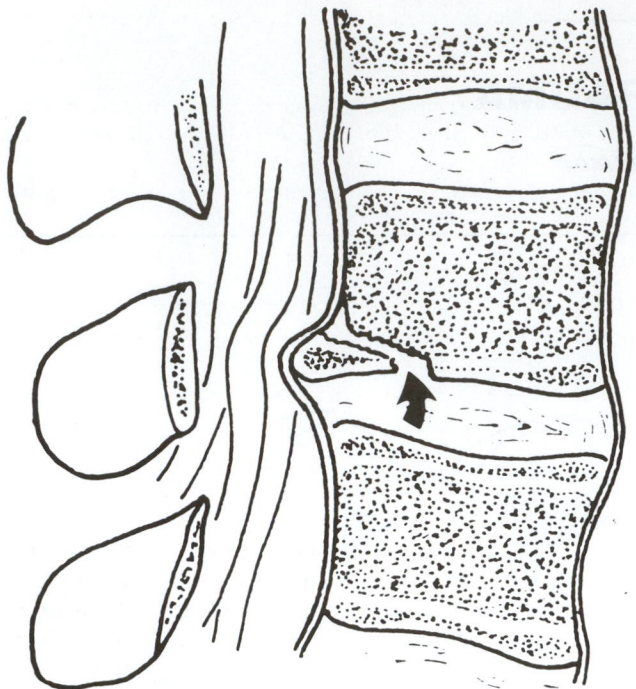

Figure 68-2
Schematic of posterior epiphyseal injury that may mimic disc hernia-tion. (Reproduced with permission from Ogden JA: Spine. In: *Skeletal Injury in the Child*. Philadelphia: WB Saunders; 1990:611.)

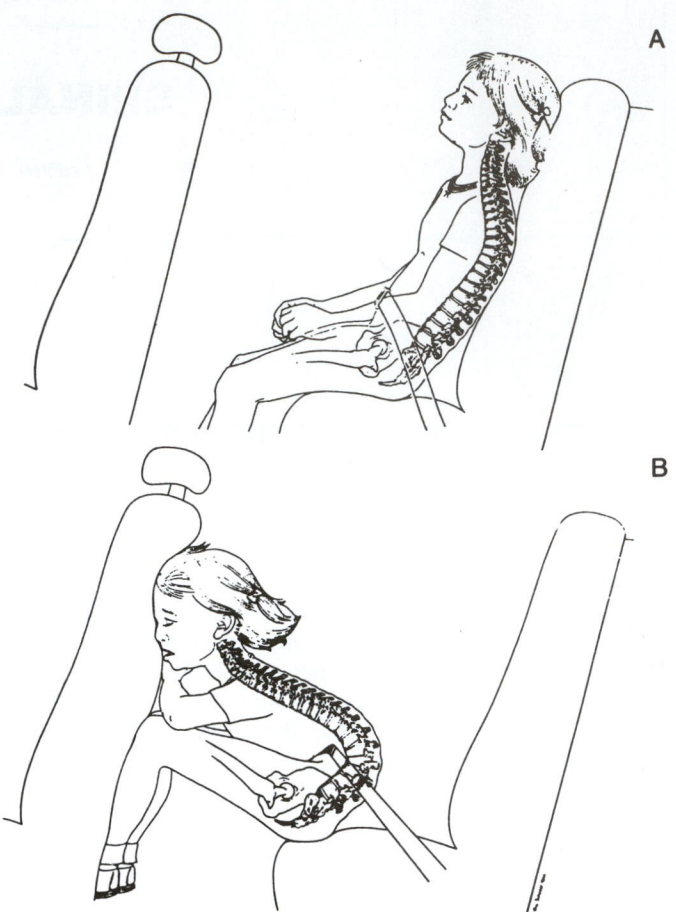

Figure 68-3
Demonstrating hyperflexion injury in a child. [Reproduced with per-mission from Chambers HG, Akbarnia BA: Thoracic, lumbar, and sacral spine fractures and dislocations. In Weinstein SL (ed): *The Pediatric Spine: Principles and Practice*. New York: Raven Press; 1994:749.]

PRESENTING SYMPTOMS

Following a trauma event, complaints of back pain, muscle spasms, or torticollis may represent significant spinal pathology in a child. In addition, if a child has multiple injuries, one should not ignore even minor-appearing fractures on radiographs. Many of these mul-tiply traumatized children will have visceral injury which may be masking a spine injury.

A slipped vertebral apophysis is usually associated with an acute traumatic event in an adolescent. The symptoms include neurologic findings such as fatigue with walking, absent reflexes, and a positive straight leg raise.

NEUROLOGIC INJURY IN CHILDREN

Children may present at the time of injury with paraplegia or they may develop it within hours or days after the injury. In children over the age of 10 years, neurologic deficit is usually associated with a fracture observable on radiograph. Most of these occur in the thoracic spine. In young children, SCIWORA may be quite common. The degree of deficit from these injuries is quite variable and the mechanism of in-jury is variable. Neurologic loss can either be complete or incomplete.

Birth injuries may present as either a floppy baby or a child with respiratory distress.

RADIOGRAPHIC STUDIES

Plain films are essential in the initial evaluation; however, these may be normal even with significant spinal cord pathology. In a child with a neurologic injury, an MRI is the preferred study. CT scan can be utilized for bony reconstructions in fracture dislocations of the spine.

TREATMENT

Compression injuries can be treated with simple bed rest and cast or brace immobilization. Children usually improve within the first few weeks. Chance fractures that are without significant kyphosis can be treated in a lordosing brace if the injury is bony in nature. If signif-icant kyphosis is present, then surgical stabilization is required. A soft tissue Chance fracture should be treated with posterior fusion.

Children with fracture dislocations of the spine are ordinarily treated as adults as these injuries are usually seen in adolescence after spinal growth is completed. However, burst fracture involving more than 25 percent of the spinal canal may injure growth plates at the upper and lower ends of the vertebrae, which may cause a progressive kyphosis. This fracture in younger children should be treated operatively in order to restore lordosis and to prevent future kyphosis.

A fracture of the vertebral apophysis ordinarily requires surgical treat-ment, including a laminectomy and removal of the apophyseal fragment.

The type of surgical instrumentation utilized to achieve fusion in children depends on patient age. Only adolescents can be treated as adults. Younger children may just require sublaminar or interbody wiring to achieve a reduction and fusion, as well as a reconstruction of the posterior elements.

There is a very high incidence of spinal deformity and scoliosis in children with traumatic paraplegia after a fracture dislocation of the spine. In children below the age of 10 years, the incidence approaches 100 percent. This curve is a neuromuscular curve and should be treated as such. The more proximal the level of paraplegia, the more likely spinal deformity will occur. Like most neuromuscular scoliosis, this should be treated surgically as the curve magnitude approaches 50 degrees. Curves of less than 40 degrees may be treated in a brace to allow for spinal growth. Segmental fixation is the method to be utilized, if possible. The child must be mobilized to prevent complications of prolonged bed rest. Deterioration of this neurologic level in a child, even years after the injury, may be secondary to syringomyelia. MRI is indicated to rule out this lesion.

CERVICAL SPINE INJURIES

Although cervical spine injuries are rare in children, they are more common than injuries of the thoracic and lumbar spine. Most of these injuries in children will occur at the atlas or axis. Adolescents have the same distribution of fractures as adults. Children under 10 years of age will be the focus of this discussion.

ANATOMY

The anatomy of the upper cervical vertebrae in children is quite complex and variable. The atlas has three ossification centers: two for the posterior aspects of the neural arches and one for the vertebral body. The posterior arch becomes complete by the third year of life. The second cervical vertebra, or C2, has four ossification centers at birth. There is again, one for the body, two for the posterior aspect of the axis, and one for the odontoid. It is important to realize that the physis of the odontoid is within the body of the axis; it is not at the base of the odontoid. Each of the lower cervical vertebrae has three ossification centers, two posterior and one anterior. The posterior neural arches close at approximately the third year of life. The vertebral body fuses with the posterior arch at approximately the age of 7 years.

MECHANISM OF INJURY

Upper cervical spine injuries are much more common in children than lower cervical spine injuries. Children may also sustain spinal cord injury without radiographic abnormality. Most injuries occur from a motor vehicle accident. However, sporting injuries increase in frequency as the child ages.

PHYSICAL EXAMINATION

Children often present with torticollis, particularly if the injury is in the upper cervical spine. The child may also complain of pain in that area. Respiratory distress can occur in an infant. Other neurologic symptoms, including headache and bladder and bowel dysfunction, may also occur. The patient should undergo active range of motion testing of the cervical spine. Passive range of motion should be avoided in acute injuries. In addition, the child should not be placed flat on a board as the head is large and this may cause a flexion of the cervical spine, even in the resting position. The shoulders can be lifted up or the child can have a special board in which there is a cutout for the head to allow positioning without flexion.

RADIOGRAPHIC EVALUATION

In the acute setting, careful evaluation of the lateral cervical spine radiograph is essential. There are a number of notable differences between children and adults regarding the lateral cervical spine x-ray:

1. The posterior spinal lamina line may not be present in a child and, therefore, there may be an absence of the cervical lordosis on this film.
2. The child, if crying, may have an increase of paravertebral soft tissue space.
3. In children, vertebral bodies may appear wedge shaped. This is secondary to the osseous structure only being the ossification center and not the true shape of the vertebral body.
4. The atlantodens interval in a child can be up to 4 to 5 mm. This compares to 3 mm in an adult.
5. Furthermore, pseudosubluxation of C2 on C3 can be seen. This pseudosubluxation can occur in C3 on C4 as well.

FRACTURES

Children, in general, are susceptible to cervical spine fractures as described before. The child may sustain neonatal trauma secondary to a difficult birth. This may occur with SCIWORA. Although fractures of the occiput to C1 may occur in children, this is quite rare and is treated in the same manner as for adults. A Jefferson fracture is also a rare fracture in children. There are few differences from its adult counterpart.

C1 AND C2 INSTABILITY

Most C1 and C2 instability is a result of chronic ailments. Acute rupture of the transverse ligament is quite rare in children. Although children who have chronic ailments are more at risk for spinal cord injury, treatment is not usually performed unless there is neurologic compromise or if the child has approximately 1 cm of instability. Treatment consists of C1 to C2 fusion.

ATLANTOAXIAL ROTARY SUBLUXATION

Atlantoaxial rotary subluxation may be traumatic or atraumatic. If traumatic, the trauma may be mild. This usually occurs after an upper respiratory infection and ordinarily resolves spontaneously. The classification has been divided into four types, depending on the severity of the subluxation and dislocation (see Fig 60-2). Ordinarily, subluxation will resolve in a few days with rest, collar, and perhaps a muscle relaxant. Over time, however, the deformity can become fixed and treatment is necessary. Children who have had prolonged instability may require reduction with halo traction, followed by spinal fusion.

ODONTOID FRACTURE

Odontoid fractures are quite common in children. These fractures in children are usually through the synchondrosis. This is essentially a physeal fracture of the odontoid. Treatment consists of immobilization in a halo vest for approximately 6 to 8 weeks. Surgery is not generally required unless reduction cannot be achieved. Os odontoideum is thought to be the nonunion of an odontoid fracture in a child. If this fracture demonstrates instability, then a C1/C2 fusion is indicated.

Other fractures in children, although seen, are similar to adult fracture types. However, the diagnosis is often delayed due to the difficult reading of the child's radiograph.

TRAUMATIC SPONDYLOLISTHESIS OF C2

Traumatic spondylolisthesis of C2 (hangman's fracture) is quite unusual in a child. The treatment has traditionally been nonoperative with a halo cast. Surgery is indicated only if chronic instability results.

SUGGESTED READINGS

Anderson JM, Schutt AH: Spinal injury in children: A review of 156 cases seen from 1950 through 1978. *Mayo Clin Proc* 1980; 55:499.

Crawford AH: Operative treatment of spine fractures in children. *Orthop Clin North Am* 1990; 21:325.

McGrory BJ, Klassen RA, Chao EY, et al: Acute fractures and dislocations of the cervical spine in children and adolescents. *J Bone Joint Surg [Am]* 1993; 75:988.

McPhee IB: Spinal fractures and dislocations in children and adolescents. *Spine* 1981; 6:533.

Chapter 69

UPPER EXTREMITY

David S. Feldman

SCAPULA FRACTURES

ANATOMY

The scapula is initially formed from intramembranous ossification and begins to ossify from a center during the eighth week of fetal growth. The body and spine of the scapula are ossified by birth. The center of the coracoid ossifies at 1 year of age and the base of the coracoid and upper one-quarter of the glenoid ossify by 10 years of age. A third center at the tip of the coracoid ossifies at a variable time, and all fuse by age 15 to 16 years. Two to five centers in the acromion begin to form during puberty, fusing by age 22. Centers for the vertebral border, inferior angle, and lower three-quarters of the glenoid also appear at puberty and also fuse by age 22.

SCAPULAR BODY FRACTURES

Although uncommon, body and neck fractures of the scapula occur by means of a direct blow. There is a high incidence of concomitant injury for this type of scapular fracture, usually involving the C-spine, clavicle, and brachial plexus. Associated ipsilateral rib fractures with pneumothorax and pulmonary contusion occur in 50 percent of these fractures. If the fracture involves the suprascapular notch, one should suspect a suprascapular nerve injury. True AP and lateral radiographs should be made with opposite-side comparison views taken in order to screen for more subtle injuries. A CT scan may be needed to identify any associated glenoid fractures. Conservative treatment is recommended.

GLENOID FRACTURES

Fractures of the glenoid are associated with scapular neck fractures and shoulder dislocations, and are often an indirect result of a fall on a flexed elbow. Treatment is nonoperative in most cases, although open reduction with internal fixation is indicated if a large anterior or posterior rim fragment is associated with glenohumeral instability.

AVULSION FRACTURES

These are avulsion-type injuries which usually occur through the common physis at the base of the coracoid and the upper one-quarter of the glenoid; a second type occurs through the tip of the coracoid. The coracoacromial ligament remains intact; however, the acromioclavicular ligaments may be stretched. The Stryker notch view is the most helpful radiograph; however, the injury may be seen through an axillary lateral view with the gantry widened to include the coracoid on the film. This injury can be treated by sling immobilization of the shoulder for 3 weeks, followed by progressive shoulder exercises.

ACROMIAL FRACTURES

This is a rare fracture that is usually the result of a direct blow to this part of the shoulder. Note that the os acromiale, an unfused ossification center, should not be mistaken for a fracture. Conservative treatment is recommended unless there is severe displacement of the acromioclavicular joint.

CLAVICLE FRACTURES

INCIDENCE

Fracture of the clavicular shaft occurs in 0.5 percent of normal deliveries and 1.6 percent of breech deliveries. It is the most frequent type of fracture in childhood. Approximately 85 percent of clavicle fractures occur in the shaft, most often just lateral to the insertion of the subclavius muscle, which protects the underlying neurovascular structures.

ANATOMY

The clavicle is the first bone to ossify. Primary centers convert to bone by intramembranous ossification. Secondary centers develop via endochondral ossification: The medial epiphysis, where 80 percent of growth occurs, ossifies between 12 to 19 years of age and fuses by age 22 to 25. The lateral end does not ossify until fusion at 19 years of age. The periosteal sleeve ordinarily remains in the anatomic position, thus remodeling is assured.

MECHANISM OF INJURY

Clavicular injury at birth often occurs during delivery of the shoulders through a narrow pelvis. A correlation has been shown for clavicular injury at birth with birth weight, midforceps delivery, and inexperience of the delivering physician. In children, indirect injury, usually from a fall onto an outstretched hand, is the most common mechanism of injury. A direct blow to the clavicle is a less common mechanism of injury; however, it carries the highest incidence of injury to the underlying neurovascular and pulmonary structures.

CLINICAL EVALUATION

The physical exam reveals a painful, palpable bump along the clavicle. In addition, there may be tenting of the skin, crepitus, and ecchymosis. In newborns, the fracture may not be detected until a lump appears over the clavicle at about 10 days following birth. Prior to 10 days, a fairly specific indication of a clavicular fracture in the neonate is an asymmetric Moro reflex. When making a diagnosis, the neurovascular and pulmonary status must be evaluated carefully, especially if a direct blow is suspected.

DIFFERENTIAL DIAGNOSIS

Cleidocranial Dysostosis

This is a defect in intramembranous ossification that most commonly affects the clavicle. It is characterized by an absence of the distal end of the clavicle, a central defect, or a complete absence of the clavicle. Treatment is conservative.

Congenital Pseudarthrosis

Congenital pseudarthrosis most commonly occurs at the junction of the middle and distal thirds of the right clavicle; the ends of the pseudoarthrosis are pointed and smooth. Pseudarthrosis most commonly affects the right clavicle although it may be bilateral in some cases. Most authors recommend repair of the pseudoarthrosis after the age of 2 years.

RADIOGRAPHIC EVALUATION

Recommended views for evaluation include an AP of the clavicle and a lordotic view (cephalic tilt of 35 to 40 degrees) which eliminates overlying structures.

TREATMENT

Newborn to Age 2 Years

Reduction is not indicated for fractures occurring at this age. A sling or figure-eight bandage is applied for 2 to 3 weeks or until the patient is comfortable. Complete fracture under the age of 2 years is unusual and is possibly caused by excessive force.

Age 2 to Maturity

Treatment is the application of a figure-eight bandage or a sling for 2 to 4 weeks, at which time union should be nearly complete.

Open Treatment

Operative treatment is rarely indicated for clavicle fractures in children; however, those with associated vascular compromise should undergo open reduction. In addition, if the skin has been opened or compromised as a result of the fracture, open reduction and fixation may be required.

COMPLICATIONS

Neurovascular complications are rare in children because of the thick periosteum that protects the underlying structures. Malunion complications are rare due to the high remodeling potential; when present, however, they are well tolerated.

CLAVICLE FRACTURES: MEDIAL END

Medial fractures of the clavicle are rare and comprise less than 1 percent of clavicle fractures. They are often seen as a birth injury. Salter-Harris type I or II fractures are common. True sternoclavicular joint dislocations are rare. Displacement is usually anterior, with swelling and tenderness. Posterior displacement may be associated with neurovascular compromise or damage to the trachea. The inferomedial periosteal sleeve remains intact and provides a scaffold for remodeling. Tomograms or lordotic radiographs may be required. Treatment is conservative: 80 percent of growth occurs at this end, thus providing great remodeling potential. Prognosis is excellent, and rapid healing can be anticipated.

CLAVICLE FRACTURES: LATERAL END

Injury to the lateral end of the clavicle is uncommon and comprises 10 to 12 percent of clavicle fractures. The mechanism of injury is direct trauma to the acromion. The coracoclavicular ligaments always remain intact and are attached to the inferior periosteal tube. The acromioclavicular ligament also remains intact and is attached to the distal fragment. Treatment is conservative for patients under 16 years of age. The fracture will heal with periosteal new bone formation and remodeling in 12 months. Surgery is reserved for open fractures.

ACROMIOCLAVICULAR JOINT INJURIES

Injury to the acromioclavicular joint is rare in children under 16 years of age. In children, unlike adults, the coracoclavicular ligaments usually remain intact. The defect is a longitudinal split in the superior portion of the periosteal sleeve.

Classification is the same as for adults: Type I injuries are nondisplaced; type II are partially displaced; type III are totally displaced; type IV injuries are totally displaced with entrapment in the trapezius; type V are subcutaneous; and type VI are infracoracoid.

Radiographic evaluation may include stress views with hanging weights and a Stryker notch view.

Treatment for types I to III is conservative, as remodeling is expected. Treatment for types IV to VI is operative, with reduction of the clavicle and repair of the periosteal sleeve. Internal fixation is often necessary.

GLENOHUMERAL DISLOCATIONS

Dislocation of the glenohumeral joint is very uncommon in children under 12 years of age. Approximately 90 percent are anterior dislocations. In neonates, radiographic appearance of a dislocation may actually represent a physeal injury. A distinction must be made between traumatic and atraumatic dislocations. Bankart lesions and Hill-Sachs deformities are often present. CT arthrography and MRI best define these lesions.

Treatment involves closed reduction and a short period of immobilization. The recurrence rate is in the range of 50 to 90 percent. Surgery is occasionally required for recurrent traumatic dislocations, but its results for children are not well documented.

PROXIMAL HUMERUS FRACTURES

INCIDENCE

Fractures of the proximal humerus account for less than 1 percent of all types of fractures in children and approximately 3 percent of epiphyseal fractures. They are most common in adolescents due to increased sports participation, followed by neonates who sustain birth trauma. For neonates and children under the age of 5 years, Salter-Harris type I injuries predominate; for children ranging from 5 to 11 years, metaphyseal injuries predominate; and for children over the age of 11, Salter-Harris type II injuries predominate.

ANATOMY

Eighty percent of humeral growth occurs at the proximal physis, giving this region significant remodeling potential. There are three centers of ossification within the proximal humerus: the humeral head (ossifies at 6 months), the greater tuberosity (ossifies at 3 years), and the lesser tuberosity (ossifies at 5 years). All three centers coalesce at age 6 to 7 years.

The physis closes at age 14 to 17 in girls and at age 16 to 18 years in boys. The proximal fragment is held by the rotator cuff muscles in a neutral position or in a position of slight abduction and external rotation. The distal fragment pierces the periosteum anterolateral to the biceps tendon. It is held in adduction by the pectoralis major and is pulled proximally by the deltoid. The thick posterior periosteum remains intact.

MECHANISM OF INJURY

Newborns usually incur this type of injury from the trauma of delivery. Injury in children is frequently the result of a fall backward onto an outstretched hand with the elbow extended and the wrist dorsiflexed. Sustaining a direct blow to the posterolateral aspect of the shoulder has also been a common mechanism of injury for children.

CLINICAL EVALUATION

When evaluating newborns, findings may range from irritability with arm movement to pseudoparalysis. In order to avoid a misdiagnosis, septic arthritis, distal clavicular injury, and brachial plexus injury should be eliminated as possibilities. Occasional fever may also be present in newborns. Pain, arm dysfunction, splinting, swelling, and ecchymosis are commonly present in older children who have sustained a proximal humerus fracture. In displaced fractures, the distal fragment may ride anteriorly and proximally. A careful neurovascular examination is required, and should include the axillary, musculocutaneous, radial, ulnar, and median nerves.

RADIOGRAPHIC EVALUATION

AP, lateral, and axillary radiographs should be obtained. If necessary, comparison views of the opposite side should be made. Ultrasound is necessary for newborns because the epiphysis is not yet ossified.

CLASSIFICATION

The Salter-Harris classification consists of four types of injury. Type I is classified as a separation through the physis. It most commonly occurs in children under the age of 5 years; however, approximately 25 percent of children over the age of 11 years also incur this type of proximal humerus fracture. In type II injuries, the metaphyseal fragment is always posteromedial. This type generally occurs in adolescents over the age of 11 years, accounting for approximately 75 percent of the proximal humerus fractures for this age group. Type III injuries have an intraarticular fracture that is commonly associated with dislocations; however, it is rarely observed in adolescents. Type IV Salter-Harris injuries have an intraarticular transmetaphyseal fracture that is associated with open fractures. As with type III fractures, type IV fractures are rarely found in adolescents.

The Neer-Horowitz classification defines four grades of proximal humerus fractures: grade I fractures have displacement less than 5 mm; grade II have displacement less than one-third the width of the shaft; grade III fractures have displacement one-third to two-thirds the width of the shaft; and grade IV fracture displacement is greater than two-thirds the width of the shaft.

TREATMENT

Newborn

The majority of proximal humerus fractures in newborns are Salter-Harris type I and the prognosis for these fractures is excellent. Ultrasound may be used for guiding reduction. The treatment of choice is closed reduction which is achieved by applying gentle traction with 90 degrees of flexion, then 90 degrees of abduction and external rotation. For a stable fracture, the arm should be immobilized against the chest for 5 to 10 days. For an unstable fracture, the arm is held abducted and is externally rotated for 3 to 4 days to allow early callus formation.

Ages 1 to 4 Years

Fractures for this age group are either Salter-Harris type I or, in rare instances, Salter-Harris type II. Treatment is by closed reduction with an angulation of up to 60 degrees and complete displacement being acceptable. The arm is placed in a sling for 10 days and progressive activity is initiated. Note that extensive remodeling is possible at this age.

Ages 5 to 12 Years

The metaphyseal fracture is most common in this age group as this area is undergoing the most rapid remodeling and is therefore weakened. Closed reduction is once again employed as treatment. In this case, 40 to 45 degrees of angulation and a displacement of one-half the width of the shaft are acceptable. For a stable fracture, a simple sling-and-swathe is used. For an unstable fracture, the arm is placed in a shoulder spica cast with the arm in the salute position for 2 to 3 weeks.

Ages 12 Years to Maturity

At the age of 12 years or beyond, fractures are either Salter-Harris type II or, in rare situations, type I. If treatment is by closed reduction, then 15 to 20 degrees of angulation and displacement of less than 30 percent are acceptable. Treatment for a stable fracture is a sling-and-swathe for 2 to 3 weeks followed by progressive range-of-motion exercises. For an unstable fracture, treatment is immobilization in a shoulder spica cast with the arm in the salute position or a closed reduction and pinning. Note that at this age there is less remodeling potential than for those patients who are under the age of 12 years.

Open reduction with internal fixation is indicated for open fractures, fractures with neurovascular compromise, Salter-Harris Type III and IV fractures, and irreducible fractures with soft tissue interposition (biceps tendon). These fractures are fixed with either percutaneous pins, smooth K-wires, or Steinmann pins.

Prognosis

Neer-Horowitz grade I and II fractures do well because of the remodeling potential of the proximal humeral physis. Fractures that are either Neer-Horowitz grade III or grade IV may be left with up to 3 mm of shortening or residual angulation; for the most part, this is well tolerated by the patient and is often clinically insignificant. As a rule, the younger the patient, the higher the potential for remodeling and the greater the acceptance of initial deformity.

HUMERAL SHAFT FRACTURES

Fractures of the shaft of the humerus are a relatively uncommon injury in children. Although these fractures may occur in adolescents, if they are seen in very young children, child abuse should be suspected. The fracture may also be associated with a simple bone cyst. Neonates may present with a birth fracture and have a pseudoparalysis of the limb.

CLASSIFICATION

Humeral shaft fractures are classified by their location (i.e., proximal, middle, distal). The proximal third ends at the pectoralis major insertion. The type of fracture (i.e., transverse, oblique, or spiral), as well as the extent of comminution and soft tissue injury, is important to specify.

BIRTH INJURIES

Humeral shaft fractures are seen at birth most commonly in large infants who are in breech presentation and delivered vaginally. A newborn may simply not move the affected arm. The infant with a suspected injury needs to be evaluated carefully for swelling, crepitus, and neurologic status. At times the entire extremity including the clavicle will need to be radiographed to determine the diagnosis.

These infants have a high potential to remodel; the limb should be treated in a neutral position of rotation with a splint and swathe around the chest holding the arm to the body. One should try to avoid excessive internal rotation as this may be a deformity that does not fully remodel. Up to 70 degrees of angulation and 2 cm of shortening can be accepted. Treatment is often required for only 2 weeks. The prognosis for this injury is excellent.

TREATMENT

Humeral shaft fractures have a high remodeling potential and therefore most are treated nonoperatively. Stable fractures such as a Torus fracture of the proximal humerus can be treated simply with a sling. For more unstable fractures or those fractures requiring manipulation, coaptation splints or a U splint, along with a collar and cuff, are often satisfactory. In open fractures with bone loss, external fixation is the preferred method. Retrograde nailing of the humerus is also a viable alternative for grossly unstable fractures that cannot be maintained with nonoperative measures. Fractures of the distal one-third of the humerus may be treated the same way as supracondylar fractures (i.e., stable fractures with simple immobilization and unstable fractures with closed reduction and percutaneous pinning). Open reduction should be reserved for irreducible fractures.

COMPLICATIONS

Complications of humeral shaft fractures include nerve palsies. Radial nerve palsy is the most common primary and secondary nerve injury. Observation is the treatment of choice for all primary closed lesions of the radial nerve. Secondary lesions may be explored immediately or observed over a period of 2 months and an EMG performed. If there is no recurrence in 2 months then exploration is indicated. Additional nerve injuries have been described and should be considered.

Other complications are unusual in children. Malunion may occur but is rarely clinically significant. Nonunion is exceptionally rare in children with humerus fractures. Limb-length inequality is usually significant if there is a greater than 3-cm discrepancy at skeletal maturity.

PEDIATRIC ELBOW

INCIDENCE

Elbow fractures make up approximately 8 to 9 percent of all fractures in children. Of all elbow fractures, 86 percent occur at the distal humerus, 69 percent of which are supracondylar. Most fractures occur at 5 to 10 years of age and are more common in males.

ANATOMY

The elbow consists of three joints: the ulnohumeral, radiocapitellar, and proximal radioulnar. The capsule defines the confines of the joint—proximal: proximal to the coronoid and olecranon fossae; and distal: beyond the tips of the coronoid and olecranon processes.

The epicondyles are extraarticular. A broad anastomotic network forms the intra- and extraosseous blood supply to the elbow. The capitellum is supplied by a posterior branch that enters the lateral crista. The trochlea is supplied by a medial branch that enters along the nonarticular medial crista and a lateral branch that crosses the physis. There is no anastomotic connection between these two vessels. These vessels are at risk after fractures. The carrying angle is influenced by the obliquity of the distal humeral physis; this averages 6 degrees in females and 5 degrees in males, and is important in the assessment of angular growth disturbances. The elbow accounts for only 20 percent of the longitudinal growth of the upper extremity.

Ossification Centers: "CRMTOL"

The rate of ossification in centers associated with the elbow varies considerably. Centers are located within the capitellum (6 months to 2 years; includes the lateral crista of the trochlea), the radial head (4 years), the medial epicondyle (6 to 7 years), the trochlea (8 years), the olecranon (8 to 10 years; often multiple centers, which ultimately fuse), and the lateral epicondyle (12 years).

RADIOGRAPHIC EVALUATION

A standard AP radiograph is important to assess Baumann's angle (normal is 15 to 20 degrees) with comparison also made to the opposite side (Fig. 69-1A). This angle is drawn between the bisector of a midhumeral line and the capitellar physis. A lateral radiograph should be obtained and an anterior humeral line drawn to transect the capitellum (Fig. 69-1B). Fat pad signs should be inspected on the lateral radiograph to detect occult fractures; the posterior fat pad being more significant. A Jones axial view with the elbow hyperflexed and the forearm supinated assists in demonstrating alignment in varus/valgus.

SUPRACONDYLAR HUMERUS FRACTURES

INCIDENCE

These fractures comprise 60 percent of all elbow fractures. Depending on the mechanism of injury, two types of supracondylar fractures occur: the extension type and the flexion type. Approximately 97 percent are the extension type with less than 3 percent the flexion type. Peak incidence occurs in children 5 to 8 years of age, after which dislocations become more frequent. This type of elbow fracture occurs twice as often in males as in females.

ANATOMY

Remodeling of bone in the 5- to 8-year-old causes a decreased AP diameter in the supracondylar region, making this area susceptible to injury. The likelihood of hyperextension injury increases because of ligament laxity in this age range. The periosteal hinge remains intact on the side of the displacement.

CLINICAL EVALUATION

The child presents with swelling and pain, as well as possible deformity over the involved elbow. A careful neurologic examination is performed, and if the extremity is pulseless, a distinction should be made of whether the hand is cold, or warm and pink. The anterior skin may be bruised and tented.

EXTENSION TYPE

Mechanism of Injury

Hyperextension occurs during a fall onto an outstretched hand, with or without a varus/valgus force.

Classification

The classification is based on degree of displacement. Type I supracondylar humerus fractures are nondisplaced. Type II fractures are partially displaced, with a broken anterior cortex but with the posterior cortex remaining intact. In this type there may be slight posterior angulation or rotation of the distal fragment. Type III fractures have complete displacement in which the distal fragment has lost continuity with the proximal fracture fragment.

Treatment

Type I fractures are treated with simple immobilization at approximately 90 degrees or less of flexion. For type II fractures, simple immobilization is usually adequate, for example, a cast applied in the same manner as that for a type I fracture. Minimal reductions of posterior angulation can be achieved. Crossed versus two lateral percutaneous pins may be required if the fracture appears to have a rotational deformity or significant posterior angulation. In type III fractures, closed reduction and pinning with two lateral pins or one medial and one lateral pin is the treatment of choice (Fig. 69-2). For rotationally unstable fractures where a closed reduction cannot be performed, for open fractures, and for those fractures with neurovascular injury, open reduction with pinning is the treatment of choice.

Complications

Neurologic Injury (7 Percent)   Traction injury from the fracture or during reduction can be due to tenting or entrapment at the fracture site. It also may result from either a Volkmann's ischemic contracture, angular deformity, or incorporation into the callus or scar. Most injuries are neurapraxias requiring no treatment; they include injury to the radial nerve (45 percent), median nerve/anterior interosseous nerve (32 percent), and ulnar nerve (23 percent).

Vascular Injury (0.5 Percent)   Although rare, direct injury to the brachial artery can occur. If the hand is cold and pulseless after reduction, exploration of the artery is required. If the hand is warm and well perfused but there is no palpable pulse, the child can simply be observed. Although compartment syndrome is rare it can occur, particularly if the elbow has been hyperflexed.

Other Complications   Loss of motion may occur secondary to a poor reduction or significant soft tissue injury. It is not common for children to lose significant motion after supracondylar humerus fractures. Myositis ossificans is a rare complication and may be seen after a too vigorous manipulation or after a delayed open reduction.

Angular deformity (varus more frequently than valgus), such as cubitus varus, is usually seen with an inadequate reduction or when there has been significant medial column comminution. The child may require a valgus osteotomy at a later date.

Avascular necrosis of the trochlea may occur up to 3 years after the fracture. Although the distal humerus may develop the characteristic fishtail deformity, the patient will often have a paucity of symptoms.

FLEXION TYPE

Mechanism of Injury

This type of flexion injury is a result of a direct blow or fall onto a flexed elbow.

Classification

The Gartland (1959) classification describes three flexion-type injuries of supracondylar fractures: type I are nondisplaced, type II are displaced with the anterior cortex intact, and type III represent complete displacement that is usually anterolateral.

Treatment

Management of type I flexion injuries is immobilization of the elbow in near-extension. In type II injuries, the fracture is manipulated into reduction followed by the insertion of percutaneous pins with either two lateral pins or crossed pins. Reduction of type III injuries is difficult, and may require open reduction. Reduction is followed by internal fixation with pins, as described.

Complications

Ulnar nerve injury is the most common complication in flexion fractures. Acute signs suggest the nerve is being tented by the medial spike of the proximal fragment. Late signs of nerve injury suggest it is secondary to progressive valgus deformity. Loss of motion is more common in this type of injury, probably due to the inability to achieve an adequate reduction. Angular deformity may also occur. Cubitus valgus is the most common residual deformity after this injury.

LATERAL CONDYLAR PHYSEAL FRACTURES

INCIDENCE

Lateral condylar physeal fractures comprise 17 percent of all distal humerus fractures and 54 percent of distal humeral physeal fractures. The frequency of this fracture peaks at the age of 6 years.

MECHANISM OF INJURY

There are two mechanism-of-injury theories for this fracture, the first being the "pull-off" theory. In this case, avulsion of the lateral condyle occurs through the extensors due to varus stress on an extended elbow. Conversely, the "push-off" theory refers to injury that is the result of a fall onto an extended hand which causes the radial head to knock off the lateral condyle.

CLASSIFICATION

The Milch (1964) classification is anatomically based. In type A fractures, the fracture line courses lateral to the trochlea and into the capitella-trochlear groove (Salter-Harris type IV). The fracture may

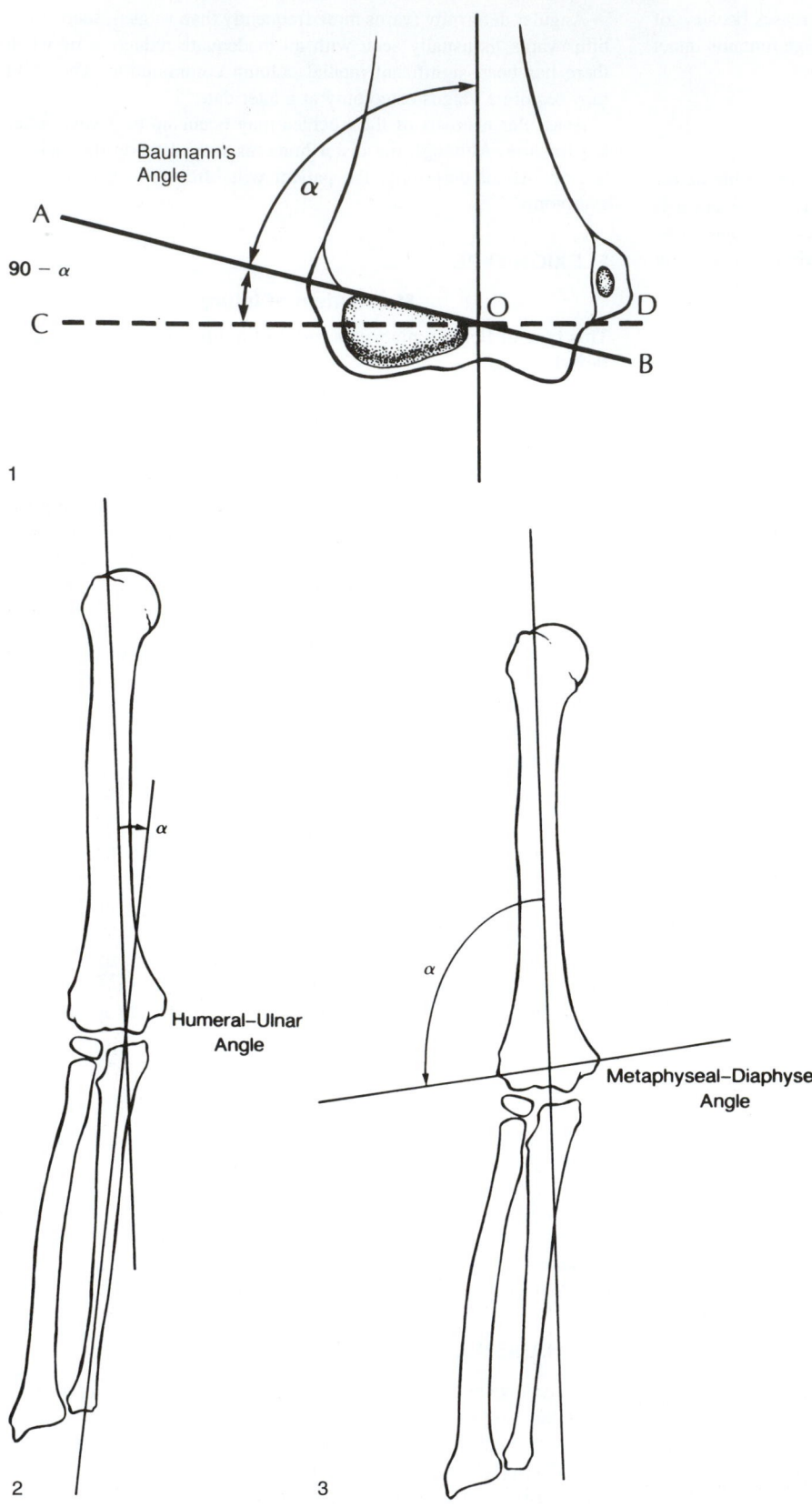

Figure 69-1

A. Anteroposterior radiograph angles of the elbow. 1. Baumann's angle. 2. The humeral-ulnar angle. 3. The metaphyseal-diaphyseal angle. [Reproduced by permission from Wilkins KE, Beaty JH, Chambers HG, et al: Fractures and dislocations of the elbow region. In Rockwood CA Jr, Wilkins KE, Beaty JH (eds): *Fractures in Children*, 4th ed. Philadelphia: Lippincott-Raven; 1996: 665.] B. (Facing page, top) Lateral radiograph lines of the distal humerus. 1. The "teardrop" of the distal humerus. 2. The angulation of the lateral condyle with the shaft of the femur. 3. The anterior humeral line. 4. The coronoid line. [Reproduced by permission from Wilkins KE, Beaty JH, Chambers HG, et al: Fractures and dislocations of the elbow region. In Rockwood CA Jr, Wilkins KE, Beaty JH (eds): *Fractures in Children*, 4th ed. Philadelphia: Lippincott-Raven; 1996: 666.]

be stable because the trochlea is intact; this is the less common type. With type B injuries, the fracture line extends into the apex of the trochlea; the loss of trochlear abutment causes the radius and ulna to be laterally displaced (Salter-Harris type II or IV). The elbow is unstable because the trochlea is not intact; this is the more common type of fracture.

A more useful classification is Jakob's (1975) classification which is based on displacement of the fragment. In stage I the fracture is nondisplaced with an intact articular surface. Stage II injury is a complete fracture that extends through the articular surface with moderate displacement. Stage III injury is complete displacement and capitellum rotation with elbow instability.

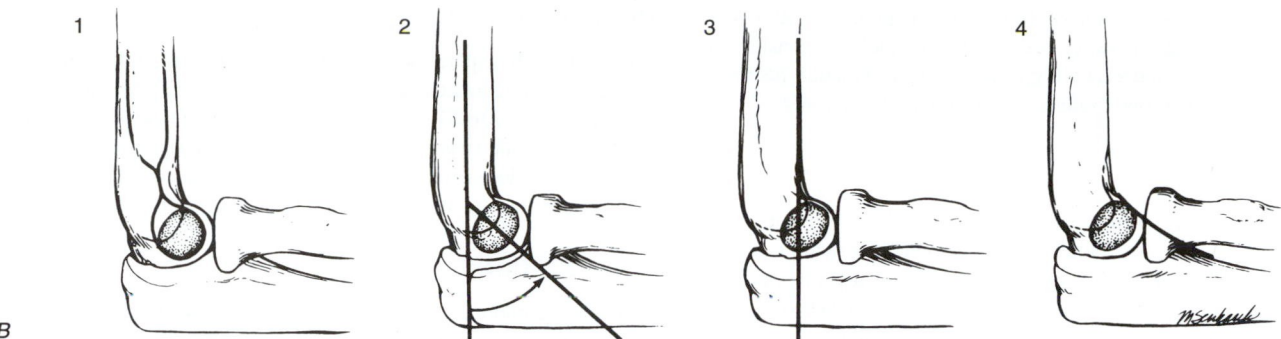

B

RADIOGRAPHIC EVALUATION

AP, lateral, oblique, and varus stress views should be obtained. An arthrogram to assess the size of the cartilaginous fragment and articular displacement will help in the evaluation of young children.

TREATMENT

Simple immobilization for 3 weeks is adequate for type I fractures with less than 2 mm displacement. To ensure that displacement does not occur, the fracture can be treated with closed pinning followed by 3 weeks of cast immobilization. If one is uncertain as to whether the fracture is truly nondisplaced, then pinning should probably be performed. After obtaining an anatomic reduction to ensure a good result, a type II fracture may be reduced, closed, and secured with percutaneous pins. In general though, displaced type II and type III fractures must be reduced anatomically; therefore, open reduction with pin fixation is usually the required method of treatment. The fragment should be secured with two smooth Kirschner pins. The pins

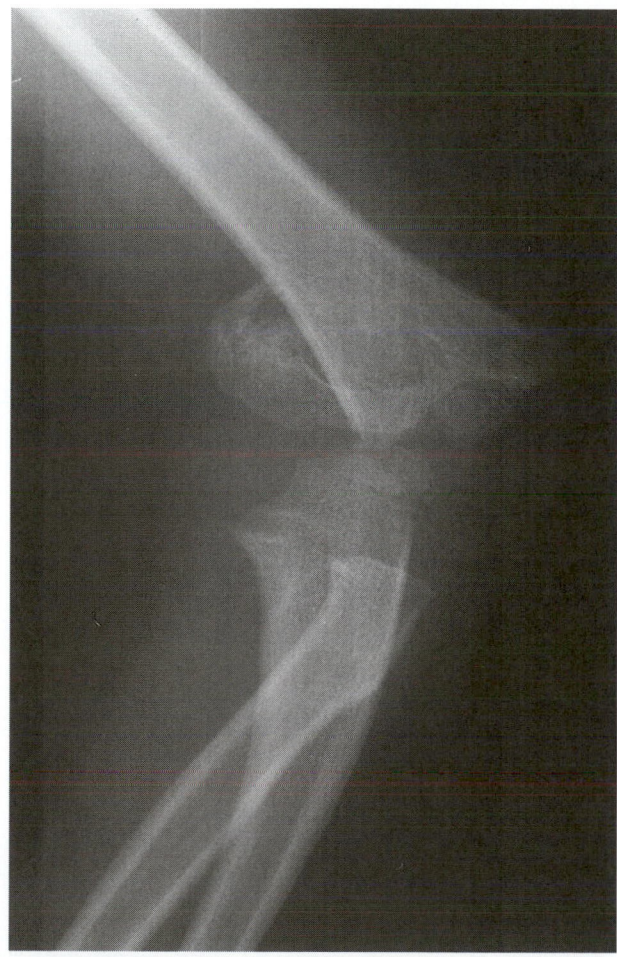

A

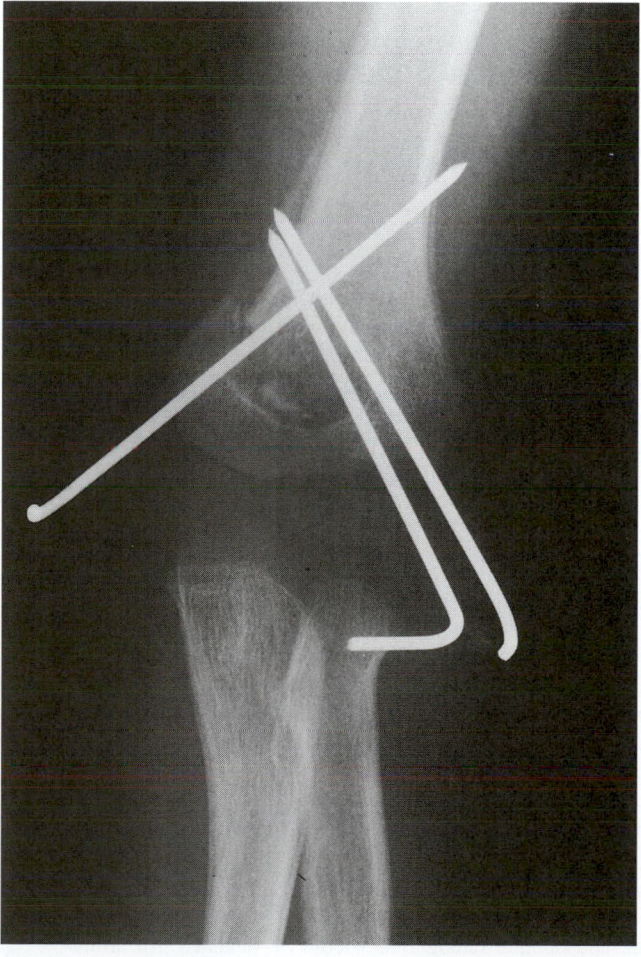

B

Figure 69-2

Five-year-old male. *A.* Type III supracondylar humerus fracture. *B.* Fracture with closed reduction and pinning. Note restoration of Baumann's angle.

are removed after 3 weeks and motion is then begun. If treatment is delayed by 6 or more weeks, closed treatment should be considered regardless of displacement as a high incidence of avascular necrosis is associated with late open reduction and internal fixation.

COMPLICATIONS

Poorer results are achieved in lateral condylar phlyseal fracture than in supracondylar humerus fractures. This is likely due to the fact that the diagnosis of lateral condylar physeal fractures is less obvious and may be missed in subtle cases, loss of motion is more severe due to intraarticular involvement, and there is a higher incidence of growth disturbance.

Lateral condylar overgrowth with spur formation (30 percent) is usually not a functional or cosmetic problem. Delayed union or nonunion (>12 weeks) may be due to the pull of extensors, inadequate internal fixation, or failure to perform it due to misdiagnosis. Valgus deformity can occur from a nonunion or malunion of a lateral condyle fracture. Only rarely has a lateral epiphysiodesis been a cause of clinically significant cubitus valgus. Acute neurologic complications are rare. The late neurologic complication of tardy ulnar nerve palsy is due to cubitus valgus. Other complications include avascular necrosis (AVN) which is usually iatrogenic, especially in delayed cases. AVN may cause "fishtail" deformity if the vessel to the lateral trochlea is disrupted posteriorly. Myositis ossificans is a rare complication of lateral condylar physeal injury.

MEDIAL CONDYLAR PHYSEAL FRACTURES

INCIDENCE

This fracture accounts for less than 2 percent of all elbow fractures, and usually occurs in children ranging from ages 8 to 12 years.

MECHANISM OF INJURY

There are two mechanisms of injury for this type of fracture, the first being direct trauma to the tip of the elbow with the olecranon splitting the trochlea. In this case, the fracture line extends proximally to the metaphysis. Indirect injury may also occur as a result of a fall onto an outstretched hand with valgus strain on the elbow. Avulsion injury ensues with the fracture line starting in the metaphysis and then propagating distally through the articular surface.

CLASSIFICATION

The anatomically based classification of Milch (1964) divides medial condylar physeal fractures into two types. In type I, the fracture line traverses the apex of the trochlea. In type II, the fracture line traverses the capitella-trochlear groove; type II fractures present infrequently.

Jakob's classification (1975), based on displacement, describes three stages. Stage I are nondisplaced fractures with the articular surface intact. Stage II fractures have a fracture line complete with minimal displacement. Stage III fractures have complete displacement with rotation of the fragment due to the pull of flexor mass.

RADIOGRAPHIC EVALUATION

AP, lateral, and oblique radiographs should be obtained. An arthrogram may be helpful in minimally displaced fractures to assess articular congruity. Stress views may help distinguish epicondylarfractures (valgus laxity) from condylar fractures (both varus and valgus laxity).

TREATMENT

For type I and II displacement, the arm should be immobilized in a long arm cast. Open reduction with internal fixation should be performed if the fracture displaces. In type III fractures, open reduction with internal fixation is the treatment of choice because rotation precludes the possibility of closed treatment. If treatment is delayed by more than 6 weeks, the fracture should not be treated with open reduction.

COMPLICATIONS

Associated complications include: missed diagnosis, nonunion (may be secondary to the pull of flexors with rotation), angular deformity (usually varus due to medial physeal arrest), and delayed union (may be due to inadequate or no fixation).

TRANSPHYSEAL FRACTURES OF THE DISTAL HUMERUS

INCIDENCE

Transphyseal fractures of the distal humerus are uncommon but not rare, most occurring by 4 years of age. Variants of this fracture may be seen in patients up to age 12 years.

ANATOMY

The epiphysis includes the medial epicondyle until age 6 to 7 years. Fractures prior to this time will therefore include the medial epicondyle. The joint surface is not involved in this injury, and the relationship between the radius and capitellum is maintained. The AP diameter of the bone in this region is wider than in the supracondylar region, and consequently there is not as much tilting or rotation.

MECHANISM OF INJURY

These are usually extension injuries with posterior displacement similar to supracondylar humerus fractures. This usually requires a rotary force to cause the fracture, and it can occur during delivery. Child abuse must be contemplated in the child with this fracture.

CLASSIFICATION

The DeLee (1980) classification is based on the degree of ossification of the lateral condyle: group A—Infant, prior to appearance of lateral condylar ossification center (birth to 7 months), diagnosis is easily missed, Salter-Harris Type I; group B—Lateral condyle ossified (7 months to 3 years), Salter-Harris Type I or II (fleck of metaphysis); and group C—large metaphyseal fragment, usually lateral (3 to 7 years).

RADIOGRAPHIC EVALUATION

AP, lateral, and oblique radiographs are recommended. In group A, evaluation must rely on the relationship of the humerus to the radius and ulna; the radius and ulna displace posteromedially (diagnostic sign). In Groups B and C, the radius and capitellum maintain a normal relationship, but the capitellum is displaced posteromedial relative to the humeral shaft; evaluation must discriminate this setting from elbow dislocation. An arthrogram can be useful for clarification.

TREATMENT

Treatment of these fractures is similar to that of a supracondylar humerus fracture. The problem is in recognizing the fracture pattern.

Nondisplaced fractures can be treated in a long arm splint in flexion for 3 weeks. If the fracture is displaced, a closed reduction and pinning is the treatment of choice within the first week after the injury. Although some authors recommend closed reduction with casting in hyperflexion, this has the associated risk of vascular compromise and loss of reduction. Pinning with two lateral pins is recommended in very young children, as well as performing the reduction and pinning with the aid of an arthrogram. Delayed treatment should be avoided due to healing of the fracture. If there is residual deformity, it is more readily treated with a late osteotomy.

COMPLICATIONS

Malunion may result in cubitus varus although it is a less common occurrence in transphyseal fracture of the distal humerus than in untreated supracondylar humerus fractures. Osteonecrosis is seen mainly in the trochlea ("fishtail" deformity).

MEDIAL EPICONDYLAR APOPHYSEAL FRACTURES

INCIDENCE

Fractures of the medial epicondyle account for over 10 percent of all elbow fractures in children. Up to one-half of these fractures are associated with elbow dislocations. The fractures usually occur between the ages of 9 and 12 years, and boys are much more commonly involved.

ANATOMY

The medial epicondyle is a traction apophysis for the medial collateral ligament (MCL) and wrist flexors but does not contribute to humeral length. It is the last ossification center to fuse with the metaphysis (15 years of age) and does so independently of the other ossification centers. The fragment is usually displaced distally and may be incarcerated in the joint about 20 percent of the time. It is often associated with other fractures such as of the proximal radius, olecranon, and coronoid.

MECHANISM OF INJURY

Medial epicondylar apophyseal fractures may occur by direct blow to the epicondyle (rare), secondary to an elbow dislocation (MCL provides avulsion force), or from an avulsion injury by the flexor mass from a valgus force during a fall onto an outstretched hand.

CLINICAL EVALUATION

There is commonly pain and swelling as well as a possible block to motion if the fragment is within the joint. Valgus instability may also be present.

RADIOGRAPHIC EVALUATION

AP, lateral, and oblique radiographs should be performed and, if needed, a stress view may be ordered.

CLASSIFICATION

The classification of this injury is a descriptive one. The extent of the displacement, the location of the fragment (i.e., incarcerated in the joint or not), and its association with an elbow dislocation are all de-

scribed. A differentiation between acute and chronic injuries should also be made. Chronic injuries, such as with repetitive throwing in children, should be differentiated from the acute injury which has been described here.

TREATMENT

Immobilization is the treatment of choice for this injury. Even displaced fractures will have a good outcome when treated nonoperatively.

Indications for open reduction include: incarceration of fragment in the joint; valgus instability in a throwing athlete; and chronic ulnar nerve irritation from a scar or callus.

COMPLICATIONS

The most common complication of this injury is loss of motion; however, this can usually be avoided with appropriately prescribed early motion exercises. Ulnar nerve dysfunction can be present in up to 15 percent of patients sustaining this fracture. Nonunion occurs in 50 percent of cases with significant displacement; this is to be expected and usually does not cause a functional problem. Myositis is rare, however, it may be present if multiple closed attempts at extracting the fragment from the joint are attempted.

RADIAL HEAD AND NECK FRACTURES

INCIDENCE

The fracture of the proximal radius will involve either the physis or neck in up to 90 percent of cases; the radial head is rarely involved. These fractures constitute less than 10 percent of all elbow fractures in children. Their peak incidence is at approximately 10 years of age.

CLASSIFICATION

Proximal radial physeal fractures can be classified according to any of the physeal fracture classifications. These fractures can be further grouped by the degree of angulation at the femoral neck or physis. O'Brien (1965) divided these into three types: type I (0 to 30 degrees), type II (30 to 60 degrees), and type III (>60 degrees).

Wilkins (1984) has divided radial head and neck fractures by mechanism of injury. Types A, B, and C are caused by a fall onto the outstretched hand (compression) with resultant valgus angular deformity: type A injuries are the Salter-Harris type I or II physeal fractures; type B injuries are the Salter-Harris type III or IV intraarticular fractures. Type C fractures are completely within the metaphysis. Two types of fractures associated with elbow dislocation are described: type D injuries, resulting from reduction injury; and type E injuries, caused by the initial dislocation.

TREATMENT

Treatment for type I injuries (<30 degrees angulation) is simple immobilization. Type II injuries (30 to 60 degrees angulation) should receive closed reduction and/or manipulation. Type III injuries (greater than 60 degrees angulation) require immediate open reduction with oblique K-wire fixation; transcapitellar pins are contraindicated due to a high rate of pin breakage.

The indications for open treatment include: greater than 60 degrees angulation, failed closed reduction, interposed soft tissue, complete displacement, and more than 4 mm translocation. Surgical correction, if possible, should include closed reduction utilizing a joy stick technique or intramedullary reduction. A formal open reduction of the fracture should be the last resort. Radial head excision should be avoided as it results in poor outcomes in children due to the high incidence of overgrowth.

Regardless of treatment, poor results can be expected in 15 to 23 percent of cases. If the fracture is associated with significant soft tissue injury, such as with an elbow dislocation, even an anatomic reduction may result in persistent stiffness.

COMPLICATIONS

Complications of radial and neck fractures include loss of ROM (pronation, supination, and possibly flexion/extension), radial head overgrowth (uncommon), premature physeal closure, and AVN of the radial head (rare, but rate increases with the amount of displacement). Valgus deformity may occur, with an average of 10 degrees. Neurologic injury is uncommon, but if present, it is usually a posterior interosseous nerve neurapraxia. Radioulnar synostosis is the most serious complication. Myositis occurs in approximately 30 percent of cases and is seen mostly within the supinator.

RADIAL HEAD SUBLUXATION

INCIDENCE

Radial head subluxation is commonly referred to as "nursemaid's elbow" or "pulled elbow." It accounts for 28 percent of all elbow injuries in children. With a peak age of occurrence between 2 and 3 years of age, females are twice as likely to develop a radial head subluxation. Up to 30 percent of children will have a second episode.

ANATOMY

The radial head subluxes beneath the annular ligament.

MECHANISM OF INJURY

Radical head subluxation is caused by longitudinal traction force on an extended elbow. This usually occurs when the child is walking while holding an adult's hand, and then falls. The force of the body against the extending elbow causes the radial head to slip under the annular ligament.

TREATMENT

Closed reduction is the treatment of choice. In stage I injuries, the forearm is supinated with pressure on the radial head. With stage II injuries, the arm is brought into maximum flexion with the forearm still in supination. A palpable "clunk" may be felt upon reduction.

ELBOW DISLOCATIONS

INCIDENCE

Elbow dislocations usually occur after skeletal maturity, peaking in the 13- to 14-year-old child. They account for less than 10 percent of all elbow injuries in children. There is a high incidence of associated fractures: medial epicondyle, coronoid, and radial head and neck.

ANATOMY

The bony stability of the elbow is augmented by the collateral ligaments and capsule. Of these, the anterior bundle of the MCL is the most important. The radial head and the anterior capsule provide some stability to valgus load in extension. The olecranon provides bony stability in extension, and the coronoid provides bony stability in flexion.

MECHANISM OF INJURY

Elbow dislocations may result from either a combination of valgus and hyperextension (posterior dislocation) or a direct blow to a flexed elbow (anterior dislocation).

CLASSIFICATION

The posterior elbow dislocation is by far the most common, caused by a combination of hyperextension and valgus stress. An anterior dislocation is much less common (<2 percent), caused by a direct blow to the posterior aspect of a flexed elbow. A divergent dislocation is extremely rare. Medial/lateral dislocations have not been reported in children.

TREATMENT

Closed reduction followed by immobilization for 7 to 10 days, and early range of motion exercises is the treatment of choice. Open reduction is indicated for unsuccessful closed reduction, open dislocation, and delayed presentation (over 7 days).

COMPLICATIONS

Elbow stiffness is always a problem following elbow dislocations. This is more common when there are associated fractures. Early motion gives the best chance of avoiding this complication. Neurologic injury (11 percent) may occur, with the ulnar nerve most commonly involved. Most are neurapraxias from stretch but entrapment is also seen. Arterial injury is rare with possible lacerations, entrapment, and Volkmann's ischemia. Myositis ossificans is not uncommon, with 3 percent in pure dislocations and 18 percent when associated with fractures, and may be caused by vigorous attempts at reduction.

FOREARM AND WRIST FRACTURES

INCIDENCE

Fractures of the forearm and wrist are very common in children and account for 45 percent of all pediatric fractures. Most fractures (80 percent) occur in children greater than 5 years of age. The peak incidence corresponds to the peak velocity of growth when the bone is weakest. Up to 15 percent of children will have an ipsilateral supracondylar fracture.

ANATOMY

Ossification

The radial and ulnar shafts ossify during the eighth week of gestation. Associated epiphyses emerge at different ages: the distal radial epiphysis appears at 1 year of age (often from two centers); the distal ulnar epiphysis appears at age 6 years; the radial head appears at age 5 to 7 years; and the olecranon epiphysis appears at age 9 to 10 years. All of these epiphyses close between the ages of 16 and 18 years.

Osteology

The radius is a curved bone, cylindrical in the proximal third, triangular in the middle third, and flat distally with an apex lateral bow. The ulna has a triangular shape throughout, with an apex posterior bow in the proximal third.

The proximal radioulnar joint (PRUJ) is most stable in supination where the broadest part of the radial head contacts the radial notch of the ulna and the interosseous membrane is most taut. The annular ligament is its major soft tissue stabilizer. The distal radioulnar joint (DRUJ) is stabilized by the ulnar collateral ligament, the anterior and posterior radioulnar ligaments, and the pronator quadratus muscle. The triangular fibrocartilage complex (TFCC) has an articular disk joined by volar and dorsal radiocarpal ligaments and by ulnar collateral ligament fibers. It attaches to the distal radius at its ulnar margin, with its apex attached to the base of the ulna styloid. This firmly unites both bones. The periosteum is very strong and thick in the child. It is generally disrupted on the convex side, while an intact hinge remains on the concave side. This is an important consideration when attempting closed reduction.

Biomechanics

The posterior distal radioulnar ligament is taut in pronation, while the anterior ligament is taut in supination. The radius effectively shortens with pronation and lengthens with supination. The interosseous space is narrowest in pronation and widest in neutral to 30 degrees of supination. Further supination or pronation relaxes the membrane. The average range of pronation/supination is 90 degrees/90 degrees (50 degrees/50 degrees for function). Malreduction of 10 degrees in the middle third limits rotation by 20 to 30 degrees. Bayonet apposition (overlapping) does not reduce forearm rotation.

Deforming Muscle Forces

Proximal third fractures result in flexion and supination of the proximal fragment due to the pull of the biceps and supinator muscles, and pronation of the distal fragment due to the pull of the pronator teres and pronator quadratus. Middle third fractures result in the neutral position of the proximal fragment (due to the pull of the supinator, biceps, and pronator teres) and pronation of the distal fragment (pronator quadratus). Distal third fractures result in dorsiflexion and radial deviation of the distal segment due to the brachioradialis, and additional deformity due to the pull of the pronator quadratus, wrist flexors and extensors, and thumb abductors.

MECHANISM OF INJURY

The cause of forearm and wrist fracture may be indirect or direct. Indirect trauma is usually from a fall onto an outstretched hand. Rotation determines the direction of angulation. Pronation results in a flexion injury (posterior angulation) and supination in an extension (anterior angulation) injury. A direct mechanism would be a blow from an object onto the radial or ulnar shaft

CLINICAL EVALUATION

The history should identify the mechanism of injury, the age of the patient, and any other areas of pain. The physical examination should identify the deformity and skin integrity (remove all bandages). A complete neurovascular exam is essential. The elbow and wrist joints should be carefully examined to rule out contiguous injuries. Compartment syndrome, while rare, is a serious complication which must be avoided at all costs.

RADIOGRAPHIC EVALUATION

AP and lateral radiographs of the forearm, wrist, and elbow are essential. The forearm should not be rotated to obtain these views; instead, the x-ray beam should be rotated to obtain a cross-table view.

The bicipital tuberosity is the landmark for identifying the rotational position of the proximal fragment: at 90 degrees supination, it points medial; at a neutral position, it points posterior; and at 90 degrees pronation, it points lateral. The bicipital tuberosity should always be 180 degrees to the radial styloid.

CLASSIFICATION

Most fractures of the forearm and wrist are described by their location and type. Locations are proximal, middle, or distal third. Types are plastic deformation, incomplete ("greenstick"), compression ("torus" or "buckle"), or complete. The presence or absence of the physeal injury, as well as the type of fracture, is described.

A *Monteggia fracture* refers to a proximal ulna fracture with dislocation of the radial head. This accounts for 0.4 percent of all forearm fractures in children. The peak incidence is between 4 and 10 years of age. The ulnar fracture is usually located at the junction of proximal/middle thirds. It is classified by Bado (1967) and based on the direction of the radial head dislocation. The apex of the ulna fracture will point to the direction of the dislocation. (see Chap. 79). Many variations exist, including those which have plastic deformities.

A *Galeazzi fracture* is a middle to distal third radius fracture with an intact ulna and disruption of the distal radioulnar joint. This is a rare injury in children. The peak incidence is between 9 and 12 years of age.

Some 4 to 13 percent of elbow fractures may have ipsilateral forearm fractures. Combinations include forearm fracture with supracondylar humerus fracture (floating elbow), distal radial epiphysis fracture with supracondylar humerus fracture (floating elbow), elbow dislocation with forearm fracture, olecranon physeal fracture with distal radial physeal fracture, forearm fracture with lateral condylar humerus fracture, and distal forearm fracture with Monteggia type I or an equivalent fracture.

TREATMENT

Initial management consists of assessing the soft tissues and neurovascular status, obtaining prereduction radiographs, correcting the gross deformity, and splinting the extremity for pain relief and for prevention of further injury if closed reduction will be delayed. The extent and type of fracture and the child's age are factors that determine whether reduction can be carried out with sedation, local anesthesia, or general anesthesia. A closed reduction is performed with application of a well-molded long arm cast or splint.

The fracture level generally determines the forearm rotation used to maintain a reduction; however, these guidelines are highly disputed, so each fracture should be treated individually. Proximal third fractures are maintained in supination, middle third fractures are held in neutral, and distal third fractures are supported in pronation. Freshly applied casts should be split initially if there is concern about swelling inside the cast.

In general, patients older than 10 years of age should be managed like adults, and no deformity should be accepted. In patients less than 10 years of age, initial deformity can be accepted based on the natural history of remodeling (Fig. 69-3). Angular correction of 1 degree per month, or 10 degrees per year due to epiphyseal growth can be expected. Exponential correction occurs over time; therefore, increased correction occurs for greater deformities. Rotational deformities do not correct; therefore, rotational alignment must be perfect. Approximately 1 cm of bayonet apposition is acceptable and will remodel if the patient is less than 8 to 10 years old. Undisplaced distal radial fractures, such as an uncomplicated torus fracture of the distal radius, may be treated in a short arm cast for 3 weeks. All other

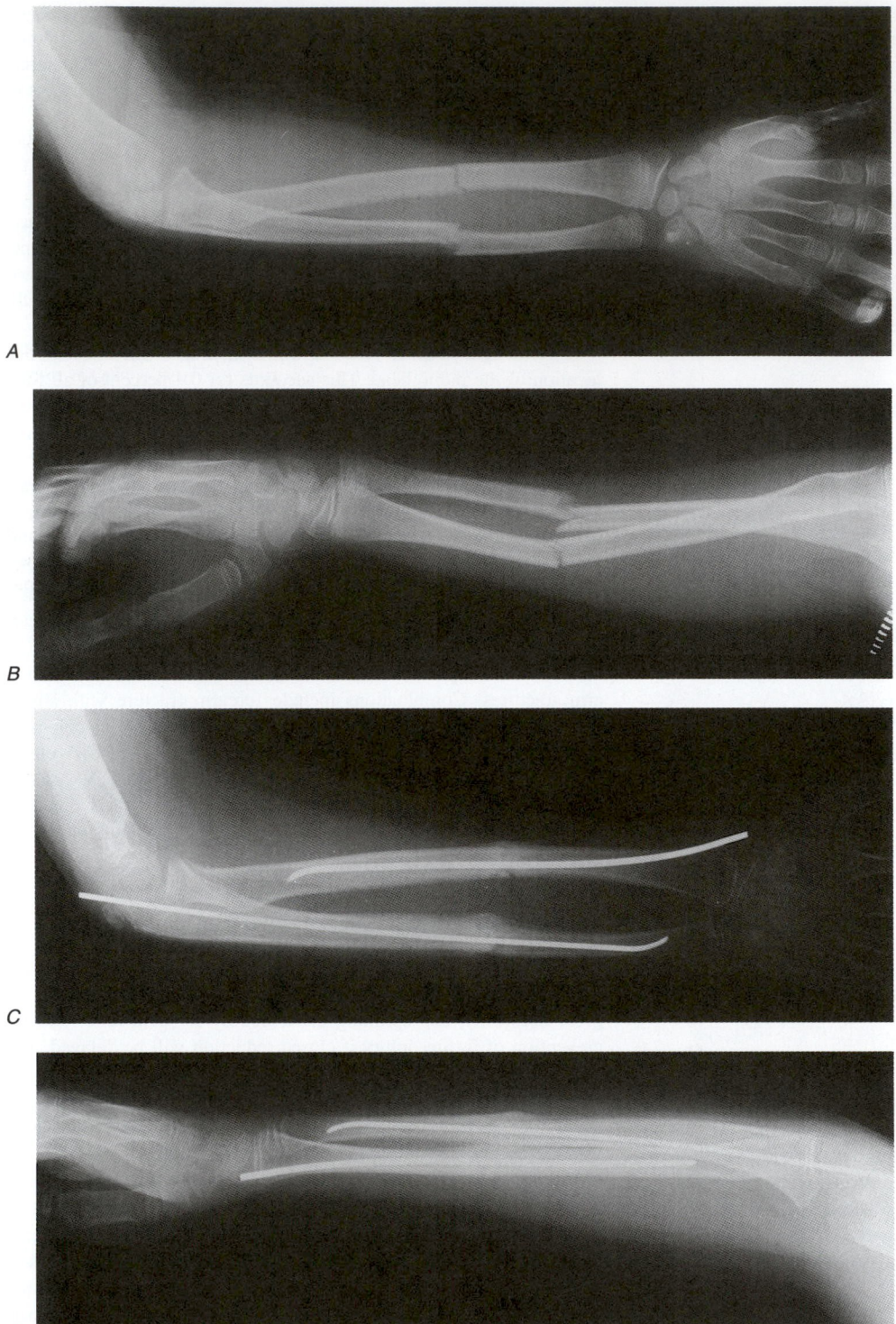

Figure 69-3
(*A*) Anteroposterior and (*B*) lateral views of 13-year-old male with inability to maintain acceptable alignment. (*C*) Anteroposterior and (*D*) lateral views of treatment with flexible intramedullary nails.

fractures should be treated in a long arm cast for 4 to 6 weeks until the fracture site is nontender and there is radiographic evidence of healing.

Plastic Deformation

Children less than 4 years of age or with deformities <20 degrees usually remodel and require only a long arm cast for 4 to 6 weeks until the fracture site is nontender. Any plastic deformation should be corrected that (1) prevents reduction of a concomitant fracture, (2) prevents full rotation in a child more than 4 years of age, or (3) exceeds 20 degrees (Fig. 69-4). General anesthesia is necessary, as forces of 20 to 30 kg are needed. The apex of the bow is placed over a well-padded wedge, a constant force is then applied for 2 to 3 min, followed by one application of a well-molded long arm cast. The correction should be within 10 to 20 degrees of anatomic angulation.

Greenstick Fractures

Nondisplaced or minimally displaced fractures should be held in a well-molded long arm cast. They should be slightly overcorrected to prevent recurrence. Completing the fracture decreases the risk of recurrence of the deformity; however, reduction of the displaced fracture may be more difficult. Therefore, it may be beneficial to carefully crack the intact cortex while preventing displacement. A well-molded long arm cast should then be applied.

Complete Displacement

Patients less than 10 years of age have greater remodeling potential; an attempt at closed reduction and casting should be performed. If the fracture is irreducible, open reduction and internal fixation may be indicated. Fractures in patients greater than 10 years of age and proximal third fractures are very difficult to manage by closed means; open reduction and internal fixation should generally be performed.

Physeal Injuries

Salter-Harris types I and II are treated by a gentle closed reduction, followed by application of a long arm cast or sugar tong splint; 50 percent apposition with no angular or rotational deformity is acceptable. Growth arrest can occur in 25 percent of patients if two or more manipulations are attempted.

In Salter-Harris type III fractures anatomic reduction must be achieved. Open reduction and internal fixation with smooth pins or screws parallel to the physis is recommended.

Salter-Harris type IV injuries are rare. Open reduction and internal fixation is performed if the fracture is displaced and growth disturbance is likely.

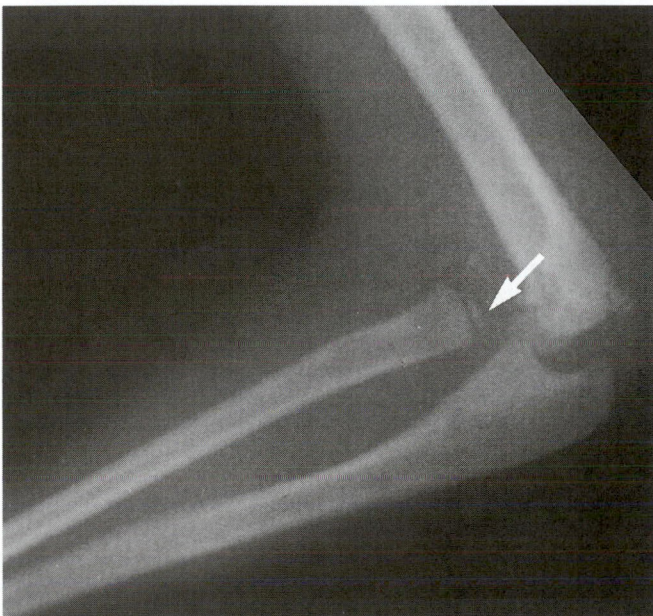

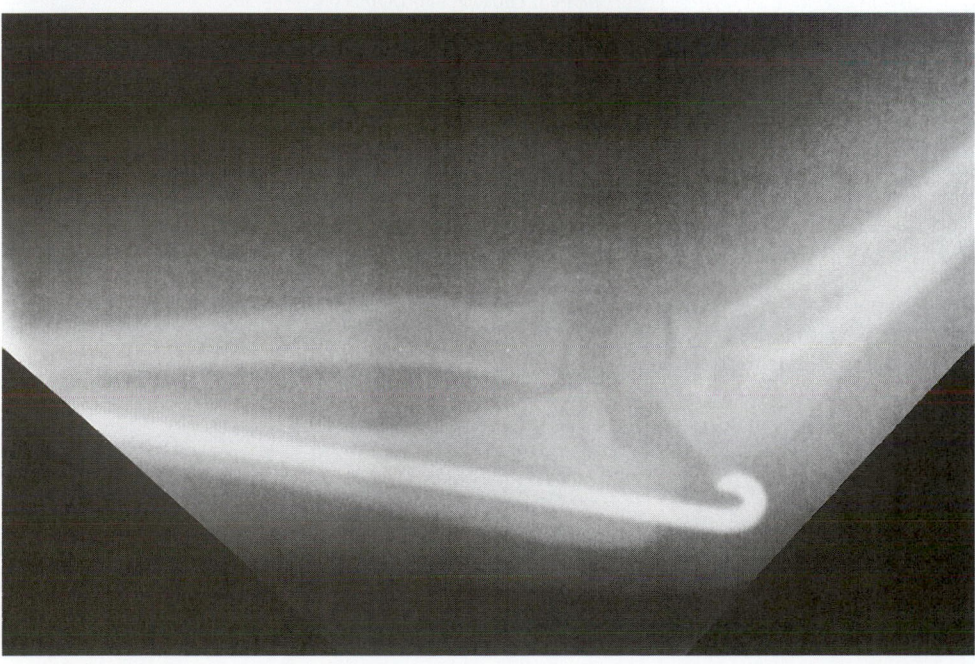

Figure 69-4
Seven-year-old female with (*A*) plastic deformation of ulna and anterior radial head dislocation (Monteggia's fracture) (*arrow*). *B*. Treatment with closed reduction and intramedullary nail of ulna.

COMPLICATIONS

Malunion

Common causes of malunion are inadequate follow-up, improper positioning in the cast, failure to perform cast changes when needed (redisplacement occurs in 7 to 13 percent of patients within the first 2 weeks), failure to correct inadequate reduction, and delay in diagnosis. Loss of pronation is more common in children (in contrast to adults). Over 60 percent have rotational losses of >20 degrees, yet more than 85 percent have satisfactory results.

Refracture

The incidence of refracture approaches 12 percent; therefore, refraining from active sports for 1 month after cast removal is recommended. Refracture may occur as late as 1 year after the initial injury.

Nonunion

Nonunion is extremely rare in children. It is more likely after high-energy trauma, open fractures, infection, or significant soft tissue loss. Ulnar nonunion occurs more commonly than radial nonunion.

Neurovascular Injuries

Direct injury to the nerves is unusual; however, anterior interosseus and median nerve injuries have been reported. Injury to the posterior interosseous nerve can be seen with Monteggia fractures (especially type III, lateral).

Compartment Syndrome

Compartment syndrome most commonly occurs after crush injuries or with an ipsilateral supracondylar humerus fracture. The cardinal symptom is pain aggravated by passive stretch of the fingers. Compartments feel tense, numbness and tingling are present in the hand, and there is a paucity of active motion of the fingers. Management includes removal of constricting bandages and splitting casts (including the padding). Compartment pressures >30 mmHg are indicative of the syndrome, at which time fasciotomies should be performed.

Infection

Infection is usually a consequence of an open fracture in which debridement is delayed more than 8 h. Contaminated fractures should undergo immediate irrigation and debridement with proper antibiotic coverage (including tetanus prophylaxis).

Reflex Sympathetic Dystrophy

Reflex sympathetic dystrophy (RSD) rarely occurs in children. Continuous burning pain, hyperesthesia, sweating, discoloration, and swelling are the cardinal signs. Aggressive physical therapy, psychological counseling, transcutaneous nerve stimulation, and stellate ganglion blocks are the mainstays of treatment. It usually resolves 6 to 12 months after the injury.

Overgrowth

Fast growth usually occurs for the first 6 to 8 months after the injury. Overgrowth averages 6 to 7 mm, which is generally insignificant.

SUGGESTED READINGS

Beaty JH: Fractures of the proximal humerus and shaft in children In Eilert RE (ed): *Instructional Course Lectures*. Park Ridge: American Academy of Orthopaedic Surgeons; 1992; 41:369.

Friberg KS: Remodeling after distal forearm fractures in children. III. Correction of residual angulation in fractures of the radius. *Acta Orthop Scand* 1979; 50(6 pt 2):741.

Hovelilus L: Anterior dislocation of the shoulder in teenagers and young adults. Five-year prognosis. *J Bone Jont Surg [Am]* 1987; 69:393.

Huber H, Gerber C: Voluntary subluxation of the shoulder in children. A long-term follow-up study of 36 shoulders. *J Bone Joint Surg [Br]* 1994; 76:118.

Jakob R, Fowles JV, Rang M, and Kassab MT: Observations concerning fractures of the lateral humeral condyle in children. *J Bone Joint Surg* 1975; 57-B:430.

Larsen CF, Kiaer T, Lindequist S: Fractures of the proximal humerus in children: Nine-year follow-up of 64 unoperated on cases. *Acta Orthop Scand* 1990; 61:255.

Milch HE: Fractures and fracture-dislocations of the humeral condyles. *J Trauma* 1964; 4:592.

O'Brien PI: Injuries involving the proximal radial epiphysis. *Clin Orthop* 1965; 41:51.

Vince KG, Miller JE: Cross-union complicating fracture of the forearm. Part II: Children. *J Bone Joint Surg [Am]* 1987; 69:654.

Wilkins KE: Fractures of the neck and head of the radius. In: *Fractures in Children*, Philadelphia: Lippincott; 1984:502.

Wilkins KE, Beaty JH, Chambers HG, et al: Fractures and dislocations of the elbow region. In Rockwood CA Jr, Wilkins KE, Beaty JH (eds): *Fractures in Children*, 4th ed. Philadelphia: JB Lippincott; 1996: chap 10.

Chapter 70

PELVIS AND HIP FRACTURES

David S. Feldman

PELVIC FRACTURES

Pelvic fractures in children are rare. They are, however, usually associated with significant injury. They often occur secondary to motor vehicle accidents, and usually result from high energy. When there is an osseous pelvic injury other structures may be involved, such as the viscera or genitourinary system. Pelvic fractures in children often do not require any treatment. This chapter will discuss these injuries specifically as they pertain to the younger child. Pelvic fractures in adolescents who are near skeletal maturity are treated as adults.

Pelvic fractures in children are unique in many respects. First, children will often have avulsion fractures of the apophyses without a break in the pelvic ring. Furthermore, injuries can occur through the triradiate cartilage in children which may have significance to the overall development of the acetabulum. The child also has elastic bone which may cause plastic deformation of the pelvis or displacement within a joint without a secondary break in the ring.

The three primary centers of ossification of the ilium, ischium, and pubis meet at the triradiate cartilage and fuse by approximately the age of 8 to 10 years. Secondary centers of ossification appear at the apophyses. Other secondary centers of ossification appear at the outer rim of the acetabulum, as well as in the ischium.

An accurate history may be difficult to obtain, and therefore, careful physical examination is important. In addition, careful examination of the neurologic status of the child, due to possible injury of the lumbosacral plexus, is quite important.

Radiographic evaluation is the same as for adults, including plain films, possible CT scan, and magnetic resonance imaging (MRI).

Due to the high incidence of concomitant injuries, the pelvic fracture may not be the life-threatening problem in the child. The mortality rate approaches 15 percent in children with a pelvic fracture; therefore, the overall child must be treated and concomitant conditions must be evaluated.

CLASSIFICATION

Classification of pelvic fractures is descriptive. The most common fracture is an avulsion fracture, and can occur at the anterior superior iliac spine, anterior inferior iliac spine, ischial tuberosity, or iliac apophyses. These injuries are quite common, and occur from a pull on the apophyses. This may be due to an eccentric load or a force that exceeds the limit of the apophyses. Patients will often be in a sporting activity such as soccer or football and will have immediate pain. They may develop limitation of motion and swelling in the region. Radiographs will demonstrate a varying amount of bony avulsion. Over time, there may be a large amount of callus formation.

Treatment consists of crutches, ice, and anti-inflammatories until, over the ensuing weeks, the fracture heals and the pain subsides.

Fractures may also occur in the sacrum or coccyx of children. Although they are difficult to diagnose, they are often treated conservatively.

The second type of fracture involves a single break in the pelvic ring and has three subtypes: a fracture of the ipsilateral inferior and superior pubic ramus; fractures near the symphysis pubis; and fractures near the sacroiliac joint. If these fractures are associated with the subluxation of the symphysis pubis or the sacroiliac joint, a pelvic sling can be utilized with progressive ambulation after approximately 4 weeks. The prognosis for these fractures is quite good and one must rule out visceral injuries.

A third type of injury is a double break in the pelvic ring. These include bilateral superior and inferior pubic rami fractures (a straddle fracture). This fracture can be treated conservatively in children as it will unite, and the children can be allowed to ambulate after approximately 4 to 6 weeks. Another fracture is a vertical shear fracture which often occurs in an older child. Treatment, once again, should tend to be conservative, with skeletal traction and possibly an external fixator if there is an open-book injury. Open reduction of these fractures should be reserved for those fractures which are not able to be maintained in an acceptable alignment closed. A subtype of fracture is a multiple-fractured pelvis. Once again, the most important problem here is massive hemorrhage and closing of the book with a fixator may be indicated. Visceral injury is quite common.

The fourth type of pelvic fracture is a fracture of the acetabulum. There are two types: a fracture associated with dislocation of the hip, and a fracture through the acetabulum, which is associated with a nondisplaced pelvic fracture. The child can also develop a central dislocation of the hip, injuring the triradiate cartilage. A fracture of the acetabulum in children usually connotes another injury. There may be an associated posterior dislocation of the hip, in which case, treatment would consist of a concentric reduction. As long as the hip is stable, no other treatment is required. Open reduction is indicated if the reduction is not concentric, and the entrapped capsule or bony fragment needs to be removed.

If the fracture consists of a pelvic fracture with an associated acetabulum fracture, treatment depends on the type of acetabular fracture seen. If it is a displaced fracture of the acetabulum with loss of weightbearing surface, this needs open reduction and internal fixation (ORIF), similar to an adult. Treatment of a central dislocation of the hip or a triradiate cartilage injury requires observation. As this child may develop subluxation of the hip later with dysplasia, it may require an acetabular reconstruction at a later date.

HIP FRACTURES

INCIDENCE

Hip fractures are uncommon in children, occurring 1/100th as often as in adults (Fig. 70-1).

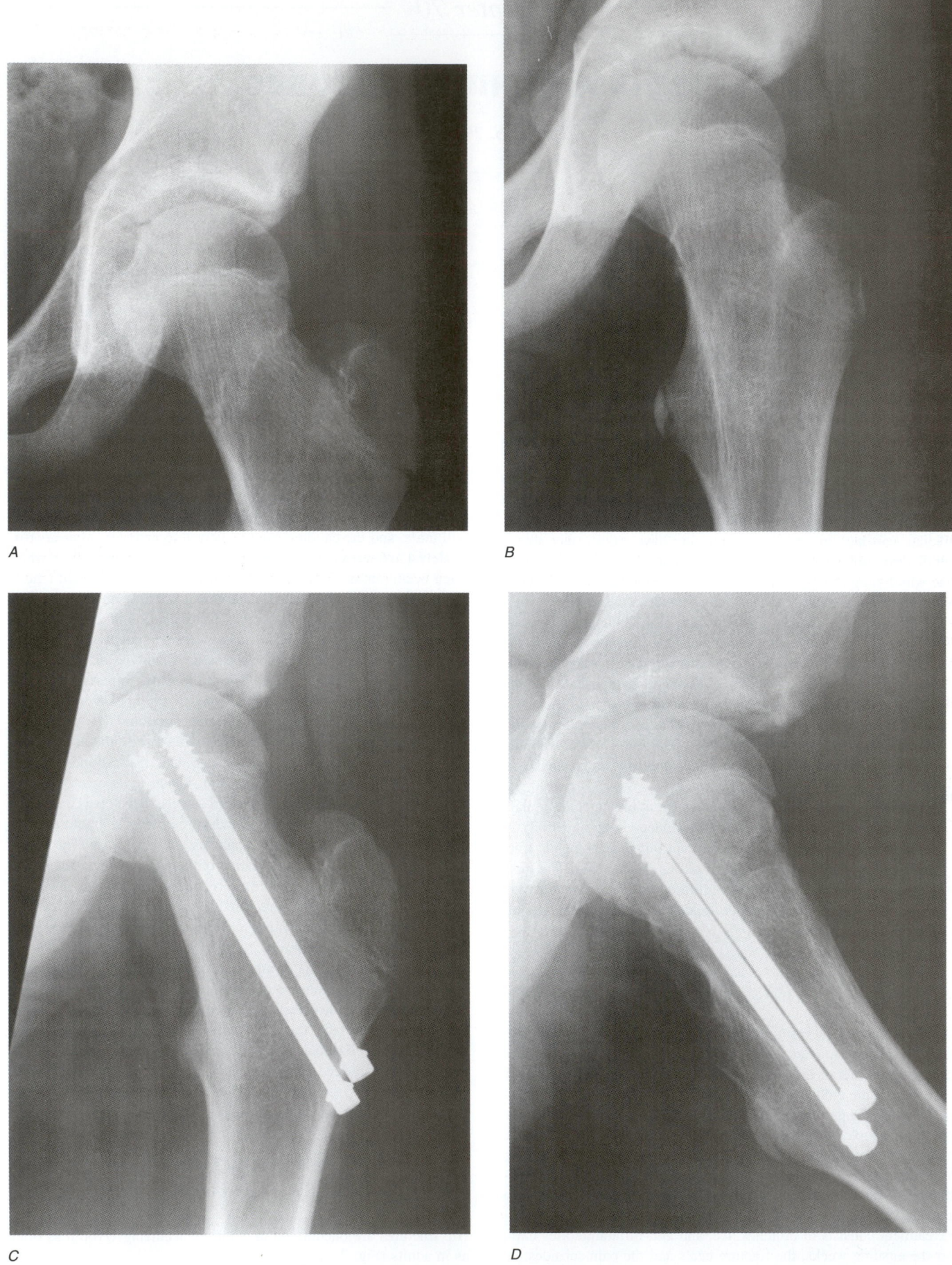

Figure 70-1
Femoral neck fracture in 13-year-old boy; (*A*) AP view, (*B*) lateral view. After ORIF; (*C*) AP view, (*D*) lateral view.

ANATOMY

Ossification of the proximal femur occurs at week 7 in utero, of the epiphysis by 4 months after birth, and of the trochanter by 4 years. Fusion of the proximal femoral epiphysis occurs by 18 years of age and of the trochanteric apophysis by 16 to 18 years.

Blood is supplied to the hip by the lateral femoral circumflex artery and, more importantly, the medial femoral circumflex artery. Anastomoses at the anterosuperior portion of the intertrochanteric groove form the extracapsular ring. Ascending retinacular vessels travel to the epiphysis. Vessels of the ligamentum teres contribute little before age 8 and approximately 20 percent in adulthood.

MECHANISM OF INJURY

Fractures of the hip in children ordinarily occur secondary to a high-energy injury such as a motor vehicle accident or child abuse. Children will also develop these fractures if their bone has been weakened by disease such as Gaucher's disease, fibrous dysplasia, or a bone cyst.

CLASSIFICATION AND TREATMENT

Type I: Transepiphyseal Fracture

Transepiphyseal fractures account for 8 percent of pediatric hip fractures. The rate of osteonecrosis approaches 100 percent. If minimal trauma occurs in a young child with this injury, hypothyroidism, hypogonadism, and renal disease should be considered. In newborns, differential diagnosis includes congenital hip dysplasia (CHD) and septic arthritis due to the nonossified femoral head mimicking a dislocation.

Treatment consists of closed reduction with pin fixation. Threaded pins should be used in the older child, smooth pins in the young child. ORIF is done if the fracture is irreducible by closed means.

Type II: Transcervical Fracture

Transcervical fractures account for 45 percent of pediatric hip fractures (most common type). Up to 80 percent are displaced, and the osteonecrosis rate approaches 50 percent.

Treatment for nondisplaced fractures consists of either an abduction spica cast or operative in situ pinning; these may evolve to coxa vara or nonunion. For displaced fractures, closed reduction (or open, if necessary) and pinning should be performed; the fixation pins should not cross the physis.

Type III: Cervicotrochanteric Fracture

Cervicotrochanteric fractures account for 30 percent of pediatric hip fractures. The rate of osteonecrosis is 20 to 30 percent.

In nondisplaced fractures traction is applied, then spica versus immediate abduction spica versus in situ pinning. In displaced fractures, ORIF should be performed (the physis must not be crossed with pins).

Type IV: Intertrochanteric Fracture

Intertrochanteric fractures account for 10 to 15 percent of pediatric hip fractures and are frequently secondary to a direct blow. This fracture has fewer complications than other hip fractures in children.

Treatment consists of 2 to 3 weeks of traction, then abduction spica casting for 6 to 12 weeks. ORIF is performed for unstable fractures or where closed reduction is achievable.

COMPLICATIONS OF PEDIATRIC HIP FRACTURES

Osteonecrosis occurs in up to 40 percent of hip fractures in children. The incidence of osteonecrosis is directly related to initial fracture displacement and the fracture location. Ratliff described three types of osteonecrosis. In type I (60 percent), there is diffuse, complete head involvement and collapse; this type has a poor prognosis. In type II (22 percent), there is localized head involvement only, with minimal collapse. Type III (18 percent) fractures have femoral neck involvement only, with sparing of the femoral head.

There is an increased incidence of premature closure of the epiphyseal plate with pins penetrating into the physis; this complication may cause femoral shortening, coxa vara, and a short femoral neck. It is frequently seen with osteonecrosis, and trochanteric arrest may be indicated for children under 8 years of age.

The incidence of coxa vara is approximately 20 percent and may be secondary to inadequate reduction. There is a reduced incidence noted with ORIF.

The incidence of nonunion is approximately 10 percent and is seen primarily with inadequate reduction or inadequate internal fixation. Treatment includes valgus osteotomy with or without bone graft.

HIP DISLOCATION

Hip dislocations are more common than hip fractures. The incidence is greater in children under 3 years of age due to joint laxity and soft pliable cartilage. Posterior dislocations occur 10 times more frequently than anterior dislocations.

TREATMENT

Treatment consists of closed reduction within 12 h, with open reduction if the dislocation irreducible. Careful attention should be given to the reduction as it is possible that soft tissue interposition may lead to a nonconcentric reduction.

COMPLICATIONS

Osteonecrosis (8 to 10 percent) is a known complication of hip dislocation. There is a decreased incidence below the age of 5 and an increased incidence with a delay in reduction. Patients should be evaluated for possible epiphyseal separation. Patients may also suffer from recurrent dislocations (due to capsular tears or capsular attenuation). Degenerative joint disease is a possible long-term complication.

SUGGESTED READINGS

Barquet A: Traumatic hip dislocation in childhood. A report of 26 cases and a review of the literature. *Acta Orthop Scand* 1979; 50:549.

Canale ST: Fractures of the hip in children and adolescents. *Orthop Clin North Am* 1990; 21:341.

Davison BL, Weinstein SL: Hip fractures in children. A long-term follow-up study. *J Pediatr Orthop* 1992; 12:355.

Heeg M, Klasen HJ, Visser JD: Acetabular fractures in children and adolescents. *J Bone Joint Surg [Br]* 1989; 71:418.

Sundar M, Carty H: Avulsion fractures of the pelvis in children: A report of 32 fractures and their outcome. *Skel Radiol* 1994; 23:85.

Chapter 71

LOWER EXTREMITY

David S. Feldman

FEMORAL SHAFT FRACTURES

MECHANISM OF INJURY

Femoral shaft fractures in children may be the result of a high-energy direct blow such as from a motor vehicle accident or it may be from a relatively minor rotational injury. One must consider physical abuse in a child presenting with a femur fracture, and particularly in children below the age of 3 years.

CLASSIFICATION

Femoral shaft fractures are classified in a descriptive manner, that is, open versus closed, level of fracture, fracture pattern, degree of comminution, and displacement, as well as the area of the bone fractured.

TREATMENT

The treatment of the fracture depends on the age and size of the child. Children between the ages of 0 and 2 years should be treated with application of a hip spica cast within the first few days after the fracture. This may require adjustment (wedging of the cast) or replacement during the treatment period. Early spica cast application may lead to malunion unless careful follow up and correction are performed if the fracture fragments shift.

Children between the ages of 2 and 10 years are treated depending on the fracture pattern. If the fracture has less than 2 cm of overriding, then the child can be treated with an early spica cast. With greater than 2 cm of overriding, traction (preferably distal femoral pin proximal to the physis) until callus has formed and then a spica cast until fracture consolidation is the treatment of choice.

In children between the ages of 10 and 15 years, with multiple injuries or open fracture, external fixation may be considered (Fig. 71-1). Adolescents may be treated with an intramedullary nail; however, this has fallen into disfavor due to the risk of osteonecrosis to the femoral head with antegrade insertion of the nail. Retrograde-inserted flexible nails may be a good alternative in the adolescent. An acceptable reduction differs by age. In ages 2 to 10 years, up to 2 cm overriding is acceptable and may be preferable. In children older than 10, up to 1 cm overriding is acceptable.

Acceptable angular deformity is approximately 30 degrees in the sagittal plane and 10 degrees in the frontal plane. Although no rotation is preferable, up to 10 degrees is acceptable with external rotation being more easily accepted.

Indications for operative intervention include patients with multiple trauma, head trauma, open fractures, vascular injury, and pathologic fractures. The method utilized to stabilize the fracture in these patients depends on the type of injury, extent of soft tissue injury, the age of the patient, and the surgeon's preference. Choices include external fixation with a monolateral frame and rigid or flexible Im rod or plate fixation.

COMPLICATIONS

Complications following femoral shaft fractures in children are unusual. Malunion may occur as remodeling will often not correct rotational malalignment. Although nonunion is rare, delayed union particularly with treatment with an external fixator has been recognized (Fig. 71-2). Overgrowth of the femur after femoral shaft fractures is always a concern in children below the age of 10 years. The overgrowth may be as great as 1.5 to 2.0 cm. Although this cannot be avoided, care should be taken not to over distract the fracture in children with femur fractures. These children should be followed through adolescence.

PEDIATRIC KNEE

ANATOMY

The knee is a hinge joint with little osseous stability. It thus relies on ligamentous integrity for most of its stability. Because ligaments in the immature skeleton are more resistant to tensile stresses than are physeal plates, trauma leads to physeal separations and avulsions not seen in the skeletally mature patient. There are three physeal plates with secondary ossification centers about the knee. The distal femur appears at the 39th week of gestation , the proximal tibia at birth, and the tibial tubercle between the seventh and ninth years. Physeal closure occurs between the ages of 15 and 19 years in all physes about the knee. The tibial tubercle may close several years earlier. The patella is a sesamoid bone, with its own ossification center, which appears at age 3 to 5 years. Two-thirds of longitudinal growth of the lower extremity is provided by the distal femoral (3/8 in. per year) and proximal tibial (1/4 in. per year) physes.

DISTAL FEMORAL FRACTURES

INCIDENCE

The distal femoral physis is the most common physeal injury about the knee. It accounts for up to 5 percent of all physeal injuries in children. Two-thirds of these fractures occur in adolescents.

ANATOMY

The distal femoral epiphysis is the largest and fastest growing physis in the body. There is no inherent protection of the physis; ligamentous and tendinous structures insert on the epiphysis. The sciatic nerve divides at the level of the distal femur. The popliteal artery gives off

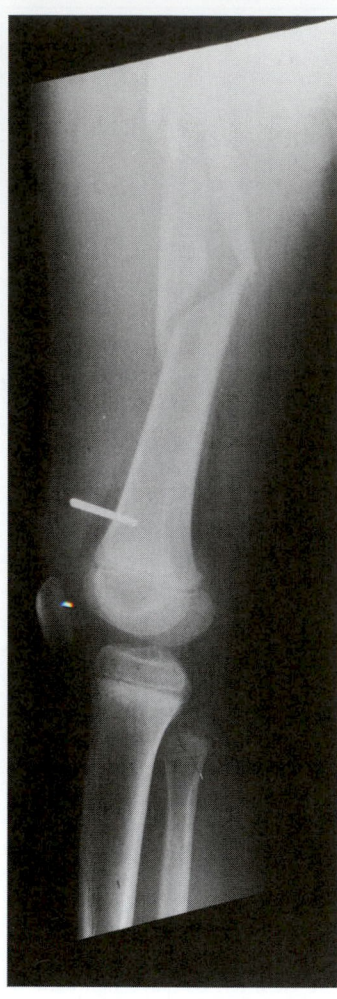

A

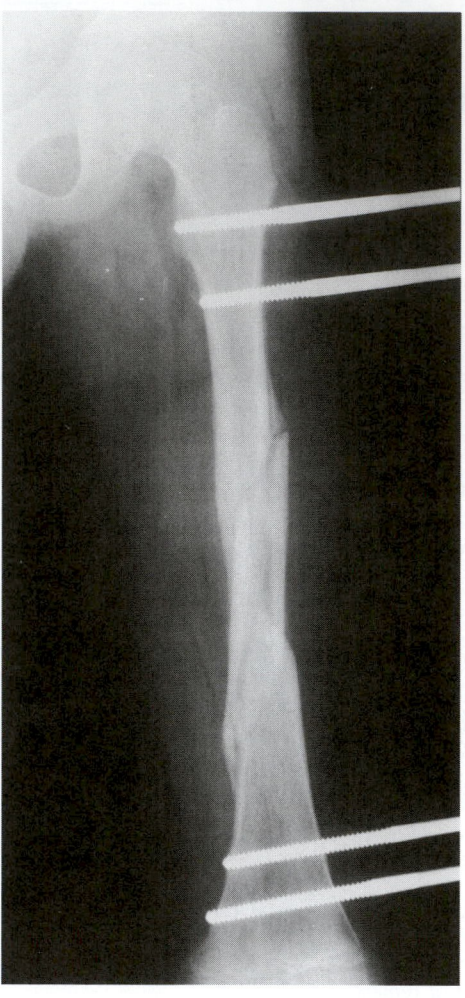

B

Figure 71-1

(*A*) Femur fracture treated with traction overnight and (*B*) then external fixation.

the superior geniculate branches to the knee just posterior to the femoral metaphysis.

MECHANISM OF INJURY

Indirect injury is the most common cause of distal femoral epiphyseal separation. Valgus is the most common force causing this injury; however, excessive varus, hyperflexion, or hyperextension can also cause this fracture. Occasionally, a difficult delivery (breech presentation) can cause this fracture. In addition, minimal trauma in conditions that cause generalized weakening of the growth plate (osteomyelitis, leukemia, myelodysplasia) may be the causative factor.

CLINICAL EVALUATION

The child will ordinarily be unable to bear weight on the extremity and will hold the knee in flexion with apparent hamstring tightness. A displaced fracture may demonstrate gross shortening or obvious angular deformity. The distal neurologic status must be carefully assessed.

RADIOLOGIC EVALUATION

AP, lateral, and oblique views of the distal femur and knee are needed with comparison views of the normal side if indicated. Stress views

should be obtained to diagnose type I or other nondisplaced separations. CT scan or tomograms can be used to assess intraarticular involvement. Angiogram should be utilized if vascular injury is suspected. An arthrogram can be used if a large chondral defect is suspected.

CLASSIFICATION

Distal femoral physeal separations are most commonly classified by the Salter-Harris classification. Type I injuries are seen in newborns and adolescents. The diagnosis can easily be missed. A key may be physeal widening on stress radiographs. Type II injuries are the most common of the distal femoral phis. Displacement is usually medial or lateral with a metaphyseal fragment on the compression side.

DISPLACEMENT

Medial displacement is caused by a valgus force and is the most common fracture encountered. Lateral displacement is caused by a varus force. These fractures most commonly represent a Salter-Harris type II physeal separation. Anterior displacement results from a hyperextension injury. There is a high incidence of neurovascular injury from stretch on the neurovascular structures, as well as the proximal metaphyseal spike being driven posteriorly. Posterior displacement is caused by a hyperflexion injury and is quite rare.

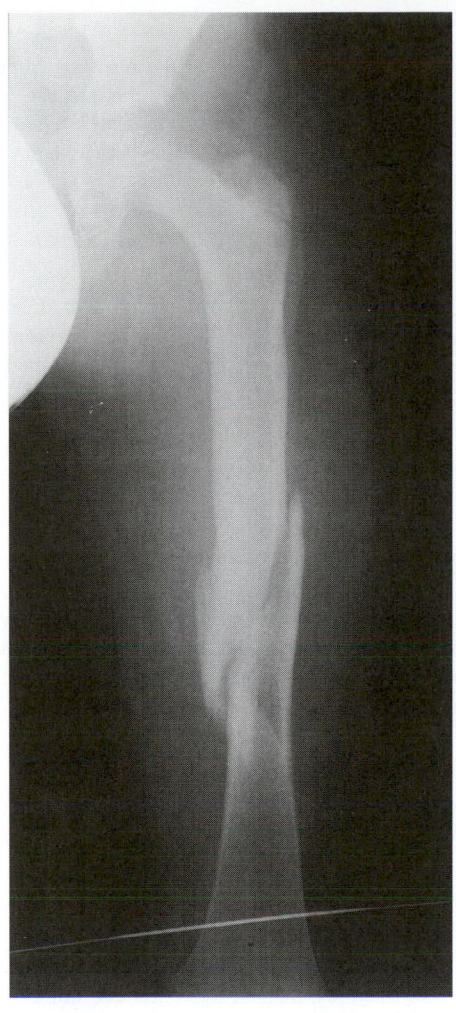
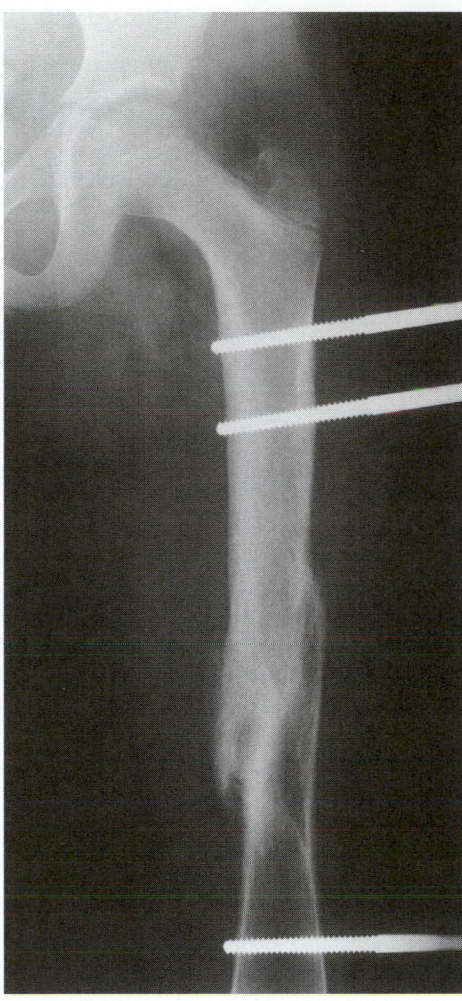

A   B

Figure 71-2
Refracture of femoral shaft fracture (A) in an 11-year-old boy with reapplication of external fixator (B).

TREATMENT

Nondisplaced fractures should be immobilized in a single leg hip spica. Displaced fractures should be treated with closed reduction with traction and gentle manipulation: medial/lateral—immobilize in 15 to 20 degrees knee flexion; anterior—immobilize first at 90 degrees, then decrease with time; and posterior—immobilize in extension.

Indications for open reduction and/or internal fixation include an irreducible Salter-Harris type II fracture with interposed soft tissue and a Salter-Harris type III or IV fracture in which joint congruity must be restored. If an unstable reduction is encountered then smooth percutaneous wires or cannulated screws avoiding the physis should be inserted. The metaphyseal fragment can be stabilized to the intact metaphysis. Crossing the physis should be avoided, if possible. If the physis must be crossed (small or no metaphyseal fragment), then smooth pins, placed as perpendicular as possible to the physis should be utilized. The fixation should be removed as soon as possible.

COMPLICATIONS

Popliteal artery injury (<2 percent) is associated with hyperextension injuries. Peroneal nerve palsy (3 percent) is caused by traction injury during fracture or reduction. Multiple attempts at reduction may further injure the physis. Angular deformity (19 percent) can be caused by asymmetric physeal closure. Leg length discrepancy (24 percent) depends on the age of the child. Knee stiffness (16 percent) is due to adhesions and involves capsular or muscular contractures.

PROXIMAL TIBIAL FRACTURES

INCIDENCE

This represents less than 1 percent of all physeal injuries and usually occurs in adolescence.

ANATOMY

The popliteal artery runs behind the posterior aspect of the upper tibia. The blood supply is from the anastomosis of the inferior geniculate arteries. The physis is well protected, which may account for the low incidence of injuries to the proximal tibia physis.

MECHANISM OF INJURY

A direct blow to the upper tibia (motor vehicle, lawnmower accident) or an indirect tibia injury due to hyperextension or abduction is the most common cause of this injury. A birth injury with hyperextension during breech delivery may also be a causative factor in a newborn.

CLINICAL EVALUATION

Pain and inability to bear weight are the most common presenting symptoms. A hemarthrosis may be present. There is tenderness over the proximal tibial physis with possible gross deformity or angulation. Popliteal artery injury and/or compartment syndrome are possible, and one must assess neurovascular status.

CLASSIFICATION

The Salter-Harris classification for proximal tibial fractures includes five types. Type I is a transphyseal injury, and the diagnosis is often missed; it may require stress or comparison views. Type II is a transphyseal injury exiting the metaphysis. One-third of type II injuries are nondisplaced; those that displace usually do so medially into valgus. Type III is an intraarticular fracture of the lateral plateau; it is more common than the medial. The fracture line exits the physis. Type IV is an intraarticular fracture of the medial or lateral plateau; the fracture line exits the metaphysis. Type V is a crush injury; the diagnosis is retrospective after growth arrest.

DISPLACEMENT

Medial displacement is caused by an abduction force. Posterior displacement is caused by a hyperextension force and has an increased incidence of popliteal artery injury. The tibial tubercle and fibula prevent anterior and lateral displacement, respectively.

TREATMENT

Salter-Harris types I and II fractures, if nondisplaced, can be treated in a long leg cast but should be monitored closely for displacement. Displaced fractures should be treated by gentle closed reduction and held with smooth pins across the physis in type I and parallel to the physis (metaphysis) in type II. Salter-Harris types III and IV require open reduction and internal fixation (ORIF) parallel to the physis; articular congruity is the goal.

COMPLICATIONS

Recurrent displacement can be seen. Popliteal artery injury is seen, particularly in hyperextension injuries. Compartment syndrome is possible, and patients need to be observed for this complication. Peroneal nerve palsy may occur from a traction injury. Physeal arrest, angular deformity, and leg length discrepancy are common late complications after fracture.

TIBIAL TUBERCLE FRACTURES

INCIDENCE

Tibial tubercle fractures represent 1 to 3 percent of all physeal injuries, and are most commonly seen in athletic males 14 to 16 years old. It is important to differentiate these fractures from Osgood-Schlatter disease.

ANATOMY

The tibial tubercle physis, which is continuous with the tibial plateau, is most vulnerable between the ages of 13 and 16 years, when it closes from posterior to anterior.

MECHANISM OF INJURY

The mechanism of injury is typically indirect, usually resulting from a sudden accelerating or decelerating force involving the quadriceps mechanism. Predisposing factors include patella baja, tight hamstrings, preexisting Osgood-Schlatter disease, and disorders with physeal abnormalities.

CLINICAL EVALUATION

There is swelling and tenderness over the affected region with an associated hemarthrosis. A palpable fragment of bone may be present. Patella alta will be evident if there is severe displacement and there is little or no ability to actively extend the knee.

CLASSIFICATION

Watson-Jones

The Watson-Jones classification describes three types of tibial tubercle fractures. In type I, a small fragment is avulsed and displaced proximally. In type II, the secondary ossification center has already coalesced with the proximal tibial epiphysis; the fracture occurs at this junction. With type III, the fracture line passes proximally through the tibial epiphysis and into the joint.

Ogden

The Ogden classification is a modification of the Watson-Jones classification (*above*) and subdivides each type into A and B categories to account for degree of displacement and comminution.

TREATMENT

For type IA tibial tubercle fractures, manual reduction and immobilization is recommended. With types IB, II, and III, ORIF with screws or tension band wiring are advocated.

COMPLICATIONS

Genu recurvatum secondary to premature closure of the anterior physis is rare because the injury occurs near skeletal maturity. There may be residual knee stiffness. Patella alta may occur if the reduction is insufficient.

TIBIAL SPINE FRACTURES

ANATOMY

There are two tibial spines: anterior and posterior. The anterior cruciate ligament (ACL) spans from the medial aspect of the lateral femoral condyle to the anterior tibial spine. Since in the immature skeleton ligaments are more resistant to tensile stresses than are physeal cartilage or cancellous bone, forces that would lead to an ACL tear in an adult cause avulsion of the incompletely ossified tibial spine in the child.

MECHANISM OF INJURY

Falls from a bicycle account for 50 percent of tibial spine fracture cases caused by rotatory, hyperextension, or valgus forces.

CLINICAL EVALUATION

Patients with tibial spine fracture present with a painful hemarthrosis. There may be a bony block to full extension. Anterior draw is positive only if there is a concomitant MCL injury.

RADIOLOGIC EVALUATION

AP, lateral, and plateau views should be obtained. CT scan may afford better appreciation of fracture displacement.

CLASSIFICATION

Meyers and McKeever (1970) described four types of tibial spine avulsion fractures. Type I has minimal or no displacement of the fragment. Type II has an angular elevation of the anterior portion with an intact posterior hinge. Type III includes complete displacement with or without rotation (15 percent). Type IV is comminuted (5 percent). Types I and II account for 80 percent of tibial spine fractures.

TREATMENT

Treatment of types I and II tibial spine fractures are immobilized in extension. The fat pad may contact the spine in extension and thus help with reduction. Types III and IV have demonstrated poor results with conservative management. Arthrotomy is recommended with debridement of the fracture site and fixation with sutures, pins, or screws. Arthroscopic fixation may be attempted in order to avoid arthrotomy. Fixation devices should be placed into the tibial epiphysis avoiding the physis.

PATELLA FRACTURES

INCIDENCE

Patella fractures are rare in children, with only 1 percent of all patella fractures seen in patients under 15 years of age.

ANATOMY

The patella is the largest sesamoid in the body. Its two functions are to protect intraarticular structures and to increase the mechanical advantage of the quadriceps. Forces generated by the quadriceps in children are not as high as adults due to a smaller muscle mass and shorter moment arm. The blood supply to the patella derives from the anastomotic ring from the superior and inferior geniculate arteries. An additional supply through the distal pole is from the fat pad. The ossification center appears between 3 and 5 years, proceeds peripherally, and is complete by 10 to 13 years. This fracture must be differentiated from the bipartite patella, which is located superolaterally.

MECHANISM OF INJURY

A direct blow or an indirect injury, such as a sudden accelerating or decelerating force on the quadriceps, is the cause of patella fractures. Marginal fractures are usually medial due to patellar subluxation or dislocation laterally.

CLINICAL EVALUATION

In patella fractures there is often swelling, tenderness, and a hemarthrosis. The extremity should be tested for active extension of the knee as well as the presence of a palpable defect. Patella alta may represent an avulsion or a sleeve fracture.

CLASSIFICATION

The classification of patella fractures is descriptive. The fracture may be transverse, complete, or incomplete. A marginal fracture may be present which results from lateral subluxation or dislocation of the patella. A sleeve fracture is unique to the immature skeleton, and consists of an extensive sleeve of cartilage pulled from the osseous patella. A stellate fracture occurs from direct trauma in the older child. The child can also have a longitudinal or avulsion fracture.

TREATMENT

For nondisplaced fractures of the patella, closed treatment with a cylinder cast in extension is the treatment of choice. Displaced fractures (>4 mm diastasis or >3 mm articular step-off) should be treated with tension band wiring, sutures, or screws, and the retinaculum must also be repaired. Sleeve fractures are treated with careful reduction of the involved pole and cartilaginous sleeve, stabilization, and retinacular repair; if this is not done, the result will be an elongated patella with extensor lag and quadriceps weakness.

COMPLICATIONS

Complications of patella fractures include compromised quadriceps function secondary to a missed diagnosis or inadequate treatment. Degenerative changes may occur if the articular surface is left unreduced.

KNEE DISLOCATION

Knee dislocations are rare in skeletally immature individuals. The trauma necessary to disrupt ligaments usually disrupts the physis first. These events are frequently associated with major disruptions of soft tissue and damage to neurovascular structures. Vascular repair must take place within the first 6 to 8 h to avoid permanent damage. The clinical evaluation and treatment are the same as for adults.

PROXIMAL TIBIAL METAPHYSEAL FRACTURES

Although these fractures are uncommon, they usually occur in the young child between ages 3 to 6 years. They mostly consist of nondisplaced greenstick fractures of the medial cortex. The fibula generally remains intact. Treatment consists of a long leg cast with the knee in full extension with a varus moment placed on the cast to prevent valgus collapse.

COMPLICATIONS

Primarily progressive valgus angulation may occur after this fracture. This may be due to primary tethering of the fibula with tibia overgrowth or initial valgus positioning of the fracture. Treatment consists of observation with gradual restoration of the mechanical axis of the limb. The natural resolution of this problem has been recently questioned by some authors.

TIBIA SHAFT FRACTURES

Tibia and fibula fractures are relatively common in children. They occur at all ages in childhood. Various age groups have specific fractures such as the young child below the age of 4 years. The most commonly fractured area is the distal one-third, accounting for approximately 50 percent of all tibia fractures.

Tibial shaft fractures in children can often be treated nonsurgically. The fracture should be reduced to obtain an angular correction within 10 degrees of anatomic and correct rotation. Apposition of the fragments should be at least 50 percent. Fractures close to the ankle usually have apex posterior angulation and may need to be treated in a cast in plantar flexion. Angulation in the sagittal plane close to the ankle is well tolerated in children.

Indications for open reduction or stabilization with an external fixator are the same as those for adults.

PEDIATRIC ANKLE

INCIDENCE

Ligamentous injuries, in general, are rare in children because their ligaments are stronger relative to bone; therefore, fractures of the ankle in children are quite common.

ANATOMY

All ligaments attach distal to the physes of the tibia and fibula; this is important in understanding fracture patterns in children. The distal tibial ossific nucleus appears between the ages of 2 and 3 years; it fuses with the shaft at about 15 years of age in girls and 17 years in boys. Over an 18-month period, the lateral portion of the distal tibial physis remains open while the medial part has closed. The distal fibular ossific nucleus appears at age 2 and unites with the shaft at age 20 years. Secondary ossification centers occur and can be confused with a fracture of either the medial or lateral malleolus; they are often bilateral.

CLINICAL EVALUATION

The entire limb should be examined in suspected ankle fracture. In particular, tenderness, swelling, ecchymosis, deformity, and neurovascular status are assessed.

RADIOGRAPHIC EVALUATION

AP, lateral, and oblique views are used initially. CT scan or tomography is often helpful with complex intraarticular fracture patterns.

CLASSIFICATION

Dias and Tachdjian

In the Dias and Tachdjian classification of ankle fractures, Lauge-Hansen principles are correlated with the Salter-Harris classification. Typology is simplified by noting the direction of physeal displacement, Salter-Harris type, and location of the metaphyseal fragment. Classification aids in determining the proper maneuver for closed reduction.

Supination–External Rotation (SER)   *Stage I*: Salter-Harris II fracture of the distal tibia with the metaphyseal fragment located posterolaterally; a long spiral fracture of the distal tibia starting laterally at the physis.

Stage II: As external rotation force continues, a spiral fracture of the fibula occurs, beginning medially and extending posterosuperiorly; this differs from an adult SER injury.

Pronation–Eversion   In *pronation–eversion* [external rotation (PER)] injuries, tibial and fibular fractures occur simultaneously. It is most commonly a Salter-Harris type II fracture of the distal tibial physis, but type I also occurs; the metaphyseal fragment is located laterally. A short oblique distal fibular fracture occurs 4 to 7 cm proximal to the fibula tip.

Supination–Plantar Flexion   *Supination–plantar flexion* (SPF) most commonly is a Salter-Harris type II fracture of the distal tibial physis with the metaphyseal fragment posterior. A fibula fracture is rare in this injury.

Supination–Inversion   *Supination–inversion* (SI) is the most common mechanism of fracture with the highest incidence of complications.

Stage I: Salter-Harris type I or II fracture of the distal fibular physis is most common; pain can be noted along the physis when radiographs are negative.

Stage II: Salter-Harris type III or IV fracture of the medial tibial physis, as the talus wedges into the medial tibial articular surface; rarely, a type I or II fracture; occasionally an open injury associated with a talus fracture (Fig. 71-3).

Juvenile-Tillaux Fractures

A juvenile-Tillaux fracture is a Salter-Harris type III fracture of the anterolateral tibial epiphysis. External rotation force causes the anterior tibiofibular ligament to avulse the fragment. This fracture occurs in the 12- to 14-year age group when the central and medial portions of the distal tibial physis have already fused and the lateral physis remains open. CT scan or tomograms are helpful in distinguishing this injury from triplane fractures.

Triplane Fractures

A triplane fracture occurs in three planes: transverse, coronal, and sagittal. It is best explained by fusion of the tibial physis from central to anteromedial to posteromedial, and finally to lateral. The peak incidence of triplane fractures is 13 to 15 years in males and 12 to 14 years in females. The mechanism of injury is thought to be external rotation of the foot and ankle. A fibular fracture is possible; usually oblique from anteroinferior to posterosuperior, 4 to 6 cm proximal to the tip. The tibia may be in two or three parts.

CT scans are invaluable in preoperative assessment. Two-part fractures are either medial, where the coronal fragment is posteromedial, or lateral, where the coronal fragment is posterolateral. Three-part fractures consist of (1) an anterolateral fragment that mimics the Juvenile-Tillaux fracture (Salter-Harris type III); (2) the remainder of the physis with a posterolateral spike of the tibial metaphysis; and (3) the remainder of the distal tibial metaphysis.

TREATMENT OF ANKLE FRACTURES

Distal Fibula Salter-Harris Type I or II

Treatment consists of closed reduction and cast management. If open reduction is necessary, a K-wire perpendicular to the physis is used.

Distal Tibia Salter-Harris Type I or II

These fractures occur predominantly in SER, PER, and SPF fractures. Closed reduction is the treatment of choice; it is usually attainable unless soft tissue interposition prevents reduction. In children less

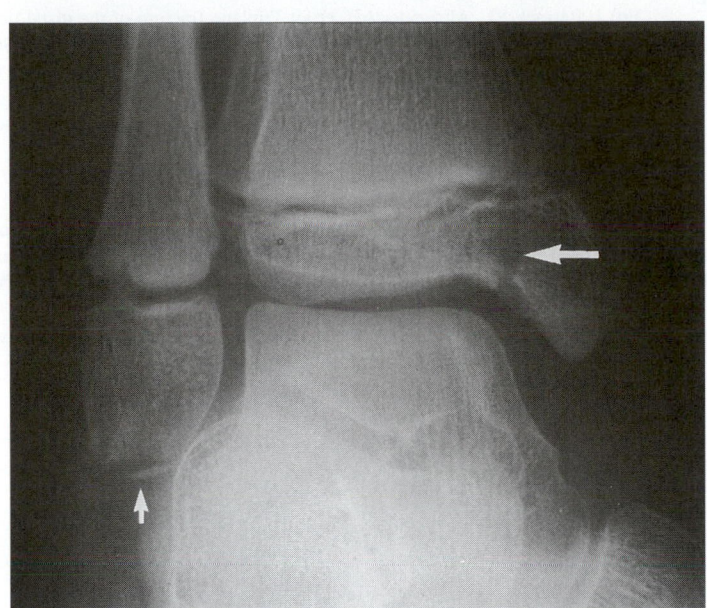

A

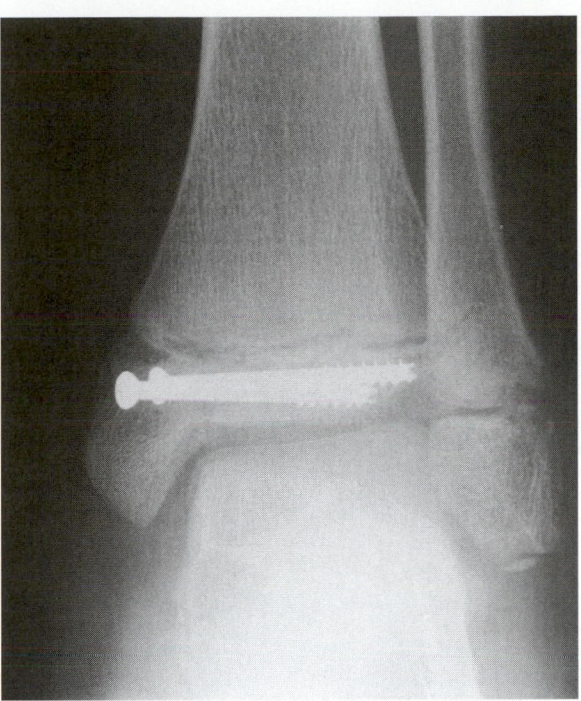

B

Figure 71-3
A. Supination: inversion fracture of the ankle with Salter-Harris type III fracture of tibia (*long arrow*) and avulsion fracture of the fibula (*short arrow*). *B.* Status post-ORIF of Salter-Harris type III fracture of the tibia.

than 10 years of age some residual angulation is acceptable since remodeling does occur. Open reduction is performed by removing the interposed periosteum or tendon and placing a transmetaphyseal lag screw or K-wire parallel and proximal to the physis. Cast immobilization is usually required for up to 6 weeks.

Distal Tibia Salter-Harris Type III or IV

This fracture is usually seen in SI injuries. These are intraarticular fractures that exhibit the highest rate of growth disturbance (i.e., bar formation). Anatomic reduction is essential, and any step-off or widening greater than a few millimeters is unacceptable and should be opened.

Juvenile-Tillaux Fracture

Treatment consists of closed reduction via internal rotation, maintained in a long leg cast. The joint surface must be congruent, otherwise ORIF is indicated. CT scan or tomography may be necessary to assess reduction.

Triplane Fracture

Once again articular restoration is the cornerstone to treating these fractures. CT scan with reconstructions should be utilized to assess reduction or to preoperatively plan the fracture reduction. These fractures may be treated closed if the joint surface has been restored, otherwise ORIF is indicated.

COMPLICATIONS

Angular deformity secondary to premature physeal arrest may be seen in Salter-Harris types III and IV injuries. Varus deformity is most common in SI injuries secondary to premature arrest of the medial tibial physis. Valgus deformity is seen with distal fibular physeal arrest; it may be due to a poor reduction or interposed soft tissue. Leg length discrepancy is related to the age of the patient. The distal tibia contributes approximately 1/8 in. per year to growth. Post-traumatic arthritis may be due to inadequate reduction of the articular surface in Salter-Harris types III and IV fractures.

FOOT

Foot injuries and fractures in children are fairly common and most are quite benign. Injuries to the pediatric foot usually correspond to the adult counterpart, and are treated similarly. There are a few exceptions, however. Young children, below the age of 6 years, rarely sustain significant hind foot injuries such as talar neck fractures or significant displaced intraarticular calcaneal fractures. Those types of fractures usually occur in the older child, and can be treated similar to adults.

Calcaneal fractures in young children are ordinarily treated nonsurgically, and only as the child reaches adolescence, do intraarticular fractures occur that are treated similar to those in an adult. Likewise, fractures of the talus do not usually occur in a young child, and the older child is usually treated the same as an adult. Fractures of Lisfranc's joint are uncommon in children. However, a Lisfranc fracture dislocation can occur, and fractures at the base of the metatarsals should alert the physician to this possibility. An open reduction may be required.

Fractures to the metatarsals in children most often can be treated nonoperatively in a short leg walking cast, however, marked displacement must be reduced. The older the child, the more accurate an alignment is required. Very young children have a remarkable propensity to remodel displaced metatarsal fractures. Phalangeal fractures in children are, for the most part, benign and are treated by taping the toes together. If there is marked displacement or angulation, then reduction is indicated.

SUGGESTED READINGS

Balthazar DA, Pappas AM: Acquired valgus deformity of the tibia in children. *J Pediatr Orthop* 1984; 4:538.

Baxter MP, Wiley JJ: Fractures of the tibial spine in chidren. An evaluation of knee stability. *J Bone Joint Surg [Br]* 1988; 70:228.

Beaty JH, Austin SM, Warner WC, et al: Interlocking intramedullary nailing of femoral-shaft fractures in adolescents: Preliminary results and complications. *J Pediatr Orthop* 1994; 14:178.

Burkhart SS, Peterson HA: Fractures of the proximal tibial epiphysis. *J Bone Joint Surg [Am]* 1979; 61:996.

Cramer KE, Limbird TJ, Green NE: Open fractures of the diaphysis of the lower extremity in children. Treatment, results, and complictions. *J Bone Joint Surg [Am]* 1992; 74:218.

Ertl J, Barrack RL, Alexander AH, et al: Triplane fracture of the distal tibial epiphysis. Long-term follow-up. *J Bone Joint Surg [Am]* 1988; 70:967.

Meyers MH, McKeever FM: Fracture of the intercondylar eminence of the tibia. *J Bone Joint Dis [Am]* 1970; 52:1677.

Ogden JA, Tross RB, Murphy MJ: Fractures of the tibial tuberosity in adolescents. *J Bone Joint Surg [Am]* 1980; 62:205.

Ray JM, Hendrix J: Incidence, mechanism of injury and treatment of fractures of the patella in children. *J Trauma* 1992; 32:464.

Salter RB, Best TN: The pathogenesis of progressive valgus deformity following fractures of the proximal metaphyseal region in the tibia in young children. In Eilert RE (ed): *Instructional Course Lectures*. Park Ridge, IL: 1992; 41:409.

Stanitski CL, Harvell JC, Fu F: Observations on acute knee hemarthrosis in children and adolescents. *J Pediatr Orthop* 1993; 13:506.

Chapter 72

ADULT ORTHOPAEDIC TRAUMA: GENERAL CONSIDERATIONS

Kenneth J. Koval

MULTIPLE TRAUMA

FIELD TRIAGE

Cowely (1974) introduced the concept of the "golden hour," defined as the first hour following critical injury within which immediate and appropriate care at a trauma center could avoid fatal shock and hemorrhage if definitive treatment were received at a trauma center. Since then, numerous evaluation tools and scales have been developed that facilitate determining which patients would benefit the most by direct transport to a specialized trauma center. The CRAMS score (Table 72-1) is one such scoring system that evaluates five areas of body function; each area is assigned a number and the five are combined for a total score. A combined score of 6 or less identifies patients who would benefit by transfer to a trauma center. Another standard for assessing trauma injury is the Revised Trauma Score (RTS) (Table 72-2), which combines separate scores for the respiratory rate, systolic blood pressure and the Glasgow Coma Scale (GCS). A score of 12 or under identifies patients for whom a trauma center would be advantageous.

The GCS (Table 72-3) is a simple system that can also be used alone to triage patients. It measures the level of and changes in consciousness, degree of brain damage, and residual brain function by evaluating eye opening and motor and verbal responses). A number is assigned to each response with the total indicating the severity of trauma sustained. Finally, the Injury Severity Score (ISS) evaluates the likelihood of surviving by mathematically manipulating high scores of the Abbreviated Injury Scale (AIS) for blunt trauma; AIS scores are derived from the degree and type of injury to six body regions (face, head/chest, abdomen, pelvis, extremities, external).

Certain observed clinical signs mandate immediate transport to a trauma center irrespective of trauma scoring (Table 72-4).

PRIMARY SURVEY

Management of trauma should follow an orderly approach as exemplified by the ABCs of trauma resuscitation: airway, breathing, and circulation, respectively; followed by a secondary survey to identify extremity-, organ-, and system-associated trauma. In general, injuries identified as the most immediately lethal are addressed as they are diagnosed.

AIRWAY

It must be established immediately whether a clear or obstructed airway exists. An obstructed airway is identified by asking the patient a question that normally would elicit a response (e.g., "Are you all right?" or "What is your name?"). A verbal response confirms the airway is unobstructed and the patient is oxygenating sufficiently. The airway should also be auscultated for gurgling, stridor, or snoring. A nonverbal response demands further investigation and possibly immediate action. Two techniques effective for clearing the airway are the chin lift and the forward jaw thrust. The oropharynx should also be examined by direct observation (with an illuminated source) for any obstruction. Once an airway is patent, it can be maintained with an oropharyngeal or nasopharyngeal airway, if necessary. If it is not possible to secure the airway by the above methods, endotracheal intubation is indicated. In general, any movement of the neck should be avoided in trauma cases until appropriate cervical support is applied.

BREATHING

Trauma patients should always receive supplemental oxygen to optimize oxygenation of tissue, and counteract metabolic acidosis and shifts in pH balance. If an adequate airway is secured, but the patient is not ventilating properly, the chest should be inspected, palpated, and auscultated for cause. A flail chest (loss of stability of rib cage associated with pulmonary contusion, multiple rib fractures, and/or sternum fracture): open pneumothorax (air enters chest cavity through open chest wound), and tension pneumothorax (inspired air from damaged lung tissue enters pleural space) must be ruled out. Left untreated the ipsilateral lung collapses; clinical signs include tracheal deviation, same side hyperresonant breath sounds, and jugular venous distension. Each of these events, should they occur, can be adequately controlled by the following emergency measures. Treatment of a flail chest (flapping chest wall) requires consistent monitoring of fluid balance (to prevent excessive hydration) and possible utilization of ventilatory support. The wound causing an open pneumothorax must be completely covered by an occlusive bandage, and appropriately taped (three sides) to allow expiration until operative treatment with a distant chest tube can be applied. If a hemopneumothorax develops (blood accumulating within the pleural cavity from injury to mediastinal or intercostal structures), a chest tube is inserted and accompanied by hemodynamic support. By placing a large-bore IV catheter in the second intercostal space (midclavicular line), a tension pneumothorax may be rapidly transformed into a simple pneumothorax, avoiding immediate catastrophic sequelae; later, a chest tube provides appropriate management.

CIRCULATION

All identified sources of bleeding need to be tamponaded using direct pressure with a sterile dressing. Blood pressure can be estimated by palpating peripheral pulses. The observance of palpable peripheral

---
Table 72-1

The CRAMS Scale

Circulation

2	Normal capillary refill and BP > 100 mmHg systolic
1	Delayed capillary refill or BP > 85–90 mmHg systolic
0	No capillary refill or BP < 85 mmHg systolic

Respiration

2	Normal
1	Abnormal (labored, shallow, or rate > 35)
0	Absent

Abdomen

2	Abdomen and thorax not tender
1	Abdomen or thorax tender
0	Abdomen rigid, thorax flail, or deep penetrating injury to either chest or abdomen

Motor

2	Normal (obeys commands)
1	Responds only to pain—no posturing
0	Postures or no response

Speech

2	Normal (oriented)
1	Confused or inappropriate
0	None or unintelligible sounds

____   Total CRAMS Score (add the five areas)

SOURCE: Reproduced with permission from Clemmer TP, Orme JF Jr, Thomas F, et al: Prospective evaluation of the CRAMS scale for triaging major trauma. *J Trauma* 1985; 25:189.

Table 72-2

The Revised Trauma Score

System	Rate	Score
A. Respiratory Rate (breaths/min)	10–29	4
	>29	3
	6–9	2
	1–5	1
	0	0
B. Systolic Blood Pressure (mmHg)	>89	4
	76–89	3
	50–75	2
	1–49	1
	0	0
C. Glasgow Coma Scale Conversion	13–15	4
	9–12	3
	6–8	2
	4–5	1
	3	0
Revised Trauma Score (A + B + C)		_____

SOURCE: Reproduced with permission from Ciraulo DL, Cowell V, Jacobs LM: Evaluation and treatment of the multiple-injured patient. In Browner BD, Jupiter JB, Levine AM, et al (eds): *Skeletal Trauma: Fractures, Dislocations, and Ligamentous Injuries*, vol 1, 2d ed. Philadelphia: Saunders; 1998:134. Modified from Champion HR, Sacco WJ, Copes et al: A revision of the Trauma Score. *J Trauma* 1989; 29:623.

Table 72-3

Glasgow Coma Scale

A. Eye opening
   Spontaneous _____ 4
   To voice _____ 3
   To pain _____ 2
   None _____ 1

B. Verbal Response
   Oriented _____ 5
   Confused _____ 4
   Inappropriate words _____ 3
   Incomprehensible sounds _____ 2
   None _____ 1

C. Motor Response
   Obeys commands _____ 6
   Purposeful movements (pain) _____ 5
   Withdraw (pain) _____ 4
   Flexion (pain) _____ 3
   Extension (pain) _____ 2
   None _____ 1

Total GCS points (A + B + C) _____ (3–15)

SOURCE: Reproduced with permission from Ciraulo DL, Cowell V, Jacobs LM: Evaluation and treatment of the multiple-injured patient. In Browner BD, Jupiter JB, Levine AM, et al (eds): *Skeletal Trauma: Fractures, Dislocations, and Ligamentous Injuries*, vol 1, 2d ed. Philadelphia: Saunders; 1998:134. Modified from Teasdale G, Jennett B: Assessment of coma and impaired consciousness. A practical scale. *Lancet* 2:81. © Lancet, Ltd, 1974.

Table 72-4

Clinical Criteria for Transport to Trauma Center

1. Blood pressure < 90 mmHg
2. Heart rate > 120 min
3. Respiratory rate > 30 min
4. Penetrating injuries to thorax, abdomen, head, or neck
5. Neurologic impairment
6. Amputation above wrist or ankle
7. Flail chest
8. Two or more long bone fractures
9. No spontaneous eye opening
10. Blunt thoracic trauma with systolic BP < 90 mmHg
11. Involvement in a motor vehicle accident with blunt abdominal trauma
12. Falling from > 15 feet
13. Age less than 5 years or greater than 65

SOURCE: Bone BL: Emergency treatment of the injured patient. In Browner BD, Jupiter JB, Levine AM, et al (eds): *Skeletal Trauma*, vol 1. Philadelphia: WB Saunders; 1972:127. Based on West JG et al: *J Trauma* 1986; 26:655, and Kane G et al: *J Trauma* 1985; 25:482.

pulses allows an approximation of systolic blood pressure in the respective region, for example; radial, at least 80 mmHg or higher; carotid, 60 mmHg or more; and femoral, 70 mmHg or greater.

Hemorrhagic shock is more probable in trauma than septic, cardiogenic or neurogenic, and should be assumed in patients who develop shock in trauma settings unless there is clinical evidence for one of the latter types. Cardiogenic shock has a very high mortality rate, up to 80 percent occurs when cardiac function is insufficient to sustain adequate tissue perfusion. Relative to acute trauma, cardiogenic shock develops with myocardial contusion, myocardial infarction, or cardiac tamponade. Increased central venous pressure, distended neck veins with hypotension, and muffled heart sounds (Beck's triad) strongly suggest cardiac tamponade. If confirmed, emergent pericardiocentesis is required; a needle is placed under the xiphoid process, through the chest cavity, and into the pericardium for removal of the fluid.

Suspected or confirmed spinal cord and/or head injury patients with hypotension, but without concomitant tachycardia or peripheral vasoconstriction and who are not responsive to fluid management may have neurogenic shock. Monitoring of venous pressure is recommended.

Hemorrhagic shock may induce neurologic change, decreased blood pressure, or cold/clammy skin. Laboratory tests will also reveal characteristic metabolic changes that lead to end-organ failure if shock is not treated. There are four classes of hemorrhagic shock, generally categorized as follows: Class I, a minimum of 15 percent of blood volume lost with few clinical findings (slight tachycardia, no change in blood pressure, pulse, capillary refill, respiratory rate, or urine output); Class II, 15 to 30 percent of blood volume lost with an increase in clinical findings (tachycardia, tachypnea, and normal systolic pressure with an increased diastolic pressure, known as narrowed pulse pressure). CNS symptoms are sometimes noted; Class II, 30 to 40 percent blood volume lost with further development of clinical signs (tachycardia, tachypnea, and decreased systolic, narrowed pulse pressure, and altered mental status); Class IV, 40 percent loss of blood volume with profoundly depressive clinical signs (tachycardia, hypotension, cold/clammy skin, obtundation, and minimal urine output).

Hemorrhagic shock is initially treated by placing two large-bore intravenous lines in the arm; the subclavian and jugular veins cannot deliver the large volume of fluid required to manage shock therapy. If venous access is not obtained, cut-downs are necessary.

Class I and II hemorrhage are usually managed with crystalloid. Fluid replacement therapy includes a bolus of Ringer's lactate; the initial patient response is then evaluated. In the event that a second response is needed, blood is administered.

Class III and IV hemorrhage management necessitates both crystalloid and blood replacement. Along with fluid replacement, pneumatic anti-shock garments (PASG) can be applied. PASGs function by increasing peripheral vascular resistance. Contraindications to PASGs include myocardial abnormality, pulmonary edema, intrathoracic hemorrhage, head injury, pregnancy, and ruptured diaphragm.

NEUROLOGIC STATUS

When resuscitation has been secured, the patient's neurologic status should be assessed. Toward this end, the GCS is useful for both initial and repeat evaluations of consciousness. It is the first GCS score performed which represents the degree and kind of incurred neurologic injury; for example, acute subdural hematoma; a GCS score of 3 to 5 has a very high fatality rate and minimal possibility of a good outcome. Pupil size and reaction are evaluated to establish the presence of intracranial injury. The neurologic status of all four extremities must be evaluated.

SECONDARY SURVEY

A secondary survey is performed to identify injuries associated with any organ system. Facial lacerations and possible facial and skull fractures are identified and evaluated.

The ears should be examined for the presence of blood, the nose for cerebral spinal fluid, and the mouth for injury and swelling. The cervical spine, in particular, should be noted for development of any expanding hematomas, as well as for swelling and crepitation, using palpation. The survey generally begins with the head and continues downward in an organized fashion (Table 72-5).

HEAD INJURY

Head injury is a serious cause of mortality in trauma patients, and accounts for 40 to 60 percent of fatalities in motor vehicle accidents. A concussive episode that includes a loss of consciousness for more than 5 min requires inpatient observation for 24 h as these patients are at high risk for convulsions. Cerebral contusion is usually associated with a period of extended unconsciousness and focal neurologic signs.

Computed tomography of the head is required to fully assess the extent and severity of head injury and intracranial bleeding (meningeal bleeding or brain hemorrhage), for which trauma patients are at high risk. Persons with a fixed, dilated pupil or who are unconscious should be evaluated for intracranial bleeding. Three types occur: epidural, subdural, and subarachnoid. The classic pattern of untreated epidural bleeding is an initially unconscious patient who wakes and appears to have recovered (i.e., they are lucid), but shortly thereafter, returns to a deeper loss of consciousness. Fractures in the temporal and parietal areas of the skull should raise an index of suspicion and a necessity for patient monitoring.

Subdural hematomas may be fatal, and can develop in the absence of skull fracture. They are caused by tears in the venous system, and evidence of them may be delayed. Management is immediate surgical decompression.

Subarachnoid hemorrhage is bleeding into the cerebrospinal fluid with irritation of the meninges, but it is not life-threatening. Serial CTs are used with therapeutic intervention, if necessary.

Parenchymal brain hemorrhage (intracranial bleeding) carries a high rate of mortality.

Avoidable perils in the assessment and management of head injury include (1) not securing a patent airway in unconscious or obtunded persons (these individuals should be intubated with hyperventilation); (2) not providing for observation of a patient during a lucid period when it was known that loss of consciousness had or might have occurred; (3) not achieving a level of absolute certainty as to whether a cord injury or cervical fracture occurred; and (4) failure to distinguish/diagnose head injury and intracranial bleeding with appropriate and timely intervention, possibly avoiding progression to an extreme cerebral emergency. For discussion of cervical and spine-related trauma, see Chaps. 74 and 75.

THORACIC INJURY

The majority of deaths occurring by blunt trauma include thoracic injury. Pleural contusions should be considered in blunt trauma patients, and cardiac contusions in those with abnormal electrocardiograms and/or arrhythmia. Chest x-rays should be examined for the following signs of aortic injury or mediastinal hematoma: deviation of the trachea or the lung margin away from the middle of the chest; change in appearance or loss of the aortic knob (transition point from ascending to descending aorta), margin may appear shaggy or enlarged; thick and

Table 72-5

Secondary Survey[a] Following ABCs of Resuscitation

Region	Evaluate
Scalp	Lacerations
Face	Lacerations, fractures, periorbital hematoma (anterior cranial fossa injury)
Cranium	Fractures (possible brain injury and neurologic deficit)
Ears	Blood in external auditory meatus
Nose	Cerebrospinal fluid
Mouth	Swelling and any injury
Maxillofacial	Fractures, deformity
Neck	Penetrating wounds
Cervical spine	Expanding hematomas, swelling, and crepitation, x-ray to rule out fracture
Chest	Fractured ribs and/or sternum, flail chest, distended neck veins (possible cardiac tamponade), and penetrating wounds (pneumothorax/tension pneumothorax)
Abdomen	Palpation and auscultation for diminished bowel sounds, distension, and abdominal sensitivity or pain with pressure
Pelvis	Palpation/compression for stability/instability (possible fractures, retroperitoneal hematoma)
Rectum	Rectal (sensation and tone), abnormal position of and injury to prostate and/or urethra
Genitourinary	Blood at opening (possible pelvic fracture or urethral injury); if found, use of Fley catheter is contraindicated
Extremities	Fractures, crepitus, swelling, abnormal passive/active movement, neurovascular status

[a]Abbreviated description.

SOURCE: Ciraulo DL, Cowell V, Jacobs LM: Evaluation and treatment of the multiple-injured patient. In Browner BD, Jupiter JB, Levine AM et al (eds): *Skeletal Trauma*, vol 1, 2d ed. Philadelphia: Saunders; 1998:131.

enlarged appearing descending aorta; rib fractures (with frequent damage to nearby organs and tissues); and mediastinal widening.

Evidence on radiographs of pneumomediastinum or pneumopericardium is indicative of chest injury. Actual injury to the trachea and esophagus may be difficult to confirm on plain films; an exception is compression of the trachea which can occur with high-energy injuries. Thoracic trauma may cause abnormal elevation of the diaphragm either from paralysis of the diaphragmatic nerves or by diaphragmatic rupture with concomitant herniation of abdominal structures; discerning between the two conditions may be problematic. CT can also document the above injuries and probably more easily, though time or access may not permit its use. Any penetrating injury to the mediastinum left untreated may lead to serious infection, thus diagnosis is critical. Additional types of chest injuries necessitating urgent treatment, such as tension pneumothorax, open pneumothorax, cardiac tamponade, and flail chest are discussed above.

ABDOMINAL INJURY

The abdomen is the most frequent site for occult bleeding in a trauma setting; however, many patients do not manifest any peritoneal signs such as rebound tenderness. Management ranges from placement of a nasogastric tube, to peritoneal lavage and the more recent use of abdominal ultrasound and CT scan. Management includes a nasogastric tube to decompress the stomach and avoid aspiration. Trauma patients who have sustained blunt abdominal injury and cannot tolerate an adequate physical exam should have a peritoneal lavage. Others who should be considered for peritoneal lavage are patients with hypotension of unknown etiology, head and spinal cord injuries, altered mental status (alcohol/drugs), pelvic fracture, and those without access to careful monitoring. Prior abdominal surgeries and indications for exploratory laparotomy are contraindications to performing abdominal lavage. Aspirate containing more than 100,000 red blood cells per mm^3, more than 500 leukocytes per mm^3, or the presence of intestinal material, such as bile or feces, represents a positive lavage.

Abdominal ultrasound has been reported diagnostically comparable to peritoneal lavage and CT for detecting peritoneal bleeding (hemoperitoneum) and to have a high sensitivity and specificity for identifying abdominal injury. Ultrasound can provide visualization of the heart, kidney, spleen, bladder, and other pelvic contents.

Abdominal CT scan retains some superiority in identifying abdominal organ injury and retroperitoneal injury; it should not be employed with patients who have not been stabilized and/or require laparotomy.

GENITOURINARY INJURY

Genitourinary injury can be caused by direct or indirect force. Blunt trauma to the abdomen, pelvic region, genital organs, or perineum suggests the possibility of genitourinary injury. Clinical findings that are suggestive include blood at the urethral meatus, hematoma of the genital organs or area, pelvis fracture, or lower rib fracture. If hematuria is present, a cystogram, intravenous pyelogram and excretory urography, or CT scan should be performed. If there is evidence of urethral injury, a retrograde urethrogram is necessary before placement of a Foley catheter.

EXTREMITY FRACTURES

Injury to the extremities must be identified and affected limbs immobilized prior to transportation to decrease the risk of fat embolization. Early stabilization of fractures of long bones and the pelvis will facilitate patient mobilization which in turn optimizes respiratory function, the main cause of morbidity and mortality in the polytrauma patient.

OPEN FRACTURES

An open or compound fracture is defined by a perforation of the skin and soft tissue that creates an open wound down to the fracture.

EVALUATION

All open fractures should receive formal debridement in the operating room; the ER is not an appropriate setting for wound exploration and debridement. The wound is covered with a saline soaked sterile dressing and the extremity is splinted. Antibiotics and tetanus prophylaxis should be administered as soon as possible. Evaluation must also rule out the possibility of compartment syndrome. The identification of wounds that communicate with joints is accomplished by injecting saline into the joint(s) of concern and noting any extravasation of the saline. AP and lateral views of the affected bone(s) should include the joints above and below the fracture. Suspicion of a vascular injury may require angiography.

CLASSIFICATION

The most accepted classification system of open fractures was initially described by Gustillo (1987), and then modified by Gustillo, Mendoza, and Williams. A type I injury is a low-energy wound which is the result of bone piercing from the inside to outside; it is usually less than 1 cm in length. Type II open fractures are defined by a laceration greater than 1 cm laceration without significant soft tissue crush injury and osseous comminution. Type III open fractures are high energy injuries with extensive soft tissue damage and high degrees of comminution. Type IIIA injuries have some soft tissue coverage over the exposed bone. Type IIIB injuries have sustained extensive periosteal stripping, and usually require plastic surgery techniques as part of the closure. Type IIIC open fractures include a major vascular injury that requires repair to salvage the limb.

TREATMENT

Adequate debridement is the most critical component of operative management; all patients with open fractures must, therefore, undergo formal debridement in the operating room. Abundant irrigation is critical. The objectives of debridement are to remove any foreign material and nonviable tissue, reduce bacterial contamination, and create a cleansed wound environment that can tolerate the remaining bacterial count, healing without infection.

Debridement is accomplished starting with the superficial tissue layers and progressing to the deeper levels. The margins of the wound are extended to better examine the area of injury. Nonviable and contaminated tissue are excised, contractility being a good indicator of tissue viability. Bone that is denuded of soft tissue attachment is excised.

Prompt fracture stabilization using internal or external fixation protects soft tissues, eases wound care, reduces wound sepsis, improves soft tissue healing, and facilitates mobilization. Traditional care for the stabilization of open fractures has been external fixation. There have been recent reports using small-diameter intramedullary nails to stabilize open diaphyseal shaft fractures; these nails are inserted without prior reaming.

The surgical wound can be closed, but the traumatic wound should be left open and covered with a saline-soaked or synthetic dressing following formal debridement. Good results have been reported using a "bead pouch" of antibiotic-impregnated cement beads that were secured beneath a nonpermeable dressing. The minimal antibiotic coverage for grade I and II open fractures is a first generation cephalosporin. Patients with grade III injuries should also be administered an aminoglycoside. In farm injuries, a cephalosporin, aminoglycoside, and penicillin are necessary. If secondary procedures are necessary, antibiotic coverage is reinstituted for 72 h. The majority of open fractures demand repeat debridement.

COMPARTMENT SYNDROME

Compartment syndrome is a condition in which increased pressure within a closed anatomical space threatens the vitality of enclosed tissues. If the compartment pressure exceeds the pressure of the small intramuscular arterioles, capillary blood flow ceases.

ETIOLOGY

The etiology of compartment syndrome consists of two possible mechanisms: reduced compartment size and/or increased compartment contents. Both mechanisms often occur together, a setting that may conceal the identification of the initial mechanism or the exact etiology. Decreased compartment size may be caused by an external compressive dressing inappropriately applied to an extremity. Severe tissue edema or a developing hematoma may result in increased compartment content sufficient to cause or contribute to compartment syndrome.

DIAGNOSIS

A high index of suspicion is central to making a diagnosis of compartment syndrome. The most important symptom in responsive and coherent patients is pain that is disproportionate to the injury. Pain with passive stretch is also symptomatic of compartment syndrome. Paresthesia associated with nerves that transverse the affected compartment is a late sign of compartment syndrome. Palpation may demonstrate a tense, firm extremity. Pallor and pulselessness are rare without an associated vascular injury. Paralysis and motor weakness are very late signs suggestive of compartment syndrome.

If the diagnosis of compartment syndrome remains uncertain or if objective data is needed, compartment pressures may be obtained; however, they are most useful when clinical symptoms are inconclusive and in polytrauma patients and patients with head injury.

The Whitesides method and the Stic catheter system are the best-known methods used to measure compartment pressures. The Stic catheter is a hand-held device that permits rapid measurement of compartment pressures. All compartments in the involved extremity must be measured during the evaluation of pressures. There is no agreement as to the exact compartment pressure at which a fasciotomy should be performed. Treatment guidelines recommend a fasciotomy when compartment pressures are within 10 to 30 mmHg of the patient's diastolic blood pressure, when compartment pressures are between 30 to 45 mmHg, or if the clinical signs and symptoms are persuasive, without regard to pressure measurements.

TREATMENT

If compartment syndrome is suspected, the cast or bandage should be removed, and the limb elevated to the heart level. Fasciotomy should be performed once a compartment syndrome has been diagnosed. The entire length of the compartment is incised, and all compartments of the extremity are released. The incisions are left open and closed at a later date or skin grafted.

GUNSHOT WOUND

The severity of injury from gunshot wounds depends primarily on the projectile's kinetic energy. Based on the equation, $KE = 1/2\ m(v)^2$, (m, mass; v, velocity), kinetic energy varies exponentially with velocity—making velocity the main determinant of a bullet's wounding potential.

Gunshot injuries are either low velocity (less than 2000 ft/s) or high velocity (greater than 2000 ft/s). Low velocity injuries are usually the result of civilian weapons (e.g., handguns); high velocity injuries are caused by military weapons, such as an M16. High velocity injuries are more likely to result in serious soft tissue and bony injury, wound contamination/infection, and neurovascular injury.

An adequate evaluation of gunshot injury must include additional attributes of the projectile, as well as of the target tissues. For example, the capacity of the projectile to transfer kinetic energy to the target tissue is a major determinant of tissue injury. A bullet that follows a straight path through a target may carry away a significant amount of energy in the form of its exit velocity. By contrast, a bullet that tumbles, deforms, or fragments has a delayed transit time as it passes through tissue, and thus it transfers more of its kinetic energy to the target. Examples representative of this phenomenon are a hollowpoint bullet, which deforms, or a "dum-dum" bullet, which fragments on impact; both cause more tissue damage than standard bullets with similar velocities.

In terms of characteristics of the target tissue, the most important determinants relative to gunshot injury are specific gravity and elasticity. In general, the higher the specific gravity of a tissue, the greater the damage it will sustain from any given projectile. Cortical bone has the highest specific gravity of any body tissue; consequently, it may suffer more damage than other tissues in the path of a projectile. In contrast, the greater the elasticity of a tissue the less likely it is to be damaged by a gunshot.

Shotgun wounds should be considered separately. The charge velocity of shotgun pellets is relatively low, and ranges from 1100 ft/s to 1350 ft/s; however, the mass of the shot in the average shotgun shell is very high (1-5/8 to 2 oz). The kinetic energy is concentrated at the muzzle; injuries that occur at close range when the shot is still tightly packed usually involve extreme tissue destruction. Shotgun injuries occurring at close range (usually under 20 ft) are generally managed as high velocity injuries. During the shotgun blast, the pellets rapidly disperse, which limits the total mass impacting the target, and the velocity of the individual pellets rapidly declines due to their poor aerodynamic properties. Therefore, shotgun injuries occurring from large distances involve significantly less kinetic energy and generally result in minimal damage to tissues. Other factors such as choke and wadding must also be considered in assessing shotgun injuries. Choke is the constriction at the end of a shotgun barrel, which acts to determine the pattern of distribution of shotgun pellets at any target range. The greater the choke, or constriction, the tighter the distribution of pellets at a given target, and the greater mass (and kinetic energy) impacting on that target. Wadding is the material situated between the powder and the shot charge, and may be paper, plastic, cork, or felt. With close range shooting, the wadding may stay in the wound, making treatment more difficult.

MECHANISM OF INJURY

There are three mechanisms by which damage to target tissue by gunshot occurs: laceration and crushing, shock waves, and cavitation. In laceration and crush injury (both low velocity and high velocity gunshot injuries), the missile crushes and forces apart material that is in its direct path. This crush injury creates a permanent cavity, and manifests as a loss of tissue along the missile tract. Shock waves are predominantly associated with high velocity gunshot injuries, and occur as the impact of the projectile compresses the tissue in front of the missile; the tissue retreats in a shock wave of spherical form that continues to be transmitted and reflected from tissue interfaces, causing tissue injury to proceed away from the direct missile tract. In cavitation (high velocity gunshot injuries), as the missile penetrates tissues, the encompassing tissues are accelerated in a radial direction away from the missile tract. The acceleration stretches surrounding tissues, creating a temporary cavity that surrounds the permanent cavity. This temporary cavity collapses rapidly, leaving behind damage caused by the sudden stretch of the tissues; the degree of damage caused is determined by tissue elasticity.

TREATMENT

Fractures caused by low velocity gunshot wounds are managed as closed fractures. Entry and exit wounds are cleansed in the emergency room and intravenous antibiotics are administered. High velocity gunshot wounds are treated with methods similar to those employed in open fractures with formal debridement in the operating room, followed by osseous stabilization, and soft tissue coverage.

HETEROTROPIC OSSIFICATION AND MYOSITIS OSSIFICANS

ETIOLOGY

Ectopic bone is mature lamellar bone situated in nonosseous tissue. Organized bone within muscle is termed myositis ossificans; bone in tissue planes outside of muscle is heterotopic ossification.

Traumatic localized myositis develops due to severe injury such as an elbow dislocation. In myositis ossificans, ectopic bone develops between the muscle fibers. The "zonal" microscopic appearance is indistinguishable from heterotopic ossification. Clinical features include tenderness, swelling, and pain on motion.

The etiology of heterotopic ossification is not well understood. It is known to develop in the presence of a variety of local and systemic factors such as ankylosing spondylitis, proliferative hip osteoarthritis, multiple trauma, thermal injury, infection, head injury, spine injury, and genetic disorders. In addition, select fractures, dislocation patterns, and surgical approaches have been associated with an increased incidence of heterotopic ossification.

Heterotopic ossification develops from unorganized proliferation of pluripotential mesenchymal cells into osteoblastic cells with sub-

Table 72-6

Brooker Classification of Heterotopic Ossification of the Hip

Stage	
0	No heterotopic bone
I	Islands of bone within the soft tissue about the hip
II	Bone spurs from the pelvis or proximal end of the femur, leaving at least 1 cm between opposing bone surfaces
III	Bone spurs reducing the space between opposing bone surfaces to less than 1 cm
IV	Apparent bony ankylosis of the hip

SOURCE: Reproduced and modified with permission from Brooker JW, Robinson JA, Riley LH Jr: Ectopic ossification following total hip replacement: incidence and a method of classification. *J Bone Joint Surg [AM]* 1973; 55:1629.

sequent transformation to mature lamellar bone. Cell proliferation usually begins within 16 h of the initial injury and is believed to be the result of unidentified biologic mediators.

PATHOLOGY AND PATHOGENESIS

The pathologic features of heterotropic ossification and myositis ossificans are identical. Microscopic findings will differ depending on the age of the lesion, but are typified by a "zoning" pattern which begins within 3 weeks of the injury. The center zone is a dense, undifferentiated zone; it contains pluripotential mesenchymal cells of variable size and shape and includes many mitotic figures. The adjacent zone consists mainly of osteoblasts and osteoid, but cartilage may be found as well. The most peripheral zone includes well-formed mineralized trabeculae whose microscopic appearance is similar to cancellous bone.

The onset and progression of heterotopic ossification is variable; its course often depends on the type of sustained injury. Radiographic evidence of heterotopic ossification following direct injury has been observed as early as 3 weeks. Clinical presentation includes local swelling, erythema, and warmth. Later, a mass may be palpated when the area calcifies. Despite clinical improvement with early physical therapy, pain and decreased range of motion may accompany the condition. An elevated serum alkaline phosphatase may appear as soon as 1 month following injury; it can be 3.5 times the normal value. Elevated alkaline phosphatase is associated with numerous other disorders, however, and is not specific for heterotopic ossification. Plain radiographs are a cost-effective method by which heterotopic ossification can be diagnosed. Heterotopic ossification about the hip has been classified by Brooker (Table 72-6) (also see Fig. 49-4).

A three-phase bone scan is a sensitive evaluation test and can be used to diagnose heterotopic ossification prior to clinical symptoms. Computed tomography scans are helpful in preoperative planning and establishing the most advantageous surgical approach.

PROPHYLAXIS

Prophylaxis of heterotopic ossification has involved adminstering either diphosphonates (etidronate disodium and ethane hydroxy diphosphonate) or nonsteroidal anti-inflammatory drugs. Diphosphonates inhibit the crystallization of hydroxyapatite, ultimately causing a reduction in the mineralization of osteoid but not in the total amount of osteoid. The effectiveness of diphosphonates is limited to active use; on cessation, mineralization of osteoid ensues. Nonsteroidal medications inhibit cyclooxygenase, and thereby decrease the synthesis of prostaglandins.

Radiation is another method of prophylactic treatment for heterotopic ossification. Low-dose external beam radiation prevents the conversion of precursor cells to bone forming cells. Therapy should be started within 24 to 72 h following the insult. Therapeutic recommendations include a single dose of 800 to 1000 centigrays or divided doses of 200 centigrays over a 4- to 5-day period.

Fully mature heterotopic ossification can be excised, if necessary. However, the timing of excision relative to the stage of the condition is critical because immature bone that remains following surgical excision will continue to develop and mature. Ectopic bone is defined as mature when there is evidence of trabeculation, size stabilization, and maturation of ossification margins on plain films.

TREATMENT

Treatment of myositis ossificans includes immobiliation of the extremity, rest, ice, compression, elevation, and non-steroidal anti-inflammatory medication during the initial active phase (days 1 to 10). Range of motion exercises can be initiated after initial symptoms have subsided. If limited range of motion, nerve irritation, or overlying skin pressure is present, surgical excision may be necessary, but should be performed only after the ectopic bone is fully matured.

NONUNIONS

A delayed union is defined as a fracture which takes a longer period of time to unite than normal. Nonunion is complete arrest of the fracture repair process.

ETIOLOGY

Nonunions may be caused by excessive fracture motion, improper alignment or gap, infection, or avascularity. Fracture gap can result from various phenomena: soft tissue interposition, fracture distraction, fracture malposition, or bone loss. Avascularity is caused by damaged nutrient vessels, excessive soft tissue stripping, or severe fracture comminution. Patient issues that predispose to nonunion are an older age, poor nutritional status, steroid or anti-coagulation medication, radiation therapy, and associated burn injury.

CLINICAL AND RADIOGRAPHIC EVALUATION

The severity of the initial osseous injury must be assessed, and should include the condition of soft tissues, knowledge of any prior treatment, previous coverage problems, and any history of prior infection. The functional status of the patient also needs to be evaluated, including mental health, family stability, work status, and possible secondary gains. The extremity is examined for tenderness, evidence of fracture motion, and range of joint motion, as well as for vascular status, limb length, and evidence of reflex sympathetic dystrophy.

Radiographic examination includes AP, lateral, and oblique views of the extremity; radiographs of the unaffected extremity may facilitate preoperative planning. Flexion and extension lateral views are helpful in detecting nonunion motion. Nuclear studies (bone, gallium, and indium scans) may help to establish the biological viability of the nonunion and any evidence of infection.

CLASSIFICATION

Weber and Cech (1976) classified nonunions based on the evaluation of plain radiographs and bone scans as vascular or hypovascular. Vascular nonunions are capable of biological reaction, and usually contain abundant callus, but there is insufficient osseous stability for union to occur. Hypovascular (avascular) nonunions are incapable of biological reaction and require osseous stability via a bone graft to stimulate a vascular response. Synovial pseudarthroses may form a false joint with a synovial lining. Infected nonunion is an additional category within this classification.

TREATMENT

Treatment objectives are union with restoration of correct limb alignment joint motion, and the absence of infection. The rationale for treatment of nonunion is the clinical value gained by decreasing nonunion motion, reduction of the nonunion gap, increased limb function (resulting in improved blood supply and decreased stiffness), and eradication and prevention of further infection. Treatment options include cast bracing, electrical/ultrasound stimulation, bone grafting, fibular osteotomy, and internal/external fixation. Functional braces and casts may be of benefit in delayed unions; however, they require prolonged use and do not correct osseous malposition.

Advocates of electrical stimulation have reported 75 to 80 percent success rates when applied to tibial nonunions. Contraindications to electrical stimulation are a nonunion gap greater than 1 cm and/or a synovial pseudarthrosis. Electrical stimulation has no impact on and does not correct deformity.

Fibular osteotomy has a reported union rate of 77 percent in the treatment of tibial nonunions. It is a simple procedure, avoids the fracture site, and allows extremity loading. However, it does not correct tibial deformity, necessitates extremity immobilization, and may cause destabilization of the tibia.

Posterolateral bone grafts for the treatment of tibial nonunions have an 80 to 90 percent success rate; poor anterior soft tissue and infection are not contraindications and the grafts may be utilized during internal/external fixation. Posterolateral bone grafting does not correct deformity, may require immobilization of the extremity, and requires an intact fibula.

Autologous bone marrow injection taken from the iliac crest has a 90-percent union rate for tibial nonunion.

Bone morphogenic proteins are osteoinductive, but remain experimental.

Compression plating has a high rate of union for diaphyseal and metaphyseal nonunions; fracture location and prior infection are not exclusion factors. Disadvantages to compression plating are the need

for dissection prior to application, the number of stress risers created, and prolonged protected weightbearing postoperatively.

Reamed intramedullary nailing is generally the implant of choice for most femoral and tibial shaft nonunions; reported union rates are between 90 to 95 percent. Reamed interlocked nails provide stable fixation of diaphyseal fractures and nonunions and osteoinductive internal reaming particles, and permit early postoperative patient weightbearing. Small diameter–wire circular fixators permit slow correction of the deformity, can be applied with a semi-closed method, and can be used to correct limb length inequality. The disadvantages of circular fixators are implant bulkiness, impalement of soft tissue, and the potential of pin tract infection.

PATHOLOGIC FRACTURES

Pathologic fractures occur when the normal integrity and strength of bone have been weakened by invasive disease or destructive process, most particularly by neoplasm or necrosis. Other etiologies include disuse, infection, iatrogenic (i.e., surgical defect), metabolic disorder, primary bone tumor, and metastatic disease.

EVALUATION

Fractures that occur with normal activity, minimal trauma, excessive pain, a primary malignancy, or in patients with a history of multiple fractures, or other select risk factors (i.e., smoking, environmental exposure to carcinogens) should raise suspicion to the possibility of pathologic fracture. Physical examination should evaluate soft tissue mass at the fracture site, look for evidence of primary disease, and examine for painful areas to identify or exclude impending pathologic fractures.

Plain radiographs should include the entire extremity. A chest radiograph is necessary to rule out primary lung tumor or metastatic disease. A bone scan can be used to demonstrate lesions which are not clinically or radiographically apparent; a 30-percent decrease in bone mineral content is required before osseous changes are apparent on x-ray. Bone scans are most reliable in detecting metastatic bone disease associated with breast, prostate, lung, and kidney tumors. In myeloma, areas of decreased radionuclide uptake are often observed.

Baseline laboratory tests should include a complete blood count with differential, peripheral smear, sedimentation rate, and blood chemistries (calcium, phosphate, blood urea nitrogen, creatinine, albumin, globulin, and alkaline phosphate). A urinalysis should be done, as well as a stool guaiac. Tests of acid phosphatase should be ordered for males with unknown primary malignancy, a SPEP and UPEP is performed if multiple myeloma is suspected, and a 24-h urine hydroxyproline is collected for Paget's disease. Thyroid function tests, CEA, and PTH levels may provide additional information.

Other useful tests in evaluating patients suspected of pathologic fracture are the following: an upper and lower GI series; endoscopy; mammography; chest CT; intravenous pyelogram; renal ultrasound; and scans of the liver, spleen, and thyroid. Primary malignancy can not be diagnosed in approximately 15 percent of patients with suspected metastatic disease even with testing.

CLASSIFICATION

Pathologic fractures can be categorized according to the existing condition compromising the affected bone. Systemic conditions leading to pathologic fracture include osteoporosis (the most common cause in the elderly), metabolic bone diseases (osteomalacia and hyperparathyroidism), and Paget's disease. Pathologic fracture is the most frequent orthopaedic complication seen in Paget's disease (10 to 30 percent).

The second most common cause of pathologic fractures is localized disease processes, such as primary benign and malignant bone tumors, hematopoietic disorders, and metastatic disease. The vast majority (80 percent) of pathologic fractures secondary to metastatic disease are associated with primaries of the breast, lung, thyroid, kidney, or prostate. Common skeletal sites of pathologic fractures associated with metastatic disease are the spine, ribs, pelvis, femur, and humerus.

Biopsy of the affected site usually permits diagnosis of the associated disease as a systemic skeletal disease, primary bone tumor, or metastatic tumor and provides histologic differentiation that can be applied toward appropriate treatment.

TREATMENT

Pathologic fractures should be initially treated like any acute fracture, with reduction and immobilization. Additional clinical and laboratory evaluation are done to identify the specific underlying pathologic processes and to evaluate and manage the patient's medical status.

Pathologic fractures require a longer healing time than normal fractures; if the patient has undergone radiation and/or chemotherapy as an adjuvant treatment, healing may be prolonged further. Fractures occurring within primary benign bone lesions will unite without surgical intervention.

The standard of care for the majority of long bone pathologic fractures is internal fixation. Treatment objectives are to prevent progression of osteoporosis due to disuse, to provide mechanical support that permits the patient to continue daily activities, to relieve pain, and to reduce the length of hospital stay. Adequate management demands interdisciplinary care and evaluation from oncologists, internists, and radiation therapists. Radiation and chemotherapy are the main treatment modalities in the treatment of pathologic fractures, and are used to decrease the size of the lesion, stop its progession, and alleviate symptoms. Because both of these therapies delay the healing of soft tissues, they should not be administered until approximately 10 to 21 days following surgery.

Contraindications to operative treatment of pathologic fractures include a medical status that suggests an inability to tolerate anaesthesia or surgery, obtunded patients, or those with altered consciousness where the need to alleviate pain is not necessary.

More than 50 percent of pathologic long bone fractures occur in the proximal femur because of the attending high weightbearing stresses. Femoral neck pathologic fractures do not achieve union, regardless of the degree of displacement, and should be managed with prosthetic replacement. If the acetabulum remains intact, hemiarthroplasty may be adequate treatment; however, with acetabular involvement, total joint replacement is indicated. Pathologic shaft fractures of the femur are usually managed with an intramedullary nail.

The humeral shaft is frequently involved with metastatic disease, increasing the possibility of pathologic fracture. Prophylactic internal fixation of the humerus is not recommended on a routine basis; however, operative stabilization of pathologic humerus fractures has been reported to support a number of treatment objectives: to allieviate pain, reduce the need for nursing care, and optimize patient independence.

Pathologic fractures in the spine are usually compression fractures of the vertebral bodies secondary to osteoporosis. They are generally managed by a temporary reduction in activity or by wearing a brace. The vertebral body is the most common site for spinal metastases. Compromise of the spinal cord or nerve root may occur from direct extension of the metastatic lesion or secondarily from spinal insta-

bility. Surgical intervention may be used to stabilize the spinal column, prevent neurologic deficit, and reduce pain.

There is significant controversy concerning prophylactic fixation of impending pathologic fractures. The associated risk for fracture is dependent on the site of the lesion, the histologic tumor type, and the amount of osseous involvement. Conditions predisposing towards prophylactic fixation include cortical bone destruction of 50 percent or more, a proximal femoral lesion of 2.5 cm or greater, pathologic avulsion of the lesser trochanter, and persistent pain in spite of adjuvant radiation and/or chemotherapy.

MUSCLE CONTUSION AND SOFT TISSUE INJURY

CONTUSION

Muscle contusion is caused by a direct blow, and is a common injury during contact sports. Contusion causes damage and partial disruption of muscle fibers, and is frequently accompanied by capillary rupture with infiltrative bleeding. The objective of treatment is to reduce inflammation and includes ice, compression, elevation, rest, and medication, followed by rehabilitation.

Muscle contusions are categorized by the degree of function remaining in the injured muscle. Mild contusions have close-to-normal joint motion, local tenderness, and generally no changes in the patient's gait. Moderate contusions permit approximately 75 percent of the normal range of motion, are swollen and tender, and patients will have a limp. Severe contusions allow only 50 percent of normal range of motion, are significantly tender and swollen, and patients walk with a limp.

Myositis ossificans may occur and complicate the management and healing of muscle contusion.

MUSCLE STRAIN

Muscle strains are an indirect injury to muscle resulting from excessive stretch or tension to the muscle. They are categorized in terms of severity: first-degree strains include minor stretching of the musculotendinous unit and do not result in permanent injury; second-degree strains have partial tearing of the musculotendinous unit; and third-degree strains have total disruption of the unit. Muscles that include two joints are more vulnerable to strain injury. Treatment is similar to that for contusion and includes rest, ice, compression, elevation, and medication, followed by rehabilitation.

SOFT TISSUE INJURY

Tscherne has described a four grade (grades 0 to 3) classification for closed fractures, based on muscle and skin trauma and fracture comminution which may assist in guiding treatment planning (Table 72-7).

BURN INJURY

Partial-thickness burns include first- and second-degree and deep dermal (third-degree) skin burns. The mechanism of injury is usually a brief contact with heat or hot liquids. These injuries have viable epithelial components that permit reepithelialization of the injury if it is protected from additional trauma or infection. The appearance of partial-thickness burns varies from pink to mottled red, is wet, and covered with vesicles and bullae; they are exquisitely painful. In full-thickness burns, all viable epithelial components have been destroyed. These injuries generally necessitate excision and always require skin

---

Table 72-7

Tscherne Classification of Soft Tissue Injuries

Grade	
0	Minimal soft tissue damage; indirect violence; simple fracture pattern.
1	Superficial abrasion of contusion caused by pressure from within; mild to moderately severe fracture configuraton.
2	Deep contaminated abrasions associated with localized skin or muscle contusion; impending compartment syndrome; severe fracture configuration.
3	Extensive skin contusion or crush; underlying severe muscle; decompensated compartment syndrome; associated major vascular injury, severe or comminuted fracture configuration.

SOURCE: Reproduced with permission from Tscherne H, Gotzen L: *Fractures with Soft Tissue Injuries.* Berlin: Springer-Verlag; 1984.

---

grafts. The mechanism of injury is contact with fire, electricity, or chemicals. They generally appear as dry and charred, sometimes translucent, and occasionally with superficial thrombosed veins.

The initial evaluation of burn patients is similar to the examination of polytrauma patients—addressing the degree and severity of injury is a crucial first step. The American Burn Association has established guidelines to assist in determining which patients need to be transferred to a burn unit (Table 72-8).

The "Rule of Nines" (Table 72-9) is also a standard tool used to estimate the extent of burn injury in adults. Burned areas are diagrammed onto figures which have been divided into body areas that collectively represent the person's total body surface area (TBSA). A person with burns covering his back (18 percent TBSA) and left arm (9 percent TBSA) would have a total burn injury of 27 percent of the TBSA. Other standards use percentages that account for growth, and are used with infants and children.

Fluid hydration in burn injury is crucial as capillary permeability is increased in burn injury and may cause tissue edema, pulmonary and peripheral vascular hypertension, acute tubular necrosis, and a decrease in cardiac output. During the second postburn day, capillary permeability returns towards normal.

Treatment

Burn wounds should always be examined with sterile technique. A sterile dressing with topical antimicrobials is applied to avoid infection. Nonviable tissue is excised. One of the most common complications is wound infection; the greatest risk being to those patients with burns greater than 30 percent of the TBSA. Epithelialization of partial thickness burns and grafting of full thickness burns may decrease the incidence of wound infection.

Electrical Burns

Factors determining the degree of severity in electrical burns are the duration of electrical contact; path of the current, voltage, and amperage; and resistance to the passage of current at the points of contact. Alternating current is potentially the most serious mechanism of injury, because it can produce tonic muscle contractions where the

---

Table 72-8

Guidelines of American Burn Association for Transfer of Patients to Burn Unit

1. Second and third degree burns of 10% or more of total body surface area (TBSA) in patients under 10 or over 50 years of age.

2. In all other age gruops, second and third degree burns involving 20% TBSA.

3. Full thickness burns of at least 5% of TBSA.

4. Burns that may result in cosmetic or functional disability, including burns of the face, hands, feet, eyes, ears, or perineum.

5. High voltage electrical injury.

6. Inhalation injury or associated trauma.

7. Significant chemical burns.

8. Burns in patients with diseases that would increase their chances of dying.

SOURCE: American Burn Association, Chicago, IL.

Table 72-9

Rule of Nines for Total Body Surface Area

%TBSA	Regions
9	Head and Neck
18	Anterior trunk (from clavicles to pubes)
18	Posterior trunk (from root of neck to and including buttocks)
9 each	Upper extremity (total, 18%)
18 each	Lower extremity (total, 36%)
1	Genitalia/Perineum
100%	Total

victim is unable to release the source of electricity. Very high voltage can result in arc burns which occur without direct contact with the body surface. Electrical burn patients are at risk for cardiac arrhythmias and for acute renal failure secondary to increased blood concentrations of hemoglobin and myoglobin; patients should receive inpatient monitoring for both these potentialities.

SNAKEBITE

The intense pain of a poisonous snake bite will distinquish it from the bite of a nonpoisonous snake. Presentation of a poisonous snake bite generally includes edema, tenderness, pain, and ecchymosis. Symptoms usually appear within 30 min of the bite; edema may continue to worsen over the next 24 h. Hemorrhagic cutaneous lesions may appear between 8 and 30 h following the injury, with subsequent thrombosis of the superficial vessels and sloughing of the skin. Systemic symptoms include muscle fasciculations (commonly the perioral area and the neck), muscle weakness, and parasthesias.

One should place a tourniquet, make an incision, and suck out the venom. The tourniquet is not removed until an IV has been started and antivenin has been prepared for administration. Surgical exploration is reserved for severe bites seen within 1 h of the incident. The most important treatment for snake bites is antivenin; however, in 30 percent of bites, envenomation does not occur and antivenin is not necessary. One should titrate the dosage of antivenin based on clinical improvement. Antivenin is administered until severe local or systemic symptoms begin to resolve. Antibiotics are needed to prevent secondary infection, and the patient's tetanus status needs to be assessed. The affected extremity must also be assessed for compartment syndrome (see Chap. 120).

SUGGESTED READINGS

GENERAL

Browner BD, Jupiter JB, Levine AM, et al (eds): *Skeletal Trauma,* 2d ed. Philadelphia: WB Saunders; 1998.

Rockwood CA Jr, Green DP, Bucholz RW: *Fractures in Adults,* 4th ed. Philadelphia: Lippincott-Raven; 1996.

Weber BG, Cech O: *Pseudarthrosis.* New York: Grune & Stratton, 1976.

MULTIPLE TRAUMA

Bone LB: Emergency treatment of the injured patient. In Browner BD, Jupiter JB, Levine AM, et al (eds): *Skeletal Trauma*. Philadelphia: WB Saunders; 1992:chap 5.

Bone LB: Management of polytrauma. In Chapman M (ed): *Operative Orthopedics* Philadelphia: Lippincott; 1993:chap 19.

Johnson KD, Cadmambi A, Seibert G, et al: Incidence of adult respiratory distress syndrome in patients with multiple musculoskeletal injuries: Effects of early operative stabilization of fractures. *J Trauma* 1985; 25:375.

MUSCLE CONTUSIONS

Arrington ED, Miller MD: Skeletal muscle injuries. *Orthop Clin North Am* 1995; 26:411.

Sullivan JB Jr, Wingert WA, Norris RL: North American venomous reptile bites. In Auerbach PS (ed): *Wilderness Medicine: Management of Wilderness and Environmental Emergencies.* St. Louis: Mosby; 1995.

OPEN FRACTURES

Chapman MW: Role of bone stability in open fractures. In Frankel VH (ed): *Instructional Course Lectures.* Park Ridge, IL: American Academy of Orthopaedic Surgeons; 1982; 31:75.

Gustilo RB: Current concepts in the management of open fractures. In Griffin PP (ed): *Instructional Course Lectures.* Park Ridge, IL: American Academy of Orthopaedic Surgeons; 1987; 36:359.

Tscherne H, Gotzen L: *Fractures with Soft Tissue Injuries.* Berlin: Springer-Verlag; 1984.

GUNSHOT FRACTURES

Adams DB: Wound ballistics: A review. *Mil Med* 1982; 147:831.

Brettler D, Sedlin ED, Mendes DG: Conservative management of low velocity gunshot wounds. *Clin Orthop* 1979; 140:26.

PATHOLOGIC FRACTURES

Harrington KD: Impending pathologic fractures from metastatic malignancy: evaluation and management. In Anderson LD (ed): *Instructional Course Lectures.* Park Ridge, IL: American Academy of Orthopaedic Surgeons. 1986; 35:357.

Chapter 73

SPINAL TRAUMA: GENERAL CONSIDERATIONS

Jeffrey M. Spivak

FIELD RESUSCITATION

In the field, emergency technicians immobilize victims of suspected spinal injury on rigid backboards for transportation. The neck is immobilized using a rigid cervical collar or sandbags. Awake patients should be questioned about any history of neck deformity. A previously normal neck (or if the patient cannot give a history) should be immobilized in a neutral position; any preexisting deformity should be recreated (if known to the emergency technician) and then the neck immobilized in that position. Special consideration must be given to the child with suspected cervical spine injury. Due to a disproportionately large head size as compared to adults, immobilization on a flat backboard places the cervical spine in a potentially dangerous amount of flexion. Pediatric backboards, therefore, have a recess for the head to fit into, maintaining a neutral cervical alignment.

CLINICAL EVALUATION

The specific directed examination of a patient with suspected spinal injury begins only after the typical ABC (airway, breathing, circulation) evaluation standard for all trauma patients. The spinal examination includes inspection and palpation of the spine and a careful and complete neurologic evaluation. A high suspicion for head, chest, and abdominal injuries, which are frequently associated with cervical, thoracic, and thoracolumbar trauma respectively, should prompt serial mental status, chest, and/or abdominal exams in the early postinjury period when a significant spinal injury is diagnosed.

The cervical collar placed in the field is maintained until the neck is cleared radiographically, but it may be opened by the examining physician during the examination for inspection and palpation. The patient is carefully log-rolled onto his or her side as the neck is maintained in a neutral position. The entire spinal column is inspected; abrasions and deep lacerations are suspicious for underlying spinal column injury. Open spinal injuries are infrequent, but failure to diagnose an open injury due to an incomplete examination must be avoided. Palpation of all spinous processes is done, feeling for areas of tenderness (in the awake, cooperative patient), fluid collection, bony crepitus, or an increase in the interspinous distance. These all signal possible injury to the posterior elements, and should be correlated with the radiographic examination.

The neurologic examination for spinal trauma includes dermatomal sensory testing, assessing cervical, lumbar, and sacral root motor function (Table 73–1), and a detailed spinal reflex examination (Table 73–2). The term "spinal shock" refers to a flaccid paralysis due to physiologic disruption of all spinal cord function at and caudal to the anatomic level of spinal cord injury. All sensory, motor, and reflex function are absent. A true assessment of the patient's neurologic status cannot be made when the patient is in spinal shock, which resolves within 24 to 48 h in over 99 percent of cases. The absence of spinal shock is confirmed by the return of spinal cord mediated reflexes below the anatomic area of injury. The bulbocavernosus is the lowest cord mediated reflex and is generally the first to return.

A "complete" neurologic injury is marked by a total absence of sensory and voluntary motor function below the anatomic level of injury in the absence of spinal shock. In incomplete lesions, residual spinal cord and/or nerve root function exists below the anatomic level of injury. The most common types of incomplete neurologic injuries are an incomplete cord lesion in cervical and thoracic spine trauma and a complete cord lesion with lumbar root sparing for injuries at the thoracolumbar junction. With the spinal cord ending generally at the L1–2 disc space level, neurologic injuries (complete or incomplete) associated with low lumbar trauma (L3–L5) are all root level injuries. Complete root level injuries result in a flaccid paralysis which has a clinical picture that may be indistinguishable from true cord-mediated spinal shock.

An incomplete spinal cord lesion is confirmed by sensory and/or voluntary motor function emanating from a cord segment below the anatomic level of injury. This must include the lowest sacral segments as defined by the American Spinal Injury Association. Low sacral sensation includes both the perianal region and deep anal sensation, and motor function testing is by digital exam palpation of voluntary contraction of the external anal sphincter.

Incomplete spinal cord lesions often follow one of four described patterns, or syndromes, based on the location of neural damage within the spinal cord (Fig. 73–1). The most common of these incomplete cord injury patterns is the central cord syndrome. Since the spatial orientation of the long tracts in the spinal cord maintains cervical function more centrally and lumbosacral function more peripherally, a central cord syndrome results in greater loss in the upper extremity motors with relative sparing of the lumbar and sacral motors. Functional motor recovery is expected in 75 percent of cases. In the anterior cord syndrome, the dorsal columns remain intact preserving proprioception, vibration, and light touch, and there is profound loss of motor function and deep pain and temperature sensation. Functional recovery is seen in only 10 percent of these cases. The posterior cord syndrome is very uncommon, characterized by isolated dorsal column loss (vibration, proprioception, and light touch sensation). The Brown-Séquard syndrome results from a unilateral hemispinal cord injury. This uncommon injury pattern is characterized by ipsilateral loss of motor function, light touch, proprioception and vibration sense, and contralateral loss of deep pain and temperature sense. Functional motor recovery occurs in over 90 percent of these patients.

The final aspect of the clinical evaluation of the spinal trauma patient involves the examination for associated internal injuries of the

Table 73-1

Cervical and Lumbar Root Level Functions

Root	Reflex	Muscles	Sensation
C5	Biceps	Deltoid/biceps	Lateral arm (deltoid patch)
C6	Brachioradialis Biceps	Wrist extensors	Radial forearm Thumb
C7	Triceps	Wrist flexors Finger extensors Triceps (elbow extension)	Middle finger
C8		Finger flexors Hand intrinsics	Little finger Ulnar forearm
T1		Hand intrinsics	Medial arm
L1		Internal oblique Transverse abdominis	Posterolateral buttocks Inguinal area above pubis
L2		Hip adductors Hip flexors	Prox anterior medial thigh
L3		Hip adductors Hip flexors	Lateral thigh
L4	Knee jerk	Quadriceps Tibialis anterior	Medial leg and foot
L5		EHL Foot inversion (Tib post)	1st web space, dorsal foot
S1	Ankle jerk	FHL, gastrocsoleus Peroneus longus/brevis	Lateral foot

head, chest, and abdomen. Significant head injury is often seen in conjunction with trauma to the cervical spine. Intrathoracic trauma, including hemopneumothorax, major vessel injury, and diaphragmatic rupture may be seen in more than one-third of patients with thoracic

spine fractures and neurologic injury. Intraabdominal trauma including liver, splenic and pancreatic lacerations, bowel rupture, major vessel injury, and injuries to the upper urinary tract are associated with flexion-distraction injuries and fracture-dislocations of the thoracolumbar junction and lumbar spine.

Table 73-2

Reflex Testing in Thoracolumbar Spine Injuries

Superficial abdominal (above umbilicus)	T7–T10
Superficial abdominal (below umbilicus)	T11–L1
Cremasteric reflex	T12–L1
Knee jerk	L3–4
Ankle jerk	S1
Anal wink	S2–S4
Bulbocavernosus reflex	S3–4
Plantar response	Brain/lumbosacral cord continuity

NEUROGENIC SHOCK

Patients with spinal shock due to spinal cord injury have an associated loss of sympathetic tone (T1–L2). The unopposed vagal parasympathetic vasodilatation causes a sudden increase in the available intravascular space, resulting in a state of relative hypovolemia and hypotension. This is known as *neurogenic shock*. It can be differentiated from *cardiogenic shock* (pump failure) or true *hypovolemic shock* (due to blood loss out of the intravascular space) based on the heart rate response to the hypotension. Neurogenic shock is characterized by bradycardia despite the hypotension resulting from the unopposed vagal output. In patients with hypotension and tachycardia, the physical examination will usually point to another cause for the circulatory compromise, such as direct cardiac injury or hypovolemia due to chest, abdominal, or extremity trauma with local hemorrhage. Hypotension is caused by neurogenic shock in about 70 percent of patients with cervical spinal cord injuries. In upper spinal thoracic injuries, the percentage of hypotension due to neurogenic shock is probably similar, but in thoracolumbar junction and lumbar injuries,

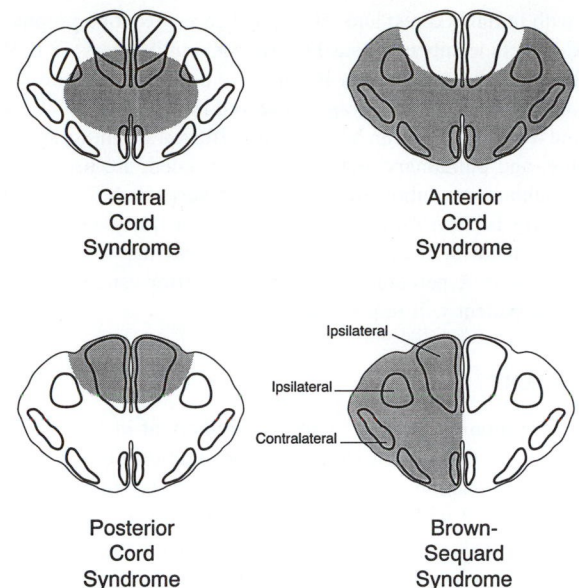

Central
Cord
Syndrome

Anterior
Cord
Syndrome

Ipsilateral

Ipsilateral

Contralateral

Posterior
Cord
Syndrome

Brown-
Sequard
Syndrome

Figure 73-1

Types of spinal cord injury (*gray zones*) which produce the four major incomplete injury patterns seen clinically. [Copyright © 1995 American Academy of Orthopaedic Surgeons. Reprinted from Spivak JM, Vaccaro AR, Cotler JM: Thoracolumbar spine trauma: I. Evaluation and classification. *Journal of the American Academy of Orthopaedic Surgeons: A Comprehensive Review,* 1995; 3(6):347, with permission.]

the majority of sympathetic tone is maintained and neurogenic shock is less common.

RADIOGRAPHIC EVALUATION

Radiographic evaluation of specific suspected spinal trauma begins only after the standard "trauma series" radiographs (lateral cervical spine, AP chest, and AP pelvis), as in all cases of blunt trauma. The chest radiograph is carefully examined for evidence of mediastinal widening. Suspicion of fullness in the mediastinum must be evaluated by computed tomography, and an aortogram may be indicated to rule out a traumatic aortic dissection, even if thoracic spinal trauma and paraspinal hematoma is clearly visible.

Regions of suspected spinal trauma based on pain complaints or the physical examination are then evaluated by AP and lateral radiographs of the spinal region in question. In patients who cannot communicate areas of pain or who are uncooperative with their examination secondary to head trauma, cervical trauma with neurologic deficit, or alcohol and drug intoxication, the entire spinal column must be imaged in the AP and lateral projections. In awake alert patients, areas of local pain and tenderness should be evaluated by coned-down views, and flexion-extension lateral radiographs may be indicated if initial radiographs show no obvious bony or ligamentous injury.

The importance of imaging the entire spine in blunt trauma situations, even if a spinal injury has already been identified, is to rule out additional spinal injuries which might be unstable, and if missed, could lead to the development or progression of neurologic injury. Multi-level noncontiguous spinal injuries have been reported in up to 17 percent of cases. The additional injury is originally missed in up to 50 percent of cases, with the delay in diagnosis averaging one week to over 50 days in various series. The development or progression of a neurologic deficit occurs in 25 percent of these missed injuries due to improper initial immobilization. Common injury patterns and sub-

patterns have been described. Upper thoracic injuries are common among patients with multilevel noncontiguous injuries.

Computed tomographic (CT) scanning continues to be important in the evaluation of spinal injuries, especially in assessing the integrity of the posterior aspect of the vertebral body and posterior bony elements. Plain CT is indicated in all cases of suspected injuries to the posterior elements and posterior vertebral body. Retropulsion of bony fragments into the spinal canal can be clearly seen on transverse sections. Sagittal and coronal reconstructions aid in evaluating the alignment of the spinal canal. Both CT scanning with sagittal and coronal reconstructions and plain tomography are useful for imaging areas of suspected injury on plain films and areas not well visualized by plain radiographs, such as the upper cervical spine and the cervicothoracic junction. Tomograms offer the benefit of direct imaging in the sagittal and coronal plane, but are becoming less and less available as an imaging modality.

Magnetic resonance imaging (MRI) provides direct visualization of the spinal cord and allows for evaluation of traumatic intervertebral disc pathology. It is indicated in all cases with neurologic deficit to assess for both intrinsic and extrinsic cord pathology. MRI is also indicated in operative cases (even without a neurologic deficit) as a preoperative exam to provide complete evaluation of the spinal canal. MRI can differentiate between intrinsic cord injuries such as edema, hematoma, and spinal cord transection (very uncommon). Edema is seen as a fusiform enlargement of the spinal cord with increased signal intensity on T2-weighted images. Hematoma demonstrates decreased signal on T2 images acutely, and is often surrounded by a halo of T2 enhancement from adjacent edema. Edema extending more than two vertebral levels and the presence of hematoma within the spinal cord are poor prognostic signs for functional motor recovery. Extrinsic cord compression secondary to spinal canal compromise by bony elements, soft tissue, or fluid collection is also readily identified using MRI.

MRI is also an important part of the evaluation of spinal cord injury without radiographic abnormalities, commonly seen in children. In these patients as well as in patients with significant bony injury, MRI can evaluate the extent of intradiscal injury and posterior ligamentous injury. MRI diagnosis of acute soft tissue injury may impact greatly on the understanding of the stability of the injury and the recommended treatment. Diffuse posterior ligamentous disruption may indicate a more unstable injury and prompt early surgical stabilization. MRI is also useful in the post-injury period, especially for evaluation of the late development or worsening of a pre-existing neurologic injury, due to a posttraumatic cyst or syrinx.

Myelography may also be as useful for many of the same indications as MRI, but is invasive and does not view the intrinsic anatomy of the spinal cord. It is indicated for cases with progressive neurologic deficit when MRI is not available. Myelography and CT scanning are particularly useful in the postoperative evaluation of possible persistent spinal cord compression, especially when spinal instrumentation has been used posteriorly.

MANAGEMENT ISSUES

There are a variety of issues to be considered in the management of patients with significant spinal trauma. Initial management issues include immobilization, medical stabilization, and achievement of spinal alignment. Definitive management decisions are based on spinal stability at the injury site and the need for decompression of neural elements. In the recovery period, appropriate rehabilitation is needed to maximize the patient's functional outcome.

IMMOBILIZATION

Experimental evidence exists from in vivo animal studies that immobilization helps to limit further damage to the injured spinal cord. Immobilization also helps in controlling the pain associated with a spinal column injury. For cervical injuries, initial immobilization is advised using a rigid cervical orthosis, usually applied in the field. This can be maintained, if desired, or converted to skeletal immobilization using a halo or Gardner-Wells tongs. Tongs are more easily applied, placed in the neutral position just 1 cm above the pinnae in line with the external auditory meatus. A more anterior placement will result in an extension moment on the neck with applied linear traction; a more posterior placement results in a flexion moment. Depending on the injury, these forces may be detrimental or beneficial to the spinal reduction and immobilization. Halo fixation can be used for traction, but not for the heavy weights that can be supported by the Gardner-Wells tongs. Halo fixation has the added advantage of being directly convertible to halo-vest immobilization, allowing the patient to be mobilized immediately or following a period of traction. Generally, four halo pins are used in adults, applied to a torque of 8 in./lb. The two anterior and posterior pins are applied directly opposing one another, and the anterior pins are applied in the region 1 cm superior to the lateral two-thirds of the eyebrow (orbital rim). The region superior to the medial third of the eyebrow is avoided to prevent inadvertent injury to the supraorbital and supratrochlear nerves and vessels, which course superiorly in this region.

For thoracic and lumbar injuries, simple bed rest with logrolling can be used. Problems may occur with improper log-rolling of the patient or miscommunication with hospital staff regarding the patient's spinal stability and activity level. An oscillating bed, such as the Roto-Rest bed, is often utilized to regularly shift the patient's body weight without moving the patient. Traction can be applied using Gardner-Well tong/bifemoral skeletal fixation, if it is deemed desirable.

MEDICAL STABILIZATION

Assessment and stabilization of the vital signs is extremely important in patients with suspected or known spinal trauma. Maintenance of an adequate blood pressure for perfusion of vital organs is the prime concern. Both neurogenic shock and hemorrhagic (hypovolemic) shock result in life-threatening hypotension which must be reversed by intravascular volume expansion using blood and other volume replacement fluids. Vasopressors may be required in addition. Critical internal organ systems must be evaluated and treated if needed.

Medical treatment of the injured spinal cord minimizes or prevents the secondary cord injury caused by both edema and ischemia. Intravenous methylprednisolone is administered routinely for all blunt spinal cord injuries, beginning with a 30 mg/kg body weight bolus followed by a continuous infusion of 5.4 mg/kg/h for a total of 23 h. The efficacy of this protocol has been established only for blunt spinal cord injury with treatment started within 8 h from the time of injury. The efficacy of intravenous steroid use is unknown for pure spinal nerve root injuries. Intravenous steroid treatment is not without risk of complications, including the development of gastric ulcers and a higher rate of postoperative wound infection. Multicenter prospective evaluation of other pharmacologic agents, including beta-glycosides and growth factors, are currently under way.

Prevention of thromboembolic disease remains an important medical consideration in patients with spinal injury. Mechanical prophylaxis using compression stockings and intermittent external pneumatic compression devices is commonly employed in all spinal injury cases with initial bed rest and all surgical cases. Routine prophylaxis may also include subcutaneous heparin 5000 units every 12 h. Real-time B-mode ultrasonography is currently utilized to diagnose deep vein thrombosis, with venography reserved for cases in which the ultrasound results are unclear. Ventilation-perfusion scanning, spinal CT scanning, and pulmonary angiography, if needed, are used to diagnose a pulmonary embolism when one is suspected. Treatment includes early heparinization and use of Coumadin (warfarin) for 6 months as medical management if the patient has a nonoperative spinal problem. A percutaneously placed inferior vena cava filter is used if the patient will require surgery.

ALIGNMENT

Early restoration of spinal alignment is important in the peri-injury period along with immobilization to remove deformity-related compression on the neural elements and minimize secondary neural injury. Realignment with reduction of cervical deformity secondary to trauma requires skeletal traction, which can be applied using Gardner-Wells tongs or a halo ring (see Chap. 74). Postural reduction of thoracic and lumbar injuries with simple bed rest and a small bolster placed at the apex of a spinal deformity may be effective in certain injury patterns. The skin beneath any padded bolster must be examined daily for evidence of skin breakdown, which could significantly compromise a posterior surgical site. Another way to improve anterior vertebral column height and reduce the degree of kyphosis is through the use of Gardner-Wells tong/bifemoral skeletal traction. Skeletal traction has the added benefit of ensuring patient compliance in terms of bed rest.

SPINAL STABILIZATION

In general terms, the spine is considered stable if it is able to withstand normally applied physiologic loads without the development of neural injury, unacceptable deformity, or chronic pain due to abnormal motion. Previously, the posterior elements were thought to be the most important structures in assessing spinal stability. More recently, CT has allowed for a more detailed analysis, visualizing the bony and ligamentous injury in conjunction with the degree of spinal canal compromise, spinal deformity, and neurologic deficit. Denis, in 1983, proposed the three column theory of stability of the thoracolumbar spine (see Chap. 75). The spine is considered to be unstable if two or more columns are injured. Denis also described three levels of instability: (1) mechanical instability, with the potential for later development of hypermobility and deformity during and after tissue healing; (2) neurologic instability, with potential for later development of neurologic injury; and (3) mechanical and neurologic instability, injuries with initial neurologic injury, unacceptable destruction of bony and ligamentous support, or unacceptable initial deformity. White and Panjabi (1990) have devised a clinical checklist for cervical, thoracic, and lumbar instability, considering radiographic criteria (subluxation, segmental angulation), neural injury, and anticipated dangerous loading to determine if a spinal injury is stable or not.

DECOMPRESSION

Decompression of the spinal canal is often needed in cases with canal intrusion by bony or soft tissue fragments. Compression more commonly occurs anteriorly, due to bone or disc fragments retropulsed from the injured posterior vertebral body or disc. Posterior compression can also occur from displaced lamina fractures. Persistent neural compression due to spinal canal compromise in patients with incomplete spinal cord deficits requires operative spinal decompression. For complete lesions of the midcervical spine, thoracolumbar junction, and lumbar spine, decompression may be indicated if significant canal compromise exists. In these regions, additional root recovery can provide important functional benefits. In cases without neurologic deficit, canal decompression may not be indicated as long as spinal stability can be assured due to eventual bony remodeling of retropulsed bony fragments. This is currently a point of some controversy.

In general, spinal decompression can be done via an anterior, posterolateral, or posterior approach. Anterior decompression via partial or complete corpectomy (removal of the vertebral body) is commonly performed for spinal canal compromise due to retropulsed bone and disc fragments from the middle column in the cervical, thoracic, and thoracolumbar spine. Vertebral body reconstruction can be performed using an autogenous anterior iliac crest strut graft, an allograft of iliac crest or diaphyseal shaft with or without inner autograft cancellous bone (fibula for cervical spine; humeral, femoral, or tibial shaft for thoracic and lumbar spine), or a prosthetic replacement (e.g., surgical cylindrical titanium mesh, ceramic block, methacrylate). Anterior vertebral body reconstruction following trauma requires additional stabilization. This may be accomplished by external immobilization such as a halo-vest, or body cast; commonly, internal fixation is utilized, which can be applied anteriorly, posteriorly, or both.

Laminectomy as a sole procedure has been shown to be ineffective in relieving anterior spinal canal compression. Indications for laminectomy include cases with neurologic deficits and accompanying lamina fractures, in order to inspect for entrapped neural elements and dural tears. Laminectomy is also occasionally needed for decompression of a compressive epidural hematoma, which is seen in some minimally displaced fractures in patients with ankylosing spondylitis. Whenever a laminectomy is performed the spinal column is further destabilized and a fusion with instrumentation should be performed.

TIMING OF SURGERY

Debate continues regarding the timing of operative decompression of spinal canal compromise. Most believe that decompression should be done urgently, not emergently. Patients are medically stabilized as active fracture bleeding slows and hematoma forms. This minimizes operative blood loss with anterior decompressive procedures, especially in the thoracolumbar spine. Emergent indications for surgery in spinal trauma include a progressive neurologic deficit and an incomplete neurologic deficit associated with an irreducible dislocation. Improved overall neurologic outcomes have not been demonstrated with emergent stabilization of unstable spinal injuries with or without neural decompression. In fact, cases with worsening neurologic deficits following emergent decompression have been attributed to further secondary spinal cord injury with increased edema. Late decompression of persistent spinal cord compression has been shown to result in late neurologic improvement.

REHABILITATION

Passive motion exercises and splinting are utilized in the early injury period in all patients with neurologic deficits in order to maintain joint flexibility and maximize functional potential. Maximal flexibility and upper body strength are essential for functional paraplegics in order to perform self-transfers and return to independence in society. The use of orthotic devices with appropriate training can allow independent ambulation in many patients with low-lumbar functional neurologic levels. The use of assistive devices and vocational retraining allows patients to regain maximal functional and financial independence.

SUGGESTED READINGS

Bohlman HH, Freehafer A, Dejak J: The results of treatment of acute injuries of the upper thoracic spine with paralysis. *J Bone Joint Surg [Am]* 1985; 67:360.

Bracken MB, Shepard MJ, Collins WF, et al: A randomized, controlled trial of methylprednisolone or naloxone in the treatment of acute spinal-cord injury. Results of the Second National Acute Spinal Cord Injury Study. *N Engl J Med* 1990; 322:1405.

Denis F: Spinal instability as defined by the three-column spine concept in acute spinal trauma. *Clin Orthop* 1984; 189:65-76.

International Standards for Neurological and Functional Classification of Spinal Cord Injury, Revised 1996. Chicago, IL: American Spinal Injury Association and The International Medical Society of Paraplegia; 1996.

Soderstrom CA, McArdle DQ, Duker TB, et al: The diagnosis of intra-abdominal injury in patients with cervical cord trauma. *J Trauma* 1983; 23:1061.

Vaccaro AR, An HS, Lin S, et al: Noncontiguous injuries of the spine. *J Spinal Disorders* 1992; 5:320.

White AA, Panjabi MM: *Clinical Biomechanics of the Spine*. Philadelphia: Lippincott; 1990.

Chapter 74

CERVICAL SPINE

Jeffrey M. Spivak

OCCIPITOCERVICAL DISSOCIATION

CLASSIFICATION

Occipitocervical injuries have been classified by Traynelis and associates based on the direction of displacement: anterior, vertical, or posterior. All patterns of injury, from a biomechanical standpoint, represent ligamentous damage to the alar ligaments and tectorial membrane, and are considered unstable. As the forces required to produce these injuries are quite high, occipitocervical injuries are usually associated with high-energy trauma; severe neurologic injury with high cervical quadriplegia is common. Associated injuries include submental and posterior pharyngeal wall lacerations, mandible fractures, and injury to the cranial nerves and vertebral artery.

In anterior dislocations (the most common type), the occipital condyles are forward to the lateral masses of C1, and the clivus points anterior to the dens tip. In posterior dislocations, the direction is opposite, and the posteriorly displaced occipital condyles result in the dens positioned anterior to the clivus. Vertical occipitocervical instability is classified into two patterns. One pattern demonstrates distraction between the occiput and C1, while the second pattern occurs between C1 and C2. The latter injury is associated with rupture of the transverse ligament. The injury that causes distraction between C1 and C2 is considered a form of occipitocervical instability because the ligamentous injury to the major stabilizers—the alar ligaments and tectorial membrane—is similar.

Power's Ratio is used as a radiographic measure of atlantooccipital translation (Fig. 74-1). Two lines are drawn and the lengths measured (BC from the basion of the skull to the anterior aspect of the posterior arch of the atlas, and AO, from the posterior border of the anterior arch of the atlas to the opisthion of the skull). The ratio BC/AO should be <1. If it is greater, an anterior atlantooccipital injury is likely.

TREATMENT

Treatment goals for injuries to the occipitocervical articulation include closed reduction, maintenance of reduction, and both acute and long-term stability. As these injuries are highly unstable, posterior occipitocervical fusion to C1 or C2 is usually required. Internal fixation with sublaminar/occipital wiring techniques or plate fixation (to C2 or below) can be utilized. Cervical traction is contraindicated because of the severe instability. Immediate application of a halo-vest to reduce and stabilize the joint can be useful. Since these injuries are primarily due to ligamentous disruption, closed treatment offers little promise for adequate long-term healing and stability.

C1 FRACTURES

CLASSIFICATION

There are three primary types of fractures of the ring of C1:

(1) Posterior arch fracture, which usually occurs at the junction of the posterior arch and the lateral mass, and can be unilateral or bilateral. These result from a hyperextension mechanism, and are associated with odontoid fractures.

(2) Lateral mass fracture, which usually occurs on one side only with the fracture line passing either through the articular surface or just anterior and posterior to the lateral mass on one side; a fracture through the posterior arch on the opposite side may also occur. These result from an axial loading and lateral bending mechanism.

(3) A "burst" fracture (a.k.a. Jefferson's fracture), which is classically described as bilateral fractures of the anterior and posterior arches. These are axial loading injuries.

One or more of the C1 fracture lines can usually be seen on the AP, lateral, and open-mouth views. On the open-mouth view, the alignment of the lateral masses of C1 and C2 is checked; combined lateral displacement of lateral masses of C1 on C2 of >6.9 mm indicates rupture of the transverse ligament and likely C1-2 translational instability. Suspected or visualized fractures of the C1 ring should be followed by CT with reconstructions to fully evaluate the C1 ring and the odontoid process.

TREATMENT

Nondisplaced atlas fractures are treated by immobilization in a rigid cervical orthosis (ring or lateral mass fractures) or a halovest (Jefferson fractures). Immobilization is recommended for 8 to 12 weeks to allow for bony healing.

In C1 fractures with combined lateral mass displacement of more than 7 mm beyond the articular surfaces of the axis, reduction of the fracture with halo traction is recommended. Continued traction to maintain the reduction may be needed for 3 to 6 weeks until the fracture becomes "sticky," after which the traction can be converted to halo-vest treatment. After bony healing, the stability of the C1-2 articulation must be checked using flexion and extension radiographs, as rupture of the transverse ligament may have occurred. If instability is demonstrated, posterior C1-2 fusion is necessary.

TRAUMATIC C1-C2 INSTABILITY

CLASSIFICATION

Generally resulting from a forced flexion injury, traumatic C1–2 instability without bony injury is uncommon. It is seen most commonly in older patients (in their 50s and 60s), and may present as simple neck pain or as a devastating, often fatal, high cervical paraplegia. Diagnosis is made on the lateral cervical radiograph, or on flexion-extension lateral radiographs, done only in a supervised setting with an awake, alert patient when no gross abnormalities were seen on initial cervical radiographs. The anterior atlanto-dens interval (AADI), the distance between the posterior aspect of the anterior arch of C1 and the anterior aspect of the odontoid, is measured. An AADI of <3 mm on maximal flexion in an adult implies intact ligamentous restraints (transverse and

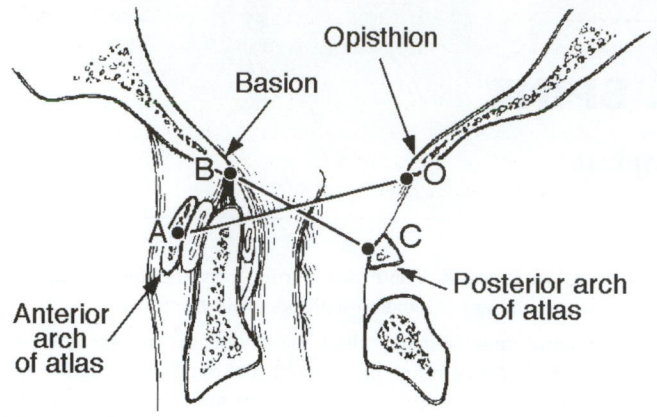

Figure 74-1
Power's ratio. [Reproduced with permission from Jarrett PJ, Whitesides TE Jr: Injuries of the cervicocranium. In Browner BD, Jupiter JB, Levine AM, et al (eds): *Skeletal Trauma*. Philadelphia: WB Saunders; 1992:668.]

alar ligaments). An AADI of 3 to 5 mm implies intact alar ligaments and an injured transverse ligament. An AADI of >5mm indicates ruptured transverse and alar ligaments.

TREATMENT

Initial immobilization in a halo-vest in relative extension will bring about reduction in most acute cases. Rarely is traction needed. Final treatment options include primary C1-2 fusion or 6 to 8 weeks of halo-vest immobilization, followed by flexion-extension radiographs to assess stability. C1-2 fusion is then done for persistent instability or chronic pain.

In general, pure ligamentous injuries are less likely to heal and become stable, so that C1-2 fusion may be the better option in cases with an AADI >5 mm. Occasionally, the transverse ligament is rendered unstable by avulsion off the lateral mass of C1 with a fragment of bone. These cases may have a higher likelihood of achieving stability with bony union.

ATLANTOAXIAL ROTATORY SUBLUXATION

CLASSIFICATION

This is a relatively uncommon injury in adults, caused by a high-velocity motor vehicle accident, and it may not be recognized initially. In children, this injury may follow a lower-velocity trauma or subluxation may occur in the absence of trauma (see also Chap. 60). Patients present with an acute painful torticollis and restricted neck motion. It is described as a distraction-rotary subluxation injury of the atlas about the odontoid process of C2, resulting in a partial dislocation of the lateral mass of C1 on C2. During the period of subluxation, the neural canal can be significantly reduced in size, but on its own, this injury rarely leads to neurologic injury. In chronic cases in young children, the deformity may present as a failure in the development in one side of the face, resulting in facial asymmetry as well as painful and decreased range of neck motion.

On an AP open-mouth radiograph, the odontoid process appears asymmetric between the lateral masses of the atlas, due to lateral gliding of C1 on C2, and can be offset as much as 2 to 4 mm. It is often difficult to distinguish between normal lateral gliding and subluxation. If there is no fracture seen, then asymmetric positioning of

the dens with lateral offset of the articular surfaces indicates a rotatory subluxation. Asymmetry of the C1 lateral masses with unilateral facet joint narrowing or overlap (known as the wink sign) is common. In older patients who have osteoarthritis involving the atlantoaxial joint, degenerative spurs may asymmetrically narrow the space between the lateral masses of the atlas and the axis.

Five types of atlantoaxial rotatory subluxations have been described (Fig. 74-2):

Type 1: The most common type, where the odontoid process acts as the point of rotation. The AADI is <3 mm.

Type II: The point of rotation is one facet, and at the opposite facet, the C1 lateral mass rotates forward. The AADI is generally <5 mm.

Type III: Anterior translation of C1 on C2 is combined with rotation of C1, such that both facet joints are anteriorly subluxed but to varying degrees. An AADI of >5 mm is common.

Type IV: Rarely seen, with both facet joints posteriorly subluxed (C1 on C2) to varying degrees. This type may be associated with a fracture of the odontoid process, allowing the posterior subluxation of C1.

Type V: Complete dislocation of both facet joints (extremely rare).

TREATMENT

In children with atlantoaxial subluxation (type I) without significant trauma, soft collar immobilization and pain medication is the initial treatment, with traction reserved for cases where the subluxation persists for 2 to 3 weeks.

The initial treatment of traumatic rotatory subluxation consists of cervical traction with progressive weights of up to 10 to 15 lb, applied via head halter or skeletal traction. Gentle manipulation may be

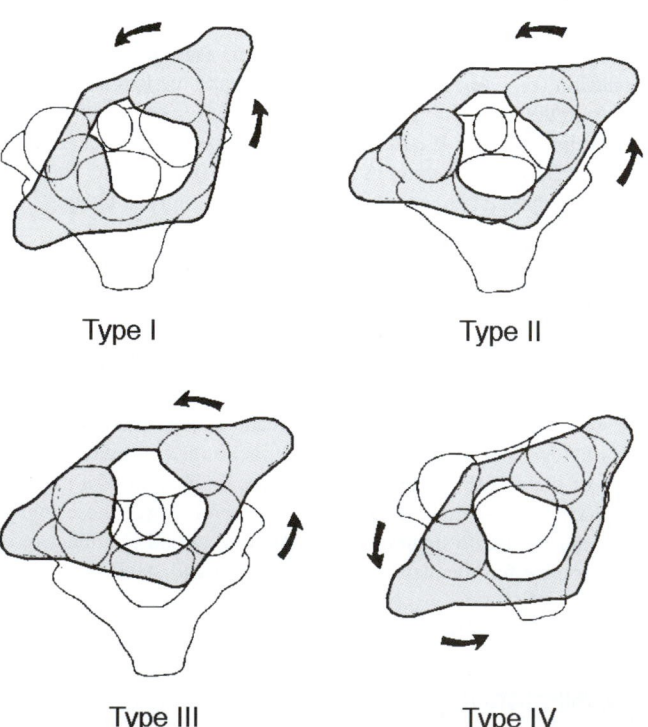

Figure 74-2
Patterns of atlantoaxial rotatory subluxation. [Reproduced with permission from Jarrett PJ, Whitesides TE Jr: Injuries of the cervicocranium. In Browner BD, Jupiter JB, Levine AM, et al (eds): *Skeletal Trauma*. Philadelphia: WB Saunders; 1992:676.]

helpful in the acute injury, but not in late cases. After reduction, halo immobilization in the reduced position for 6 weeks is utilized.

In acute cases of rotary C1-2 subluxations which do not reduce with traction, closed manipulative reduction can be attempted. The patient is maintained awake or given general anesthesia (with spinal cord monitoring utilized), and a halo ring is applied to control the head. With gentle traction applied, the halo ring is used to derotate the skull and C1 while posteriorly directed pressure is placed on the anteriorly displaced lateral mass of C1 through the posterior pharynx. If a stable reduction is achieved and satisfactory alignment is maintained on radiographs and a CT scan, halo-vest immobilization is maintained for 4 to 6 weeks.

In unstable subluxations (types III to V), early C1-2 stabilization and fusion should be considered. Surgical fusion is also indicated in cases of instability and chronic pain, and (with open reduction) in cases which do not reduce in traction. Open reduction is more commonly attempted via a posterior approach, but an anterior transoral reduction of the C1-2 facets may also be considered in chronic cases.

ODONTOID PROCESS (DENS) FRACTURES

CLASSIFICATION

Dens fractures are classified according to the anatomic level of injury and the amount of displacement. The anatomic classification of Anderson and D'Alonzo (1974) is most frequently used (Fig. 74-3):

Type I: An oblique fracture of the tip of the dens, where the alar ligament attaches and may have pulled off.

Type II: A fracture through the lower portion and at the base of the dens, up to the junction of the dens with the central body of the axis.

Type III: A fracture caudal to the base of the dens, into the cancellous bone of the C2 body.

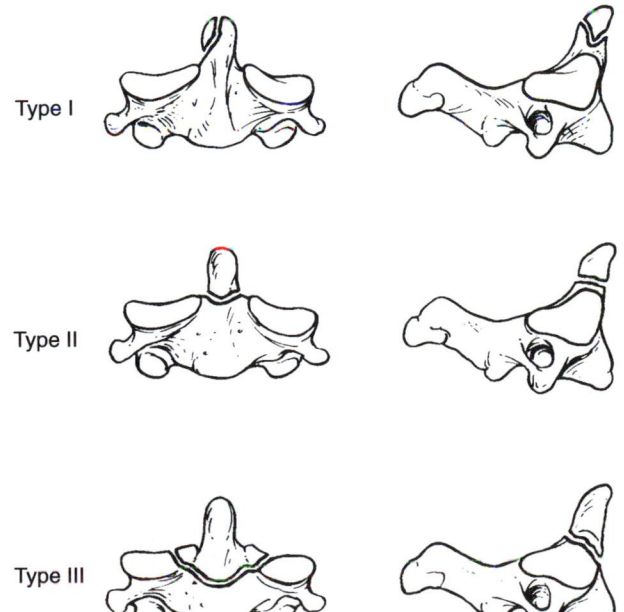

Figure 74-3
The Anderson and D'Alonzo classification of odontoid fractures. [Reproduced with permission from Schneider PL, Dzenis PE, Kahanovitz N: Spinal Trauma. In Zuckerman JD (ed): *Comprehensive Care of Orthopaedic Injuries.* Baltimore: Urban & Schwarzenberg; 1991:223.]

Each of these types is further classified as displaced or nondisplaced, with displacement measured in terms of angulation and translation.

Nonunion is most frequent in type II fractures and in fractures displaced more than 5 mm. Other factors felt to be important in the development of nonunion include patient age, the adequacy of the reduction, and the type of immobilization.

TREATMENT

Type I fractures are rare, and are treated by simple external immobilization until symptoms abate. Nonunion is not a significant problem since the fracture is located too high on the odontoid to cause C1-2 instability. Type I fractures can be associated with atlantooccipital dislocation, and this potentially fatal instability may need to be ruled out by a stretch test after a complete radiographic evaluation.

Type II fractures are the most common and the most difficult to treat. These fractures have a nonunion rate of up to 36 percent when treated nonoperatively for a number of reasons. First, the base of the odontoid is a watershed area of two blood supplies, coming from caudal for the vertebral body and from cephalad for the apex of the dens. Also, the odontoid is surrounded by a bursa posteriorly and articular cartilage anteriorly, and healing must occur surrounded by joint fluid (similar to a talar neck fracture). Finally, movement between C1 and C2 is difficult to control externally. External orthoses are rendered ineffective by jaw motion, and halo-vest fixation spans eight mobile levels in the neck, allowing significant motion to occur within this stabilized segment. Atlantoaxial motion is restricted by 75 percent with halo immobilization compared to about 45 percent with other rigid orthoses.

Type II fractures are initially treated by closed reduction (when necessary) and halo immobilization. Late C1-2 fusion (or anterior odontoid repair with bone grafting and screw fixation) should be considered in cases of nonunion, especially if instability is demonstrated on flexion-extension radiographs or if pain persists. Early operative treatment of type II fractures should be considered in cases with displacement exceeding 5 mm (especially posteriorly) and in patients >60 years old. The most common method of operative treatment for type II dens fractures is posterior C1-2 fusion. Postoperatively, following C1-2 fusion, approximately 50 percent of neck rotation and 20 percent of flexion/extension will be lost. Anterior screw fixation of the odontoid is a newer surgical option, which has the added benefit of preserving C1-2 motion. With this fixation technique, one or two cancellous screws are inserted through the anterior inferior border of the C2 vertebral body superiorly into the odontoid using biplanar fluoroscopy. The approach is the standard anterior approach to the cervical spine at about the level of C5–6, and the screws are inserted over or following guide pin placement. This technique can only be used for fracture fixation in situ; reduction of a displaced fracture must first be accomplished by closed manipulation, traction, or positioning (and confirmed radiographically) prior to beginning the procedure.

In type II fractures of the dens, it is important to determine if the displacement is anterior or posterior. Anteriorly displaced fractures are the least stable. Posterior wiring using the modified Gallie (C1 sublaminar wire and C2 spinous process wire over an H-shaped graft) or Brooks (bilateral C1-2 sublaminar wires enclosing separate wedge-shaped bone grafts) techniques, or posterior compression interlaminar clamp instrumentation are most commonly used to reduce and stabilize the spine. Transarticular C1-2 screw fixation and anterior odontoid screw fixation are other surgical techniques which can be used in this clinical situation. After adequate surgical stabilization, the patient is maintained in a hard cervical collar until healing occurs.

Posterior wiring techniques tend to further displace posteriorly displaced type II fractures, and should be used with care. The Gallie fusion causes a posteriorly directed force that maintains reduction by a tension band. This posterior force may cause a loss of reduction of an initially posteriorly displaced fracture. A bone block technique, like the Brooks-Jenkins method, will lessen the posteriorly directed vector force, and maintain reduction of posteriorly displaced odontoid fractures. Bilateral lateral mass C1-2 transarticular fixation, despite being more technically demanding, provides neutral and strong fixation, and can be combined with midline Gallie-type wiring to provide the most biomechanically sound construct in these cases.

Patients with posteriorly displaced fractures are more likely to also have fractures of the ring of C1. If a concomitant C1 posterior arch fracture exists, posterior C1-2 wiring techniques cannot be utilized. Treatment options include: halo (with/without traction) immobilization until healing of the C1 fracture, followed by C1-2 posterior fusion if an odontoid nonunion occurs; halo (with/without traction) immobilization until healing of the C1 fracture, followed by anterior repair of the odontoid nonunion; immediate posterior C1-2 fusion using bilateral C1-2 transarticular screw fixation; or immediate anterior odontoid fixation, followed by halo immobilization until healing of the C1 fracture. Early posterior occiput-C2 fusion is also a surgical treatment option, but is rarely utilized due to the large postoperative motion restrictions in both rotation and flexion-extension.

Type III fractures through the body of the axis may be displaced or non-displaced. Nondisplaced fractures are considered to be stable injuries that will heal with 8 to 12 weeks of immobilization in either a halo-vest or rigid cervical collar. The goal of treatment for displaced dens fractures is the correction of angulation in a halo-vest, while permitting the fracture to settle until union occurs. If nonunion does occur, a fusion of C1 and C2 should be considered to prevent possible late myelopathy, especially if significant motion is demonstrated on late flexion-extension radiographs.

SPONDYLOLISTHESIS OF THE AXIS (HANGMAN'S FRACTURE)

CLASSIFICATION

Traumatic spondylolisthesis is classified by both displacement and angulation of the vertebral bodies on each other (Fig. 74-4). Type I fractures are displaced less than 3 mm and have no significant angulation. They are considered a stable injury. Neurologic injury is uncommon in type I fractures. The mechanism of injury is a combination of a hyperextension and axial loading force that fractures the neural arch through the pedicles. This force, however, is not strong enough to disrupt the disk or compromise the posterior ligaments. There is a significant association with other axial loading injuries, such as Jefferson fractures of C1.

Type II fractures have more than 3 mm of anterior translation and significant angulation. This is a bipedicular fracture, where the anterior longitudinal ligament is elevated but not disrupted. These fractures are caused by initial hyperextension and axial loading which cause the neural arch to fail with a predominantly vertical fracture line, followed by flexion resulting in stretching and/or disruption of the posterior annulus and posterior longitudinal ligament at the C2–3 level and eventual significant anterior translation and angulation. A subset of these fractures, designated type IIa, show severe angulation between C2 and C3 with minimal translation. The IIa fracture line

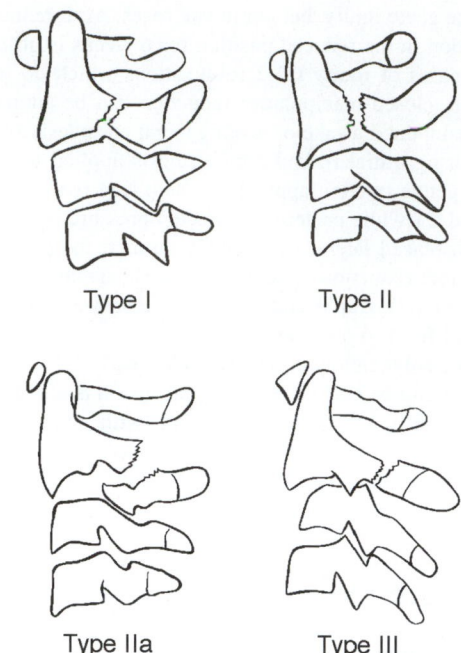

Figure 74-4
Classification of traumatic spondylolisthesis of C2. (Reproduced with permission from Levine AM, Edwards CC: The management of traumatic spondylolisthesis of the axis. *J Bone Joint Surg [Am]* 1985; 67:219–220.)

through the arch of C2 is usually more horizontal than vertical. The anterior disc space is not widened due to hinging on the anterior longitudinal ligament. The predominant force in these injuries is a combination of flexion and distraction.

Type III injuries are characterized by the bipedicular fractures in addition to damage to one or both of the posterior facet joints. They exhibit severe angulation and displacement of the neural arch fracture and an associated unilateral or bilateral facet dislocation at C2–3. These fractures are frequently associated with neurologic deficits. The predominant force here is flexion combined with compression.

TREATMENT

Type I fractures are generally considered stable, and are treated with 8 to 12 weeks of immobilization in a rigid cervical orthosis. Frequent radiographic evaluation is required early in the course of treatment to detect possible early displacement. If the fracture becomes displaced, it is considered unstable and is treated as a type II fracture. Following orthotic treatment, healing and stability are assessed by flexion-extension radiographs.

Treatment of type II fractures consists of application of a halo-vest and attempted closed reduction under fluoroscopy. If reduction can be achieved and maintained in the halo-vest, continued treatment consists of early ambulation and halo-vest immobilization for 12 weeks. Again, frequent radiographs in the early healing period are needed to confirm that reduction is maintained. If a stable closed reduction cannot be achieved, halo traction is applied through an extension moment to achieve reduction. Traction is maintained for 4 to 6 weeks until the fracture becomes "sticky," followed by conversion to halo-vest immobilization to complete 12 weeks of halo treatment. These fractures frequently unite with an initial gap in the neural arch and develop a spontaneous anterior fusion at C2-3.

The importance of recognizing type IIa fractures becomes evident in the treatment of these injuries. As this is a distraction injury, traction acts to worsen the displacement and can be dangerous. This subgroup is treated by application of a halo-vest and fluoroscopy-guided closed reduction using mainly compression with some extension. Once reduction is obtained, halo-vest immobilization is continued for 12 weeks until union occurs.

Type III fractures are extremely unstable. Reduction of the facet dislocation should be attempted immediately by applying skeletal traction. However, closed reduction often fails since the pedicular fractures leave the facets free floating. Also, any fracture of the neural arch posterior to the facets makes maintenance of any closed facet reduction difficult. Operative intervention is generally needed to obtain and maintain reduction of the facet dislocation. This makes type III injuries the only type of hangman's fracture that commonly require surgical stabilization. The lamina and spinous process of C2 are a free-floating fragment; bilateral oblique wiring of C2-3 can be employed to achieve a stable reduction of the C2-3 facets. Posterior fusion maintains the long-term stability of the C2-3 facet. The anterior structures are the only elements with anatomic integrity and in general should not be disrupted. After this type of fixation of the C2-3 level, external immobilization in a halo vest is necessary for 3 months to treat the bipedicular fracture and for consolidation of the fusion mass. A newer alternate fixation method, which provides complete stabilization in this injury, employs the use of lateral plate fixation with pedicle screws in C2 (the fractures should be reduced) and lateral mass screws in C3. Following this fixation method, immobilization with a hard cervical collar for 8 to 12 weeks is adequate, and halo-vest immobilization is not usually necessary.

LOWER CERVICAL SPINE INJURIES

CLASSIFICATION

The mechanistic classification of Allen and Ferguson (1982) is most commonly used to classify injuries of the lower cervical spine. Six common mechanistic injury patterns are described as follows; each is subdivided into stages based on the degree of injury to the osseous and ligamentous structures.

Compressive Flexion ("teardrop fractures")

CF Stage 1: Blunting of the anterosuperior vertebral margin to a rounded contour, and no evidence of failure of the posterior ligamentous complex.

CF Stage 2: Obliquity of the anterior vertebral body with loss of some anterior height of the centrum, plus the changes seen in stage 1. The anteroinferior vertebral body exhibits a "beak" appearance, concavity of the inferior end plate may be increased, and the vertebral body may have a vertical fracture.

CF Stage 3: Fracture line passing obliquely from the anterior surface of the vertebra through the centrum and extending through the inferior subchondral plate, and a fracture of the beak, in addition to the components of a stage 2 injury.

CF Stage 4: Deformation of the centrum and fracture of the beak with mild (less than 3 mm) displacement of the inferoposterior vertebral margin into the spinal canal.

CF Stage 5: Bony injuries as in stage 3 but with greater than 3 mm of displacement of the posterior portion of the vertebral body posteriorly into the spinal canal. The vertebral arch is intact, the articular facets are separated, and the interspinous process space is increased at the level of the injury, suggesting a posterior ligamentous disruption in a tension mode.

Vertical Compression (burst fractures)

VC Stage 1: Fracture of the inferior or superior end plate with a "cupping" deformity. The failure of the end plate is central as opposed to anterior, and posterior ligamentous failure is not apparent.

VC Stage 2: Fracture of both vertebral end plates with cupping deformities. Fracture lines through the centrum may be present, but displacement is minimal.

VC Stage 3: Progression of vertebral body damage as described in stage 2. The centrum is fragmented, and the displacement is peripheral in many directions. Most often the centrum fails with significant impaction and fragmentation. The posterior aspect of the vertebral body is fractured and may be displaced into the spinal canal. The vertebral arch may be intact with no sign of ligamentous failure of the posterior ligamentous complex; the ligamentous disruption is between the fractured vertebra and the vertebra caudal to it.

Distractive Flexion (dislocations)

DF Stage 1: Failure of the posterior ligamentous complex, as evidenced by facet subluxation in flexion, with splaying of the spinous processes at the level of injury.

DF Stage 2: Unilateral facet dislocation. Subluxation of the facet on the side opposite the dislocation suggests a more severe and unstable ligamentous injury. In addition, a small piece of bone may be displaced from the posterior surface of the articular process, which is displaced anteriorly. Widening of the uncovertebral joint on the side of the dislocation and displacement of the tip of the spinous process toward the side of the dislocation may be seen.

DF Stage 3: Bilateral facet dislocations, with about 50 percent anterior subluxation of the vertebral body. Blunting of the anterior-superior margin of the inferior vertebra to a rounded corner may or may not be present.

DF Stage 4: Full vertebral body width displacement anteriorly or a grossly unstable motion segment, both giving the appearance of a "floating" vertebra.

Compression Extension

CE Stage 1: Unilateral vertebral arch fracture, with or without anterior rotatory vertebral displacement. Posterior element failure may consist of a linear fracture through the articular process, ipsilateral pedicle and lamina fractures causing a "transverse facet" appearance on the anterior-posterior roentgenograms ("floating lateral mass"), or a combination of same-sided pedicle and articular process fractures.

CE Stage 2: Bilaminar fractures without evidence of other tissue failure. Usually, the laminar fractures occur at multiple contiguous levels.

CE Stage 3: Bilateral vertebral arch fractures with fracture of the articular processes, pedicles, lamina, or some bilateral combination, without vertebral body translation.

CE Stage 4: Bilateral vertebral arch fractures with partial anterior vertebral body subluxation.

CE Stage 5: Bilateral vertebral arch fracture with complete anterior vertebral body displacement. The posterior part of the vertebral arch of the fractured vertebra does not displace, and the anterior portion of the arch stays with the centrum. Ligament failure posteriorly occurs between the fractured vertebra and the one caudal to it. Classically, the anterior-superior portion of the caudal vertebra is sheared off by the anteriorly displaced centrum.

Distractive Extension

DE Stage 1: Either failure of the anterior ligamentous complex or a transverse fracture of the centrum. The injury usually is ligamentous, but there may be an associated fracture of the adjacent anterior vertebral margin. The typical radiographic finding associated with this injury is abnormal widening of the disc space.

DE Stage 2: Evidence of failure of the posterior ligamentous complex, with posterior translation of the vertebral body into the spinal canal, plus the changes seen in stage 1 injuries. The displacement tends to reduce spontaneously when the head is placed in a neutral position, so that the subluxation may be minimal (rarely more than 3 mm) on the initial radiographs with the patient supine.

Lateral Flexion

LF Stage 1: Asymmetric compression fracture of the centrum and same-sided vertebral arch fracture, without displacement of the arch on the anterior-posterior view. Compression of the articular process or comminution of the corner of the vertebral arch may be seen.

LF Stage 2: Lateral asymmetric compression of the centrum and either ipsilateral displaced vertebral arch fracture or distractive ligamentous failure on the contralateral side with separation of the articular processes. Both of these displaced ipsilateral compressive and contralateral distractive vertebral arch injuries may be present.

Additional miscellaneous lower cervical spine fractures with commonly used eponyms include the *Clay Shoveler's* fracture and the *Sentinel* fracture. The clay shoveler's fracture is a spinous process avulsion, most commonly at C7, due to a flexion mechanism. It can also be seen at C6 and T1. It is a stable injury by itself, requiring only symptomatic treatment. The Sentinel fracture describes a fracture through both sides of the lamina surrounding a spinous process. This creates a loose posterior element which may impinge on the spinal canal.

TREATMENT

The goals of treatment of these lower cervical injuries include:

1. Maintenance or restoration of normal spinal alignment
2. Maintaining or obtaining spinal stability
3. Maximizing recovery of neurologic dysfunction (includes decompression of any compressed neural elements)
4. Maximizing the speed and extent of functional recovery

Stable injuries with minimal displacement and no neural element compression can be treated by immobilization in a rigid cervical brace or halo-vest for an 8 to 12 week period, resulting in a stable, painless spine without residual deformity. Stable compression fractures of the vertebral bodies and nondisplaced fractures of the laminae, lateral masses, or spinous processes can be treated by immobilization in a rigid cervical orthosis. Unilateral facet dislocations that are reduced in traction can be immobilized in a halo-vest for 8 to 12 weeks. Persistent pain due to instability or arthritic facet changes may require spinal fusion. Any nonoperative treatment of these lower cervical spine fractures needs to be followed by serial radiographs, weekly for the first 3 weeks, then subsequently at 6 weeks, 3 months, 6 months, and 1 year. The radiographic evaluation should include flexion/extension lateral films beginning at 12 weeks to assess for late instability.

Displaced fractures and subluxations are stabilized and reduced using Gardner-Wells tong or halo-ring traction. The neutral axis for longitudinal traction is at the level of the external auditory meatus. Tongs placed posterior to this will provide a slight flexion moment with longitudinal pull, which is advantageous for reduction of facet dislocations. Ten pounds of traction is initially applied, and a lateral radiograph is taken; weight is then added in 5- to 10-lb increments, with lateral roentgenograms after each addition until spinal realignment is achieved. In unstable injuries (excluding dislocations), a rough estimation for weight needed to realign the spine is 10 lb for the head and 5 lb for every additional level of injury. Once spinal realignment is achieved using traction and is documented radiographically, the traction is continued to maintain alignment and stability until the final course of treatment is determined.

The use of high weight reduction of facet dislocations (greater than 100 lb of traction) has been described, but requires frequent neurologic reevaluation with each weight addition made in an awake, cooperative patient. Any loss of neurologic function is treated by immediately decreasing the applied weight; and no permanent worsening of neurologic function has been reported using this technique. Once the dislocation is reduced, the weight is decreased (usually to 20 to 30 lb) but maintained until definitive treatment is carried out. The more unstable bilateral facet dislocations usually require less traction weight for reduction than unilateral facet dislocations, which tend to have more intact ligamentous support.

One report of five cases of postreduction neurologic worsening associated with disc herniations has prompted some to recommend prereduction MRI or CT-myelography, with prereduction anterior discectomy in cases of documented disc herniations. This approach is also indicated in all patients with significant head injury or who are uncooperative due to substance abuse.

If spinal realignment fails via traction, then open reduction and stabilization is indicated. As the patient will be anesthetized during the open reduction, neurologic function cannot be serially assessed. Therefore, preoperative MRI or CT-myelography is used to examine for coexisting disc herniation at the site of the subluxation. If found, the disc herniation is treated by initial anterior discectomy followed by either anterior reduction and plate fixation, anterior reduction and posterior stabilization, or anterior bone grafting with posterior reduction and stabilization. In the absence of a disc herniation (most cases), a posterior approach for open reduction and stabilization is utilized.

Decompression of the spinal canal, when needed, is performed on the side of the compression, which is almost always anterior. Occasionally, posterior decompression is indicated for compression due to a displaced laminar fracture or a rotated lateral mass fracture. Posterior decompression performed for anterior compressive pathology should not be done, as it does not adequately address the problem and may add to clinical instability and neurologic deficit.

Stabilization of the unstable cervical spine or following decompression and vertebral reconstruction can be performed anteriorly, posteriorly, or both. Following anterior decompression via corpectomy, iliac reconstruction and plate fixation is the most common surgical procedure. Despite biomechanical evidence to the contrary, anterior cervical plate fixation alone seems to provide adequate stability and good clinical results, even in cases with additional significant posterior column injury. Additional posterior plate or wire fixation may also be performed, and is needed if anterior plate fixation is not utilized.

Following reduction of simple dislocations without persistent spinal cord compression, posterior stabilization using spinous process wire fixation such as the modified triple wire technique of Bohlman (central Rogers spinous process wire with overlying bone plate fixation to the spinous processes using two additional wires) or the Dewar technique (bone plate fixation to the spinous processes by transverse Kirshner wires connected by an overlying figure-eight tension band wire) can be utilized. More rigid fixation can be achieved by lateral plate fixation, with screws generally 16 to 18 mm in length directed approximately 25 degrees laterally and parallel to the facet joint into the lateral masses of C3-C6, and pedicle screws 20 to 25 mm in length directed 20 to 25 degrees medially into the pedicles of C2, C7, T1, and T2 as needed. The triple wire technique is the only one of these which provides initial posterior compression and can be used to complete reduction of a flexion deformity.

CERVICAL FRACTURES IN ANKYLOSING SPONDYLITIS

The prevalence of ankylosing spondylitis in the general population is about 1.4 percent. The rigidity of the spondylitic cervical spine unprotected by ribs or abdominal musculature renders it particularly vulnerable to trauma. Patients with ankylosing spondylitis have a 3.5 times greater incidence of traumatic cervical spine trauma as compared to the nonaffected population.

The classic pathologic lesions of ankylosing spondylitis include vertebral body osteoporosis, ankylosis of the apophyseal joints, intervertebral disc calcification, and ligamentous ossification. Stress fractures may occur in the vertebra, as severe osteoporosis weakens the ankylosed spine. Calcification of the annulus fibrosis reduces the movement and elasticity of the intervertebral disc. The force of a trauma cannot be absorbed by mobile cervical segments and the ankylosed spine behaves in a manner similar to long bone. The fractures are commonly transverse, occurring at the level of a disc space in the lower cervical spine (C5-T1). Hyperextension is the most common mechanism of injury. Since there is a degree of osteoporosis, the spine may fracture easily with minimal pain, and the patient may not recall the injury. Patients with ankylosing spondylitis who experience a recent increase in neck pain or an acute change in neurologic status, even without trauma, require a detailed radiographic evaluation, including plain radiographs and possibly CT scanning and/or MRI.

Appropriate initial immobilization of the patient with ankylosing spondylitis and acute cervical trauma is essential to a successful outcome. The routinely recommended neutral position with the head secured on a back board may be hazardous to these patients, resulting in worsening of neurologic status. Previous neck deformity, if known, should be recreated and the neck maintained with cushions. If unknown, the neck is maintained in mild cervical flexion, a position more common in patients with ankylosing spondylitis. After radiographic confirmation of fracture/dislocation, traction is applied through a halo using appropriate vectors (usually directed superiorly and anteriorly) to realign the spine in the patient's preinjury alignment. Further neurologic deterioration can still occur, even with the neck correctly aligned in traction, due to rotation or development of a compressive epidural hematoma.

Definitive treatment can be via prolonged traction or early surgery. Traction is generally required for 6 to 8 weeks, until the fracture ends become "sticky," at which time conversion to a halo-vest for an additional 6 to 12 weeks is done. Problems of continued motion in traction and delayed or nonunion have led many to recommend early surgical stabilization with internal fixation via an anterior or posterior approach. This approach allows early mobilization in a halo brace or rigid cervicothoracic orthosis, lessening respiratory complications. Respiratory complications seen in spinal cord injury are more frequent in patients with ankylosing spondylitis, as their lungs are frequently fibrotic and the rib excursion is diminished due to rib-vertebral ankylosis.

SUGGESTED READINGS

Allen BL Jr, Ferguson RL, Lehmann TR, et al: A mechanistic classification of closed, indirect fractures and dislocations of the lower cervical spine. *Spine* 1982; 7:1.

Amamilo SC: Fractures of the cervical spine in patients with ankylosing spondylitis. *Orthop Rev* 1989; 18:339.

Anderson LD, D'Alonzo RT: Fractures of the odontoid process of the axis. *J Bone Joint Surg [Am]* 1974; 56:1663.

Browner BD, Jupiter JB, Levine AM, et al: *Skeletal Trauma: Fractures, Dislocations, Ligamentous Injuries.* Philadelphia: WB Saunders; 1992.

Detwiler KN, Loftus CM, Godersky JC, et al: Management of cervical spine injuries in patients with ankylosing spondylitis. *J Neurosurg* 1990; 72:210.

Duncan RW, Esses SI: Dens fractures: Specifications and management. *Semin Spine Surg* 1996; 8:19.

Effendi B, Roy D, Cornish B, et al: Fractures of the ring of the axis. A classification based on the analysis of 131 cases. *J Bone Joint Surg [Br]* 1981; 63:319.

Fast A, Parikh S, Marin EL: Spine fractures in ankylosing spondylitis. *Arch Phys Med Rehabil* 1986; 67:595.

Laxer EB, Aebi M: Management of subaxial cervical spine injuries with internal fixation: The anterior approach. *Semin Spine Surg* 1996; 8(1):27.

Levine AM, Edwards CC: The management of traumatic spondylolisthesis of the axis. *J Bone Joint Surg [Am]* 1985; 67:217.

Rizzolo SJ, Cotler JM: Unstable cervical spine injuries: Specific treatment approaches. *J Am Acad Orthop Surg* 1993; 11:57.

Steinmann JC, Anderson PA: Subaxial cervical spine fractures with internal fixation: The posterior approach. *Semin Spine Surg* 1996; 8(1):35.

White AA, Southwick WO, Panjabi MM: Clinical instability in the lower cervical spine. A review of past and current concepts. *Spine* 1976; 1:15.

Chapter 75

THORACOLUMBAR SPINE

Jeffrey M. Spivak

CLASSIFICATION

HISTORICAL

Classifications of thoracolumbar spine fractures have traditionally been based on theories of spinal stability. In Holdsworth's (1963) mechanistic classification (flexion, flexion-rotation, extension, and compression injuries), stability was based on the intactness of the posterior ligament complex. In the two-column theory of spinal stability of Kelly and Whitesides (1968), the anterior vertebral column provides a primary weightbearing function while the posterior neural arch column primarily resists tension; stability is also based on the intactness of the posterior column.

DENIS

Based on a review of CT scans in thoracolumbar injuries, Denis (1984) devised a new classification based on a three column theory of the spine. The anatomic spine is divided into three columns (Fig. 75-1):

Anterior column: The anterior longitudinal ligament and anterior two-thirds of the annulus and vertebral body.

Middle column: The posterior one-third of the vertebral body and annulus and the posterior longitudinal ligament.

Posterior column: The bony neural arch, the interspinous and supraspinous ligaments, and the ligamentum flavum.

Spinal stability is based on the intactness of at least two of the three described columns. Minor (about 15 percent overall) and major injuries are described. Minor injuries involve partial injury of one column, and include fractures of the spinous and transverse processes, the pars interarticularis, and the facet articulations. Major spinal injuries involve complete injury of at least one column, and are divided into compression fractures, burst fractures, seatbelt injuries, and fracture-dislocations.

1. Compression fractures (Fig. 75-2): Compression failure of the anterior column with an intact middle column and a posterior column which is intact or disrupted in tension. Posterior column failure occurs with greater than 40 to 50 percent loss of anterior vertebral body height. Four subtypes are described based on endplate failure:

    Type A: Failure of both endplates (16 percent of compression fractures)

    Type B: Failure of superior endplate (62 percent, most common)

    Type C: Failure of inferior endplate (6 percent)

    Type D: Both endplates remain intact (15 percent)

2. Burst fractures (Fig. 75-3): Compression failure in the anterior and middle columns with or without injury to the posterior column. Retropulsion of bone from the middle column into the spinal canal is common. Five types are described:

    Type A: Fracture of both endplates (24 percent of burst fractures)

    Type B: Fracture of only the superior endplate (49 percent, most common)

    Type C: Fracture of only the inferior endplate (7 percent)

    Type D: Burst/rotation injury (15 percent)

    Type E: Burst/lateral flexion injury (5 percent)

3. Seat-belt injuries (Fig. 75-4): These result from flexion about an axis near the anterior longitudinal ligament, with tension failure of the posterior and middle columns through bone and/or soft tissue. The anterior longitudinal ligament is usually not disrupted although there may be compression failure of the anterior column. Four types are described:

    Type A: One-level bony injury (47 percent, the so-called Chance fracture)

    Type B: One-level ligamentous injury (11 percent)

    Type C: Two-level injury through bone in middle column (26 percent)

    Type D: Two-level injury through ligamentous middle column (16 percent)

4. Fracture-dislocations (Fig. 75-5): Three subtypes are described. In each subtype all three columns fail, either in compression, tension, rotation, or shear. Resulting sagittal or lateral vertebral translation causes narrowing of the spinal canal at the site of injury and a high incidence of neurologic deficits.

    Type A: *Flexion-Rotation* fracture-dislocation. The posterior and middle columns fail in tension and rotation, while the anterior column fails in compression and rotation. Seventy-five percent have neurologic deficits, more than half of which are complete.

    Type B: *Shear* fracture-dislocation. All three columns fail in shear, most commonly in the postero-anterior direction. All cases suffered complete neurologic injury.

    Type C: *Flexion-Distraction* fracture-dislocation. The posterior and middle columns fail in distraction with anterior tearing of the annulus fibrosus and stripping of the anterior longitudinal ligament. The anterior column may be narrowed

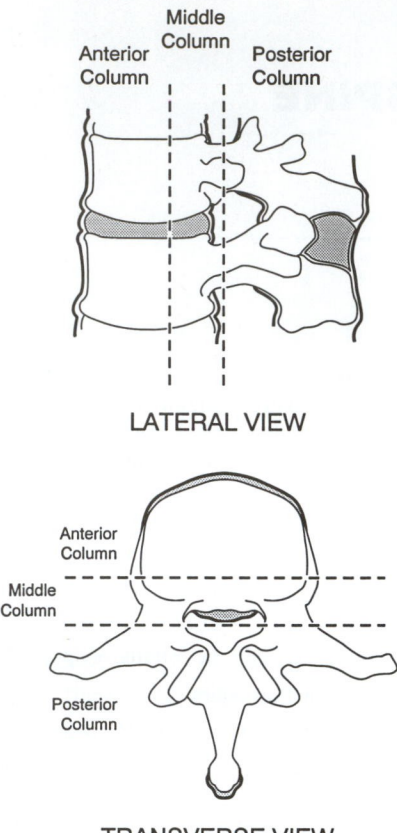

LATERAL VIEW

TRANSVERSE VIEW

Figure 75-1

The three columns of the spine. [Reprinted with permission from Spivak JM, Vaccaro AR, Cotler JM: Thoracolumbar spine trauma: I. Evaluation and classification. *J Am Acad Orthop Surg* 1995; 3:350.]

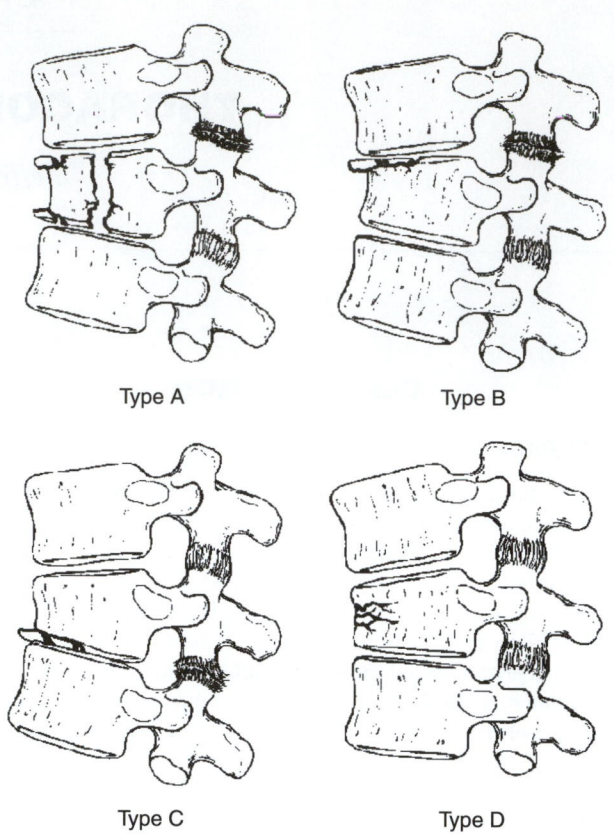

Type A   Type B

Type C   Type D

Figure 75-2

Compression fracture subtypes. [Reproduced by permission from Eismont FJ, Garfin SR, Abitbol JJ: Thoracic and upper lumbar spine injuries. In Browner BD, Jupiter JB, Levine AM, et al: *Skeletal Trauma*. Philadelphia: WB Saunders; 1992:746.]

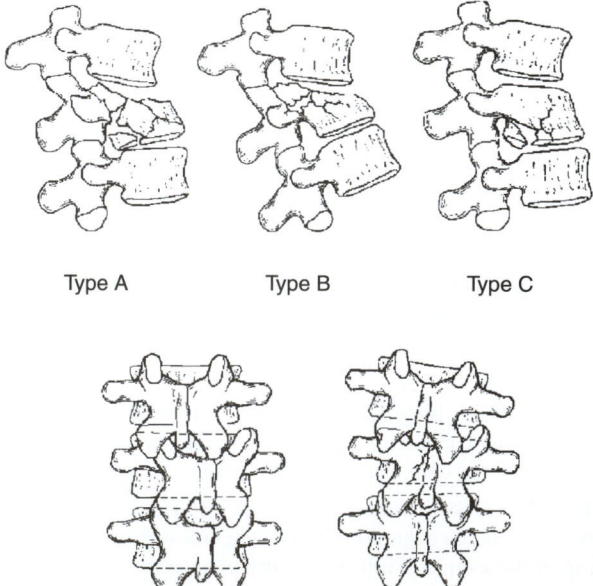

Type A   Type B   Type C

Type D   Type E

Figure 75-3

Burst fracture subtypes. [Reproduced by permission from Eismont FJ, Garfin SR, Abitbol JJ: Thoracic and upper lumbar spine injuries. In Browner BD, Jupiter JB, Levine AM, et al: *Skeletal Trauma*. Philadelphia: WB Saunders; 1992:753.]

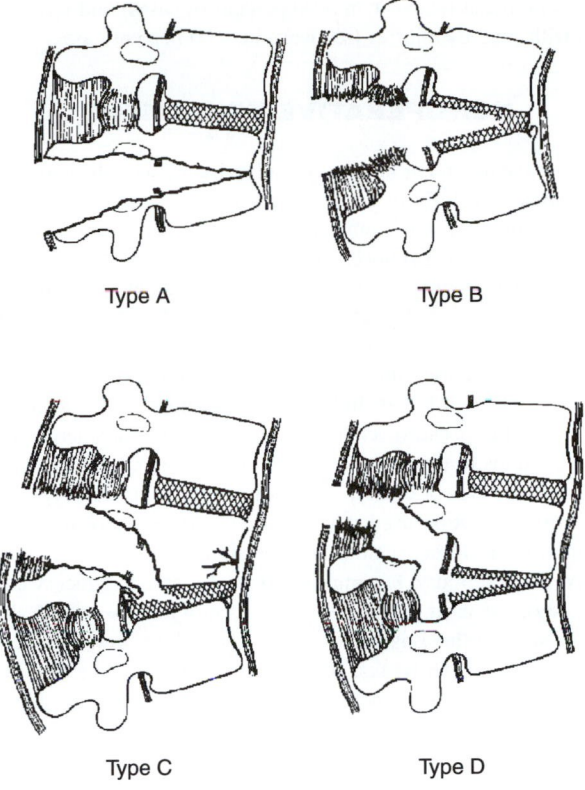

Type A   Type B

Type C   Type D

Figure 75-4
Seatbelt injury subtypes. [Reproduced by permission from Eismont FJ, Garfin SR, Abitbol JJ: Thoracic and upper lumbar spine injuries. In Browner BD, Jupiter JB, Levine AM, et al: *Skeletal Trauma.* Philadelphia: WB Saunders; 1992:754.]

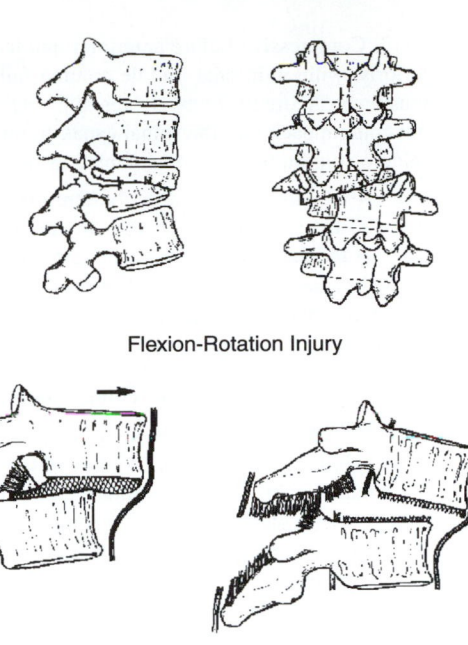

Flexion-Rotation Injury

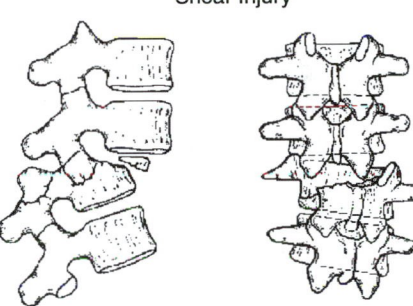

Shear Injury

Flexion-Distraction Injury

Figure 75-5
Fracture-Dislocation subtypes. [Reproduced by permission from Eismont FJ, Garfin SR, Abitbol JJ: Thoracic and upper lumbar spine injuries. In Browner BD, Jupiter JB, Levine AM, et al: *Skeletal Trauma.* Philadelphia: WB Saunders; 1992:758.]

indicating compression, possibly during the recoil or settling of the fractured vertebrae. Seventy-five percent of cases had neurologic deficits; all were incomplete.

McAFEE

McAfee (1983) also used CT scan analysis to devise a classification of six fracture types based on the failure mode of the middle column:

1. Compression fractures (anterior column compression failure)
2. Stable burst fractures (both anterior and middle column compression failure)
3. Unstable burst fractures (anterior and middle column compression failure with failure of the posterior column, either in compression, lateral flexion, or rotation)
4. Chance fractures (similar to flexion-distraction injuries of Denis)
5. Flexion-distraction injuries (similar to Denis' seat-belt injuries with compression failure of the anterior column and distraction failure of the middle and posterior columns)
6. Translational injuries (failures in shear or rotation, primarily in combination with the other injury types)

Factors such as a progressive neurologic deficit, greater than 20 degrees of progression of kyphosis, greater than 50 percent loss of vertebral body height, and free bone fragments within the spinal canal were indicative of instability in burst fractures.

FERGUSON AND ALLEN

The mechanistic classification of Ferguson and Allen (1984) describes seven injury patterns of thoracolumbar injury. The injuries are categorized by the inciting forces, which is useful in guiding both nonoperative and operative treatment. Within a number of the categories, progressively more severe injuries are described:

1. *Compressive Flexion* (CF) injuries:

    CF 1: Anterior column failure in compression.

    CF 2: Compression failure of the anterior column combined with tension failure of the posterior column, with the axis of the flexion moment within the middle column.

CF 3: Compressive failure anteriorly and tension failure posteriorly, with additional middle column failure due to either tension or "hydraulic blowout" resulting in rotation of the middle column back into the spinal canal. In this mechanism, the middle column height is maintained or increased.

2. *Distractive Flexion* injuries describe tension failure of all three columns of the spine resulting from flexion about an axis at or anterior to the anterior longitudinal ligament. Within this category are the seat-belt injuries and flexion-distraction fracture dislocations described by Denis.
3. *Lateral Flexion* (LF) injuries:

LF 1: Anterior and middle column failure unilaterally in compression.

LF 2: Unilateral compression failure of the anterior and middle columns with posterior column injury. On the ipsilateral side, posterior element fracture in compression occurs, and on the contralateral side, tension failure is seen, including bony element fracture and facet joint subluxations and dislocations.

4. *Translation* injuries result from shear forces, either in the sagittal or coronal plane. Translational displacement can be anterior, posterior, or lateral depending on the direction of the shear force. Pure translational injuries are uncommon, but a translational injury component is commonly associated with other injury mechanisms.
5. *Torsional Flexion* injuries result in anterior and middle column failure in compression and rotation and posterior element failure in tension and rotation. These are among the most unstable thoracolumbar injuries, with the highest propensity for paraplegia.
6. *Vertical Compression* injuries are characterized by vertebral body shortening due to compression failure of the anterior and middle columns. The posterior elements may also fail in compression due to fracture. Neurologic injuries and progression of deformity are uncommon in these injuries.
7. *Distractive Extension* injuries, rare in the thoracolumbar spine, result in tension failure of the anterior column and compression failure of the posterior column.

DALL AND STAUFFER

Burst fractures at the thoracolumbar junction with partial neurologic injury and canal compromise have been further classified by Dall and Stauffer (1988) based on the degree of regional kyphosis and the location of maximal canal compromise. The purpose of this classification is to correlate fracture pattern with neurologic injury and recovery. Four fracture patterns are described:

Type I: Kyphosis >15 degrees with maximal canal compromise at the level of the ligamentum flavum.

Type II: Kyphosis >15 degrees with maximal canal compromise at the level of the posterior bony neural arch.

Type III: Kyphosis ≤ 15 degrees with maximal canal compromise at the level of the posterior bony neural arch.

Type IV: Kyphosis ≤ 15 degrees with maximal canal compromise at the level of the ligamentum flavum.

The authors found that the severity of initial neurologic injury did not correlate with the fracture pattern or with the amount of spinal canal compromise. Neurologic recovery did not correlate with the treatment method or the amount of spinal canal decompression. Neurologic recovery was greatest in patients with type I and II injuries (significant recovery in >90 percent of cases) and least in patients with type III injuries (recovery in <50 percent cases).

NONOPERATIVE TREATMENT

Nonoperative treatment in thoracolumbar trauma is indicated for stable injuries with little or no potential for progressive deformity or neural compromise with ambulatory treatment and external immobilization. Significant kyphosis, especially at the thoracolumbar junction, is a poor prognostic factor for optimal outcome with nonoperative treatment. A multicenter prospective study of spine fractures found that patients with a kyphotic deformity of greater than 30 degrees had an increased incidence of significant back pain.

One-column injuries, including wedge compression fractures and fractures of the posterior elements, are generally considered stable. These fractures heal well when treated with external immobilization using a plaster cast or orthotic and early ambulation. The type of external immobilization used must provide a force vector opposite of the initial injury force, such as an extension cast or brace for a compressive flexion injury. For injuries above T_7, an occipitocervicothoracic orthosis is used; healing is expected in 8 to 12 weeks. A thoracolumbosacral orthosis is used for injuries at T_7 or below, with healing expected in 12 to 16 weeks. In low lumbar injuries, the cast or orthosis should include immobilization of one thigh for the first 6 to 12 weeks in order to stabilize the pelvis.

Nonoperative treatment is also indicated for some injuries with bony instability and no neurologic deficits. Flexion-distraction injuries through bone (Chance fractures) will heal when immobilized in an extension cast or thoracolumbosacral orthosis. Also, vertical compression fractures with minimal middle column comminution or shortening and minimal kyphosis ("stable" burst fractures) can usually be treated by early ambulation in an external cast or brace.

OPERATIVE TREATMENT

INDICATIONS

Operative treatment of thoracic and lumbar spine fractures is indicated for:

1. Grossly unstable injuries, regardless of the neurologic status.
2. Patients with incomplete spinal cord injury and significant spinal canal compromise and cord compression.
3. Fracture-dislocations requiring open reduction for spinal realignment.
4. Complete neurologic injuries at the conus or cauda level with persistent neural element compression, where additional root recovery may provide a significant functional improvement.

Even in patients with complete neurologic deficits, surgical stabilization of an unstable injury allows for more rapid mobilization and commencement of physical rehabilitation, often without a brace or cast, and should be considered.

Some controversy remains regarding operative treatment of unstable spinal column injuries in patients without neurologic injury. Proponents of initial nonoperative treatment feel that good results can be obtained in most cases, and late neurologic injury, bony deformity, and instability can be corrected if they occur. Many, however, feel that early surgical stabilization is important for protection of neural elements at risk and for the most rapid functional return and reintegration into society for patients with unstable fractures. Operative stabilization also prevents the late complications of neurologic injury, deformity, and painful instability. The surgical methods needed to correct the sequelae of late instability and fixed deformity are quite complex and fraught with significant morbidity.

GENERAL PRINCIPLES

The choice of operative procedure for thoracolumbar spine injuries must address all of the goals of treatment of the specific injury. Significant spinal canal compromise and neurologic injury are addressed by decompression and/or correction of any causative deformity. Unacceptable spinal deformity must be corrected. The unstable spinal column must be left stable by the use of spinal instrumentation and fusion. In many cases, anterior, posterior, or a combined approach may all be acceptable alternatives for operative treatment. In these cases, the final decision by the treating surgeon may be based on personal experience and familiarity with operative techniques.

The optimal timing for operative treatment of thoracolumbar injuries remains unclear. Proponents of immediate emergent treatment (within 8 to 12 h from injury) believe that early decompression and stabilization is beneficial to the spinal cord and preventing other injury complications. Proponents of urgent treatment (within 2 to 3 days from injury) feel that medical stabilization and fracture hematoma formation are beneficial, and more emergent treatment may worsen neurologic function by further compromising the acutely injured spinal cord. Two indications for emergent surgical intervention are a progressive neurologic injury with proven spinal canal compromise and an incomplete neurologic injury associated with an irreducible dislocation.

DECOMPRESSION

Spinal canal decompression may be direct or indirect, and may be done through an anterior or posterior approach. Anterior decompression is always direct, with removal of compressive bone and disc material via thoracotomy, thoracolumbotomy, or a retroperitoneal approach. This is the most commonly used method of spinal canal decompression in thoracic and thoracolumbar injuries with anterior spinal cord compression due to retropulsed middle column elements. Following anterior decompression, vertebral reconstruction is accomplished and anterior support provided using a rigid structural graft. Common reconstruction options include tricortical autologous iliac crest, allograft femoral or tibial shaft filled with autograft (vertebral body bone, morselized rib, or cancellous iliac crest), and surgical titanium mesh filled with autograft. Rib graft alone may not provide enough structural support in cases of significant vertebral body compromise, but may be adequate in certain uncommon situations where the majority of the anterior and middle columns are intact (in addition to rigid anterior or posterior instrumentation).

Posterior decompression may be direct or indirect. Indirect posterior decompression through distraction and lordosis forces can be used in the thoracic region and at the thoracolumbar junction. Distraction instrumentation has been shown to be effective in reducing retropulsed middle column fragments in the spinal canal, especially when done within 72 h of the injury. Polyethylene sleeves around distraction rods, described by Edwards, provides a three-or four-point bending moment maintaining lordosis in the setting of posterior distraction. Transpedicular screw constructs can also apply distraction and lordosing forces, and can also be used for indirect canal decompression. Failures of short segment pedicle screw constructs, however, have been reported in the setting of poor anterior column support.

Following indirect posterior decompression and stabilization, patients with persistent neurologic deficits should be considered for postoperative examination of the spinal canal via myelogram and post-myelogram CT scanning. Persistent canal compromise and neural compression should be treated by a second stage anterior decompression and vertebral reconstruction.

In vitro experimentation has shown that indirect reduction results from the insertion of the posterior annulus fibrosis into the superior vertebral endplate, not from traction along the posterior longitudinal ligament. Distraction, not lordosis, was found to be the major reduction force; a combination of distraction and lordosis provides the optimal indirect reduction forces necessary for spinal realignment.

Direct posterior decompression with removal or anterior impaction of retropulsed middle column fragments is recommended only below the conus medullaris, in the region of the cauda equina. Retraction of the dural sac is generally needed for direct posterior decompression; this can damage the spinal cord and conus medullaris. The safe region for direct posterior decompression is typically at the level of L2 and caudally, and can be easily confirmed with a preoperative MRI. Direct posterior decompression is indicated at all levels of the thoracolumbar spine if the spinal canal compression is caused by anteriorly displaced posterior element fragments.

Direct decompression at the thoracolumbar junction can also be safely accomplished posterolaterally through the use of a modified costotransversectomy approach by removal of the transverse process and pedicle. Although this approach can also be used for posterior spinal stabilization through the same incision, structural grafting of the anterior column is difficult because of the limited anterior exposure. Another uncommon method of direct posterolateral decompression which can be used at the level of the conus medullaris involves removal of the medial half of the pedicle at the injured level, undercutting anterior to the retropulsed bone fragment, and impaction of the fragment anteriorly without retraction of the dura.

Posterior surgery is an important part of the operative treatment of burst fractures with associated lamina fracture and neurologic deficits. A number of reports have documented dural tears and entrapment of neural elements within the lamina fracture. The initial splaying of the pedicles and posterior element displacement is followed by a recoiling to the stable position seen on initial radiographic evaluation. The dura and neural elements can become trapped within the fractured posterior elements and compressed or torn during the recoil. Full recognition of trapped neural elements can only be accomplished through direct exploration posteriorly.

During the approach, special care must be taken as the dura and neural elements may be encountered before the lamina. Exposure of the lamina above and below the injury level is done first, and then the injury level is exposed by careful blunt dissection. Visualization of the dura or neural elements is an indication for a more complete exploration via hemi- or total laminectomy to explore the surrounding dura. Identified tears are repaired if possible. Hemilaminectomy and dural exploration may also be useful in patients without posteriorly visible neural elements, as neural entrapment along the inner aspect of the lamina is possible. This might be particularly important in patients with definite neural deficits and minimal anterior compression; in this case, occult neural injury secondary to lamina entrapment is more likely.

STABILIZATION

Operative stabilization of thoracic and lumbar spine injuries can be accomplished using anterior or posterior spinal instrumentation, or both.

Following anterior decompression and/or anterior vertebral reconstruction, a variety of vertebral body screw and plate or rod fixation systems are available to anteriorly stabilize one or more motion segments. Due to lateral screw placement, these can be used with safety along the thoracolumbar junction to the L3 level. Caudal to this, especially at L5, the overlying iliac vessels may present an anatomic constraint to safe screw positioning. Some of the available systems have a smoother contour and lower profile and may result in less irritation to the psoas muscle and less risk to the major vessels at caudal levels.

Posterior spinal instrumentation can be used following anterior decompression and reconstruction (with or without anterior instrumentation) or as part of an isolated posterior procedure. The choice of specific instrumentation and the method of application (specific construct used) is based on a variety of factors. The mechanism of injury and resultant fracture pattern determine the forces which must be supplied through the instrumentation system chosen. Generally, distraction constructs are used for compression injuries with intact posterior elements. Distraction and lordosing constructs are also used for indirect decompression of the spinal canal narrowed by retropulsion of a fracture fragment from the middle column. Distraction can be achieved using either hooks, pedicle screws, or combinations of both connected to longitudinal rods. One or two pairs of polyethylene rod sleeves can be used to provide a three- or four-point lordosing bending moment.

Compression constructs are used for flexion distraction injuries if the middle column is not comminuted. Compression constructs are also used following anterior vertebral reconstruction. The posterior compressive force restores lordosis and locks in the rigid anterior structural graft, creating the most stable overall construct.

Segmental stabilization using hooks, sublaminar wires, and transpedicular screws are always used in the most unstable injuries, caused by flexion-rotation and translation. The rigid and separate hold of spinal elements above and below the injury can be set in neutral, without additional forces, or used in combination with compressive or distractive forces if needed.

Low lumbar (L3-L5) injuries requiring surgical stabilization are managed by transpedicular segmental screw instrumentation, fusing one level above and one level below the injury. Distraction hook constructs are avoided, as these can severely reduce the physiologic lordosis of this region and because of the need to instrument additional levels above and below the injury site. Caution must be exercised in using short segment instrumentation in the setting of loss of anterior or middle column support due to the potential for screw failure. Transpedicular bone grafting of the injured level may be of benefit in these cases.

SUGGESTED READINGS

Bradford DS, McBride GG: Surgical management of thoracolumbar spine fractures with incomplete neurologic deficits. *Clin Orthop* 1987; 218:201.

Cammisa FP Jr, Eismont FJ, Green BA: Dural laceration occurring with burst fractures and associated laminar fractures. *J Bone Joint Surg [Am]* 1989; 71:1044.

Dall BE, Stauffer ES: Neurologic injury and recovery patterns in burst fractures at the T12 or L1 motion segment. *Clin Orthop* 1988; 233:171.

Denis F: Spinal instability as defined by the three-column spine concept in acute spinal trauma. *Clin Orthop* 1984; 189:65.

Denis F: The three column spine and its significance in the classification of acute thoracolumbar spinal injuries. *Spine* 1983; 8:817.

Ferguson RL, Allen BL Jr: A mechanistic classification of thoracolumbar spine fractures. *Clin Orthop* 1984; 189:77.

Fredrickson BE, Edwards WT, Rauschning W, et al: Vertebral burst fractures: An experimental morphologic, and radiographic study. *Spine* 1992; 17:1012.

Gertzbein SD: Scoliosis Research Society multicenter spine fracture study. *Spine* 1992; 17:528.

Holdsworth FW: Fractures, dislocations and fracture-dislocations of the spine. *J Bone Joint Surg [Br]* 1963; 45:6.

Kelly RP, Whitesides TE Jr: Treatment of lumbodorsal fracture-dislocations. *Ann Surg* 1968; 167:705.

McAfee PC, Yuan, HA, Fredrickson BE, et al: The value of computed tomography in thoracolumbar fractures. An analysis of one hundred consecutive cases and a new classification. *J Bone Joint Surg [Am]* 1983; 65:461.

McLain RF, Sparling E, Benson DR: Early failure of short-segment pedicle instrumentation for thoracolumbar fractures. A preliminary report. *J Bone Joint Surg [Am]* 1993; 75:162.

Chapter 76

SHOULDER

Kenneth J. Koval

SHOULDER DISLOCATION

ANATOMY

The shoulder is composed of four articulations. Three of these, the glenohumeral, acromioclavicular, and sternoclavicular joints, are true diarthrodial (synovial) joints. The remaining scapulothoracic articulation is the muscular attachment of the scapula to the thorax. The combined function of the four articulations provides a wide range of shoulder motion with a potential forward elevation of 180 degrees. Approximately two-thirds of the 180-degree range is accounted for by the glenohumeral joint and one-third by the scapulothoracic articulation.

CLASSIFICATION

Shoulder dislocations are classified based on the direction, degree, frequency, and acuteness of the dislocation, as well as on the anatomic location of the humeral head with respect to the glenoid. Anterior and posterior dislocations are classified separately.

ANTERIOR DISLOCATION

Incidence and Mechanism of Injury

Anterior dislocations represent more than 95 percent of glenohumeral dislocations. They are usually caused by a fall onto the outstretched arm. This results in a complex movement of combined abduction, external rotation, and extension which drives the humeral head anteriorly. Subcoracoid dislocation is the most common presentation. Subglenoid dislocation is the second most common, and results from increasing amounts of abduction of the arm. Subclavicular and intrathoracic dislocations are caused by high-energy injuries which drive the humeral head medially.

Clinical and Radiographic Evaluation

Patients with an acute anterior dislocation often complain of significant shoulder pain. However, some patients may be quite comfortable, particularly if the dislocation is a recurrent episode. The patient may maintain the injured arm in a position of abduction and external rotation. The normal contour of the shoulder alters as the lateral acromion becomes more prominent; an anterior fullness and a posterior depression become apparent about the shoulder. Efforts at motion are usually painful. A neurovascular examination with evaluation of axillary nerve function is mandatory to identify any deficits.

Radiographic evaluation includes an AP and lateral of the scapula, and an axillary view (Fig. 76–1). After closed reduction, repeat radiographs should be done to confirm the reduction and identify any associated injuries.

Treatment

Shoulder reduction is performed with the patient in a supine position, and gentle traction applied in line with the humeral shaft. Counter traction is applied by means of a sheet wrapped around the patient's chest. If necessary, the thumb can be used simultaneously to gently reduce the humeral head.

If postreduction radiographs confirm an adequate reduction, the shoulder can be immobilized. In patients over 60 years of age for whom this is a first dislocation, immobilization is maintained from 7 to 10 days and then discontinued; pendulum exercises and isometric deltoid and rotator cuff strengthening can be started, followed by an active range of motion program.

Acute anterior dislocations can usually be successfully reduced. If a closed reduction with sedation is not successful and the axillary radiograph does not indicate a chronic problem, closed reduction with general or regional anesthesia should be attempted. If this approach is also not successful, open reduction is indicated. It may be achieved through an anterior approach with release or by removal of the obstructing structure and repair of the rotator cuff or capsule.

Complications

Complications associated with primary anterior shoulder dislocation are recurrent instability, rotator cuff tear, brachial plexus injury, and axillary nerve injury. Fractures commonly associated with anterior dislocations include greater tuberosity fractures, anterior glenoid frac-

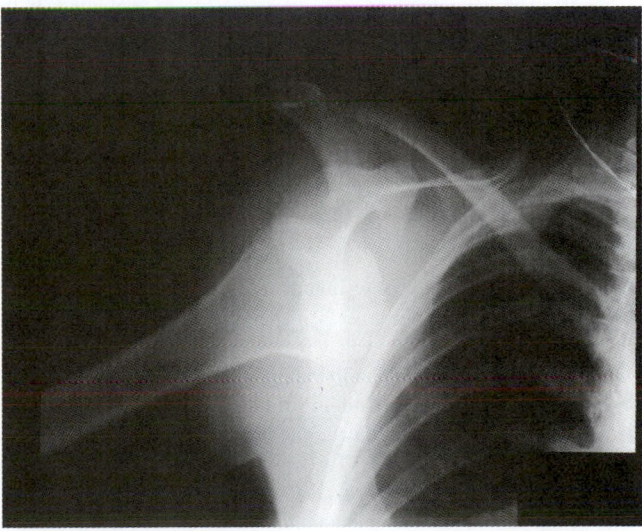

Figure 76-1
Anterior dislocation of right shoulder.

tures, and compression fractures of the humeral head. In the elderly, rotator cuff tears are a more common occurrence than fractures which occur following anterior dislocation.

POSTERIOR DISLOCATION

Incidence and Mechanism of Injury

Posterior glenohumeral dislocations are uncommon; the incidence is reported to be 1 to 3.7 percent. The most common presentation is the subacromial type; subglenoid and subspinous dislocations are extremely rare.

Posterior dislocations may result from either direct or indirect mechanisms. The direct mechanism would be a posteriorly directed blow to the front of the shoulder. Indirect mechanisms occur more commonly and consist of a force directed toward the abducted, flexed, and internally rotated humerus—a position which occurs during a fall onto the outstretched arm. Accidental electrical shock, seizures, and electroconvulsive therapy are also classic causes of posterior shoulder dislocations.

Clinical and Radiographic Evaluation

When dislocation occurs, the posterior aspect of the shoulder becomes more prominent with flattening anteriorly. The coracoid process may also protrude on the affected side compared to the unaffected shoulder. The arm is usually held in an abducted and internally rotated position; efforts at motion are usually painful.

Radiographic evaluation is used to identify any associated fractures. Anteromedial impression fractures of the humeral head are caused by forced contact between the posterior glenoid rim and the anteromedial portion of the humeral head. Lesser tuberosity fractures are produced by avulsion of the subscapularis muscle.

Treatment

Closed reduction is accomplished with the application of traction along the humerus in line with the deformity. A hand may be utilized to gently reposition the humeral head laterally and anteriorly, returning it to the glenoid fossa. If the humeral head is locked onto the posterior glenoid rim, additional lateral traction may be necessary. Following the reduction, shoulder stability is evaluated. If the shoulder is stable with the arm placed over the chest, a simple sling may be used for immobilization. If the shoulder is unstable in this position, immobilization will be required with the arm placed in neutral to 20 degrees of external rotation. Irreducible acute posterior dislocations are rare.

INFERIOR DISLOCATION

Inferior shoulder dislocations (luxatio erecta) are the result of hyperabduction of the humerus with impingement on the lateral edge of the acromion; a movement that forces the humeral head to dislocate inferiorly. It is a high-energy injury which can result in disruption of the capsule, avulsion of the rotator cuff, proximal humeral fracture, and neurovascular injury. The affected arm is held in an abducted position (greater than 110 degrees). Neurovascular compromise is generally present, however, it usually resolves following reduction. Closed reduction is accomplished by applying traction upward along the humerus with countertraction directed downward through a folded sheet across the top of the shoulder. After closed reduction, sling immobilization is started and should be continued for 1 to 3 weeks. If closed reduction is not successful, open reduction

may be necessary to clear the humeral head which has buttonholed through a perforation in the inferior capsule.

SCAPULOTHORACIC DISSOCIATION

INCIDENCE AND MECHANISM OF INJURY

Scapulothoracic dissociation is a rare and frequently fatal closed injury. It includes lateral displacement of the scapula with associated neurovascular injury and either acromioclavicular or sternoclavicular separation or clavicle fracture. The mechanism of injury is a violent force directed to the anterolateral aspect of the shoulder. The associated brachial plexus injury is generally complete; the vascular injury usually occurs at the level of the subclavian vessels and can produce a pulseless extremity.

CLINICAL AND RADIOGRAPHIC EVALUATION

The diagnosis of scapulothoracic dissociation should be considered in any patient who has suffered massive trauma to the upper extremity associated with a neurovascular deficit. Diagnosis is made by comparing the anatomic locations of the two scapulae on chest radiograph; the affected scapula is significantly displaced laterally. Immediate evaluation of the ipsilateral vascular structures using angiography is mandatory to prevent fatal internal hemorrhage. Careful neurologic examination is required to evaluate the level and degree of injury.

TREATMENT CONSIDERATIONS

Once the level of vascular injury has been established, emergent surgical exploration is necessary to restore vascularity to the ischemic limb. Complete brachial plexus root avulsions result in a flail limb; there is no potential for neurologic recovery. The resultant injuries are probably best treated with a shoulder arthrodesis and an above or below elbow amputation. In partial root avulsions or postganglionic lesions limb salvage should be attempted.

SCAPULA FRACTURES

INCIDENCE AND MECHANISM OF INJURY

Scapula fractures are relatively uncommon and represent 3 to 5 percent of all shoulder fractures and 0.5 to 1 percent of all fractures. They are generally the result of high-energy trauma; 80 to 90 percent of scapula fractures have associated injuries. The thorax, ribs, or clavicle are most commonly involved; brachial plexus and vascular injuries occur with less frequency. Because these associated injuries can be life-threatening, their assessment and management should take priority over the scapula fracture. A fracture of the scapula with an associated underlying fracture of the first rib is a particularly serious and critical event due to the potential for associated pulmonary and neurovascular injury.

CLINICAL AND RADIOGRAPHIC EVALUATION

Clinical findings may be subtle, however, the severity of the associated injuries frequently leads to a delayed diagnosis of the scapula fracture. Radiographic evaluation includes a chest film, scapula AP, scapular Y, and axillary view. A 45-degree cephalic tilt is helpful in the evaluation of coracoid fractures. CT scanning can provide further information and is particularly useful in the evaluation of intraarticular glenoid fractures.

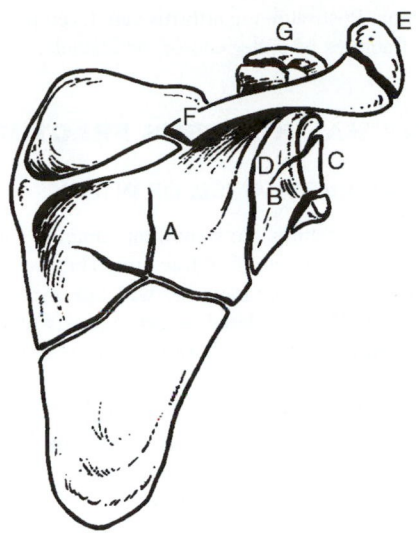

Figure 76-2
Anatomic classification of scapula fractures. *A*, Scapula body; *B, C*, glenoid; *D*, scapula neck; *E*, acromion; *F*, scapula spine; and *G*, coracoid. [Reproduced by permission from Alpert SW, Ben-Yishay A, Koval KJ, et al (eds): Scapula. In: *Fractures and Dislocations.* New York: Hospital for Joint Diseases Orthopaedic Institute; 1994:48.]

CLASSIFICATION

Scapula fractures are classified by anatomic location as being either body, neck, glenoid, acromion, spine, or coracoid fractures (Fig. 76–2). Glenoid fractures have been further classified based on their location and the direction of the fracture line(s): type I, avulsion fracture of the anterior margin; type IIA, transverse fracture through the glenoid fossa exiting inferiorly; type IIB, oblique fracture through the glenoid fossa exiting inferiorly; type III, oblique fracture through the glenoid exiting superiorly and often associated with an acromioclavicular joint injury; type IV, transverse fracture exiting through the medial border of the scapula; and type V, a combination of a type II and type IV pattern (Fig. 76–3).

TREATMENT CONSIDERATIONS

The great majority of scapula fractures are treated nonoperatively with ice, sling support, and early range of motion. Operative management is usually indicated for: (1) intraarticular glenoid fractures with subluxation and instability of the humeral head; (2) depressed acromion fractures which encroach upon the subacromial space and interfere with rotator cuff function; (3) coracoid fractures with an associated A-C separation that compromises the overlying skin; and (4) scapular neck fractures with severe angulation of the glenoid articular surface, a condition that predisposes to glenohumeral instability.

RESULTS

The results of nonoperative treatment of scapular fractures have been relatively good. In a series reported by McGinnis and coworkers (1989) of 40 scapula fractures managed nonoperatively, 73 percent had good to excellent results with a 16-month average follow-up. The study used the criteria of pain, strength, and range of motion. Hardegger and associates (1984) reported on the outcome of operative treatment in 37 patients who had displaced scapula fractures. Seventy-nine percent had good to excellent results, using the criteria of pain, muscle strength, and range of motion.

COMPLICATIONS

Complications associated with fracture of the scapula are suprascapular nerve injury, nonunion, and malunion. Suprascapular nerve injury results from fractures of the coracoid and scapula body that involve the suprascapular notch. Nonunion is rare because of the vascular supply and the ample soft tissue that covers the scapula. Malunion is rarely symptomatic.

CLAVICLE FRACTURE

INCIDENCE AND MECHANISM OF INJURY

Clavicle fractures are common and are caused by direct trauma or a fall onto the outstretched hand. Less than 3 percent have associated injuries.

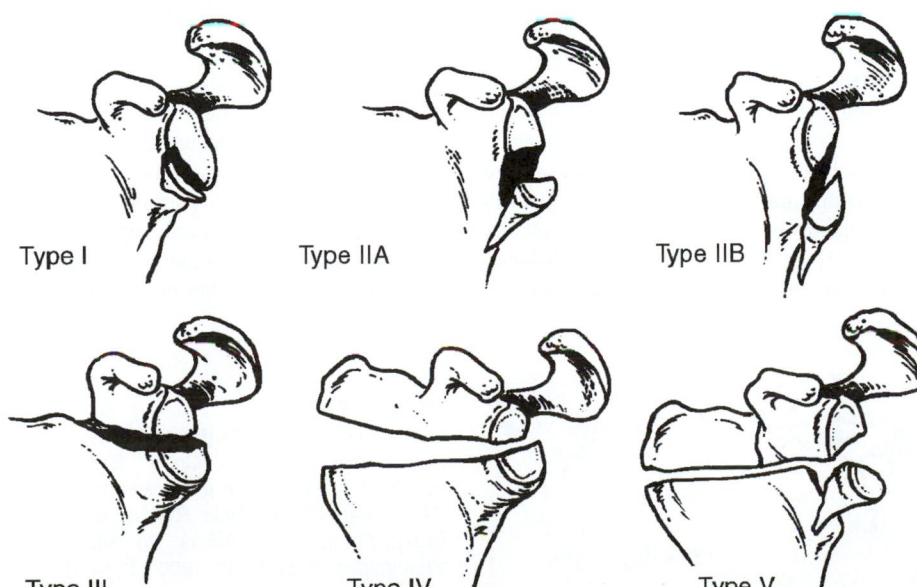

Type I   Type IIA   Type IIB

Type III   Type IV   Type V

Figure 76-3
Ideberg classification of glenoid fractures. [Reproduced by permission from Alpert SW, Ben-Yishay A, Koval KJ, et al (eds): Scapula. In *Fractures and Dislocations.* New York: Hospital for Joint Diseases Orthopaedic Institute; 1994:49.]

RADIOGRAPHIC EVALUATION

Radiographic evaluation includes an AP and a 45-degree cephalic tilt view to evaluate superior–inferior and anterior–posterior displacement. Weighted radiographic views can be useful to assess the status of the coracoclavicular ligaments in lateral-third fractures.

CLASSIFICATION

Clavicle fractures are classified according to location as medial-third, middle-third, and lateral-third fractures. In displaced middle-third fractures, the medial fragment is generally displaced upward by the pull of the sternocleidomastoid and trapezius muscles. The lateral fragment is displaced downward by the weight of the arm. Lateral-third fractures are further classified based on the functional status of the coracoclavicular ligaments. Type I distal clavicle fractures are minimally displaced and the coracoclavicular ligaments are functionally attached to the medial fragment (Fig. 76–4). Type II fractures are displaced and the coracoclavicular ligaments are functionally detached from the medial fragment. Type III fractures include the articular surface of the lateral clavicle.

TREATMENT CONSIDERATIONS

Treatment approach depends on fracture location, displacement, and associated injuries. The majority of middle-third fractures are managed nonoperatively with a figure-of-eight bandage or arm sling. Regardless of the type of immobilization applied, residual deformity and shortening will occur, but it is usually painless and does not obstruct shoulder function. Indications for operative intervention in middle-third fractures are open fractures, displaced fractures that compromise the overlying skin, and fractures that involve neurovascular injury. Internal fixation devices include an intramedullary pin or plate and screws. Comminuted fractures should be evaluated for bone grafting.

Types I and III lateral-third fractures are usually managed with sling support and early range of motion. Management of type II fractures is controversial, due to a higher rate of nonunion. Both primary open reduction (with intramedullary or coracoclavicular stabilization) and nonoperative management have been advocated.

COMPLICATIONS

Complications related to clavicle fracture are uncommon and include nonunion, malunion, neurovascular compromise, and posttraumatic arthritis. Predisposing factors for nonunion are inadequate immobilization, fracture location (lateral third), trauma severity, soft tissue interposition, refracture, and primary open reduction and internal fixation.

Malunion is rarely symptomatic. Angulatory deformities are essentially a cosmetic problem, however, significant shortening may occur and could result in muscular dysfunction. Acute neurovascular complications may occur secondary to fracture displacement or be delayed secondary to compromise by exuberant fracture callus or

mobile nonunion. Posttraumatic arthritis can develop associated with intraarticular fractures of either end of the clavicle.

PROXIMAL HUMERUS FRACTURES

INCIDENCE AND MECHANISM OF INJURY

Proximal humerus fractures are somewhat common and account for approximately 4 to 5 percent of all fractures. They occur twice as often in females. The incidence increases with age, especially after age 50; they are generally considered as osteoporosis-related fractures. Proximal humeral fractures are caused by indirect and direct mechanisms of injury. In young patients, these mechanisms frequently result in dislocation rather than fracture because the strength of the bone is significantly greater than that of the supporting ligaments. In elderly people with osteoporosis, the bone is often considerably weaker than the ligaments, and a fracture results.

CLINICAL AND RADIOGRAPHIC EVALUATION

Fracture stability must be assessed to determine if the fracture segments move as a unit. Appropriate radiographic evaluation includes a chest film, a scapula AP, a scapular Y, and an axillary view.

CLASSIFICATION

The proximal humerus fracture classification most often referred to was described by Neer (Fig. 76–5). It is organized around the four major anatomic segments: the articular segment, the greater tuberosity, the lesser tuberosity, and the proximal shaft (beginning at the level of the surgical neck). Fracture types are based on the degree of displacement of one or more of the four segments. By definition, a segment is displaced if it is displaced more than 1 cm or if it is angulated greater than 45 degrees from its normal anatomic position. The number of fracture lines does not have significance in the Neer classification system.

Displaced fractures may involve two-part, three-part, and four-part fractures. A two-part fracture is characterized by displacement of one of the four segments; the remaining three are not fractured or do not fulfill the criteria for displacement. There are four types of two-part fractures: greater tuberosity, lesser tuberosity, anatomic neck, and surgical neck. A three-part fracture is characterized by displacement of two of the segments from the remaining two nondisplaced segments. There are two types of three-part fracture patterns. In the more commonly encountered pattern, the greater tuberosity and the shaft are displaced from the lesser tuberosity, the latter remaining with the articular segment. The less commonly encountered three-part fracture pattern involves displacement of the lesser tuberosity and shaft from the greater tuberosity which remains with the articular segment. A four-part fracture features displacement of all four segments.

Fracture dislocations consist of displaced two-, three-, or four-part proximal humeral fractures associated with either anterior or poste-

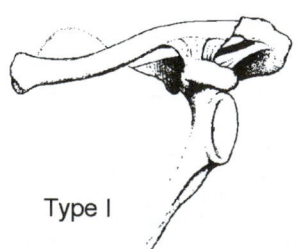
Type I

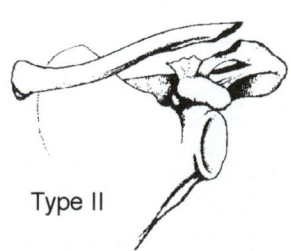
Type II

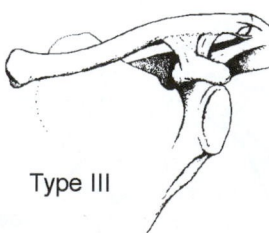
Type III

Figure 76-4
Distal clavicle fractures. [Reproduced by permission from Craig EV: Fractures of the clavicle. In Rockwood CA, Green DP, Bucholz RW, et al (eds): *Fractures in Adults*, 2d ed. Philadelphia: Lippincott; 1996:1117–1119.]

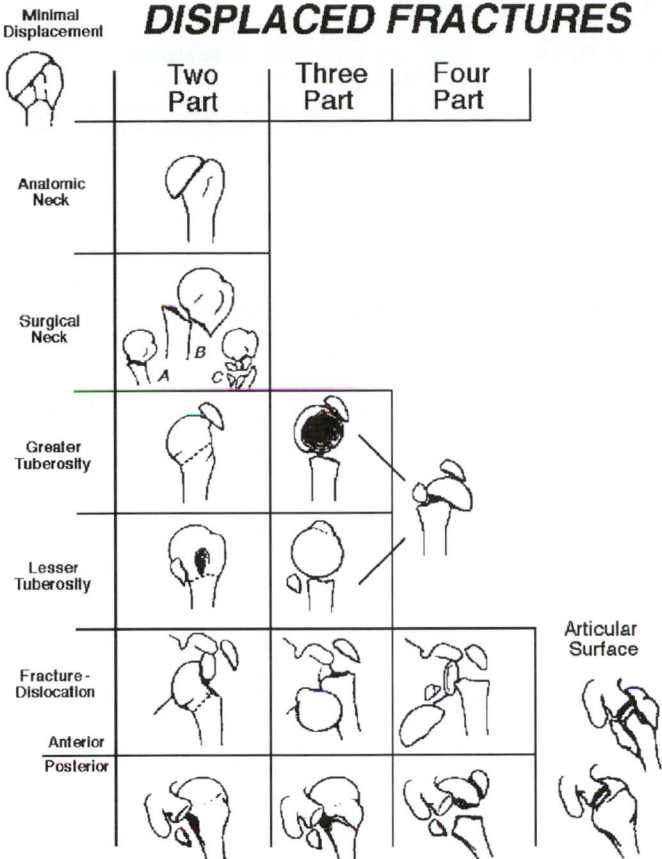

Figure 76-5
Neer classification of proximal humerus fractures. (Reproduced by permission from Neer CS II: Displaced proximal humeral fractures. Part I. Classification and evaluation. *J Bone Joint Surg [Am]* 1970; 52:1079.)

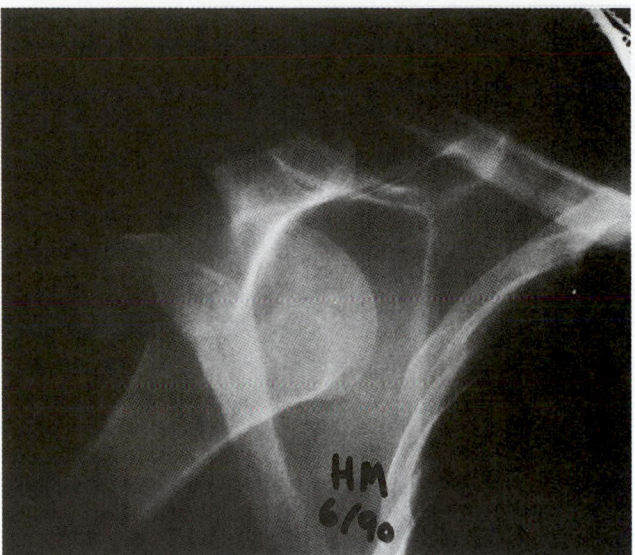

Figure 76-6
Two-part fracture dislocation of right shoulder with displacement of greater tuberosity.

rior dislocation of the articular segment (Fig. 76–6). Six types of fracture-dislocation patterns may occur. Articular surface fractures are categorized as either impression fractures or head-splitting fractures. An impression fracture usually occurs in association with chronic dislocation. As such, they may be termed as either anterior or posterior and involve varying amounts of the articular surface. Head splitting fractures are generally associated with other displaced fractures of the proximal humerus in which the disruption or "splitting" of the articular surface is the most clinically significant component.

TREATMENT PRINCIPLES

Eighty percent of proximal humerus fractures present with minimal displacement, and can be managed with protective immobilization and early range of motion, depending on fracture stability.

Two-part fractures that involve the anatomic neck are rare, however, they carry a high risk of osteonecrosis. Closed reduction is problematic; younger patients should be treated with open reduction and internal fixation and older patients should be managed with hemiarthroplasty. Isolated two-part lesser tuberosity fractures are also rare; they usually occur in association with a posterior glenohumeral dislocation. Small fragments may be managed nonoperatively; larger fragments should be internally stabilized. Two-part greater tuberosity fractures are usually associated with longitudinal rotator cuff tear; they tend to retract superiorly, interfering with forward elevation and abduction. Displaced greater tuberosity fractures should receive open

reduction and be internally stabilized with a tension band technique or screw fixation. Two-part surgical neck fractures are either impacted (stable) but malpositioned, or completely displaced and unstable. Treatment options are closed reduction with or without percutaneous pinning, or open reduction with internal fixation.

Three-part fractures generally necessitate open reduction as closed reduction is both difficult to achieve and maintain. Hemiarthroplasty is indicated in elderly patients, in severely osteoporotic bone, or in comminuted fractures. In four-part fractures, the articular segment is deficient in soft tissue attachment, and has a subsequent high risk of osteonecrosis. Open reduction and internal fixation should be attempted in young patients who have strong bone stock; most remaining patients should have a hemiarthroplasty.

Fracture dislocations are high-energy injuries. Operative management is indicated following careful patient selection and proper preoperative planning and includes either open reduction and internal fixation or hemiarthroplasty. Head-splitting fractures usually occur in association with other injuries. The degree and percentage of articular injury should be assessed. Large fragments in young patients ought to be reduced and stabilized; comminuted fractures and fractures within osteoporotic bone should be managed with hemiarthroplasty. Articular impression fractures occur with chronic dislocations; treatment approach is based on the percent of articular surface involved.

RESULTS

The outcome following treatment of a proximal humerus fracture is dependent on the severity of the injury, fracture displacement, bone quality, and the degree of comminution. One-part proximal humerus fractures generally have a good result; the vast majority of elderly patients have 50 to 75 percent of normal shoulder motion restored. However, most series of displaced proximal humerus fractures report a significant number of fixation failures, irrespective of the type of implant used. Jaberg and coworkers (1992) reported a study of 54 proximal humerus fractures managed with closed reduction and percutaneous fixation using three terminally threaded 2.5-mm pins. Forty-eight fractures were followed for an average of 3 years. Eighteen of twenty-nine (62 percent) two-part surgical neck fractures, all eight three-part fractures, and three of five (60 percent) four-part fractures had a good or excellent result. Hawkins and associates (1986) reported a study of 14 patients who were stabilized with a tension band wiring. At an average of 6 weeks follow-up, all fractures achieved union without loss of fixation; on follow-up, active forward elevation averaged 126 degrees, external rotation averaged 29 degrees, and abduction averaged 81 degrees. Osteonecrosis developed in two patients, one of whom required a hemiarthroplasty.

COMPLICATIONS

Complications associated with proximal humerus fractures are decreased range of shoulder motion, nonunion, malunion, and osteonecrosis. Loss of shoulder motion is dependent on the severity of injury, fracture pattern, length of immobilization, fracture reduction, and status of the rotator cuff. Nonunion is not uncommon after two-part surgical neck fractures and may be secondary to soft tissue interposition or inadequate immobilization. Malunion may be related to either inadequate initial reduction or loss of reduction. Osteonecrosis is most commonly associated with four-part fractures and fracture-dislocations.

SUGGESTED READINGS

SHOULDER DISLOCATIONS

Hawkins RJ, Neer CS II, Pianta RM, et al: Locked posterior dislocation of the shoulder. *J Bone Joint Surg [Am]* 1987; 69:9.

Rowe CR: Acute and recurrent anterior dislocation of the shoulder. *Orthop Clin North Am* 1980; 11:253.

SCAPULA FRACTURES

Hardegger FH, Simpson LA, Weber BG: The operative treatment of scapular fractures. *J Bone Joint Surg [Br]* 1984; 66:725.

McGinnis M, Denton JR: Fractures of the scapula: A retrospective study of 40 fractured scapulae. *J Trauma* 1989; 29(11):1488.

CLAVICLE FRACTURES

Allman FL: Fractures and ligamentous injuries of the clavicle and its articulation. *J Bone Joint Surg [Am]* 1967; 49:774.

Anderson K, Jensen PO, Lauritzen J: Treatment of clavicular fractures: Figure-of-eight bandage versus a simple sling. *Acta Orthop Scand* 1987; 58:7174.

Neer CS II: Fractures of the distal third of the clavicle. *Clin Orthop* 1968; 58:43.

Neviaser JS: Injuries to the clavicle and its articulations. *Orthop Clin North Am* 1980; 11:233.

ACROMIOCLAVICULAR JOINT INJURIES

Tossy JD, Mead NC, Sigmond HM: AC separations: A useful and practical classification for treatment. *Clin Orthop* 1963; 28:111.

Williams GR, et al: Classification and radiographic analysis of AC dislocations. *Appl Radiol* 1989; Feb:29–34.

STERNOCLAVICULAR JOINT INJURIES

DeJoeng KP, Dinesh MK: Anterior sternoclavicular dislocation: A long-term follow-up study. *J Orthop Trauma* 1990; 4:420.

Selesnick FH, Jablon M, Frank C, Post M: Retrosternal dislocation of the clavicle. *J Bone Joint Surg [Am]* 1984; 66:287.

PROXIMAL HUMERUS FRACTURES

Hawkins RJ, Bell RH, Gurr K: The three part fracture of the proximal part of the humerus: Operative treatment. *J Bone Joint Surg [Am]* 1986; 68:1410.

Jaberg H, Warner JJ, Jakob RP: Percutaneous stabilization of unstable fractures of the humerus. *J Bone Joint Surg [Am]* 1992; 74:508.

Neer CS II: Displaced proximal humerus fractures. I. Classification and evaluation. *J Bone Joint Surg [Am]* 1970; 52:1077.

Neer CS II: Four-segment classification of displaced proximal humeral fractures. In: *Instructional Course Lectures.* (American Academy of Orthopaedic Surgeons) St. Louis: Mosby; 1975; 24:160.

Tanner MW, Cofield RH: Arthroplasty for fractures and fracture: Dislocations of the proximal humerus. *Clin Orthop* 1983; 179:116.

Chapter 77

HUMERUS

Kenneth J. Koval

HUMERAL SHAFT FRACTURES

ANATOMY

The humeral shaft lies between the upper border of the pectoralis major insertion and the supracondylar ridge. The configuration of muscle origin and insertions combine to act on the shaft and produce characteristic fracture deformities. A humeral fracture that is proximal to the pectoralis major insertion creates abduction and internal rotation of the proximal fragment, secondary to the pull of the rotator cuff. When a fracture is proximal to the deltoid insertion and distal to the pectoralis major insertion, the distal fragment is displaced laterally by the deltoid. The pectoralis major, latissimus dorsi, and teres major act to medially displace the proximal fragment. If a fracture is distal to the insertion of the deltoid, the proximal fragment becomes abducted as well as flexed; the distal fragment is proximally displaced.

INCIDENCE AND MECHANISM OF INJURY

Three percent of all humeral fractures involve the humeral shaft. They can result from either direct or indirect trauma. Mechanisms of injury include falls onto an outstretched hand, motor vehicle accident, and direct load to the arm.

RADIOGRAPHIC EVALUATION

For humeral shaft injury AP and lateral views taken at 90 degrees to each other are standard; however, these views should be extended to include the shoulder and elbow joint but obtained without moving the injured extremity. Technicians should be advised to move the patient and not the injured extremity in obtaining the radiographic views.

CLASSIFICATION

There is no generally agreed upon classification system for humeral shaft fractures. Historically, these fractures have been classified instead on select clinical factors that influence treatment. Factors include: (1) location of fracture; (2) character/direction of the fracture line; (3) related soft tissue injury; (4) associated periarticular injury that includes the glenohumeral or elbow joint; (5) associated nerve injury; and (6) inherent condition of the bone, whether it is normal or pathologic.

The AO/ASIF classification describes the fracture patterns of comminution: type A are simple (noncomminuted), type B include a butterfly fragment, and type C are comminuted. Each fracture type is then further divided by fracture pattern.

TREATMENT PRINCIPLES

The majority of humeral shaft fractures are treated with nonsurgical methods and have a 90 to 100 percent rate of union. Current closed treatment methods include: (1) hanging arm cast; (2) coaptation or U-shaped brachial splint; (3) Velpeau dressing; (4) abduction humeral splint/shoulder spica cast; (5) skeletal traction; and (6) functional brace. In spite of the fact that satisfactory to excellent results can be achieved with each of these treatment modalities, functional fracture bracing has become the standard treatment for closed humeral shaft fractures. The humeral fracture brace may be applied immediately post-injury as part of acute care or after 1 to 2 weeks after application of a hanging arm cast or a coaptation splint.

Indications for surgical treatment of humeral shaft fractures are: open fractures, fractures associated with vascular injury, floating elbow, segmental humerus fractures, pathologic fractures, bilateral humerus fractures, polytrauma patients, radial nerve dysfunction after fracture manipulation, neurologic loss after penetrating injury, fractures in which one cannot maintain an acceptable alignment, and fractures associated with intraarticular fracture extension. Up to 3 cm shortening, 20 degrees of anterior or posterior angulation, and 30 degrees of varus are acceptable. Obese patients and women with large pendulous breasts are at greater risk of varus angulation. However, malrotation is adequately tolerated secondary to compensatory shoulder motion.

Plates and screws have proven to be effective devices which allow anatomic fracture reduction and provide stable fixation of the humeral shaft; futhermore, use of plates and screws avoids encroachment on the rotator cuff. A broad (4.5 mm) dynamic compression plate is generally chosen for management of midshaft fractures (Fig. 77-1).

Flexible intramedullary devices currently used in the management of humerus fractures include: Ender pins, Hackethal nails, and Rush rods. Multiple pins and rods should be added to ensure fracture stability. They can be inserted retrograde through the distal humerus, or antegrade through the rotator cuff.

Interlocked nails can be used to stabilize fractures which occur 2 cm distal to the surgical neck to 3 cm proximal to the olecranon. With antegrade insertion, the humeral nail should be embedded below the rotator cuff to avoid nail impingement beneath the acromion. Despite placement of the nail below the rotator cuff, however, there remains a significant risk of shoulder pain following antegrade nail insertion.

OPEN FRACTURE—TREATMENT

Gustillo grade I open fractures can be managed as closed fractures following adequate debridement (Gustilo and colleagues, 1969). Humerus fractures with more significant soft tissue damage should be stabilized surgically to permit better soft tissue management. While external fixators as well as plates and screws have been used successfully to manage open humerus fractures, more recently, interest has increased in using interlocked humeral nails.

PATHOLOGIC FRACTURE

The humeral shaft is frequently involved with metastatic disease, a setting conducive to pathologic fracture. While prophylactic measures

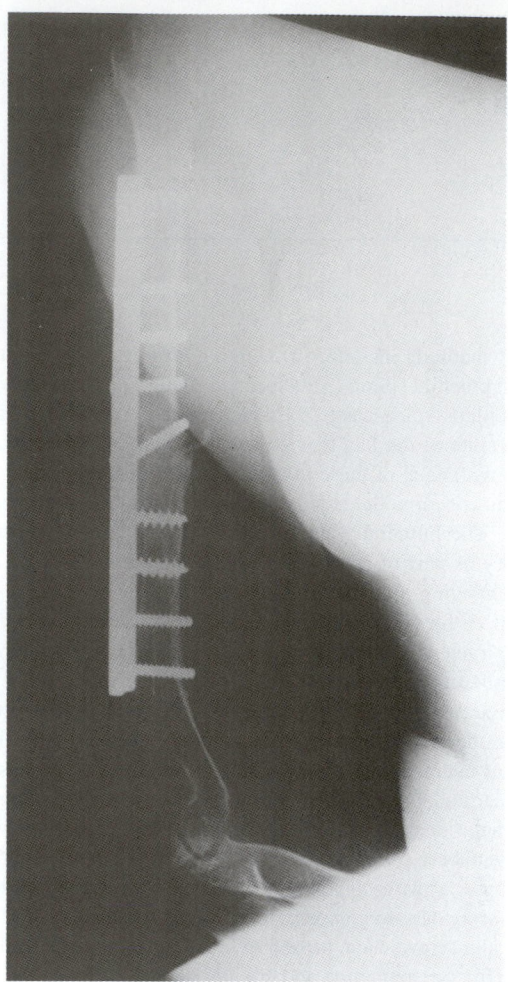

Figure 77-1
Humeral shaft fracture in osteopenic bone treated with plate and screws.

such as internal fixation of the humerus are not recommended on a routine basis, surgical stabilization of pathologic fractures remains the currently best known way to lessen patient pain, ease nursing care, and support patient independence.

RESULTS

Both nonoperative and operative management of humeral shaft fractures yields good to excellent results. Zagorski and coworkers reported in 1988 on 170 patients with humeral shaft fractures who were treated using a functional brace; 98 percent of the fractures achieved union and 95 percent had an excellent functional result with virtually full range of motion of the elbow and shoulder. Hall and Pankovich reported in 1987 on a prospective study of 89 humeral shaft fractures that were stabilized with Ender nails. Ninety-nine achieved union by an average of 7.2 weeks. Russell and colleagues (1990) reported on another prospective series of 51 consecutive interlocked humeral nailings where union was accomplished in all acute fractures and eight out of ten nonunions.

COMPLICATIONS

According to the literature, up to 18 percent of humeral shaft fractures are associated with a radial nerve injury. While the Holstein-

Lewis fracture (oblique, distal third) is well known for associated neurologic injury, radial nerve palsy most frequently occurs in middle-third humerus fractures. The majority of nerve injuries are a neuropraxia or axonotmesis; 90 percent of these injuries will resolve in 3 to 4 months. Monitoring of the degree of nerve injury and the rate of nerve regeneration can be achieved through electromyography and nerve conduction studies. Radial nerve palsy that is related to an open fracture or that occurs after fracture manipulation is an indication for early nerve exploration.

The nonunion rate associated with humeral shaft fracture ranges from 0 to 15 percent. Proximal and distal humeral areas are at a higher risk for nonunion than those which occur on the humeral shaft. Clinical and surgical issues pertinent to nonunion include a transverse fracture pattern, fracture distraction, soft tissue interposition, and ineffective immobilization. When shoulder motion is limited, the risk of humeral nonunion is further increased. Higher rates of nonunion have been reported after operative treatment than with nonoperative management though the cause is uncertain.

DISTAL HUMERUS FRACTURES

ANATOMY

The humeral shaft flattens at its distal segment to form triangular medial and lateral columns. Within the sagittal plane, the columns distally form a 40-degree angle anteriorly. The distal humeral articular surface has a 10- to 15-degree valgus angulation.

INCIDENCE/MECHANISM OF INJURY

Distal humerus fractures usually occur from a fall onto the outstretched arm and are relatively rare; they account for less than 1 percent of all humeral fractures.

RADIOGRAPHIC EVALUATION

AP and lateral views of the elbow are the standard initial radiographs in distal humeral fractures. If there is significant fracture shortening or deformity, traction radiographs are particularly useful to evaluate intercondylar fracture extension, but may be beneficial in that setting even without shortening or deformity.

CLASSIFICATION

The Riseborough and Radin classification (Fig. 77–2) describes distal humerus fractures with intercondylar extension and consists of 4 types: type I are nondisplaced; type II are fractures with the trochlea and capitellum displaced but not rotated; type III fractures have the

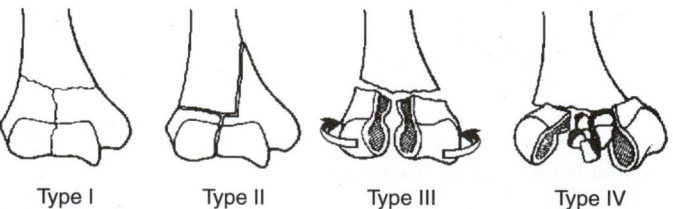

Type I   Type II   Type III   Type IV

Figure 77-2
Riseborough and Radin classification of distal humerus fractures. (Reproduced by permission from Henley MB, Bone LB: Operative management of intraarticular fractures of the distal humerus. *J Orthop Trauma* 1987; 1:24.)

trochlea and capitellum both displaced and rotated; and finally, type IV are type III fractures with significant intercondylar comminution. A more comprehensive classification is the AO/ASIF classification which divides distal humerus fractures into three dominant classes: type A, extraarticular; type B; unicondylar; and type C, bicondylar. The groups are subdivided again into further subgroups which represent the severity of the fracture.

TREATMENT PRINCIPLES

Minimally displaced and impacted distal humerus fractures can be treated with plaster immobilization. Patients are allowed progressive passive-assisted range of elbow motion as healing progresses.

Displaced intraarticular distal humerus fractures require anatomic joint reduction with stable fixation to permit early range of motion. Open fractures and those with neurovascular injury and/or compartment syndrome require emergent treatment. An olecranon osteotomy is often needed for distal humerus visualization. The articular surface is reduced and stabilized with lag screws. The metaphysis is stabilized using double plates, preferably oriented 90 degrees from each other. The olecranon osteotomy is stabilized with either k-wires or a lag screw, supplemented with tension band wiring.

RESULTS

Approximately 75 percent of intraarticular distal humerus fractures have a good to excellent outcome following surgical treatment. Evidence of a successful result after low energy distal humerus fracture is a postoperative 15- to 140-degree range of elbow motion. Higher energy injuries with greater soft tissue injury generally have greater restriction of elbow motion.

COMPLICATIONS

Distal humerus fracture complications include heterotopic ossification, infection, ulnar nerve palsy, failure of fixation, and nonunion.

High energy injuries, repeat attempts at closed reduction, delayed surgery, and postoperative passive motion are all associated with higher rates of heterotopic ossification.

SUGGESTED READINGS

HUMERAL SHAFT

Balfour GW, Mooney V, Ashby M: Diaphyseal fractures of the humerus treated with a ready made fracture brace. *J Bone Joint Surg [Am]* 1982; 64:11.
Brumback RJ, Bosse MJ, Poka A, et al: Intramedullary stabilization of humeral shaft fractures. *J Bone Joint Surg [Am]* 1986; 68:960.
Foster RJ, Dixon GL, Bach AW, et al: Internal fixation of fractures and nonunions of the humeral shaft. *J Bone Joint Surg [Am]* 1985; 67:857.
Pollack FH, Drake D, Bovill EG, et al: Treatment of radial neuropathy associated with fractures of the humerus. *J Bone Joint Surg [Am]* 1981; 63:239.
Russell TA, Simard J, Taylor JC, et al: *Interlocking Intramedullary Nailing of Humeral Fractures. Orthop Trans* 1992; 16:334.
Sarmiento A, Kinwan PB, Calvin EG: Functional bracing of fractures of the shaft of the humerus. *J Bone Joint Surg [Am]* 1977; 59:596.

DISTAL HUMERUS

Grantham SA, Norris TR, Bush DC: Isolated fracture of the humeral capitellum. *Clin Orthop* 1981; 161:262.
Gustilo RB, Simpson L, Nixon R, et al: Analysis of 511 open fractures. *Clin Orthop* 1969; 66:148.
Jupiter JB, Neff U, Holzach P, Allgoewer M: Intercondylar fracture of the humerus. *J Bone Joint Surg [Am]* 1985; 67:226.
Milch HE: Fractures and fracture-dislocations of the humeral condyles. *J Trauma* 1964; 4:592.
Riseborough EJ, Radin EL: Intercondylar "T"-fractures of the humerus in the adult. *J Bone Joint Surg [Am]* 1969; 51:130.

Chapter 78

ELBOW

Kenneth J. Koval

ELBOW DISLOCATION

ANATOMY

The elbow is one of the more stable but highly constrained joints in the body. The major stabilizing and constraining forces are the medial and lateral collateral ligaments. The lateral collateral ligament passes from the lateral humeral epicondyle to the annular ligament which invests the radial head and the ulna. The lateral ligament complex is additionally reinforced by the anconeus muscle and the extensors of the wrist and hand. Principle ligamentous support of the elbow is provided by the medial collateral ligament complex, traditionally characterized as composed of three parts: the anterior oblique ligament which is the primary stabilizer (runs from the medial epicondyle to the coronoid process); the fan-shaped posterior oblique ligament which functions only in flexion (origin is the medial epicondyle; insertion is to the olecranon); and a small transverse ligament which extends from the coronoid to the olecranon (no known significance).

INCIDENCE AND MECHANISM OF INJURY

Elbow dislocation occurs most frequently in adolescents and young adults. The mechanism is often a fall onto an outstretched arm. Tearing of the brachial artery has occasionally been reported with elbow dislocation, and requires an index of suspicion confirmed by arteriography. Twenty percent of elbow dislocation cases report neuropraxia, usually involving ulnar or median nerves. However, the majority of neurologic deficits are transient and will resolve without treatment.

CLASSIFICATION

Simple dislocations of the elbow do not involve a fracture. They are classified according to the direction of the dislocation: posterior, posterolateral, posteromedial, lateral-medial, or divergent (Fig. 78–1). Dislocations of the elbow associated with a fracture are termed complex and represent approximately 50 percent of all elbow dislocations. The pathoanatomy of simple posterior elbow dislocation includes rupture of the anterior capsule, the medial collateral ligament, and the flexor pronator mass to a variable degree, as well as injury to the brachialis muscle and possible chondral damage.

TREATMENT

The elbow should be managed with gentle closed reduction; postreduction treatment includes protected early range of motion. Repeat attempts at manipulation should be avoided. A congruent reduction is generally achieved by longitudinal traction followed by flexion of the elbow. Passive motion to within 20 degrees of full extension without subluxation suggests a stable reduction. Open repair of the medial

collateral ligament for simple elbow dislocations has not been documented to have an improved outcome.

Treatment of complex dislocations usually involves surgery. Adequate stability must be achieved during open reduction to allow early range of motion. Fractures associated with an elbow dislocation may involve the medial epicondyle, coronoid process, or the radial head. Open reduction and internal fixation of a displaced medial epicondyle fracture is indicated when displacement exceeds 10 mm,

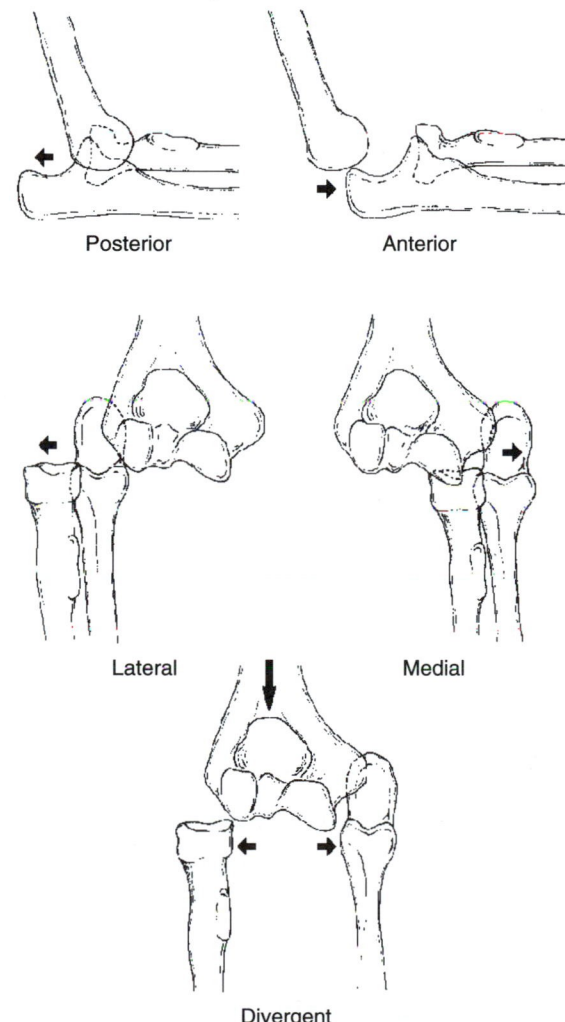

Figure 78-1

Elbow dislocations. [Reproduced by permission from Jupiter JB: Part 1. Trauma to the adult elbow and fractures of the distal humerus. In Browner BD, Jupiter JB, Levine AM, et al (eds): *Skeletal Trauma*. Philadelphia: WB Saunders; 1992:1142.]

if there is severe valgus instability, associated ulnar nerve symptoms are present, or there is incarceration of the fragment within the ulno-humeral joint.

Elbow dislocations that include a large coronoid fragment are usually unstable, are associated with high redislocation rates, and require open reduction and internal fixation to reestablish stability. Treatment of elbow dislocations with associated radial head fractures are controversial. The radial head is an important secondary stabilizer; salvage with open reduction and internal fixation is preferable to excision. If radial head excision is indicated due to severe comminution, then use of a Silastic or metallic radial head prosthesis may be necessary as a temporary spacer. There have been recent reports of the use of hinged elbow distractors that provide both stability and controlled elbow motion.

RESULTS

Management of simple elbow dislocations usually has a good outcome with a return to full range of motion, normal strength, minimal pain, and restored stability. Poor results are usually associated with complications and can be anticipated in 15 percent of simple elbow dislocations. Mild loss of extension is a common sequela; delayed immobilization over two weeks is associated with greater flexion contracture. Recurrent dislocation is uncommon and implies disruption of the medial collateral ligament and flexor forearm muscles.

COMPLICATIONS

Common complications following elbow dislocation are heterotopic calcification, loss of elbow motion, recurrent dislocation, instability, and posttraumatic arthritis. The ulnar nerve is the most commonly injured, primarily from valgus stretching.

OLECRANON FRACTURES

ANATOMY

The greater sigmoid notch is formed by the olecranon and coronoid and articulates with the trochlea of the distal humerus. The triceps inserts onto the upper aspect of the olecranon with medial and lateral extensions onto the proximal ulna.

INCIDENCE AND MECHANISM OF INJURY

Olecranon fractures can result from direct or indirect force. Indirect force usually results in transverse fractures, secondary to eccentric loading of the triceps when the person falls onto the outstretched hand.

CLINICAL AND RADIOGRAPHIC EVALUATION

It is important to evaluate the status of the triceps extensor mechanism; if intact, the elbow will be able to actively extend against gravity. Both AP and lateral radiographic views of the elbow should be taken. A lateral radiograph will most clearly identify and locate the fracture as well as reveal the direction and extent of articular disruption. A lateral radiograph at 90 degrees flexion may confirm fracture stability in minimally displaced fractures.

CLASSIFICATION

Olecranon fractures were classified by Colton (1973) into nondisplaced (<2 mm displacement with the elbow 90 degrees flexed) and

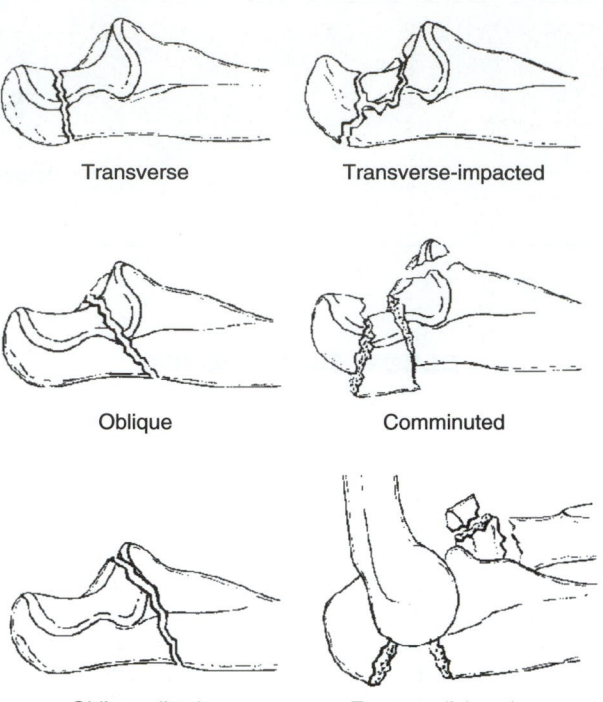

Figure 78-2
Schatzker classification of olecranon fractures. [Reproduced by permission from Jupiter JB: Part 1. Trauma to the adult elbow and fractures of the distal humerus. In Browner BD, Jupiter JB, Levine AM, et al (eds): *Skeletal Trauma*. Philadelphia: WB Saunders; 1992:1137.]

displaced. Displaced fractures were further subdivided into avulsion, oblique or transverse, comminuted, or fracture-dislocation. Schatzker classified olecranon fractures as either transverse, transverse-impacted, oblique, comminuted, oblique-distal, or fracture-dislocation (Fig. 78-2).

TREATMENT PRINCIPLES

Olecranon fractures that are nondisplaced are immobilized for 3 to 4 weeks in a long arm splint or cast with the elbow flexed 90 degrees. Indications for operative treatment include displacement greater than 2 mm, articular stepoff, or an inability to actively extend the elbow against gravity. Transverse olecranon fractures should be stabilized with a tension band technique (Fig. 78–3). Depressed articular fragments should be elevated and bone grafted. Lag screws should be placed across oblique fractures and protected with a tension band wire or plate. Fractures extending beyond the coronoid require plate application, as tension band wires will not provide sufficient rotational control.

COMPLICATIONS

Common complications following olecranon fracture are loss of elbow motion, malunion, nonunion, and posttraumatic arthritis.

RADIAL HEAD FRACTURES

ANATOMY

The radial head articulates with the capitellum and also acts as a stabilizer to valgus stress.

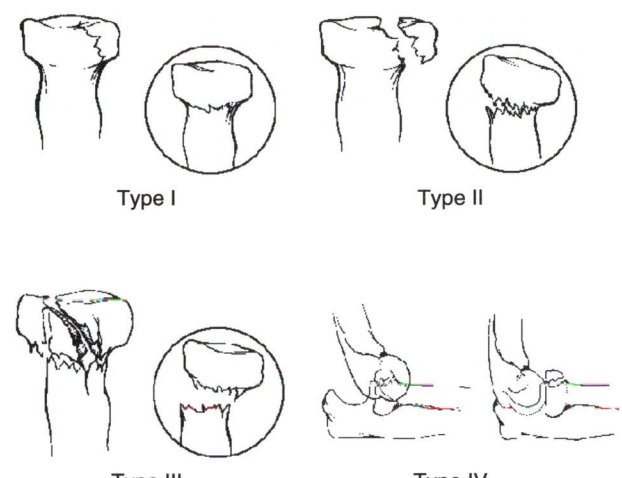

Figure 78-4
Mason classification of radial head and neck fractures. [Reproduced by permission from Broberg MA, Morrey BF: Results of treatment of fracture-dislocations of the elbow. *Clin Orthop* 1987; 216:109.]

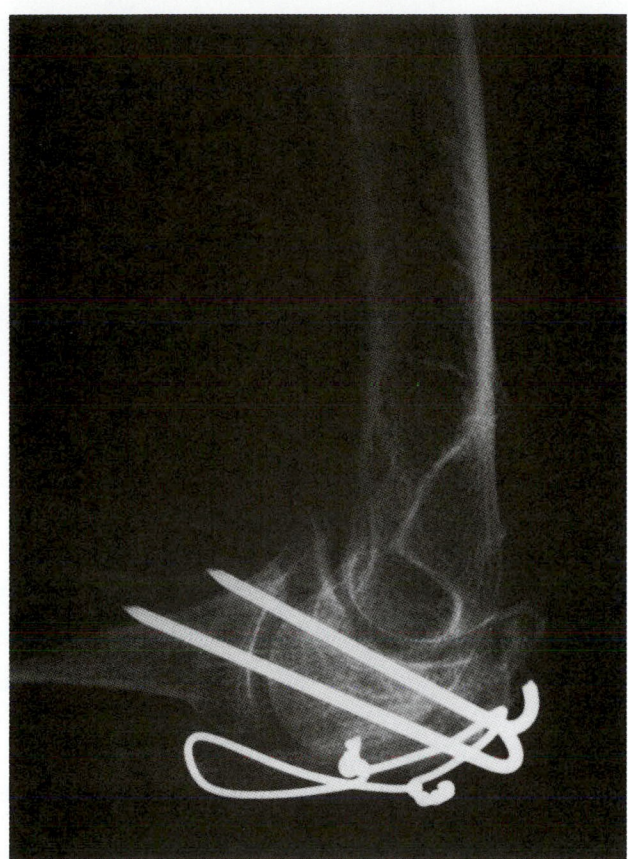

Figure 78-3
Displaced olecranon fracture with tension band wiring.

Static loading studies suggest as much as 60 percent of the force across the elbow is transmitted through the radiocapitellum articulation.

INCIDENCE AND MECHANISM OF INJURY

Almost 20 percent of all elbow injuries involve fractures of the radial head, making this a common injury. Radial head fractures are caused by axial load during a fall onto the outstretched hand.

CLINICAL AND RADIOGRAPHIC EVALUATION

Patients with radial head fracture often present with a hemarthrosis that is palpable in the triangular space bordered by the olecranon, radial head, and lateral epicondyle. In the presence of hemarthrosis, joint aspiration shows evidence of fat globules and indicates fracture. One needs to confirm that patients with a radial head fracture are able to fully extend their elbow; complete evaluation may require joint aspiration and injection of lidocaine. Less than full extension secondary to a bony block is an indication for operative management. The distal forearm should also be examined for injury to the radioulnar joint.

Radiographic evaluation includes AP and lateral views of the elbow, with visualization of the distal radioulnar joint. On radiographs of patients without a fracture, an anterior fat pad is evident. A posterior fat pad is suggestive of capsular distraction. If radial head fracture is suspected, a radio-capitellum radiograph which isolates the radial head and capitellum should be taken.

CLASSIFICATION

Radial head fractures were classified by Mason as: type I, nondisplaced; type II, a displaced split fragment; and type III, comminuted. A fourth type of radial head fractures associated with an elbow dislocation also has been added (Fig. 78–4).

TREATMENT

Following a brief period of immobilization, nondisplaced radial head fractures should be treated with early range of motion. Operative indications include: patients with loss of elbow extension secondary to a bony block, associated disruption of the interosseous membrane, and distal radioulnar joint (Essex-Lopresti lesion), or unstable elbow dislocation. Fractures with a single displaced large fragment should have open reduction and internal fixation to restore articular congruity. Management of comminuted radial head fractures remains controversial. There are advocates of nonoperative treatment with early range of motion and proponents of early radial head excision. Studies have demonstrated that the outcome of patients with delayed excision of the radial head is equivalent to that of patients who undergo early excision. If there is associated soft tissue injury (elbow dislocation, Essex-Lopresti lesion), a temporary radial head spacer is necessary to provide stability and proximal radial shaft migration. Prosthetic fragmentation, however, can result in silicone synovitis.

CORONOID FRACTURES

ANATOMY

The coronoid functions as an anterior buttress of the greater sigmoid notch of the olecranon, and is the site of attachment for the brachialis muscle, the anterior bundle of the medial collateral ligament, and the anterior elbow capsule.

MECHANISM OF INJURY

Coronoid fracture can be associated with an elbow dislocation or result from forceful eccentric contraction of the brachialis muscle.

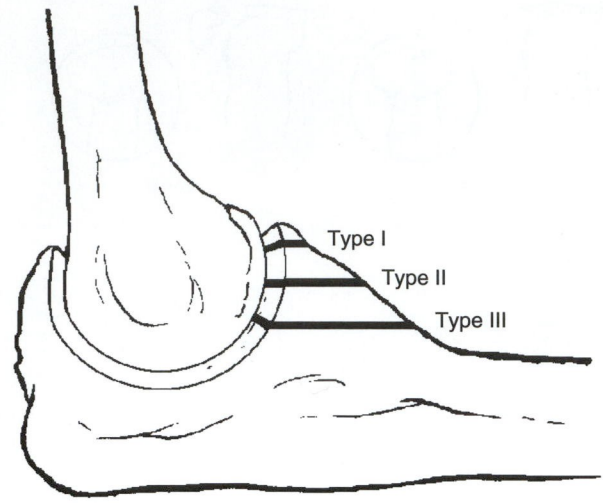

Figure 78-5
Coronoid fractures. [Reproduced by permission from Regan W, Morrey B: Fracture of the coronoid process of the elbow. *J Bone Joint Surg [Am]* 1989; 71:1349.]

CLINICAL AND RADIOGRAPHIC EVALUATION

In the presence of coronoid fracture, elbow stability should be evaluated. Radiographic evaluation should include AP and lateral radiographs of the elbow, with the coronoid best seen on the lateral view.

CLASSIFICATION

Coronoid fractures were classified by Regan and Morrey into: type I, tip avulsion; type II, a single or comminuted fracture involving <50 percent of the coronoid; and type III, a single comminuted fracture involving >50 percent of the coronoid (Fig. 78-5).

TREATMENT PRINCIPLES

Displaced coronoid fractures require open reduction and internal fixation, particularly those which present a block to full elbow extension or are associated with an elbow dislocation.

CAPITELLUM FRACTURES

Capitellum fractures are rare. They account for only 1 percent of all elbow fractures and 6 percent of all distal humerus fractures. Coronal fractures of the capitellum are caused by shear. The fragment can involve a varying amount of osseous bone (Fig. 78–6). Type I fractures (Hahn-Steinthal) have a large osseous component. The fracture hinges anteriorly between the radial head and the radial fossa, acting as a block to motion. Excellent results have been reported with open reduction and internal fixation of the fracture with screw fixation, followed by early range of motion. Excision is recommended if the fracture is comminuted. The type II or Kocher-Lorenz fracture is a sleeve fracture of the articular surface with little osseous bone; healing potential is low, and excision is recommended.

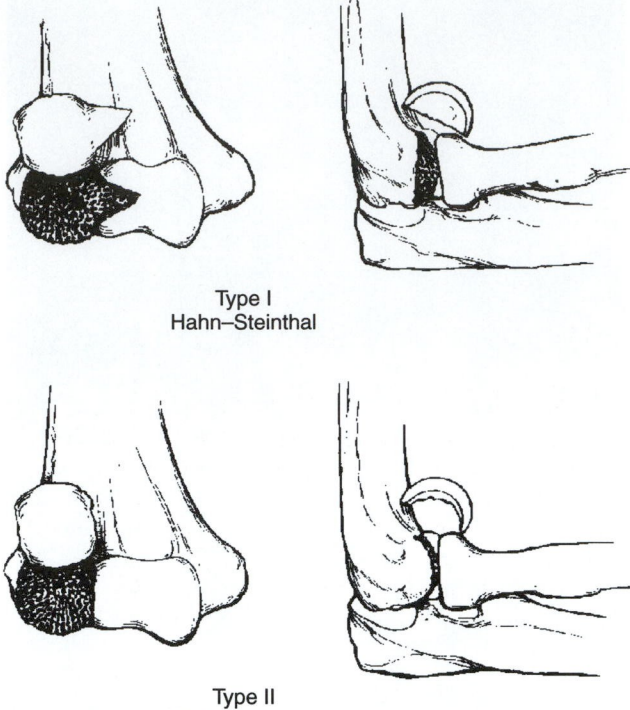

Type I
Hahn–Steinthal

Type II
Kocher–Lorenz

Figure 78-6
Capitellar fractures. [Reproduced by permission from Hotchkiss RN: Fractures and dislocations of the elbow. In Rockwood CA, Green DP, Bucholz RW (eds): *Fractures in Adults*, 4th ed. Philadelphia; Lippincott-Raven: 1996:960.]

SUGGESTED READINGS

ELBOW DISLOCATIONS

O'Driscoll SW, Morrey BF, Korinek S: Elbow subluxation and dislocation: A spectrum of instability. *Clin Orthop* 1992; 280:17.

Regan W, Morrey B: Fractures of the coronoid process of the ulna. *J Bone Joint Surg [Am]* 1989; 71:1348.

OLECRANON AND RADIAL HEAD

An KN, Morrey BF, Chao EYS: The effect of partial removal of the proximal ulna on elbow constraint. *Clin Orthop* 1986; 209:270.

Broberg MA, Morrey BF: Results of delayed excision of the radial head after fracture. *J Bone Joint Surg [Am]* 1986; 68:669.

Colton CL: Fractures of the olecranon in adults: Classification and management. *Injury* 1973–74; 5:121–129.

Mason ML: Some observations on fractures of the head of the radius with a review of one hundred cases. *Br J Surg* 1954; 42:123.

Wolfgang G, Burke F, Bush D, et al: Surgical treatment of displaced olecranon fractures by tension band wiring technique. *Clin Orthop* 1987; 224:192.

Chapter 79

FOREARM

Kenneth J. Koval

FRACTURES OF THE RADIUS AND ULNA

CLINICAL AND RADIOGRAPHIC EVALUATION

Clinical evaluation of patients with forearm fractures should include a detailed inspection of the skin for open wounds, as the subcutaneous location of the ulna predisposes to open fractures. A careful neurovascular examination is essential to identify any deficits that may have resulted from the injury. Radiographic evaluation should include AP and lateral views of the entire forearm. Radiographic evaluation of the elbow and wrist is mandatory to identify associated injuries.

CLASSIFICATION

To date there is no established classification system for fractures of the radial and ulnar shafts. Location of the fracture, extent of comminution, and degree of displacement and angulation are criteria used to determine an appropriate treatment plan.

TREATMENT

Nondisplaced fractures of the radius and ulna are rare in adults. Treatment is usually a long-arm cast worn for 6 to 12 weeks with the elbow flexed 90 degrees and the forearm in neutral rotation. Since these fractures may displace, weekly radiographs should be taken to confirm that displacement has not occurred. If displacement does occur, internal fixation is required to restore the normal anatomic relationship of the radius and ulna. Compression plating using a 3.5-mm dynamic compression plate is currently the preferred technique.

Surgical approach depends on the fracture location. Fractures of the proximal and middle third of the radius are exposed through a dorsal approach, while fractures of the distal third of the radius are more easily exposed using a volar approach. Ulnar shaft fractures can be directly accessed through an incision along the ulnar subcutaneous border, centered over the level of the fracture. The need for primary bone grafting is controversial; it is usually performed in cases where there is comminution greater than 33 percent of the circumference of the involved bone. Range of motion can be started several days postsurgery.

Open forearm fractures are generally grade I injuries caused by relatively low energy and have minimal soft tissue damage. The site of the open wound usually overlies the subcutaneous border of the ulna. Less frequently, it overlies the dorsal or volar aspect of the distal radius. Management includes debridement, followed by open reduction and internal fixation. Primary closure of the open wound should be delayed 3 to 5 days. In higher grade open fractures with extensive soft tissue injury, an external fixation device can be used; it may be preferable to delay internal fixation until soft tissue healing has occurred.

COMPLICATIONS

Complications of both-bones forearm fractures include nonunion, malunion, infection, neurovascular injury, compartment syndrome, and radioulnar synostosis. Nonunion and malunion occur much less frequently as compression plating has become the standard treatment. Chapman and coworkers (1989) reported a union rate of 98 percent in forearm fractures treated by immediate open reduction and internal fixation using AO/ASIF principles of fracture fixation and bone grafting of all open and comminuted fractures. Surgical approaches include a moderate risk of neurovascular injury to the posterior interosseous nerve (the dorsal approach to the proximal radius) and to the radial artery and superficial radial nerve (the volar approach to the distal radius). Compartment syndrome is rare following low-energy injury. Radioulnar synostosis is also uncommon, and generally occurs with fractures that are the result of a high-energy injury. Refracture of forearm bones has been observed after plate removal, particularly when 4.5-mm plates and screws were the implants. Therefore, routine plate removal is not recommended following forearm fracture. If plate removal is necessary, cortical remodeling should be apparent and confirmed by radiography; remodeling may require as many as 18 to 24 months postsurgery.

ISOLATED ULNAR SHAFT FRACTURE

Isolated ulnar shaft fractures are usually caused by a direct blow to the ulnar aspect of the forearm. The eponym "night stick" fracture reflects this as the dominant mechanism of injury for these fractures. Radiographic examination of the entire forearm, elbow, and wrist are necessary to identify any associated fractures. Treatment depends on the location of the fracture and the degree of displacement and angulation. Nondisplaced fractures are best managed by short-term immobilization in a long arm splint. When the acute symptoms subside (approximately 7 to 10 days), a removable posterior splint is applied and range of motion is initiated. A similar approach is used for fractures which have less than 50 percent shaft displacement and up to 10 degrees of angulation. Radiographs should be repeated every week for the first 3 weeks to confirm that further displacement or angulation has not occurred.

Open reduction and internal fixation should be carefully considered for isolated ulnar shaft fractures with more than 50 percent displacement or greater than 20 degrees of angulation. The preferred treatment is compression plating followed by early range of motion.

ISOLATED RADIAL SHAFT FRACTURE

Isolated fractures of the radial shaft are rare. The surrounding musculature protects the radius from trauma secondary to a direct blow. The anatomic position of the radius during common activities also makes injury to the radial shaft less likely compared to the ulna. When an isolated radial shaft fracture does occur, it is virtually always located in the proximal two-thirds.

Fracture displacement is common. Nondisplaced fractures can be treated in a long arm cast with the forearm in supination. Radiographs should be repeated weekly for 2 to 3 weeks to be certain that displacement has not occurred. Immobilization should be continued until there are radiographic signs of healing. Displaced fractures should be treated by open reduction and internal fixation using plate and screws. An exception is a very proximal radius fracture in which adequate fixation of the proximal fragment cannot be obtained. These fractures should be treated in a long arm cast with the forearm in supination.

Bone grafting should be considered for comminuted fractures being treated with open reduction and internal fixation. If stable fixation is achieved, range of motion can be started several days postoperatively.

GALEAZZI FRACTURE

A Galeazzi fracture is a radial shaft fracture with subluxation or dislocation of the distal radioulnar joint (Fig. 79–1).

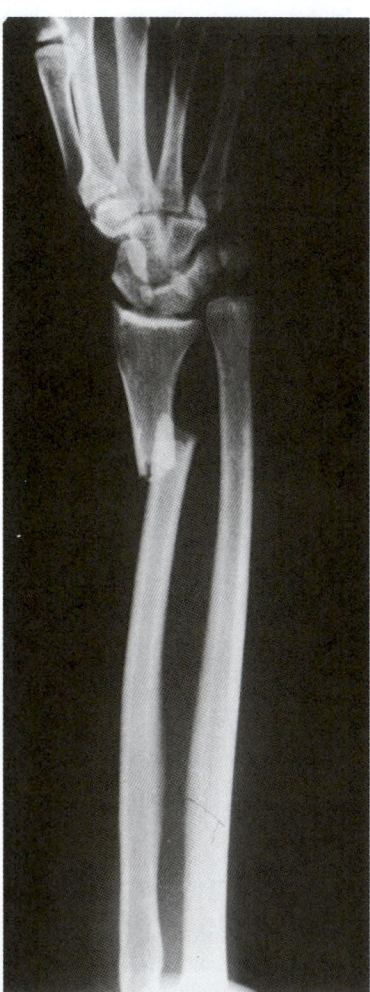

Figure 79-1
Galeazzi fracture in a 40-year-old male.

INCIDENCE AND MECHANISM OF INJURY

Galeazzi fractures are a rare injury. The incidence varies from 3 to 6 percent of all forearm fractures. They are caused by a blow to the dorsolateral aspect of the wrist or occur as a result of a fall onto the outstretched hand with forced pronation of the forearm.

CLINICAL AND RADIOGRAPHIC EVALUATION

Clinical evaluation is based on the degree of fracture displacement and disruption of the distal radioulnar joint. Generally, the fracture site is tender to palpation and some degree of deformity. Tenderness is also present over the distal radioulnar joint. The distal ulna is usually displaced into a dorsal position. Required radiographs include AP and lateral views of the elbow, forearm, and wrist. A lateral wrist view may facilitate assessing the degree of disruption of the distal radioulnar joint. The four most dependable radiographic signs of disruption of the distal radioulnar joint are: (1) fracture of the base of the ulnar styloid; (2) widening of the joint space as demonstrated on an AP view; (3) dislocation of the radius relative to the ulna as evidenced on a lateral radiograph; and (4) greater than 5 mm shortening of the radius.

CLASSIFICATION

Classically, a Galeazzi fracture is defined by a fracture of the middle to distal radius associated with subluxation or dislocation of the distal radioulnar joint. A Galeazzi equivalent in adults, as described by Reckling, is a fracture of the radius 6 to 8 cm proximal to the wrist with an additional fracture of the distal 2 cm of the ulna.

TREATMENT

Operative management is required of all Galeazzi fractures. A 92 percent failure rate for closed treatment was reported by Hughston in a 1957 review of the mismanagement of distal radial shaft injuries. In that series, loss of reduction was common and attributed to specific factors such as: (1) pull of the brachioradialis, resulting in shortening of the radius; (2) pull of the pronator quadratus, causing rotation of the distal fragment toward the ulna; and (3) weight of the hand acting as a deforming force, causing dorsal angulation of the radius and subluxation of the distal radioulnar joint.

Treatment includes open reduction and internal fixation of the radius with stabilization of the distal radioulnar joint. Comminuted fractures should be considered for bone grafting. Clinical and radiographic evaluation of the distal radioulnar joint is done after internal fixation is accomplished. If the joint is stable during forearm rotation, some authors suggest the arm not be immobilized and the patient be allowed early forearm and wrist motion. If the distal radioulnar joint is successfully reduced but remains unstable, the arm may be immobilized in full supination or the joint may be pinned. If the distal radioulnar joint cannot be reduced, an open reduction is necessary using a dorsal approach.

RESULTS

Successful treatment of Galeazzi fractures depends on adequate reduction of the fracture and distal radioulnar joint. Satisfactory treatment results were reported by Reckling (1982) in a group of 17 patients whose fractures were managed by open reduction and internal fixation of the fractured radius with immobilization of the forearm in full supination for 6 to 8 weeks. Moore and colleagues also reported satisfactory results using compression plating techniques and 4 weeks immobilization in a 1985 study.

COMPLICATIONS

Malunion of the radius will result in significant loss of forearm rotation. Residual displacement of the distal radioulnar joint may result in painful pronation and supination; resection of the distal ulna may be necessary. The incidence of nonunion is very low. In Moore's series of 36 patients, superficial radial nerve injuries occurred in 17 percent.

MONTEGGIA FRACTURE

A Monteggia fracture is a fracture of the proximal ulna with dislocation of the radial head.

INCIDENCE

Monteggia fractures are uncommon. The incidence varies between 1 to 2 percent of all forearm fractures.

CLINICAL AND RADIOGRAPHIC EVALUATION

Patients with Monteggia fractures present with pain and tenderness around the elbow. A neurologic exam should be performed with particular attention to assessment of the posterior interosseous nerve, as it is the most common neurologic injury associated with Monteggia fracture.

Radiographic evaluation includes AP and lateral views of the complete forearm, elbow, and wrist. If a Monteggia lesion is suspected, additional radiographs of the elbow should be taken. Normally, the radial shaft and capitellum lie in a straight line on any radiographic view. If this is not observed, a radial head dislocation should be suspected. Evidence of a proximal ulnar shaft fracture in the absence of a radial shaft fracture raises suspicion for the presence of a Monteggia lesion.

CLASSIFICATION AND MECHANISM OF INJURY

Originally, a Monteggia fracture was defined as a fracture of the proximal third of the ulna with associated anterior dislocation of the radial head. This description was expanded on by Bado (1967) to include all ulna fractures associated with dislocations of the radiohumeral articulation; fractures were termed "Monteggia lesions" (Fig. 79–2). The Bado classification of Monteggia lesions includes: type I, fracture of the ulnar diaphysis with anterior angulation and anterior dislocation of the radial head; type II, fracture of the ulnar diaphysis with posterior angulation and posterior or posterolateral dislocation of the radial head; type III, fracture of the ulnar metaphysis with lateral or anterolateral dislocation of the radial head; type IV, fracture of the proximal third of the radius with the fracture of the ulna at the same level and anterior dislocation of the radial head.

The type of Monteggia lesion is determined by the mechanism of injury. Type I lesions occur either as a result of a fall onto the pronated forearm or by a direct blow to the posterior aspect of the ulna. Type II lesions occur with a mechanism similar to those which produce a posterior elbow dislocation. Although the radial head dislocates posteriorly, the ligamentous attachment of the proximal ulna prevents dislocation, and a proximal ulnar fracture results. Type III lesions probably result from direct trauma over the inner aspect of the elbow, with or without forearm rotation. Type IV injuries may result from a type I mechanism in association with a second blow over the radial aspect of the forearm.

TREATMENT

In adults, closed treatment of Monteggia lesions has not produced satisfactory results. Recommended treatment is open reduction and internal fixation of the ulna fracture and closed or open reduction of the radial head fracture. Comminuted fractures are best treated with bone grafting. Reduction of the ulna fracture generally allows reduction of the radial head. If closed reduction is attempted and unsuccessful, open reduction must be performed. A posterolateral approach to the radial head provides excellent exposure. Division of the annular ligament or removal of an unfolded portion may be necessary for reduction of the radial head. In some type II fractures, an associated fracture of the radial head occurs which could require separate treatment. If the fracture includes just a small portion of the radial head, then excision of the fragment is recommended. However, if a comminuted fracture is present instead, radial head excision is indicated. In type IV lesions, open reduction and internal fixation of the radius fracture is necessary.

Postoperative immobilization prevents redislocation of the radial head, and is usually necessary. Types I, III, and IV injuries should be immobilized in a long arm cast with approximately 110 degrees of elbow flexion and moderate supination. Type II injuries should be immobilized with approximately 70 degrees of elbow flexion.

RESULTS

Reported outcomes of treatment in Monteggia lesions in adults have been variable. Boyd and Boals (1969) published that 77 percent of cases had from good to excellent results with a variety of treatment approaches. More recently, in a large series of Monteggia lesions in adults reviewed by Reckling (1982), the best results were with type I lesions. Treatment was open anatomic reduction and internal fixation

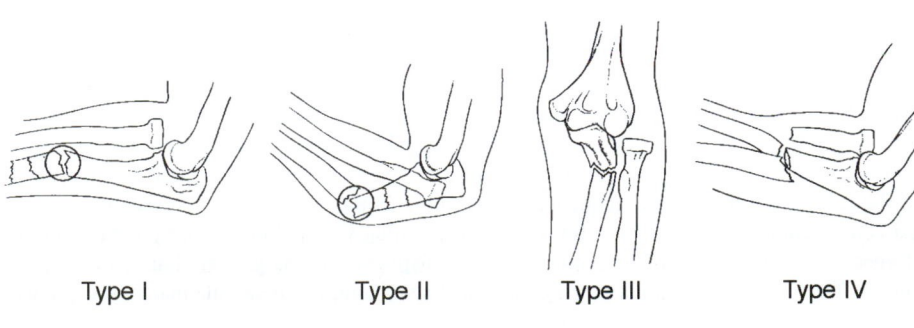

Type I   Type II   Type III   Type IV

Figure 79-2
Bado classification of Monteggia fractures. [Reproduced by permission from Kellam JF, Jupiter JB: Diaphyseal fractures in the forearm. In Browner BD, Jupiter JB, Levine AM, et al (eds): *Skeletal Trauma*. Philadelphia: WB Saunders; 1992:1117.]

of the ulna fracture with closed reduction of the radial head. Poor results in type I lesions were attributed to failure to achieve an anatomical reduction of the ulna, heterotopic ossification resulting in synostosis of the proximal radius and ulna, and persistence or recurrence of dislocation of the radial head. Most treatment results following types II, III, and IV injuries were fair, with some loss of elbow and forearm motion. However, the majority of patients were restored to a preinjury level of function and did not need secondary procedures.

COMPLICATIONS

Complications of Monteggia lesions include recurrent subluxation or redislocation of the radial head, injury to the posterior interosseous nerve, and delayed diagnosis. Recurrent subluxation or dislocation of the radial head is often associated with loss of fixation of the ulna fracture, inadequate postoperative immobilization, or both. With early recognition, repeat open reduction and internal fixation and radial head reduction should result in a successful resolution. Posterior interosseous nerve injuries usually resolve without further treatment.

The most serious underlying reason for the potential development of complications is a delayed diagnosis from inadequate radiographic evaluation, misdiagnosis of a Monteggia lesion as an isolated ulna fracture, or a lack of access to timely and appropriate medical attention. If the diagnosis is recognized prior to complete healing of the ulna fracture, open reduction and internal fixation should be performed. The radial head may be reduced by closed or open approaches. If the radial head remains unstable, reconstruction of the annular ligament may be required. A radial head resection may be a better option in select cases, most particularly in the elderly. If the ulna fracture has healed and the radial head is still dislocated, treatment is determined by the patient's symptoms, functional requirements, and the degree of residual ulna angulation.

DISTAL RADIUS FRACTURE

ANATOMY

The metaphysis of the distal radius is primarily cancellous bone with thin cortices. The bi-concave articular surface articulates with the proximal carpal row. The scaphoid and lunate fossae are two concave articular surfaces separated by a dorsal-volar ridge, which defines a clear articulation for the scaphoid and lunate, respectively. The radial inclination of the distal radius averages 23 degrees (range, 13 to 30 degrees), radial length averages 13 mm (range, 8 to 18 mm), and volar tilt averages 11 degrees (range, 1 to 21 degrees). The distal radius supports approximately 80 percent of the axial load; the ulna/triangular fibrocartilage complex (TFCC) supports the remaining 20 percent. A reversal of the normal palmar tilt causes load transfer onto the ulna/TFCC.

INCIDENCE AND MECHANISM OF INJURY

Distal radius fracture is a relatively common injury and accounts for an estimated 17 percent of all fractures presenting to emergency rooms. In one study, distal radius fractures comprised 75 percent of all forearm fractures.

The most frequent mechanism of injury is a fall onto the hyperextended hand. In this setting the palmar aspect of the radius fails in tension with the fracture propagating dorsally and causes compressive failure of the dorsal surface. The amount of energy associated with a distal radius fracture determines the amount of fracture displacement and comminution.

CLINICAL AND RADIOGRAPHIC EVALUATION

Patients present with pain, swelling, and often a classical "dinner fork" deformity at the wrist. Tenderness on palpation and crepitus at the fracture site also occur, as well as decreased range of finger motion. A sensory deficit may be demonstrated in the median nerve distribution.

Radiographic examination includes AP, lateral, and oblique views which will generally reveal a distal radius fracture with dorsal displacement and compression of the dorsal cortex. The latter is best seen on the lateral view. The AP view documents shortening and radial deviation of a varying degree. Additional fracture lines may continue into the radiocarpal or distal radioulnar joint.

CLASSIFICATION

Distal radius fractures have many eponyms. A *Colles' fracture* is a fracture of the distal radius with the distinguishing deformity of dorsal angulation, radial displacement, and shortening. A *Smith's fracture* is a distal radius fracture with palmar displacement. A *Barton's fracture* is a dorsal or volar lip fracture of the distal radius. A *Chauffeur's fracture* is an avulsion fracture of the radial styloid.

Distal radius fractures may be classified by the biomechanics of the injury pattern. In *bending*, the metaphysis fails in tension and the result is a Colles' or Smith's fracture. *Compression* causes a fracture of the articular surface with impaction of the subchondral and metaphyseal bone ("die-punch" fracture), *Shear* results in a fracture of the articular lip (Barton's fracture). *Avulsion fractures* occur at the site of ligamentous attachments. Combinations of the above forces result in high-energy injuries.

The most widely utilized classification was described by Frykman (1967) and is based on the type of the fracture pattern (intraarticular versus extraarticular) and the presence of a distal ulna fracture. As the numerical fracture type increases, so does the complexity and difficulty in management of the fracture: types I and II include extraarticular distal radius fracture; types III and IV involve the radiocarpal joint; types V and VI involve the distal radioulnar joint; and types VII and VIII include both radiocarpal and radioulnar joints. Types I, III, V, and VII have an intact ulnar styloid, while types II, IV, VI, and VIII have a fractured ulnar styloid.

Melone classified intraarticular distal radius fractures based on a consistent mechanism, lunate impaction injury (Fig. 79–3). Within this classification, he introduced the concept of a die-punch fragment, the impacted medial fragment of the distal radius articular surface.

TREATMENT

The approach for the treatment of distal radius fracture is determined by displacement and stability. The degree of initial displacement impacts on fracture stability. An unstable fracture is classified by some authors as having one or more of the following: greater than 20° dorsal angulation, more than 10 mm radial shortening, and marked dorsal comminution. Stable fractures should be treated by closed reduction and immobilization; however, the forearm position, duration of immobilization, and need for a long arm cast remain controversial. A position of extreme wrist flexion should be avoided as it increases carpal canal pressure (and thus medial nerve compression) and limits normal function of the flexor tendons. The criteria for an acceptable reduction either after initial reduction or subsequent radiographics remains unclear; studies have documented poorer outcome when residual articular displacment was greater than 2 mm, radial shortening was greater than 5 mm, or dorsal angulation was greater than 20 degrees.

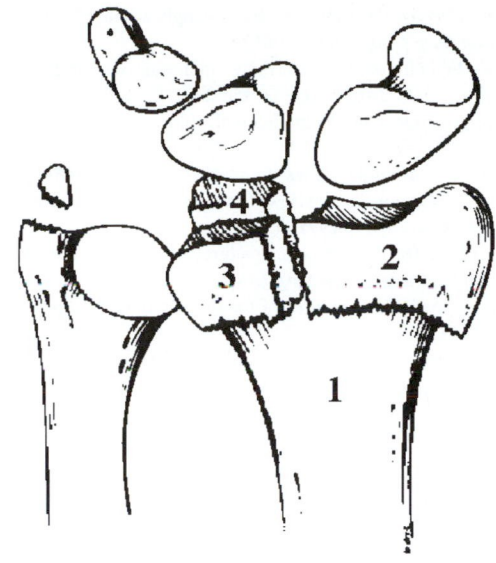

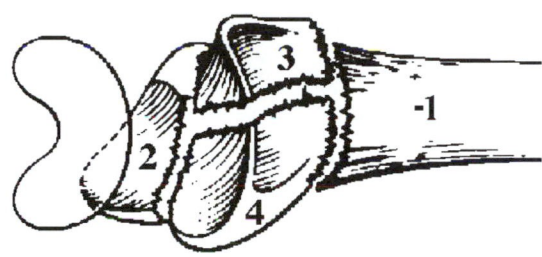

Figure 79-3
Intraarticular distal radius fractures. (Reproduced by permission from Melone CP Jr: Open treatment for displaced articular fractures of the distal radius. *Clin Orthop* 1986; 202:103.)

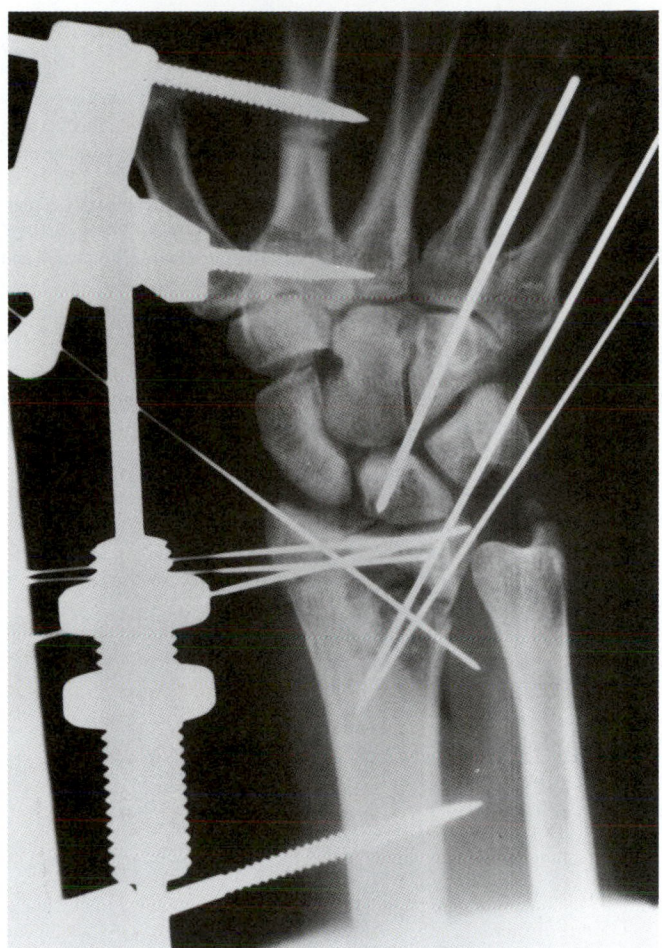

Figure 79-4
Distal radius fracture treated with external and internal fixation.

While unstable fractures may also be treated with closed reduction, they must be monitored closely in anticipation of loss of reduction. Some authors recommend primary internal or external fixation for unstable fractures. Surgical options include: percutaneous pinning, pins and plaster, external fixation, and open reduction. The majority of external fixators include a half frame positioned on the radial side of the wrist. The proximal pins should be inserted using an open technique to avoid injury to the superficial radial nerve. External fixation is maintained for 6 to 8 weeks. Open reduction is recommended for articular lip fractures, displaced radial styloid fractures, and when residual joint incongruity is greater than 2 mm (Fig. 79–4).

Rehabilitation following distal radius fracture is mandatory regardless of treatment option. The metacarpal-phalangeal joint must not be immobilized by the cast, and the patient should be encouraged to do full active range of motion with the digits, shoulder, and elbow from the day of injury.

COMPLICATIONS

Early complications of distal radius fractures include median nerve dysfunction, compartment syndrome, incomplete reduction, and iatrogenic neurovascular injury secondary to pin placement. Later complications include malunion, carpal tunnel syndrome, distal radioulnar derangement, reflex sympathetic dystrophy, and extensor tendon rupture, most commonly the extensor pollicis longus.

A frequent complication is entrapment of the median nerve at the wrist (carpal tunnel syndrome), which may occur at any time after wrist fracture. Management of median nerve entrapment after distal radius fracture remains controversial. Surgical exploration and decompression are recommended for patients with complete lesions that do not improve following reduction. If nerve entrapment develops after fracture reduction, the splint/cast should be released and the wrist placed in a neutral position. If there is no improvement, exploration and release of the nerve are indicated. With incomplete lesions in fractures requiring operative intervention from the outset, most authors advocate release.

Rapid post-fracture swelling under an unyielding circular cast can compromise circulation. This perilous clinical setting is marked by increasing pain, cyanosis, diffuse numbness, and motor deficit. It is critical to evaluate any symptom of a tight cast with urgency; treatment is cast splitting or removal to prevent limb-threatening ischemia.

Disruption of the distal radioulnar joint is common following a displaced distal radius fracture. Despite anatomic reduction, injury to the complex ligaments of the distal radioulnar joint may result in distal radioulnar dysfunction.

SUGGESTED READINGS

FOREARM

Bado JL: The Monteggia lesion. *Clin Orthop* 1967; 50:71.

Boyd HB, Boals JC: The Monteggia lesion: A review of 159 cases. *Clin Orthop* 1969; 66:94.

Chapman MW, Gordon JE, Zissimos AG: Compression plate fixation of acute fractures of the diaphyses of the radius and ulna. *J Bone Joint Surg [Am]* 1989; 71:159.

DeLuca PA, Lindsey RW, Ruwe PA: Refracture of bones of the forearm after removal of compression plates. *J Bone Joint Surg [Am]* 1988; 70:1372.

Hughston JC: Fractures of the distal radial shaft: mistakes in management. *J Bone Joint Surg [Am]* 1957; 39:249-264,402.

Moore TM, Klein JP, Patzakis MJ, Harvey JP Jr: Results of compression plating of closed Galeazzi fractures. *J Bone Joint Surg [Am]* 1985; 67:1015.

Reckling, F.W.: Unstable fracture-dislocations of the forearm (Monteggia and Galeazzi lesions). *J Bone Joint Surg [Am]* 1982; 64:857.

DISTAL RADIUS

Bradway J, Amadio PC, Cooney WP: Open reduction and internal fixation of displaced comminuted intraarticular fractures of the distal end of the radius. *J Bone Joint Surg [Am]* 1989; 71:839.

Cooney WP, Dobyns JH, Linscheid RL: Complications of Colles' fractures. *J Bone Joint Surg [Am]* 1980; 62:613.

Frykman G: Fracture of the distal radius including sequelae: Shoulder-hand-finger syndrome, disturbance in the DRUJ, and impairment of nerve function. A clinical and experimental study. *Acta Orthop Scand* 1967; 108(supp 1).

Jenkins NH: The unstable Colles' fracture. *J Hand Surg [Br]* 1989; 14:149.

Jupiter JB: Current concepts review: Fractures of the distal end of the radius. *J Bone Joint Surg [Am]* 1991; 73:461.

Knirk JL, Jupiter JB: Intraarticular fractures of the distal end of the radius in young adults. *J Bone Joint Surg [Am]* 1986; 68:647.

Melone CP Jr: Articular fractures of the distal radius. *Orthop Clin North Am* 1984; 15:217.

Riis J, Fruensgaard S: Treatment of unstable Colles' fractures by external fixation. *J Hand Surg [Br]* 1989; 14:145.

Chapter 80

WRIST

Salvatore R. Lenzo

FRACTURES OF THE SCAPHOID

ANATOMY AND MECHANISM OF INJURY

The mechanism of injury, described by Weber and Chao (1978) and based on the cadaver studies, is hyperextension of the wrist greater than 100 degrees associated with a force applied to the radial aspect of the palm. The blood supply of the scaphoid, described separately by Taleisnik (1966) and Gelberman (1980), is through its ligamentous attachments. It is comprised of a dorsal blood supply, which is the main source to the bone, and supplies approximately 80 percent of the scaphoid and the entire proximal pole. In addition, there is a volar branch off the radial artery which supplies the distal tuberosity. Therefore, there is a poor blood supply to the proximal pole.

CLINICAL EVALUATION

Usually there is tenderness within the radial snuff box. Radiographic evaluation should include an ulnar deviation PA view of the wrist. This projects the scaphoid in a longitudinal view and will depict the fracture. In addition, an oblique and a lateral radiographic view are necessary. The lateral view is important to assess possible associated ligamentous instability patterns associated with a scaphoid fracture, (i.e., a trans-scaphoid perilunate dislocation). On occasion, despite having positive tenderness within the radial snuff box with an acute injury, an initial radiograph will be negative. It is prudent to immobilize this patient, and have them return in approximately two weeks for subsequent radiographs. In addition to the standard radiograph views, the use of a tomogram and/or CT scan can give further analysis to the fracture site, (i.e., if there is significant bony loss or angulation at the fracture site). Finally, as Stordahl (1984) has noted, bone scans are helpful in making a definitive diagnosis, if, despite subsequent negative radiographs, there is a question of a fracture.

CLASSIFICATION

Two classifications, one developed by Russe in 1960 (Table 80-1) and the other by Herbert in 1984 (Table 80-2), have received considerable attention with regard to scaphoid fractures.

TREATMENT

Acute Fractures

Nondisplaced acute fractures of the scaphoid can be treated with cast immobilization. The level of the fracture will dictate the type of cast. If the fracture is in the distal third, the patient can be treated with a short arm-thumb spica cast. If the fracture is in the middle third, or more proximal to this, the initial six weeks of immobilization should be in a cast that blocks pronation and supination at the elbow in addition to the thumb spica component. Subsequent to this initial six week period, the patient can be placed in a short arm-thumb spica cast until there is evidence of radiographic consolidation and healing

of the fracture. The recommended position for immobilization is gentle radial deviation and flexion of the wrist.

Operative treatment is indicated in acute fractures in which there is greater than 1 mm of displacement between fracture fragments, or there is significant angulation of the fracture fragments with an associated abnormal carpal alignment.

In acute fractures, operative treatment is done via a volar approach in order to reduce and stabilize the scaphoid fracture. Fixation of the scaphoid involves either Herbert screws or Kirschner wires, depending on the surgeon's expertise and/or preference. In either case, anatomic fracture reduction is critical. Contraindications to the Herbert screws are avascular necrosis within the proximal pole, or a very small proximal pole fragment which will not accommodate the leading threads of the screw. In acute injuries involving ligamentous damage about the wrist, an additional dorsal approach is needed to realign any instability pattern (i.e., typically a DISI pattern at the mid carpal joint). Bone grafting can also be done at the time of fixation of the scaphoid fracture, but usually is not indicated unless there is significant comminution.

Delayed or Nonunions of Scaphoid

All displaced delayed unions and all nonunions should be reduced and bone grafted regardless of symptoms. For the stable nondisplaced delayed union, a trial at immobilization should be given. Mack and colleagues (1984) found, that if nonunion of the scaphoid was not

Table 80-1

Location of Fracture and Approximate Time for Union

	Location	Union
	Distal Third 10 %	6-8 weeks
	Middle Third 70 %	6-8 weeks
	Proximal Third 20 %	10-12 weeks

SOURCE: Reproduced and modified with permission from Russe O: Fracture of the carpal navicular. Diagnosis, non-operative treatment and operative treatment. *J Bone Joint Dis [Am]* 1960; 42:760.

Table 80-2

Classification of Scaphoid Fractures

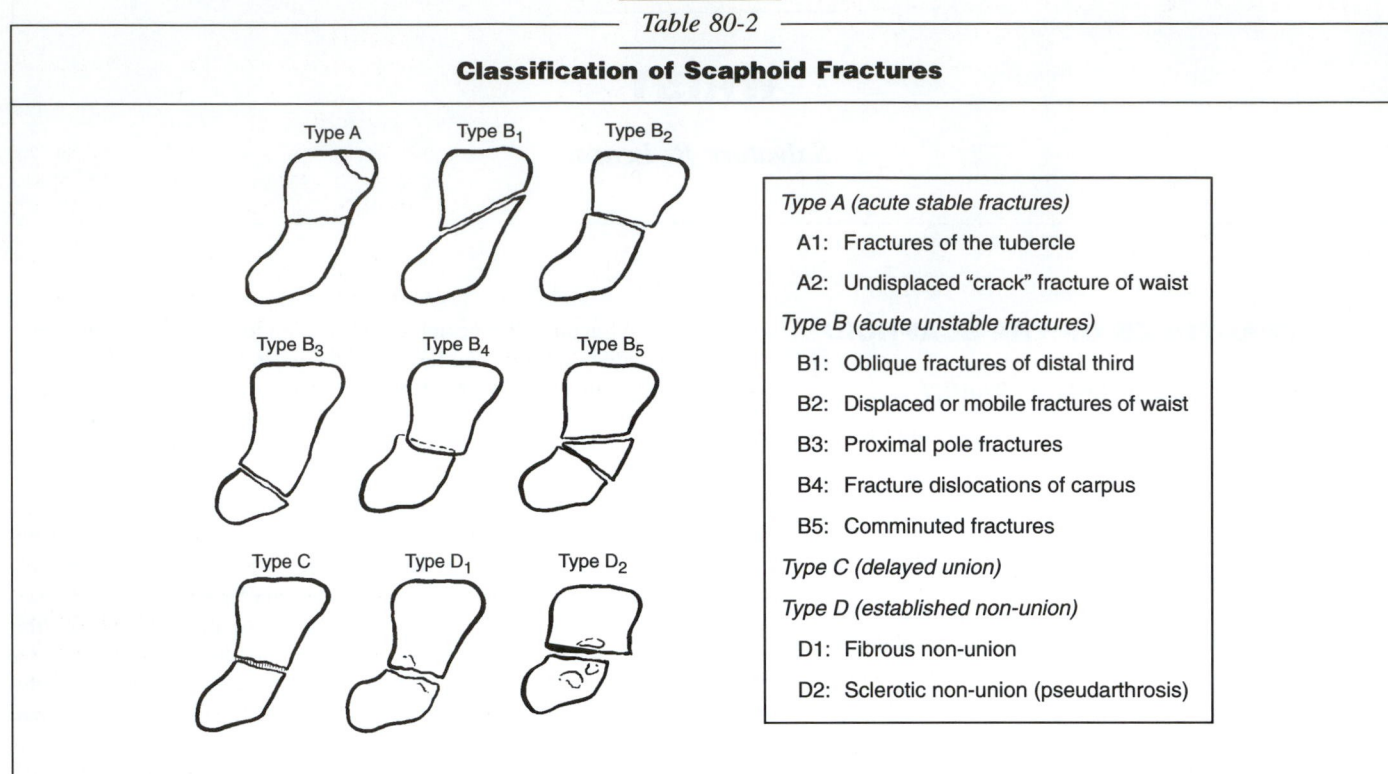

Type A   Type B₁   Type B₂

Type B₃   Type B₄   Type B₅

Type C   Type D₁   Type D₂

Type A (acute stable fractures)

   A1: Fractures of the tubercle

   A2: Undisplaced "crack" fracture of waist

Type B (acute unstable fractures)

   B1: Oblique fractures of distal third

   B2: Displaced or mobile fractures of waist

   B3: Proximal pole fractures

   B4: Fracture dislocations of carpus

   B5: Comminuted fractures

Type C (delayed union)

Type D (established non-union)

   D1: Fibrous non-union

   D2: Sclerotic non-union (pseudarthrosis)

SOURCE: Reproduced and modified with permission from Herbert JJ, Fisher WE: Management of the fractured scaphoid using a new bone screw. *J Bone Joint Dis [Br]* 1984; 66:119.

---

addressed, the wrist would go on to develop degenerative changes in a predictable pattern [e.g., as with scapholunate advanced collapse (SLAC) wrist deformity]. Initial degenerative changes begin at the radioscaphoid joint and are subsequently followed by changes at the mid-carpal joint, and finally at the radiolunate joint. The gold standard for treatment of scaphoid nonunion was described by Russe. He used a volar approach in an effort not to disturb the vascular supply of the scaphoid and created a trough in both the proximal and distal poles for acceptance of a cortical cancellous strut graft. This graft can either be fixed via a Kirschner wire or, in appropriate situations, with a Herbert's screw. With proximal third fractures, special situations arise when there is a very small proximal pole with advanced avascular changes. In these cases, preference for excision of this small scaphoid pole with insertion of soft tissue in the subsequent deficit is preferred. This allows early mobilization and avoids the high possibility of nonunion, despite the bone grafting technique.

Salvage Procedures

Proximal row carpectomy is indicated in older patients who do not wish to undergo the long-term immobilization necessary for healing of the scaphoid nonunion or in those patients who have already developed radioscaphoid arthritis. In these patients, care must be taken to assess whether there is advanced degenerative arthritis at the level of the capitate head or at the level of the lunate fossa. An advantage of the proximal row carpectomy is that early mobilization can be initiated after a short period of splinting and/or casting (approximately three to four weeks).

Limited wrist arthrodesis is indicated for patients who do heavy labor. If there are advanced degenerative changes at the radial scaphoid joint, an associated four-corner fusion (i.e., at the level of the capitate, lunate, hamate, and triquetrum) is done. This is a so-called SLAC wrist procedure. It was initially described with place-

ment of a silicone implant for the scaphoid, but is now employed just with the surgical excision of the scaphoid.

Another option in cases where there has been a failed attempt at surgical union of the scaphoid is fusion of the proximal and distal poles to the capitate. This would prevent further collapse of the wrist into an unsatisfactory alignment.

Total wrist arthrodesis is indicated in the patient with advanced SLAC wrist deformity, secondary to the scaphoid nonunion (i.e., in the patient that has already developed degenerative changes at the radioscaphoid, mid carpal, and radiolunate joint levels).

KIENBÖCK'S DISEASE

MECHANISM OF INJURY

A. A single severe compressive force.

B. Repetitive loading strains such as seen in those patients with ulnar negative variance.

C. Those patients with vascular risk.

STAGING OF KIENBÖCK'S DISEASE

Lichtman (1982) has developed four clinical and radiographic stages:

Stage I is a linear or compressive fracture, but *with* normal architecture and density within the lunate. Often, however, there is a stage that precedes a compressive fracture in which there will be a normal radiograph, but an abnormal MRI and/or bone scan.

Stage II is abnormal density within the lunate, but *without* lunate or carpal collapse.

Stage IIIA is fragmentation within the lunate with associated collapse, but *without* rotation of the scaphoid with its associated carpal collapse.

Stage IIIB is both fragmentation and collapse of the lunate, as well as rotation of the scaphoid with associated carpal collapse.

Stage IV is panosteoarthritic changes within the joint.

DIAGNOSIS

Physical examination often reveals the patient to have pain over the dorsal aspect of the wrist in the area of the lunate associated with stiffness. Diagnosis is made initially with radiographs and/or the use of bone scans and MRIs (these are especially useful in the earliest stages of the disease).

TREATMENT

Kienböck's disease is a *surgical* disease. Studies have shown that there is a continuing progression of lunate collapse and wrist degeneration if this problem is not addressed in a surgical fashion.

Surgical treatment is predicated on:

1. Stage of Kienböck's disease
2. Presence or absence of ulnar neutral variance.

In Stages I through III, joint leveling procedures are in vogue. If there is an ulnar minus variance, either a radial shortening or an ulnar lengthening can be done. Radial shortening has a lesser incidence of postoperative complications. Studies have shown that only a shortening of 2 mm of the radius is indicated in order to unload the lunate. Care must be taken, however, to make sure there is no distal radioulnar joint derangement in either procedure. With the radial shortening, if there is loss of rotation after shortening of the radius, then the distal radial fragment should be translated radially in order to ensure there is full pronation and supination at the distal radioulnar joint.

Other options include the use of intercarpal arthrodesis. Two of the more popular procedures to unload the lunate are either the scaphotrapezium trapezoid arthrodesis, or the scaphocapitate arthrodesis. In addition, if there is significant fragmentation of the lunate and associated synovitis, such as seen in Stage III, then another option would be to excise the lunate in addition to doing the above outlined arthrodesis. Proximal row carpectomy can also be a treatment for Stage III disease. Indications would be similar to those described above for treatment of scaphoid nonunion. Finally, for Stage IV Kienböck's disease, the most common procedure is a total wrist arthrodesis. This is because of the panarthritic picture within the wrist.

ISOLATED FRACTURES OF CARPAL BONES, EXCLUDING THE SCAPHOID

A. Fracture of the *triquetrum* is typically seen with a hyperextension injury and ulnar deviation force to the wrist. The most common triquetrum fracture is the dorsal lip fracture. It is best seen on a lateral view. Usual treatment is a splint for approximately four weeks, and then early mobilization. Other types of fractures of the triquetrum are those within the body itself and the avulsion fracture seen with perilunate dislocations (to be described later.)

B. Fracture of the *pisiform* is usually secondary to direct trauma to the hypothenar area. Initial treatment is splinting for comfort. If secondary pisotriquetral arthritis develops, then excision of the bone is indicated. Diagnosis is made with special radiographic views (i.e., carpal tunnel views and/or the supination oblique view).

C. Fracture of the *trapezium* can involve:
1. The body of the trapezium
2. Intraarticular fractures at the level of the carpometacarpal Joint
3. Fractures of the trapezial ridge

Fractures of the body, as long as they are not intraarticular, are treated with either splinting or casting. Fractures of the trapezium, which are intraarticular at the level of the carpometacarpal joint and are displaced, require surgical intervention. Fractures of the trapezial ridge are best diagnosed by the carpal tunnel view. They can either occur within the base of the trapezial ridge or at the tip. Treatment is immobilization for approximately four weeks. If they remain symptomatic and/or cause median nerve compression, then surgical intervention is warranted, with excision of the fracture fragment.

D. Fractures of the *capitate* can be isolated fractures but are more commonly involved with other carpal bone fractures (i.e., the scaphocapitate syndrome). In isolated fractures, it is possible to develop avascular necrosis at the proximal pole in light of the precarious blood supply to this area of the capitate. If the patient becomes symptomatic, then consideration for bone grafting is indicated and/or the possibility of midcarpal arthrodesis at later stages. In the scaphocapitate syndrome, there is a displaced fracture of the neck of the capitate associated with a fracture of the scaphoid. In these cases, open reduction and internal fixation of both fractures is indicated.

E. Fractures of the *hamate*. There are two main hamate fractures: Those involving the body and/or dorsal lip, and those involving the hook of the hamate. Isolated body fractures are typically stable, and can be treated with splinting and/or immobilization. Those involving the dorsal lip of the hamate body are often associated with a dislocation at the level of the carpometacarpal joint at the base of the fourth and fifth metacarpals. If this involves a significant amount of the lip, then open reduction for the dislocation, and proper stabilization of the dorsal lip, in order to give stability to the joint, is indicated. The second most common area of fracture is that involving the hook of the hamate. This fracture is seen in baseball players, tennis players and golfers. Typically, there is pain over the hypothenar eminence on deep palpation over the hook of the hamate and/or over the dorsoulnar aspect of the wrist.

Complications include ulnar nerve compression at the level of Guyon's canal, and ruptures involving the flexor tendons of the small and ring finger. Diagnosis can be made from a carpal tunnel view, but it is better evaluated on either a CAT scan and/or a spinal tomogram. The recommended treatment for this is excision of the hook of the hamate. Care is indicated to prevent damage to the motor branch of the ulnar nerve, which comes around the hook of the hamate, and dives deep to innervate the intrinsic muscles of the hand.

LIGAMENT INJURIES ABOUT THE WRIST WITH ASSOCIATED CARPAL INSTABILITY PATTERNS

ANATOMY OF THE WRIST

Columnar Carpus Concept (Taleisnik's Concept)

Taleisnik's (1976) concept is that of a central flexion extension column, formed by the lunate, hamate, capitate, trapezium and trape-

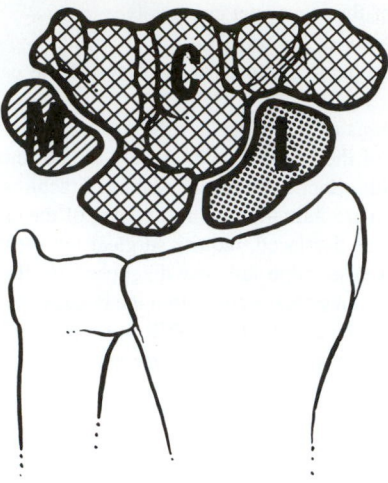

Figure 80-1
Columnar carpus. L, lateral or mobile column (scaphoid); C, central or flexion-extension column (lunate and distal carpal row); M, medial or rotation column (triquetrum). (Reproduced with permission from Taleisnik J: Carpal kinematics. In *The Wrist.* New York: Churchill Livingstone; 1985:41.)

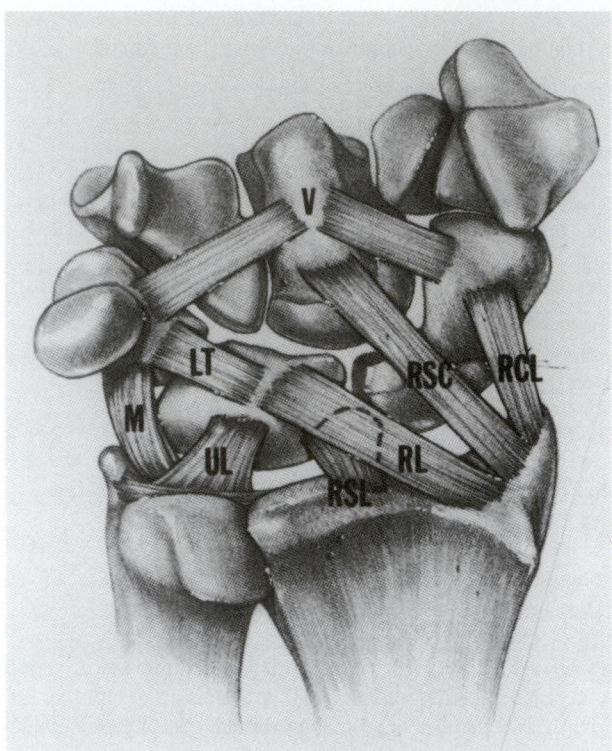

Figure 80-2
Extrinsic ligaments. RCL, radial collateralligament; RSC, radioscaphocapitate ligament; RL, radiolunate ligament; RSL, radio-scapholunate ligament; UL, unlnolunate ligatment; M, ulnocarpal meniscus homologue; LT, lunotriquetral ligament; V, V or deltoid ligament. (Reproduced with permission from Taleisnik J: The ligaments of the wrist. In *The Wrist.* New York: Churchill Livingstone; 1985:14.)

zoid, a lateral column formed by the scaphoid, and a medial column formed by the triquetrum (Fig. 80-1).

Lichtman (1982) felt that the wrist should be conceptualized as an oval ring. The proximal and distal rows were linked at the scaphoid trapezoid joint and rotatory triquetral hamate joint. Any break in the so-called link system would cause a carpal instability.

LIGAMENTOUS ANATOMY ABOUT THE WRIST

The major stabilizers of the carpal bones consist of the volar ligamentous structures (Fig. 80-2). The major stabilizers at the level of the scapholunate joint consists of the radioscapholunate ligament and the scapholunate interosseous ligament. The midcarpal joint is stabilized by the arcuate ligament, with its ulnar arm from the capitate to the triquetrum, and its radial arm from the capitate to the scaphoid. At the level of the midcarpal joint, there is an area of ligamentous weakness called the space of Poirier in which midcarpal dislocations occur. The ulnar aspect of the wrist is stabilized by the ulnar lunate and ulnar triquetral ligamentous structures, as well as by the lunotriquetral interosseous structures. On the dorsal aspect of the wrist, there are weaker ligamentous structures. The two main structures are the dorsal radiocarpal ligament coursing from the radius over the lunate to the triquetrum, and the dorsal intercarpal ligament connecting the distal row of the carpal bones (Fig. 80-3).

KINEMATICS OF WRIST MOTION

In order to understand the various carpal instabilities, it is necessary to comprehend the normal relationship of the carpal bones with various wrist motions.

Radial Deviation of the Wrist

With radial deviation of the wrist, the scaphoid volar flexes; on the PA view, it appears foreshortened. Through the scapholunate interosseous ligaments, the lunate volar flexes with the scaphoid. With the radial deviation, the triquetrum rides up the slope of the hamate to its high position, pulling the lunate into volar flexion as well.

Ulnar Deviation

In ulnar deviation, the scaphoid takes a dorsiflexed position; with this movement the lunate also dorsiflexes through the scapholunate interosseous ligamentous structures. The triquetrum migrates distally, and takes a low position on the hamate. This also dorsiflexes, and through the lunotriquetral ligaments, causes the dorsiflexion of the lunate as well.

DIAGNOSIS

Most ligamentous injuries about the wrist are due to a hyperextension type of injury. This happens most frequently from a fall, but can also occur from more serious injuries, such as motor vehicle accidents or a fall from a height. Clinical examination is essential in evaluating a patient for dislocations about the wrist. Neurovascular assessment is especially important in acute injuries. In order to assess ligament injuries, it is important to have an understanding of the basic normal carpal anatomy. Several views are useful in assessing a patient with ligamentous instability. These include: a PA view in ulnar deviation, a PA view in radial deviation, a lateral view, and an oblique view of the wrist. There are several normal angles present which are altered in various instability patterns. The radioscaphoid and scapholunate angles are on the average 47 degrees (Fig. 80-4*A* and *B*). The radiolunate angle is normally zero degrees (Fig. 80-4*C*). Finally, the capitolunate angle is also normally zero degrees. Deviations from the normal values are indicative of ligamentous instabilities patterns. Other radiographic assessments include carpal height as described by Youm (1978). Youm's ratio is calculated by

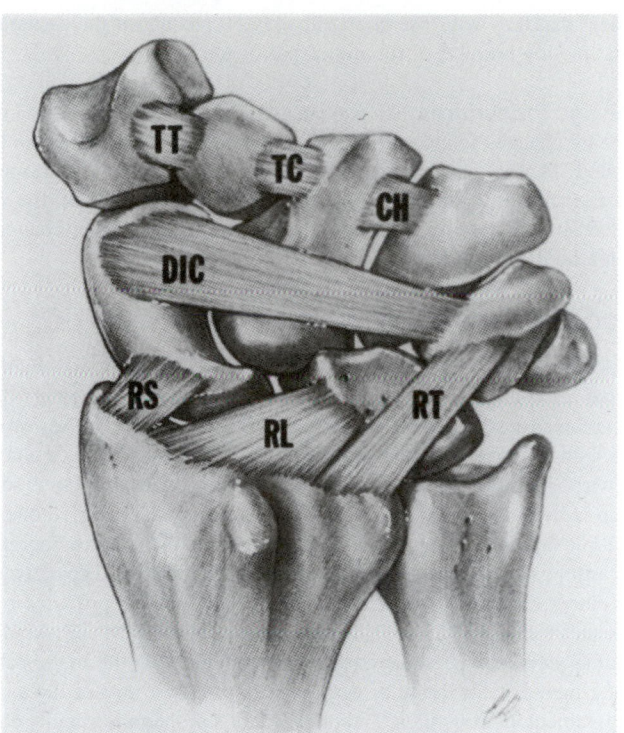

Figure 80-3
Dorsal ligaments. TT, trapeziotrapezoid; TC, trapeziocapitate; CH, capitohamate; DIC, dorsalinter arpal; RS, RL, RT, radioscaphoid, radiolunate, and radiotriquetral fascicles of the dorsal radiocarpal ligament. (Reproduced with permission from Taleisnik J: The ligaments of the wrist. In *The Wrist.* New York: Churchill Livingstone; 1985:23.)

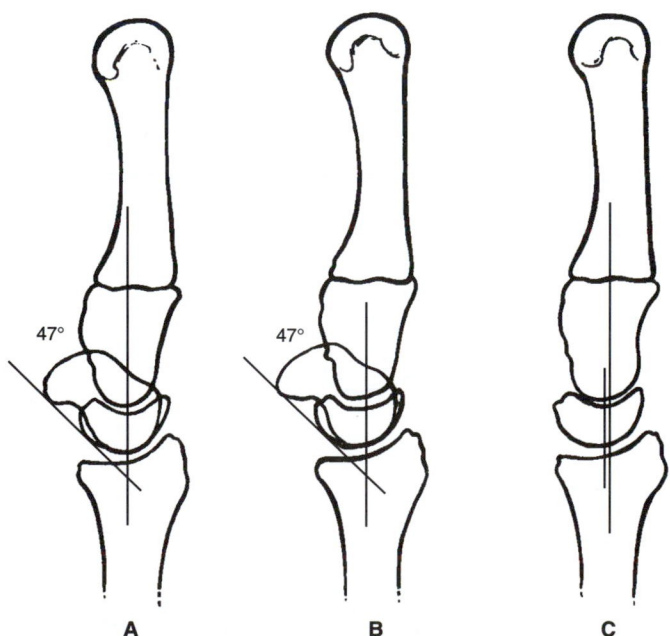

Figure 80-4
Normal values of the (*A*) radioscaphoid angle, (*B*) the scapholunate angle, and (*C*) the radiolunate angle. [Reproduced and modified with permission from the American Society for Surgery of the Hand (ASSH): Part III—Distal radial fractures. In: *ASSH 1996 Regional Course Syllabus.* Englewood, CO: ASSH; 1996:12 (source illustration by Gary Schnitz, A.M.I.).]

dividing the carpal height L2, which extends from the base of the third metacarpal to the distal articular surface of the radius, by the length of the third metacarpal. A normal height ratio is 0:54.

Additional Radiographic Tests

Cineradiographs are especially helpful in patients who have clunking with radial and/or ulnar deviation of the wrist. The cine test is especially helpful in assessing midcarpal instabilities. Usually, as the examiner asks the patient to ulnarly deviate the wrist, at the termination of this deviation, there will be a sudden dorsiflexion of the lunate and associated clunking at the midcarpal joint. This is helpful in diagnosing damage to the ulnar arm of the arcuate ligamentous structure.

Arthrograms are most helpful in chronic ligamentous injuries. It is especially important to evaluate the flow of dye either from the midcarpal or from the radiocarpal joints. Tri-phase arthrograms are the examination of choice. However, separate studies by Belsole (1990) and Herbert (1990) show that there can often be poor correlation between the patient's symptoms and arthrographic findings.

With the advent of more sophisticated techniques in wrist *arthroscopy*, examination of the radial carpal and midcarpal joint and ligamentous tears, in both the acute and chronic situations, can be better evaluated.

CARPAL INSTABILITY PATTERNS

SCAPHOLUNATE DISASSOCIATION

This injury can represent an isolated injury such as that seen in Stage I injuries as described by Mayfield, be associated with distal radius fractures, or represent the initial stage of a more serious ligamentous injury, such as a perilunate and/or lunate dislocation. *Physical examination* in the more chronic and isolated cases reveals tenderness in the dorsal aspect of the wrist over the scapholunate joint area. Watson (1988) described a test that takes advantage of the changes in the orientation of the scaphoid when the wrist is deviated from an ulnar to a radial position. He applies pressure on the distal pole of the scaphoid as the wrist is moved from ulnar to radial deviation. This prevents the scaphoid from taking a volar flexed attitude. If there is ligamentous damage of the scapholunate joint area, then the proximal pole of the scaphoid displaces dorsally.

Radiographic Diagnostic Features of Scapholunate Disassociation

Increase in scapholunate gap. This is best elicited radiographically with supination clench fist view and the AP view. Greater than 3 mm of diastasis is indicative of a scapholunate ligament tear. If there is less dissociation with clinical suspicion, then comparison views of the uninjured hand are indicated. There will be a cortical ring shadow because of the abnormal orientation of the foreshortened scaphoid. On the lateral view, there is increased palmar flexion of the scaphoid with an increase in the scapholunate angle typically greater than 80 degrees. In addition, there is often a dorsiflexed orientation of the lunate (Fig. 80-5). As discussed in the section on kinematics, normally with the scaphoid palmarly flexed, the lunate should follow and also be positioned in a volar flexed orientation. However, with the loss of "influence" of the scaphoid on the lunate orientation, the triquetrum tends to dorsiflex the lunate, thus giving the DISI orientation to the lunate. This rotatory subluxation of the scaphoid can also be seen in stage III Kienböck's disease as described above, and/or in nonunions of the scaphoid.

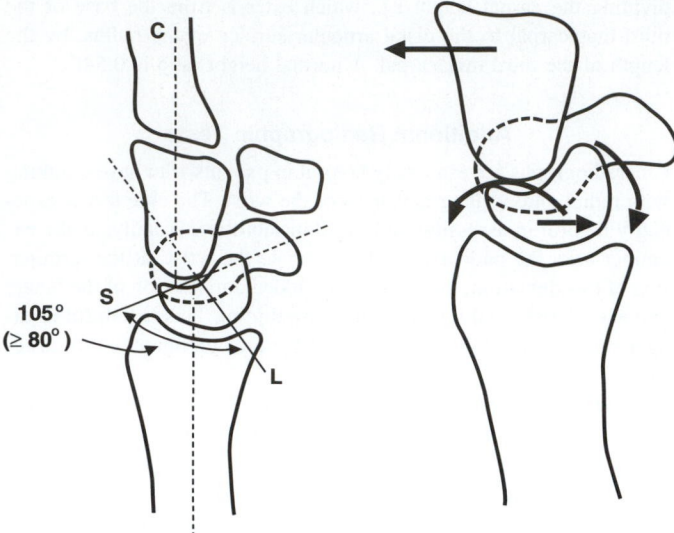

Figure 80-5
Change in carpal angle secondary to scapholunate dissociation.

Treatment of Scaphoid Lunate Disassociations

Acute cases are usually those in which the injury is less than 4 weeks old. In these cases, definitive interosseous ligamentous structures can be identified. Studies have shown that closed reduction with cast immobilization and/or closed reduction with percutaneous pin fixation does not afford adequate treatment for this injury. Consensus for the best technique is that outlined by Taleisnik. This technique employs a dorsal approach to identify the ligamentous damage to the scapholunate interosseous ligamentous structures. The scaphoid is reduced into its normal orientation and pinned to both the lunate and capitate. The interosseous ligamentous structures are identified and repaired through drill holes usually in the lunate. Post-operative immobilization is for approximately 8 weeks. If, however, there is no significant interosseous ligament to be found, then more reconstructive techniques must be employed.

Soft tissue reconstructions   The procedure described by Blatt (1987) is now in vogue, and represents a dorsal capsulodesis technique. The highlights of this procedure are the reorientation of the scaphoid into a more horizontal position (i.e., correcting the scapholunate angle and insertion of a dorsal flap harvested from the dorsal capsular structures distal to the mid axis rotation of the scaphoid). Although, as described by Blatt, this technique does not necessarily close down the scapholunate diastasis as seen on the PA view of the wrist; it does reorient the scaphoid into its proper position, such as to hopefully preclude development of the SLAC wrist arthritic changes. Usually with this technique, however, the patient does lose palmar flexion of the wrist. Postoperative immobilization is for approximately 2 months, but Blatt leaves the Kirschner wire in, transfixing the scaphoid to the capitate for approximately three months time.

Intercarpal Arthrodeses   The scapho-trapezium-trapezoid (STT) arthrodesis, described by Watson (1980), has also become a procedure for late reconstructive treatment. With this procedure it is important to reorient the scaphoid into its proper orientation.

Scaphocapitate Arthrodesis   Like the STT fusion, it reorients the scaphoid to proper orientation. In either of the above procedures, it is imperative to make certain that there are no degenerative changes at the radioscaphoid joint. In addition, it is important to inform the

patient that they will lose approximately 50 percent of their existing wrist motion because of the midcarpal fusion.

Salvage Procedures   In patients who have already developed the arthritic changes found with SLAC, wrist-salvage procedures are indicated. These can take the form of either a proximal row carpectomy, excision of the scaphoid and a midcarpal arthrodesis, the so-called SLAC wrist operation, or if there are more panarthritic changes, then a total wrist arthrodesis.

MIDCARPAL INSTABILITY

Midcarpal instability has also been classified as a nondissociative carpal instability by Dobyns et al. (1975) or a triquetral hamate dissociation as described by Lichtman and Martin (1988). The key problem with this type of instability, despite the nomenclature, is a clunking wrist with radial or ulnar deviation. Usually, this problem is seen in an individual with lax ligamentous structures who suffered one or multiple injuries to the wrist. It is best diagnosed on a cine radiograph. An arthrogram and routine radiographs will be normal. Typically, on the cine radiograph there will be a sudden shift of the proximal row as a unit into the VISI or DISI pattern (Fig. 80-6) with active radial or ulnar deviation. Cadaver studies have shown that the main stabilizing ligament for the midcarpal joint is the ulnar arm of the arcuate ligamentous structures. Treatment for this problem is initially conservative, using splinting and steroid injections; but if continuing problems persist, then a midcarpal arthrodesis is indicated. This would involve fusing the lunate, capitate, hamate, and triquetral bones.

CARPAL DISLOCATIONS DORSAL PERILUNATE DISLOCATION

Perilunate dislocations occur with either a purely ligamentous injury or with an associated scaphoid fracture, and/or radial styloid fracture, i.e., a greater arc injury (Fig. 80-7). In either case, there is a dislocation of the lunocapitate joint with the capitate usually dorsal to the lunate. This dislocation represents a spectrum of injuries. In stage II, the capitate is usually displaced dorsal to the lunate. In stage III, there is ligamentous injury at the triquetral-lunate joint. In stage IV, there is ligamentous injury with the spilled teacup sign of the lunate (Fig. 80-8).

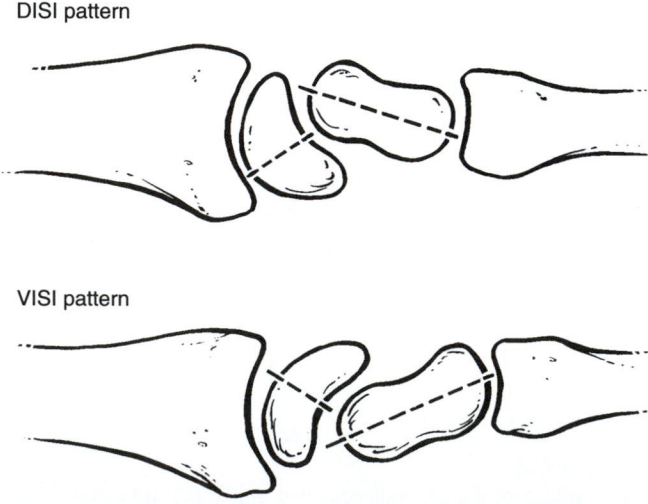

Figure 80-6
Volar intercalated segmental instability (VISI) and dorsal intercalated segmental instability (DISI). [Reproduced and modified with permission from the American Society for Surgery of the Hand (ASSH): Part III—Distal radial fractures. In: *ASSH 1996 Regional Course Syllabus.* Englewood, CO: ASSH; 1996:12–13.]

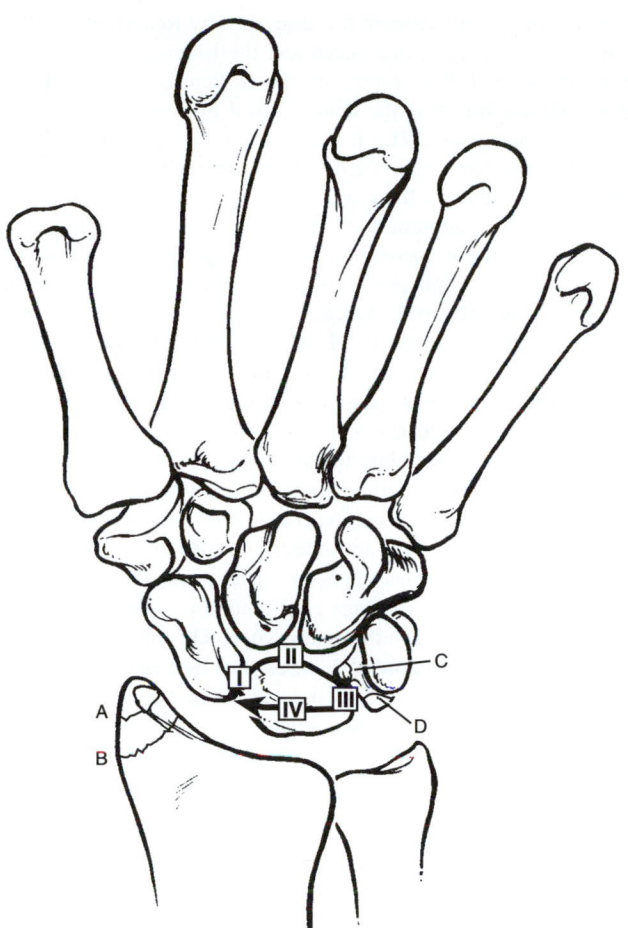

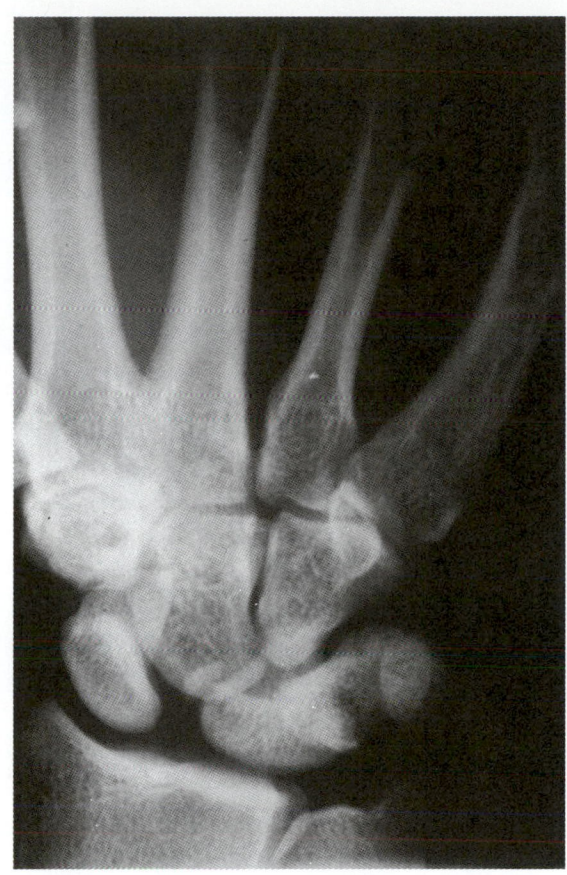

A

Figure 80-7
Greater or lesser arc injuries (Mayfield classification). Associated fractures: A, B, C, D. Stages: I, II, III, IV. [Reproduced and modified with permission from Mayfield JK: Mechanism of carpal injuries. *Clin Orthop* 1980; 149:50.]

Treatment for dorsal perilunate dissociation involves both volar and dorsal approaches. Initially, in the emergency room, dislocations at the midcarpal joint (i.e., between the capitate and lunate), can be reduced. However, even after closed reduction, open reduction in both the dorsal and volar approaches is warranted. The dorsal approach is utilized in order to reduce the scaphoid to its proper orientation with regard to the lunate (i.e., correct the scapholunate angle), and in addition, the midcarpal joint is assessed such that the capitolunate angle is 0 degrees. These bones are transfixed and pinned in the proper orientation. A volar approach is then undertaken in order to decompress the carpal tunnel, and also to assess the volar ligamentous structures. There will always be a transverse rent of the wrist capsule and ligamentous structures in these injuries. Although it is impossible to repair the individual ligaments, the capsule themselves and the transverse rent should be repaired. In those injuries in which there is a spilled teacup sign (stage IV, Mayfield classification) that has not been reduced, the lunate will be seen extruded through the transverse rent; causing compression on the structures within the carpal tunnel. Postoperative management in these cases requires approximately 8 weeks of immobilization in the cast, and then subsequent therapy after removal of the pins at the 2-month period. In those injuries, in which there is a transscaphoid perilunate dislocation, attention must also be turned to the scaphoid injury. The scaphoid injury may be approached either through a volar or dorsal approach. In greater arc injuries, if there is an associated radial styloid fracture, it should be

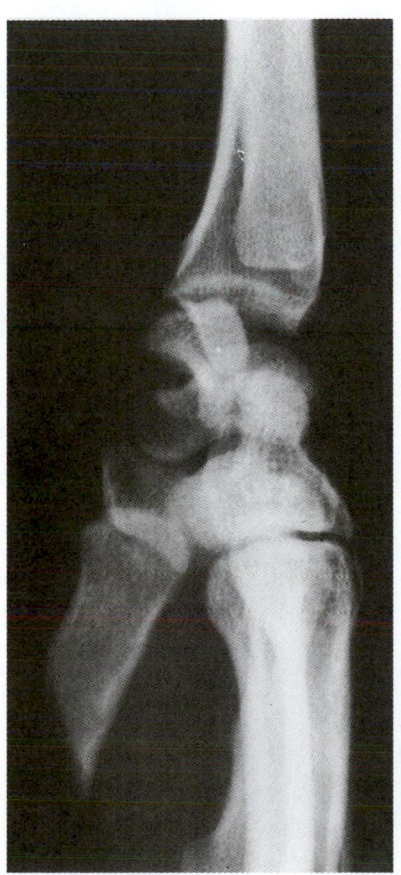

B

Figure 80-8
A. PA view of perilunate dislocation. *B.* Lateral view of perilunate dislocation.

reduced and stabilized. This represents the origin of the major volar ligamentous structures on the radial aspect of the wrist.

Treatment for these fracture dislocations is predicated on the healing of the scaphoid. Thus, immobilization should be continued until the scaphoid is healed. Again, a postoperative regimen of therapy will be needed after the pins are removed. In chronic cases of a dorsal perilunate dislocation and/or trans-scaphoid perilunate dislocation, it is often impossible to reduce the dislocation or the fracture (Fig. 80-9); a proximal row carpectomy is the best surgical alternative. Other considerations would be an arthrodesis of the wrist. However, if there are not significant degenerative changes at the head of the capitate and also within the radial fossa, then the proximal row carpectomy is a viable alternative in chronic cases that have been missed. Usually, it is necessary to pin the capitate to the radius in order to stabilize the wrist while the capsulorraphy procedure associated with this proximal carpectomy heals.

TRIQUETROLUNATE DISSOCIATIONS

Triquetrolunate dissociations result from a supination-type injury and fall on the hypothenar aspect of the wrist. These can be isolated injuries or associated with a broader peri-lunate dislocation. With regard to the isolated injury, typical symptoms are pain on the dorsal aspect of the left wrist. On physical examination, the tests for as-

sessment are the ballottement test described by Reagan et al (1984). In this test the lunate is stabilized and the triquetrum and pisiform are rocked up and down on the lunate. If there is pain, this is consistent with a problem at the lunotriquetral joint. Initial radiographs may or may not reveal a VISI pattern, as well as degenerative changes in the lunotriquetral joint. Further tests can include an arthrogram (Fig. 80-10), although, there are often asymptomatic tears seen on arthrogram. More importantly, ulnar impingement must also be assessed since it is not uncommon for lunotriquetral tears to be associated with ulnar impingement. Conservative treatment is the best management initially with injection of cortisone preparation in the area of the wrist. However, in advanced cases or significantly symptomatic cases, treatment can include a triquetrolunate arthrodesis (Fig. 80-11). However, there is a high rate of failure with this arthrodesis, approximately 40 percent. In contemplating this type of arthrodesis, evaluation of a possible ulnar impaction syndrome must also be assessed. In these cases, an ulnar shortening and/or the Wafer type of procedure, as described by Feldon et al (1990), can be used as an adjunct to the triquetrolunate arthrodesis in order to unload the ulnar aspect of the wrist. Arthroscopy is increasingly utilized to debride associated triangular fibrocartilage tears, and also to perform a Wafer type of procedure through the arthroscope. The ulnar head is shortened, thus taking impaction loads off on the ulnar aspect of the wrist. With the arthroscope, synovitis and degenerative tears can also be debrided on the ulnar aspect of the wrist.

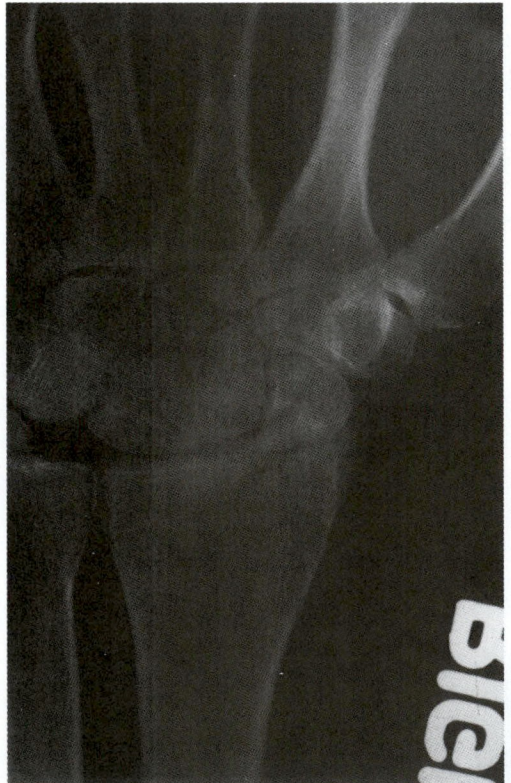

A

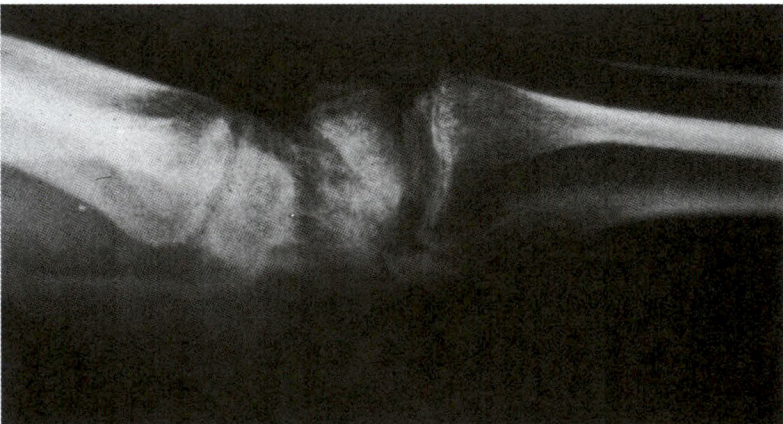

B

Figure 80-9
A. PA degenerative changes after chronic volar perilunate dislocation. *B.* Lateral degenerative changes after chronic volar perilunate dislocation.

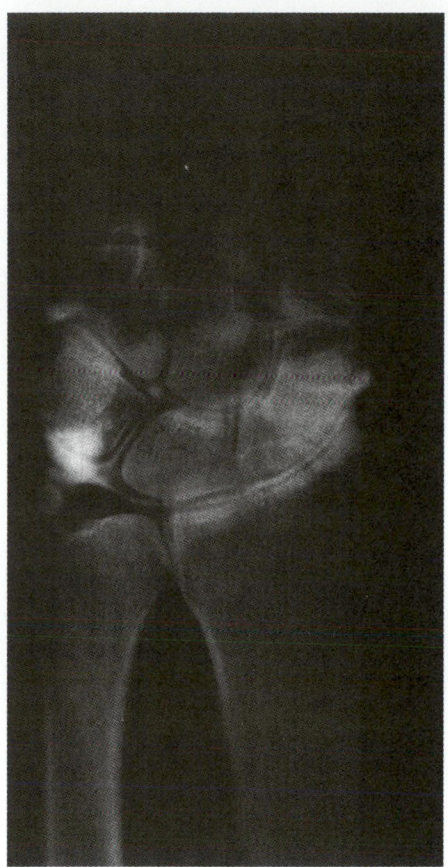

Figure 80-10
Arthrogram indicating triquetrolunate ligament tear.

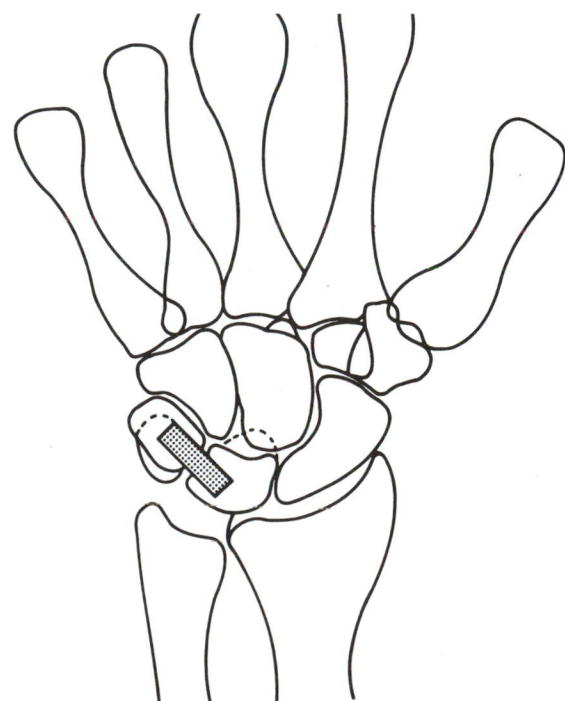

Figure 80-11
Technique for triquetrolunate. [Reproduced and modified with permission from Alexander CE, Lichtman DM: Triquetrolunate instability. In: *The Wrist and Its Disorders*, 2d ed. Philadelphia: Saunders; 1997:313.]

SUGGESTED READINGS

SCAPHOID FRACTURES

Cooney WP, Dobyns JH, Linscheid RL: Fractures of the scaphoid: A rational approach to management. *Clin Orthop* 1980; 149:90.

Gelberman RH, Menon J: Vascularity of the scaphoid bone. *J Hand Surg [Am]* 1980; 5:508.

Herbert TJ, Fisher WE.: Management of the fractured scaphoid using a new bone screw. *J Bone Joint Surg [Br]* 1984; 66:114.

Mack GR, Bosse MJ, Gelberman RH, et al: The natural history of scaphoid non-union. *J Bone Joint Surg [Am]* 1984; 66:504.

Russe O: Fracture of the carpal navicular. Diagnosis, nonoperative treatment and operative treatment. *J Bone Joint Surg [Am]* 1960; 42:759.

Stordahl A, Schjoth A, Woxholt G, et al: Bone scanning of the fractures at the scaphoid. *J Hand Surg [Br]* 1984; 9:189.

Talesnik J, Kelly PJ: The extraosseous and intraosseous blood supply of the scaphoid bone. *J Bone Surg [Am]* 1966; 48:1125.

Weber ET, Chao EY: Experimental approach to the mechanism of scaphoid waist fracture. *J Hand Surg [Am]* 1978; 3:142.

KIENBÖCK'S DISEASE

Gelberman RH, Bauman TD, Menon J, et al: The vascularity of the lunate bone and Kienböck's disease. *J Hand Surg [Am]* 1980; 5:272.

Lichtman DM, Alexander AH, Mack GR, et al: Kienböck's disease—update on silicone replacement arthroplasty. *J Hand Surg [Am]* 1982; 7:343.

Mikkelsen SS, Gelineck J: Poor function after nonoperative treatment of Kienböck's disease. *Acta Orthop Scand* 1987; 58:241.

LIGAMENT INJURIES AND CARPAL INSTABILITY PATTERNS

Alexander CE, Lichtman DM: Ulnar carpal instabilities. *Orthop Clin North Am* 1984; 15:307.

Taleisnik J: The ligaments of the wrists. *J Hand Surg [Am]* 1976; 1:110.

CARPAL INSTABILITY PATTERNS

Belsole RJ, Quinn SF, Greene TL, et al: Digital subtraction arthrography of the wrist. *J Bone Joint Surg [Am]* 1990; 72:846.

Blatt G: Capsulodesis and reconstructive hand surgery. Dorsal capsulodesis for the unstable scaphoid and volar capsulodesis following excision of the distal ulna. *Hand Clin* 1987; 3:81.

Dobyns HJ, Linscheid RL, Chao EYS, et al: Traumatic instability of the wrist. In *Instructional Course Lectures (American Academy of Orthopaedic Surgeons)*. St. Louis: CV Mosby; 1975; 24:182.

Hebert TJ, Faithfull RG, McCann DJ: Bilateral arthrography of the wrist. *J Hand Surg [Br]* 1990; 15:233.

Lavernia CJ, Cohen M, Taleisnik J: Treatment of scapholunate dissociation by ligamentous repair and capsulodesis. *J Hand Surg [Am]* 1992; 17:354.

Lichtman DM, Martin RA: Introduction to the carpal instabilities. In Lichtman DM (ed): *The Wrist and Its Disorders*. Philadelphia: WB Saunders; 1988:244.

Mayfield JK: Mechanism of carpal injuries. *Clin Orthop* 1980; 149:45.

Watson HK: Examination of the scaphoid. *J Hand Surg [Am]* 1988; 13:657.

Watson HK: Limited wrist arthrodesis. *Clin Orthop* 1980; 149:126.

Youm Y, McMurtry RY, Flatt AE: Kinematics of the wrist. I. An experimental study of radial-ulnar deviation and flexion-extension. *J Bone Joint Surg [Am]* 1978; 60:423.

TRIQUETROLUNATE DISSOCIATIONS

Reagan DS, Linscheid RL, Dobyns JH, et al: Lunotriquetral sprains. *J Hand Surg [Am]* 1984; 9:502.

Feldon P, Belsky MR, Terrono AL: Partial ("wafer") distal ulna resection for triangular fibrocartilage tears and/or ulnar impaction syndrome (abstract). *J Hand Surg [Am]* 1990; 15:826.

Chapter 81

HAND

Salvatore Robert Lenzo

EVALUATION

It is important to obtain an accurate history to determine the mechanism of injury in hand and ligament trauma; for example, aggressive surgical debridement would be indicated in a metacarpal head fracture which was associated with a human bite.

On physical evaluation, assessment of both rotational and angulatory deformity is critical. This will dictate whether a reduction of a fracture is required and if stabilization is needed. Range of motion of the fingers and assessment of flexor and extensor tendon function is also critical. Neurovascular status must be evaluated to test for possible nerve compressions and/or lacerations associated with soft tissue injury. Finally, swelling and local tenderness must be assessed, and the treating physician must always be cognizant of the possibility of a compartment syndrome within the hand after significant trauma and/or crush injury.

Radiographic evaluation of metacarpal fractures includes PA, lateral, and oblique views. In evaluating carpometacarpal joint Injuries, a 30-degree supination view is also helpful to assess the fourth and fifth carpometacarpal joints.

CLASSIFICATION OF METACARPAL FRACTURES

Metacarpal head fractures are usually secondary to direct trauma to the metacarpal head such as in clinch fist injury. While routine x-rays are used in evaluating these injuries, Elaine (1977) has reported using the Brewerton view (MP joint flexed 65 degrees with dorsum of fingers lying flat on the x-ray plate and tube angled 15 degrees ulnar to radial) to facilitate fracture detection.

There are several different types of metacarpal head fractures:

1. *Oblique intraarticular fractures* with significant step off are treated with open reduction and screw internal fixation to allow for prompt immobilization, in order to avoid intraarticular adhesions and/or tendon adhesions about the fracture site.
2. *Markedly comminuted fractures* distal to ligament origin are treated with immobilization for a limited period, that is, 2 to 3 weeks, followed by subsequent mobilization. These fractures can also be treated with skeletal traction, especially if there is significant soft tissue injury associated with them. Finally, as a salvage procedure, a silicone arthroplasty can be done at a later date.
3. *Collateral ligament avulsion fractures* also require open reduction and fixation if there is involvement of approximately 30 percent of the joint surface. Screw fixation is used to allow early immobilization. Complications of metacarpal head fractures: extensor mechanism and intraarticular adhesions result in dorsal

capsular contracture and degenerative arthritic changes. Treatment for these problems include tenolysis of the extensor mechanism, dorsal capsulectomy, and implant arthroplasty. Finally, two rarer complications are avascular necrosis (AVN) of the metacarpal head and damage to the epiphyseal growth plate with associated arrest and shortening of the metacarpal.

4. *Metacarpal neck fractures* are usually caused by a direct blow. Such an injury results in volar comminution of the metacarpal neck and associated dorsal angulation. The flexed position of the metacarpal head is accentuated by the pull of the intrinsics which are volar to the axis at the level of the metacarpophalangeal (MP) joint. The amount of angulation that can be accepted depends on which metacarpal is fractured. Greater degrees of angulation can be accepted in the ring and small fingers because the fourth and fifth carpometacarpal joints have 20 to 30 degrees of mobility and can thus compensate for any angulatory deformity more distally. This is not the case in the middle and index fingers, in which there is a limited mobility at the carpometacarpal joints. Treatment with less than 15 degrees of angulation in a splint or a cast is adequate. This should last for approximately 3 weeks, and then initiation of early motion is instituted with protective splinting. With 15 to 40 degrees of angulation, an attempt at reduction should be made. Immobilization is maintained with the MP joint flexed at a maximum of 90 degrees and the interphalangeal (IP) joints at 0 degrees. More aggressive treatment is needed if there is greater than 40 degrees of angulation within the ulnar border digits, or greater than 15 degrees in the radial two digits, otherwise a reciprocal hyperextension deformity develops at the MP joint. Such aggressive treatment can consist of closed reduction and a percutaneous pinning. If this is unsuccessful, then an open reduction would be indicated.
5. *Metacarpal shaft fractures* can be transverse, spiral oblique, or comminuted (Fig. 81–1). Transverse fractures often angulate dorsally, secondary to the pull of the interosseous muscles. Less angulation is tolerated with the second and third metacarpals than with the fourth and fifth metacarpals. Spiral oblique fractures are often caused by a twisting injury to the fingers. Evaluation of rotational deformity is critical in these fractures. Comminuted fractures are often associated with significant soft tissue loss. A minimal amount of shortening can be tolerated if there is no rotational deformity.

Treatment of closed, stable metacarpal shaft fractures (i.e., transverse fracture less than 10 degrees of dorsal angulation, spiral oblique fracture with less than 3 to 4 mm of shortening and no rotational deformity) can consist of splinting and/or casting for approximately 3–1/2 weeks. Treatment of unstable transverse fractures is usually either a closed reduction and percutaneous pinning or open reduction and plating.

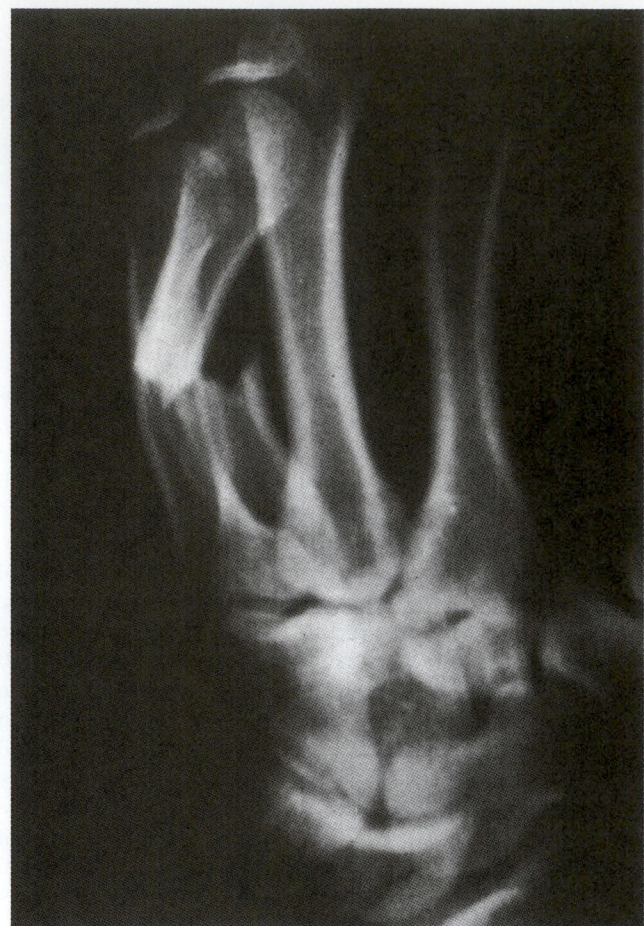

Figure 81-1
Unstable transverse fracture of metacarpal shaft.

Other indications for open reduction and internal fixation (ORIF) include those in which there are multiple fractures with or without significant soft tissue injury. In severe crush injuries and/or open injuries, early fixation allows for stabilization of the osseous architecture, and thus permits the surgeon to address the associated soft tissue injuries. External fixation, for example, with a mini-external fixateur as described by Seitz (1987) is another option in open crush injuries of the fingers. It is especially appropriate in cases of bone loss.

Complications of metacarpal fractures include malunion, nonunion, and soft tissue adhesions.

THUMB: METACARPAL FRACTURES

Thumb metacarpal fractures can be intraarticular at the MP joint, at the carpometacarpal joint, or may be a shaft fracture. Shaft fracture can be either transverse, oblique, or markedly comminuted.

1. *Thumb metacarpal fractures* at the level of the MP joint can be condylar fractures associated with either an ulnar or radial collateral ligament injury, or more rarely can be avulsions of the collateral ligaments. More often, however, these avulsions occur distally at the ligamentous insertion into the proximal phalanx. Any significant displacement of these avulsed fractures would require ORIF in order to regain ligamentous stability to the MP joint. Osteochondral fractures, if large enough, should also be fixed if there is a significant intraarticular displacement.

2. *Extraarticular metacarpal shaft fractures* are associated with deforming forces that are important to understand relative to treatment. Typically, there is a dorsal angulation of the metacarpal shaft fracture. The abductor pollicis longus tendon extends the proximal fragment while the short muscles around the MP joint, that is, the abductor pollicis brevis, adductor pollicis brevis, and flexor pollicis brevis, tend to flex the distal fragment. In addition, the distal fragment becomes supinated. Therefore, a closed reduction of the fracture is performed by volar pressure on the dorsal angulation and also pronation of the thumb. If there is less than 20 degrees of angulation, reduction of the shaft fracture is acceptable. However, if there is greater than 20 degrees of angulation, then fixation is indicated.

THUMB INTRAARTICULAR FRACTURES AT THE CARPOMETACARPAL JOINT

Bennett's fracture is a fracture-dislocation at the level of the thumb carpometacarpal joint. The major stabilizing structure of the carpometacarpal joint is the anterior oblique ligament which connects the base of the first metacarpal to the trapezium, and the second metacarpal. The metacarpal shaft displaces proximally, radially, and dorsally, secondary to the pull of the abductor pollicis longus. In addition, there is a flexion deformity of the shaft secondary to the pull of the adductor pollicis brevis.

Fixation is necessary to prevent continuing deformity and posttraumatic arthritic changes at the carpometacarpal joint. If the intraarticular fracture is less than 20 percent, then a closed reduction and percutaneous pinning can be adequate. The patient is then immobilized in a cast for approximately 5 to 6 weeks. If the fracture fragment is greater than 20 percent, then ORIF is warranted.

Rolando's fracture is an intraarticular fracture at the carpometacarpal joint of the thumb; it is often markedly comminuted. If there are large fracture fragments, then ORIF is a suitable method of treatment. There may be some bone loss at the metaphyseal level, and one should consider bone grafting. If there is marked comminution, open reduction is not warranted; rather, oblique skeletal traction is indicated or external fixation with a limited open reduction.

PROXIMAL AND MIDDLE PHALANGEAL FINGER FRACTURES

EVALUATION

With physical examination, one must assess rotational alignment and extensor and flexor tendon function. Finally, neurovascular status and soft tissue assessment are essential. Radiographic evaluation is done with PA, lateral, and oblique views.

CLASSIFICATION

Proximal Phalanx Transverse Fractures

The deforming forces in these fractures are the lateral bands which flex the proximal fragment and the central slip mechanism which extends the distal fragment, causing a hyperextension deformity. Transverse fractures can be treated closed if they are reduced properly. These fractures can then be maintained in a cast and/or splint with the MP joints flexed at 90 degrees to keep the collateral ligaments at their greatest length and also to reduce the deforming forces of the interossei. The proximal interphalangeal (PIP) joint is immobilized in 0 degrees of extension. If the fracture pattern is still un-

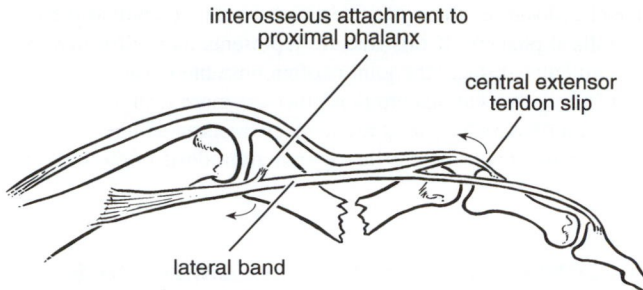

interosseous attachment to proximal phalanx

central extensor tendon slip

lateral band

Figure 81-2

Forces causing unstable proximal phalanx fracture. [Redrawn with permission from the American Society for Surgery of the Hand (ASSH): Fractures of the hand. In *ASSH 1996 Regional Review Course Syllabus.* Englewood, CO: 1996; 9–6.]

stable after this, then percutaneous pinning is indicated (Fig. 81–2). In addition, buddy taping to an adjacent digit can correct any rotational deformity. Kirschner wire fixation, however, must be supplemented by casting for approximately 3–1/2 to 4 weeks.

Proximal Phalanx Oblique Fractures

Rotationally unstable, oblique fractures cannot be held with a closed reduction (Fig. 81–3). Open reduction with miniscrew fragment fixation is indicated.

Transverse Middle Phalanx Fractures

Deforming forces at this level depend on the site of the fracture. If fracture is proximal to the flexor digitorum sublimis insertion, these fractures will tend to angulate dorsally. If the fracture is distal to the flexor digitorum sublimis insertion, these fractures will angulate volarly. Treatment often requires fixation, as these fractures tend to be unstable.

Special Children's Fractures in Fingers

Supracondylar Type Fracture Level of Proximal or Middle Phalangeal Head This fracture is best assessed by a lateral view. Often the phalangeal head is angulated at approximately 90 degrees to the phalangeal shaft. Treatment requires ORIF.

Salter Harris Fractures Salter Harris type II fractures can be treated like the oblique type fractures. If there is a rotational deformity, then fixation should be indicated, usually with Kirschner wires. Salter Harris type III fractures are treated similarly to intraarticular fractures and/or ligamentous avulsion type fractures. If there is significant displacement, then ORIF is indicated (Fig. 81–4).

COMPLICATIONS OF PROXIMAL OR MIDDLE PHALANGEAL SHAFT FRACTURES

Extraarticular complications include: rotational deformity, angulatory deformity, shortening of a phalangeal fracture, loss of finger motion

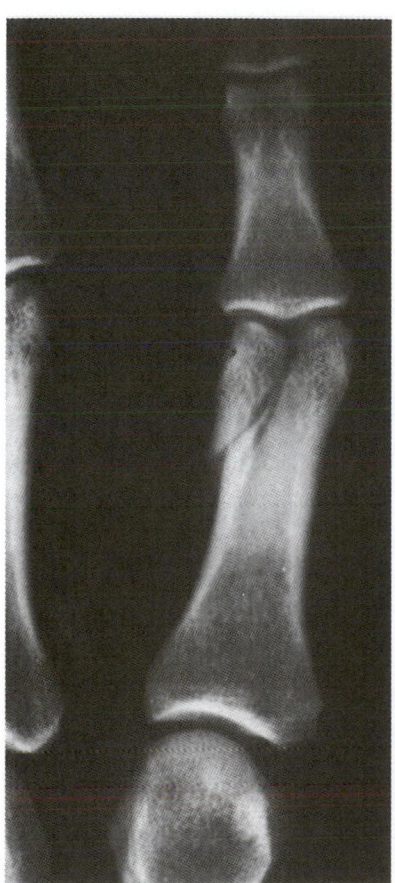
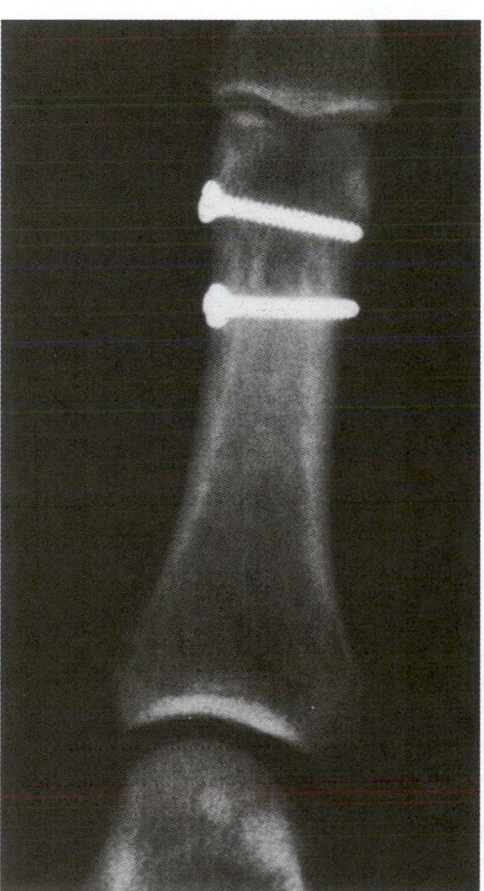
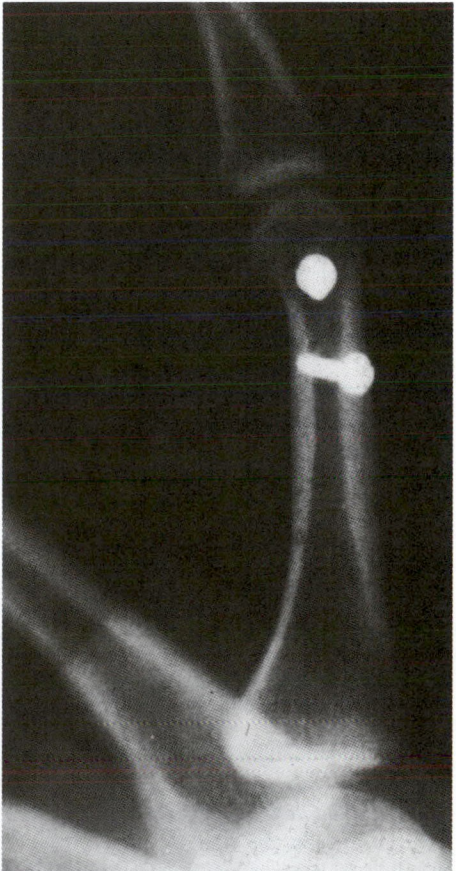

A   *B*   *C*

Figure 81-3

A. Oblique fracture of proximal phalanx with intraarticular component. *B.* PA view of open reduction internal fixation of an oblique proximal phalanx fracture. *C.* Lateral view of open reduction internal fixation of an oblique proximal phalanx fracture.

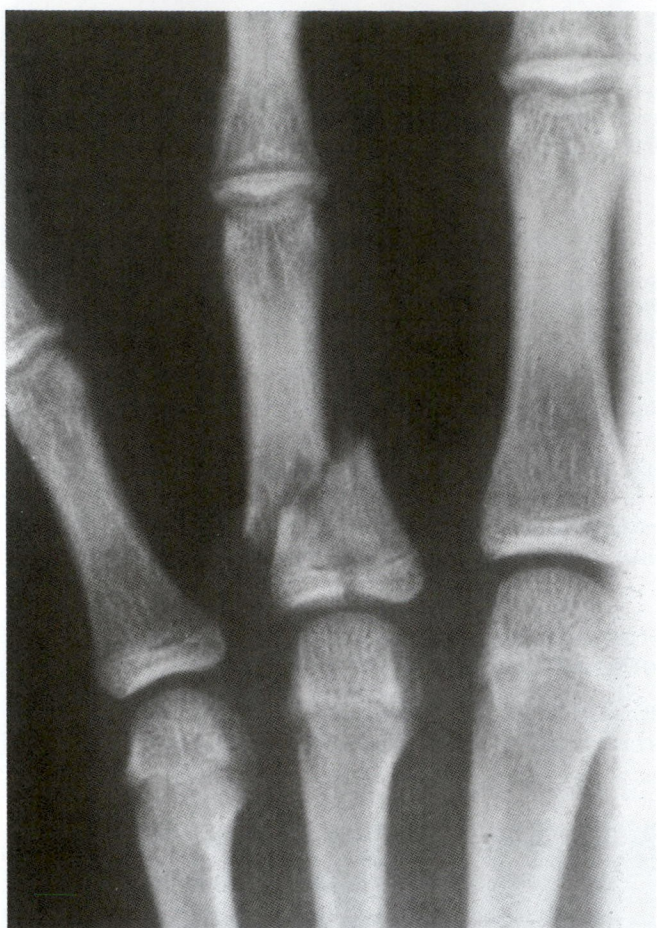

Figure 81-4
Salter type IV fracture of proximal phalanx.

(secondary to either extensor or flexor tendon adhesions and/or contractures around the metacarpal or proximal interphalangeal joints), and infection from either open wounds or pins.

DISTAL PHALANX INJURIES AND DISTAL JOINT INJURIES OF THE THUMB AND FINGERS

FRACTURES OF DORSAL LIP DISTAL PHALANX

These fractures are divided into two groups: first, small avulsion fractures involving the extensor tendon at the level of its insertion into the distal phalanx; and second, intraarticular fractures. The avulsion fracture is not associated with any joint subluxation or treated as an extensor tendon injury, and is splinted in extension for approximately 6 weeks. Intraarticular fractures that comprise more than 40 percent of the articular surface result in subluxation of the distal phalanx on the middle phalangeal head, and require ORIF.

Dislocations of the distal interphalangeal (DIP) joints are rare and usually dorsal. Because of the relative rigidity of the soft tissues about the distal joints, these injuries are frequently compound injuries with tearing of the volar skin. Treatment includes debridement of the wound along with irrigation and longitudinal traction. Subsequent to the reduction of a dorsal dislocation, a protective extension block splint is applied, blocking the terminal 15 degrees of extension. With

a dorsal dislocation, there is an associated volar fracture at the base of the distal phalanx. If this fracture represents more than one-third of the articular surface, the joint is often unstable despite the reduction. Chronic dislocations are those that are more than 4 weeks old. Usually an open reduction is required. If the time of injury is more than a few months prior, a primary joint arthrodesis of the DIP joint is indicated.

DISLOCATIONS AND LIGAMENTOUS INJURIES ABOUT THE METACARPOPHALANGEAL JOINTS OF THE FINGERS AND THUMB

ANATOMY OF THE FINGER METACARPOPHALANGEAL JOINT

The metacarpal head is narrowed dorsally and is wider volarly. The ligamentous structures extend from the metacarpal neck and insert onto the base of the proximal phalanx. They are most taut in flexion and loose in extension. Thus, when immobilizing the MP joint, it should be immobilized in 90 degrees of flexion, with certain exceptions (i.e., immobilization for extensor tendon repairs).

Volarly, the MP joint is supported by the transverse metacarpal ligamentous structures. In addition, the sagittal bands, which initiate from the extensor tendon mechanism, course volarly to insert onto the volar plates and give further secondary support. Finally, the intrinsic musculature, which courses along the lateral aspect of the respective MP joints, also adds support to the joint.

DORSAL METACARPOPHALANGEAL JOINT DISLOCATIONS

The most commonly involved MP joints are those of the index and small fingers. The mechanism of injury is a hyperextension injury with avulsion of the volar plate off its insertion on the metacarpal head (Fig. 81–5); often the dislocation is irreducible (complete dislocation). On physical examination, the index or small finger is deviated to the central finger of the hand and prominence of the

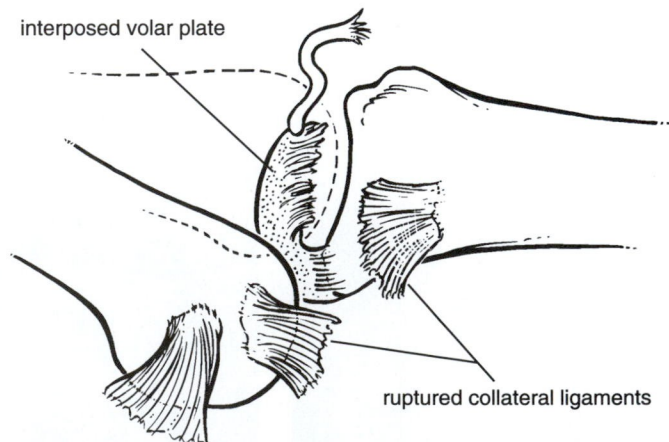

Figure 81-5
Complex dorsal dislocation MP joint with interposition Volar plate. [Redrawn and modified with permission from the American Society for Surgery of the Hand (ASSH): Articular fractures and joint injuries. In *ASSH 1996 Regional Review Course Syllabus.* Englewood, CO: 1996; 9–14.]

metacarpal head can be felt in the palm. In addition, there is an inability to both actively and/or passively flex the MP joint.

TREATMENT

Management requires an open reduction. It is usually recommended to go through a volar approach. The joint is reduced, and the MP joint immobilized in approximately 30 to 40 degrees of flexion for approximately 2 to 3 weeks.

LIGAMENT INJURIES ABOUT THE THUMB METACARPOPHALANGEAL JOINT

INJURIES TO THE ULNAR COLLATERAL LIGAMENT

The mechanism of injury is a radial deviation force to the thumb at the level of the MP joint. This injury can either result in an avulsion of the ligament, usually off its insertion in the proximal phalanx or a midsubstance tear. Rarely is the ligament avulsed off of the metacarpal head. It is important to differentiate between the partial ulnar collateral ligament tear versus the complete tear. In the complete tear, one often sees a so-called Stener lesion in which the ligament retracts proximally and the adductor aponeurosis is interposed between the ligament and its insertion into the proximal phalanx (Fig. 81–6). Thus, in this case, open repair of the ligament is necessary.

In differentiating the partial from a complete tear, the MP joint is assessed in full extension and also in 30 degrees of flexion. If the joint is more than 30 degrees unstable, as compared to the normal contralateral thumb with radial deviation, then a complete tear of the ligament can be inferred. However, before performing any examination about the MP joint, a radiograph should be obtained. This would avoid the possibility of making a nondisplaced avulsion fracture of the proximal phalanx into a displaced one that would then subsequently require surgical intervention. As noted, if there is gross instability, then surgical intervention is warranted because of the interposition of the adductor aponeurosis.

On the lateral view, if there is significant palmar subluxation of the proximal phalanx on the metacarpal head, this is indicative of a dorsal capsular tear as well. With surgical intervention, care must also be taken to repair this ligament. After injecting the joint with a local anesthetic, stress views on x-ray can be of help. If the proximal phalanx subluxates radially greater than 33 percent of the metacarpal head, then a Stener lesion can be inferred.

Proper treatment for a partial ligament tear is immobilization in a splint for at least 4 and up to 6 weeks. If there is a complete tear,

then an open repair is warranted. Usually, if the ligamentous tear is addressed within 3 to 4 weeks, then a direct and/or secondary repair is possible.

CHRONIC ULNAR COLLATERAL LIGAMENT INJURIES

If the ligament injury is more than 4 to 5 weeks old, it is often difficult to do a secondary repair of the ligamentous structures. In this case, the most reliable reconstructive procedure is a tendon graft reconstruction of the ligament.

RADIAL COLLATERAL INJURIES OF THE METACARPOPHALANGEAL JOINT

The mechanism of injury to the radial aspect of the joint is an adduction force. Typically, the joint is also flexed at the time of the injury; often with radial collateral ligament injuries there is significant damage to the dorsal capsule. In a similar fashion if there is greater than 30 degrees of instability on stressing the joint in ulnar deviation, then surgical intervention is warranted (Fig. 81–7).

DORSAL METACARPOPHALANGEAL JOINT DISLOCATIONS OF THE THUMB

This injury occurs with a hyperextension force to the MP joint. Usually, the volar plate is avulsed proximally off its insertion into the metacarpal head. In addition, there is often a tear of the collateral ligaments. Most commonly, this injury can be reduced with a closed reduction. Subsequent to the reduction, however, testing of the stability of the collateral ligaments both on the radial and ulnar aspect of the joint should be performed. Usually, however, they are quite stable and hyperextension block splinting is indicated subsequent to the closed reduction for approximately 4 weeks. Occasionally, a closed reduction cannot be achieved due to interposition of the volar plate, sesamoid bones and their associated muscular attachments, or the flexor pollicis longus tendon. Release of the flexor pollicis longus sheath or interposed volar plate is performed in an open reduction. The joint can be pinned at approximately 25 degrees of flexion for approximately 3 to 4 weeks.

THUMB CARPOMETACARPAL JOINT DISLOCATIONS

The major stabilizer of the carpometacarpal joint of the thumb is the so-called volar beak ligament which attaches from the trapezium to the base of the first metacarpal. If this ligament is damaged, the thumb metacarpal tends to subluxate and/or dislocate in a dorsal direction.

Treatment

In acute cases, a dislocation should be reduced. If there is stability after the reduction, then consideration for casting can be done for approximately 6 weeks. More often, however, there is significant instability despite the reduction and/or subsequent subluxation after the reduction of the dislocation, and patients are better treated with a pinning after the reduction, transfixing the first metacarpal into the trapezium. Immobilization should be for at least 6 weeks. In cases of chronic instability, Eaton (1984) and colleagues have described a reconstruction of the volar beak ligament using a strip of the flexor carpi radialis.

FINGER CARPOMETACARPAL JOINT INJURIES

The most commonly injured carpometacarpal joint of the fingers is on the ulnar aspect, that is, the fourth and fifth carpometacarpal joints.

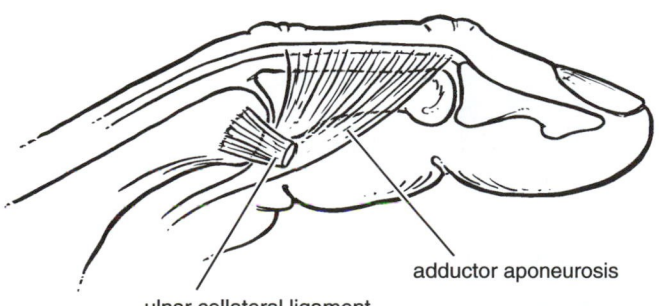

Figure 81-6
Stener lesions (interposition of adductor aponeurosis). [Redrawn and modified with permission from the American Society for Surgery of the Hand (ASSH): Articular fractures and joint injuries. In *ASSH 1996 Regional Review Course Syllabus.* Englewood, CO: 1996; 9–16.]

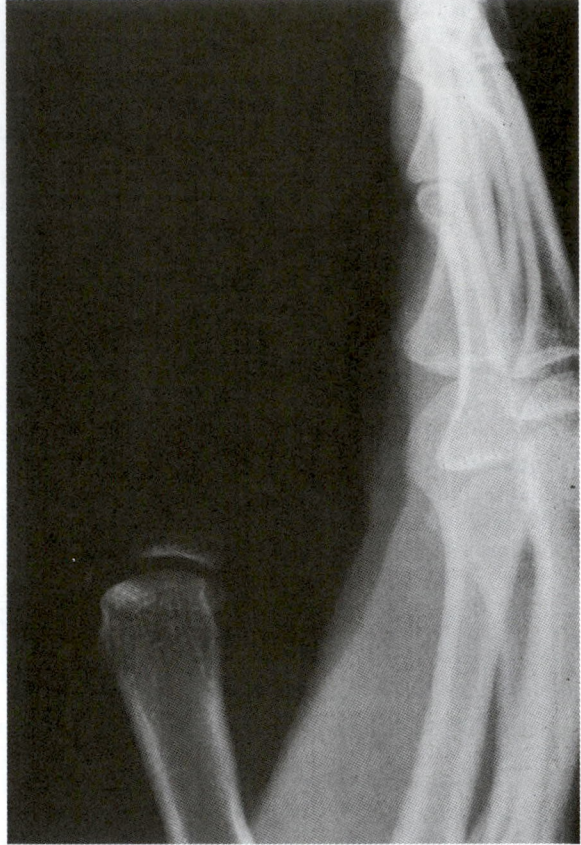

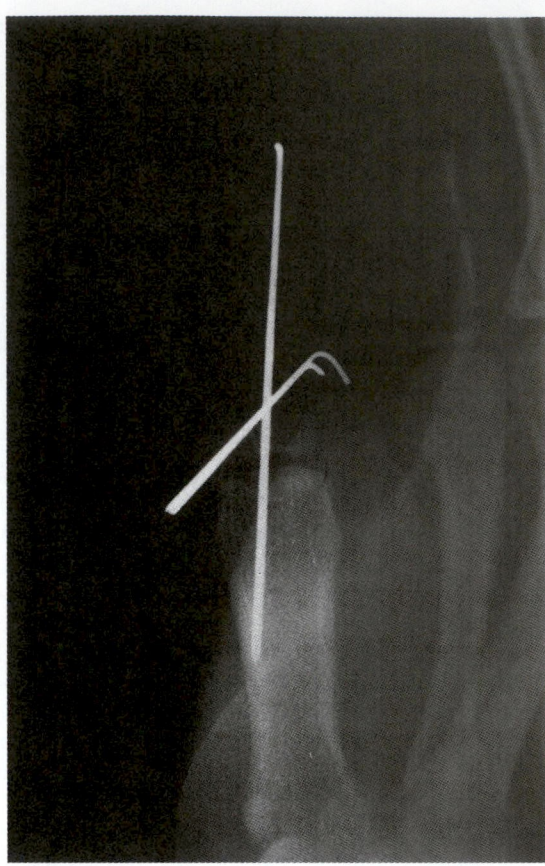

A   B

Figure 81-7
A. Avulsion radial collateral ligament thumb MP joint. *B.* Open reduction of radial collateral ligament thumb MP joint.

Typically, there is a fracture dislocation associated with a direct blow to the hand. Often, there is an avulsion of the dorsal lip of the hamate associated with a fracture and/or possibly just a dislocation of the fourth and or fifth metacarpal (Fig. 81–8). On the PA view, one will see an overlap of the base of the fifth carpal onto the hamate with loss of the joint space at this level. The best view from which to make the diagnosis is the so-called Brewerton view which is a 30-degree pronated lateral view (Fig. 81–9).

If there is no significant fracture and/or avulsions, these injuries can be treated with a closed reduction and a percutaneous pinning. However,

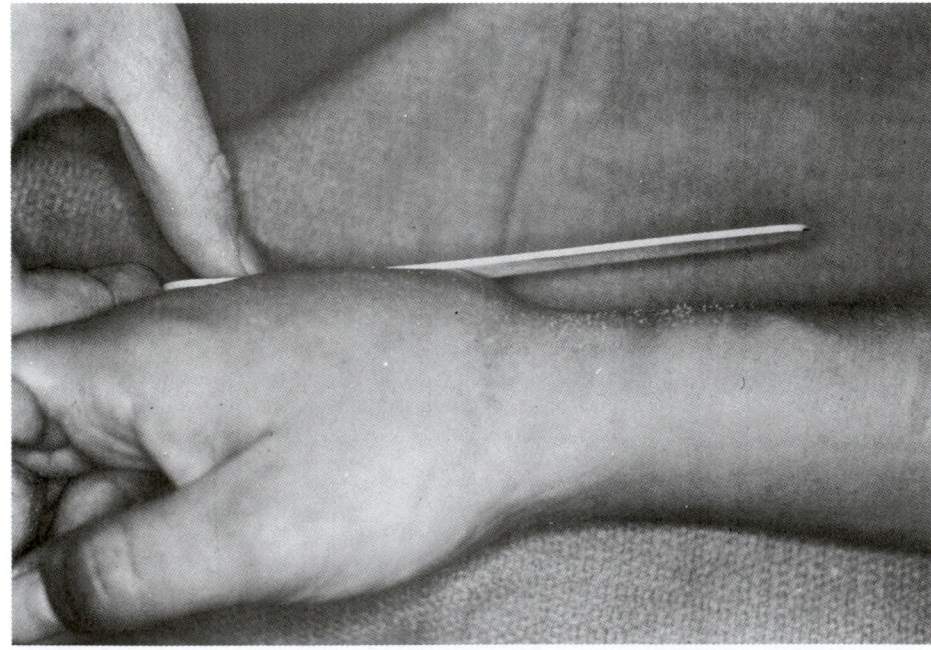

Figure 81-8
Appearance of hand with carpal-metacarpal joint dislocation. Notice dorsal displacement of metacarpals.

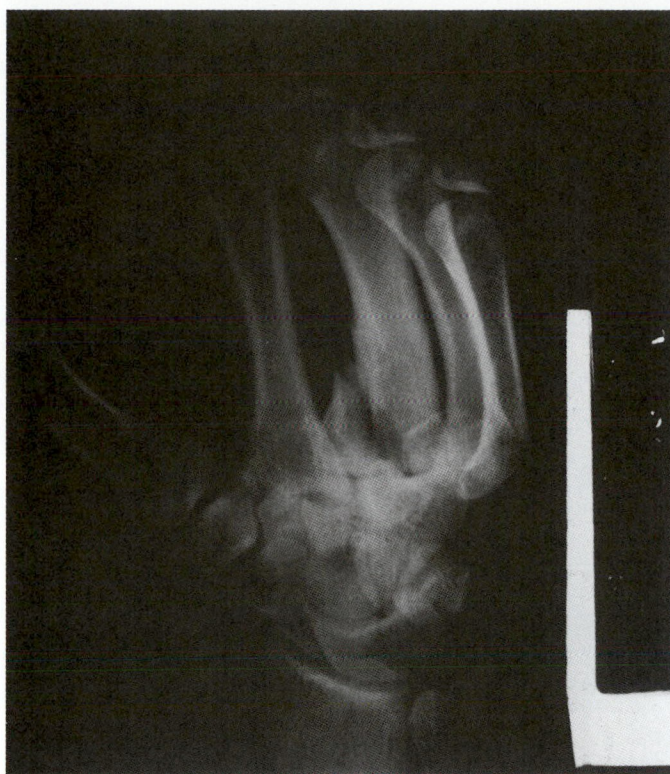

Figure 81-9
Oblique view showing fracture dislocation at third, fourth, and fifth carpometacarpal joints.

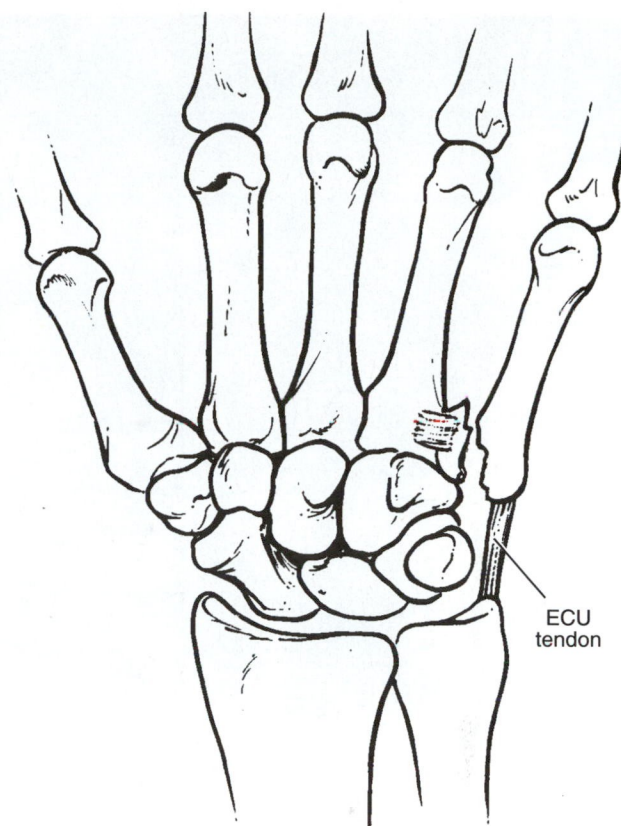

Figure 81-10
Deforming forces in reverse Bennet's fracture. [Redrawn and modified with permission from the American Society for Surgery of the Hand (ASSH): Articular fractures and joint injuries. In *ASSH 1996 Regional Review Course Syllabus.* Englewood, CO: 1996; 9–15.]

if there is a significant avulsion of the hamate and/or a significant intraarticular step off of the fracture, then an open reduction is indicated.

A reverse Bennett's fracture is a fracture through the base of the fifth metacarpal which is oblique in nature (Fig. 81–10). Specifically, it is an intraarticular fracture with displacement of the majority of the shaft of the fifth metacarpal secondary to the pull of the extensor carpi ulnaris. Treatment consists of traction, along with a closed reduction and pinning of the fracture. If there is a large intraarticular fracture pattern, then an open reduction is warranted.

DISLOCATIONS AND LIGAMENT INJURIES IN THE HAND

PROXIMAL INTERPHALANGEAL JOINT

The stability of the PIP joint is maintained by its articular contours, ligamentous integrity (both at the level of the collateral ligaments and volar plate structures), and tendon insertions about the joint. Passive testing such as stress testing can be used in association with radiographic evaluation. The radiographic examination includes PA, lateral, and oblique views. Stability of the joint can be tested both actively and passively. The most common dislocation about the proximal PIP joint is that associated with hyperextension and longitudinal compressive forces. Dorsal dislocations have been classified by Eaton and Littler (1976) into three types.

Type I

In type I injuries, hyperextension of the volar plate is avulsed from the base of the middle phalanx with minor longitudinal splits in the collateral ligaments. The articular surface of the proximal phalangeal head and middle phalanx base remain intact.

Type II

Type II is a true dorsal dislocation. It consists of an avulsion of the volar plate, associated with a major bilateral split in the collateral ligaments. Thus, the middle phalangeal base lies dorsal to the proximal phalangeal head in a bayonet deformity. In this type of deformity there is no contact between the associated articular surfaces.

Type III

Type III injuries are fracture dislocations about the PIP joint. These injuries are either stable or unstable. Typically, a stable fracture dislocation will involve an avulsion fracture at the base of the middle phalanx involving less than 40 percent of the articular surface of the middle phalanx (Fig. 81–11). The majority of the collateral ligaments remain attached to middle phalangeal shaft. In the unstable fracture dislocation situation, there is a fracture involving greater than 40 percent of the volar articular surface of the middle phalanx. In addition, all of the stabilizing ligamentous structures, that is, the volar plate and collateral ligaments, are attached to the fracture fragment. Thus, there are no further ligamentous structures attached to the middle phalangeal shaft, and therefore there is gross instability to this dislocation. Treatment of acute dorsal PIP dislocations is predicated on whether the injury is a stable or unstable situation. In a stable setting, the joint can be treated with a hyperextension block splint at approximately 25 to 30 degrees of flexion of the joint. Typically, this is utilized for approximately 10 to 14 days, and then subsequent mobilization is initiated. These injuries, while not affecting the stability of the joint, often cause residual swelling and soreness within the PIP

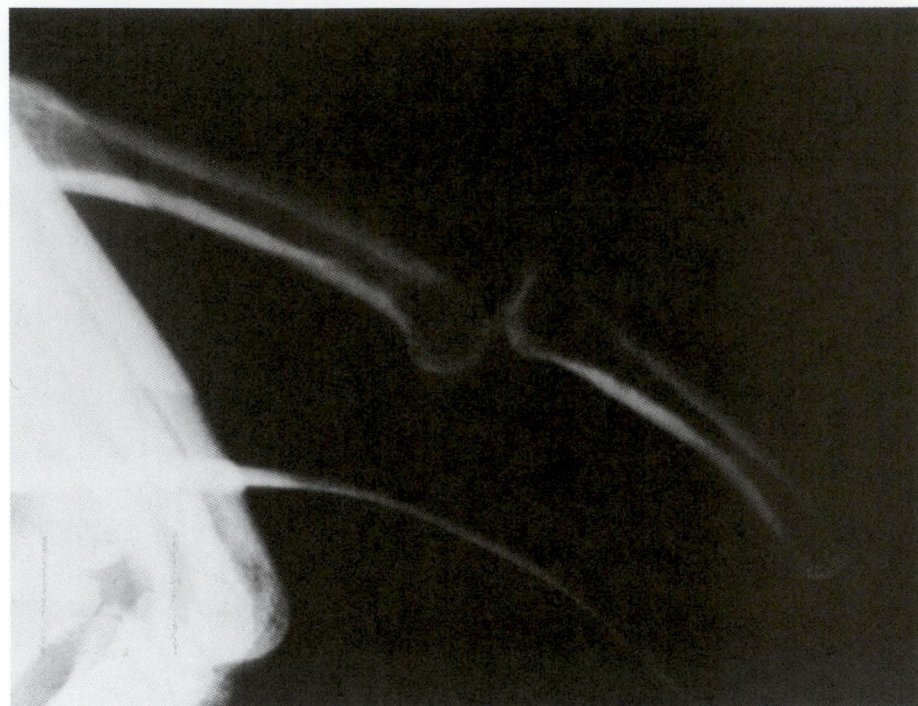

Figure 81-11
Dorsal fracture dislocation of the PIP joint.

joint. They are best treated after the short period of immobilization with aggressive therapy and Cobanning of the joint to decrease edema in the finger. The unstable fracture dislocation of the PIP joint necessitates surgical intervention. Most commonly, the volar fracture fragment of the middle phalanx is comminuted in nature, and thus, cannot be repaired. Therefore, a volar plate arthroplasty is indicated in this situation (Fig. 81–12). Specifically, excision of the comminuted fracture fragments is performed, and the volar plate is advanced into the deficit in the middle phalanx. Typically, the PIP joint is pinned in approximately 30 degrees of flexion for approximately 3 weeks to allow the volar plate to heal into the base of the middle phalanx. Subsequent to this hyperextension block splinting is initiated and active range of motion of the PIP joint is begun.

TREATMENT FOR CHRONIC PIP HYPEREXTENSION SUBLUXATIONS

Chronic PIP hyperextension subluxation injuries require surgical intervention, and are best treated with either volar plate advancement or flexor superficialis tenodesis of the proximal interphalangeal joint (Fig. 81–13).

TREATMENT FOR CHRONIC PIP DORSAL FRACTURE DISLOCATIONS

Chronic PIP dorsal fracture dislocations can be treated with a volar plate arthroplasty if there are no significant changes within the joint. This technique, however, requires release of the collateral ligament, and possibly a dorsal capsulectomy.

OTHER TYPES OF DISLOCATIONS

Lateral PIP dislocations involve an injury to the collateral ligament and the volar plate. In acute injuries the ligamentous structures re-

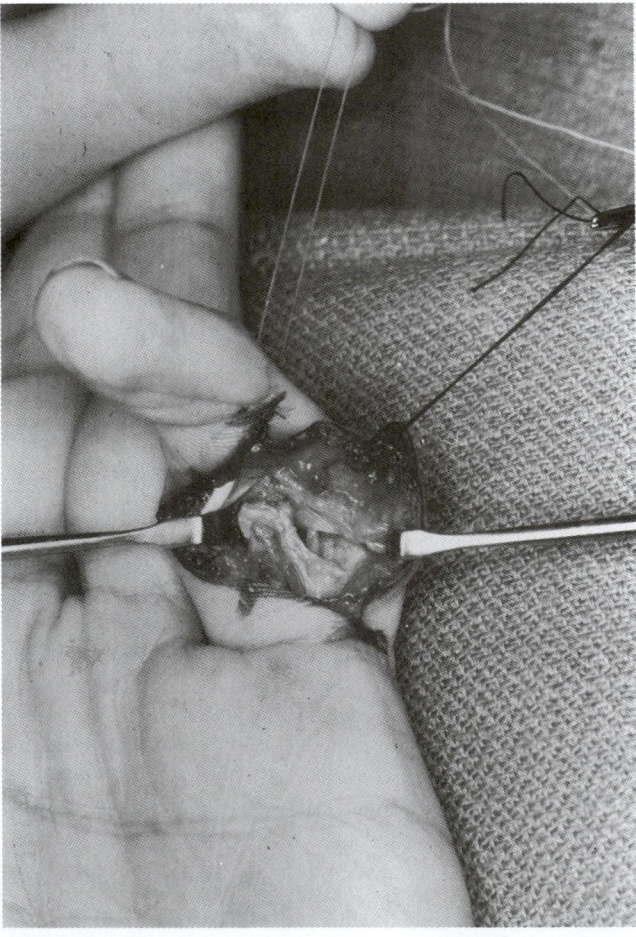

Figure 81-12
Technique of volar plate arthroplasty.

turn to their normal alignment and can be treated with protective splinting. If there is a chronic instability to the joint, then consideration for tendon grafting reconstruction an be given. However, problems with this technique often involve loss of joint motion (Fig. 81–14).

Volar PIP dislocations result from compressive and rotatory forces when the PIP joint is flexed. The proximal phalangeal condyle is buttonholed between the central slip and its lateral band. Reduction of this deformity is performed by traction while both the MP joint and PIP joints are flexed. Assessment of the central slip mechanism is then performed. If there is loss of full, active extension of the joint, the dislocation must be treated like a boutonniere deformity with the PIP joints splinted in extension for a period of approximately 6 weeks with the DIP joint free. If a closed reduction is unsuccessful, then an open reduction is indicated (Fig. 81–15).

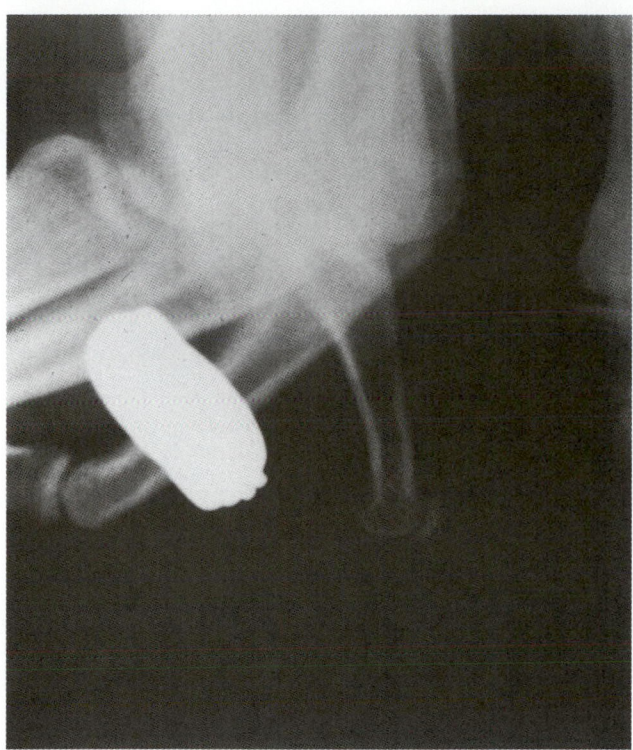

Figure 81-13
Chronic hyperextension laxity of the PIP joint.

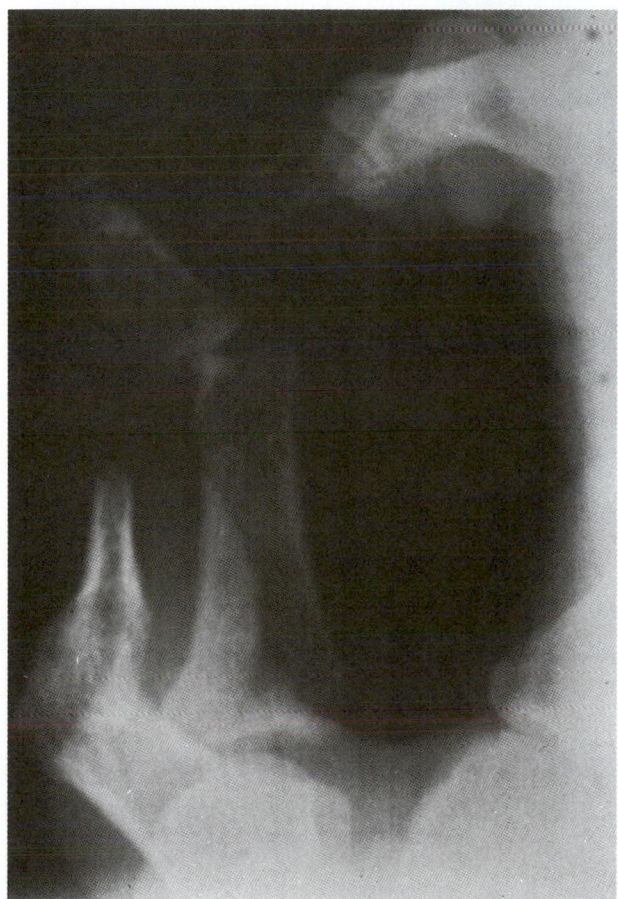

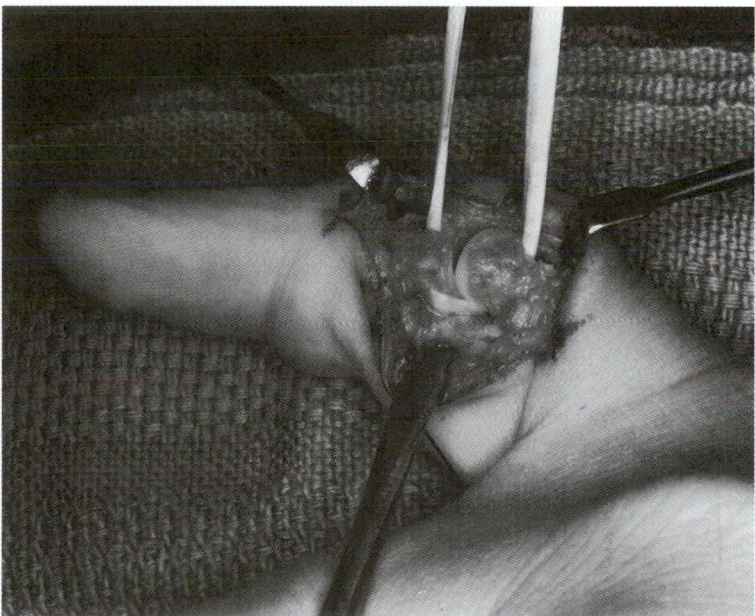

B

A

Figure 81-14
A. Chronic lateral instability of the PIP joint. *B.* Ligament reconstruction for chronic lateral instability of the PIP joint.

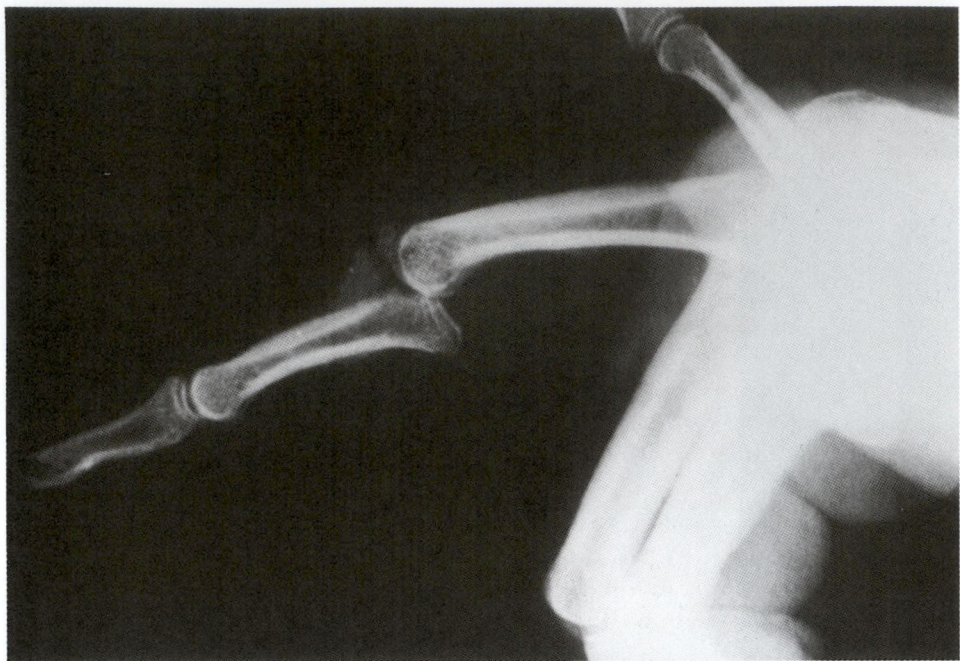

A

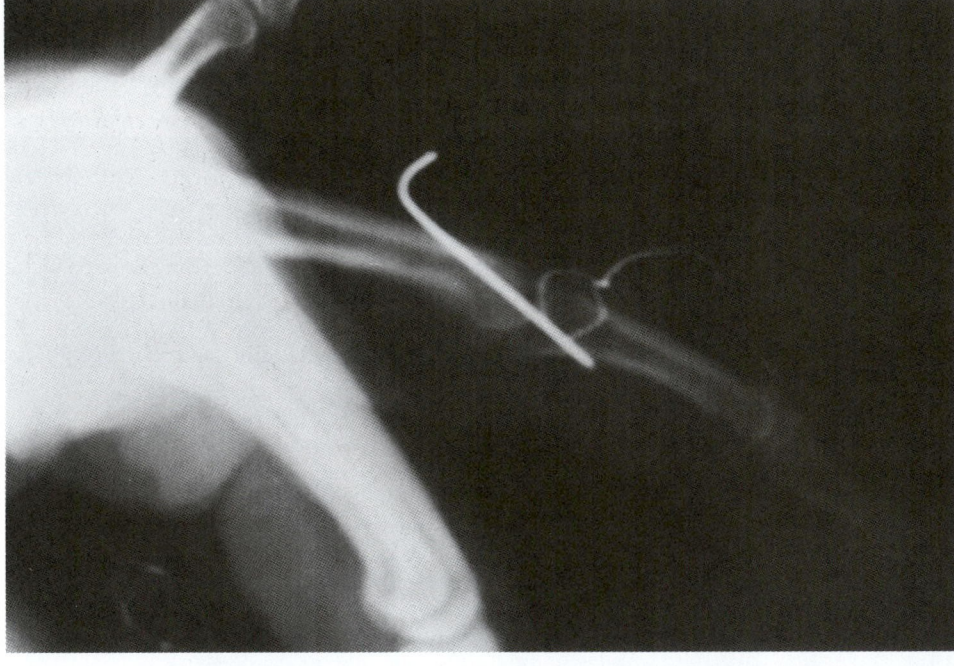

B

Figure 81-15
A. Palmar dislocation PIP joint with avulsion of extensor mechanism. *B.* Open reduction of PIP joint with avulsion of extensor mechanism.

SUGGESTED READINGS

FRACTURES/METACARPALS

Elaine CS: Detecting occult fractures of the metacarpal head: The Brewerton view. *J Hand Surgery [Br]* 1977; 2:131.

Seitz WH, Gomez W, Putnam MD, et al: Management of severe hand trauma with a mini external fixateur. *Orthopedics* 1987; 10:601.

PROXIMAL OR MIDDLE PHALANGEAL SHAFT FRACTURES

Eaton RG, Littler JW: Joint injuries and their sequelae. *Clin Plast Surg* 1976; 3:85.

DISTAL PHALANX INJURIES

Lenzo SR: Distal joint injuries of the thumb and fingers. *Hand Clin* 1992; 8(4):769.

LIGAMENT INJURIES ABOUT THE THUMB METACARPOPHALANGEAL JOINT

Eaton RG, Lane LB, Littler JW, et al: Ligament reconstruction for the painful thumb carpometacarpal joint: A long term assessment. *J Hand Surg [Am]* 1984; 9:692.

Chapter 82

PELVIS

Kenneth J. Koval

PELVIS FRACTURES

ANATOMY

The pelvis is formed by two innominate bones and the sacrum. Pelvic stability is dependent on ligamentous support to resist the pressures of normal physiologic stresses. The posterior pelvis ligaments join the sacrum and innominate bones, and are considered among the strongest ligaments in the body. They include the sacroiliac, sacrospinous, sacrotuberous, iliolumbar, and iliosacral ligaments. The anterior pelvis is joined by the symphysis pubis. Fractures of the pelvis and acetabulum place the superior gluteal vessels at particular risk for injury as they pass through the greater sciatic foramen (see Chap. 18).

INCIDENCE/MECHANISM OF INJURY

Most pelvis fractures are stable and result from a simple fall. Higher energy injuries result from a motor vehicle accident or a fall from a height. Unstable pelvis fractures often have associated injuries; 1 to 12 percent include a neurologic injury.

Bladder and urethral injury occur frequently with pelvic fracture, and are most likely caused by direct laceration from a fracture fragment or pressure-intentioned stresses during deformation of the pelvic ring. Intravenous pyelograms, transurethral cystograms, and retrograde urethrograms may be necessary to arrive at a definitive diagnosis. Gynecologic injury may involve laceration of the vagina, usually caused by dislocation of the symphysis pubis or fracture of the pubic rami. Gastrointestinal injury such as tearing and/or puncture of the rectum, or less frequently, perforation of the small and/or large bowel is possible. If rectal laceration occurs, a diverting colostomy with thorough irrigation and debridement of the fracture is mandatory.

CLINICAL AND RADIOGRAPHIC EVALUATION

The primary objective of evaluation is to determine whether the pelvis fracture is stable or unstable. The clinical examination should also document the presence of pelvic asymmetry, bruising, and open wounds. Physical examination must also assess areas of pain, crepitation, and signs of abnormal movement. Caution during the physical examination is important as repeat stressing of an unstable pelvis may increase retroperitoneal bleeding secondary to clot disruption. The penile urethral meatus should be inspected for blood. Examination of the rectum and vagina is necessary to determine if an open pelvis fracture has occurred.

Radiologic examination includes an AP, a 40-degree caudad or inlet projection, and a 40-degree cephalad or outlet projection. An inlet projection demonstrates anterior-posterior displacement of the hemipelvis, and the outlet view superior/inferior migration.

Radiographic signs of pelvis instability are: superior and/or posterior displacement of the hemipelvis and fracture of the L5 transverse process. Judet films may facilitate evaluation of iliac wing fractures. CT scans assist in defining the posterior pelvis to include the sacroiliac joint and sacrum. The decision to perform angiography is based on evidence of need.

CLASSIFICATION

Pelvis fractures may be classified based on mechanism of injury; types include fractures caused by lateral compression, anterior-posterior compression, or vertical shear. Lateral compression produces an implosion of the ipsilateral hemipelvis and an internal rotation deformity. These injuries generally result in sacral compression with impaction of the cancellous bone. Lateral compression injuries are generally stable (Fig. 82-1). Anterior directed lateral force may cause a fracture of the iliac wing or fracture dislocation of the sacroiliac joint. Anterior-posterior injuries cause external rotation of the ipsilateral hemipelvis and disruption of the symphysis, followed by tearing of the anterior and posterior sacroiliac ligaments. Anterior diastasis in excess of 2.5 cm indicates some degree of posterior disruption; separation greater than 6 cm suggests complete posterior disruption. Vertical shear injuries are high energy injuries, resulting in complete posterior pelvic disruption with superior displacement of the hemipelvis.

Tile (1980) divided pelvic injuries into an A, B, and C classification. Type A injuries are stable. A1 fractures of the pelvis do not involve the pelvic ring. A2 injuries are minimally displaced fractures of the pelvic ring. Type B fractures are rotationally unstable but are vertically stable. B1 are open book fractures with external rotation deformity. B2 fractures are lateral compression ipsilateral injuries with internal rotation deformity. B3 fractures are lateral compression contralateral injuries and are bilaterally rotationally unstable. Type C fractures are rotationally and vertically unstable injuries. C1 injuries are unilateral, C2 are bilateral, and C3 are associated with an acetabular fracture.

TREATMENT PRINCIPLES

Most pelvic ring injuries are stable. Management consists of bedrest for initial comfort followed by protected ambulation until full weight-bearing can be tolerated.

Unstable pelvis fractures must be assessed for hemodynamic instability. Observed or suspected bleeding is usually venous from the cancellous fracture surfaces; patients with pelvis fractures rarely have a major vessel injury. Pelvic bleeding can be controlled through military antishock trousers (MAST), external fixation, angiography, or exploration. MAST are simple to apply, rapid, and reversible; however, they also lower visibility and restrict access to the abdomen and extremities. Protracted use of MAST is reported to be associated with compartment syndrome and a decrease in the patient's vital lung

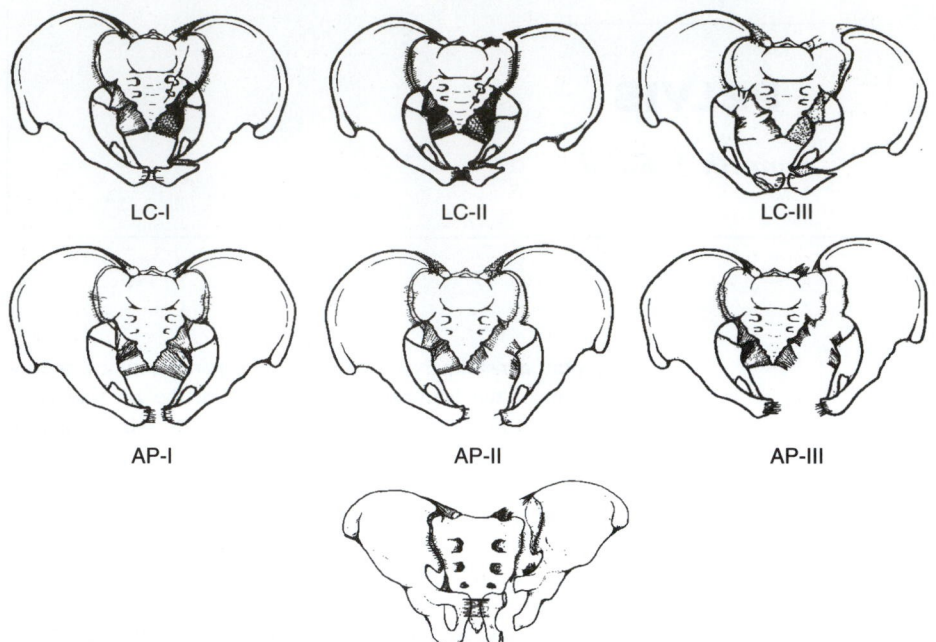

LC-I   LC-II   LC-III

AP-I   AP-II   AP-III

Vertical Shear

Figure 82-1
Young and Burgess classification of pelvic ring fractures. See text for details. [Reproduced by permission from Young JWR, Burgess AR: *Radiologic Management of Pelvic Ring Fractures.* Baltimore: Urban & Schwarzenberg, (now Lippincott Williams & Wilkins); 1987: 17–55.]

capacity. MAST are contraindicated if a history of congestive heart disease exists. External fixation will control the pelvic volume, allow access to the abdomen and extremities, promote mobilization of the patient, and control bleeding of vessels that are less than 3 mm in diameter. Angiography is only indicated for continued arterial bleeding; embolization is effective to control bleeding from vessels less than 5 mm in diameter and requires specialized resources and personnel.

Stabilization of rotationally unstable but vertically stable pelvis fractures is accomplished with either internal or external fixation. Internal fixation devices can be applied during laparotomy by extending the general surgery incision or through an ilioinguinal or Pfannenstiel approach. Posterior stabilization is used to restore stability to vertically unstable pelvis fractures. Acute stabilization for vertically unstable pelvis fractures can be achieved using external fixators; however, regardless of frame configuration, external fixation does not provide adequate posterior pelvic stabilization.

The decision to use internal fixation and the choice of surgical approach to the posterior pelvis is based on the fracture type, associated injuries, and condition of the soft tissue. The *anterior approach* allows direct visualization and access to the sacroiliac joint. However, this approach places the L5 nerve root at risk as it passes over the sacral alae. The *posterior approach* to the posterior pelvis is associated with a higher risk of infection and wound slough. Iliac wing fractures are stabilized with plates and screws. Sacroiliac dislocations are generally stabilized with sacroiliac lag screws, transiliac bars or plates, or anterior plates. Sacroiliac lag screws must be placed under radiographic control to prevent misplacement of screws into the sacral foramen or the vertebral canal. Sacral fractures may also be stabilized using sacroiliac lag screws or transiliac bars or plates.

RESULTS AND COMPLICATIONS

Management of vertically stable pelvis injuries is generally associated with few major long-term problems. Vertically unstable pelvis fractures have a worse prognosis regarding function and pain relief,

regardless of the type of treatment. Failure to recognize significant displacement or instability can result in nonunion and subsequent sacroiliac pain, leg-length discrepancy, difficulty in sitting, and functional impairment. Women may have further difficulties relating to parturition and dyspareunia.

ACETABULAR FRACTURES

ANATOMY

The acetabulum is supported within the arms of a bony inverted-Y that is formed by aspects of the anterior and posterior columns. The anterior column (iliopubic) consists of iliac, acetabular, and pubic components, and is the longer of the two major columns, extending from the iliac crest to the pubic symphysis. The posterior column (ilio-ischial) is more massive, with a triangular cross-section. The anterior and posterior columns join around the midpoint of the anterior column and form an angle of approximately 60 degrees; the acetabulum lies within this angle.

INCIDENCE/MECHANISM OF INJURY

Acetabular fractures are high energy injuries resulting from a force directed to the acetabulum from the femoral head. The fracture pattern is determined by the position of the femoral head in the acetabulum at the time of impact and the magnitude and direction of the related force. Acetabulum fractures may also be associated with other injuries such as sciatic nerve palsy.

CLINICAL AND RADIOGRAPHIC EVALUATION

Patients with an acetabular fracture must be evaluated for possible neurologic injury. The skin overlying the pelvis and hip should also be inspected for evidence of injury. A shearing injury to the skin, termed a Morel-Lavelle lesion, can occur and separate the subcutaneous fat from the deep fascia; necrosis of the subcutaneous fat subsequently occurs.

Four radiographic views are recommended: a standard AP view of the entire pelvis; a standard AP view centered on the injured hip; and two oblique views taken exactly at 45 degrees (Judet views). The obturator oblique view demonstrates the posterior wall and anterior acetabular column; the iliac oblique view depicts the anterior wall and posterior acetabular column. CT scans are indicated in the majority of cases and can help evaluate the presence of depressed segments, fractures involving the quadrilateral plate, rotational displacement of the anterior-posterior columns, and fragments between the femoral head and the wall of the acetabulum.

CLASSIFICATION

Letournel's classification of acetabular fractures describes ten fracture types (Fig. 82-2). The five *simple* fracture patterns are: (1) posterior wall, (2) posterior column, (3) anterior wall, (4) anterior column, and (5) transverse. Posterior wall fractures of the acetabulum involve the posterior articular surfaces; the ilioischial line (posterior column) remains intact. In contrast, posterior column fractures include not only the posterior articular surface, but also the ilioischial line. Anterior wall fractures involve the central aspect of the anterior column, whereas anterior column fractures involve varying amounts of anterior column. In both settings, the ilioinguinal line is involved in the fracture. Transverse fractures include the anterior and posterior acetabulum, and divide the acetabulum into a superior component containing the acetabular roof and an inferior component.

The five *complex* fracture types include: (1) combined posterior wall and posterior column fracture, (2) posterior wall and transverse fracture, (3) T-shaped fracture, (4) anterior column and (5) posterior hemitransverse fracture, and both-column fracture. The T-shaped fracture is a transverse fracture associated with a vertical component that separates a lower ischial segment into anterior and posterior fragments. An anterior column and posterior hemitransverse fracture is an anterior column or anterior wall fracture with a transverse component that involves the posterior column. In both-column fractures, all segments of the articular surface are separated from the ilium.

TREATMENT PRINCIPLES

Residual fracture displacement, even as small as 1 to 2 mm, can lead to degenerative changes in the hip; this is especially true with weight-bearing surfaces. Deciding which fractures are best managed by operative treatment requires both plain radiographs and CT scans. Measuring the amount of intact acetabular dome is of particular importance. Three radiographic measurements (medial, anterior, and posterior roof arc) are used to determine this value. The medial roof arc measurement is determined from the anterior-posterior radiograph. A vertical line is drawn from the roof of the acetabulum to the geometric center of the femoral head. A second line is drawn from the fracture to the geometric center. The angles attended by these lines form the medial roof arc. Similar measurements are made to determine the anterior and posterior roof arcs. The former is determined on the obturator oblique view and the latter on the iliac oblique view.

A candidate for nonoperative treatment should satisfy the following criteria: (1) the anterior roof, medial roof, and posterior roof arcs are each greater than 45 degrees; (2) the posterior acetabulum wall is adequate; (3) the femoral head is congruent with the acetabular roof when traction is removed; and (4) there are no incarcerated intraarticular fracture fragments. Fracture patterns that are considered amenable to nonsurgical treatment include very low transverse fractures that do not involve the weightbearing dome- and both-column fractures without wide displacement, as determined by three arc measurements. If nonoperative management is the treatment of choice, traction should be maintained from 4 to 8 weeks to allow adequate healing and bony union.

Immediate surgical attention must be given to an acetabular fracture with an anterior or posterior dislocation that cannot be reduced by closed means. For other fractures, waiting 2 to 3 days with the

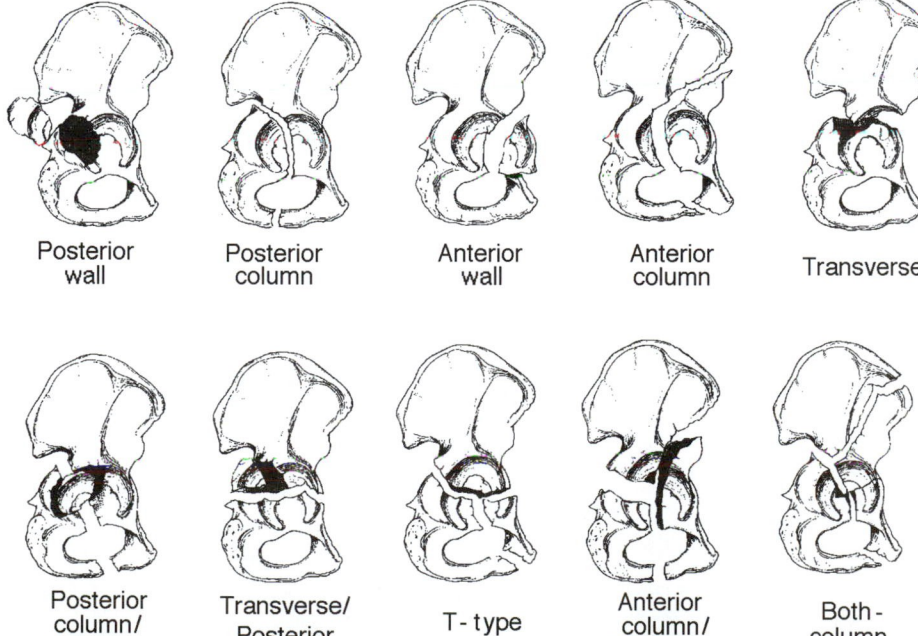

Posterior wall

Posterior column

Anterior wall

Anterior column

Transverse

Posterior column/ Posterior wall

Transverse/ Posterior wall

T-type

Anterior column/ Posterior hemitransverse

Both-column

Figure 82-2
Judet and Letournel classification of acetabular fractures. [Reproduced by permission from Matta J: Surgical treatment of acetabulum fractures. In Browner BD, Jupiter JB, Levine AM, et al (eds): *Skeletal Trauma*. Philadelphia, Saunders, 1992:902–903.]

patient in distal femoral traction is appropriate. A delay of more than 10 days will make reduction more difficult; a 3 week delay will likely have callus formation which will significantly complicate the reduction.

The incision approach is based on location and direction of the fracture lines and surgical strategy. Options include the Kocher-Langenbeck, ilioinguinal, extended iliofemoral, and tri-radiate approaches. The extended iliofemoral and triradiate approaches are extensile. Fracture stabilization employs lag screws and plates.

RESULTS

Successful outcome following acetabular fracture is highest when there is less than 3 mm residual displacement of the articular surface. However, a significant number of patients still develop osteonecrosis and require total hip arthroplasty, even with anatomic reduction. Factors associated with a poorer outcome following acetabular fracture include: younger patient age, hip dislocation upon injury, significant heterotopic ossification, and residual subluxation of the femoral head. Poor results may also be associated with extensile approaches.

COMPLICATIONS

Common complications following acetabular fracture include: infection, thromboembolism, nerve injury, heterotopic ossification, osteonecrosis, and post-traumatic arthritis. The risk of infection is significantly increased by concomitant urologic or GI injury, as well as skin laceration or degloving lesions. The most common cause of nerve palsy is retraction of the sciatic nerve during the posterior approach. Adjusting the operative position so the patient's knee is flexed to 60 degrees reduces the risk of this complication. Ectopic bone most commonly occurs with the extensile approaches; it is negligible with the ilioinguinal approach. Prophylaxis includes postoperative irradiation or indomethacin.

SUGGESTED READINGS

PELVIS

Browner BD, Cole JD: Initial management of pelvic ring disruptions. In Bassett FH III (ed): *Instructional Course Lectures,* vol 37. Park Ridge, IL: American Academy of Orthopaedic Surgeons; 1988; 37:129.

Dalal SA, Burgess AR, Siegel JH, et al: Pelvic fracture in multiple trauma: Classification by mechanism is key to pattern of organ injury, resuscitative requirements, and outcome. *J Trauma* 1989; 29:981.

Mears D: Trauma to the pelvis and acetabulum. *Curr Opin Orthop* 1990; 1:222.

Peters PC, Bucholz RW: Assessment of pelvic stability following pelvic ring disruptions. *Tech Orthop* 1990; 4:52.

Tile M: Pelvic fractures: Operative versus nonoperative treatment. *Orthop Clin North Am* 1980; 11:423.

Young WR, Burgess AR: *Radiological Management of Pelvic Ring Fractures.* Baltimore: Urban & Schwarzenberg; 1987.

ACETABULUM

Brumback AJ, Holt ES, McBride MS, et al: Acetabular depression fracture accompanying posterior fracture dislocation of the hip. *J Orthop Trauma* 1990; 4:42.

Heeg M, Oostvogel HJM, Klasen HJ: Conservative treatment of acetabular fractures: The role of the weightbearing dome and anatomic reduction in the ultimate results. *J Trauma* 1987; 27:555.

Letournel E: Classification and evaluation of acetabular fractures. *Tech Orthop* 1990; 4:5.

Matta J, Anderson L, Epstein H, et al: Fractures of the acetabulum: A retrospective analysis. *Clin Orthop* 1986; 205:230.

Matta J, Merritt PO: Displaced acetabular fractures. *Clin Orthop* 1988; 230:83.

Mayo KA: Surgical approaches to the acetabulum. *Tech Orthop* 1990; 4:24.

Mears D: Trauma to the pelvis and acetabulum. *Curr Opin Orthop* 1990; 1:222.

Routt CL, Swiontkowski ML: Operative treatment of complex acetabular fractures. *J Bone Joint Surg [Am]* 1990; 72:897.

Chapter 83

HIP

Kenneth J. Koval

HIP FRACTURES: GENERAL CONSIDERATIONS

RISK FACTORS

Hip fracture incidence increases with age, doubling every 10 years after 50 years of age. Females are affected 2 to 3 times more frequently than males; incidence in white females is reported to be more than twice that of black and Hispanic women. Risk factors for hip fracture include living in a metropolitan/urban setting, excessive use of caffeine and/or alcohol, lack of physical exercise, prior hip fracture, use of psychotropic agents (hypnotics-anxiolytics, tricyclic antidepressants, and antipsychotics), and senile dementia. In the elderly, osteoporosis should not be viewed as the cause of a hip fracture, but as a potential contributing factor along with other risk factors. There is no evidence to suggest that osteomalacia is a risk factor for hip fractures. Coxarthrosis of the ipsilateral hip is rarely associated with intracapsular femoral neck fracture; however, intertrochanteric fractures can occur when degenerative changes are present.

A simple fall is responsible for approximately 90 percent of hip fractures in the elderly; body habitus and protective responses have been implicated as co-factors impacting the risk of hip fracture following a fall. Changes in age-related neuromuscular function may also increase the probability that a hip fracture will occur after a fall. Additional age-related changes include decreased rate of ambulation (point of impact will be closer to the hip) and delayed reaction time (potential for an effective protective response is reduced).

IMAGING STUDIES

Standard radiographic evaluation for hip fractures includes an AP view of the hip and pelvis and a cross-table lateral view. Nondisplaced fractures can be difficult to identify on standard AP and lateral views. To improve the probability of detecting a nondisplaced fracture, an AP view with the lower extremity internally rotated 15 degrees may be helpful. When a fracture is suspected, but not identified on standard radiographs, an MRI or bone scan may be performed. Two to three days may be necessary for bone scintigraphy to become positive in the elderly hip fracture patient. MRI has been demonstrated to be as accurate as bone scanning in the assessment of occult fractures of the hip and can be employed within 24 h of the initial injury.

MORTALITY

In elderly patients, the overall mortality rate one year post hip fracture ranges from 14 to 36 percent. The highest mortality risk appears to occur within the first 4 to 6 months. After one year, the mortality rate is similar to age and gender-matched controls.

TREATMENT PRINCIPLES

Hip fractures should be treated surgically. Nonoperative methods result in excessive rates of morbidity and mortality, malunion, and nonunion. Nonoperative management is appropriate in nonambulators who have minimal discomfort from their injury. However, these patients should be quickly mobilized to prevent complications associated with recumbency.

If possible, all coexisting medical conditions must be evaluated, controlled, or corrected, prior to surgery. Hip fracture patients can usually undergo operative treatment within 24 h of the injury. Medically unstable patients have a significantly increased mortality risk if they undergo surgery. Regional versus general anesthesia has not been reported to significantly impact the rate of postoperative confusion or mortality in elderly hip fracture patients. In general, the objectives of postoperative management should be directed towards and support of early patient mobilization.

HIP DISLOCATIONS

Hip dislocations are generally a consequence of high-energy trauma. Associated musculoskeletal and soft tissue injuries are common and often severe; they may include craniofacial, chest, and abdominal injuries. Hip dislocations are divided into anterior and posterior types. Treatment principles include: (1) evaluation to detect associated injuries; (2) immediate closed reduction, or, if necessary, open reduction with assessment and management of hip stability; and (3) radiographic and CT evaluation for adequacy of reduction and identification of related femoral head or acetabular fracture.

If a concentric stable reduction is achieved, patients can be mobilized with protective weightbearing for 4 to 6 weeks. A nonconcentric reduction, resulting from either intraarticular osteochondral fragments, interposed soft tissue, or malreduction of associated fracture, requires open reduction with joint exploration. Management of related femoral head or acetabular fractures will be guided by the size and location of fragments and the stability of the reduction.

ANTERIOR DISLOCATIONS

Anterior dislocations can be classified as either superior or inferior and are a consequence of abduction and external rotation. These dislocations are uncommon and account for only 10 to 18 percent of all hip dislocations. Superior anterior hip dislocations occur during extension and are far more common than inferior dislocations which occur in flexion. Closed reduction is achieved by traction followed by extension and internal rotation.

Associated femoral head fractures occur in 22 to 77 percent of cases and are classified as transchondral or indentation. Transchondral fractures with nonconcentric reduction require open reduction with either excision or internal fixation; the choice is based on the fragment size and location. Indentation fractures are typically located on the superior femoral head, and do not require specific treatment. However, fracture location has important implications for prognosis.

Osteonecrosis occurs in 10 percent of anterior dislocations. Two noted risk factors are a time delay in reduction and repeated reduction attempts. Risk factors associated with posttraumatic degenerative arthritis include transchondral fracture, osteonecrosis, and indention fracture greater than 4 mm in depth.

POSTERIOR DISLOCATIONS

Posterior dislocations account for the vast majority of hip dislocations (up to 90 percent), and are caused by an axial force applied to the flexed knee. A simple dislocation occurs if the hip is in a neutral or adducted position at the time of injury. If the hip is abducted, a posterior acetabular rim fracture/dislocation occurs. Posterior dislocations as classified by Epstein are based on the presence or absence of associated acetabular and/or femoral head fracture (Fig. 83-1). Type I has no fracture or only a minor "chip" fracture. Type II has a large, single fragment of the posterior acetabular rim. Type III is a comminuted fracture of the posterior rim. Type IV has a fracture of both the acetabular rim and floor. Type V is a fracture of the femoral head with or without additional fractures.

Closed reduction consists of traction on the adducted and flexed hip. CT may be helpful to assess stability following reduction of posterior wall fracture-dislocations. Stability is inversely related to the size of the posterior acetabular fragment.

The acetabular depression fracture is a rotated, impacted osteocartilaginous fragment of the posteromedial acetabulum that occurs as a result of posterior fracture dislocation. CT evaluation has documented a 23 percent incidence. This type of depression fracture should be elevated and bone grafted.

Osteonecrosis of the femoral head occurs in over 50 percent of fracture-dislocations and in 10 percent of simple posterior dislocations. Risk is related to severity of the injury, a delay in reduction (greater than 6 to 12 h), and repeated closed reduction attempts. Risk factors for posttraumatic degenerative arthritis are a higher energy initial injury, a nonconcentric reduction, a time delay between injury and reduction, and the presence of osteonecrosis.

POSTERIOR DISLOCATIONS WITH FEMORAL HEAD FRACTURE

Posterior dislocation with associated fracture of the femoral head or neck (approximately 10 percent) was categorized by Pipkin (1957) into four types: type I are fractures of the femoral head caudal to the fovea; type II are fractures of the femoral head cephalad to the fovea; type III are type I or type II fractures plus femoral neck fracture; and type IV are type I, II, or III fractures plus fracture of the acetabular rim. Femoral head fractures are caused by an axial force applied to the flexed knee with the hip adducted and flexed less than 50 degrees.

CT scanning is preferred over standard radiographs to identify and size the femoral head fragment. Gentle closed reduction should be attempted for Pipkin types I, II, and IV; type III injuries require open

reduction. Radiographs and CT scanning following reduction should be used to evaluate concentricity and adequate reduction of the femoral head fragment.

Open reduction is mandatory for unsuccessful or nonconcentric closed reduction even if general anesthesia was used. Type III fractures in active young patients should be managed first with open reduction and internal fixation of the femoral neck fracture, followed by internal fixation of the femoral head fracture. For elderly or low functional demand patients, prosthetic replacement is indicated. Treatment of type IV injuries depends on the stability and concentricity of the reduction. Open reduction and fixation of the femoral head and acetabulum fracture are indicated if the reduction is unstable or nonconcentric.

Patients with posterior hip dislocations and associated femoral head fractures are at increased risk for developing osteonecrosis and posttraumatic degenerative arthritis; prognosis for these injuries is variable. Pipkin type I and II fractures are reported to have a prognosis similar to a simple dislocation. Pipkin type IV injuries have a prognosis similar to posterior fracture-dislocations without a femoral head fracture. Pipkin type III injuries have a poor prognosis.

FEMORAL NECK FRACTURES

ANATOMY

The femoral neck rises from the intertrochanteric line and extends to the base of the femoral head. The cylindrical neck forms an angle of 125 to 140 degrees with the femoral shaft in the anteroposterior plane and 10 to 15 degrees (anteversion) in the lateral plane. The complete anterior aspect of the femoral neck and the proximal half of the posterior aspect lie within the hip joint capsule.

The femoral artery serves as the blood supply of the femoral head. A branch, the profunda femoris, divides into the medial and lateral femoral circumflex arteries. The medial femoral circumflex and the ascending branch of the lateral femoral circumflex form the extra-capsular arterial ring at the base of the femoral neck. Ascending cervical arteries branch off this arterial ring and traverse the neck proximally. Finally, small branches of the ascending cervical arteries descend into the femoral neck and anastomose with the intramedullary nutrient artery of the femur. As the ascending cervical arteries approach the junction of the head and neck, they create the intracapsular ring, the branches of which then penetrate the femoral head and function as its primary blood supply. In adults, an artery that travels within the ligamentum teres has a limited role in supplying blood to the femoral head.

CLASSIFICATION

The most commonly referred-to classification of femoral neck fractures is the Garden classification (Fig. 83-2). Femoral neck fractures are divided into four types depending on the degree of displacement of fracture fragments. A type I fracture is an incomplete or valgus impacted fracture. A type II fracture is a complete fracture without displacement. A type III fracture is a complete fracture with partial displacement of fracture fragments. A type IV fracture is a complete

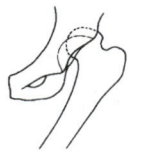 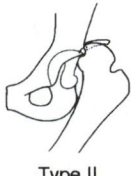 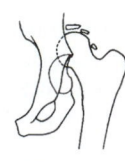 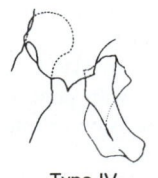 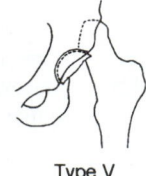

Type I   Type II   Type III   Type IV   Type V

Figure 83-1

Thompson and Epstein classification of posterior hip dislocations. [Reproduced by permission from DeLee JC: Fractures and dislocations of the hip. In Rockwood CA, Green DP, Bucholz RW, et al (eds): *Fractures in Adults*, 4th ed. Philadelphia: Lippincott; 1996:1761–1763.]

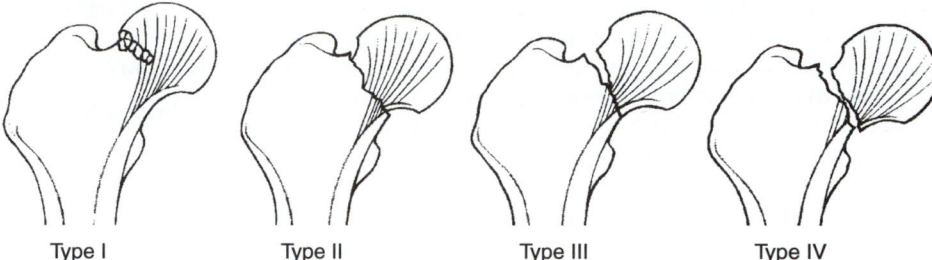

Figure 83-2
Garden classification of femoral neck fractures. [Reproduced by permission from Swiontkowski MF: Hip dislocations and femoral head fractures. In Hansen S, Swiontkowski MF (eds): *Orthopaedic Trauma Protocols*. New York: Raven Press; 1993:238.]

Type I   Type II   Type III   Type IV

fracture with total displacement of the fragments which allows the femoral head to rotate back to an anatomical position. In practice, it is difficult to differentiate among the four types. Therefore, classifying femoral neck fractures as nondisplaced (Garden I and II) or displaced (Garden III and IV) may facilitate arriving at an accurate diagnosis.

TREATMENT PRINCIPLES

Nondisplaced femoral neck fractures (Garden types I and II) should be internally stabilized using multiple lag screws or pins placed in parallel (Fig. 83-3). Most authors have reported a successful outcome with three or four pins/screws for both nondisplaced and displaced fractures.

Treatment of the displaced femoral neck fracture is controversial. Generally, closed/open reduction and internal fixation is the preferred treatment in active younger patients and primary prosthetic replacement in less active older patients. There appears to be general consensus that when internal fixation is employed, achieving anatomic reduction is probably the single most important factor that contributes to preventing postoperative healing complications. An adequate reduction may have up to 15 degrees of valgus angulation and less than 10 degrees of anterior or posterior angulation. Although immediate reduction of displaced fractures has been consistently recommended, this approach has not consistently decreased the rate of nonunion or osteonecrosis. If closed reduction is not satisfactory, open reduction through an antero-lateral approach may be required. Hemiarthroplasty is an alternative treatment for displaced femoral neck fractures in older, less active patients. Historically, a one-piece Austin Moore or Thompson endoprosthesis was utilized in the treatment of these fractures. Although successful in select patient populations, use of these prostheses has been reported to be associated with increased rates of acetabular erosion and loosening of the femoral stem. The availability and use of methyl methacrylate has reduced the incidence of femoral stem loosening; however, acetabular wear has remained a problem. Factors which best correlate with the development of severe acetabular erosion are patient activity level and duration of follow-up.

The bipolar prosthesis is a self-articulating device. It was designed to reduce the incidence of acetabular erosion by encouraging hip motion at a low friction inner bearing. However, controversy remains regarding indications and the amount of actual motion occurring at the outer and inner surfaces of the prosthesis.

Primary total hip arthroplasty has a role in the treatment of acute femoral neck fractures for patients with preexisting acetabular disease (rheumatoid arthritis, osteoarthritis, Paget's disease).

STRESS FRACTURES

Stress fractures of the femoral neck are uncommon injuries, which usually occur in athletes and military recruits. They are classified as either tension or compression fractures. Tension fractures are found on the superior aspect of the femoral neck, are potentially unstable, and require surgical stabilization. Compression fractures occur on the inferior aspect of the femoral neck. They are more stable than tension fractures, and can be managed nonoperatively. Treatment recommendations are a brief period of rest followed by protected weightbearing and frequent serial radiographs to monitor changes in fracture pattern or displacement. Indications for internal fixation are radiographic documentation of a fracture widening or disruption of both cortices.

COMPLICATIONS OF FEMORAL NECK FRACTURES

Postoperative complications associated with internal fixation of femoral neck fractures include loss of fixation, infection, nonunion and osteonecrosis. Early failure of fixation occurs in 12 to 24 percent

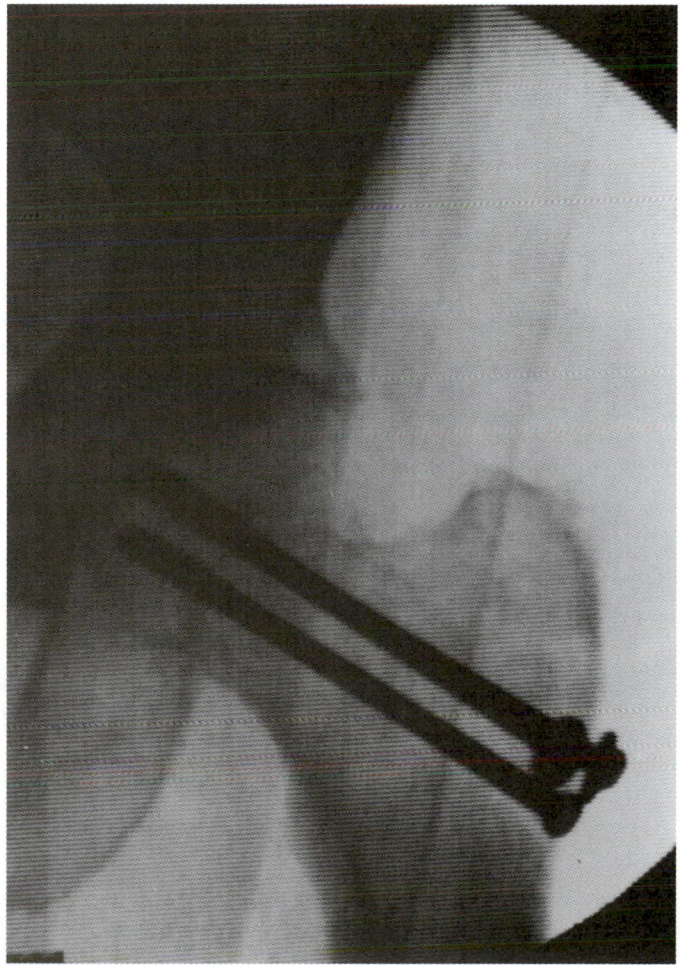

Figure 83-3
Nondisplaced femoral neck fracture treated with multiple screws.

of displaced femoral neck fractures. The incidence of nonunion is related to the type of fracture. Nonunion occurs in 0 to 5 percent of cases in nondisplaced fractures and 9 to 35 percent in displaced fractures. The osteonecrosis rate following nondisplaced femoral neck fracture is usually reported as 5 to 8 percent; however, some authors have reported a rate as high as 15 percent. The osteonecrosis rate following displaced femoral neck fracture has been as high as 9 to 35 percent, with most series reporting 20 to 35 percent. Factors influencing the development of osteonecrosis include a time delay in reduction, inadequate reduction, and use of sliding hip screw or nail plate devices.

Postoperative complications after primary prosthetic replacement for acute femoral neck fracture are infection, dislocation, and pain related to acetabular erosion and prosthetic loosening. Recent series of prosthetic replacements (usually bipolar endoprostheses) have reported infection rates of 2 to 8 percent. The incidence of infection varies with the surgical approach; rates are higher with a posterior approach. The reported incidence of postoperative dislocation after prosthetic replacement varies from 1 to 10 percent, the posterior approach being associated with a higher dislocation rate than the anterior. Dislocation seems to occur less frequently after bipolar hemiarthroplasty; however, closed reduction of a dislocated bipolar endoprosthesis is more difficult to achieve than a dislocated unipolar hemiarthroplasty.

INTERTROCHANTERIC FRACTURES

ANATOMY

The intertrochanteric region is extracapsular. It includes the greater and lesser trochanters as well as the transitional bone between the femoral neck and shaft. The bone in this region is primarily dense trabecular bone that transmits and distributes stresses. The calcar femorale is a vertical wall of dense bone arising from the posteromedial aspect of the femoral shaft and extending to the posterior portion of the femoral neck. It functions as an internal trabecular strut within the inferior portion of the neck and intertrochanteric region, acting as a conduit for significant stresses in this area. Cancellous bone in the calcar femorale is highly vascularized. As a result, nonunion and osteonecrosis after intertrochanteric fracture rarely occurs.

CLASSIFICATION

The most commonly used classification system devised for intertrochanteric hip fractures was introduced by Evans in 1949. Hip fracture types are based on fracture stability and the ability to achieve a stable reduction (Fig. 83-4). Evans recognized the key contribution to a stable reduction was the restoration of posteromedial cortical continuity. In stable fracture patterns, the posteromedial cortex re-

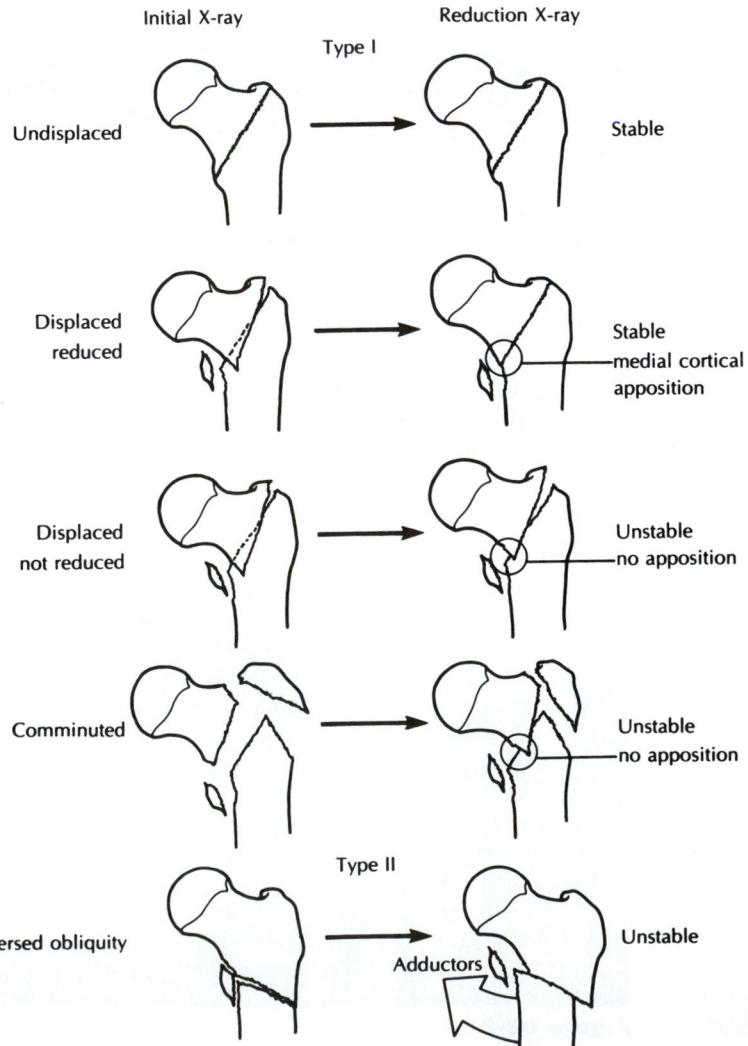

Figure 83-4

The Evans classification of intertrochanteric fractures. [Reproduced by permission from DeLee JC: Fractures and dislocations of the hip. In Rockwood CA, Green DP, Bucholz RW, et al. (eds): *Fractures in Adults,* 4th ed. Philadelphia: Lippincott; 1996:1721.]

mained intact and a stable reduction could be achieved. Unstable fracture patterns were characterized by comminution of the posteromedial cortex in the region of the calcar femorale. Although these fractures were inherently unstable, they could be converted to a stable reduction, if medial cortical opposition was obtained. Evans also realized that the reverse obliquity pattern was inherently unstable due to the tendency for medial displacement of the shaft. The development of this system of classification was important, because it differentiated stable and unstable fracture patterns and also helped to define the characteristics of a stable reduction. Later studies using the Evans classification, however, have reported poor reproducibility. Therefore, it may be more prudent to classify intertrochanteric fractures as either stable or unstable, dependent on the status of the posteromedial cortex. Unstable fracture patterns are fractures with comminution of the posteromedial cortex, intertrochanteric fractures with subtrochanteric extension, and reverse obliquity fractures.

TREATMENT PRINCIPLES

Virtually all intertrochanteric hip fractures need operative stabilization in order to allow early patient mobilization. The vast majority of intertrochanteric hip fractures can be managed by a closed reduction and internal fixation. If an acceptable closed reduction cannot be achieved after several attempts with gentle manipulation and traction, more aggressive manipulation should not be applied. An open reduction is then preferred. With release of traction and limited fracture site exposure, the fragments can generally be manipulated into an acceptable position.

The most suitable implant for fixation of intertrochanteric fractures is the sliding hip screw (Fig. 83-5). The need for medial displacement osteotomy using the sliding hip screw remains controversial. Because the sliding hip screw provides for controlled fracture collapse, unstable fractures that are anatomically aligned can be expected to spontaneously settle to a stable and often medially displaced position. The result is less shortening of the extremity than in a formal medial displacement osteotomy.

The most significant step in sliding hip screw insertion is secure placement of the screw within the proximal fragment. The screw should be placed within 1 cm of the subchondral bone. A central position between the femoral head and the neck is the usual recommendation. A posteroinferior position is preferred if a central position is not possible. Because the bone is weakest in the anterosuperior aspect, screw placement should be avoided in this region. The likelihood of superior screw cut-out is, therefore, less likely. If a large posteromedial fragment exists, an effort should be made to internally stabilize the fragment in a near anatomical position with a lag screw or cerclage wire.

A modified approach is used for basilar neck fractures. These fractures are extracapsular and are located just proximal to the intertrochanteric line. Insertion of the sliding hip screw into the head and neck may cause the proximal fragment to rotate. To avoid this, two wires are inserted; the first is placed in an inferior position and the second more superiorly. The hip screw is inserted over the inferior guide wire, and an "anti-rotation" cancellous screw is inserted over the superior guide wire. This technique prevents rotation of the head and neck fragment during reaming and screw insertion.

Reverse obliquity fractures are unstable fractures. They are characterized by an oblique fracture line that extends from the medial cortex laterally and slightly distally. The position and direction of the fracture line results in a tendency towards medial displacement due to the pull of the adductor muscles.

The controlled impaction that is characteristic of the sliding hip screw will not occur in this setting due to the location and angle of

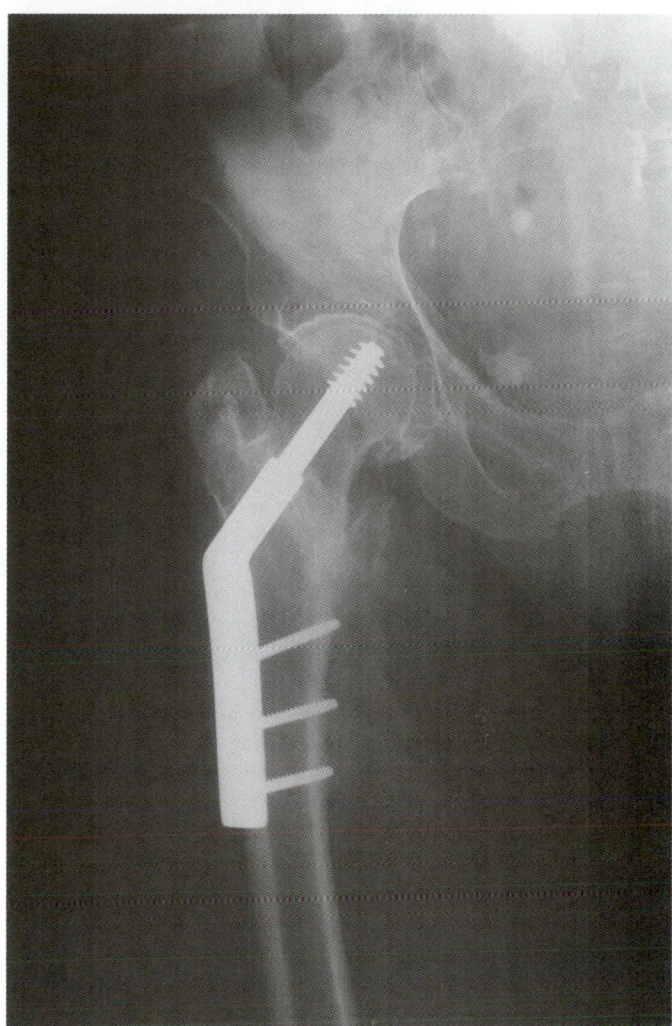

Figure 83-5
Intertrochanteric hip fracture treated with sliding hip screw.

the fracture line. The sliding portion of the device is located completely within the proximal fragment; the plate and screws stabilize the distal fragment. These types of fracture are most suitably managed similar to subtrochanteric fractures using an intramedullary nail, an intramedullary hip screw, or a 95-degree fixed-angle device.

Intramedullary devices have been used for the management of intertrochanteric fractures, most particularly Ender nails. Complication rates have varied widely, from 16 to 71 percent; the most common events are varus deformity, knee pain caused by distal migration of the nails, and external rotation deformity. Reoperation has been reported to be necessary in up to 19 percent of cases; the highest complication rate occurs in the treatment of unstable fractures.

Intramedullary hip screws combine the features of both a sliding hip screw and an intramedullary nail and have recently been applied to the treatment of intertrochanteric fractures. Theoretically, they can be inserted in a virtually closed manner with limited fracture exposure, decreased blood loss, and less tissue damage than with a sliding hip screw. These devices are also subjected to a lower bending moment than the sliding hip screw due to the intramedullary location. Despite these apparent advantages, recent studies have not documented a clinical advantage of the intramedullary hip screw compared to the sliding hip screw.

Prosthetic replacement has been successfully used with intertrochanteric fractures to manage postoperative fixation loss when repeat open reduction and internal fixation is not feasible or desired. A calcar replacement prosthesis is also required due to the fracture level. Primary prosthetic replacement for comminuted, unstable fractures has been successfully applied in patients. However, this is a larger, more extensive surgical procedure, and there is a potential for dislocation. Its usefulness in the management of acute intertrochanteric fractures has not been defined, and the procedure has no apparent advantages over a properly inserted sliding hip screw.

COMPLICATIONS

Varus displacement following internal fixation is generally associated with unstable fractures because of inadequate posteromedial support. In varus displacement, the screw typically "cuts out" through the anterosuperior aspect of the femoral head. Other complications include implant breakage or bending, screw penetration into the joint and disassociation of the plate from the shaft (screws breaking or pulling out). These problems are less likely to occur with the sliding hip screw than with fixed nail-plate devices. The latter complications occur as a result of other factors including: (1) insertion of the screw into the anterosuperior portion of the femoral head; (2) improper reaming (creates a second channel); (3) inability to achieve a stable reduction; (4) excessive collapse of the fracture (sliding capacity of the device is exceeded); (5) inadequate screw-barrel engagement (prevents sliding); and (6) severe osteoporosis (precludes secure fixation).

SUBTROCHANTERIC FRACTURES

ANATOMY

The subtrochanteric region extends distally 5 cm from the lesser trochanter. It is primarily thick, dense cortical bone and forms the cylindrical shape of the femoral shaft. The subtrochanteric region transmits both axial and torsional loads, and functions as a region of high stress concentration.

INCIDENCE AND MECHANISMS OF INJURY

Approximately 15 percent of all proximal femur fractures are subtrochanteric fractures (Fig. 83-6), and are generally seen in three types of patients: (1) young patients with normal bones who are involved in high-energy trauma; (2) older patients with weakened bone whose fracture occurred as a result of a minor fall; and (3) older patients with pathological or impending pathological fractures associated with metastatic lesions.

CLASSIFICATION

Various classification systems have been proposed, but none have been universally accepted. Determining fracture stability is essential in planning treatment. Fracture stability depends on the presence or absence of a posteromedial buttress, similar to intertrochanteric fractures. In stable fractures, medial and posteromedial cortical support remains intact or can be reestablished. In unstable fractures, comminution causes a loss of medial cortical continuity; these fractures are at the highest risk for postoperative complications and implant failure.

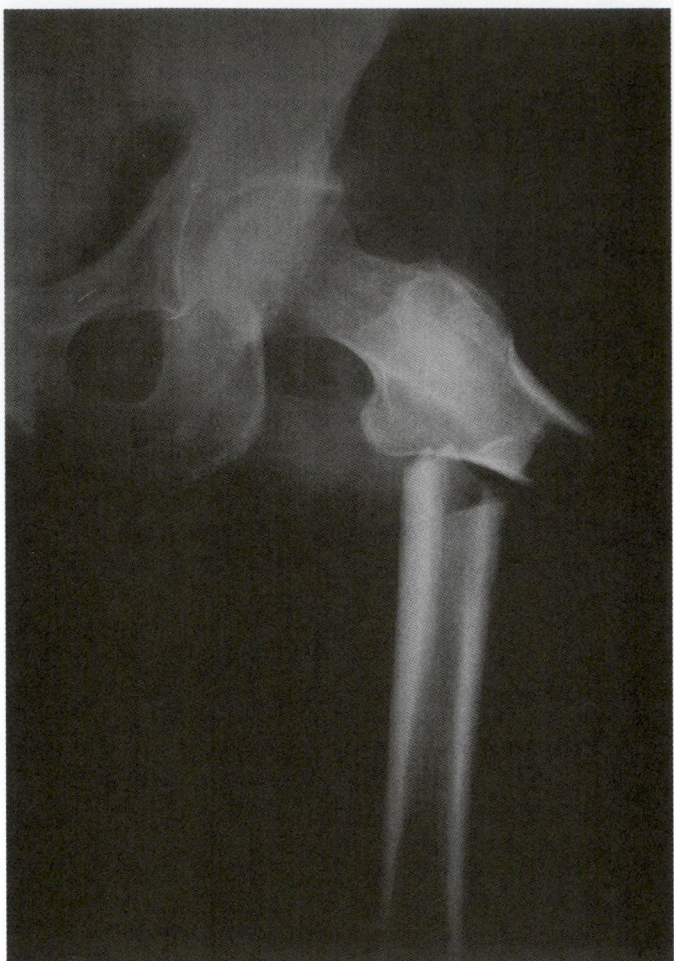

Figure 83-6
Left subtrochanteric femur fracture.

TREATMENT PRINCIPLES

Operative stabilization is required for virtually all subtrochanteric fractures. Interlocked nails are the implant of choice in subtrochanteric fractures. Regardless of the fracture pattern or degree of comminution, virtually all nonpathologic subtrochanteric fractures can be stabilized by interlocked nails. Their favorable mechanical and functional characteristics have obviated the need to surgically reconstitute the medial femoral cortex. Use of interlocked nails has produced high rates of union in large series of subtrochanteric femur fractures.

When the fracture line in subtrochanteric fractures extends toward the piriformis fossa, plate and screws are the best implant devices. Intramedullary nailing is more problematic. In elderly patients with low-energy subtrochanteric fractures, good results have been reported using a sliding hip screw. One series reported a 95 percent union rate. For optimal function, the sliding component of the device must cross the fracture site. Alternatively, a 95-degree fixed-angle device such as a blade plate or condylar screw can also be used. If the medial cortex is not broken, these devices provide enhanced fixation of the proximal fragment and function as a lateral tension band. The condylar screw is technically simpler to insert than the blade plate. Recent studies documenting the treatment of subtrochanteric fractures have reported similar positive results with either device. The 95-degree devices appear to offer the greatest advantage when an anatomic reduction is possible. Complication rates of up to 20 percent have been reported; problems are usually related to difficulties in restoring the medial femoral cortex. It is possible to reduce complications with indirect reduction techniques that minimize soft tissue stripping. Bone grafting should be performed if significant medial cortical comminution or soft tissue stripping exist.

SUGGESTED READINGS

HIP AND FEMORAL HEAD

Brumback RJ, Kenzora JE, Levitt LE, et al: Fractures of the femoral head. In Brand RA (ed): *The Hip. Proceedings of the 14th Open Scientific Meeting of the Hip Society, 1986.* St. Louis: Mosby; 1987:181.

DeLee JC, Evans JA, Thomas J: Anterior dislocations of the hip and associated femoral head fractures. *J Bone Joint Surg [Am]* 1980; 62:960.

Epstein HC: Posterior fracture dislocations of the hip: Long-term follow-up. *J Bone Joint Surg [Am]* 1974; 56:1103.

Epstein HC: Traumatic dislocations of the hip. *Clin Orthop* 1973; 92:116.

Epstein HC, Wiss DA, Cozen L: Posterior fracture dislocations of the hip with fractures of the femoral head. *Clin Orthop* 1985; 201:9.

Hougard K, Thomsen PB: Traumatic posterior fracture dislocation of the hip with fracture of the femoral head or neck or both. *J Bone Joint Surg [Am]* 1988; 70:233.

Pipkin G: Treatment of grade IV fracture dislocation of the hip. *J Bone Joint Surg [Am]* 1957; 39:1027.

Thompsen VP, Epstein HC: Traumatic dislocation of the hip. *J Bone Joint Surg [Am]* 1951; 33:746.

INTERTROCHANTERIC HIP

Boyd HB, Griffin LL: Classification and treatment of trochanteric fractures. *Arch Surg* 1949; 58:853.

Chang WS, Zuckerman JD, Kummer FJ, et al: Biomechanical evaluation of anatomic reduction versus medial displacement osteotomy in unstable intertrochanteric fractures. *Clin Orthop* 1987; 225:141.

Evans EM: The treatment of trochanteric fractures of the femur. *J Bone Joint Surg [Br]* 1949; 31:190.

Kyle RF, Gustilo RB, Premer RF: Analysis of six hundred and twenty-one intertrochanteric hip fractures. *J Bone Joint Surg [Am]* 1979; 61:216.

Zuckerman JD, Schon LC: Hip fractures. In Zuckerman JD, ed: *Comprehensive Care of the Elderly.* Baltimore: Urban & Schwarzenberg; 1990:69–90.

SUBTROCHANTERIC HIP

Fielding JW, Magliato HJ: Subtrochanteric fractures. *Surg Gynecol Obstet* 1966; 122:555.

Johnson KD: Current techniques in the treatment of subtrochanteric fractures. *Tech Orthop* 1988; 3:14.

Seinsheimer F: Subtrochanteric fractures of the femur. *J Bone Joint Surg [Am]* 1978; 60:300.

Chapter 84

FEMORAL SHAFT

Kenneth J. Koval

FEMORAL SHAFT FRACTURES

ANATOMY

The femoral shaft is apportioned into four areas: subtrochanteric, isthmal, infraisthmal, and supracondylar. The *isthmus* is the region where the intramedullary canal is narrowest. The medullary canal widens within the *infraisthmal area*. The *supracondylar* area flares out to become the distal femoral condyles. Three fascial compartments (anterior, medial, posterior) contain the entire thigh musculature. The blood supply to the femoral shaft is predominately from the profundus femoral artery.

MECHANISM OF INJURY

Femoral shaft fractures are generally high energy injuries. A first priority in these patients is to rule out the presence of other life-threatening injuries. Femoral shaft fractures in the elderly caused by low-energy trauma characteristically have spiral and oblique fracture patterns.

RADIOGRAPHIC EVALUATION

Radiographic views include an AP of the pelvis, and AP and lateral radiographs of the complete femur, including the hip and knee. The possibility of concurrent fractures, such as ipsilateral femoral neck and shaft fractures, must be excluded.

CLASSIFICATION

Classification of femoral shaft fractures is based on fracture location, fracture pattern, degree of comminution, associated soft tissue injury, and mechanism of injury. Winquist (1984) classified the degree of comminution by type (Fig. 84-1): type I is a small butterfly fracture involving less than 25 percent of the width of the bone; type II is a larger butterfly fragment or comminution involving 50 percent or less of the circumference of the bone; type III is a butterfly fragment or comminution involving more than 50 percent of the circumference of the bone; and type IV are comminuted fractures with segmental comminution and no contact within major proximal distal fragments. Types III and IV fractures are unstable in length and rotation.

TREATMENT PRINCIPLES

Prompt stabilization of the femoral shaft, particularly in the polytraumatized patient, is important to optimize patient mobility and pulmonary function. The implant used for practically all femoral shaft fractures is an interlocked nail (Fig. 84-2). Interlocked nails have both mechanical and biological advantages over plates and screws in that the intramedullary location brings less stress to the implant, they have the potential for load sharing, and they can be inserted with minimal tissue dissection.

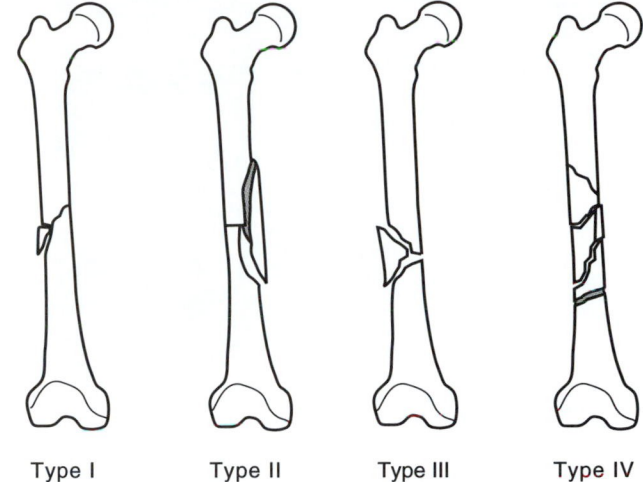

| Type I | Type II | Type III | Type IV |

Figure 84-1

Winquist and Hansen classification of femoral shaft fractures. [Reproduced by permission from Johnson KD. Femoral shaft fracture. In Browner BD, Jupiter JB, Levine AM: et al, eds: *Skeletal Trauma*. Philadelphia: WB Saunders; 1992:1537.]

Closed interlocked nailing is preferred over open nailing, but an open technique will achieve similar results if the incision is primarily for reduction and there is minimal soft tissue dissection. Reaming the femoral canal allows a larger diameter nail to be used which enhances fixation stability. Inserting unreamed smaller diameter nails has been recommended in open femur fractures and in patients with associated pulmonary injury where emboli created by reaming may result in further lung injury. Femoral nails should be routinely locked proximally and distally; a 10 percent loss of reduction was reported by Brumback and coworkers (1988) when femoral nails were dynamically locked. There is no need for routine dynamization of statically locked femoral nails

OPEN FRACTURES

All open fractures must be thoroughly debrided. Following debridement, fractures of Gustilo grade I, II, and IIIA may undergo immediate intramedullary nailing, whether the patient has multiple injuries or an isolated fracture (Gustilo, 1993). Patients with the settings of grade IIIB and IIIC fractures require individual approaches. The use of unreamed nails for open fractures should be considered.

Compartment syndrome of the thigh is relatively rare. It occurs in patients with multiple injuries and those presenting with systemic hypotension, coagulopathy, vascular injury, and thigh trauma with or without fracture.

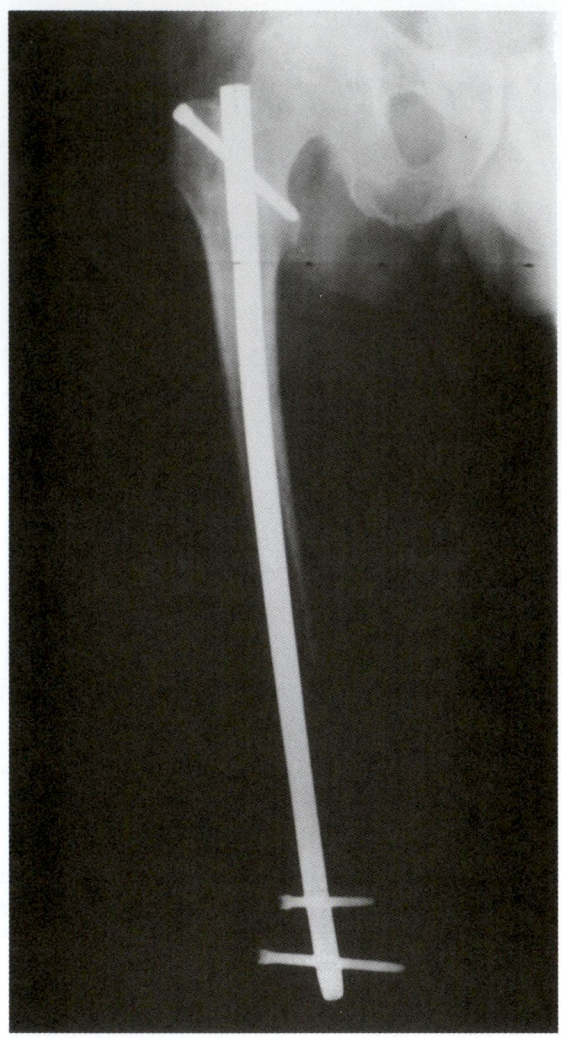

Figure 84-2
Femoral shaft fracture using an interlocked intramedullary nail.

GUNSHOT FRACTURES

Femur fractures which are the result of low-velocity gunshot wounds are treated as closed fractures following debridement of the entrance and exit wounds. Wounds secondary to close-range shotgun blasts and high velocity rifles are managed similar to type III open fractures.

IPSILATERAL FEMORAL NECK AND SHAFT FRACTURE

Ipsilateral femoral neck and shaft fractures occur in up to 5 percent of femoral shaft fractures; they are frequently overlooked on initial examination. The best clinical results are obtained by simultaneous stabilization of the hip and shaft.

FEMORAL SHAFT AND ASSOCIATED KNEE LIGAMENT INJURY

The incidence of ipsilateral femoral shaft and knee ligament injury is approximately 5 percent. Following stabilization of all femoral shaft fractures, ligamentous stability should be assessed intraoperatively.

RESULTS

Closed femoral nailing has a union rate of approximately 98 percent; healing time to union ranges from 16 to 20 weeks. Almost 90 percent of patients will achieve a preinjury range of knee motion.

COMPLICATIONS

The infection rate following closed intramedullary femoral nailing ranges from 0.5 to 1.5 percent. The infection rate following nailing of open femur fractures ranges from 0 to 4 percent. Delayed union and nonunion occurs in 0 to 2 percent of cases. The most frequent postoperative complication of femoral shaft fracture is malunion, particularly with use of a dynamically locked nail.

DISTAL FEMUR FRACTURES

ANATOMY

The supracondylar area of the distal femur extends from the infraisthmus to the femoral condyles. This region of the distal femur is metaphyseal; its characteristics include a wide intramedullary canal, thin cortices, and poor bone stock. The anatomic axis of the femur has an average valgus angulation of 9 degrees (range is 7 to 11 degrees). Muscle attachments associated with the distal femur produce characteristic fracture deformities. The gastrocnemius muscle produces posterior condyle displacement with apex posterior angulation. When intercondylar fracture extension exists, rotational malalignment occurs from the pull of the medial and lateral heads of the gastrocnemius. The superficial femoral artery enters the popliteal fossa approximately 10 cm proximal to the knee, passing through the adductor magnus muscle.

INCIDENCE AND MECHANISM OF INJURY

With hip fractures excluded, fractures of the distal femur represent 30 percent of all fractures of the femur. They occur mainly within two populations: in the young, following high-energy trauma and in the elderly, after a low-energy fall. Relative to the younger population, the mechanism of injury is generally one of direct impact on the flexed knee. In the elderly, axial loading together with varus/valgus or rotational forces is the mechanism of injury.

RADIOGRAPHIC EVALUATION

Radiographic evaluation includes an AP and lateral view of the distal femur. Oblique radiographs at 45 degrees may help to establish the extent of intercondylar extension. With highly comminuted or displaced fractures, traction radiographs may improve fracture definition. Tomograms and CT may be employed to further define intraarticular involvement.

CLASSIFICATION

No single classification system of distal femur fractures is universally accepted; however, virtually all distinguish between extraarticular and intraarticular fractures. The most widely accepted was described by Müeller and coworkers (1991) and divides distal femur fractures into three groups: type A is extraarticular; type B is unicondylar; and type C is bicondylar (Fig. 84-3). The three types are further separated into three subgroups. These latter subgroups represent severity of the fracture and the impact on treatment and prognosis.

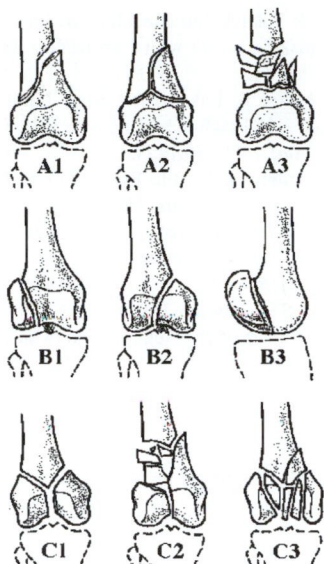

Figure 84-3
AO classification of distal femur fractures. [Reproduced by permission from Müller ME. The comprehensive classification of fractures of long bones. In Müller ME, Allgöwer M, Schneider R, et al eds: *Manual of Internal Fixation,* 3d ed. New York: Springer-Verlag; 1991:141.]

TREATMENT PRINCIPLES

A splint should be applied to the injured lower extremity immediately following the initial assessment. If surgery will be delayed for several or more hours, a proximal tibial traction pin should be inserted in a location away from the planned operative field. Skeletal traction is then applied with the knee flexed to relax the gastrocnemius muscle.

A knee immobilizer or cast may be used for impacted or minimally displaced fractures in which intercondylar displacement does not occur. The immobilizer or cast may be replaced later with a fracture brace or cast brace once the pain and swelling have subsided. The patient should mobilize with partial weightbearing ambulation on the involved extremity. Fracture alignment must be monitored for fracture displacement until union has occurred.

Displaced supracondylar and intercondylar distal femur fractures mandate anatomic articular restoration and stable fixation, followed by early range of knee motion. Absolute surgical indications are: open fracture, fractures with vascular compromise, and fractures associated with compartment syndrome.

The distal femoral articular surface requires anatomical reduction and stabilization. Large cancellous screws with washers are the best treatment option to achieve definitive stability. Screw location depends on the choice of fixation device for shaft stabilization.

Implants used for stabilization of supracondylar fractures are: (1) 95-degree fixed-angle condylar blade-plates or screws (Fig. 84-4); (2) condylar buttress plates; (3) interlocked intramedullary nails, placed either antegrade or retrograde; (4) flexible intramedullary nails; and (5) external fixators.

UNICONDYLAR FRACTURES

Displaced unicondylar fractures require anatomic reduction and internal fixation to restore joint congruity and permit early range of knee motion. Coronal fractures of the medial or lateral condyle (Hoffa

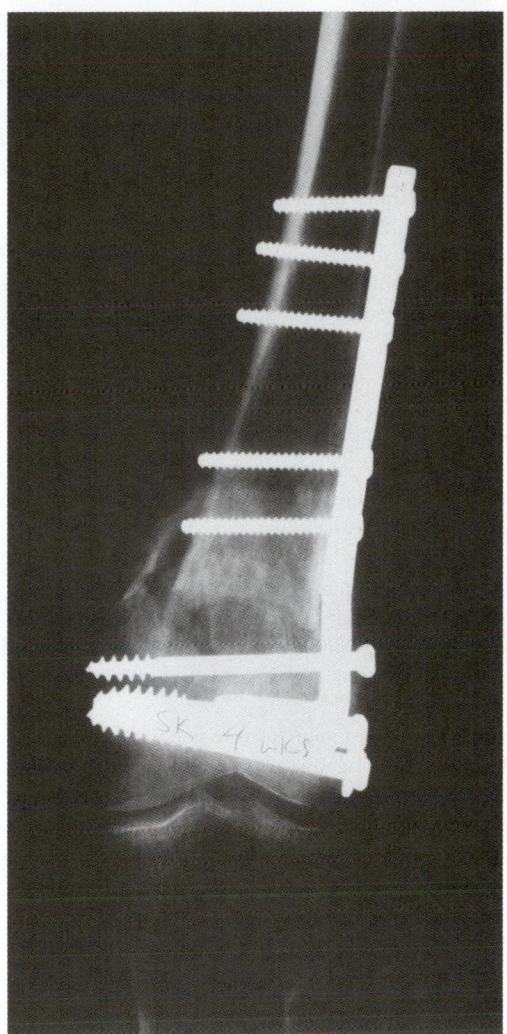

Figure 84-4
Distal femur fracture stabilized with a 95-degree dynamic condylar screw.

fractures) ought to be stabilized with cancellous lag screws countersunk below the articular surface. Medial and lateral sagittal unicondylar fractures need to be stabilized with cancellous lag screws and washers. Depending on the bone quality, an antiglide plate is applied to enhance stability.

BONE GRAFTING

Medial fracture comminution or fracture sites involving soft tissue stripping should be bone grafted, especially when the fracture is stabilized using a lateral plate. Studies have recently suggested bone grafting may not be necessary if the medial aspect of the distal femur and the associated soft tissue attachments are left undisturbed by using indirect reduction techniques.

RESULTS

The outcome of operative and nonoperative treatments depends on the degree of severity of the fracture and the quality and stability of the reduction. Good to excellent results can be anticipated with nonoperative treatment of minimally displaced and impacted distal femur fractures. The percentage of good to excellent results following displaced distal femur fracture are more variable. A series of 30 distal femur fractures stabilized with a 95-degree condylar blade plate was reported by Mize and colleagues (1982). Eighty percent had good to excellent results at an average follow-up of 28 months. Sanders and coworkers (1989) reported a study of 35 distal femur fractures that were stabilized with a 95-degree dynamic condylar screw. With an average follow-up of 28 months, 71 percent of patients had good to excellent results. Leung and coworkers (1991) published findings from a series of 37 supracondylar and intercondylar femur fractures using interlocked intramedullary nailing. All fractures achieved union, and 94 percent (31) achieved a good or excellent result.

COMPLICATIONS

The most common complications following distal femur fracture include: infection, nonunion, malunion, loss of fixation, and loss of knee motion. Recent studies show the range of infection and nonunion rates following operative stabilization of distal femur fractures is 0 to 6 percent. Conditions that influence infection and nonunion include: (1) high energy injuries, particularly fractures with significant osseous devascularization; (2) open fractures; (3) extensive surgical dissection which compromises osseous vascularity; (4) an inexperienced operating team with a prolonged open wound time; and (5) inadequate fixation.

Malunion after distal femur fracture is more frequent with nonoperative than operative treatment. The most common deformity observed with distal femoral malunion is varus and recurvatum. Distal femur fractures are in close proximity to the knee, and frequently result in limited knee motion. Possible etiologies for the loss of knee motion are: protruding intraarticular hardware, articular malreduction, intraarticular adhesions, ligamentous or capsular contractures, quadriceps or hamstring scarring, and post-traumatic arthritis.

SUGGESTED READINGS

FEMORAL SHAFT

Brumback RJ, Ellison PS, Poka A: Intramedullary nailing of femoral shaft fractures. III. Long term effects of static interlocking fixation. *J Bone Joint Surg [Am]* 1992; 74:106.
Brumback RJ, Ellison PS, Poka A, et al: Intramedullary nailing of open fractures of the femoral shaft. *J Bone Joint Surg [Am]* 1989; 71:1324.
Brumback RJ, Reilly JP, Poka A: Intramedullary nailing of femoral shaft fractures. I. Decision making errors with interlocking fixation. *J Bone Joint Surg [Am]* 1988; 70:1441.
Brumback RJ, Uwagie-Ero S, Lakatos RP, et al: Intramedullary nailing of femoral shaft fractures. II. Fracture healing with static interlocking fixation. *J Bone Joint Surg [Am]* 1988; 70:1453.
Gustilo RB, Open Fractures. In Gustilo RB, Kyle RF, Templeton DC (eds): *Fractures and Dislocation.* St. Louis: Mosby, 1993:169.
Gustilo RB, Anderson JT: Prevention of Infection in the treatment of one thousand and twenty-five open fractures of long bones: Retrospective and prospective analyses. *J Bone Joint Surg [Am]*, 1976; 58:453.
Winquist RA, Hansen ST, Clawson DK: Closed intramedullary nailing of femoral fractures: A report of five hundred and twenty cases. *J Bone Joint Surg [Am]* 1984; 66:529.

FEMORAL NECK

Barnes JT, Brown JT, Garden RS, et al: Subcapital fractures of the femur: A prospective review. *J Bone Joint Surg [Br]* 1976; 58:2.
Frandsen PA, Andersen E, Madsen F, et al: Gardens classification of femoral neck fractures: An assessment of interobserver variation. *J Bone Joint Surg [Br]* 1988; 70:588.
Pauwels F: *Biomechanics of the Normal and Diseased Hip.* New York: Springer-Verlag; 1976.
Swiontkowski MF: Intracapsular fractures of the hip. *J Bone Joint Surg [Am]* 1994; 76;129.

DISTAL FEMUR

Johnson KD, Hicken G: Distal femoral fractures. *Orthop Clin North Am* 1987; 18:115.
Leung KS, Shen WY, So WS, et al: Interlocking intramedullary nailing for supracondylar and intercondylar fractures of the distal part of the femur. *J Bone Joint Surg [Am]* 1991; 73:332.
Mize RD, Bucholz RW, Grogan DP: Surgical treatment of displaced, comminuted fractures of the distal end of the femur. *J Bone Joint Surg [Am]* 1982; 64:871.
Neer CS II, Grantham SA, Shelton ML: Supracondylar fracture of the adult femur. *J Bone Joint Surg [Am]* 1967; 49:591.
Sanders R, Regazzoni P, Ruedi TP: Treatment of supracondylar-intercondylar fractures of the femur using the dynamic condylar screw. *J Orthop Trauma* 1989; 3:214.
Schatzker J, Lambert DC: Supracondylar fractures of the femur. *Clin Orthop* 1979; 138:77.
Seinsheimer F: Fractures of the distal femur. *Clin Orthop* 1980; 153:169.
Siliski JM, Mahring M, Hofer HP: Supracondylar-intercondylar fractures of the femur: Treatment by internal fixation. *J Bone Joint Surg [Am]* 1989; 71:95.

Chapter 85

KNEE

Kenneth J. Koval

KNEE DISLOCATION

INCIDENCE AND MECHANISM OF INJURY

Knee dislocations are rare but represent an orthopaedic emergency secondary to the possibility of vascular disruption within the popliteal fossa. The majority occur due to motor vehicle accidents.

CLASSIFICATION

Knee dislocations are classified based on position of the tibia relative to the femur. There are five types described: anterior, posterior, medial, lateral, and rotatory. An anterior dislocation is caused by a hyperextension injury; sequential disruption of the posterior capsule, posterior cruciate, and anterior cruciate ligaments occur. Anterior dislocations may secondarily produce a traction injury to the popliteal artery, causing acute intimal tear and possibly an intraluminal thrombosis. Posterior knee dislocation generally results from a posteriorly directed force, such as the leg striking the dashboard during a motor vehicle accident. Both cruciate ligaments are disrupted with a posterior dislocation; posterior dislocation can cause complete laceration of the popliteal artery. A medial dislocation is caused by a varus force to the thigh with disruption of the lateral supporting structures. A lateral dislocation is caused by valgus stress and results in disruption of the medial supporting structures and often both cruciate ligaments. Rotatory dislocations rarely occur. Fifty to seventy percent of dislocations are anterior or posterior; 20 to 30 percent of dislocations are open.

TREATMENT

Closed reduction should be performed as soon as possible after knee dislocation. Injury to the popliteal artery occurs in 10 to 50 percent of dislocations. Therefore, arteriography is advocated as part of early management. If the leg appears ischemic, an arteriogram may be bypassed and exploration and repair of the popliteal artery, as well as fasciotomy, should be performed directly. Vascular flow must be restored within 6 to 8 h to reduce the possibility of an amputation. Twenty to forty percent of knee dislocations include associated peroneal nerve injury; approximately half of all neurologic injuries become permanent. In all types of knee dislocations, both cruciate ligaments and at least one, if not both, collateral ligaments are disrupted. Surgical repair and/or reconstruction is recommended with early postoperative range of knee motion to prevent knee stiffness.

PATELLA FRACTURES

ANATOMY

The patella is the largest sesamoid bone in the body, and serves as the attachment for the quadriceps and patella tendons. The medial and lateral patella retinaculum are confluences of the deep investing layer of the thigh with the aponeurotic fibers of the vastus medialis and lateralis, and serve as additional knee extensors. The articular surface of the patella is composed of seven facets divided by several ridges.

The patella increases the mechanical advantage of the quadriceps tendon, protects the femoral condyles from injury, and aids in nutritional support to the articular cartilage of the knee joint.

INCIDENCE/MECHANISM OF INJURY

Patella fractures represent approximately 1 percent of all skeletal injuries. They result from either direct or indirect forces. A direct blow to the knee will typically result in a comminuted or stellate fracture but without significant fracture displacement, as the patella retinaculum generally remains intact. Patella fractures due to indirect forces occur when the osseous strength of the patella is overcome by the muscle forces of the quadriceps; these fractures usually have a tear in the retinaculum, as well as significant fracture separation.

EVALUATION

It is important to evaluate the ability of the patient to actively extend the knee against gravity. Full active extension suggests an intact extensor mechanism. Lidocaine may be injected into the knee if the patient has significant knee pain that interferes with an effective clinical evaluation.

Initial radiographs include an AP, lateral, and sunrise views of the knee. The patella fracture is generally best revealed on the lateral radiograph. The sunrise view assists in ruling out vertical marginal fractures of the patella.

CLASSIFICATION

Patella fractures are classified based on fracture type, displacement, and location (Fig. 85-1). Types include transverse, stellate (comminuted), vertical, and osteochondral. Transverse fractures occur most frequently, representing 50 to 80 percent of patellar fractures; those involving the proximal or distal patella are called "polar."

TREATMENT

Nonoperative treatment is appropriate for minimally displaced patella fractures with an intact extensor mechanism. A long leg or cylinder cast is worn for 4 to 6 weeks, and the patient is permitted partial to full weightbearing. Compliant patients can be treated with a knee immobilizer or knee brace. Isometric quadriceps exercises and straight leg raising are prescribed as pain decreases.

Indications for operative intervention include: fractures with more than 2 mm articular displacement, more than 3 mm fragment separation, loss of extensor mechanism function, and displaced osteo-

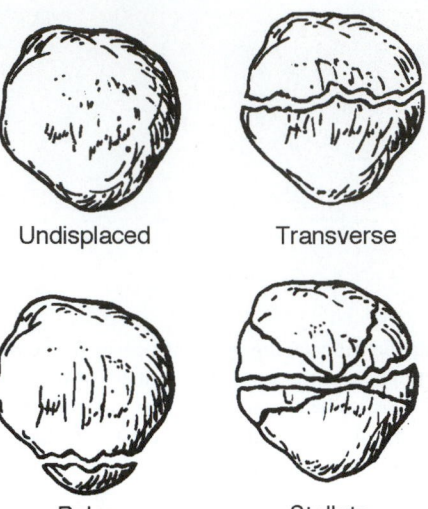

Undisplaced   Transverse

Polar   Stellate

Figure 85-1
Patella fractures. [Reproduced by permission from Perry CR, Pankovich AM: Thigh, knee, and leg fractures. In Zuckerman JD (ed): *Comprehensive Care of Orthopaedic Injuries in the Elderly.* Baltimore: Urban and Schwartzenberg; 1990:151.]

chondral fractures. The majority of internal fixation techniques apply a form of cerclage wiring in conjunction with Kirschner wires or lag screws (Fig. 85-2). Partial patellectomy is done if a portion of the articular surface cannot be reconstructed, or if the distal/proximal polar fractures are too small or comminuted for adequate fixation. Total patellectomy is reserved for severely comminuted fractures in which there are no large fragments remaining. It is essential to repair associated retinacular tears, regardless of fixation technique used.

RESULTS

Minimally displaced patella fractures have a long-term good functional outcome. Results following operative treatment of displaced patella fractures depend on the fracture type and whether the articular surface, as well as the extensor mechanism, can be adequately restored. More than 80 percent are reported to have good to excellent results with the application of modified tension-band wiring. Results following a partial patellectomy approach those after open reduction and internal fixation. Total patellectomy has varying degrees of clinical success.

COMPLICATIONS

Possible complications following patella fracture include: infection, loss of fixation, refracture, wire breakage, delayed and nonunion, loss of knee motion, posttraumatic arthritis, and tendon rupture. The rate of nonunion following patella fracture is 2 to 3 percent. Pain from retained hardware is not uncommon and is generally the result of irritation of the extensor mechanism by a protruding wire.

TIBIAL PLATEAU FRACTURES

MECHANISM OF INJURY

Tibial plateau fractures are caused by indirect coronal and/or direct axial compressive forces. The combination of a varus position and

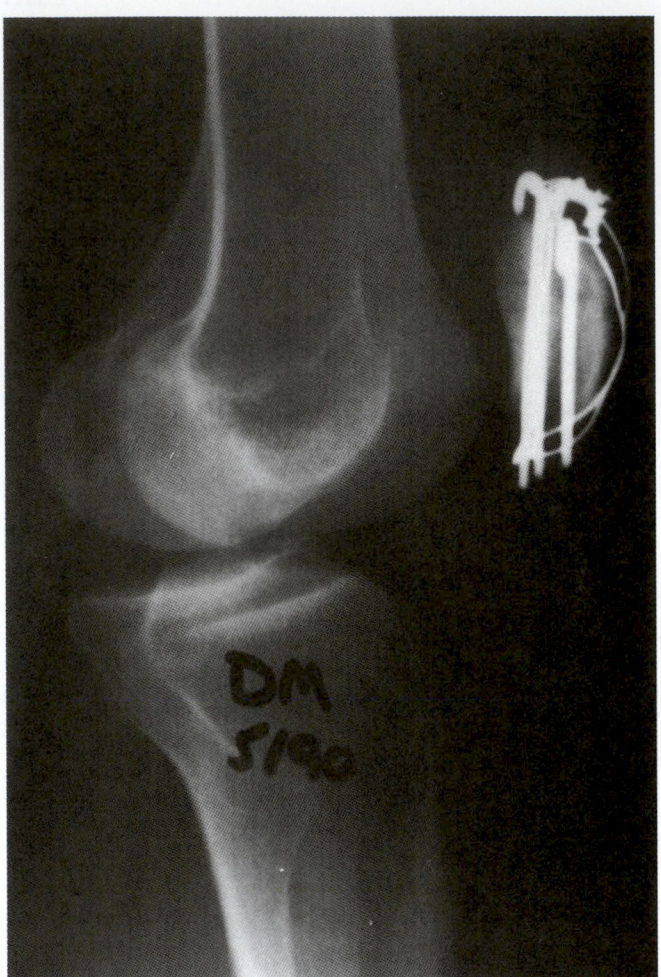

Figure 85-2
Patella fracture stabilized with tension-band wire technique.

compression results in a medial plateau fracture; valgus stress and compression combine to produce a lateral fracture pattern. Lateral plateau fractures are related to the valgus inclination of the anatomic axis and the usual lateral direction of the applied force.

Patient age and quality of bone influence the resultant fracture pattern and associated ligament injury. Younger patients with stronger bone usually develop split fractures and have a high rate of ligamentous disruption. With increasing age, the subchondral bone is more likely to succumb to axial loading; patients typically develop depression or split-depression fractures. As the bone compresses, the force is diffused, thereby protecting the opposite collateral ligament from injury.

RADIOGRAPHIC EVALUATION

Radiographic views include an AP, lateral, two obliques, and a 15-degree caudal plateau view. The degree of condylar depression should be measured from the intact articular surface on either the 15-degree caudal or lateral radiographs. Stress radiographs of the knee can be used to identify any indication of collateral ligament rupture.

CLASSIFICATION

The Schatzker classification is the most widely accepted. Type I is a wedge (split) fracture of the lateral tibial plateau (Fig. 85-3). Type II

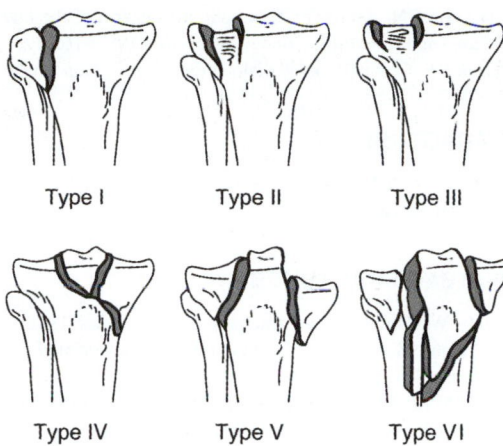

Type I   Type II   Type III

Type IV   Type V   Type VI

Figure 85-3

Schatzker classification of tibial plateau fractures. [Reproduced by permission from Benirschke SK, Swiontkowski MF: Knee. In Hansen ST Jr, Swiontkowski MF (eds): *Orthopaedic Trauma Protocols*. New York: Raven Press; 1993:315.]

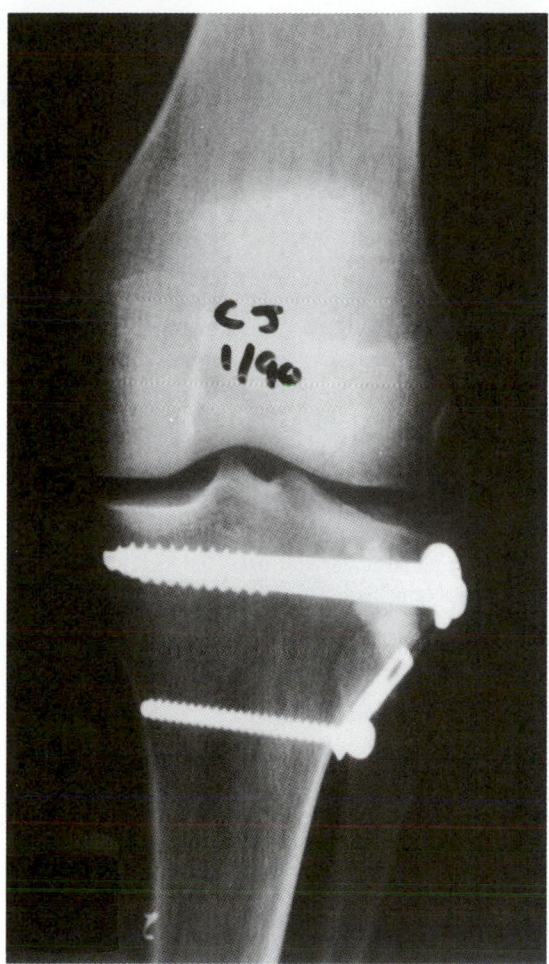

Figure 85-4

Displaced tibial plateau fracture treated with limited open reduction and lag screw fixation.

is a split-depression fracture of the lateral plateau. Type III is a pure central depression fracture of the lateral plateau but without an associated split. Type IV is a fracture of the medial tibial plateau, and generally involves the entire condyle. Type V is a bicondylar fracture that typically is comprised of split fractures of both the medial and lateral plateaus without articular depression. Type VI is a tibial plateau fracture with an associated proximal shaft fracture.

TREATMENT CONSIDERATIONS

A hinged cast brace can be used for minimally displaced, stable, tibial plateau fractures. Patients are permitted isometric quadriceps exercises and progressive passive, active, and active-assisted range of knee motion. Partial weightbearing is necessary for 8 to 12 weeks.

Indications for open and closed management of tibial plateau fractures are controversial. Some authors have advocated nonoperative management for tibial plateau fractures with up to 1 cm of depression. Others accept only minimal displacement of the articular surface. There is consensus, however, that an instability of greater than 10 degrees (compared to the uninvolved knee) of the nearly extended knee is an indication for operative intervention. Plateau fractures associated with a tibial shaft fracture are generally not responsive to closed treatment, since traction frequently causes separation of the shaft component rather than reduction of the articular surface. Open tibial plateau fractures or fractures presenting with a compartment syndrome or vascular insufficiency require emergent care.

Operative principles include anatomic joint reduction and stable fixation to permit early range of knee motion. Fractures with tibial shaft separation can generally be stabilized using cancellous screws (Fig. 85-4). Buttress plates or external fixators are required to best manage Schatzker type VI fractures.

OPEN FRACTURES

At the time of initial irrigation and debridement, limited internal fixation of the articular surface may be performed. If additional stability is required, temporary external fixation can be placed across the knee. Alternatively, a definitive thin-wire external fixator may be applied.

RESULTS

There is general agreement that minimally displaced tibial plateau fractures do well with nonoperative treatment; most series report approximately 90 percent of cases achieve good to excellent results. Treatment results of displaced tibial plateau fractures are difficult to evaluate since there are no universally accepted classifications, surgical indications, or follow-up grading system. Furthermore, patients whose injured tibial plateau has an abnormal radiologic appearance may still have a good clinical result, because the lateral meniscus bears almost the entire load carried by the lateral plateau. Conversely, patients may complain of pain associated with degenerative joint disease without significant radiologic changes.

A series of seventy tibial plateau fractures with an average follow-up of 28 months was reported by Schatzker (1979). Fractures treated with open reduction and internal fixation, elevation of the plateau "en masse," bone grafting, and early motion had an 89 percent acceptable outcome rate. In a series of 52 tibial plateau fractures that received operative treatment, Savoie and colleagues (1987) reported an 87 percent satisfactory outcome rate with an average follow-up of 24 months. Lansinger and coworkers (1986) reported a 90 percent good to excellent result rate in 102 patients using clinical instability of the nearly extended knee joint as the main indication for surgical treatment; patients were followed for an average of 20 years.

COMPLICATIONS

Infection following tibial plateau fracture is reported to occur in up to 12 percent of cases; it may be related to the initial fracture condition or iatrogenically introduced. Skin slough is a risk factor for later infection and a specific concern in the proximal leg secondary to poor soft tissue coverage. Significant predisposing factors for skin slough are poor surgical timing, improper soft tissue handling, and the use of bicondylar implants.

Appropriate pre-operative planning may prevent fixation loss. Stabilization of tibial plateau fractures using only lag screws should be reserved for patients with good bone quality and noncomminuted fractures. Fractures associated with metaphyseal-diaphyseal dissociation and those occurring in osteopenic bone require buttress plate fixation.

Posttraumatic arthrosis may occur as a result of cartilage damage from the initial injury or be related to residual joint incongruity. Preservation of the meniscus is important to avoid excessive load bearing by the underlying plateau. Some loss of joint motion may occur secondary to periarticular soft tissue injury. With prolonged immobilization, problems associated with loss of joint motion may be compounded.

SUGGESTED READINGS

KNEE DISLOCATION

Montgomery JB: Dislocation of the knee. *Orthop Clin North Am* 1987; 18:149.
Moore TM: Fracture-dislocation of the knee. *Clin Orthop* 1981; 156:128.
Roman PD, Hopson CN, Zenni EJ: Traumatic dislocation of the knee: A report of 30 cases and literature review. *Orthop Rev* 1987; 16:917.
Sisto DJ, Warren RF: Complete knee dislocation. *Clin Orthop* 1985; 198:94.

PATELLA FRACTURES

Carpenter JE, Kasman R, Matthews LS: Fractures of the patella. *J Bone Joint Surg [Am]* 1993; 75:1550.

TIBIAL PLATEAU FRACTURES

Anglen J, Healy W: Tibial plateau fractures. *Orthopaedics* 1988; 11:1527.
Delamarter R, Hohl M, Hopp E: Ligament injuries associated with tibial plateau fractures. *Clin Orthop* 1990; 250:226.
Gausewitz S, Hohl M: The significance of early motion in the treatment of tibial plateau fractures. *Clin Orthop* 1986; 202:135.
Helfet DL, Koval KJ: The management of fractures of the tibial plateau. *Int J Orthop Trauma* 1991; 1:148.
Lansinger O, Bergman B, Andersson GB: Tibial condylar fractures. A twenty-year follow-up. *J Bone Joint Surg [Am]* 1986; 68:13.
Schatzker J, McBroom R, Bruce D: The tibial plateau fracture: The Toronto experience, 1968–1975. *Clin Orthop* 1979;138:94.
Savoie FH, Vander Griend RA, Ward EF, et al: Tibial plateau fractures: A review of operative treatment using AO technique. *Orthopedics* 1987; 10:745.

Chapter 86

LEG FRACTURES

Kenneth J. Koval

TIBIAL SHAFT FRACTURES

ANATOMY

On cross section, the tibia has a triangular shape reflecting its anteromedial, anterolateral, and posterior surfaces. The anterior subcutaneous border of the shaft is virtually without muscular attachments, making it a readily palpable structure. The position of its anterior border is subcutaneous. A nutrient artery derives from the posterior tibial artery and perforates the middle third of the tibia at the origin of the soleus muscle. The blood supply of most of the tibial diaphysis is provided by the medullary arterial system. Following fracture, periosteal vessels (peripheral blood supply) increase to revascularize necrotic areas.

The leg is divided into four compartments (anterior, lateral, superficial posterior, deep posterior) by fibrous septa. The *anterior compartment* contains the tibialis anterior, extensor hallucis longus, and extensor digitorum communis muscles, the anterior tibial artery and vein, and the deep peroneal nerve. The *lateral compartment* includes the peroneal longus and brevis muscles and the superficial peroneal nerve. The *superficial posterior* compartment includes the gastrocnemius, soleus and plantaris muscles, and sural nerve. The *deep posterior compartment* comprises the flexor digitorum longus, flexor hallucis longus, and tibialis posterior muscles, the posterior tibial artery and vein, and the tibial nerve.

MECHANISM OF INJURY

Tibial shaft fractures are the most common long bone fracture. They result from low- or high-energy trauma. The superficial subcutaneous location of the tibia makes it vulnerable to injury; fractures of the tibia are therefore frequently open.

CLASSIFICATION

Tibia fractures are generally classified by fracture location, fracture pattern, the amount of comminution, the presence or absence of an associated fibula fracture, and the amount of soft tissue injury (Fig. 86-1).

EVALUATION

Examination of the injured leg should include identification and evaluation of any accompanying soft tissue injury, neurovascular status, and determination of an imminent, impending, or established compartment syndrome. Small puncture wounds should be assumed to communicate with the underlying fracture. Radiographs include AP and lateral views inclusive of the knee and ankle.

TREATMENT PRINCIPLES

The majority of closed tibial shaft fractures are able to be treated nonoperatively with closed fracture reduction and a long leg cast. Rotational alignment, however, must be carefully assessed following closed reduction. The knee is positioned to almost full extension and the patient instructed to weightbear as pain decreases. Studies have confirmed that the fracture will not shorten more than the amount observed on initial radiographs. A snugly fitting short leg cast or fracture brace can replace the long leg cast after 4 to 6 weeks. These fractures must be closely monitored to detect loss of reduction.

Indications for immediate surgical intervention include patients with an open fracture, vascular compromise, or compartment syndrome. Other indications for surgery are: fractures in which an adequate reduction (<5 degree varus/valgus angulation, <10 degree anterior/posterior angulation, <10 degree malrotation, and <1 cm shortening) cannot be obtained or maintained; bilateral tibia fracture; ipsilateral tibia and femur fracture (floating knee); and fractures with intraarticular extension.

An intramedullary nail is the implant of choice for the majority of tibial shaft fractures. Flexible nails are best suited for transverse fractures with minimal comminution; interlocked nails are the choice for unstable fractures (Fig. 86-2). Intramedullary nailing of proximal tibia fractures, however, has been associated with angular malreduction. Interlocked nails may be inserted with or without prior reaming; the need to ream a closed tibia fracture prior to insertion of intramedullary nails is controversial. Fractures of the proximal and distal tibia appear to be best treated by plates.

OPEN TIBIA FRACTURES

Open tibia fractures must receive immediate debridement. Repeat debridements should be done at intervals of 36 to 48 h until the wound has been thoroughly cleansed. Four compartment fasciotomies are required in approximately 5 to 10 percent of open tibial fractures. The choice of implant for stabilization is controversial; both external fixators and unreamed small diameter interlocked nails have been advocated. Although the use of plates with open tibial shaft fractures has been reported to have good results, the infection rate and secondary complications (implant failure, nonunion) are unacceptably high. The majority of open wounds can be closed on a delayed primary basis using a split-thickness skin graft. Open fractures with large soft tissue defects require flap coverage. A gastrocnemius flap is used to cover proximal leg wounds, a soleus flap will provide adequate cover for soft tissue defects extending toward the mid aspect of the tibia, and a free flap is necessary for more distal defects. Higher energy injuries with fracture comminution should be treated with early bone grafting.

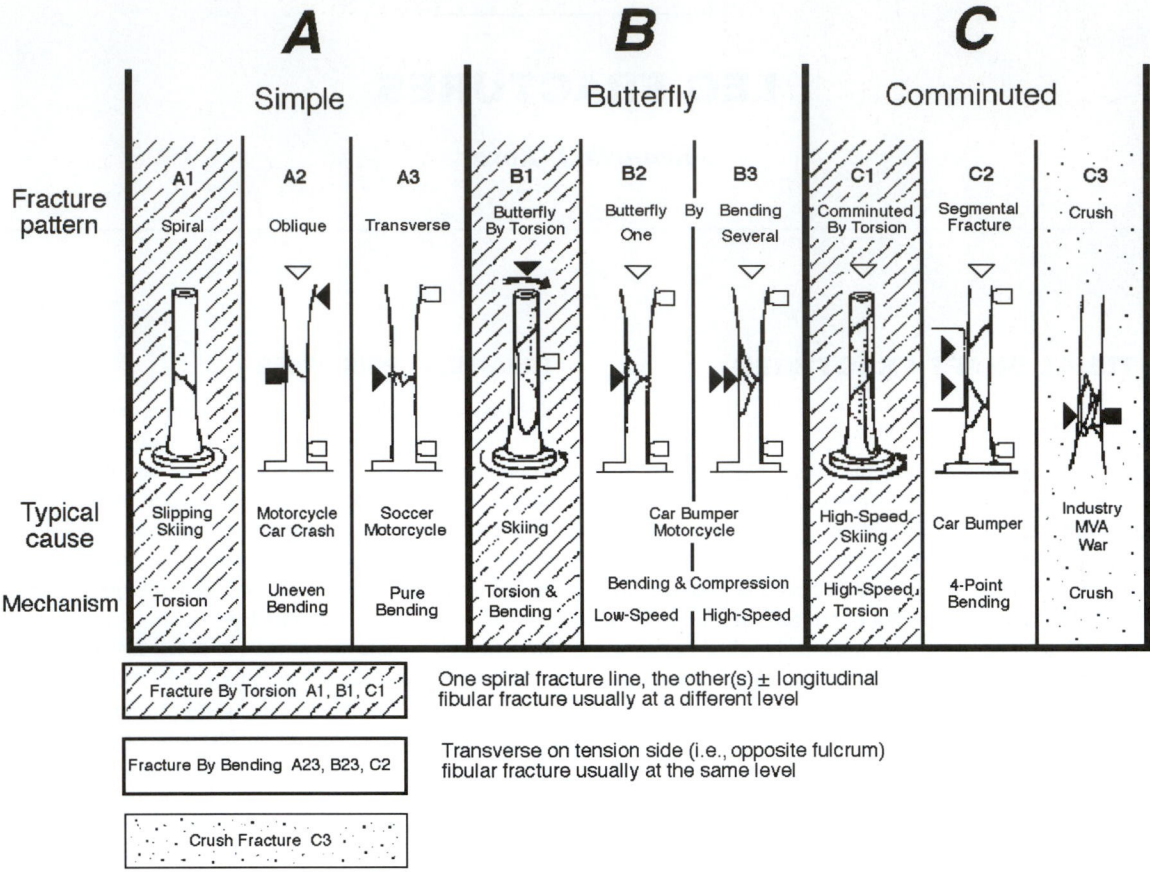

Figure 86-1
AO (Johner-Wruhs) classification of tibial shaft fractures. (Reproduced by permission from Johner R, Wruhs O: *Clin Orthop* 1983: 178:9.)

RESULTS

The time to union for closed low-energy tibia fractures ranges from 10 to 13 weeks. Higher-energy fractures unite in 13 to 20 weeks. Open tibia fractures take 16 to 26 weeks.

COMPLICATIONS

Complications after tibia fracture include: infection, delayed union, nonunion, loss of reduction, fixation failure, refracture, wound slough, nerve injury, vascular compromise, compartment syndrome, loss of joint motion, and functional disability. Delayed union is defined as a fracture that takes longer to unite than expected. A nonunion is an arrest of the fracture repair process. For the tibia, a nonunion is defined at 9 months after fracture. Treatment options for tibial nonunion include: electrical stimulation, fibula osteotomy, anterior or posterolateral bone grafting, and internal/external fixation. Refracture can occur after plate removal.

FIBULA SHAFT FRACTURES

The majority of fibula shaft fractures take place in association with a tibia fracture and are treated in the same manner as the tibia. Isolated fibula shaft fracture without tibia fracture or ankle injury are rare and usually result from the impact of a direct force on the lateral leg.

TREATMENT

Isolated fibula shaft fractures are managed symptomatically; a short leg walking cast or brace can be applied for 4 to 6 weeks if needed for relief of pain. Alternatively, the leg can be supported with an elastic bandage and the patient permitted to weightbear with a cane or crutches. Nonunion of fibula shaft fracture is rare; internal fixation and bone grafting are performed based on clinical need.

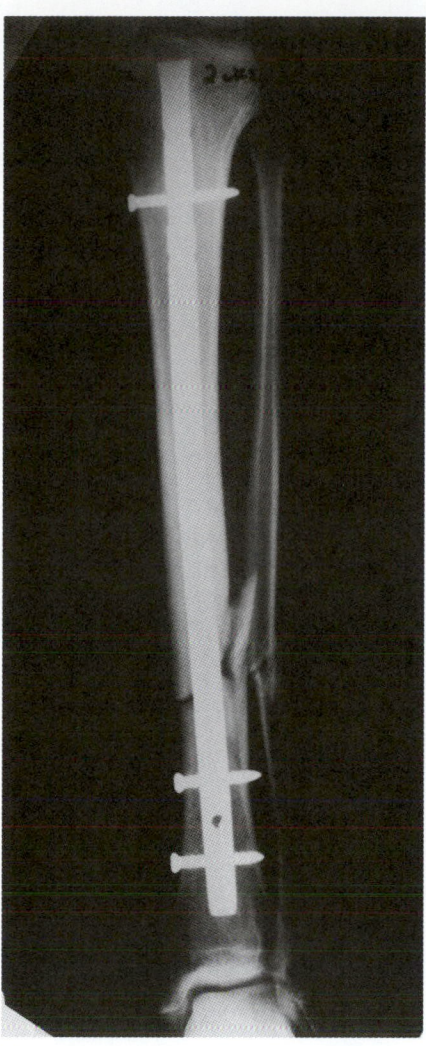

Figure 86-2
Tibial fracture stabilized with interlocked intramedullary nails.

SUGGESTED READINGS

TIBIAL AND FIBULAR SHAFTS

Johner R, Wruhs O: Classification of tibial shaft fractures and correlation with results after rigid internal fixation. *Clin Orthop* 1983; 178:9.

Sarmiento A, Gersten LM, Sobol PA, et al: Tibial shaft fractures treated with functional braces: Experience with 780 fractures. *J Bone Joint Surg [Br]* 1989; 71:602.

Chapter 87

ANKLE

Kenneth J. Koval

ANKLE FRACTURES

ANATOMY

The ankle is a modified hinge joint. The distal region of the medial malleolus of the tibia is divided into two prominences, the anterior and the posterior colliculi. The lateral malleolus protrudes approximately one centimeter distal and posterior to the medial malleolus. The talus is covered largely by cartilage; the body of the talus is wider anteriorly than posteriorly and is matched to the distal tibial articular surface and thereby forms a congruent joint.

The deltoid ligament is a thick triangular band made up of superficial and deep fibers. A majority of the superficial fibers arise from the anterior colliculus of the medial malleolus and continue in the sagittal plane as one sheet to attach to the navicular, the sustentaculum tali, and the talus. The intra-articular and more horizontal deep fibers course from the intercollicular notch and posterior colliculus to the medial surface of the talus. The deep fibers of the deltoid ligament provide important medial stability to the joint.

The lateral side of the ankle has three ligaments which collectively comprise the lateral collateral ligament: (1) the anterior talofibular ligament; (2) the calcaneofibular ligament; and (3) the posterior talofibular ligament.

The most distal aspects of the fibula and tibia are bound together by four ligaments plus the interosseous membrane. The ligaments are the anterior inferior tibiofibular ligament, the posterior inferior tibiofibular ligament, the inferior transverse ligament, and the interosseous ligament. Together they stabilize the distal articulation of the tibia and fibula.

INCIDENCE/MECHANISM OF INJURY

Patterns of injury to the ankle are based on many factors, including: patient age, bone quality, position of the foot at time of injury, and direction, magnitude, and rate of loading force. The majority of ankle fractures are caused by an external rotational force. The mechanism of injury in ankle fracture is also discussed in the classification section.

CLINICAL AND RADIOGRAPHIC EVALUATION

Areas of tenderness around the ankle should be identified and evaluated. Medial ankle tenderness suggests possible deltoid ligament rupture with a resultant unstable ankle. Radiographic examination includes an AP, lateral, and mortise view. The medial clear space, evaluated on the 15 degree internal rotation mortise view, should be less than 4 mm. When there is medial side tenderness without evidence of fracture, an external rotation stress view, performed with the ankle dorsiflexed, is helpful to evaluate ankle stability.

CLASSIFICATION

Lauge-Hansen developed a detailed classification of ankle fractures (Fig. 87-1). In this classification, the first word (*Supination*-adduction) refers to the position of the foot at the time of the injury, and the second word (Supination-*adduction*) to the direction of the force of the injury.

In supination-external rotation injuries, stage I is a tear of the anterior inferior tibiofibular ligament or equivalent osseous avulsion from the tibia or fibula. Stage II includes an associated spiral oblique fracture of the lateral malleolus. Stage III has an added fracture of the posterior lip of the tibia. Stage IV has either an associated fracture of the medial malleolus or a deltoid ligament rupture.

In supination-adduction injuries, stage I is either a transverse fracture of the lateral malleolus or disruption of the lateral collateral ligaments. Stage II includes an associated fracture of the medial malleolus.

In pronation-abduction injuries, stage I is either a fracture of the medial malleolus or a tear of the deltoid ligament. Stage II has an associated disruption of the anterior inferior tibiofibular, posterior inferior tibiofibular ligament, and the transverse ligament with a fracture of the posterior lip of the tibia. Stage III has an associated oblique supra-malleolar fracture of the fibula.

In pronation-external rotation fractures, the stage I pattern is the same as stage I of the pronation-abduction injury. Stage II has an associated tear of the anterior inferior tibiofibular and interosseous ligaments. Stage III has an associated interosseous membrane tear and a spiral fracture of the fibula 7 to 8 cm proximal to the tip of the lateral malleolus. Stage IV has an associated fracture of the posterior lip of the tibia secondary to ligamentous avulsion by the posterior and inferior transverse tibiofibular ligaments.

The Danis-Weber classification (Fig. 87-1) emphasizes the fibular fracture; the more proximal the fibular fracture, the more severe the syndesmotic injury. The interosseous membrane is torn up to the level of the fibula fracture. Three separate types of fibular fractures are described. Type A is a transverse fracture below the joint line. Type B is a fracture at the level of the joint line. Type C fractures are proximal to the joint line.

TREATMENT PRINCIPLES

Treatment objectives for ankle fractures include: maintenance of the anatomic position of the talus in the mortise, a joint line that is parallel to the ground, and a congruous articular surface. Stable injuries (e.g., nondisplaced isolated medial or lateral malleolar fractures) which do not require reduction are immobilized for comfort and protection. A short leg cast is applied and the patient is permitted to gradually weightbear as tolerated. Alternatively, the ankle can be immobilized with an aircast.

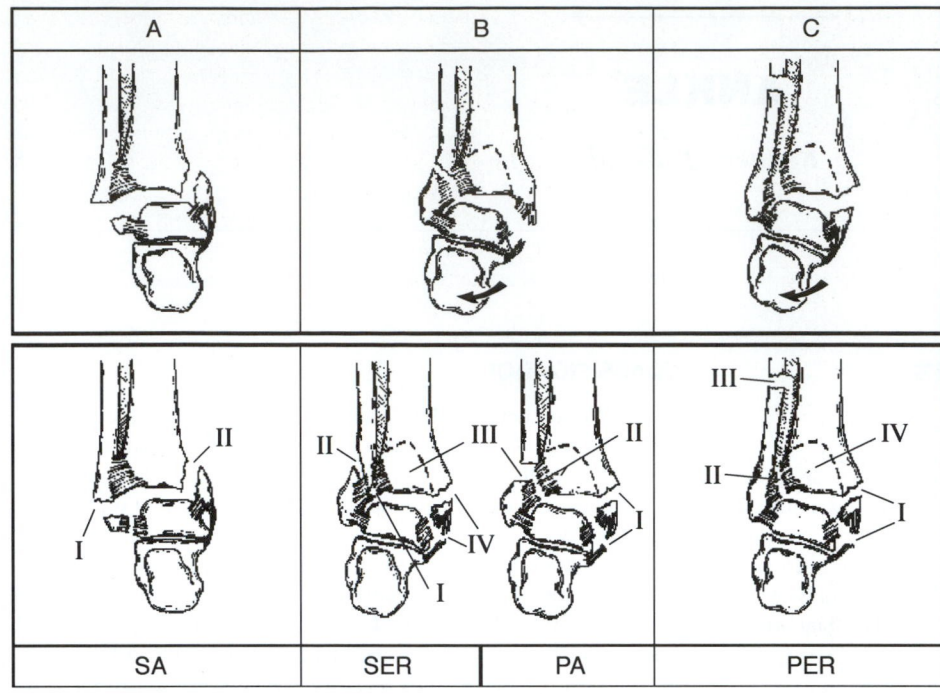

Figure 87-1
Weber (*top*) and Lauge-Hansen (*bottom*) classification of ankle fractures. [Reproduced by permission from Trafton PG, Bray TJ, Simpson LA: Fractures and soft tissue injuries of the ankle, In Browner BD, Jupiter JB, Levine AM, et al (eds): *Skeletal Trauma*. Philadelphia: WB Saunders; 1992:1891.]

Unstable injuries or fractures associated with lateral displacement of the talus must be reduced so that the talus is positioned anatomically beneath the tibial plafond. Even a slight talar shift could result in joint incongruity and eventual degenerative changes. Ramsey and Hamilton (1976) have demonstrated that a lateral shift of the talus of just 1 mm can result in significantly increased pressure on the tibiotalar joint.

Displaced fractures can be treated by closed reduction, but maintaining an anatomic position is frequently difficult once swelling has subsided. The reduction is accomplished by reversing the mechanism of injury; a long leg cast is applied with the knee flexed for 6 to 8 weeks. Close follow-up is required to monitor for loss of reduction.

Open reduction and internal fixation is usually recommended if the patient is medically cleared for surgery. Lag screws and plates are used to stabilize the lateral malleolus (Fig. 87-2). Cancellous screws or tension band wire are used to stabilize medial malleolus fractures. Open reduction and internal fixation of the posterior fragment are indicated depending on the size of the fragment and joint stability. Fragments that represent greater than 25 to 30 percent of the articular surface need to be internally stabilized.

The necessity of a syndesmotic screw is based on fracture pattern and intraoperative evaluation of syndesmotic stability. The syndesmotic screw is a positioning screw as opposed to a lag screw and should be inserted with the foot dorsiflexed. It is generally removed 8 weeks postsurgery. If the syndesmotic screw is not removed, screw loosening or breakage may result. Recent clinical and mechanical studies have demonstrated that a syndesmotic screw is not generally required if the fibula fracture is less than 4 cm from the ankle joint and is anatomically reduced.

A Maisonneuve fracture is a proximal fracture of the fibula associated with disruption of the ankle, and is caused by external rotation. The injury can be divided into five stages of severity: stage I, rupture of the anterior tibiofibular ligament or avulsion of its osseous insertion, usually associated with rupture of the interosseous ligament; stage II, fracture of the posterior malleolus or rupture of the posterior tibiofibular ligament; stage III, rupture of the anteromedial joint capsule or avulsion fracture on its osseous insertion; stage IV, fracture of the fibula in the proximal third; and stage V, rupture of the deltoid ligament or medial malleolus fracture. Treatment includes reduction and stabilization of the mortise with placement of a syndesmotic screw and stabilization of the medial malleolus, if fractured. If there is fracture shortening, the proximal fibula fracture should also be reduced and stabilized.

RESULTS

The outcome of fracture of the ankle is determined by multiple factors including severity of the initial injury and adequacy of reduction. Stable ankle fractures with minimal displacement usually have a good long-term result. Unstable ankle fractures with displacement are dependent on the quality of reduction for a successful result. In a series reported by Lindsjö (1985), 87 percent of 217 patients with adequate reduction of their displaced ankle fracture had good to excellent results compared to 68 percent of 89 patients who had good to excellent results with residual displacement.

COMPLICATIONS

Complications following ankle fracture include: nonunion, malunion, soft tissue slough, infection, posttraumatic arthritis, and reflex sympathetic dystrophy. Most nonunions include the medial malleolus. The infection rate following internal fixation of closed ankle fractures is under 2 percent.

ANKLE DISLOCATION

INCIDENCE/MECHANISM OF INJURY

Ankle dislocations rarely present without an associated fracture; the mechanism of injury is a force applied to the plantarflexed foot.

lon: rotation and axial compression. Rotational fractures are lower energy injuries of the distal tibia extending into the ankle joint; they are usually produced by falls or sporting accidents, most particularly skiing. Compression fractures are higher energy injuries caused by axial loading forces that drive the talus into the distal tibia; the result is impaction of the distal tibia articular surface and comminution of the metaphyseal bone. Associated fractures of the calcaneus, tibial plateau, pelvis, acetabulum, and spinal fractures must be identified and assessed during evaluation. The region of the tibial plafond most damaged by the loading force is determined by the position of the foot at the time of impact.

RADIOGRAPHIC EVALUATION

Radiographs include AP, lateral and oblique views of the distal tibia. In complex and/or comminuted injuries of the tibial pilon, tomography and/or CT scanning may assist in defining the extent of involvement of the articular surface and to identify all fracture fragments.

CLASSIFICATION

A classification by Rüedi and Allgöwer (1979) is based on the degree of articular and metaphyseal displacement and comminution (Fig. 87-3). A type I fracture has minimal displacement. A type II fracture has articular displacement, with minor displacement. A type III fracture has significant articular displacement and comminution.

A more prognostic classification, based on mechanism of injury, was described by Kellam and Waddell (1979). In this classification, type A fractures are rotational, and are usually associated with a short oblique or transverse fibular fracture above the level of the plafond. Type A fractures generally have a good prognosis. Type B, or compression fractures, have severe anterior tibial cortical comminution, multiple articular fragments, and metaphyseal impaction. They frequently do not have an associated fibular fracture, but do have a significantly worse prognosis than type A injuries.

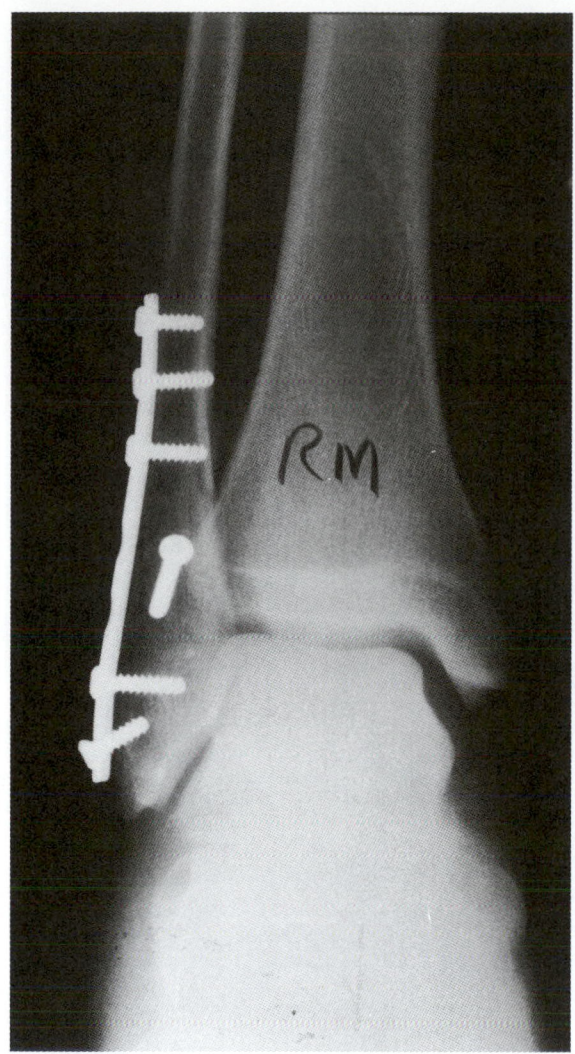

Figure 87-2
Displaced lateral malleolus fracture stabilized with plate and screws.

CLASSIFICATION

Ankle dislocations are classified based on the position of the talus in relation to the tibia: medial, lateral, posteromedial, posterior, rotational.

TREATMENT

A dislocated ankle must be reduced emergently. Generally, a closed reduction under sedation is successful. An open reduction may be necessary if the fibula is also dislocated. The leg is immobilized in a short leg cast for 6 to 8 weeks, and the patient is permitted partial weightbearing ambulation. Dislocated ankles have a good prognosis; the majority of poor results occur in open dislocations.

PILON FRACTURES

INCIDENCE/MECHANISM OF INJURY

Fractures of the distal tibia with extension into the ankle joint (pilon fracture) represent less than 1 percent of fractures of the lower extremity. Two separate mechanisms result in fractures of the tibial pi-

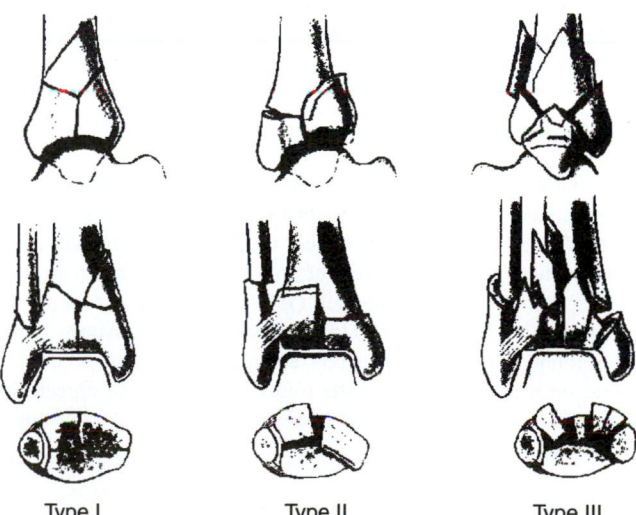

| Type I | Type II | Type III |

Figure 87-3
Rüedi-Allgöwer classification of distal tibial (pilon) fractures. (Reproduced by permission from Müller ME, Allgöwer M, Schneider R, et al: *Manual of Internal Fixation,* 2d ed. New York: Springer-Verlag; 1979:279.)

Müller and coworkers (1990) have proposed the most detailed and prognostic classification. It divides pilon fractures into three types, each type with further subgroups. Type A is an extraarticular fracture with a simple metaphyseal fracture. Type B is a partial articular fracture, and type C is a complete articular fracture. Each type is subdivided based on the fracture obliquity, fracture location, and amount of comminution.

TREATMENT CONSIDERATIONS

Plaster immobilization may be used for minimally displaced or nondisplaced intraarticular fractures. Patients are permitted progressive passive, active, and active-assisted range of ankle motion as healing progresses; partial weightbearing is necessary for 8 to 12 weeks.

Displaced intraarticular pilon fractures require anatomic joint reduction with stable fixation in order to allow early active and functional range of motion. The principles for operative intervention in pilon fractures were described by Rüedi and Allgöwer (1979): (1) restore length by open reduction and internal fixation of the fibula; (2) reconstruct the articular surface of the distal tibia using the intact "chaput" fragment as the key fragment; (3) bone graft any metaphyseal defect; and (4) medial buttress plate the tibia. Length is usually established by reconstructing the fibula. In order to prevent skin slough, an 8 cm (minimal acceptable length) skin bridge between the medial and the lateral approaches should be planned.

The distal tibia articular surface must be anatomically restored to optimize the potentiality of long-term clinical success. Joint reduction is generally achieved by working through the split fracture fragments to preserve soft tissue attachments. The metaphyseal defect should be bone grafted and the tibia buttressed with a plate or external fixator (Fig. 87-4).

OPEN FRACTURES

Open fractures need emergent irrigation and debridement without attempting primary wound closure. At the time of debridement, however, if the articular surface is readily visible the joint can be anatomically reduced with definitive internal fixation, as long as it does not require additional soft tissue stripping. The metaphyseal fracture can be definitively treated with an external fixator, or it can be plated at a later time.

RESULTS

The anticipated clinical result appears to be dependent on the fracture type. Bourne et al. (1989) report better than 80 percent satisfactory results in the operative treatment of Rüedi and Allgöwer type I and II fractures. Only 44 percent of type III fractures had a satisfactory outcome. Kellam and Waddell (1979) published that 84 percent of rotational fractures had good to excellent results while only 53 percent of higher energy compression fractures had good to excellent results at an average of 18 months follow-up. They also agreed that posttraumatic arthritis, should it occur, would manifest itself within one year of the initial fracture.

COMPLICATIONS

Skin slough may occur after the injury or following surgery. The major surgeon-controlled predisposing factors to skin loss are poor timing of the definitive procedure, rough handling of the soft tissue, and a too narrow skin bridge between the medial and lateral incisions.

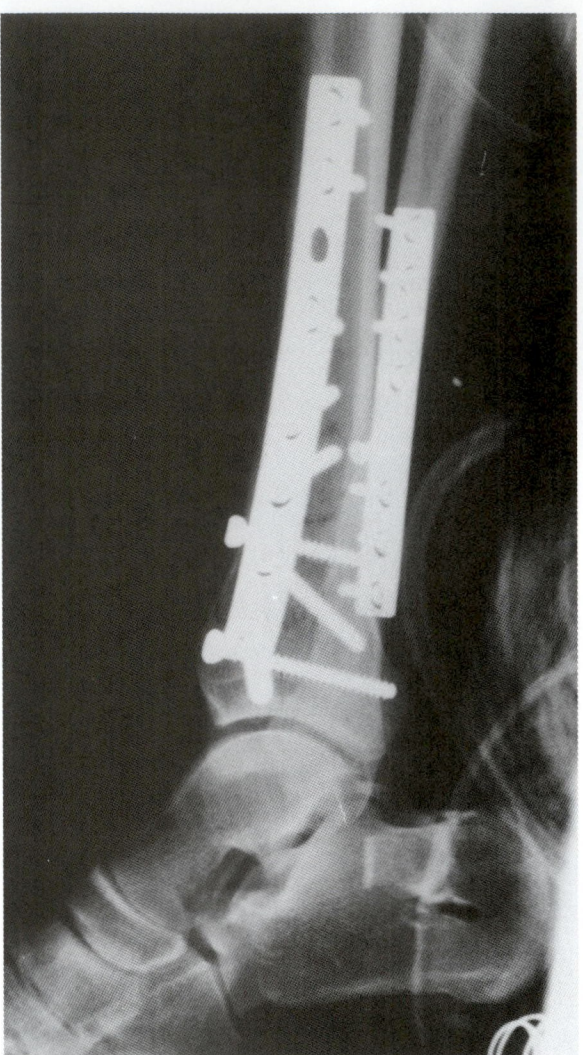

Figure 87-4
Pilon fracture stabilized with plate and screws.

Some loss of joint motion can be expected secondary to periarticular soft tissues injury and can be compounded by prolonged immobilization. Post-traumatic arthrosis may occur due to cartilage damage or residual joint incongruity. Varus malunion is the most frequent axial deformity observed and can be prevented by medial buttressing, especially in fractures with a medial or anterior-medial cortical defect. Nonunion is rare but can be managed with open reduction, internal fixation, and bone grafting, as with all metaphyseal nonunions.

SUGGESTED READINGS

ANKLE

Lauge-Hansen N: Fractures of the ankle: Analytic historic survey as basis of new experimental roentgenologic and clinical investigations. *Arch Surg* 1948; 56:259.

Lauge-Hansen N: Fractures of the ankle. II. Combined experimental-surgical and experimental-roentgenologic investigation. *Arch Surg* 1950; 60:957.

Lindsjö U: Operative treatment of ankle fracture-dislocations. A follow-up study of 306/321 consecutive cases. *Clin Orthop* 1985; 199:28.

Mast JW, Teipner WA: A reproducible approach to the internal fixation of adult ankle fractures: Rationale, technique, and early results. *Orthop Clin North Am* 1980; 11:661.

Pankovich AM: Maisonneuve fracture of the fibula. *J Bone Joint Surg [Am]* 1976; 58:337.

Ramsey P, Hamilton W: Changes in the tibiotalar area of contact caused by lateral talar shift. *J Bone Joint Surg [Am]* 1976; 58:356.

PILON

Bone LB: Fractures of the tibial plafond. The pilon fracture. *Orthop Clin North Am* 1987; 18:95.

Brennan MJ: Tibial pilon fractures, in Greene WB (ed): *Instructional Course Lectures.* Park Ridge, IL: American Academy Orthopaedic Surgeons; 1990; 39:167.

Kellam JF, Waddell JP: Fractures of the distal tibial metaphysis with intraarticular extension: The distal tibial explosion. *J Trauma* 1979; 19:593.

Mast JW, Speigel PG, Pappas JN: Fractures of the distal pilon. *Clin Orthop* 1988; 230:68.

Müller ME, Nazarian S, Koch P, et al: Tibia/Fibula. In *The Comprehensive Classification of Fractures of Long Bones.* Berlin/New York: Springer-Verlag; 1990:171–179.

Rüedi TP, Allgöwer M: The operative treatment of intraarticular fractures of the lower end of the tibia. *Clin Orthop* 1979; 138:105.

OPEN FRACTURES

Bourne RB: Pylon fractures of the distal tibia. *Clin Orthop* 1989; 240:42.

Chapter 88

FOOT

Kenneth J. Koval

CALCANEUS FRACTURES

ANATOMY

The calcaneus includes articular surfaces for the talus and cuboid, a large extraarticular body, and a sustentaculum tali that supports the neck of the talus medially. Superiorly, the calcaneus has three facets (anterior, middle and posterior) which articulate with the talus. The posterior facet is the major weightbearing surface. The middle facet is located on the sustentaculum tali, and is often confluent with the anterior facet. The flexor hallucis longus courses beneath the sustentaculum tali. The Achilles tendon inserts onto the posterior aspect of the tuberosity.

Two important angles can be demonstrated on a lateral radiograph of the calcaneus: Bohler's tuber joint angle and the "crucial angle" of Gissane (Fig. 88-1). The tuber angle of Bohler is a measure of calcaneal height, and is normally 20 to 40 degrees. It is formed by the complement of the angle made by the intersection of two lines. The

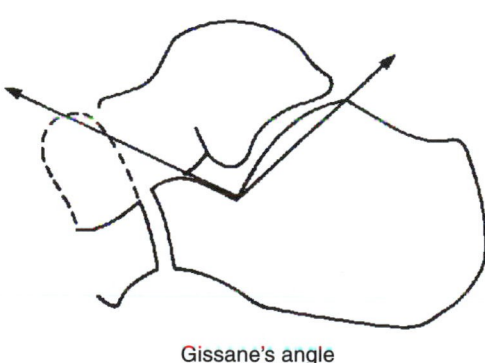

Gissane's angle

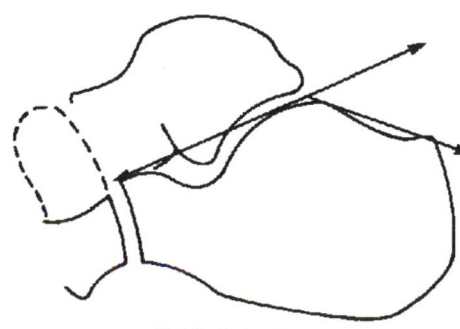

Bohler's angle

Figure 88-1

Radiographic measurements in calcaneal fractures that assess the posterior facet. [Reproduced by permission from Sanders R, Hansen ST Jr, McReynolds IS: Trauma to the calcaneus and its tendon. In Jahss MH (ed): *Disorders of the Foot and Ankle,* vol 3, 2d ed. Philadelphia: WB Saunders; 1991:2327.]

first line is drawn from the highest point of the anterior process and the highest point of the posterior articular surface. The second line runs from the same point on the posterior articular surface to the upper edge of the tuberosity.

Laterally, the angle of Gissane is formed by two cortical struts that are inferior to the lateral process of the talus. The first strut is positioned along the lateral border of the posterior facet, and the second strut extends anteriorly to the anterior process of the calcaneus. The struts create an obtuse angle.

INCIDENCE AND MECHANISM OF INJURY

Calcaneal fractures are rare. They account for 2 percent of all fractures. A fall from a height is usually the cause of injury; however, calcaneus fractures also frequently happen during motor vehicle accidents as the foot strikes the floor board. Seventy-five percent of these fractures are displaced. Other commonly associated fractures include pilon, tibial plateau, and spinal compression fractures.

Calcaneus fractures are classified as extraarticular or intraarticular. Extraarticular avulsion fractures are usually caused by twisting forces. Intraarticular fractures are typically the result of axial compressive forces produced as the lateral process of the talus is driven into the calcaneus, disrupting the subtalar joint and distorting the angle of Gissane. Because the center of the calcaneal tuberosity is lateral to the center of the talus, a shear fracture is created and is known as the primary fracture line. Laterally, the primary fracture line typically exits through the angle of Gissane; however, it may also exit as far anteriorly as the calcaneo-cuboid joint. The fracture generally divides the posterior facet and runs medially, producing a sustentaculum and a tuberosity fragment. As the force continues at the time of injury, the talus and sustentaculum fragment are driven plantar and medial, creating a shortened and widened heel and rotating the tuberosity fragment into adduction and varus. The sustentaculum fragment maintains a constant relationship to the talus due to strong ligamentous attachments.

During higher energy injuries, the talus impacts the lateral aspect of the posterior facet which comminutes the facet and creates a blowout of the lateral wall. Secondary fracture lines are produced in the posterior facet; they may exit just posterior to the facet and create a "joint depression" fracture, or exit through the posterior aspect of the tuberosity, forming a "tongue" type fracture (Fig. 88-2).

The resulting deformities include: a loss of calcaneal height, increased calcaneal width, decreased calcaneal length, incongruity of the posterior subtalar facet, and lateral calcaneal wall bulge. The tuberosity fragment is rotated into adduction and varus.

CLINICAL AND RADIOGRAPHIC EVALUATION

A displaced calcaneus fracture is usually associated with acute pain, hindfoot swelling and ecchymosis, and pain on subtalar motion. One must be aware of the possibility of compartment syndrome.

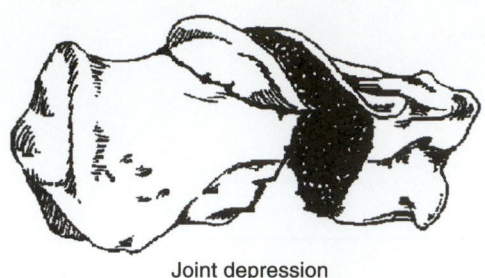

Joint depression

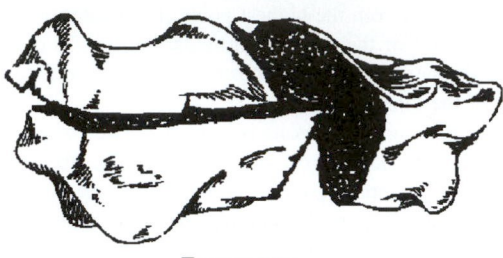

Tongue-type

Figure 88-2
Primary and secondary fracture patterns in intraarticular calcaneal fractures. (Reproduced by permission from Kozin SH, Berlet AC: *Handbook of Common Orthopaedic Fractures,* 2d ed. Medical Surveillance, West Chester, PA, 1992.)

Plain radiographs include AP and lateral views of the foot, as well as a Harris axial view of the heel. The lateral view will document the intraarticular involvement of the posterior facet as well as demonstrate secondary fracture lines. The posterior facet should be assessed for joint incongruity. The AP view will assist in evaluating the involvement of the calcaneo-cuboid joint. The Harris axial view demonstrates the posterior and middle facets as well as the tuberosity.

Broden's views are an approach to demonstrate the articular surface of the posterior facet with conventional radiography. The patient is placed in a supine position with the ankle in neutral flexion and the extremity internally rotated 30 to 40 degrees. The radiograph is centered over the lateral malleolus, and a series of views are taken with the tube angled 0, 10, 20, 30, and 40 degrees cephalad. The resulting radiographs depict various aspects of the posterior facet. The angled radiographs progressively demonstrate more posterior aspects of the subtalar joint.

CT revolutionized the understanding of calcaneal fractures. Articular congruity, the number and displacement of fragments, heel width and height, peroneal and fibula impingement, and tuberosity malposition can be accurately assessed. CT should be performed in the coronal and axial planes. The coronal view depicts information relating to the posterior facet, to include the number and displacement of fracture fragments. The size of the sustentaculum fragment, position of the tuberosity, width and height of the heel, presence of a lateral wall bulge, and status of the peroneal and flexor hallucis tendons are clearly depicted and should be evaluated. The axial view shows the status of the calcaneo-cuboid joint, the antero-inferior aspect of the posterior facet, the sustentaculum, and heel length.

CLASSIFICATION

Both extraarticular and intraarticular calcaneus fractures can be classified by anatomic location. Extraarticular fractures involve the ante-

rior process of the calcaneus, posterior tuberosity fractures, and calcaneal body fractures not involving the posterior facet. Intraarticular fractures can be classified as tongue-type or joint depression. In tongue-type fractures (Essex-Lopresti), the intraarticular fracture exits posteriorly with a large fragment of the posterior facet. In joint depression fractures, the fracture line is slightly more horizontal than tongue type fractures; the line exits just posterior to the posterior facet with a smaller piece of bone.

The commonly used CT classification described by Sanders (Fig. 88-3) is based on the number and location of posterior facet fracture fragments demonstrated on the CT coronal view. The posterior facet is divided into three anatomical areas: medial, central, and lateral. These areas may break into three fragments during the injury; when added to the sustentaculum tali, the result is a total of four potential pieces. All nondisplaced fractures are considered to be type I. Type II fractures are two-part fractures which can be further defined as type A, B, or C based on the location of the primary fracture line. Type III fractures are three-part fractures and can be subdivided as type AB, AC, or BC, depending on the location of the fracture lines. Type IV fractures are highly comminuted.

TREATMENT

The majority of extraarticular fractures can be treated nonoperatively. Anterior process fractures are treated with a short leg cast or rigid shoe; the choice is based on patient symptoms. Large fragments may develop a pseudarthrosis; if so, they require late excision. Displaced tuberosity fractures require open reduction and internal fixation. Displaced calcaneal body fractures which do not involve the posterior facet should have a closed or open reduction and internal rotation.

Nondisplaced intraarticular calcaneus fractures should be managed with restricted weightbearing and early range of motion exercises. The treatment of displaced calcaneus fractures is controversial. Some authors advocate nonoperative treatment (restricted weightbearing and early range of motion) while others recommend operative treatment (open reduction and internal fixation).

Indications for nonoperative treatment are: nondisplaced fractures, open fracture, soft-tissue compromise that contraindicates surgery, severe peripheral vascular disease or diabetes, and severe infirmity.

Advocates for operative fixation of displaced intraarticular calcaneus fractures assert that the calcaneus is a weightbearing joint and that anatomic restoration of the posterior facet is necessary in order to minimize the risk of posttraumatic arthritis. Additionally, restoring the calcaneal anatomy facilitates later reconstructive surgery, if needed. Timing of surgical intervention is based on soft-tissue swelling. The surgery should be done within 3 weeks of the injury; if it is not, significant osseus healing will have already occurred. The surgical approach is generally lateral; however, the sural nerve is at risk with this approach. The subtalar joint is anatomically reduced and stabilized with lag screws. The body of the calcaneus is subsequently reduced (along with restoration of Bohler's and Gissane's angle) and stabilized using a buttress plate (Fig. 88-4). The necessity of bone grafting is controversial.

RESULTS

Minimally displaced calcaneus fractures have a good prognosis. It is not easy to evaluate the outcome of operative interventions in displaced calcaneus fractures because fracture classification and reports of postoperative assessment are not consistent. However, the best op-

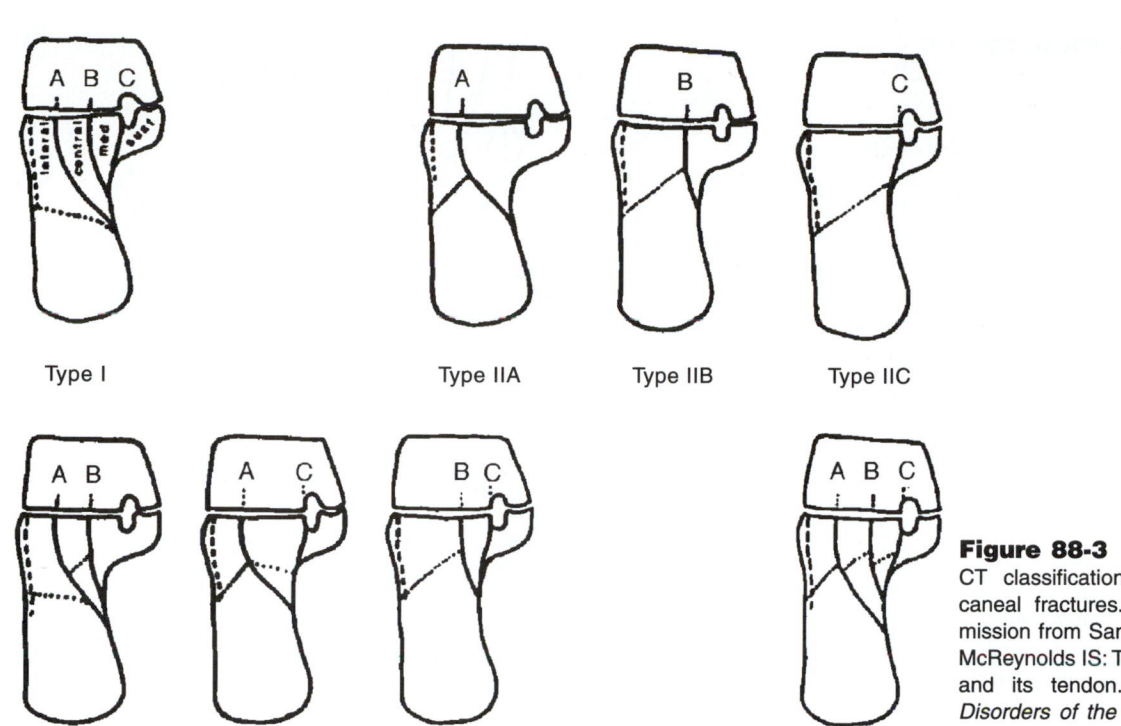

Type I

Type IIA Type IIB Type IIC

Type IIIAB Type IIIAC Type IIIBC

Type IV

Figure 88-3
CT classification of intraarticular calcaneal fractures. [Reproduced by permission from Sanders R, Hansen ST Jr, McReynolds IS: Trauma to the calcaneus and its tendon. In Jahss MH (ed): *Disorders of the Foot and Ankle,* vol 3, 2d ed. Philadelphia: WB Saunders; 1991:2336–2337.]

erative results seem to occur in the simpler fracture patterns with minimal comminution.

COMPLICATIONS

The most common complications following calcaneus fracture are wound dehiscence, subtalar arthritis, calcaneal osteomyelitis, lateral impingement syndrome, heel spur, and difficulty with shoe wear. Proper handling of soft tissue at surgery is the key to preventing wound healing complications. Subtalar arthritis may subsequently result from articular incongruity or cartilage necrosis suffered at the initial injury. Lateral wall impingement is caused by a displaced lateral wall fragment and requires resection of the lateral wall or removal of hardware.

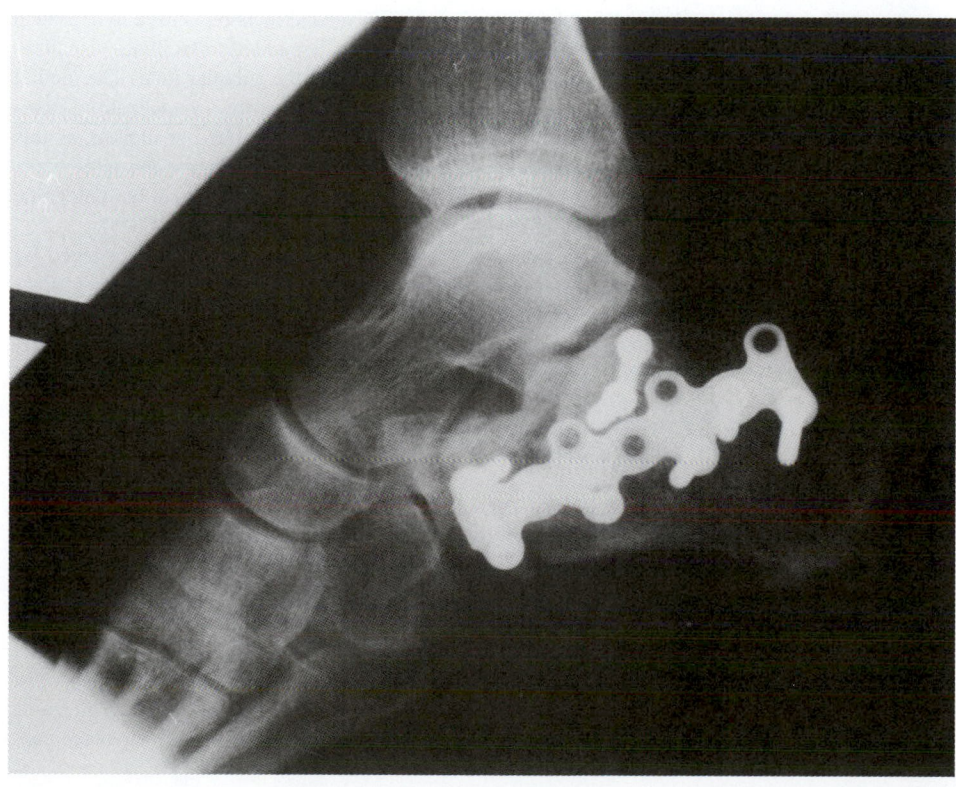

Figure 88-4
Displaced calcaneus fracture stabilized with plate and screws.

TALUS FRACTURES

ANATOMY

Sixty-percent of the talus is covered by articular cartilage. At the superior aspect, the talar dome articulates with the tibial plafond. Medially and laterally, the articular surface extends plantar to articulate with the medial and lateral malleoli. Inferiorly, the body of the talus articulates with the calcaneus through the posterior facet. The neck of the talus deviates 15 to 20 degrees medial, and articulates at the inferior aspect with the sustentaculum tali of the calcaneus via the middle facet. The head of the talus articulates anteriorly with the navicular and inferiorly with the calcaneus via the anterior facet. There are two bony processes, the posterior and lateral processes. The posterior process of the talus has medial and lateral tubercles, separated by a groove for the flexor hallucis longus tendon.

The talus does not have any muscle attachments; therefore, it is at risk for osteonecrosis following injury. The vascular supply includes: a branch from the artery to the sinus tarsi (originating from the peroneal and dorsal pedis arteries), the artery of the tarsal canal (a branch of the posterior tibial artery), the deltoid artery (a branch of the posterior tibial artery) which supplies the medial talar body, capsular/ligamentous vessels, and intraosseous anastomoses.

INCIDENCE AND MECHANISM OF INJURY

Thirty percent of talus fractures involve the talar neck. A talar neck fracture is caused by hyperdorsiflexion of the foot; the neck of the talus becomes wedged against the anterior margin of the distal tibia. Historically, talar neck fractures were caused by the foot resting on the rudder bar of an aircraft at impact; hence the name "aviator's astragalus." Most talus fractures today are caused by a motor vehicle accident or a fall from a height.

CLINICAL AND RADIOGRAPHIC EVALUATION

Fifteen to twenty percent of talar body fractures present as open injuries. In closed talus fractures, the skin may be tented over the displaced fracture fragments and become ischemic; The fracture must be promptly reduced to minimize the risk of skin slough. Twenty to twenty-five percent of talar neck fractures have an associated malleolar fracture (generally, medial malleolus).

Radiographic evaluation should include AP, oblique, and lateral views of the foot as well as the Canale view. This view demonstrates the complete talar neck in the anteroposterior direction; the foot is positioned on the x-ray cassette in 15-degree pronation, and the ankle is in maximum equinus. The x-ray beam is then directed cephalad 15 degrees from the vertical.

CLASSIFICATION

Talus fractures are classified based on fracture location: talar body, talar neck, talar head, lateral process, and/or osteochondral. Hawkins classified talar neck fractures according to the amount of fracture displacement (Fig. 88-5); it is useful to assess the likelihood of osteonecrosis of the talar body following talar neck fracture. Type I is a minimally displaced fracture. Type II is a displaced talar neck fracture with disruption of the subtalar joint. Type III is a displaced talar neck fracture with disruption of both the subtalar and ankle joints. Type IV (added by Canale and Kelly, 1978) is a displaced talar neck fracture with dislocation and extrusion of the talar body.

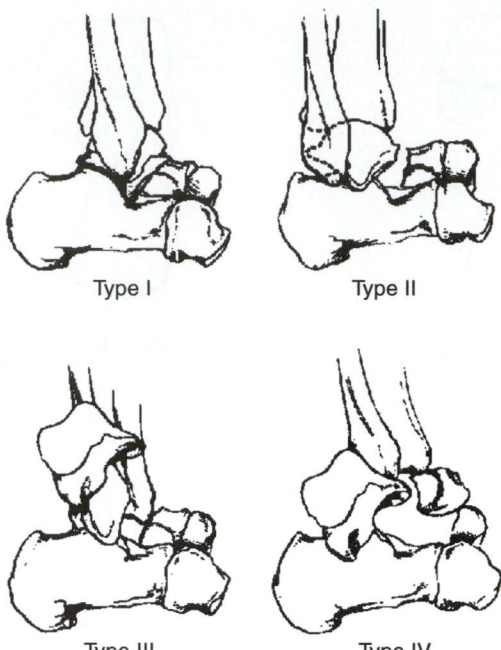

Type I   Type II

Type III   Type IV

Figure 88-5
Hawkins classification of talar neck fractures. (Reproduced by permission from Mann RA, Coughlin MJ: *Surgery of the Foot and Ankle,* 6th ed. St. Louis, MO:Mosby Year-Book, 1993:1550–1551.)

TREATMENT

Nondisplaced talar neck fracture (Hawkins type I) are best managed with a short leg cast and immobilization for 6 to 8 weeks with close monitoring during follow-up to detect loss of reduction.

Displaced talar neck fractures need anatomic joint reduction and internal fixation. Surgery should be done emergently, in order to help lower the risk of osteonecrosis. A medial incision is used to approach the talar neck; a lateral incision is often added to facilitate visualization of the ankle and posterior facet of the subtalar joint. The medial malleolus can also be osteotomized to improve visualization; however, the deltoid ligament should not be detached or incised, as this ligament contains an important vascular supply for the talar body. Following reduction, the talar neck is stabilized with either antegrade or retrograde insertion of cancellous lag screws (Fig. 88-6).

Displaced talar body and head fractures should be managed by open reduction and internal fixation employing cancellous lag screws. Adequate fracture exposure of the talar body may require a medial malleolus osteotomy. Lateral process fractures involving large fragments of bone should be stabilized.

REHABILITATION

Postoperatively, the leg is splinted and the patient is allowed non-weightbearing mobility or foot flat weightbearing and foot and ankle range of motion exercises. Once union has occurred (6 to 8 weeks), the patient is allowed progressive weightbearing as long as there are no indications of osteonecrosis. Osteolysis (disuse osteopenia, Hawkins' sign) in the subchondral bone of the dome of the talus at 6 weeks indicates that the talar body has vascularity. With evidence of osteonecrosis at 6 weeks, treatment becomes controversial. Some authors recommend progressive weightbearing; others advocate con-

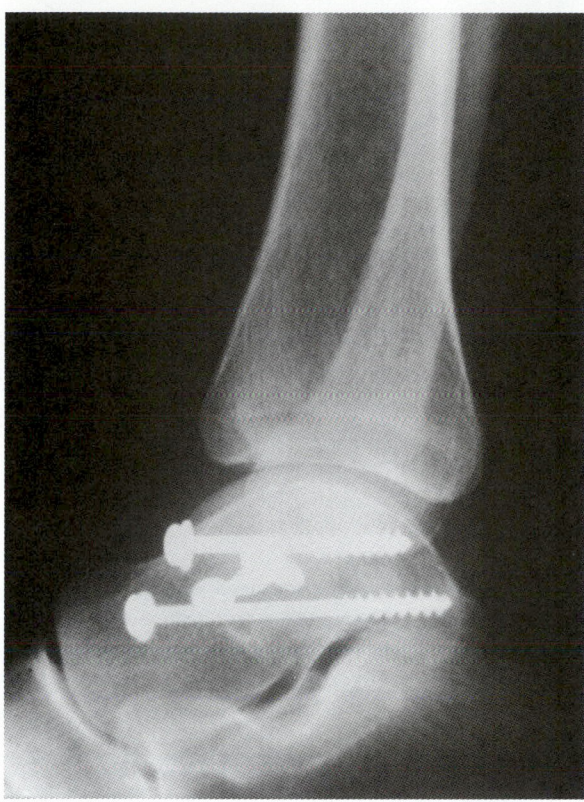

Figure 88-6
Displaced talar neck fracture stabilized with multiple lag screws.

tinuing nonweightbearing ambulation until there is evidence of revascularization.

COMPLICATIONS

The most frequent and severe complication following talar neck fracture is osteonecrosis. The risk of osteonecrosis can be predicted by the Hawkins classification (1970): Hawkins' type I has less than 10 percent risk; type II has less than 40 percent risk; type III has under a 90 percent risk; and type IV has a 100 percent risk. The incidence of posttraumatic arthritis ranges from 40 to 90 percent. Up to 15 percent of talar neck fractures have been reported to have delayed union for longer than six months.

FRACTURES OF THE MIDFOOT

ANATOMY

The midfoot includes the talonavicular and calcaneocuboid joints (transverse tarsal or Chopart's joint). The midfoot functions with the subtalar joint in both inversion and eversion. The transverse tarsal joint is mobile during pronation of the heel and fixed during supination.

CLASSIFICATION AND TREATMENT

Main and Jowett (1975) described five patterns of midfoot injury based on the direction of the applied injury force and the direction of displacement of the forefoot—medial, lateral, longitudinal, plantar, or crush. Medial stress injuries caused by inversion with adduc-

tion of the forefoot produce sprains, fracture subluxations, and dislocations. In a swivel dislocation, a medially directed force dislocates the talonavicular joint, leaving the calcaneocuboid joint intact and subluxing the subtalar joint. Midfoot sprains are generally managed with protected weightbearing. Fracture subluxations and dislocations are caused by medial displacement of the forefoot. Such injuries are generally unstable and need open reduction and internal or external fixation.

Lateral stress injuries are caused by lateral forces while the foot is in pronation. Usually, this results in an avulsion of the navicular tuberosity associated with a compression fracture of the cuboid. Immobilization and protected weightbearing are used to manage these injuries. Higher energy injuries result in subluxation of the talonavicular joint and comminution of the calcaneus or cuboid ("nutcracker fracture") which collapses the lateral longitudinal arch. Injuries such as these have a worse prognosis; open reduction and internal or external fixation may be needed.

The largest percentage of midfoot injuries are caused by longitudinal forces. The foot may be in varying degrees of plantarflexion, with lateral force applied through the metatarsal heads. Fractures usually take place vertically through the navicular along the line of force. If the fractures are not displaced, they can be treated nonoperatively; if displaced, internal fixation is required.

NAVICULAR FRACTURES

There are four types of navicular fractures: cortical avulsion, tuberosity, body, and stress fractures. Cortical avulsion fractures represent 50 percent of presenting navicular fractures. If they are displaced and involve more than 20 percent of the articular surface, these fractures require open reduction and internal fixation.

Tuberosity fractures represent 20 to 25 percent of navicular fractures and result from eversion of the foot, with avulsion through the posterior tibial tendon or anterior fibers of the deltoid ligament. Displaced fractures need excision or open reduction and internal fixation for larger fragments.

Navicular body fractures frequently occur in association with other midfoot injuries. They have been classified by Sangeorzan into three categories (Fig. 88-7): in type I, the transverse fracture line is in the coronal plane with no angulation of the forefoot; in type II, which is the most common, the fracture line extends from dorsolateral to plantarmedial with the forefoot displaced medially; and in type III, there is a comminuted fracture pattern with the forefoot displaced laterally. Nondisplaced navicular body fractures are managed nonoperatively. Displaced fractures need open reduction and internal or external fixation in order to preserve anatomic reduction.

Stress fractures of the navicular body happen mainly in athletes secondary to the absorption of repetitive force and bone fatigue. Stress fractures may not be initially visible on plain radiographs; bone scans may be needed to confirm the diagnosis. Fractures can be complete or incomplete, and typically occur in the sagittal plane. If diagnosed early, they may be treated with cast immobilization (6 to 8 weeks).

CUBOID AND CUNEIFORM FRACTURES

Cuboid fractures are often associated with a Lisfranc fracture-dislocation or avulsion fracture of the navicular. Those with minimal displacement may be treated with a short leg walking cast. If significant comminution or displacement exists, calcaneocuboid arthrodesis may be necessary. Cuneiform fractures generally present in association with midtarsal or tarsometatarsal joint injuries; isolated cuneiform injuries can occur by direct force.

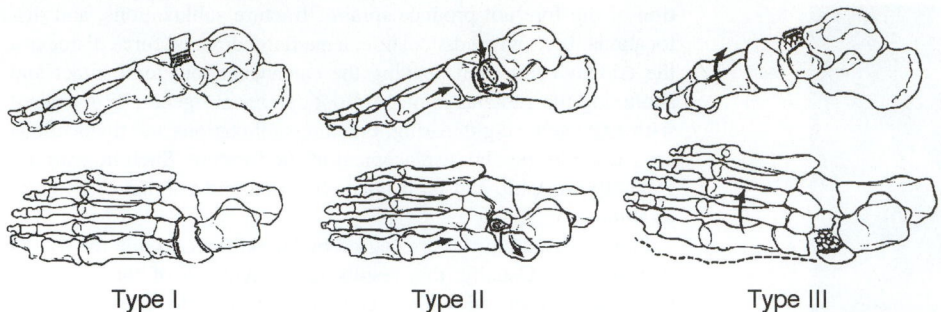

Type I   Type II   Type III

Figure 88-7
Sangeorzan classification of navicular body fractures. (Reproduced by permission from Sangeorzan BJ, Benirschke, SK, Mosca V, et al: Displaced intraarticular fractures of the tarsal navicular. *J Bone Joint Surg [Am]* 1989; 71:1504–1508.)

INJURIES TO THE TARSOMETATARSAL JOINT

ANATOMY

The tarsometatarsal joint (Lisfranc's joint) is immobile. Osseo-ligamentous attachments and the bony architecture are responsible for its intrinsic stability. The base of the second metatarsal is recessed between the three cuneiforms. Lisfranc's ligament is a strong ligament and joins the second metatarsal base to the medial cuneiform. The metatarsal heads are stabilized by the transverse metatarsal ligaments; the lateral 4 metatarsal bases are also connected by strong ligamentous attachments.

MECHANISM OF INJURY

Fracture-dislocations of Lisfranc's joint are the result of either direct or indirect forces. Forefoot twisting, axial loading of the fixed foot, and crushing are the three most common mechanisms of injury.

EVALUATION

AP, lateral, and oblique radiographs are required for evaluation of the tarsometatarsal joint. Normally, the medial border of the second metatarsal is in line with the medial border of the middle cuneiform on the AP view, and the medial border of the fourth metatarsal is in line with the medial border of the cuboid on the oblique view. If an injury is suspected on clinical examination but cannot be confirmed by radiographs, a stress roentgenogram should be taken. The most reliable radiographic sign of Lisfranc injury is a widening between the first and second metatarsal bases.

CLASSIFICATION

Quenu and Kuss described a simple classification system of tarsometatarsal joint injury; it divides Lisfranc fracture dislocations into three types (homolateral, isolated, divergent) based on the pattern of injury (Fig. 88-8). In homolateral dislocations, all five metatarsals are displaced in the same direction. In isolated dislocations, one or two metatarsals are displaced from the remaining metatarsals. In divergent dislocations, displacement of the metatarsals occurs in both the sagittal and/or coronal planes.

Myerson and coworkers described a classification system using joint incongruity to distinguish among Lisfranc injuries (Fig. 88-9). Type A is total joint incongruity which may occur in any plane or direction. Type B1 is partial joint incongruity where the displacement effects only the medial ray. In type B2, also partial incongruity, the displacement effects one or more of the lateral metatarsals in any plane or direction. Type C1 injuries have a divergent pattern; the first

metatarsal is displaced medially and the lateral metatarsals have partial incongruity. Last, type C2 injuries have a divergent pattern with total incongruity.

TREATMENT

Sprains of Lisfranc's joint should be managed with immobilization to optimize proper ligament healing. Anatomic reduction and stable fixation using wires, pins, or screws are required for subluxation or dislocation of this complex.

METATARSAL FRACTURES

Fractures of the first metatarsal usually result from direct trauma. First metatarsal fractures that are nondisplaced are treated with immobilization. Displaced fractures need internal fixation. Second, third and fourth metatarsal fractures are the result of either direct trauma, indirect twisting forces, or repetitive stress. Nondisplaced fractures can be managed with a short leg cast or by orthosis. Displaced fractures with more than 2 to 4 mm shortening or elevation should be treated by internal fixation.

Fifth metatarsal fractures include either the metatarsal neck, shaft, and/or base. Fifth metatarsal neck and shaft fractures are managed similar to fractures of the lesser metatarsals. Fifth metatarsal base fractures are either an avulsion fracture of the tuberosity (pseudo-

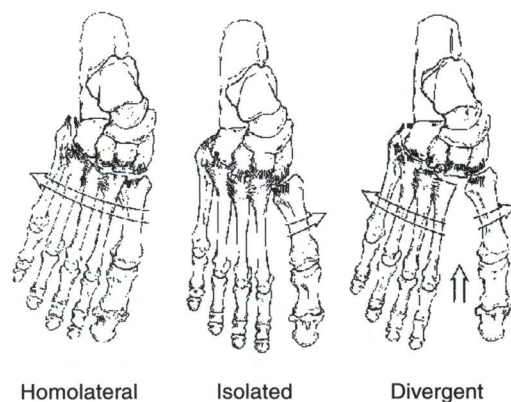

Homolateral   Isolated   Divergent

Figure 88-8
Quenu and Kuss classification of Lisfranc fracture-dislocations. [Reproduced by permission from Adelaar RS: The treatment of tarsometatarsal fracture-dislocation. In Greene WB (ed): *Instructional Course Lectures.* Park Ridge, IL: American Academy of Orthopaedic Surgeons; 1990; 39:142.]

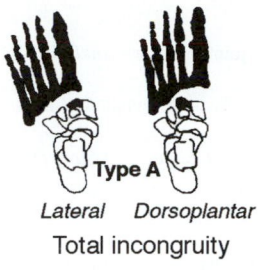

Type A

Lateral   Dorsoplantar

Total incongruity

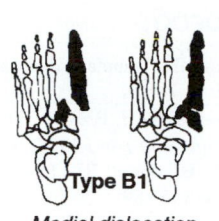

Type B1

Medial dislocation

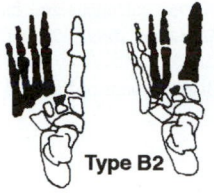

Type B2

Lateral dislocation

Partial incongruity

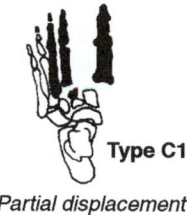

Type C1

Partial displacement

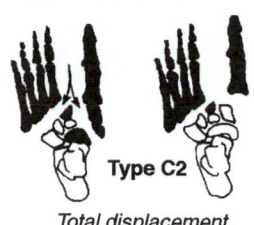

Type C2

Total displacement

Divergent

Figure 88-9
Myerson classification of Lisfranc fracture-dislocations. (Reproduced by permission from Myerson MS, Fisher RT, Burgess AR, et al: Fracture dislocation of tarsometatarsal joints. *Foot and Ankle* 1986; 6:228.)

Jones fracture) or fracture of the proximal shaft at the diaphyseal/metaphyseal junction (Jones fracture).

Avulsion fracture of the fifth metatarsal tuberosity is caused by acute inversion with plantarflexion of the foot; avulsion occurs due to the pull of the lateral plantar aponeurosis. This injury is managed nonoperatively applying a walking cast or boot. Fractures involving significant displacement can be reduced and stabilized with a lag screw or tension band construct.

Fractures at the proximal diaphyseal/metaphyseal junction of the fifth metatarsal commonly result from either an acute traumatic injury or repetitive stress. Acute fractures are managed with a short leg cast and nonweightbearing (6 weeks). Stress fractures require a prolonged period of time for union and may need operative treatment. Operative management should include intramedullary screw fixation.

METATARSAL STRESS FRACTURES

Stress fractures generally occur in the second and third metatarsals. Patients complain of discomfort and prodromal pain prior to the acute onset of localized pain. Radiographs can be negative for 1 to 2 months; radioisotope scanning is recommended if there is a high index of suspicion from the clinical examination. Nondisplaced stress fractures are managed with application of a short leg cast or orthosis and limitations on physical activity. Displaced metatarsal stress fractures require internal fixation.

METATARSOPHALANGEAL JOINTS

Metatarsophalangeal joint (MTP) motion is important for normal gait. Sprains of the first MTP joint (turf toe) often occur as the result of football injury. Treatment includes: rest, ice, compression, elevation with protective taping, and a gradual return to activity. Dislocation of the first MTP is caused by high energy trauma and forced hyperextension; treatment includes joint reduction and protective taping/splinting. Dislocations that cannot be reduced require open reduction. Intraarticular fractures of the first MTP also require open reduction and internal fixation. Dislocation of the lesser MTP joints is usually caused by lower energy trauma; treatment is joint reduction with toe

traction and buddy taping to the adjacent toe. Intraarticular fractures of the lesser MTP joints are managed using open reduction and internal fixation, fragment excision, or benign neglect, depending on the size the fragment and amount of comminution.

FRACTURES OF THE SESAMOIDS

The tibial and fibular sesamoid bones are located within the medial and lateral tendon slips of the flexor hallucis brevis muscle. The medial sesamoid supports a larger percentage of weight than the lateral sesamoid, and is therefore fractured more frequently. These fractures are typically transverse or comminuted and must be distinguished from a bipartite sesamoid. Treatment is a short leg walking cast or orthosis for 3 to 4 weeks. If nonoperative treatment is unsuccessful, a sesamoidectomy should be considered.

PHALANGEAL FRACTURES

Nondisplaced great toe phalangeal fractures may be treated symptomatically with protective splinting. Fractures that are displaced require reduction with buddy taping to the adjacent toe. Open reduction may be necessary if the fracture is intraarticular or nonreducible. Symptomatic treatment is also appropriate for lesser toe fractures of the proximal and middle phalanges; moderate displacement is generally of little significance. Intraarticular fractures of the interphalangeal joint are treated in a similar nonoperative manner unless they are open or have significant displacement. If lesser toe phalangeal fractures should unite with significant angulation, a lateral prominence could develop with a resultant interdigital corn.

SUGGESTED READINGS

CALCANEUS FRACTURES

Essex-Lopresti P: The mechanism, reduction technique, and results in fractures of the os calcis. *Br J Surg* 1952; 39:395.

Hammesfahr JFR: Surgical treatment of calcaneus fractures. *Orthop Clin North Am* 1989; 20:679.

Sanders R, Hansen ST Jr, McReynolds IS: Trauma to the calcaneus and its tendon. In Jahss MH (ed): *Disorders of the Foot and Ankle,* 2d ed. Philadelphia: WB Saunders; 1991; 3:2326.

Souer R, Remy R: Fractures of the calcaneus with displacement of the thalamic portion. *J Bone Joint Surg [Br]* 1975; 57:413.

TALUS FRACTURES

Adelaar RS: The treatment of complex fractures of the talus. *Orthop Clin North Am* 1989; 20:691.

Canale ST, Kelly FB: Fractures of the neck of the talus. *J Bone Joint Surg [Am]* 1978; 60:143.

Hawkins LG: Fractures of the neck of the talus. *J Bone Joint Surg [Am]* 1970; 52:991.

Mayo KA: Fractures of the talus: Principles of management and techniques of treatment. *Tech Orthop* 1987; 2:42.

Mulfinger GL, Trueta J: The blood supply of the talus. *J Bone Joint Surg [Br]* 1970; 52:160.

MIDFOOT

Jahss MH: Traumatic dislocation of the first MTP joint. *Foot and Ankle* 1980; 1:15.

Kavanaugh JH, Brower TD, Mann RV: The Jones fracture revisited. *J Bone Joint Surg [Am]* 1978; 60:776.

Main BJ, Jowett RL: Injuries of the midtarsal joint. *J Bone Joint Surg [Br]* 1975; 57:89.

Myerson MS: The diagnosis and treatment of injuries to the Lisfranc joint complex. *Orthop Clin North Am* 1989; 20:655.

Rodeo SA, O'Brien S, Warren RF, et al: Turf-toe: An analysis of metatarsophalangeal joint sprains in professional football players. *Am J Sports Med* 1990; 18:280.

Sangeorzan BJ, Benirschke SK, Mosca V, et al: Displaced intraarticular fractures of the tarsal navicular. *J Bone Joint Surg [Am]* 1989; 71:1504.

Chapter 89

POSTTRAUMATIC OSTEOMYELITIS

Kenneth J. Koval

PATHOGENESIS

In posttraumatic osteomyelitis, bacteria gain access to the bone by direct inoculation. Local tissues, compromised by edema and necrotic debris, present an ideal environment for bacterial growth. Bone, stripped of its periosteum, has exposed collagen and hydroxyapatite, which provide metabolites for bacteria and surfaces for adherence. Host defenses, such as leukocytes and macrophages, are mobilized but cannot penetrate the avascular focus of infection. Antibiotics are ineffective because the lack of a local blood supply prevents the uptake of bacteriocidal levels.

MICROBIOLOGY

Historically, gram-positive aerobic organisms (*Staphylococcus* and *Streptococcus*) were the most common pathogens known to cause osteomyelitis. Recent reports, however, have documented the increasing frequency of gram-negative, anaerobic, and mixed infections.

CLINICAL AND RADIOGRAPHIC EVALUATION

One should assess whether the patient had an open or closed fracture, a history of previous infection, and prior attempts at treatment. In the acute situation, the extremity may exhibit the typical signs of inflammation, such as erythema, warmth, swelling, and tenderness. These signs are characteristically absent in chronic osteomyelitis.

The osseous integrity (infected union vs. nonunion) should be determined for its impact on prognosis. With nonunion, there may be gross motion at the fracture or simply pain on weightbearing and tenderness to palpation.

In addition to the often-present draining sinus, the condition of the soft tissues and adjacent joints should be carefully assessed. Skin quality may be poor due to scarring; muscle tissue may be inadequate either from actual tissue loss at the time of the original injury or from fibrosis.

The neurovascular status of the involved limb has significant impact on the treatment plan. Particular attention should be addressed towards the vascularity of the extremity; the quality of the distal pulses and any skin changes suggestive of vascular insufficiency, such as venous stasis ulcers, should be noted. Concerns which arise regarding the vascular status of the extremity should be addressed by a vascular consultant or arteriography. This is mandatory if one is considering performing a free tissue transfer.

One must assess the general medical and metabolic condition of the patient. Systemic disorders such as diabetes, malnutrition, renal failure, liver failure, and hypoxia from chronic pulmonary disease all impact on the prognosis. Other factors to be considered are alcohol and tobacco abuse, steroid use, immune deficiency, and concomitant malignancy. All of the above factors have in common an effect on host metabolism, immune surveillance, and local vascularity, which, in turn, has direct bearing on the ability to "cure" osteomyelitis. Finally, one must evaluate the activity level of the patient. An extensive surgical reconstruction may not be warranted in a marginal ambulator with multiple medical problems and chronic osteomyelitis.

Laboratory tests to be obtained as part of the initial workup should include the leukocyte count with differential, erythrocyte sedimentation rate (ESR), and C-reactive protein (CRP). In chronic osteomyelitis, the leukocyte count may be normal. The ESR and CRP, both acute phase reactants, are nonspecific markers of inflammation and are usually elevated. However, serial determinations may help assess the response of infection to treatment. Chemistries, albumin, total protein, renal function tests, and liver function tests should also be included as part of a metabolic analysis.

Sinus tract cultures have little place in the bacteriologic diagnosis of chronic osteomyelitis. They may not accurately reflect the bacteriology of the underlying infection because *Staphylococcus* and gram-negative bacilli often colonize sinus tracts. Operative specimens are the only acceptable source for bacteriologic diagnosis.

Radiographic evaluation includes an AP and lateral of the extremity. One should note the status of the fracture (union versus pseudarthrosis) and the presence and type of retained hardware. Necrotic bone (sequestrum) is the hallmark of chronic osteomyelitis and can be recognized radiographically as an area of sclerosis surrounded by new bone formation (involucrum). Even in the presence of these findings, radionucleotide scans (technetium, gallium, and indium) should be obtained in order to identify "skip lesions," determine the extent of osseous involvement, and to help plan the surgical approach. Osteomyelitis presents as an area of increased uptake on the delayed image of a technetium bone scan. This phase reflects active osteoblastic activity, and therefore, increased uptake is not specific for osteomyelitis. Gallium scanning is often used in conjunction with three-phase bone scanning to localize inflammatory lesions. Its exact mechanism of uptake is unclear. As in technetium scans, increased uptake is nonspecific. The combination of gallium and technetium scans, however, increases diagnostic specificity. In noninflammatory conditions, technetium uptake will be more intense than that of gallium. In areas of inflammation, such as osteomyelitis, the gallium uptake will either exceed that of technetium, or differ in its distribution. Indium scanning is more specific for acute infection than either bone or gallium scanning. The patient's leukocytes are directly labeled with indium-111; leukocytes are not usually incorporated into areas of increased bone turnover.

Computed tomography (CT) and magnetic resonance imaging (MRI) are other modalities useful in the evaluation of chronic osteomyelitis. CT is superior to MRI in delineating cortical abnormalities, abscesses, sinus tracts, cloacae, and sequestra. MRI is useful for the detection of soft tissue and bone marrow pathology.

CLASSIFICATION

The Cierny and Mader (1989) classification of adult osteomyelitis is based on the anatomic osseous involvement and the physiologic condition of the host. These two factors are combined to form clinical stages which can be used to determine treatment and prognosis.

There are four anatomic types, based on the site and extent of osseous involvement: type I is medullary osteomyelitis; type II is superficial osteomyelitis limited to the surface of the bone; type III is localized osteomyelitis with full-thickness cortical involvement; and type IV is diffuse osteomyelitis with circumferential cortical involvement. Types I and II represent straightforward conditions while Types III and IV are complex disease states often involving massive osseous and soft tissue reconstruction.

The physiologic class of the host is related to the systemic and local factors that affect patient response to infection and treatment. Class A persons have normal systemic defenses, metabolic capabilities and vascularity. Class B patients have local and or systemic factors which affect immune surveillance, metabolism, or local vascularity. Included in the B category are patients suffering from malnutrition, renal or liver failure, or "extremes of age." Therefore, many elderly patients with chronic osteomyelitis would be considered class B hosts. Class C patients have anticipated treatment morbidity worse than the presenting condition with a poor prognosis for cure.

TREATMENT

Successful treatment of osteomyelitis must fulfill the following criteria: (1) adequate debridement of necrotic and infected soft tissue and osseous structures, (2) the preservation or creation of bony stability, (3) ablation of dead space, and (4) soft-tissue coverage.

Debridement of dead and infected tissue is the most important factor in the treatment of chronic osteomyelitis. All dead and infected tissue must be excised. Because of the difficulty in determining bone viability, multiple debridements may be necessary to excise all necrotic tissue. Preservation or creation of bony stability is vital to the treatment of osteomyelitis. Dead-space management is crucial to control bacterial growth. Open-wound management with packing and dressing changes, as well as whirlpool therapy, performs local debridement, prevents hematoma collection, and allows the growth of granulation tissue. Methylmethacrylate acts as a spacer to prevent hematoma formation and preserves room for later bone graft placement. Culture specific antibiotics can be added to the methylmethacrylate to increase local antibiotic delivery.

Bone grafting can be performed as an open or closed technique, and can involve the use of pure cancellous bone, vascularized free tissue transfer, or bone transport. Closed-wound bone grafting should be performed once all necrotic tissue has been eradicated and a healthy tissue bed remains. It is advisable to use pure cancellous bone as it will not form a sequestrum if infection persists. Free fibular grafts can be used for the treatment of large osseus defects. Because the graft is vascularized, there are fewer complications with host incorporation than with conventional grafting techniques. The use of distraction histogenesis allows bone transport without bone grafting. There is, theoretically, no limit to the distance one can span using this technique.

Muscle transposition obliterates dead space and may improve vascularity through delivery of a new permanent blood supply. This improved vascularity may increase local antibiotic concentration and provide the cellular, noncellular, and oxygen environment necessary to help control infection, promote wound healing, and provide a soft tissue envelope resistant to further breakdown. Antibiotic therapy should be based on intra-operative cultures and sensitivities. The length of antibiotic therapy is controversial.

RESULTS

Weiland and coworkers (1984) reported on the efficacy of free tissue transfer in 33 cases of osteomyelitis, 25 involving the tibia. Twenty (59 percent) had successful treatment at an average follow-up of 41.4 years. Fifty percent of the failures were the result of unsuccessful microvascular anastomosis. Kelly (1990) reported on the treatment of 425 cases of osteomyelitis, 124 involving the tibia. All wounds were debrided and closed over suction drainage, received suction irrigation, and/or had a rotational or free muscle flap. Patients were followed for a minimum of 2 years; 84 percent were successfully treated.

SUGGESTED READINGS

Cierny G 3d, Mader JT: Approach to adult osteomyelitis. *Orthop Rev* 1987; 16:259.

Kelly PJ, Fitzgerald RH Jr, Cabanela ME, et al: Results of treatment of tibial and femoral osteomeylitis in adults. *Clin Orthop* 1990; 259:295.

Moore JR, Weiland AJ: Vasularized tissue transfer in the treatment of osteomyelitis. *Clin Plastic Surg* 1986; 13:657.

Pellegrini VD Jr, Reid JS, Evarts CM: Complications: osteomyelitis. In Rockwood CA Jr, Green DP, Bucholz RW, et al (eds): *Fractures in Adults,* 4th ed. Philadelphia: Lippincott-Raven; 1996:467, 505.

Weiland AJ, Moore JR, Daniel RK: The efficacy of free tissue transfer in the treatment of osteomyelitis. *J Bone Joint Surg [Am]* 1984; 66:181.

Chapter 90

SEPTIC ARTHRITIS

Kenneth J. Koval

ETIOLOGY

Septic, or pyogenic, arthritis is typically monoarticular and the result of microorganisms entering the joint space. It can result from hematogenous seeding, contiguous spread, direct inoculation via trauma, or an iatrogenic mechanism through therapeutic procedures.

Staphylococcus aureus is the most common causative agent in adults. *Neisseria gonorrhoeae* is a common causative microorganism in sexually active adults. In children, *Hacmophilus influenzae* is frequently the cause of infection. A significant percentage (50 percent) of older patients diagnosed with infectious arthritis concomitantly have underlying rheumatoid arthritis; these infections are generally caused by *Streptococcus pyogenes, Streptococcus pneumoniae,* and gram-negative bacilli. Intravenous drug abuse is associated with an increased incidence of bacteremia, endocarditis, and septic arthritis. Higher rates of joint infection can also be seen in patients with diabetes and those with compromised immunity.

CLINICAL EVALUATION

The most common sites for septic arthritis are the knee (40 to 50 percent), hip (20 to 25 percent), ankle, shoulder, elbow, and hand. Classically, patient presentation is characterized by an erythematous joint that is acutely painful, swollen, warm to the touch, tender to palpation, and has a limited range of motion; however, manifestations may vary widely.

Joint aspiration is necessary to diagnose septic arthritis. The aspirate should be evaluated by gram stain with WBC, culture and sensitivity, and fluid chemistry determinations. If there are >50,000 cell/mm^3 with 90 percent polymorphs, septic arthritis should be suspected. A complete blood count with differential and measurement of serum glucose for comparison with synovial fluid should be done. Normal synovial fluid glucose concentration is approximately two-thirds that of serum glucose concentration. In septic arthritis, glucose level in the joint decreases relative to that of the serum. Increased protein levels in synovial fluid are generally within a range of 3 to 7 g/dl. Diagnostic confirmation is by microscopic examination of the synovial fluid and identification of the offending microorganisms.

TREATMENT

If started early in the course of the disease, effective management can be achieved using serial joint aspirations coupled with appropriate antibiotic therapy. Therapeutic response can be assessed by observing if the fluid volume and percent of neutrophils declines with successive aspirations. Surgical drainage is necessary if antibiotics and repeated aspirations are not effective over the first 3 to 5 days of treatment, or if treatment was started late in the course of the disease and the exudate was loculated or too thick to be aspirated. Hip joint infection virtually always requires surgical drainage because joint aspiration is difficult. No demonstrable benefit has been found using local antibiotics or continuous through and through irrigation of the joint.

Parenteral antibiotic therapy should be started based upon the probable causative organism and the gram stain. In adults, a cephalosporin or nafcillin are usually effective; if gonococcus is suspected, ceftriaxone should be used. Antibiotic therapy should be changed or adjusted based on susceptibility data. Usual recommendations are 6 weeks of antibiotic therapy for nongonococcal infections and 2 weeks for gonococcal arthritis. Oral antibiotics may be started with signs of clinical improvement as demonstrated by decreased joint pain, swelling, and fever. The role of continuous passive motion of the affected joint remains a controversial aspect of management.

SUGGESTED READINGS

Brower AC: Septic arthritis. *Radiol Clin North Am* 1996; 34:293.

Cunningham R, Cockayne A, Humphreys H: Clinical and molecular aspects of the pathogenesis of Staphylococcus aureus bone and joint infections. *J Microbiol* 1996; 44:157.

Dubost JJ, Fills I, Denis P, et al: Polyarticular septic arthritis. *Medicine* 1993; 72:296.

Jeroasch J, Hoffstetter I, Schroder M, et al: Septic arthritis: Arthroscopic management with local antibiotic treatment. *Acta Orthop Belg* 1995; 61:126.

Norman DC, Yoshikawa TT: Infections of the bone, joint, and bursa. *Clin Geriatr Med* 1994; 10:703.

Chapter 91

INDICATIONS, TECHNIQUES, AND COMPLICATIONS OF ARTHROSCOPY

Andrew S. Rokito

ARTHROSCOPY OF THE ELBOW

INDICATIONS

Common indications for arthroscopic surgery of the elbow include: (1) the removal of loose bodies, (2) the evaluation and treatment of osteochondritis dissecans of the capitellum, (3) the treatment of chronic synovitis that is either posttraumatic or inflammatory, such as in rheumatoid arthritis, and (4) the excision of osteophytes that can be painful and limit flexion or extension of the elbow. Other indications include: (1) debridement of posttraumatic adhesions and articular surface defects, (2) evaluation of the articular surfaces following subtle intraarticular fractures, and the (3) evaluation of the chronically painful elbow of undetermined etiology.

Contraindications to elbow arthroscopy include: (1) ankylosis of either a bony or fibrous nature that would prevent introduction of the arthroscope into the joint, and (2) altered anatomy that would place the neurovascular structures at an increased risk for injury, such as following ulnar nerve transposition.

SURGICAL TECHNIQUE

Patient Positioning

Arthroscopy of the elbow can be successfully performed with the patient in the supine, prone, or lateral decubitus positions. Elbow arthroscopy was originally described with the patient supine. This position allows access to both the medial and lateral sides of the elbow which can be freely pronated and supinated to identify the bony landmarks. It, however, requires the use of an overhead traction system, which may limit flexion and extension of the elbow. The extremity is also somewhat unstable in this position as it tends to swing like a pendulum, requiring the arm to be stabilized by an assistant. Access to the posterior compartment is somewhat difficult in that the instruments are positioned beneath the operative field forcing the surgeon to operate "upside down" in an awkward fashion.

Arthroscopy of the elbow with the patient in the prone position eliminates the need for an overhead traction system. This allows for improved mobility and stability and utilizes gravity to maintain the elbow in approximately 90 degrees of flexion. In this position, the olecranon faces the surgeon allowing direct access to and more normal orientation of the posterior compartment. Patient positioning, however, may be somewhat more inconvenient for both the surgeon and the anesthesiologist.

The lateral decubitus position for elbow arthroscopy allows ready access to all of the various portal sites without the inconvenience of positioning the patient prone or using an overhead traction system for the supine position. In addition, the lateral decubitus position, like the prone position, provides optimum mobility and stability of the

extremity, and facilitates surgery within the posterior compartment. The upper arm is supported on a well-padded bolster which is secured to the side of the operating table. The forearm is allowed to hang free with the elbow flexed 90 degrees. This affords unlimited elbow flexion, extension, pronation, and supination.

Anatomy

The bony anatomic landmarks are outlined with a marking pen prior to the procedure, as fluid extravasation and soft tissue swelling can make later identification very difficult. The course of the ulnar nerve as it passes across the posteromedial aspect of the elbow, is also marked to avoid inadvertent injury.

Laterally, the bony landmarks include the radial head and the lateral epicondyle. The medial epicondyle is identified on the medial side, and the olecranon can be located posteriorly. The ulnar nerve courses through the cubital tunnel on the posteromedial aspect of the elbow.

Portals and Arthroscopic Anatomy

Several portals have been described for arthroscopy of the elbow. Those most commonly used include the: (1) proximal medial, (2) anterolateral, (3) midline posterior, and the (4) posterolateral portals.

Prior to insertion of the arthroscope, the elbow joint is distended with fluid. The entry point for initial capsular distention is located at the "soft spot" in the center of the triangle formed by the lateral epicondyle, radial head, and olecranon tip.

The proximal medial portal is located 2 cm proximal to the medial epicondyle, just anterior to the metaphyseal ridge and the medial intermuscular septum. With the arm held in 90 degrees of flexion, the arthroscopic sheath and trocar are inserted and directed toward the center of the joint (Fig. 91-1). Only the skin is penetrated with the scalpel blade to avoid injury to the medial antebrachial cutaneous nerve. Care must be taken to keep the arthroscopic sheath and trocar anterior to the intermuscular septum to avoid injury to the ulnar nerve. The trocar should be guided along the distal humerus until the capsule is pierced, to avoid the median nerve and the brachial artery.

The capitellum and radial head can best be visualized from the proximal medial portal. By pronating and supinating the forearm, visualization of the radial head is facilitated, and approximately 75 percent of it can usually be seen. Flexion and extension allow a more complete inspection of the articular surface of the capitellum. Slow, careful retraction of the arthroscope, while directing it toward the ulna, allows visualization of the coronoid process.

An anterolateral portal is established using an "inside-out" maneuver. This technique involves passing a Wissinger rod through the proximal medial arthroscopic sheath and directing it to a point on the

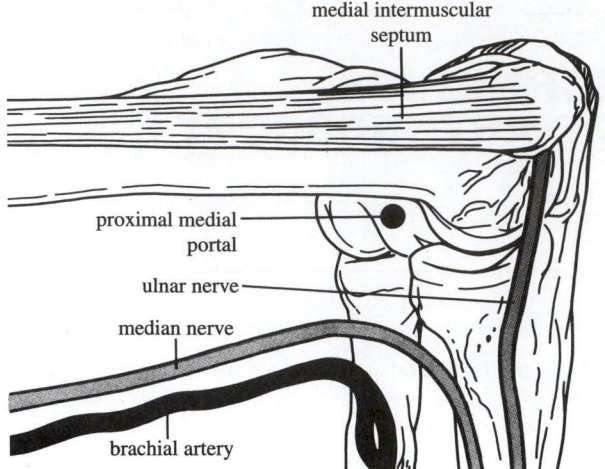

Figure 91-1
Proximal medial portal. The patient is in the prone position. [Reproduced by permission from Parisien JS: The elbow. In: *Techniques in Therapeutic Arthroscopy*, 2d ed. New York: Raven Press (now Lippincott Williams & Wilkins); 1993:21.7.]

inner aspect of the joint adjacent to the anterior border of the capitellum at the level of the radiocapitellar articulation. The rod is advanced through the capsule into the subcutaneous tissue. A cannula is then placed over the rod and arthroscopic sheath, and all three are then retracted into the joint. The arthroscope can now be inserted to complete the evaluation of the anterior compartment.

The extensor carpi radialis brevis muscle is pierced when establishing the anterolateral portal. Structures at risk for injury include the lateral and posterior antebrachial cutaneous and radial nerves. Cadaveric dissections have demonstrated that the arthroscope can come within 7 mm of the radial nerve. Thus, precise placement of this portal is critical.

The intraarticular structures that can be visualized through the anterolateral portal include the distal humerus and trochlear ridges and the coronoid process of the ulna. Careful retraction of the arthroscope with rotation also allows a small portion of the radial head to be visible. Flexion and extension of the elbow allow a more complete inspection of the articular surfaces.

The midline posterior portal is established approximately 3 cm proximal to the tip of the olecranon directly through the triceps tendon. This portal should also be established with the elbow in 20 to 30 degrees of flexion. A viewing space is created by clearing intraarticular adhesions and fatty tissues with gentle side to side movement of the arthroscopic sheath and trocar.

The posterolateral portal entry point is located approximately 1 1/2 to 3 cm proximal to the olecranon tip, just superior and posterior to the lateral epicondyle, adjacent to the lateral border of the triceps muscle. This portal is also best established with the elbow in 20 to 30 degrees of flexion to allow relaxation of the triceps.

In establishing the posterior portals, the triceps tendon and muscle are pierced. Structures to be avoided when making these portals include the posterior antebrachial cutaneous nerve which courses over the posterolateral distal humerus, and the ulnar nerve located approximately 2 1/2 cm medial to the center of the elbow joint.

The arthroscopic anatomy visualized from the posterior portals include the olecranon fossa located over the posterior aspect of the distal humerus, and the tip of the olecranon. By flexing and extending the elbow, a more complete inspection of the distal humerus and olecranon can be performed.

COMPLICATIONS

Complications associated with elbow arthroscopy include injury to neurovascular structures, iatrogenic injury to articular surfaces, and infection.

Neurovascular injury can occur either by direct means or from compression secondary to fluid extravasation. Injuries to the sensory nerves are more common. Most fluid extravasation is subcutaneous and will resolve spontaneously with elevation of the extremity. Extravasation can be minimized by avoiding multiple attempts at establishing portals and maintaining them throughout the procedure. Local anesthetic should not be injected into the elbow postoperatively, as this has been associated with a transient sensory nerve block interfering with the assessment of postoperative neurological status. Significant injury to motor nerves, although rare, has been reported. A subluxating or dislocating ulnar nerve is at particular risk for injury, particularly with the elbow flexed, and the existence of this entity should be determined preoperatively. In general, maintaining elbow flexion of 90 degrees and keeping the joint maximally distended, while paying careful attention to portal placement, minimizes the risk of neurovascular injury.

Inadvertent injury to chondral surfaces is perhaps the most common complication of elbow arthroscopy, and once again, strict attention to detail and maintaining maximal joint distention becomes critical.

The incidence of infection following elbow arthroscopy is low and should be no higher than that associated with arthroscopy of the knee and shoulder.

ARTHROSCOPY OF THE SHOULDER

INDICATIONS

Indications for shoulder arthroscopy can be categorized into intraarticular and subacromial procedures. Intraarticular procedures include (1) the removal of loose bodies, (2) the debridement of rotator cuff tears, (3) the repair or debridement of superior labral lesions, (4) the repair of Bankart lesions, and (5) the lysis of adhesions as in adhesive capsulitis. Subacromial or extraarticular procedures include: (1) subacromial decompression, (2) lateral clavicle resection, (3) the debridement or repair of rotator cuff tears, and (4) the treatment of calcific tendinitis.

SURGICAL TECHNIQUE

Patient Positioning

Shoulder arthroscopy can be performed with the patient in either the sitting or lateral decubitus positions. There are several advantages of the sitting, or beach-chair, position. These include the following: (1) ease of patient positioning, (2) ability to convert directly to an open procedure without repositioning, (3) more anatomic orientation, (4) ability to manipulate the arm during the procedure, (5) lower risk of neuropraxia from traction, and (5) ability to perform the procedure under regional anesthesia with the patient awake. Proponents of the lateral decubitus position feel that it provides optimum exposure for instrument placement and allows for distraction as the arm is held in traction.

Anatomy

The important anatomic landmarks include: (1) the spine of the scapula, (2) the acromion, (3) the acromioclavicular joint, (4) the coracoid process, (5) the humeral head, (6) the glenoid rim, and (7) the glenohumeral joint. These can be outlined with a surgical marker prior to the procedure.

Portals and Arthroscopic Anatomy

Shoulder arthroscopy begins with the posterior portal. This is the primary viewing portal and is located approximately 2 cm inferior and 1 cm medial to the posterolateral corner of the acromion. Only the skin is pierced with a knife and the arthroscopic sheath and blunt trocar are directed toward the coracoid process as they are advanced into the glenohumeral joint (Fig. 91-2). An anterior working portal is created with an "inside-out" technique using a Wissinger rod which is advanced across the triangular interval formed by the biceps and subscapularis tendons and the anterosuperior glenoid margin. The Wissinger rod should be directed lateral and superior to the coracoid to avoid neurovascular injury. A systematic arthroscopic examination of the shoulder is then performed.

The biceps tendon is one of the first intraarticular structures encountered. It attaches to the superior glenoid labrum at the supraglenoid tubercle. Its intraarticular course can be followed as it enters the bicipital groove. The superior labrum should be carefully assessed for the presence of a SLAP lesion. This refers to an injury to the superior labrum that extends both anterior and posterior to the biceps and includes the biceps tendon anchor to the glenoid. This lesion should not be confused with normal mobility of the superior labrum or a normal hiatus of the anterior labrum at approximately the 2 o'clock position.

The subscapularis recess is then examined and the presence and integrity of the superior and middle glenohumeral ligaments are assessed along with the subscapularis tendon. Loose bodies can also be found in this region. The anterior band of the inferior glenohumeral ligament and the anterior-inferior glenoid labrum are carefully inspected for laxity and detachment (i.e., Bankart lesion). The ligament should tighten with abduction and external rotation of the shoulder. The ability to pass the arthroscope directly across the joint into the

anteroinferior cavity, or "drive-through" sign, indicates excessive capsular laxity. The axillary pouch is then checked for loose bodies and excess volume.

The undersurface of the rotator cuff is next evaluated with careful attention paid to its insertion on the greater tuberosity. The presence or absence of partial or full-thickness rotator cuff tears is noted. The articular surfaces of the humeral head and glenoid are inspected for post-traumatic or degenerative disease. The posterolateral aspect of the humeral head, in particular, should be examined for a defect or Hill-Sachs lesion. Switching sticks can be used to place the arthroscope into the anterior portal. This enables visualization of the entire posterior glenoid labrum as well as the extent of a Bankart lesion, particularly during an arthroscopic stabilization procedure.

The arthroscopic sheath and blunt trocar can be redirected from the posterior viewing portal into the subacromial space. A lateral working portal is created approximately 3 cm lateral to the anterolateral corner of the acromion in line with the anterior border of the acromion. An accessory posterolateral portal can be made approximately 3 cm lateral to and 3 cm inferior to the posterolateral corner of the acromion. This portal can be used for visualization or as an accessory inflow portal. Visualization of the subacromial space can be obscured by bursal tissue. Once this tissue is excised the inferior surface of the acromion, the coracoacromial ligament, and the bursal surface of the rotator cuff can be seen. Epinephrine can be added to the arthroscopy fluid to minimize bleeding. The acromioclavicular joint is covered with a thick capsule. Large osteophytes may protrude from the undersurface of the distal clavicle and should be excised.

COMPLICATIONS

Complications associated with shoulder arthroscopy include neurologic injury, articular cartilage injury, and infection. Neurologic injury most commonly occurs indirectly through prolonged traction in the lateral decubitus position which can result in a brachial plexus neuropraxia. This usually resolves spontaneously. Traction time

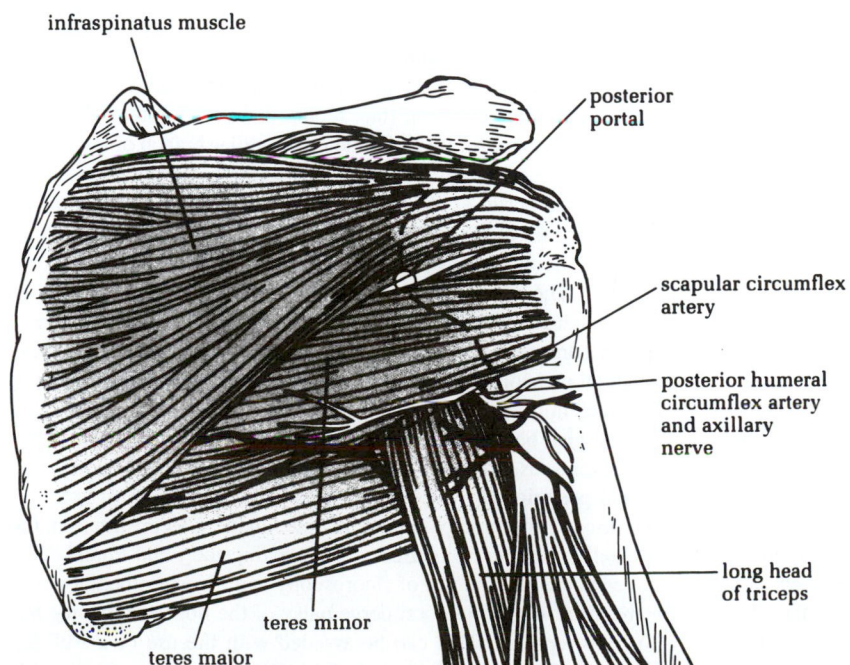

infraspinatus muscle

posterior portal

scapular circumflex artery

posterior humeral circumflex artery and axillary nerve

long head of triceps

teres minor

teres major

Figure 91-2

Relationship of posterior portal location to associated neurovascular structures. [Reproduced by permission from Parisien JS: The shoulder. In: *Techniques in Therapeutic Arthroscopy*, 2d ed. New York: Raven Press (now Lippincott Williams & Wilkins); 1993:11.3.]

should be limited to 2 h. The most common nerve that can be directly injured during shoulder arthroscopy is the suprascapular nerve as it passes near the posterior glenoid rim. This nerve is especially vulnerable to injury during arthroscopic transglenoid capsulorrhaphy for instability. Although very uncommon, the axillary nerve can also be injured during shoulder arthroscopy, particularly if the surgeon is unaware of the anatomy and instruments are directed inferiorly. Injury to the articular cartilage during the percutaneous placement of instruments into the joint. This is avoided by having a thorough knowledge of the bony and soft tissue anatomy, using a blunt trocar, and inflating the joint with fluid prior to insertion of the arthroscope. As in the knee, the incidence of infection is low (less than 1 percent) and can be minimized with strict aseptic technique. The routine use of prophylactic antibiotics is still somewhat controversial and under investigation.

ARTHROSCOPY OF THE KNEE

INDICATIONS

The basic indications for knee arthroscopy include: (1) meniscal lesions which can be treated with either meniscectomy or repair, (2) anterior and posterior cruciate ligament reconstruction, (3) chondral or osteochondral lesions which can be treated with internal fixation, chondroplasty, abrasion or "microfracture" arthroplasty, or more recently, with cartilage cell transplantation or osteochondral transfer procedures, (4) removal of osteochondral loose bodies, (5) synovectomy, (6) correction of patellar maltracking, (7) release of intraarticular adhesions, and (8) the evaluation and treatment of intraarticular fractures (i.e., tibial eminence, osteochondral, and tibial plateau).

SURGICAL TECHNIQUE

Patient Positioning

Knee arthroscopy is performed with the patient in the supine position. A leg holder can be used to maintain control of the extremity and assist the surgeon in applying varus or valgus stress during the procedure. The knee is flexed at the end of the table. Alternatively, a lateral post or kidney rest can be used for valgus stress. This technique, however, requires a figure-of-four position for access to the lateral compartment. A tourniquet is applied to the upper thigh and can be used if the surgeon desires. An adequate inflow of fluid is important to maintain joint distention. This can be accomplished either with gravity flow or any one of several infusion pumps that are commercially available.

Portals and Arthroscopic Anatomy

The procedure usually begins with the creation of an anterolateral portal located approximately 1 cm superior to the joint line and 1 cm lateral to the patellar tendon. This is the primary viewing portal and provides excellent visualization of most of the knee joint with the exception of the anterior horn of the lateral meniscus. The anteromedial portal located approximately 1 cm superior to the joint line and 1 cm medial to the patellar tendon can be either created directly with a knife at the beginning of the procedure, or it can be localized with the use of a spinal needle while viewing from the anterolateral portal. This is the primary working portal for most arthroscopic procedures. Suprapatellar portals, either lateral or medial, are placed 1 cm above the patella and are used for inflow or outflow cannulas. The superolateral portal is also used to evaluate patella tracking. A posteromedial portal can be created 1 cm above the joint line and 1 cm

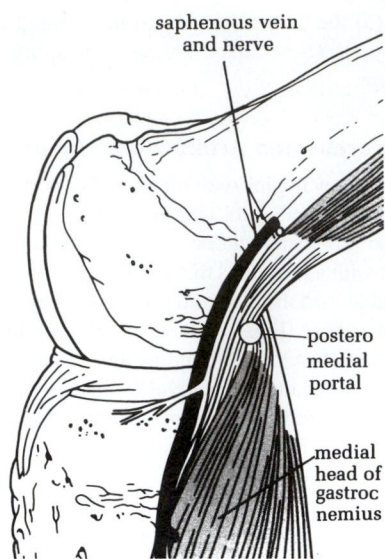

Figure 91-3
Posteromedial portal. [Reproduced by permission from Parisien JS: The knee. In: *Techniques in Therapeutic Arthroscopy*, 2d ed. New York: Raven Press (now Lippincott Williams & Wilkins); 1993:1.5.]

posterior to the medial femoral condyle (Fig. 91-3). This portal is often used during posterior cruciate ligament reconstruction procedures, for the removal of loose bodies, and occasionally to address tears of the posterior horn of the medial meniscus.

The specific arthroscopic techniques are well reviewed in other sections of this book and are beyond the scope of this chapter.

COMPLICATIONS

The rate of infection following arthroscopy of the knee is low (<0.1 percent). There is no consensus concerning the use of preoperative antibiotics, however, several recent studies have failed to demonstrate an increased rate of infection when they are not used for routine arthroscopic knee procedures.

Neurovascular complications following arthroscopic knee surgery are probably more common than reported. Several authors have reported the potential for injury to the infrapatellar branch of the saphenous nerve causing neuropraxia and neuroma formation. Placement of the medial portal above the joint line and avoiding injury to the vein that passes along the joint line will assist in avoiding injury to the nerve. Meniscal repair surgery can also lead neurovascular complications. The saphenous and peroneal nerves are at risk for injury during medial and lateral meniscal repairs, respectively. Most surgeons recommend inside-out repairs with posteromedial and posterolateral incisions and tying the sutures directly over the capsule to avoid such injuries. The posterior tibial nerve and popliteal artery and vein can also be injured during repairs of the posterior horn of the lateral meniscus if needles are passed through the lateral portal and directed posteriorly.

During arthroscopic posterior cruciate ligament reconstruction, the popliteal artery can be injured while creating the tibial tunnel. This can be avoided by the use of fluoroscopy and a posteromedial portal for the arthroscope. Femoral nerve palsy of the nonoperative leg has also been reported. This can be avoided with the use of a well-leg holder that flexes and abducts the hip. Compartment syndrome can also occur after arthroscopy or cruciate ligament reconstruction. This is especially a risk if arthroscopy is performed acutely after combined ligamentous injuries, such as following a knee dislocation. In this case, capsular disruption allows fluid extravasation into the leg compartments. Tourniquet-related complications can also occur and most often consist of transient paresthesias. Some investigators have indicated that tourniquets can cause muscle and nerve damage under the cuff; however, such damage is believed to be transient and reversible. Nevertheless, tourniquet time should be kept to under 2 h with a minimal pressure that will block arterial flow, but that will not cause venous congestion.

Iatrogenic articular cartilage injury is also a potential risk during all arthroscopic procedures. A thorough knowledge of the anatomy and accurate portal placement are critical in avoiding such injuries. Vigorous distraction of the knee, especially while using a leg holder, can cause femoral fractures and ligament disruption, in particular, the medial collateral ligament. The most common complication following arthroscopic knee surgery is hemarthrosis. These can be avoided with adequate hemostasis during the procedure, the use of drains and a compression dressing if significant bleeding is expected, such as following a lateral release. Although rare, thromboembolic complications such as deep venous thrombosis and pulmonary embolism have been reported following arthroscopic knee surgery. These can be minimized by emphasizing early mobilization and prophylaxing those patients at risk. Arthrofibrosis after arthroscopic knee surgery is a significant problem. Factors that increase the risk for developing knee stiffness include a large effusion, hemarthrosis, prolonged postoperative immobilization, infection, multiple procedures, and acute ligament reconstruction. Early recognition followed by aggressive physical therapy and manipulation when necessary are used to treat this condition. Synovial fistulas at portal sites result in persistent drainage of synovial fluid. These are rare and usually resolve spontaneously with a brief course of immobilization.

ARTHROSCOPY OF THE ANKLE

INDICATIONS

Indications for ankle arthroscopy include the evaluation and treatment of (1) osteochondral lesions (osteochondral fractures and osteochondritis dissecans), (2) loose bodies, (3) impingement lesions (anterolateral or posterior), (4) adhesions, (5) degenerative joint disease (osteophyte removal, chondroplasty), (6) synovitis (post-traumatic, inflammatory, pigmented villonodular, and synovial chondromatosis) (7) infection, and (8) chronic ankle pain of uncertain etiology.

SURGICAL TECHNIQUE

Patient Positioning

Ankle arthroscopy can be performed with the patient supine and the affected extremity secured in an arthroscopic leg holder. This position allows access to the anterior aspect of the ankle. Distraction can be applied either manually by a surgical assistant or with a kerlex loop placed around the patient's ankle and then around the surgeon's foot. There are also commercially available distraction devices although these are often unnecessary. The patient can also be positioned in a semi-lateral decubitus position with the leg holder supporting the extremity in internal rotation. This allows easier access to the posterior aspect of the joint. Alternatively, the patient can be positioned supine with the hip and knee flexed over a deflated bean bag with the foot in a plantigrade position.

Anatomy

The two malleoli provide fixed bony landmarks for arthroscopy of the ankle. The anterior articular margin is located 2 cm proximal to the tip of the medial malleolus. A 3- to 5-mm notch of the anterior articular margin of the tibia allows for passage of arthroscopic instruments. The talar dome is wider anteriorly than it is posteriorly and is concave in the coronal plane and convex in the sagittal plane. Prominent medial and lateral margins help to produce osteochondral injuries. The three sensory nerve systems include the saphenous which runs with the greater saphenous vein just anterior to the medial malleolus, the superficial peroneal which runs anterolaterally and bifurcates into medial and lateral branches, and the sural nerve which runs posterior to the lateral malleolus and peroneal tendons. The dorsalis pedis artery and the deep peroneal nerve run between the extensor digitorum longus and extensor hallucis longus tendons.

The medial malleolus is the site of attachment for the deltoid ligament which consists of superficial and deep intraarticular fibers. Lateral stabilizing structures include the anterior inferior tibiofibular, the anterior talofibular, and the calcaneofibular ligaments. Posterior stabilizing structures are the posterior inferior tibiofibular ligament, the posterior talofibular ligament, and its extension, the transverse ligament.

Portals and Arthroscopic Anatomy

There have been ten arthroscopic portals to the ankle described, which can be placed within three major groups: (1) anterior, (2) posterior, and (3) transmalleolar. Most arthroscopic procedures can be performed using only anterior portals.

Anterior portals include the following: (1) anterolateral, (2) anteromedial, (3) anterocentral, (4) accessory anterolateral, and (5) accessory anteromedial portals. Posterior portals consist of the (1) posterolateral, (2) posteromedial, and (3) transachilles portals (Fig. 91-4). Transmalleolar portals may be created either on the (1) medial or (2) lateral sides.

The anterolateral portal is located 5- mm below the joint line just lateral to the extensor tendons and peroneus tertius and medial to the lateral cutaneous branch of the superficial peroneal nerve. This portal is the primary diagnostic portal used for initial placement of the arthroscope. Through this portal the medial, central and most of the lateral portions of the tibiotalar joint can be visualized. The medial gutter, medial malleolus, deep deltoid ligament, and the central aspect of the joint at the notch of Hardy, are inspected. The procedure is usually begun by first identifying the location of this portal with an 18-gauge spinal needle. The joint is then distended with normal saline using a 60-cc syringe and intravenous extension tubing.

The anteromedial portal is created just medial to the tibialis anterior tendon 5 mm distal to the joint line and lateral to the saphenous nerve and greater saphenous vein. This portal is used initially as a working portal for placement of a motorized shaver or probe to clear synovium that can often block visualization. Transillumination with the arthroscope anterolaterally can be performed to help avoid injury to the greater saphenous vein and saphenous nerve when establishing the portal. From this portal one can visualize the talus, tibia, and fibula bones, and the lateral stabilizing ligaments.

The anterocentral portal is created 5 mm distal to the joint line, lateral to the extensor hallucis longus tendon and through or just medial to the extensor digitorum longus. This portal is usually not recommended due to its close proximity to the deep peroneal nerve and dorsalis pedis artery.

The accessory anterolateral and anteromedial portals are located 5 mm inferior to their respective anterolateral and anteromedial por-

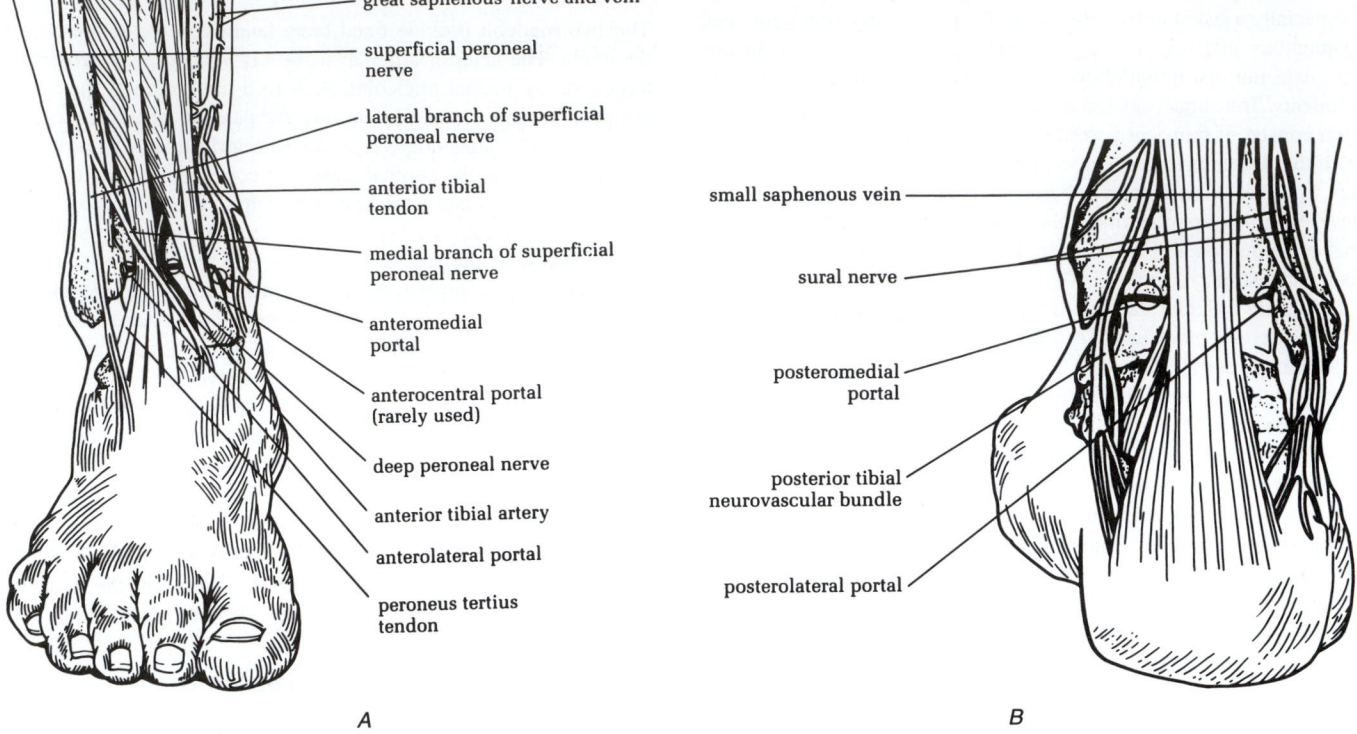

Figure 91-4
A. Anterior portals. *B*. Posterior portals. [Reproduced by permission from Parisien JS: The ankle. In: *Techniques in Therapeutic Arthroscopy*, 2d ed. New York: Raven Press (now Lippincott Williams & Wilkins); 1993:17.5.]

tals. Accessory portals are not routinely used, especially when there is adequate distraction.

The posterolateral portal is made in the triangular space between the Achilles and peroneal tendons 1.5 cm distal to the level of the anterolateral portal. The portal should be made just adjacent to the lateral border of the Achilles tendon to avoid injury to the sural nerve and short saphenous vein. This portal is used for instrumenting the posterior compartment when this area is inaccessible from an anterior portal.

A transachilles portal can be created just distal to the posterior joint line directly through the Achilles tendon. The advantage of this portal over other posterior portals is the avoidance of the neurovascular structures.

The posteromedial portal is made just medial to the Achilles tendon. This portal is not recommended due to the high potential for injury to the contents of the tarsal tunnel.

Transmalleolar portals may be created either on the medial or lateral sides. These portals may be used to drill or internally fix an osteochondral lesion of the talar dome which is not accessible by anterior or posterior approaches.

Instrumentation

Most arthroscopic procedures can be performed with a standard 4-mm 30-degree oblique-viewing arthroscope and standard size instruments. Occasionally, a small joint scope and small instruments are necessary.

COMPLICATIONS

Complications of ankle arthroscopy include nerve injury or neuroma formation, vascular injury, infection, sinus tract formation, instrument breakage, iatrogenic chondral injury, traction injury, and fluid ex-

travasation with possible compartment syndrome. As always, strict attention to detail can minimize the frequency of these complications.

ARTHROSCOPY OF THE WRIST

INDICATIONS

Indications for wrist arthroscopy include: (1) the assessment and treatment of tears of the triangular fibrocartilage (debridement verses repair), (2) the removal of loose bodies, (3) the evaluation and debridement of articular cartilage defects, (4) the resection of bone (e.g., distal ulna), and (5) the visualization and treatment of intraarticular fractures, and (6) the evaluation and treatment of wrist pain of undetermined etiology.

SURGICAL TECHNIQUE

Patient Positioning

The patient is positioned supine and with the hand placed in sterile finger traps which are used to supply 5–10 pounds of distraction. The arm is stabilized with a wrist holder or countertraction weighted sling around the upper arm. A small 2.5 to 3-mm, 25 to 30-degree angled arthroscope is routinely used along with small arthroscopic probes, baskets, and shavers.

Portals and Arthroscopic Anatomy

Several portals for wrist arthroscopy have been described. In order to assess the radiocarpal joint, three portals are commonly used. The first portal is created between the third and fourth dorsal compartments, 1 cm distal to Lister's tubercle. Insertion of the arthroscope is made easier by first distending the joint with fluid by needle puncture at this

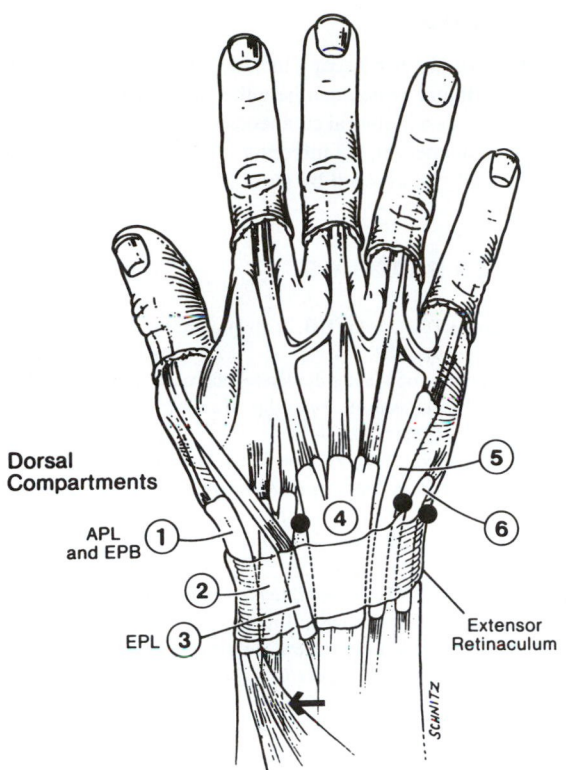

Figure 91-5

Dorsal compartments (6) of the wrist. In de Quervain's tenosynovitis, the first dorsal compartment containing the abductor pollicis longus and extensor pollicis brevis is inflamed. Inflammation also occurs at the intersection of the first and third dorsal compartments (arrow), observed clinically as intersection syndrome or "sneakers." (Courtesy Gary Schnitz, MD. Modified and reproduced by permission from Jacobson MD, Plancher KD: Evaluation of hand and wrist injuries in athletes. *Operative Techn Sports Med* 1996; 4:214.)

portal site. A second portal which can be used for inflow or instrumentation is created just volar to the extensor carpi ulnaris and below the triquetrum. A third portal is placed between the fifth and sixth dorsal compartments distal to the triangular fibrocartilage (Fig. 91-5).

After the arthroscope has been placed into the radiocarpal joint, orientation is initially achieved by visualizing the scapholunate interval including the radioscapholunate ligament with its characteristic overlying tuft of synovium. The scope is then moved along the articular surfaces visualizing the scaphoid, lunate, triquetrum, radius, and volar ligaments. The triangular fibrocartilage complex, including the ulnolunate and ulnotriquetral ligaments, and the scapholunate and lunotriquetral ligaments can be seen. The scope may be placed through one of the ulnar portals for a different perspective.

The midcarpal joint can be examined through a portal that is created just distal to the radiocarpal portal between the third and fourth dorsal compartments along the radial edge of the third metacarpal in a soft spot just proximal to the capitate. The articular surfaces of the capitate, hamate, and triquetrum can be visualized through this portal.

COMPLICATIONS

Complications of wrist arthroscopy include: (1) nerve injury (pressure on the median nerve from fluid extravasation can cause carpal tunnel-like symptoms); (2) articular cartilage injury, (3) infection, and (4) synovial fistula formation.

ARTHROSCOPY OF THE HIP

INDICATIONS

Indications for arthroscopy of the hip include: (1) the removal of loose bodies, (2) debridement of osteoarthritis, in particular, localized degenerative disease, (3) treatment of osteochondritis dissecans, (4) irrigation and lavage for chondrolysis, (5) assessment of the articular cartilage prior to corrective osteotomy for selected cases of slipped capital femoral epiphysis, (6) synovectomy and evaluation of the articular cartilage in juvenile idiopathic arthritis (formerly termed juvenile rheumatoid arthritis), (7) treatment of labral tears, and (8) evaluation of the persistently painful hip following trauma.

SURGICAL TECHNIQUE

Anatomy

The hip joint is a ball-and-socket joint covered by a strong fibrous capsule which is attached superiorly to the acetabular rim and inferiorly to the femoral neck. The fibrocartilaginous labrum deepens the acetabulum and is continuous inferiorly with the transverse ligament which is connected only at its ends, the proximal edge being free of any attachments. The ligamentum teres, which inserts on the fovea of the femoral head is attached to both sides of the acetabular notch and to the fossa of the acetabular floor.

Anteriorly, the capsule reaches the base of the femoral neck, whereas posteriorly, it attaches more proximally, such that the distal third of the neck is extracapsular. The capsule is reinforced by the iliofemoral, ischiofemoral, and pubofemoral ligaments, named for their pelvic attachments. The strongest of the three is the iliofemoral ligament or the ligament of Bigelow, which covers the anterior aspect of the joint.

The muscles that immediately surround the hip joint include the iliopsoas, reflected head of the rectus femoris, and gluteus minimus, anteriorly; the obturator externus and pectineus, medially; and the piriformis, gemelli, obturator internus, and quadratus femoris, posteriorly. The important bony landmarks include the greater trochanter, anterior superior iliac spine, and the pubic symphysis.

Patient Positioning and Approaches

Traditionally, the anterolateral approach has been the one most commonly used. The patient is positioned supine on a fracture table with the involved hip in slight abduction and flexion so as to relax the anterior capsule. Traction is used as well as an image intensifier. A spinal needle is directed medially and posteriorly at a 45-degree angle, at a point intersected by a vertical line drawn from the anterosuperior iliac spine crossing a horizontal line drawn approximately 3 cm above the greater trochanter (Fig. 91-6). The capsule is distended with 20 to 30-ml of normal saline. The arthroscope and blunt obturator are then directed parallel to the needle into the hip joint.

Arthroscopic evaluation of the hip joint begins with inspection of the anterolateral aspect of the femoral head. The arthroscope is then advanced medially to evaluate the anteromedial aspect of the head and the acetabulum. The different regions of the femoral head along with the anterior aspect of the acetabulum, labrum, and ligamentum teres can be seen. A working portal can be created lateral to the arthroscope; however, care must be taken to avoid injury to the lateral femoral cutaneous nerve which runs over the sartorius approximately 2.5 cm below the anterosuperior iliac spine.

Glick (1987) has popularized the lateral approach to hip arthroscopy in which the arthroscope is introduced laterally, directly above the tip of the greater trochanter. The patient is placed in the lateral

COMPLICATIONS

Complications of hip arthroscopy include: (1) iatrogenic chondral injury, (2) nerve injury which can be either direct while making a lateral portal (i.e., lateral femoral cutaneous nerve) or indirect from traction (i.e. pudendal nerve), (3) infection, and (4) instrument breakage. These can usually be avoided by strict attention to detail.

SUGGESTED READINGS

Glick JM, Sampson TG, Gordon RB, et al: Hip arthroscopy by the lateral approach. *Arthroscopy* 1987; 3:4.

Glick JM: Hip arthroscopy using the lateral approach. In Basset FH III (ed): *Instructional Course Lectures.* Parkridge, IL: American Academy of Orthopaedic Surgeons; 1988; 37:223.

Parisien JS: *Arthroscopic Surgery.* New York: McGraw-Hill; 1988.

Parisien JS: *Techniques in Therapeutic Arthroscopy.* New York: Raven Press; 1993.

Parisien JS: *Current Techniques in Arthroscopy,* 2d ed. Philadelphia: CM Medicine; 1996.

Warner Jon JP, Iaonnotti JP, Gerber C (eds): *Complex and Revision Problems in Shoulder Surgery.* Philadelphia: Lippincott-Raven; 1997.

Snyder SJ: *Shoulder Arthroscopy.* New York: McGraw-Hill; 1994.

Jobe FW (ed): *Operative Techniques in Upper Extremity Sports Injuries.* St. Louis: Mosby; 1996.

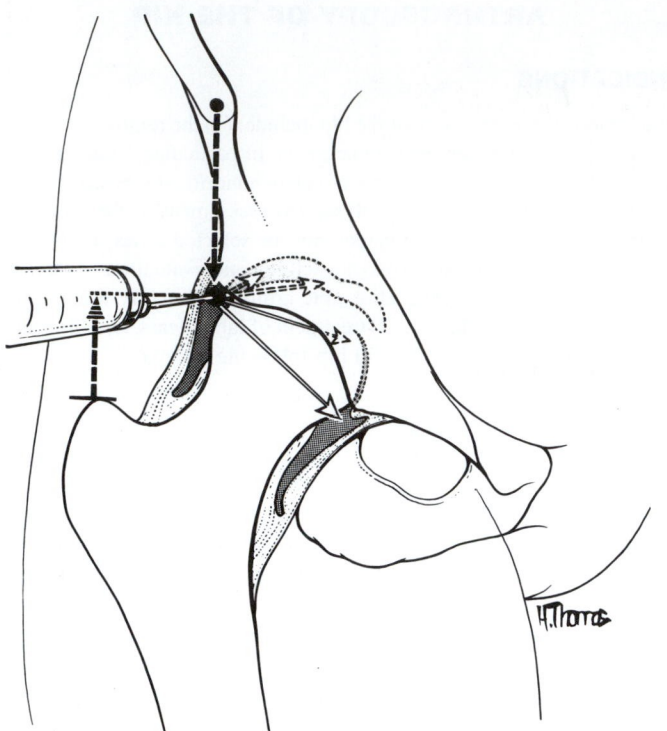

Figure 91-6
Landmarks and area of needle insertion for hip arthroscopy. (Reproduced by permission from Parisien JS: *Arthroscopic Surgery.* New York: McGraw-Hill; 1988:23.6.)

position with the involved leg in 45 degrees of abduction and 10 degrees of flexion using traction. A spinal needle is directed over the greater trochanter directly into the hip joint. The joint is then distended and the arthroscope is inserted. Free back flow of fluid confirms entry into the joint. Additional portals for inflow and instrumentation can be created anterior and posterior to the greater trochanter.

Chapter 92

ACROMIOCLAVICULAR JOINT

Andrew S. Rokito

ACROMIOCLAVICULAR JOINT DISLOCATION

Acromioclavicular (AC) joint injuries typically occur in young athletes participating in contact sports. The usual mechanism of injury is a direct blow to the top of the shoulder. This results in failure of the AC and/or the coracoclavicular (CC) ligaments.

Patients with these injuries will usually present with pain and swelling over the AC joint. The degree and direction of displacement of the distal clavicle encountered is dependent upon the severity of the injury. In addition to a routine shoulder trauma series, a 15-degree cephalic tilt view of the AC joint should also be obtained. Some authors also recommend AP stress views with 10 to 15 lb of weight suspended from each arm by wrist straps to evaluate the integrity of the CC ligaments.

Six types of injuries to the AC joint have been described (Fig. 92-1). Type I injuries involve a sprain of the AC ligaments in which the joint remains intact. In type II injuries, the AC ligaments are completely torn and the CC ligaments are sprained, resulting in slight displacement of the AC joint. Type III injuries are complete tears of both the AC and CC ligaments with detachment of the deltoid and trapezius from the distal clavicle. This results in an actual dislocation of the AC joint with relative upward displacement of the clavicle of 25 to 100 percent. Type IV injuries are also complete AC joint dislocations; however, the clavicle is displaced posteriorly into the trapezius. Type V injuries are severe type III injuries with extensive detachment of the deltoid and trapezius from the distal clavicle, resulting in upward clavicular displacement of 100 to 300 percent. Type VI injuries, which are extremely rare, involve inferior dislocations of the AC joint, in which the clavicle is displaced into a subcoracoid or subacromial position.

The treatment for incomplete injuries (i.e., types I and II) is nonoperative, consisting of an initial period of ice to reduce swelling and rest in a sling, followed by early range of motion. Types IV, V, and VI injuries, however, involve severe displacement of the distal clavicle with extensive soft tissue disruption, and operative intervention is usually recommended.

The treatment of type III injuries remains controversial with a trend toward initial nonoperative treatment in most cases. This is particularly the case in patients who participate in contact sports (e.g., football, hockey, soccer, and lacrosse) where the risk of reinjury is quite high. Some patients, however, with type III injuries initially treated nonoperatively will present with persistent pain and mechanical symptoms that interfere with their ability to perform their usual sport or job. In these cases, operative intervention has been successful in reducing pain and improving function.

With concern over pin migration and fixation failure, most authors recommend "coracoclavicular" reconstructive techniques (fixation between the coracoid and the clavicle), rather than "acromioclavicular" repairs (fixation across the AC joint). Various methods of CC fixation have been used including: sutures, suture tapes, stainless steel wires, lag screws, Dacron grafts, and fascia lata, as well as dynamic muscle transfers. Coracoclavicular repairs are combined with CC ligament transfer as popularized by Weaver and Dunn (1972). In addition, with symptomatic, chronic complete AC dislocations, as well as in acute dislocations in which there is significant joint damage, an excision of the distal clavicle may also be performed.

ACROMIOCLAVICULAR JOINT ARTHRITIS

Arthritis of the AC joint can develop after trauma as in intraarticular distal clavicle fractures or after AC joint dislocations. More often, however, this condition is idiopathic. Inferior AC joint osteophytes may reduce the size of the subacromial space and can be associated with subacromial impingement. A painful AC joint is often found in association with impingement syndrome.

Patients with this condition will have pain and tenderness localized to the AC joint as well as pain with horizontal adduction. Radiographs may show degenerative changes at the AC joint, but do not necessarily correlate with the symptoms. A selective lidocaine injection into the AC joint can help confirm the diagnosis.

Many patients with AC joint arthritis will respond to nonoperative treatment including activity modification, nonsteroidal anti-inflammatory medications, ice, and corticosteroid injections. Multiple injections should be avoided. Surgical treatment involves resection of 1.5 to 2.0 cm of the distal clavicle (Munford procedure). This can be accomplished either as an open procedure or arthroscopically.

DISTAL CLAVICLE OSTEOLYSIS

Distal clavicle osteolysis is most commonly the result of repetitive microtrauma, such as weight lifting. Other causes include acute trauma, rheumatoid arthritis, and hyperparathyroidism. Patients with this condition present with pain and tenderness localized to the AC joint as well as the characteristic radiographic features of distal clavicle osteopenia, cystic changes, and sometimes cupping. As with AC joint arthritis, most patients will respond to nonoperative treatment, which includes avoidance of those activities that cause pain, such as weight lifting, nonsteroidal anti-inflammatory medications, and corticosteroid injections. When these measures are unsuccessful, surgical resection of the distal clavicle is usually recommended.

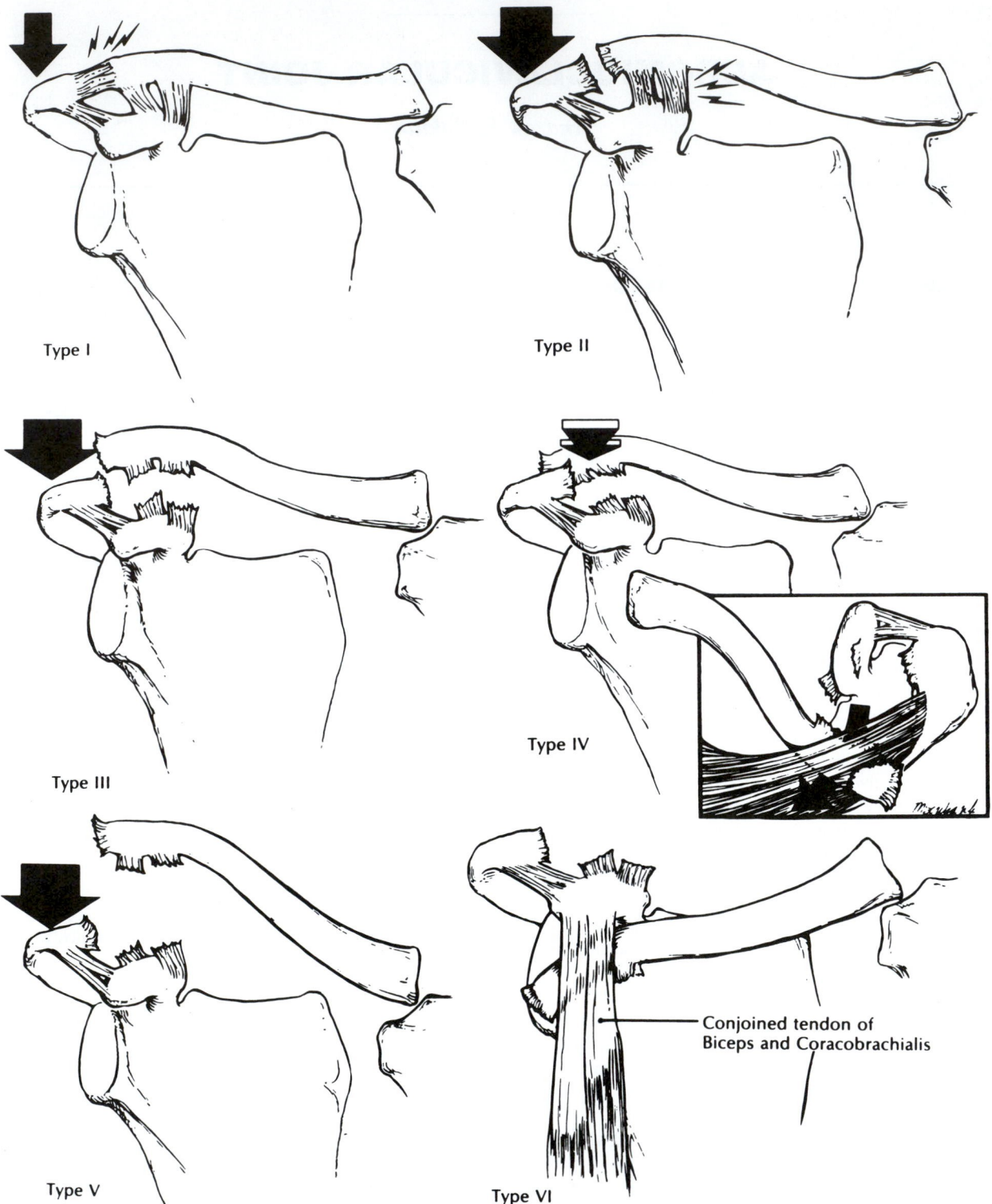

Figure 92-1

Schematic drawings of the classification of ligamentous injuries to the acromioclavicular joint. (*Top left*) In the type I injury, a mild force applied to the point of the shoulder does not disrupt either the acromioclavicular or the coracoclavicular ligaments. (*Top right*) A moderate to heavy force applied to the point of the shoulder will disrupt the acromioclavicular ligaments, but the coracoclavicular ligaments remain intact. (*Center left*) When a severe force is applied to the point of the shoulder, both the acromioclavicular and the coracoclavicular ligaments are disrupted. (*Center right*) In a type IV injury, not only are the ligaments disrupted, but the distal end of the clavicle is also displaced posteriorly into or through the trapezius muscle. (*Bottom left*) A violent force applied to the point of the shoulder not only ruptures the acromioclavicular and coracoclavicular ligaments, but also disrupts the muscle attachments and creates a major separation between the clavicle and the acromion. (*Bottom right*) This is an inferior dislocation of the distal clavicle in which the clavicle is inferior to the coracoid process and posterior to the biceps and coracobrachialis tendons. The acromioclavicular and coracoclavicular ligaments are also disrupted. [Reproduced by permission from Rockwood CA Jr, Williams GR, Young CD: Injuries to the acromioclavicular joint. In Rockwood CA Jr, Green DP, Bucholz RW, et al (eds): *Fractures in Adults,* 4th ed. Philadelphia: Lippincott-Raven; 1996:1354.]

SUGGESTED READINGS

Rockwood CA Jr, Williams GR, Young DC: Injuries to the acromioclavicular joint. In Rockwood CA Jr, Green DP, Bucholz RW, et al (eds): *Fractures in Adults*, vol 2, 4th ed. Philadelphia: Lippincott-Raven; 1996:1341.

Rockwood CA Jr, Young DC: Disorders of the acromioclavicular joint. In Rockwood CA Jr, Matsen FA 3d (eds): *The Shoulder*, vol 1. 2d ed Philadelphia: WB Saunders; 1998:483.

Rokito AS, Zuckerman JD, Cuomo F: Acromioclavicular joint dislocation. In Fu FH, Ticker JB, Imhoff AB (eds): *An Atlas of Shoulder Surgery*. London: Martin Dunitz; 1998:287.

Weaver JK, Dunn HK: Treatment of acromioclavicular injuries, especially complete acromioclavicular separation. *J Bone Joint Surg [Am]* 1972; 54:1187.

Williams GR Jr, Rockwood CA Jr: Injuries to the acromioclavicular joint. In DeLee JC, Drez D Jr: *Orthopaedic Sports Medicine: Principles and Practice*, vol 1. Philadelphia: WB Saunders; 1994:481.

Chapter 93

SUBACROMIAL IMPINGEMENT SYNDROME

Andrew S. Rokito

Mechanical impingement of the bursal surface of the rotator cuff on the coracoacromial arch is a common source of shoulder pain that is frequently seen in middle-aged patients. In general, subacromial impingement is believed to result from a reduction of available space. The anterior one-third of the acromion, coracoacromial ligament, subacromial bursa, and acromioclavicular joint all have been implicated as contributing to "outlet stenosis" and impingement of the rotator cuff.

CLASSIFICATION

This disorder has traditionally been classified by Neer (1983) into three progresssive stages based on the degree of involvement of the rotator cuff. Stage I consists of inflammation and edema. Stage II involves fibrosis and tendinitis while stage III involves an actual rotator cuff tear which may be either partial or full-thickness.

HISTORY

The most common complaint on presentation is that of pain which often begins gradually. Pain is frequently difficult to localize and patients often complain of radiation into the upper arm to the region of the deltoid tuberosity. Patients may also present with pain anteriorly along the biceps tendon that radiates along the muscle toward the elbow. Night pain with an inability to sleep on the involved side is a very common symptom associated with subacromial impingement syndrome. Difficulty with overhead activities, weakness, fatigue, and stiffness are also typical symptoms. Activities of daily living that can be affected include dressing, washing, eating, and toileting.

PHYSICAL EXAMINATION

A comprehensive approach to the physical examination is critical to establishing the diagnosis and consists of inspection, palpation, range of motion, strength testing, neurologic assessment, and special testing.

On inspection of the shoulder girdles, the examiner should look for muscle wasting which may occur in the infraspinatus or supraspinatus fossae and is characteristic of a chronic rotator cuff tear. Rupture of the long head of the biceps tendon results in a characteristic bulge in the arm as the muscle is retracted distally with contraction.

Tenderness over the acromioclavicular joint may indicate pathology specific to this region. The bicipital groove should also be palpated to evaluate for associated bicipital tendinitis. The insertion of the supraspinatus tendon can be palpated through the deltoid just distal to the anterolateral edge of the acromion with the shoulder extended and internally rotated.

Active and passive range of motion of both shoulders should be measured with a goniometer. In patients with isolated subacromial impingement, there is, typically, limited active, but full, passive range of motion. Ranges of motion that should be recorded include forward elevation, external rotation with the arm at the side, and internal rotation as the highest posterior vertebral anatomy that can be reached with the hitchhiking thumb. External rotation should also be recorded in the more functional position of 90 degrees of scapular plane abduction, especially in the athletic population.

Manual muscle testing is used to grade strength on a scale from 0 to 5. It is important to distinguish actual weakness beyond that considered secondary to pain, as this is considered to be a specific sign of rotator cuff deficiency.

It is important to assess shoulder stability, as rotator cuff pain can be secondary to underlying glenohumeral instability. This is especially true in overhead athletes in whom anterior subluxation can cause secondary impingement of the rotator cuff.

There are several special tests that should be performed in the evaluation of a patient with suspected subacromial impingement. These include: (1) the classic painful arc between 60 and 120 degrees of abduction; (2) pain on forced forward elevation causing impingement between the greater tuberosity and the anterior acromion; and (3) pain on forced internal rotation of the 90 degree abducted arm causing impingement against the coracoacromial ligament. Involvement of the biceps tendon can be assessed by eliciting pain in the area of the bicipital groove with resisted forward elevation of the humerus or with resisted supination with the elbow flexed to 90 degrees. The lidocaine impingement test, as described by Neer (1983) can be very helpful in the evaluation of the painful shoulder (see Fig. 23-4). This test is considered positive if after an injection of local anesthetic into the subacromial space there is relief of pain and reversal of previously positive impingement signs. It should be pointed out, however, that while this test can supply additional information about the source of pain, it is not specific and can be positive in patients with primary or secondary impingement.

IMAGING STUDIES

Plain films should include at least three views of the shoulder directed 90-degrees to one another. These consist of an anteroposterior film at right angles to the scapular plane, a lateral or supraspinatus outlet view in the scapular plane with the beam tilted 10 degrees caudally to look at acromial shape and slope, and an axillary view. These films are often times normal, especially in younger patients during the earlier stages of impingement. The typical radiographic signs of more advanced rotator cuff disease include sclerosis and cyst formation in the greater tuberosity, osteophytes on the undersurface of the acromion and acromioclavicular joint, and sometimes in the presence of a cuff tear, a narrowed acromiohumeral distance.

Recently, much attention has been focused on acromial morphology with three variations of acromial shape described: type I (flat), type II (curved), and type III (hooked). It has been theorized that in those individuals with a type III acromion there is a higher incidence of rotator cuff disease. It is important to distinguish, however, between a type III acromion and the presence of a subacromial osteophyte. Subacromial osteophytes are more likely an acquired phenomenon, rather than a preexistent or primary condition that predisposes one to rotator cuff disease. As such, they develop over time and are likely to be secondary to chronic compression of the humeral head and rotator cuff against the undersurface of the acromion.

Single or double contrast arthrography is a very sensitive technique for detecting full-thickness rotator cuff tears. The extravasation of contrast material into the subacromial space confirms the presence of a tear. Although it is considered to be the "gold standard," arthrography is an invasive test and as such is associated with complications. While ultrasonagraphy is noninvasive, allows comparison with the contralateral shoulder, and is especially useful in evaluating patients who have previously undergone a rotator cuff repair. Sensitivity of results can be related to the examiner's experience.

Recently, magnetic resonance imaging (MRI) has been used in the evaluation of rotator cuff pathology. As technology has improved, increasing sensitivities and specificities have been reported. MRI is a noninvasive test that can provide information on rotator cuff characteristics, tear size, and location. Studies using contrast-enhanced MRI with gadolinium (MR arthrography) are currently being performed. This technique may have a role in the evaluation of patients having undergone previous rotator cuff repairs and in the delineaton of partial versus full-thickness tears. Validation of the use of contrast, however, requires further investigation.

TREATMENT

The vast majority of patients with subacromial impingement syndrome can be successfully managed nonoperatively. Nonoperative treatment includes: activity modification, nonsteroidal anti-inflammatory medications, subacromial corticosteroid injections, and stretching and strengthening exercises. It is important to consider the specific etiology of the condition when deciding on a specific course of treatment. A patient with an acute traumatic episode, for instance, is more likely to respond to a brief course of rest followed by an exercise program as opposed to a patient with a full-thickness rotator cuff tear who presents with chronic pain and weakness. In the latter situation, earlier consideration would be given towards surgical intervention.

Initially, a period of rest with avoidance of those activities that produce pain is recommended. This is especially important in athletes in whom overuse is the common mechanism of injury. During this time, patients are encouraged to substitute other activities to maintain endurance and muscle tone. Nonsteroidal anti-inflammatory medications may provide symptomatic relief and help alleviate acute pain to allow rehabilitation. Subacromial injections consisting of 40 to 80 mg of triamcinolone or methylprednisolone combined with 5 to 6 cc of lidocaine are usually reserved for those patients with chronic pain that does not respond to other forms of nonoperative treatment. These injections can be effective in alleviating pain and improving shoulder range of motion for impingement syndrome in the short-term. Multiple injections, however, should be avoided, as their deleterious effects have been well documented.

Specific rotator cuff stretching and strengthening exercises can be both therapeutic and preventative for impingement syndrome. The goal of stretching is to maintain shoulder range of motion and to prevent or correct any muscle imbalances or capsular contractures. Secondary adhesive capsulitis is commonly encountered in patients with long-standing subacromial impingement. While stretching should be generalized to include forward elevation, internal and external rotation, abduction, and adduction, specific attention should be directed toward internal rotation and cross-chest adduction to correct posterior capsular tightness which often occurs with this condition.

Strengthening is the mainstay of treatment for patients with rotator cuff disease. The goal of strengthening is to rehabilitate a compromised, weakened musculotendinous unit. Rotator cuff strengthening exercises are commonly performed with the use of rubber tubing or free weights. The external rotators (i.e., infraspinatus and teres minor) can be exercised with the arm at the side as can the subscapularis for internal rotation strength.

Specific strengthening of the supraspinatus is commonly acheived by abducting the arm in the scapular plane with the forearm and shoulder internally rotated. Elbow flexion and forearm strengthening exercises are performed to strengthen the biceps. A well-constructed shoulder strengthening program must also include the scapular stabilizers (i.e., rhomboids, trapezius, serratus anterior, and latissimus dorsi) as scapular lag can lead to secondary impingement. These muscles can be strengthened by doing push-ups with the arms adducted (scapular rotators), sitting rows (serratus and rhomboids), shrugs (trapezius), and pull-downs (latissimus).

Surgical management is reserved for those patients in whom nonoperative treatment is unsuccessful. Surgical approaches can be divided into open, arthroscopic, and combined procedures. The primary goals of surgery are pain relief and restoration of function; the procedures used are subacromial decompression and rotator cuff repair. The choice of procedure depends predominantly on the underlying etiology and the extent of the abnormality.

If a full-thickness rotator cuff tear is not present, a subacromial decompression alone is usually performed. Anterior acromioplasty was first described by Neer (1972) as an open procedure; however, today it is most commonly performed arthroscopically. This procedure involves resection of bursa, release of the coracoacromial ligament from its attachment to the acromion, and anterior acromioplasty. It can be combined with resection of the distal clavicle for concomitant acromioclavicular joint arthritis.

If there is a full-thickness rotator cuff tear, arthroscopic subacromial decompression can also be combined with a "mini-open" repair through a lateral deltoid-splitting incision. The advantage of this procedure, which is usually reserved for relatively small, mobile tears, is that it does not require detaching the deltoid from the acromion, as is normally done during open surgical repairs.

For full-thickness rotator cuff tears, open surgical repair is usually recommended. In most instances the cuff defect is repaired to bone. In some cases of chronic, large, retracted rotator cuff tears, it is not possible to fully close the defect. In these circumstances the surgeon can either perform just a debridement of the cuff or a muscle transfer using the subscapularis and/or the latisssimus dorsi. The overall results of the latter, however, have not been good, particularly in terms of function. Debridement alone, on the other hand, can provide significant pain relief, and be performed either as an open procedure or arthroscopically. In the case of massive rotator cuff tears that cannot be repaired, the coracoacromial ligament should be preserved, as resection may allow the humeral head to sublux arteriorly and superiorly. Finally, techniques are currently being developed to perform arthroscopic rotator cuff repairs using suture anchors.

SUGGESTED READINGS

Hawkins RJ, Mohtadi NGH: Rotator Cuff Problems in Athletes. In: DeLee JC, Drez D Jr (eds): *Orthopaedic Sports Medicine: Principles and Practice,* vol 1. Philadelphia: WB Saunders; 1994:623.

Matsen FA III, Arntz CT, Lippitt SB: Rotator cuff. In: Rockwood CA Jr, Matsen FA III (eds): *The Shoulder,* 2d ed, vol 2. Philadelphia: WB Saunders; 1998:755.

Neer CS II: Impingement lesions. *Clin Orthop* 1983; 173:70.

Neer CS II: Anterior acromioplasty for the chronic impingement syndrome in the shoulder: A preliminary report. *J Bone Joint Surg [Am]* 1972; 54:41.

Chapter 94

ADHESIVE CAPSULITIS

Andrew S. Rokito

OVERVIEW

Frozen shoulder is a condition of uncertain etiology characterized by significant restriction of both active and passive shoulder motion. Most studies report a cumulative risk for at least one episode as 2 percent. It is most common in patients who are between their fourth and sixth decades of life, with a higher incidence in women than men.

Different pathologic mechanisms have been proposed to explain the etiology of frozen shoulder, all of which remain largely theoretical. The most common theories include an autoimmune response, biochemical changes in the capsule, neurological dysfunction, endocrine disorders (i.e., diabetes mellitus, thyroid disease), trivial trauma, and psychological factors.

The term "adhesive capsulitis" was coined to describe an avascular, tense capsule that it is markedly adherent to the humeral head and associated with decreased joint volume and synovial fluid. Histologically, changes consistent with chronic inflammation, fibrosis, and perivascular infiltration in the subsynovial layer have been found.

Frozen shoulder associated with a known underlying disorder is considered "secondary" and may include intrinsic, extrinsic, or systemic disorders. Intrinsic shoulder pathology includes rotator cuff tendinitis, rotator cuff tears, tendinitis of the long head of the biceps tendon, calcific tendinitis, and acromioclavicular arthritis.

Extrinsic disorders, which represent pathology remote from the shoulder region, include ischemic heart disease, pulmonary disorders, cervical disc disease and radiculopathy, cerebral vascular hemorrhage, previous coronary artery bypass graft surgery, previous breast surgery, lesions of the midhumerus, and central nervous system disorders, such as Parkinson's disease. Systemic disorders represent generalized medical conditions that are known to occur in association with frozen shoulder, such as diabetes mellitus, hypothyroidism, hyperthyroidism, and hypoadrenalism.

SIGNS AND SYMPTOMS

Patients with this condition will report a gradual loss of function associated with vague discomfort about the shoulder following minimal or no trauma at all. These symptoms, which often are worse at night, will usually begin insidiously. Overhead and behind the back activities become especially difficult to perform as motion is diminished. These symptoms closely resemble those found in patients with rotator cuff problems, thereby requiring a careful physical examination to consider frozen shoulder as either the primary condition or one that is secondary to specific shoulder pathology.

CLINICAL EXAMINATION

Physical examination of the cervical spine, opposite shoulder, and trunk should always be performed to exclude any associated pathology. The clinical hallmark is the limitation of both active and passive range of glenohumeral motion. The degree of motion, including forward elevation, internal rotation, and external rotation must be documented accurately. A firm endpoint is appreciated with pain at the extremes of motion. Except for osteopenia associated with disuse, radiographs are usually negative.

MANAGEMENT

The overall goal in the treatment of patients with frozen shoulder is to relieve pain and restore motion and function. Ideally, efforts should be directed toward prevention by identifying those patients at risk, and initiating early intervention. This is best accomplished by emphasizing early motion in potential secondary cases (following trauma and surgery) whenever possible.

In general, all patients with frozen shoulder should be placed on an exercise program with the aim of maintaining and regaining range of motion. Each patient should begin an active and active-assisted range of motion program combined with gentle passive (stretching) exercises. These exercises should include motion in four directions: forward elevation, external rotation, internal rotation, and cross-body adduction.

Manipulation under anesthesia (MUA) is generally considered for patients who have not improved despite compliance with a structured, supervised exercise program for a period of at least three months. Manipulation should be performed in a gentle, controlled manner to avoid complications. Complications that can occur include humeral fracture, glenohumeral dislocation, rotator cuff tears, and radial nerve injuries. Manipulation is contraindicated in patients with severe osteopenia because of the increased risk of fracture.

Arthroscopy has been used in the evaluation and, more recently, in the treatment of frozen shoulder. It offers the possibility of releasing contracted structures. It is usually performed in association with some type of manipulation. This procedure allows for precise, selective capsular release, thereby avoiding the potential morbidity associated with an open procedure. It has been used in patients with frozen shoulder who have failed physical therapy and/or closed manipulation.

An open surgical release is reserved for those patients who fulfill one or more of the following criteria: (1) significant osteopenia or rotator cuff thinning or tears; (2) failed manipulation or arthroscopic release; or (3) attempted manipulation or arthroscopic release that was unsuccessful in regaining range of motion.

When performing an open release, it is critical to identify those tissues which are contracted and how their release should increase range of motion. Specifically, those structures usually released include: (1) subacromial and subdeltoid bursal adhesions; (2) the coracohumeral ligament and rotator interval; (3) the capsule, either circumferentially or selectively around the glenoid; and (4) the subscapularis, which is often lengthened, then securely repaired to maintain anterior stability.

SUGGESTED READINGS

Harryman DT II, Lazarus MD, Rozencwaig R: The stiff shoulder. In Rockwood CA Jr, Matsen FA III: *The Shoulder,* vol 2, 2d ed. 1998:1064.

Rokito AS, Cuomo F, Zuckerman JD: Frozen shoulder. In Warner JP, Iannotti JP, Gerber C (eds): *Complex and Revision Problems in Shoulder Surgery.* Philadelphia: Lippincott-Raven; 1997:119.

Chapter 95

BICEPS TENDON INJURIES

Andrew S. Rokito

Pathologic conditions affecting the long head of the biceps tendon include tenosynovitis, rupture, subluxation, dislocation, and superior labral detachment.

BICEPS TENDON RUPTURE (PROXIMAL)

Biceps tendonitis is usually secondary to subacromial impingement. The long head of the biceps tendon lies directly beneath the supraspinatus within the area of impingement and is therefore subject to the same attritional process as the rotator cuff. Inflammation of the biceps tendon will eventually lead to weakening and possible rupture. In many cases, this process is insidious and patients will present with signs of a biceps tendon rupture without a history of previous pain or injury. In other cases, patients will present with a history that is characteristic of impingement syndrome.

With an acute rupture, patients will often describe performing an activity that involves loading of the upper extremity with the elbow in flexion and the forearm in supination. Pain is localized to the anterior aspect of the shoulder and the midportion of the upper arm. On physical examination, ecchymosis is often present from the upper arm down to the elbow. The classic "Popeye muscle," a bulge in the anterior compartment of the upper arm, will also be present. There is usually pain with shoulder and elbow motion, as well as with resisted elbow flexion. This maneuver will also allow a defect to be palpated in the upper arm secondary to retraction of the long head of the biceps tendon. A careful evaluation of rotator cuff function should be performed. Radiographs may show signs of chronic rotator cuff disease. On MRI the biceps tendon will often not be visualized within the bicipital groove, as this is where most of these ruptures occur.

The treatment of proximal ruptures of the biceps tendon is dependent upon the patient's level of activity and functional requirements. The vast majority of these can be managed nonoperatively. In young, active patients tenodesis of the tendon in the bicipital groove can be considered. The remaining intraarticular portion of the tendon should be excised to prevent the possibility of mechanical symptoms such as locking or catching. If there is a rotator cuff tear, a repair is performed along with an acromioplasty and resection of the coracoacromial ligament.

BICEPS TENDON DISLOCATION

Subluxation or dislocation of the long head of the biceps tendon commonly occurs following an injury that places the shoulder in a position of extreme abduction and external rotation. This may cause disruption of the rotator interval and rotator cuff, especially the subscapularis.

Two mechanisms for medial dislocation of the biceps tendon have been described. In the first type, the dislocation occurs following disruption of the coracohumeral and transverse humeral ligaments, and the biceps tendon slides over an intact subscapularis tendon. More commonly, the tendon displaces medially following a complete rupture with retraction of the subscapularis. The second type of dislocation occurs when the biceps tendon slides under an internally ruptured subscapularis tendon. In this type, the subscapularis is partially ruptured on its articular side.

Patients will often have pain and tenderness over the anterior aspect of the shoulder that may be localized to the bicipital groove. The subscapularis lift-off test is used to clinically determine whether this tendon is intact. MRI can provide valuable information concerning the location of the biceps tendon, as well as the integrity of the rotator cuff. Biceps tendon dislocations are generally treated with tenodesis in the bicipital groove and repair of the subscapularis tendon.

SUPERIOR LABRAL DETACHMENT

Injuries to the superior glenoid labrum are relatively uncommon. This area has significant functional importance because it serves as the anchor for the long head of the biceps tendon on the glenoid rim. Injuries in this region begin posterior and extend anterior to the biceps tendon and are termed SLAP (superior labrum anterior and posterior) lesions.

The mechanism of injury for these lesions most commonly involves a fall onto the shoulder or a direct blow to the joint. Traction to the superior labrum by the biceps tendon during throwing has also been described as a mechanism of injury. These patients may complain of painful catching or popping, although this is inconsistent, and no clinical examination or imaging modality has been found to accurately identify these lesions. A high clinical suspicion is therefore necessary to make the diagnosis which is then confirmed arthroscopically.

Four types of SLAP lesions have been described (Fig. 95-1). Type I lesions involve fraying and degeneration of the superior labrum with an intact biceps anchor and are treated with debridement. In Type II lesions the superior labrum and biceps anchor are detached from the glenoid rim. These are generally treated with arthroscopic fixation (i.e., bio-absorbable tack versus sutures). In Type III lesions, there is a bucket-handle tear of the superior labrum with the remaining labral tissue and biceps tendon anchored to the glenoid rim. In these lesions, the bucket-handle portion of the labral tear is excised. Type IV lesions involve a superior labral bucket-handle tear that extends into the biceps tendon. These are treated with excision of the torn labral tissue and biceps tear versus arthroscopic suturing of the split biceps tendon and labrum, depending upon the degree of biceps involvement.

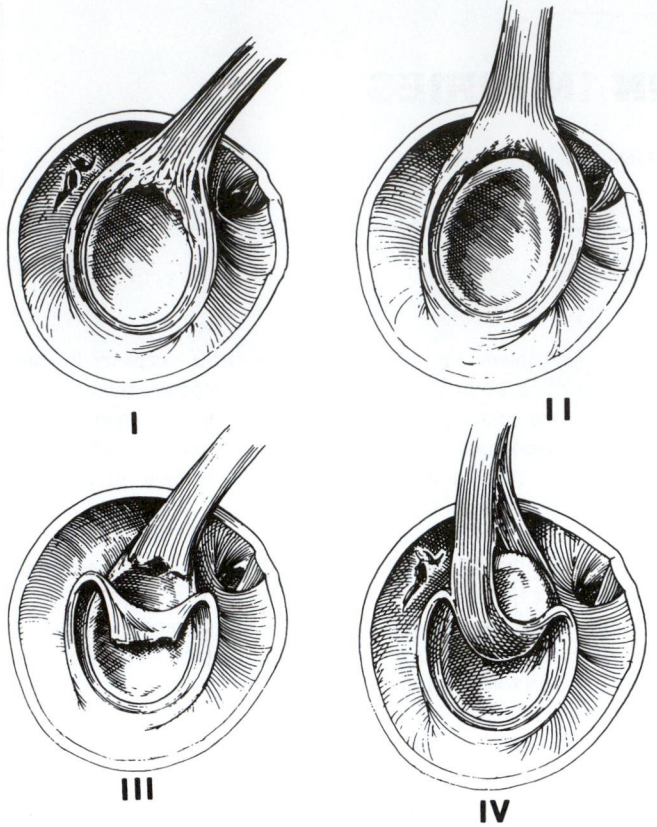

Figure 95-1

Types of SLAP lesions. Type I: Fraying and degeneration of the superior labrum with normal biceps tendon anchor. Type II: Detachment of the labrum and biceps anchor from the superior glenoid. Type III: Vertical tear through the superior labrum producing a bucket-handle lesion which may displace into the glenohumeral joint. The biceps anchor remains intact. Type IV: A bucket-handle tear of the superior labrum with expansion into the biceps tendon. The biceps anchor and remainder of the superior labrum are well attached. [Reproduced with permission from Snyder SJ: Labral lesions (non-instability and SLAP lesions). In *Shoulder Arthroscopy*. New York: McGraw-Hill; 1994:121,122.]

SUGGESTED READINGS

Burkhead WZ Jr, Arcand MA, Zeman C, et al: The biceps tendon. In Rockwood CA Jr, Matsen FA III (eds): *The Shoulder*. Vol 2, 2d ed. Philadelphia: WB Saunders; 1998:1009.

Snyder SJ, Banas MP, Belzer JP: Arthroscopic evaluation and treatment of injuries to the superior glenoid labrum. In Pritchard DJ (ed): *Instructional Course Lectures*. Rosemont, IL: American Academy of Orthopaedic Surgeons; 1996; 45:65.

Snyder SJ, Banas MP, Karzel RP: An analysis of 140 injuries to the superior glenoid labrum. *J Shoulder Elbow Surg* 1995; 4:243.

Chapter 96

SHOULDER INSTABILITY

Howard J. Luks and Andrew S. Rokito

Instability of the glenohumeral joint is a common problem faced by the orthopaedist in clinical practice. In order to properly comprehend the pathomechanics present in all forms of instability, it is necessary to possess a basic understanding of the static and dynamic restraints present about the shoulder and how they interact to maintain the glenohumeral joint in its anatomic location.

BIOMECHANICS

The superior (SGHL), middle (MGHL) and inferior glenohumeral (IGHL) ligaments along with the bony geometry and negative intra-articular pressure, comprise the *static* stabilizers of the shoulder. The role of each ligament is highly complex and varies with the position of the arm and with the direction of the translating force. The SGHL resists inferior subluxation of the shoulder joint and provides anterior stability in the neutral or adducted position. The MGHL provides anterior stability in mid-ranges of abduction. The most important anterior static stabilizer of the shoulder is the inferior glenohumeral ligament. This ligament forms a complex (IGHLC) that is composed of anterior and posterior bands with an intervening axillary pouch (Fig. 96-1). It is the anterior band of the IGHLC that provides the greatest restraint to anterior translation with the arm in abduction and external rotation. The posterior band of the IGHLC, as well as the SGHL, provides resistance to posterior translation of the humeral head with the arm in the abducted position. Inferior translation is resisted by the SGHL in the neutral or adducted position and the IGHLC in the abducted extremity. The rotator interval is located between the superior border of the subscapularis and the anterior border of the supraspinatus. The coracohumeral ligament, which travels within this interval, also aides in resisting inferior translation. Recent attention has been given to the rotator interval and its role in inferior and anterior/posterior translation when a defect is present. The bony geometry, in combination with the glenoid labrum, provides additional resistance to translation and the negative intraarticular pressure aids in resisting inferior subluxation of the humeral head.

The rotator cuff and the biceps tendon provide the *dynamic* restraints necessary to resist excessive humeral translation. It is likely that the muscles of the rotator cuff act by adjusting the tension present in the capsuloligamentous complex. By contracting, the muscles of the rotator cuff compress the humeral head against the glenoid, and thus, increase the force necessary for translation to occur. The role of the scapular stabilizers, the rhomboids, and the serratus anterior in glenohumeral instability should not be underestimated. The scapula controls the position of the glenoid with changing arm positions. Patients with shoulder instability often display scapulohumeral asymmetry between the affected and contralateral extremity.

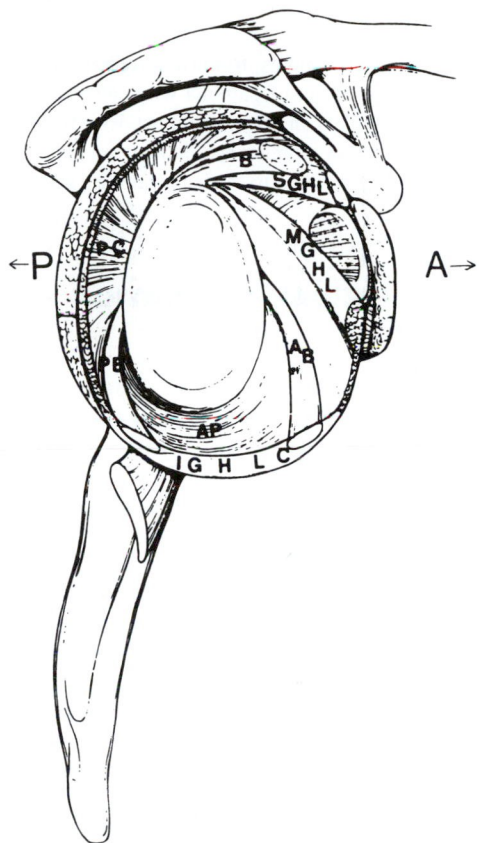

Figure 96-1
Capsuloligamentous complex of the shoulder. A, anterior; P, posterior; B, biceps tendon; SGHL, superior glenohumeral ligament; MGHL, middle glenohumeral ligament; AB, anterior band of inferior glenohumeral ligament complex (IGHLC); PB, posterior band of IGHLC; AP, axillary pouch; PC, posterior capsule. (Reproduced with permission from O'Brien SJ, Neves MC, Arnoczky SP, et al: The anatomy and histology of the inferior glenohumeral ligament complex of the shoulder. *Am J Sports Med* 1990; 18:451.)

CLASSIFICATION

Instability of the shoulder can be classified in terms of direction(s), degree, chronicity or frequency, etiology, and volition. The instability pattern present can be anterior, posterior, inferior, or multidirectional, and can be of an acute, chronic, fixed, or recurrent nature. The etiology of the initial occurrence may be traumatic or atraumatic,

Figure 96-2

A. Capsular exposure. B. Capsular separation is extended medially to allow placement of a retractor along the glenoid neck. A second retractor is then placed to retract the humeral head. C. Currently, suture anchors are used for suture fixation at the glenoid margin. The anchors should be placed near the glenoid margin rather than medially along the glenoid neck. The capsule is then pulled superomedially and reattached to the bony glenoid so that it obliterates the medial defect in the capsulolabral complex. D. A T-plasty is performed if excess capsular laxity is noted. When capsular laxity is accompanied by a Bankart lesion, the vertical limb of the T should be created medially at the glenoid margin. [Images A and C reproduced with permission from O'Brien SJ, Warren RF, Schwartz E, et al: Anterior shoulder instability. Orthop Clin North Am 1987: 18:395. Images B and D reproduced with permission from Pagnani MJ, Galinat BJ, Warren RF: Glenohumeral instability. In DeLee JC, Drez D Jr, et al. (eds): Orthopaedic Sports Medicine: Principles and Practice. Philadelphia: WB Saunders; 1994:602.]

---

such as that which is secondary to chronic repetitive microtrauma. Finally, there exists a subset of patients who can voluntarily sublux or dislocate their shoulder. The clinician must determine whether this is a positional problem or whether the patient can actively sublux or dislocate the shoulder due to behavioral or attention-seeking pathology.

CLINICAL EVALUATION

A careful history and physical examination is crucial in this patient population. The age of the patient, activity level, and the activities associated with symptoms provide important clues for proper diagnosis and classification. Younger patients (<21 years) have an increased incidence of recurrent dislocation; older individuals have a greater incidence of coexistent rotator cuff pathology. The most common complication following an anterior shoulder dislocation in the younger patient is an injury to the axillary nerve, whereas the most common complication in the older patient is a concomitant tear of the rotator cuff. Pain during the late cocking or early acceleration phases of the overhead throwing motion is associated with anterior instability, while pain during the deceleration or follow-through phases is generally associated with posterior instability.

A proper examination begins with visual inspection of the shoulder assessing for signs of asymmetry at rest and with active motion. Atrophy of the rotator cuff musculature or asymmetry of the scapulothoracic articulation is commonly present in the instability patient. The cervical spine is carefully assessed for range of motion and symptoms referable to nerve entrapment. Range of motion, the presence or absence of active and passive arcs of motion, and muscle strength are noted.

Many tests have been described to evaluate shoulder instability. It should be stressed that all tests must be compared to the contralateral extremity. In order to assess the degree of translation of the humeral head on the glenoid, various drawer tests are performed. The *sulcus sign* is assessed by placing downward traction on the adducted, neutrally aligned extremity; the distance between the lateral acromion and the humeral head is assessed. If a large gap or sulcus is produced in a symptomatic patient, inferior instability exists; this is considered to be pathognomonic for multidirectional instability (MDI). The *drawer test* is performed with the patient in the supine position with the arm in 90 degrees of abduction and neutral rotation. The examiner translates the head anteriorly and posteriorly on the glenoid. The resultant translation is then graded. The *load and shift test* is performed with the patient in a seated position. The examiner stabilizes the scapular spine and clavicle with one hand while using the other hand to apply a "load and shift" and assess the amount of translation present. *Anterior apprehension* is assessed by placing the patient's affected shoulder in 90 degrees of abduction and then slowly externally rotating the arm. Apprehension in this position is considered a positive test and diagnostic of anterior instability. This can be combined with the relocation test in which the examiner then imparts a posteriorly directed force to the upper arm. In the patient with anterior instability, this will result in a relief of symptoms. Posterior instability is assessed by placing the arm in a position of flexion, adduction, and internal rotation, while a posteriorly directed load is simultaneously applied to the humerus. Pain in this position occurs in patients with posterior instability. Assessing the patient's overall degree of ligamentous laxity is also important in the evaluation of instability. The examiner should check for the presence of metacarpophalangeal, elbow and knee hyperextension and the ability of the patient to bring the thumb to the volar forearm and the little finger to the dorsal forearm.

Diagnosing recurrent anterior shoulder subluxation is more difficult than recurrent anterior dislocation. The onset of symptoms in this population can be acute or chronic. These patients typically complain of pain with overhead activity that often resembles impingement. During the overhead throwing motion, pain is experienced during the late cocking or early acceleration phases. This may be due to secondary or internal impingement, as the rotator cuff is impinged between the greater tuberosity and the posterior superior labrum with anterior subluxation of the humeral head. On physical examination, these patients often do not have a positive apprehension sign. They will, however, have a positive relocation test, as this maneuver will center the humeral head on the glenoid, and thus, relieve the impingement. A lidocaine impingement test can aid in differentiating the patient with subacromial impingement from the patient with impingement secondary to instability.

Patients with MDI will have a sulcus sign and demonstrate pathological translation on anterior and posterior drawer tests. These patients often present with signs of bilateral shoulder instability, and classically, there is no history of trauma.

DIAGNOSTIC IMAGING

A trauma series of radiographs should be obtained on any patient with a presumed dislocation of the shoulder. This series includes an anterior-posterior of the shoulder in internal and external rotation, a scapular Y view, and an axillary view. The axillary view is particularly important in the evaluation of a possible posterior dislocation. The axillary view will also help delineate a bony component of a Bankart lesion if it is present.

Radiologic evaluation of the patient with shoulder instability should also begin with a trauma series, which will usually be normal. Special views, such as the Stryker notch and West Point axillary, can be obtained to assess for Hill-Sachs and osseous Bankart lesions, respectively. Further biplanar evaluation may be performed with CT evaluation of the glenoid in patients with suspected glenoid fractures or dysplasia. MRI techniques are becoming more precise in their appli-

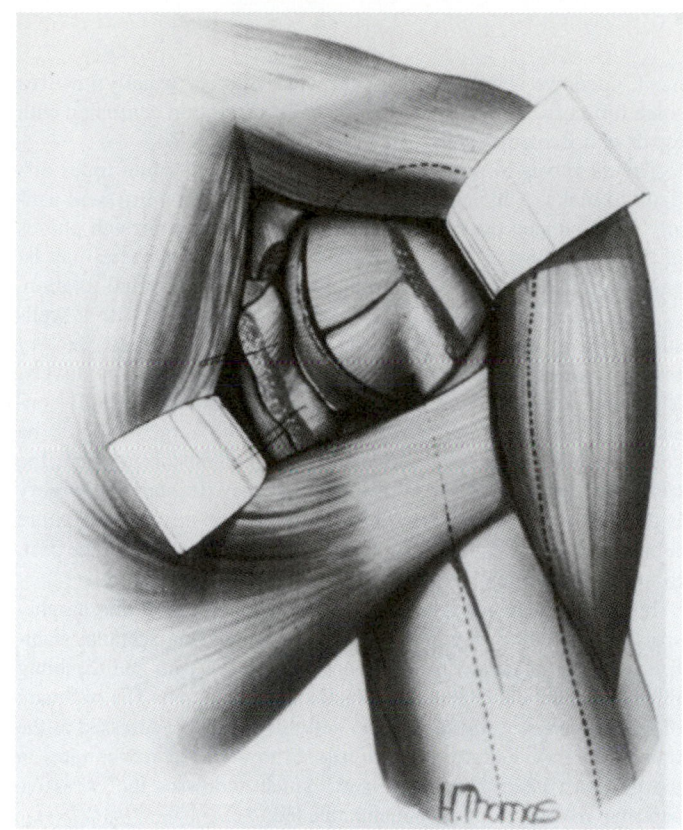

A

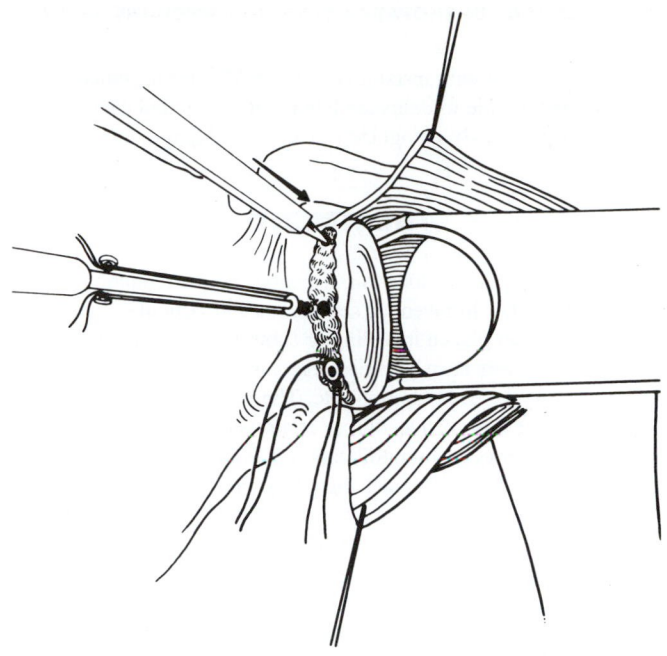

B

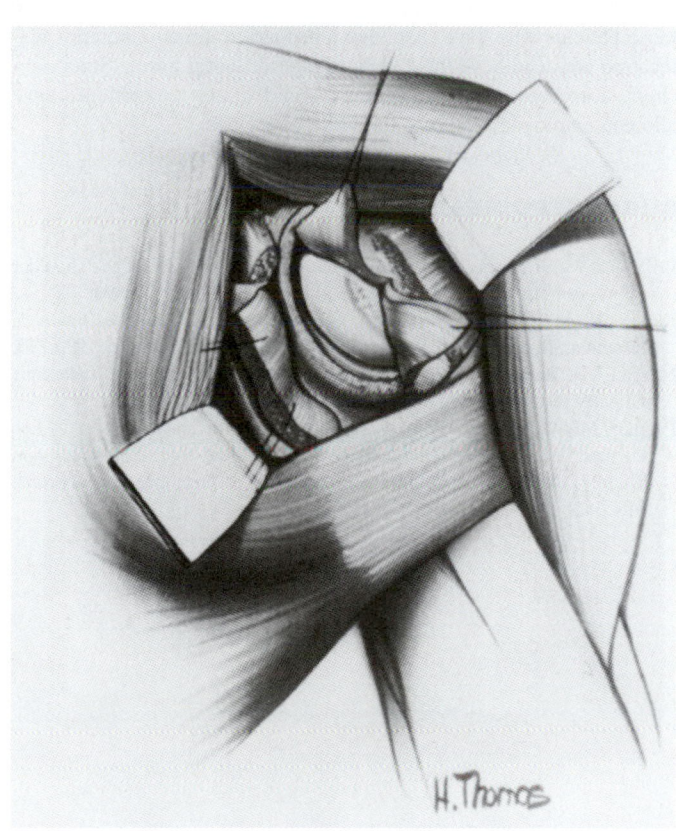

C

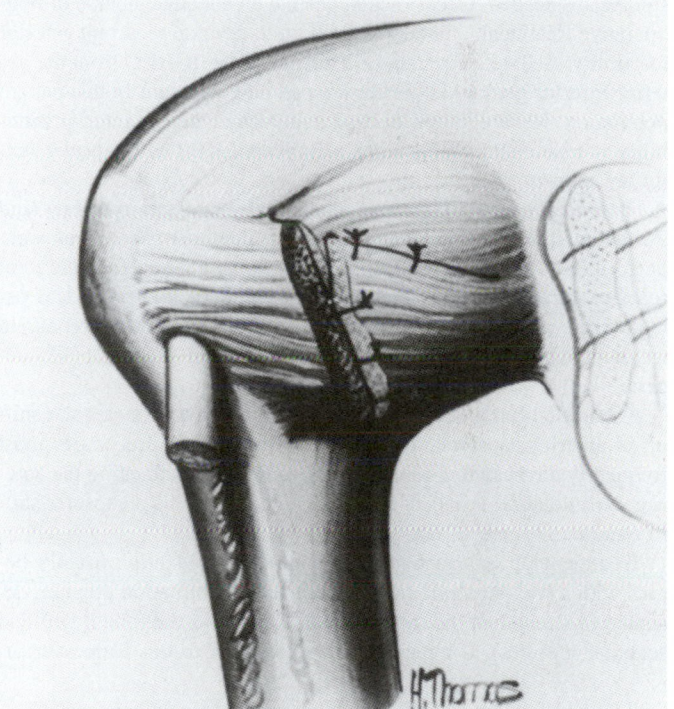

D

cation to the patient with instability. MRI or MR arthrograms, in particular, are better able to delineate labral pathology and capsular disruptions not previously recognized by other imaging modalities.

TREATMENT

Following a shoulder dislocation, a gentle closed reduction is performed using either intravenous sedation or intraarticular anesthesia. The patient is then placed in a sling or shoulder immobilizer. Several reduction maneuvers have been described, including traction-countertraction, gravity-assisted traction, etc. The period of immobilization following a first time dislocation is controversial. Most authors advocate 4 to 6 weeks of immobilization followed by a course of rehabilitation. In patients younger than 21 years of age, the risk of recurrence approaches 75 percent in some series. Older patients, greater than 50 years of age have a much lower incidence of recurrence, and some authors advocate simply the use of a sling until the pain subsides.

In general, recurrent instability may be independent of immobilization. A formal rehabilitation program and modification of activity for 2 to 3 months may lessen the incidence of recurrence, but more studies are needed. Occasionally, despite an adequate course of nonoperative treatment, a patient will go on to develop recurrent anterior instability. A Bankart lesion, or avulsion of the IGHLC from the anterior inferior glenoid is the classic pathology present in this patient population. Rehabilitation of a patient with recurrent anterior instability is rarely successful when a Bankart lesion and capsular laxity are present.

Historically, the Magnuson-Stack (subscapularis transfer) and Putti-Platt (subscapularis and capsular plication) procedures were performed to limit external rotation. By doing so, however, the joint reactive forces increased, leading to a high incidence of late osteoarthritis. Bone block procedures, such as the Bristow (coracoid transfer), have also been advocated with overall good rates of success.

A modified Bankart procedure in combination with a capsular shift or an anterior capsulolabral reconstruction are the procedures most frequently advocated. These procedures involve reattaching the anterior capsulolabral complex to the glenoid as well as a capsular shift to eliminate excessive laxity.

Treatment of recurrent anterior shoulder subluxation usually begins with a well-structured and supervised rehabilitation program designed to strengthen the dynamic stabilizers (i.e., the rotator cuff and scapular muscles). If a patient fails to respond to this form of treat-

ment, operative stabilization is warranted. Surgery usually involves some form of an open capsular shift or reconstruction combined with repair of a Bankart lesion, if present.

The diagnosis of primary posterior instability is often times difficult to make. Athletes with primary posterior instability will usually describe pain during the deceleration or follow-through phases of their throwing motion. On physical examination, there may be pain or apprehension with flexion, adduction, and internal rotation, of the shoulder. Once again, treatment should begin with a well-supervised rehabilitation program. Studies have shown satisfactory results in upwards of 75 percent of patients treated nonoperatively. If nonoperative treatment fails, surgery is indicated and usually consists of a posterior, inferior capsular shift. The surgeon should be cognizant of coexistent multi or bidirectional instability, and the treatment plan should be adjusted accordingly. In general, surgery is directed toward the most symptomatic site of instability. Failure to recognize a patient with a component of MDI has led, in the past, to high failure rates for posterior reconstructive procedures.

Initial treatment consists of a rehabilitation program that emphasizes strengthening exercises for the rotator cuff and scapular stabilizers. When patients with MDI continue to have pain and disabling instability, surgical alternatives should be considered. The hallmark of MDI is *inferior capsular laxity* and this must be addressed at the time of surgery. Failure to do so has led to high recurrence rates in the past. An inferior capsular shift, which addresses the excessive capsular volume, is usually recommended.

Arthroscopic treatment of shoulder instability has become a topic of much interest. A high rate of success can usually be achieved in those patients who have sustained a primary traumatic, anterior dislocation and who have thick, robust anterior labral tissue. Suture anchors, absorbable tacks, and trans-glenoid suturing techniques have all been employed to secure the labrum in place.

SUGGESTED READINGS

Burkhead WZ Jr, Rockwood CA Jr: Treatment of instability of the shoulder with an exercise program. *J Bone Joint Surg [Am]* 1992; 74:890.

Kasser JR (ed): Shoulder: instability. In *Orthopaedic Knowledge Update* 5. Rosemont, IL: American Academy of Orthopaedic Surgeons; 1996:233.

Morgan CD, Bodenstab AB: Arthroscopic Bankart suture repair: Technique and early results. *Arthroscopy* 1987; 3:111.

Pagnani MJ, Galinat BJ, Warren RF: Glenohumeral instability. In DeLee JC, Drez D Jr, (eds): *Orthopaedic Sports Medicine: Principles and Practice*. Rosemont, IL: American Academy of Orthopaedic Surgeons; 1994:580.

Chapter 97

ELBOW

Andrew S. Rokito and Howard J. Luks

TENDINOPATHIES

LATERAL EPICONDYLITIS (TENNIS ELBOW)

Lateral epicondylitis (i.e., tennis elbow) was originally described by Major in 1883. The condition has been attributed to angiofibroblastic hyperplastic changes of the extensor carpi radialis brevis (ECRB), a consistent finding in pathological specimens. Although 95 percent of cases of lateral epicondylitis do not occur in tennis players, it is estimated that 50 percent of tennis players will suffer at least one episode during their playing careers.

Lateral epicondylitis can occur from an acute injury; however, more commonly, it is the result of overuse in which continuous flexion/extension of the elbow in combination with pronation/supination of the forearm results in repetitive microtrauma. In tennis, it often occurs in recreational athletes with poor technique. Pain on contact with the ball while hitting groundstrokes is commonly noted. It has been attributed to improper backhand form in which "leading" with the elbow in combination with excessive pronation stresses the extensor muscle mass, placing it at risk for injury.

Lateral epicondylitis is characterized by pain over the lateral epicondyle that may radiate into the forearm. Patients may complain of weakness in the wrist and hand with grasping. As symptoms progress, they can be exacerbated by picking things up such as a cup of coffee, carrying a briefcase, or shaking hands.

The most consistent finding on physical examination is point tenderness just distal and anterior to the midpoint of the lateral epicondyle over the insertion of the ECRB. The distribution of pain, however, can be of a more diffuse nature and there may be tenderness over the proximal radial aspect of the forearm. The pain is often intensified with resisted wrist and finger (especially the middle finger) extension when the elbow is in full extension and the forearm is in full pronation. The "coffee-cup" test, which assesses for pain by grasping or pinching with the wrist in extension, is often positive. Range of motion and strength are usually normal; however, loss of active elbow extension and wrist extension weakness may be present secondary to pain. In long-standing cases, muscle atrophy or rupture may be present.

Radiographs are usually normal. However, in 22 to 25 percent of cases, punctate calcification within the soft tissues adjacent to the lateral epicondyle may be seen. The differential diagnosis includes entrapment of the radial nerve within the radial tunnel, cervical radiculopathy, intraarticular pathology such as osteochondritis dissecans, degenerative joint disease, or loose bodies, and posterolateral rotatory instability. In cases of radial tunnel syndrome, patients typically complain of pain more distally over the corresponding nerve, usually 4 to 5 cm distal to the epicondyle. A 5 percent incidence of coexistent radial nerve entrapment and lateral epicondylitis has been reported.

Lateral epicondylitis can most often be successfully treated nonoperatively. Nonoperative treatment begins with attempts to relieve pain and inflammation. Avoidance of the aggravating activity, ice, and NSAIDs (if not medically contraindicated), should all be instituted initially. If these measures are not successful, a corticosteroid injection can be administered. A maximum of two to three injections is recommended. Once the initial pain and inflammation are relieved, a well-supervised exercise program that emphasizes wrist extensor stretching and strengthening is started. A careful assessment of the patient's swing mechanics and proper racquet grip size should be performed at this time. The use of counterforce bracing, which potentially inhibits full muscular expansion and thus decreases the force experienced by the extensor tendon, is controversial.

Surgery is indicated for those patients whose symptoms persist despite compliance with a well-managed nonoperative program for at least 6 months. Fewer than 10 percent of patients with lateral epicondylitis will require operative intervention for resistant symptoms. Several surgical techniques have been described. These include tenotomy of the extensor origin, lengthening of the extensor carpi radialis brevis, release of the tendon with excision of the pathologic tissue and subsequent reattachment of the tendon, or any combination of these procedures. Most authors report favorable results following surgery.

MEDIAL EPICONDYLITIS

Medial epicondylitis is much less common than lateral epicondylitis. It is characterized by inflammation of the flexor pronator mass, in particular, the pronator teres and the flexor carpi radialis. Nirschl and Pettrone (1979) have suggested that vascular compromise and altered nutritional status result in angiofibroblastic hyperplasia and ultimately macroscopic tissue disruption. Valgus forces generated along the medial aspect of the elbow during throwing can create significant stress in the flexor pronator origin and the medial collateral ligament.

As in lateral epicondylitis, the onset of symptoms can be acute; however, more often it is of an insidious nature. Medial epicondylitis is usually characterized by pain that radiates along the medial elbow. Typically, patients present with an ache over the flexor/pronator mass and a weakness in grip strength. In cases of concomitant ulnar nerve irritation, patients may describe a vague tingling in the ring and little fingers.

On physical examination, there is tenderness over the flexor pronator origin, and more specifically, over the pronator teres and flexor carpi radialis. Pain is exacerbated with resisted wrist flexion and forearm pronation. Coexistent ulnar neuropathy may be present in upward of 50 percent of cases. These patients may exhibit subluxation of the ulnar nerve with elbow flexion as well as a positive Tinel's sign at the cubital tunnel. Radiographs are usually normal. However, in patients with associated chronic medial collateral ligament strain there may be medial ulnar traction spurs or calcification within the ligament.

The differential diagnosis of medial epicondylitis includes primary ulnar neuropathy and primary medial collateral ligament insufficiency. These are discussed below.

Most patients with medial epicondylitis will respond to nonoperative treatment. This includes an initial period of rest, NSAIDs, local modalities, and possibly a corticosteroid injection. This is followed by a therapeutic exercise program that emphasizes wrist flexor and forearm pronator stretching and strengthening. An evaluation of technique and equipment should also be performed.

Surgery is reserved for those patients whose symptoms persist despite compliance with a well-supervised nonoperative treatment program. As in lateral epicondylitis, surgical procedures are aimed at excising the inflammatory tissue with subsequent reapproximation of the tendon with most studies reporting good results and a high rate of return to sport activity and work. Some surgeons have advocated concurrent ulnar nerve decompression.

TENDON RUPTURE

DISTAL BICEPS TENDON RUPTURE

Distal biceps tendon ruptures are relatively rare injuries, comprising only 3 percent of all biceps tendon ruptures. These injuries are usually the result of a single traumatic event with the elbow flexed 90 degrees, involving a sudden contracture against a significant load. This typically occurs in the dominant extremity of males between the fourth and fifth decades of life. Complete ruptures usually occur at the tendo-osseous junction, leaving no distal tendon stump at the radial tuberosity. Partial ruptures of the distal biceps tendon are especially uncommon with very few cases reported in the literature.

When complete ruptures occur, patients usually present with acute pain and swelling in the antecubital fossa. This is often associated with a popping or tearing sensation. Clinically, there is often localized tenderness, swelling, a palpable defect, and weakness of elbow flexion and forearm supination. The contour of the distal biceps is usually altered and a deformity may be present as the muscle belly retracts proximally. Patients will maintain the ability to flex the elbow owing to an intact brachialis and lacertus fibrosus, but supination strength will be considerably decreased. The clinical findings associated with partial rupture of the distal biceps tendon are similar but more subtle when compared with those found in cases of complete tears. Radiographs are usually normal, but subtle hypertrophic changes at the radial tuberosity are sometimes present. Magnetic resonance imaging, although usually not necessary to make the diagnosis, can occasionally be helpful in distinguishing partial from complete ruptures. Other causes of pain in the antecubital fossa that should be considered include biceps tendinitis, bicipital bursitis, and pronator syndrome.

Treatment of complete ruptures of the distal biceps tendon is surgical, with the aim of restoring flexion and supination strength. Morrey (1994) found only 61 percent and 65 percent strength in flexion and supination, respectively, in cases that went unrepaired. Partial ruptures of the distal biceps tendon can also result in significant loss of flexion and supination strength, leaving the patient with a disabling functional deficit. Although the tendon is not completely avulsed from its insertion site, the intratendinous failure that accompanies a partial rupture leads to persistent weakness.

Surgical repair of complete distal biceps tendon ruptures involves reinsertion of the torn end into the radial tuberosity. This is usually performed through a two-incision approach, so as to minimize the risk of radial nerve injury (Fig. 97-1). The posterior incision involves a muscle-splitting approach through the extensor mass, avoiding periosteal elevation, to decrease the chances of radio-ulnar synostosis. This same technique has been advocated for the repair of partial ruptures.

TRICEPS TENDON RUPTURE

Rupture of the triceps tendon is rare. The mechanism of injury usually involves a deceleration force, such as a fall on an outstretched hand. It has been found in weight lifters with a possible association with anabolic steroid use. Most tears occur at the tendon insertion. Patients usually present with pain and ecchymosis over the triceps insertion, a palpable defect, and weakness on extension. Radiographs may demonstrate a "fleck sign" which represents avulsed bone from the olecranon. Treatment involves immediate repair using transosseous suture.

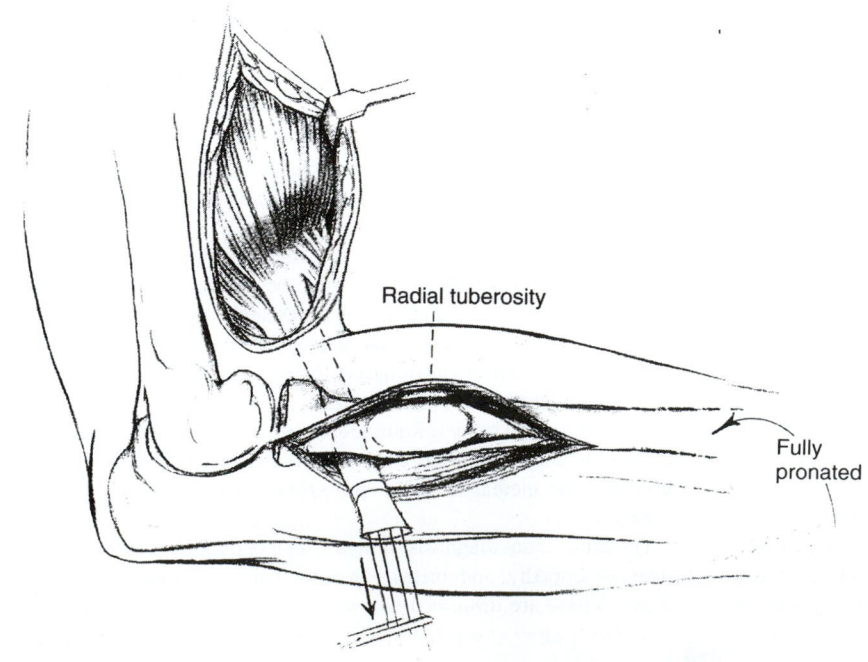

Radial tuberosity

Fully pronated

Figure 97-1

Double incision approach for repair of distal biceps tendon rupture. (Reproduced with permission from Mayo Foundation; Morrey BF, Askew LJ, An KN, et al: Rupture of one distal tendon of the biceps brachii. *J Bone Joint Surg [Am]* 1985; 67:418.)

ULNAR NEUROPATHY

Ulnar nerve mobility, combined with the repetitive valgus stress and forceful extension withstood by the elbow during throwing, may result in ulnar neuritis in this location.

The ulnar nerve is a terminal branch of the medial cord of the brachial plexus and is composed of fibers from the eighth cervical and first thoracic nerve roots. Approximately 8 cm proximal to the medial epicondyle, the ulnar nerve passes into the posterior compartment of the brachium by piercing a thick fibrous raphe of the medial intermuscular septum known as the arcade of Struthers. The nerve now lies anterior to the medial head of the triceps brachii muscle and may be palpable, as it passes downward toward the medial epicondyle. Typically, the nerve gives off no muscular branches in the arm.

At the elbow, the nerve travels posterior to the medial epicondyle into a fibroosseous canal known as the cubital tunnel whose boundaries are the medial collateral ligament of the elbow, the medial edge of the trochlea, and the medial epicondylar groove. The roof of this tunnel is formed by the cubital tunnel retinaculum or arcuate ligament, which extends from the medial epicondyle to the medial border of the olecranon (Fig. 97-2). The ulnar nerve continues into the forearm passing between the two heads of the flexor carpi ulnaris muscle supplying it with numerous motor branches.

During the act of pitching, the elbow is subjected to considerable medial tensile and lateral compression forces. The acceleration and early follow-through phases of the throwing motion are accompanied by rapid, forceful elbow extension and forearm pronation. Ulnar neuritis represents one syndrome in a spectrum of disorders that result from repeated valgus stress at the elbow. Those athletes commonly at risk include baseball pitchers, javelin throwers, tennis players, gymnasts, and football quarterbacks.

Ulnar nerve entrapment may result from both pathologic (tensile and compressive forces on the medial side of the elbow) and physiologic (osseous, muscular, or ligamentous hypertrophy) responses to repetitive trauma. Three types of pathologic stresses may eventually lead to ulnar neuritis: compression, friction, and traction. These may occur in isolation, or more commonly, in combination.

Compression of the ulnar nerve may result from physiologic hypertrophy of the medial head of the triceps, cubital tunnel retinaculum, or flexor carpi ulnaris muscles. Intrinsic masses such as ganglia or lipomas may also compress the ulnar nerve. Traction neuritis occurs when an attenuated or ruptured medial collateral ligament allows the elbow joint to "open up," excessively placing tension on the

ulnar nerve and creating a valgus deformity. Recurrent subluxation or dislocation of the ulnar nerve anterior to the medial epicondyle as the elbow moves from extension to flexion may cause friction neuritis. As much as 16 percent of the population may have recurrent ulnar nerve dislocation that is often secondary to congenital or developmental laxity of the soft tissue restraints that normally maintain the nerve in the epicondylar groove.

The first presenting symptom will often be intermittent medial elbow pain that is associated with or exacerbated by overhand activities. As the inflammation of the nerve becomes more severe, pain and paresthesias radiating down the ulnar aspect of the forearm to the hand may become apparent. Paresthesias of the ring and little fingers will be present in a majority of patients and usually precede any detectable motor weakness of the intrinsic muscles of the hand. A painful popping or snapping sensation at the elbow with flexion and extension is suggestive of a dislocating ulnar nerve.

The most consistent physical finding is the presence of a *Tinel's sign* over the cubital tunnel. Palpation of the inflamed nerve will often reveal tenderness along its course in the epicondylar groove and its passage into the forearm musculature. The nerve itself may have a thickened or "doughy" consistency and can often be subluxed or dislocated manually from the groove. True motor weakness of the flexor carpi ulnaris and flexor digitorum profundus is rarely encountered as the motor fibers to these muscles are well protected, being located deep within the cubital tunnel. Findings of diminished sensation, hypesthesias, and intrinsic muscle wasting are usually absent in the athlete. The *elbow flexion test,* which is performed with the elbow maximally flexed and the wrist in full extension for 3 min, is positive if symptoms of pain, numbness, and paresthesias occur in the ulnar nerve distribution.

A complete roentgenographic series of the elbow, including a cubital tunnel view, should be performed to assess for the presence of osteophytes or loose bodies in the region of the ulnar nerve which may be causes of pain.

Abnormalities in nerve conduction velocity testing of the ulnar nerve or in electromyographic recordings of the muscles it innervates, are helpful in making the diagnosis, when present. Negative electrodiagnostic studies, however, do not rule out the diagnosis of ulnar neuritis, which in most cases is based upon the history and physical examination.

Excessive valgus stress and tension overload secondary to repetitive, high-velocity throwing results in a spectrum of medial elbow pathology of which ulnar neuritis is one component. Associated pathology such as medial collateral ligament laxity, medial epicondylitis, loose bodies, and degenerative changes must be considered by the clinician as potential sources of nerve irritation when evaluating the athlete with elbow pain. Entrapment at other sites such as in cervical disc protrusion, thoracic outlet syndrome, and compression at Guyon's canal can all produce symptoms along the ulnar nerve distribution and should be ruled out by the clinical presentation and electrodiagnostic studies, if necessary.

Ulnar neuritis in which symptoms are mild and muscle atrophy is not present may respond to nonoperative treatment. A period of rest from the inciting activity, followed by a gradual return that includes a warm-up period and ice after the activity have been reported to be helpful. If this is unsuccessful, splint immobilization for 2 to 3 weeks is often effective in reducing the acute symptoms. Corticosteroid injections into the cubital tunnel are not recommended. Surgical intervention is indicated for the patient with persistent ulnar neuritis that is unresponsive to nonoperative treatment.

While simple decompression or cubital tunnel release may be sufficient for the nonathletic population, it does not address the possibility for continued traction or subluxation of the nerve. Others have

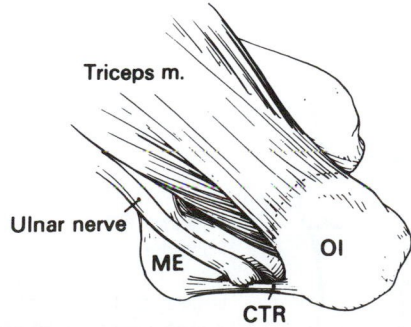

Figure 97-2

Cubital tunnel. Olecranon (OI), medial epicondyle (ME), cubital tunnel retinaculum (CTR). (Reproduced with permission from O'Driscoll SW, Horil E, Carmichael SW, et al: The cubital tunnel and ulnar neuropathy. *J Bone Joint Surg [Br]* 1991; 73:613.)

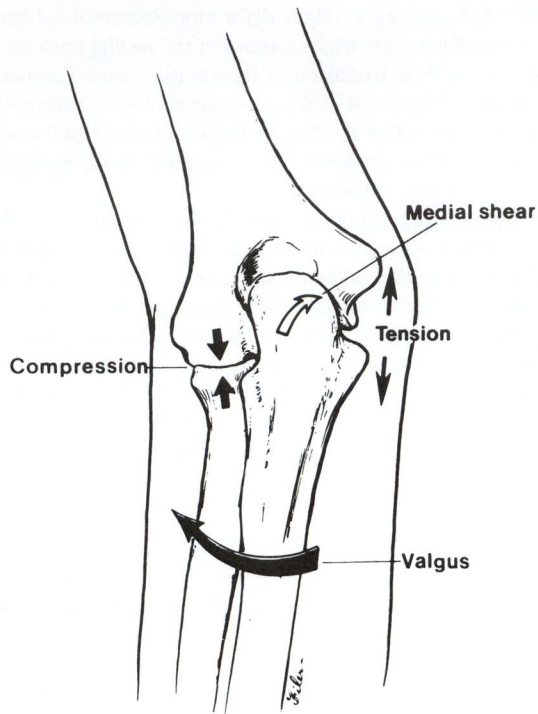

Figure 97-3
Forces generated about the elbow during throwing: medial tension overload, lateral compression, and posteromedial shear. [Reproduced with permission from Harnar CD, Bradley JP, McMahon PJ, et al: Baseball. In Fu FH, Stone DA (eds): *Sports Injuries: Mechanisms, Prevention, and Treatment*. Baltimore: Lippincott Williams & Wilkins; 1994.]

advocated medial epicondylectomy. This procedure is also discouraged in athletes as it carries with it the risk of injuring the humeral origin of the medial collateral ligament and altering the flexor-pronator origin. Subcutaneous transfer has also been recommended; however, as the nerve is left in a superficial, relatively unprotected position, the procedure may not be suitable for the overhead athlete or manual laborer. This procedure also does not address the unstable nerve. Some authors have adopted the use of a fasciodermal sling to stabilize the nerve. However, this may become a site of nerve compression. Anterior submuscular transposition of the ulnar nerve deep to the flexor muscle group decompresses all potential sites of entrapment and provides protection from both direct and indirect trauma that occurs during sports.

THROWING INJURIES

The five phases of throwing motion include wind-up, early and late cocking, acceleration, and follow-through. The tremendous forces generated by the upper extremity during late cocking and early acceleration leads to medial tension overload, lateral compression, and posteromedial shear injuries (Fig. 97-3).

Isolated medial collateral ligament (MCL) insufficiency secondary to attenuation of the anterior band of the ligament occurs in throwers as a result of repetitive microtrauma. Those who present with problems referable to the MCL are usually baseball pitchers or javelin throwers who have experienced months to years of symptoms associated with throwing. Occasionally, a sudden event occurs that forces the athlete to stop playing immediately. In the majority, however, a slow deterioration in function of the elbow occurs, accompanied by increasing pain and loss of control.

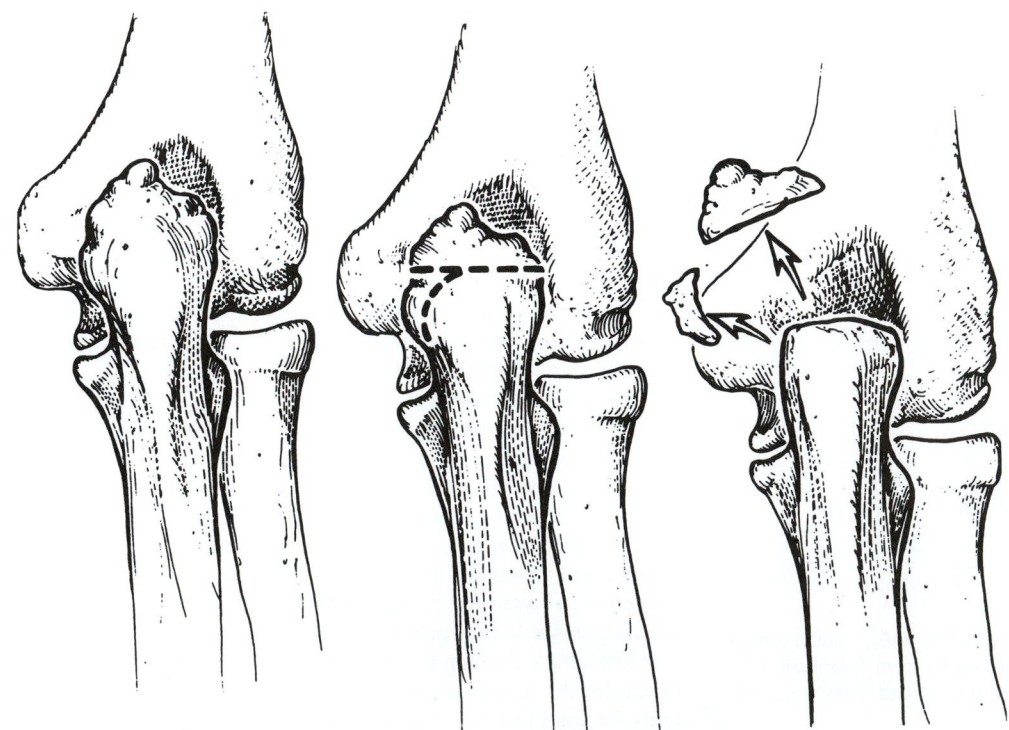

Figure 97-4
Posterior compartment debridement including removal of loose bodies and resection of osteophytes. [Reproduced with permission from Bennet JB: Articular injuries in the athlete. In Morrey BF (ed): *The Elbow and Its Disorders*, 2d ed. Philadelphia: WB Saunders; 1993:592.]

These athletes usually present with pain associated with the late cocking and acceleration phases of the throwing motion. Tenderness is typically localized to the ulnar aspect of the MCL because the ligament usually tears off the coronoid process. Valgus stress testing in 25 degrees of flexion may show evidence of laxity and reproduce symptoms of pain or apprehension. Radiographs may show evidence of calcification in the ligament. Stress radiographs may show evidence of MCL insufficiency. MR scans and CT arthrograms are also useful in visualizing the torn or attenuated ligament.

Nonsurgical treatment involves rest until the swelling settles, application of ice, anti-inflammatory medication, a stretching and strengthening program, and a gradual return to throwing. Cortisone injections should be avoided.

Surgical management for those patients who fail nonoperative treatment consists of reconstruction using a free tendon graft. The graft most commonly used is the palmaris longus tendon. Favorable results have been reported with a high rate of return to competitive throwing by 9 to 12 months.

Valgus extension overload occurs when the medial tip of the olecranon abuts against the posteromedial aspect of the olecranon fossa during forced extension. This results in posteromedial osteophyte and loose body formation as well as fibrous deposition in the olecranon fossa. Overhead athletes with excessive medial laxity and valgus alignment are prone to developing this syndrome.

Athletes present with pain over the posterior aspect of the elbow during follow-through. Complaints of catching or popping may also be present. On physical exam, there is usually tenderness over the tip of the olecranon process, crepitus, pain with forced terminal extension, and a flexion contracture. Radiographs including AP, lateral, and axial views may demonstrate the posterior osteophyte formation and loose bodies.

Treatment initially consists of rest and evaluation of throwing mechanics. Surgery involves removal of the loose bodies and resection of the osteophytes (Fig. 97-4). This can be accomplished by open or arthroscopic means.

Lateral compression injuries include osteochondritis dissecans, loose bodies, and osteochondral defects. As with medial injuries, these may occur as a result of a single traumatic event; however, more often, they result from chronic overuse. Lateral compression injuries can occur with or without medial tension overload. Advances in surgical technique have allowed many of these injuries to be treated arthroscopically.

SUGGESTED READINGS

Boyd HD, Anderson LD: A method for reinsertion of the distal biceps brachii tendon. *J Bone Joint Surg [Am]* 1961; 43:1041.

Conway JE, Jobe FW, Glouseman RE, et al: Medial instability of the elbow in throwing athletes: Surgical treatment by ulnar collateral ligament repair or reconstruction. *J Bone Joint Surg [Am]* 1992; 74:67.

Jobe FW: *Operative Techniques in Upper Extremity Sports Injuries*. St. Louis: Mosby; 1996.

Morrey BF, Regan WD: Tendinopathies about the elbow. In DeLee JC, Drez D Jr (eds): *Orthopaedic Sports Medicine: Principles and Practice*, vol 1. Philadelphia: WB Saunders; 1994:860.

Morrey BF, Regan WD: Fractures about the elbow in sports and their sequelae. In DeLee JC, Drez D Jr (eds): *Orthopaedic Sports Medicine: Principles and Practice*, vol 1. Philadelphia: WB Saunders 1994:824.

Morrey BF: Distal biceps tendon rupture. In Morrey BF (ed): *Master Techniques in Orthopaedic Surgery, the Elbow*. New York: Raven Press; 1994.

Morrey BF: Elbow dislocation in the athlete. In DeLee JC, Drez D Jr (eds): *Orthopaedic Sports Medicine: Principles and Practice*, vol 1. Philadelphia: WB Saunders; 1994:836.

Nirschl RP, Pettrone FA: Tennis elbow: The surgical treatment of lateral epicondylitis. *J Bone Joint Surg [Am]* 1979; 61:832.

Regan WD, Morrey BF: Entrapment neuropathies about the elbow. In DeLee JC, Drez D Jr (eds): *Orthopaedic Sports Medicine: Principles and Practice*, vol 1. Philadelphia: WB Saunders 1994:844.

Rokito AS, McLaughlin JA, Gallagher MA, et al: Partial rupture of the distal biceps tendon. *J Shoulder Elbow Surg* 1996; 5:73.

Chapter 98

HAND AND WRIST INJURIES IN THE ATHLETE

Nader Paksima, Daniel S. Zapson, and Steven M. Green

History and physical examination are the cornerstones of diagnosis of athletic injuries. When assessing the athlete with an injured hand or wrist, the history should include the mechanism of injury, the onset, the type and location of pain, any preexisting condition, and the athlete's sport activity. Frequently, the first line of treatment has been provided on the sidelines and the subsequent treating physician must then learn the full nature and extent of the injury and prior treatment.

WRIST DISORDERS

FRACTURES

Scaphoid Fractures

The scaphoid is the most commonly fractured carpal bone. The mechanism of injury is a fall on an outstretched dorsiflexed hand. The athlete will present with pain in the radial side of the wrist. Patients with tenderness in the anatomic snuff box should be considered to have a scaphoid fracture until proven otherwise. Appropriate radiographs include a PA, an ulnar deviation PA, a supinated clenched fist, and lateral views. The ulnar deviation view extends the scaphoid to provide better visualization of cortical disruption while the clenched fist view can depict a scapholunate ligament injury.

If a fracture is not identified and the athlete has tenderness in the snuff box, a thumb spica splint should be applied and the athlete reexamined in a week. If tenderness persists, a bone scan or CT scan should be obtained.

Nondisplaced scaphoid fractures are usually treated in a long or short arm thumb spica cast until radiographic evidence of union. Union may take longer in a short arm cast but a long arm cast is more difficult for the athlete to tolerate.

If there is more than 1 mm displacement or if the fracture pattern is unstable (a vertical oblique fracture or comminution), open reduction and internal fixation (ORIF) of the scaphoid is warranted. Some authors have recommended immediate screw fixation of nondisplaced fractures in the high level athlete to allow earlier return to sports.

If the fracture is amenable to treatment with a compression screw, postoperative immobilization is not necessary. However, unprotected return to contact sports should be restricted until union is achieved.

Previously unrecognized scaphoid nonunions may become symptomatic after an acute episode of trauma. The patient may or may not recall a history of previous wrist trauma. The radiographic findings that differentiate a scaphoid nonunion from an acute fracture include sclerosis of the fracture line, smooth rounded edges at the fracture, cyst formation, pseudoarthrosis formation, and scaphoid collapse with radiocarpal arthritis. Scaphoid nonunions are usually treated with ORIF and bone grafting.

Repetitive wrist trauma can lead to a stress fracture of the scaphoid. This condition is usually seen in gymnasts. The athlete will present with pain in the snuff box and limitation of motion. Radiographs and bone scan confirm the diagnosis. Nondisplaced stress fractures are treated with immobilization; displaced fractures need an ORIF.

Another condition related to repetitive loading of the wrist in gymnasts is physeal growth arrest. Usually, the distal radius is involved. The resultant deformity is relative overgrowth of the ulna which can lead to ulnar impaction syndrome.

Hamate Fractures

Hook of the hamate fractures occur most commonly from direct trauma to the hypothenar eminence from the handle of a golf club, bat, or racquet. The athlete will present with pain over the hook of the hamate, which is one finger breadth distal and radial to the pisiform.

Although these fractures can be identified by obtaining a carpal tunnel view radiograph of the wrist, the CT scan provides the best depiction of the fracture anatomy.

Nondisplaced fractures can be treated in a cast which immobilizes the fourth and fifth metacarpophalangeal (MCP) joints in 90 degrees flexion. Large displaced fragments can be treated by ORIF, and small fragments can be excised. There is a high incidence of delayed diagnosis and nonunion associated with this fracture.

Late sequelae of nonunion include rupture of the fifth finger profundus tendon from attrition wear at the fracture surface and ulnar nerve irritation in Guyon's canal.

Fractures of the body of the hamate usually involve a dislocation of the carpometacarpal joint. Reduction and fixation is required to prevent painfull posttraumatic arthritis.

Lunate Fractures

Isolated lunate fractures are rare. Displaced fractures require anatomic reduction and internal fixation. Kienböck's disease refers to osteonecrosis of the lunate which may occur subsequent to a fracture of this carpal bone. There is an association between repetitive trauma and osteonecrosis of the lunate.

Triquetrum Fractures

The triquetrum is the second most commonly fractured carpal bone. The dorsal marginal fracture is a result of ligamentous avulsion of the dorsal radiotriquetral ligament or impingement of the triquetum against the dorsal margin of the radius when the wrist is hyperextended. Despite its high nonunion rate, this fracture is seldom problematic and is usually treated in a short arm cast for 4 weeks. A gradual return to play can then be started as symptoms permit.

Fractures through the body of the triquetrum are associated with perilunate dislocations. These are serious disruptions of carpal stability and require operative intervention.

Trapezium Fractures

There are two patterns of trapezium fractures. The vertical body fracture is the mirror image of a Bennett's fracture subluxation and requires ORIF. The anterior ridge fracture is an avulsion fracture of the transverse carpal ligament which is usually treated with immobilization. Late sequelae of the anterior ridge fracture include flexor carpi radialis tendonitis and median nerve irritation and may require excision of the fragment with decompression of the tendon or nerve.

LIGAMENTOUS INJURIES

Carpal Instability

Scapholunate Ligament Tears   The most commonly injured intrinsic ligament of the wrist is the scapholunate interosseous. This U-shaped ligament stabilizes the scaphoid to the lunate. Injuries to this ligament can produce a dorsal intercalated segmental instability (DISI) pattern. In this situation the scaphoid will volarflex and the lunate will dorsiflex. The scapholunate angle will be increased to greater than 70 degrees (normal 30 to 60 degrees, average 47 degrees). The distal pole of the scaphoid will appear as a cortical ring sign on the PA radiograph, the scapholunate interval will be increased to greater than 3 mm, and the lunate will lose its trapezoidal appearance. The Watson test is performed by bringing the wrist from ulnar to radial deviation while the examiner's hand is on the scaphoid tubercle to stabilize it and prevent volar flexion. A painful clunk is palpable when the scaphoid reduces and is indicative of scapholunate instability. One must check the unaffected wrist because a clunk can be a normal finding in ligamentously lax individuals.

Acute injuries with instability require open repair. Symptomatic partial tears without evidence of instability can initially be treated with splinting. If symptoms persist, arthroscopic debridement of the flap tear can be carried out.

Chronic tears can lead to a progressive pattern of carpal collapse and arthritis which has been termed scapholunate advanced collapse (SLAC wrist). Prior to the onset of arthritis, treatment options include ligamentous reconstruction and intercarpal fusion. Surgical techniques for the arthritic (SLAC) wrist are proximal carpectomy, scaphoid excision with intercarpal fusion, and total wrist fusion. Treatment of chronic tears with instability remains controversial; options include soft tissue reconstruction, resection of the proximal carpal row, intercarpal fusion, and total wrist fusion.

Lunotriquetral Ligament   Acute lunotriquetral ligament tears can be isolated or occur as part of a perilunate dislocation. Degeneration of this ligament often occurs in patients whose ulna is longer than the radius (ulnar plus variant).

The treatment for acute injuries in the absence of carpal instability, is cast immobilization, whereas with intercarpal instability, surgery is recommended. Symptomatic chronic cases can be treated with intercarpal fusion, ligament reconstruction, and shortening of the ulna.

TFCC Disorders   The triangular fibrocartilage complex (TFCC) stabilizes the distal radioulnar joint (DRUJ) and helps in load transfer between the carpus and the forearm. The TFCC is commonly injured in athletes, especially golfers and gymnasts. The differential diagnosis of ulnar-sided wrist pain in the athlete includes TFCC tears, DRUJ instability, extensor carpi ulnaris (ECU) subluxation, ulnar impaction syndrome, flexor carpi ulnaris (FCU) tendonitis, and pisotriquetral instability.

Symptoms of TFCC tears include pain with forearm rotation, ulnar deviation, and forceful grip. Examination will reveal tenderness over the ulnar styloid and in cases of complete tears of the TFCC from its peripheral attachment, DRUJ instability. Stability testing of the DRUJ is performed by translating the distal ulna on the radius in supination, pronation, and midrotation of the forearm. The exam should be compared to the noninjured side. A PA radiograph (taken with the shoulder abducted to 90 degrees, elbow flexed to 90 degrees, and the forearm in neutral rotation) will demonstrate the ulnar variance. Positive variance (ulna head is distal to the medial radius articular margin) has been correlated with TFCC tears because a greater percentage of the forces across the wrist are transmitted through the TFCC to the prominent ulnar head. MRI provides the best noninvasive method of imaging the TFCC. Triple injection arthrography can also demonstrate TFCC and other ligamentous tears, by showing dye extravasation into the DRUJ or midcarpal joint. Acute TFCC tears are initially treated by immobilization in a long arm splint or cast. Arthroscopy is an excellent diagnostic and therapeutic method of evaluating and treating TFCC injuries. Patients with chronic symptoms can be addressed surgically. Peripheral tears can be repaired by both arthroscopic and "open" techniques. Central tears are debrided arthroscopically. Associated large ulnar styloid avulsion fragments are treated by ORIF.

Central tears associated with ulnar impaction syndrome can be addressed via arthroscopic debridement and distal ulnar resection or ulnar shortening osteotomy, which may provide the added advantage of tightening the ulnocarpal ligament complex.

TENDONITIS

FCU / ECU Tendonitis

ECU tendon subluxation is another cause of ulnar-sided wrist pain which can result from traumatic or degenerative tearing of the extensor sheath. The diagnosis is made by palpating the tendon as the forearm is supinated and pronated. Reconstruction of the ECU sheath with a strip of extensor retinaculum is effective for treatment of this chronic condition. Tendonitis of the ECU is seen in squash and racquet ball players and usually responds well to nonoperative measures such as stroke modification, rest, anti-inflammatories and steroid injection.

FCU tendonitis presents as pain along the volar ulnar aspect of the distal forearm. FCU tendonitis is caused by repetitive wrist flexion, as in tennis or golf. Since the FCU inserts onto the pisiform, this attachment can become painful. Treatment is rest, splinting, and anti-inflammatory medication.

Pisotriquetral instability can be very painful; it is diagnosed by grasping the pisiform between the thumb and index finger and translating it on the triquetrum. This condition can lead to posttraumatic arthritis which is amenable to excision of the pisiform, preserving FCU function.

Intersection Syndrome

Intersection syndrome, or "squeakers" is caused by friction of the first compartment muscle tendon unit (abductor pollicis longus or APL, extensor pollicis brevis or EPB) on the second compartment muscle tendon unit (extensor carpi radialis brevis or ECRB, extensor carpi radialis longus or ECRL). The athlete will present with discomfort in the distal radial forearm, especially with extension of the thumb and wrist against resistance. Weight lifters and oarsmen are among the athletes most affected by this condition. There is a characteristic sound that is produced which has been described as a squeak or "footsteps in fresh snow." Rest and anti-inflammatory medications are usually effective.

de Quervain's Tenosynovitis

de Quervain's tenosynovitis refers to inflammation of the tendons of the first dorsal compartment—the abductor pollicis longus and the extensor pollicis brevis. Patients present with pain over the radial aspect of the wrist, which is exacerbated with ulnar deviation of the wrist with the thumb flexed (Finkelstein's test). Treatment involves rest, anti-inflammatory medications, thumb spica splinting, and cortisone injection. Surgical decompression of the entire first compartment is indicated for chronic symptoms.

FCR Tendonitis

The distal FCR may be inflamed as it passes through a tunnel which is formed by fascial tissue and the trapezium. This condition can be seen in tennis players and athletes involved in wrist flexion activities. Rest, splinting, and anti-inflammatory medication are usually effective, but surgical release of the tendon tunnel may be necessary.

EPL Rupture

Spontaneous rupture of the EPL can occur in tennis players. Attrition of the tendon as it passes around Lister's tubercle can lead to tendon rupture. Ruptures are usually treated with transfer of the EIP tendon.

METACARPOPHALANGEAL JOINT INJURIES

COLLATERAL LIGAMENT INJURIES

Thumb

Acute disruption of the ulnar collateral ligament of the thumb MP joint is often labeled skier's thumb (game keeper's thumb more properly refers to chronic instability).The mechanism of injury involves severe radial deviation of the thumb MP joint. Examination will reveal tenderness on the ulnar aspect of the MP joint. Stability is assessed under gentle examination with the MP joint slightly flexed. The Stener lesion is caused by extreme radial deviation which displaces the collateral ligament, superficial to the adductor aponeurosis. If the instability is less than 30 degrees, the injury can be treated with a thumb spica cast, molded so that the MP joint is in slight ulnar deviation. Instability of the joint to greater than 30 degrees indicates total disruption and should be repaired. Surgery carried out more than 3 weeks after injury often requires use of a tendon graft to reconstruct the ligament.

Radial collateral ligament injuries are a result of an ulnar deviation force at the MP joint. Complete tears, with instability, are best treated by direct operative repair whereas partial tears are treated with a thumb spica cast.

Fingers

Isolated radial collateral ligament injury of the fingers usually involves the ulnar three digits. The mechanism is a forced ulnar deviation which may result in a lateral dislocation. These injuries generally heal with immobilization of the joint in extension for 3 weeks followed by buddy taping. Persistent instability is rare.

DISLOCATION

MP dislocations are simple (reducible) or complex (irreducible). "Simple" dislocations present with the MP joint in 60 to 80 degrees of hyperextension. Reduction is accomplished by hyperextending the proximal phalanx, then applying traction to the hyperextended phalanx until it slides over the metacarpal head, and finally gently flexing the proximal phalanx. A dimple in the palmar skin over the MP joint is a sign of an irreducible dorsal dislocation. Complex dislocations require surgery to extract the volar plate which is found interspersed between the head of the metacarpal and the proximal phalanx. The dorsal approach is favored to minimize danger to the digital neurovascular bundle.

PIP JOINT DISORDERS

INSTABILITY

Stability of the proximal interphalangeal (PIP) joint is dependent on ligamentous support, dynamic stabilization provided by the FDS, and the geometry of the bony architecture (Chap. 17). All of which provide the PIP joint with great stability, while allowing mobility.

There are three types of PIP instability: (1) dorsal instability with hyperextension indicating volar plate injury; (2) lateral instability, indicating collateral ligament tears often associated with volar plate disruption; and (3) volar instability, indicating a tear of the central slip, with or without collateral ligament tears.

Dorsal Instability

Hyperextension of the PIP joint can result from volar plate injuries. Pain on the volar aspect of the joint should alert the physician to the diagnosis. Stress testing may demonstrate instability. Incomplete tears (no instability) can be treated with buddy taping and immediate motion. Complete tears can be treated in a splint with the digit flexed to 30 degrees for 3 weeks, followed by buddy taping. Complete tears associated with dislocations require reduction and immobilization (see Chap. 81). A complication of a volar plate injury is the pseudoboutonniere deformity. In these cases the volar plate scars down so that full extension at the PIP joint is not possible. Unlike in a true boutonniere deformity, DIP motion is unaffected.

Lateral Instability

Lateral instability is a result of collateral ligament injury. Grade 1 injuries present with pain and no instability and can be treated with buddy taping. Grade 2 injuries represent partial tears with minor instability with an end point. These are treated with 10 days of splinting with the PIP joint in slight flexion. Grade 3 tears are complete tears that may involve the volar plate, and are splinted with the joint flexed to 30 degrees for 2 to 3 weeks, followed by protected motion and buddy taping.

Volar Instability

Volar instability occurs when the dorsal support is insufficient to maintain proper joint alignment. The important stabilizers are the extensor apparatus (central slip and lateral bands), the dorsal articular surface of the middle phalanx, and the collateral ligaments. Forced volar flexion of the PIP joint and contusions can disrupt these tissues, causing volar subluxation/dislocation or boutonniere deformity.

X-rays can be misleading, since a dislocation may have already been reduced on the playing field. Therefore, careful examination of the mobility, stability, and extensor power of the injured joint is of paramount importance. Although volar dislocation can usually be effectively treated with manipulative reduction and 6 weeks of constant splinting with the PIP joint in full extension, soft tissue interposition may necessitate open reduction. If the dorsum of the joint is swollen and tender or if there is weakness of extension (in spite of the digital anesthetic block), the physician should assume that the central slip has been disrupted and treat the injury as a volar dislocation. Displaced articular fractures that cause subluxation/dislocation are best treated via ORIF.

Dorsal PIP dislocations can be associated with fractures of the middle phalanx. Avulsion fractures usually involve a variable portion of the volar articular margin of the middle phalanx. The volar plate is attached to the avulsed fragment. If the articular fracture involves less than 15 percent of the joint, treatment is as for a simple dislocation. Articular fractures of 15 to 30 percent of the joint surface are treated with a dorsal block splint. The digit is flexed to a position 20 degrees beyond the point of reduction. The athlete is followed weekly and the amount of flexion is decreased gradually as the injury heals. Each splint adjustment should be followed by radiographs to demonstrate a congruent reduction. Articular fragments of greater than 30 percent may be treated with ORIF.

DIP JOINT INJURIES

MALLET FINGER

Disruption of the terminal extensor tendon to the distal phalanx results in a mallet finger deformity. The DIP joint assumes a flexed position and cannot be actively extended. This injury is frequently the result of a blow to the tip of the finger, as from a basketball. Treatment involves full-time splinting of the DIP joint for 6 weeks, followed by 6 weeks of night splinting. Skin maceration can be a problem and must be monitored. Disruption of the extensor mechanism may also be the result of an intraarticular fracture, the mallet fracture. Articular fractures involving less than 30 percent of the joint and without subluxation are treated the same way as a tendonous mallet finger. Larger articular fragments or joint subluxation are treated with ORIF.

JERSEY FINGER

Avulsion of the flexor digitorum profundus from its insertion is referred to as Jersey finger. The mechanism is forced extension of a flexed DIP joint, as may occur when grabbing a football jersey. The ring finger is most commonly involved. The condition is frequently overlooked by the player and coach, to whom it appears as a "jammed finger." Inability to flex the DIP joint confirms the diagnosis. Radiographs should be obtained to look for a bony avulsion fragment. Leddy and Packer (1977) have described three types of FDP avulsion. Type 1: the tendon retracts into the palm with disruption of both the long and short vinculum. Operative repair should be carried out within 10 days. Type 2: associated with a slender avulsion fracture; the long vincula remains attached, preserving some blood supply to the tendon. Type 2 injuries require operative repair and reattachment of the tendon/bone. Type 3: involve a large intraarticular bony fragment. The tendon does not retract proximal to the A4 pulley. Type 3 avulsions are amenable to repair up to several months postinjury.

NEUROLOGIC DISORDERS

ULNAR NEURITIS

Cubital tunnel syndrome is often seen in athletes that are in throwing sports or activities that cause a valgus stress on the elbow. If there is medial instability, a valgus stress will put the ulnar nerve on stretch as it passes through the cubital tunnel. Weight lifters can have compression of the ulnar nerve at the two heads of the FCU. Sensory symptoms include decreased sensation of the dorsal-ulnar aspect of the hand, the palmar surfaces of the little finger, and the ulnar half of the ring finger. Motor findings include weakness of the adductor pollicis, the interossei, the hypothenar muscles, the ulnar two lumbricals, and the ulnar two FDP units. Treatment methods include splinting, activity modification, ulnar nerve decompression with or without transposition, and medial collateral ligament reconstruction (see Chap. 113).

The ulnar nerve can be injured at Guyon's canal by a compressive force such as "handle bar" palsy in bicyclists, or by repetitive trauma on the hypothenar eminence (the hypothenar hammer syndrome). Hypothenar hammer syndrome can also be caused by ulnar artery thrombosis. Hook of the hamate fractures can irritate the ulnar nerve as it passes through Guyon's canal. Treatment initially involves activity modification. Persistent cases require decompression of the ulnar nerve.

CARPAL TUNNEL SYNDROME

Carpal tunnel syndrome refers to a compression of the median nerve within the carpal canal. In the athlete this is primarily related to flexor tendon inflammation. Symptoms include numbness in the radial three digits, and in advanced cases atrophy of the thenar muscles. Electro-diagnostic testing studies can be an aid in diagnosis. Nonoperative treatment is successful in the majority of cases and includes splinting, NSAIDs, tendon gliding exercises, and cortisone injection. Resistant cases are treated by operative decompression (see Chap. 113).

BOWLERS THUMB

The digital nerves to the thumb (especially the ulnar digital nerve) can be compressed at the edge of the thumb hole in the bowling ball. Treatment can include filling in the opening (ensuring that less of the thumb will go in the hole), padding the thumb, and rest. Operative intervention is rarely indicated.

SUGGESTED READINGS

Leddy JP: Soft-tissue injuries of the hand in the athlete. In Cannon WD Jr (ed): *Instruction Course Lectures.* Rosemont, IL: AAOS; 1998; 47:181.

Leddy JP, Packer JW: Avulsion of the profundus tendon insertion in athletes. *J Hand Surg [Am]* 1977; 2:66.

Mandelbaum BR, Bartolozzi AR, Davis CA, et al: Wrist pain syndrome in the gymnast; pathogenetic, diagnostic, and therapeutic considerations. *Am J Sports Med* 1989; 17:305.

McCue FC III, Bruce JF Jr: The wrist. In DeLee JC, Drez D Jr (eds): *Orthopaedic Sports Medicine: Principles and Practice.* Philadelphia: WB Saunders; 1994:913.

Mooney JF 3d, Siegel DB, Koman LA: Ligamentous injuries of the wrist in athletes. *Clin Sports Med* 1992; 11(1):129.

Raab DJ, Fischer DA, Quick DC: Lunate and perilunate dislocations in professional football players. A five-year retrospective analysis. *Am J Sports Med* 1994; 22(6):841.

Smail DF: Handlebar Palsy (letter). *N Engl J Med* 1975: 292:322.

Chapter 99

HIP

Geoffrey I. Phillips.

Severe athletic injuries to the hip joint and pelvis are relatively unusual owing to their durable construction. The hip is an intrinsically stable ball and socket joint surrounded by powerful musculature while the large pelvic bones primarily facilitate mechanical transfer of body weight from the trunk to the appendicular skeleton and prevent traumatic injury to the abdominal viscera. Forces exceeding six times body weight are transmitted through the hip joint during walking, with larger stresses generated by running and contact sports. Most sports injuries referable to the hip and pelvis involve the enveloping soft tissues. Injury may result either from direct trauma or from repetitive overuse. Management of the painful hip or pelvis in the athlete necessitates an adequate understanding of the anatomic and biomechanical factors predisposing to injury.

RUNNING INJURIES TO THE HIP JOINT

The dynamics of running have been implicated in the cause of numerous hip disorders, including gluteus medius muscle strain, greater trochanteric bursitis, iliotibial band syndrome, adductor tendinitis, hamstring strain, iliac and ischial apophysitis, sacroiliitis, osteitis pubis, piriformis syndrome, and femoral neck stress fracture. Abnormal pelvic tilt secondary to a leg length discrepancy, poor gait, running on banked surfaces or roadside curbs, and an increased Q angle are frequent etiologies of lateral hip pain. These may all contribute to strain at the distal attachments of the abductor musculature, particularly the gluteus medius insertion onto the greater trochanter, and to inflammation of the bursa deep to the gluteal muscles. Iliotibial band friction syndrome represents an overuse injury associated with running, cycling, and other athletic activities that involve repetitive knee flexion. Extending from the iliac crest to Gerdy's tubercle, the iliotibial band is the second most common cause of knee pain among runners and a less frequent source of lateral hip pain. Conservative measures usually suffice in the management of these three conditions, including stretching and strengthening exercises of the hip abductor muscles and iliotibial band as well as an occasional local corticosteroid injection. Leg length discrepancy and associated anatomic variants should be assessed and corrected, if possible, to prevent recurrence.

Shearing forces transmitted across the pelvis during running may result in sacroiliitis, osteitis condensans ilii, and osteitis pubis, with referred pain arising from the sacroiliac and pubic symphyseal joints. Physical examination demonstrates tenderness over the affected joints and radiographs may reveal localized sclerosis, although a bone tumor should be excluded. Rest from the aggravating activity often ameliorates the symptoms associated with these disorders. Strain injuries tend to occur in speed athletes with the hamstrings, which cross multiple joints with a lengthy musculotendinous junction. Muscle strains and tendinitis are best managed conservatively, although total proximal avulsion of the hamstring muscle complex from the ischial tuberosity may represent an indication for surgery in the elite athlete population. Improper rehabilitation of a minor muscle strain can often lead to a far more disabling injury.

CONTACT AND COLLISION SPORTS

Hip injuries may also arise during contact and collision sports. Both hip dislocations and fractures have been reported among football players, representing less than 3% of football-specific injuries. The more common injuries sustained by these athletes include iliac crest contusion and iliopsoas strain, with apophyseal avulsion fractures occurring in the adolescent age group. Myositis ossificans of the hip following a direct blow to the joint during a soccer game has been reported.

SPECIAL CONSIDERATIONS: THE SKELETALLY IMMATURE ATHLETE

In evaluating a skeletally immature athlete with hip pain, the physician must carefully consider a variety of special disorders in the differential diagnosis, including slipped capital femoral epiphysis, Salter-Harris physeal fractures, labral tears, transient synovitis, Perthes' disease, osteomyelitis, and septic arthritis. Fortunately, most athletic injuries to the hip and pelvis are soft-tissue in nature as the inherent durability of the osseous structures enhances their ability to withstand the transmission of large weightbearing and contact loads. The majority of athletic injuries affecting the hip respond favorably to a program of nonoperative management and rehabilitation.

SUGGESTED READINGS

Gross ML, Nasser S, Finerman GAM: Hip and pelvis. In DeLee JC, Drez D Jr (eds): *Orthopaedic Sports Medicine Principles and Practice.* Philadelphia: WB Saunders; 1994:1063.

Kaeding CC, Sanko WA, Fischer RA: Myositis ossificans: Minimizing downtime. *Physician Sports Med* 1995; 23(2):77.

Sim FH, Rock MG, Scott SG: Pelvis and hip injuries in athletes: Anatomy and function. In Nicholas JA, Hershman EB (eds): *The Lower Extremity and Spine in Sports Medicine.* New York: Mosby; 1995:1025.

Chapter 100

KNEE: PATELLOFEMORAL JOINT DISORDERS

Mark I. Pitman and Howard J. Luks

OVERVIEW

Problems of the patellofemoral joint in both males and females, athletic and non-athletic, are a difficult challenge. Interest in and understanding of patellofemoral pathomechanics and pathoanatomy has been increasing in recent years. Anatomic malalignment and muscle imbalance are recognized as the primary causes of pain, instability, and pathologic changes within the patellofemoral joint. In addition to these well-recognized anatomic predispositions, there are, however, many other causes of patellofemoral (anterior knee) pain.

Accurate diagnosis of anterior knee pain is essential if attempts at treatment are to be successful. Prior to defining this as a "patellofemoral syndrome," other causes of pain must be ruled out. These include:

1. "Referred Knee Pain": Complaints of anterior knee pain may be the initial symptom of pathology within the hip joint or the spine. In the young, problems such as Legg-Perthes disease, slipped capital femoral epiphysis, and hip dysplasia, or, in older individuals, the onset of arthritic change within the hip joint, must be ruled out.
2. Synovial plica: Medial synovial plica, if pathologic, may be a cause of anterior knee pain and may mimic mechanical problems such as meniscal tear, and patellar snapping and subluxation.
3. Extensor mechanism tendinitis: This includes patellar tendinitis and quadriceps tendinitis.
4. Cruciate ligament insufficiency: Chronic ligamentous injuries, both to the anterior cruciate ligament (ACL) and posterior cruciate ligament (PCL), may go unrecognized for a prolonged period of time and may present as anterior knee pain.
5. Bursitis: Prepatellar bursitis, retropatellar bursitis, and pes anserine bursitis may present as anterior knee pain.
6. Inflammatory synovitis
7. Neoplasms within the joint or within adjacent structures.
8. Reflex sympathetic dystrophy (RSD): This is a frequently overlooked cause of anterior knee pain that is extremely resistant to treatment. It may lead to severe and permanent disability. Diagnosis is often missed or delayed.

All these entities must be considered, evaluated, and recognized before concentrating on the patellofemoral joint. Incorrect diagnosis leads to incorrect therapeutic choice and to poor results.

ANATOMY

Anatomic structures causally implicated in patellofemoral disorders include the tibia, the femur, and the patella, as well as soft tissues about the knee joint. The pathoanatomy of patellofemoral disorders includes bony abnormalities with angulation and torsion and soft tissue abnormalities or imbalances with resultant angulation and torsion due to improper force distribution.

BONY STRUCTURES

The patellofemoral joint consists of the patella, the femoral trochlea, the medial and lateral condyles, and the supratrochlear sulcus.

Patella

The patella is a sesamoid bone within the extensor mechanism of the knee connecting the quadriceps tendon to the patellar tendon. Its articular surface basically has two facets, medial and lateral, separated by the medial ridge. The lateral facet, longer and with less of a slope, articulates with the larger and higher lateral femoral condyle. The most medial articular surface of the patella consists of what is called the "odd" facet.

Femoral Articular Surface of the Patellofemoral Joint

The femoral surface articulating with the patella consists of the medial condyle, lateral condyle, trochlea, and the supratrochlear sulcus. The lateral facet is larger than the medial facet. It extends further anteriorly and further proximally than does the medial facet. The trochlea is the concave groove separating the two convex condyles. A dysplastic, or shallow, trochlear sulcus has been recognized as a cause of patellofemoral malalignment. Either the medial or lateral femoral condyle may be dysplastic, or the trochlea may be dysplastic and, rather than being concave, it is either flat or convex. This is most easily demonstrated on CT scans.

In full extension, the lower pole of the patella articulates with the sulcus. As the knee flexes, the contact area between the patella and the femur moves superiorly on the patella and inferiorly on the femur. After 10 degrees of flexion, the patella begins to articulate with the trochlea. The more distal portion of the patella articulates with the more proximal portion of the trochlea. As the knee continues to flex, the area of articulation moves more distally on the femur and, at 90 degrees, most of the articular surface of the patella lies within and articulates with the trochlea. There is debate concerning at what degree of flexion the patella may dislocate. It is our feeling that dislocation occurs at or near the start of full extension. Signs associated with a dislocating patella such as the apprehension test and the J-sign, which will be discussed later, occur in full or near extension. For this reason, the shape of the proximal trochlea and supratrochlear sulcus are important.

Femoral and Tibial Torsion

Certain torsional deformities can affect the line of pull on the patella or the Q angle. Anteversion of the femoral neck is often combined with external torsion of the tibia, and with increased valgus of the knee. These torsional abnormalities change the vector of forces upon the patella, causing it to displace laterally in relation to the trochlea. This is reflected in the Q angle, which is increased in this patient population. Collectively, these torsional abnormalities are referred to as the miserable malalignment syndrome.

SOFT TISSUE STRUCTURES

The lateral patellar retinaculum consists of superficial fibers attaching to the iliotibial band and deeper fibers attaching to the lateral epicondyle. The medial retinaculum attaches the patella superiorly to the medial femoral epicondyle and more inferiorly to the anterior margin of the medial meniscus. Both of these attachment sites are passive stabilizers but may be influenced by the active stabilizers. The forces created by the iliotibial band (ITB) affect the lateral retinaculum and the forces created by the vastus medialis obliquus (VMO) affect the medial retinaculum.

Active Stabilizers

The quadriceps muscle is the major active stabilizer of the patella. The rectus femoris inserts into the anterior portion of the superior aspect of the patella and extends down to the patellar tendon. The vastus intermedius attaches to the posterior portion of the superior surface of the patella. The vastus lateralis inserts into the lateral portion of the quadriceps tendon and the lateral portion of the patella and forms the lateral portion of the patellar ligament. There appears to be a separate vastus lateralis obliquus (VLO) which interdigitates with the lateral intramuscular septum and inserts laterally onto the patella. The vastus medialis extends more distally onto the patella than does the vastus lateralis. The most distal portion of the vastus medialis consists of more oblique fibers and is the VMO. These fibers appear to be both neurologically and functionally separate from the vastus medialis itself, and provide a medially directed force on the patella which actively resists the tendency towards lateral displacement of the patella.

EVALUATION OF ANTERIOR KNEE PAIN

HISTORY

The onset may be acute or chronic and the injury reported at onset may be direct or indirect. Acute trauma may be direct such as a dashboard injury to the patella or indirect such as an athletic pivoting maneuver. Chronic symptoms may progress slowly and insidiously. The patient may note a sensation of "slipping" but may not be able to localize this feeling to the patella. Locking is also a frequent complaint of patellar problems. This is not a mechanical locking but usually a momentary "catching" in full extension. Crepitus or clicking behind the patella may be noted and it may be palpable or audible. Crepitus is frequently encountered in the absence of anterior knee pain and may not be significant. Precise localization of the pain may be difficult and is often increased by immobility such as prolonged sitting. It is often worse on stairs, especially descending, and with weather changes.

The patient may localize the pain superiorly to the patella about the quadriceps mechanism, or inferiorly to the patella about the patellar tendon. Either of these suggest the presence of patellar or quadriceps tendinitis rather than intraarticular pathology.

RSD is classically characterized by severe pain out of proportion to the injury sustained or to the pathology found (see Chap. 157). Anterior knee pain due to RSD is frequently moderate rather than se-

vere as in the classical symptoms of advanced RSD. RSD may occur after knee surgery, following knee trauma, or without any specific onset. Symptoms, which the patient may notice and which must be probed for, include hyperesthesia, in addition to pain present day and night. This may be clinically manifested by increased pain on wearing tight slacks, especially jeans, by the rubbing of bed clothes, by washing the leg, or in difficulty shaving about the knee in females. The presence of any of these symptoms should raise a high degree of suspicion that RSD may be the underlying cause.

PHYSICAL EXAMINATION

Standing

The patient should be examined while standing and walking. Overall alignment and gait should be systematically evaluated. Observation for the presence of excessive valgus or varus of the knees, of anteversion of the neck of the femur, of tibial torsion, and hyperpronation of the feet should be noted.

Ligamentous laxity is assessed by asking the patient to try to place the palms of the hands on the floor while standing, by checking for upper extremity signs of laxity such as excessive recurvatum of the elbow, a positive thumb to forearm test, and increased hyperextension of the metacarpophalangeal and interphalangeal joints. Lower extremities may reveal increased recurvatum as well as increased rotatory motion of the hips and of the knees. The position of the patella should be evaluated. In cases of excessive femoral antetorsion and external tibial torsion, the patellae may point inward (squinting patellae).

Sitting

The patient is next examined while sitting over the side of the table with the knees flexed to 90 degrees. Patellar alignment is visualized at this time. Dynamic alignment may be assessed as the knees are slowly extended. As the knee goes into full extension, the patella may move laterally or even subluxate and this produces the visible "J-sign." In addition, this movement often elicits painful crepitus.

Supine

Overall alignment of the extremity should be checked. Range of motion of the hip must be carefully evaluated. Any limitation of range of motion of the hip is highly suggestive of hip joint pathology. Such limitations may be subtle; the one most frequently observed is limitation of internal rotation.

The quadriceps musculature is evaluated. Quadriceps atrophy is frequently seen in this population. The VMO should be carefully visualized and palpated to evaluate its position relative to the patella and for the presence of any hypoplasia or atrophy. Following an acute injury, a defect may be palpable at the insertion of the VMO onto the patella. The Q angle (the angle between the anterior superior iliac spine, mid-portion of the body of the patella, and the tibial tubercle) is evaluated (see Fig. 27-1). The Q angle measures the angle between the pull of the quadriceps and of the patellar tendon. In males, this angle should be 10 degrees or less and, in females, 15 degrees or less. Ligamentous or meniscal injuries and range of motion are evaluated prior to proceeding to examination of the patella.

The patella is examined last. Evaluation of the patella includes examination for fluid within the knee, either the presence of a palpable effusion, a ballottable patella, or a fluid wave. The patella and the peripatellar tissues are palpated next. The patellar tendon is palpated and tenderness may be elicited, especially when the patella itself is displaced distally. Similarly, the quadriceps tendon is palpated. Tenderness of either of these locations suggests a patellar or quadriceps tendinitis, respectively.

The lateral retinaculum is palpated. This is most satisfactorily done with the patella displaced laterally in order to relax the retinaculum. The medial retinaculum and the VMO are also palpated. The articular surface is palpated by palpating the medial facet with the patella displaced medially and the lateral facet with the patella displaced laterally, although lateral palpation is usually not as revealing as medial palpation. The medial facet is often tender.

Mobility of the patella is evaluated by measuring the number of quadrants in which the patella can be displaced (one quadrant, four quadrants, etc.). Forced lateral displacement, especially in patients with subluxation or dislocation, may cause an "apprehension sign," manifested by anxiety, sudden quadriceps contraction, or resistance by the patient. It strongly suggests the presence of patellar subluxation or dislocation. Patellar tilt is then evaluated. With the patient supine and the leg in neutral position, the patella should be parallel to the floor. If the lateral side is more posterior, then patellar tilt is present. Attempts should then be made to lift the lateral side of the patella anteriorly, to make the patella parallel to the floor. If this is not possible, then the lateral retinaculum is excessively tight. Due to the dynamic component of lateral subluxation provided by the ITB, the Ober test is performed to assess for a tight ITB.

Direct compression of the patella against the underlying femur may elicit pain or crepitus. Crepitus with pain, which reproduces this patient's symptoms, is significant. Crepitus without pain is probably not significant.

RSD is evaluated by noting an increase or decrease in hair growth, skin temperature, sensitivity to light touch, pin prick, or percussion about the tissues of the anterior knee, especially the area of the infrapatellar branch of the saphenous nerve.

RADIOGRAPHS

Routine radiographs provide information concerning the presence of bony pathology, the shape, and the location of the patella. Routine AP radiographs may show the presence of accessory ossification centers, and the relative heights of the patellae of both knees. The lateral view may be used to determine the presence of patella alta or patella baja. It also may be used to demonstrate the depth of the trochlear groove and the presence of trochlear dysplasia. Axial views (skyline) reveal the position of the patella within the trochlear groove. Several measurements are made on this view, such as the congruence angle and the lateral patellofemoral angle. However, the pathology noted with these views is extremely dependent on the angle of knee flexion at which the radiograph is taken. The most important views are those taken nearest full extension. The Laurin view is taken at 20 degrees of flexion and the Merchant view at 45 degrees. Schutzer and coworkers have shown pathology is best demonstrated between 0 and 30 degrees of flexion. By 30 degrees, even the abnormally tracking patella usually rides normally within the groove.

Computed tomography, as described by Schutzer, Ramsby and Fulkerson (1986), is the most informative imaging modality. Recommended axial views of the patellofemoral joint are taken with the knee at 0, 10, 20, and 30 degrees flexion. Measurements are made through the center of the patella to determine the amount of patellar tilt and patellar subluxation (Figs. 100-1 and 100-2).

Magnetic resonance imaging provides similar information but also can provide evidence of pathology such as articular cartilage injuries, chondromalacia, osteochondritis dessicans, and, on the sagittal view, pathology within the patellar or quadriceps tendons.

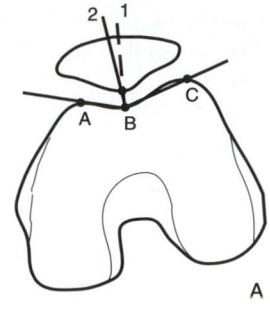

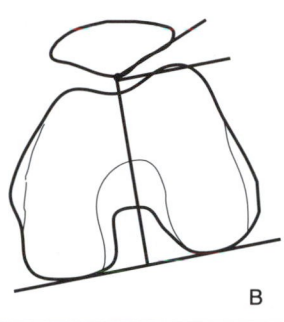

Figure 100-1
A. Measurement of congruence angle for patellar subluxation. Congruent angle is determined by connecting points A, B, and C. Points A and C represent the highest points on the trochlea and point B the depth of the trochlea. Line 1 is drawn bisecting this angle. Line 2 is drawn to connect point B with the apex of the patella. The angle between these two lines is measured. If line 1 lies medial to line 2, the angle is negative; if lateral to line 2, the angle is positive. A positive angle suggests lateral displacement. *B.* Measurement of angle of patellar tilt. A line is drawn along the posterior surface of the femoral condyle. A second line is drawn along the lateral articular surface of the patella. The angle between these two lines should be greater than 8 degrees. An angle lesser than 8 degrees suggests patellar tilt. [Reproduced with permission from Walsh MW: Patellofemoral joint. In DeLee JC, Drez D Jr (eds): *Orthopaedic Sports Medicine: Principles and Practice.* Philadelphia: WB Saunders; 1994; 1190.]

Bone scanning is useful to demonstrate metabolic activity within the patella. However, it has not been shown to be of definitive diagnostic or prognostic value. Its greatest value appears to be in the diagnosis of RSD.

TREATMENT

Treatment depends upon proper diagnosis. Most treatment for anterior knee pain is nonsurgical in nature.

REST

Initial treatment consists of modification of activity or rest. A careful history will elicit the predisposing activities, such as downhill running or uphill bicycling. These are diminished or modified, and performed, if at all, only in a pain-free method.

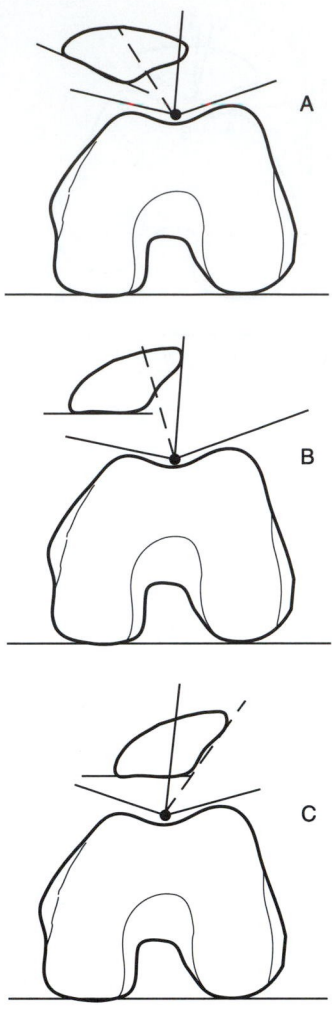

Figure 100-2
Measurements of patellofemoral incongruity. *A.* Patellar subluxation alone. *B.* Patellar tilt and subluxation. *C.* Patellar tilt alone. [Reproduced with permission from Walsh MW: Patellofemoral joint. In DeLee JC, Drez D Jr (eds): *Orthopaedic Sports Medicine: Principles and Practice.* Philadelphia: WB Saunders; 1994:1191.]

STRETCHING

Stretching of tight lateral structures, the hamstrings, the gastrocnemius, the ITB band, and the quadriceps is important.

EXERCISES

Active exercises are performed cautiously. Those that stress the patellofemoral joint must be avoided. These are basically isotonic quadriceps exercises. Quadriceps exercise should, initially, be isometric, that is straight leg raising exercises and quadriceps contraction with the knee in extension. Hip abduction, hip extension, and hip adduction are useful. Isotonic or isokinetic hamstring and gastrocnemius exercises are started early. Closed chain exercises, such as a leg press machine, a bicycle (with the seat raised to decrease the amount of knee flexion and with tension on the chain low), and well-supervised stair climbing exercises are useful. Later, isotonic or isokinetic short arc quadriceps exercises are added. These are done within the

painless range of motion which is usually 0 to 30 degrees but, in some patients, 60 to 90 degrees. These exercises must be individualized. Attempts have been made to selectively strengthen the VMO. Methods include hip adduction, electric stimulation, and biofeedback approaches. Ice massage and patellar mobilization with lateral retinacular stretches are helpful.

BRACES

Bracing during activity may reduce symptoms, although little clinical data exists to support their use.

SURGICAL TREATMENT

Surgical treatment is reserved for patients with significant symptoms who have not responded to a prolonged course of carefully controlled and supervised, nonoperative therapy. Fulkerson has attempted to guide the practitioner in regard to operative treatment for patellofemoral pathology by categorizing the pathology noted into one of three groups. Fulkerson type I patients have patella subluxation, type II have subluxation and tilt, and type III have only tilt.

Decision making with regard to surgery about the patellofemoral joint depends on the degree and type of alignment abnormality present. A lateral retinacular release attempts to correct lateral patellar tilt in the Fulkerson type III patient. It is not, however, without significant complications, including continued pain, weakness, hemarthrosis (most common), excessive release of the vastus lateralis, transection of the quadriceps tendon, and RSD. In patients with a normal Q angle and subluxation +/- patella tilt, a proximal realignment with a lateral release, VMO advancement, and imbrication of the medial retinaculum should suffice. In the presence of a markedly increased Q angle, we perform both a proximal and distal realignment to compensate for the abnormal Q angle. The distal component of the surgery is an anteromedialization of the tibial tubercle as described by Fulkerson. This procedure accomplishes the goals of realigning the Q angle and decompressing the patellofemoral joint with a single osteotomy.

SUGGESTED READINGS

Brattström H: Shape of the intercondylar groove normally and in recurrent dislocation of the patella. *Acta Orthop Scand* 1964; suppl 68.

DeLee JC, Drez D Jr (eds): The knee. In *Orthopaedic Sports Medicine Principles and Practice.* Philadelphia: WB Saunders; 1994:1113.

Fulkerson JP, Hungerford DS: *Disorders of the Patellofemoral Joint,* 2d ed. Baltimore: Williams & Wilkins; 1990.

Goodfellow JW, Hungerford DS, Zindel M: Patello femoral mechanics and pathology: I. functional anatomy of the patellofemoral joint. *J Bone Joint Surg [Br]* 1976; 58:287.

Henry JH: The patellofemoral joint. In Nicholas JA, Hershman EB (eds): *The Lower Extremity and Spine in Sports Medicine,* 2d ed. St. Louis: Mosby; 1995:935.

Malghem J, Maldague B: Depth insufficiency of the proximal trochlear groove on lateral radiographs of the knee: Relation to patellar dislocation. *Radiology* 1989; 170:507.

Peterson L, Karlsson J, Brittberg M: Patellar instability with recurrent dislocation due to patellofemoral dysplasia. Results after surgical treatment. *Bull Hosp Joint Diseases* 1988; 48:130.

Schutzer SF, Ramsby GR, Fulkerson JP: Computer tomographic classification of patellofemoral pain patients. *Ortho Clin North Am* 1986; 17:235.

Chapter 101

KNEE: INSTABILITY

Howard J. Luks and Andrew S. Rokito

The knee is the largest and most complex joint in the body. Injury to the ligamentous or capsular structures about the knee is very common because of the large moments created by the tibia and femur and their respectively long lever arms. Knee motion cannot be likened to that of a simple hinge but is instead a series of complex coupled motions with 6 degrees of freedom.

EXPERIMENTAL STUDIES AND BIOMECHANICS OF LIGAMENTS

There are a multitude of methodologies by which the function of each of the ligamentous and capsular structures within the knee can be delineated. The *flexibility approach* involves applying a load to the knee joint, observing the displacement, sectioning a certain ligament, and then assessing any change that may have taken place. This method is analogous to clinical laxity measurements such as the anterior draw test. The *stiffness approach* ascertains the function of a ligament by measuring the load in a joint as a function of the application of a predetermined displacement. Following sectioning of the structure under investigation, the load is again assessed and any decrease noted. A decrease indicates the relative importance of the structure sectioned. The concept of primary and secondary stabilizers about the knee was developed by applying the stiffness approach to human cadavers. These studies demonstrated that the anterior cruciate ligament (ACL) is the primary restraint to anterior translation and acts as a secondary restraint to internal rotation. The posterior cruciate ligament (PCL) was found to be the primary stabilizer against posterior translation of the tibia and a secondary stabilizer that resisted external rotation. Both cruciate ligaments also function as secondary stabilizers against varus/valgus stresses.

Many authors have utilized the flexibility approach to document the function of the various other ligamentous and capsular structures. The posterolateral structures [lateral collateral ligament (LCL), arcuate ligament, and popliteus tendon] were found to be the primary restraint to lateral joint opening, especially at 30 degrees of flexion, which relaxes the various other capsular and tendinous secondary stabilizers. In addition, pathological tibial external rotation at 30 degrees of knee flexion was seen with sectioning of the posterolateral structures. If the PCL is sectioned, pathological external rotation will also occur at 90 degrees of flexion. Combined sectioning of the ACL and the posterolateral structures lead to pathological anterior translation and internal-external rotation, respectively. Similarly, combined sectioning of the ACL and medial collateral ligament (MCL) produces a pattern of excessive anterior translation and internal rotation. Due to the complexity in determining the instability patterns present in some patients, proper understanding and interpretation of the relevant biomechanical testing is necessary in order to accurately assess the knee joint.

ANTERIOR CRUCIATE LIGAMENT INJURY

Patients with instability due to incompetence of the ACL may possess a significant functional impairment. In addition, these patients are at risk for developing significant meniscal pathology and possibly late osteoarthritic changes. Active patients are at particular risk, especially those involved in sports which require cutting, pivoting, twisting, and rapid deceleration. The estimated incidence of ACL rupture is 0.6/1000 player days in football players and 0.4/1000 health members/year in a typical HMO patient population. The coexistence of meniscal pathology is between 50 and 75 percent and increases with the chronicity of the instability present. Acute ACL ruptures are more commonly associated with lateral meniscal pathology, whereas patients with chronic ACL instability have a higher incidence of medial meniscal pathology.

PHYSICAL EXAMINATION

The patient with an acute rupture of the ACL will have a hemarthrosis and limited range of motion. These patients generally report a noncontact cutting or pivoting injury and will frequently state they heard a "pop." There is a 75 percent chance that this history will reveal an acute ACL rupture. Initially, the patient should be treated with rest, ice, compression, and elevation. Accurate examination is possible, but difficult in the acute stage. After the pain has resolved, ROM activities and weightbearing is allowed as tolerated. Clinical examination is directed towards demonstrating pathological anterior translation of the tibia. The Lachman test is performed with the knee at 30 degrees of flexion while the examiner stabilizes the femur and imparts an anteriorly directed force on the tibia. The examiner needs to determine the amount of translation as well as the presence or absence of a firm endpoint. Increased excursion in comparison to the contralateral extremity and/or the lack of a firm endpoint are diagnostic of an ACL tear. The absence of an ipsilateral rupture of the PCL must be confirmed because this, if present, will give the impression of increased tibial translation even though the endpoint may be normal.

The pivot shift test is another physical examination technique used to diagnose an incompetent ACL. When performing the pivot shift, the examiner grasps the foot of the patient and internally rotates the tibia with the knee in extension. In the ACL-deficient knee this anteriorly subluxes the anterolateral portion of the tibia. The examiner then flexes the knee slowly. This causes the iliotibial band (ITB) to tighten and to change from a position anterior to the flexion axis of the knee joint to a position posterior to that axis. This, in turn, causes the tibia to reduce with a characteristic "pivot shift." Several factors, however, can cause a false assessment of the pivot shift test. An acute MCL tear will allow the leg to fall into valgus and will thus decrease the ability of the ITB to generate tension, and this will dampen the reduction achieved with knee flexion. Instrumented testing with a KT-1000 arthrometer is not necessary to diagnose an ACL rupture, but if performed properly, it can aid in standardizing information necessary for published reports. On manual maximum anterior displacement testing a 3-mm side to side difference or more than 5 mm total displacement is considered diagnostic of an ACL disruption.

TREATMENT

Nonsurgical treatment

Treatment recommendations for patients with an ACL deficient knee vary depending on the age of the patient, the degree of disability, and the presence of any associated meniscal or ligamentous pathology. In the patient with an acute tear of the ACL with no associated abnormalities, a trial of rest is warranted until the acute symptoms are relieved. The patient should next undergo a strengthening program directed towards hamstring and quadriceps balancing. It is often not possible to accurately judge the degree of disability that may be present for at least a few months following the initial injury. After full strength and motion are regained, the patient is allowed to return to sports but is advised to avoid those activities that require cutting, pivoting, or rapid deceleration. If patients can tolerate such activity modification and are willing to alter their lifestyle accordingly, continued nonoperative management is warranted. If patients are unwilling to modify their activities and continue to experience instability, surgical reconstruction of the ACL is indicated. In a patient with a repairable meniscus tear, concomitant reconstruction of the ACL results in a much higher rate of healing of the meniscal lesion.

Surgical Treatment

Many surgical techniques have been developed to reconstruct the ACL. Similarly, several different types of graft material have been utilized. The two most common types of grafts are an autogenous bone-ligament-bone graft involving the central one-third of the posterior ligament and an autogenous graft involving the hamstring tendons (semitendinosus and gracilis). Particular attention must be paid to tunnel placement in order to minimize stretching of the graft and decrease the risk of blocking extension (Fig. 101-1). The most common mistake during reconstruction of the ACL is to place the femoral tunnel too far anteriorly. This placement will lead to difficulty obtaining flexion and cause the graft to stretch and fail prematurely. Anterior placement of the femoral or tibial tunnels may cause impingement of the graft and formation of scar tissue or a cyclops lesion.

POSTOPERATIVE COMPLICATIONS

One of the most serious complications of ACL reconstructive surgery is infrapatellar contracture syndrome (IPCS) or arthrofibrosis. Increased understanding of the pathogenesis of this condition and its relationship to the lack of an aggressive postoperative therapy regimen has recently led to a decreased incidence. Aggressive ROM must be instituted immediately following reconstruction and the progress of the patient must be frequently assessed by the surgeon. Failure to achieve full range of motion within 2 weeks of the reconstruction will lead to an increased incidence of IPCS. Treatment varies according to the stage of the disease, which is a function of the time it has been present. Within 6 weeks of reconstruction, aggressive physical therapy, including extension bracing, can relieve the symptoms. After 6 to 8 weeks, these pathological processes become more recalcitrant to

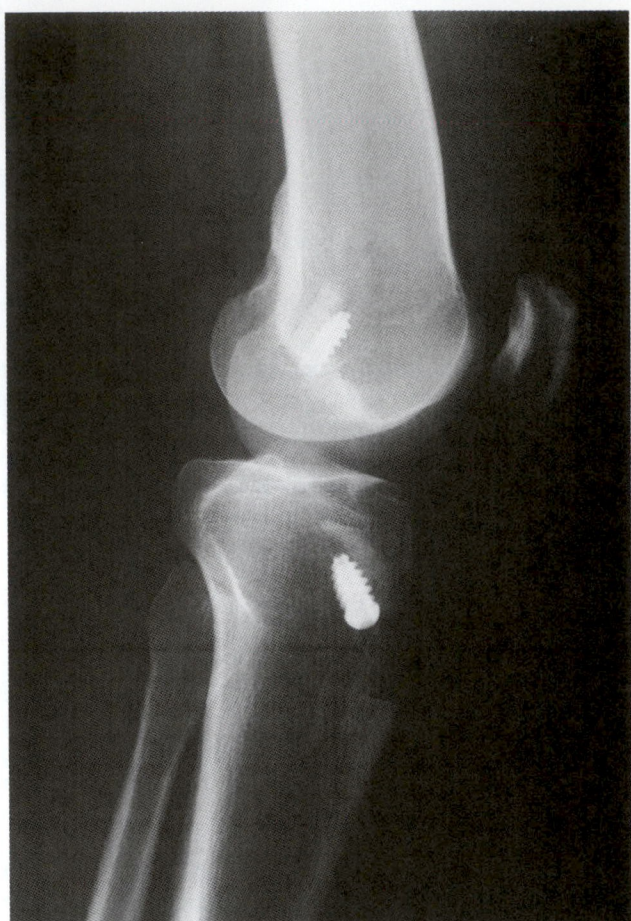

Figure 101-1
Postoperative lateral radiograph demonstrating the correct placement for the femoral and tibial tunnels.

treatment and will require manipulation under anesthesia and a possible arthroscopic lysis of adhesions. In severe cases it is sometimes necessary to debride the graft itself in order to restore motion. Prevention remains the best treatment available.

MEDIAL COLLATERAL LIGAMENT INJURY

The MCL is one of the most commonly injured knee ligaments. Injury usually occurs with valgus stress. The most common associated injuries include tears of the MCL, ACL, and lateral meniscus. O'Donoghue's triad refers to tears of the ACL, MCL, and peripheral medial meniscus.

CLINICAL EVALUATION

On physical examination, the site of ligament injury (femur, tibia, midsubstance) is usually tender to palpation, and there may be a palpable defect. Injuries are graded I (0-5 mm), II (5-10 mm), or III (10-15 mm) based on the degree of medial joint line opening with abduction stress at 30 degrees and the firmness of the endpoint.

TREATMENT

Isolated grade I and II tears are treated nonoperatively. Grade II tears are protected with a rigid brace. Rehabilitation consists of pain control, ROM exercises, weightbearing, and progression to strengthening and sport-specific drills with a return to athletic activity in approximately 2 to 6 weeks.

Isolated grade III injuries are protected in a hinged knee brace locked at 30 degrees of flexion for 2 weeks and then allowed 30 to 90 degrees of flexion for a total of 6 weeks. Combined ACL and MCL injuries are treated with reconstruction of the ACL. Intraoperatively, after the ACL is reconstructed, if there is residual instability (2+ or greater), the medial structures are repaired.

POSTERIOR CRUCIATE LIGAMENT INJURY

Isolated rupture of the PCL is much less common than injury to the ACL. The force needed to rupture the PCL is on the magnitude of 3 to 4 times greater than that necessary to rupture the ACL. Consequently, these patients have typically suffered a high-energy blow to the anterior tibia from a motor vehicle accident or sporting activity. Dashboard injuries, falls on the knee with the foot plantarflexed, knee hyperflexion, and open field tackles on an extended knee are common mechanisms of PCL injury. Due to the high energy needed to rupture the PCL, additional ligamentous injuries or combined injuries are common (see below).

CLINICAL EVALUATION

Initial assessment of the patient with an acute PCL rupture should include a meticulous physical examination, assessing the other capsuloligamentous structures to rule out a spontaneously reduced dislocation of the knee joint. In such circumstances, particular attention to the neurovascular status of the limb is imperative and an angiogram should usually be obtained. Once a knee dislocation has been ruled out, the patient can be treated initially with rest, ice, compression, and elevation of the limb to limit the discomfort associated with an acute injury. The tense effusion commonly associated with rupture of the ACL is frequently absent, and the injury is often dismissed as minimal by an injured athlete. When pain-free motion has been achieved, a more thorough physical examination can follow. Radiographs will occasionally reveal the presence of a bony avulsion of the PCL insertion from the tibia.

Physical examination of the patient with a suspected PCL rupture is performed with the patient supine and in a relaxed state. As previously stated, the hemarthrosis associated with injuries to the ACL is usually absent. Range of motion and stability are then assessed. Next, the examiner should flex both hips and knees to 90 degrees and observe the tibial-femoral contours from the side of the examining table. In a knee with a ruptured PCL, the involved tibia will sag posteriorly, and the normal silhouette will be lost. Additionally, palpation of the anteromedial portion of the tibia, with respect to the medial femoral condyle, will demonstrate loss of the normal relationship, in which the tibia is anterior to the femoral condyle. The degree of posterior displacement can be graded. A posterior drawer test is then performed with the patient's knee flexed 90 degrees and the tibia in neutral or external rotation. The examiner should stabilize the patient's foot and place a posteriorly directed force on the tibia. The presence of excessive excursion and the loss of a firm endpoint is noted and graded. With the knee flexed 90 degrees, the examiner sup-

ports the patient's thigh and stabilizes the foot. The patient is then asked to slide the foot down the table. In a patient with a ruptured PCL and resultant posterior tibial displacement, the quadriceps contraction will reduce the tibia. This is termed a positive quadriceps active test. It should be noted that patients with a ruptured PCL might appear to have a positive Lachman test due to the posterior starting position of the tibia. In actuality, the examiner is simply reducing the posteriorly subluxed tibia to a neutral position. Close attention to the endpoint achieved is essential to correct assessment of the ACL.

TREATMENT

Long-term natural history studies of isolated PCL injuries do not exist. Studies have not been able to define adequately which patients with an isolated PCL rupture will progress to develop symptomatic instability and resultant arthrosis. Therefore, treatment of the patient with an isolated PCL rupture should be tailored to the individual and the symptoms experienced. Rehabilitative efforts will probably suffice in the treatment of most patients with isolated PCL ruptures.

Operative indications for chronic posterior cruciate ligament injuries include demonstrable posterior laxity, disabling instability, and early degenerative disease (medial and patellofemoral compartments). Currently advocated techniques include an arthroscopically assisted reconstruction with the use of an Achilles tendon or bone-patellar tendon-bone allograft. Prospective randomized trials of the various methods used to reconstruct the PCL have not been done; therefore, there is no known "gold-standard" operative technique.

POSTEROLATERAL ROTATORY INSTABILITY

Injury to the PCL, arcuate complex, LCL, and popliteus tendon, or a combination thereof, results in posterolateral rotatory instability (PLRI) of the knee. Patients with PLRI possess a very disabling condition that is very difficult to treat. In most series, only a small percentage of patients were able to return to their previous level of activities.

CLINICAL EVALUATION

Proper diagnosis of these severe injuries and the institution of prompt treatment remain the cornerstone to the management of PLRI. These injuries are usually the result of high-energy trauma imparted to the anteromedial tibia such as via a car bumper or tackler in football. Meticulous examination to rule out an occult knee dislocation is also needed in these situations. The presence of a peroneal nerve deficit in this setting may help to confirm the examiner's suspicion of the injury pattern present. Due to the severe nature of the injury, the resultant guarding, and the need to treat this injury early if it is present, it is recommended that an examination under anesthesia be performed as soon as possible. Careful assessments of the PCL and ACL are carried out as previously outlined. The examiner can then assess the knee for the presence of varus instability. This will be most pronounced at 30 degrees of knee flexion, but will also be present in full extension if the PCL is also ruptured. The external rotation recurvatum test is performed by lifting both of the patient's legs by the heels or great toes. The test is positive if the affected leg falls into varus, external rotation, and recurvatum. The posterolateral drawer test has also been used to assess the posterolateral corner. This test is performed by first flexing the patient's knee to 90 degrees and stabilizing the foot on the examination table. A routine posterior drawer then performed with the tibia in neutral rotation. Then, with increasing increments of external rotation of the tibia, the posterior drawer is repeated. If the degree of posterior drawer is increased with external rotation, then the test is considered positive, indicating rupture of the posterolateral complex (Fig. 101-2). The examiner should then assess for pathological external rotation of the involved extremity. This is done by first holding the patient's feet while an assistant stabilizes both knees in 30 degrees of flexion. The examiner then attempts maximal external rotation of both feet. In the knee with disruption of the posterolateral corner, increased external rotation will be observed in comparison to the uninjured extremity at 30 degrees of flexion. The test is repeated in 90 degrees of flexion; if increased external rotation is again evident, a concomitant rupture of the PCL should be suspected. The reverse pivot shift may also be used to test for PLRI. The examiner lifts the ankle of the injured extremity and externally rotates the leg. The knee is flexed 70 to 90 degrees, which causes the lateral plateau to sublux posteriorly. The examiner then allows the leg to extend as a valgus, and axial load is applied to the leg. In cases of PLRI, at approximately 20 degrees of flexion, the tibia will relocate and a palpable reduction will be witnessed by the examiner.

TREATMENT

Acute repair of PLRI should be performed within 2 weeks of the injury. A lateral approach is advocated by most authors and will allow visualization of most of the pathology. The posterolateral corner is explored and the pathology present is evaluated. Fixation or reconstruction of the PCL is performed. The popliteus tendon, arcuate complex, and LCL are all repaired primarily side to side or via transosseous sutures, depending on the site of disruption (Fig. 101-3).

Chronic PLRI can be a very disabling problem that does not respond well to treatment. Unfortunately, most patients with acute PLRI escape detection and the chronic form of PLRI instability is more commonly seen in clinical practice. These patients may need a bony realignment procedure prior to ligamentous reconstruction because of the varus deformity present. Following correction of any malalignment, reconstruction of the deficient structures can be carried out. Many different complex procedures have been described for reconstruction of the posterolateral corner without consensus as to the treatment regimen most appropriate for chronic PLRI. Procedures advocated include biceps tenodesis and allograft reconstruction of the LCL.

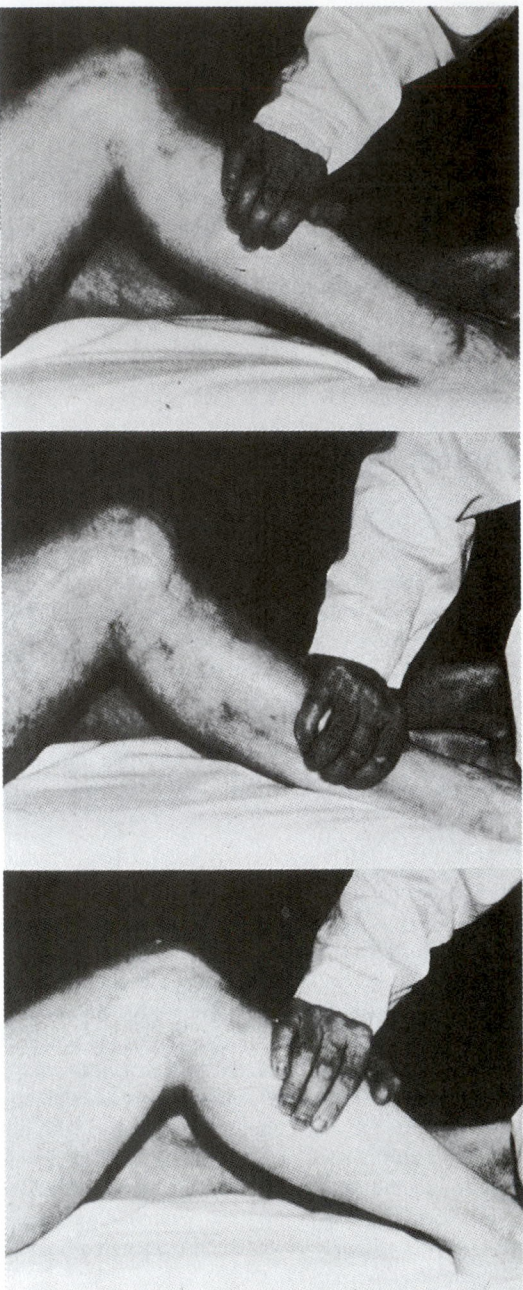

Figure 101-2
Posterior drawer sign in severe PLRI in neutral rotation *(top)* is 2+; in external rotation *(center)*, it is 3+, and in internal rotation *(bottom)*, it is 0. (Reproduced with permission from Jakob RP, Hassler H, Staubli HU: Observations on rotary instability of the lateral compartment of the knee. *Acta Orthop Scand* 1981; 191:27.)

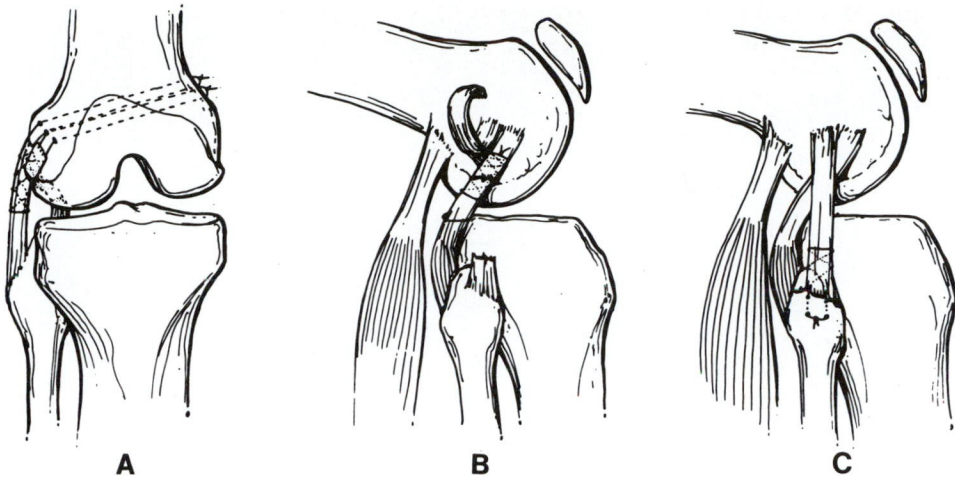

Figure 101-3

A. Repair of femoral attachment avulsion of fibular collateral ligament and popliteal tendon using transosseous drill holes. *B*. Repair of midsubstance tear of popliteal tendon with Bunnell-type suture. *C*. Repair of avulsion of fibular attachment of fibular collateral ligament using Bunnell-type sutures. [Reproduced and modified with permission from Jakob RP, Warner JP: Lateral and posterolateral rotatory instability of the knee. In DeLee JC, Drez D Jr (eds): *Orthopaedic Sports Medicine: Principles and Practice.* Philadelphia: WB Saunders; 1994:1299. Original source is Sisk TD: Knee injuries. In Crenshaw AH (ed): *Campbell's Operative Orthopaedics.* St. Louis: CV Mosby; 1987:2352.]

SUGGESTED READINGS

Butler DL, Noyes FR, Grood ES: Ligamentous restraints to anterior-posterior drawer in the human knee: A biomechanical study. *J Bone Joint Surg [Am]* 1980; 62:259.

Daniel DM, Fritschy D: Anterior cruciate ligament injuries. In DeLee JC, Drez D Jr (eds): *Orthopaedic Sports Medicine: Principles and Practice.* Philadelphia: WB Saunders; 1994; vol 2:1313.

DeLee JC, Bergfeld JA, Drez D Jr, et al: The posterior cruciate ligament. In DeLee JC, Drez D Jr (eds): *Orthopaedic Sports Medicine: Principles and Practice.* Philadelphia: WB Saunders; 1994; vol 2:1374.

Feagin JA Jr, Curl WW: Isolated tear of the anterior cruciate ligament: 5-year follow-up study. *Am J Sports Med* 1976; 4:95.

Fowler PJ, Messieh SS. Isolated posterior cruciate ligament injuries in athletes. *Am J Sports Med* 1987; 15:553.

Jackson RW: The torn ACL: Natural history of untreated lesions and rationale for selective treatment, 2nd ed. In Feagin JA (ed): *The Crucial Ligaments.* New York: Churchill Livingstone; 1994:485.

Jakob RP, Warner JP: Lateral and posterolateral rotatory instability of the knee. In DeLee JC, Drez D Jr (eds): *Orthopaedic Sports Medicine: Principles and Practice.* Philadelphia: WB Saunders; 1994; vol 2:1275.

Chapter 102

KNEE: CRUCIATE LIGAMENT INJURIES

David S. Menche and Andrew Harrison

ANTERIOR CRUCIATE LIGAMENT INJURIES

EPIDEMIOLOGY

In a large population-based study the incidence of anterior cruciate ligament (ACL) injury over a 3-year period was found to be 0.38 per thousand per year. In this study, 78 percent of the sports-related injuries were from football, baseball, soccer, skiing, and basketball. Recent studies have shown a higher incidence of ACL injury among women basketball players. This may be related to anatomic variations in the intercondylar notch of the distal femur, ligament size, muscular strength, neuromuscular control, and hormonal influences.

ANATOMY

The ACL is an intraarticular extrasynovial structure that courses obliquely from its origin on the posterolateral femoral condyle to the tibia. It is composed of multiple fascicles and has a reported average length ranging from 31 to 38 mm. The location and orientation of the fibers determine a twisting of the ligament as the knee goes from an extended to a flexed position. It has been determined that the most isometric portion of the anterior cruciate ligament is the anteromedial bundle (Fig. 102-1). The major blood supply to the anterior cruciate ligament arises primarily from ligamentous branches of the

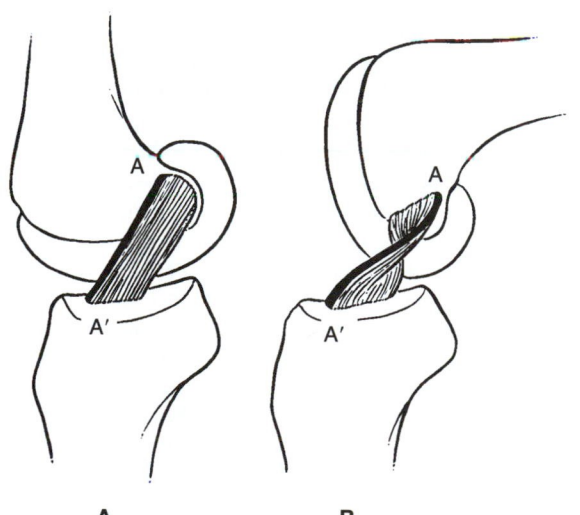

Figure 102-1
ACL components representing changes in shape and tension during (*A*) extension and (*B*) flexion. The A-A' band is considered the most isometric component of the ACL. (Reproduced and modified with permission from Girgis FG, Marshall JL, Monajem ARS: The cruciate ligaments of the knee joint; anatomical functional, and experimental analysis. *Clin Orthop* 1975; 106:229.)

middle geniculate artery. It also receives some blood supply from terminal branches of the medial and lateral inferior geniculate arteries. The cruciate ligaments are covered by a synovial fold which forms an envelope around the ligament. The ligament consists of fibroblasts forming an extracellular matrix of mainly type I collagen and water. The neural anatomy of the ACL has been described as consisting of both nerve fibers and sensory receptors which often accompany the vessels.

FUNCTION

The anterior cruciate ligament is the primary restraint to anterior displacement of the tibia. The ACL also acts as a secondary stabilizer of the knee, resisting varus/valgus rotation and internal/external rotation.

HISTORY

When determining whether a patient has sustained an ACL injury, as in most cases in orthopaedic surgery, the history and physical examination are extremely important in ascertaining the correct diagnosis. Most patients will give a history of a twisting injury to the knee. In many instances this will be a deceleration injury that involves valgus, rotation, and hyperextension. The patient may report a feeling of a snap or a pop in the knee, the inability to bear weight, and swelling. The incidence of ACL injury with the above history and a hemarthrosis is approximately 70 to 80 percent. One must differentiate an ACL injury from other causes of hemarthrosis.

PHYSICAL EXAMINATION

The physical examination of the knee should always include inspection, palpation, range of motion, and ligamentous stability testing. It is important to examine the patient's normal knee first, in order to get a baseline assessment of the patient's normal ligamentous laxity. Another benefit of examining the normal knee is that it will tend to relax and reassure the patient that the examination of the injured knee will be relatively comfortable. Active range of motion should be assessed and recorded. If there is a block to active extension, one should try to ascertain whether the difficulty in attaining full extension is a mechanical block, such as that due to a meniscal tear or whether this is due to pain or disruption of the extensor mechanism. Palpation of the joint should be performed in order to identify areas of tenderness and potential concomitant injuries (e.g., meniscal tears and MCL sprain). An accurate neurovascular examination should always be performed.

In the acute setting, definitive ligamentous stability testing may not be possible. The Lachman test is the most sensitive test in the acute setting to assess ACL integrity. This is performed with the knee in approximately 20 to 30 degrees of flexion. A subtle side-to-side difference in the Lachman test could mean that the ACL was significantly injured. The quality of the end-point should be assessed (i.e., firm, marginal, or soft). Performing a pivot shift test in the acute setting may be difficult as this is painful, and the patient guards. Varus and valgus instability testing should be performed at both 0 and 30 degrees of flexion. The integrity of the PCL should also be assessed as will be discussed later in this chapter.

DIAGNOSTIC STUDIES

All acute knee injuries should have a complete set of radiographic examinations in order to assess for osteochondral injuries, loose bodies, or avulsion injuries. The Segond fracture, a lateral capsular avulsion injury from the lateral edge of the tibia, is pathognomonic for an ACL tear of the knee. An MR scan can be performed; this diagnostic test, however, is often not necessary as the diagnosis should be made in the great majority of cases by the history and physical examination.

The KT-1000 arthrometer is a device which measures the amount of anterior tibial displacement in millimeters at 15- and 20-lb loads and when performing a manual maximum test. A side-to-side difference of 3 mm or more during a manual maximum test is associated with ACL disruption.

TREATMENT

In deciding whether to treat a patient with an ACL disruption operatively or nonoperatively, many factors must be considered. The type of treatment must be individualized to the patient, based on the extent of injury as well as taking into consideration functional goals and expectations. A primary objective of treatment is the prevention of re-injury of the knee after an ACL disruption in the hope of preventing additional ligamentous injuries, meniscal injuries, and possible deterioration of the knee with degenerative changes. If this can be accomplished by nonoperative means including physical therapy, bracing, and activity modification, then nonoperative treatment is a viable option.

Surgical options in the past included direct repair, extraarticular reconstructions, and various intraarticular reconstructions. An arthroscopic-assisted bone-patellar tendon-bone autograft technique is probably the most widely used procedure in the United States today.

In regard to graft selection, autograft tissue is the tissue of choice for most surgeons. The most commonly used autograft tissues include the patellar tendon, semitendinosus and gracilis, and iliotibial band. Some surgeons prefer to use allograft tissue, especially in revision cases. The risk of HIV transmission has been calculated at being approximately one in a million.

The key for a successful operative technique is proper graft placement. The recommended point of placement on the tibia is posterior central, just anterior to the posterior cruciate ligament. Posterior placement of this tunnel avoids the problem of anterior or roof impingement of the graft as the knee is extended. The femoral tunnel is placed along the posterior aspect of the lateral femoral condyle within 2 mm of the posterior cortex, at the eleven o'clock position on the right knee and one o'clock position on the left knee.

Most failures of ACL reconstruction are due to improper graft placement, which will cause excessive laxity or restriction in range of motion. In acute injuries surgical reconstruction is delayed until the patient has essentially full range of motion and no effusion as several studies have shown an increased incidence of postoperative stiffness if surgery is performed in the acute setting.

POSTOPERATIVE TREATMENT

Postoperatively, an accelerated approach to rehabilitation of ACL injuries has been advocated over the last several years. In the initial postoperative phase, efforts are made to control pain and swelling and to achieve full passive extension. Immediate weightbearing with crutches is allowed. Patella mobilization exercises are taught to the patient, as patella immobility can lead to restrictions of motion in both extension and flexion. Muscle strengthening exercises and sports-specific training are an integral part of the rehabilitation process.

POSTERIOR CRUCIATE LIGAMENT INJURIES

EPIDEMIOLOGY

Posterior cruciate ligament (PCL) injuries are rare, accounting for 3 to 20 percent of all knee ligament injuries. However, the true incidence of PCL injuries has been difficult to ascertain, because many isolated PCL disruptions are undetected or missed on initial examination. A PCL injury rate of 2 percent has been noted among asymptomatic college football players. Sixty percent of all PCL injuries are usually combined ligamentous injuries and the remainder are isolated tears. The most common combined ligamentous injury is a posterior cruciate ligament and posterolateral complex disruption, followed by combined PCL and ACL tears. Meniscal pathology is much less commonly associated with PCL tears compared with ACL tears.

ANATOMY

The PCL has a large semicircular origin on the lateral wall of the medial femoral condyle, beginning approximately 1 to 3 mm from the anterior articular edge. It is located at the 10:30 (left knee) and 1:30 (right knee) intercondylar notch positions. The PCL inserts on the posterior aspect of the tibia approximately 1 cm below the articular surface onto an inclined, recessed shelf (fovea) which is located centrally. The PCL is surrounded by a synovial sleeve. It has a broad cross-sectional area proximally that tapers at its distal aspect. The PCL diameter is approximately 1.5 times larger than that of the ACL from its femoral origin to its mid-substance. Seventy percent of knees possess either a meniscofemoral ligament of Humphrey which is anterior to the PCL or, more commonly, a ligament of Wrisberg which is posterior to the PCL. Both of these meniscofemoral ligaments merge with the PCL at its femoral origin. The PCL consists of two bundles, a larger anterolateral bundle which tightens with flexion and relaxes with extension, and a smaller posteromedial bundle which relaxes with flexion and tightens with extension (Fig. 102-2). Further studies have shown that the PCL origin consists predominantly of anterior and central fiber regions with the remainder of the ligament composed of posterior-longitudinal and posterior-oblique fibers. The PCL receives its major blood supply from the ligamentous branches of the middle geniculate artery and terminal branches of the medial and lateral inferior geniculate arteries. The PCL is innervated by the popliteal plexus which is derived primarily from the posterior tibial nerve. In addition, it possesses axons and receptors for maintaining proprioceptive reflex arcs, as well as afferent nerve endings which serve as pain receptors.

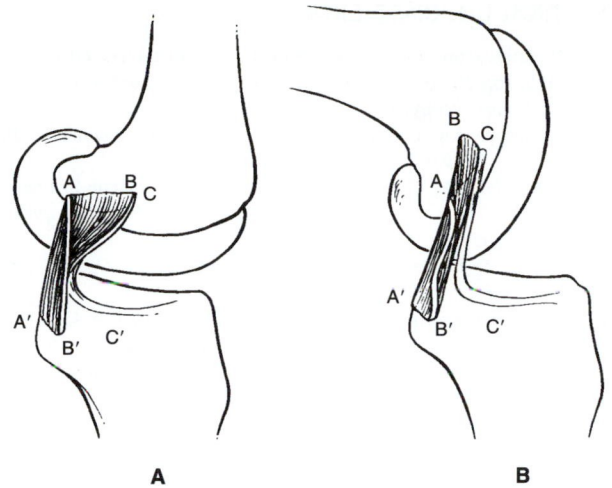

Figure 102-2
PCL components representing changes in shape and tension during (*A*) extension and (*B*) flexion. In flexion, there is lengthening of the bulk of the ligament (B-B') and shortening of a small band (A-A'). C-C' is the anterior meniscofemoral ligament (ligament of Humphry) attached to the lateral meniscus. (Reproduced and modified with permission from Girgis FG, Marshall JL, Monajem ARS: The cruciate ligaments of the knee joint; anatomical, functional, and experimental analysis. *Clin Orthop* 1975; 106:229.)

FUNCTION

Biomechanically, the posterior cruciate ligament is the primary restraint to straight posterior translation of the tibia in nearly all positions of flexion. Additional functions of the PCL are to regulate the "screw-home" mechanism in which the tibia externally rotates on the femur as the knee goes from flexion to extension in combination with the anterior cruciate ligament. It also acts as a secondary restraint to varus/valgus stress and external tibial rotation. Isolated PCL ruptures have a minimal effect on rotation or varus/valgus stability. However, a combined PCL and posterolateral complex rupture increases posterior translation, as well as varus angulation and tibial external rotation. The majority of PCL fibers are anisometric. Chronic PCL insufficiency with resultant increased posterior tibial translation shifts the tibiofemoral contact forces to the medial compartment and the patella, resulting in degenerative changes in those areas.

HISTORY

Most posterior cruciate ligament injuries are the result of vehicular trauma (50 percent) and sports activities (40 percent). The mechanism of injury includes a fall on a flexed knee, hyperflexion of the knee such as with a dashboard injury, knee dislocation, and forced hyperextension of the knee. The types of posterior cruciate ligament injuries include isolated mid-substance PCL tears, combined ligamentous PCL mid-substance tears, a PCL bony avulsion from the femoral, or more commonly tibial attachment site, and PCL soft tissue attachment avulsion injuries. In the acute injury, patients will usually give a history of gradual swelling and pain. They will usually be able to bear weight on the injured leg and will not usually recall an audible or palpable "pop" as with ACL injuries. In the chronic, isolated injury, patients usually will complain of increasing disability over time with retro-patellar knee pain during long-distance ambulation and unsteadiness on stairclimbing. They ususally do not complain of instability.

PHYSICAL EXAMINATION

Physical examination findings in the acute setting may include evidence of soft tissue trauma around the tibial tubercle, mild hemarthrosis, and passive range of motion which is usually well tolerated between 0 and 90 degrees with flexion beyond 90 degrees eliciting pain. Neurovascular injury should be ruled out, especially in the setting of a knee dislocation. In this case an urgent arteriogram should be performed to rule out popliteal artery injury. Specific physical exam tests for PCL instability include the posterior drawer test at 90 degrees, the posterior sag sign, and the quadriceps active test. The quadriceps active test is performed with the knee in 90 degrees of flexion. Active contraction of the quadriceps muscle will pull the tibia forward in a posterior cruciate deficient knee. One should direct particular attention to detecting the presence of other ligamentous injuries. Diagnostic work-up can include a plain radiograph knee series, MRI, and diagnostic arthroscopy.

TREATMENT

Indications for nonoperative treatment of PCL injuries include acute grade I isolated PCL tears and acute grade II isolated PCL tears, except in high demand athletes, and minimal or nondisplaced bony avulsions. Indications for operative treatment include PCL injuries with combined ligamentous instability patterns, grade III PCL tears, and failure of nonoperative treatment. Other indications for operative treatment include bony avulsions with significant displacement and greater than grade I laxity. Nonoperative treatment primarily consists of a rehabilitation program that emphasizes quadriceps muscle strengthening.

For acute displaced PCL tibial avulsion injuries, open reduction and internal fixation are performed.

Acute PCL (soft tissue) attachment avulsion injuries can be treated by a direct primary repair; however, this mode of treatment remains controversial. At present, the standard of care is a direct surgical recontruction using autograft or allograft. Chronic PCL avulsions and ruptures usually require posterior cruciate ligament reconstruction.

Arthroscopic-assisted posterior cruciate ligament reconstruction has recently become popular. Potential complications include neurovascular injuries (popliteal artery and peroneal nerve), recurrent instability, stiffness, avascular necrosis of the medial femoral condyle, compartment syndrome, deep venous thrombosis, and infection. Postoperative rehabilitation protocols usually involve an initial period of 2 to 3 weeks in immobilized bracing, followed by range of motion exercises while protecting the proximal aspect of the posterior lower leg against sag, protected weightbearing (3 to 6 weeks), and a total lower extremity strengthening program initially emphasizing quadriceps muscle strengthening. Patients are usually able to return to sports between 9 to 12 months postoperatively.

SUGGESTED READINGS

ANTERIOR CRUCIATE LIGAMENT

Daniel DM, Fritschy D: Anterior cruciate ligament injuries. In DeLee JC, Drez D Jr (ed): *Orthopaedic Sports Medicine: Principles and Practice.* Philadelphia: WB Saunders; 1994:1313.

DeLee JC, Drez D Jr: Anterior cruciate ligament injuries. *Op Tech Sports Med* 1993; 1(1):1.

Fu FH: The anterior cruciate ligament. *Clin Sports Med* 1994; 12(4):625.

Fanton GS, Thabit G: Orthopaedic uses of arthroscopy and lasers. In Griffin LY (ed): *Orthopaedic Knowledge Update: Sports Medicine*. Rosemont, IL: American Academy of Orthopaedic Surgeons; 1994:52–53.

Wheaton MT, Molnar TJ: Overuse injuries of the lower extremities. In Griffin LY (ed): *Orthopaedic Knowledge Update: Sports Medicine*. Rosemont, IL: American Academy of Orthopaedic Surgeons; 1994:258–259.

Jackson DW, Kurzweil PR: Anterior cruciate ligament reconstruction. In Jackson DW (ed): *Reconstructive Knee Surgery: Master Techniques in Orthopaedic Surgery*. New York: Raven Press; 1995:101.

Johnson RJ, Beynnon BD, Nicholas CE, et al: The treatment of injuries of the anterior cruciate ligament. *J Bone Joint Surg [Am]* 1992; 74:140.

Larson RL, Taillon M: Anterior cruciate ligament insufficiency: principles of treatment. *J Am Acad Orthop Surg* 1994; 2(1):26.

Sapega AA: Arthroscopically assisted reconstruction of the anterior cruciate ligament. In Torg JS, Shepard RJ (eds): *Current Therapy in Sports Medicine*, 3d ed. St. Louis: Mosby; 1995:332.

Shelbourne DK, Klootwyk TE: Nonoperative management of medial collateral ligament tears with anterior cruciate ligament reconstruction. In Torg JS, Shepard RJ (eds): *Current Therapy in Sports Medicine*, 3d ed. St. Louis: Mosby; 1995:353.

POSTERIOR CRUCIATE LIGAMENT

Covey DC: Arthroscopically assisted reconstruction of the posterior cruciate ligament. In Torg JS, Shepard RJ (eds): *Current Therapy in Sports Medicine*, 3d ed. St. Louis: Mosby; 1995:367.

Covey DC, Sapega AA: Injuries of the posterior cruciate ligament. *J Bone Joint Surg [Am]* 1993; 75:1376.

DeLee JC, Bergfeld JA, Drez D Jr, et al: The posterior cruciate ligament. In DeLee JC, Drez D Jr (eds): *Orthopaedic Sports Medicine: Principles and Practice*. Philadelphia: WB Saunders; 1994:1374.

DeLee JC, Drez D Jr: Posterior cruciate ligament injuries. *Op Tech Sports Med* 1993; 1:86.

Clancy WG Jr: The posterior cruciate ligament. *Clin Sports Med* 1994; 13(3):509.

Fanton GS, Thabit G: Orthopaedic uses of arthroscopy and lasers. In Griffin LY (ed): *Orthopaedic Knowledge Update: Sports Medicine*. Rosemont, IL: American Academy of Orthopaedic Surgeons; 1994:54.

Mooney MF, Paulos LE: Arthroscope-assisted posterior cruciate ligament repair/reconstruction. In Jackson DW (ed): *Reconstructive Knee Surgery: Master Techniques in Orthopaedic Surgery*. New York: Raven Press; 1995:117.

Veltri DM, Warren RF: Isolated and combined posterior cruciate ligament injuries. *J Am Acad Orthop Surg* 1993; 1:67.

Wheaton MT, Molnar TJ: Overuse injuries of the lower extremities. In Griffin LY (ed): *Orthopaedic Knowledge Update: Sports Medicine*. Rosemont, IL: American Academy of Orthopaedic Surgeons; 1994:258.

Chapter 103

KNEE: COLLATERAL LIGAMENT INJURIES

Mark I. Pitman and Howard J. Luks

MEDIAL COLLATERAL LIGAMENT

The medial collateral ligament (MCL) consists of two parts, the superficial medial collateral ligament itself and the deep medial capsule, consisting of the meniscotibial and the meniscofemoral ligaments. Anteriorly, the medial collateral ligament is thin and provides little support. Posteriorly, the thickened posterior medial capsular ligament is defined as the posterior oblique ligament (POL). The tibial collateral ligament is the primary restraint to valgus stress, especially in flexion when the POL and the cruciate ligaments are relaxed. In extension, the POL and the anterior cruciate ligament (ACL) provide a restraint to valgus forces. The deep capsular ligaments are attached to the medial meniscus, and tearing of these ligaments may produce a laceration at the meniscal capsular junction.

EXAMINATION

The integrity of the MCL is tested by applying a valgus stress to the knee in full extension and in 30 degrees of flexion. Testing in flexion relaxes the POL and the ACL and thus tests primarily the MCL. Laxity in full extension signifies injury to the ACL and POL as well as the MCL. The presence of hyperextension and of valgus laxity in hyperextension also suggests disruption of the posterior cruciate ligament (PCL). Sprains of the MCL may be graded as Grade 0, no laxity but with tenderness, often localized to the area of the medial femoral epicondyle. Grade I (1 to 5 mm laxity) suggests tearing of the MCL but not of the capsular ligament. Grade II (5 to 10 mm laxity) suggests rupture of the deep and superficial components of the MCL; and grade III (over 10 mm of medial opening) suggests concomitant rupture of the ACL.

Examination for location of tenderness may reveal the anatomic site of the lesion. In cases of grade I tears, the tenderness is often at the medial epicondyle and may be used to differentiate this from a meniscus injury. grades I and II have a palpable, firm end point; grade III does not.

RADIOGRAPHS

Routine radiographs are usually normal, but may show bony injury. In young patients with open epiphyses, valgus stress views should be performed to rule out the presence of an epiphyseal fracture which may be misinterpreted as an MCL tear on clinical exam. MRI may aid in identifying associated injuries to the menisci or to the cruciate ligaments.

TREATMENT

Treatment is evolving into aggressive nonoperative therapy with early protected motion. For grade I injuries, a simple knee immobilizer may be used as tolerated, with crutches and weightbearing; the immobilizer may be removed for early range of motion activities.

For the more severe grades II and III ruptures, a long leg brace hinged at the knee may be applied which will allow active flexion and extension but prevent excessive valgus forces. When the patient is able to actively fully extend the knee and flex to over 90 degrees, and as pain and tenderness diminish, more active functional exercises are begun. Patients should be progressed with closed chain exercises such as a bicycle, an underwater treadmill, or a leg press machine. As motion and strength increase, more strengthening exercises to the quadriceps and hamstrings, as well as to the hip and ankle musculature, may be instituted. Functional exercises, such as jogging, sprinting, and pivoting, are instituted as the patient tolerates.

Treatment for severe MCL injury in combination with an ACL injury is still being defined. The ACL should be reconstructed, but this reconstruction delayed until all signs of inflammation subside and until the MCL has healed enough to allow full, painless range of motion. There have been reports of excellent results in this combined injury with surgical treatment of the ACL and nonsurgical treatment of the MCL (Shelbourne and Porter, 1992). Again, obtaining full range of motion and allowing early healing of the MCL prior to surgery is important and may be key to a successful outcome.

In summary, recent evidence has shown that the vast majority of MCL injuries may be treated with protected early motion. Surgery is only necessary to reconstruct a concomitant ACL injury and should be delayed until the MCL has had time to heal.

LATERAL COLLATERAL LIGAMENT

The lateral (fibular) collateral ligament (LCL) is the primary restraint to varus instability of the knee. Isolated LCL injury is uncommon. Injuries to the associated structures, especially to the posterolateral corner of the knee, are becoming more frequently recognized and a more complete understanding of the biomechanics of the posterolateral corner is developing. The structures of the posterolateral corner include the LCL, the arcuate complex (which includes the arcuate ligament and the posterolateral joint capsule), the popliteal tendon, and the popliteo-fibular ligament.

The lateral head of the gastrocnemius, the biceps femoris, and the iliotibial band (ITB) all provide dynamic support to the posterolateral corner. The popliteus tendon passes through and attaches to the capsular structures providing attachment to the lateral meniscus, the fibula, the lateral epicondyle, and the fabellofibular ligament. The fabellofibular ligament, a portion of this complex, attaches to the fabella. The popliteus muscle is the major internal rotator of the tibia and dynamically opposes posterolateral rotatory instability.

Due to the severe force with which these injuries occur, injury to the lateral side of the knee is frequently accompanied by rupture of the posterior cruciate ligament and in very severe injuries to the ACL as well. If a combined injury to the LCL, the posterolateral corner, and the PCL is identified, a high index of suspicion should arise with regard to a spontaneously reduced knee dislocation. In such circumstances, a careful neurovascular exam, with routine close follow-up, is necessary to rule out injury to the popliteal artery and the peroneal nerve.

EXAMINATION

Isolated injury to the LCL usually allows only mild varus laxity on testing, both in 20 degrees and in full extension. The LCL may be difficult to palpate but if the knee is placed in the Figure 4 position, the intact ligament can usually be identified. Localized tenderness suggests injury to this ligament. Examination for signs of posterior laxity and posterolateral rotatory instability must follow, to rule out a more severe complete corner disruption (see Chap. 101).

RADIOGRAPHS

Radiographs may show avulsion of the fibular head, and/or of the mid-third of the lateral capsule with a small avulsion of the tibial attachment (Segond's fracture) which usually indicates an associated lesion of the ACL, or an avulsion of Gerdie's tubercle from the ITB. MRI is often indicated and most helpful in preoperative planning. It can be especially useful to confirm a clinical impression of the integrity or lack of integrity of the ACL and PCL.

TREATMENT

Treatment of the isolated LCL injury remains controversial. Isolated LCL injuries can probably be treated nonoperatively with early protected range of motion. Clinical evidence to support nonoperative treatment of isolated LCL injuries is not as well delineated as it is with respect to the MCL. Prior to instituting a nonoperative treatment regimen, the examining physician must be sure that the injury is truly isolated.

SURGERY

With combined injuries, surgery is the treatment of choice and consists of attempts at early anatomic repair. The peroneal nerve must be protected during the initial approach. The biceps tendon and the ITB, if torn, must be repaired. The LCL and the popliteus tendon are isolated and repaired, either by intrasubstance suture or repair to bone. The arcuate ligament, posterolateral complex, and the lateral capsule should be repaired; laceration of the lateral meniscus at its synovial margin must be repaired as well. The cruciate ligaments must also be inspected, by arthroscopy or arthrotomy. In severe, combined injuries, the PCL, if torn from its bony attachments, should be reattached; otherwise, primary reconstruction of the PCL should be performed.

In chronic injuries of the lateral side of the knee, involved structures should be reconstructed or substituted biomechanically. An examination under anesthesia is performed to delineate the full extent of the injury. Arthroscopically, reconstruction of the torn PCL and ACL is performed as needed. Open reconstruction of the LCL and the posterolateral corner has been described in detail by many authors and is beyond the scope of this review (Fig. 103-1).

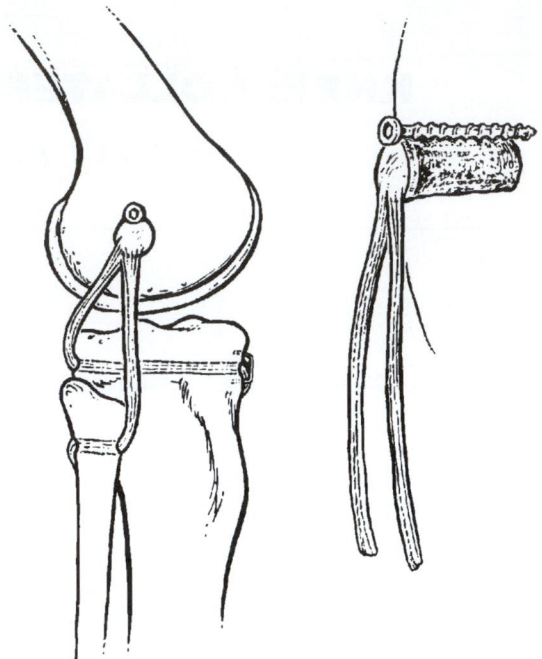

Figure 103-1
"Two-tailed graft" reconstructing lateral collateral ligament and posterolateral corner (*left*). Bone plug fixed to lateral femoral condyle by interference screw (*right*). One tail reproduces the popliteus tendon and the other tail reproduces the LCL.

SUGGESTED READINGS

DeLee JC, Drez D Jr (eds): *Orthopaedic Sports Medicine: Principles and Practice.* Philadelphia: WB Saunders; 1994.

Gollehon DL, Torzilli PA, Warren RF: The role of the posterolateral and cruciate ligaments in the stability of the human knee. *J Bone Joint Surg [Am]* 1987; 69:233.

Grood ES, Noyes FR, Butler DL, et al: Ligamentous and capsular restraints preventing straight medial and lateral laxity in intact human cadaver knees. *J Bone Joint Surg [Am]* 1981; 63:1257.

Hershman EB, Nicholas JA: *The Lower Extremity and Spine in Sports Medicine*, vol 2. St. Louis: Mosby; 1995.

Hughston JC, Jacobson, KE: Chronic posterolateral rotatory instabiilty of the knee. *J Bone Joint Surg [Am]* 1985; 67:351.

Hughston JC, Norwood L Jr: The posterolateral drawer test and external rotation recurvatum test for posterolateral rotatory instability of the knee. *Clin Orthop* 1980; 147:82.

Indelicato PA, Hermasdorfer J, Huegel M: The nonoperative management of complete tears of the medial collateral ligament of the knee in intercollegiate football players. *Clin Orthop* 1990; 256:174.

Indelicato PA: Non-operative treatment of complete tears of the medial collateral ligament of the knee. *J Bone Joint Surg [Am]* 1983; 65:323.

Jakob RP, Hassler H, Staubli, HU: Observations on rotatory instability of the lateral compartment of the knee. *Acta Orthop Scand* 1981; 191:6.

Muller W: *The Knee: Form, Function, and Ligament Reconstruction.* New York: Springer-Verlag; 1983.

Peterson L, Pitman MI, Gold J: The active pivot shift: The role of the popliteal muscle. *Am J Sports Med* 1984; 12:313.

Seebacher JR, Ingles AE, Marshall JL, et al: The structure of the posterolateral aspect of the knee. *J Bone Joint Surg [Am]* 1982; 64:536.

Shelbourne KD, Porter DA: Anterior cruciate ligament-medial collateral ligament injury: Nonoperative management of medial collateral ligament tears with anterior cruciate ligament reconstruction. A preliminary report. *Am J Sports Med* 1992; 20:283.

Chapter 104

KNEE: MENISCAL TEARS

David S. Menche and Andrew Harrison

EPIDEMIOLOGY

A torn meniscus is one of the more common causes of knee pain in an active individual, especially in an athlete. The incidence of acute meniscal tears has been reported to be as high as 61 per 100,000. Meniscal tears occurring in sports account for one-third of all meniscal tears, with the medial meniscus torn more frequently than the lateral meniscus in all sports except wrestling. Moreover, football, basketball, and wrestling are responsible for the greatest number of tears. Overall, the most common site of all tears is the posterior horn of the medial meniscus, in both acute and chronic injuries. Knees with chronic anterior cruciate ligament insufficiency have an incidence of associated meniscal tears of 80 to 90 percent.

FUNCTION AND ANATOMY

The functions of the meniscus include primarily tibiofemoral load sharing, passive stabilization, increasing joint congruity, shock absorption, lubrication, nutrition, prevention of synovial impingement at the joint periphery, and possibly to aid in limiting the extremes of flexion and extension.

The menisci are semilunar wedges of fibrocartilage that have direct bony attachments to the tibia at the anterior and posterior horns. Both menisci have an average thickness of 3 to 5 mm. The medial meniscus has a larger diameter and forms a C-shaped incomplete semicircle, with an average width of 9 to 10 mm. The lateral meniscus is more U-shaped with an average width of 10 to 11 mm. They are primarily composed of extracellular matrix that contains 70 percent water and 30 percent organic components. These organic components are predominantly composed of type 1 collagen. The central region of the meniscus is subjected to the greatest compressive forces. In this region there is an abundant chondroid area of aggregating proteoglycans that makes the meniscus viscoelastic and significantly contributes to its weightbearing function. The fiber orientation is unique in that the peripheral third exhibits predominantly circumferential fibers which act to resist "hoop stresses" that develop from radially-directed tensile strains occurring with axial comprehensive loads. The architecture of the remaining two-thirds of the meniscus consists of radial-transverse as well as circumferential fibers. Some of these transverse fibers act as "tie fibers" between the circumferential fibers and assist in resisting longitudinal splitting. Last, there is the "middle perforating bundle," with fibers oriented parallel to the tibial plateau, traversing the inner two-thirds of the meniscus.

The meniscus is innervated by nerve fibers consisting of free nerve endings from the popliteal plexus, and corpuscle-type mechanoreceptors penetrating the peripheral third of its substance. The meniscus receives nutrition from synovial fluid as well as from the perimeniscal capillary vascular plexus. Both the superior and inferior medial and lateral geniculate arteries branch and form this perimeniscal capillary vascular plexus which passes through the meniscosynovial junction forming smaller radial branches which in turn supply essentially the peripheral 25 to 33 percent of the meniscus. The vascular anatomy of the meniscus has resulted in a classification of meniscal tears based on location or zones of potential healing. The red-red zone, within 3 mm from the meniscocapsular junction, is a vascular area which has excellent healing potential. The red-white zone, 3 to 5 mm from the meniscocapsular junction, has variable vascularity and adequate healing potential. The white-white zone, greater than 5 mm from the meniscocapsular junction, is an avascular area which has poor healing potential.

BIOMECHANICS

With flexion of the knee, the lateral meniscus displays more mobility than the medial meniscus, exhibiting an average excursion of 11.2 mm and 5.1 mm respectively. In both compartments the mean excursion of the anterior horn is greater than the posterior horn.

Knee position is a major determinant of load transmission across the meniscus, with the posterior horn receiving the greater percentage of load as the knee is flexed. In general, the menisci increase the tibiofemoral surface contact area thereby decreasing peak articular contact stresses. Given its greater width and therefore greater surface area, the lateral meniscus carries the majority of the lateral compartment load, transmitting 65 to 75 percent of the axial compressive load compared to 40 to 50 percent by the medial meniscus. A torn meniscus disrupts the normal gliding mechanism of the tibiofemoral joint. Meniscectomy increases peak articular contact stresses at least two- to threefold, leading to the development of early degenerative osteoarthritis.

PATHOPHYSIOLOGY

Meniscal injuries are classified based on the plane of the tear, the direction of propagation, shape, location within the meniscus, and degree of thickness. Eight main types of meniscal tear patterns have been described (Fig. 104-1). Younger, more active patients are more likely to sustain a traumatic, sports-related injury which usually results in a peripheral longitudinal tear. Older patients usually incur degenerative meniscal injuries with complex and/or horizontal cleavage patterns.

The mechanism of injury for meniscal tears is usually rotation with or without axial compression. This commonly occurs during a twisting injury to the knee or a rapid change in direction. As a result, radially directed tensile strains are propagated about the meniscal fibers and exceed the capacity of the meniscus to resist them, thereby causing a tear.

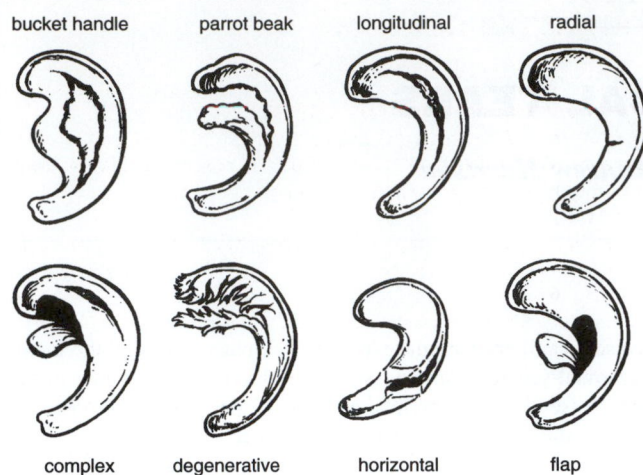

Figure 104-1
Schematic illustration of the main types of meniscal tears.

CLINICAL PRESENTATION

In the acute setting, the patient commonly gives a history of sudden onset of joint-line pain with associated persistent swelling or effusion in the knee. True locking, the inability to actively or passively attain full extension from a flexed position, remains a significant symptom and sign, elicited in as much as 81 percent of patients with bucket-handle tears. This finding combined with a history of persistent effusion and knee buckling is highly suggestive of a meniscal tear.

On physical examination, joint-line tenderness is considered the most significant and accurate finding, present in 77 to 86 percent of cases with torn menisci. Provocative tests one can utilize to detect a torn meniscus include most commonly, the flexion McMurray's test (~58 percent accuracy), followed by the Apley Grind test, and Helfet maneuver. Authors of all of these tests manipulate the knee into positions that force the torn meniscus into a displaced position, thereby recreating the patient's symptoms of pain and locking.

If the diagnosis remains uncertain after a thorough history and physical examination, then one should consider further diagnostic workup. Every patient with a history of knee injury should have a complete set of plain radiographs to rule out bony injury and assess for degenerative disease. MRI has replaced arthrography and has a greater accuracy, sensitivity, and specificity in diagnosing meniscal tears. The reported accuracy of MRI in detecting medial and lateral tears is 93 to 99 percent and 90 to 96 percent, respectively. MRI findings of meniscal lesions follow a grading system of I to III. Grade I signal intensity is intrameniscal, focal, and does not extend to the meniscal surface. Grade II signal is intrameniscal, linear, and does not extend to the meniscal surface. These signals are believed to represent either normal variants, early degeneration, or the results of minor trauma. Grade III signals are linear, extending to the meniscal surface, representing a definitive tear, which would be visible at the time of arthroscopy.

TREATMENT

The decision to manage a patient nonoperatively versus operatively should be individualized to the patient. Nonoperative treatment includes therapeutic modalities for reduction of swelling, obtaining full range of motion, and completing a balanced strengthening program.

Operative treatment of meniscal tears is performed utilizing arthroscopic techniques. Indications for arthroscopy include failure of nonoperative treatment with persistent symptoms or a locked knee. Meniscal tears that are stable should be left alone. When performing arthroscopy, partial, subtotal, or total meniscectomy may be required. The technique of partial meniscectomy involves removing all torn, abnormal, and unstable (>3 mm displacement on probing) meniscal tissue. This is followed by a "balanced resection" of the residual meniscus which involves removing additional meniscal tissue anterior and posterior to the tear site. A "balanced resection" creates a smooth transition from abnormal to normal tissue thus preventing stress concentration which could lead to further tearing. Postoperatively, the patient is treated with ice, immediate full weight-bearing as tolerated, range of motion exercises, and a balanced strengthening program. Many patients are able to return to full activity by 3 to 4 weeks postoperatively.

The indications for performing an isolated meniscal repair include vertical-longitudinal, full-thickness, peripheral tears within 3 mm of the meniscocapsular junction, that are greater than 10 mm in length. Multiple techniques are available for meniscal repair. Open repairs can be performed for very peripheral tears located less than 3 mm from the meniscocapsular junction. Arthroscopic inside-out repairs are best suited for body and posterior horn tears while the arthroscopic outside-in technique has been used successfully for anterior horn tears. Recently, the all-inside arthroscopic technique using either suture anchors or bioabsorbable implants has become popular. The incidence of successful healing of isolated meniscal tears has been reported to range from 50 to 80 percent as compared to repairs performed concomitantly with anterior cruciate ligament reconstruction where results are approximately 90 percent. An increased rate of healing has been suggested to have been found with insertion of exogenous fibrous clot, meniscal trephination, and synovial abrasion.

The biology of the meniscal repair process has been described by many investigators. At 6 weeks, fibrovascular scar forms and anchors the repair. By 8 weeks, circumferential collagen fiber orientation develops at the repair site. At 3 months, the fibrovascular scar is transformed to fibrocartilage which then matures by 6 months.

The postoperative physical therapy regimen is individualized according to the type of tear and quality of repair. Immediate goals would be full range of motion, weightbearing as tolerated, and strengthening. Return to sports is not recommended until 6 months postoperatively.

ACL-DEFICIENT KNEE WITH MENISCAL TEARS

Lateral meniscal tears are more commonly associated with acute ACL tears while medial meniscal tears are often associated with chronic ACL insufficiency. Two-thirds of all repairable meniscal tears occur in ACL-deficient knees. Recent clinical studies have shown that vertical-longitudinal lateral meniscal tears that are posterior to the popliteus tendon, or avulsed at the posterior horn, may be left in situ after ACL reconstruction with no demonstrable detrimental effects. The treatment of the meniscal tear usually does not alter the standard postoperative ACL rehabilitation protocol.

MENISCAL CYSTS

Meniscal cysts are usually associated with degenerative meniscal tears. These cysts are rare and most commonly are located at the periphery of the lateral meniscus. Clinically, a meniscal cyst presents as a tender, visible, and palpable mass at the joint line, which decreases in size with knee flexion. The diagnosis can be confirmed with an MRI. Nonoperative treatment is offered to the patient initially, but if symptoms persist, operative treatment is indicated. Operative management options include knee arthroscopy with partial meniscectomy if required, combined with intraarticular cyst decompression, or open cyst excision.

MENISCAL TRANSPLANTATION

Meniscal transplantation is currently being performed in certain centers. Current indications include a nonfunctional or absent meniscus in a knee with minimal degenerative changes, without ligamentous instability or lower extremity malalignment. The transplantation is currently performed utilizing an arthroscopically assisted fixation technique. To date, the long-term efficacy of this procedure has not been documented.

SUGGESTED READINGS

Belzer JP, Cannon WD Jr: Meniscus tears: Treatment in the stable and unstable knee. *J Am Acad Orthop Surg* 1993; 1:41.

DeLee JC, Drez D Jr: Meniscal surgery. *Op Tech Sports Med* 1994; 2:151.

Fitzgibbons RE, Shelbourne KD: "Aggressive" nontreatment of lateral meniscal tears seen during anterior cruciate ligament reconstruction. *Am J Sports Med* 1995; 23(2):156.

Fu FH, Baratz M: Meniscal injuries. In DeLee JC, Drez D Jr (eds): *Orthopaedic Sports Medicine: Principles and Practice.* Philadelphia: WB Saunders; 1994:1146.

Ivey FM: Acute knee injuries. In Griffin LY (ed): *Orthopaedic Knowledge Update: Sports Medicine.* Rosemont, IL: American Academy of Orthopaedic Surgeons; 1994:255.

Kuhlman JR: Meniscal repair. In Torg JS, Shepard RJ (eds): *Current Therapy in Sports Medicine*, 3d ed. St. Louis: Mosby; 1995:295.

Newman AP, Daniels AU, Burks RT: Principles and decision making in meniscal surgery. *Arthroscopy* 1993; 9:33.

Singer KM (ed): Meniscal injuries. *Clin Sports Med* 1990; 9(3):523.

Chapter 105

ANKLE

Brian C. Toolan and Daniel S. Zapson

ANKLE SPRAINS

Sprain of the lateral ligaments of the ankle is one of the most common injuries sustained with sporting activities. These injuries occur when athletes "roll over" their foot, applying an inversion force to a plantar flexed ankle. The anterior talofibular ligament (ATFL), the primary restraint to translation and rotation of the talus under these conditions, fails first. Continued inversion of the foot disrupts the calcaneofibular ligament (CFL). The posterior talofibular ligament (PTFL) is the strongest of the lateral ligaments and is the least often injured. Involvement of all three ligaments occurs under extreme circumstances and usually as a result of a complete dislocation of the ankle. Isolated sprains of the CFL or PTFL rarely occur. These injuries require internal rotation or inversion of the foot, respectively, with full dorsiflexion of the ankle to disrupt the particular ligament.

Isolated sprains of the syndesmosis or the deltoid ligament are rare. The mechanism of injury required to produce such a ligamentous injury often disrupts both structures. External rotation with eversion of the dorsiflexed ankle stresses the deep deltoid ligament and the anterior-inferior tibiofibular ligament, the most commonly injured portion of the syndesmosis. Except in severe injuries causing a wide diastasis of the ankle, the interosseous membrane, the posterior-inferior tibiofibular ligament and the transverse tibiofibular ligament remain intact. Syndesmotic and deltoid disruptions with a fracture of the fibula above the level of the joint are unstable ankle injuries that necessitate operative management.

A thorough history and physical examination are essential to the proper evaluation of all ankle sprains. The mechanism of injury, chronicity, ability to bear weight on the affected extremity, appreciation of a "pop" or "snap" at the time of injury, and initial treatment should be elicited during the interview of the patient. A history of previous injuries and residual symptoms involving the ankle should also be included. The physical examination begins with an inspection of the lower extremity to identify the location of swelling and ecchymosis. The exam continues with palpation of the bony and ligamentous anatomy to identify tenderness. The entire fibula and foot must be included in the exam to determine the extent of involvement and the presence of associated injuries. Active and passive range of motion should be measured and the anterior drawer and inversion stress (talar tilt) test should be performed and compared to the uninjured extremity to assess the stability of the ankle.

Based upon the results of the "Ottawa rules" multicenter study, it has been recommended that radiographs of the ankle be obtained only in the presence of pain in association with tenderness to palpation over the distal six centimeters of the lateral or medial malleolus, or when the patient is unable to bear weight. In the absence of these criteria, the risk of missing a clinically significant fracture is no different than if radiographs had been obtained. Persistent symptoms warrant diagnostic radiographs. Stress radiographs of the ankle with comparison views of the intact side may aid in the diagnosis of unstable ligamentous injuries (Figs. 105-1 and 105-2). Fracture of the distal fibular physis should be suspected when the skeletally immature athlete presents with a presumed "ankle sprain."

Classically, lateral ankle sprains have been classified under a three-stage scheme. Mild grade 1 injuries represent stretching of the ligament without tearing. Often a single ligament is involved. The patient demonstrates minimal swelling and point tenderness without loss of function or ankle stability. Partial tearing of the ligament describes a grade 2 injury. Usually, the ATFL and CFL are injured. Physical examination reveals significant swelling, tenderness, and loss of motion. The anterior drawer or talar tilt test may elicit mild ligamentous laxity. Complete disruption of the ligament and involvement of two or more lateral ligaments defines a grade 3 sprain. Examination finds extensive soft tissue edema, ecchymosis, and tenderness to palpation about the ankle. The patient will not be able to bear weight through the extremity. There may have been dislocation of the joint at the time of injury and instability is present, although difficult to demonstrate on stress testing due to guarding, pain, and muscle spasm.

Initial treatment of ankle sprains includes rest, ice, compressive bracing, and elevation. The patient should be prescribed crutches and restricted weightbearing if gait is painful. Nonsteroidal anti-inflammatory drugs (NSAIDs) will alleviate pain and soft tissue swelling. A progressive, controlled program of physical therapy begins once initial symptoms have subsided and the patient can tolerate weightbearing. Active assisted, passive, and resisted range of motion with gait, balance, and proprioceptive training should be gradually instituted, along with isolated strengthening of the peroneal muscles as the patient is weaned from immobilization. Rehabilitation of syndesmotic sprains may require a longer period of time to achieve functional recovery. The majority of patients will be able to return to full activity within six weeks of their injury.

CHRONIC LATERAL ANKLE INSTABILITY

Instability of the ankle may develop from a lack of appropriate rehabilitation or a cumulative effect of repetitive trauma. It has been described as two distinct entities that may present separately or coexist. Functional instability describes the "unreliable" ankle that presents with recurring episodes of giving way, but no discrete, anatomical lesion on physical examination. Mechanical instability correlates to an anatomic laxity that may or may not be associated with a functional deficit. A diagnostic work-up to exclude an osteochondral fracture, peroneal tendon injury, neuromuscular imbalance, cavovarus deformity of the foot or rotational malalignment of the lower extremity, should precede the diagnosis of chronic ankle sprain.

A program of physical therapy directed toward proprioceptive training, peroneal strengthening, and range of motion exercises can

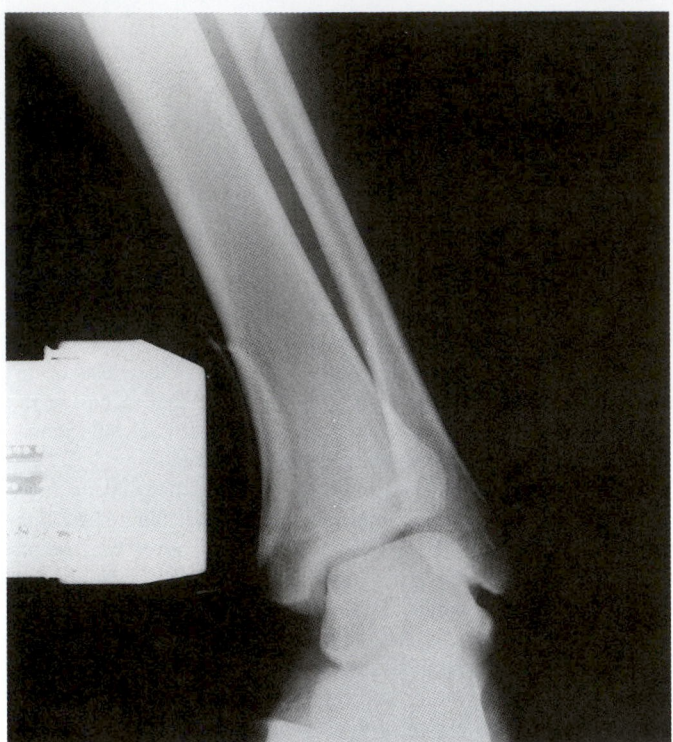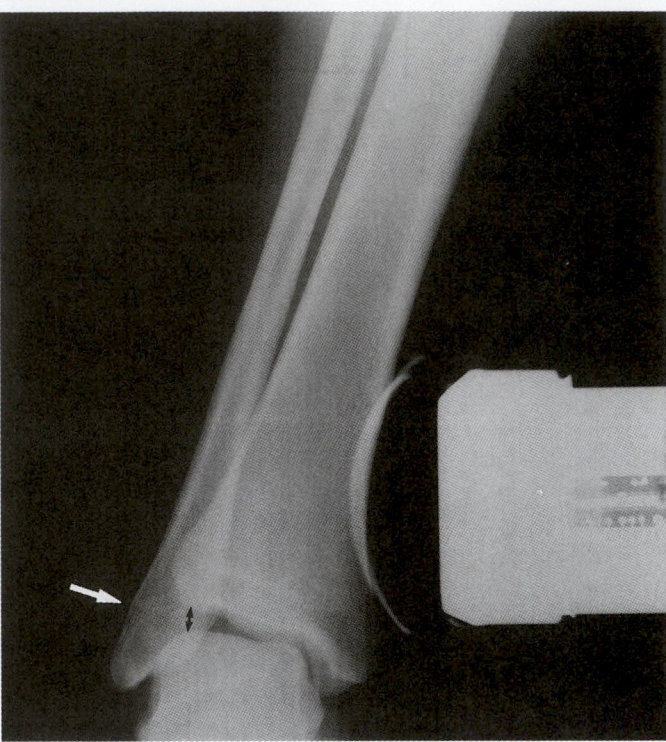

Figure 105-1

Ankle sprain. Stress radiographs were obtained in a 24-year-old male who complained of twisting his ankle severely while playing basketball. *A* is normal. *B* demonstrates abnormal talar tilt. This is seen because of an injury to the calcaneofibular ligament. The incompetence of the ligament allows for a widening of the distance between the lateral talar surface and the tibia (*arrow*).

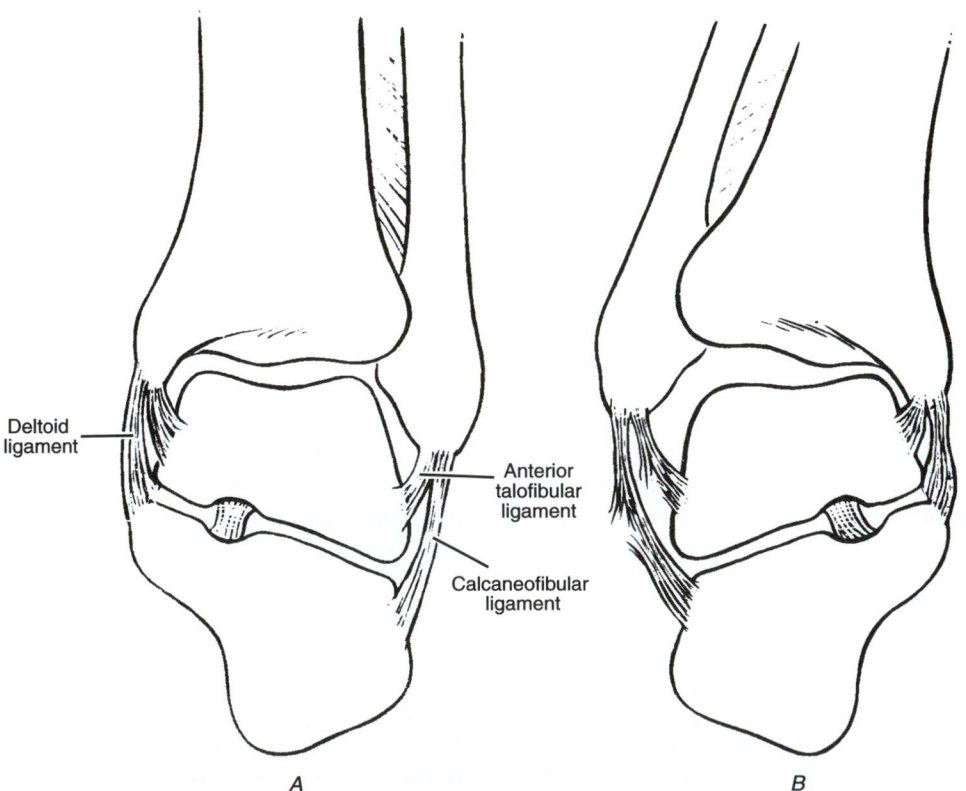

A   *B*

Figure 105-2

Ankle sprain diagram. *A* depicts a normal ankle. *B* is a diagrammatic representation of the torn calcaneofibular ligament referred to in Fig. 105-1*B*. Fibers of the anterior talofibular ligament are also shown to be torn. Again, a positive talar tilt test is demonstrated.

be effective treatment in many cases. Patients with functional instability demonstrate the best results with this approach. An assessment for mechanical factors contributing to instability may identify specific problems to be addressed in therapy or by surgical management.

Surgical options to address chronic instability include an anatomic repair of the involved ligaments or a tenodesis to serve as a lateral checkrein. Direct repair shortens and imbricates the elongated or disrupted ATFL and CFL (Brostrum technique). Advancement of the anterolateral aspect of the ankle retinaculum to the lateral malleolus can be performed to augment the strength of the repair (Gould modification). These procedures restore the static restraints through an anatomical reconstruction without restricting motion of the ankle. The presence of generalized ligamentous laxity may comprise the success of the repair. Tenodesis procedures employing local tendon grafts, fascia lata, or synthetic materials through drill holes in the fibula and calcaneus have been used successfully to substitute for damaged ligaments. In the most popular procedures, the peroneus brevis is split and rerouted to substitute for the repaired ATFL and CFL (Chrisman-Snook technique). All tenodesing procedures will limit talar tilting to varying degrees, at the expense of physiological motion of the ankle or subtalar joints. Some procedures increase nonphysiologic motions of the talus in order to control talar tilting. The compromise of dynamic stabilization provided by intact peroneal tendons to achieve improved static restraint may detrimentally affect the long-term results of tenodesing procedures.

The benefit of prophylactic bracing and taping to prevent ligamentous injury during sporting activity and to protect the ankle after surgical reconstruction remains unclear. Taping effectively supports the ankle, however, its effect diminishes rapidly with activity. Bracing has not been demonstrated to be superior to taping in maintaining ankle stability. The intended goals of externally stabilizing the ankle without limiting motion may be difficult to achieve in most circumstances. Bracing and taping may offer some benefit through proprioceptive cues facilitating decreased reaction times.

TENDINOPATHIES

POSTERIOR TIBIAL TENDON

Johnson and Strom (1989) classified posterior tibial tendon insufficiency into a three-stage scheme that describes degree of tendon dysfunction and associated foot deformity. Stage 1 posterior tibial tendon dysfunction (PTTD) defines tenosynovitis of the tendon sheath with no elongation of the tendon or change in the alignment of the hindfoot. Stage 2 tendinopathy describes intratendinous degeneration characterized by longitudinal tearing, thickening, and elongation of the tendon. The foot acquires a supple planovalgus deformity with loss of the medial longitudinal arch of the foot and excessive valgus alignment of the hindfoot. Stage 3 PTTD involves a fixed, manually uncorrectable planovalgus deformity of the foot derived from long-standing, untreated disease with elongation, and in some cases, complete rupture of the tendon.

The treatment of stage 1 disease begins with activity modification, use of NSAIDs, and an orthosis with medial posting. A brief period of immobilization may provide quicker relief of symptoms. Continued symptoms, despite prolonged nonoperative management, may warrant surgery which includes tenosynovectomy, tendon debridement, and possible flexor digitorum longus tendon transfer.

The management of stage 2 PTTD remains controversial. Soft tissue debridement and tendon transfers without bony stabilization will relieve symptoms, but may not provide lasting correction of the as-

sociated foot deformity. A variety of midfoot fusions and calcaneal osteotomies performed alone or in various combinations have been advocated as the best treatment for stage 2 PTTD; however, an individualized assessment of the particular components of each patient's deformity is the best approach.

Stage 3 disease necessitates arthrodesis. The fixed subluxations of the joints of the midfoot and hindfoot will not correct without realignment and fusion. Triple arthrodesis involving fusion of the talonavicular, calcaneocuboid, and subtalar joints can restore anatomic alignment at the expense of accommodative motion of the hindfoot. Recently, selective fusion(s) have gained in popularity in an effort to limit the restriction of motion associated with triple arthrodesis.

PERONEAL TENDONS

Tendinitis of the peroneus brevis and longus may occur following lateral ankle sprain or in association with chronic instability. In the acute setting, the immobilization, rest, ice and elevation, and subsequent physical therapy directed at the treatment of the sprain will suffice as management for the tendon injury. The management of tendinitis with chronic instability is not as simple. Identification and treatment of the underlying cause of ankle instability is often most effective. Acute, complete rupture of one or both of the peroneal tendons rarely occurs; however, if this is the case, they should be directly repaired or tenodesed to one another.

Dislocation of these tendons may occur as an isolated injury or in association with an ankle sprain. The superior peroneal retinaculum holds the peroneal tendons in a shallow groove behind the fibula. The mechanism of injury is unclear, but disruption or attenuation of the retinaculum will permit recurrent subluxation or dislocation of the tendons. Acute injuries usually heal with immobilization. Surgery should be reserved for recurrent, symptomatic dislocations. Direct repair, reconstruction of the retinaculum, or deepening the peroneal groove on the fibula with sliding bone blocks, have yielded excellent results.

OSTEOCHONDRAL FRACTURE AND OSTEOCHONDRITIS DISSECANS OF THE TALUS

Osteochondral fracture of the talus should be considered when pain, joint effusion and mechanical symptoms persist after acute lateral ankle sprain. Often initially overlooked because their signs and symptoms are attributed to the concomitant ankle sprain, radiographs should be obtained to identify a large, displaced fragment; however, initial radiographs may not reveal a subtle injury. If symptoms persist and physical findings localize to the joint, repeat radiographs, which include oblique views of the plantarflexed ankle, may show the lesion. A magnetic resonance imaging (MRI) will identify an osteochondral fracture and determine its exact size, location, and stability. This information will guide the indication and approach for surgery.

Berndt and Harty (1959) classified osteochondral fractures into four stages based upon displacement and stability of the fragment on plain radiographs. A stage 1 injury represents a discrete area of impacted subchondral bone. Stage 2 and 3 lesions are partially or completely detached from the bony bed, but not displaced. A stage 4 lesion is unstable; the fragment is detached from its bony bed and displaced.

The form of treatment depends upon the stability of the osteochondral fragment. Unstable lesions justify operative intervention. Open or arthroscopic excision of the fragment, combined with drilling of the subchondral bed to foster fibrocartilaginous healing, is indicated for stage 4 and persistently symptomatic stage 3 lesions. A medial malleolar osteotomy may be required for posteromedial lesions. Stage 1 and 2 lesions usually heal with casting and protected weight-bearing. Large fragments without deformation or comminution may be internally fixed if an anatomic reduction is obtained.

Osteochondritis dissecans describes a chronic, non-united osteochondral fracture. These patients describe a gradual onset of activity–related pain, swelling, and stiffness with or without a remote history of ankle trauma. Similar to the acute situation, the work-up assesses the stability of the lesion. MRI determines the stability of the lesion through the absence of synovial fluid or granulation tissue between the lesion and its bed. The mode of treatment follows the assessment of stability and the nature of the symptoms. Immediate surgical management of a stable, but symptomatic lesion may be justified when ankle complaints are long-standing.

ANKLE IMPINGEMENT SYNDROMES

The os trigonum represents the failure of an ossicle to unite to the posterolateral processs of the talus. Instead, it forms a stable fibro-ligamentous attachment to this structure and generally remains an asymptomatic radiographic finding. Repetitive, forced plantarflexion will impinge an os trigonum between the posterior lip of the tibia and the calcaneus. Kickers and ballet dancers are susceptible to posterior ankle impingement because they generate the requisite force with sufficient frequency to induce a symptomatic injury. They present with vague posterior ankle pain. Forced, passive plantarflexion with an axial load applied through the heel will reproduce the symptoms of impingement. A careful exam to distinguish impingement from flexor hallucis longus, peroneal or Achilles tendinitis is crucial. Restriction of activity, NSAIDs, therapeutic modalities, and physical therapy comprise the initial management. Persistent symptoms despite treatment and a work-up with a bone scan, MRI, or anesthetic injection to confirm the diagnosis is an indication for surgical excision.

Anterior ankle impingement refers to soft tissue entrapment between traction exostoses which form on the anterior lip of the tibia and the neck of the talus from repetitive traumatic avulsions of the anterior joint capsule (footballer's ankle). The impingement with dorsiflexion of the ankle incites inflammation of the surrounding synovial and capsular tissues. Patients present with pain with decreased range of motion. NSAIDs and a heel lift to limit dorsiflexion combined with activity restriction may provide symptomatic relief. Persistent pain despite these measures is an indication for exostectomy.

SUGGESTED READINGS

Berndt AL, Harty M: Transchondral fractures (osteochondritis dissecans) of the talus. *J Bone Joint Surg [Am]* 1959; 41:988.

Conale TS: Osteochondrosis and related problems of the foot and ankle. In DeLee JC, Drez D Jr (eds): *Orthopaedic Sports Medicine:* vol 2. *Principles and Practice*, Philadelphia: WB Saunders; 1994:1940.

Eiff MP, Smith AT, Smith GE: Early mobilization versus immobilization in the treatment of lateral ankle sprains. *Am J Sports Med* 1994; 22:83.

Keene JS: Tendon injuries of the foot and ankle. In DeLee JC, Drez D Jr (eds): *Orthopaedic Sports Medicine: Principles and Practice*, vol 2. Philadelphia: WB Saunders; 1994:1768.

Johnson KA, Strom DE: Tibialis posterior tendon dysfunction. *Clin Orthop* 1989; 239:197.

Jones DC, Singer KM: Soft tissue conditions of the ankle and foot. In Nicholas JA, Hershman EB (eds): *The Lower Extremity and Spine in Sports Medicine,* vol 1, 2d ed. St. Louis: Mosby; 1995:441.

Liu SH, Baker CL: Comparison of lateral ankle ligamentous reconstruction procedures. *Am J Sports Med* 1994; 22:313.

Liu SH, Jason WJ: Lateral ankle sprains and instability problems. *Clin Sports Med* 1994; 13:793.

Renstrom PAFH, Kannus P: Injuries of the foot and ankle. In DeLee JC, Drez D Jr (eds): *Orthopaedic Sports Medicine: Principles and Practice*, vol 2. Philadelphia: WB Saunders; 1994: 1705.

Shapiro MS, Kabo JM, Mitchell PW, et al: Ankle sprain prophylaxis: An analysis of the stabilizing effects of braces and tape. *Am J Sports Med* 1994; 22:78.

Singer KM, Jones DC, Taillon MR: Ligament injuries of the ankle and foot. In Nicholas & Hershman (eds): *The Lower Extremity and Spine in Sports Medicine*, vol 1, 2d ed. St. Louis: Mosby; 1995:423.

Stiell I, Wells G, Laupacis A, et al: Multicenter trial to introduce the Ottawa ankle rules for use of radiography in acute angle injuries. *Br Med J* 1995; 311:594.

Surve I, Schwellnus MP, Noakes T, et al: A five-fold reduction in the incidence of recurrent ankle sprains in soccer players using the Sports-Stirrup orthosis. *Am J Sports Med* 1994; 22:601.

Wredmark T, Carlstedt CA, Bauer H, et al: Os trigonum syndrome: A clinical entity in ballet dancers. *Foot Ankle* 1991; 11:404.

Chapter 106

FOOT

Brian C. Toolan
Daniel S. Zapson

HEEL PAIN

ACHILLES TENDINITIS, RETROCALCANEAL BURSITIS, PLANTAR FASCIITIS

There are numerous pathological processes which can cause pain and swelling about the heel. These can lead to an inability to perform daily functional and recreational activities. Within this anatomic region the symptoms can be divided into plantar-medial and posterior-superior heel pain. The evaluation of these patients should be directed towards distinguishing the location and nature of the pain to determine its exact etiology.

Most cases of plantar heel pain arise from plantar fasciitis. Chronic tensile strain incites a localized inflammatory response at the origin of the plantar fascia at the plantar medial aspect of the calcaneus. Presumably, microruptures and age-related degeneration of the collagen fibrils induce fibrosis of the fascia and an associated periostitis of the calcaneus. The condition presents in middle-aged individuals who may report the onset of symptoms which coincide with a change in shoewear or activity level, a gain in weight or an episode of mild trauma. Classically, they will complain of intense pain at the plantar medial aspect of the heel when arising from bed in the morning or after a period of sitting. This intense pain abates rapidly. Often an achy, throbbing pain which intensifies throughout the day replaces this sharp pain.

Tenderness to palpation over the plantar medial aspect of the calcaneal tuberosity confirms the diagnosis of plantar fasciitis. Radiographs to rule out tumor or stress fracture should be obtained if symptoms do not relent with treatment. The clinical significance of a calcaneal spur seen on x-ray has not been determined, but it is not the source of symptoms. Bone scan and MRI offer little benefit in the diagnosis of plantar fasciitis.

Plantar fasciitis is a self-limiting disease. In most cases, symptoms resolve within one year. Supportive measures to minimize repetitive re-injury and alleviate symptoms provide varying degrees of relief to the majority of patients. Nonsteroidal anti-inflammatory drugs (NSAIDs), heel cord stretching exercises and orthotics that cushion or cup the heel comprise the initial approach to management. If intense morning or start-up pain are the predominating complaints, splints can be used to prevent fascial contracture from equinus positioning of the foot during the night. A steroid injection may facilitate pain relief, however, multiple or frequent injections can cause atrophy of the fat pad or complete rupture of the plantar fascia.

Clinical studies have not provided clear indications for surgery or a reliable prediction of outcome. Surgical release of the plantar fascia may alleviate symptoms in recalcitrant cases, however the consequences of disabling the windlass mechanism and altering foot function remain unknown. A thorough work-up to exclude compression of the first branch of the lateral plantar nerve, tumor, stress fracture, infection, and rheumatological causes for heel pain should precede surgery.

Insertional Achilles tendinitis, retrocalcaneal or adventitial bursitis, or a combination of these clinical entities are all causes of posterior heel pain. These disorders are often difficult to separate clinically due to anatomic proximity and overlap in presenting signs and symptoms, and may restrict activity and shoewear.

Insertional tendinitis arises from intrasubstance degeneration and replacement with fibrous scar tissue. Intratendinous calcifications may develop and will appear on a lateral radiograph of the heel. The area of pathologic change in the tendon often lies within the zone of relative avascularity, found between two and six centimeters above its insertion on the calcaneus.

Retrocalcaneal bursitis and Achilles tendinitis often occur together in patients complaining of posterior heel pain. The retrocalcaneal bursa lies between the anterior margin of the Achilles tendon and the superior prominence of the posterior calcaneal facet. Inflammation due to overuse or impingement will cause symptoms.

Adventitial bursitis relates to the body's response to mechanical irritation from the rubbing of the shoe counter over the posterolateral calcaneal prominence. Commonly referred to as a "pump bump", the bursa which forms over this bony ridge becomes inflamed and enlarged with fluid, making shoewear painful.

Haglund's syndrome combines these three pathologic entities into the clinical presentation of posterior heel pain. Management focuses upon reducing inflammation with rest, NSAIDs, and shoe modification. A shoe lift to limit ankle dorsiflexion with padding of the shoe counter will remove the mechanical irritant while physical therapy addresses the soft tissues. Casting the lower extremity may be successful in severe cases when these initial measures fail to control the symptoms. Judicious use of steroid injections may hasten relief. If the symptoms fail to improve with prolonged nonoperative management, excision of the bursa and bony prominence with tendon debridement may be indicated. Care must be taken not to compromise the insertion of the Achilles tendon onto the calcaneus.

RUPTURE OF THE ACHILLES TENDON

The Achilles tendon may rupture secondary to an eccentric contraction of the gastrocnemius-soleus complex. Active muscle contraction shortening the muscle-tendon unit during forceful dorsiflexion of the ankle can create a powerful tensile strain within the tendon, causing it to fail. This situation commonly arises during recreational activities in otherwise non-athletic, middle-aged individuals. These patients present with pain and difficulty ambulating. They may experience a "pop" or the sensation of having been struck in the back of the ankle. Physical examination reveals a palpable gap in the continuity of the tendon and an inability to actively plantarflex the ankle. A positive Thompson's test confirms disruption of the Achilles mechanism in nearly all cases. The clinical diagnosis is usually extremely reliable and obviates the need for an MRI.

In deciding how to best manage a ruptured Achilles tendon, the physician should consider each patient's functional requirements and expectations. Surgical treatment offers an anatomic reapproximation of the tendon ends, presumably limiting the extent of fibrous scar tissue that may be prone to rerupture. Generally, younger, more active patients who are desirous of a return to sporting activities should undergo surgery. Excellent functional results have been demonstrated with the use of casts, although a higher rate of rerupture, and loss of plantarflexion strength and muscle endurance have been reported. Sedentary, older patients who are reluctant to accept the morbidity associated with surgery may be managed successfully in a cast.

SPRAIN OF THE FIRST METATARSOPHALANGEAL JOINT (TURF TOE)

Forced hypersdorsiflexion of the first metatarsophalangeal (MTP) joint during axial loading of the forefoot may lead to a sprain of the plantar capsuloligamentous complex. This injury often occurs in athletes playing on hard artificial surfaces, hence the term, "turf toe". The plantar soft tissue disruption may be associated with an avulsion of the plantar base of the proximal phalanx or an impaction of the articular surface and subchondral bone of the dorsal aspect of the first metatarsal head.

These injuries may be classified into three grades based upon the degree of soft tissue disruption and bony injury. A grade 1 injury describes an isolated stretch of the plantar capsule. Grade 2 and 3 injuries represent partial and complete tears of these structures, respectively. A grade 3 injury also includes an impaction injury to the articular cartilage or complete dorsal dislocation of the MTP joint.

Treatment of these injuries involves rest, ice, NSAIDs, and protective taping (to foster an early return to sporting activity) for grade 1 and 2 injuries or prolonged restricted weightbearing, use of an orthotic with a rigid toe extension, and surgery for loose bodies or repair of the capsuloligamentous injury for more severe grade 3 injuries.

INTERDIGITAL (MORTON'S) NEUROMA

Entrapment and subsequent compression of the interdigital nerve between the leading edge of the transverse metatarsal ligament and the plantar aspect of the foot can cause perineural fibrosis and degeneration. This condition predominately affects the interdigital nerve of the third dorsal webspace. Two theories may explain this predisposition to injury. Only this interdigital nerve receives branches from the medial and lateral plantar nerves which, therefore, may be subject to an increased "tethering" effect as the MTP joints of the forefoot dorsiflex during gait. Also, the third webspace demarcates the relatively rigid medial rays of the forefoot from the two mobile lateral rays, causing the structures located in this transitional zone to experience increased motion and shearing during gait.

Initial treatment entails the use of metatarsal pads to off-load this region and splay apart the metatarsal heads. This effect may be facilitated further with the use of wide toebox shoes. Injection of steroids, with and without local anesthetic, may prove therapeutic as well as diagnostic in many cases. Surgical excision should be reserved for patients with persistent symptoms despite prolonged nonoperative management.

FREIBERG'S INFRACTION

Freiberg's infraction refers to avascular necrosis of the metatarsal head. This process usually involves the second ray, but can also be seen in the third or fourth metatarsals. Freiberg's infraction may arise from the cumulative effect of repetitive microtrauma compromising the blood supply to the metatarsal head.

The approach to treatment depends upon the degree of symptoms. A metatarsal pad to off-load the affected metatarsal may succeed in the mildly symptomatic patient with minimal deformity of the metatarsal head. More severe symptoms warrant immobilization and restricted weightbearing. Extensive destruction of the head and joint degeneration with pain are indications for surgery. Resection of the metatarsal head should be avoided as this may overload the adjacent metatarsal. A metatarsal shortening osteotomy or modified condylectomy may achieve symptomatic relief.

SUGGESTED READINGS

Baxter DE: The heel in sport. *Clin Sports Med* 1994; 13(4):683.

Bordelon RL: Heel pain. In DeLee JC, Drez D Jr (eds): *Orthopaedic Sports Medicine: Principles and Practice*. Philadelphia: WB Saunders; 1994:1806.

Clanton TO, Ford JJ: Turf toe injury. *Clin Sports Med* 1994; 13(4):731.

Canale ST: Osteochondrosis and related problems of the foot and ankle. In DeLee JC, Drez D Jr (eds): *Orthopaedic Sports Medicine: Principles and Practice*. Philadelphia: WB Saunders; 1994:1940.

Coughlin MJ: Conditions of the forefoot. In DeLee JC, Drez D Jr (eds): *Orthopaedic Sports Medicine: Principles and Practice*. Philadelphia: WB Saunders; 1994:1842.

Jones DC, Singer KM: Soft tissue conditions of the ankle and foot. In Nicholas JA, Hershman EB (eds): *The Lower Extremity and Spine in Sports Medicine*. New York: Mosby; 1995:441.

Kay DB: Forefoot pain in the athlete. *Clin Sports Med* 1994; 13(4):785.

Keene JS: Tendon injuries of the foot and ankle. In DeLee JC, Drez D Jr (eds): *Orthopaedic Sports Medicine: Principles and Practice*. Philadelphia: WB Saunders; 1994:1768

Mann RA: Entrapment neuropathies of the foot. In DeLee JC, Drez D Jr (eds): *Orthopaedic Sports Medicine: Principles and Practice*. Philadelphia: WB Saunders;. 1994:1831.

Soma CA, Mandelbaum BR: Achilles tendon disorders. *Clin Sports Med* 1994; 13(4):811.

Chapter 107

SPINE

Donald J. Cally

HEAD AND CERVICAL SPINE INJURIES

CONCUSSIONS

Head and cervical spine injuries occur frequently with contact sports. Early diagnosis and management of these injuries are essential. Appropriate management, rehabilitation, and subsequent return to sports are the goals of the treating physician.

A number of principles need to be followed during the initial management. One individual should be designated as the captain of the medical team. Appropriate equipment should be available including a spine board, a stretcher, and equipment necessary for CPR. Transportation with an appropriately equipped ambulance needs to be available, as well as telephone communication with the hospital emergency room where the athlete will be taken.

Prevention of further injury is the most important initial objective. The first step in management is to immobilize the head and neck so they are supported in a stable position. Next, the ABCs of CPR should be addressed and evaluated along with the patient's level of consciousness.

If the patient is prone, he needs to be moved into the supine position; the movement should be a log roll maneuver to a spine board with the team leader controlling the head while other team members maintain the body in line with the patient's head and spine during the roll.

If the athlete is not breathing or stops breathing, an airway must be established. If he is wearing a helmet with a face mask, the helmet need not be removed, but the face mask must be taken off. The type of mask that is attached to the helmet determines the method of removal. Bolt cutters are used with the older single and double bar masks. The newer masks that are attached with plastic loops should be removed by cutting the loops with a sharp knife or scalpel. Removal of the mask allows one to obtain access to the airway and begin CPR. Once an airway has been established and circulation is adequate, the patient can be transported to the hospital for further evaluation. Lifting and carrying the athlete requires five individuals: four to lift, and the team leader to maintain immobilization of the head. Using these precautions, an athlete can be safely managed and transported to a medical facility.

Athletes who receive direct blows to the head can experience a sudden acceleration and deceleration force and sustain a concussion. An initial on-field examination should include evaluation of the patient's orientation to person, place, and time, his facial expression, evaluation of his memory both prior to and following the event, and evaluation of gait.

Three categories of brain injury have been recognized: (1) a mild concussion, in which there is temporary disturbance of neurologic function without loss of consciousness; (2) a classic cerebral concussion where there is a temporary loss of consciousness and reversible neurologic deficiency; and (3) diffuse axonal injury which presents with prolonged traumatic brain coma with loss of consciousness that lasts more than 6 h. Residual deficits are usually present with this type of injury.

Mild cerebral concussions are the most common type of head injury seen with contact sports. A grade I mild concussion is the mildest form of head injury which results in some confusion and disorientation without amnesia. This injury is completely reversible with no long-term sequela. The athlete is usually confused, has a dazed look, and may exhibit some unsteadiness of gait. Amnesia is not usually associated with this injury.

A grade II mild concussion is characterized by confusion with retrograde amnesia, which usually develops 5 to 10 min following the injury. When initially seen on the field, the player may recall all of the events immediately prior to the impact. However, reexamination 5 to 10 min later will demonstrate retrograde amnesia.

A grade III mild concussion presents with confusion and amnesia, which are present from the time of impact. There is some posttraumatic amnesia with this type of concussion, as well as retrograde amnesia. Athletes with grade I concussions may resume sport activity the same day, as soon as they become asymptomatic. Those with grades II and III concussions should not return to play on the same day.

A classic cerebral concussion is seen in a player who states he has been "knocked out." In this situation, the athlete is temporarily in a paralytic coma, usually recovering after a few seconds or several minutes. The patient will then pass through stages of stupor, confusion with or without delirium, and an almost lucent state with automatism before becoming fully alert. These individuals almost certainly have retrograde, as well as posttraumatic amnesia. If the patient's loss of consciousness lasts more than several minutes or there are other signs of neurologic deterioration, the patient should be immediately transferred to a hospital for neurosurgical evaluation. An athlete who has sustained a cerebral concussion should not return to play that day, and observation in a hospital overnight should be considered.

Intracerebral hematoma and contusion can occur in athletes who sustain a head injury. These patients may present without a loss of consciousness or any focal neurologic findings. They will, however, continue to complain of headaches and periods of confusion after their initial injury, as well as posttraumatic amnesia. These patients should be seen by a neurosurgeon and undergo a CT scan or MRI to evaluate the possibility of a hematoma or cerebral contusion.

Cantu has developed a simplified classification of cerebral concussion, as well as criteria for returning to play following a concussion (see Table 107–1).

BURNERS

Cervical spine injuries also occur frequently in athletes, especially to those involved in contact sports or athletic activities involving a high rate of speed. The spectrum of injuries can run from a cervical sprain to a fracture dislocation with permanent paralysis.

Table 107-1

Guidelines for Return to Play After Concussion

	First Concussion	Second Concussion	Third Concussion
Grade 1 (mild)	May return to play if asymptomatic[a]	Return to play in second week if asymptomatic at that time for 1 week	Terminate season; may return to play next season if asymptomatic
Grade 2 (moderate)	Return to play after being asymptomatic for 1 week	Minimum of 1 month; may return to play then if asymptomatic for 1 week; consider terminating season	Terminate season; may return to play next season if asymptomatic
Grade 3 (severe)	Minimum of 1 month; may then return to play if asymptomatic for 1 week	Terminate season; may return to play next season if asymptomatic	

[a]No headache, dizziness, or impaired orientation, concentration, or memory during rest or exertion. Grade 1 (mild): no loss of consciousness; posttraumatic amnesia <30 min. Grade 2 (moderate): loss of consciousness; <5 min or posttraumatic amnesia >30 min. Grade 3 (severe): loss of consciousness; >5 min or posttraumatic amnesia >24 h.

SOURCE: Reproduced and modified with permission from Cantu R. In Torg JS (ed): *Athletic Injuries to the Head, Neck and Face,* 2d ed. St. Louis: Mosby-Year Book; 1991:324, 327.

The most common cervical injury is the pinch-stretch neuropraxia of the nerve roots or brachial plexus, referred to as stingers or burners. These typically occur following axial loading of the head, neck, or shoulder with the athlete experiencing a unilateral sharp burning pain in the neck; the pain may radiate through one shoulder and down into the arm and hand. There may also be associated weakness and paraesthesias of the affected upper extremity, lasting from several seconds to several minutes. Weakness usually involves elbow flexion and external rotation of the shoulder. If symptoms are bilateral and/or involve the legs, central spinal cord contusion needs to be ruled out with an MRI.

Symptoms of persistence of paraesthesia, weakness, or limitation of cervical motion lasting more than 2 weeks require further work-up which should include a neurologic evaluation, MRI of the cervical spine, and EMG.

The above constellation of findings is typically seen in football players and may be a result of traction injury to the brachial plexus, usually involving the upper trunk, which is a result of depression of the shoulder with forceful deviation of the head in the opposite direction. Another proposed mechanism is preexisting neuroforaminal narrowing with axial force causing compression of a cervical nerve root, usually C5 or C6.

When a patient experiences a burner, the initial evaluation consists of evaluation of the patient's neck for tenderness and range of motion, and a neurologic examination of the involved upper extremity. If the results are normal, there is no neck pain, and symptoms are resolved, the athlete may return to his activity. However, if there is pain with range of motion of the neck, or the patient's upper extremity symptoms have not completely resolved, he should be removed from the playing field. Plain radiographs of the cervical spine should be obtained at that time to rule out pathology. Further work-up may be necessary depending on the resolution of the patient's symptoms.

SPRAINS

Athletes involved in collision sports are also prone to sustaining acute cervical sprains. The athlete will frequently complain of having "jammed" his neck and complain of pain in the cervical spine region;

presentation will usually include some muscle spasm with limitation of motion but without radicular or neurologic complaints. The athlete who does not have pain-free range of motion or has persistent paresthesia or weakness should be removed from his activity and undergo further evaluation. Initially, the patient should have AP and lateral views of the cervical spine, and when acute symptoms have subsided, lateral flexion extension views. In the case of persistent radicular symptoms or neurologic findings, an MRI may be necessary to evaluate the possibility of a herniated nucleus pulposus.

DISC DISEASE

The intervertebral discs of the cervical spine are also prone to injury. Acute cervical disc herniation is rare, but has been reported in the athlete sustaining transient quadriplegia after head impact.

Chronic loading of the cervical discs can also result in degeneration over time. A study of football players from the University of Iowa demonstrated that 32 percent of the freshmen football class had one or more of the following: occult fracture, vertebral body compression fractures, intervertebral disc space narrowing, or other degenerative changes. Acute and chronic cervical disc injury without herniation and neurologic findings is observed with considerable frequency in athletes who participate in contact sports. MRI of these patients frequently demonstrate degenerative changes within the cervical discs, as well as mild diffuse bulging, but without herniation. These athletes can generally be managed conservatively with a return to sports when asymptomatic and a full range of motion of the cervical spine has returned.

FRACTURES

Fractures and dislocations of the cervical spine may also occur and should be treated in the athlete as they would in any other trauma patient. The initial evaluation and management of the patient is crucial to prevent further injury, similar to the trauma setting. The goals of initial management are protection of the spinal cord from further injury, early reduction of the fracture or dislocation, and stabilization (depending on the type of injury, either with a cervical collar, a halo-vest or surgery). An early rehabilitation program can then begin to return the patient to his or her daily activities, and depending on the extent of injury, to his or her sport (see Chaps. 68, 73, 74, and 75).

CERVICAL SPINAL STENOSIS

Cervical cord neuropraxia and transient quadriplegia can occur in patients with cervical spinal stenosis. The athletes will usually experience an acute transient neurologic episode of cervical cord origin with sensory changes and paresis; symptoms may involve both arms, both legs, or all four extremities. The mechanism of injury is usually forced hyperextension, hyperflexion, or axial loading. The episodes are usually transient; complete recovery normally occurs within 10 to 15 min. There have been some cases, however, where complete resolution did not occur for 36 to 48 h. Evaluation should include plain radiographs with flexion extension views. A CT or MR scan may also be necessary. Routine radiographs in these patients may identify cervical stenosis. Torg and Pavlov (1986) described what is now referred to as the Torg ratio. This ratio was used to evaluate the size of the spinal canal within the cervical spine. Measurements are made from a lateral radiograph of the cervical spine by taking the distance from the mid-point of the posterior aspect of the vertebral body to the nearest point on the corresponding spinal laminar line, and dividing this by the AP width of the vertebral body (see Fig. 107–1). A ratio of less than 0.8 is indicative of cervical stenosis. One should note, however, that the Torg ratio has a very low predictive value and should not be used as a screening tool.

In a review of this type of injury, Torg and coworkers concluded that the presence of uncomplicated developmental narrowing of a stable cervical spine represents neither a harbinger of nor a predisposition to permanent neurologic injury.

CRITERIA FOR RETURN TO ACTIVITIES

With regard to activity restrictions, no firm principles based on scientific information are available. However, it is recommended that individuals with cervical cord neuropraxia and canal stenosis be restricted from contact sports if they have concurrent ligamentous instability, intervertebral disc disease and cord compression, significant degenerative changes, cervical cord defects or swelling, neurologic symptoms which last more than 36 h, and more than one recurrence.

Some criteria have been proposed for return to contact activities in the presence of cervical spine abnormalities or following injury or surgery. These criteria are not based on scientific data, and for the most part, are recommendations derived from anecdotal experience.

Spina bifida occulta can occur in the cervical spine, although this is rare and is not a contraindication to sports participation. Atlanto-occipital fusion, however, is an absolute contraindication. Other absolute contraindications to resuming contact sports activity are anomalies of the odontoid (for example, os odontoideum, hypoplasia of the odontoid, and odontoid agenesis) and atlantoaxial instability from ligamentous injury or destruction.

The Klippel-Feil anomaly refers to congenital fusion of cervical vertebral motion segments. Fusion of more than three segments is a contraindication to contact sports; fusion of one or two segments with full cervical range of motion and no other abnormality is not a contraindication.

Review of the National Football Head and Neck Registry has provided information on the description of "spear tacklers spine." This entity consists of developmental narrowing, loss of normal cervical lordosis, subtle torticollis, and radiographic evidence of prior injury in an individual who employs spear tackling techniques. This com-

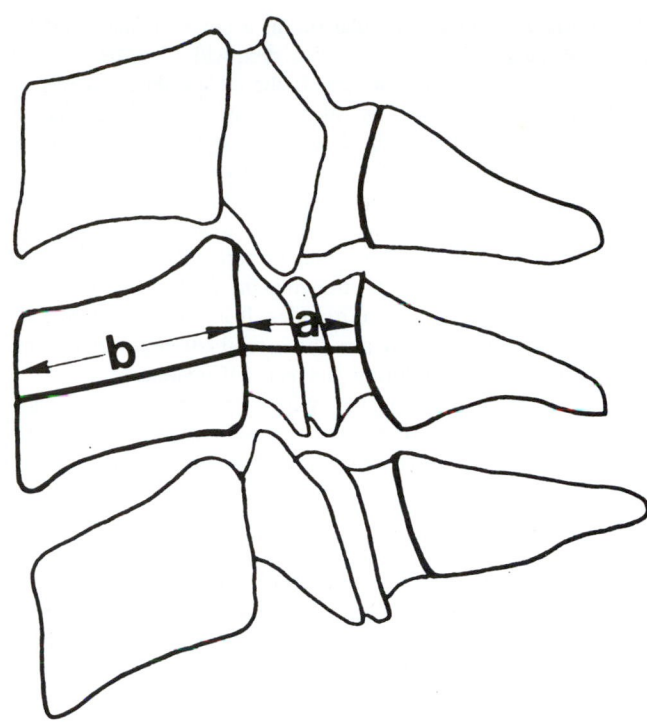

Figure 107-1
The ratio of the spinal canal to the vertebral body is the distance from the mid-point of the posterior aspect of the vertebral body to the nearest point on the corresponding spinolaminar line (a) divided by the anteroposterior width of the vertebral body (b). [Reproduced by permission from Torg JS, Pavlov H, Genuario AT, et al: Neurapraxia of the cervical spinal cord with transient quadriplegia. *J Bone Joint Surg [Am]* 1986; 68:1355.]

bination of features constitutes an absolute contraindication to further participation in contact sports.

Other absolute contraindications to participation in contact sports include: athletes with acute central disc herniations or chronic hard disc herniations with associated neurologic findings; those with pain and/or significant limitation of motion; and patients with symptoms of cord neuropraxia due to compression from a hard or soft disc. An athlete who has a herniated disc with full range of motion and no neurologic symptoms may return to contact sports. An athlete who undergoes a one-level anterior or posterior disc fusion and is pain free with normal range of motion may also return to contact sports. A relative contraindication is present for a person with a stable two- or three-level fusion who is asymptomatic, neurologically normal, and has pain-free full range of motion. More than a three-level anterior or posterior fusion, however, is a contraindication to return to contact sports. In addition, a C1-C2 fusion is an absolute contraindication to return to contact sport.

THORACOLUMBAR SPINE

STRAINS AND SPRAINS

Muscular or ligamentous tears can result in local pain and tenderness. Frequently, there is a history of injury, a direct blow, or a forceful movement. In the absence of a specific incident, the athlete may recount pain that occurs with a change or increase in training intensity or duration.

Diagnostic imaging in muscular strains is controversial. If the history and physical examination are consistent with a soft tissue injury, it is acceptable to begin treatment. If the athlete does not respond quickly, anteroposterior and lateral radiographs should be obtained. Treatment should include a short period of cold therapy and control of the muscle spasm. Use of a lightweight corset and a muscle relaxant will help during the acute injury phase.

Once the initial pain and spasm subside, treatment is directed toward rehabilitation and a return to athletic participation. The program involves stretching and muscle strengthening for both the paraspinal musculature and the abdominal muscles. It is crucial that the hamstring musculature be included in the rehabilitation program. Moist heat may also be helpful during this phase of treatment.

The athlete may return to sports participation as soon as the pain has subsided sufficiently to allow it, and sufficient motion regained to allow the athlete to protect himself in contact activities.

DISC DISEASE AND RING APOPHYSIS FRACTURE

Disc disease is very common in athletes and may cause low back pain; if a true disc herniation has occurred, leg pain may be the predominant symptom. A thorough history and physical examination will help to narrow the diagnosis. Differentiating between referred and radicular pain may be difficult.

Plain radiographs may be obtained; however, they are frequently not helpful. Interpretation of findings may be problematic; for example, degenerative changes seen may represent the actual source of pain or just the normal aging process.

The treatment of lumbar degenerative disc disease in athletes is no different than in nonathletes. It is aimed at reducing pain, increasing range of motion, and strengthening. The mainstay of treatment is an active exercise program.

Return to sports by an athlete with disc degeneration is based on the patient's pain and range of motion. Disc herniation with production of radicular leg pain is common. The patient may initially complain of back pain secondary to an annular tear and then develop leg pain with herniation. The presence of bilateral leg numbness or weakness may represent the early stages of cauda equina syndrome. Similarly, any bowel or bladder dysfunction should alert one to a cauda equina syndrome. Examination, including neurologic assessment, should be performed to make the diagnosis and determine the level of herniation. Initial treatment is conservative, combining a short course of bedrest, nonsteroidal anti-inflammatories, and analgesics. Once adequate pain relief has been achieved, an exercise program is begun. If significant pain persists, epidural steroid injections may be considered.

Early surgery is indicated for the patient with a cauda equina syndrome or progressive neurologic deficit.

The duration of nonoperative treatment varies with no scientific evidence to support a specific period of time. However, the results of discectomy diminish when symptoms have been present for 6 months or longer. In general, if resumption of day to day activities is not possible by 6 weeks, operative intervention should be considered. The standard surgical procedure is a laminotomy and discectomy.

There have been reports in the literature of traumatic displacement of the lumbar vertebral ring apophysis into the spinal canal with associated disc herniation. The majority of these injuries have occurred at the L4 level; less commonly at L3 and L5. This type of injury typically follows a traumatic incident such as weight lifting, gymnastics, or shoveling. Initial signs and symptoms are that of a central herniated disc. If the condition goes untreated, it can present chronically as spinal stenosis. Radiographically, cases demonstrate a small bony fragment involving the inferior edge of the vertebral end plate which is displaced into the spinal canal.

An MRI will demonstrate a large anterior extradural impression with signal characteristics of a disc, as well as cortical bone; however, on an MRI it may be difficult to differentiate these two. A myelogram may demonstrate a complete block, with the CT myelogram demonstrating the block, as well as a large anterior extradural impression and bone within the canal.

These patients are initially treated nonoperatively, similar to treatment for a herniated disc. If the patient does not have significant resolution of his pain and discomfort or significant neurologic findings persist, surgery can be recommended. Treatment is removal of the herniated disk as well as the bony ridge; this can be accomplished with laminotomy or laminectomy depending on the size of the bony fragment and the position of these fragments.

Following lumbar discectomy, the athlete should be able to return to his sport. The criteria for return is adequate strength to protect oneself in the chosen activity and relief of pain to a level allowing participation. Typically, patients return to limited workouts approximately 1 month following surgery, and are then able to return to full participation between 6 and 8 weeks.

SPONDYLOLYSIS AND SPONDYLOLISTHESIS

Spondylolysis is a stress defect in the pars interarticularis. Spondylolisthesis is the anterior slippage of one vertebrae in relation to the vertebrae below it. Wiltse (1983) classified spondylolisthesis into etiologic groups. The groups are congenital or dysplastic, isthmic, degenerative, traumatic, and pathologic. Similarly, the amount of slippage was graded by Meyerding (1932). Grade I represents 0 to 25 percent slippage, grade II is 25 to 50 percent slippage, grade III is 50 to 75 percent slippage, and grade IV is 75 to 100 percent slippage.

Spondylolysis and spondylolisthesis typically occur in younger athletes. However, affected individuals can remain asymptomatic until adulthood, at which time, the condition may be incidentally found when obtaining radiographs.

Stress reaction of the pars interarticularis, spondylolysis, and spondylolisthesis are part of a disease continuum. These injuries most frequently occur at the fifth and fourth lumbar levels. The proposed cause is repetitive hyperextension, causing a pincer effect on the pars. Athletes normally develop this lesion in late childhood and adolescence, and will complain of back pain and occasionally leg pain when a spondylolisthesis is present. This is usually the result of L5 nerve root irritation with an L5-S1 spondylolisthesis.

Initially, plain radiographs are normal. Approximately 3 to 6 weeks after the onset of pain, a stress reaction can be seen on oblique radiographs. With further stress, spondylolysis occurs, and in some cases, the condition progresses to a spondylolisthesis.

The diagnosis can be made early with a technetium bone scan and SPECT imaging. This can be performed after several weeks of unresolved low back pain in an athlete in order to arrive at the diagnosis before the lysis appears on radiographs. The other instance where imaging may be helpful is when a spondylolysis exists and one needs to determine if it is acute or chronic, as this would play a role in the choice of management.

A review of sports medicine literature reveals a number of treatment options, although none have scientifically proved superior. Options range from participation in prior activity with modification to a thoracic-lumbosacral orthosis (TLSO) with a pantaloon.

Athletes with a stress reaction or lysis can be treated with activity modification with no sports activity for at least 3 months and a rehab program. The other option is activity modification and bracing with a rehabilitation program and a return to athletic activities once the patient is pain free during his activities of daily living. Bracing is continued for up to 3 months. If pain persists out of the brace at 3 months, an additional 3 months of bracing is recommended. If pain persists beyond 6 months, surgical intervention should be considered. There is no literature to support or refute a return to sports activity after surgical repair.

Athletes with spondylolysis and a cold bone scan have a very low probability of healing. Therefore, they are treated using a less rigid warm and form orthosis with a gradual return to activities supported by a rehabilitation program.

The majority of symptomatic spondylolysis patients are adolescents; however, older recreational athletes will occasionally present with back pain and a spondylolytic defect noted on plain radiographs. These individuals are treated the same as patients with chronic spondylolytic lesions. Bone scanning is not routinely ordered as this defect is felt to develop prior to skeletal maturity. The treatment program is a lumbar orthosis and physical therapy with return to activities when the pain has subsided.

A symptomatic grade I or II spondylolisthesis is treated with a brace and a rehabilitation program. Return to sports activity occurs when the patient is pain free. There is no documentation that sports will cause progression of a grade I or II slip. Activity restriction in these patients is not necessary.

Symptomatic and asymptomatic grade III and IV spondylolisthesis in skeletally immature athletes requires restriction of contact sports; consideration should be given to fusion to prevent progression and/or to control the patient's pain and discomfort. If surgical intervention is necessary for a grade III or IV spondylolisthesis, the fusion should extend from L4 to S1. The role of reduction of these high grade slips has yet to be completely defined. One risk with reduction of an L5/S1 spondylolisthesis is injury to the L5 nerve root. This is frequently transient but can be permanent with loss or weakness of motor function in the L5 innervated musculature (see Chap. 65).

SUGGESTED READINGS

Bridwell KH, DeWald RL (eds): *The Textbook of Spinal Surgery,* 2d ed. Philadelphia: Lippincott-Raven, 1997.

Cantu RC: Criteria for return to competition after a closed head injury. In Torg JS (ed): *Athletic Injuries to the Head, Neck and Face*, 2d ed. St Louis: Mosby-Year Book; 1991:323.

Hensinger RN: Spondylolysis and spondylolisthesis in children and adolescents. *J Bone Joint Surgery [Am]* 1989; 71:1098.

Lowrey JJ: Dislocated lumbar vertebral epiphysis in adolescent children. Report of three cases. *J Neurosurg* 1973; 38:232.

Meyerding HW: Spondylolisthesis. *Surg Gynecol Obstet* 1932; 54:371.

Micheli L: Low back pain in the adolescent: Differential diagnosis. *Am J Sports Med* 1979; 7:362.

Nicholas JA, Hershman EB (ed): *The Lower Extremity and Spine in Sports Medicine,* 2d ed. St. Louis: Mosby-Year Book, 1995.

Teasdale G, Mathew P: Mechanisms of cerebral concussion, contusion, and other effects of head injury. In Youmans JR (ed): *Neurological Surgery,* vol 3, 4th ed. Philadelphia: WB Saunders; 1995:1533.

Torg JS, Pavlov H, Genuario SE, et al: Neuropraxia of the cervical spinal cord with transient quadriplegia. *J Bone Joint Surg [Am]* 1986; 68:1354.

Wiltse LL, Newman PH, MacNab W: Classification of spondylolysis and spondylolisthesis. *Clin Orthop* 1976; 117:23.

Chapter 108

STRESS FRACTURES

Geoffrey I. Phillips and Daniel S. Zapson

Stress fractures are ubiquitous in the athletic population, comprising between 0.7 to 15.6 percent of all sports-related injuries, most notably in track and field. Running accounts for 69 percent of all stress fractures, many of which are implicated in the diagnosis of unexplained leg or foot pain. These injuries typically arise as a consequence of repetitive microtrauma in normal or weakened bone, and are best viewed within the context of "overuse injuries." Those skeletal locations undergoing activity-related mechanical loading are susceptible to stress fracture. For example, track and field athletes overall sustained 0.7 stress fractures per 1000 training hours, with power athletes having substantially more stress fractures of the foot. Long bone and pelvic stress fractures were more common among endurance athletes. Although stress fractures most frequently occur in the weightbearing sites of the lower extremity, nonweightbearing areas may also be affected such as the olecranon or hamate in baseball players (Table 108–1).

EPIDEMIOLOGY

Among runners, 76 percent of stress fractures occur in the tibia, fibula, and metatarsals. Tibial stress fractures are the most common, ranging from 34 to 49 percent of all injuries, with the shaft usually involved at the junction of the middle and distal thirds. Additional sites of tibial stress fractures include the medial tibial plateau, medial malleolus, and anterior midshaft tibia, with the latter having a more ominous prognosis. Fibula and metatarsal stress fractures comprise 7 to 24 percent and 9 to 20 percent of the total cases, respectively.

Prospective and retrospective studies of stress fractures among military recruits reported a cumulative incidence of 0.99 to 2.0 percent for males. Female recruits generally sustained stress fractures at a rate of over three times that of their male counterparts, while blacks maintained a lower risk for developing this condition. Other retrospective studies have documented stress fracture rates of 13 to 52 percent among female distance runners and 22 to 45 percent among ballet dancers. Prospective studies have confirmed higher recurrence rates. In one year-long study approximately 60 percent of track and field athletes presenting with stress fracture had a prior history of this condition. Female athletes with a history of multiple stress fractures should be evaluated for a hypoestrogenic state with ensuing osteoporotic bone, predisposing them to exercise-induced pathologic fracture.

FEMALE ATHLETE TRIAD

Several studies have identified competitive female distance runners as having later menarche, menstrual irregularities with diminished circulating reproductive hormones, and a reduced peak bone mass. The female athlete triad, describing an association between amenorrhea, anorexia, and osteoporosis, is a relatively prevalent condition among elite female athletes with a reported incidence ranging from 15 to 62 percent. While mechanical loading has a positive effect on the bone mineral density of estrogen-replete female distance runners, amenorrheic athletes have a significantly lower bone mineral density, even compared with a control group of sedentary eumenorrheic females. There should be a high index of suspicion for this condition among female competitors in all sports, particularly distance running, gymnastics, figure-skating, and ballet. Once the diagnosis of female athlete triad is suspected, a multidisciplinary approach should be taken besides orthopaedic care of the stress fracture, with consideration of gynecologic and psychological issues. While pharmacologic treatment has displayed promising results for the partial reversibility of osteoporosis, prevention remains crucial for management of this condition affecting the female athletic population.

HISTORY AND PHYSICAL EXAMINATION

Typically, the athlete presenting with a stress fracture has a history of a recent change in training schedule or footwear, or has an abrupt increase in intensity of activity. The onset of a stress fracture may be insidious in nature as the athlete initially complains of localized pain at the conclusion of running. Although the pain is generally relieved by rest from the inciting activity, continuation of a running program exacerbates the condition, increasing the severity of pain and hastening its onset. While physical examination may be nonspecific, local point tenderness is the most consistent clinical finding in the diagnosis of a stress fracture.

IMAGING STUDIES

Plain radiographs obtained within the first 2 to 3 weeks are almost universally negative. Only half of the affected athletes will present with positive radiographs displaying evidence of a stress fracture, such as callus formation, endosteal thickening, and a radiolucent line (Fig. 108-1). Technetium pyrophosphate bone scan is the most sensitive and earliest indicator of a stress fracture, revealing a focal area of intense radionuclide uptake within the first 2 to 7 days. Consequently, a negative bone scan virtually eliminates the diagnosis of stress fracture from a differential. Although not supplanting nuclear medicine techniques, the use of magnetic resonance imaging has emerged for the early identification of stress fractures.

Table 108-1

Sports and Activities Commonly Associated with Different Stress Fracture Sites

Site of Stress Fracture	Sport or Activity
Coracoid process of scapula	Trapshooting
Scapula	Running with hand-held weights
Humerus	Throwing, racquet sports
Olecranon	Throwing, pitching
Ulna	Racquet sports (especially tennis), gymnastics, volleyball, swimming, softball, wheelchair sports
Ribs	
First	Throwing, pitching
Second to 10th	Rowing, kayaking
Pars interarticularis	Gymnastics, ballet, cricket, fast bowling, volleyball, springboard diving
Pubic ramus	Distance running, ballet
Femur	
Neck	Distance running, jumping, ballet
Shaft	Distance running
Patella	Running, hurdling
Tibia	
Plateau	Running
Shaft	Running, ballet
Fibula	Running, aerobics, race-walking, ballet
Medial malleolus	Basketball, running
Calcaneus	Long-distance military marching
Talus	Pole vaulting
Navicular	Sprinting, middle-distance running, hurdling, long-triple jumping, football
Metatarsal	
General	Running, ballet, marching
Base second	Ballet
Fifth	Tennis, ballet
Sesamoid bones of foot	Running, ballet, basketball, skating

SOURCE: Reproduced with permission from Brukner PD, Khan KM: *Clinical Sports Medicine*. Sydney: McGraw-Hill; 1991:17.

HIP

Compressive, tensile, and shearing forces all contribute to the development of stress fractures in a dynamic model. The direction of the biomechanical load, associated fracture pattern, and specific location of the fracture all have implications for management. Nondisplaced stress fractures occurring on the compression surface of the femoral neck can be treated nonoperatively with nonweightbearing and close radiographic scrutiny. However, transverse or tension-type fractures which begin as a cortical defect on the superior aspect of the femoral neck are best treated with internal fixation, primarily using multiple screws. Displaced femoral neck fractures represent another indication for surgery.

LEG AND ANKLE

The majority of tibial shaft stress fractures are best managed with a nonoperative regimen. Analgesics or nonsteroidal anti-inflammatory medications combined with relative rest usually suffice for early relief of pain. The athlete may later engage in low-impact conditioning activities such as swimming and bicycling, with progression to walking, while the stress fracture heals. Although immobilization of the lower extremity is rarely necessary, it is recommended for treating stress fractures of the medial malleolus. A structured program of strengthening and flexibility exercises usually facilitates complete resolution by 6 to 8 weeks with a graduated return to full activity. Open reduction and internal fixation of medial malleolar stress frac-

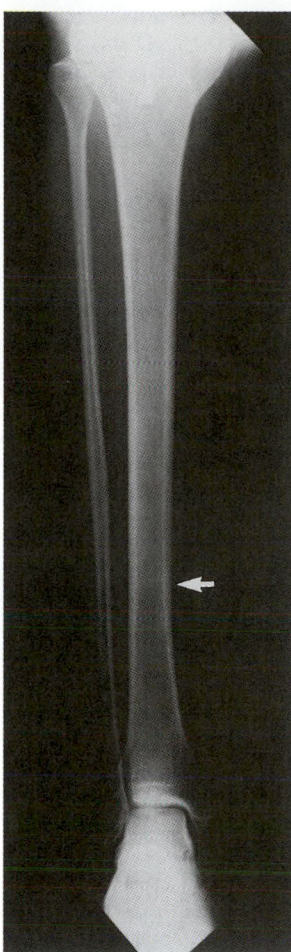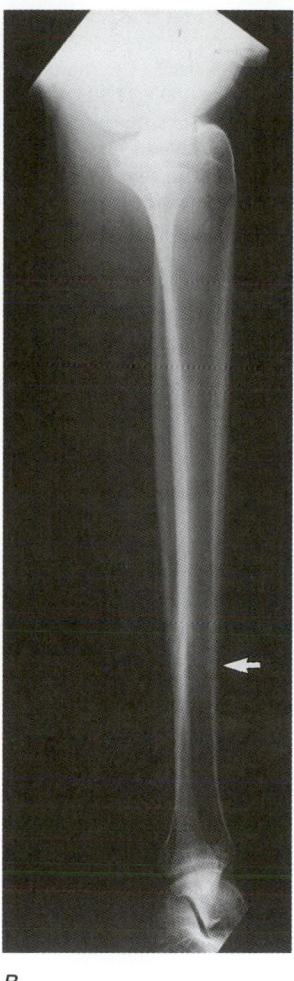

A   *B*

Figure 108–1

Stress fracture. AP (*A*) and lateral (*B*) views of the tibia and fibula were obtained in a 15-year-old boy with activity-related shin pain that was worsening over time. No specific injury was known. The radiographs demonstrate cortical thickening of the distal one-third of the medial tibia. Linear intramedullary sclerosis to the cortex can also be seen. These findings are consistent with a stress fracture.

tures have been advocated by some surgeons for high-level athletes desiring an accelerated return to competition.

Persistence of the "dreaded black line" (signifying a stress fracture) on plain radiographs for greater than 6 months (pathognomonic for a delayed union or nonunion) is an indication for lesion excision, bone grafting, and possible internal fixation. Transverse anterior tibial stress fractures are particularly susceptible to delayed union and may fracture completely, often necessitating surgical intervention. Moderate success has been reported with the use of pulsating electromagnetic fields and prolonged immobilization for the specific treatment of anterior midshaft tibial stress fractures.

FOOT

Stress fractures of the tarsal navicular bone are prone to nonunion and are initially managed with cast immobilization and nonweightbearing for a period of 6 to 8 weeks. Internal fixation or bone grafting is recommended for displaced fractures or established nonunions.

Metatarsal stress fractures are found among runners and military recruits, typically occurring in the diaphysis of the second and third metatarsals. Treatment can be symptomatic, and a walking cast or orthosis is rarely necessary. Stress fractures at the relatively avascular proximal metaphyseal-diaphyseal junction of the fifth metatarsal are common in jumping sports and may progress to a nonunion if inappropriately treated. This so-called "Jones fracture" should be managed with cast immobilization and nonweightbearing for 6 to 8 weeks. Treatment of calcaneus and distal fibula stress fractures involves relative rest for at least 3 weeks with maintenance of a conditioning program.

UPPER EXTREMITY

High-repetition loading of the wrist complex may lead to a variety of upper extremity injuries, including carpal scaphoid stress fractures and distal radial physis stress syndrome. Nondisplaced scaphoid stress fractures are treated with protected rest until healing is completed. Distal radial physis stress syndrome occurs in young gymnasts and appears radiographically as widening and irregularity of the distal radial physis with marginal sclerosis.

Stress fractures of the humerus have been reported in athletes participating in throwing and racquet sports with associated high acceleration forces. Young pitchers may be predisposed to sustaining diaphyseal fractures. Olecranon stress fractures can occur in throwing athletes secondary to extension overload during the motion of pitching. Ulna shaft stress fractures have been noted in a tennis player, a volleyball player, and a softball player. The aforementioned cases all healed uneventfully with 4 to 6 weeks of rest followed by a progressive return to athletic participation.

SUMMARY

Treatment of stress fractures in the athletic population must be individualized, although relative rest from the offending activity and continuation of aerobic conditioning represent common approaches. The athlete's desire for an early return to competition must be balanced with the treating physician's knowledge regarding the particulars of the fracture location, the nature of the biomechanical forces, and the specific patterns of bone healing. The relatively high incidence of menstrual dysfunction and concomitant osteoporosis in female athletes predisposes to stress fracture. Among distance runners, the physician should carefully consider alterations in the athlete's training routine and type of footwear, coupled with potential anatomic variations in the lower extremity, as contributing factors in the generation of a stress fracture. Efforts at reducing the morbidity associated with stress fracture should largely be directed towards prevention of this overuse injury in the athletic population.

SUGGESTED READINGS

Barrett GR, Grondel RJ, Papendick L, et al: Sports medicine. In Kasser JR (ed): *Orthopaedic Knowledge Update 5*. Rosemont, IL: American Academy of Orthopaedic Surgeons; 1996:96–99.

Bennell KL, Brukner PD: Epidemiology and site specificity of stress fractures. *Clin Sports Med* 1997; 16:179.

Blue JM, Matthews LS: Leg injuries. *Clin Sports Med* 1997; 16:467.

Brukner PD, Bradshaw C, Bennell KC: Managing common stress fractures: Let risk level guide treatment. *Physician Sports Med* 1998; 26:34.

Caborn DNM, Grollman LJ, Nyland JA, et al: Running. In Fu FH, Stone DA (eds): *Sports Injuries: Mechanisms, Prevention, Treatment*. Baltimore: Williams & Wilkins; 1994:572–573.

Caine D, Roy S, Singer KM, Broekhof J: Stress changes of the distal radial growth plate: A radiographic survey and review of the literature. *Am J Sports Med* 1992; 20:290.

Clanton TO, Solcher BW: Chronic leg pain in the athlete. *Clin Sports Med* 1994; 13:743.

Fredericson M, Bergman AG, Hoffman KL, et al: Tibial stress reaction in runners: Correlation of clinical symptoms and scintigraphy with a new magnetic resonance imaging grading system. *Am J Sports Med* 1995; 23:472.

Fullerton LR Jr, Snowdy HA: Femoral neck stress fractures. *Am J Sports Med* 1988; 16:365.

Hershman FB, Mailly T: Stress fractures. *Clin Sports Med* 1990; 4:183.

James SL: Running injuries of the knee. In Cannon WD Jr (ed): *Instructional Course Lectures*. Rosemont, IL: American Academy of Orthopaedic Surgeons; 1998; 47:407.

Johansson C, Ekenman I, Tornkvist H, et al: Stress fractures of the femoral neck in athletes: The consequence of a delay in diagnosis. *Am J Sports Med* 1990; 18:524.

Marky KL: Stress fractures. *Clin Sports Med* 1987; 6:405.

McBryde AM Jr: Stress fractures in runners. *Clin Sports Med* 1985; 4:737.

Meyer SA, Saltzman CL, Albright JP: Stress fractures of the foot and leg. *Clin Sports Med* 1993; 12:395.

Murakami Y: Stress fracture of the metacarpal in an adolescent tennis player. *Am J Sports Med* 1988; 16:419.

Myburgh KH, Hutchins J, Fataar AB, et al: Low bone density is an etiologic factor for stress fractures in athletes. *Ann Intern Med* 1990; 113:754.

Pecina M, Bojanic I, Dubravcic S: Stress fractures in figure skaters. *Am J Sports Med* 1990; 18:277.

Teitz C: The female athlete triad. In Teitz C (ed): *The Female Athlete*. AAOS Monograph Series. Rosemont, IL: American Academy of Orthopaedic Surgeons: 1997:75.

Teitz C: Stress fractures. In Teitz C (ed): *The Female Athlete*. AAOS Monograph Series. Rosemont, IL: American Academy of Orthopaedic Surgeons: 1997:81.

Weiker GG: Hand and wrist problems in the gymnast. *Clin Sports Med* 1992; 11:189.

Chapter 109

MEDICAL PROBLEMS IN ATHLETES

Daniel S. Zapson

EXERCISE INDUCED ILLNESS

A wide variety of medical problems can affect athletes. As the benefits of exercise continue to be realized, individuals who previously did not participate in athletic activities are now being encouraged to do so. Medical conditions may be precipitated by exercise or preexisting conditions may be aggravated by exercise.

Asthma is a chronic condition associated with acute exacerbations. It is characterized by reversible airway obstruction, inflammation, and increased airway reactivity. There are numerous stimuli that can cause varied reactions in different individuals. These include allergens, infectious organisms, and pollutants. In some individuals exercise alone can trigger an asthma attack.

Exercise induced asthma (EIA), recently referred to as exercise induced bronchoconstriction (EIB), can cause a variety of symptoms. These include: chest pain or tightness, cough, shortness of breath, endurance problems, or wheezing. The severity of the symptoms vary with the individual and with differing climatic conditions. Cold, dry air is often responsible for causing an asthmatic exacerbation. Some athletes will be more affected by the air condition than others. The severity of symptoms within an individual will often depend on that person's ability to warm and humidify inspired air. The athlete's minute ventilation and hydration status will therefore be important variables with regard to EIA. Minute ventilation is the total volume of new air entering the lung each minute. It is a factor of both the respiratory rate and tidal volume, both of which increase with exercise. Increases in minute ventilation lead to incomplete warming and humidification of inspired air, especially when exercise is first initiated. Symptoms often spontaneously improve, presumably as pulmonary blood flow increases, helping to warm and humidify inspired air.

Symptoms of EIA typically peak within the first 15 min of exercise. For many athletes, if exercise can be continued, the symptoms will spontaneously resolve. Others will require treatment. In some, the onset of symptoms may be delayed up to 8 h after exercise.

The most effective treatment is prevention. When possible, athletes with EIA should choose sports that can be performed in warm moist climates (i.e., swimming). Regardless of the sport, these athletes should undertake a vigorous warm-up of 15 to 30 min prior to competition.

Inhaled β-2 agonists (i.e., albuterol) are very effective in the treatment of EIA, for most athletes, when used 5 to 15 min prior to exercise. The medication may be repeated if necessary for intense exercise lasting longer than 2 h. Use of a long-acting β-2 agonist such as salmeterol may provide relief beyond 2 h. This medication may be more helpful for those exercising longer than 1 h or for those that wish to use their inhaler hours before participation. The duration of action in EIA is not clearly defined but the medication should be used at least 30 min prior to exercise.

Cromolyn sodium is generally used for the treatment of chronic asthma. Its efficacy is less than the β-2 agonists when used sporadically to treat EIA. Common side effects present with the use of β-2 agonists are related to their stimulant properties. Tremor, nervousness, palpitations, tachycardia, and increased blood pressure can occur. All of which would be much less common with cromolyn; however, cromolyn does have adverse effects including throat irritation or dryness, cough, wheeze, or nausea. The dose timing for this medication, when used for EIA, is 30 min prior to competition. There is an additive effect when cromolyn is used together with albuterol in those athletes who have incomplete relief from symptoms with the β-2 agonists alone.

Leukotriene-receptor agonists offer a different approach to the treatment of EIA. These drugs work to mediate the inflammatory component of the condition. Recent research has demonstrated beneficial effects for some, but not all, participants in a study on the effects of montelukast taken once daily for the treatment of this disease. This oral medication has no known side effects or drug interactions. In those who benefited from this medication the positive effects lasted at least 20 h. The National Collegiate Athletic Association (NCAA) and the U.S. Olympic Committee (USOC) have approved this drug for use in their athletes.

Corticosteroids are the best treatment for chronic, severe asthma. In some individuals with EIA, inhaled steroids are used when β-2 agonists and cromolyn, alone or in combination, are not sufficiently controlling the symptoms.

Exercise-induced anaphylaxis is characterized by a constellation of potentially life-threatening symptoms following the onset of physical activity, with no known contact or ingestion of an allergen. Usually the exercise-induced reaction is relatively minor, with most symptoms resolving within hours. The more common minor symptoms, however, such as pruritus, urticaria, and excessive cutaneous flushing, may be accompanied by airway findings and respiratory distress. Exercise-facilitated urticaria or pruritus may occur from exposure to an allergen, during exercise, that does not otherwise cause symptoms in the individual. Many affected athletes have a personal or family history of atopy.

An anaphylactic reaction is a medical emergency. Treatment includes airway and vascular support, epinephrine, corticosteroids, antihistamines, and other medications as needed, with emergency transfer to an appropriate health care facility.

In situations where an *allergic reaction* is facilitated by exercise, the etiologic agent should be identified. If a food or medication is responsible, it should be avoided for several hours prior to exercise. Other causative factors, such as a particular fabric, should be avoided during exercise. Exercise modification or change in environment may be necessary. The use of nonsedating antihistamines or cromolyn may be helpful prophylactically and in the treatment of mild reactions. Individuals with known reactions involving exercise should carry an epinephrine kit, wear or carry medical alerting information, and avoid exercising alone. These athletes should be advised against participation in scuba diving and other high risk activities.

Sudden death at an athletic event in a previously healthy individual is a rare, but devastating occurrence. In younger athletes (<30 years old) anatomic cardiovascular abnormalities are usually found at autopsy. The most common abnormalities are hypertrophic cardiomyopathy and anomalous origin or number of coronary arteries. Many of the structural cardiac problems have a known inheritance pattern and, therefore, all athletes should be questioned during their preparation physical examination with regard to sudden death in a family member. As the most common causes of sudden death in this age group, consisting of previously healthy individuals, are unlikely to be diagnosed on physical examination, referral to a cardiologist should be made in any individual with a history suggestive of cardiac problems.

In athletes over 30 years old, atherosclerotic coronary artery disease (CAD) is responsible for the majority of sudden deaths. This is true even though regular exercise reduces the risk of a fatal cardiac event secondary to CAD. This dichotomy underlines the fact that well-conditioned athletes are not protected from CAD.

MEDICAL CONDITIONS AFFECTED BY EXERCISE

Individuals with *sickle cell disease or trait* often participate in organized sports without any problems. In conditions of extreme oxygen deprivation or dehydration tissue ischemia may occur secondary to vasoocclusive events. Prompt administration of oxygen and fluid resuscitation is indicated. Arbitrary exclusion of these individuals from athletic activities is not indicated, although those with sickle cell disease should be considered for exercise stress testing prior to participation in strenuous activities.

Insulin dependent diabetes mellitus (IDDM) is a chronic, autoimmune disease in which antibodies are made against pancreatic islet cells. These antibodies act mostly on β-islet cells leading to subhomeostatic production of insulin. The α-islet cells are affected to a lesser extent, causing a partial glucagon deficiency and, therefore, a decreased response to hypoglycemia.

Insulin is necessary for glucose uptake into myocytes, but the need for insulin as a facilitator of glucose transport is diminished during exercise. This increased muscle sensitivity to insulin may last up to 24 h after physical activity. This potential for excess insulin effect is also enhanced by a greater absorption of injected insulin during exercise. Thus, increased muscle sensitivity combined with increased absorption of insulin during exercise may lead to hypoglycemia.

Glucagon and epinephrine are released in response to hypoglycemia. Release of epinephrine, however, may be reduced as a result of neurologic damage that may exist after several years of diabetes. The decrease in epinephrine release may blunt the symptoms that an individual had previously recognized as being associated with hypoglycemia.

The risk of severe hypoglycemia is greatest in the hours following strenuous activity. The increased glucose uptake into myocytes and hepatocytes following exercise, which is necessary for glycogen replenishment, also contributes to potential hypoglycemia. The nadir in the diabetic athlete's blood sugar is often reached 6 to 15 h after exercise. Profound hypoglycemia can, therefore, occur while the individual is asleep, potentially resulting in severe morbidity or mortality. Diabetic athletes, therefore, need to check their blood sugars often, including before, during, and after periods of intense activity, especially while in the unconditioned state. Prior to the commencement of exercise the athlete should be euvolemic, relatively euglycemic, and nonketonuric. Carbohydrate intake should be increased before, during, and after exercise.

Insulin should be given at least 1 h prior to exercise. The dose should be timed so as not to a have peak effect during strenuous activity. Glucagon should always be available as an emergent diagnosis treatment for hypoglycemia where the severity of symptoms precludes oral treatment. Glucagon can be administered intramuscularly and will cause a breakdown of stored glycogen (increasing circulating glucose) within minutes of injection. Hypoglycemia should always be considered to be the cause of a seizure or altered mental status in a known diabetic; glucagon should be administered emergently. High risk activities are to be avoided. Would make emergent diagnosis and treatment very difficult. Examples would be rock-climbing, race-car driving, or scuba diving.

The major benefits of exercise in the person with IDDM are the same as those for the general population, including maintenance of ideal body weight, improved self-image, and an improved cardiogenic risk profile.

In *non-insulin dependent diabetes mellitus* (NIDDM) insulin resistance, rather than production, is the problem. In this condition exercise is a part of the treatment regimen, as it will help to maintain euglycemia. The risk of hypoglycemia is low in athletes with NIDDM unless insulin is being used as part of the treatment.

The sequelae of diabetes may preclude participation in specific activities. A careful preparticipation examination should be undertaken assessing for conditions such as hypertension, peripheral neuropathy, and retinopathy. Exercise guidelines based on exam findings can then be provided.

OTHER MEDICAL PROBLEMS ASSOCIATED WITH EXERCISE

Drug abuse. In athletes, drugs have been used to enhance performance by improving strength, speed, or fine motor control. Narcotics may be used to mask pain inappropriately. Diuretics may be used to "make weight" in wrestling or boxing by causing water weight loss. The use of such drugs may lead to dehydration or disturbance in electrolyte balance, which can cause further problems including seizures and death.

Many properly used, prescribed medications are illegal for competitive athletes. The NCAA and the USOC each have specified legal and illegal drugs for athletes. Lists of these drugs, as well as testing protocols, have been published (Knopp et al, 1997). It is the physician's responsibility to be aware of the signs of illegal drug use, particularly for the adverse health effects that many drugs have, and to not prescribe a medication that is illegal in competition.

The misuse of *anabolic steroids* continues to be a problem for both the competitive and recreational athlete. Individuals use anabolic steroids for a variety of reasons including the hope of increasing muscle mass and strength, and increasing endurance. Steroids may be taken orally or injected intramuscularly. Many athletes self-administer these drugs cyclically and will often "stack" (use multiple drugs at once). The pattern of increasing the dose through a cycle is known as "pyramiding."

Side effects of anabolic steroid use are numerous. They include increased rate of muscle strains and ruptures, premature physeal closure, hypertension, thrombosis, hypercholesterolemia, decrease in HDL cholesterol, hepatitis (both infectious and noninfectious), severe acne, alteration in gonadotropic hormones which can lead to testicular atrophy, decreased testosterone, and decreased spermatogenesis. Gynecomastia may also occur. In females masculinizing effects such as hirsutism, voice deepening, clitoral hypertrophy, and male pattern baldness may occur. Individuals also may experience mood swings, irritability, aggressiveness, and altered libido. Depression and other symptoms may occur with withdrawal.

The incidence of use of anabolic steroids has been difficult to study because of the illegality of the issue. However, the rate of new female use is thought to be increasing relative to new male use in high school students.

Anorexia, amenorrhea, and osteoporosis are the constellation of problems defining the *female athlete triad*. Disturbed self image or the notion that being thin will make one more competitive are often the initiating issues leading to abnormal eating patterns. Anorexia nervosa is characterized by a distorted self image, fear of gaining weight or becoming fat (despite being underweight), loss of 15 percent body weight or falling 15 percent below recommended ideal weight for height and age, and missing three consecutive menstrual cycles. Athletes who start vigorous training prior to puberty may experience primary amenorrhea, that is, not having any mentrual periods by 16 years of age. Bulimia nervosa is characterized by binge eating and purging, on average at least twice a week for 3 months, in conjunction with a distorted self image.

Bone loss and lack of new bone formation often follow oligomenorrhea or amenorrhea. Return of normal menstrual cycles does not appear to cause bone density to return to normal. Therefore, emphasis on prevention is extremely important. In addition, cardiac arrhythmias may be precipitated by eating disorders.

Physical examination findings in those with insufficient caloric intake may include: weight loss or decreased percentile on a standardized growth curve, fat and muscle loss, dry hair and skin, cold extremities, decreased core temperature, lanugo (fine, soft hair that normally covers a fetus), lightheadedness, or bradycardia.

SUGGESTED READINGS

American Psychiatric Association: *Diagnostic and Statistical Manual of Mental Disorders*, 4th ed. Washington D.C.: American Psychiatric Association; 1994.

Briner WW: Physical allergies and exercise. Clinical implications for those engaged in sports activities. *Sports Med* 1993; 15(6):365–373.

Burke AP, et al: Sports related and not-sports related sudden cardiac death in young athletes. *Am Heart J* 1991; 121:568–575.

Finney TP, D'Ambrosia RD: Sudden cardiac death in an athlete. In DeLee, Drez (eds): *Orthopaedic Sports Medicine Principles and Practice*. Philadelphia, WB Saunders; 1994:404.

Jarjour NN, Lemanske RF: Management of exercise-induced asthma. In DeLee, Drez (eds): *Orthopaedic Sports Medicine Principles and Practice*. Philadelphia, WB Saunders; 1994:320.

Johnson MD: Disordered eating in active and athletic women. *Clin Sports Med* 1994; 13(2):355–369.

Kark JA, Ward FT: Exercise and hemoglobin. *Semin Hematol* 1994; 31(3):181–225.

Knopp WD, Wang TN, Bach BR Jr: Ergogenic drugs in sports. *Clin Sports Med* 1997; 16(3): 375.

Landry GL, Allen DB: Diabetes mellitus and exercise. *Clin Sports Med* 1992; 11(2):403–418.

Leff JA, et el: Montelukast, a leukotriene-receptor antagonist, for the treatment of mild asthma and exercise induced bronchoconstriction. *N Engl J Med* 1998; 339:147.

McFadden ER Jr, Gilbert IA: Exercise induced asthma. *N Engl J Med* 1994; 330:1362.

National Asthma Education Program Expert Panel Report: *Guideline for the Management of Asthma*. National Institutes of Health, Publication #91–3042, 1991.

Nattiv A, et al: The female athlete triad: The inter-relatedness of disordered eating, amenorrhea, and osteoporosis. *Clin Sports Med* 1994; 13(2): 405–418.

Nelson JA, et al: Effect of long-term salmeterol treatment on exercise-induced asthma. *N Engl J Med* 1998; 339:141.

Nichols AW: Exercise-induced anaphylaxis and urticaria. *Clin Sports Med* 1992; 11(2):303–312.

Taunton JE, McCargar L: Managing activity in patients who have diabetes. *Physician Sports Med* 1995; 23(3):41–52.

Van Camp SP: Sudden death. *Clin Sports Med* 1992; 11(2):273–289.

Chapter 110

CONGENITAL ANOMALIES

Lester Silver

GENERAL CONCEPTS

The accepted classification of congenital abnormalities of the hand falls into seven categories (Table 110–1). The etiology of congenital hand abnormalities can either be genetic in 30 percent of the cases or non-genetic in 10 percent of the cases, the other 60 percent being from an unknown cause. The genetic etiology can be a single mendelian gene, multiple gene disorders, or a chromosomal abnormality. The nongenetic etiology can include environmental teratogens alone or in combination with genetic factors, usually with exposure between days 25 and 50 after conception.

Embryologically, the upper limb development precedes development of the corresponding lower limb. The sequence of limb development is proximal to distal and is as follows: On day 26 the arm bud appears, on day 33 the hand paddle appears, on day 41 digital rays appear, on day 47 finger separation begins, and on day 54 finger separation is complete.

The goals of surgery in congenital hand problems are to preserve and/or to improve function. Consideration must be given to the ability to place and maneuver the hand in space, and to the aesthetic appearance of the hand and limb.

The timing of surgery varies but generally can be considered in four categories:

1. First few days of life: if the viability of the limb is threatened (such as a digit constricted by a congenital band syndrome)
2. Before 1 year of age: if deformity is increasing by a tethering effect with growth (such as a radial club hand)
3. Within approximately 3 years of age: if the developmental patterns of limb use will be influenced by surgery (such as with a pollicization)
4. Age 4 years or more: if the cooperation of the child in rehabilitation is critical to success of the procedure (such as with a tendon graft)

Table 110-1

Classification of Congenital Abnormalities of the Hand

1. Failure of formation of parts
2. Failure of differentiation of parts
3. Duplication of parts
4. Undergrowth
5. Overgrowth
6. Congenital constriction ring syndrome
7. Generalized skeletal abnormalities with hand involvement

The most common malformations are syndactyly, which is more common in Caucasians, and polydactyly, which is more common in people of African ancestry due to a high incidence of postaxial (ulnar) polydactyly.

FAILURE OF FORMATION OF PARTS

Failure of formation of parts is either transverse or longitudinal. The transverse ranges from a complete amputation (Fig. 110–1) to merely short fingers (brachydactyly). Longitudinal failure of formation of parts can range from phocomelia (Fig. 110–2), in which the whole upper extremity is missing and the hand may be attached to the shoulder, to distal deficiencies of the radial side (radial club hand), the ulnar side (ulnar club hand), or the central distal hand (a cleft hand).

If there is a short below-elbow deficiency or amputation, the treatment of choice is to fit the patient with a passive type of prosthesis prior to one year of age and then increase the level of sophistication of the prosthesis as the child grows. In phocomelia, surgery is rarely indicated for any stabilization or limb lengthening procedures.

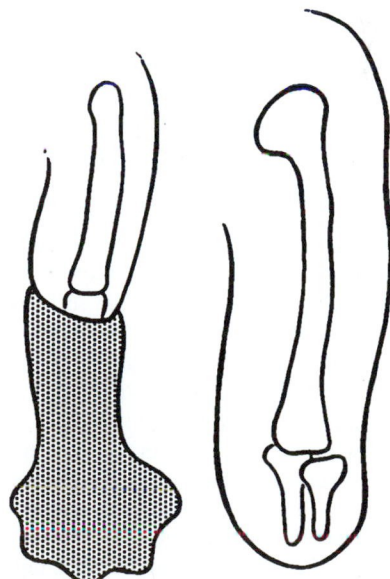

Figure 110-1
Failure of formation of parts: transverse (short below elbow amputation). [Reproduced and modified with permission from the American Society for Surgery of the Hand (ASSH): Congenital anomalies. In: ASSH 1996 Regional Review Course Syllabus. Englewood, CO: ASSH; 1996:17-2.]

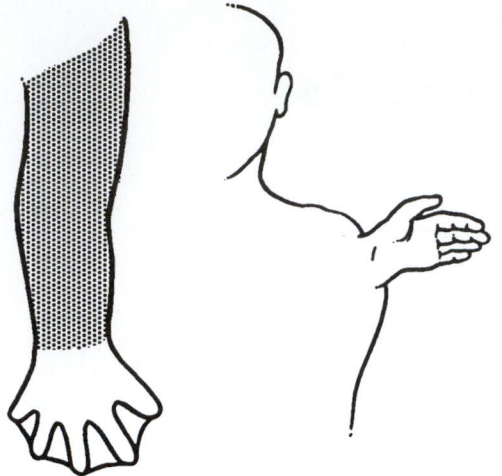

Figure 110-2
Failure of formation of parts: longitudinal (phocomelia). [Reproduced and modified with permission from the American Society for Surgery of the Hand (ASSH): Congenital anomalies. In: ASSH 1996 Regional Review Course Syllabus. Englewood, CO: ASSH; 1996:17-2.]

BRACHYDACTYLY (SHORT DIGIT)

If the digits are so short that they represent only useless tiny nubbins, amputation of the nubbins is the treatment of choice. Other options include a nonvascularized toe proximal phalanx transfer to fill the empty digital skin sleeve of the nubbin if it is of sufficient size, or a vascularized toe transfer(s) usually using the second toe, although the latter has limited indications. These short digits frequently represent symphalangism as well (discussed under "Failure of Differentiation of Parts").

RADIAL DEFICIENCY (LONGITUDINAL ABSENCE: DISTAL) RADIAL CLUB HAND

Radial deficiency is often associated with multi-system abnormalities. Some of these include hematopoietic (anemia and thrombocytopenia); gastrointestinal (tracheoesophageal fistula; imperforate anus); vertebral (hemivertebrae); cardiac; and other associated abnormalities, such as in the TAR (*thrombocytopenia and *absent *radius) syndrome and VATER (*vertebral defects, *anal atresia, *tracheoesophageal fistula with *esophageal atresia, and *radial and renal anomalies) association, as well as certain specific problems such as Fanconi anemia. In radial deficiency, the entire limb should obviously be evaluated because a stiff elbow, which is occasionally found, may contraindicate a distal centralization procedure. Digital mobility here is usually best in the ulnar digits. The treatment regime consists of stretching of the soft tissues on the radial aspect of the forearm beginning at birth with serial casting or splinting, followed by centralization of the hand and wrist on the distal ulna before 1 year of age. This may require an osteotomy of the ulna if it is angulated, and necessitates rebalancing the musculotendinous forces. A pollicization, usually of the index digit, is often necessary for an absent or hypoplastic thumb (usually at 2 to 3 years of age).

Various radiologic stages have been used to classify a radial club hand deformity: Stage 1—deficiency of the distal epiphyses. Stage 2—the radius is complete but short (hypoplasia). Stage 3—The radius is present proximally (partial aplasia), Stage 4—complete absence (total aplasia) of the radius. Often there are concomitant changes in the ulna, humerus and the carpus.

ULNA DEFICIENCY (LONGITUDINAL ABSENCE: DISTAL) ULNA CLUB HAND

In ulna deficiency, unlike the radial clubhand, associated systemic abnormalities are uncommon although other musculoskeletal abnormalities can be found. The elbow joint is primarily responsible for how the hand will be positioned in space, and in this condition problems with the elbow are common. The forearm and wrist will be ulnar deviated, the ulnar digits are often syndactylous, and the wrist tends to be stable.

In treating this deficiency, consideration must first must be given to the elbow where, if there is a severe flexion contracture, a release and splinting will be needed. A synostosis can be present between the humerus and radius, and this may require rotational osteotomies to improve the position of the hand. The wrist, although usually stable, may need to be released if there is progressive ulnar deviation.

CENTRAL DEFICIENCY (LONGITUDINAL ABSENCE: DISTAL) CLEFT HAND

Central deficiency represents a longitudinal absence where the distal central portion is missing (often referred to as a lobster-claw hand). It is often autosomal dominant and tends to be bilateral along with similar foot deformities. The defect varies from a simple cleft between the middle and ring fingers to hypoplasia of the radial digits and syndactylies, which are usually of the ulnar digits. A tight first web space is often found as well. Treatment of this disorder includes one or more of the following: closure of the central intermetacarpal defect with a skin revision, metacarpal osteotomy, ray transposition, and reconstruction of the transverse intermetacarpal ligament. If tight, the first web space needs to be released, and syndactylies, when present, should also be released. If extra transverse bones are present, which are usually at the metacarpal level, these should be excised with care to preserve the metacarpophalangeal joints.

FAILURE OF DIFFERENTIATION OF PARTS

RADIOULNAR SYNOSTOSIS

This is usually a proximal synostosis where the rotation of the forearm is affected and fixed; it is bilateral in over half the cases (Fig. 110–3A). In these instances, a rotational osteotomy or ostectomy is needed for the fixed elbow pronation deformity.

SYNDACTYLY

Syndactyly, along with polydactyly of the digits, are the most common congenital abnormalities of the hand (Fig. 110–3B). Syndactyly is spoken of as being either complete or incomplete in that either the full length of the interdigital space is involved or it only extends the partial length of the interdigital space. Also, it is classified as either being complex, where there is a bony union between the involved digits (usually of the distal or nail level), or simple syndactyly, where there is no union of the nail or the bone but just a skin union. There is a type of syndactyly referred to as acrosyndactyly, but this is not a true syndactyly. In this case, the fusion is present between the distal portion of the digits but there is an opening or tract between the proximal portion of the digits near the web space. That is because this is not a true failure of differentiation of parts but is, rather, secondary to a constriction band syndrome.

True syndactyly is most common between the middle and the ring fingers and then in decreasing order of frequency, between the ring and small fingers, the index and middle fingers, and the thumb and index fingers. The more complete and complex the syndactyly is, usu-

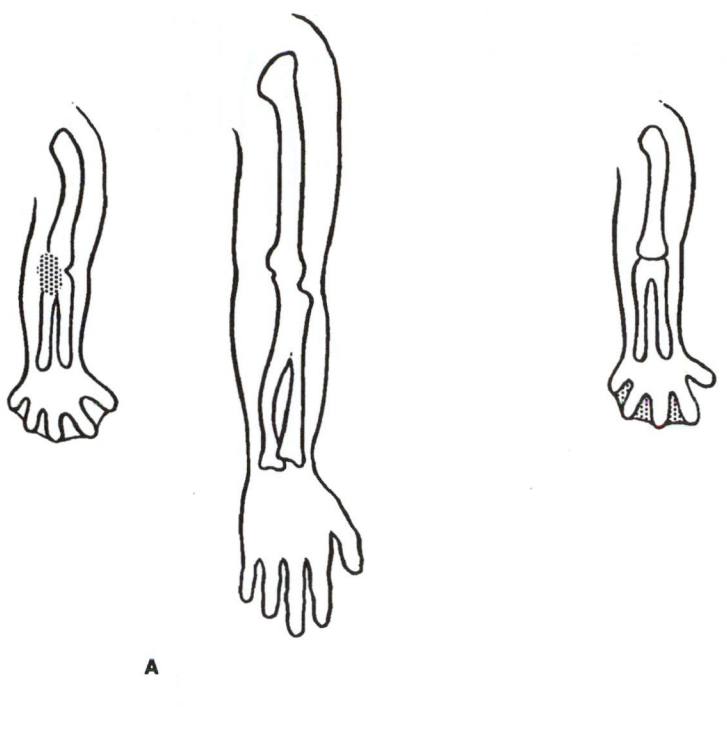

A

B

Figure 110-3
Failure of differentiation of parts: *A.* Synostosis. *B.* Syndactyly. [Reproduced and modified with permission from the American Society for Surgery of the Hand (ASSH): Congenital anomalies. In: ASSH 1996 Regional Review Course Syllabus. Englewood, CO: ASSH; 1996:17-2.]

ally the greater the chances are for an abnormality of other components of the digits.

Syndactyly is often found with certain syndromes; two of the best known are Poland's syndrome and Apert's syndrome. In Poland's syndrome the shortness of the digits tends to be due to a decrease in the size of the middle phalanx, and these shorter digits are usually totally syndactylous. There is often a general hypoplasia of the hand and noteworthy in this abnormality is an absence of the sternocostal head of the pectoralis major muscle on the same side.

In Apert's syndrome (also known as acrocephalosyndactyly) there is an associated hypertelorism with a bilateral complex syndactyly, often with symphalangism.

Treatment principles in syndactyly include the following: (1) Early separation is important when there is a distal adhesion in acrosyndactyly and whenever the syndactyly involves digits of unequal length; this could be done by six months of age. (2) Usually, only one side of a digit is released during each procedure because of the higher incidence of possible vascular abnormalities. (3) The web should always be created with a local skin flap. (4) Skin grafts are almost always needed, and full-thickness skin grafts are preferable. (5) The releasing incisions used are usually of a zig-zag type to decrease the incidence of postoperative linear scar contraction.

SYMPHALANGISM

Symphalangism is a congenital stiffness of the finger that can occur at any joint although it is usually at the proximal interphalangeal joint. The shortness tends to be due to shortness of the middle phalanx. This has been described as either a hereditary type, which is more common in the ulnar digits, or a nonhereditary type, which can be found in association with other abnormalities such as syndactyly. When treating this type of symphalangism, if it is to be treated, one usually waits until the epiphysis is fused and then an angulation osteotomy is considered.

CLINODACTYLY

Clinodactyly represents an angular digital deformity or curvature in the radioulnar plane. It is most commonly seen in the small finger

and can also be observed in a triphalangeal thumb. The curvature is usually toward the midline of the hand and is a result of a deformity of the middle phalanx which tends to be somewhat irregular or trapezoidal in shape. One cause is a so-called delta or triangular shaped phalanx which is due to an abnormal epiphyses. Most cases of clinodactyly of the small finger tend to be mild and are usually not treated. However, if the defect is severe the treatment will entail an osteotomy of the involved triangular shaped phalanx, usually of an opening wedge type.

CAMPTODACTYLY

Camptodactyly represents a flexion deformity of the digit which is usually at the proximal interphalangeal joint, and primarily affects the small finger. There are basically two types: one is found in infancy in males or females, and the second occurs in adolescent females. The function of these digits tends to be satisfactory. The etiology of the condition is basically unknown, but what has been described are abnormal insertions of the lumbrical and/or the superficial flexor tendon in the involved digit. Many of these are not treated because they represent only a mild deformity; however, when treatment is indicated it is directed towards the anomalies of the lumbrical or the superficial flexor tendon. The imbalance of the flexor, extensor, and intrinsic forces have to be addressed. It is noteworthy that camptodactyly is often seen in the fingers of patients with arthrogryposis.

ARTHROGRYPOSIS

Arthrogryposis is a motor unit defect between the anterior horn cell and the muscle. In this condition, because of the severity of the muscle weakness, the joints become immobile, and without appropriate therapy, lead to joint contractures. The disorder can be mild or extremely severe involving both upper and lower extremities. A peripheral as well as a general form of the disorder have been described. Treatment in mild cases is directed at correcting the isolated deformities that exist. In complex cases, treatment is directed at overcoming the severe contractures and in trying to substitute for the absent essential motor units.

FLEXED THUMB

The flexed thumb could either be the common type of trigger thumb in which the interphalangeal (IP) joint alone is involved, or a more complicated type of clasped thumb with more than just IP joint involvement. In the trigger type of thumb, where the deformity is at the IP joint, therapy and splinting is recommended, with surgical release of the first annular pulley if the condition is not improved as the infant approaches 12 months of age. The more complex variety of flexed thumb is a clasped thumb, which can be due to several factors. These can include one or all of the following: hypoplastic and/or weak extensor tendons, metacarpophalangeal joint flexion contracture, laxity of the ulnar collateral ligament, hypoplasia of the thenar muscles, and a tightness of the first web space. A clasped thumb, especially the more complex type, is often found in association with arthrogryposis and certain other pediatric syndromes.

In treating this disorder in infants, therapy and splinting is carried out initially, especially with the more supple thumbs. If the thumb remains supple but is weak, eventually a tendon transfer (such as transferring the extensor indices proprius) may be indicated. In the more complex clasped thumb, a series of procedures may have to be performed depending on the nature of the particular problem. These procedures may include: a release of all contractures on the palmar side, lengthening of the flexor pollicis, releasing the web space with a web space resurfacing with either a flap or graft, and tendon transfers as indicated on the extensor side.

DUPLICATION OF PARTS

POLYDACTYLY

When polydactyly involves the little finger, it tends to be genetic and is often bilateral. When polydactyly involves the thumb, it is usually more of a sporadic problem unless it involves a triphalangeal thumb which does have a genetic component. The least common type of polydactyly is the central type.

THUMB DUPLICATION

Thumb duplication is a type of polydactyly (Fig. 110–4) which can occur at any level. The accepted classification is the so-called Wassel classification (Fig. 110–5), wherein there are seven types of duplicated thumb abnormalities.

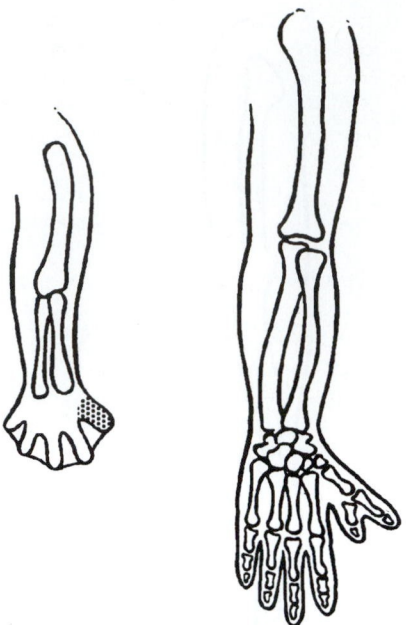

Figure 110-4
Duplication of parts. [Reproduced and modified with permission from the American Society for Surgery of the Hand (ASSH): Congenital anomalies. In: ASSH 1996 Regional Review Course Syllabus. Englewood, CO: ASSH; 1996:17–3.]

The treatment for duplication varies with the type. If the thumbs are of relatively equal size, such as is often the case in types 1 and 2, a procedure that shares components of both thumbs (Bilhaut-Cloquet) can be used where slightly more than half of each of these hypoplastic thumbs is used. It is not unusual in the treatment of these to have residual nail deformities and occasional unintentional epiphysiodesis. In more proximal types, the choice of treatment is based on the size, deviation, function, and mobility of the involved digit. On occasion, the decision as to the procedure cannot be made until the time of surgery when the anatomy becomes clear. As outlined by Lister (1994), the principles to be followed in the most common type of thumb duplication (type 4) are as follows: Try to retain the ulnar thumb if possible, as this avoids the need to reconstruct the ulnar collateral ligament; explore and realign the flexor and extensor tendon insertions; divide the anomalous connections between the flexor and

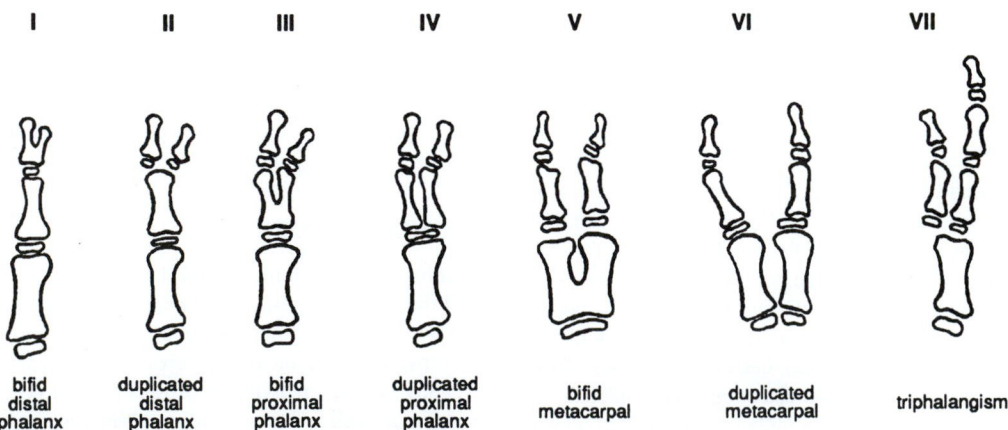

I	II	III	IV	V	VI	VII
bifid distal phalanx	duplicated distal phalanx	bifid proximal phalanx	duplicated proximal phalanx	bifid metacarpal	duplicated metacarpal	triphalangism

Figure 110-5
Wassel classification. [Reproduced and modified with permission from the American Society for Surgery of the Hand (ASSH): Congenital anomalies. In: ASSH 1996 Regional Review Course Syllabus. Englewood, CO: ASSH; 1996:17–3.]

extensor tendons; shave the metacarpal head on the side of the excision of the duplicate to avoid a postoperative prominence in this area; reconstruct the collateral ligaments; and reattach the intrinsics.

If there is a triphalangeal thumb, it can be an isolated abnormality or part of a type 7 duplication. The extra phalanx is between the proximal and distal phalanges and may often be a so-called *delta* or triangular phalanx. This delta phalanx may need to be excised early. If not seen until later the combination of one-joint arthrodesis and wedge osteotomy often is necessary. If the triphalangeal thumb approaches a true five-fingered hand, then the operation of choice is a pollicization.

A central polydactyly is the least common type and often found with syndactyly. This is the most difficult type to treat because of the intimate involvement between the involved digits with syndactyly, and it is not unusual following surgery in this instance that stiff or deviated digits will result. Often, not all of the fingers in a central polysyndactylous mass can be preserved.

UNDERGROWTH

Undergrowth primarily refers to hypoplasia or aplasia of the thumb and has been classified by Blauth from grades one through five. *Grade one* is a minor hypoplasia where all elements are present and the thumb is just slightly smaller than normal. Further stages progress to include web contractures, decreased muscles, decreased intrinsics, and further skeletal hypoplasia, up until *grade five* which is a total absence of the thumb. Hypoplasia of the thumb can therefore be seen in association with many other findings.

Treatment options, in the milder forms of hypoplasia, include an opponensplasty (often done by a hypothenar muscle transfer), collateral ligament and capsular advancement and reinforcement, and a web space release with local flaps. In the more severe hypoplastic/absent thumbs, it is recommended that the useless hypoplastic thumb be ablated and that a pollicization of the index finger to the thumb position be carried out. When doing a pollicization, the principles involve the following: local skin flaps to establish the first web space, skeletal shortening with rotation of the bone, preservation of neurovascular structures, and rebalancing the musculotendon forces wherein the extensors are shortened and the intrinsics are reinserted. The timing of a pollicization operation should take into consideration that the developmental pattern of the limb use will be affected by the surgery. Consequently, many authors have been doing this procedure at a progressively younger age, but the surgery generally is performed at approximately 3 years of age.

OVERGROWTH

MACRODACTYLY

An overgrowth can be due to a particular disorder, such as a vascular malformation, a hemangioma, or a lymphangioma. However, within this discussion, the primary concern is the disorder known as *macrodactyly*. In the true type of macrodactyly all of the structures are involved. This is a congenital enlargement, not usually hereditary, usually unilateral, and in most instances more than one digit is involved. The involved digits tend to correspond to a peripheral nerve territory (usually the median), leading certain authors to refer to this disorder as a nerve territory oriented overgrowth. Consequently, a neurogenic influence has been postulated as to the etiology of the overgrowth of the affected tissue.

There are basically two types of macrodactyly. The first is a static type which is present at birth wherein the growth keeps pace with the growth of the remainder of the hand. The second is a progressive type which may not be noted at birth but where the growth is faster than that of the adjacent parts of the extremity. This growth can be dramatic and result in stiffness, deviation, and impairment of the neurovascular status of the involved part. Although the etiology of this true type of macrodactyly generally is unknown, if patients are followed for a period of time some cases will eventually fall into the category of neurofibromatosis as other manifestations of this disorder make themselves apparent. Also, macrodactyly of the true type must be differentiated from various types of fibromatoses, many of which are fairly aggressive, and some approach a sarcoma-like presentation. Also, macrodactyly is described in conditions where the overgrowth is due primarily to fatty tissue (that is, a lipomatosis, such as in the Proteus syndrome). Treatment tends to follow certain guidelines in these enlarged digits and hands. If the affected digit is severe and is a single digit, it is often best to ablate it. However, if it is not severe and/or if there are multiple digits involved, treatment options include: epiphysiodesis, bone shortening, debulking to keep up with the growth, or nerve stripping. It should be noted that despite all of the aforementioned treatment options, scarred and stiff digits are not an unusual outcome in these cases.

CONSTRICTION RING SYNDROME

Constriction ring syndrome is also known as annular band syndrome (Fig. 110–6), and occurs sporadically. The results of the congenital constriction bands are variable, ranging from a superficial ring constriction alone to a more constrictive ring with lymphedema of the segment distal to the ring. With further constriction, there will be necrosis of the digital parts which then necrose causing distal syndactyly; however, when an opening remains proximally near the web

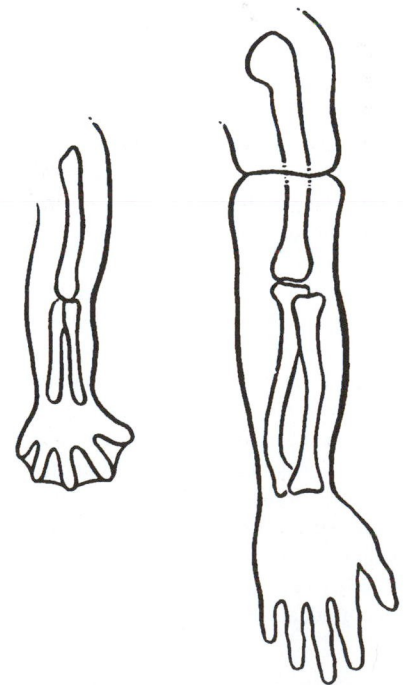

Figure 110–6
Constriction band. [Reproduced and modified with permission from the American Society for Surgery of the Hand (ASSH): Congenital anomalies. In ASSH 1996 Regional Review Course Syllabus. Englewood, CO: ASSH; 1996:17–6.]

between the digits, that is acrosyndactyly. The final presentation of a constriction ring is an amputation where the ring was so severe that the segment distal to the ring did not survive, resulting in a congenital amputation. In these cases, there is a tapered appearance at the point of amputation and often the bone is tapered as well.

The treatment of these constriction rings involves a release of the tight ring or band as well as all of the structures beneath it and closure with interposed flaps such as a Z-plasty or W-plasty. The release should include the skin and subcutaneous tissue and the fascia. If the constriction ring is severe at birth, with impairment of both the circulation and neurological function distal to the ring, an early release is advised. It was initially thought that only a portion of the circumference of the part should be done at one operative procedure in order to preserve the circulation to the distal portion; however, more recent magnification techniques make it reasonable to do multiple Z-plasties in a circumferential fashion at the same operative procedure. The annular band could result in acrosyndactyly or thumb amputation. These conditions are treated as already noted.

GENERALIZED SKELETAL ABNORMALITIES

In addition to the classification of intrinsic congenital hand abnormalities, there is a category of hand problems wherein the hand involvement is only one aspect of a generalized skeletal abnormality. Examples of this would include diastrophic dwarfism, Marfan's syndrome, and multiple hereditary exostoses. In these, and in other generalized skeletal abnormalities, the hand problem will fit into one of the previously noted categories in which case the hand abnormality is treated as already discussed. The difference is that what needs to be done for the hand as well as the timing of the procedure will often be dictated by the patient's generalized abnormality and what, if any, treatment is indicated for that. In many instances, hand procedures can be done concomitantly with other skeletal operations.

FUTURE DIRECTIONS

Technology has changed the way diagnosis and treatment proceed regarding congenital hand anomalies. Present technology allows the diagnosis of some anomalies to be made in utero as a result of more liberal use of newer imaging techniques. At present, hand anomalies do not fit into the category of those surgeries likely to be done in utero although this would take advantage of the fetus's potential for scar-free healing. The techniques currently available in radiology regarding scanning and imaging the hand and upper extremity have also been of assistance for earlier diagnosis and planning for treatment. This, along with the evolution of microsurgical techniques, has resulted in a tendency towards performing earlier surgery and applying procedures to these small structures at an age that was previously thought unsuitable. Lastly, certain new technologies continue to evolve, which to some degree does change the outlook for treatment. One example of this is the Ilizarov technique that has become common in orthopaedics for limb lengthening in recent years. This technique has applicability in congenital deformities not only for lengthening but also for gradual correction of angulation and contraction

deformities of the hand and wrist. A significant amount of cooperation is needed for this labor intensive procedure so the patient probably should be almost school age before the technique is applied.

It should be noted regarding the treatment of congenital hand anomalies that the decision as to what is to be done with the hand is made by the surgeon in conjunction with the parents, with the result setting the stage for the usage pattern of the hand and extremity. This plays a large part in the future as to what that child will be able to do. Unlike an adult who sustains an injury where the usage pattern and needs of the person are already known and the surgical procedure can be adapted to the needs of the patient, when dealing with infants and children, this decision is made for them without knowledge of prior usage patterns. Consequently, all decisions managing congenital hand problems should be made only after full discussion with the parents, as well as consideration of the child's general condition and suitability for surgery.

SUGGESTED READINGS

Barsky AJ: Cleft hand: classification, incidence, and treatment. *J. Bone Joint Surg [Am]* 1964; 46:1707.

Brons JT, van der Harten HJ, Van Geijn HP, et al: Prenatal ultrasonographic diagnosis of radial-ray reduction malformations. *Prenat Diagn* 1990; 10:279.

Broudy AS, Smith RJ: Deformities of the hand and wrist with ulnar deficiency. *J Hand Surg [Am]* 1979; 4:304.

Buck-Gramcko D: Congenital malformations. In Nigst N, Buck-Gramcko D, Millesi H, et al (eds): *Hand Surgery*. New York: Thieme; 1988:chap 12.

Buck-Gramcko D: Pollicization of the index finger. Method and results in aplasia and hypoplasia of the thumb. *J Bone Joint Surg [Am]* 1971; 53:1605.

Buck-Gramcko D: Radialization as a new treatment for radial club hand. *J Hand Surg [Am]* 1985; 10(6 pt 2):964.

Cheng JC, Chow SK, Leung PC: Classification of 578 cases of congenital upper limb anomalies with the IFSSH system—10 years' experience. *J Hand Surg [Am]* 1987; 12(16):1055.

Dobyns JH, Wood VE, Bayne LG, Frykman GK: Congenital hand deformities, In Green DP (ed): *Operative Hand Surgery*, vol II. New York: Churchill Livingstone; 1982:213.

Flatt AE: *The Care of Congenital Hand Anomalies*, 2d ed. St. Louis: Quality Medical Publishers; 1993.

Ledesma-Medina J, Bender TM, Oh KS: Radiographic manifestations of anomalies of the limbs. *Radiol Clin North Am* 1991; 29:383.

Light TR (ed): The pediatric upper extremity. *Hand Clin* 1990; 6(4).

Light TR, Manske PR: Congenital malformations and deformities of the hand. In Barr JS Jr (ed): *Instructional Course Lectures*. Park Ridge, IL: American Academy of Orthopaedic Surgeons. 1989; 38:31.

Lister GD. Congenital. In Manske P (ed): *Hand Surgery Update*. Englewood, CO: American Society for Surgery of the Hand; 1994.

Manske PR (ed): Thumb reconstruction. *Hand Clin* 1992; 8(1).

Netscher DT, Scheker LR: Timing and decision-making in the treatment of congenital upper extremity deformities. *Clin Plast Surg* 1990; 17:113.

Siegert JJ, Cooney WP, Dobyns JH: Management of simple camptodactyly. *J Hand Surg [Br]* 1990; 5(15):181.

Smith RJ, Lipke RW: Treatment of congenital deformities of the hand and forearm. Parts I and II. *N Engl J Med* 1979; 300:344, 402.

Smith RJ: Congenital deformities of the hand. *Hand Clin* 1985; 1(3):371.

Tsuge K: Treatment of macrodactyly. *J Hand Surg [Am]* 1985; 10(pt 2):968.

Upton J, Tan C: Correction of constriction rings. *J Hand Surg [Am]* 1991; 16(5):947.

Chapter 111

ARTHRITIS OF THE HAND AND WRIST

Jamie R. Wisser, Jose M. Santiago-Figueroa, and Steven A. Stuchin

This chapter will review the general aspects, diagnoses, and management of arthritic conditions affecting the hand and wrist. The clinical aspects of rheumatoid arthritis are emphasized. Osteoarthritis and other arthritides will be reviewed to complete the overview of inflammatory and degenerative joint diseases affecting the hand and wrist.

RHEUMATOID ARTHRITIS

One out of four surgical procedures performed on the arthritic patient involves the hand and wrist areas. Hand reconstruction can improve function and appearance but will never restore complete premorbid status. Weakness and limited dexterity remain significant disabilities. A multidisciplinary approach and candid discussions with patients concerning prognosis and expectations are essential facets of surgical management. The multidisciplinary team should include rheumatologists, physical and occupational therapists, as well as hand and orthopaedic surgeons, who can perform reconstructive operative procedures in the arthritic patient.

Rheumatoid arthritis is a chronic, systemic, autoimmune inflammatory disease without known etiology. The joint synovial folds are the site of an antibody-antigen and antibody-antibody reaction producing complement-level reduction, changes in vascular permeability, and white blood cell infiltration. Inflammatory changes produce joint cartilage destruction, effusions, instability, and tendon degeneration. Deformities and imbalance of the joints secondary to this pathologic process aggravate the destruction of articular cartilage. The pannus is granulation tissue of the synovium which, in turn, fuels further progression in cartilage erosion. Rheumatoid synovitis infiltrates tenosynovium, the joint capsule, and stabilizing ligaments. Rheumatoid synovitis can cause primary tendon rupture by attenuation, or produce tendon rupture secondarily by affecting tendon gliding and nutrification at impingement points aggravated by bone and joint destruction. The most common site of tendon involvement is at the extensor retinaculum of the dorsal ulnar wrist.

SURGICAL TREATMENT IN RHEUMATOID ARTHRITIS

The indications for surgical management in rheumatoid patients are: (1) progression of disease and synovitis despite appropriate medical management, (2) severe pain, (3) nerve entrapment and tendon rupture, and (4) deformities causing impairment of function. Operative priorities are to control pain, delay the progression of the disease, restore function, and correct cosmetic deformities. Patient expectations prior to operative intervention must be clarified and modified through patient education. Patients need to be aware that postoperative restoration of function and dexterity will never reproduce the prediseased state.

A thorough preoperative evaluation is invaluable in reducing the patient's risk of suffering intraoperative or perioperative complications. A thorough cervical spine evaluation should be performed in all rheumatoid patients to rule out instability. Temporomandibular pathology should also be assessed in order to reduce the risk of perioperative anesthetic complications. Rheumatoid patients being treated with gold, D-penicillamine, or aspirin (ASA) may have depressed platelet function and are susceptible to perioperative bleeding. Aspirin should be discontinued 10 to 14 days prior to surgery to allow platelets with *irreversibly* inhibited cyclooxygenase to be replaced with newly produced, untreated platelets. Nonsteroidal anti-inflammatory drugs (NSAIDs) affect cyclooxygenase *reversibly* and should therefore be discontinued prior to surgery at a time period equal to five times the particular medication's dosage interval to reverse the platelet effect. NSAIDs are typically stopped 5 to 7 days prior to surgery in most clinical practices.

Surgical treatment options can be classified as preventive, corrective, or as salvage procedures. As a *preventive* option, synovectomy has proven to lower the incidence of tendon rupture and is considered most effective when performed in the early stages of rheumatoid arthritis with one or two joint involvement in patients under effective medical control. Some have extended the indications of synovectomy to include those patients with moderate disease and have achieved fair results. *Corrective* procedure options include tendon transfer, nerve decompression, soft tissue reconstruction, and synovectomy as well. *Salvage* procedures are performed in those patients with advanced disease and include total joint arthroplasty and arthrodesis.

Rheumatoid nodules occur in 20 to 25 percent of patients with rheumatoid arthritis, but can also be seen in systemic lupus erythematosus. Rheumatoid nodules are commonly seen in the olecranon area and posterior forearm, but occur in the digits as well. Patients who develop rheumatoid nodules have strong seropositivity and aggressive forms of the disease. Digital nodules are unsightly in appearance and can mechanically compress digital nerves producing pain. Operative removal requires meticulous hemostasis to avoid hematoma and draining sinus formation; both are difficult to manage. *Rheumatoid nodulosis* is a separate entity comprised of multiple rheumatoid nodules with only intermittent polyarthralgias and minimal joint destruction.

The Rheumatoid Wrist

The wrist is the cornerstone to the balanced hand. The wrist should always be considered prior to, or at the same time as, any distal region in the hand when contemplating surgery. The pathomechanics of the rheumatoid wrist are critical to understanding the principles of surgical management.

The inflammatory process creating synovitis of the wrist joint creates attenuation of the distal radio-ulnar joint, and the volar radiocarpal and ulnocarpal ligaments. The outcome is a dissociation of the distal radioulnar joint with dorsal migration of the ulna, supination of the carpus, scapholunate dissociation, rotatory scaphoid displacement, and carpal collapse. The extensor carpi ulnaris dislocates volarly aggravating both carpal supination and wrist collapse. The final wrist and hand deformity is a radially and volarly deviated carpus (supination), carpal collapse, metacarpal radial shifting, and ulnar drifting of the fingers. This creates a non-functional intrinsic plus hand with a caput ulna and the propensity for fixed digital deformity and tendon ruptures to occur.

RADIOCARPAL JOINT The indications for wrist synovectomy are not well established as synovectomy has not clearly been demonstrated to alter the natural course of the disease. The wrist joint is composed of multiple articulations making total synovectomy technically impossible. This may affect operative outcome. Synovectomy has been shown to improve pain and preserve grip strength, but carpal collapse and ulnar translocation of the digits are not prevented.

On the other hand, patients who suffer from persistent wrist pain under stable medical management and demonstrate slow disease progression with minimal carpal collapse are good candidates for total wrist synovectomy. A dorsal approach to the wrist through either the fourth or sixth extensor compartment is commonly utilized. Curvilinear incisions and elevation of thick cutaneous flaps reduce the risk of skin sloughing. A volar approach to the wrist is indicated when there is clinical evidence of flexor tenosynovitis, median nerve compression, or flexor tendon rupture. Although a functional range of motion is preserved, the overall range of motion is decreased following wrist synovectomy.

Equilibrium of forces across the wrist joint is important for function. Tendon relocation and transfer of the wrist extensors is indicated when deforming forces are identified early and articular cartilage of the wrist joint is preserved. Extensor carpi ulnaris (ECU) relocation and transfer of the extensor carpi radialis longus (ECRL) to the ECU insertion is an effective soft tissue procedure to balance the wrist.

A soft tissue stabilization, or "shelf procedure," can be performed on a painful, volarly, and radially subluxed wrist with successful alleviation of pain while preserving some degree of radiocarpal motion. Motion is preserved through resecting the distal radius and relocating the carpus to intentionally create a pseudoarthrosis. Pain relief is obtained once the pseudoarthrosis has formed. Unintended radiocarpal fusion is the most common complication of this procedure.

Partial wrist arthrodesis can be used successfully in patients who have severe radiocarpal disease with midcarpal articular preservation. Radioscapholunate or radiolunate fusion can prevent a progression of ulnar translation and preserve 25 to 50 percent of wrist motion. Rapidly progressive disease is a contraindication to radiolunate fusion.

Total wrist arthrodesis has been and still is the procedure of choice for advanced rheumatoid arthritis. This salvage procedure is predictable, provides stability, and provides excellent pain relief. The optimal wrist position in a unilateral arthrodesis should be in neutral or slight extension with some ulnar deviation. Radial deviation should be avoided. In patients undergoing bilateral wrist arthrodeses one wrist may be positioned in flexion to help with personal hygiene. The single intramedullary rod technique is used when wrist arthrodesis is combined with metacarpophalangeal (MP) joint replacement. The dual intermetacarpal-intramedullary technique is also used. Both techniques minimize surgical exposure and have very low non-union rates.

Patients with advanced disease in whom wrist motion must be preserved may undergo wrist arthroplasty as a salvage procedure. Ideal patients for this procedure typically: (1) have low demand, (2) do not use assisting devices for ambulation, (3) have good bone stock, and (4) have minimal tendon imbalance. Resection arthroplasty with interposition of a silastic implant is the most common technique. Studies have shown that results deteriorate over time with a high incidence of implant fracture and synovitis. The use of grommets for protection of the implant has decreased the incidence of synovitis and

breakage. The total post-operative arc of motion should be limited to 80 degrees. Bilateral wrist arthroplasties are contraindicated.

Caput ulna syndrome is the clinical entity created by a combination of joint swelling, instability, pain, and limitation of pronation and supination. If severe, this condition can cause the Vaughan-Jackson injury in which the extensor digitorum communis (EDC) tendons of the ring and little fingers and the extensor digiti minimi (EDQ) tendon rupture at the dorsal ulnar side of the wrist. Early treatment with tenosynovectomy and ECU relocation can avoid rupture of these extensor tendons. Once ruptured, the little finger extensors are reconstructed by transferring the extensor indicis proprius (EIP) tendon to the EDQ. A side-to-side tenoplasty of the extensor communis tendon of the ring finger to the intact extensor communis tendon of the long finger reconstructs a tendon motor for ring finger extension.

DISTAL RADIO-ULNAR JOINT (DRUJ) The traditional method for reconstructing the DRUJ in the rheumatoid patient has been the resection of the distal ulna, or Darrach procedure. Ulnar stump instability is the most common complication of the Darrach procedure and is more likely to occur when greater than 2 cm of the distal ulna is resected. Carpal collapse can similarly worsen with loss of bony support of the ulnar side of the wrist.

A hemiresection interposition technique of the distal ulna (HIT) has been described by Bowers and is utilized in the management of rheumatoid DRUJ pathology. The articular surface of the ulnar head is resected to match the sigmoid notch of the radius followed by soft tissue stabilization. The HIT procedure should be done in patients with mild to moderate degeneration of the DRUJ. A prerequisite in patient selection is that the triangular fibrocartilage complex (TFCC) is either intact, or at least reconstructable.

The Sauve-Kapandji procedure involves fusing the DRUJ and creating a pseudoarthrosis in the ulna distally. This procedure is recommended for young rheumatoid patients with DRUJ involvement. Formation of an ulnar pseudoarthrosis typically improves wrist pronosupination. Components of the procedure critical to maintaining the pseudoarthrosis include the length and location of the ulnar resection (a 1.2- to 1.5-cm segment is removed just below the ulnar head) as well as complete resection of any periosteum within the gap. Proximal ulnar stump instability is a potential complication of the Sauve-Kapandji procedure. Excess bone resection can lead to instability. Attaching the proximal ulnar segment to the pronator quadratus fascia during the initial operation can reduce the risk of instability and bone bridging. Non-union of the radioulnar fusion site and decreased wrist flexion and extension are additional complications of this procedure.

THE RHEUMATOID HAND

Metacarpophalangeal Joint Deformities

Proliferative synovitis at the metacarpophalangeal joint (MP) produces joint capsular and ligamentous attenuation. Forces due to tendon imbalance across the wrist result in volar and ulnar forces at the MP joint. Nalebuff and Millender stage MP rheumatoid joint involvement which is used to govern treatment. Stage I disease is limited to synovitis and is treated nonoperatively with local steroid injections and splinting. Stage II disease involves cartilage and bony erosions and surgical synovectomy is indicated. In stage III disease, volar and ulnar joint subluxation takes place, but the hand remains moderately functional. Splinting and medication are the mainstay of treatment, but soft tissue joint reconstruction is beneficial provided some degree of cartilage preservation is maintained on both sides of the joint. Soft tissue procedures include: crossed intrinsic transfer, extensor tendon relocation, capsular reefing, synovectomy with intrinsic release, and division of the junctura tendinae. Stage IV disease is classified by advanced joint destruction with fixed deformity and loss of function. MP arthroplasty is the procedure of choice provided fixed wrist deformities are addressed and corrected prior to, or simultaneously with, MP joint replacement surgery. Total joint arthroplasty is complemented by capsular reefing, crossed intrinsic transfer, and extensor tendon relocation at the time of surgery. Following MP arthroplasty, patients experience good pain relief, cosmetic improvement, and bone remodeling rather than absorption. Grip strength does not appreciably improve with this procedure. A regimented postoperative splinting protocol (static followed by dynamic) is critical to successful outcome.

Proximal Interphalangeal Joint

Proximal interphalangeal joint (PIP) involvement in rheumatoid patients involves synovial proliferation, ligamentous and tendinous attenuation, and tendon force imbalance. Boutonniere deformities (PIP flexion/DIP extension) can occur due to attenuation of the central slip and palmar lateral band migration. Ultimately contracture of the transverse and oblique retinacular ligaments produces a fixed deformity. Tendon imbalance at the terminal tendon results in DIP extension. Stage I disease, in which there is synovitis but mild deformity, is correctable with splinting, synovectomy, central slip reconstruction, lateral band repositioning dorsal to the rotation axis, or terminal tendon tenotomy. Stage II disease is manifested by a 35- to 45-degree flexion contracture able to be corrected with passive extension. Surgical options for stage II disease are similar to those listed for stage I. Stage III disease is classified by a fixed PIP flexion contracture unable to be passively corrected. Salvage procedures for stage III disease include arthroplasty or arthrodesis.

Swan-neck deformities may occur in the involved PIP joints. Superficialis tendon rupture or palmar plate attenuation can produce PIP hyperextension primarily. Secondary PIP hyperextension can result from terminal tendon attenuation or rupture at the DIP joint producing a Mallet deformity with proximal tendon imbalance, or intrinsic tightness secondary to MP subluxation similarly producing tendon imbalance at the PIP joint. Type I deformities have full PIP passive mobility despite MP positioning. Splinting can be successful

in treating type I deformities. Surgical options are flexor tenodesis to limit PIP hyperextension, and DIP fusion. Type II deformities are due to MP joint destruction and intrinsic tightness limiting PIP passive motion with MP extension. Intrinsic release or MP reconstruction are indicated for type II deformities. Type III deformities represent limited PIP flexion despite MP positioning with radiographic joint preservation. Lateral band mobilization from the central slip, closed manipulation with PIP joint k-wire fixation, and dorsal skin releases have been described as surgical options for type III deformities. Type IV deformities involve PIP joint destruction with loss of mobility. Joint arthrodesis is the most predictable surgical option and is recommended in index and middle fingers for pinching. Arthrodesis of the ring and little fingers is again most predictable, but PIP joint arthroplasty remains a surgical option for gripping.

Distal Interphalangeal Joint

Distal interphalangeal (DIP) joint deformities in rheumatoid patients may be due primarily to DIP joint disease or secondarily to proximal joint involvement. Primary DIP joint disease is best treated with arthrodesis. Surgical options for secondary joint involvement have been previously discussed in the context of PIP joint pathology.

Thumb Deformities

Rheumatoid disease of the thumb carpometacarpal (CMC), metacarpophalangeal (MP), or interphalangeal (IP) joints is due to an inflammatory proliferative synovitis that produces attenuation of ligamentous, capsular, and tendinous structures, and ultimately destroys cartilage and bone. Nalebuff classified rheumatoid thumb joint disease as a guideline for assessment and treatment (Fig. 111-1).

The Nalebuff type I thumb involves a boutonniere-like MP flexion deformity and secondary IP hyperextension. Joints are passively mobile. Attenuation of the extensor hood with volar and ulnar extensor pollicus longus (EPL) tendon subluxation produces the flexed MP posture with secondary intrinsic imbalance producing IP hyperextension. Soft tissue repair of the extensor hood and reinsertion of the EPL into the base of the proximal phalanx is acceptable for early Nalebuff type I deformities, but there is a relatively high rate of de-

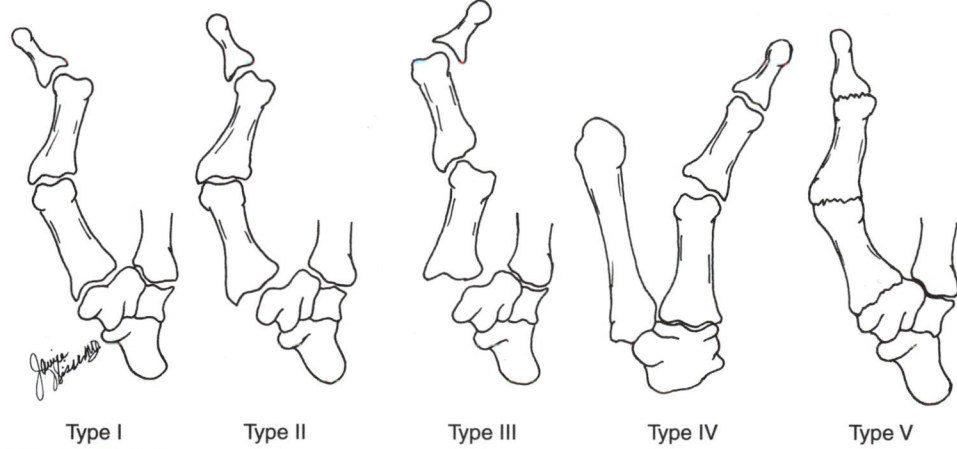

| Type I | Type II | Type III | Type IV | Type V |

Figure 111-1

A schematic depiction of bone and joint deformities of the rheumatoid thumb as described by Nalebuff. The Nalebuff type I deformity involves a boutonniere-like MP flexion deformity with secondary DIP hyperextension. All joints are passively correctable. Type II deformity is identical to type I with the addition of CMC radial subluxation. Type III deformities mimic swan neck deformities with CMC radial subluxation, MP hyperextension, and passively correctable DIP flexion. The type IV deformity (drawn as a radial side view) involves MP joint UCL laxity and a metacarpal adduction deformity. Finally, the type V deformity involves multilevel joint destruction with a fixed boutonniere-like deformity.

formity recurrence. Moderately advanced type I deformities involve a fixed MP deformity. MP arthrodesis is most suitable for the high demand patient while MP arthroplasty can be performed for the low demand patient. Advanced type I deformities involve fixed IP and MP deformities. Metacarpophalangeal arthroplasty with IP fusion, or fusion of both MP and IP joints are acceptable surgical alternatives. Minimal involvement and good functional status of the CMC joint are critical in combined fusion procedures.

Nalebuff type II deformities are rare and involve a type I boutonniere thumb deformity with CMC joint radial subluxation. CMC arthroplasty and potentially adductor fascial release are important surgical adjuncts in managing type II deformities.

Nalebuff type III thumb deformities mimic swan neck deformities with CMC radial subluxation, first metacarpal adduction, MP hyperextension, and passively correctable IP flexion. Early stages may be treated with CMC splinting or arthroplasty. Moderately advanced disease with passively correctable joints requires CMC arthroplasty with MP joint volar plate advancement or arthrodesis. Advance disease involves fixed joints and a first metacarpal adduction contracture which requires a CMC hemiarthroplasty, adductor fascial release, and MP arthrodesis.

Nalebuff type IV deformities are due to attenuation of the MP joint ulnar collateral ligament (UCL) due to synovitis with a resultant first metacarpal adduction deformity. Early surgical intervention involves UCL reconstruction with adductor fascial release and MP synovectomy. Late intervention includes UCL reconstruction with MP arthroplasty, or simply MP arthrodesis.

Nalebuff type V deformities involve multilevel joint destruction in the thumb (MP, IP) with a boutonniere-like deformity that is fixed. Surgical options include IP and MP arthrodesis in patients with an uninvolved CMC joint, or IP arthrodesis with MP arthroplasty.

JUVENILE RHEUMATOID ARTHRITIS

Inflammatory arthritis that begins before the age of 16 is considered juvenile rheumatoid arthritis (JRA), often referred to today as juvenile idiopathic arthritis (JIA). Three modes of JIA onset have been classified: (1) systemic, (2) polyarticular, and (3) pauciarticular. *Systemic* onset has variable joint involvement and no particular immunologic testing correlation. *Polyarticular* onset involves inflammatory synovitis and arthritis in more than four joints and is associated with IgM rheumatoid factor in 5 to 20 percent of cases and a positive Anti-nuclear antibody test (ANA) in 25 to 75 percent of cases. *Pauciarticular* onset involves arthritis in one to four joints and has a 60 to 80 percent ANA immunologic marker correlation, while IgM rheumatoid factor presence is rare. Medical treatment involves high level ASA treatment maintaining serum blood levels of 20 to 30 mg/dl but has been associated with gastronintestinal, hepatic complications, and a concern over potential development of Reye's syndrome. Tolmetic sodium and Naproxen are FDA approved NSAIDs for use in treating JIA.

Joint involvement in the hand and wrist is most commonly seen in the polyarticular form of JIA. Distal upper extremity joint involvement is usually symmetrical and manifested by wrist flexion with ulnar deviation, accompanying stiffness of the MP joints, and PIP extension. Flexor tenosynovitis is more common than extensor tenosynovitis. Open physes of affected joints are subject to growth arrest. The mainstay of treatment is corrective splinting and medical management.

Operative intervention is indicated for disease progression despite medical management. Synovectomy provides pain relief but does not alter joint motion. Flexor tenosynovectomy can improve joint motion and should be undertaken if local synovial steroid injections fail to improve motion. Spontaneous fusion of the carpometacarpal and in-

tercarpal joints of the wrist with limited radiocarpal motion is common. Should the ankylosis not occur in a position of function, corrective osteotomy should be performed. A painful DRUJ due to ulnar shortening can be treated by a hemiresection interposition arthroplasty as described by Bowers.

OSTEOARTHRITIS

Osteoarthritis (OA) is a slowly progressive degenerative condition affecting diarthrodial joints. Osteoarthritis is a primary disorder of hyaline cartilage. The hand and large weight-bearing joints are most commonly affected. The most commonly affected hand joints are the finger DIP, PIP, and thumb CMC joints.

Osteoarthritis of the hand is classified as primary or secondary. Primary OA most commonly affects women, has a familial predisposition, and is often characterized by the formation of osteophytic nodules at the base of the distal phalanx known as Heberden's nodes. Erosive inflammatory OA is a subgroup of primary OA typically seen in postmenopausal women and is manifested by acute onset of pain and swelling of the PIP and DIP joints. Erosive joint destruction occurs within a short period of time and may mimic the clinical picture of rheumatoid arthritis. Secondary OA is a degenerative joint process caused by trauma, prior inflammatory processes, avascular necrosis, or metabolic disorders.

The diagnosis of osteoarthritis in the hand is based on clinical evaluation and confirmed radiographically. Patients generally complain of pain, weakness, loss of mobility, and joint deformities. Limited deformity without pain or functional disability is rarely an indication for surgery. Clinical evaluation should include accurate measurement of joint motion arcs, pinch, and grip strength for each joint that is involved. The overall function of the hand should be carefully assessed and each joint's deformity and relative stability should be carefully documented. Distal interphalangeal joint examination should include the extent and distribution of Heberden's nodes and mucous cysts. The presence of osteophytic nodules at the base of the middle phalanx, or Bouchard's nodes, should be evaluated and noted. Thumb trapeziometacarpal joint evaluation should include assessing subluxation, adduction deformity, and pain secondary to metacarpophalangeal joint hyperextension. Provocative stress testing of the thumb CMC joint involves axial loading and repeated rotation of the thumb, otherwise known as "grind" testing, and helps to clinically assess the degree of degeneration. Correlation of clinical findings with plain radiographs generally completes patient assessment and guides treatment plans.

The majority of patients with osteoarthritis can be treated nonoperatively. Initial management should include resting the affected joint with activity restriction and/ or splinting. Immobilization or rest should be followed by a controlled regimen of stretching and strengthening exercises to functionally stabilize and improve motion of the affected joint. Nonsteroidal anti-inflammatory drugs (NSAIDs) and acetaminophen have not been proven to be more effective than rest. They can, however, provide symptomatic relief, although they do not affect the natural progression of osteoarthritic joint degeneration.

SURGICAL TREATMENT IN OSTEOARTHRITIC PATIENTS

Distal Interphalangeal Joint

Indications for surgical management of osteoarthritic DIP joints are: (1) intractable pain, (2) deformity with instability, and (3) existence of a problematic mucous cyst. Arthrodesis of the DIP joint is the most frequently performed and reliable operative procedure for OA. Joint position for fusion varies from 10 to 15 degrees of flexion for the index finger, progressing to 30 degrees of flexion for the small finger. Arthroplasty of the DIP is infrequently indicated due to the relatively high rate of complications and failures. Mucous cysts are most often associated with an osteophyte that can cause progressive enlargement of the cyst, nail plate deformity, pain, or infection. Treatment should be debridement of the associated osteophyte and synovial tissue. If joint degeneration is advanced with a limited motion arc, arthrodesis may be a preferable treatment option for mucous cysts.

Proximal Interphalangeal Joint

Surgery for PIP joint osteoarthritis is most commonly performed for pain refractory to medical therapy. Proximal interphalangeal joint deformity, or instability with functional impairment are also operative indications. Stiffness and cosmesis are generally not indications for surgery. Stabilizing the index and long fingers for lateral pinch with the thumb is important. In the ring and small fingers preservation of motion of the PIP joint is crucial for power grip strength. This approach is translated into performing PIP arthrodesis in the index and long fingers and arthroplasty in the ulnar digits. Arthrodesis of the ulnar digits should be considered in a young manual worker. The position of PIP arthrodesis should be 40 degrees in the index, 45 degrees in the long, and 50 degrees in the ring and little fingers.

Trapeziometacarpal Joint

Operative indications for trapeziometacarpal joint reconstruction are: (1) pain, or (2) deformity associated with functional limitation. Asymptomatic patients with severe radiographic degeneration of the trapeziometacarpal joint should not be candidates for surgery. The specific operative procedure described for treatment of basal joint arthritis of the thumb varies depending upon the degree of joint degeneration. Painful instability with preservation of joint cartilage is successfully treated by reconstruction of the oblique volar ligament with a slip of flexor carpi radialis (FCR) tendon as described by Eaton and Littler. Patients with mild degenerative changes can be treated with a closing wedge extension osteotomy to unload the joint.

Advanced degenerative changes in the trapeziometacarpal joint are best treated by a salvage procedure. Joint arthrodesis has declined in popularity due to the high incidence of pseudoarthrosis, progression of arthritis in adjacent joints, and the inability to manipulate the hand into restricted areas or on a flat surface. Arthrodesis may be indicated in a young patient with high demands. The most commonly performed salvage procedure is trapeziometacarpal arthroplasty. Excisional arthroplasty was described by Gervis in 1949. The major drawbacks are weakness and CMC instability. Excisional arthroplasty is a good option to treat failed infected implant arthroplasties. Interposition arthroplasty with a silastic or metal implant have presented various types of complications and failures. The compromise between excisional and implant arthroplasties is a ligament reconstruction and interposition arthroplasty (LRIA) described by Burton and Pelligrini in 1986. The trapezium is excised through a volar approach and the volar oblique ligament is reconstructed with a slip of the flexor carpi radialis tendon. Utilizing harvested tendon as a "space filler" following trapezium excision has been described and is known as the anchovie procedure.

OTHER ARTHRITIDES

PSORIATIC ARTHRITIS

The clinical hallmarks of psoriatic arthritis (PA) are psoriasis associated with a typical asymmetrical polyarthritis producing fusiform "sausage swelling" of the digits with absence of subcutaneous nod-

ules or resorptive changes on plain radiographs. DIP joints, unlike in rheumatoid arthritis, are commonly involved. Psoriatic arthritic patients are typically seronegative and are found in familial aggregates. The incidence of specific haplotypes HLAB27, HLADR7, and HLA DR4 is quite high in these patients. There is a slightly higher incidence of PA in men. Rheumatoid disease occurs more frequently in women. The average age of onset is in the third decade and flare-ups may be initiated by trauma.

Psoriatic skin lesions usually antedate joint involvement, but may occur simultaneously in few cases. Four clinical subgroups of the disease are: (1) pseudorheumatoid psoriatic arthritis, (2) oligoarthritis, (3) spondyloarthropathy, and (4) distal interphalangeal joint psoriatic arthritis. *Pseudorheumatoid psoriatic* arthritis produces less virulent, symmetrical, distal joint involvement when compared to RA. Nodules are generally absent and flexor tenosynovitis of the wrist and digital flexor tendons is common. *Oligo-articular* psoriatic arthritis tends to involve one to three joints, is slowly progressive, and produces boutonniere digital deformities. The *spondyloarthropathy* form is hand sparing. The *distal interphalangeal joint* form produces IP joint swelling, pain, and redness. Radiographically this form of the disease can be differentiated from OA by *widening* of the joint space, and subsequent development of the pencil-in-cup deformity (see below). The DIP form can be rapidly progressive in patients with HIV infections.

Joint involvement in psoriatic arthritis differs from RA in that synovial inflammatory changes and edema produce fibrosis and erosion of articular margins which often progresses to the adjacent bone shaft. A synovial pannus is not typically present. The radiographic findings demonstrate marginal erosions along the phalangeal shafts producing a scalloped appearance while the joint space is maintained. Whittling of the phalangeal distal end with associated bony overgrowth at the tendon insertion site produces the pencil-in-cup radiographic sign. Periostosis of adjacent ligamentous insertions and nail calcifications can also be seen along with terminal phalangeal tuft erosion. The *mutilans* form of psoriatic arthritis can produce PIP joint osteolysis radiographically and is seen clinically by digital shortening. The mutilans form can occur in both the pseudorheumatoid and oligoarthritis forms of the disease.

Medical management includes topical medications for skin lesions, ASA, NSAIDs, systemic corticosteroids, DMARDs (i.e., sulfasalazine and gold), and immunosuppressive agents (i.e., methotrexate and azathioprine). A hierarchal approach to medical management is effective when combined with hand therapy. Operative intervention at the wrist is indicated if the wrist does not spontaneously fuse in a functional position. Total wrist arthrodesis with or without ulnar shortening is the procedure of choice. Interphalangeal joints generally remain mobile. Painful interphalangeal joints with minimal mobility are most reliably treated with arthrodesis. Interphalangeal joint arthroplasty is difficult to perform due to phalangeal bony erosion, but has been performed as an alternative to joint fusion.

SCLERODERMA

Scleroderma or systemic sclerosis is a connective tissue disorder with the hallmark of skin and visceral fibrosis. The diagnosis is made based on easily recognized findings of thickened skin. Skin fibrosis is preceded by an inflammatory phase in which prominent vascularity is seen. Treatment in the inflammatory phase can retard fibrotic progression. The two disease classifications are: (1) diffuse cutaneous systemic sclerosis (dSSc) involving truncal skin, widespread visceral fibrosis, rapid progression, and has the worst prognosis; and (2) limited cutaneous systemic sclerosis (lSSc) which has a more indolent course with less visceral disease and contains the subgroup of patients with CREST syndrome (calcinosis, Raynaud's phenomenon, esophageal hypomotility, sclerodactyly, telangiectasia). Sclero-70 antibody testing is seropositive in 40 to 50 percent of patients with systemic disease, and 80 percent of patients with CREST syndrome.

Scleroderma often affects the hand in the form of Raynaud's phenomenon, soft tissue calcifications, skin ulcers, PIP joint flexion deformities, and septic arthritis. Raynaud's *phenomenon* occurs in 90 percent of patients with scleroderma and is associated with painful cutaneous ulcerations of the distal digits. Raynaud's *disease*, in contrast, is a reversible vasospastic entity common in young women which seldom produces permanent deformities. Raynaud's phenomenon is associated with proper and common digital arterial occlusion, with or without vasospasm, and frequently involves the superficial arch and ulnar artery. Local skin care and temperature protection, in combination with calcium channel blockers (i.e., Nifedipine), is effective in 60 percent of cases. Operative intervention is indicated when environmental protection and medical interventions fail. Preoperative evaluation includes pulse volume recordings (PVR) performed before and after stellate ganglion anesthetic blockade to determine the presence of signal augmentation and potential effectiveness of surgical sympathectomy. Failure of abnormal digital PVR augmentation is followed by arteriography to determine the level and location of fixed lesions for arterial reconstruction considerations. Operative choices include sympathectomy as well as palmar arch and ulnar artery reconstruction. Necrotic fingertips may be left to autoamputate or may be surgically amputated.

Severe, fixed flexion deformities of 90 degrees of the PIP joint are best treated with arthrodesis. Calcific deposits should be debrided if they erode through the skin or are painful. The skin is left open to heal secondarily in these circumstances. Good pain relief is usually obtained.

SYSTEMIC LUPUS ERYTHEMATOSUS

Systemic lupus erythematosus (SLE) is a multisystemic immune disease with variable aggressiveness and characteristic periods of remission and exacerbation. SLE primarily affects females with a prevalence of 1 in 1000. There is genetic association with HLADR2, and a familial aggregation. SLE is characterized by the production of autoantibodies (i.e., ANA), and more specifically anti-DNA antibodies. Clinical evidence suggests SLE flare-ups may be initiated by environmental, chemical, hormonal, infectious, or stress factors. Clinical manifestations are multisystemic involving the spleen, heart, lungs, kidneys, thymus, lymphatics, and synovium.

Over 90 percent of patients with SLE have arthritis which frequently involves the hand in a rheumatoid-like fashion. The inflammatory changes can occur with SLE flare-ups and changes can often be temporary without permanent affect. Some patients develop progressive rheumatoid-like deformities of the hand clinically, but these tend to be pain-free and joint erosion is not seen on plain radiographs. Patients with fixed arthritic changes have *joint laxity* at the MP joints known as Jacoud's arthritis. The rheumatoid-like findings include ulnodorsal subluxation, palmar distal radius subluxation, ulnar subluxation of the extensor tendons at the MP joints with extensor lag, ulnar deviation of the MP joints, and PIP swan neck deformities. Trapeziometacarpal laxity with radial subluxation, secondary thumb MP hyperextension, and an IP flexion deformity can occur. The joints, however, tend to be hyperflexible rather than fixed early on during the disease process. Although splinting may be corrective during medical treatment with corticosteroids, disease progression can lead to fixed deformities.

Surgical intervention includes distal ulna resection for painful DRUJ symptoms or tendon erosion at the extensor retinaculum. Although frequently asymptomatic, painful intercarpal instability is predictably treated with wrist arthrodesis. Soft tissue reconstructions are less reliable. If interphalangeal joints are passively correctable, arthroplasty is a reasonable option to arthrodesis for management of pain or instability. Success has been limited with digital joint arthroplasty when joint deformities have become fixed.

CRYSTAL-INDUCED ARTHRITIS

Crystal-induced arthritides are produced by deposition of sodium urate crystals (gout) or calcium pyrophosphate crystals (pseudogout) in upper extremity joints. The wrist and hand joints are frequently involved in crystal-induced arthritides. Acute forms of the disease may mimic infectious arthritis while indolent disease forms may mimic rheumatoid arthritis. Joint aspiration for crystal analysis and fluid culture is invaluable as a diagnostic tool. Sodium urate chrystals are strongly negative birefringent needle-shaped crystals found in polymorphonuclear (PMN) white blood cells. Calcium pyrophosphate crystals are negative or weakly positive birefringent crystals under plane polarized light.

Attacks of acute gouty arthritis most often occur in the first metatarsophalangeal joint (podagra) or the knee, but can present in wrist or hand joints. Wrist involvement in the elderly can produce diffuse hand edema in both gout and calcium pyrophosphate deposition disease (CPPD). Tendinitis is rare, but olecranon bursitis is common. Acute attacks of gout are produced by PMN crystal phagocytosis and the release of lysosomal enzymes. Acute gouty attacks may include tenosynovitis and tendon rupture. Management is medical with NSAID therapy (i.e., Indomethacin), or may consist of 40 U intramuscular injections of adrenocorticotropin (ACTH). Colchicine has been found to have undesirable side effects and is the third line of treatment for acute gouty arthritis attacks. Temporary usage of resting splints can reduce symptoms.

Chronic gouty arthritis is produced by the release of collagenase and stromelysin by cells in the tophi periphery resulting in pathognomonic erosive bone lesions adjacent to moderately radio-dense, partially calcified, soft-tissue masses (tophi) seen on plain radiographs. Recurrent acute attacks warrant prophylactic treatment against chronic disease using Probenecid or Allopurinol.

Surgical management involves diagnostic aspiration, and is otherwise reserved for patients in whom medical management has failed. Operative procedures include carpal tunnel release, tenosynovectomy, tophi debridement, and hand or wrist arthroplasty or arthrodesis.

Pseudogout or calcium pyrophosphate deposition disease (CPPD) has a propensity to involve the wrist, occurs aggressively and spontaneously, and is easily confused with septic arthritis. Joint aspiration is critical in making the diagnosis. Fusiform swelling of the hand occurs distal to the involved wrist. Digital joints can be involved in a form of the disease known as *pseudorheumatoid CPPD*. Pseudorheumatoid CPPD should be considered in patients with new onset, spontaneous signs of RA who are rheumatoid factor seronegative. Calcification of the TFCC and the carpal bone cartilage are hallmark radiographic findings in CPPD. Scapholunate dissociation is a common finding; disease advancement produces narrowing of the radiocarpal and intercarpal joint spaces. Joint splinting is typically successful in relieving symptoms concomitant with medical management with ACTH, NSAIDs, or Colchicine. Surgical intervention outside of joint aspiration or synovial biopsy is uncommon and is generally limited to joint arthrodesis.

SUGGESTED READINGS

Albright JA, Chase RA: Palmar-shelf arthroplasty of the wrist in rheumatoid arthritis: A report of nine cases. *J Bone Joint Surg [Am]* 1970; 52:896.

Belsky MR, Feldon P, Millender LH, et al: Hand involvement in psoriatic arthritis. *J Hand Surg [Am]* 1982; 7:203.

Bowers WH: Distal radioulnar joint arthroplasty: The hemiresection-interposition technique. *J Hand Surg [Am]* 1985; 10:169.

Brumfield R Jr, Kuschner SH, Gellan H: Results of dorsal wrist synovectomies in the rheumatoid hand. *J Hand Surg [Am]* 1990; 15:733.

Burton RI, Pellegrini VD Jr.: Surgical management of basal joint arthritis of the thumb. Part II: Ligament reconstruction with tendon interposition arthroplasty. *J Hand Surg [Am]* 1986; 11:324.

Calabro JJ, Hogerson WB, Sonpal GM, et al: Juvenile rheumatoid arthritis: A general review and report of 100 patients observed for 15 years. *Semin Arthritis Rheum* 1976; 5:257.

Clawson MC, Stern PJ: The distal radioulnar joint complex in rheumatoid arthritis: An overview. *Hand Clin* 1991; 7(2):373.

Dray GJ: The hand in systemic lupus erythematosus. *Hand Clin* 1989; 5(2):145.

Eaton RG, Lane LB, Littler JW, et al: Ligament reconstruction for the painful thumb carpometacarpal joint: A long-term assessment. *J Hand Surg [Am]* 1984; 9:692.

Fleisher A, McGrath MH: Rheumatoid nodulosis of the hand. *J Hand Surg [Am]* 1984; 9:404.

Hamerman D: The biology of osteoarthritis. *N Engl J Med* 1989; 320:1322.

Jones NF, Imbriglia JE, Steen VD, et al: Surgery for scleroderma of the hand. *J Hand Surg [Am]* 1987; 12:391.

Katz WA: Psoriatic arthritis. In Katz WA, (ed): *Diagnosis and Management of Rheumatic Diseases,* 2d ed. Philadelphia: JB Lippincott; 1988:433.

Linscheid RL, Dobyns JH: Rheumatoid arthritis of the wrist. *Orthop Clin North Am* 1971; 2:649.

Parke A, Rothfield NF: Systemic lupus erythematosus. In Katz WA, (ed): *Diagnosis and Management of Rheumatic Diseases,* 2d ed. Philadelphia: JB Lippincott; 1988:448.

Posner MA, Ambrose L: Excision of the distal ulna in rheumatoid arthritis. *Hand Clin* 1991; 7:383.

Resnick CS, Miller BW, Gelberman RH, et al: Hand and wrist involvement in calcium pyrophosphate dihydrate crystal deposition disease. *J Hand Surg [Am]* 1983; 8:856.

Simmons BP, Nutting JT: Juvenile rheumatoid arthritis. *Hand Clin [Am]* 1989; 5:157.

Swanson AB, Poitevin LA, de Groot Swanson G: Bone remodeling phenomena in flexible implant arthroplasty in the metacarpophalangeal joints. Long-term study. *Clin Orthop* 1986; 205:254.

Terrono A, Millender LH, Nalebuff EA: Boutonniere rheumatoid thumb deformity. *J Hand Surg [Am]* 1990; 15:999.

Vaughan-Hackson OJ: Attrition ruptures of tendons in rheumatoid hands. *J Bone Joint Surg [Am]* 1958; 40:1431.

Yu T: Gout. In Katz WA, (ed): *Diagnosis and Management of Rheumatic Diseases,* 2d ed. Philadelphia: JB Lippincott; 1988:544.

Chapter 112

DUPUYTREN'S DISEASE

Stephen J. Eshman and Steven M. Green

Dupuytren's disease is characterized by pathologic changes of unknown etiology in palmar fascia and its digital prolongations. Typically, it affects males in the fifth to seventh decades of life and individuals of Northern European and Celtic descent. It is inherited as an autosomal dominant trait with variable penetrance. Male to female ratios vary from 2:1 to 10:1; females present at a later age and with less severe disease. Dupuytren's disease is associated with chronic alcoholism, diabetes mellitus, smoking, and chronic pulmonary disease. Typical clinical presentation begins with one or several pathognomonic nodules (often tender) in the palmar fascia of the ring and little fingers with adjacent skin dimpling. As the disease progresses, involvement of the palmar and digital fascia may produce flexion contractures of the MCP and PIP joints and occasionally the DIP joint. Additional anatomic sites of involvement include the dorsum of the PIP joint (knuckle pads), the dorsum of the penis (Peyronie's disease), and the plantar fascia (Ledderhose's disease). Dupuytren's diathesis represents a subset of patients with a strong positive family history and with aggressive early onset of disease afflicting both hands especially the radial side, the feet, and the penis.

ANATOMY AND PRESENTATION

Knowledge of the anatomy of the fascia of the palm and digits is crucial to understanding the pathology of Dupuytren's disease. By convention, normal fascia is termed "bands" and diseased fascia designated as cords. Figure 112-1A demonstrates the components of the palmar fascia that may become diseased. The palmar pretendinous bands are the most commonly affected structures. As the thickened band contracts and becomes cordlike, it produces a flexion contracture of the MCP joint. The transverse fibers of the palmar aponeurosis (superficial transverse metacarpal ligament) lie deep to the pretendinous band and are only affected in the first web space. The natatory ligament is frequently involved, and may cause adduction contractures.

Components of the normal digital fascia involved in Dupuytren's disease are illustrated in Figure 112-1B. The spiral band is a continuation of the pretendinous band of the palmar aponeurosis which is attached to skin and bifurcates distal to the MP joint to continue as a spiral band on either side of the digit. The band passes deep and then superficial to the neurovascular bundle as it proceeds distally. The lateral digital sheet is a condensation of superficial fascia on either side of the finger. Grayson's ligament functions to hold the skin in position during motion of the digit; it originates from the fibrous tendon sheath volar to the neurovascular bundle and attaches to the lateral digital sheet. Of note, Cleland's ligament is unaffected. Changes in normal fascia bands to diseased cords are illustrated in Figure 112-1C.

Three cords (central, spiral, and lateral) cause PIP contractures. The *central cord* is a midline structure often in continuity with a pretendinous cord and attaches to either side of the middle phalanx or flexor tendon sheath. The *spiral cord* arises from the spiral band or the abductor digiti minimi, the lateral digital sheet, and Grayson's ligament. With contracture, the spiral cord displaces the neurovascular bundle toward the midline, proximally and superficially. The *lateral cord* arises from the lateral digital sheet and is a contributor to PIP contracture. The retrovascular cord lies dorsal to the neurovascular bundle. It arises from the periosteum of the proximal phalanx, attaches to the distal phalanx, and is the main cause of DIP contracture. The *abductor digiti minimi cord* arises from the musculotendon junction of the abductor digiti minimi and inserts into the ulnar base of the middle phalanx of the fifth digit. The *first web space intercommissural cord* arises from the thumb pretendinous band, transverse fibers of the palmar aponeurosis, and natatory ligament and can cause a flexion and adduction contracture.

Luck grouped the histopathology of Dupuytren's disease into three stages in which the myofibroblast plays a central role. The cell of origin of the myofibroblast is unknown but three possibilities exist: fibroblast, smooth muscle cell, or pericyte. In the first stage (proliferative), large myofibroblasts predominant with numerous cell to cell connections; the nodules are vascular with numerous pericytes. The second stage (involutional) is characterized by dense myofibroblast network aligned to collagen bundles and an increased ratio of type III to type I collagen. In stage three (residual), the myofibroblasts disappear and fibrocytes predominate. It is theorized that these changes occur because of cellular oxygen free radicals produced from damaged microvasculature due to pericyte proliferation. Platelet-derived growth factor has also been implicated in this process.

TREATMENT AND FOLLOW-UP

Splinting and vitamin E treatment have been shown to be ineffective and chemical or enzymatic fasciotomy is experimental and unproven. Prior to the onset of contracture, steroid injection of painful nodules or knuckle pads has been advocated. The cornerstone of treatment is surgical fasciectomy. Surgical intervention is recommended for MCP contractures of 20 to 30 degrees and any loss of PIP mobility. Excellent exposure of all diseased fascia with complete visualization of the neurovascular bundle prior to excision of diseased fascia is imperative. Additional procedures to improve PIP correction include opening the tendon sheath, releasing the check rein ligament, the accessory collateral ligaments, and the volar plate. Popular incisions include longitudinal with Z-plasty, transverse, and zig-zag (Brunner). Fasciotomy is rarely employed because of a high recurrence rate and a high risk to the neurovascular bundle. Regional fasciectomy, in which only diseased fascia is removed, is the most commonly performed procedure. Dermofasciectomy (skin and all fascia removed) is reserved by some for recurrent disease and increased diathesis. Closure under tension is to be avoided due to the high incidence of

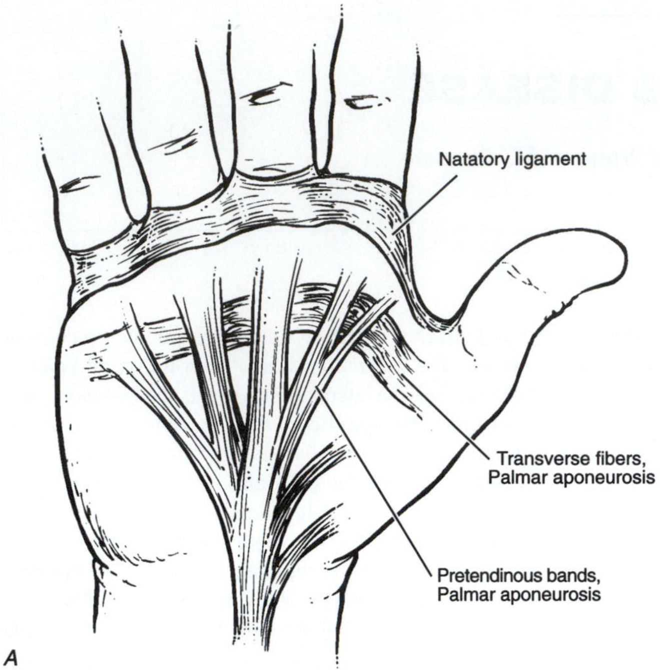

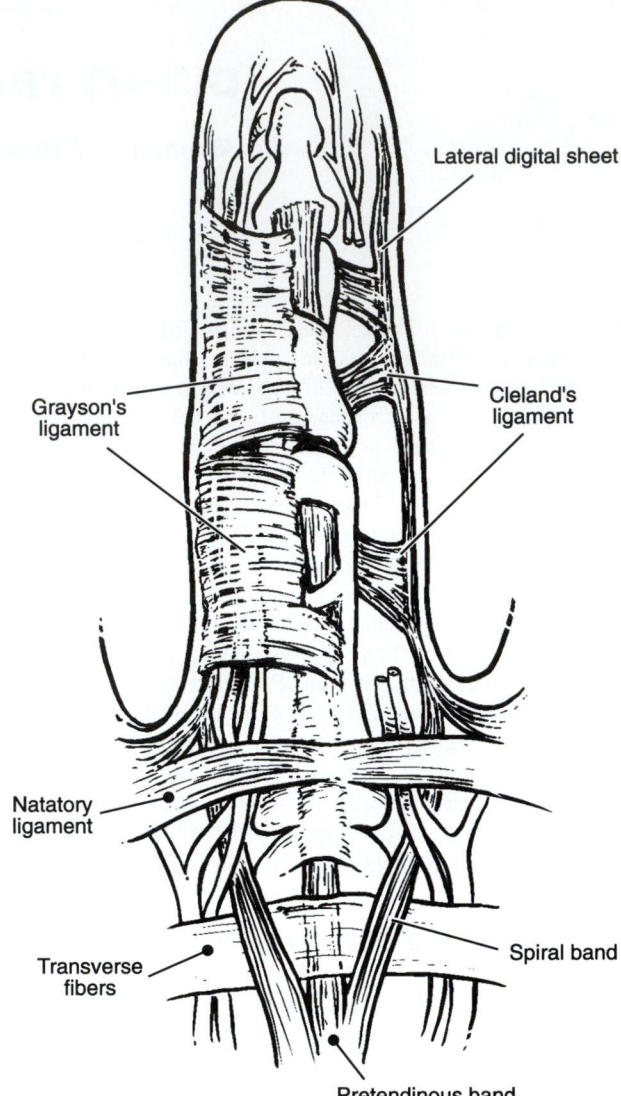

A. Natatory ligament

Transverse fibers, Palmar aponeurosis

Pretendinous bands, Palmar aponeurosis

A

B. Lateral digital sheet

Grayson's ligament

Cleland's ligament

Natatory ligament

Transverse fibers

Spiral band

B

Pretendinous band

C. Grayson's ligament

Spiral cord

Lateral cord

Central cord

Natatory cord

Pretendinous band

Intrinsic muscle

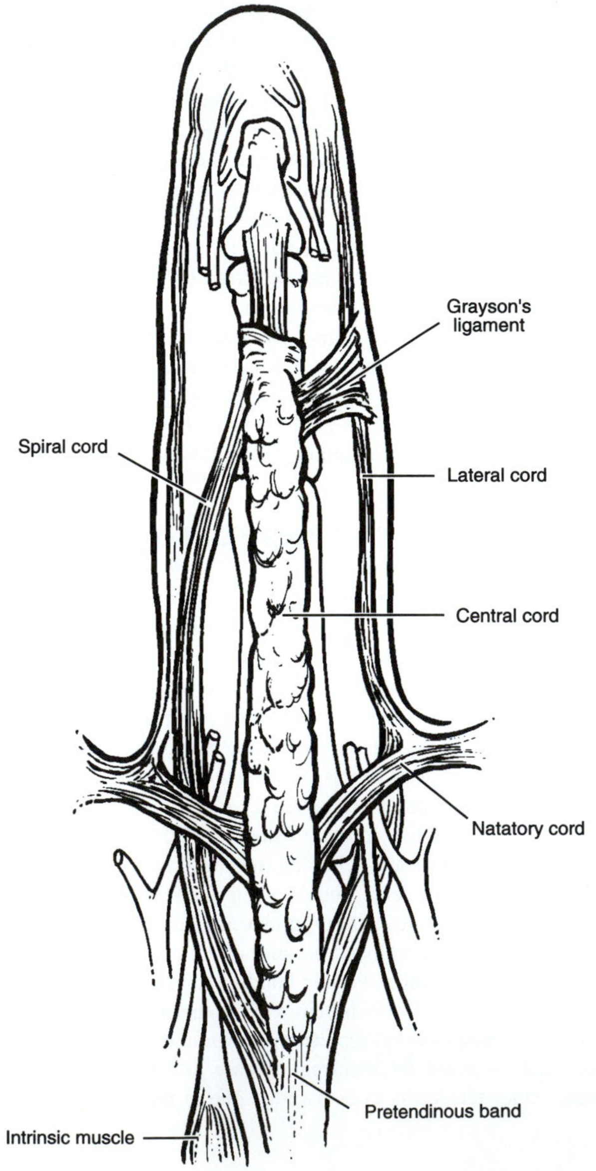

C

Figure 112-1

A. Components of the palmar fascia associated with Dupuytren's contracture. *B.* Normal digital fascia affected by Dupuytren's contracture. *C.* Depiction of normal facia bands progressing to diseased cords. [Reproduced and modified with permission from McFarlane RM: Dupuytren's contracture. In Green DP (ed): *Operative Hand Surgery*, 3d ed. New York: Churchill Livingstone; 1993:564, 565, 567.]

hematoma formation. Z and Y to V skin plasties and skin grafts can avoid tension in wound closure. The open palm technique of McCash has many advantages: no hematoma formation, less pain and swelling, and early motion. However, the wound takes 4 to 6 weeks to heal and requires daily dressing. Prior to closure, release of the tourniquet and meticulous hemostasis will avoid hematoma formation and subsequent loss of skin and infection.

Postoperative care consists of three to six months of extension splinting to lessen scar and flexion contractures and to tighten stretched digital extensors with active and passive exercises (often supervised by hand therapists). Surgical complications include: hematoma formation, neurovascular damage, reflex sympathetic dystrophy (RSD), and the flare reaction. Hematomas should be evacuated; neurovascular damage should be repaired intraoperatively. RSD occurs in 4 percent of males and 8 percent of females; if treated early with stellate sympathetic blocks and intensive hand therapy, a good result can usually be expected. The flare reaction, an unusually red color of the incision or the entire palm, and generally seen several weeks postoperatively in females, usually disappears by 6 weeks but must be followed closely for the occurrence of RSD.

OUTCOME

Early results of MCP correction are excellent; lesser degrees of correction are obtained at the PIP joint, especially in the fifth digit. With the exception of recurrent disease and marked PIP contracture, approximately 80 percent will achieve normal range of motion initially. Although long-term studies indicate a 20 to 80 percent recurrence of disease, only a small subset of patients, that is, young patients with a diathesis, usually have recurrences severe enough to require additional surgery. In those cases, loss of correction usually occurs at the PIP joint. Surgical options in severe recurrence include repeat fasciectomy, dermofasciectomy and skin grafting, PIP joint arthroplasty or joint fusion, and digit amputation.

SUGGESTED READINGS

Hurst LC: Dupuytren's disease. In Manske PR (ed): *Hand Surgery Update* (developed by American Society for Surgery of the Hand). Rosemont, IL: American Academy of Orthopaedic Surgery; 1996:271.

McFarlane RM: Dupuytren's contracture. In Green DP (ed): *Operative Hand Surgery*, vol 1, 4th ed. New York: Churchill Livingston; 1993:563.

Seyfer AE, Hueston JT (eds): Dupuytren's contracture. *Hand Clin* 1991; 7(4).

Chapter 113

COMPRESSION NEUROPATHIES

Martin A. Posner

ANATOMY OF A NERVE

PERIPHERAL NERVE FIBER

A nerve fiber consists of a central core of *axoplasm* surrounded by a multilayered sheath of *Schwann cells.* Axoplasm is an extension of perinuclear cytoplasm in the nerve cell body on which it is dependent for survival. The term *axon* is commonly used to describe any extension from a cell body, although technically, it applies only to an extension from anterior horn cells in the spinal cord or from sympathetic ganglia. Those extensions connected to dorsal root ganglia are termed *dendrites.* Nerve fibers (motor, sensory, and sympathetic) are classified as either *myelinated* or *nonmyelinated* fibers depending on the presence or absence of a *myelin sheath.* Motor fibers are *all* myelinated, and range in thickness from 2 to 30 μm in diameter. Sensory fibers also range from 2 to 30 μm in thickness, and include both myelinated and nonmyelinated fibers, with nonmyelinated fibers predominating. Sympathetic fibers are all nonmyelinated.

CONNECTIVE TISSUE COMPONENTS (Fig. 113-1)

1. Epineurium: The investing sheath around a nerve trunk which delineates it from surrounding structures. It also comprises the areolar connective tissue between *fascicles* (also referred to as *funiculi*) which holds them loosely together. The percentage of epineurium in a cross section of a nerve varies from 30 to 75 percent. However, the ulnar nerve at the elbow has less (22 percent),

and the sciatic nerve in the gluteal area has considerably more (88 percent). The percentage of epineurium depends on the number of fascicles; the more fascicles, the higher the percentage of epineurium.

2. Perineurium: The investing sheath around each fascicle. It has three functions: protection, maintenance of intrafascicular pressure necessary for axoplasmic flow, and resistance to longitudinal stretch. The perineurium also serves as a barrier to the spread of infection.

3. Endoneurium: The supporting connective tissue within each fascicle. In addition to the packing it provides around the nerve fibers, it forms a thin limiting membrane around each fiber, the *endoneurial tube.*

PATHOPHYSIOLOGIC EFFECTS OF COMPRESSION

Nerve injuries result from a variety of factors including: *mechanical, thermal, ischemic,* and *chemical.* Mechanical factors are *compression, severance* and *stretch.* The least damage is caused by local compression of intraneural circulation and results in a *metabolic conduction block.* A common example is when our foot falls asleep after our legs are crossed for a prolonged period of time. In this situation, pressure on the peroneal nerve results in local ischemia and a block in sensory conduction. The conduction block is usually transient and is rapidly reversed after pressure is removed. However, if pressure is prolonged, the motor fibers are also affected and actual structural changes develop in the nerve fibers and connective tissue supporting components.

Nerve injuries are classified using either of two systems. The first system was introduced by Herbert Seddon (1975) and comprises three categories: *neurapraxia, axonotmesis,* and *neurotmesis.* The second system was introduced in 1951 by Sydney Sunderland who graded nerve damage in terms of degrees of injury, of which there are five.

First degree: physiologic block in axon conduction.

Second degree: loss of axon continuity, but the endoneurium remains intact.

Third degree: loss of nerve fiber continuity (axon and endoneurium), but the perineurium around the fascicles remains intact.

Fourth degree: loss of perineurium (fascicular disorganization), but the epineurium around the entire nerve trunk remains intact.

Fifth degree: loss of continuity of the entire nerve trunk (axons, endoneurium, perineurium and epineurium).

While Seddon's system is the more widely used, Sunderland's provides a clearer description of the pathophysiology. Seddon's *neurapraxia* corresponds to Sunderland's *first degree injury.* There is local myelin damage without any damage to the underlying axons. Since larger motor fibers are generally more vulnerable to compression than

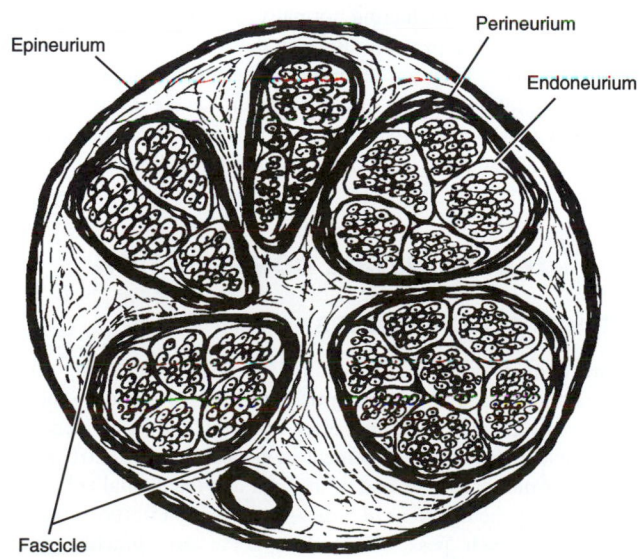

Figure 113-1
Cross section of a peripheral nerve.

Epineurium

Perineurium

Endoneurium

Fascicle

thinner sensory fibers, this type of injury usually results in paralysis, but spares sensation. An example is "Saturday night palsy" which is paralysis of the extensor muscles caused by external pressure on the radial nerve in an inebriated individual who collapses after a night of drinking and whose arm is wedged against the hard edge of a chair or bed post. It also occurs in addicts who become unconscious after ingesting or injecting drugs. Since myelin damage is confined to the site of compression, the nerve can still be electrically stimulated further distally. Usually, the injured axons "awaken" and complete function is restored.

Seddon's *axonotmesis* corresponds to Sunderland's *second degree injury* and indicates axonal disruption, but the endoneurial tubes remain intact. *Wallerian degeneration,* a process of myelin fragmentation and digestion by the Schwann cells, occurs in these injuries. Since the endoneurial tubes remain intact, normal function can be expected to return with axonal regeneration. The time necessary for recovery depends on several factors including: the age of the patient, the level of the injury, and the rate of advance of regenerating axons. While neuropraxic lesions recover in weeks, axonotmetic lesions usually take months. Surgery is rarely necessary for these injuries.

Neurotmesis is loss of continuity of not only the axons, but all the structures of the nerve; endoneurial tubes, perineurium and epineurium. Seddon used this term to describe a nerve "that has either been completely severed or is so seriously disorganized by scar tissue that spontaneous regeneration is out of the question." Most neurotmetic injuries are the result of lacerations, but they can also follow severe and prolonged compression. Sunderland subdivided neurotmesis into third, fourth and fifth degrees of injury, depending on the continuity or discontinuity of the endoneurium, perineurium and epineurium. In a *third degree injury,* the endoneurial tubes are disrupted, but the perineurium and epineurium are preserved. Intrafascicular fibrosis develops, which interferes with the regenerating axons. While some axons get past the injured nerve segment, their rate of regeneration is delayed and they are often diverted from traveling down their original endoneurial tubes. The end result is reinnervation that is not only different from the original, it is also often of marginal quality. The scarred portion of the nerve is commonly referred to as a "neuroma in continuity." It generally must be resected, with care taken to protect the intact fascicles which are separated from the damaged ones by intrafascicular dissection. After the damaged fascicles are repaired, the intact fascicles are looser than the repaired fascicles and bulge out, which gives that portion of the nerve the appearance of a "caterpillar."

In a *fourth degree injury,* the perineurium is destroyed in addition to the endoneurium, resulting in complete disorganization of the fascicles. Only the investing epineurium of the nerve remains intact. This injury is also referred to as a "neuroma in continuity," but it is much more severe than a third degree injury since all the critically important parts of the nerve have been destroyed. Surgical excision of the entire nerve segment is required with end-to-end repair or an interposition nerve graft. Similar treatment is required for a *fifth degree injury,* which is a nerve that is no longer in continuity.

The effects of nerve compression depend on *external factors* such as the magnitude of the force and the duration of its application, as well as *internal factors* related to the size of the fiber and its location within the nerve trunk. Large fibers are more vulnerable to compression and ischemia than small fibers, as are fibers that are located superficially in a nerve trunk as compared to those situated more centrally. The connective tissue composition of the nerve is another important factor. The greater the amount of epineurial and perineurial tissue, the better the protection. Therefore, a nerve consisting of multiple small fascicles is less vulnerable to the deleterious effects of compression than a nerve containing a few large fascicles. Nerves usually have a greater number of fascicles in areas where they are subjected to stretch, such as around joints, than in other areas. An exception is the ulnar nerve at the elbow, which explains the frequency of neuropathies at that location.

Nerve compressions usually occur at specific anatomical sites where they pass through confined areas. These sites may be bony (for example, epicondylar groove), muscular (for example, pronator teres muscle) or fibrous (for example, arcade of Frohse). Not uncommonly, the compression is at more than one site. When neural function is compromised at one level, the axons of that nerve are susceptible to damage at another level, probably on the basis of impaired axoplasmic flow. Upton and McComas in 1973 termed this condition, "double crush syndrome." The second "crush" is usually more proximal at the cervical roots, but occasionally it is distal, resulting in a "reversed double crush syndrome." Occasionally, there is a "triple crush syndrome." Recognizing that there can be more than a single site of nerve compression is obviously important in making an accurate diagnosis and formulating an effective treatment program.

Regardless of the nerve involved or its site of compression, all neuropathies require a detailed history of the onset, symptoms and aggravating factors, as well as a thorough physical examination. When evaluating sensibility, both *threshold* and *innervation density* are tested (Table 113-1). *Threshold* tests measure a single nerve fiber innervating a single receptor or a group of receptors, while *innervation density* tests measure the density of innervation. Changes in threshold always precede changes in innervation density. This sequence of events is analogous to compression of a motor nerve which begins with mild weakness (without any axonal loss) and progresses to severe weakness and eventually muscle atrophy where there is a loss of axons. With compression of a sensory nerve, the first symptoms are numbness and paresthesias. These changes are measured by testing *pressure threshold* in *slowly adapting* nerve fibers with Semmes-Weinstein nylon monofilaments or von Frey hairs, or by testing *vibratory threshold* in *quickly* adapting fibers with a tuning fork or vibrometer.

When nerve compression is chronic, damage may progress to actual loss of axons which affects *innervation density*. This is measured using *static* two-point discrimination for slowly adapting fibers, and *moving* two-point discrimination for quickly adapting fibers. Both static and moving two-point discrimination can be intact, even if only a few nerve fibers are conducting normally. The tests are not sensitive to a gradual decrease in nerve function that is common in compressive neuropathies. They are abnormal only when compression is of such long duration that it has resulted in severe nerve damage. Innervation density tests are therefore most useful for diagnosing lacerating injuries and for assessing regeneration following nerve repairs.

MEDIAN NERVE COMPRESSION

SUPRACONDYLAR PROCESS

A supracondylar process is an anomalous bony spur arising on the anteromedial surface of the humerus, 3 to 5 cm proximal to the medial epicondyle. It is congenital, often bilateral, and its incidence has been estimated at 0.7 to 2.7 percent in Caucasians and 0.01 percent in African-Americans. The end of the spur and the medial epicondyle are spanned by the *ligament of Struthers,* forming a fibroosseous tunnel through which pass the median nerve and brachial artery. Frequently, the brachial artery divides proximal to the spur and in such cases, the median nerve is accompanied by the ulnar artery. A

Table 113-1

Summary of Sensibility Testing for Threshold and Innervation Density

Nerve Fiber	Peripheral Receptor	Sensation	Test
Threshold			
Slowly adapting	Merkel cell-neurite complex	Pressure	Semmes-Weinstein monofilament nylons or von Frey hairs
Quickly adapting	Meissner corpuscle	Moving touch or flutter	30 cps tuning fork, or vibrometer
	Pacinian corpuscle	Moving touch or vibration	256 cps tuning fork, or vibrometer
Innervation Density			
Slowly adapting	Merkel cell-neurite complex	Tactile gnosis (static)	Static two-point discrimination
Quickly adapting	Meissner corpuscle Pacinian corpuscle	Tactile gnosis (moving)	Moving two-point discrimination

---

supracondylar process rarely causes clinical problems, although median nerve symptoms may appear after local trauma to that area. In most cases, the neuropathy resolves with nonoperative care.

PRONATOR SYNDROME

Pronator syndrome is entrapment of the median nerve in the proximal forearm. Typically, there is local pain and numbness in the median nerve distribution of the hand, and muscle weakness. As with any compressive neuropathy, the sensory deficits in the anatomical distribution of the nerve may not be uniform. Some digits may have less feeling than others and sometimes, one or more digits may even have normal sensibility. The same is true for motor deficits. Not all of the extrinsic and intrinsic muscles supplied by the median nerve may be weak to the same degree and some, particularly the extrinsics, may be totally spared. In some patients, the sensory complaints predominate and in other patients the motor deficits are more severe.

The site of compression is usually where the nerve passes between the two heads of the pronator muscle, hence the name of the syndrome. The compression may be due to hypertrophy of the muscle, pressure from an aponeurotic band on the deep surface of the superficial head of the muscle, or less commonly, a band on the superficial surface of the deep head of the muscle. There are two other potential sites for nerve entrapment, one proximal to the pronator muscle at the lacertus fibrosis, and the other distal to the muscle at the arch of the flexor digitorum superficialis muscle. Identifying the site of entrapment depends on a careful physical examination. Localizing the Tinel sign to a specific area is helpful as well as reproducing or aggravating the symptoms by certain provocative maneuvers. When forearm pain is caused or worsened by resisted flexion of the elbow with the forearm in pronation, the problem is probably at the pronator muscle. If, however, the discomfort occurs with resisted flexion of the elbow, but with the forearm supinated, the problem is at the lacertus fibrosus. Pain with resisted flexion of the superficialis tendon to the middle finger indicates that the compression is at the arch of the superficialis (Fig. 113-2). Compression at a supracondylar

process is sometimes considered the fourth site of compression. Regardless of location, a pronator syndrome requires surgery if muscle weakness persists despite nonoperative care. If the site of compression cannot be determined by preoperative examination, it is important to explore and decompress the nerve at the three sites distal to the humerus. A more proximal exploration is indicated only when preoperative radiographs show a supracondylar process.

ANTERIOR INTEROSSEOUS SYNDROME

An anterior interosseous syndrome, like a pronator syndrome, is a neuropathy of the median nerve in the proximal forearm, but it affects only its anterior interosseous division. This is purely a motor nerve which when compressed results in a motor deficit without any sensory complaints or deficits in the hand. However, patients frequently complain of vague aching pain in their forearms. The classical finding on physical examination is loss of pinch between the thumb and index finger due to paralysis of the flexor pollicis longus and flexor digitorum profundus (to the index), two muscles supplied by the anterior interosseous nerve. In many cases the two muscles are not weakened to the same degree and active flexion of either the thumb or index finger may remain strong. A third muscle supplied by the anterior interosseous nerve is the pronator quadratus whose strength is evaluated by resisted pronation of the forearm with the elbow in full flexion in order to weaken the stronger pronator teres. The flexor profundus to the middle finger is also supplied by the anterior interosseous nerve, but it is rarely weakened because its muscle belly is dually innervated by the ulnar nerve. An anterior interosseous syndrome is primarily diagnosed by clinical examination. Although electrodiagnostic studies can be helpful, they should not be used as the sole factor in deciding on surgery. If muscle weakness persists with no sign of clinical improvement for more than 3 months, surgical exploration of the median nerve and its anterior interosseous branch are necessary, regardless of any improvement in the electrical activity of the affected muscles. The surgeon may encounter a variety of anatomic variations involving vascular structures, muscles, and tendons.

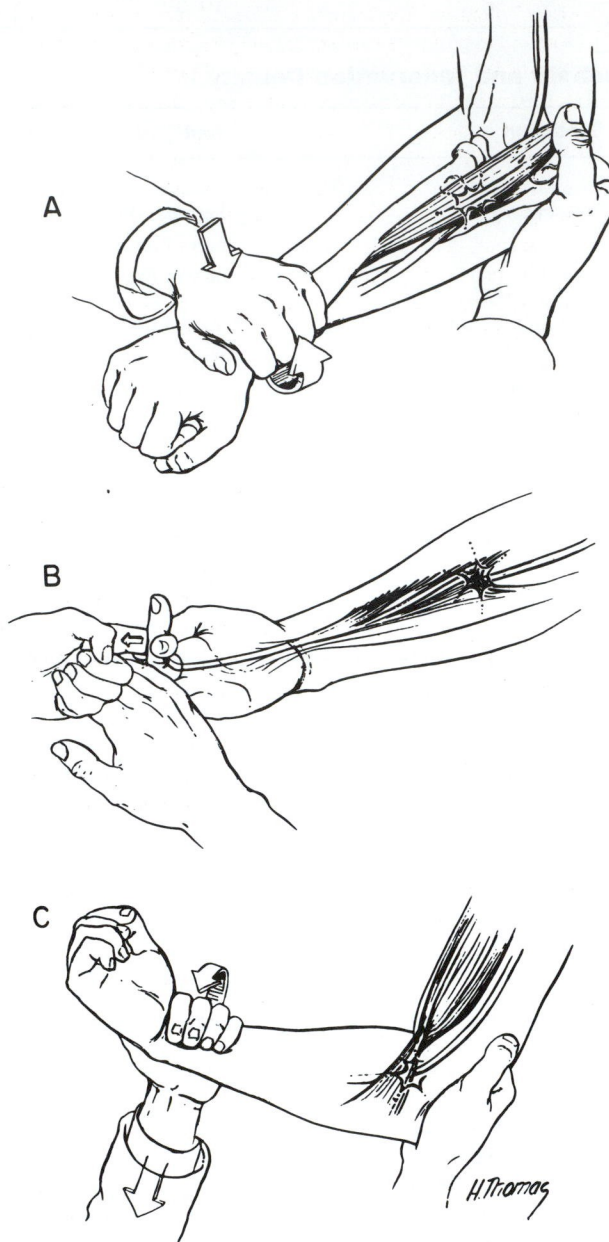

Figure 113-2
Locating the site of compression in a pronator syndrome by physical examination. *A*. At the pronator teres muscle when pain is aggravated by resisted elbow flexion and forearm *pronation*. *B*. At the lacertus fibrosus when pain is aggravated with resisted elbow flexion and the forearm in *supination*. *C*. At the arch of the flexor superficialis when pain is aggravated with resisted flexion of the proximal interphalangeal joint of the middle finger. [Reproduced with permission from Spinner M: Principles of tendon transfers. In Omer G, Spinner M, (eds): *Management of Peripheral Nerve Problems.* Philadelphia WB Saunders; 1980, p. 579.]

CARPAL TUNNEL SYNDROME

Carpal tunnel syndrome is compression of the median nerve in the carpal tunnel, and is the most common compressive neuropathy in the upper extremity. Anatomically, the carpal tunnel is formed posteriorly and laterally by a rigid convex arch of the carpal bones, and anteriorly by the thick *transverse carpal ligament* which spans the

arch. The carpal tunnel is an unyielding tunnel and any pressure within it is transmitted to its contents. The median nerve is the most vulnerable structure within the carpal tunnel. Initially, the increased pressure is more likely to cause nerve ischemia than nerve deformation. A wide variety of space-occupying lesions within the tunnel can cause increased pressure, with nonspecific tenosynovitis of the flexor tendons being the most common. Other conditions include tumor, ganglion, gouty tophus, fracture fragment, dislocated carpal bone, foreign body, and anatomic anomalies such as an aberrant muscle or a persistent median artery. Many medical conditions are also associated with carpal tunnel syndrome such as diabetes mellitus, amyloidosis, collagen diseases, and hormonal changes as seen in menopause, myxedema, acromegaly, and pregnancy. In recent years, occupational activities have been implicated, but rarely is there conclusive evidence that the activity itself is the primary causative factor.

Patients commonly complain of nocturnal paresthesias in their hands and digits, which frequently awaken them from sleep. They usually obtain some relief by shaking their hands or rubbing them together. The paresthesias also occur during the daytime hours and often radiate proximally into their forearms and occasionally, into their shoulders. Numbness within the median nerve distribution is another common symptom, but less so than paresthesias. Patients sometimes have difficulty in describing their complaints and may report that their hands feel "swollen" or "full." Regarding muscle strength, patients may not be aware of any actual weakness, and instead complain that their hands feel "tired" and fatigue easily with activities. They may also report difficulty in holding objects which fall from their grasp.

The physical examination is important to confirm that the patient's subjective complaints are consistent with median nerve compression in the carpal tunnel. Provocative tests such as tapping over the median nerve (Tinel test), the wrist flexion test (Phalen's test), and the tourniquet test should elicit paresthesias into all or at least a portion of the median nerve distribution of the hand. Phalen's test is carried out by the patient allowing his or her wrists to simply drop into flexion. The test is positive if paresthesias occur within 60 s. Usually, the paresthesias occur much earlier, sometimes within 5 to 10 s. It is important that the patient's wrists are not forced into flexion, because this will produce many false positive results. Phalen's test is more sensitive than the Tinel test, but it is not as specific. The tourniquet test involves inflation of a pneumatic tourniquet wrapped around the upper arm to above the systolic pressure. In a normal individual, the test causes paresthesias in the ulnar nerve distribution but in a carpal tunnel syndrome, the paresthesias are in the median nerve distribution. The tourniquet test is not as sensitive as the Phalen's test.

Regarding sensibility, testing for *threshold* will generally yield more significant results than testing for *innervation density*. Since all clinical tests for sensibility require a conscious awareness of the stimulus being applied, none are totally objective. The only objective test is a measurement of sensory nerve conduction. A distal latency greater than 3.5 ms or asymmetry in conduction times between the two hands greater than 0.5 ms is abnormal. Since sensory fibers comprise more than 95 percent of the fibers in the median nerve in the carpal tunnel and are situated more superficial than the motor fibers, sensory conduction times are generally more sensitive to early nerve damage than motor conduction times. The motor conduction time should still be measured and a distal latency greater than 4.5 ms is abnormal.

Evaluating muscle strength is critically important. There should be no weakness of the extrinsic muscles innervated by the median nerve unless there is a concomitant compression of the nerve proximal to the carpal tunnel. Thenar muscle strength is tested by resisted thumb abduction which primarily evaluates the most important thenar muscle, the abductor pollicis brevis. Both thumbs are tested and strength of the thenar muscles is compared to the strength of the ulnar innervated first dorsal interossei. Thenar muscle weakness is a clear indication for surgery, regardless of electrodiagnostic findings, which may be falsely negative in up to 20 percent of cases. When there is no muscle weakness, conservative measures including rest, a wrist splint, and nonsteroidal anti-inflammatory medication (NSAIDs) can be tried. A steroid injection into the carpal tunnel can also be effective. It is important to always use a soluble steroid such as dexamethasone rather than an insoluble steroid which will leave a deposit that may cause additional nerve damage. Pyridoxine (vitamin B_6) has not proved to be of any benefit.

Carpal tunnel syndrome is bilateral in about 50 percent of patients and, frequently, there is a concomitant stenosing tenosynovitis of one or more flexor tendon sheaths ("trigger finger" and/or "trigger thumb"). Even if none is present, patients should be alerted that it can occur at some future time since the etiology of most carpal tunnel syndromes is a nonspecific tenosynovitis.

When surgery is necessary, an incision is made along the thenar crease in the palm, stopping just short of the wrist flexion crease. The palmar fascia is incised, avoiding any branches of the palmar cutaneous branch of the median nerve. The surgeon must be aware that there are normal anatomic variations of the median nerve, particularly the course of its motor branch to the thenar muscles. While the branch is usually at the distal end of the transverse carpal ligament, it can arise proximal to the ligament and, on rare occasions, even penetrate it. An awareness of these variations will avoid an iatrogenic injury. Once the ligament is sectioned, the entire median nerve and the tunnel are visualized. Although medical opinions differ, many surgeons advocate an epineurolysis (epineurotomy or epineurectomy) if the nerve is severely constricted and its epineurium thickened. Greater controversy exists concerning the benefits of endoscopic carpal tunnel releases. Advocates of the procedure claim there is less pain and morbidity than following a conventional open technique. However, these purported benefits are temporary and, many believe, they are far outweighed by the hazards of the procedure. Although statistically, the risk of injury to the median nerve with an endoscopic release is rare, it is still far greater than with the open technique.

ULNAR NERVE COMPRESSIONS

ENTRAPMENT AT THE ELBOW

The relationship of the ulnar nerve to its surrounding anatomy predisposes it to injury in its path across the elbow. There are five potential sites for compression.

1. The most proximal site is the *arcade of Struthers* (in contradistinction to the *ligament of Struthers* which is attached to a supracondylar process and is associated with median nerve compressions) which is a musculofascial band that extends from the medial head of the triceps to the medial intermuscular septum. It is located 6 to 10 cm proximal to the medial epicondyle and is 1.5 to 2 cm in width. In the absence of an arcade, the medial intermuscular septum can cause compression, but generally this occurs as a postoperative complication following anterior transposition of the nerve.

2. The second site is at the distal end of the humerus, proximal to the epicondyles, when there is an angulatory or cubitus valgus deformity. This deformity occurs as a consequence of an old epiphyseal injury to the lateral condyle or a malunited supracondylar fracture. An ulnar nerve compression at this site was first described by Mouchet in 1914, and in Europe the condition was called the "maladie de Mouchet". In 1916, Hunt described the

same problem in this country and called it "tardy ulnar palsy."

3. The third area for potential nerve compression is the fibrosseous epicondylar, or olecranon groove. The groove is formed anteriorly by the medial epicondyle, laterally by the olecranon, and its roof is a fibroaponeurotic band that extends to the two heads of the flexor carpi ulnaris muscle. Compressions within the groove can result from a wide variety of conditions that can be categorized into *space occupying lesions* (i.e., fracture fragment, arthritic spur, tumor), *direct pressure on the nerve* (i.e., truck drivers who rest their elbows on the window ledge of their vehicle, poor positioning of the upper extremity in patients undergoing surgery), and *habitual subluxation of the nerve* (i.e., congenital laxity of the fibroaponeurotic roof of the groove, bony abnormalities, trauma).

4. The fourth area, which together with the third area are the most common sites for compression, is where the ulnar nerve passes between the two heads of the flexor carpi ulnaris muscle. This site is spanned by the *arcuate ligament,* also known as *Osborne's ligament.* Feindel and Stratford (1958) referred to this site as the "cubital tunnel." Therefore, the diagnosis of a "cubital tunnel syndrome" should be reserved for those ulnar neuropathies at this specific anatomic site. With elbow flexion, Osborne's ligament stretches and becomes taut, narrowing the tunnel and compressing the nerve. The medial collateral ligament also bulges medially which causes additional nerve compression. Normally, there is a seven-fold increase in pressure on the nerve with elbow flexion, which increases to tenfold when contraction of the flexor carpi ulnaris is added. Scarring of the nerve in the cubital tunnel and/or epicondylar groove interferes with its normal gliding action and increases the traction effect on the nerve with elbow flexion.

5. The fifth and most distal site for compression is where the ulnar nerves leaves the flexor carpi ulnaris and penetrates a fascial layer to lie between the flexor digitorum superficialis and profundi muscles. This site, located approximately 5 cm distal to the medial epicondyle, has been termed the "flexor pronator aponeurosis."

Regardless of site of compression, the most common symptoms are numbness and paresthesias in the ulnar nerve distribution of the hand. Tenderness over the nerve is also common and an effort should be made to isolate it to one of the five potential sites of compression where there is often a positive Tinel. Sometimes the nerve is compressed at more than one site. Muscle weakness can affect both the extrinsic and intrinsic muscles supplied by the nerve, although generally the weakness is confined to the intrinsics. When there is extrinsic muscle weakness, it is usually the flexor digitorum profundus to the little finger.

Nonoperative treatment primarily involves avoiding direct pressure on the nerve and avoiding prolonged elbow flexion. Temporarily immobilizing the elbow in about 30 degrees of flexion is usually effective and this can best be achieved by a splint fabricated out of a lightweight thermoplastic material. The splint is worn for 3 to 4 weeks, but removed several times each day for active range of motion exercises to prevent elbow stiffness. NSAIDs can also be used, but local steroid injections around the nerve should be avoided. If symptoms persist and particularly when they are accompanied by muscle weakness, surgery is warranted.

Operations are divided into two main categories, decompressions *without* transposing the nerve, and decompressions *with* transposing the nerve. The first category includes *neurolyses in situ* and *medial epicondylectomies.* A neurolysis in situ is indicated in those rare cases of snapping of a hypertrophied medial head of the triceps muscle with elbow flexion that is sometimes seen in body builders. It is also indicated when there is an anconeus epitrochlearis muscle, an anomalous muscle that arises from the medial border of the olecranon and inserts into the medial epicondyle. In humans, the muscle is probably atavistic and is replaced by a fibrous band, the epitrochleoanconeus ligament. Medial epicondylectomies, although recommended by some, are not popular procedures. They fail to relieve the traction effect on the nerve that occurs with elbow flexion even though the channel in which the nerve travels has been enlarged and the nerve is allowed to subluxate. The procedure also risks damage to the medial collateral ligament of the elbow joint.

Ulnar nerve decompressions *with* transposition have been described using one of three methods, *subcutaneous, intramuscular* or *submuscular.* In all three methods, the medial intermuscular septum is excised in order to eliminate any sharp fibrous edge over which the nerve glides in its new path volar to the axis of the elbow. *Subcutaneous transpositions* are the simplest and the most commonly performed of the three methods. After the nerve is shifted, a fasciodermal sling is fashioned to prevent it from shifting back into the epicondylar groove. The operation is indicated for elderly inactive patients, and in obese patients who have a thick layer of fat tissue in their upper arm. Opinions differ concerning its effectiveness in other patients. *Intramuscular transpositions* are generally condemned because they risk additional damage to the nerve which is placed at right angles to the direction of the fibers of the pronator teres muscle and is subjected to traction forces of the muscle. These transpositions have a high failure rate. *Submuscular transpositions* have enjoyed popularity since they were first described by Learmonth in 1942. It is the only method that insures that all five potential sites of compression are released. The ulnar nerve is placed in an anatomic plane on the unscarred bed of the brachialis muscle where it is no longer subjected to compressive or traction forces. By virtue of being placed deep to the entire flexor-pronator muscle mass, the nerve is well protected and it cannot shift back to its original position. Submuscular transpositions are effective procedures even when prior subcutaneous and intramuscular transpositions have failed.

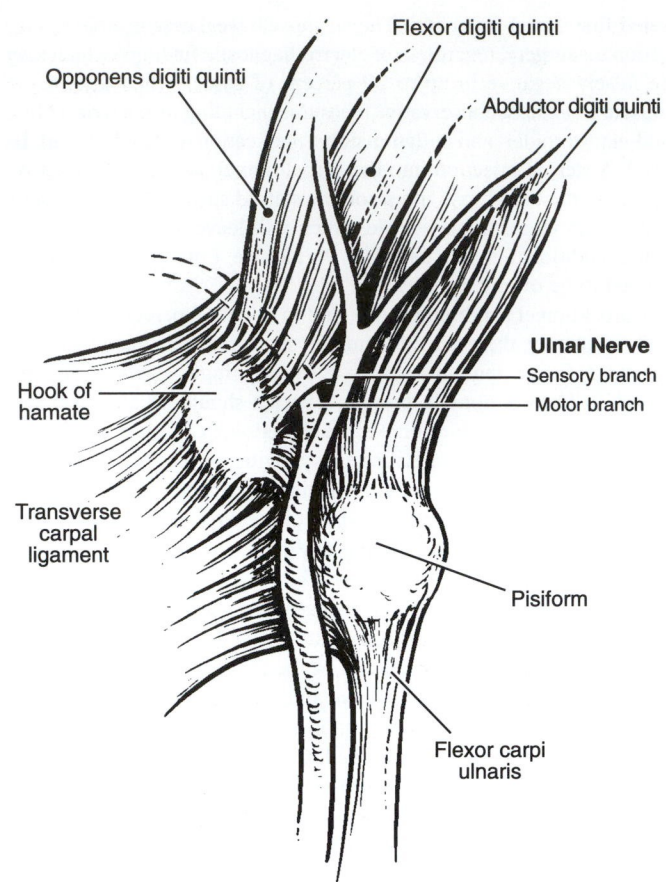

Figure 113-3
The canal of Guyon. [Original illustration by Elizabeth Roselius © 1988. Reprinted (modified) with permission from Green DP. *Operative Hand Surgery;* New York: Churchill Livingstone; 1988:1453.]

ENTRAPMENT AT THE WRIST (ULNAR TUNNEL SYNDROME)

Since Guyon's description in 1861 of the ulnar tunnel in the wrist that bears his name, compressive neuropathies in this area have been well documented. Anatomically, Guyon's canal is triangular in shape and contains the ulnar nerve and artery (Fig. 113-3). The nerve enters the canal medial to the artery, and then divides into a superficial sensory branch and a deep motor branch. The motor branch, along with a branch of the ulnar artery, passes through a tendinous arch between the origins of the abductor digiti quinti and flexor digiti quinti brevis muscles to supply the interossei muscles to the fingers, the adductor pollicis, and the deep head of the flexor pollicis brevis to the thumb. The sensory branch passes superficial to the arch in the distal part of the canal. Three types of ulnar nerve compressions within Guyon's canal have been described.

Type I - The entrapment is at or just proximal to the canal. Since the nerve has not yet bifurcated, there are both motor and sensory deficits. The motor weakness affects all the ulnar innervated intrinsic muscles, including those in the hypothenar eminence. The sensory deficit involves the entire palmar surface of the little finger and ulnar one half of the ring finger. Sensibility is intact on the dorsal surfaces of the two fingers because the dorsal cutaneous branch of the nerve has already split from the main trunk, 5 to 6 cm proximal to the wrist.

Type II - The compression is within the canal at the hook of the hamate and origin of the abductor and flexor digiti quinti muscles.

Only the motor branch of the nerve is affected, resulting in a purely motor deficit. The hypothenar muscles are spared because they are innervated at a more proximal level. When severe and chronic, a type II compression results in marked weakness and even paralysis of the interossei and adductor pollicis muscles. Clinically, there is clawing of the ring and little fingers, and positive Froment's and Jeanne's signs in the thumb.

Type III - The compression is at the distal end of the canal and affects only the sensory branch of the nerve. There is no weakness of the intrinsic muscles.

Ulnar nerve compression in Guyon's canal can be caused by a ganglion, thrombosis or aneurysm of the ulnar artery, tumors, fractures and/or dislocations of the adjacent metacarpal and carpal bones, and anatomic abnormalities involving the intrinsic muscles. A history of the patient's work and leisure time activities can sometimes aid in making the diagnosis. The use of a pneumatic drill can lead to ulnar artery thrombosis and injury to the nerve. Sports activities which involve forceful pressure on the heel of the palm, such as cycling and weight lifting, can also cause nerve compression. The most common cause is a ganglion which can sometimes be palpated in the hypothenar eminence. An Allen test should always be carried out, and if circulation via the ulnar artery is impaired, a thrombosis or aneurysm should be suspected. In addition to conventional radiographs, CT is indicated if a fracture of the hook of the hamate bone is suspected. MRI is performed if a ganglion or other space-occupying mass is thought to be the problem.

Treatment depends on the etiology of compression. If it is due to occupational or recreational activities, cessation of the activity is usually effective combined with wrist splinting. Nonoperative treatment is also indicated for a neuropathy that follows closed trauma. If the neuropathy does not resolve in 6 to 8 weeks, surgery is indicated. The entire canal of Guyon is explored and both motor and sensory branches of the nerve are identified and decompressed.

RADIAL NERVE COMPRESSIONS

HIGH RADIAL NERVE

Compression of the radial nerve in the upper arm usually occurs at the lateral head of the triceps or at the lateral intermuscular septum. In most cases it is due to local trauma, either from stretch or local pressure. Stretch injuries are common because the nerve is relatively fixed in its passage through the spiral groove of the humerus. The nerve is also vulnerable to the pressure of a narrow tourniquet that remains in place for a prolonged period of time, or the edge of a chair or bed post in the patient who develops a "Saturday night palsy."

Most closed injuries to the radial nerve result in a neurapraxia or axonotmesis (first- or second-degree injury) and resolve spontaneously. Surgery is indicated when there is no recovery in four months or sooner if damage is at a more distal level (i.e., supracondylar area).

RADIAL TUNNEL SYNDROME

The radial tunnel is an anatomical area that extends from the radial head to the supinator muscle and is the most common area for radial nerve compressions. There are five potential sites for compression:

1. At the entrance to the tunnel by fibrous bands which lie anterior to the radial head.
2. The radial recurrent vessels (the leash of Henry) that lie across the nerve.
3. The tendinous proximal edge of the extensor carpi radialis brevis.
4. The arcade of Frohse, a fibrous band at the proximal margin of the supinator muscle. This is the most common site of compression.
5. The distal edge of the supinator muscle.

Radial tunnel syndrome is a painful condition without sensory or motor deficits. Patients typically complain of pain over the lateral aspect of their forearms and elbows. It is important to rule out a lateral epicondylitis (tennis elbow) which frequently coexists and possibly predisposes to a radial tunnel syndrome because of inflammation it causes in the area. The location and quality of the tenderness in the two conditions are usually distinctive. In tennis elbow, the tenderness is over the lateral epicondyle and/or radial head and is often described as "sharp" or "knifelike," while in a radial tunnel syndrome, it has a duller quality and is directly over the nerve, either laterally between the brachioradialis and extensor carpi radialis brevis, or further proximally and anteriorly between the brachialis and the mobile wad. An injection of a local anesthetic into the epicondyle can be a useful diagnostic test to differentiate between the two conditions. Pain can sometimes be provoked or aggravated by resisted extension of the middle finger and/or resisted forearm supination with the forearm extended. Electrodiagnostic studies are usually negative or inconclusive.

Treatment is aimed at relieving the inflammatory process, which is best achieved by immobilizing the patient's elbow and wrist with an above-elbow splint. The splint, fabricated out of a lightweight thermoplastic material and held in place with several Velcro fasteners, is

worn for about one month. It is removed only for bathing, during which times active range of motion exercises are carried out to prevent elbow or wrist stiffness. Once the inflammation subsides, a graduated program of active resistive exercises is begun to strengthen the muscles. Beginning the exercise program before there is a significant improvement in pain will only worsen the problem. If nonoperative measures fail, and generally 4 to 6 months is a reasonable time to wait, surgery is warranted. The tunnel is explored by a posterior surgical approach, either splitting the brachioradialis muscle or going in the interval between the extensor digitorum communis and extensor carpi radialis brevis muscles (Fig. 113-4). It is important to explore

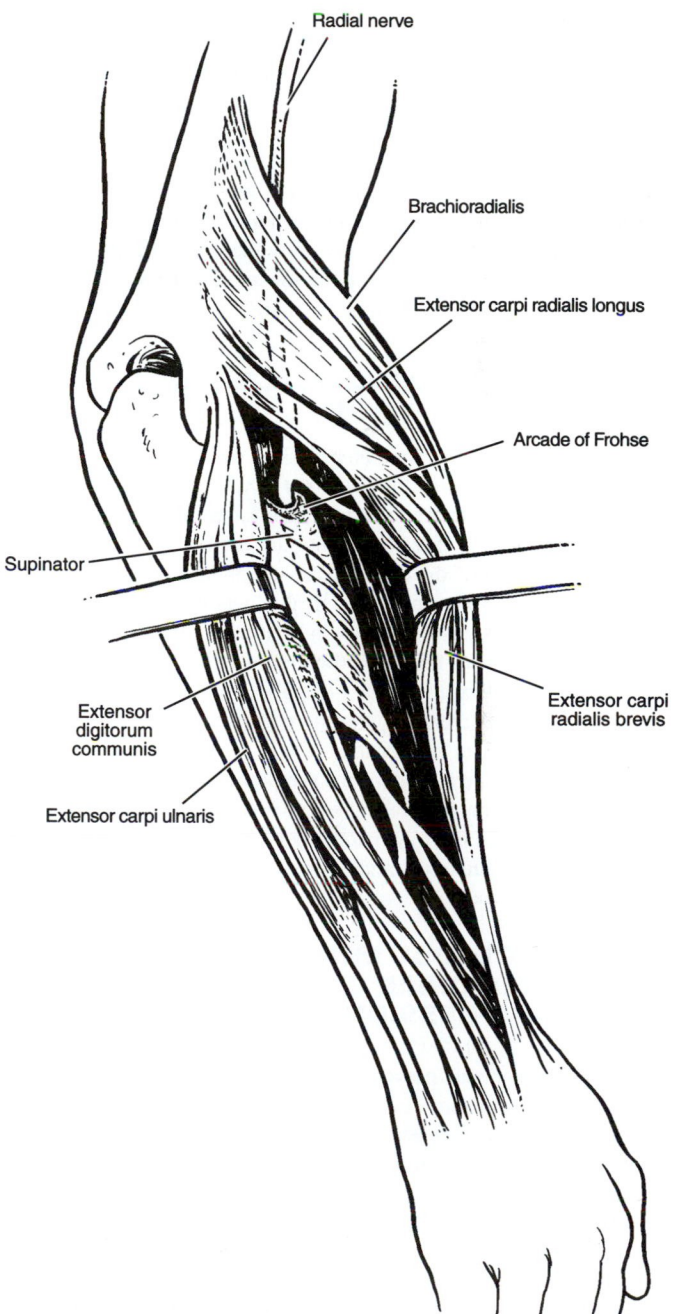

Figure 113-4
Posterior surgical approach to the radial tunnel. [Original illustration by Elizabeth Roselius © 1988. Reprinted (modified) with permission from Green DP. *Operative Hand Surgery*; New York: Churchill Livingstone; 1988:1457.]

all potential sites for compression. The disadvantage of a posterior surgical approach is that it permits only a limited anatomic exposure. If on preoperative examination, tenderness is not localized to the radial tunnel, it is preferable to use an anterolateral approach in order to visualize the radial nerve at a more proximal level, between the brachioradialis and brachialis muscles.

POSTERIOR INTEROSSEOUS NERVE SYNDROME

Compression of the posterior interosseous nerve, for which the syndrome is named, results in a pure motor deficit that affects the muscles innervated by that nerve. Unlike a radial nerve paralysis, wrist extension remains because the extensor carpi radialis longus, and sometimes the extensor carpi radialis brevis, are innervated by the radial nerve. However, wrist extension is in a radial direction because the extensor carpi ulnaris, which is innervated by the posterior interosseous nerve, is paralyzed. There is also loss of extension of the metacarpophalangeal joints of the thumb and all fingers, although the digital extensor muscles may not all be affected to the same degree and active extension of one or more digits may remain. Extension of the proximal and distal interphalangeal joints of the fingers are not affected because those movements are carried out by the intrinsic muscles. Generally, surgical exploration of the nerve is indicated when paresis or paralysis persists for more than 3 months.

RADIAL NERVE COMPRESSION AT THE WRIST (WARTENBERG'S SYNDROME)

Wartenberg in 1932 described compression of the sensory branch of the radial nerve. He called the condition "cheilalgia paresthetica" because it resembled the neuropathy of the lateral cutaneous nerve in the thigh, which is called "meralgia paresthetica." Compression of the sensory branch of the radial nerve commonly occurs where the nerve pierces the forearm fascia, in the interval between the brachioradialis and extensor carpi radialis longus tendons. These two tendons converge with forearm pronation which results in a scissoring effect on the nerve. Patients typically complain of forearm pain and dysesthesias. Percussion over the nerve will usually elicit distal paresthesias. A useful provocative test is forceful pronation of the forearm which should reproduce the symptoms within 60 s. Treatment consists of restricting the patient's activities, splinting the wrist and forearm, and NSAIDs. If symptoms persist for months, the forearm fascia is surgically released and a neurolysis carried out.

MUSCULOCUTANEOUS (LATERAL ANTEBRACHIAL CUTANEOUS) NERVE COMPRESSION AT THE ELBOW

The musculocutaneous nerve originates from the lateral cord of the brachial plexus and supplies motor branches to the coracobrachialis, biceps, and brachialis muscles. The nerve then continues distally and penetrates the brachial fascia 2 to 5 cm proximal to the flexion crease of the elbow where it lies lateral to the biceps tendon and medial to the brachioradialis muscle. It is at this point that the nerve becomes the *lateral antebrachial cutaneous nerve of the forearm* and it is at this site that it can be compressed. This is a rare nerve compression that is characterized by pain over the anterolateral aspect of the elbow and dysesthesias along the radial aspect of the forearm. On examination, there is point tenderness lateral to the biceps tendon at the elbow flexion crease. In the acute phase, patients complain of pain with active elbow extension and their forearms fully pronated. In the subacute and chronic phases, pain occurs as they move their forearms from supination to pronation with the elbow held in full extension. A local anesthetic nerve block is a useful diagnostic test. If conservative measures are not successful, surgical decompression is required.

SUGGESTED READINGS

Amadio PC, Beckenbaugh R: Entrapment of the ulnar nerve by the deep flexor-pronator aponeurosis. *J Hand Surg [Am]* 1986; 11:83.

Bassett FH 3d, Nunley JA: Compression of the musculocutaneous nerve at the elbow. *J Bone Joint Surg [Am]* 1982; 64:1050.

Dellon AL, Mackinnon SE; Radial sensory nerve entrapment in the forearm. *J Hand Surg [Am]* 1986; 11:199.

Dellon AL: Review of treatment results for ulnar nerve entrapment at the elbow. *J Hand Surg [Am]* 1989; 14:688.

Dellon AL: Patient evaluation and management considerations in nerve compression. *Hand Clin* 1992; 8:229.

Eaton RG, Crowe JF, Parkes JC 3d: Anterior transposition of the ulnar nerve with a non-compressing fasciodermal sling. *J Bone J Surg [Am]* 1980; 62:820.

Eversmann WW Jr: Entrapment and compressive neuropathies. In Green DP (ed): *Operative Hand Surgery,* vol 1, 3d ed. New York: Churchill Livingstone; 1993:1341.

Feindel W, Stratford J: The role of the cubital tunnel in tardy ulnar palsy. *Can J Surg* 1958; 1:287.

Lanz U: Anatomical variations of the median nerve in the carpal tunnel. *J Hand Surg [Am]* 1977; 2:44.

Lundborg G: Structure and function of the intraneural microvessels as related to trauma, edema formation, and nerve function. *J Bone Joint Surg [Am]* 1975; 57:938.

Lundborg G, Gelberman RH, Minteer-Convery M, et al: Median nerve compression in the carpal tunnel-functional response to experimentally induced controlled pressure. *J Hand Surg [Am]* 1982; 7:252.

Moneim MS; Ulnar nerve compression at the wrist. Ulnar tunnel syndrome. *Hand Clin* 1992; 8:337.

Omer GE Jr: Median nerve compression at the wrist. *Hand Clin* 1992; 8:317.

Roles NC, Maudsley RH: Radial tunnel syndrome: Resistant tennis elbow as a nerve entrapment. *J Bone J Surg [Br]* 1972; 54:499.

Schrader PA, Reina CR. Struther's ligament neuropathy in a juvenile. *Orthopedics* 1994; 17:723.

Seddon H: *Surgical Disorders of the Peripheral Nerves.* 2d ed. Edinburgh: Churchill Livingstone; 1975.

Shea JD, McClain EJ: Ulnar-nerve compression syndromes at and below the wrist. *J Bone Joint Surg [Am]* 1969; 51:1095.

Spinner M: Management of nerve compression lesions of the upper extremity. In Omer G, Spinner M (eds): *Management of Peripheral Nerve Problems.* Philadelphia: WB Saunders; 1980:569.

Sunderland S: *Nerve and Nerve Injuries.* 2d ed. Edinburgh: Churchill Livingstone; 1978.

Tanzer RC: The carpal tunnel syndrome. A clinical and anatomical study. *J Bone Joint Surg [Am]* 1959; 41:626.

Teleisnik J, Szabo RM: Compression neuropathies of the upper extremity. In Chapman MW (ed): *Operative Orthopaedics,* vol 2, 2d ed. Philadelphia: JB Lippincott; 1993:1419.

Upton AR, McComas AJ: The double crush in nerve entrapment syndromes. *Lancet* 1973; 2:359.

Chapter 114

NERVE LACERATIONS: ACUTE AND CHRONIC

Martin A. Posner

Following laceration of a peripheral nerve, metabolic and structural changes occur both in the trunk and cell body. The portion of the trunk distal to the laceration undergoes *Wallerian degeneration,* a process usually completed by 3 weeks. The endoneurial tubes shrink and eventually close, which blocks axon regeneration. Changes also occur in the denervated muscles. The muscle spindles and muscle cells shrink and connective tissue components, the endomysium and perimysium, thicken. This deterioration can only be reversed by reinnervation, which must occur within 18 months (up to 24 months in children); otherwise, muscle damage is irreversible. Sensory end organs, unlike muscle cells, are not dependent on innervation for their survival. Sensibility can therefore be restored years after an injury, although the longer the period of denervation, the poorer the quality of recovery.

A variety of factors influence the timing of nerve repairs including the general medical condition of the patient and the nature of the injury. Seriously ill or injured patients are obviously not candidates for primary nerve repairs. Regarding the injury itself, skin loss, vascular compromise, and skeletal defects and/or instability are the first priorities for treatment. When a nerve has been cleanly cut, the damage is confined to the immediate areas of the two ends. However, when a nerve is disrupted by a ripping injury (i.e., power saw) or missile (i.e., bullet), or avulsed, the damage is much more extensive. It extends further proximally in the proximal stump and further distally in the distal stump for distances that can be considerable. For this reason a primary repair should be deferred until Wallerian degeneration is complete and neuromas, which delineate the true extent of damage at both ends, have developed. This generally occurs within 3 to 4 weeks. Primary treatment for these injuries consists of wound debridement and approximation of the nerve ends with a single mattress suture to prevent retraction.

PRIMARY NEURORRHAPHIES

A primary neurorrhaphy is preferred when a nerve has been sharply lacerated, the wound is free of severe contamination, there are no other more severe injuries, the patient's general medical condition is good, and an experienced operating staff is available. The surgical techniques for repair include:

1. *Epineurial repair* is the standard method of nerve repair. Proper alignment of the two ends is important and is facilitated by lining up the blood vessels on the surface of the epineurium and matching the fascicles in each cut end. Magnification is helpful, using either loupes or the operating microscope, depending on the personal preference of the surgeon. Monofilament nylon is used for suture material; generally 8-0 for large nerves and 9-0

or 10-0 for smaller nerves. The two nerve ends are brought together using as few sutures as possible. While no fascicles should be allowed to protrude, the epineurium should not be closed so tightly that it will cause bunching and malalignment of the fascicles.

2. In a *fascicular repair,* the epineurium is dissected away from both nerve ends for a distance that approximates the diameter of the nerve. The individual fascicles are then sutured together, generally using 10-0 nylon sutures placed in the interfascicular epineurium and the perineurium. In theory, fascicular repairs are more precise than epineurial repairs. However, in practice they are technically more demanding and they can result in greater damage because of the extensive dissection that is required. Placement of sutures within the nerve trunk can also lead to fibrosis. Fascicular repairs are usually reserved for those nerves which have fewer than five fascicles, such as the ulnar nerve at the elbow.

3. A *grouped fascicular repair* is, as its name suggests, a nerve repair that joins together recognizable groups of fascicles rather than individual fascicles. It requires less handling of the nerve and fewer sutures than a fascicular repair, and it is therefore less likely to cause damage. Proper fascicular identification is important for both fascicular and grouped fascicular repairs and the anatomic dissections of Sunderland, who studied the intraneural topography of the major nerves in the upper and lower extremities, are helpful. Histochemical techniques have been developed to identify motor and sensory fascicles by staining for two enzymes, *acetylcholinesterase* and *carbonic anhydrase.* Acetylcholinesterase staining will distinguish highly reactive motor axons from less reactive sensory fibers. The problem with the stain is that it requires between 12 and 36 h of incubation which necessitates a two-stage operative procedure carried out on successive days. Staining for carbonic anhydrase activity is a newer technique which shows that axoplasmic staining is predominately a feature of sensory fibers, while myelin staining is characteristic of motor fibers. Although the technique takes less time (3 to 4 h) than staining for acetylcholinesterases, it is still a lengthy process which limits its clinical applications.

Electrical stimulation has also been used intraoperatively to distinguish between motor and sensory fascicles. In the distal stump, the motor fascicles are identified by observing for muscle contractions. This electrical activity persists for only a few days after the injury, until Wallerian degeneration begins. In the proximal stump, identifying sensory fascicles requires that the patient remain awake during the operation in order to be able to report when a sensory fascicle has been stimulated. Obviously, patient cooperation is critically important and the procedure, which must be carried out under local anesthesia, can take many hours, two reasons why it has never been widely accepted.

4. A *combined epineurial* and *fascicular repair* utilizes the best qualities of the two approaches. It is particularly useful when repairing a median nerve laceration at the wrist, where a grouped fascicular repair of the motor fibers is combined with an epineurial repair of the sensory fibers.

SECONDARY NEURORRHAPHIES

A late or secondary neurorrhaphy involves resecting the neuroma until normal-appearing fascicles appear at both cut ends. This is generally carried out using loupe magnification or the operating microscope. Loupe magnification of $4.5\times = 9\times$ microscopic magnification. Fascicular or grouped fascicular repairs are rarely possible in secondary neurorrhaphies, and in almost all cases epineurial repairs are performed. It is important to avoid tension on the sutures. Generally, if the ends cannot be brought together with an 8-0 suture, the tension is too great. Eliminating tension can be accomplished by a variety of techniques and frequently two or more are used concurrently. These techniques include:

1. *Stretching.* Ony a slight increase in length (1 to 2 cm) is achieved when a nerve is stretched to the limit of its capacity. Further stretching should be avoided because it can result in damage.
2. *Mobilization.* This is the simplest and most common method of gaining length of both nerve segments. Opinions differ as to the size of the gap that can be overcome. Some claim it is as little as 2.5 cm, but most accept that it is up to 4 cm. The extent of mobilization depends on the location of the neuroma. Mobilization is limited if it is near motor branches.
3. *Positioning of Joints.* By flexing the digit, wrist, and/or elbow, several additional centimeters in length can be gained. Wrist flexion will gain about 2.5 cm, and when combined with elbow flexion, 7.5 cm. It is important not to flex any joint too acutely because it can result in a traction injury on the nerve after the joint(s) is extended. Generally, digital joints and the wrist should not be flexed more than 45 degrees, and the elbow not more than 70 to 80 degrees.
4. *Nerve Transposition.* By transposing the ulnar nerve at the elbow, as much as a 13-cm gap can be overcome with elbow flexion. The median nerve in the proximal forearm can be rerouted anterior to the pronator teres, which when combined with elbow flexion will gain about 8 cm in length, and the radial nerve can be rerouted anterior to the humerus. In the palm, the motor division of the ulnar nerve can be routed through the carpal tunnel. This technique sacrifices reinnervation of the intrinsic muscles in the hypothenar eminence and to the ring and little finger, to achieve reinnervation of the more important intrinsic muscles to the index finger and thumb.
5. *Bone Shortening.* This method is rarely indicated except in situations when surgery on the bone is required, such as repair of a nonunion.

NERVE GRAFTING

When the gap between nerve ends is large, generally more than 4 cm, a nerve graft is required. Grafting techniques include:

1. *Grouped Fascicular Nerve Graft.* This is the most common and effective type of graft. It is interposed between groups of fascicles that are dissected out and identified at each nerve end. The epineurium, which is the primary source of connective tissue, is resected at both nerve ends in order to minimize scarring. For repair of a major nerve, several grafts are required. The donor nerve is usually the sural nerve in the calf because it is accessible, has a tight fascicular pattern, and the sensory deficit it leaves on the lateral side of the foot is not disabling. The medial and lateral antebrachial cutaneous nerves can also be used for grafts, but they have more interfascicular tissue than the sural nerve; sacrificing either nerve results in a significant sensory deficit. The terminal portion of the posterior interosseous nerve in the distal forearm is useful for grafting digital nerves.
2. *Cable Nerve Graft.* A cable graft unites two or three strands of grafts into a unit which is then interposed in the gap between the nerve ends. The technique is not as precise as a grouped fascicular graft.
3. *Trunk Nerve Graft.* A trunk graft uses an entire segment of a nerve. The problem with the procedure is that the thickness of the graft interferes with revascularization of its central portion which results in fibrosis, thereby interfering with axon regeneration. The procedure has limited applications such as a severe injury to both the median and ulnar nerves; a segment of the distal portion of the ulnar nerve is used to repair the median nerve.
4. *Pedicle Nerve Graft.* A pedicle nerve graft was described by Strange whose name is appropriate for this unusual procedure. It can be used for avulsion injuries of both median and ulnar nerves in the forearm when the gaps between the nerves are too large (usually greater than 10 to 12 cm) to be bridged by conventional grafts. The objective of the procedure is to restore protective sensibility in the median nerve distribution using the proximal portion of the ulnar nerve as a vascularized pedicle. The procedure requires two operative stages. In the first stage, the neuromas at the proximal ends of the median and ulnar nerves are resected, and the two nerves are sutured together by means of an epineurial repair to form a U. At the same time, the ulnar nerve is divided proximally in the upper arm at a distance that is slightly greater than the size of the defect in the median nerve. The proximal cut in the ulnar nerve allows Wallerian degeneration to occur further distally. Regenerating axons from the median nerve can now cross the suture site and travel up the ulnar nerve. At the second stage, weeks or months later, the proximal segment of ulnar nerve is turned down and sutured to the distal stump of the median nerve after the neuroma at that end is resected. The two-stage procedure maintains the longitudinal circulation in the proximal segment of the ulnar nerve.
5. *Free Vascularized Nerve Graft.* There are only a few reports of vascularized nerve grafts in the literature. It is a procedure that should be considered only when a long graft is required and the bed is so scarred that it is unacceptable for conventional grafting.

SUGGESTED READINGS

Braun RM: Epineurial nerve repair. In Omer GE, Spinner M (eds): *Management of Peripheral Nerve Problems.* Philadelphia, WB Saunders; 1980; 366.

Gruber H, Zenker W: Acetylcholinesterase: Histochemical differentiation between motor and sensory nerve fibers. *Brain Res.* 1973; 51:207.

Hakstian RW: Funicular orientation by direct stimulation. An aid to peripheral nerve repair. *J Bone J Surg [Am]* 1968; 50:1178.

Jabaley ME, Wallace WH, Heckler FR: Internal topography of major nerves of the forearm and hand: A current review. *J Hand Surg [Am]* 1980; 5:1.

Millesi H, Meissl G, Berger A: The interfascicular nerve-grafting of the median and ulnar nerves. *J Bone Joint Surg [Am]* 1972; 54:727.

Millesi H, Meissl G, Berger A: Further experience with interfascicular grafting of the median, ulnar and radial nerves. *J Bone J Surg [Am]* 1976; 58:209.

Riley DA, Lang DH: Carbonic anhydrase activity of human peripheral nerves: A possible histochemical aid to nerve repair. *J Hand Surg [Am]* 1984; 9:112.

Schultz RJ.: Management of nerve gaps. In Omer GE, Spinner M, (eds): *Management of Peripheral Nerve Problems*, Philadelphia: WB Saunders; 1980:388.

Strange FG StC: Case report on pedicled nerve graft. *Br J Surg* 1950; 37:331.

Sunderland S: *Nerve and Nerve Injuries*, 2d ed. Edinburgh: Churchill Livingstone; 1978.

Wilgis EFS, Brushart TM: Nerve repair and grafting. In Green DP, (ed): *Operative Hand Surgery*, 3d ed. New York: Churchill Livingstone; 1993:1315.

Chapter 115

TENDON TRANSFERS

Martin A. Posner

A tendon transfer shifts the insertion of a tendon to a different location, either to another tendon(s) or to a bone. It is a procedure that is commonly used to substitute for a muscle that is irreversibly paralyzed, or is so weak that it is no longer functional. Muscle paralysis is usually the result of irreparable nerve injury, but it can also be due to neurological conditions such as poliomyelitis. Tendon transfers are also used to replace ruptured or avulsed tendons that cannot be repaired, as substitutions for congenitally aplastic muscles and/or tendons, and to correct muscle imbalance caused by spasticity.

PRINCIPLES OF TENDON TRANSFERS

1. *Patient Education.* Patients must understand the limited objectives of the procedure. Rarely will a tendon transfer restore normal mobility or strength. Patient's motivation is important because *effective* postoperative exercises are essential for the success of the procedure.
2. *Timing.* All joints should be free of significant contractures. A tendon transfer cannot be expected to actively move a joint more than the joint can be moved passively. The bed through which the tendon glides should be supple, including the overlying skin. Steindler thought tissues should be in "equilibrium" which indicates soft tissue induration has resolved and scarring has reached a point of maximum improvement. In some situations, scarred or previously grafted skin must be replaced by means of a pedicle flap or a free vascularized flap. If necessary, a silicone rod is inserted in the subcutaneous tissues as a preliminary procedure in order to form a gliding channel for the later tendon transfer.
3. *Muscle Strength.* The donor tendon must have sufficient power to carry out its new function. The term *muscle strength* has been used to describe both *muscle force* and *muscle work capacity* which are different measures of muscle function.

Muscle force measures the *pressure* that a muscle exerts at its insertion. It is at its maximum when the muscle is at its resting length which is midway between maximum stretch (just short of rupture) and maximum contraction. Muscle force decreases when fibers are either lengthened or shortened from their resting length. The maximum potential *force* of a muscle has been calculated to be 3.65 kg/cm^2 of its physiologic cross-section. In addition to the *contractile force* of a muscle, there is a *viscoelastic force* which is the resistance to stretch imparted by muscle cells and connective tissue components. The viscoelastic force, which is small, is the force exerted by totally paralyzed muscles when they are stretched. While the viscoelastic force increases with passive stretch of a muscle past its resting length, the contractile force decreases. The Blix curve represents the summation of the contractile and viscoelastic forces of a muscle (Fig. 115-1). Both forces are at a minimum when the muscle fibers are contracted. At its resting length, the contractile force is at its maximum, while

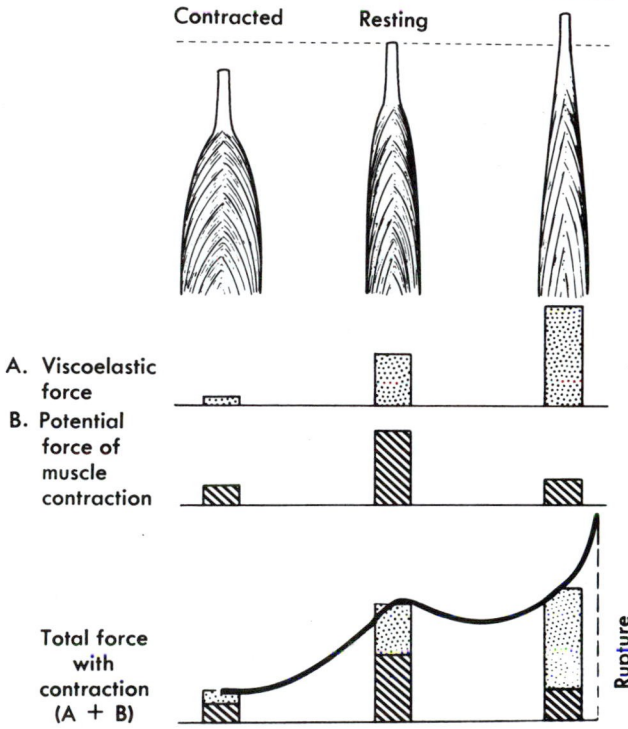

Figure 115-1

Blix curve. [Reprinted with permission from Smith RJ, Hastings H: Principles of tendon transfers to the hand. In: *Instructional Course Lectures. American Academy of Orthopaedic Surgeons.* St. Louis: CV Mosby; 1980; vol 29:133.]

the viscoelastic force is at 50 percent of its maximum. At maximum stretch, the contractile force is zero and the viscoelastic force is at its peak. Therefore, the greatest potential force for contraction of a muscle is at its resting length, and it is at that position that its tendon is sutured when transferred.

Work capacity (Table 115-1) is the ability of a muscle to exert force over a distance. It is related to the *cross-sectional area* of the muscle and the *length of its fibers,* which together represents muscle *volume* or *mass.* When comparing the flexor digitorum profundi (FDP) and interossei muscles, they both have similar cross-sectional areas, and therefore similar force potentials. However, the muscle fibers of the profundi are 3.5 times the length of the fibers of the interossei; its mass is therefore 3.5 times that of the interossei which means that its work capacity is 3.5 times greater. Combining the approximate equal masses of the flexor digitorum profundi and flexor digitorum superficialis (FDS) results in a work capacity that is 7 times that of the interossei.

Table 115-1

Work Capacity of Forearm and Hand Muscles (Mkg)

BR	2.0	ECU	1.0
FCU	2.0	APL	1.0
PT	1.5	EIP	0.5
FPL	1.0	EDQP	0.5
FDS (each)	1.0	EDC (each)	0.5
FDP (each)	1.0	EPB	0.1
ECRL	1.0	PL	0.1
ECRB	1.0	Interossei (all)	2.7

NOTE: APL, abductor pollicis longus; BR, brachioradialis; ECRL, extensor carpi radialis longus; ECU, extensor carpi ulnaris; EDC, extensor digitorum communis; EDQP, extensor digiti quinti proprius; EIP, extensor indicis proprius; EPB, extensor pollicis brevis; FCU, flexor carpi ulnaris; FDP, flexor digitorum profundi; FDS, flexor digitorum superficialis; FPL, flexor pollicis longus; PT, pronator teres; ECRB, extensor carpi radialis brevis; PL, palmaris longus.

4. *Amplitude.* The definition of amplitude is the excursion of a muscle and is directly related to the resting length of its fibers. Muscle fibers contract about 40 percent of their length *(contractile length),* which can be determined by faradic stimulation at surgery. They also can be stretched about 40 percent *(stretch length)* by putting traction on the tendon until the "spring" in the muscle is exhausted. The sum of contractile and stretch lengths represents the total amplitude of the muscle/tendon unit (Table 115-2).

The *true* amplitude of a muscle/tendon can be effectively increased by changing the position of the intercalary joints over which it passes. Normal wrist motions increase the amplitude by 25 mm. Therefore, when a wrist motor tendon with an average amplitude of 33 mm is transferred to finger extensors that require 50 mm of amplitude, full flexion and extension of the metacarpophalangeal (MP) joints can be achieved, provided the wrist remains mobile. Contraction of the wrist motors (33 mm) added to the normal tenodesis effect of wrist motions (25 mm) results in an *effective* amplitude of 55 mm. When active wrist motions are severely limited, the tendon transfer provides about 65 percent of normal amplitude (33 mm of excursion in the wrist motor vs. 50 mm required for digital extension).

The amplitude of some muscle/tendon units can be significantly increased by releasing their fascial attachments. An example is the brachioradialis (BR) muscle whose amplitude can

be more than tripled by mobilizing its fascial attachments in the proximal forearm.

5. *Direction.* A tendon transfer should pass in as straight a line as possible. This is not always possible or even desirable, as when carrying out an opposition tendon transfer using a flexor superficialis tendon. The direction of the tendon is deliberately altered by passing it through a pulley constructed near the pisiform so that it can pass across the palm, paralleling the pull of the abductor pollicis brevis (APB).

6. *Integrity.* The functional integrity of the donor tendon must be preserved. It cannot be split and transferred into tendons that move joints in opposite directions or into tendons that have different excursions. A tendon transferred to tendons with different excursions will effectively pull only on the tendon with the lesser amplitude. However, a donor tendon can be attached to multiple tendons, provided they perform similar functions, such as transfer of a single wrist tendon to all four finger extensors. Some tendon transfers maintain their original function in addition to their new function. For example, transfer of the pronator teres (PT) into the extensor carpi radialis brevis (ECRB) for wrist extension will not significantly reduce forearm pronation because the PT continues to pull in the same direction. Similarly, the brachioradialis transferred into the flexor digitorum profundi continues to act as an elbow flexor.

7. *Synergy.* *Synergistic* muscles are those that contract simultaneously to achieve a particular function such as the extrinsic finger flexors functioning together with the wrist extensors and the extrinsic finger extensors with the wrist flexors. *Antagonistic* muscles are those that have opposite actions such as the wrist flexors and wrist extensors. While in the lower extremities synergistic and antagonistic muscle functions are clearly defined, the same is not true in the upper extremities. For example, the extensor pollicis longus (EPL) and flexor pollicis brevis (FPB) muscles are considered synergistic because they both extend the thumb interphalangeal joint. However, they carry out that function under different circumstances; the EPL contracts with active MP joint extension, and the FPB with active MP flexion and when the thumb is in opposition. Antagonistic muscles can sometimes function together, such as the extensor carpi radialis longus (ECRL) and flexor carpi ulnaris (FCU). Both muscles contract simultaneously when using a hammer in order to control its speed and force on the up and down strokes. Each muscle functions as a brake for the other.

In the lower extremity, antagonistic muscles are never transferred, but the same is not true in the upper extremity. While retraining following a synergistic transfer is generally easier than after an antagonistic transfer, antagonistic transfers can be effective procedures in the upper extremities. For example, transferring a flexor digitorum superficialis tendon which is a proximal interphalangeal joint flexor into lateral bands which are extensors of those joints, is frequently used to

---

Table 115-2

Average Amplitude of Forearm Muscle/Tendon Units

Wrist flexors and extensors	33 mm (3.5 cm)
Finger extensors and flexor pollicis longus	50 mm (5.0 cm)
Finger flexors	70 mm (7.0 cm)

Table 115-3

**Planning Tendon Transfers in a Patient
with an Irreparable High Radial Nerve Injury**

Muscles Present	Muscles Available for Transfer	Functions Required
Pronator teres (PT)	PT	Wrist extension
Flexor carpi radialis (FCR)	FCR or FCU	Thumb extension/ Finger extension
Flexor carpi ulnaris (FCU)	(use only one)	
Flexor pollicis longus (FPL)	—	
Flexor digitorum profundi (FDP 2–5)	—	
Flexor digitorum superficialis (FDS 2–5)	FDS (middle and/or ring)	Thumb extension/ Finger extension
Palmaris longus (PL) absent in 10–15%	PL	Thumb extension
Thenar intrinsics	—	
Finger intrinsics	—	

---

restore *intrinsic* function. However, transferring the same tendon to the *extrinsic* extensor digitorum communis (EDC), which extend the metacarpophalangeal joints, sometimes results in retraining problems.

Planning tendon transfers is facilitated by making three columns (Table 115-3). The first column is a list of the extrinsic and intrinsic muscles in the extremity and their strengths, which are graded 0 to 5. The second column are those muscles in the first column that are available for transfer. Some muscles are *not* expendable; one flexor and one extensor must be retained for each digit as well as for the wrist, unless that joint is arthrodesed. The third column lists those functions that must be restored. The surgeon then matches the available muscles in the second column with the functions in the third column, taking into consideration muscle force, amplitude, direction, and integrity. If both wrist flexors are available, generally the flexor carpi radialis (FCR) is transferred and the more powerful FCU retained because it is the more effective flexor and it also provides for ulnar deviation of the wrist. Regarding the three wrist extensors (ECRL, ECRB, and ECU), if only one is required for transfer, the more central ECRB is used and the ECRL and extensor carpi ulnaris (ECU) are retained for extension as well as for radial and ulnar deviation of the wrist. If, however, two wrist extensors are required, the ECRL and ECU are used and the ECRB retained for wrist extension. The donor tendon does not become weaker after it is transferred since there is no change in the muscle itself, its nerve supply, or its circulation. However, the muscle does lose some of its elasticity as a consequence of unavoidable scarring.

Tendon transfers sometimes require two or more stages. Those transfers that require the wrist to be positioned in flexion postoperatively are generally performed in the first stage and those that require postoperative wrist extension, in the second stage. Tenodeses, capsulodeses, and arthrodeses are frequently carried out in conjunction with tendon transfers or are used as alternative procedures.

RADIAL NERVE PALSY

It is important to distinguish between a *radial* and *posterior interosseous palsy*. In a *radial palsy*, all the muscles supplied by the radial nerve, with the exception of the triceps, are paralyzed. The pa-

tient has complete loss of both wrist and digital (thumb and finger) extension. In a *posterior interosseous palsy*, the brachioradialis and extensor carpi radialis longus are intact since they are innervated more proximally by the radial nerve. Active wrist extension remains intact, although it is in a radial direction.

COMPLETE RADIAL PALSY

Many combinations of tendon transfers have been described for the treatment of a high radial nerve palsy. There is general agreement on only one transfer and that is the use of the pronator teres for restoring wrist extension. The procedure was first described by Sir Robert Jones who transferred the PT into both radial wrist extensors, the ECRL and ECRB. The preferred procedure is to transfer it only into the ECRB in order to minimize radial deviation of the wrist (Fig. 115-2).

Four combinations of tendon transfers for a complete radial palsy will be described.

1. PT to ECRB
   FCU to EDC (2-5)
   PL to rerouted EPL
   These combinations are sometimes referred to as the "standard" set of transfers (Fig. 115-3).

Disadvantages:
a. Nothing is done to replace the paralyzed extensor pollicis brevis (EPB) or the more important abductor pollicis longus (APL). The APL is a misnamed muscle because it only weakly abducts the thumb. Rather, by virtue of its origin on the dorsal aspect of the radius and insertion into the base of the first metacarpal, it extends the first metacarpal which is necessary to maintain the longitudinal arch of the thumb. It would be more appropriate to call this muscle the "extensor metacarpus primus." Failure to restore function of the APL results in the first metacarpal assuming a flexed position at the trapeziometacarpal joint. A zigzag or swan-neck deformity develops at the other two joints with hyperextension of the MP joint and flexion of the interphalangeal joint.

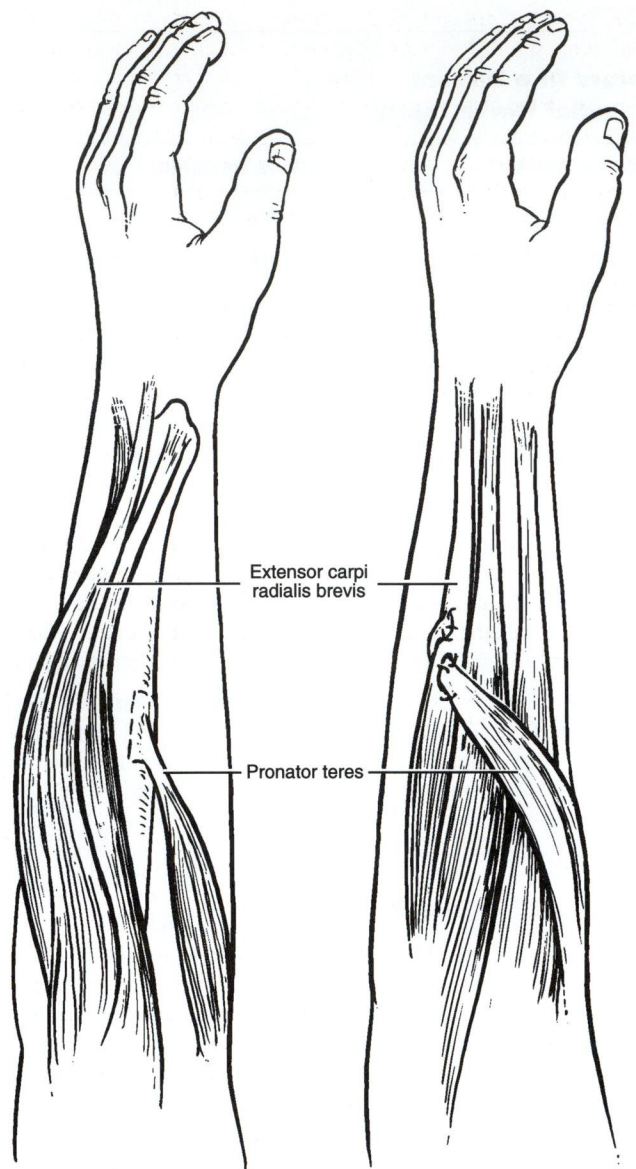

Figure 115-2
Transfer PT to ECRB. [Original illustration by Elizabeth Roselius ©
1988. Reprinted (modified) with permission from Green DP. *Operative
Hand Surgery.* New York: Churchill Livingstone; 1988:1488.]

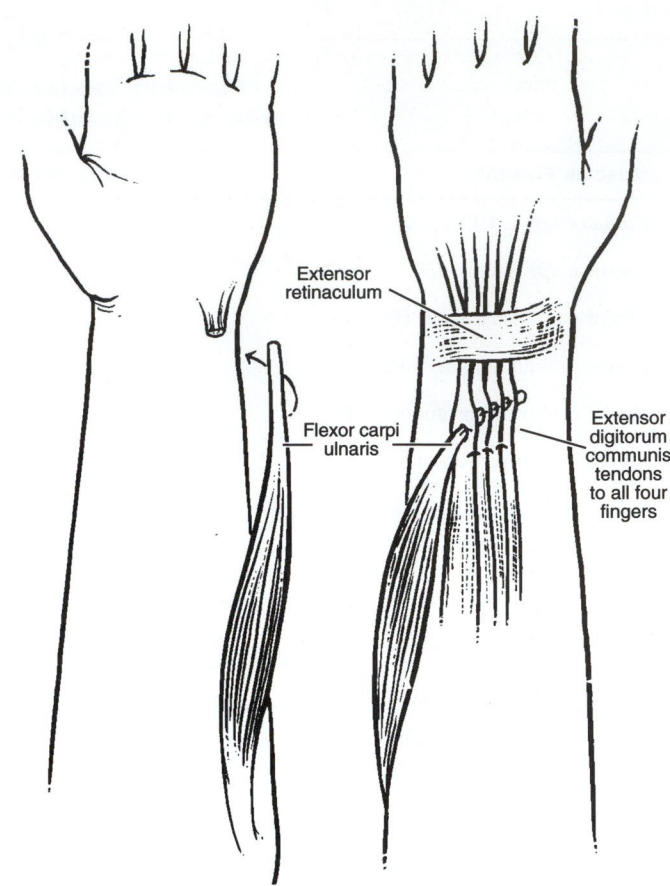

Figure 115-3
Transfer FCU to EDC. The FCU must be mobilized into the proximal
forearm in order that its pull is in as straight a line as possible. If necessary, the EDC tendons can be cut proximal to the tendon junctions.
[Original illustration by Elizabeth Roselius © 1988. Reprinted (modified) with permission from Green DP. *Operative Hand Surgery.* New
York: Churchill Livingstone; 1988:1488.]

b. Using the FCU removes the strongest flexor of the wrist
whose force is twice that of the FCR. In addition, normal
wrist motions pass through an oblique plane from volar-
ulnar to dorsal-radial, and removing the FCU weakens
flexion-ulnar deviation which is important in many manual
activities.

2. PT to ECRB
FCR to EDC (2-5)
PL to EPL (In patients whose thumbs have considerable MP flex-
ion, the EPB is first sutured into the EPL to prevent the joint
from falling into flexion)
APL tenodesis

Disadvantages:
a. Not suitable if the palmaris longus (PL) is absent

b. The limited excursion of the FCR requires that wrist motions
are excellent in order to achieve a full range of finger motions. This is also true when the FCU is used.
c. Can result in mild ulnar deviation of the wrist
3. Boyes' tendon transfers/Smith's tendon transfers
Both Boyes' and Smith's transfers have the following in *common:*
PT to ECRB
FDS (ring) through the interosseous membrane to EDC
FDS (middle) through the interosseous membrane to the extensor indicis proprius (EIP) and EPL
They *differ* in the tendon transferred to the APL. In Boyes'
transfers, the FCR is transferred to the APL and EPB, and in
Smith's transfers, the PL is transferred to the APL. If the
PL is absent, the APL is tenodesed.

Advantages of Boyes' and Smith's transfers:
a. Since the FDS muscles have greater excursion than either
the FCR or FCU, better digital excursion is restored if wrist
motions are limited.
b. Separates thumb-index extension from extension of the ulnar three fingers.

c.   Since Smith's transfers does not use a wrist motor, the normal flexion/ulnar deviation and extension/radial deviation of the joint are maintained.

d.   The length of FDS tendons permits them to reach the MP joints if there is scarring or a loss of extensor tendon substance on the dorsum of the hand.

e.   Passing FDS tendons through the interosseous membrane results in a direct line of pull and avoids any tendency for lateral deviation of the fingers which sometimes occurs when the tendons are passed around the radial or ulnar side of the forearm. However, the technique is not applicable in patients with rheumatoid wrist disease. In that condition, the tendons are passed around the *radial* aspect of the forearm to avoid increasing any ulnar deviation of the fingers that may exist or may develop in the future.

Disadvantages of Boyes' and Smith's transfers:

a.   Some patients have trouble relearning that the transferred FDS tendons are no longer finger flexors, but finger extensors. Instead of contracting the transferred tendons when attempting to actively extend their finger MP joints, they contact their intrinsic muscles which has the opposite effect on the MP joints. In order to reduce this tendency, patients are instructed to actively extend their MP joints while keeping both interphalangeal joints flexed.

b.   The procedure weakens the grip of the two donor fingers, although this is rarely a clinical problem.

c.   The two FDS tendons can become scarred in their path through the interosseous membrane.

d.   Leaving both wrist flexors intact in Smith's transfers may overpower the PT transfer into the ECRB.

POSTERIOR INTEROSSEOUS NERVE PALSY

The main disability of a posterior interosseous palsy is loss of finger and thumb extension. Wrist extension remains via the intact ECRL, but it is unbalanced, and since the ECRL originates proximal to the elbow, its power decreases significantly with elbow flexion. Radial deviation of the wrist can be improved by suturing the ECRB under sufficient tension into the functioning ECRL. If the ECRL and ECRB are both functioning, which sometimes occurs in a posterior interosseous palsy, and the wrist is radially deviated, the ECU is sutured to the ECRB. The options for restoring active finger and thumb extension are the same as for a complete radial palsy, with one exception. The FCR should not be used because it will exaggerate the radial deviation of the wrist.

MEDIAN NERVE PALSY

LOW MEDIAN NERVE PALSY

In a low median nerve palsy the forearm muscles are normal, but the thenar muscles, the abductor pollicis brevis, the radial head of the flexor pollicis brevis and the opponens pollicis are paralyzed. (The adductor pollicis is sometimes referred to as a "thenar muscle," but it is not situated in the thenar eminence and therefore should not be considered as such.) The lumbricals to the index and middle fingers are also paralyzed, but their loss rarely causes a problem because the interossei muscles to those two fingers, which are innervated by the ulnar nerve, remain intact.

The thenar intrinsic muscles provide *opposition* which is the position the thumb achieves when its pulp is opposite the pulp of the mid-

dle finger and its nail parallel to the volar surfaces of the fingers. *Opposition* is different from *apposition* which is when the thumb is simply in contact with the radial side of a finger and its nail is at 90 degrees to the plane of the palm. Opposition is a combination of three movements, *abduction, flexion,* and *pronation,* which all occur at the trapeziometacarpal joint. The metacarpophalangeal joint provides some flexion and a very limited degree of abduction. Opposition is not a type of grasp, but rather a *preparatory* position to grasp which when combined with the actions of the intrinsic adductor pollicis and the extrinsic flexor pollicis longus (FPL), *achieves* grasp. It is those two muscles that provide the *force* of grasp; the adductor pollicis for *pulp-to-side* or *key pinch,* and the flexor pollicis longus for *pulp-to-pulp tip pinch* (thumb and index finger) and *three-point chuck pinch* (thumb, index finger and middle finger). The position of the interphalangeal joint varies, depending on the type of pinch that is required. With *key pinch* it is extended, with *tip pinch* it is flexed, and with *three-point chuck pinch* it is midway between extended and flexed.

The most important of the thenar muscles for opposition is the *abductor pollicis brevis,* because it abducts, flexes and pronates the first metacarpal. In addition, by virtue of its insertion into the proximal phalanx and lateral band, it flexes and abducts the proximal phalanx, and extends the distal phalanx. The flexor pollicis brevis is not nearly as effective as the APB for abduction, and the opponens pollicis (OP), which inserts only on the metacarpal, has no effect on either the proximal or distal phalanx. Its action is limited to the metacarpal, similar to that of the APB, but much weaker. Therefore, when surgery is required for paralysis of the thenar intrinsic muscles, the objective is to restore function of the APB and not the other two intrinsic muscles, particularly the OP which is the least important of the thenar muscles. It was for that reason that Emanuel Kaplan preferred the term "opposition tendon transfer" to "opponensplasty", because it more accurately described the objective of the operation.

Since opposition is a *preparatory* movement, it does not require great force. Any muscle strong enough to move a thumb that is passively mobile, particularly at its trapeziometacarpal joint, can be used. An opposition tendon transfer should *not* attempt to strengthen grasp. If *force* of grasp is unsatisfactory, and generally this is due to paralysis of the flexor pollicis longus in a high median palsy and/or paralysis of the adductor pollicis in an ulnar palsy, tendon transfers for those muscles would be required. These transfers are discussed in later sections.

Since the APB muscle is the most important thenar muscle for opposition, the most effective tendon transfer is one that will parallel its fibers which are in line with the pisiform. Directing the tendon transfer from the pisiform to the thumb results in maximum abduction, flexion, and pronation which are the three movements of opposition. Directing the transfer from a more distal or ulnar location in the palm results in greater thumb flexion and pronation, but less abduction.

A variety of insertions into the thumb have been described. Generally, inserting the transfer into the tendon of the APB has been favored, but in patients with mobile MP joints, this attachment may cause unwanted flexion of the joint and have little or no effect on interphalangeal joint extension. In these situations, the tendon or a slip of the transferred tendon is attached to or passed around the extensor pollicis longus. If the objective of surgery is to obtain the maximum amount of thumb pronation, which is usually desirable, the tendon is attached into the base of the proximal phalanx just to the ulnar side where the tendon forms a tangent to the thumb. With this method of insertion, care must be taken not to cause a hyperextension deformity of the MP joint.

Common Opposition Tendon Transfers

1. *Flexor digitorum superficialis.* Described by Stirling Bunnell in 1938, this has become the "standard" opposition transfer. The flexor digitorum superficialis tendon of the ring finger is passed through a pulley constructed out of one half of the flexor carpi ulnaris tendon near its insertion, and then rerouted across the palm to the thumb, paralleling the paralyzed APB. The advantages of an FDS transfer are that the tendon has sufficient length to reach the dorsal aponeurosis of the thumb, and the muscle has excellent amplitude. It also has excellent strength, although, as previously noted, strength is not important for opposition. The procedure requires that there is no scarring on the volar aspect of the wrist and palm which might interfere with tendon gliding. Obviously, it can not be used in a high median nerve palsy.

2. *Extensor indicis proprius.* The extensor indicis proprius transfer is an excellent procedure that can be used for either a low or high median palsy, or for a combined median and ulnar palsy. The advantages of the procedure are that there is no loss of grip strength, the FDS is spared to use for restoring intrinsic tendon function in the fingers (in a combined median and ulnar palsy), and it is not necessary to construct a pulley. Disadvantages are that the tendon may not reach the thumb, and the patient may lose independent extension of the index MP joint, which is rarely a significant problem.

3. *Abductor digiti quinti.* This transfer was described separately by Huber and Nicolaysen in 1921. It is a technically more difficult procedure than other opposition transfers because, in addition to detaching the muscle distally at its insertion, it also must be detached proximally where there is risk of damaging its neurovascular bundle. The origin of the muscle is detached in order to rotate it 180 degrees and is then passed in a subcutaneous tunnel to the tendon of the APB. The advantages of the procedure are that it can be carried out when there is extensive scarring at the wrist (since all the dissection is within the palm), it provides excellent thumb pronation and flexion (but little abduction), and it restores the aesthetic bulge to the thenar eminence. The main disadvantage is the potential problem of injuring the neurovascular bundle which can result in muscle necrosis and denervation.

4. *Palmaris longus.* This transfer, described by Camitz in 1929, is the least complicated of all opposition tendon transfers. At surgery, the tendon is *not* detached at its insertion into the palmar fascia. Rather, it is dissected into the palmar fascia where a strip 1.5 cm in width and 4 to 5 cm in length is mobilized. This fascial strip effectively "lengthens" the tendon which is then inserted into the APB. The procedure is most applicable in older patients undergoing surgery for long standing carpal tunnel syndrome who have thenar muscle wasting. Since the PL lies radial to the median nerve, it will not compress the nerve after a carpal tunnel release. The transfer provides good abduction, but no pronation and for that reason it has been referred to as an "abductorplasty" rather than an opposition tendon transfer.

5. *Extensor carpi ulnaris.* This transfer utilizes the normal insertion of the extensor pollicis brevis as a point of attachment on the thumb. The EPB is divided at its *musculotendinous junction* in the forearm. The tendon is then rerouted across the palm and attached to the ECU which has been divided at its insertion into the base of the fifth metacarpal. The procedure, described by Phalen and Miller (1947), is not commonly performed because the excursion of the ECU is limited and the length of the EPB tendon is short which makes it difficult to suture to the ECU.

HIGH MEDIAN NERVE PALSY

In addition to paralysis of the thenar intrinsic muscles to the thumb, a high median nerve palsy results in paralysis of all the extrinsic muscles on the volar surface of the forearm, with the exception of the FCU and the FDP to the ring and little fingers. Since the FDS muscles are paralyzed, active flexion of both interphalangeal joints of the index finger is lost. However, flexion of the distal interphalangeal joint of the middle finger usually remains (although weakened), because its profundus muscle receives cross-innervation from the ulnar nerve.

The objectives of surgery are to restore opposition and active flexion (with power) to the thumb, index, and middle fingers. For opposition, the EIP can be used. Active flexion of the index and middle fingers can be restored simply by suturing their profundi tendons into the adjacent profundi to the ring and little fingers in the forearm (Fig. 115-4).

An alternative procedure is transfer of the ECRB to the profundi tendons and the brachioradialis to the FPL. The BR must be extensively mobilized in order to increase its excursion. Another disadvantage is its effect on thumb flexion which weakens with elbow flexion. This may cause a problem with some activities such as using a hammer. The worker may notice that his grip on the tool weakens on the upswing. An alternative procedure is to transfer the ECRB to the FPL and attach the profundi tendons of the index and middle fingers into the adjacent profundi of the middle and ring fingers.

ULNAR NERVE PALSY

The effects of an ulnar nerve palsy are profound and result in significant loss of grip strength and dexterity. Sterling Bunnell eloquently

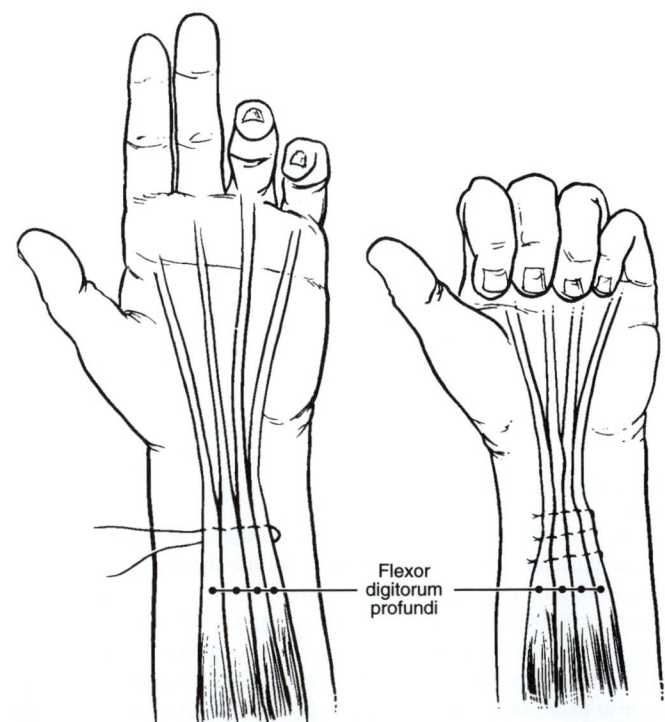

Figure 115-4
The tendons of the FDP (index and middle) are attached to the adjacent FDP tendons (ring and little). [Original illustration by Elizabeth Roselius © 1988. Reprinted (modified) with permission from Green DP: *Operative Hand Surgery.* New York: Churchill Livingstone; 1988:1551.]

described these changes; "The muscle balance in the hand will be so upset from loss of action of the intrinsic muscles that the hand will have lost its skill and be awkward at work."

CLINICAL SIGNS

Paralysis of the ulnar innervated muscles in the hand results in many deformities of the fingers and thumb. The number of eponymous signs that describe these deformities far exceeds those for any other neuropathy.

The signs associated with *finger* deformities include:

1. *Duchenne's sign: Clawing* of the fingers which is hyperextension of the MP joints and flexion of the interphalangeal joints. Normally, finger flexion is initiated at the MP joints and then all three finger joints flex simultaneously. With intrinsic paralysis, flexion at the MP joints occurs *after* flexion at both interphalangeal joints is complete. As a consequence, the fingers curl into the palm, and objects placed in the palm tend to be pushed away rather than grasped.

   For clawing to occur, *two* conditions must be present in addition to paralysis of the intrinsic muscles. The profundi tendons must be intact and the MP joints must be capable of passively hyperextending. Without intact profundi, such as occurs in a *high* ulnar palsy, the interphalangeal joints will not be flexed, and if the MP joints do not passively hyperextend, which is normally encountered in many individuals, the interphalangeal joints will only be slightly flexed. The greater the degree of passive MP joint hyperextension, the greater the degree of clawing. In a low ulnar nerve palsy, clawing is confined to the ring and little fingers because the lumbrical muscles to the index and middle fingers are innervated by the median nerve.

   If hyperextension of the MP joints is passively blocked, the extrinsic extensor digitorum communis and extensor digiti quinti, proprius (EDQP) will normally actively extend the interphalangeal joints. This is *Bouvier's maneuver* and is present in all patients with early ulnar neuropathies, regardless of etiology. The maneuver is the physiologic basis for a *lumbrical bar splint* which is commonly used following an ulnar nerve repair while waiting for reinnervation of the intrinsic muscles. The splint, which consists of a bar across the dorsal surfaces of the proximal finger segments, passively blocks MP joint extension. The MP joints are blocked in sufficient flexion to permit the extrinsic extensors to exert their normal extension force on the interphalangeal joints.

   When clawing is allowed to persist, the extensor tendon mechanism may become stretched and attenuated over the proximal interphalangeal joints. Bouvier's maneuver will no longer achieve active interphalangeal joint extension. The PIP joints may also develop fixed flexion *contractures* which are sometimes confused with *clawing. Flexion contracture* result from injury or disease to those anatomical structures that physically prevent the interphalangeal joints from passively extending (i.e., Dupuytren's disease or scarring of the skin, tendon sheath, flexor tendons and/or joint capsule). Clawing can lead to flexion contractures if a lumbrical bar splint is not used and if the interphalangeal joints are not periodically passively extended.

2. *André-Thomas sign:* Palmar flexion of the wrist which frequently accompanies clawing. It is a patient's unintentional attempt to improve finger extension by tenodesing the extrinsic extensor tendons. However, it is usually not effective and tends to increase the clawing.

3. *Masse's sign:* Flattening of the transverse metacarpal arch of the palm due to paralysis of the opponens digiti quinti, the prime flexor of the fifth carpometacarpal joint.

4. *Wartenberg's sign:* Inability to *adduct* the little finger to the extended ring finger. This is often a presenting complaint of patients with ulnar neuropathies and results from paralysis of the third volar interosseous. The abducted position of the little finger is due to the action of the functioning extensor digiti quinti proprius and/or the flexor carpi ulnaris which pulls on the paralyzed abductor digiti minimi into which it is partially inserted.

5. *Sunderland's sign:* Inability to rotate the little finger.

6. *Egawa's sign:* Inability to abduct and adduct the middle finger due to paralysis of the 2d and 3d dorsal interossei, respectively.

7. *Mumenthaler's sign:* The loss of dimpling in the skin over the hypothenar eminence with resisted abduction of the little finger. This obscure sign, which results from paralysis of the palmaris brevis muscle, has no clinical significance.

The signs associated with *thumb* deformities include:

1. *Froment's sign:* Froment described the "signe du journal" or "paper sign" which is characterized by acute flexion of the interphalangeal joint of the thumb with pinch. It is an attempt by the flexor pollicis longus to compensate for paralysis or weakness of the adductor pollicis and, to a lesser extent, the first dorsal interosseous muscle. Flexion of the interphalangeal joint is also a compensatory maneuver to increase the tension on the extensor pollicis longus tendon which, in addition to extending the interphalangeal joint, adducts the thumb.

2. *Jeanne's sign:* Hyperextension of the MP joint with pinch due to paralysis of the adductor and flexor pollicis brevis muscles which normally flex the MP joint. The sign is present only in patients with normal laxity of their MP joints.

SURGICAL TREATMENT FOR INTRINSIC PARALYSIS OF THE FINGERS

Static Procedures

Static procedures are all based on the normal function of the extrinsic extensor tendons to actively extend the interphalangeal joints *provided* that they do not hyperextend the metacarpophalangeal joints. Thus if hyperextension of the MP joints is blocked, clawing of the fingers will be corrected (Bouvier's maneuver). Static procedures are useful in clinical situations where there are a paucity of active tendons available for transfer, such as in patients with brachial plexus injuries. They are not effective in chronic cases when the extensor tendons have become stretched over the PIP joints or when flexion contractures have developed at those joints.

The *Dorsal Bone Block* procedure, described by Mikhail 1964, involved inserting a wedge of iliac bone into the dorsal aspect of the metacarpal head in order to block full extension of the proximal phalanx. The procedure has never gained wide acceptance because the bone graft sometimes resorbs or is dislodged, and there is risk of later arthritis due to injury to the articular surface of the metacarpal head.

Volar Capsulorrhaphy was introduced in 1957 by Zancolli who tightened the volar plate as a method to prevent MP joint extension. The problem with the original technique was that it had a tendency to stretch, and MP joint hyperextension recurred. A reliable technique that minimizes the risk of recurrence, is to detach the proximal membranous portion of the plate and anchor it into a slot in the neck portion of the metacarpal.

Tenodeses have been described and they can be divided into two groups, depending on whether they begin *distal* or *proximal* to the wrist. Tenodeses that begin distal to the wrist are inserted either into the *proximal phalanx* when they simply prevent MP joint hyperextension, or into the *lateral band* when they function as *active tenodeses* since they extend the PIP joints when the MP joints are extended. Three examples are the Sling, Parkes, and Riordan tenodeses:

1. The *Sling tenodesis* is a short tendon graft that is attached to the ulnar lateral band of one digit, passed around the deep transverse metacarpal ligament, and attached to the radial lateral band of the adjacent finger. The graft is sutured with the MP joints in 30 degrees of flexion and the PIP joints in complete extension. It is not a complicated procedure, but it tends to cause mild scissoring between the two fingers.

2. *Parkes tenodesis* is a tendon graft that is sutured proximally to the transverse carpal ligament and distally to the lateral bands of the fingers. Its proximal attachment is distal to the wrist joint and therefore, it is not influenced by motions of the wrist.

3. The *Riordan tenodesis* is similar to Parkes tenodesis, except the tendons have a dorsal route. The ECRL and ECU tendons are each split longitudinally and one half of each tendon is divided proximally. The divided portion of each tendon is then split again longitudinally which provides a total of four tendon slips; two remain attached to the base of the second metacarpal and two to the base of the fifth metacarpal. The four slips are then passed between the metacarpals volar to the deep transverse metacarpal ligaments in order that they are volar to the axis of motion of the MP joints. The two slips from the ECU are sutured to the *radial* lateral bands of the ring and little fingers. The two slips from the ECRL are sutured to the *radial* lateral band of the middle finger and the *ulnar* lateral band of the index finger. The slip to the index finger cannot be sutured to its radial lateral band because there is no deep transverse metacarpal ligament on the radial side of the index finger. The method of attachment to the index finger is the same for all active tendon transfers that arise from the *dorsal* aspect of the hand and wrist. Since the proximal origins of the four tendon slips remain attached to the bases of the metacarpals, the tenodeses are not affected by wrist movements.

The only tenodesis that begins *proximal* to the wrist is the *Fowler tenodesis*. Two free tendon grafts (the plantaris tendons are best suited because of their long length), are each split longitudinally to form four tendon slips. They are passed through the extensor retinaculum and each is tunneled through one of the intermetacarpal spaces and attached to the lateral band of each finger (Fig. 115-5). Since the four tendon slips begin proximal to the wrist they function as "active" tenodeses; with active wrist flexion they tighten resulting in MP joint flexion and interphalangeal joint extension.

Tendon Transfers

Tendon transfers are preferable to static procedures (if active donors are available) because in addition to correcting clawing, they also improve grip strength (slightly) and restore synchronous motions at the MP and interphalangeal joints. As with tenodeses, tendon transfers must pass *volar* to the axis of motion of the MP joints. Intrinsic tendon transfers utilize the following motors.

Flexor Superficialis Transfers

Stiles-Bunnell Tendon Transfer A flexor superficialis tendon is divided, split longitudinally and each slip is passed through the

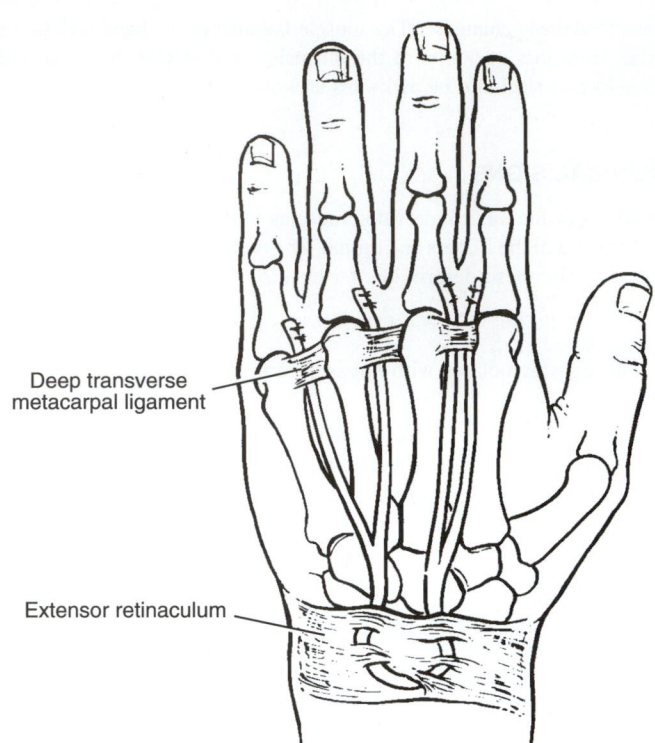

Figure 115-5
Fowler tenodesis to correct clawing. [Original illustration by Elizabeth Roselius © 1988. Reprinted (modified) with permission from Green DP: *Operative Hand Surgery.* New York: Churchill Livingstone; 1988:1541.]

lumbrical canal of the ring and little fingers and sutured to the lateral band of that finger (Fig. 115-6). Generally, the FDS tendon of the middle finger is used. In combined low median and ulnar neuropathies, two FDS tendons are required for all four fingers. Disadvantages of the procedure are that the force of flexion of the donor finger(s) is diminished and patients with supple joints sometimes develop postoperative hyperextension or swan neck deformities of the proximal interphalangeal joint.

Transfer to the Proximal Phalanx To avoid the risk of postoperative swan-neck deformities, the FDS is attached to the proximal phalanges rather than to the lateral bands (Fig. 115-7). This will only

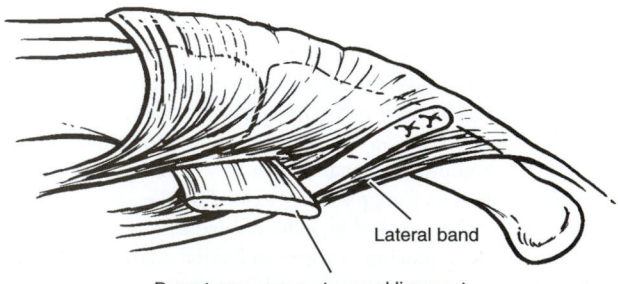

Figure 115-6
The lateral band is the common point of attachment for an intrinsic tenodesis or active tendon transfer. [Original illustration by Elizabeth Roselius © 1988. Reprinted (modified) with permission from Green DP: *Operative Hand Surgery.* New York: Churchill Livingstone; 1988:1542.]

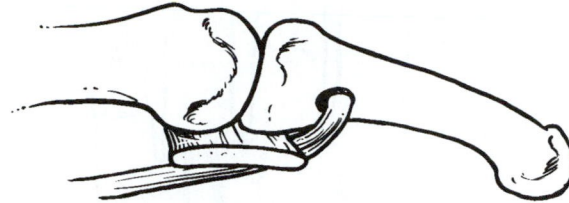

Figure 115-7
Attachment of the tendon into the proximal phalanx. [Original illustration by Elizabeth Roselius © 1988. Reprinted (modified) with permission from Green DP: *Operative Hand Surgery*. New York: Churchill Livingstone; 1988:1542.]

be effective if Bouvier's maneuver remains intact. Otherwise, the FDS must be transferred into the lateral bands.

Zancolli Lasso Procedure   The FDS of each clawed finger is divided, passed through a window made in the A-2 pulley of the flexor tendon sheath, and looped back and sutured to itself in the distal palm (Fig. 115-8). If the FDS are paralyzed, as in a high median neuropathy, it can still be used to make a "lasso," but the proximal end of the tendon must be transferred into an available wrist motor. The FDS tendon in these situations functions as a free tendon graft.

Extensor Carpi Radialis Longus and Brevis Transfers

Brand Transfer   Paul Brand noted that FDS intrinsic transfers often caused swan neck deformities, particularly in his patients who had leprosy and tended to be loose jointed. Instead of using the FDS, he recommended that the ECRL or ECRB be used as a motor, or if either was unavailable, the ECU. The wrist tendon is "lengthened" with a "four-tail" tendon graft, preferably a plantaris tendon because of its long length. If a plantaris tendon is absent, multiple toe extensors or two palmaris longus tendons that are each split, can be used. The four tendon slips are transferred *volarly* through the carpal tunnel, and each is passed through the lumbrical canal of a finger and sutured into the lateral band (Fig. 115-9). The problem with routing the tendon slips volarly is that it can result in median nerve compression. This was not a problem in Brand's patients who had chronic leprosy and generally had insensate hands due to their underlying disease. Most Brand transfers now involve passing the tendon slips dorsally through the intermetacarpal spaces and then volar to the deep transverse metacarpal ligaments. The slips are attached to the radial

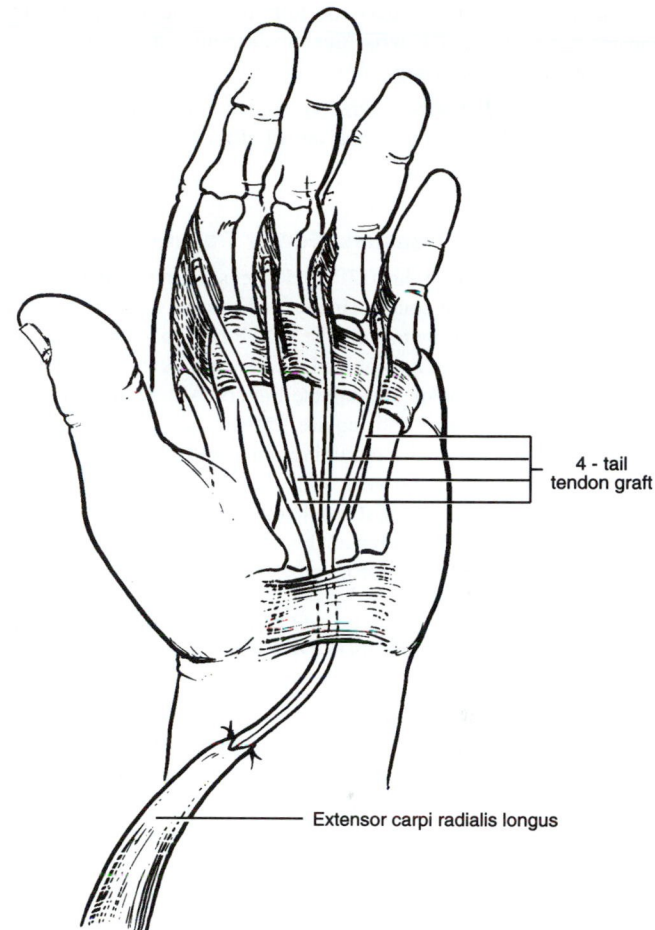

Figure 115-9
Brand intrinsic transfer utilizing the ECRL. Since the 4 tendon grafts are volar, each is passed through a lumbrical canal to the radial lateral band of that finger. [Original illustration by Elizabeth Roselius © 1988. Reprinted (modified) with permission from Green DP: *Operative Hand Surgery*. New York: Churchill Livingstone; 1988:1545.]

lateral bands of the middle, ring and little fingers and the ulnar lateral band of the index finger. The main advantage of a Brand transfer is that it improves grip strength. However, it risks increasing wrist flexion which is common in patients with claw deformities.

Burkhalter Transfer   This transfer is similar to a Brand transfer except the tendon slips are attached to the proximal phalanges rather than to the lateral bands. The advantage of attaching the tendons to the phalanges is that the force of the transfer is concentrated at the bones which supposedly increases power grip. The disadvantage is that it does not restore active PIP joint extension and it cannot be used if Bouvier's maneuver is negative.

Flexor Carpi Radialis Transfers

Riordan Transfer   Instead of using a wrist extensor, as advocated by Brand, the flexor carpi radialis tendon is the motor. It is "lengthened" with a "four-tailed" graft which is passed *dorsally* and inserted into the lateral bands in the same method as described by Brand. The advantage of using the FCR is that it is normally in phase with the

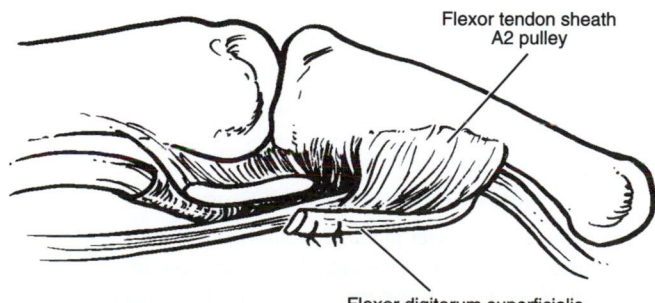

Figure 115-8
Zancolli lasso procedure. [Original illustration by Elizabeth Roselius © 1988. Reprinted (modified) with permission from Green DP: *Operative Hand Surgery*. New York: Churchill Livingstone; 1988:1542.]

intrinsic muscles to the fingers and little retraining is required. The transfer also corrects the wrist flexion deformity that is present in many patients with clawing.

Brooks-Jones Transfer   The four tendon slips from the FCR are passed *volarly* through the carpal tunnel. This risks compression of the median nerve.

Extensor Proprius Transfers (Fowler Transfer)

The extensor indicis proprius (EIP) and extensor digiti quinti proprius (EDQP) are each split longitudinally and passed deep to the deep transverse metacarpal ligaments. The EDQP is transferred to the ring and little fingers, and in a combined median and ulnar palsy, the EIP is transferred to the index and middle fingers. Although these transfers are not complicated and require few incisions, they are out of phase at the MP joints and retraining may be difficult. In addition, the two donor tendons are weak and will not significantly improve grip strength. Another potential problem is that the EDQP may be the only extensor of the MP joint of the little finger, which obviously should be determined before it is transferred.

Palmaris Longus

The palmaris longus is lengthened with a four-tailed plantaris graft that is passed through the carpal tunnel and inserted into the lateral bands. As with any transfer through the carpal tunnel, there is risk of median nerve compression. The procedure has been successful in patients with leprosy who generally have very supple hands. In other patients, it is not as effective because of the limited power and excursion of the palmaris longus.

SURGICAL TREATMENT FOR THUMB DEFORMITIES IN ULNAR PALSY

With paralysis of the ulnar innervated intrinsic muscles, the effects on power grip are profound. In contradistinction to *precision handling* when only modest power of the thenar muscles is necessary to place the thumb in opposition, *power grip* requires strength of the adductor pollicis muscle to hold the thumb in an adducted position. The cross-sectional area of the adductor pollicis muscle is large which accounts for its great force. Its muscle fiber length is short which limits its amplitude, but amplitude is unnecessary for power grip. The radial head of the first dorsal interosseous also contributes to thumb adduction, but it is not nearly as powerful as the adductor pollicis. When both muscles are paralyzed, adduction of the thumb is reduced more than 75 percent. The extrinsic extensor pollicis longus weakly adducts the thumb, since its tendon courses dorsal to the trapeziometacarpal joint which is the axis of abduction-adduction movements. The flexor pollicis longus neither adducts nor abducts the thumb, because its path is close to the axes of motion of the trapeziometacarpal and metacarpophalangeal joints. It is a pure flexor of the thumb.

The surgical procedures that have been described for the treatment of weakness of power grip and pinch can be divided into those which improve thumb adduction and those that strengthen index finger abduction.

Thumb Adduction Procedures (Adductorplasties)

These procedures attempt to restore function of the adductor pollicis muscle. In order to be most effective, the transfers should pass on the volar surface of the transverse head of the adductor muscle and be

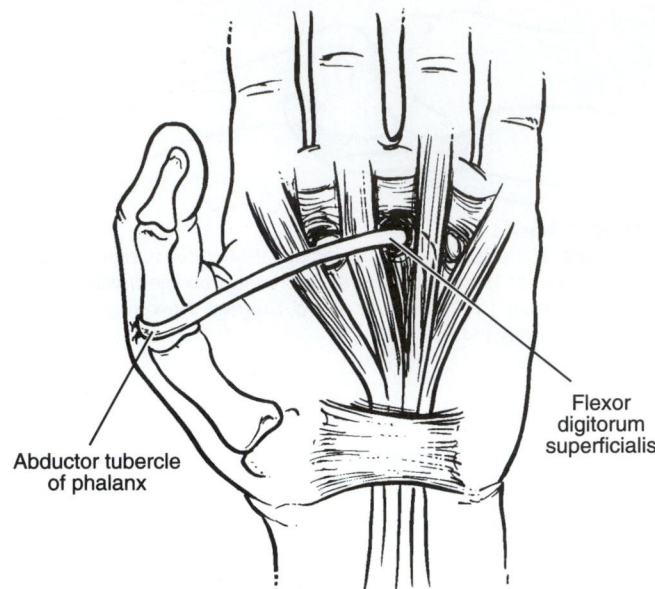

Figure 115-10
Transfer of FDS tendon ring finger to the abductor tubercle. [Original illustration by Elizabeth Roselius © 1988. Reprinted (modified) with permission from Green DP: *Operative Hand Surgery*. New York: Churchill Livingstone; 1988:1547.]

sutured at its insertion. The only donor muscles whose tendons are of sufficient length and do not require lengthening with free tendon grafts are the extensor indicis proprius and flexor digitorum superficialis. The problem with the EIP is its limited strength. Flexor superficialis transfers are usually routed through a hole in the palmar fascia and then directed toward the thumb and sutured into the *adductor* tubercle of the proximal phalanx (Fig. 115-10). In combined median and ulnar palsies, the attachment is sometimes into the *abductor* tubercle of the proximal phalanx. The FDS tendon can also be routed to the dorsum of the wrist, through the interosseous membrane proximal to the pronator quadratus. The tendon is then passed around the extensor carpi ulnaris tendon, which acts as a pulley, and then across the dorsal aspect of the palm in line with the EPL and deep to the other extensor tendons, and is sutured into the ulnar base of the proximal phalanx of the thumb.

Other muscles used for thumb adduction are the brachioradialis and extensor carpi radialis brevis (Fig. 115-11). Both are effective transfers because of their power, but both must be lengthened with a free tendon graft in order to reach the insertion of the adductor pollicis muscle.

Index Finger Abduction Procedures

The components of power pinch are thumb adduction and index finger abduction. A variety of transfers have been described to improve abduction of the index using the EIP, a slip of the abductor pollicis longus, or the extensor pollicis brevis. Of the three, the APL requires lengthening with a tendon graft in order to be of sufficient length to reach the tendon of the first dorsal interosseous muscle at its insertion into the radial base of the proximal phalanx of the index finger.

SUGGESTED READINGS

Brand PW: Principles for restoration of muscle balance after forearm and hand paralysis. In Chapman MW (ed): *Operative Orthopaedics.* 2d ed. Philadelphia: JB Lippincott; 1993; vol 2:1445.

Green DP: Radial nerve palsy. In Green DP (ed): *Operative Hand Surgery* vol 2, 3d ed. New York: Churchill Livingstone; 1993:1401.

Green SM: Reconstruction for ulnar nerve palsy. In Peimer CA (ed): *Surgery of the Hand and Upper Extremity.* New York: McGraw-Hill; 1996:1399.

Imbriglia JE, Hagberg WC, Baratz ME: Median nerve reconstruction. In Peimer CA (ed): *Surgery of the Hand and Upper Extremity.* New York: McGraw-Hill; 1996:1381.

Mannerfelt L: Studies on the hand in ulnar nerve paralysis. A clinical-experimental investigation in normal and anomalous innervation. *Acta Orthop Scand.* 1966 (suppl 87).

Mikhail IK: Bone block operation for clawhand. *Surg Gynecol Obstet* 1964; 118:1077.

Phalen GS, Miller RC: The transfer of wrist extensor muscles to restore or reinforce flexion power of the fingers and opposition of the thumb. *J Bone Joint Surg [Am]* 1947; 29:993.

Smith RJ: *Tendon Transfers of the Hand and Forearm.* Boston: Little, Brown and Co; 1987.

Zancolli EA: Claw-hand caused by paralysis of the intrinsic muscles. A simple surgical procedure for its correction. *J Bone Joint Surg [Am]* 1957; 39:1076.

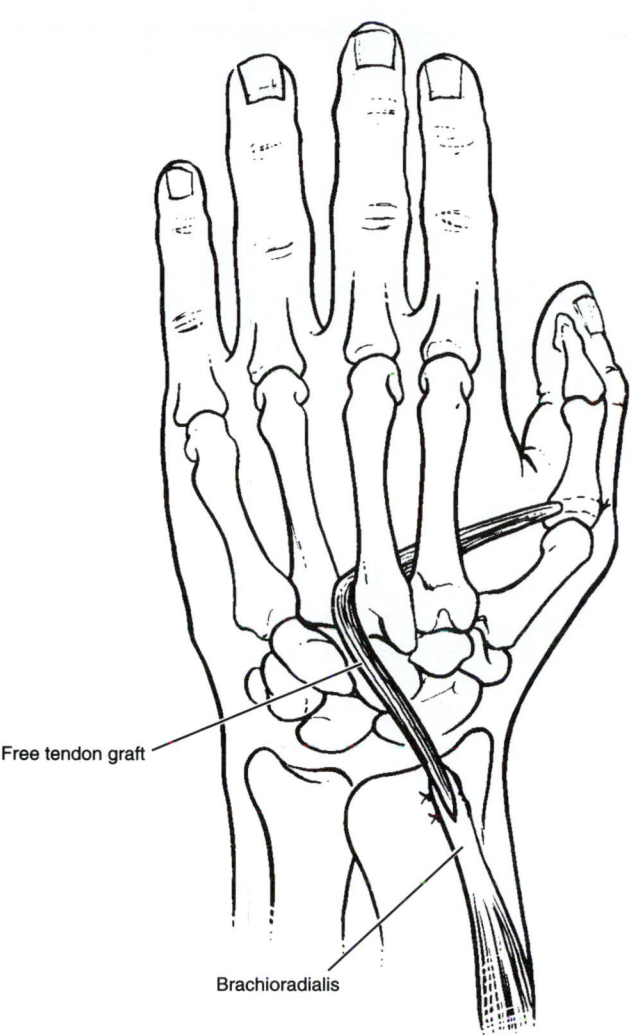

Free tendon graft

Brachioradialis

Figure 115-11

Transfer of BR prolonged with a free tendon graft that is passed through an intermetacarpal space and inserted on the adductor tubercle. [Original illustration by Elizabeth Roselius © 1988. Reprinted (modified) with permission from Green DP: *Operative Hand Surgery.* New York: Churchill Livingstone; 1988:1546.]

Chapter 116

TENDON INJURIES

Steven M. Green

FLEXOR TENDON INJURIES

Until about 20 years ago, repair of flexor tendon lacerations within the digit was so unsatisfactory that such surgery was not recommended. Since then, new information concerning the anatomy, physiology, biomechanics, and intrinsic healing of the flexor tendon system has led to improved surgical technique and post-operative therapy so that primary repair of flexor tendons is now the norm.

ANATOMY

The flexor tendons begin in the mid-forearm as the continuation of the flexor muscles, which arise from the distal humerus, the radius, the ulna, and the radioulnar interosseous membrane. There are three wrist flexors: flexor carpi radialis (FCR), palmaris longus (PL), and the flexor carpi ulnaris (FCU). The FCR enters its individual tunnel at the wrist, passes around the trapezium, and then inserts on the index metacarpal. The palmaris longus, when present (80 percent), merges with the palmar facia and is a weak flexor of the wrist. The FCU, a strong wrist flexor and ulnar deviator inserts on the pisiform. The digital flexors include the flexor pollicis longus (FPL), the flexor digitorum superficialis (FDS), and the flexor digitorum profundus (FDP). Whereas the FPL and the FDS have independent muscles, the FDP shares a common muscle which is innervated by both the median and ulnar nerves. At the wrist level the digital flexors enter the carpal canal and then pass into a fibroosseous digital sheath. At the proximal phalanx the FDS divides into two slips (the decussation) which loop around the profundus tendon, then rejoin at the Chiasm of Camper only to divide again into two tendons which insert onto the middle phalanx. The primary function of the FDS is independent flexion of the proximal interphalangeal joint (PIP). The FPL and the FDP pass along the entire length of the digit inserting into the distal phalanx. The FPL flexes the thumb interphalangeal joint and the FDP flexes both finger interphalangeal joints.

The fibroosseous tunnel is composed of a series of retinacula, bands that arise from the phalanges and the volar plates of the metacarpophalangeal (MP), PIP, and DIP joints. This tunnel begins at the MP joint and covers the digital flexors from this level to the distal phalanx. Those portions of the sheaths which lie transversely are called annular pulleys while those that are composed of an oblique or crisscrossing fibers are called cruciate pulleys (see Fig. 17-1). Without an adequate pulley system the flexor tendons would bowstring upon flexion. This displacement, which increases the flexor moment arm, would adversely affect active flexion and eventually lead to a flexion contracture. The finger A-2 (proximal phalanx) and A-4 (middle phalanx) and the thumb C-1 (proximal phalanx) are the essential pulleys and must be preserved or reconstructed during surgery.

Within the digital sheath the flexor tendons are surrounded by a double layer tenosynovium. The tenosynovium of the thumb (radial bursa) extends proximally to the wrist. The ulnar bursa is the proximal continuation of the small finger tenosynovium which also surrounds the finger flexors within the carpal canal and continues proximally to the wrist where it may communicate with the radial bursa.

A popular classification system localizes the digital flexor tendons into five anatomic zones (Fig. 116-1.)

PHYSIOLOGY

Until recently flexor tendons were considered to be inert, incapable of intrinsic healing. It is now accepted that healing can occur by both ingrowth from peripheral tissues into the tendon (extrinsic) and directly from one edge of the tendon laceration to the other (intrinsic). The proportion of extrinsic versus intrinsic healing depends upon the site and cause of the injury, individual variation, and the method of postoperative rehabilitation. Extrinsic healing begins with the ingrowth of capillaries and fibroblasts. Collagen formation then follows. Remodeling begins after 21 days. Intrinsic healing is initiated by tenocytes at the tendon periphery; tenocytes within the tendon

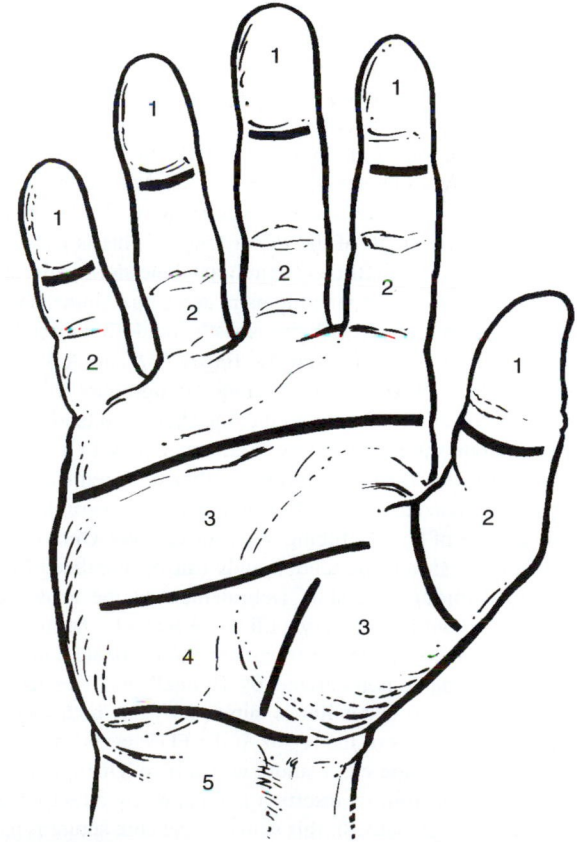

Figure 116-1
Flexor tendon zones.

(endotenon) become active 2 to 3 weeks later. By 2 months this process is completed.

Tendons are metabolically active structures which are nourished by both the tenosynovial fluid and a vascular network. Within the digital sheath diffusion of nutrients from tenosynovial fluid is of primary importance. Of lesser importance is an arterial system which is both extra- and intratendinous. The extratendinous vessels called vincula are branches of the digital arteries. Usually each tendon has both a short vinculum near its insertion and a long vinculum more proximally. The FDP long vinculum arises from or adjacent to the FDS short vinculum. Therefore excision of the FDS may affect the vascularity of the FDP.

Blood enters the dorsal surface of the tendons via the vinculae and flows axially within its substance, ending in closed capillary loops. Flexor tendons not covered with tenosynovium are totally dependent upon vascular nutrition.

FLEXOR TENDON REPAIR

Primary repair of lacerated flexor tendons should not be attempted in an emergency room setting. Instead, the skin wound should be cleansed and closed (unless grossly contaminated), and the tendon repair accomplished in the operating room. Closed rupture of the FDP is another cause of flexor disruption and occurs when a flexed digit is forcefully extended. A classic example is the football player who ruptures the ring finger FDP while attempting a one-hand tackle. Since the profundus avulsion may be associated with a fracture of a distal phalanx, a radiograph is required when evaluating this injury.

Flexor tendon repair accomplished within 24 h of injury is classified as primary and delayed primary if carried out 1 to 14 days thereafter. Direct secondary repair can often be accomplished up to 3 to 4 weeks from injury. After 1 month, muscle contracture and tendon shortening usually precludes direct repair. Because the tendons usually retract after injury, the skin laceration will usually not provide sufficient exposure to permit tendon repair. If the digits were in extension when the tendon was lacerated, the skin and tendon injury will be at the same site. If the injury occurred with the digits flexed, the tendon will have been cut distal to the skin wound. In the operating room, surgical incision should be planned to allow full visualization of the entire length of the flexor tendon. This is usually accomplished using zig-zag (Bruner) or mid-axial incisions in the digits, with proximal extension through the palm and carpal tunnel and into the forearm as necessary. The digital sheath should be opened judiciously, preserving at a minimum the finger A-2 and A-4 and the thumb C-1 pulleys. Flexing and extending the digit may aid in visualizing the tendon ends and help predict the site of the tendon repair. Retracted tendons should be retrieved atraumatically to avoid additional damage to the tendons and digital sheath. A retracted flexor tendon may be passed up the sheath with a grasping instrument, a suture, or some type of flexible tubing or plastic catheter. Once replaced within the digital sheath the tendon ends can be stabilized by fine needles passed through the skin. Debridement of the tendon ends should be carried out if necessary, utilizing a scalpel. The most popular suturing methods utilize a 3-0 or 4-0 nonabsorbable core suture which were originally popularized by Bunnell and Kessler (Fig. 116-2). A running 6-0 epitendinous suture provides both increased strength and smoothness of the repair. If the FDS has been lacerated near its insertion, a figure-eight suture will suffice. Disruption of the FDP less than 1 cm from its insertion is repaired by direct reattachment into the distal phalanx. In this situation the core suture is passes through the bone with a Keith needle and tied over a cotton pad or button on the finger nail. If both tendons have been lacerated within the finger but cannot be simultaneously repaired, suture of the FDP

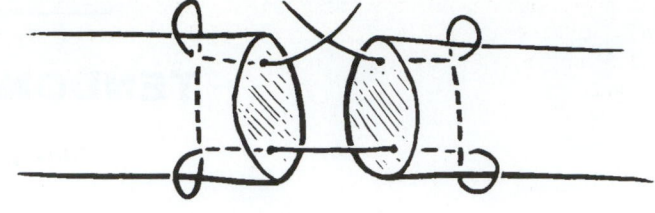

modified Kessler

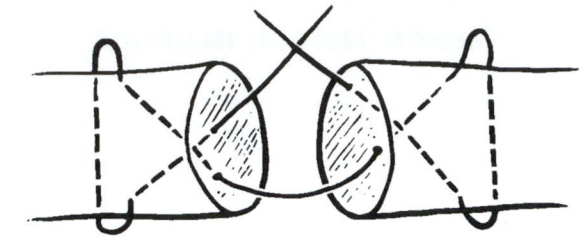

modified Bunnell

Figure 116-2
Modified Kessler and Bunnell tendon suture techniques.

is carried out and one or both slips of the FDS is excised. Under no circumstances should an intact FDS be sacrificed in the attempt to repair the FDP. Partial flexor lacerations that amount to less than 50 percent of the tendon usually do not profit from repair. The intact portion is strong enough to permit gentle early mobility exercises and suturing actually weakens the uninjured portion. A partial flap-type laceration in Zone II (usually the profundus) which causes "triggering" should be treated by either debridement or suturing depending upon the severity of the tendon injury.

Although early mobilization after flexor tendon surgery generally improves tendon glide and strength, the surgeon's preference and the type of patient are important considerations. Early mobilization can be accomplished in several fashions. The Kleinert method utilizes a dorsal splint with the wrist in 45 degrees of flexion, the MPs in 70 degrees of flexion, and the interphalangeal joints fully extended. An elastic string or rubber band is attached to the finger nail and to the distal forearm and maintains a flexed posture of the digit. Each hour the patient is instructed to actively extend the digit up to the splint to a count of 10. It is theorized that with active extension the flexor muscles relax allowing passage of the repaired tendon through the sheath without tension. Such gliding inhibits adhesions and the gentle load on the flexor tendon aids in healing without disrupting the repair. The patient is cautioned not to actively flex the digit. Flexion contractures occur if the patient does not properly exercise or if the elastic tension is excessive, preventing full digital extension. After 3 to 4 weeks the elastic traction is discontinued and active flexion is added to the program. A removable protective splint is continued until the sixth postoperative week. The Duran method also utilizes a dorsal splint but does not involve dynamic traction. Instead, passive flexion and extension of the digit is undertaken to inhibit spot welding of the repair site. This is done with the wrist and MP joint in flexion while the digit is mobilized. Some surgeons believe that with modern suture techniques immediate active flexion is possible, but this philosophy is not widely accepted. Blocking exercises are begun 6 weeks postoperatively. By 8 weeks strengthening can be instituted with hand putty as necessary. Dynamic splinting can be used at this time if a joint contracture exists.

Recovery of mobility is best accessed with a goniometer. The total active motion system (TAM) measures the total degrees of active MP and IP flexion minus any extension deficit. Recovery is graded as follows:

Excellent   220 degrees or more
Good   200 degrees to 219 degrees
Fair   180 degrees to 199 degrees
Poor   Less than 180 degrees

Despite the best efforts of the surgeon and patient, flexor tendon surgery is not predictably effective in restoring mobility. Unsatisfactory recovery may be the result of disruption of the repair, adhesions, or joint contractures. Tenolysis can be considered 3 to 4 months after tenorrhaphy if adhesions inhibit mobility. Such surgery is often more extensive than the initial repair procedure and requires immediate postoperative therapy to prevent the reformation of peritendinous scar. Tenolysis is commonly carried out under local anesthesia so that the active function of the flexor system can be accurately evaluated. During the tenolysis the critical pulleys must be preserved to prevent postoperative bowstringing. A small catheter can be inserted near the digital nerves to deliver bupivacaine (Marcaine) during the first postoperative days, reducing postoperative pain and promoting rehabilitation. The major complication of tenolysis is delayed rupture of a tendon whose nutrition may have been adversely affected.

FLEXOR TENDON RECONSTRUCTION

A flexor tendon reconstruction is undertaken when direct repair is not possible or following a failed tendon repair. Success is dependent upon joint mobility, digital sensibility, pulley integrity, and adequate skin coverage. If these are all present, surgery is accomplished in one stage with removal of the lacerated tendon(s) and replacement with a free flexor graft. The flexor system is exposed preserving the pulley system to permit excision of the tendon remnants. A tendon graft is harvested (palmaris longus, plantaris or toe extensor) and passed through the digital sheath and fixed into the distal phalanx with a pullout suture or suture anchor. The proximal juncture, usually in the palm is accomplished with an interweaving technique as popularized by Pulvertaft. This method requires passing the graft through a slit in the larger flexor tendon. This is repeated one or two more times with each slit 90 degrees from the adjacent one. Tension is set so that the digit rests at the physiological cascade. If the tension is excessive the patient may be unable to fully extend the digit. If the reverse, the patient may be unable to make a fist either because the graft is too long or because of increased lumbrical muscle tension. This so-called lumbrical plus deformity produces a paradoxical interphalangeal extension when the patient attempts to make a fist. This occurs when the FDP contracts transmitting force to the lumbrical which is under greater tension than the lax tendon graft. Several methods of postoperative management have been described and closely resemble those for flexor tendon repair.

Staged reconstruction is required in cases where skin resurfacing, capsulectomy, pulley reconstruction, and nerve repair are necessary in addition to tendon grafting. During the first stage the remnants of the damaged tendons are excised and the additional reconstruction procedure is accomplished as indicated. If the critical pulleys are not adequate they must be reconstructed utilizing either the excised flexor tendons, free tendon grafts or portions of the extensor retinaculum. The edges of the existing sheath can be used to anchor the new pulleys or the tissue used for the pulley reconstruction, passed into holes in the phalanx, looped under the extensor at the proximal interphalangeal level or over the extensor at the middle phalanx. A silicone rod is then passed through the pulley system and secured to either the profundus stump or distal phalanx. Traction on the rod should produce flexion without displacement (bow string) of the flexor rod. If this occurs then additional pulleys should be reconstructed.

The rod is then passed through the carpal canal and placed between the deep and superficial flexors in the distal forearm. Passive digital motion begins 7 to 10 days after surgery and continues until the digit is ready for flexor tendon grafting (approximately three months postoperatively). At this time the silastic rod is exchanged for a flexor tendon graft utilizing the technique as previously described.

EXTENSOR TENDON INJURIES

Although more attention has been paid to flexor than extensor injuries, the result of extensor repair are certainly not predictably successful. This may be because they are often treated by junior surgeons who are not aware of the complex anatomy, the techniques of repair and the principles of post-operative rehabilitation. In addition, extensor disruptions are more often associated with fractures. Postoperative adhesions are frequently encountered and the resultant loss of digital flexion can be rather disabling. An anatomical "Zone" classification has been proposed to aid in the diagnosis and treatment of extensor tendon injuries.

ZONE 8—FOREARM

Lacerations at this level often cause simultaneous disruption of extensor muscles and tendons. Often there is an associated injury to the radial nerve. Fine epimysial sutures should be applied rather than large strangulating sutures which cause muscle necrosis. Tenorrhaphy is accomplished with 3-0 or 4-0 sutures using the Kessler, modified Bunnell, figure-eight, or horizontal mattress suture technique. If the laceration is close to the elbow, the posterior interosseous branch of the radial nerve should be explored and if disrupted, repaired microsurgically. During the first postoperative month, the wrist is immobilized in 45 degrees of extension, the thumb in radial abduction with the MP and interphalangeal joints extended, and the finger MP joints in 15 degrees of flexion with the finger interphalangeal joints free to move. After one month, the digits are mobilized and the wrist protected for an additional 2 weeks in a wrist splint. If repair is delayed beyond 3 weeks, muscle contracture and fibrosis will probably preclude direct repair. In such situations tendon transfers as described for radial nerve palsy are indicated.

ZONE 7—WRIST

At this level the extensor tendons lie within a retinacular tunnel which is divided into six compartments:

1st compartment   Abductor pollicis longus, extensor pollicis brevis
2d compartment   Extensor carpi radialis brevis and longus
3d compartment   Extensor pollicis longus
4th compartment   Extensor indicis proprius, extensor digitorum communis
5th compartment   Extensor digiti quinti
6th compartment   Extensor carpi ulnaris

Repair at this level often requires retrieval of tendons which may have migrated proximally and often requires unroofing the compartments through judicious division of the retinaculum. If a large segment of the retinaculum is opened in order to afford tendon repair, it should be repaired; if not, annoying bowstringing may result. Kessler or Bunnell sutures are recommended utilizing 4-0 nonabsorbable material. Although most surgeons utilize 4 weeks of postoperative immobilization there is a trend towards early dynamic splinting to minimize adhesions within the compartments. Attrition ruptures of the extensor pollicis longus occasionally occur in the vicinity of Lister's tubercle. This may occur spontaneously or subsequent to injury, especially after Colles' fractures. Direct repair of the ruptured tendon is rarely possible. Treatment usually entails a transfer of the extensor indicis proprius.

ZONE 6—DORSUM HAND

At this level the extensors are subcutaneous and prone to laceration. Juncture tendinea, which interconnect the finger extensors, may prevent retraction after laceration, providing the possibility of repair many weeks after injury. A juncture may transmit extensor force to a tendon distal to its laceration confusing the diagnosis. Therefore, if incomplete active digital extension is noted a tendon injury should be suspected. Since thumb interphalangeal joint extension is provided by both the extensor pollicis longus as well as the thumb intrinsics the ability to extend this terminal joint should not exclude disruption of the extensor pollicis longus. The best diagnostic method is to place the palm down on the examining table and ask the patient to lift the thumb dorsal to the hand. If this can not be accomplished, then laceration of the extensor pollicis longus has occurred. Repair and postoperative treatment is the same as described for Zone 7.

ZONE 5—MP JOINT

The finger extensor is stabilized at the MP joint by sagittal fibers which arise from the tendon and pass volarly towards the volar plate and intermetacarpal ligament. Finger MP extension is affected by this sling and not a direct insertion into the proximal phalanx. The thumb MP joint is extended by both the extensor hood as well as the extensor pollicis brevis which inserts onto the proximal phalanx. Disruption of the sagittal fibers can produce subluxation or dislocation of the extensor which inhibits or prevents MP joint extension. Damage to the sagittal fibers is usually the result of a closed twisting injury. This is usually successfully treated with immobilization of the MP joint in full extension for one month.

Laceration of the extensor tendon at the MP joint is a common injury since the tendon is rather superficial. Direct repair utilizing 4-0 suture can often be accomplished in the emergency room since the junctures tend to prevent retraction. A radiograph should be obtained prior to tenorrhaphy to preclude bony injury or foreign body penetration. If a human bite is suspected the region should be inspected with the MP joint in flexion. An injury to the extensor hood or joint may be unrecognized if the digit is examined in extension. The area should be thoroughly irrigated and the patient given prophylactic antibiotics. A delayed repair of both the skin and the tendon is carried out several days later assuming no infection ensues. Following repair, the hand is immobilized for one month with the wrist in 30 to 45 degrees of extension and the MP joints in slight flexion.

ZONE 4—PROXIMAL PHALANX

In this region the continuation of the extrinsic extensor (central slip) coalesces with the ulnar and radial intrinsic tendons. Lacerations in this area are repaired with fine nonabsorbable sutures. In such cases it is necessary to immobilize the proximal interphalangeal joint as well as the MP and wrist for approximately one month. Extensor pollicis lacerations are similarly repaired and immobilized.

ZONE 3—PIP JOINT

The most complex injuries are at the PIP joint level where laceration, volar dislocation, or closed crushing injuries can disrupt the central slip from its insertion at the middle phalanx with subsequent volar migration of the lateral bands. This produces the typical boutonniere (PIP flexion and DIP hyperextension). Prompt recognition and treatment usually prevent such a deformity. Closed injuries are usually treated by splinting the PIP joint in full extension for 4 to 6 weeks leaving the distal joint free to prevent adherence of the lateral bands. Open injuries can be managed either by primary repair of the tendon or splinting. Because a disrupted central slip does not retract very far from its insertion, good recovery can be obtained using a splinting program even in those patients who present several weeks or a few months after the injury in this zone. Chronic boutonniere deformities usually require surgical correction. If the PIP joint is not contracted a delayed repair of the central slip and mobilization of the lateral bands is usually possible. If a flexion contracture of the proximal interphalangeal joint is present, it must be addressed first either by splinting or surgical release prior to reconstruction of the extensor mechanism.

ZONE 2—MIDDLE PHALANX

The extensor at the middle phalanx is the confluence of the two intrinsic tendons. Primary repair or splinting of injuries at this level usually effect a good recovery unless dense adhesions ensue which restrict DIP joint flexion.

ZONE 1—DISTAL INTERPHALANGEAL JOINT

These "mallet" injuries are very common and usually occur as a consequence of a sudden flexion force upon an extended distal joint. The tendon may be avulsed with a portion of the dorsal distal phalanx. Closed rupture is best managed with a splint immobilizing the distal joint in extension for 8 weeks. Hyperextension is avoided since this actually diminishes the local blood supply and may cause skin necrosis. Surgical repair may be considered if the tendon has been lacerated or avulsed with a large piece of bone causing subluxation of the distal joint. Chronic mallet deformities rarely cause pain but the flexed attitude may interfere with function, necessitating either secondary extensor repair or distal joint fusion.

SUGGESTED READINGS

FLEXOR TENDONS

Boyes JH, Stark HH: Flexor-tendon grafts in the fingers and thumb. A study of factors influencing results in 1000 cases. *J Bone Joint Surg Am* 1971; 53:1332.

Duran RJ, Houser RG, Coleman CR, et al: A priliminary report in the use of controlled passive motion following flexor tendon repair in zones II and III. Proceedings: 31st Annual Meeting of the American Society for Surgery of the Hand, New Orleans, 1976. *J Hand Surg Am* 1976; 1:79. Abstract.

Hunter JM, Salisburg RE: Flexor tendon reconstruction in severely damaged hands. A two stage procedure using a silicone dacron reinforced gliding prosthesis prior to tendon grafting. *J Bone Joint Surg Am* 1971; 53:829.

Hunter JM, Schneider LH, Mackin EJ (eds): *Tendon Surgery in the Hand*. St. Louis: CV Mosby; 1987.

Kleinert HE, Smith DJ: Primary and secondary repair of flexor and extensor tendon injuries. In Jupiter JB (ed): *Flynn's Hand Surgery*, 4th ed. Baltimore: Williams & Wilkins; 1991:241.

Leddy JP: Flexor tendons-acute injuries. In Green DP (ed): *Operative Hand Surgery*, 3d ed. New York: Churchill Livingstone; 1993:1823.

Lister GD, Kleinert HE, Kutz JE, et al: Primary flexor tendon repair followed by immediate controlled mobilization. *J Hand Surg [Am]* 1977; 2:441.

Lundborg G, Rank F: Experimental intrinsic healing of flexor tendons based upon synovial fluid nutrition. *J Hand Surg [Am]* 1978; 3:21.

Schneider LH, Hunter JM: Flexor tendons-late reconstruction. In Green DP (ed): *Operative Hand Surgery,* 3d ed. New York: Churchill Livingstone; 1993:1853.

Strickland JW (ed): Flexor tendon surgery. *Hand Clin* 1985; 1(1).

EXTENSOR TENDONS

Burton RI: Extensor tendons-late reconstruction. In Green DP (ed): *Operative Hand Surgery,* 3d ed. New York: Churchill Livingstone; 1993:1955.

Doyle JR: Extensor tendons-acute injuries. In Green DP (ed): *Operative Hand Surgery,* vol 2, 3d ed. New York, Churchill Livingstone, 1993:1925.

Eversman W: Complications of extensor tendon injuries. In Boswick J (ed): *Complications in Hand Surgery.* Philadelphia: WB Saunders; 1986:38.

Hunter JM, Schneider LH, Mackin EJ (eds): *Tendon Surgery in the Hand.* St. Louis: CV Mosby, 1987.

Kleinert HE, Smith DJ: Primary and secondary repair of flexor and extensor tendon injuries. In Jupiter JB (ed): *Flynn's Hand Surgery,* 4th ed. Baltimore: Williams & Wilkins; 1991:241.

Newport ML, Williams CD: Biomechanical characteristics of extensor tendon suture techniques. *J Hand Surg Am* 1992; 17:1117.

Schneider LH (ed): Extensor tendon injuries. *Hand Clin* 1995; 11(3).

Chapter 117

AMPUTATIONS: SOFT TISSUE MANAGEMENT AND MICROSURGICAL APPLICATIONS

Francis Rockland Pelham

AMPUTATION AND REPLANTATION SURGERY

Amputations occur as a result of trauma or surgically created as in treatment of malignant tumors. This chapter will include three aspects of managing an upper extremity traumatic amputation: optimizing the stump site when replantation is not feasible, replantation of the amputated part when indicated, and last, later reconstructions to improve function. Soft tissue coverage and microsurgical applications will be emphasized.

Initially, the amputated part should be examined for feasibility of reattachment. This includes meeting the basic tenets of providing improved function without pain as compared to only completing the amputation. When replantation is not recommended, goals in treatment include maximization of function and providing a comfortable stump site. In addition, one must keep in mind the anticipated need for and early fitting of a prosthesis. Hand therapy is integral and should be implemented as early as possible to maximize function.

AMPUTATION COMPLETIONS

If a part is simply unable to be replanted or it will not improve long-term function then techniques to avoid later sequelae in managing the stump site should be implemented. Symptomatic neuroma formation can often be avoided by placement of the nerve ending in a protected location away from a tactile surface. This includes simple resection to allow retraction out of the zone of injury and subsequent dense scar tissue formation. Other options include placement in muscle and bone.

Adequate well-vascularized soft tissue at the site is useful in avoiding a painful stump. This requires adequate bone debridement and a tension-free closure with local tissue, regional flaps, or placement of distant tissue utilizing microsurgical techniques.

FINGER AMPUTATIONS

Thicker volar skin with good sensibility is better than dorsal skin. Tension can be avoided by cutting the dorsal flap with the joint in flexion and the volar flap with the joint in extension. Contouring the flap "dog ears" should not jeopardize vascularity. Maximum bone length should not be achieved at the expense of stable soft tissue coverage. Condyles should be contoured to avoid a bulbous tip and cartilage may be removed to allow for better adherence of the overlying tissue.

The ulnar three flexor digitorum profundus tendons share a common muscle belly. If not allowed to freely retract, *quadriga*

syndrome, or the limitation of flexion of the uninvolved digits, can develop. *Lumbrical plus* fingers usually do not develop with significance as a result of proximal retraction of the lumbrical attachment to the profundus tendon. Otherwise, with more proximal amputations, preservation of or reinsertion of flexor tendons can improve strength and motion. Examples include the flexor pollicis longus and the flexor digitorum superficialis at both the middle and proximal phalanx levels.

Digital Tip Amputations

Management of amputations of the fingertips varies depending on the amount of skin lost, the depth of soft tissue defect, and whether bone has been exposed or partially amputated. Long-term results of allowing finger tip wounds to heal by secondary intention are good when less than one centimeter of skin is lost and no bone is exposed. However, it can take 3 or more weeks to heal. Sensibility and contour often can be excellent. Primary closure, if performed under tension, increases the rate of dysesthesia and subsequent disability.

Split skin grafts provide poor padding and sensibility and are a lesser option. They do achieve a closed wound and with time contract, bringing normal tissue into the area. Both secondary healing and skin grafted wounds can lead to cold sensitivity and the latter is more likely to cause hypesthesias.

When bone is exposed, well-padded tissue is required. Often, the amputated part of the finger is recovered; however, replacing it as a free graft composite is not recommended except in children. One can harvest a full-thickness graft from the part to cover a defect where there is no bone exposed. Local flaps are ideal for these larger defects with deeper tissue loss and exposed bone. The geometry of the defect dictates which local flap offers the best coverage. The local flap is chosen based on where the relative surplus of tissue exists.

V-Y advancement techniques utilizing a simple volar flap or bilateral ulnar and radial flaps have been described (Fig. 117-1). Key points on both these techniques include making a broad-based flap, not crossing the joint crease, and completely releasing the fascial attachments to the underlying flexor sheath and bone to allow for a tension-free closure. The volar advancement (Moberg) flap is most often used for thumb tip amputations. Bilateral midaxial incisions are made at the glabellar-dorsal skin junction. Sensibility is restored but flexion contracture deformities can occur, especially with greater than one centimeter advancement.

Additional regional flaps can be useful, providing new tissue to the injured areas (Fig. 117-2). The cross finger flap provides coverage and preserves length when local tissue is not sufficient. Most commonly, the adjacent ulnar digit dorsum overlying the middle phalanx is utilized as the donor site. The flap is based laterally on the digital vessel branches on the side of the injured digit. The flap is turned

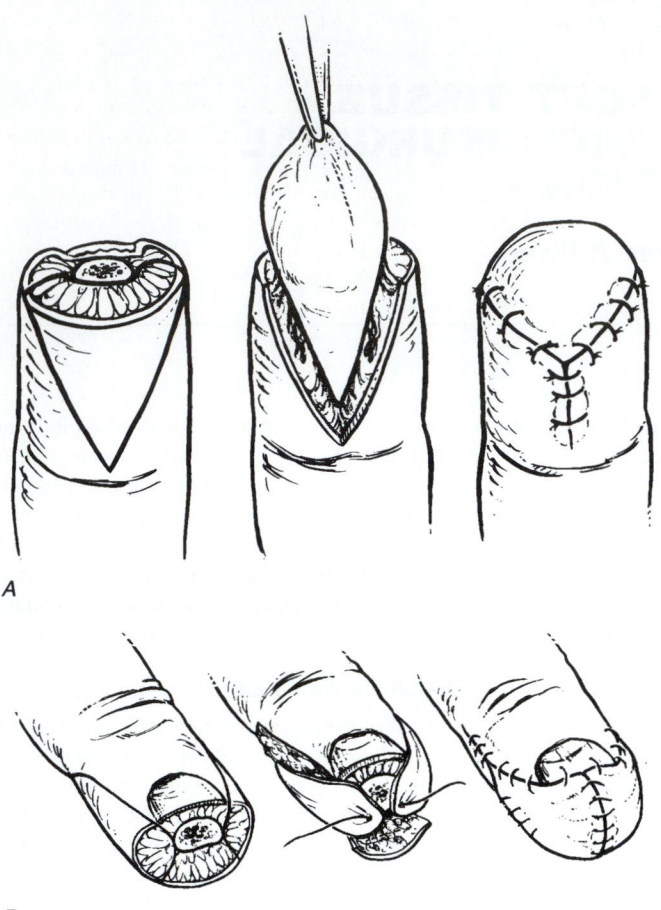

Figure 117-1

A. Atasoy-Kleinert volar V-Y advancement flap. The fibrous septae are divided, permitting free mobilization on end branches of the neurovascular pedicles and adjacent adipose tissue. B. Kutler double lateral V-Y advancement flaps. The fibrous septae are divided, permitting free mobilization on end branches of the neurovascular pedicles and adjacent adipose tissue. [Reproduced and modified with permission from Louis DS: Amputations. In Green DP (ed): *Operative Hand Surgery,* vol 1, 3d ed. New York: Churchill Livingstone; 1993:56.]

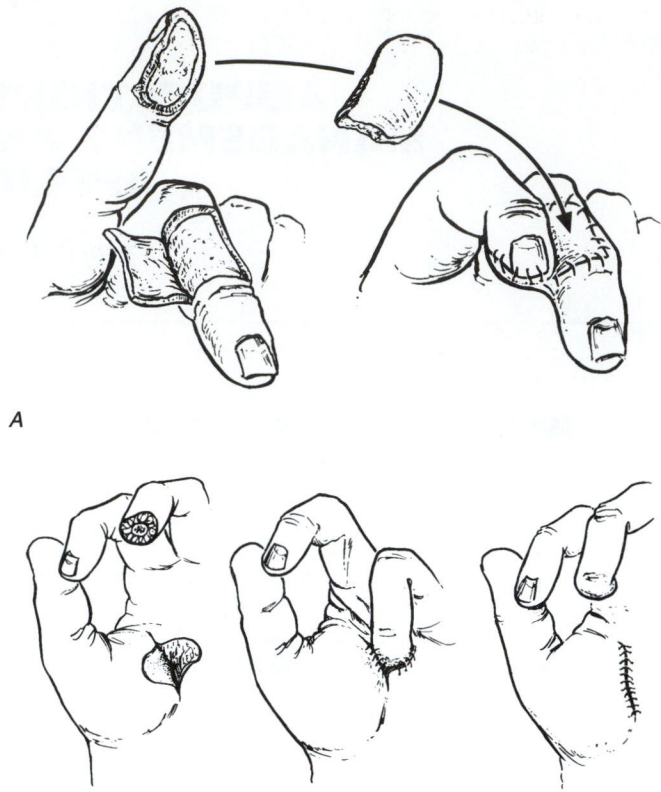

Figure 117-2

A. Cross-finger flap technique. The cross-finger flap has been elevated on a radial-based pedicle over the dorsum of the adjacent middle finger. The full-thickness skin flap, either taken from the amputated part or from an independent site, is sutured onto the dorsum with a bed of extensor paratenon. [Reproduced and modified with permission from Lister GD: Skin flaps. In Green DP (ed): *Operative Hand Surgery,* vol 2, 3d ed. New York: Churchill Livingstone; 1993:1768.] B. Thenar two-staged flap coverage utilizing palmar skin and underlying subcutaneous tissue at the thenar crease level. (Modified from Smith, Albin: *J Trauma* 1976; 16:778.]

down and tacked into position on three sides. At 2 to 3 weeks, the flap is separated and contoured.

The thenar flap is another choice when local tissue is insufficient. The flap is marked at the point where the injured finger tip touches the thenar eminence with effort to minimize proximal interphalangeal (PIP) joint flexion. PIP joint flexion increases as the involved digit moves from the small finger towards the index finger, increasing the risk of later stiffness and loss of motion. Additional drawbacks of both of these flaps include involvement of either an uninvolved finger or the working palm surface, respectively, and a resultant flap which has the sensory drawbacks of a full-thickness skin graft.

Proximal Finger Amputations

The index finger is utilized in pinch and is the radial most component in grasping. With injury, however, it can hinder hand function as the long finger is used preferentially. The presence of the proximal phalanx stump may provide improved grasp function. If it becomes detrimental then a ray amputation at the base of the metacarpal bone is performed. An alternative is to disarticulate the metacarpophalangeal (MP) joint and contour the radial condyle, providing

for an intact transmetacarpal ligament. Similar options are available for the small finger.

Long and ring finger amputations with a short proximal phalanx create a gap in which small objects can escape grasp. Excision of the metacarpal bone and apposition of its border digits with repair of the transverse metacarpal ligament closes the space but scissoring can result due to the rotational differences of each finger. A ray transfer by osteotomy of the base of the border digit of the metacarpal bone and transposition of the finger also closes the space. This can prevent scissoring but adds the additional complexity of an osteotomy. Both of these procedures are accomplished at the expense of grip strength due to a narrowed hand. A narrowed palm reduces the breadth of grasp during such torque producing actions as swinging a hammer or fly fishing.

TRANSCARPAL AND WRIST ARTICULATION

A transcarpal amputation provides a mobile wrist with better performance with a prosthesis than more proximal amputations in that the wrist itself supplies the power, avoiding a cumbersome shoulder harness. A wrist disarticulation provides improved rotation with an intact radioulnar joint including the triangular fibrocartilage. The prominent styloid processes require contouring for prosthetic fitting. In children, preservation of the growth potential is an added advantage.

REPLANTATION SURGERY

Replantation of a completely amputated part offers different immediate and long-term nuances than an incompletely amputated part requiring *revascularization*. Venous outflow and sensibility may be intact affecting both ease of repair and long-term outcome, respectively.

PREOPERATIVE MANAGEMENT

The amputated part should be wrapped in moist saline gauze and placed into a sealed plastic bag and into an iced saline container. Direct contact with ice causes frostbite and to be submerged in saline would cause the tissue to become waterlogged. The stump site should be dressed with a sterile, moist gauze and elevated. Antibiotics, tetanus, and x-rays of both stump site and amputated part should be obtained.

An initial trauma triage followed by a more detailed workup should not be bypassed. More proximal injuries relate to higher likelihood of major life-threatening trauma requiring immediate care. In addition, specific effects of proximal amputations include hyperkalemia, significant blood loss, and myoglobinuria which can promote renal failure. Diagnosis and early treatment should be implemented including to alkalinize the urine by bicarbonate infusion. The amputated part can be taken to the operating room for exploration on a separate table in advance of the patient.

INDICATIONS

The replanted part must improve hand function above that achieved by amputation completion with or without prosthesis. The *younger* the patient the better the likelihood of improved long-term function. This relates to both nerve regeneration and joint stiffness. Patient's occupation and motivation are important as well. Technical factors include the *mechanism of injury* in that both crush and avulsion cause much larger injury zones as compared to guillotine cuts. Another factor is *ischemia time*. With proximal amputations, muscle necrosis becomes significant with warm ischemia of 4 to 6 h. Ischemia time can be extended to 12 h if the part is cooled appropriately. A cooled distal digit or hemihand can be successfully replanted at 24 h.

Single digit amputations which occur between the origin of the fibroosseous canal at the distal palmar crease and the insertions of the flexor digitorum superficialis are absolute contraindications at many replant centers. However, these *zone two* amputations can become indicated replantations when multiple digits are involved due to the improved grasp function often obtained. The *thumb* should be salvaged even if stiffness and altered sensation are present, since its role as a stable post provides usefulness and reconstructive options are complex and with equivalent results. *Segmental* injuries portend to a poor prognosis. These injuries as with proximal injuries at times do allow replantation of a portion of the part to improve function or provide stable stump coverage. An example includes use of a radial free forearm flap with an unreplantable arm amputation.

INTRAOPERATIVE MANAGEMENT

Most procedures can be done under brachial plexus block anesthesia using an indwelling catheter. The catheter can be utilized during the postoperative period for both pain relief and help with vasodilatation of the extremity. Intraoperative precautions to avoid pressure sores including a water or air mattress should be implemented, and a heating blanket used to help prevent hypothermia.

Dissection of the amputated part is performed on a towel over ice to maintain cold ischemia. Initial debridement followed by identification and labeling of all structures with microclips or sutures is accomplished under the microscope. The sequence of repair may vary but, in general, for more distal amputations, skeletal fixation followed by the repair of gross structures including tendons are done prior to the microneurovascular repairs. For more proximal injuries with significant muscle bulk, either a shunt placement initially or a vascular repair immediately after skeletal fixation should be done to minimize myonecrosis.

Bone shortening is done both to provide clean bone edges and to allow a tension-free repair of all vital structures. Skeletal fixation should be as rigid as possible to allow early motion without impinging on joints in close proximity. K-wire fixation is most expedient but may block nearby joints. Interosseous wires avoid this but require more dissection and time. Plates are less often used in fingers due to the extensive dissection and added time. In more proximal amputations, especially in the forearm, compression plates provide the required rigid internal fixation. Amputations through joints are usually managed with shortening and primary arthrodesis. In severely comminuted fractures with segmental bone loss and in badly contaminated injuries, external fixation provides skeletal stabilization.

Tendons should be minimally shortened to clean the edges and compensate for bone reduction. Sometimes tendon shortening can be performed away from the fracture line to prevent later dense scarring and subsequent loss of tendon gliding. Usually, the fingers are not moved for 10 days due to the neurovascular anastomoses. Silastic tendon rods as with silastic joints placed at initial injury can increase the risk of infection.

The arteries are debrided proximally to the level where good pulsatile flow is observed. Distal debridement is taken out of the zone of injury as noted by microscopic evaluation of the arterial walls. Signs include "cobwebbing," and "telescoping" of the intima which represent intimal damage. Another sign of intimal damage is thrombus which is difficult to irrigate away. The "ribbon" sign represents avulsion injury to the vessel. Lidocaine-soaked gauze on the vessels can help relieve spasm. If needed a vein graft harvested from the dorsum of the foot or forearm can be utilized. Vessels under 1 mm in diameter can be successfully repaired utilizing 10.0 and sometimes 11.0 suture material. At the wrist, however, 9.0 suture material is satisfactory.

LEVELS OF AMPUTATION

Zone I amputations, distal to the insertion of the flexor digitorum superficialis, have an excellent expectation with regard to sensory recovery, motion (significant pip joint motion is preserved), and appearance (Fig. 117-3).

Zone II replantation or injuries along the flexor sheath beginning at the distal palmar sheath carry a poor expectation with regard to functional outcome. This is due to loss of motion related to tendon scarring in the fibroosseous canal and PIP joint injury and stiffness. A single stiff finger is bypassed or hinders function. With multiple digits, both flexor tendons in each finger should be repaired if possible and the best fingers can be put on the best stumps to maximize length and joint function.

The thumb should be replaced even in severe crush and avulsion injuries. The thumb can be quite useful as a post and later reconstructive procedures such as a neurovascular island pedicle flap can be used for sensory improvement. An interposition vein graft from the snuff box to the princeps pollicis offers a technically less challenging vascular anastomoses.

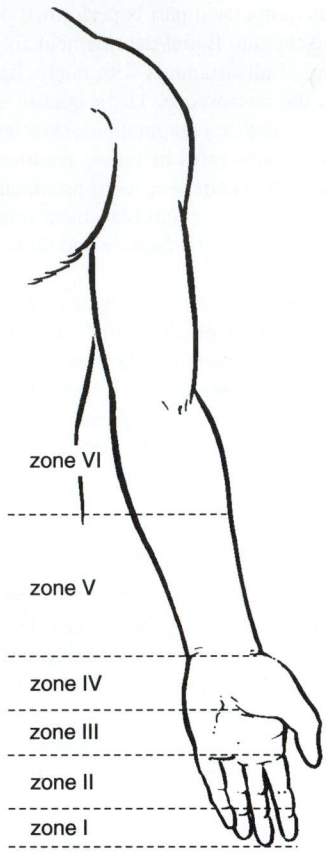

Figure 117-3
Zones of amputations. Each zone has specific features which help predict outcomes, and therefore better define indications. [Reproduced with permission from Gallico, 1990.]

Ring avulsion injuries can be revascularized with good results but they are technically challenging and again depends on degree of damage to the flexor tendons and PIP joint with regard to later functional outcome. Nerve recovery in the finger is usually better than protective sensation.

Zone III injuries should be managed with efforts to maintain MP joint motion when applying skeletal fixation. If the joint is injured, resection with arthrodesis is straight forward. However, silastic implant arthroplasty can be performed; this is better as a staged procedure due to the risk of infection. The metacarpal bones allow for rapid pinning using either axial or crossed k-wires. Single large dorsal and volar flaps provide good exposure. Using the pedicled superficial arch allows for good arterial mobilization in performing the arterial repair and dorsal veins are usually large and multiple.

In zone IV, the region of the carpal tunnel, the transverse carpal ligament and distal intrinsic spaces should be released. A proximal row carpectomy with radiocarpal fusion offers an excellent way of achieving skeletal fixation and avoiding tension on the repairs including skin closure.

Zone V amputations offer a reasonable functional return given an intact wrist joint and minimal injury to the forearm musculature.

Zone VI replantation requires rigid compression plate fixation. An arterial shunt provides rapid revascularization of musculature if needed. Carpal canal, intrinsic muscle, and forearm compartments require fasciotomies.

Amputations about the elbow offer less reliable results with significant muscle loss by direct trauma and greater distances for nerve regeneration and protective sensory return. Intrinsic muscle loss is

likely. Nonavulsing amputations in young patients allow for best nerve regeneration. Segmental level and proximal nerve avulsions, especially involving the brachial plexus should not be replanted. Injury to the elbow joint or significant forearm muscle loss also portend to a poor outcome.

At each level of injury reference has been made towards utilizing expendable or "spare parts" to maximize later function. One is reconstructing the thumb with an amputated index finger if the latter is in better condition. Another is replanting the best digits onto the best stump. With proximal injuries, the opportunities to utilize parts of a nonsalvageable arm amputation become even more varied. The most common example is to utilize a radial free forearm to preserve stump length or less commonly to use the uninjured wrist joint to reconstruct the elbow joint.

POSTOPERATIVE MANAGEMENT

At the completion of surgery a loose fitting, bulky dressing is recommended. Elevation helps both decrease edema and augment venous outflow. The height can be adjusted if arterial insufficiency is noted. Medications include aspirin in low dose, low molecular weight dextran, and in extenuating circumstances such as severe crush etiology and compromised vascular anastomoses, heparin infusion can be started.

Constant monitoring is required by staff observing capillary refill and evidence of appearance changes. An example would be a rapid refill with a distended appearance and a deep ruddy hue consistent with venous congestion. Pricking the finger in this case would produce dark blood. On the other hand, trace capillary refill, an empty pulp and a pale appearance is evidence for arterial insufficiency; little to no bleeding at the needle stick site would be seen.

Additional monitoring includes a skin temperature probe that demonstrates readings which should parallel the normal control finger. A precipitous drop or in general a temperature which falls below 30° implies a failing replant. Doppler ultrasound monitoring of the pulsatile flow is useful but at times can be misleading and should not be relied upon in isolation of other findings. If a failing replant is diagnosed, initial management includes adjusting the elevation of the part and loosening the blood soaked dressing. The best opportunity of salvaging a failing replant is immediate return to the operating room for reexploration. If promptly returned after making an early diagnosis, as many as half of these parts can be salvaged.

LATE RECONSTRUCTION OF STUMP SITE AND REPLANTATION

Hand therapy is implemented in an effort to decrease scarring, regain motion and decrease pain. After 6 months of intensive therapy the extremity begins to demonstrate its long-term functional outcome. The most common procedures performed after digital replantation are flexor tenolyses and capsulotomies to improve motion. Tendon elongation often follows injuries to the muscle bellies with later scar contraction.

In general, the traumatized stump must have stable skin and soft tissue covering. If this has not been achieved at the initial operative sitting, then efforts geared towards this prior to any further reconstructive procedures must be implemented. For example, an unstable metacarpal hemihand stump site would require a regional or distant flap coverage prior to attempts of microvascular transfer of toes to the hand.

Local flaps add injury to the already debilitated hand but often can still be accomplished. Examples include the radial forearm flap based on the radial artery and the volar forearm skin territory and utilized in either retrograde flow fashion for hand coverage or antegrade flow for elbow coverage. Less frequently used options at the forearm level include the posterior interosseous artery flap and the ulnar artery flap. At the upper arm level options include a lateral arm flap based on the radial collateral blood flow in a retrograde direction to cover elbow defects.

Free tissue transfer brings healthy tissue into the traumatized area and choices include fascial, fasciocutaneous, and muscle flap coverage. The temporoparietal fascial flap based on the temporal artery provides thin coverage, avoiding a bulky flap. However a skin graft would be required. A free radial forearm flap from the contralateral extremity provides skin coverage and remains relatively thin. Muscle flaps when taken with skin are quite bulky and usually not indicated.

THUMB RECONSTRUCTION

Thumb reconstruction involves efforts to improve sensation, length, and motion. Amputations that retain most of the proximal phalanx will usually maintain adequate length without the need for bone lengthening or web space deepening procedures. More proximal amputations result in inadequate pinch and grasp, and require reconstruction procedures to improve function.

DISTRACTION LENGTHENING

Amputations at the MP joint level require additional length but maintain the thenar cone of musculature. Distraction lengthening with progressive elongation of the thumb post adds valuable length to a thumb with sensation and fingers which can move into satisfactory opposition with it. At this level, distraction lengthening can reliably improve function, especially when more complex reconstructions are not an option. After metacarpal osteotomy, the desired amount of gradual lengthening is achieved, and a corticocancellous bone graft is inserted with internal fixation. Relative length can further be augmented by web space deepening procedures at the time of bone grafting.

TRANSFER OF AN INJURED DIGIT

Not infrequently, other digits especially the index finger are partially amputated and provide ideal donors for thumb reconstruction at the MP joint level. These digits can provide both length and sensory perception. Given that the injured index finger often becomes an obstacle to hand function this technique can be very useful and also serves to widen and deepen the first web space.

PRIMARY BONE GRAFTS WITH SOFT TISSUE COVERAGE

Other techniques which are no longer routinely considered include the "cocked-hat flap," osteoplastic thumb reconstruction, and the composite radial forearm island flap. All of these procedures involve fixation of an iliac crest bone graft at the distal aspect of the thumb stump. The "choked-hat" flap as originally described by Gilles involves the mobilization of dorsal and lateral soft tissue over the proximal stump site and rotation is based on the volar circulation to cover up to 2 to 3 cm of bone graft. A skin graft is then applied over the donor site. Drawbacks include that sensory perception in the lengthened thumb is often marginal because dorsal skin is being transferred. Bony erosion over time and bone graft nonunion can occur.

Osteoplastic reconstruction includes placement of an iliac crest bone graft in conjunction with flap coverage such as a tubed groin flap. At 3 weeks, the superficial circumflex artery can be ligated as a delay technique prior to division of the tube flap at 4 to 6 weeks as necessary. This plan requires an additional sensory restoration procedure such as a neurovascular island flap to provide tactile sensation over the ulnar border working surface.

POLLICIZATION

For amputations proximal to the MP joint, pollicization is an excellent reconstruction alternative (Fig. 117-4). Pollicization of an injured digit or a normal index finger can significantly improve the grasp and pinch potential of the hand, and has the advantage of being a one-stage procedure that maintains joint motion and normal sensation.

The skin incisions for thumb pollicization should attempt to retain normal first web space skin. The neurovascular pedicles are dissected at the base of the finger with care to preserve the dorsal veins. The vertical septae of the palm are incised to achieve straight line excursion of the flexor tendons. The second metacarpal requires resection at its base and at the region of the MP joint. The level of resection is based on the amputation level. Extensor tendon length needs to be primarily shortened and flexor tendon shortening may be staged. The

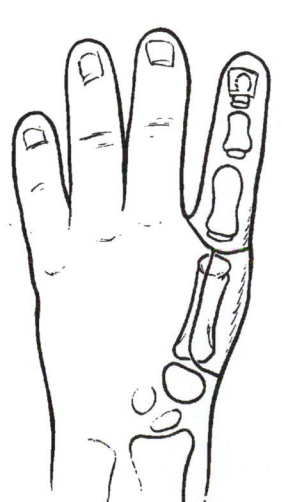
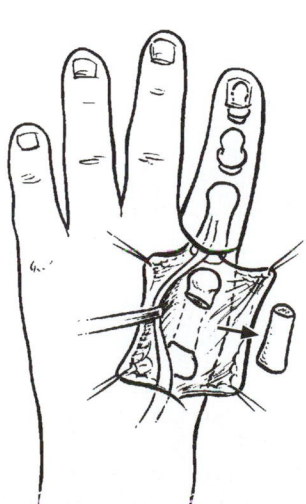
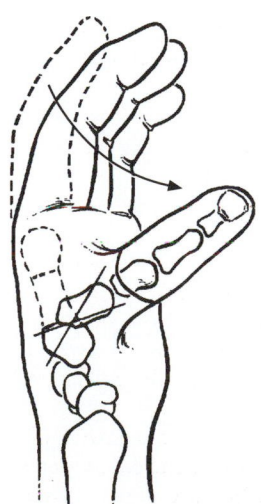

Figure 117-4
Pollicization utilizing the index digit. After adequate exposure is attained, a portion of metacarpal bone is excised with repositioning of the digit into palmer abduction, radical abduction, and rotation to achieve a position better opposing the ulnar three digits. [Reproduced and modified with permission from Strickland JW, Kleinman WB: Thumb reconstruction. In Green DP (ed): *Operative Hand Surgery*, vol 2, 3d ed. New York: Churchill Livingstone; 1993:2047.]

obvious disadvantage of using a normal index or ring finger is related to further injury and concomitant loss in strength to a hand which has already been traumatized.

TOE TO THUMB TRANSFERS

The great toe and thumb have similar skeletal lengths and appearances, however, the former has increased bossing giving it a heavier broader appearance. Its functional attributes and esthetics have led to great toe to thumb transfers becoming a popular means of reconstruction of a thumb amputated proximal to the MP joint. When there is preservation of the thenar cone of musculature even better appearance and function can be expected. This technique offers optimal reconstruction without sacrifice of additional digits of the hand.

Although the great toe is more closely matched, the donor site morbidity is also greater in that it is much more noticeable than second toe transfers and causes weight distribution changes during ambulation. The donor foot during ambulation will weight shift to provide minimal gait abnormalities unless stressed during vigorous exercise. Despite the further mismatch in skeletal length and appearance, some authors prefer the second toe to thumb transfer due to the lessened morbidity at the foot donor site. Female patients, patients wishing to wear open or thong style shoes, and athletes may opt for a second toe transfer. Preoperative angiograms of both foot and hand are a helpful adjuvant to pulse exam. Doppler exams can often be useful if an angiogram is not performed. A long arterial pedicle can be obtained in the dorsal-dominant arterial supplied foot. The plantar arterial dominated foot has a shorter pedicle and may require vein graft interposition.

SUGGESTED READINGS

Gallico GG III: Replantation and revascularization of the upper extremity. In McCarthy JG, May JW, Littler JW (eds): *Plastic Surgery*, vol 7. Philadelphia: WB Saunders; 1990:4355.

Goldner RD, Urbaniak JR: Replantation. In Green DP, Hotchkiss RN, Pederson WC (ed): *Green's Operative Hand Surgery*, vol 1, 4th ed. New York: Churchill Livingstone; 1999:1139.

Kleinman WB, Strickland JW: Thumb reconstruction. In Green DP, Hotchkiss RN, Pederson WC (ed): *Green's Operative Hand Surgery*, vol 1, 4th ed. New York: Churchill Livingstone; 1999:2068.

Louis DS, Jebson JL, Graham TJ: Amputations. In Green DP, Hotchkiss RN, Pederson WC (ed): *Green's Operative Hand Surgery*, vol 1, 4th ed. New York: Churchill Livingstone; 1999:48.

May JW: Microvascular great toe to hand transfer for reconstruction of the amputated thumb. In McCarthy JG, May JW, Littler JW (eds): *Plastic Surgery*. Philadelphia: WB Saunders; 1990:536.

McKee NH: Amputation stump management and function preservation. In McCarthy JG, May JW, Littler JW (eds): *Plastic Surgery*. Philadelphia: WB Saunders; 1990:92.

Russell RC, Casas LA: Management of fingertip injuries. *Clin Plast Surg* 1989; 16:405.

Strauch B, Greenstein B, Goldstein R, Liebling RW: Problems and complications encountered in replantation surgery. *Hand Clin* 1986; 2:389.

Valauri FA, Buncke HJ: Thumb reconstruction—great toe transfer. *Clin Plast Surg* 1989; 16:475.

Chapter 118

VASCULAR DISORDERS OF THE UPPER EXTREMITY

Yosef Eidelman[†] and Francis Rockland Pelham

Vascular disorders of the hand and upper extremity are relatively uncommon. The central theme on presentation tends to be ischemia, with pain being the most common complaint. Other findings at presentation include masses, thrills, or a bruit and ischemia of the digits. The differential includes arterial thrombosis, aneurysms, fistulas, emboli, trauma, and Raynaud's phenomenon.

ARTERIAL ANATOMY

In the majority of cases the ulnar artery is the dominant source of blood flow to the hand and enters at the wrist through Guyon's canal. Within the canal, thrombosis and aneurysm can affect the companion nerve and after emerging from the canal, all the structures are vulnerable to blunt injury.

The ulnar artery forms the superficial palmar arch in cases where it is dominant, and thus feeds the volar digital arteries. The arch may be complete (80 percent of hands), with all five paired digital arteries arising from it, or any combination of incomplete arch may occur. The deep arch is fed by a dorsally coursing deep radial artery, running deep to the first dorsal compartment tendons through the snuff box (where it is palpable), and ends in the deep palmar arch, the princeps pollicis artery and often a large branch to the index finger.

DIAGNOSTIC TECHNIQUES

HISTORY AND PHYSICAL EXAMINATION

The initial history and physical exam can provide the most valuable information to diagnosis in most cases. A history of smoking, use of vasoconstrictive drugs, systemic disorders, cold exposure, or chemical or traumatic exposure is important. Physical findings such as soft and compressible masses (hemangioma); a pulsatile mass with systole (aneurysms); continuous thrill (arteriovenous fistula); or a tender lesion (thrombosed arteries) suggests or indicates the diagnosis. Blood pressure measurements should be done bilaterally. The digital to brachial pressure index (DBI) is a valuable measure to use (normal: 0.78 to 1.27). Low DBI indicates obstruction at some level between the brachial and digital vessels.

ALLEN TEST

The Allen test evaluates the relative contribution of the radial and ulnar arteries to the hand's vascular anatomy. The ulnar and radial arteries of each wrist are compressed, the subject makes a fist several times to exsanguinate the hand, and the patient then opens the hand. Each artery is released individually and the time to filling is assessed. A positive test shows no filling or flush in the palm of the hand within a period of 1.5 s.

NONINVASIVE TESTS

The hand-held Doppler is a most useful device to evaluate blood flow. Absent audible or recordable frequency indicates obstructed flow or very low flow. This modality can also be used to standardize the Allen test. Plethysmography is useful to measure the DBI.

INVASIVE TESTS

Arteriography and radionuclide imaging are discussed below where appropriate. Generally, they are performed through femoral approaches.

ARTERIAL THROMBOSIS

Thrombosis and aneurysm of the ulnar artery are commonly associated with repeated blunt trauma to the hypothenar area. There may also be an association with anomalous musculature in the area or fracture of the hamate.

The presentation involves one or more of the following:

1. Tenderness and a painful mass in the hypothenar area
2. Ischemic symptoms with pain and pallor or early gangrene
3. Numbness due to nerve compression in one or more branches of the ulnar nerve
4. Raynaud's phenomenon (cold sensitivity and intolerance)

Most patients are working-age males with work-related repeated blunt trauma. The radial artery is less prone to this problem but the snuff box is a typical location for compression from a ganglion. An anomalous median artery can thrombose and present with carpal tunnel type symptoms or digital ischemia.

The diagnosis of these lesions is suspected from the history. The Allen test and Doppler are crucial to confirm thrombosis. Angiography is rarely needed. The differential diagnosis includes ganglia, aneurysm, or embolus. The history is most helpful to exclude emboli. Ganglia and aneurysms are managed surgically.

In general, the treatment is direct surgical resection of the involved segment of the thrombosed artery and interposition vein graft. Thrombectomy is rarely successful. Even if thrombosis of a repair occurs, the result may be good because the symptoms of nerve compression and ischemia that can accompany this are relieved.

[†]Deceased.

ANEURYSMS

The majority of aneurysms are traumatic. Mycotic aneurysms are uncommon and usually embolic in origin; atherosclerotic aneurysms are even more rare. The most common sites are at wrist level and in the digital arteries.

TRUE ANEURYSM

True aneurysms include some elements of all three layers of the arterial wall. They arise as a result of weakness in the arterial wall from trauma, in most cases due to hypothenar hammer syndrome with repeated blunt trauma on the ulnar side at the wrist level. They may also be related to granulomatous arteritis.

FALSE ANEURYSM

Pseudoaneurysms occur as a result of penetrating injury to the vessel wall with arterial perforation. These are more common in the hand than true aneurysms, and over a period of months the cavity becomes lined with endothelium.

Patients tend to complain of a mass at the wrist which is pulsatile and often tender and painful. As with a thrombosis, emboli, nerve compression, and Raynaud's phenomenon can be seen. The exam may show a systolic bruit or thrill. The appearance may be erythema simulating an abscess.

A pulse exam, an Allen test, and a Doppler test are helpful, whereas arteriography is usually not needed. Treatment involves resection and ligation of the ends or an interposition vein graft. If the noninvolved artery supplies flow to the hand, resection and ligation provide as good a result as interposition vein grafting.

ACQUIRED ARTERIOVENOUS FISTULAE

Traumatic or surgically created arteriovenous (AV) fistulae are usually amenable to surgical correction, especially if done early. A direct approach for correction of the fistula requires proximal and distal control, excision, and repair or replacement as needed.

EMBOLI

Fifteen percent of all emboli lodge in the upper extremity. The sources are either cardiac or large arteries. Cardiac emboli are twice as common as arterial. The usual associated problems are atrial fibrillation or a recent myocardial infarction. Arterial thrombi with showers of emboli can originate in thoracic outlet syndrome, arteriosclerotic plaques, aneurysms, or mechanical problems with grafts.

Emboli from the heart are macroemboli, causing sudden, acute obstruction proximally with the classic five *P*s: pain, pallor, pulselessness, paresthesias, and paralysis. Emboli from arteries are atheroemboli or thromboemboli and are likely to shower microemboli with more subtle symptoms. These may mimic Raynaud's phenomenon and therefore all patients with Raynaud's phenomenon need evaluation initially for mechanical causes such as microembolic.

Arteriography is crucial. Treatment is usually surgical, with proximal arteriotomy and embolectomy. Fogarty balloon catheters small enough to pass to the arches of the hand are available. Fibrinolysis in small vessels is unlikely to work but can be used as a last adjunct. Streptokinase and plasminogen are given directly into the involved artery. Following this, the patient should be anticoagulated with heparin for 7 to 10 days. Bleeding complications, although rare, must be watched for.

VASCULAR COMPRESSION AND OTHER PROBLEMS IN THE NECK

In cases of obscure causes of digital ischemia, or when venous occlusion of the upper extremity is present, vascular constriction in the neck must be considered, such as in the rare condition of thoracic outlet syndrome where symptoms of nerve compression are more common than vascular symptoms. There are three points at which the arteries in the neck may become obstructed. The most proximal is at the crossing of the first rib at the exit of the thoracic cavity. The artery is posterior to the scalenus anticus muscle at this point, and the vein is anterior. A fibrous band attaching the first rib to a cervical rib can squeeze the artery at this point. The next level is between the clavicle and the first rib, and the third level is posterior to the pectoralis minor muscle origin. The spectrum of presentation can range from Raynaud's phenomenon to severe digital gangrene. For compression to occur, a bony or fibrous abnormality must exist, the scalenus anticus muscle must be hypertrophied, or an abnormal stress must be placed on these structures. Aneurysms or thrombosis of the subclavian vein complex may occur. Diagnosis is by maneuvers that elicit signs of neurovascular compression in the neck. The following are a few:

Adson's maneuver: The arm of the affected side is placed on the thigh of the sitting patient with the forearm supinated. The patient turns his or her head to the affected side and extends the neck. A positive test is obliteration of the radial pulse.

Wright maneuver: The patient places the extremity at full abduction and reaches back as far as possible. The test is done both passively and actively. Loss of the radial pulse with reproduction of symptoms is a positive test. If a bruit is created in the supraclavicular space, further evidence has been added.

"At attention" test: The patient thrusts his shoulders back and down narrowing the costoclavicular space. Radial pulse obliteration is positive. Along with these maneuvers, routine vascular workup is warranted.

Asymptomatic patients with positive tests should be wary of inciting maneuvers or actions/tasks. A plain AP cervical spine film is important to check for a cervical rib. Angiography or venography are often needed for a final diagnosis. Treatment is surgical removal of the offending structure (cervical rib, first rib, scalenus muscle, or fibrous band). If arterial obstruction is seen, thromboendarterectomy or interposition graft is needed. If symptoms persist, cervicodorsal sympathectomy may help with pain and ischemia in the hand. In venous thrombosis, thrombectomy is likely to fail, and long-term anticoagulation may be necessary.

RAYNAUD'S PHENOMENON AND RELATED PROBLEMS

This group of disorders is generally managed nonsurgically except in extreme cases in which cervicodorsal sympathectomy may alleviate symptoms. The hand surgeon may have these patients referred for management of end stage gangrene by amputation of the digits or hand.

RAYNAUD'S PHENOMENON

Raynaud's phenomenon presents with pallor of the digits with or without cyanosis on exposure to cold. Paresthesia or hypesthesia is common in involved digits, with the thumb usually spared. On rewarming, intense hyperemia follows with a gradual return to normal appearance which remains so between these attacks. Episodes of vasospasm occur due to one of the following: (1) decreased blood pressure and flow ceases at a critical closing pressure of the vessel, (2) vessel constriction reaches a point where blood flow ceases, (3) increased blood viscosity causes sluggish flow with final ceasing of flow. These three factors work individually or together to cause an attack. Proximal vascular obstruction is an example of the first mechanism. Idiopathic Raynaud's phenomenon or collagen vascular disorders is an example of the second mechanism, and cryoglobulinemia is an example of the third.

RAYNAUD'S DISEASE

Primary Raynaud's phenomenon is referred to as Raynaud's disease. This is mainly seen in young females versus males in a ratio of 3.5 to 1 with onset late in the teen years. Attacks are induced by cold exposure or emotional upset. To confirm the diagnosis the following are needed: (1) intermittent attacks of acral discoloration, (2) symmetrical or bilateral involvement, (3) absence of clinical occlusion of peripheral arteries, (4) gangrene or trophic changes limited to distal digital skin, (5) symptoms for at least 2 years, (6) absence of organic disease accounting for the vasomotor changes, and (7) strong female predilection. Cold always induces the attacks and emotional upset does it 60 percent of the time. The symptoms almost always disappear after menopause.

RAYNAUD'S SYNDROME

Secondary Raynaud's phenomena occurs in conjunction with other underlying disease processes, predominantly connective tissue disorders and is referred to as Raynaud's syndrome. In the connective tissue type, females predominate, otherwise the sex ratio is equal. Other diseases associated include: neurovascular compression syndromes, obstructive arterial diseases, and vibrational occupational disease. Among the collagen diseases, the symptom complex of the CREST form of scleroderma is found: calcinosis, Raynaud's, esophageal motility disorders, sclerodactyly, and telangiectasias. Digital nerve calcifications may be seen and meticulous care of ischemic digits is most important. In systemic lupus erythematosus, up to 50 percent of patients whose hands are affected can be disabled by Raynaud's syndrome. Polyarteritis, mixed connective tissue diseases, rheumatoid arthritis, dermatomyositis, and polymyositis can all exhibit Raynaud's phenomenon. Diseases with increased blood viscosity often are associated with Raynaud's. Polycythemia and cryoglobulinemia are the main ones, and the latter may result in enough ischemia to require amputation. Specialty laboratory studies include erythrocyte sedimentation rate (ESR), protein electrophoresis, antinuclear antibody (ANA), rheumatoid factor (RF), cryoproteins, and cold agglutinins.

Features suggesting the syndrome versus the disease include: (1) age of onset greater than forty and no gender predilection, (2) decreased peripheral pulses, (3) nail and nail fold changes, (4) marked progression of distal ischemia, (5) asymmetrical digital involvement, (6) systemic symptoms, (7) anemia with increased ESR, (8) other skin changes (purpura, telangiectasias). When symptoms are not due to correctable lesions, treatment involves cessation of smoking, as for all vasospastic disorders. Pentoxifylline (Trental) may help by increasing red cell deformability and decreasing viscosity. Reserpine has been used intraarterially with good results by some. Sympathetic blocking drugs have had some effects as have calcium channel blockers. In acute limb-threatening ischemia, nitroprosside may be used intravenously and can be limb saving. Other options include low-molecular-weight dextran, plasmapheresis, and biofeedback. Selective sympathectomy with preservation of the upper two-thirds of the stellate ganglion can avoid Horner's syndrome while relieving pain and other symptoms. Approaches for this include posterior, cervical, transthoracic, and axillary with first rib resection. Raynaud's phenomenon due to collagen diseases will not respond well to sympa-

thectomy, but cases of obstructive vascular disease (Buerger's, embolic, thrombotic) tend to do well (must remove T1 to T5 segment of sympathetics). Digital sympathectomy with stripping of 3 to 4 mm of length of the proper digital artery has been proposed by some, but these patients must first show improvement with digital blockade. Overall, the results are mixed at best.

OTHER VASOSPASTIC DISEASES

Buerger's disease (thromboangiitis obliterans) is uncommon in the upper extremity. It is usually an inflammatory thrombosis common in the young male patient who is a smoker. The ischemic changes reverse if smoking is stopped.

FROSTBITE INJURY

Frostbite is defined as damage to tissue from exposure to low temperatures. This differs from the other group of cold injuries in which exposure is to wet environments with temperatures above freezing (e.g., trench foot). The latter represents a small problem in civilian medicine and is more common in warfare. There are two mechanisms of injury at work on exposure to extreme cold. The first is direct cellular injury by formation of ice crystals in extracellular fluid, producing an osmotic gradient with subsequent cell dehydration. The second group involves vascular injury with endothelial cell damage, thrombosis, hemoconcentration, and increased viscosity as a result of endothelial cell susceptibility to cold. Also, there is increased sympathetic tone with vasoconstriction and shunting. This results from reflex redistribution of blood to the body core.

The degree of cold, duration of exposure, wind velocity, and factors such as clothing, local medical or circulatory problems of the patient, smoking, and alcohol ingestion play a role. Acute management should follow the advanced trauma life support protocol. Steps include restoration of normal body temperature by external warming (e.g., emersion of body part in a warm bath) and oral warm fluids, management of shock, and protection of the frostbitten hand by careful handling and bulky dressings. The most important step is rapid rewarming (see above) at 40 to 44°C to salvage tissue and function. Later, avoidance of secondary infection is critical to tissue preservation. Surgical debridement should be delayed, often for several weeks, to preserve digital length. The only indication for early surgical intervention is when escharotomy is required. Tetanus prophylaxis is needed but antibiotics are withheld until infection occurs locally. Physical therapy twice a day for range of motion and whirlpool for debridement are helpful. In children, frostbite may lead to premature closure of the phalangeal epiphyses by direct injury of chondrocytes. Children of intermediate age are most susceptible to injury. Radiation injury appears 6 to 12 months later and surgical intervention such as arthrodesis or osteotomy is rarely required.

SUGGESTED READINGS

Koman LA, Ruch DS, Smith BP, et al: Vascular disorders. In Hotchkiss RN, Pederson WC, Green DP (ed): *Green's Operative Hand Surgery*, vol 2, 4th ed. New York: Churchill Livingston: 1999:2254.

Machleder H: Vaso-occlusive disorders of the upper extremity. *Curr Prob Surg* 1988; 25:1.

Pin PG, Sicard GA, Weeks PM: Digital ischemia of the upper extremities: A systematic approach for evaluation and treatment. *Plast Reconstr Surg* 1988; 82:653.

Wilgis EFS: *Vascular Injuries and Diseases of the Upper Limb*. Boston: Little, Brown; 1983.

Wilgis EFS (ed): Vascular disorders. *Hand Clin* 1993; 9(1).

Chapter 119

TUMORS

Neal L. Hochwald and Steven M. Green

BENIGN SOFT TISSUE TUMORS OF THE HAND AND WRIST

Benign soft tissue tumors comprise approximately 95 percent of all hand and wrist masses, many of which are asymptomatic. Diagnosis is largely based on: size, location, mobility, degree of firmness, and color of the overlying skin. However, no physical findings can definitively distinguish benign from malignant tumors and, therefore, a biopsy should be performed.

GANGLIONS

In the hand and wrist, nearly 50 to 70 percent of all benign soft tissue tumors are ganglions. Ganglions are more prevalent in women (3:1), and the majority (70 percent) occur between the second and fourth decades. They can originate from tendon, bone, or any joint in the hand and wrist. Presenting symptoms in adults include pain, discomfort, weakness, restricted motion, and/or disfigurement. Children generally present with a painless hand mass. The mass tends to be firm and immobile and fluctuates in size. Transillumination of the mass with a bright light aids in the diagnosis of a ganglion. The precise etiology of ganglions remains unknown. The most current theory postulates that tissue trauma or irritation of supportive joint structures stimulates the production of hyaluronic acid. This process originates at the synovial-capsular interface. The formed mucin dissects through the attached joint ligament and capsule to form capsular ducts and the main cyst.

The dorsal wrist ganglion accounts for 60 to 70 percent of all hand and wrist ganglions, and usually arises from the scapholunate ligament. Though less common, the cyst may be located between the extensor tendons and communicate with the ligament via a long pedicle (Fig. 119-1). Treatment with needle aspiration of the cyst aids in diagnosis although recurrence rates are high. Proper surgical excision of the base or the pedicle of the cyst requires removal of a portion of the capsule and has a recurrence rate of less than 10 percent.

The volar wrist ganglion is the second most common, constituting 18 to 20 percent of hand and wrist ganglions. The majority present at the wrist crease between the flexor carpi radialis tendon and the radial artery. Though clinical appearance is small, the multiloculated cysts may extend under the thenar muscles, into the carpal tunnel, or as far distal as the first web space. Effective palpation can reveal these extensions preoperatively. Since the main cyst may be situated between the bifurcating branches of the radial artery, it is essential to ascertain the patency of the radial and ulnar arteries preoperatively (with Allen's test) if surgical excision is being considered.

The volar retinacular ganglion of the hand is the third most common (10 to 12 percent), and originates from the proximal flexor tendon sheath. It is palpated as a small, firm, tender mass in the area of the digitopalmar flexion crease. Needle rupture and digital massage can delay or negate the need for surgery.

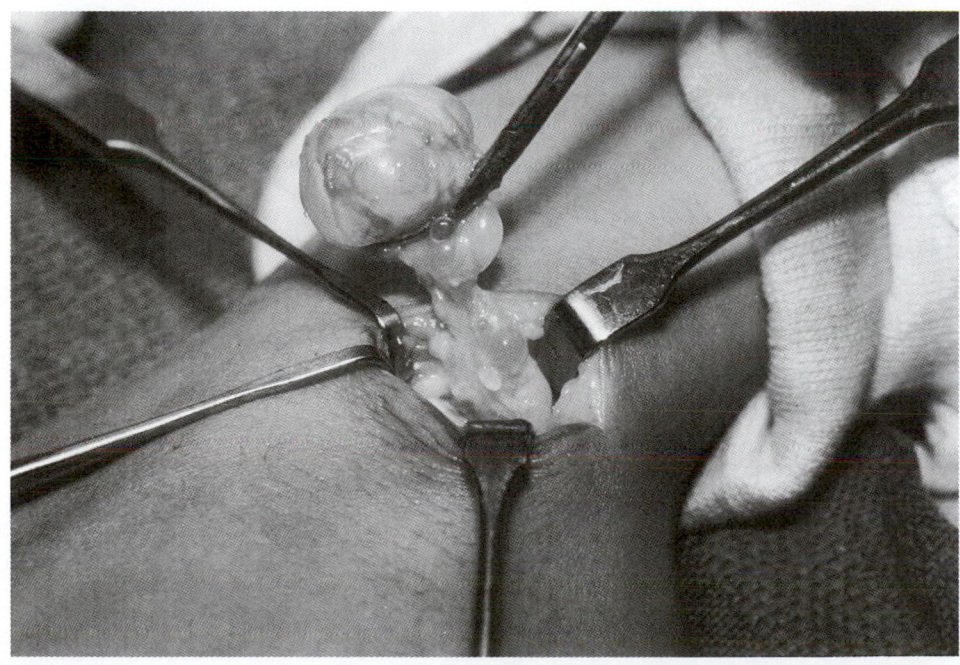

Figure 119-1
Ganglion cyst of the dorsal wrist with its stalk extending from the wrist capsule.

The mucous cyst is a ganglion of the DIP joint, and is usually located to one side of the extensor tendon between the dorsum of the joint and the eponychium. They are most common between the fifth and seventh decades and are associated with osteoarthritic changes of the joint. Treatment requires excision of the cyst and osteophyte resection or fusion of the DIP joint.

GIANT CELL TUMOR OF TENDON SHEATH

This is the second most common tumor in the hand and presents as a slowly enlarging, painless mass. The mass is multilobulated, tends to occur on the palmar surfaces of the fingers, is affixed to underlying tissue rather than skin, and is considered to be a reactive lesion. The tumor may displace normal tissues commonly causing nerve compression and bone or joint invasion. Also known as a fibroxanthoma, or localized pigmented villonodular tenovagosynovitis, the name, giant cell tumor of tendon sheath, may be a misrepresentation of this lesion which may not involve a tendon sheath, and may have only a few giant cells. Grossly, the lesion has a characteristic yellow-orange or brown color. Treatment by excision with opening of the joint or tendon sheath minimizes recurrence (Fig. 119-2). Higher recurrence rates are found at the distal interphalangeal joint or with osseous erosion by the tumor, which may indicate residual tumor left behind.

EPIDERMAL INCLUSION CYST

Inclusion cysts in the hand are usually painless, slightly mobile, firm masses on the palmar surface. If symptoms occur they are largely limited to cosmesis and the resultant mass effect of the growing cyst. However, if the lesion becomes large enough, function can be impaired. There usually is a history of an open injury or laceration in the location of the tumor that caused the epidermis to enter the subcutaneous tissue. No transillumination is seen and the lesion may cause tendon or bone erosion. The cyst contains a keratinizing squamous epithelial lining and inflammatory infiltrate. Surgical excision, including curettage of an intraosseous portion is usually curative.

LIPOMA

Lipomas are common, soft tissue masses of encapsulated fat that tend to occur in middle-aged women. These tumors are usually mobile, nontender, and often involve the thenar area (Fig. 119-3). These masses can surround or displace vessels and tendons, and although generally painless and asymptomatic, the tumors can compress nerves causing weakness and hyperesthesia. Lipoma have no tendency to undergo malignant change and the sole treatment is local excision. However, tumors that arise from intrinsic muscles often require at least partial removal of musculature to obtain adequate excision. Recurrence rates are low.

VASCULAR LESIONS

The glomus, or neuromyoarterial apparatus, normally functions to regulate temperature and exists in large numbers under nails, in finger pads, and in lesser amounts elsewhere in the hands and feet. Patients with a *glomus tumor* present with the initial complaint of severe pain around the distal finger, which is later accompanied by point specific tenderness and cold insensitivity. Physical examination may also reveal a localized, discrete area of extreme hypersensitivity associated with a burning sensation. The tumor may cause ridging of the nail, and radiographs may reveal a pressure-induced indentation of the distal phalanx. They are more common in adults than children, and have a male-to-female ratio of almost 2:1. Histology shows an encapsulated tumor with well-formed vascular channels and non-myelinated nerve endings. Treatment of the lesion is surgical excision. With subungual lesions, the nail should be removed and the nail bed incised and repaired after tumor removal (Fig. 119-4).

Pyogenic granulomas are vascular tumors commonly seen at the ends of a digit, involve the nailbed, and often clinically present as a pedunculated red, raised mass. A previous history of trauma with a puncture wound or retained foreign body is common. These wounds fail to heal, resulting in an inflammatory bed of granulation tissue with recurrent bleeding. Histology shows abundant vascular channels and endothelial cells, but no foreign body giant cells. Treatment is cauterization, usually with silver nitrate or excision.

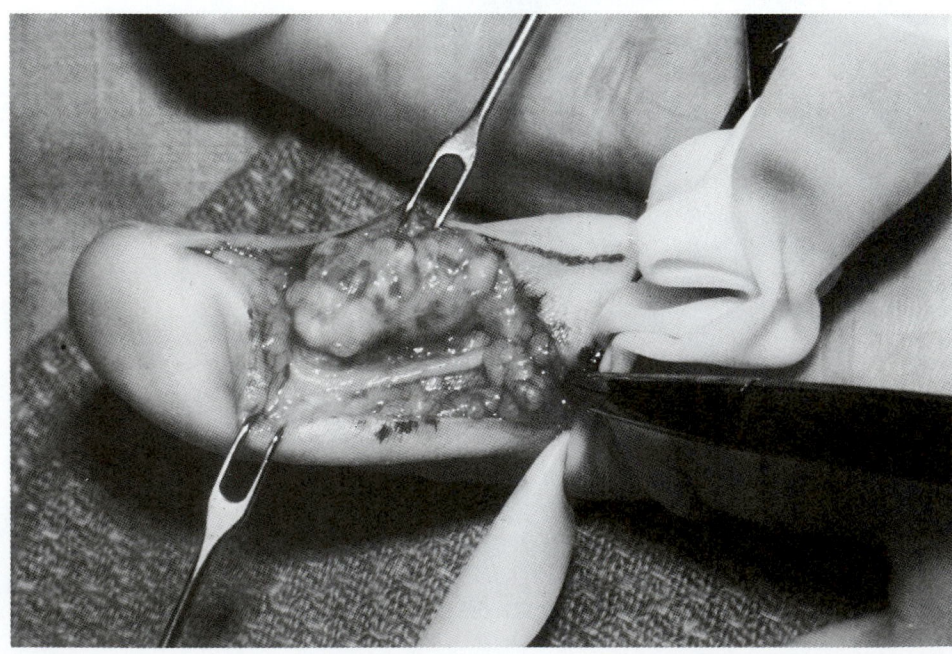

Figure 119-2
Giant cell tumor of tendon sheath dissected from a digital nerve.

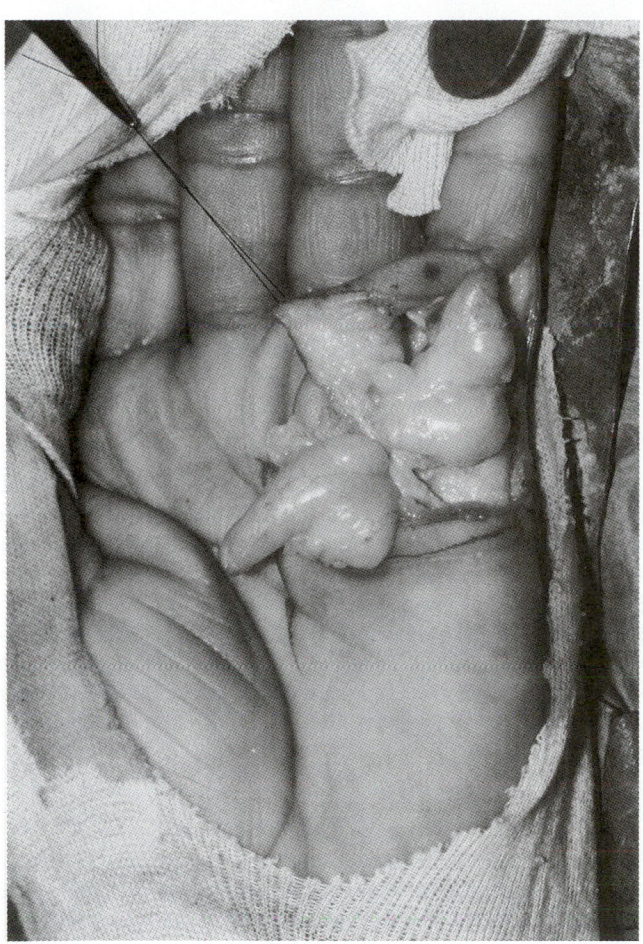

Figure 119-3
Lobulated lipoma of the distal palm.

Hemangiomas are tumors of independently growing blood channels that were likely formulated as embryonic elements of mesodermal tissue. There are three basic types of hemangiomas: cavernous, capillary, and mixed. Hemangiomas may also be classified into involuting and noninvoluting. Involuting lesions are present at birth and grow rapidly for 4 to 6 months, at which time they begin to involute and generally disappear by age 7. The involuting type may be either cavernous, capillary, or mixed. The noninvoluting type may be either capillary (port wine stain) or cavernous and is seen commonly on the face and extremities.

The most common symptoms of hemangiomas are pain or fullness in the area. Cutaneous lesions will appear reddish, subcutaneous lesions will appear to have a bluish hue. The mass may be boggy or firm, and an increase in size may be associated with warm weather or menstruation. If the hemangioma is situated in a muscle belly, diminished function may be evident. Radiographs depict a soft tissue mass with calcifications. Treatment of hemangiomas is often dependent upon the time of appearance. Those that appear either at or soon after birth should be left alone since most will involute. Noninvoluting lesions should be surgically excised, with the exception of capillary hemangiomas (port wine stains) which are almost impossible to remove, except possibly with laser surgery. Subcutaneous hemangiomas or well-localized lesions are easily excised. Infiltrative or intramuscular lesions usually require excision of muscle or bone and may recur.

Simple *lymphangiomas* are small and wartlike in appearance. They have little tendency to grow and may be locally excised. Cavernous lymphangiomas are the most common variety and appear at or shortly after birth. They consist of dilated lymphatic sinuses and have the potential to become so extensive that the entire upper extremity may be involved. Removal of this lesion can be quite difficult, occasionally requiring extensive amputation. Recurrences are common and may be curtailed with radiation.

Hemangioendothelioma are very rare vascular tumors that may represent a low-grade malignant lesion. It may be confused with angiosarcoma, thus blurring the distinction between benign and

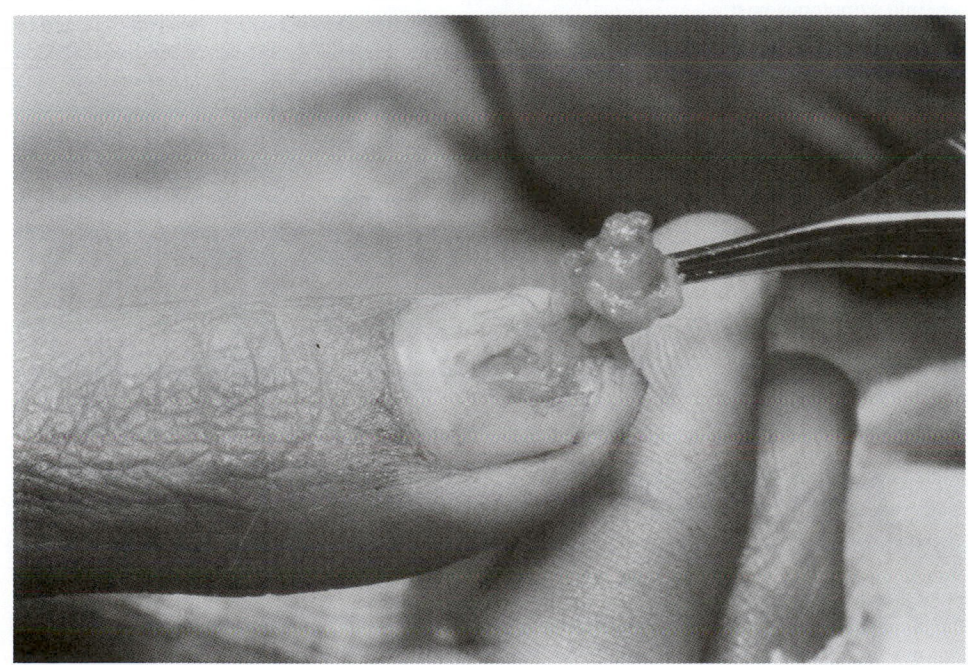

Figure 119-4
Subungual glomus tumor removed from the distal phalanx.

malignant. There is no age specificity and patients may present with a lytic bone lesion. Treatment is surgical excision.

Vascular malformations consist of various vascular anomalies including arteriovenous fistulae, aneurysms, or ectases. Complex combined vascular type malformations that involve the hand and other regions are associated with various syndromes (Klippel-Trenaunay, Parkes-Weber, Proteus, and Maffuci). Clinical findings include a painful mass, enlarged blood vessels, or enlargement of the limb. Skin stasis and trophic changes are present when a vascular steal phenomenon is ongoing. Bruits and thrills seen with an arteriovenous fistula may be present. The etiology of these uncommon lesions of the hand can be congenital or acquired. Congenital vascular malformations are uncommon, usually appear within the first two to five years of life, grow proportionally with the child, and rarely involute. Malformations are classified by their cell type (arterial, venous, capillary, or lymphatic) and flow (low or high). Radiographs may show a soft tissue mass with calcified phleboliths, new bone formation, and erosions. Symptoms of pain may be controlled with compression garments. Surgical indications include pain, intralesional thrombi, episodic bleeding, recurrent infection, and functional problems. Ligation of feeding arteries and communicators may be attempted, however, amputation of digits or even the hand may be necessary.

Acquired arteriovenous fistulas are seen after penetrating injury to the hand. Symptoms include a mass with fullness and discomfort. Distal ischemia is possible as is a bruit and thrill. Arteriograms often show a large single feeder vessel with shunting. Treatment is with single-stage ligation or reconstruction with good results expected.

A true *aneurysm* arises as a consequence of weakness in the arterial wall and contains all the elements of the wall. Hypothenar hammer syndrome, where the hand is subjected to repetitive blunt trauma may cause a true ulnar artery aneurysm. Symptoms may include a painful mass in the hypothenar area, ischemia, and numbness due to ulnar nerve compression. Treatment is resection of the involved ulna artery with reconstruction if the radial artery does not vascularize the entire hand.

Pseudoaneurysms are more common and occur from penetrating trauma with arterial puncture. Several weeks after the initial injury a slowly enlarging pulsatile mass with a bruit presents and the arterial hematoma becomes a cavity lined with endothelium and collagen. Treatment is resection or reconstruction if ischemia symptoms exist.

FIBROUS LESIONS

Nodular fasciitis is thought to be a fibrous reactive process found in the subcutaneous tissues. It is seen most commonly in the second to fourth decades. Symptoms may be due to rapid growth presenting as pain and tenderness overlying a firm, fixed mass. Pathology may show immature fibroblasts with active mitotic activity. Treatment is marginal excision, with limited recurrence.

Infantile digital fibroma is a fibrous lesion appearing as a mass along the dorsal surface or the side of the ulnar three digits, usually before the age of four. Multiple digital involvement is often seen. Histology shows fibroblastic proliferation and intracytoplasmic inclusion bodies which may contain a virus that has not been identified. Recurrence is common even after wide local excision.

Juvenile aponeurotic fibroma (calcifying aponeurotic fibroma) presents as a hard, painless mass over the thenar or hypothenar surface. Radiographs may show stippled calcification. Treatment is wide local excision but recurrence is common.

Fibroma of tendon sheath is a well-encapsulated lesion which may be periungual, or arise from a tendon or its sheath. They occur in the second to the fifth decades, are slow growing and usually painless.

Fibromas are white or tan colored and are comprised of dense fibroblastic tissue. Treatment is excision with low recurrence rates.

Found in young adults, *dermatofibroma* is a small fibrous tissue tumor involving the skin and possibly deeper tissues. Symptoms include a painless, elevated lesion which is attached to the skin. Histology shows differentiated fibroblastic tissue and histiocytic cells with foreign body multinucleated giant cells. Treatment is excision with recurrence possible.

Desmoplastic fibroma is also known as desmoid. These aggressive, fibrous tumors tend to occur in young males, and rarely affect the hand. Slow, progressive growth with deep extension is common. Treatment is wide local excision. Amputation may be required in recurrent, progressive cases.

KERATOACANTHOMA

This lesion occurs in the middle aged to elderly on the dorsum (hair-bearing area) of the hand and in the subungual area. Keratoacanthomas are nodular lesions with a central umbilication which may appear suddenly and grow rapidly. They can resemble or be premalignant precursors to squamous call carcinoma, especially when the lesion is persistent or ulcerated. Histology shows abundant keratin with squamous epithelium which may appear atypical. Excisional biopsy is usually curative. Long-term follow-up is essential secondary to the possibilities of recurrent benign lesions or conversion to squamous cell carcinoma.

NEVI

Nevi, or moles, are collections of melanocytes that are possibly genetically determined. They usually develop early in life and continue to appear throughout the aging process. Most benign moles have a uniform tan to dark brown color and sharply outlined borders. Nevi are commonly characterized by their clinical appearance and histological presentation which reveals the level of dermal invasion. Junctional nevi are flat lesions; compound nevi are slightly raised tumors; and blue nevi are uniform in color and have a smooth surface. These benign lesions are frequently found on the dorsum of the hand and foot and only rarely undergo malignant change. Senile lentigo lesions appear on exposed areas of the body. They are tan to dark brown, uniform in color, flat, and variable in size. Congenital melanocytic nevi are usually large lesions (several centimeters), present from birth and may contain numerous hairs. These lesions have a significant risk to undergo malignant transformation into melanoma. Treatment of most moles is observation if no suspicion of melanoma exists. A nevus that has changed in color or size, or has begun to bleed should be excised. An atypical nevus (also referred to as a dysplastic nevus) is large, irregular, and may have mixed shades of tan, brown, black, or red, and should also be excised.

KERATOSES

Actinic keratosis and cutaneous horns are commonly found on the dorsum of the hands or fingers in areas of sun exposure. Actinic keratoses tend to be scaly and erythematous, while cutaneous horns tend to be thick, firm, raised lesions and are thought to be premalignant squamous cell carcinomas. Histology shows hyperkeratosis and atypical appearing keratinocytes. Excisional biopsy has a good prognosis.

NERVE TUMORS

Neurofibroma is reported to be the most common benign nerve tumor and is an essential component of von Recklinghausen's disease, although the tumor can occur in absentia of the disease. There are three configurations of neurofibroma: localized, diffuse, and plexiform. The localized neurofibroma may be a single or multicentric lesion, and tends to be centrally located within a nerve. The diffuse neurofibroma is speculated to arise from nerve endings within the skin and infiltrate the dermis and subcutaneous tissue. These lesions create ill-defined, plaquelike swellings of the skin, typically found on the dorsum of the hands and fingers. The plexiform growth is often multicentric, involves small cutaneous nerves or larger deep nerves, and produces an irregular thickening of the nerve. Plexiform neurofibromas associated with von Recklinghausen's disease have a high propensity for malignant degeneration.

Neurofibromas are more centrally located than schwannomas and can have fascicles within the lesion. Even though it may not be well-encapsulated, the lesion should not be adherent to the adjacent soft tissue. Histology shows Schwann cells, axons, perineural cells, and fibroblasts. Isolated tumors involving cutaneous nerves can be surgically excised. Incisional biopsy for diagnosis is appropriate for deep plexiform neurofibromas. However, excision by microdissection is usually not possible. If the decision is to remove the entire lesion, primary nerve repair or nerve grafting for large defects is required. If malignancy is confirmed, surgical management entails either an en bloc excision of the compartment or an amputation.

Originating from Schwann cells, the *schwannoma* is considered the second most common benign nerve tumor. These lesions usually present in adults as soft-tissue masses that are round or oval in shape and typically less than 3 cm in diameter. They are usually solitary tumors that are asymptomatic and slow growing. Up to 20 percent are associated with the median, ulnar, or radial nerves. Typically the lesion is eccentrically located on the nerve and is well encapsulated. Nerve fascicles do not enter the lesion. There may be areas of hemorrhage, necrosis, and cystic degeneration within the lesion. Malignant degeneration of a true schwannoma is rare. Schwannomas are occasionally seen in association with von Recklinghausen's disease (neurofibromatosis). Surgical management involves excisional biopsy. Since fascicles do not enter the lesion, it can be microsurgically removed from the nerve and recurrence following surgical excision is rare. If a schwannoma is not encapsulated and/or it is adherent to the adjacent soft tissue, malignancy must be considered.

Granular cell tumor was previously referred to as a granular cell myoblastoma. This nontender, subcutaneous lesion has been recently identified to be of Schwann-cell origin. Upwards of 20 percent present in the upper extremity and 75 percent of these tumors are solitary lesions. Surgical management is excisional biopsy. If the lesion is involved with a nerve, fascicular dissection may be necessary.

Lipofibromatous hamartoma is usually seen within the median nerve at the wrist and its digital branches. Patients often present with symptoms of carpal tunnel syndrome or swelling at the wrist and may include an associated macrodactyly or distal tissue overgrowth. Histology of this lesion shows nerve bundles surrounded by adipose and fibrous tissue. Treatment usually consists of nerve release since attempts to remove the fibrofatty tissue from between nerve fascicles is difficult and risks nerve injury. Recurrent painful lesions can be treated with nerve resection and grafting.

Neurothekeoma is a benign nerve tumor thought to be of either Schwann or perineural cell origin. It typically presents as a slow-growing, asymptomatic soft-tissue mass. The lesion is usually solitary and less than 1 cm in diameter. Histology shows epithelioid, stellate, or spindle-shaped cells arranged in a fascicular pattern or in concentric whirls similar to a pacinian corpuscle. Treatment is excisional biopsy and recurrence is unusual.

MALIGNANT SOFT TISSUE TUMORS OF THE HAND AND WRIST

MALIGNANT SKIN TUMORS

Squamous cell carcinoma is the most common hand malignancy. Appearance can vary from a small rough, red, slightly elevated lesion with varying degrees of scale/crust to a large, ulcerated lesion. Lesions are usually located on the dorsum of the hands and fingers, interdigital skin, dorsal wrist, and subungual areas. These carcinomas occur in the elderly with a peak incidence in the sixth decade and favor men to women by a 4:1 ratio. Risk factors include sun exposure, immunosuppression, ionizing radiation, and Marjolin ulcers. Since these tumors have the potential to metastasize (3 percent of all cases), it is imperative to evaluate the regional lymphatic system.

Bowen's disease is squamous cell carcinoma in situ. This dyskeratotic tumor is a slow-growing, scaly papular lesion. Since this early form of squamous cell carcinoma is not yet invasive, excision is curative. Squamous cell tumors are highly curable when detected early and treated appropriately. Small tumors may be locally excised with a margin of normal tissue. Skin grafts or flaps are usually required. Lesions that are ulcerated, recurrent, large, or invade deeper structures require extensive excision and possible amputation of digits, rays, or the entire hand. Subungual tumors may be locally excised, although amputation may be required if late diagnosis has allowed for deep invasion. Lymph node dissection may be warranted if there are palpable nodes and in lesions that are fixed, recurrent, or located over moving parts. Radiation therapy should be considered as a palliative treatment for surgical failures or if surgery is contraindicated.

Basal cell carcinoma is the second most common skin malignancy in the hand and typically appears as a raised erythematous tumor with a pearly border on sun-exposed areas. They are usually slow-growing and behave similar to a benign tumor; however, basal cell tumors may be locally destructive, and in rare cases metastasize. Like squamous cell carcinoma, they occur mainly in middle-aged and elderly men with fair complexion. Upper extremity lesions are generally treated by surgical excision with a 5-mm normal marginal tissue. Recurrence of basal cell carcinoma is less than 1 percent.

Malignant melanoma is a common skin malignancy of the upper extremity and tends to involve the fingertips and subungual areas. Clinical findings include a pigmented lesion that may have undergone a change in color, size, or regularity of the border. Moles or dysplastic nevi that are greater than 5 mm in size are more likely to undergo a malignant transformation. Varied shades of brown, tan, or black are often the first sign of malignancy. As melanomas progress, pink/red, white and blue areas may become visible. Nail deformities may also be present. These findings help to differentiate melanoma from a benign nevus. Patients are usually middle-aged. The etiology is not completely known but sunlight, genetic predisposition, and the presence of certain dysplastic nevi are all felt to be contributing factors. Treatment of melanoma depends on its level of invasion (Clark's classification), measured depth of tumor extension, and lymph node involvement. Finger involvement is treated with either partial amputation or ray resection. Wide excision may be used for dorsal hand lesions. Prognosis is good for early superficial resected lesions, but poor for late diagnosed lesions.

Dermatofibrosarcoma protuberans is rare tumor of the dermis and is seen more commonly in men in their third and fourth decades. It most commonly presents as a variably colored, slow-growing nodule that infiltrates the subcutaneous tissue. Treatment is wide local excision with a high recurrence rate.

SWEAT GLAND TUMORS

These rare tumors involve the fingers of middle to elderly aged patients. Clinical findings usually reveal a slowly enlarging, painless, fixed mass. Regional lymph nodes must be carefully checked for potential metastases. Histology varies from low malignant carcinoma, aggressive digital papillary adenoma, and adenoid cystic carcinoma to higher malignant potential eccrine poroma, malignant cylindroma, and apocrine carcinoma. Treatment is ray amputation or wide excision with prognosis uncertain due to lymph node involvement.

SARCOMAS

Epithelioid sarcoma is an aggressive malignancy that has a predisposition for fingers, hands, and forearms. It is the most common malignant soft tissue sarcoma of the hand. It predominantly occurs during adolescence and early adulthood and affects males twice as often as females. The cell of origin is purported to be related to synovial cells. It presents as a painless, slow-growing mass or nodule that can become ulcerated with a sinus. It can be misdiagnosed as granulomatous inflammation, chronic ulcer, infected warts, nodular tenosynovitis, and nodular fasciitis.

Radiographs may show a soft tissue mass with speckled calcifications. Single or multiple nodules may be attached to fascia or tendons. There is a high incidence of proximal extension along fascial planes, tendon sheaths, and subcutaneous lymphatics. Treatment of epithelioid sarcoma distal to the metacarpal-phalangeal (MP) joint and web space is either MP disarticulation or ray resection. For sarcoma of the web space, dorsal or palmar hand and wrist, wide excision or amputation is preferred including any involved neurovascular structures. Prognosis is guarded since metastases may already be present when the diagnosis is made. Recurrence is possible several years after initial excision, and there is insufficient data on the efficacy of adjuvant chemotherapy.

Synovial sarcoma is a soft tissue sarcoma of unknown etiology and tissue origin which occurs in the second to fifth decades and is slightly more common in males. It presents as a painless, firm, deep, slow-growing mass usually close to a joint. Radiographs may show periosteal reaction or bone erosion and focal calcification. Histopathology reveals a pseudocapsule or poorly defined mass often attached to tendons, the tendon sheath or the joint capsule. It is composed of different types of mono- or biphasic cells and there may be a mix of spindle and epithelial type cells. Lymphatic spread is common. Treatment is either wide or radical excision with radiation or chemotherapy. The prognosis is guarded since metastasis is possible even after several years.

Clear cell sarcoma is also called malignant melanoma of soft parts and affects young adults, more often females. The mass tends to be located deep in the hand, next to tendons and aponeuroses. Histology shows round or fusiform cells with clear cytoplasm. Treatment is wide resection but recurrence and metastasis are common.

Rhabdomyosarcoma is a malignant tumor which originates from the primordial cell of striated muscle. It is one of the common soft-tissue sarcomas of childhood and is more common in males. Rhabdomyosarcoma is a slow-growing, painless mass and the potential for lymphatic or hematogenous spread is significant. There are four basic cell types: embryonal; pleomorphic; alveolar; and botryoid (uncommon in the hand). The recommended treatment is surgical ablation followed by adjuvant chemotherapy but the prognosis is grave.

The incidence of diagnosis of *malignant fibrous histiocytoma* has increased because many tumors once thought to be liposarcomas and fibrosarcomas are now classified as malignant fibrous histiocytoma.

Patients are usually males in the fifth to seventh decades. The mass may involve soft tissue or bone and is usually painless. Histology usually shows a pleomorphic cell population of spindle histiocytes and giant cells in a storiform pattern. Treatment is wide local excision and either preoperative or postoperative radiation treatment. Radical resection of removing the entire compartment decreases incidence of local recurrence but not overall survival rates. Local recurrence and lymphatic metastases are common.

Liposarcoma is uncommon in the hand and has a variable clinical and histologic presentation. The well-differentiated and myxoid forms are low-grade lesions that rarely metastasize, while the anaplastic, pleomorphic lesions are aggressive and tend to metastasize. Treatment is wide excision with radiotherapy.

MALIGNANT VASCULAR LESIONS

There are two types of malignant hemangiomas: *angiosarcoma* and *Kaposi's sarcoma*. Both are predominant in adult white males and present in the extremities. Angiosarcomas are red vascular tumors that metastasize and can be cured with wide excision. Kaposi's sarcoma presents as bluish-red to dark brown plaques or nodules that are painless. This lesion is seen more frequently in HIV-infected patients and has a variable clinical course with chemotherapy often the best treatment option.

MALIGNANT NERVE TUMORS

Malignant schwannoma has also been referred to as a neurofibrosarcoma, and is the most common malignant nerve tumor. Since the Schwann cell is the origin, this is a neuroectodermal tumor and no longer should be classified as sarcoma. Malignant schwannomas usually occur between the third and fifth decades and are most common in patient's with von Recklinghausen's disease. Nearly 20 percent of malignant schwannomas occur in the upper extremity and usually involve deep, large nerves. The primary symptom is pain and the predilection for deep nerve involvement frequently hinders early detection. Rapid growth of a neurofibroma is suspicious for malignant degeneration. The lesion appears fusiform or oblong in shape, contains fascicles, and may be adhered to the adjacent soft tissue or have a pseudocapsule. Histopathology reveals neoplastic Schwann cells and nerve fascicles invaded by the lesion. If the lesion is greater than 5 cm in diameter, or has ill-defined borders, malignancy should be suspected and prompt an incisional biopsy. If confirmed, either en bloc resection or amputation is necessary. Metastasis is typically by hematologic route and most commonly to the lung. Adjuvant radiation and chemotherapy have not been definitively proved to prevent recurrence or distant metastases.

BENIGN TUMORS OF BONE AND CARTILAGE

ENCHONDROMA

Enchondroma is the most common primary skeletal tumor of the hand, and usually involves the phalanges or metacarpals, rarely affecting the carpal bones. It usually occurs in young adults who often present with a pathologic fracture. Radiographs reveal a radiolucent mass in the metaphyseal-diaphyseal area with a thinned cortex and specks of calcification. Controversy exists whether to treat the tumor and pathologic fracture with fixation and bone grafting at the time of presentation, or to allow the fracture to first heal and then address the enchondroma. Surgery entails curettage through a dorsal or dorsolateral incision with or without bone grafting. Internal fixation is recommended for unstable fractures. In patients with Ollier's disease (multiple enchondromatosis) lesions tend to be larger, unilateral, and associated with deformities of the axial skeleton. Maffucci's syndrome is the combination of multiple enchondromas and venous-lymphatic vascular malformations (angiomas). It is extremely rare for a solitary enchondroma to undergo a malignant change to chondrosarcoma. Lesions that become painful and enlarged with the sudden onset of symptoms should be suspected of undergoing malignant degeneration and an incisional biopsy performed. Rates for degeneration of the enchondromas into chondrosarcomas is higher in Maffucci's syndrome than Ollier's disease.

OSTEOCHONDROMA

Osteochondroma results from distorted cartilaginous areas that produce a subungual or metaphyseal bony mass by endochondral ossification, and are frequently found in the radius and ulna. Although the hand is rarely a site for solitary lesions, it is always a site in patients with multiple osteochondromas (multiple hereditary exostosis). The lesions are usually asymptomatic and appear in the first and second decades with a slightly higher predilection for males. These tumors may cause pain, angular growth deformities, mechanical blockage of joint motion, and/or inhibition of normal longitudinal growth. Radiographs and pathology show normal cortex, a cartilaginous cap, and the medullary cavity extending into the lesion. Surgical excision is performed to treat deformity or loss of motion. Malignant transformation (chondrosarcoma) is extremely unusual for isolated hand lesions, but is more common in cases of multiple exostoses.

CHONDROMYXOID FIBROMA

This rare lesion affects young adolescents and adults, and is commonly eccentric and metaphyseal in location. It is more common in the forearm than hand and is sharply demarcated from the normal bone. Histology differentiates this tumor from giant cell tumor of bone which may have a similar radiologic presentation. Chondromyxoid fibroma contains variable amounts of chondroid, myxoid, and fibromatoid elements. Curettage and bone graft is usually curative.

OSTEOID OSTEOMA

Osteoid osteoma is a benign primary bone tumor and is found in the metaphyseal–diaphyseal area of the short tubular bones or in the carpal bones, especially the scaphoid. It occurs in the first and second decades and presents as bone pain with local swelling and tenderness. The pain is classically described as nocturnal and relieved by aspirin. Radiographs reveal an eccentric area of cortical sclerosis, often with a radiolucent nidus. Since the mass is no more than 1 cm in diameter and may be missed on plain radiographs, a bone scan or CT scan may aid in diagnosis. Surgical treatment is windowing of the cortical bone with curettage of the nidus. If the entire nidus is removed the procedure is curative, but if removal is incomplete symptoms may persist and local recurrence is possible.

OSTEOBLASTOMA

This tumor is differentiated from osteoid osteoma by its larger size (greater than 2 cm) and more common location in the medullary portion of small tubular bones. Radiographs show an expanding radiolucent lesion with irregular areas of opacification. Histology shows islands of mature bone in osteoid tissue which must be differentiated from the malignant appearing osteogenic sarcoma. Treatment is curet-

tage and bone grafting. In the occasional instances of recurrence or local destruction, resection with more extensive auto- or allografting may be required.

UNICAMERAL BONE CYST

Unicameral bone cyst is a benign lesion that is more common in the distal radius than the metacarpals or phalanges. Its radiolucent, eccentric, metaphyseal appearance is ordinarily discovered following pathologic fracture. The principal manifestation is usually pain or swelling. Treatment is either intraosseous injection of methylprednisolone or curettage and bone grafting.

ANEURYSMAL BONE CYST

Although aneurysmal bone cyst is a benign tumor, it is rapid growing and locally invasive with a potential to cause peripheral nerve impingement. Occurring in the second and third decades, it is a very rare tumor in the hand. This cystic and hemorrhagic lesion appears radiolucent and expansile on radiographs. Treatment is resection and bone grafting. Recurrence is high when curettage or resection is inadequate.

GIANT CELL TUMOR OF BONE

Although this tumor is infrequently seen in the hand, it is often seen in the distal radius of young adults. Symptoms include pain and swelling, especially if associated with a pathologic fracture. Radiographs show a radiolucent, expansile, eccentric lesion of the epiphysis and subchondral region of a tubular bone. Histology shows many giant cells with similar appearing nuclei as the proliferating mononuclear cells. Treatment of these lesions ranges from extensive curettage with an adjuvant therapy of liquid nitrogen, phenol, or cementing, to en bloc resection or amputation for more aggressive tumors.

MALIGNANT TUMORS OF BONE AND CARTILAGE

CHONDROSARCOMA

Chondrosarcoma is an uncommon skeletal tumor in the hand, occurs after the fourth decade, and is found equally in men and women. Tumor locations mimic those of enchondromas with a predilection for the proximal phalanx. The usual presenting symptoms are pain and swelling. Radiographs reveal radiolucent areas with cortical destruction of the margins to a greater extent than with enchondromas. Differentiation of enchondroma and chondrosarcoma can be quite difficult and necessitates clinical, radiographic, and histologic findings to confirm the diagnosis. The favored treatment is resection with wide margins, frequently accomplished with ray resection. Chemotherapy has not been found to be helpful. When the primary treatment is appropriate, the prognosis is very good.

OSTEOGENIC SARCOMA

This is an extremely rare tumor in the hand, usually located at the metacarpals and proximal phalanges that commonly occurs in the first and second decades. It presents as a progressively painful, swollen mass. Radiographs show a sclerotic, expansile, destructive bone lesion. Treatment after appropriate surgical biopsy involves adjuvant chemotherapy, en bloc excision, or ray amputation.

EWING'S SARCOMA

Ewing's sarcoma is a very rare skeletal malignancy in the hand, usually affecting the metacarpals and phalanges. It usually occurs in the first decade of life. Presentation is usually that of an inflammatory process with pain, swelling, erythema, and possibly fever. The sedimentation rate is often elevated. Radiographs show a destructive lytic lesion with a soft tissue component. Treatment is incisional biopsy followed by a wide en bloc resection or amputation. Radiotherapy and adjuvant chemotherapy are effective treatment modalities. Survival of patients with Ewing's sarcoma of the hand may be better than other locations possibly due to earlier recognition.

METASTASES

Lung, breast, colon, and kidney are the most common primary malignancies that metastasize to the hand. Lesions occur most commonly in the distal phalanx. Common symptoms are pain, swelling, and erythema which mimic infection. Radiographs show a destructive process. Treatment after diagnostic biopsy involves palliative digit or ray amputation or radiotherapy.

SUGGESTED READINGS

Akelman E (ed): Tumors of the hand and forearm. *Hand Clin* 1995; 11(2).

Amadio PC, Lombardi RM: Metastatic tumors of the hand. *J Hand Surg [Am]* 1987; 12:311.

Amadio PC, Reiman HM, Dobyns JH: Lipofibromatous hamartoma of nerve. *J Hand Surg [Am]* 1988; 13:67.

Ambrosia JM, Wold LE, Amadio PC: Osteoid osteoma of the hand and wrist. *J Hand Surg [Am]* 1987; 12:794.

Angelides AC: Ganglions of the hand and wrist. In Green DP (ed): *Operative Hand Surgery*, 3d ed. New York: Churchill Livingstone; 1993:2157.

Averill RM, Smith RJ, Campbell CJ: Giant-cell tumors of the bones of the hand. *J Hand Surg [Am]* 1980; 5:39.

Dick HM, Angelides AC: Malignant bone tumors of the hand. *Hand Clin* 1989; 5:373.

Fleegler EJ: Skin tumors. In Green DP (ed): *Operative Hand Surgery*, 3d ed. New York: Churchill Livingstone; 1993:2173.

Frassica FJ, Amadio PC, Wold LE, et al: Primary malignant bone tumors of the hand. *J Hand Surg [Am]* 1989; 14:1022.

Moore JR, Weiland AJ, Curtis RM: Localized nodular tenosynovitis: Experience with 115 cases. *J Hand Surg [Am]* 1984; 9:412.

Nelson DL, Abdul-Karim FW, Carter JR et al: Chondrosarcoma of small bones of the hand arising from enchondroma. *J Hand Surg [Am]* 1990; 15:655.

Newmeyer WL: Vascular disorders. In Green DP (ed): *Operative Hand Surgery*, 3d ed. New York: Churchill Livingstone; 1993:2251.

Peimer CA, Moy OJ, Dick HM: Tumors of bone and soft tissue. In Green DP (ed): *Operative Hand Surgery*, 3d ed. New York: Churchill Livingstone; 1993:2225.

Steinberg BD, Gelberman RH, Mankin HJ, et al: Epithelioid sarcoma in the upper extremity. *J Hand Surg [Am]* 1992; 74:28.

Upton J 3d: Pediatric hand tumors. In Hand Surgery Update Committee (eds): *Hand Surgery Update* (developed by the American Society for Surgery of the Hand, 1994; revised 1996), *Orthopaedic Knowledge Update*. Rosemont, IL: American Academy of Orthopaedic Surgeons; 1996:357.

Chapter 120

INFECTIONS

William L. King

GENERAL CONSIDERATIONS

Infection of the hand may occur following injury or elective surgery. Complications associated with infection of the hand range from minor functional compromise to major tissue loss and a nonfunctional limb. Effective treatment depends on a knowledge of infectious organisms, the diagnostic techniques used to identify those organisms, and the appropriate, specific treatment for the identified infection. There are also a variety of factors influencing the course of infection including: the host and bacterial response which is relevant to the incidence and severity of the infection; the extent of the injury; the patient's age and general medical health; the time of the injury as well as the wound environment; and the patient's immunologic status. Hypotension may increase the likelihood of infection by favoring bacterial proliferation. The setting of local ischemia prevents delivery of protective inflammatory cells and antimicrobial agents to sites of microbial growth and proliferation. Ischemic tissue sites favor a more rapid proliferation of infectious organisms and extension of the infection.

Local ischemia is particularly problematic in burn cases where systemic antibiotics are ineffective. Immunologic competence in burn patients is a key factor in susceptibility to infection. Antibody response to new antigens is diminished, although the ability to mount an anamnestic response is unimpaired. Burn patients also have changes in their levels of circulating immunoglobulin which may increase their susceptibility to bacterial invasion. Impairment of cellular defense mechanisms may also predispose burn patients to infection.

Patients with preexisting diseases, such as neoplasias, diabetes, malnutrition, and renal disease, or immunosuppressed individuals also have increased susceptibility to infection. Sepsis may suppress, not only the granulocytes, but also the bone marrow production of granulocytes. Microbial factors which can influence sepsis are the size of the initial wound and the net bacterial proliferation rate which determines the wound's bacterial density. The degree of virulence and the invasiveness of infections appear to be strain- or type-related for both bacteria and fungi.

Staphylococci continue to be the most frequent cause of postoperative and posttraumatic musculoskeletal infection. Coagulase negative staphylococci account for more than 50 percent of infections. Increasingly, these organisms are resistant to methicillin. Anaerobic organisms are more prevalent in wounds of compromised hosts including: elderly persons, patients undergoing multiple-revision surgery, diabetic patients, and persons with conditions involving retained foreign substances, necrotic tissue, or dead space.

Optimal antibiotic treatment depends on prompt, accurate isolation of the organism and determination of its antibiotic sensitivity patterns. It is well known that resistance is conferred by production of certain enzymes like penicillinase that alter the cell wall protein binding site (preventing the antibiotic from attaching) or by a change in the cell wall that precludes antibiotic penetration.

Interactions of bacteria within the host can also be complex. Synergism is two organisms surviving and growing together. Synergistic infection occurs when two or more infectious agents act together to produce an infection worse than if either agent existed independently. For example, *Staphylococcus aureus* and group A beta-hemolytic strep may act synergistically, causing an abscess or cellulitis more severe than if either organism acted independently. In addition, aerobic and anaerobic organisms in combination can cause resistant infections.

PYOGENIC INFECTIONS

FELON

A felon or whitlow is a closed infection of the pulp space of the terminal phalanx. The pulp area is fatty and interspersed by fascial strands which prevent spontaneous drainage of the abscess. This infection usually results from a puncture wound of the fat pad on the volar aspect of the distal phalanx. *Staphylococcus* is virtually always the offending organism occupying the tissue. In rare instances, a felon may result from herpes. A history of exposure to herpes and the presence of vesicles help to confirm the diagnosis of herpetic whitlow.

Treatment consists of incision and drainage (I&D), using a longitudinal dorsal or volar incision with disruption of the septa, and IV antibiotics. Caution is exercised to avoid the digital nerves and vessels and the flexor tendon sheath. If longitudinal dorsal incisions are chosen, they should be placed on the radial side of the thumb and small digit; incisions for other digits are on the ulna margin (Fig. 120-1). I&D of a herpetic whitlow is contraindicated as this may cause local or systemic spread of the infection.

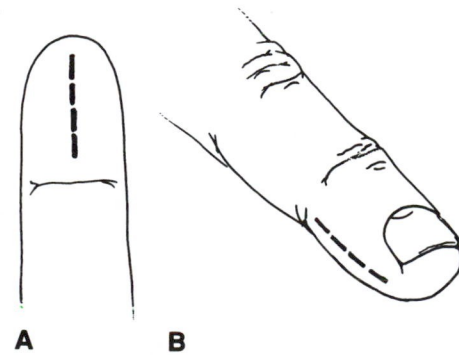

A   **B**

Figure 120-1

Incisions recommended for the drainage of felons. *A.* Midvolar. *B.* High lateral. [© 1996 American Academy of Orthopaedic Surgeons. Reprinted from the *Journal of the American Academy of Orthopaedic Surgeons: A Comprehensive Review*, Volume 4 (4), pp. 219–230 with permission.]

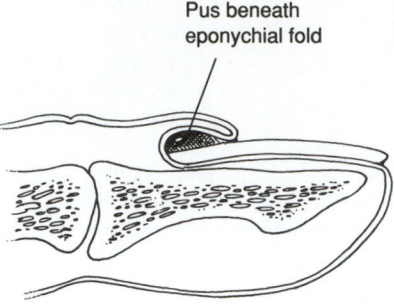

Pus beneath
eponychial fold

Figure 120-2
Sagittal section of the digital tip demonstrating the space beneath the eponychial fold under which an abscess (paronychia) can develop. [© 1996 American Academy of Orthopaedic Surgeons. Reprinted from the *Journal of the American Academy of Orthopaedic Surgeons: A Comprehensive Review*, Volume 4 (4), pp. 219–230 with permission.]

Postoperative care is as important as correct procedure to achieve infection resolution. Drains or gauze packing facilitate keeping the wound cavity open and preventing premature closure. When the incised area is clean, packing is discontinued. Complications include the need for repeat I&D, direct extension of infection to the flexor tendon sheath, and necrosis with osteomyelitis of the terminal phalanx.

PARONYCHIA/EPONYCHIA

A paronychia is an infection of the nail bed involving the soft tissue directly adjacent to the fingernail, usually caused by *Staphylococcus aureus* (Fig. 120-2). An eponychia is an infection of the tissue overlying the nail base. It typically results from direct extension of a paronychia.

Paronychia may be classified as acute or chronic. A developing acute paronychia may be treated early on by splinting, local heat, and antibiotics. If the spontaneous drainage does not occur, then I&D is necessary which may require partial removal of the nail (Fig. 120-3). A subungual abscess can occur as an extension of a deep paronychia. When this occurs the nail needs to be removed in order to eradicate the infection.

Chronic paronychia are usually caused by yeast or fungi or indolent bacterial contamination. Neoplasms may mimic paronychias. Any chronic lesion should be subjected to radiographic analysis to rule out osteomyelitis. Diagnosis may require culture, Gram stain, or biopsy. Chronic paronychia are treated with antimicrobials, avoidance of occlusive dressings and moisture, and occasionally, excision of the affected paronychium and nail.

FLEXOR TENOSYNOVITIS

Flexor tenosynovitis classically presents on the palmar aspect of the hand with Kanavel's four cardinal signs: pain on passive extension,

flexed positioning, exquisite tenderness along the tendon sheath, and fusiform swelling. For the best outcome, diagnosis must be early and treatment instituted immediately.

Infection results from either direct inoculation of the tendon sheath or delayed inoculation in which infection spreads from a neighboring pathologic process. Although puncture wounds are the most common injury associated with suppurative tenosynovitis, infection is also seen following laceration, open dislocations, abrasions, and human bites. *Staphylococcus aureus* is the most common causative agent.

The radial bursa is an extension of the tendon sheath of the flexor pollicis longus. It extends through the carpal canal into the distal forearm. The ulnar bursa is effectively an extension of the sheath of the flexor digitorum profundus of the little finger. There is an hourglass constriction in the palm at the proximal end of the respective tendon sheaths which may function as a temporary barrier to infection spreading into the bursae. These infections should be treated promptly or else they will extend into the adjacent bursa and require separate treatment in addition to the original distal infection. There may be a proximal connection which permits spread of infection from one bursa to the others.

The ulna bursa is exposed along the radial margin of the hypothenar eminence. Its proximal end is exposed through a 5 cm incision at the ulnar aspect of the wrist, proximal to the wrist flexion crease at the dorsal margin of the flexor carpi ulnaris. This tendon is retracted volarly along with the ulna artery nerve and the dorsal branch of the nerve. The bursa is found between the flexor tendons and the pronator quadratus. The infection is cleared by opening the bursa at both ends and irrigating thoroughly. Drains are placed in the bursa, brought out through the skin, and removed after 48 h. Motion exercises are prescribed for immediate postop care. For operative drainage of both the radial and ulna bursa, the open technique where drains are placed in the wound for 48 h, or the closed irrigation technique utilizing irrigation catheters, is acceptable.

Incisions are planned to expose the proximal and distal portions of the flexor sheath. After cultures are obtained the sheath is irrigated with the aid of a small catheter which is left in place for a few days to promote drainage. If extensive necrosis is evident, the entire length of the digit is surgically explored and debrided as necessary. Mobility is encouraged as soon as possible to prevent permanent loss of motion. Amputations may be necessary if the infection cannot be controlled or for residual dysfunction.

Intravenous antibiotics are usually curative if begun within 48 h of the onset. After that time I&D of the flexor sheath will be necessary.

WEB SPACE INFECTION

Web space deep abcess usually occurs through a fissure in the skin between the fingers—either from a distal palmar callous or an infection of the proximal segment of the finger. The term "collar button," used to describe these web space infections, is derived from the hourglass configuration of the abscess. The infection develops in one of

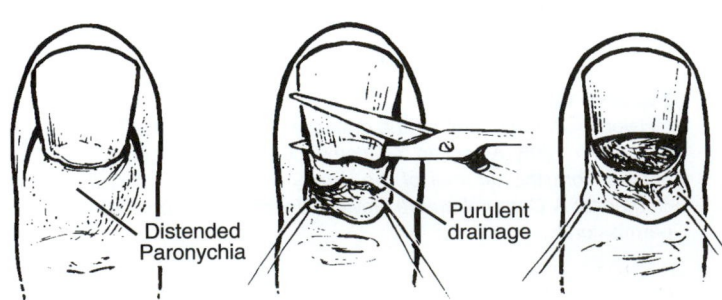

Distended
Paronychia

Purulent
drainage

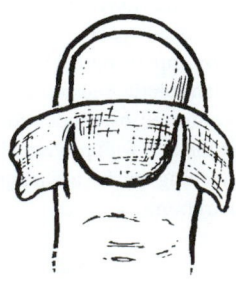

Figure 120-3
Incision and drainage of paronychia.

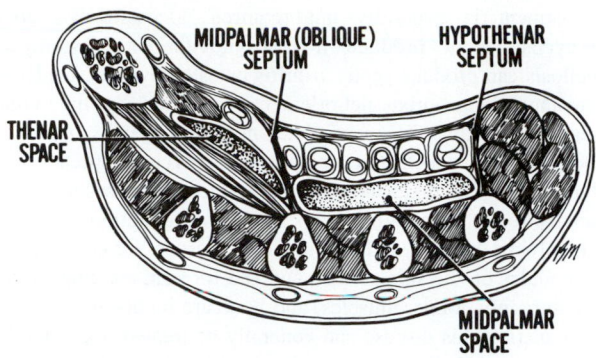

Figure 120-4
Cross section through the hand depicts the thenar and deep palmar spaces. [Illustration by Elizabeth Roselius © 1993. Reproduced by permission from Neviaser RJ: Infections. In Green DP (ed): *Operative Hand Surgery*, vol 1, 3d ed. New York: Churchill Livingstone; 1993:1028.]

two ways. One instance is where a collection of pus develops within a palmar callosity. The second method is through a distal puncture in the palmar fascia in the region of the superficial transverse metacarpal ligament. The developing infection creates palmar and dorsal abscesses that are connected through the fascia. Despite the greater dorsal swelling, the volar component should never be overlooked. After drainage of the abscesses, these wounds are never closed. Postoperative management includes removal of the gauze drain or wicks 24 to 48 h after surgery, followed by early motion with soaks and oral antibiotics.

DEEP SPACE INFECTION

The mid-palmar space lies deep to the flexor tendons and extends dorsally to the fascia over the second and third volar interossei and the third and fourth metacarpals (Fig. 120-4). It is bordered on the radial side by a vertical septum between the third metacarpal and the sheath of the long finger profundus and ulnarly by the fascia of the hypothenar muscles. The distal margins of the mid-palmar space are the vertical septa of the palmar fascia, which are approximately 2 cm proximal to the web spaces, and is limited proximally by a thin fascial layer at the distal end of the carpal canal.

Mid-palmar space infections can result from a penetrating wound, from rupture of a flexor tenosynovitis of the middle, ring or small finger, or from distal palmar abscesses extending proximally through the lumbrical canal. Motion of the middle and ring fingers is painful and limited, and there is tenderness over the space with loss of palmar concavity. As with all palmar infections, the swelling may be most prominent dorsally, however, this should not be mistaken for the prime area of infection. Transverse and longitudinal incisions, or

combinations of these, may adequately drain mid-palmar space infections (Fig. 120-5). Often an irrigation catheter is placed through the proximal incision to provide continuous irrigation for 48 h. Upon catheter removal, active digital motion is encouraged.

The thenar space is located radial to the mid-palmar space. Its borders are the vertical septum between the third metacarpal and lateral edge of the abductor pollicis. Such infections can result from a penetrating injury, an abscess of the thumb or index finger, or a flexor tenosynovitis of the thumb or index finger. Clinical presentation includes swelling of the thenar eminence and the thumb-index web space which forces the thumb into abduction. Surgically, this can be drained dorsally as well as volarly.

The hypothenar space contains the hypothenar muscles, and is enveloped by their fascia. It is bordered radially by the fibrous septum from the 5th metacarpal to the palmar fascia. Hypothenar space infections are quite rare and typically present with swelling and considerable tenderness. The approach for drainage is through a palmar incision.

NECROTIZING FASCIITIS

Necrotizing fasciitis is a rapidly progressive soft tissue infection which can be limb- and life-threatening. It is commonly caused by streptococci and clostridia. Meleney's infection is caused by the synergistic action of microaerophilic nonhemolytic strep and aerobic hemolytic staphylococcus. The most characteristic features are a widening ulceration rimmed by undermined gangrenous skin that extends down to the fascia. The degree of surrounding cellulitis and constitutional symptoms may vary. The important aspects of management are IV antibiotics, wide excision of the affected skin and subcutaneous tissue down to the fascia, and local applications of hydrogen peroxide or saline dressings.

Gangrene may develop rapidly with clostridia, another anaerobic or microaerophilic pathogen, causing a myositis or myonecrosis (gas gangrene). Necrotizing and hemolytic toxins are released together with degradative enzymes producing the damage. Treatment is immediate and aggressive with wide I&D, supplemented by IV antibiotics. In some cases, amputation and hyperbaric oxygen are necessary.

MYCOBACTERIAL INFECTIONS

TYPICAL MYCOBACTERIA

Tuberculosis may cause dactylitis in children (spinaventosa), tenosynovitis extensor or flexor, and arthritis.

Carpal tuberculosis usually begins at the carpometacarpal joint or in the proximal metacarpals and at the distal row of the carpus. It extends proximally involving the radiocarpal and radioulnar joints. It is

Figure 120-5
Recommended incisions for drain-age of deep-palmar infections. *A.* Transverse distal palmar incision. *B.* Approach through the third lumbrical canal. *C.* Combined longitudinal-transverse approach. *D.* Oblique longitudinal approach. [© 1996 American Academy of Orthopaedic Surgeons. Reprinted from the *Journal of the American Academy of Orthopaedic Surgeons: A Comprehensive Review*, Volume 4 (4), pp. 219–230 with permission.]

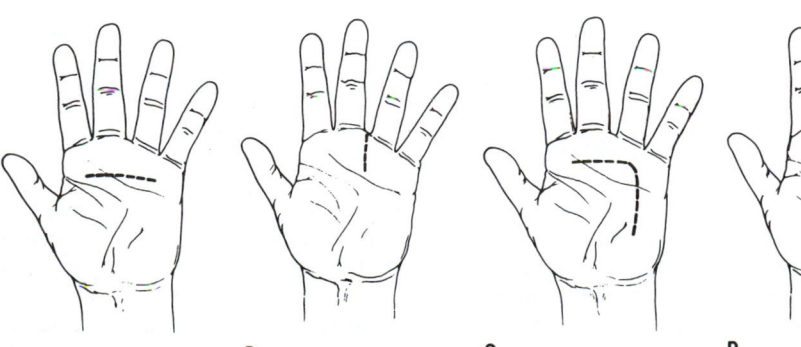

A   B   C   D

more visible dorsally than volarly, and may be accompanied by diffuse tenderness, swelling, and stiffness of the digits and the wrist. Bone absorption may cause mottling and atrophy of the proximal end of the metacarpals and marked atrophy of the carpal bones. Loss of joint space of the carpometacarpal and intercarpal joints are seen early in the course of the infection. Sinus formation is frequent. If osteomyelitis is treated prior to involvement of the radiocarpal joint, it can usually be managed successfully by splints and medication. With more severe involvement, sequestrae will require excision and intercarpal synovectomy; occasionally, radiocarpal and radioulnar synovectomy will be necessary.

Tuberculosis osteitis in adults occurs at the epiphyseal ends of bones, most commonly the radius and the ulna. Synovitis of the adjacent joint is frequently associated with epiphyseal disease. Gradually, granulation tissue in the synovitis separates cartilage from underlying bone and may advance over its free borders, causing the articular cartilage to thin, soften, and finally necrose. Pieces of cartilage may then go on to produce sequestrae. If the tuberculosis is not arrested and cartilage is reabsorbed, granulation tissue at both sides of the wrist joint will gradually coalesce to form a bony ankylosis. In addition, tuberculosis arthritis, synovitis, and tenosynovitis may result, requiring tenosynovectomy and adjunctive antituberculous treatment. When there is only minor damage to articular cartilage, synovectomy can usually restore function. However, with severe joint destruction, carpectomy or arthrodesis should be performed.

ATYPICAL MYCOBACTERIA

Atypical mycobacteria often produce wound infections. The most common are *Mycobacterium marinum, M. kansasii, M. avium,* and *M. intracellularis. M. marinum* infections occur from a penetrating wound that occurred in a marine environment, in a warm freshwater lake, or from tropical fish tanks. Signs and symptoms may include a prolonged, somewhat nonpainful swelling of the digit, palm, or wrist. Diagnosis is established by synovial biopsy on a Lowenstein-Jensen medium at a temperature of 30 to 32° C rather than the usual cultures at 37° C. Microscopically, noncaseating granulomas are visualized as well as acid-fast bacilli. Minocycline is the antibiotic of choice. Other atypical mycobacteria may cause chronic swelling, tenosynovitis, or a nonhealing ulcer. Although antituberculous medication is quite successful, I&D may be required.

LEPROSY

Mycobacterium leprae (Hansen's bacillus) is an acid-fast bacillus which does not cause tuberculosis, but may cause skin, nerve, and tendon sheath infection. It seems to have a predilection for cooler parts of the body. It commonly affects the hands and produces a neuropathy most frequently involving the ulna nerve at the elbow and the median nerve at the wrist. Intrinsic atrophy, clawing, and weakness of pinch may result. Various surgical procedures are utilized to reconstruct the limb deformities.

FUNGAL INFECTIONS

Fungal infections of the hand fall into two categories: dermatomycoses (fungus infections of the skin) and systemic mycotic infections, the hand being one area involved. The dermatomycosis infections are typically of the *Trichophyton* and *Epidermophyton* variety.

Fungal infections of the hand are treated by systemic or local antifungal agents, and except for biopsy for diagnostic purposes, surgical treatment is generally not required. Occasionally, coccidioidomycosis may produce a tenosynovitis or blastomycosis. Brucellosis can produce septic arthritis or osteomyelitis. Under such circumstances appropriate debridement is required, but the mainstay of treatment remains the appropriate antifungal agent.

Sporotrichosis is a chronic, subcutaneous mycosis, spread through the lymphatics. The majority of infected patients handle soil or plants, especially roses. Inoculation leads to chronic granulomatous infection involving the skin and subcutaneous tissues. Discoloration and small nodules on the skin of the hand and forearm are characteristic. Less commonly, joints, muscles, and bone are involved.

If cutaneous, this disease can generally be treated orally with saturated potassium iodine solution. Those with a deep infection require amphotericin or ketoconazole.

BITES

HUMAN AND ANIMAL

Bites inflicted by humans frequently come about during violence when the patient's clenched fist comes into contact with another person's mouth and teeth. This is the so-called "fight bite" infection, commonly caused by *S. aureus* and *Eikenella corrodens,* a Gram-negative anaerobic.

Animal bites may produce rapid cellulitis and lymphocytic response, especially *Pasteurella multocida.* Surgery should be performed for any joint or flexor sheath involvement and adjunctive antibiotics employed. These bite wounds should never be sutured, and if there is tendon involvement, secondary repair is done after stabilizing the infection.

Treatment includes incision, drainage, and irrigation with adjuvant IV antibiotics. It is important to allow for secondary tendon repair after the wound is well established.

VIPER BITES

Approximately 98 percent of venomous snake bites are inflicted by Pit vipers, with the remaining 2 percent inflicted by Coral snakes and foreign venomous snakes. Treatment of snake bites is quite controversial, and some authors think that surgery has no place in the management of these patients. Those physicians taking care of these patients must be familiar with physiologic problems that can arise and must be capable of handling them medically as well as surgically. Problems that may arise when treating Pit viper bites may require experience in hematologic, cardiovascular, renal, respiratory, neurologic, and electrolyte management.

Rattlesnakes, Cottonmouth or Water moccasins, Copperheads, Pigmy rattlesnakes, and Massasaugas are the Pit viper snakes (*Crotalidae*). They are characterized by heat-sensitive pits located between the eyes and the nostril. With these heat-sensitive pits they can make a direct hit on warm-blooded animals that they cannot see. The Pit vipers can be further identified by eyes that have elliptical pupils and a single row of subcaudal scutes, or scales. The genus *Crotalus* is further characterized by horny segments on the tail, known as rattles.

Envenomation is a term implying sufficient venom being introduced into the body to cause either local signs at the site of injury or systemic signs. The venom consists of many enzymes, with proteins, peptides, and other unidentified substances. The venom also contains hemotoxins, neurotoxins, venotoxins, cardiotoxin, and necrotizing factors. It can almost instantly alter blood vessel permeability, leading to loss of plasma into the tissue and breakdown of blood cells, resulting in immediate tissue edema and ecchymosis. This produces the cardinal signs of local envenomation which are severe burning pain, rapid swelling, and local necrosis with sloughing about the fang marks. These signs occur fairly quickly, within 10 min of a bite. If symptoms and signs do not occur within 4 h, it is probable that envenomation has not occurred.

Systemic signs that may occur are secondary to toxic effects on the cardiovascular, hematological, nervous, and respiratory systems. These can produce a rapid fall in blood pressure and a decrease in circulating blood volume, which also may occur with pulmonary edema. Death, although rare, is associated with destruction of red blood cells and the intimal lining of blood vessels, particularly those of the pulmonary system. Systemic signs of envenomation include weakness, sweating, faintness, nausea, and vomiting. Paresthesias and numbness about the extremities may occur, as well as periorbital and perioral musculofasciculation.

Treatment may be divided into two phases, that immediately following the snake bite and that administered at the hospital. Some modifications of a treatment protocol are: keep the patient physically and emotionally still; if possible, kill the snake and identify the type; and tourniquet application at the site proximal to the bite which is often helpful in occluding lymphatic and intracellular drainage. This tourniquet should not be tight enough to block venous or arterial circulation. A small incision is made into each fang mark, and cup suction started. Mouth suction could be dangerous if there is any mucosal injury. However, suction of snake bite wounds is one of the oldest forms of treatment, being recorded as early as 200 B.C. Radioisotope studies have demonstrated that 50 percent of tagged venom injected subcutaneously into dogs could be removed by suction if instituted within 3 min of injection. The benefit of suction decreases 30 min after the bite, and is probably of little value after one hour. The affected part should be immobilized, but not iced or cooled.

Once the patient has reached the hospital, the appropriate identification can occur as well as the laboratory tests that will help in sustaining the patient. Intravenous lines are begun, one for blood pressure support and one for administering antivenin after skin tests for sensitivity. Almost all authorities agree that antivenin is the single most important therapeutic measure recommended as the initial treatment of all serious envenomations. Studies have shown that radiolabeled antivenin accumulates at the site of the bite faster after intravenous administration then by intramuscular or subcutaneous injection. Antivenin should never be injected into a finger or toe and probably not locally. Antivenin is available through Wyeth Laboratories, in the United States. The dosage given is based on the degree of envenomation as suggested by the American College of Surgeons Committee on Trauma. Broadspectrum antibiotic should also be administered as well as tetanus prophylactic. Although some authorities have utilized corticosteriods, little has been shown that this prevents tissue damage. Ice should not be used and many authorities, including the Red Cross, the AMA, the Boy Scouts, and Wyeth Laboratories, have recommended against cooling in the first-aid treatment of snake bite. Cryotherapy was once thought to prevent dissemination of the venom, but it has been a significant factor leading to amputation of extremities. Careful monitoring is instituted at the hospital, measuring the circumference of the extremity, and obtaining serial hemoglobin, hematocrit, platelet counts and blood coagulation studies, as well as monitoring kidney function and respiratory and circulatory status, and repeating electrograms and electrolyte studies. The importance of having normal coagulation studies before fasciotomy cannot be overemphasized, as demonstrated by one patient who received over 16 units of blood before fibrinogen was given to control the bleeding.

There is disagreement as to the surgical treatment of snake bite. Some believe that immediate excision or exploration should be car-

ried out or a fasciotomy is needed. Others, however, state that the incidence and degree of necrosis in edematous limbs following Pit viper bite is not altered by fasciotomy. One physician treating more than 600 cases of snake venom poisoning states he has never had to do a fasciotomy. The use of fasciotomy, he says, usually reflects an insufficient dosage of antivenin or no antivenin during the first 12 h following the bite. Other authors point out the difficulty in differentiating between an acutely swollen limb from a true compartment syndrome and acute swelling of the snake bite. For this reason, these authors recommend intracompartmental pressure monitoring to help make the correct diagnosis. If a compartment syndrome is suspected, then fasciotomy is carried out without delay.

The guideline for decompression of soft tissues outside of a compartment is a nebulous one and based on past experience; however, the question of when a closed compartment is open should be settled by measuring the intracompartmental pressures.

OSTEOMYELITIS

Osteomyelitis is virtually always a direct bony involvement from an adjacent wound, joint, or tenosynovial infection. Hematogenous osteomyelitis of the hand is rare because of the widespread use of antibiotics. The most common pathogen is *S. aureus*. Early cases may be cured with antibiotics alone, but in chronic cases or where diagnosis is in doubt, surgical exploration is necessary. The affected bone is curetted or drill holes are used to allow decompression of the infection. All infected bone and sequestra must be removed. The wounds should be left open and allowed to heal by secondary intention after removal of the packing. An alternative regimen is continuous irrigation of the infected site with sterile saline after primary wound closure over a polyethylene catheter. For severe, extensive involvement, amputation may be the most expeditious treatment to prevent stiffness and major disability of the other parts of the extremity.

SEPTIC ARTHRITIS

Although joint infections usually result from penetrating trauma, they can also develop from extension of an adjacent bony or soft tissue infection, or hematogenously. The infected joint is warm, swollen, and tender. Motion is markedly restricted and painful. Immediate drainage is imperative to prevent lysosomal destruction of articular cartilage. The joint is debrided, irrigated, and packed open for 48 to 72 h. As soon as the packing is removed, motion exercises are initiated. Catheter irrigation can be used in very early cases of pyogenic arthritis via two butterfly IV needles at opposite sides of the joint. Motion is begun as soon as the catheter and drain are removed.

SEPTIC BOUTONNIERE

This is a complication of pyogenic arthritis of the proximal interphalangeal (PIP) joint. It generally arises in patients who have experienced delayed treatment. Intraarticular purulent material reaches a volume which can no longer be contained and the path of least resistance for the spread of the infection is dorsally. The PIP joint is supported by the strong volar plate on the volar aspect which blends with the collateral ligaments. These structures are thick and much more unyielding than the thin dorsal capsule. The infection destroys the extensor mechanism over the dorsal aspect, producing a boutonniere deformity.

The first priority is to treat the infection before performing reconstructive surgery for the boutonniere deformity. If the joint is not severely involved, the extensor tendon can be reefed or tightened to bring the lateral bands more dorsal relative to the PIP joint. The joint is then splinted in full extension for 6 to 8 weeks, allowing free motion at both the metacarpophalangeal and the distal interphalangeal joints. However, if there is significant joint involvement, fusion is the treatment of choice.

SUGGESTED READINGS

Abrams RA, Botte MJ: Hand infections: Treatment recommendations for specific types. *J Am Acad Orthop Surg* 1996; 4(4):219.

Arons MS, Fernando L, Polayes IM: *Pasteurella multocida:* The major cause of hand infections following domestic animal bites. *J Hand Surg [Am]* 1982; 7:47.

Burkhalter WE: Deep space infections. *Hand Clin* 1989; 5:553.

Fitzgerald RH Jr, Cooney WP 3d, Washington JA 2d, et al: Bacterial colonization of mutilating hand injuries and its treatment. *J Hand Surg [Am]* 1977; 2:85.

Francel TJ, Marshall KA, Savage RC: Hand infections in the diabetic and the diabetic renal transplant recipient. *Ann Plast Surg* 1990; 24:304.

Freeland AE, Senter BS: Septic arthritis and osteomyelitis. *Hand Clin* 1989; 5:533.

Glass KD: Factors related to the resolution of treated hand infections. *J Hand Surg [Am]* 1982; 7:388.

Goldstein EJ, Citron DM, Wield B, et al: Bacteriology of human and animal bite wounds. *J Clin Microbiol* 1978; 8:667.

Gunther SF, Elliott RC, Brand RL, et al: Experience with atypical mycobacterial infection in the deep structures of the hand. *J Hand Surg [Am]* 1977; 2:90.

Hausman MR, Lisser SP: Hand infections. *Orthop Clin North Am* 1992; 23:171.

Hurst LC, Amadio PC, Badalamente MA, et al: *Mycobacterium marinum* infections of the hand. *J Hand Surg [Am]* 1987; 12:428.

Kanavel AB: *Infections of the Hand,* 7th ed. Philadelphia: Lea & Febiger, 1939.

Mann RJ, Peacock JM: Hand infections in patients with diabetes mellitus. *J Trauma* 1977; 17:376.

Reyes FA: Infections secondary to intravenous drug abuse. *Hand Clin* 1989; 5:629.

Schecter W, Meyer A, Schecter G, et al: Necrotizing fasciitis of the upper extremity. *J Hand Surg [Am]* 1982; 7:15.

Siegel DB, Gelberman RH: Infections of the hand. *Orthop Clin North Am* 1988; 19:779.

Wilkerson R, Paull W, Coville FV: Necrotizing fasciitis: Review of the literature and case report. *Clin Orthop* 1987; 216:187.

Zubowicz VN, Gravier M: Management of early human bites of the hand: A prospective randomized study. *Plast Reconstr Surg* 1991; 88:111.

Chapter 121

GREAT TOE DEFORMITIES

Donna J. Astion

HALLUX VALGUS

A *bunion* is an enlargement of the medial eminence of the first metatarsal with inflammation and swelling of the underlying soft tissue bursa. *Hallux valgus* is a lateral deviation of the great toe at the first metatarsophalangeal (MTP) joint. In societies where shoes are not worn, there is an equal incidence of hallux valgus among females and males. However, in societies with Western-style shoes, the prevalence of hallux valgus among women exceeds that in men by anywhere from 3:1 to 15:1.

ANATOMY

The sesamoid bones of the great toe, which are within the tendons of the flexor hallucis brevis, articulate with two grooves on the plantar surface of the first metatarsal head. The tendons of the flexor hallucis brevis, the abductor and adductor hallucis, the plantar aponeurosis, and the joint capsule all condense on the plantar aspect of the MTP joint to form the plantar plate (Fig. 121-1). The flexor hallucis brevis tendons attach to the plantar plate, as well as the base of the proximal phalanx.

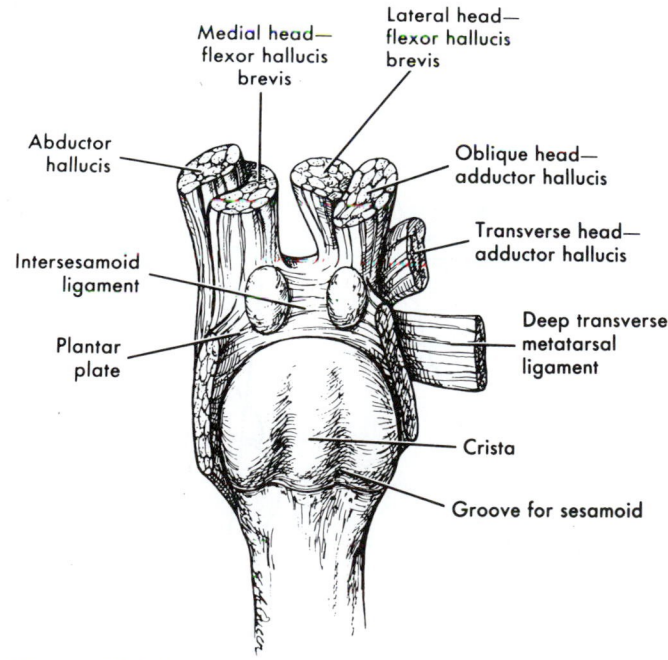

Figure 121-1
Plantar surface of the first metatarsal head with the joint capsule opened to visualize the plantar structures. [Reproduced with permission from Richardson EG: Disorders of the hallux. In Crenshaw AH (ed): *Campbell's Operative Orthopaedics*, vol 4, 8th ed. St. Louis: Mosby-Year Book; 1992:2617.]

There are four groups of tendons around the MTP joint which move the great toe (Fig. 121–2). The extensors hallucis longus and brevis pass dorsally over the joint. The tendon of the flexor hallucis longus courses on the plantar aspect of the sesamoid complex, which contains the tendons of the flexor hallucis brevis. The tendons of the abductor and adductor hallucis are positioned medially and laterally, respectively; both of these tendons are near the plantar surface of the joint. The abductor hallucis muscle acts to push the first metatarsal head towards the second metatarsal. There are no muscular insertions on the first metatarsal head and, therefore, its position is influenced by the position of the proximal phalanx.

The base of the first metatarsal articulates with the medial cuneiform. The joint is inclined slightly medial plantarly and is stabilized by caps or ligaments. Many surgeons feel that laxity of this joint exists in less than 5 percent of patients with hallux valgus.

PATHOPHYSIOLOGY

Stable MTP joints have a flatter articulation while those with a rounded articulation can progress to a hallux valgus deformity.

Patients with a rounded MTP joint have a relatively unstable joint. In these cases, when a hallux valgus deformity occurs, it is usually progressive. As the proximal phalanx moves laterally, it places pressure against the metatarsal head, which pushes the metatarsal head medially and increases the metatarsal proximal phalangeal angle (the hallux valgus angle). Over time the medial joint structures become attenuated and the lateral joint structures contract. Since the sesamoids are anchored laterally to the adductor hallucis tendon, the sesamoids remain in place and the rest of the structures of the joint rotate around this point (Fig. 121–3).

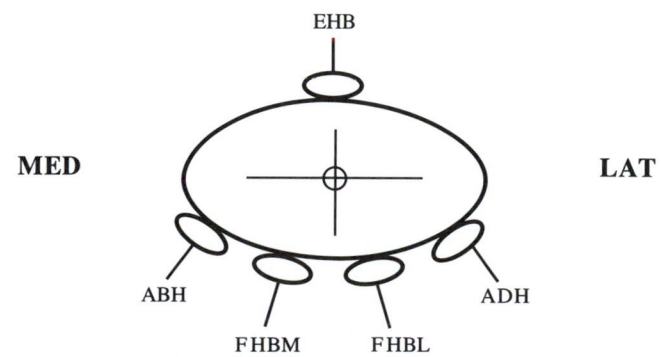

Figure 121-2
Schematic of the normal alignment of tendons around the first metatarsal head. EHB, extensor hallucis brevis; ABH, abductor hallucis; ADH, adductor hallucis; FHBM, flexor hallucis brevis medial head; FHBL, flexor hallucis brevis lateral head. [Reproduced with permission from Mann RA, Coughlin MJ: Adult hallux valgus. In Mann RA, Coughlin MJ (eds): *Surgery of the Foot and Ankle*. St. Louis: Mosby-Year Book; 1993:186.]

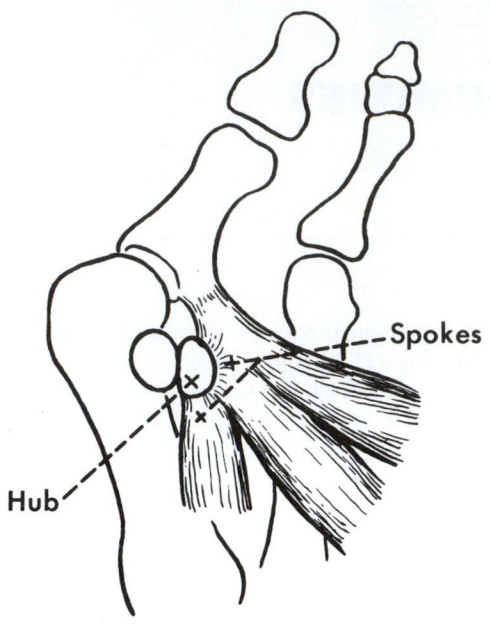

Figure 121-3
Severe hallux valgus deformity with rotation of the medial structures about the sesamoid complex. [Reproduced with permission from Mann RA, Coughlin MJ: Adult hallux valgus. In Mann RA, Coughlin MJ (eds): *Surgery of the Foot and Ankle.* St. Louis: Mosby-Year Book; 1993:187.]

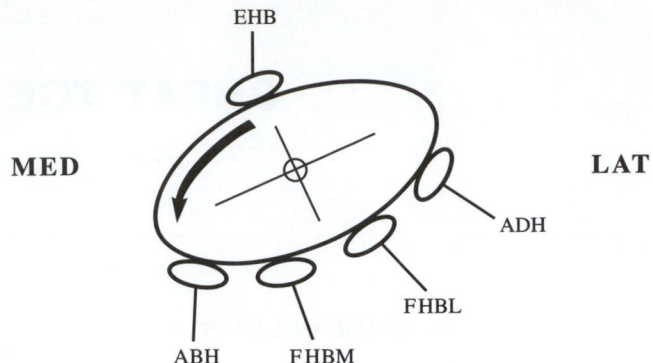

Figure 121-4
Schematic of the alignment of tendons around the first metatarsal head in a hallux valgus deformity. EHB, extensor hallucis brevis; ABH, abductor hallucis; ADH, adductor hallucis; FHBM, flexor hallucis brevis medial head; FHBL, flexor hallucis brevis lateral head. [Reproduced with permission from Mann RA, Coughlin MJ: Adult hallux valgus. In Mann RA, Coughlin MJ (eds): *Surgery of the Foot and Ankle.* St. Louis: Mosby-Year Book; 1993: 186.]

As the structures rotate, the adductor tendon moves plantarly and no longer stabilizes the metatarsal head (Fig. 121–4). The adductor tendon thus becomes an additional deforming force that pronates the proximal phalanx. Plantarly the flexor hallucis longus tendon moves laterally with the sesamoid and pulls the proximal phalanx laterally. In a marked hallux valgus deformity the extensor hallucis longus tendon is displaced laterally and adducts the proximal phalanx on the metatarsal head to further aggravate the deformity. As the deformity progresses, the great toe pronates and the sesamoid displaces laterally. The final result is that the hallux can no longer carry its share of the body weight and the weight is transferred laterally to the lesser toe metatarsal heads.

A congruous first MTP joint occurs where the articular surface of the proximal phalanx is parallel to the articular surface of the metatarsal head (Fig. 121–5). A congruous joint is relatively stable. Patients with congruous joints can still develop an enlarged medial eminence from pressure caused by shoe wear, and the overlying bursa may become enlarged and painful.

An incongruous first MTP joint occurs where the articular surfaces of the proximal phalanx and the metatarsal head are no longer parallel. The congruency of the first MTP joint becomes important when determining the optimal surgical approach for correction of the deformity.

PATIENT EVALUATION

Most patients complain of pain over the medial eminence and some complain of pain in the first MTP joint. Patients may also complain of pain under the second metatarsal head and/or a nearby callus if their weight has been transferred laterally. A careful history should reveal if the patient has any underlying systemic diseases which may aggravate or cause a painful hallux valgus. It is important to know when and under what circumstances the hallux is painful and if the pain is related to shoe wear.

Physical examination should include observation of the patient's gait, as well as examination of the weightbearing foot. With the pa-

tient standing, any deformity of the hallux and the lesser toes should be noted. Many deformities are frequently not visible in the non-weightbearing foot. If the patient has a unilateral flat foot ipsilateral to the hallux valgus during weightbearing, causes of the adult-acquired flat foot (such as posterior tibial tendon insufficiency and hindfoot arthritis) should be ruled out. With the patient sitting, the range of motion of the first MTP joint should be evaluated in its resting position and with the hallux valgus corrected as much as possible. The dorsal medial cutaneous nerve of the great toe should be palpated to rule out irritability of the nerve as the cause of the patient's pain. The mobility of the first metatarsal cuneiform joint should also be evaluated. In addition, the plantar aspect of the foot should be assessed for intractable plantar keratoses, which are most frequently located beneath the second metatarsal head. The lesser toes should be evaluated for evidence of hammer toes or mallet toes. Finally, the in-

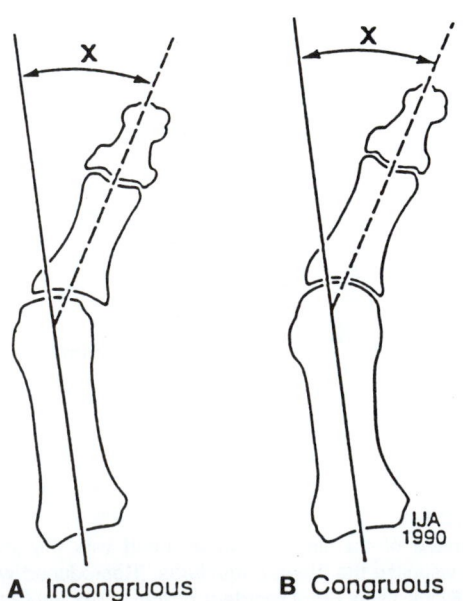

Figure 121-5
A. Incongruous first metatarsophalangeal joint. *B.* Congruous first metatarsophalangeal joint. (Courtesy of American Orthopaedic Foot Ankle Society Review Course. Baltimore: Williams & Wilkins; 1990:8.)

termetatarsal spaces should be palpated for evidence of an interdigital neuroma.

RADIOGRAPHIC EXAMINATION

AP and lateral radiographs of the foot should always be taken with the patient weightbearing. A nonweightbearing oblique radiograph of the foot should also be included. The following information should be obtained from the AP and lateral views. (Fig. 121–6):

1. The hallux valgus angle (normally less than 15 degrees)
2. The intermetatarsal angle (normally less than 9 degrees)
3. The distal metatarsal articular angle (normally less than 10 degrees of lateral deviation)
4. The joint congruency should be determined
5. The hallux interphalangeal angle
6. The metatarsal cuneiform joint angle (normally less than 10 degrees of medial angulation)
7. The size of the medial eminence
8. The sesamoid congruency

All three views should be used to evaluate the presence of arthrosis at the first MTP joint; the remainder of the foot is evaluated radiographically for the presence of other potential pathology.

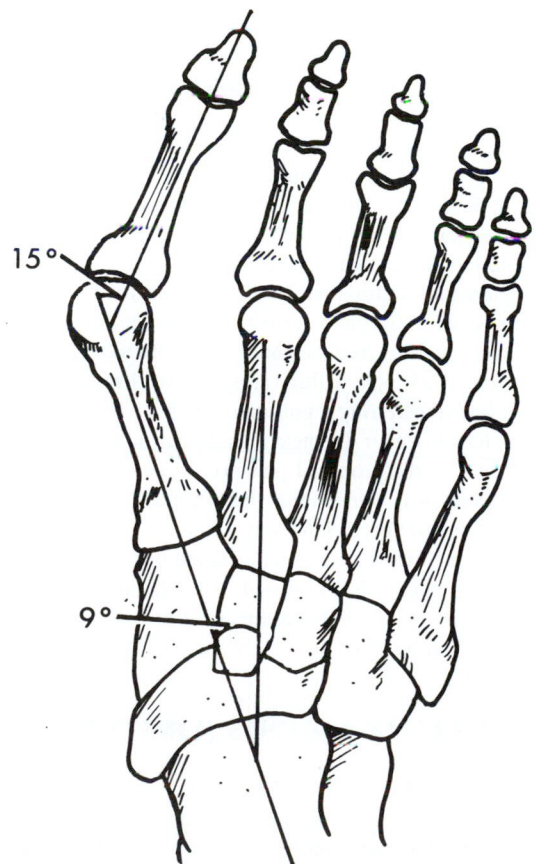

Figure 121-6
Normal alignment of the first metatarsophalangeal joint should be less than 15 degrees of valgus. The intermetatarsal angle between the first and second metatarsals should be 9 degrees or less. [Reproduced with permission from Mann RA, Coughlin MJ: Adult hallux valgus. In Mann RA, Coughlin MJ (eds): *Surgery of the Foot and Ankle.* St. Louis: Mosby-Year Book; 1993:181.]

CLASSIFICATION

Hallux valgus deformities can be classified as mild, moderate, and severe. In mild bunion deformities, the MTP joint is congruous but there is usually an enlarged painful medial eminence. The hallux valgus angle is less than 20 degrees and the intermetatarsal angle (the angle between the first and second metatarsals) is less than or equal to 11 degrees. The position of the sesamoid bones is usually anatomic; however, the fibular sesamoid may be subluxed up to 50 percent. A moderate hallux valgus deformity usually has an incongruent MTP joint. The hallux valgus angle is in the range of 20 to 40 degrees and the intermetatarsal angle is widened (11 and 18 degrees). The fibular sesamoid is displaced between 75 and 100 percent. In a severe hallux valgus deformity, the MTP joint is usually incongruent, the hallux valgus angle is greater than 40 degrees, and the metatarsal angle is usually greater than 16 degrees. The fibular sesamoid is subluxed laterally 100 percent. In these cases, there are often concomitant problems with the second toe.

TREATMENT

Initially, hallux valgus should be conservatively managed. The first recommendation is shoes that relieve pressure over the medial prominence. The shoes should be of sufficient width, with a soft leather upper and no stitching over the medial eminence. This often gives the patient significant relief of symptoms. Custom-made footwear is indicated for patients with severe hallux valgus deformities who are reluctant to undergo surgical correction.

Surgery is indicated when nonoperative measures fail. A decrease in patient function and an inability to tolerate shoes are good guidelines by which to measure the need for operative treatment. The goals of surgery are to relieve pain, correct the deformity, and retain adequate motion at the first MTP joint. There are more than 100 surgical procedures described in the literature for the correction of a hallux valgus deformity. To determine which procedure to perform for a given patient, it is important to understand that not all hallux valgus deformities are equal. Mann and Coughlin (1993) developed an algorithm to help clinicians logically approach treatment for the patient with the hallux valgus deformity. They divided the hallux deformity into three main groups:

1. Patients with a congruent joint
2. Patients with an incongruent joint
3. Patients with arthrosis of the first MTP joint

To use the algorithm, the congruence of the first MTP joint must be evaluated first. Patients with a congruent joint often have pain over the medial eminence. These patients may benefit from a distal soft tissue procedure that removes the medial eminence, tightens the medial capsule, and releases the lateral structures. In patients with a congruous joint and an intermetatarsal angle between 10 and 14 degrees, a distal chevron osteotomy may be performed.

If the first MTP joint is not congruent, then the surgical procedure must reestablish a congruent joint. Patients less than 50 years of age, with a mild hallux valgus deformity (a hallux valgus angle of less than 30 degrees and an intermetatarsal angle of less than 15 degrees) may undergo a distal chevron osteotomy with tightening of the medial capsule. There is some controversy about whether a lateral soft tissue release can be performed with a distal chevron osteotomy without increasing the risk of avascular necrosis of the metatarsal head. Some authors now report success with distal chevron osteotomies in 50 years of age. Alternative approaches are a distal soft tissue procedure with a proximal metatarsal osteotomy or a Mitchell procedure.

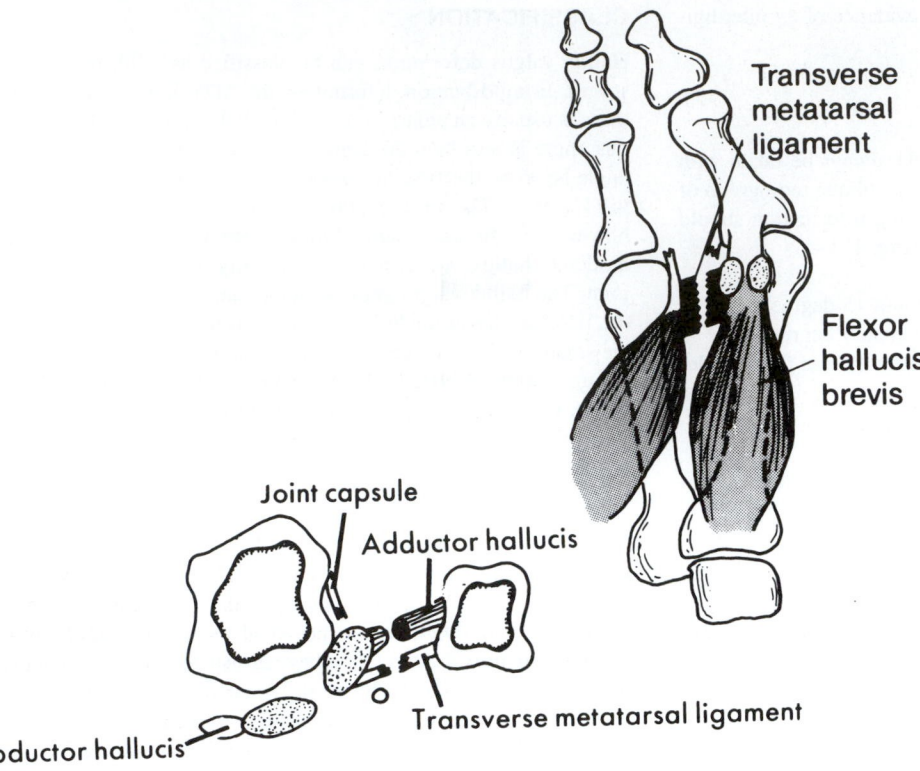

Figure 121-7
Lateral structures released in the distal soft tissue procedure for correction of a moderate or severe hallux valgus deformity. [Repro-duced with permission from Mann RA, Coughlin MJ: Adult hallux valgus. In Mann RA, Coughlin MJ (eds): *Surgery of the Foot and Ankle*. St. Louis: Mosby-Year Book; 1993:207.]

Patients with a moderate hallux valgus deformity (a hallux valgus angle of less than 40 degrees and an intermetatarsal of greater than 15 degrees) should undergo a distal soft tissue procedure with a proximal metatarsal osteotomy or a Mitchell procedure. If the hallux valgus deformity is severe (a hallux valgus angle of greater than 40 degrees and an intermetatarsal angle of greater than 20 degrees), the deformity can be corrected with a distal soft tissue procedure and a proximal metatarsal osteotomy or with an arthrodesis of the first MTP joint. The distal soft tissue procedure entails releasing the adductor hallucis tendon, the joint capsule, and the transverse metatarsal ligament laterally, while medially the eminence is removed and the capsule tightened (Fig. 121–7).

If there is significant arthrosis of the first MTP joint, it should be fused which will correct the hallux valgus deformity. Patients with a hypermobile first metatarsal cuneiform joint (about 5 percent of patients with hallux valgus deformity) should undergo an arthrodesis of the metatarsal cuneiform joint with a distal soft tissue procedure to correct the hallux valgus deformity.

Prior to undergoing any surgical procedure, the patient should understand the potential complications of the surgery. These include recurrence of the hallux valgus deformity, hallux varus deformity, avascular necrosis of the metatarsal head (reported to be 0 to 20 percent for distal Chevron osteotomies and 8 to 12 percent for Mitchell osteotomies) and metatarsalgia (reported to be 0 to 33 percent for distal osteotomies and 0 to 52 percent in proximal osteotomies). The patient should also understand that there may be some residual stiffness, pain, or deformity after the surgery, which could limit their shoe selection.

Surgery to correct a hallux valgus deformity is contraindicated in patients with vascular insufficiency, a neuropathic foot, and for cosmetic correction of a hallux valgus deformity that is not painful. Surgery is also contraindicated in children with open physis. Hallux valgus surgery is contraindicated in patients with a spastic muscular condition and relatively contraindicated in patients with a severely pronated foot because of a high recurrence rate after surgical correction.

HALLUX VARUS

Hallux varus is a medial deviation of the great toe at the MTP joint and is most commonly a complication of hallux valgus surgery. It may present immediately postoperatively or years after the index surgery. Other rare causes of hallux varus include trauma, inflammatory rupture of the conjoined tendons (which may be seen in psoriatic or rheumatoid arthritis patients), or deformity after excision of the fibular sesamoid. Surgical correction of the hallux varus is indicated only if it is painful and the patient has difficulty wearing shoes. Surgery to correct a supple hallux varus involves lengthening the medial capsule and transferring a portion of, or the whole, extensor hallucis longus tendon under the metatarsal ligament and through a drill hole at the base of the proximal phalanx. If the entire extensor hallucis longus tendon is transferred, the interphalangeal (IP) joint of the great toe must be fused; however, if half of the extensor hallucis longus is used, or if the extensor hallucis brevis tendon is used, then the IP joint does not need to be fused. If the hallux varus deformity is fixed, or if there is significant arthrosis of the joint, then fusion of the MPT joint is indicated.

HALLUX RIGIDUS (LIMITUS)

Hallux rigidus is the painful loss of motion in the great toe MTP joint. It is usually caused by arthrosis of the joint which brings about the development of osteophytes on the dorsal metatarsal head and proximal phalanx (Fig. 121–8). These bony prominences cause painful, restricted dorsiflexion of the joint. Patients often complain of pain in the joint with any activity that involves dorsiflexion of the great toe such as walking, running, or standing on their toes. Radiographically, dorsal osteophytes are present at the MTP joint at the metatarsal head and the proximal phalanx of the great toe. The sesamoid metatarsal head joints are rarely involved. Serial radiographs may show progressive narrowing of the joint space.

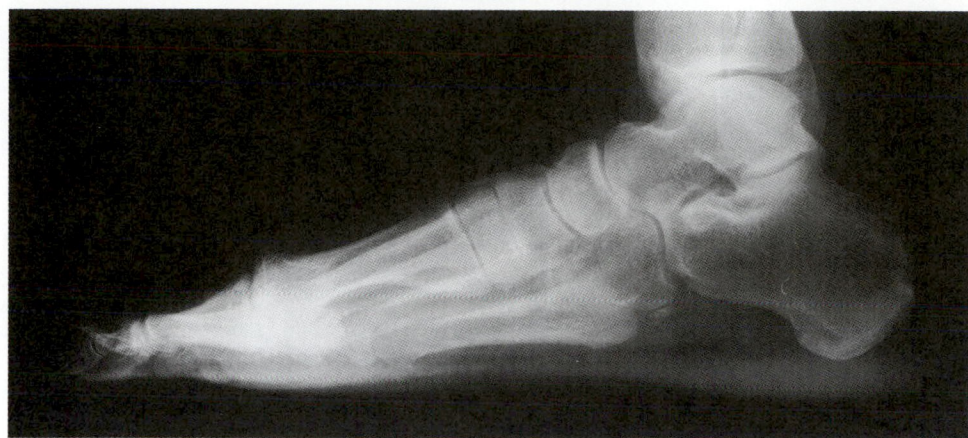

Figure 121–8
Lateral radiograph of a patient with hallux rigidus.

The initial nonoperative treatment of hallux rigidus is aimed at reducing motion at the first MTP joint and relieving the pressure on the dorsal prominence. These goals can be accomplished with a stiff-soled shoe and stretching the shoe in the area of the dorsal prominence. If these minor measures are not helpful, a steel shank or other rigid inserts can be placed in a shoe with a rocker sole. Nonsteroidal anti-inflammatory medications may also be helpful in the nonoperative management of this condition.

If nonoperative measures fail, then surgery is indicated. The surgical treatment chosen should take into consideration the patient's age, sex, and lifestyle, as well as their radiographic presentation. Patients with lateral weightbearing radiographs that show preservation of at least one-half to one-third of the plantar joint spaces are candidates for cheilectomy. In this procedure, the dorsal osteophyte and the upper 30 percent of the metatarsal head articular surface are excised with the periarticular osteophyte on the base of the proximal phalanx. Postoperatively, in an attempt to preserve the motion obtained intraoperatively, range of motion exercises are started once the skin wound is healed. If the patient has advanced arthrosis or has had a failed cheilectomy, an arthrodesis of the first MTP joint is indicated. An arthrodesis is also indicated in patients with hallux rigidus secondary to gouty arthritis. Older and relatively inactive patients are candidates for a Keller procedure (resection of the base of the proximal phalanx). The Keller procedure shortens the great toe, leaving patients at risk of developing a transfer metatarsalgia or a cock-up or angular deformity of the great toe. Some authors recommend an interpositional arthroplasty in selected patients.

CLAW HALLUX

A claw hallux deformity is defined as hyperextension of the MTP joint with flexion of the IP joint. This deformity may occur iatrogenically after cutting both slips of the flexor hallucis brevis tendon. Patients with neurologic disorders such as Charcot-Marie-Tooth disease may present with a claw hallux which is secondary in muscular imbalances. The deformity may also be seen as a late sequela of compartment syndromes in the leg or foot.

The work-up of a patient who presents with a claw hallux deformity of the great toe should include a careful orthopaedic and neurologic examination, as well as appropriate electrodiagnostic tests. Weightbearing and nonweightbearing radiographs of the foot should be obtained to determine the flexibility of the deformity. The nonoperative treatment of this condition is shoe modifications to decrease pressure from the shoe on the toe. If this fails, then surgery should be considered.

The flexibility of the affected toe determines which surgical procedure should be performed. If the patient has a cavus deformity of the foot and the claw hallux is supple, then correction of the cavus deformity with a mid-foot or proximal metatarsal osteotomy often corrects the claw hallux. The claw hallux may occur in association with a plantarflexed first metatarsal in patients with tibialis anterior weakness. In this case, if the toe is supple, the extensor hallucis longus is transferred to the neck of the first metatarsal and the IP joint of the great toe is fused (Jones procedure). Younger active patients with a rigid claw hallux are candidates for an arthrodesis, while older patients with a lower activity level are candidates for a Keller resection.

THE SESAMOIDS

The medial and lateral sesamoid bones of the first MTP joint are within the two heads of the flexor hallucis brevis tendon. The sesamoids are connected to each other by the intermetatarsal ligament and stabilized by the ligament complex of the first MTP joint. The sesamoids are usually injured by direct trauma, repetitive stress, or forced dorsiflexion. When there is injury to one or both of the sesamoids, the patient often presents with a decreased range of motion at the first MTP joint, pain on palpation of the injured sesamoid, and decreased strength of the plantar flexion of the great toe.

Standard radiographs to evaluate the sesamoids include AP and oblique views of the forefoot, as well as an axial sesamoid view. It is important to know that 25 percent of the population have a bipartite sesamoid, 80 percent of which involve the tibial sesamoid. Changes in the sesamoid may be seen over time with sequential radiographs. A bone scan may be necessary to adequately evaluate a painful sesamoid observed in a normal radiograph.

Pain in the area of the sesamoid may be secondary to sesamoiditis, osteonecrosis, acute fracture, stress fracture, or bursitis. Sesamoiditis is an acute or chronic inflammation of the sesamoid. Patients complain of pain in the area of the sesamoid with weightbearing. On physical examination there is pain with palpation of the involved sesamoid. The radiographs are usually negative and the initial treatment includes pads to unweight the sesamoid and nonsteroidal anti-inflammatory medications. In the presence of continuing symptoms for greater than one year, surgical excision may be considered.

Osteonecrosis of the sesamoid initially presents like sesamoiditis; however, sequential radiographs demonstrate fragmentation of the involved bone. The treatment consists of unweighting the sesamoid.

Acute fractures of the sesamoid will usually present after a traumatic event. These fractures are more frequently seen in the tibial

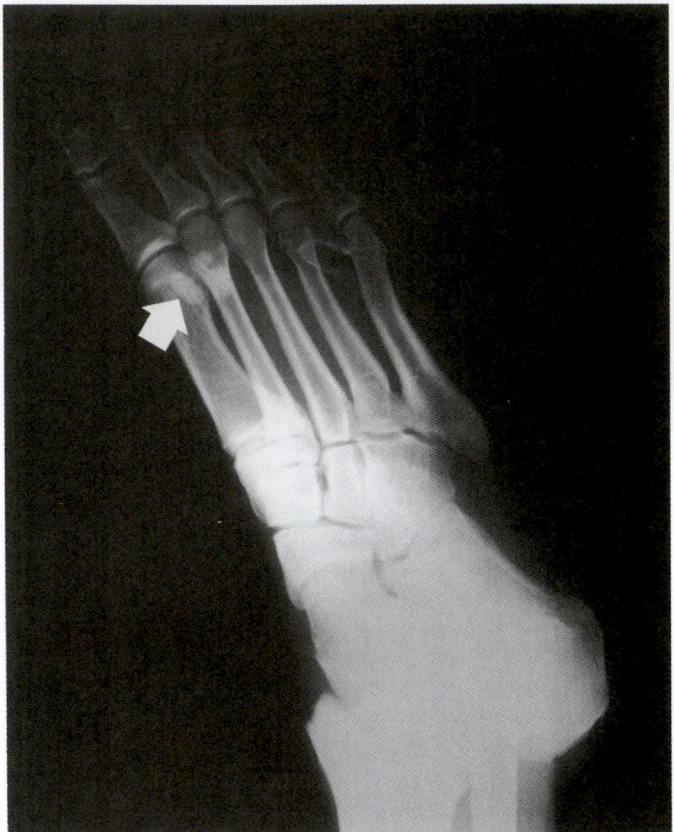

Figure 121–9
Radiograph of sesamoid fracture.

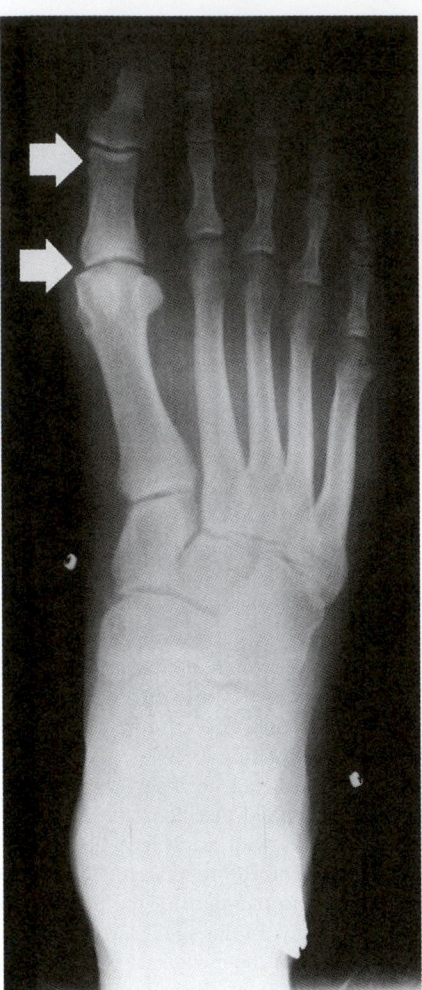

Figure 121–10
AP radiograph of the foot demonstrating periarticular erosions in gouty arthritis about the joint with maintenance of the joint spaces.

sesamoid and can be distinguished from a bipartite sesamoid because the acute fracture will have rough irregular edges between the two fragments (Fig. 121–9). If confirmation is needed, a bone scan can differentiate a bipartite sesamoid from an acute fracture. Initial treatment of a sesamoid fracture is aimed at limiting the motion at the MTP joint and minimizing the pressure on the sesamoid. This can be accomplished with a short leg cast with a toe plate or with a stiff-soled shoe and a relief under the involved sesamoid. The morbidity after a sesamoid fracture is prolonged, and it may take up to 1 year for the pain to subside. If conservative measures fail, then the involved sesamoid or portion of the sesamoid may be excised.

Sesamoid stress fractures usually occur in the tibial sesamoid and can be diagnosed by standard radiographs or, if necessary, a bone scan. The diagnosis of this condition is often delayed, since radiographs are frequently normal. These should initially be treated with immobilization, and if symptoms persist then excision is indicated.

A chronic bursitis may develop below a sesamoid and may be the cause of pain under both the medial and lateral sesamoids. Treatment is aimed at decreasing the weight on the bursal area and limiting the motion at the first MTP joint in order to decrease inflammation in the area. On rare occasions when symptoms are refractory to these measures, surgery is indicated to remove the bursa.

GOUTY ARTHRITIS

Fifty percent of first attacks of gouty arthritis involve the MTP joint of the great toe. Of patients with gout, 90 percent experience one or more attacks of this joint in their lifetime. Up to 30 percent of attacks may occur during a postoperative period. The attack is caused by the

precipitation of monosodium urate crystals in the joint fluid and the coincident inflammatory response. The attack usually begins in the evening with progressive pain and redness and warmth of the joint, and the symptoms intensify over the ensuing 2 to 3 days. Initially, radiographs demonstrate soft tissue swelling; however, after multiple attacks, periarticular erosions develop medially and laterally at the MTP joint and the articular surface remains intact (Fig. 121–10). If medical treatment does not prevent multiple episodes, the first MTP joint becomes sclerotic and arthritis develops. The accurate diagnosis of gouty arthritis depends on the recovery of monosodium urate crystals from the joint fluid. Once the diagnosis is made, treatment should begin immediately. Initial treatment consists of nonsteroidal anti-inflammatory drugs, as well as splinting of the toe. Surgery for the chronically painful and deformed MTP joint may include a Keller procedure in older patients with low demand or an arthrodesis in more active patients.

SUGGESTED READINGS

Coughlin MJ, Abdo RV: Arthrodesis of the first metatarsophalangeal joint with vitallium plate fixation. *Foot Ankle* 1994; 15:18.

Coughlin MJ, Mann RA: The pathophysiology of the juvenile bunion. In Griffin PP (ed): *Instructional Course Lectures.* Park Ridge, IL: American Academy of Orthopaedic Surgeons; 1987; 36:123.

Coughlin MJ: Sesamoid pain: causes and surgical treatment. In Greene WB (ed): *Instructional Course Lectures.* Park Ridge, IL: American Academy of Orthopaedic Surgeons; 1990; 39:23.

Frey C, Thompson F, Smith J, et al: American Orthopaedic Foot and Ankle Society women's shoe survey. *Foot Ankle* 1993; 14:78.

Jahss M: Disorders of the hallux and the first ray. In Jahss M (ed): *Disorders of the Foot and Ankle: Medical and Surgical Management,* vol 2, 2d ed. Philadelphia: WB Saunders; 1991:943.

Johnson JE, Clanton TO, Baxter DE, et al: Comparison of Chevron osteotomy and modified McBride bunionectomy for correction of mild to moderate hallux valgus deformity. *Foot Ankle* 1991; 12:61.

Johnson KA, Spiegl PV: Extensor hallucis longus transfer for hallux varus deformity. *J Bone Joint Surg [Am]* 1984; 66:681.

Mann RA: Decision-making in bunion surgery. In Greene WB (ed): *Instructional Course Lectures.* Park Ridge, IL: American Academy of Orthopaedic Surgeons; 1990; 39:3.

Mann RA, Clanton TO: Hallux rigidus: Treatment by cheilectomy. *J Bone Joint Surg [Am]* 1988; 70:400.

Mann RA, Coughlin MJ: Adult hallux valgus. In Mann RA, Coughlin MJ (eds): *Surgery of the Foot and Ankle,* vol 1, 6th ed. St. Louis: CV Mosby 1993:167.

Mann RA, Katcherian DA: Relationship of metatarsophalangeal joint fusion on the intermetatarsal angle. *Foot Ankle* 1989; 10:8.

Mann RA, Rudicel S, Graves SC: Repair of hallux valgus with a distal soft-tissue procedure and proximal metatarsal osteotomy. *J Bone Joint Surg [Am]* 1992; 74:124.

O'Doherty DP, Lowrie IG, Magnussen PA, et al: The management of the painful first metatarsophalangeal joint in the older patient. Arthrodesis or Keller's arthroplasty? *J Bone Joint Surg [Br]* 1990; 72:839.

Peterson DA, Zilberfarb JL, Greene MA, et al: Avascular necrosis of the first metatarsal head: Incidence in distal osteotomy combined with lateral soft tissue release. *Foot Ankle Int* 1994; 15:59.

Sangeorzan BJ, Hansen ST Jr: Modified Lapidus procedure for hallux valgus. *Foot Ankle* 1989; 9:262.

Shereff MJ, Bejjani FJ, Kummer FJ: Kinematics of the first metatarsophalangeal joint. *J Bone Joint Surg [Am]* 1986; 68:392.

Shereff MJ, Jahss MH: Complications of silastic implant arthroplasty in the hallux. *Foot Ankle* 1980; 1:95.

Thompson FM: Complications of hallux valgus surgery and salvage. *Orthopedics* 1990; 13:1059.

Chapter 122

LESSER TOE DEFORMITIES

Donna J. Astion

Deformities of the lesser toes can occur in isolation or in association with other forefoot deformities such as hallux valgus. The most common cause is poor footwear; however, lesser toe deformities may also have a congenital or neuromuscular etiology.

HAMMER TOE, MALLET TOES, AND CLAW TOE

ANATOMY

The position of each toe depends on both the active and passive stabilizers of the toe. The passive stabilizers consist of the collateral ligaments of each joint, the plantar aponeurosis and the volar plate, and the capsule. The dynamic stabilizers include both the extrinsic and intrinsic muscles of the foot. The flexor digitorum longus inserts on the distal phalanx while the extensor digitorum longus inserts on the extensor hood at the level of the proximal phalanx and then continues on to insert into the distal phalanx. The intrinsic muscles act to support and balance the extrinsic muscles. The extensor digitorum brevis inserts onto the middle phalanx while the lumbricales and interossei tendons course plantarly to the center of rotation of the metatarsophalangeal (MTP) joint and insert into the extensor hood. The lumbricales' function is to plantarflex the MTP joint and extend the interphalangeal (IP) joints. There are no direct tendinous insertions on the proximal phalanx (Fig. 122–1).

PATHOPHYSIOLOGY

Lesser toe deformities result from an imbalance between the intrinsic and extrinsic muscles of the foot. The position of the proximal phalanx at the MTP joint is determined by the pull of the extensor digitorum longus and the antagonistic pull of the weaker intrinsic muscles. The position of the middle and distal phalanges is determined by the pull of the long and short flexors. At each joint, there is a mismatch between the strong extrinsic muscles and the weaker intrinsic muscles.

All lesser toe deformities can be rigid or flexible. Classification is generally by the position of the IP joints (Fig. 122–2). With a hammer toe the proximal phalangeal joint is flexed, and with a mallet toe the distal interphalangeal (DIP) joint is flexed. A claw toe is flexed at both the proximal and distal interphalangeal joints and extended at the MTP joint.

Mallet toes and hammer toes are usually the result of poorly fitting shoes and are more frequently seen in women than in men. The second toe is most commonly affected because it is often the longest ray and, therefore, most affected by pressure from the shoe. These deformities usually develop over a prolonged period of time. Lesser toe deformities can be associated with inflammatory arthritides such as rheumatoid arthritis or psoriatic arthritis or with neuromuscular diseases such as Charcot-Marie-Tooth disease, Freidrich's ataxia, cerebral palsy, multiple sclerosis, degenerative disc disease, or myelodysplasia. Progressive hammer toe or claw toe deformities may also be seen as a late finding of compartment syndrome of the calf or the foot. Claw toe deformities may be associated with the same arthritic deformities and neuromuscular diseases that cause hammer toe deformities; however, in some patients the etiology of the claw toe deformity cannot be identified. Claw toe deformities usually involve multiple toes, frequently in both feet. As a claw toe deformity becomes more rigid, the toe strikes the top of the shoe and the metatarsal head is forced plantarly. Eventually, the proximal phalanx subluxes dorsally at the MTP joint and the plantar fat pad migrates distally. This deformity exposes the metatarsal heads plantarly and results in metatarsalgia and painful plantar keratoses under the metatarsal heads.

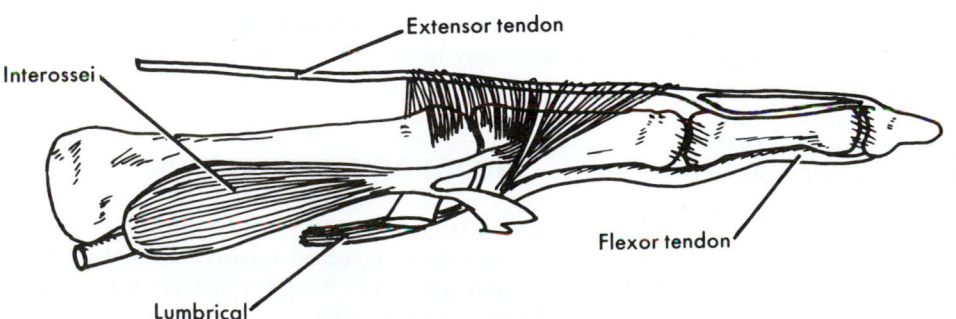

Figure 122-1
Lateral view of a lesser toe (a portion of the extensor tendon is removed). [Reproduced with permission from Mann RA, Coughlin MJ: Lesser toe deformities. In Mann RA, Coughlin MJ (eds): *Surgery of the Foot and Ankle*. St. Louis: Mosby-Year Book; 1993: 347.]

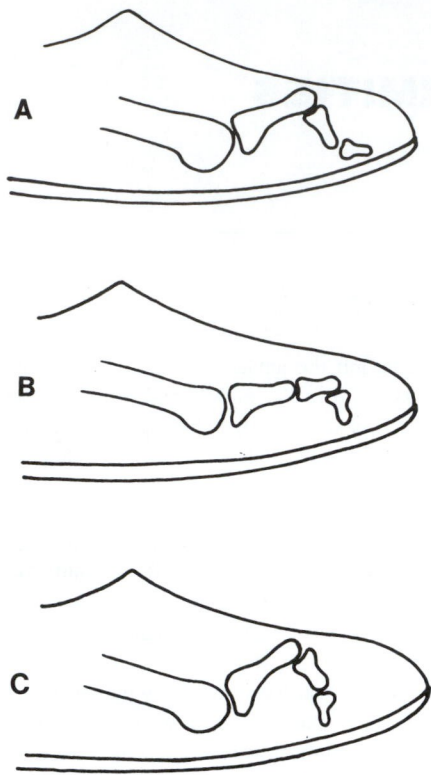

Figure 122-2
Hammer toe deformity in a shoe (*A*). Mallet toe deformity in a shoe (*B*). Claw toe deformity in a shoe (*C*). [Reproduced with permission from Frey CC: Osteoarthritis and static deformity of the forefoot. In Sammarco GJ (ed): *Foot and Ankle Manual*. Philadelphia: Lea & Febiger/Lippincott Williams & Wilkins; 1991:142.]

CHIEF COMPLAINT

Patients often complain of pain and callus in the areas where the toe hits the shoe. In hammer toe and claw toe deformities this is usually the dorsal aspect of the PIP joint, and in mallet toe deformities it is typically the tip of the toe or the dorsal aspect of the DIP joint. Patients with claw toe deformities with subluxation or dislocation of the MTP joint may complain of pain plantarly in the area of the metatarsal heads. Some of these patients may have painful calluses in the area.

PHYSICAL EXAMINATION

In addition to the standard examination of the foot, several additional areas are important to evaluate. Each digit should be examined for callosities over the IP joints, as well as the tip of the toe and the plantar aspect of the foot. In addition, the area between the toes should be inspected for callosities. Medial or lateral deviation of the toes at the MTP joint should be noted, as well as any hyperextension of the MTP joint. The laxity of the MTP joint should also be evaluated with a drawer test (stressing and subluxing the base of the proximal phalanx dorsally). Toe deformities should be evaluated with the patient sitting as well as standing. It is important to determine if the toe deformities are flexible or rigid. It is also important to determine if there is sufficient space for the involved toe when it is reduced to a normal position.

RADIOGRAPHIC EVALUATION

Weightbearing AP and lateral radiographs of the foot are helpful in evaluating the MTP joints. A diminished joint space at the MTP joint

on the AP radiograph may indicate subluxation at the joint; overlapping of the base of the proximal phalanx over the metatarsal head indicates dislocation of the joint. Medial or lateral deviation of the MTP joint also can be determined on the AP radiograph. Lateral radiographs are helpful in assessing the magnitude of the contracture of the IP joints.

TREATMENT

The initial management of all lesser toe deformities is nonsurgical. Pain in calluses at the tips of mallet toes can be alleviated by toe crests which lift the tip of the toes and prevent weightbearing on the calluses. Pain over the proximal IP joint maybe relieved by high toe-boxed shoes which will not press down on the PIP joints. Metatarsal pads in the shoe relieve pressure on the metatarsal heads. Flexible toes can be strapped and padded to diminish dorsiflexion at the MTP joint.

If these nonsurgical measures fail, then surgery is indicated. If surgery is required, the procedure should be carefully selected depending on the specific cause and nature of the deformity of the toe and the MTP joint. In cases of flexible deformities, tenotomies or tendon transfers may be sufficient, whereas in fixed deformities more extensive surgery would be necessary. With a flexible hammer toe deformity, the toe straightens when the ankle is in equinus or when a dorsiflexion force is applied to the plantar aspect of the metatarsal heads. In these cases, the flexor digitorum longus tendon is released plantarly and brought dorsally through the medial and lateral tunnels and sutured to the extensor hood with the ankle in neutral position and the toe slightly plantar-flexed. With a fixed hammer toe deformity, the PIP joint is contracted. In these cases, a DuVris arthroplasty (resection of the distal head of the proximal phalanx) is recommended. This procedure causes a fibrous union at the PIP joint which usually allows some motion.

A flexible mallet toe deformity can be treated by tenotomy of the flexor digitorum longus tendon at the level of the distal IP joint. If the mallet deformity is rigid, it can be corrected by partial phalangectomy of the distal portion of the proximal phalanx.

Claw toe deformities require more complex surgical solutions. If the deformity is flexible, soft tissue balancing is possible with a flexor digitorum longus to extensor hood tendon transfer. If the deformity is semiflexible, without bony deformity, then lengthening the extensor digitorum longus, releasing the dorsal capsulotomy of the MTP joint, and releasing the collateral ligaments can be performed in conjunction with the tendon transfer. If, however, the claw toe deformity is rigid at the PIP joint, then the distal aspect of the proximal phalanx is excised (DuVris arthroplasty) and the extensor tendon is lengthened. To surgically correct a subluxation or dislocation of the MTP joint, the extensor digitorum longus tendon is lengthened and a dorsal capsulotomy of the MTP joint is performed with release of the collateral ligaments. If the toe is medially deviated, the lateral capsule is tightened to realign the toe. The plantar capsule may need to be released in order to reduce the hyperextended MTP joint. If necessary, an MTP joint arthroplasty (removal of a portion of the metatarsal head) may be performed to preserve function while allowing relocation of the joint.

FREIBERG'S INFRACTION

Freiberg's infraction is thought to be a vascular insult to the metatarsal head. It is most common in the second metatarsal and usually occurs in the early teenage years. The condition presents with pain and swelling of the involved joint. The radiographic appearance of the metatarsal head is consistent with osteonecrosis. Osteophytes may form around the joint which limit motion and cause discomfort.

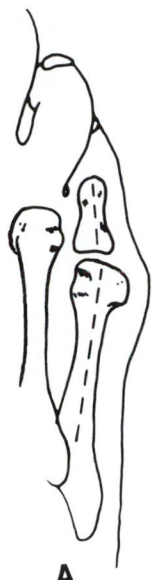 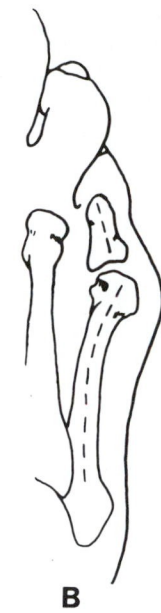 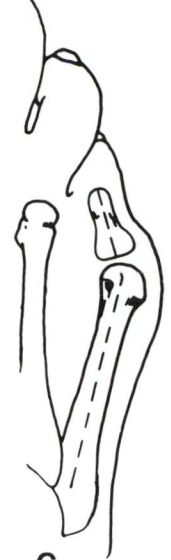

A   B   C

Figure 122-3
Bunionette deformity may be due to a prominent fifth metatarsal head condyle (*A*), angulation of the distal fifth metatarsal shaft (*B*), or an increased 4–5 intermetatarsal angle (*C*). [Reproduced with permission from Coughlin MJ: The bunionette deformity: Etiology and treatment. In Gould JS (ed): *Operative Foot Surgery*. Philadelphia: WB Saunders; 1994:54.]

Treatment of this entity depends on the degree of destruction of the metatarsal head. If the normal architecture of the joint is maintained, then symptomatic treatment is indicated. This usually consists of a rocker bottom sole to prevent motion at the joint and a metatarsal pad inside the shoe to relieve pressure on the metatarsal head plantarly. In addition, the patient's activities should be reduced. If osteophytes are present which block motion at the joint, then debridement of the osteophytes and a synovectomy are indicated. If the articular surface is damaged, then a portion of the metatarsal head may be resected to regain motion. A complete resection of the metatarsal head is not indicated as it will change the weight distribution in the plantar aspect of the foot and cause a transfer lesion.

BUNIONETTE DEFORMITIES

With a bunionette (Taylor's bunion), the lateral aspect of the small toe is prominent at the level of the metatarsal head (Fig. 122–3). Shoe pressure on this prominence can cause formation of a bursa or a callus, which can be painful. The metatarsal head may be prominent from an enlargement of the metatarsal head itself, a lateral curving of the metatarsal shaft, or an increased fourth/fifth metatarsal shaft angle. A splay foot occurs when the bunionette deformity is present with a hallux valgus deformity.

The initial treatment of a painful bunionette is nonsurgical. Patients should be advised to purchase shoes with a wider toebox with a soft leather upper. If the deformity is associated with a pronated foot, then an orthotic which supinates the foot may be helpful to relieve pressure on the lateral fifth metatarsal head.

When nonoperative treatment has not been successful, surgery is indicated. The surgery indicated depends on the etiology of the deformity. If the metatarsal head is enlarged or there is a large lateral eminence, a partial lateral condylectomy is indicated. If the metatarsal shaft is laterally deviated, then a distal osteotomy will be necessary. If there is an increase in the angle between the fourth and fifth metatarsals, then the osteotomy can be performed proximally or distally. Many different distal osteotomies have been described, but most

commonly, a distal chevron osteotomy is performed. When performing a proximal osteotomy it is important to be aware of the prolonged healing time required because the proximal metaphyseal diaphyseal junction is a relatively avascular area.

CORNS

A corn is the accumulation of keratotic layers of the epidermis over a bony prominence. When a shoe exerts extrinsic pressure over a bony prominence, this thickened epithelium accumulates. A hard corn is most commonly found on the lateral aspect of the fifth toe. Soft corns form over the condyle of the phalanx between the toes. Usually palliative measures, such as reducing the keratotic accumulation and changing footwear are most effective in relieving the symptoms. For soft corns, lamb's wool, soft gauze, or a pad may be placed between the toes to prevent the buildup of this keratotic tissue. If this is not successful, then surgical excision of the prominent condyle or the deformity may be indicated.

SUGGESTED READINGS

Coughlin MJ: Etiology and treatment of the bunionette deformity. In Greene WB (ed): *Instructional Course Lectures*. Park Ridge, IL: American Academy of Orthopaedic Surgeons; 1990; 39:37.

Janecki CJ, Wilde AH: Results of phalangectomy of the fifth toe for hammertoe: The Ruiz-Mora procedure. *J Bone Joint Surg [Am]* 1976; 58:1005.

Kitaoka HB, Holiday AD Jr, Campbell DC 2d: Distal Chevron metatarsal osteotomy for bunionette. *Foot Ankle* 1991; 12:80.

Mann RA, Coughlin MJ (eds): *Surgery of the Foot and Ankle,* vol 1, 6th ed. St. Louis: CV Mosby; 1993.

Mizel MS: Correction of hammertoe and mallet toe deformities. *Operative Tech Orthop* 1992; 2:1889.

Thompson FM, Deland JT: Flexor tendon transfer for metatarsophalangeal instability of the second toe. *Foot Ankle* 1993; 14:385.

Thompson FM, Hamilton WG: Problems of the second metatarsophalangeal joint. *Orthopedics* 1987; 10:83.

Chapter 123

TENDON DISORDERS

Donna J. Astion

ANATOMY OF TENDONS

Tendons are composed of mature fibroblasts embedded in an extracellular matrix of mucopolysacarides, mostly type I collagen and glycoproteins. The cells and collagen fibers are aligned in compact bundles surrounded by layers of collagen (endotenon) which are then covered by loose connective tissues (epitenon). The whole tendon is enclosed by an outer paratenon which is penetrated by a series of transverse vinculae (mesotenon) which bring blood vessels to the tendon. The mesotenon is a mesentery-like structure on the nonfriction side of the tendon. The blood supply to the tendon comes from the musculotendinous junction and the tendoosseous junction, as well as along its length by means of the paratenon, mesotenon, and tendon sheath.

PATHOLOGY

An inflammatory process around a tendon without a sheath is termed "peritendinitis." If the tendon has a sheath, then inflammation about the tendon is termed "tenosynovitis." Tendonosis is a degenerative lesion of the tendon. In the foot and ankle, partial or complete rupture of a tendon usually occurs in tendons with underlying tendonosis. Chronic tendon ruptures are usually an age-related phenomenon and generally occur in an area of high friction, where there is a change in the tendon direction, in an area of poor vascularity, or any site of injury or disease.

ACHILLES TENDON

The gastrocnemius and soleus tendons blend into one tendon before inserting into the posterior process of the calcaneus. The tendon is covered by a paratenon and its blood supply comes from the musculotendinous junction, the osseous insertion, and the mesotendon vessels. The blood supply of the tendon is poorest 2 to 6 cm proximal to its osseous insertion.

Patients usually present with a gradual onset of pain, swelling, and warmth about the Achilles tendon. These symptoms usually start after strenuous exercise. In cases of acute peritendinitis, crepitation may be felt with palpation of the Achilles tendon. Partial rupture can occur in cases of chronic peritendinitis with or without tendonosis and may present as an acute episode of pain and swelling. An MRI is helpful to differentiate between inflammation, tendonosis, or partial rupture of the Achilles tendon.

The initial management of these inflammatory processes is nonoperative and consists of rest, stretching exercises, nonsteroidal antiinflammatory medications (NSAIDs), and a heel lift. As the symptoms subside, the patient may gradually return to activities with some modifications. If these initial treatments are not successful, then a pe-

riod of immobilization may be necessary. Injections of steroids should be avoided since they have been associated with tendon rupture and subcutaneous atrophy. If symptoms persist, then surgery may be indicated to release the affected paratenon. If there is associated tendonosis or a partial rupture, then the diseased areas of the tendon should be debrided or the partial tendon rupture repaired. If a large portion of the tendon is debrided, then the defect should be augmented with either a flexor digitorum longus tendon transfer, a plantaris augmentation, or a turned-down flap of the gastrocnemius soleus aponeurosis.

A patient who has sustained an acute rupture of the Achilles tendon usually recalls a sharp tearing sensation and an immediate onset of pain and swelling behind the ankle. On physical exam there is a palpable defect in the Achilles tendon. The rupture usually occurs 2 to 6 cm proximal to the insertion of the tendon into the calcaneus. With the patient prone, when the superficial calf muscles are squeezed just distal to the area of its maximal girth, the foot does not plantarflex (a positive Thompson test). The patient usually will be able to actively plantarflex the ankle against resistance by recruitment of the other extrinsic plantar flexors. The reported rate of misdiagnosis of an acute Achilles tendon rupture is between 20 and 25 percent. If there is any doubt of the diagnosis from the history or physical examination, then an MRI may be useful for confirmation.

There is controversy concerning the treatment of acute Achilles tendon rupture. Nonoperative treatment consists of gravity equinus casting for eight to twelve weeks with cast changes at monthly intervals to gradually increase the amount of dorsiflexion at the ankle. After the cast is removed, a heel lift is used for an additional 4 to 8 weeks. Acute ruptures of the Achilles tendon can be treated satisfactorily nonoperatively when the diagnosis is made within 48 h of the injury. Surgical repair of the acutely ruptured Achilles tendon involves a direct end-to-end repair using one of a variety of described techniques.

The literature suggests a higher rerupture rate and decreased power of the Achilles tendon complex with nonoperative treatment as compared to surgical repair. Another advantage of operative treatment includes early physical therapy and weightbearing on the reapproximated tendon. However, surgical treatment carries with it the risks of anesthesia, as well as the possible complications of open surgery, including skin and tendon necrosis and deep infections. The choice of treatment depends on the physician and the patient. Young active individuals or high performance athletes will probably benefit the most from operative treatment.

Neglected or undiagnosed Achilles tendon ruptures present a difficult problem because of retraction of the proximal tendon and excessive scarring at the ruptured site. In these cases, end-anastomosis may not be possible and other methods need to be employed to span the gap between two tendon ends; these include flexor digitorum longus tendon transfer, turned down-strip of the tendon aponeuroses, fascia lata graft, or V–Y lengthening of the musculotendinous junction.

If the plantaris is present and intact, it can be incorporated in the repair. In older or ill patients with a chronic rupture of the Achilles tendon where surgery is not a viable option, a brace with a dorsiflexion stop and a shoe with a rocker bottom may be used.

FLEXOR HALLUCIS LONGUS TENDONS

Stenosing tenosynovitis of the flexor hallucis longus can occur at one of three anatomic sites: proximally at the start of the fibroosseous tunnel between the medial and lateral talar tubercles, within the flexor sheath behind the medial malleolus, or between the sesamoids of the hallux. This condition is associated with repetitive impact or activities requiring excessive plantar flexion. Patients with flexor hallucis longus tenosynovitis of the ankle present with pain, swelling, and crepitation posterior to the medial malleolus.

On physical examination there is demonstrable tenderness and occasionally triggering in the tendon sheath with active or passive motion of the great toe. Tenosynovitis of the flexor hallucis longus can usually be managed nonsurgically with nonsteroidal anti-inflammatory medication (NSAIDs), rest, stretching, and modification of activities. If these treatments are not successful, then a steroid injection into the tendon sheath can be helpful. If symptoms persist, then surgical release of the fibroosseous tunnel can be performed. If there is concomitant posterior impingement of the ankle from a large posterior lateral process of the talus or an os trigonum, then both conditions should be treated if surgery is necessary.

Most disruptions of the flexor hallucis longus tendon are lacerations. Such lacerations of this tendon are usually treated nonoperatively with minimal to no loss of function.

PERONEAL TENDONS

The peroneus longus and brevis tendons pass in a common synovial sheath that begins proximal to the lateral malleolus. The tendons are held in place by an overlying superior retinaculum and a fibrocartilagenous ridge in the posterior lateral aspect of the distal fibula. The peroneus longus makes three turns before inserting on the base of the first metatarsal. This first turn is at the tip of the lateral malleolus, second around the trochlear process of the calcaneus, and finally, the third, at the lateral aspect of the cuboid. The os peroneum is the fibrocartilaginous tissue, and sometimes bone, seen within the tendon as it turns at the lateral aspect of the cuboid. Nonspecific and posttraumatic peroneal tenosynovitis can occur in several places along the peroneal tendons. Usually, trauma is the major precipitating factor which causes tenosynovitis. The patient complains of pain and swelling in the area. When the foot is brought into plantar flexion and inversion, the symptoms are increased. The patient often walks with an antalgic gait.

Treatment is usually nonoperative and includes NSAIDs, immobilization, stretching, physical therapy, and possibly the addition of a lateral wedge to the shoe. If nonoperative treatments fail, then surgical exploration with tenolysis or debridement may be necessary.

Chronic longitudinal tears of the peroneus brevis are relatively common and usually occur over the distal tip of the fibula. Patients present with pain and swelling in the lateral retromalleolar area; the pain can be reproduced by passive inversion of the ankle or resisted eversion. Suspected peroneal pathology can be evaluated with MRI. Nonsurgical treatment includes NSAIDs, stretching, and a lateral heel wedge. If this is not helpful, then cast immobilization may be used. If symptoms persist, then surgical exploration of the tendon with tenolysis or debridement may be indicated. In addition, if there is

chronic lateral ankle instability, this can be surgically repaired at the same time as the peroneal tendon pathology is addressed.

Pain along the peroneus longus tendon as it turns beneath the cuboid is called painful os peroneum (POP) syndrome. Pain in this area of the tendon may be due to fracture of the os, a partial or complete rupture of the tendon, or degenerative arthritis between the os peroneum and the cuboid. On physical examination, patients are tender over the os peroneum and experience pain with passive hindfoot inversion or resisted plantar flexion of the first metatarsal. Most often, this condition can be successfully treated nonsurgically with a period of cast immobilization. If the symptoms persist, then surgical excision of the os and debridement of the tendon may be indicated.

Traumatic dislocation of the peroneal tendons is usually associated with activities such as skiing, soccer, skating, and rollerblading. Acute peroneal dislocations are frequently unrecognized and may be misdiagnosed as a lateral ankle sprain. If not treated acutely, they may result in chronically dislocating peroneal tendons. On physical examination, the pain and swelling are over the lateral malleolus at the level of the superior retinaculum. Radiographs of the ankle may show a small avulsion fracture from the lateral aspect of the lateral malleolus. The incidence of this type of fracture in peroneal tendon dislocations is 10 to 50 percent.

The treatment of acute dislocations is controversial. Nonoperative treatment includes nonweightbearing in a short leg cast positioned in slight plantar flexion for 6 weeks. In general, stable injuries can be treated nonoperatively and unstable peroneal dislocations should be treated surgically. Young active patients may also benefit from early surgical repair. The repair involves reattaching the retinaculum to the periosteum of the lateral margin of the distal fibula and inspection of the peroneal tendons. Occasionally, a longitudinal split of the peroneus brevis tendon may be seen. In these cases the tendon should be repaired or debrided as necessary.

Patients who present with recurrent subluxation or dislocation complain of painful snapping over the lateral malleolus. Their symptoms can be reproduced by resisted eversion with the foot in dorsiflexion or by asking them to circumduct their foot and ankle. Many procedures have been described for the repair of chronic dislocations of the peroneal tendons and include using a slip from the Achilles tendon to reconstruct the superior retinaculum, sliding bone blocks from the distal fibula, groove deepening procedures in the posterior distal aspect of the lateral malleolus, and rerouting the tendons under the calcaneal fibular ligament.

EXTENSOR TENDONS

The extensor tendons of the foot are subject to less wear and tear than the flexor tendons because they primarily function during the unloaded phases of gait and they do not course around anatomic pulleys. Tenosynovitis of the tibialis anterior and the extensor digitorum longus tendons is the most common. The tenosynovitis is usually secondary to irritation from shoes and shoe modifications usually resolve the problem. Degenerative rupture at the anterior tibial tendon as well as the extensor hallucis longus tendon has been reported. Weakness from a ruptured tendon must be differentiated from a neurologic lesion. Treatment for a ruptured anterior tibial tendon depends on the age and activity of the patient. The tendon should be surgically repaired in a young active patient who presents within 3 to 4 months of the injury. Older patients can be treated nonoperatively with or without a brace.

Rupture of the extensor hallucis longus tendon is usually caused by lacerations, and most authors advocate primary repair of the laceration.

POSTERIOR TIBIAL TENDONS

The posterior tibial tendon has multiple tendinous insertions in the hindfoot, midfoot, and forefoot; the largest insertion is into the navicular tuberosity. The principal function of the posterior tibial muscle is to invert the subtalar joint during the heel rise portion of gait. This helps lock the transverse tarsal joint and allow the gastrocnemius soleus to act on a rigid foot. The posterior tibial tendon lies in a shallow groove in the posterior tibia and is held in place by the retinaculum. Just below the medial malleolus, the tendon suddenly changes direction and becomes more parallel to the plantar surface of the foot.

There are several anatomic factors that predispose the tendon to inflammation or degeneration. During gait, the tendon is exposed to repetitive motion and compressive forces in the region behind the medial malleolus. The tendon lacks mesotendon behind the medial malleolus and there is a hypovascular zone approximately 1 to 1.5 cm distal to the medial malleolus. Systemic conditions such as hypertension, obesity, diabetes, previous medial foot surgery, trauma, and steroid exposure are often seen in patients with posterior tibial tendon dysfunction.

Posterior tibial tendon dysfunction can be divided into three clinical stages. Stage I involves pain and swelling along the posterior tibial tendon with mild weakness of the muscle without secondary deformity of the foot. Stage II posterior tibial tendon dysfunction refers to elongation of the posterior tibial tendon (tendon insufficiency) or disruption of the tendon with flexible flat foot deformity. In these cases, if the tendon is intact, it is not functional. In stage III posterior tibial tendon dysfunction, patients present with a rigid flat foot deformity.

Tenosynovitis, or stage I disease, may be secondary to overuse and repetitive stress. Occasionally it is associated with an ankle sprain.

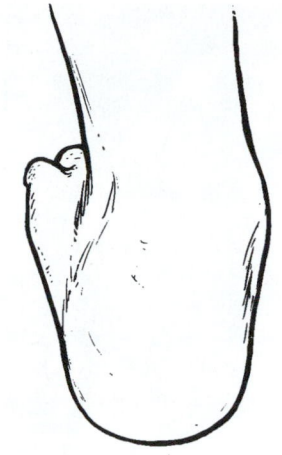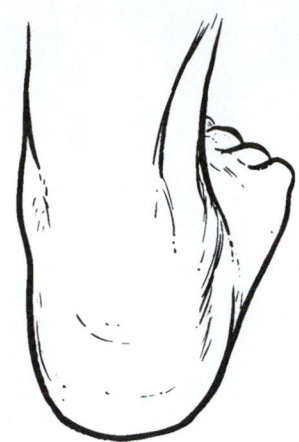

Figure 123-1
"Too many toes" sign.

In chronic dysfunction (stage II and stage III) the posterior tibial tendon symptoms may be present for several months or years before presentation, in which case the symptoms will not correlate with the degree of deformity. Patients often present with complaints of pain and swelling in the medial ankle with or without lateral pain (due to impingement). Complaints of difficulty walking, especially on uneven surfaces, are common. In addition, many patients note a progressive flat foot deformity.

On physical examination the patient will have a unilateral flat foot deformity and when viewed from behind they will have increased forefoot abduction (too many toes) and increased heel valgus (Fig. 123–1). The patient may be unable to perform a single leg heel raise on the affected side or they will have pain on attempting this maneuver. When the patient attempts a heel raise, the hindfoot stays in valgus; with a normal posterior tibial tendon, the heel moves into varus.

Weightbearing radiographs of the foot are helpful in assessing the flat foot deformity and evaluating for arthritic changes. The anterior posterior weightbearing view of the foot will often demonstrate lateral subluxation of the talonavicular joint, while the lateral weightbearing view demonstrates sagging at the talonavicular or navicular medial cuneiform joint with flattening of the longitudinal arch (Fig.

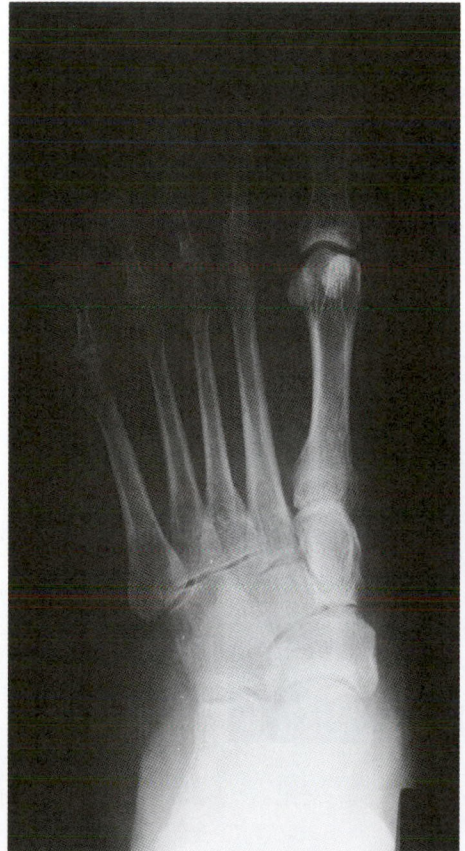

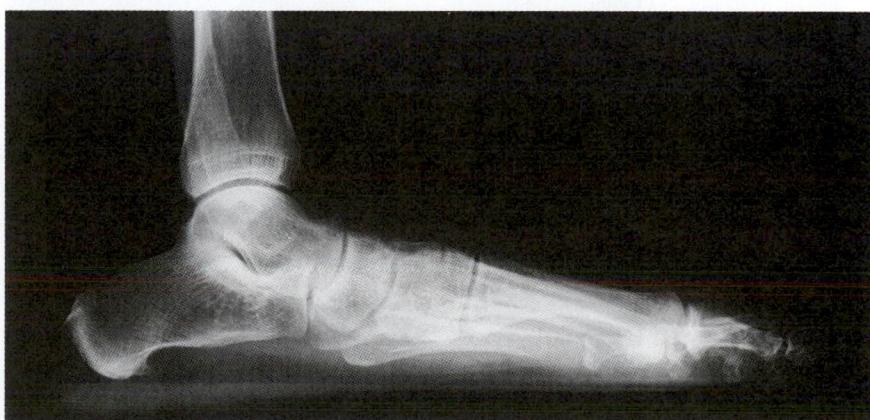

Figure 123-2
AP and lateral weightbearing radiographs of a patient with posterior tibial tendon insufficiency. Subluxation of the talonavicular joint is seen on the AP radiograph and sagging of the talonavicular joint is seen on the lateral radiograph.

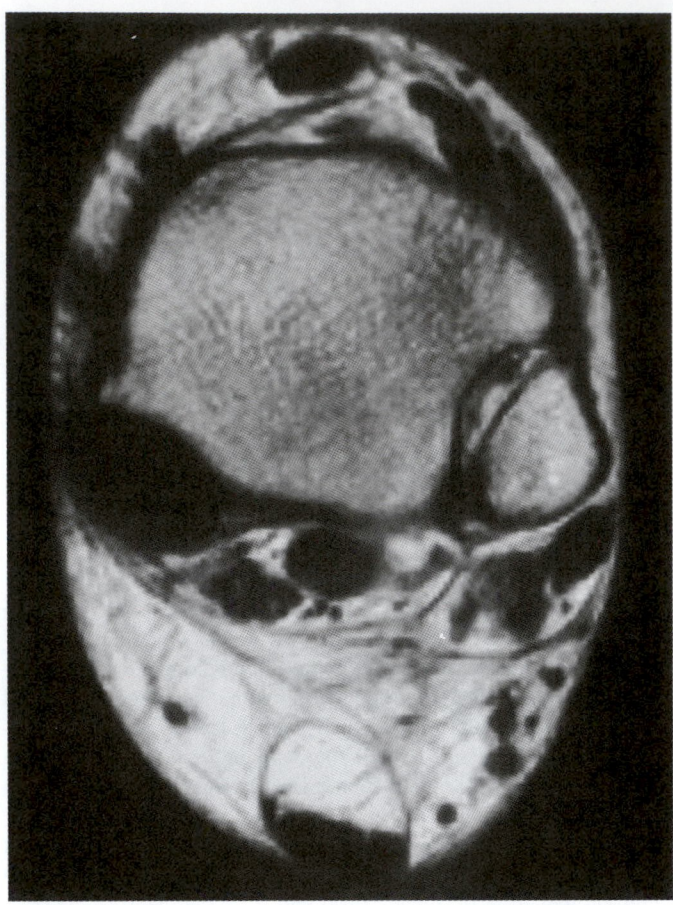

Figure 123-3
MRI demonstrating thickening and intertendinous changes in the posterior tibial tendon.

123–2). MRI is currently used to evaluate intertendinous changes such as longitudinal splits, enlargement of the posterior tibial tendon, and inflammation around the tendon (Fig. 123–3).

Tendinitis or mild tendon insufficiency (stage I disease) can be treated with NSAIDs, casting, a medial heel wedge, a University of California Biomechanics Lab (UCBL) heel cup, or an ankle-foot orthosis (AFO). If pain persists, then surgical exploration and a synovectomy may be indicated. If a longitudinal split is seen in the tendon, it should be repaired. Stage II posterior tibial tendon dysfunction (a flexible flat foot deformity with an insufficient or ruptured tendon) can be treated initially with immobilization using an AFO. If this is not helpful in relieving the patient's symptoms, surgery is recommended. Surgical treatment includes debridement of the tendon and flexor digitorum longus tendon transfer to the navicula through the posterior tibial tendon sheath. Long-term follow-up of patients with flexor digitorum longus tendon transfers shows that the results deteriorate with time and patients may eventually require an arthrodesis to stabilize the hindfoot. There are several techniques used to augment the transfer with the hope of improving the long-term results. These procedures include a lateral column lengthening with a bone block fusion through the calcaneal-cuboid joint, medial sliding calcaneal osteotomy (Fig. 123–4), and reconstruction of the spring ligament. If necessary, the Achilles tendon should be lengthened. Patients with stage III posterior tibial tendon dysfunction can be treated nonoperatively with an AFO. If this is not successful, then the patient generally requires a hindfoot arthrodesis. Posterior tibial tendon dysfunction has been treated successfully with subtalar fusion, talonavicular fusion, and triple arthrodeses.

SUGGESTED READINGS

Gabel S, Manoli A 2d: Neglected rupture of the Achilles tendon. *Foot Ankle Int* 1994; 15:512.

Hamilton WG: Stenosing tenosynovitis of the flexor hallucis longus tendon and posterior impingement upon the os trigonum in ballet dancers. *Foot Ankle* 1982; 3:74.

Johnson KA: Tibialis posterior tendon rupture. *Clin Orthop* 1983; 177:140.

Kaye RA, Jahss MH: Tibialis posterior: A review of anatomy and biomechanics in relation to support of the medial longitudinal arch. *Foot Ankle* 1991; 11:244.

Ma GWC, Griffith TG. Percutaneous repair of acute closed ruptured achilles tendon: A new technique. *Clin Orthop* 1977; 128:247.

Mann RA, Holmes GB Jr: Seale KS, et al: Chronic rupture of the Achilles tendon: A new technique of repair. *J Bone Joint Surg [Am]* 1991; 73:214.

Mann RA, Thompson FM: Rupture of the posterior tibial tendon causing flat foot. *J Bone Joint Surg [Am]* 1985; 67:556.

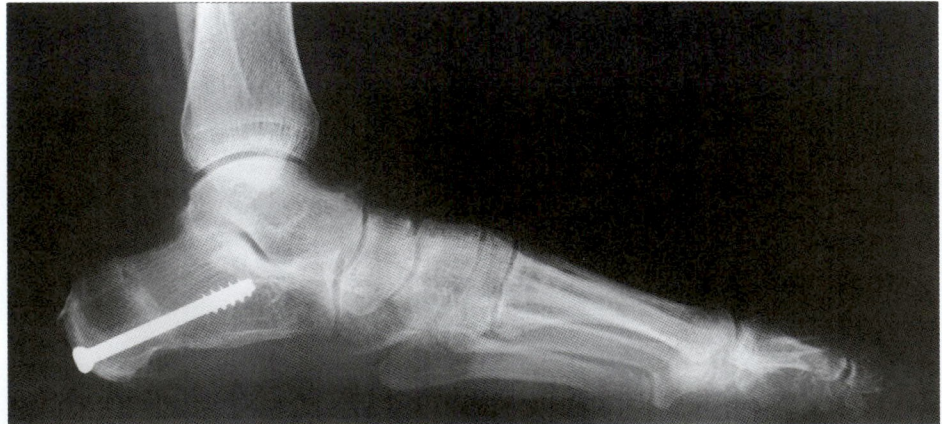

Figure 123-4
Lateral radiograph of a patient who underwent a medial sliding calcaneal osteotomy with an FDL tendon transfer for posterior tibial tendon insufficiency. Note the more normal arch to the foot.

Myerson MS, Corrigan J, Thompson F, et al: Tendon transfer combined with calcaneal osteotomy for treatment of posterior tibial tendon insufficiency: A radiological investigation. *Foot Ankle Int* 1995; 16:712.

Puddu G, Ippolito E, Postacchini F: A classification of Achilles tendon disease. *Am J Sports Med* 1976; 4:145.

Thompson FM, Patterson AH. Rupture of the peroneus longus tendon: Report of three cases. *J Bone Joint Surg [Am]* 1989; 71:293.

Troop RL, Losse GM, Lane JG, et al: Early motion after repair of Achilles tendon ruptures. *Foot Ankle Int* 1995; 16:705.

Wapner KL, Pavlock GS, Hecht P, et al: Repair of chronic achilles tendon rupture with flexor hallucis longus tendon transfer. *Foot Ankle* 1993; 14:443.

Zoellner G, Clancy W Jr: Recurrent dislocation of the peroneal tendon. *J Bone Joint Surg [Am]* 1979; 61:292.

Chapter 124

ARTHRITIS

Donna J. Astion

Arthritides of the ankle or foot can be very disabling due to the pain and deformity which accompany these conditions. There are many types of arthritis which affect the ankle and foot including crystal-induced arthritis, sero-negative arthritis, spondyloarthropathies, osteoarthritis, and posttraumatic arthritis.

ARTHRITIC CONDITIONS

GOUT AND PSEUDOGOUT

Gout and pseudogout are the two crystal-induced arthritides which affect the foot and ankle. Painful gouty arthritis results from the precipitation of sodium urate crystals in synovial fluid. These crystals, which are needle-shaped and negatively birefringent when viewed with a polarized microscope, cause an acute inflammatory reaction when they precipitate in the synovial fluid. The involved joint becomes swollen and painful, and often the overlying skin becomes hypersensitive.

Gout occurs more frequently in men than in women. Approximately 50 to 75 percent of the initial gouty attacks involve the great toe. In the foot, gout can also affect the plantar fascia, the tendons, and occasionally other joints of the foot and ankle. It is not uncommon to observe acute gouty attacks after the stress of a surgical procedure; therefore, the patient who complains of foot pain postoperatively should be evaluated for gout.

Diagnosis of gout can be inferred by the patient's history and clinical examination. The diagnosis can be confirmed by the presence of sodium urate crystals in aspirated joint fluid. Serum levels of uric acid may be normal or elevated in patients with an acute attack of gout. Radiographically, the involved joint may show no changes or may show severe destruction of the involved joint. Characteristically, radiographs also demonstrate periarticular erosion proximal to the involved joint with sparing of the articular cartilage (Fig. 124–1). Often, there are destructive bone lesions remote from the articular surface. Calcification of tophaceous deposits in the area of the joint may also be seen.

Once the diagnosis is established, the medical treatment can be assumed by the patient's internist or rheumatologist. Initial attacks can be treated with indomethacin. If the involved joint is destroyed, then surgical fusion is a treatment option.

Pseudogout results from calcium pyrophosphate dihydrate crystal precipitation in the joint fluid. These crystals are positively birefringent under polarized microscope and have a variable shape. The symptoms of pseudogout are very similar to those of gout. The attacks of pseudogout should be treated with rest, elevation, and nonsteroidal anti-inflammatory medications (NSAIDs). Once the involved joint is destroyed, fusion may be required.

SERONEGATIVE SPONDYLOARTHROPATHIES

The seronegative spondyloarthropathies which affect the ankle and foot include ankylosing spondylitis, psoriatic arthritis, and Reiter's syndrome. Ankylosing spondylitis can manifest as an enthesopathy. In addition, bony ankylosis or capsular ossifications of the metatarsophalangeal (MTP) joints may occur.

With psoriatic arthritis, there is often symmetric involvement of the distal interphalangeal (DIP) joints of the hands and feet in conjunction with psoriatic changes of the adjacent nails. Patients may also develop heel pain syndrome, which is refractory to the usual conservative treatment measures. Radiographically, resorption of the distal tuft is seen with soft tissue atrophy. As the bone atrophies at the joint, "cup and saucer" appearance develops.

Approximately half the patients with Reiter's syndrome have ankle involvement and half of these cases are bilateral. Ankle involvement is characterized by a painful, nonerythematous effusion. Radiographically, erosions of the talus can be seen which may be confused with osteochondritis dessicans of the talus. Patients may also present with heel pain or pain in the small toe joints. Persistent heel pain from Reiter's syndrome may have a characteristic radiographic appearance of fluffy calcification at the insertion of the plantar fascia, with small erosions around the spur. Radiographs of involved interphalangeal and MTP joints may show intraarticular and extraarticular erosions.

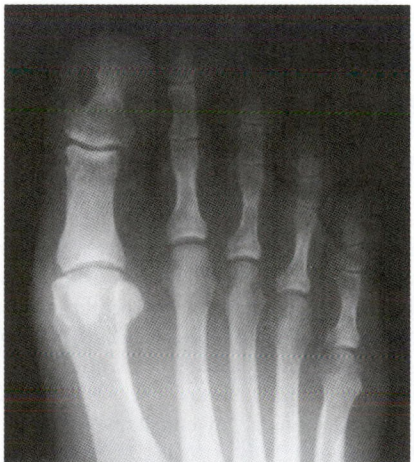

Figure 124–1

AP radiograph of patient with a history of gouty arthritis of the first metatarsophalangeal joint. Note the periarticular erosions proximal to the joint and the normal-appearing articular surfaces.

Lyme disesase may also cause foot and ankle arthritides. A high index of suspicion is necessary when evaluating patients from endemic areas. In patients with positive Lyme titers, treatment with the appropriate antibiotics results in resolution of their symptoms.

DEGENERATIVE ARTHRITIS

Degenerative joint disease of the ankle and foot usually occurs in middle age and elderly persons but can occur in younger individuals as the end stage of a posttraumatic condition. While it can occur in any joint of the ankle and foot, the most common sites are the first MTP joint and the first metatarsal cuneiform joint. Structural changes occur in the involved joint which, over time, result in loss of function and destruction of the articular cartilage. In general, the symptoms of degenerative joint disease are worse in the morning and may be aggravated by increased activity, such as prolonged walking and standing. On physical examination, the affected joint is tender, swollen, and warmer than nonaffected joints. Motion at the joint is often painful, limited, and may be associated with crepitation. Radiographically, the joint space may be decreased and subchondral cysts may be present. The margins of the affected joint may be sclerotic and osteophytes may be seen peripherally.

Initial treatment of degenerative arthritis in the ankle or foot includes nonsteroidal anti-inflammatory medication and stress reduction of the involved joint. Shoe modifications may be necessary to relieve friction over bony prominences and decrease stress on a particular joint. A rocker bottom sole can decrease the stress at the ankle, the midtarsal joints, or distal joints of the foot. Orthoses may be needed to decrease stress and support painful areas. If the ankle is affected, a molded leather ankle brace or ankle-foot orthosis (AFO) may be helpful. Weight loss and activity modification should also be recommended. If these nonsurgical measures fail, then surgery may be indicated. Surgical options for each joint are discussed later in the chapter.

RHEUMATOID ARTHRITIS

Rheumatoid arthritis begins in the feet in approximately 17 percent of the reported cases and it is generally believed that the forefoot is more commonly involved than the hindfoot. The pathologic changes in the foot occur from persistent synovitis which invades and destroys the bone and the joint cartilage. The synovitis distends the joint capsule and weakens the ligamentous structure around the joint. As the supporting structures become progressively weakened, mechanical pressures act to disrupt the anatomy and produce deformity. Large synovial cysts or rheumatoid nodules may form in various areas of the forefoot. When in weightbearing areas, they can be very painful and may create difficulties with shoe wear.

In rheumatoid arthritis, the ankle is the least often involved major weightbearing joint. Other conditions such as tenosynovitis, talonavicular arthritis, or subtalar arthritis may be mistaken for ankle problems. When the ankle joint is affected, however, the subtalar and midtarsal joint are often involved as well. As a rule, rheumatoid arthritis does not produce any significant deformity of the ankle joint. In the early stages of ankle joint involvement, radiographs usually show minimal erosive changes. In later stages, soft tissue deformity occurs without significant erosive changes at the joint. Ultimately, in the more advanced stages, there is significant articular destruction and reconstructive procedures such as arthrodeses are usually required.

Treatment of rheumatoid arthritis is directed towards relief of pain, prevention of deformity, correction of deformity, preservation of function, and restoration of function. The surgical management of rheumatoid arthritis includes early intervention during the proliferative phase

of synovial tissue. Synovectomy at this time may prevent destruction of the supporting tissues and the articular cartilage. However, once deformity or articular destruction has occurred, synovectomy is no longer indicated.

When the hindfoot is involved, the medial longitudinal arch often collapses and the heel goes into valgus. Conservative treatment with a University of California Biomechanics Laboratory (UCBL) insert or an AFO is occasionally useful; however, surgical intervention is often necessary. If there is isolated talonavicular joint involvement, then an isolated talonavicular fusion may be performed. If there is isolated subtalar involvement, then an isolated subtalar arthrodesis may be performed. However, if any two hind-foot joints are involved, then a triple arthrodesis is indicated. Arthrodesis of the hind foot is very effective in restoring the plantargrade position of the foot, restoring function, and relieving pain. Degenerative changes can be seen in the ankle when increased stress is placed on the joint due to a rigid hindfoot deformity or after a hindfoot fusion. Patients with ankle involvement can often be treated successfully with a rocker bottom shoe and an ankle foot orthosis, as long as there is no significant varus or valgus deformity present.

Deformities of the tarsometatarsal joints are uncommon in rheumatoid arthritis. Occasionally, there is instability of the first metatarsal cuneiform joint, which may cause a hallux valgus deformity. In these cases, if the patient is symptomatic despite shoe modifications, a first metatarsal-cuneiform arthrodesis is indicated.

In the forefoot, the typical deformities include a hallux valgus with subluxation or dislocation of the lesser toe MTP joints and hammering of the toes. Persistent synovitis of the MTP joints causes distension of the joint capsule and weakening of the ligaments. The constant dorsiflexion force during walking causes a progressive subluxation and eventual dislocation of the MTP joints. As the deformity progresses, the metatarsal heads are pushed more plantarly, the plantar fat pad migrates distally, and callus forms beneath the metatarsal heads. The resultant intrinsic and extrinsic muscle imbalance leads to progressive hammer-toe deformities. With these toe deformities, the forefoot is painful with weightbearing and fitting shoes becomes difficult.

Conservative treatment begins with shoewear modifications. Patients require shoes with a high, wide toebox which will accommodate the hammer toe and hallux valgus deformities. In addition, to relieve pressure on the metatarsal heads, a metatarsal pad with a cushioned insole is useful. If conservative treatment fails, surgical treatment is directed at reestablishing the alignment of the lesser toe MTP joints, restoration of padding in the forefoot, and correcting the deformity at the interphalangeal joints. While resection arthroplasty of the first MTP joint or silicon implant arthroplasty of the first MTP joint have been recommended in the past, the long-term results of these surgical corrections have been poor. At the present time, the preferred method of forefoot reconstruction includes arthrodesis of the first MTP joint, and, if the lesser toes are affected, metatarsal head resection of the lesser toes with correction of the hammer-toe deformity (Fig. 124–2). Results after first MTP joint, fusion with resection of the lesser metatarsal heads, and correction of the hammer toes has been very good. If the first MTP joint is spared while the lesser toes are afflicted, then metatarsal head resection of the lesser toes can be performed alone. However, in these patients, the hallux should be observed over time for the formation of the hallux valgus deformity.

ANKLE ARTHRITIS

Painful and disabling arthrosis of the ankle may be related to rheumatoid arthritis, degenerative joint disease, traumatic arthritis, chronic instability, osteochondral lesions, synovial osteochondromatosis, avas-

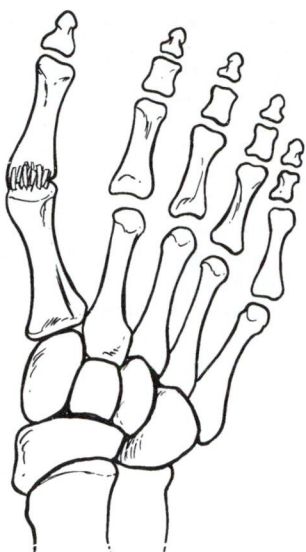

Figure 124-2
Fusion of the first MTP joint and resection of the lesser toe metatarsal heads and correction of hammer-toe deformities to correct a rheumatoid forefoot deformity. [Reproduced with permission from Sculco TP, Geppert MJ, Sobel M: The forefoot. In Sculco TP (ed): *Surgical Treatment of Rheumatoid Arthrities*. St. Louis: Mosby-Year Book; 1992:336.]

cular necrosis of the talus, tumor, hemophilia, infection, or neuropathy. The underlying disease process can often be determined from the patient's history. While obtaining the history, it is important to determine the patient's response to previous treatments for the ankle pain. During the physical examination, it is also important to examine the joints proximal and distal to the ankle. If it is difficult to localize the symptomatic area during the physical examination, diagnostic selective injections with Lidocaine can be useful in localizing the painful area.

To determine the condition of the ankle joint, weightbearing radiographic views of the ankle should be obtained. If the area causing the pain cannot be accurately localized by physical examination or plain radiographs, a bone scan is often helpful in defining the area of pathology. Nuclear medicine studies are also helpful in evaluating the likelihood of infection, stress fractures, avascular necrosis, and tumors.

The nonsurgical management of ankle arthritis includes NSAIDs, judicious use of intraarticular corticosteroid injections, bracing, and shoe modifications. The bracing options include a double upright ankle brace, a laced ankle support, or an AFO. Shoe modifications can include a rocker bottom sole and a solid ankle cushion heel.

If the patient presents with restricted ankle dorsiflexion, tenderness at the anterior joint line, and pain with passive dorsiflexion of the ankle, the arthrosis may be limited to the anterior portion of the ankle joint. In these cases, radiographically, the joint space is maintained and anterior osteophytes on the distal tibia and on the talar neck are seen in the lateral projection. If these patients fail nonsurgical treatment, then symptomatic pain relief and improved range of motion can be obtained by removing these osteophytes.

In patients with advanced arthrosis who have failed nonsurgical treatment, an ankle arthrodesis can be considered. There are many different ways to perform an ankle arthrodesis. Fixation for an ankle arthrodesis can be obtained with internal compression screws, plates and screws, staples, and external fixation devices. To achieve an arthrodesis in cases without a varus or valgus deformity, several au-

thors advocate arthroscopic debridement of the joint and percutaneous screw fixation of the bony surfaces. Regardless of the surgical approach or the type of fixation used, the alignment of the arthrodesis is critical. The preferred alignment for an ankle fusion is 0 degrees of dorsiflexion (neutral) with approximately 5 degrees of valgus and 5 to 10 degrees of external rotation and mild posterior translation of the talus with respect to the tibia. The posterior translation helps to decrease the anterior lever arm of the foot which, in turn, reduces the loading of the midfoot joints during ambulation.

Ankle arthrodesis in patients with insulin-dependent diabetes should be approached cautiously because the complication rate in this patient population is high. Arthrodesis of the ankle in patients who smoke is associated with a higher risk of nonunion and some authors advocate postponing the arthrodesis until the patient has discontinued smoking. Complications following ankle fusion include nonunion, malunion, infection, subtalar arthritis, and neurovascular injury. Nonunion can be successfully salvaged by a revision arthrodesis with bone graft. If the ankle is fused in excessive equinus, the patient may develop problems with ambulation because of difficulty clearing the foot from the floor, a "back knee" gait, and metatarsalgia. A varus malalignment of the arthrodesis can cause painful callus formation in the fifth metatarsal head area while an excessive valgus alignment can cause callus formation on the first metatarsal head area. Excessive varus or valgus of the ankle may lead to subtalar arthrosis.

HINDFOOT ARTHRITIS

Isolated subtalar joint arthritis is common in rheumatoid arthritis and after fractures of the calcaneus or talus. Patients complain of lateral ankle and hindfoot pain, as well as pain with walking and difficulty ambulating on uneven surfaces. On physical examination, there is often tenderness in the area of the sinus tarsus and painful restriction of hindfoot motion. The nonsurgical treatment of isolated subtalar arthritis includes NSAIDs, orthotic devices designed to restrict hindfoot motion, an AFO, and the judicious use of corticosteroid injections. If nonsurgical treatment fails, then the surgical treatment is a subtalar arthrodesis. If there is an associated malalignment from the arthritis, the malalignment can be addressed at the time of the arthrodesis.

Isolated talonavicular arthrodesis is indicated with isolated talonavicular joint arthritis. Patients will often complain of pain with weightbearing and difficulty walking on uneven surfaces. On physical examination, they have painful restriction of hindfoot motion and tenderness in the area of the talonavicular joint. The nonoperative treatment includes the use of NSAIDs and the judicious use of corticosteroid injections into the joint. An AFO may be helpful in restricting hindfoot motion. If nonoperative treatment fails, then surgical treatment would consist of fusion of the talonavicular joint. Many authors advocate isolated talonavicular arthrodesis which has shown favorable long-term results while other authors favor a triple arthrodesis (fusion of the talonavicular, subtalar, and calcaneocuboid joints) because fusion of the talonavicular joints will eliminate motion of the subtalar and calcaneocuboid joints.

Isolated arthritis of the calcaneocuboid joint is very rare, but this joint may be affected by posttraumatic arthritis or rheumatoid arthritis. If an isolated calcaneocuboid joint fusion is performed, most of the motion in the subtalar and talonavicular joints is retained.

Triple arthrodesis is indicated when there is arthritic involvement of at least two of the joints and may also be indicated in patients with hindfoot deformities due to neuromuscular disease. The goal of the triple arthrodesis is to relieve pain, improve function, and provide the patient with a well-aligned plantargrade foot. Complications of a triple arthrodesis include: nonunion (most commonly of the talonavicular joint), acceleration of degenerative changes of the ankle and the tarsometatarsal joints, ankle instability, and—very rarely—osteonecrosis of the talus.

Tibiotalocalcaneal arthrodeses is indicated in patients with arthrosis of the ankle and subtalar joints that is unresponsive to bracing, injections, and NSAIDs. Tibiocalcaneal arthrodeses is indicated when the talar body is deficient, infected, or necrotic. Pantalar arthrodeses is indicated for pantalar arthrosis.

MIDFOOT ARTHRITIS

Arthritic changes in the midfoot may be severe or subtle. Arthritis of the midfoot can involve any joint in isolation or in combination. Patients usually complain of pain in the midfoot or arch area and difficulty with ambulation. Some patients present with problems related to shoe pressure on osteophytes which form at the arthritic joints. The physical examination is often helpful in determining which joints of the midfoot are involved. Weightbearing radiographs of the foot are necessary to assess the alignment of the foot and to identify arthritic changes of particular joints. Narrowing of the joint spaces may be apparent on the AP radiograph, while the weightbearing lateral radiograph may demonstrate dorsal osteophytes and plantar spurring. In more severe cases, plantar gaping of the tarsometatarsal joint may be seen on the lateral radiograph. Lateral, AP, and oblique radiographs of the foot should also be used to assess the bony alignment in the midfoot. Nonsurgical treatment of midfoot arthritis includes NSAIDs and an orthotic device which supports the transverse and medial arch of the foot. Shoe modifications, including pressure relief from dorsal osteophytes, may also be helpful. If these nonoperative measures fail, then arthrodeses of the involved joints is indicated.

SUGGESTED READINGS

Cierny G, Cook W, Mader J: Ankle arthrodesis in the presence of ongoing sepsis: Indications, methods and results. *Orthop Clin North Am* 1989; 20;709.

Fogel GR, Katoh Y, Rand JA, et al: Talonavicular arthrodesis for isolated arthrosis: 9.5-year results and gait analysis. *Foot Ankle* 1982; 3:105.

Graves SC, Mann RA, Graves KO: Triple arthrodesis in older adults: Results after long-term follow-up. *J Bone Joint Surg [Am]* 1993; 75:355.

Guerra J, Resnick D. Arthritides affecting the foot: Radiographic-pathological correlation. *Foot Ankle* 1982; 2:325.

Holt ES, Hansen ST, Mayo KA, et al: Ankle arthrodesis using internal screw fixation. *Clin Orthop* 1991; 268:21.

Kirkpatrick JS, Goldner JL, Goldner RD: Revision arthrodesis for tibiotalar pseudarthrosis with fibular onlay-inlay graft and internal screw fixation. *Clin Orthop* 1991; 268:29.

Kitaoka HB, Anderson PJ, Morrey BF: Revision of ankle arthrodesis with external fixation for non-union. *J Bone Joint Surg [Am]* 1992; 74:1191.

Kitaoka HB, Romness DW: Arthrodesis for failed ankle arthroplasty. *J Arthroplasty* 1992; 7:277.

Mann RA, Baumgarten M: Subtalar fusion for isolated subtalar disorders. Preliminary report. *Clin Orthop* 1988; 226:260.

Mann RA, Van Manen JW, Wapner K, et al: Ankle fusion. *Clin Orthop* 1991; 268:49.

Marcus RE, Balourdas GM, Heiple KG: Ankle arthrodesis by Chevron fusion with internal fixation and bone-grafting. *J Bone Joint Surg [Am]* 1983; 65:833.

Mazur JM, Schwartz E, Simon SR: Ankle arthrodesis. Long-term follow-up with gait analysis. *J Bone Joint Surg [Am]* 1979; 61:964.

Mears DC, Gordon RG, Kann SE, et al: Ankle arthrodesis with an anterior tension plate. *Clin Orthop* 1991; 268:70.

Moeckel BH, Patterson BM, Inglis AE, et al: Ankle arthrodesis. A comparison of internal and external fixation. *Clin Orthop* 1991; 268:78.

Moran CG, Pinder IM, Smith SR: Ankle arthrodesis in rheumatoid arthritis. 30 cases followed for five years. *Acta Orthop Scand* 1991; 62:538.

Myerson MS, Quill G. Ankle arthrodesis. A comparison of an arthroscopic and an open method of treatment. *Clin Orthop* 1991; 268:84.

Papa JA, Myerson MS: Pantalar and tibiotalocalcaneal arthrodesis for post-traumatic osteoarthritis of the ankle and hindfoot. *J Bone Joint Surg [Am]* 1992; 74:1042.

Russotti GM, Johnson KA, Cass JR: Tibiotalocalcaneal arthrodesis for arthritis and deformity of the hind part of the foot. *J Bone Joint Surg [Am]* 1988; 70:1304.

Sangeorzan BJ, Veith RG, Hansen ST Jr: Salvage of Lisfranc's tarsometatarsal joint by arthrodesis. *Foot Ankle* 1990; 10:193.

Trevino SG, Licht N: Degenerative problems of the midtarsal joints. In Gould J (ed): *Operative Foot Surgery*. Philadelphia: WB Saunders; 1994:163.

Unger AS, Inglis AE, Mow CS, et al: Total ankle arthroplasty in rheumatoid arthritis: A long-term follow-up study. *Foot Ankle* 1988; 8:173.

Chapter 125

HEEL PAIN

Donna J. Astion

The term "heel pain" can sometimes be confusing because it may refer to one or both of two distinct anatomic areas. "Heel pain" can be plantar medial heel pain or posterior superior heel pain. The etiology of the pain in each area is different. It is important to realize that both of these conditions can present independently or coexist.

PLANTAR HEEL PAIN (HEEL PAIN SYNDROME, PLANTAR FASCIITIS)

ANATOMY

The posterior plantar aspect of the calcaneus is the main weight-bearing area of the heel. The plantar aponeurosis arises from the medial tuberosity of the calcaneus and inserts into the toes. Hyperextension of the toes and the metatarsophalangeal (MTP) joints makes the plantar fascia taut. The tightened plantar fascia raises the longitudinal arch of the foot, inverts the hind foot, and externally rotates the leg. This passive mechanism has been termed the "windlass mechanism."

Just under the plantar fascia lies the flexor digitorum brevis, which inserts onto the medial tuberosity of the calcaneus. In some patients, the insertion of the flexor digitorum brevis is calcified and forms a "heel spur" that can be seen on the lateral radiograph (Fig. 125–1). The skin over the weightbearing portion of the calcaneus is thickly keratinized and covers a large, intricate fat pad. This fatty tissue is compartmentalized by multiple fibrous septa which attach to both the skin plantarly and the bone superiorly. The arrangement of the septa within the heel fat pad helps it absorb compression and torsion forces.

The posterior tibial nerve is located on the medial side of the ankle behind the medial malleolus. Its two major branches are the medial and lateral plantar nerves. At the level of the medial malleolus or distal to it, the medial calcaneal nerve arises from the posterior tibial nerve and passes superficial to the flexor retinaculum to innervate the skin of the heel. This nerve then travels into the subcutaneous tissue between the plantar fascia and the skin. The nerve to the abductor digiti quinti is a branch of the lateral plantar nerve; it passes deep to the plantar fascia and to the flexor digitorum brevis insertion (Fig. 125–2).

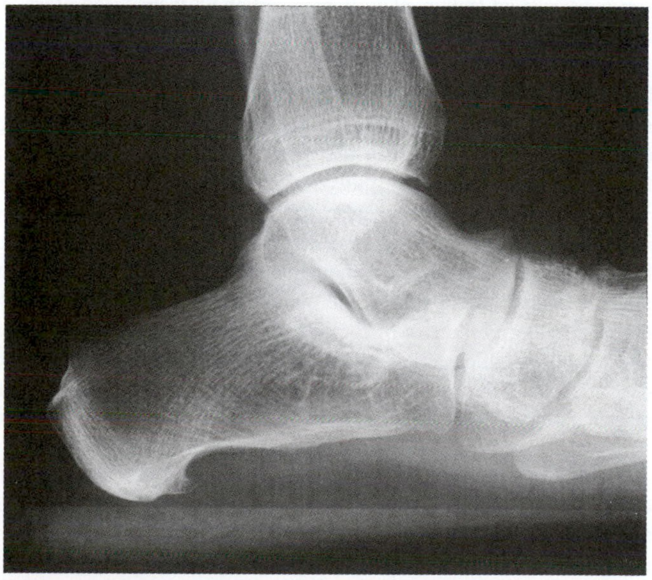

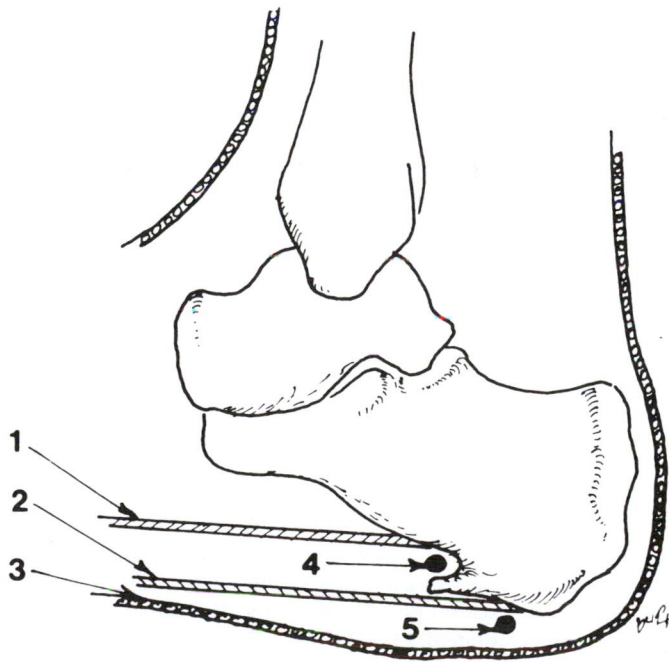

Figure 125-2
Lateral drawing of the hindfoot demonstrating the relationship of the plantar structures and nerves. (1) Long plantar ligament, (2) plantar fascia, (3) skin, (4) nerve to the abductor digiti quinti, and (5) medial calcaneal nerve. [Reproduced with permission from Bordelon RL: Heel pain. In Mann RA, Coughlin MJ (eds): *Surgery of the Foot and Ankle.* St. Louis, MO: Mosby-Year Book; 1993:840.

Figure 125-1
Lateral radiograph demonstrating the calcification of the flexor digitorum brevis insertion into the calcaneus (i.e., "the heel spur").

PATHOPHYSIOLOGY

There are many theories regarding the etiology of subcalcaneal pain. The pain has been attributed to microtrauma from the repetitive pull of the plantar fascia at its insertion into the calcaneus. The pain may be from a periostitis of the calcaneus or chronic inflammation near the insertion of the plantar fascia. Heel pain has also been attributed to entrapment of the nerve to the abductor digiti minimi between the abductor hallucis and the medial margin of the medial head of the quadratus plantae, or to irritation of the medial calcaneal branch of the posterior tibial nerve.

Abnormalities of the fat pad and its attachment to the calcaneus may also be a cause of heel pain. The entire fat pad may not be well attached to the calcaneus, and therefore function ineffectively as a cushion. The fat within the heel pad itself may become injured, with the inflammatory response being one cause of pain. Injury to fat within the septa of the heel pad may also result in atrophy in that area and thereby diminish the cushioning effect of the heel pad.

DIAGNOSIS

Patients usually describe a history of gradual onset when presenting with pain in the subcalcaneal region of the heel. The pain is usually worse when the patient takes the first few steps in the morning and after sitting for a prolonged period of time; it usually diminishes with additional walking, although it may return after prolonged activity. Occasionally, heel pain does begin after an acute trauma. Patients can occasionally recall an incident such as wearing a new pair of shoes, an increase in the level of physical activity, or recent acute weight gain.

The patient's foot type should be determined since this can impact treatment of heel pain syndrome. A supple flat foot will have more stress on the plantar fascia at its origin because the windlass mechanism is more important to maintain the arch of the foot. With a cavus foot, there is decreased heel valgus at heel strike, which diminishes the shock absorption ability of the foot and places more stress on the plantar heel when the foot hits the ground.

In patients with subcalcaneal heel pain, a careful examination of the foot will usually demonstrate localized tenderness over the plantar fascial insertion at the medial plantar aspect of the calcaneal tuberosity. The plantar fascia should also be palpated more distally to discern whether there is tenderness along its course. The course of the posterior tibial nerve and its branches should be palpated and percussed to elicit any tenderness or a Tinel's sign. In addition to testing the passive motion of the joints of the ankle and hindfoot, the length of the Achilles tendon should be assessed. In patients with heel pain syndrome, there is often an associated Achilles tendon tightness on the ipsilateral side.

Radiographs are taken to rule out other causes of heel pain such as a fracture, a foreign body, or a tumor. A weightbearing lateral radiograph of the foot and ankle is usually sufficient to evaluate patients with heel pain. An axial view of the os calcis may be taken if information in a second plane is necessary. The lateral radiographic view will demonstrate if a heel spur is present. About 50 percent of patients with heel pain syndrome have a plantar heel spur and, conversely, about 15 percent of asymptomatic patients will demonstrate a heel spur. The exact relationship between heel pain and a heel spur is not well established.

Tarsal tunnel syndrome may present with pain referred to the heel and sole of the foot. If the patient has a positive Tinel's sign along the tarsal tunnel, electromyographic and nerve conduction studies should be obtained to rule out tarsal tunnel syndrome. Heel pain may also be referred from lumbar spine pathology. If this appears to be

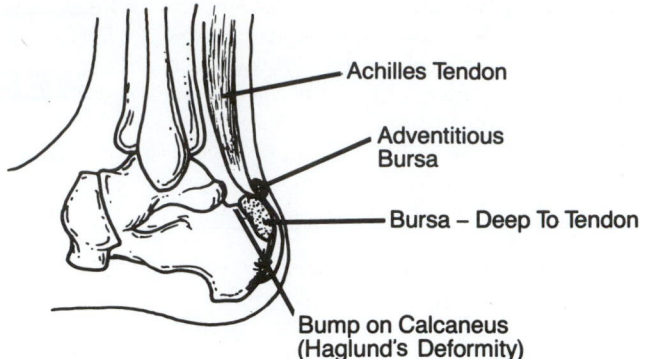

Figure 125-3

Illustration of the structures of the posterior superior heel. In this illustration, the posterior superior aspect of the calcaneous is prominent (Haglund's deformity). The retrocalcaneal bursa is between the superior calcaneous and the Achilles tendon. In some people an adventitial bursa develops between the skin and the Achilles tendon. [Reproduced with permission from Bordelon RL: Heel pain. In Mann RA, Coughlin MJ (eds): *Surgery of the Foot and Ankle.* St. Louis, MO: Mosby-Year Book; 1993:848.]

the case then appropriate diagnostic studies should be performed.

If the subcalcaneal heel pain is persistent, systemic disorders such as seronegative arthropathies should be considered. If confusion exists about the etiology of the heel pain or the diagnosis needs to be confirmed, a two-phase bone scan may be helpful to rule out a stress fracture of the calcaneus. At present MRI does not have a role in the diagnosis of subcalcaneal heel pain.

TREATMENT

There are many different treatment plans for heel pain syndrome. Nonoperative treatment begins with patient education. It is important for patients to realize that over 95 percent of patients treated receiving conservative treatment will have relief of their discomfort, although it may take several months. Conservative measures include Achilles tendon stretching and plantar fascial stretching exercises, heel cushion orthotics, night splints, and nonsteroidal anti-inflammatory medication (NSAIDs). An Achilles tendon which is not contracted theoretically decreases the stress on the plantar surface of the foot by improving ankle mobility in dorsiflexion during the gait cycle. Heel cushions can be an effective aid and come in two types: one is made of a viscoelastic material which provides an additional cushion effect; the other type is a hard plastic heel cup which supports the medial and lateral side of the plantar fat pad and helps improve the cushioning properties of the natural heel pad. Custom-made orthotic devices which relieve pressure at the heel and toward the medial arch are indicated in patients with heel pain and concomitant plantar fasciitis. Plantar fascial stretching exercises are helpful in patients who also have a component of plantar fasciitis.

Patients who do not respond to an initial course of nonoperative treatment may be candidates for dorsiflexion night splints. These have been found to be useful in up to 90 percent of cases. The night splint holds the foot in a neutral or slightly dorsiflexed position which decreases the natural contraction of the plantar fascia during periods of rest and allows the plantar fascia to mend itself in an elongated position. This often significantly reduces the heel pain felt with the first few steps in the morning. NSAIDs are helpful for acute episodes of pain but are not recommended for prolonged use.

The role of corticosteroid injection remains unclear. Risks include plantar fascial rupture and atrophy of the plantar fat pad. Despite these risks, limited use of corticosteroid injections can be considered for cases of acute tenderness. The injection should be given from the medial side and directed away from the fat pad.

In severe cases of plantar fasciitis and heel pain syndrome, the patient may benefit from immobilization in a walking cast for 3 to 4 weeks. This reduces the pressure on the heel and holds the plantar fascia in an elongated position.

The role of physical therapy is mainly to instruct patients in stretching exercises. Ultrasound and whirlpools, contrast baths, phonophoresis, and massage usually provide short-lived relief of pain and are generally not therapeutic. In patients whose symptoms persist for greater than 6 months, a work-up to rule out other systemic causes of heel pain should be undertaken including blood tests for seronegative arthropathies and Lyme disease. In these cases, treatment should be aimed at the systemic disease.

If heel pain continues despite adequate nonoperative treatment for a minimum of 9 to 12 months, surgical intervention may be considered. Less than 5 percent of all patients with heel pain syndrome require surgery. In the literature, some authors report good to excellent results from surgical release of the plantar fascia, while other authors show unpredictable results with success rates as low as 50 percent. Prior to surgery, the patient should be informed of the possible failure of operative treatment and the possibility of residual pain. Surgery for heel pain may include partial or total release of plantar fascia from the medial tuberosity of the calcaneus with or without removal of the calcaneal heel spur and release of the nerve to the adductor digiti minimi. Patients with symptoms of posterior tibial nerve involvement or patients who have failed previous surgery should also undergo exploration of the branches of the posterior tibial nerve.

Patients who have spontaneous plantar fascial ruptures or who underwent release of the entire plantar fascia may develop problems of the longitudinal arch of the foot because the windlass mechanism no longer functions. These patients often notice a flattening of the arch of the involved foot and may complain of arch pain and fatigue. Another complication of surgery is injury to the medial calcaneal nerve which may form a neuroma and produce numbness of the plantar fat pad.

SUPERIOR HEEL PAIN (RETROCALCANEAL, BURSITIS, HAGLUND'S DISEASE, AND INSERTIONAL ACHILLES TENDINITIS)

ANATOMY

The posterior heel area consists of the posterior calcaneus, Achilles tendon, the retrocalcaneal bursa, and an adventitial bursa (Fig. 125–3).

The major portion of the Achilles tendon inserts into the middle third of the posterior calcaneal surface. The retrocalcaneal bursa is a horseshoe-shaped bursa between the Achilles tendon and posterior superior aspect of the calcaneus. It can be identified as a lucency on the lateral radiographs. The adventitial bursa is located between the skin and the Achilles tendon and may be absent in some people. The adventitial bursa is generally produced by irritation from the counter of a shoe.

PATHOPHYSIOLOGY

Pain in the superior portion of the calcaneus can be caused by retrocalcaneal bursitis, enlargement of the superior tuberosity of the calcaneus, Achilles tendinitis, adventitial bursitis, or any combination of these. Retrocalcaneal bursitis occurs most often from overuse, repetitive trauma, and impingement of the calcaneus. It may, however, represent a focal manifestation of a systemic condition such as inflammatory arthritis or gout. Chronic strain of the Achilles tendon insertion can cause insertional tendinitis. As the body attempts to repair the overused tendon, the tendon thickens and hypertrophic calcifications may occur. Adventitial bursitis occurs as a soft tissue response due to pressure from the shoe counter against the bony projection of the lateral calcaneus at the Achilles tendon insertion (the so-called pump bump). Haglund's syndrome is a combination of insertional tendinitis, retrocalcaneal bursitis, and adventitial bursitis in patients who have an enlarged posterior superior aspect of the calcaneus (Fig. 125–4). The retrocalcaneal bursa becomes inflamed from progressive impingement between the Achilles tendon and the posterior superior aspect of the calcaneus with chronic repetitive activity or pressure from a shoe counter against the tendon pushing it towards the bone.

DIAGNOSIS

Patients with superior caneal heel pain generally complain of pain which is aggravated with activity and with certain shoewear. The onset may be slow or sudden. If the condition is due primarily to an acutely swollen retrocalcaneal bursa, the pain is usually constant and aggravated with activity. Acute pain may be associated with a traumatic incident.

The physical examination may help to localize the origin of the pain and swelling. A swollen retrocalcaneal bursa can be palpated just anterior to the Achilles tendon and will be painful medially and laterally. Dorsiflexion of the ankle will cause pain by increasing the pressure in a retrocalcaneal bursitis while plantar flexion will relieve the pain. When there is inflammation of the Achilles tendon in association with the retrocalcaneal bursitis, the tendon is usually painful just proximal to its insertion. If an adventitial bursa is present, it is usually located between skin and the os calcis on the lateral side.

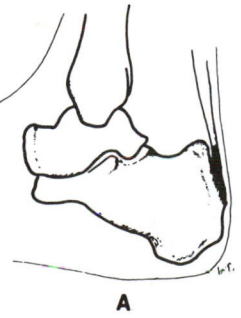

A

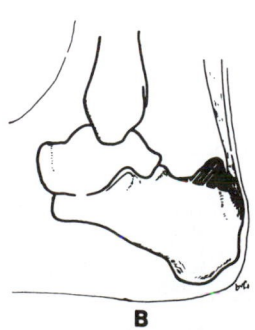

B

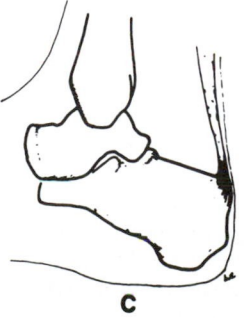

C

Figure 125-4
Haglund's deformity is a prominence of the posterior superior portion of the calcaneus. [Reproduced with permission from Bordelon RL: Heel pain. In Mann RA, Coughlin MJ (eds): *Surgery of the Foot and Ankle.* St. Louis, MO: Mosby-Year Book; 1993:854.

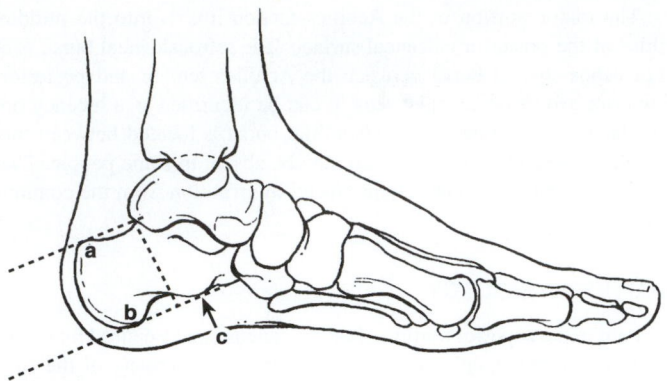

Figure 125-5
The parallel pitch lines determine the extent of the prominence of the posterior superior calcaneus. (a) Posterior superior calcaneal tuberosity margin. (b) Medial plantar tubercle. (c) Anterior plantar tubercle. The lower line is drawn connecting the anterior and posterior plantar tubercles (b and c). A line from the top of the posterior talar facet is drawn perpendicular to this lower line. The upper parallel pitch line is drawn parallel to the lower line at the length of the perpendicular line which ends at the top of the posterior talar facet. The posterior superior calcaneal tuberosity margin should be at or below the upper pitch line.

A lateral weightbearing radiograph of the foot is used to evaluate all of these conditions. Patients with insertional tendinitis may have calcification and bony enlargement at the calcaneal insertion of the Achilles tendon as well as soft tissue inflammation. Normally, the retrocalcaneal bursa appears as a space anterior to the Achilles tendon. When the bursa is inflamed, the normal lucency is obliterated on the lateral radiograph. In Haglund's syndrome, the lucency from the retrocalcaneal bursa is absent and the Achilles tendon soft tissue shadow is thickened (greater than 9 mm wide at a distance of 2 mm above the calcaneal projection).

An enlarged prominence of the posterior superior calcaneus is defined as a bony projection above the parallel pitch line. The parallel pitch line is measured on the lateral radiographs of the foot; it is a line parallel to the line between the anterior and medial tuberosities that bisects the posterior margin of the posterior facet (Fig. 125-5).

TREATMENT

Nonoperative treatments for all conditions of posterior heel pain include reduction of activity, NSAIDs, and a 1/8- to 1/2-in. heel lift. Heel elevation decreases the stress on the insertion of the Achilles tendon and decreases the pressure placed on the retrocalcaneal bursa

by plantar flexing the ankle. For Haglund's syndrome as well as for an adventitial bursitis, local application of ice and modification of the shoe by softening or eliminating the shoe counter are often helpful. Recalcitrant cases may be helped by ankle immobilization in a short leg walking cast for 4 weeks.

Steroid injection into the Achilles tendon should be avoided since it may promote the degeneration of the tendon or cause a rupture. In selective cases of retrocalcaneal bursitis, a small amount of steroid may be injected directly into the retrocalcaneal bursa, but care must be taken to avoid injection into the Achilles tendon.

Surgical treatment is indicated only if nonoperative measures fail to control these conditions. For patients with insertional tendinitis, the tendon can be debrided and any bony prominence removed. If the continuity of the tendon is disrupted or the tendon is weakened by the debridement, it may be necessary to reattach the tendon to the calcaneus with a tendon or fascial reinforcement. Extreme care should be taken to prevent rupture of the tendon at surgery and during the postoperative period. If excessive debridement of the Achilles tendon or a tendon augmentation is performed, dorsiflexion should be limited postoperatively for a minimum of 3 weeks.

Surgical treatment of recalcitrant retrocalcaneal bursitis and Haglund's syndrome includes removal of the bursa and ostectomy of the posterior superior aspect of the calcaneus. Enough bone must be removed to prevent contact between the prominence and the tendon. The tendon is also inspected and debrided if necessary. Postoperatively, the patient should wear a 1-cm heel lift for approximately 8 weeks. As always, if the Achilles tendon is weakened, it should be protected in a cast postoperatively.

SUGGESTED READINGS

Baxter DE, Pfeffer GB: Treatment of chronic heel pain by surgical release of the first branch of the lateral plantar nerve. *Clin Orthop* 1992; 279:229.

Baxter DE, Thigpen CM: Heel pain—operative results. *Foot Ankle* 1984; 5:16.

Bordelon RL: Subcalcaneal pain: A method of evaluation and plan for treatment. *Clin Orthop* 1983, 117:49.

Bordelon RL: Heel pain. In Mann RA, Coughlin MJ (eds): *Surgery of the Foot and Ankle*, vol 2, 6th ed. St. Louis: CV Mosby; 1993:837.

Daly PJ, Kitaoka HB, Chao EYS: Plantar fasciotomy for intractable plantar fascitis: Clinical results and biomechanical evaluation. *Foot Ankle* 1992; 13:188.

Frey C, Rosenberg Z, Shereffet MJ, et al: The retrocalcaneal bursa: Anatomy and bursography. *Foot Ankle* 1992; 13:203.

Pavlov H, Heneghan MA, Hersh A, et al: The Haglund syndrome: Initial and differential diagnosis. *Radiology* 1982; 144:83.

Pfeffer GB, Baxter DE: Surgery of the adult heel. In Jahss MH (ed): *Disorders of the Foot and Ankle: Medical and Surgical Management*, vol 2, 2d ed. Philadelphia: WB Saunders; 1991:1396.

Rubin G, Witten M: Plantar calcaneal spurs. *Am J Orthop* 1963; 5:38.

Chapter 126

INFECTIONS OF THE FOOT

Donna J. Astion

The principles of diagnosis and management of infections of the foot are similar to those of infections which occur elsewhere in the body. Infections of the foot can be bacterial, mycobacterial, or fungal and can present in soft tissues, joints, or bones. Foot infections, particularly in patients with diabetes or peripheral vascular disease, can be challenging to treat.

BACTERIAL INFECTIONS

SOFT TISSUE INFECTIONS

Infections from superficial lesions caused by certain skin conditions, infected blisters, or scratches usually present as cellulitis, with or without lymphangitis. Most commonly, *Staphylococcus aureus* causes cellulitis and abscess formation, while *beta hemolytic streptococci* will cause cellulitis and lymphangitis. Since both organisms are frequently combined in soft tissue infections, treatment of both organisms is recommended. Treatment with oral antibiotics is usually sufficient.

A *felon* is a painful collection of pus in the pulp space adjacent to the distal phalanx of the toe near the nail. A felon is usually caused by *hemolytic streptococci,* but in compromised hosts, such as diabetics, gram-negative organisms may cause this collection of pus. Felons should be drained under digital or regional block, with an incision extending from one side of the toe to the other (Fig. 126-1). The wound should be packed lightly for 24 h and then left open and allowed to drain. If the felon is not incised and drained, the infection may penetrate the underlying bone and cause osteomyelitis.

Puncture wounds to the foot are most common in children. These injuries are frequently due to nails, splinters, and tacks. If a sneaker or a sock is on the foot at the time of injury, material can be carried into the wound by the puncturing object. Initially, cellulitis or abscess formation can occur. Later, osteomyelitis, osteochondritis, or septic arthritis can develop. *Pseudomonas aeruginosa* is the most common infecting organism in puncture wounds, and osteomyelitis occurs in about 1 percent of puncture wounds to the foot. The initial treatment of a puncture wound to the foot is cleaning the wound with iodoform solution and, if possible, probing the wound to remove any retained foreign material that may be present. It is also important to attempt to determine if the puncture penetrated the bone or cartilage. Radiographs should be taken to determine if a foreign body is present in soft tissue or bone and to rule out any bone defects.

Tetanus prophylaxis should be given to all patients who have deep puncture wounds. The role of initial antibiotics is controversial. If the wound is clean, no antibiotics are indicated; however, if the wound is contaminated or reaches the bone, cartilage, or joint, then oral an-

tibiotics should be prescribed. The drug of choice should be effective against *Staphylococcus* and *Streptococcus*. The efficacy of treatment with antipseudomonal medications has not been adequately studied. Patients who have sustained a puncture wound of the foot should be monitored for later signs of deep infection.

Trauma which results in open wounds on the foot should be cleaned and the devitalized tissue debrided. Antibiotics which cover both *Staphylococcus* and *Streptococcus* are recommended whenever foreign material is present in the wounds. If an infection develops after a trauma, particularly if antibiotics have been used, culture results should be used to determine the antibiotics to be administered. Deep infection of the foot from penetrating wounds and massive trauma can result in abscess formation and osteomyelitis.

Cat and dog bites can introduce *Pasteurella multocida,* which behaves aggressively and quickly leads to cellulitis, tissue destruction, and abscess formation. After these wounds are debrided and irrigated, prophylactic antibiotics such as penicillin, ampicillin, cephalosporins, or amoxicillin-clavulanic acid should be administered to prevent deep infection. If the patient is allergic to penicillin, then a combination of tetracycline and Clindamycin can be used. In addition, patients with cat or dog bites should receive tetanus toxoid.

Infections of the tendon sheath or bursa may result from spread of adjacent cellulitis or from direct inoculation. Infected tenosynovitis is treated with drainage and antibiotics, while infected bursitis can usually be treated by antibiotics and, if necessary, surgical drainage.

Deep compartment abscesses in the foot can result from the spread of local infection. Clinically, the foot appears swollen and erythematous. Usually, the foot is warm and painful to palpation of the plantar aspect. Surgical drainage of the deep compartments of the foot is necessary to adequately treat this type of infection. Adequate drainage can be performed either through two parallel dorsal incisions (Fig. 126-2A) or through a single incision parallel to and just superior to the medial border of the plantar aspect of the foot (Fig. 126-2B).

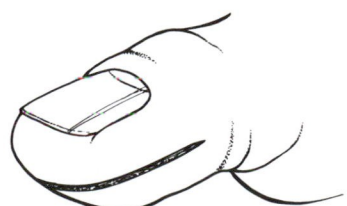

Figure 126-1

Incision for drainage of a felon. [Reproduced with permission from Johnson JE, Hall RL: Management of foot infections. In Gould JS (ed): *Operative Foot Surgery*. Philadelphia: Saunders; 1994:270.]

JOINT INFECTIONS

Joint infections can arise from systemic bacterial illness, direct inoculation, or spread from adjacent infection. Most commonly, joints are infected by *Staphylococcus aureus*. However, *Neisseria gonorrhoeae* is a common cause of septic arthritis in sexually active young adults.

In the foot, septic arthritis presents as a painful, red, and swollen joint. The differential diagnosis should include gout, Reiter's syndrome, and neuropathic joints. Radiographs often show soft tissue swelling and may show adjacent osteomyelitis. The diagnosis of septic arthritis can be confirmed by aspiration of the involved joint.

Medical management of most acute joint infections of the foot entail repeated aspiration and parenteral antibiotics. Antibiotic therapy should be started empirically before culture results are available, and modified once the culture results are obtained. If the condition does not improve in five days or if there is evidence of osteomyelitis, then the joint should be surgically opened and drained and the antibiotics continued.

BONE INFECTIONS

Osteomyelitis can develop from direct inoculation of the bone after trauma or surgery, from blood-borne organisms, or spread from an adjacent soft tissue or joint infection. Osteomyelitis from trauma, surgery, or adjacent infection may be caused by a number of different organisms. Blood-borne infections are commonly due to *Staphylococcus aureus* and occur mostly in children. The clinical presentation of osteomyelitis is variable.

Accurate diagnosis of osteomyelitis and identification of the infective organism is essential for successful treatment. Clinically, the involved area may be painful, swollen, warm, and tender to palpation. The white blood cell count may be elevated. Radiographically, the bone may appear normal or may appear moth-eaten with periosteal

reaction. The radiographic findings of osteomyelitis can take up to 1 week to appear. MRI can be used to diagnose osteomyelitis earlier than plain radiographs. A triple phase bone scan is also helpful in diagnosing osteomyelitis of the foot, especially when performed with an Indium scan.

Treatment of acute osteomyelitis depends on the presence of an abscess in the bone or adjacent soft tissue. If an abscess exists, it should be surgically drained and intravenous antibiotics administered. If there is no abscess, intravenous antibiotics should be administered and no surgery is necessary. Antibiotic treatment of gram-positive organisms should be continued for about 4 to 6 weeks, while treatment of gram-negative organisms continues for 6 weeks. In cases of chronic osteomyelitis, appropriate intravenous antibiotics along with surgical debridement of the infected bone with removal of all necrotic bone is essential.

LYME DISEASE

Lyme disease is caused by the Spirochete *Borrelia burgdorferi* and is transmitted by Ixodic ticks. Lyme disease can have a variable presentation in the foot, including heel pain, metatarsalgia, tendinitis, or synovitis. The diagnosis is usually made with a high clinical suspicion, a history of erythema chronicum nigrans, and by serology. This condition is best treated with the appropriate antibiotics.

TUBERCULOSIS

Mycobacterium tuberculosis infection of the ankle and foot is uncommon, but tuberculosis of the ankle occurs more frequently than tuberculosis in the foot proper. This is usually a blood-borne infection; however, a prior history of trauma is not uncommon. Radiographically, soft tissue swelling is seen early, but later, sub-

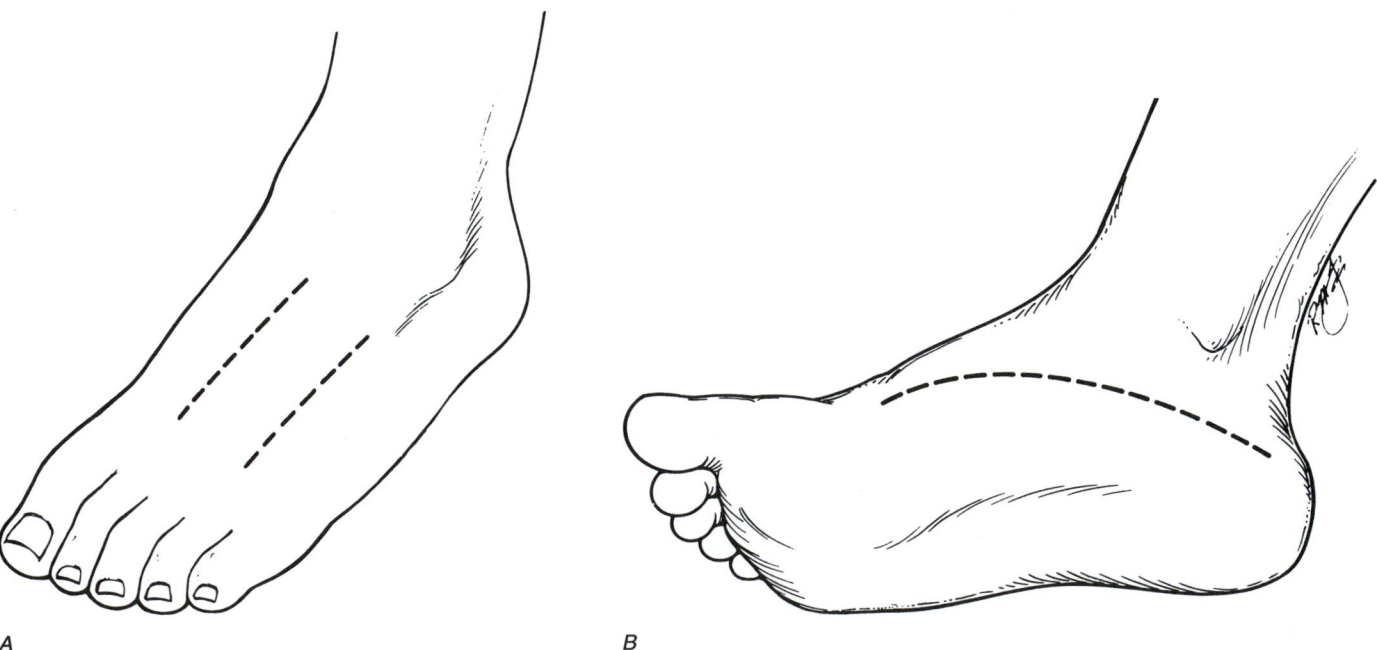

A   *B*

Figure 126-2
Incisions for drainage of deep-space infections. *A.* Parallel dorsal incisions along the 2d and 4th metatarsal shafts. *B.* Single incision along the medial border of the plantar aspect of the foot, followed by excision of a segment of plantar aponeurosis. [Reproduced with permission from Richardson EG, Landaker SD: Foot infections. In Sammarco GJ (ed): *Foot and Ankle Manual.* Philadelphia: Lea & Febiger; 1991:244, 245.]

chondral osteoporosis and bone destruction are observed. Eventually, thickening of the periosteum and cartilage destruction can occur. Tuberculosis should be suspected in cases of single lesions of the bone or joints in high-risk groups. This condition is treated with chemotherapy, and surgery is not usually necessary.

FUNGAL INFECTIONS

Tinea pedis (athlete's foot) is a very common fungal infection of the skin and nails of the foot. Patients can present with varying degrees of skin itching, cracking, scaling, and blister formation. The soles and interdigital spaces are most often affected. Fungal infections are best treated with topical antifungal agents.

Deeper tissues can be affected by other fungi, but this is uncom-mon. In the Southwestern United States, *Coccidioides immitis* may cause chronic ulceration of the skin and underlying soft tissue in the foot. *Cryptococcus neoformans* can cause bone infections in the foot.

SUGGESTED READINGS

Frierson JG, Pfeffinger LL: Infections of the foot. In Mann RA, Coughlin MJ (eds): *Surgery of the Foot and Ankle*, vol 2, 6th ed. St. Louis, MO: CV Mosby; 1993:859.

Loeffler RD Jr, Ballard A: Plantar fascial spaces of the foot and a proposed surgical approach. *Foot Ankle* 1980; 1:11.

Riegler HF, Routson GW: Complications of deep puncture wounds of the foot. *J Trauma* 1979; 19:18.

Chapter 127

COMPRESSIVE NEUROPATHIES

Donna J. Astion

ANATOMY

Knowledge of the anatomic course of the nerves as well as the peripheral nerve distribution is essential to the diagnosis and treatment of peripheral nerve conditions of the foot. While the sensory innervation about the foot and ankle is variable, in general, the saphenous nerve innervates the medial ankle area, and the sural nerve innervates the dorsolateral forefoot. The superficial peroneal nerve usually innervates the remainder of the dorsum of the foot except the area of the first web space, which is innervated by the deep peroneal nerve. The plantar surface of the foot and the toes is usually innervated by the medial and lateral plantar nerves, which are branches of the posterior tibial nerve (Fig. 127-1). The posterior tibial nerve is posterior to the medial malleolus between the flexor digitorum longus and flexor hallucis longus, and these structures are covered by the flexor retinaculum medially. The four major branches of the posterior tibial nerve are the medial calcaneal branch which innervates the medial heel, the medial plantar branch, the lateral plantar branch, and the motor branch to the abductor digiti minimi (Fig. 127-2). Aside from supplying the sensation to the plantar surface of the foot, the medial and lateral plantar nerves also innervate the intrinsic muscles of the foot.

When evaluating neurologic problems of the foot, it is important to rule out systemic disorders such as diabetes and Charcot-Marie-Tooth disease, proximal nerve injuries, local inflammatory conditions which may irritate the nerve, and local bony abnormalities.

COMPRESSIVE NERVE INJURIES

Chronic nerve compression injuries may be caused by the cumulative effects of traction or repetitive compressive pressure on the nerve. Local inflammation can reduce the normal glide of the nerve and lead to edema, scarring, stretching, and possibly permanent nerve injury. This pathoanatomic process can cause damage to the posterior tibial nerve in the tarsal tunnel. Nerves can also be damaged from excessive friction at a rigid edge of fascia, such as the interdigital nerves at the transverse metatarsal ligament. Ischemia from a tourniquet can also lead to nerve damage.

SUPERFICIAL NERVE ENTRAPMENT

Superficial nerves about the foot and ankle are prone to repeated injury and prolonged compression because of the decreased subcutaneous tissue and tight retinacular structures in this area. The dorsal and medial cutaneous branches of the superficial peroneal nerves, the deep peroneal nerve, and the lateral dorsal cutaneous nerves are most commonly affected (Fig. 127-3). Entrapment of any of these nerves can occur after blunt trauma, chronically tight footwear, or excessive activity.

Complaints of paraesthesias, burning, or foot ache are the usual presenting symptoms. These symptoms may intensify with certain footwear or with certain activities. On physical examination, there is usually a demonstrable Tinel's sign over the involved area of the nerve; and the patient may have decreased sensation or hypersensitivity distally in the cutaneous distribution of the irritated nerve.

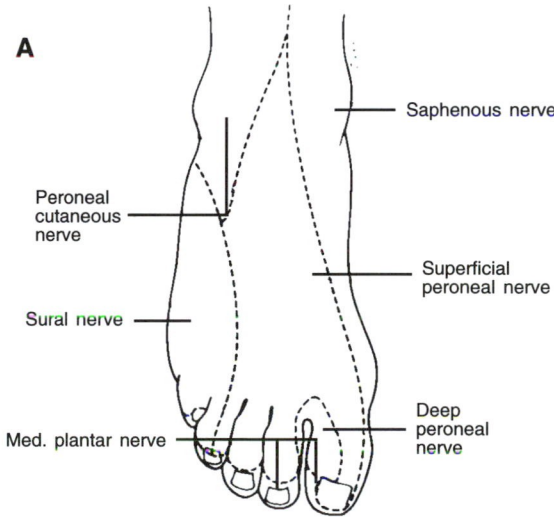

A

Peroneal cutaneous nerve

Sural nerve

Med. plantar nerve

Saphenous nerve

Superficial peroneal nerve

Deep peroneal nerve

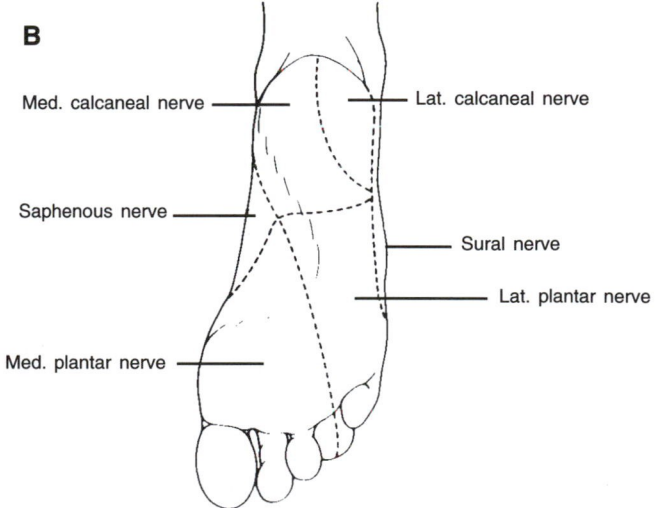

B

Med. calcaneal nerve

Saphenous nerve

Med. plantar nerve

Lat. calcaneal nerve

Sural nerve

Lat. plantar nerve

Figure 127-1

A and *B*. Sensory distribution of cutaneous nerves of the foot. [Reproduced with permission from Sammarco GJ: Anatomy and examination. In Sammarco GJ (ed): *Foot and Ankle Manual.* Philadelphia: Lea & Febiger; 1991:23.]

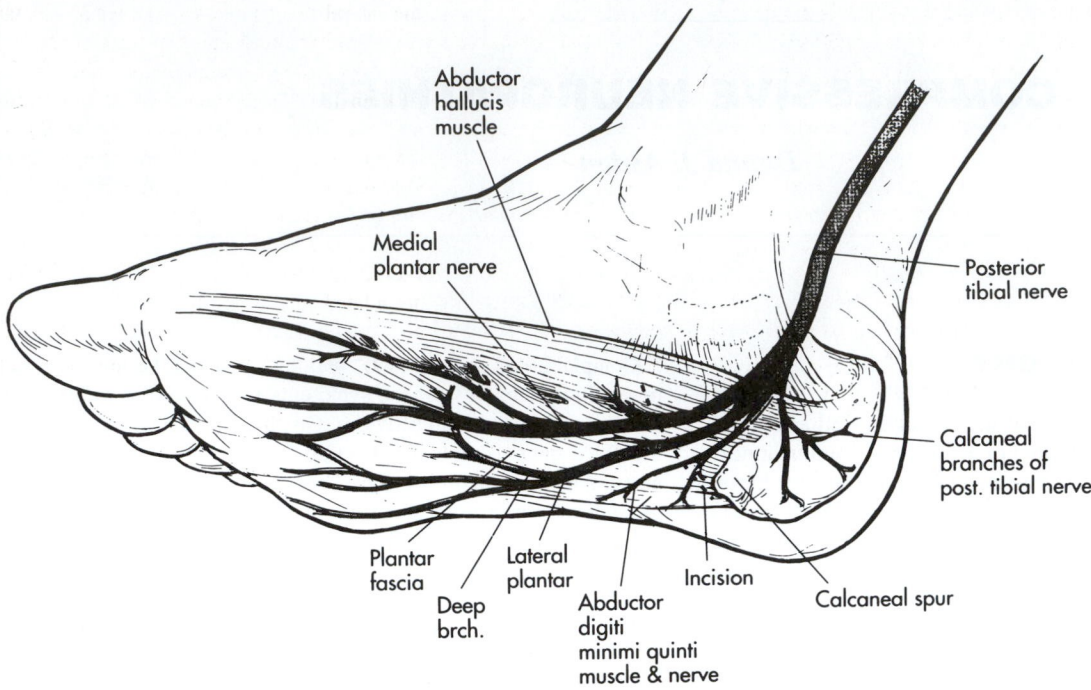

Figure 127-2
Branches of the posterior tibial nerve. [Reproduced with permission from Baxter DE: Subcalcaneal pain. In Lutter LD (ed): *Atlas of Adult Foot and Ankle Surgery.* St. Louis, MO: Mosby-Year Book; 1997:183.]

Superficial nerve entrapments are best treated nonoperatively. The patient should be advised to avoid constrictive shoes or dressings and to place pads in the shoes on each side of the entrapment area to decrease pressure on the nerve. Physical therapy is often helpful in desensitizing the hypersensitive area and in mobilizing the nerve from any surrounding scar tissue. In addition, the judicious use of cortisone injections about the nerve can be helpful. If nonoperative measures are not successful, surgery should first be directed to relieve the cause of the entrapment. Resection of the superficial nerve should be avoided because this can lead to a painful neuroma and a poor result. If the nerve is resected, the proximal stump should ideally

be placed in a well-padded, nontraumatized area. Unfortunately, it is difficult to find such an area in the subcutaneous tissue in the foot or ankle.

INTERDIGITAL NEUROMAS

An interdigital neuroma, or Morton's neuroma, is a scarring of the interdigital nerve as the nerve passes beneath the deep transverse metatarsal ligament when the toes dorsiflex. Most commonly, these neuromas occur in the third web space; the second web space is next most common. Interdigital neuromas in the first and fourth web spaces

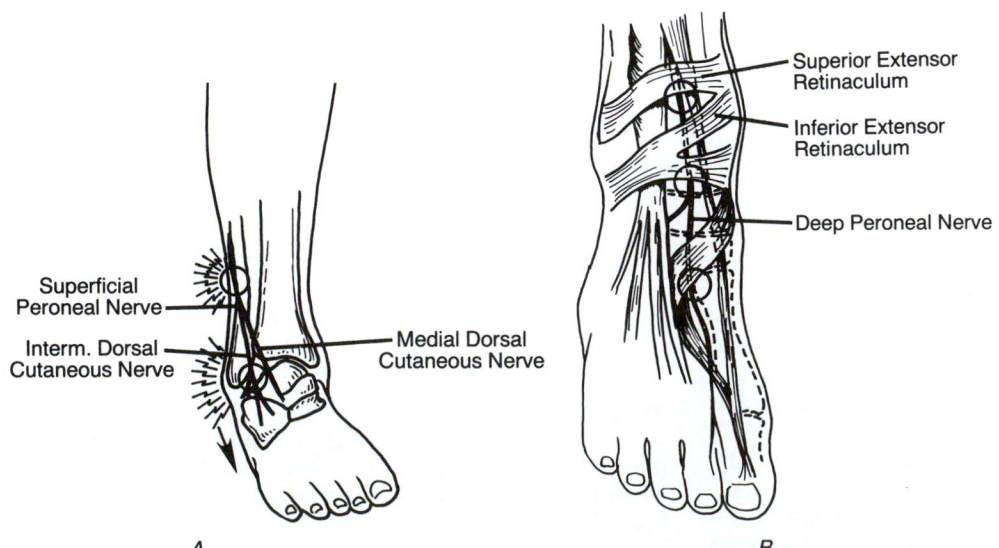

Figure 127-3
A. Area of superior peroneal nerve entrapment. *B.* Areas of deep peroneal nerve entrapment. [Reproduced with permission from Baxter DE: Functional nerve disorders. In Mann RA, Coughlin MJ (eds): *Surgery of the Foot and Ankle.* St. Louis, MO: Mosby-Year Book; 1993: 568, 570.]

are extremely rare. It is believed that the third webspace is more commonly involved because a branch of the lateral plantar nerve joins the medial plantar nerve to form a relatively larger third common digital nerve. The female-to-male predominance of interdigital neuroma is approximately 4 to 1, and the average age of presentation is 55 years.

Patients commonly complain of plantar forefoot pain with burning in the third and fourth toes while walking in shoes. The symptoms are often worse with narrow shoes and shoes with a higher heel. The pain is often relieved by rest or removing the shoe. On occasion, patients are more comfortable in shoes with a heel.

On physical examination, there is often localized tenderness with palpation of the invovled web space. A click is sometimes palpable when pressure is applied to the forefoot plantar between the metatarsal heads while simultaneously compressing all the metatarsal heads together. A diagnostic injection of Lidocaine near the nerve can be used to confirm the diagnosis. The differential diagnosis of this condition includes metatarsalgia, tendonitis, metatarsophalangeal, (MTP) joint synovitis or subluxation, and a more proximal nerve compression, such as tarsal tunnel syndrome or lumbar disc disease. MTP joint synovitis or subluxation can produce inflammation and traction of the interdigital nerve. Treatment of these MTP joint problems will often relieve the nerve symptoms.

The nonoperative treatment of Morton's neuroma includes shoe modifications such as lower heels and a wider toebox. In addition, a metatarsal pad can be used to widen the space between the metatarsal heads and minimize compression on the nerve. Corticosteroid injection into the web space is sometimes helpful in the more acute cases. If these nonopervative measures fail, then surgical excision of the entrapped nerve can be carried out through a dorsal or plantar incision. Approximately 90 percent of patients who undergo incision of the Morton's neuroma report a good result.

TARSAL TUNNEL SYNDROME

The posterior tibial nerve lies between the flexor digitorum longus and the flexor hallucis longus beneath the flexor retinaculum (lacunate ligament). The four main branches of the posterior tibial nerve are the

medial calcaneal nerve, the lateral plantar nerve, the medial plantar nerve, and the nerve to the abductor digiti quinti (Fig. 127-4). The branching pattern of these nerves within the tunnel is variable.

The symptoms of tarsal tunnel syndrome can occur due to compression of the nerves from a space occupying lesion in the tarsal tunnel, such as a ganglion, lipoma, or accessory soleus muscle, or from local inflammation related to tenosynovitis of the posterior tibial tendon or the flexor hallucis longus tendon. The nerve may also be compressed by a bony lesion following fracture of the tibia, talus, or calcaneous. Individuals with severe hindfoot valgus or pronation develop tarsal syndrome symptoms related to tension on the nerve. The diagnosis of tarsal tunnel syndrome can be controversial, and the onset of this condition is usually insidious. Patients may complain of paraesthesias, cramping, and burning in the medial ankle and foot; and the pain is often more intense at night.

On physical examination, patients usually demonstrate some sensitivity to palpation around the tarsal tunnel, and percussion of the nerve in the involved area usually reveals symptoms referable to the involved nerve branch distribution. The neurologic examination is otherwise normal. During the examination, it is important to rule out other peripheral nerve pathology as well as a more proximal compressive neuropathy. Radiographs or CT scans may be necessary to rule out a bony compression as the etiology of the symptoms and an MRI may be necessary to rule out a space-occupying lesion within the tarsal tunnel. Electromyogram and nerve conduction velocity studies are essential in the diagnosis of tarsal tunnel syndrome; however, these studies may be normal in some patients.

Treatment of tarsal tunnel syndrome includes the use of nonsteroidal anti-inflammatory medications, orthotics to decrease pronation, local steroid injection, and treatment of an associated pathology such as tenosynovitis, peripheral neuropathy, or a more proximal nerve lesion. Surgical release of the tarsal tunnel, through incision of the flexor retinaculum, is indicated for patients with persistent symptoms despite an adequate course of nonoperative treatment. If there is no specific pathology identified, then the tarsal tunnel is released. Postoperatively, patients are maintained in a compressive dressing, and orthotics should be used to support the longitudinal arch and decrease any hindfoot valgus.

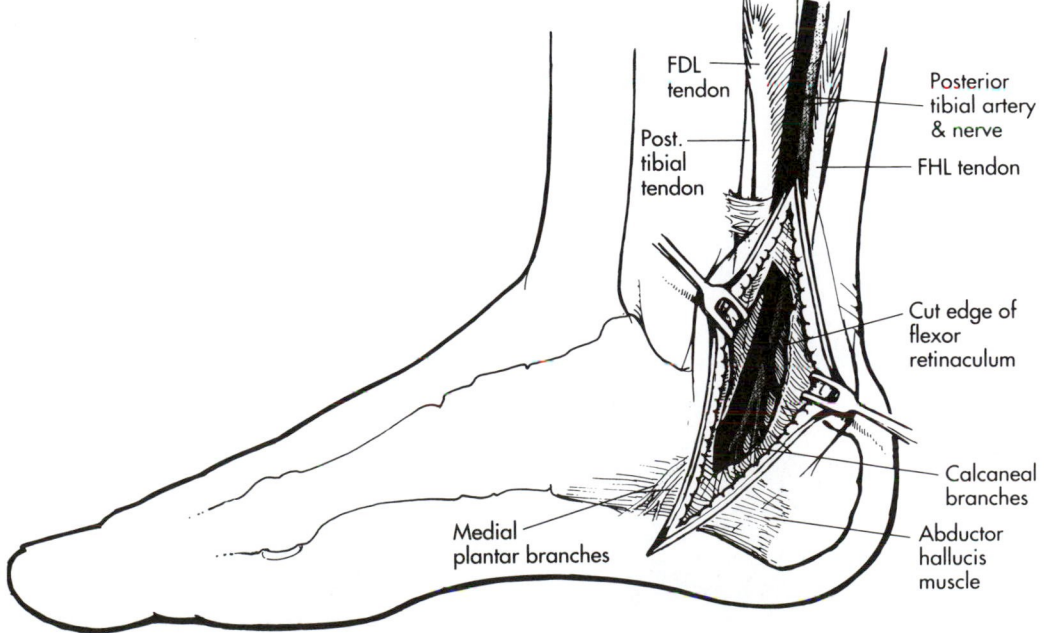

Figure 127-4
Contents of the tarsal tunnel. [Reproduced with permission from Lutter LD: Anatomy and examination. In Lutter LD (ed): *Atlas of Adult Foot and Ankle Surgery.* St. Louis, MO: Mosby-Year Book; 1997:209.]

SUGGESTED READINGS

Beskin JL, Baxter DE: Recurrent pain following interdigital neurectomy—a plantar approach. *Foot Ankle* 1988; 9:34.

Dellon AL: Deep peroneal nerve entrapment on the dorsum of the foot. *Foot Ankle* 1990; 11:73.

Greenfield J, Rea J Jr, Ilfield FW: Morton's interdigital neuroma. Indications for treatment by local injections versus surgery. *Clin Orthop* 1984; 185:142.

Kaplan PE, Kernahan WT Jr: Tarsal tunnel syndrome: An electrodiagnostic and surgical correlation. *J Bone Joint Surg [Am]* 1981; 63:96.

Kenzora JE: Symptomatic incisional neuromas on the dorsum of the foot. *Foot Ankle* 1984; 5:2.

Mann RA: Tarsal tunnel syndrome. *Orthop Clin North Am* 1974; 5:109.

Pringle RM, Protheroe K, Mukherjee SK: Entrapment neuropathy of the sural nerve. *J Bone Joint Surg [Br]* 1974; 56:465.

Radin EL: Tarsal tunnel syndrome. *Clin Orthop* 1983; 181:167.

Sarrafian S: Nerves. In Sarrafian S (ed): *Anatomy of the Foot and Ankle: Descriptive, Topographic, Functional.* Philadelphia: JB Lippincott; 1993:356.

Styf J: Entrapment of the superficial peroneal nerve. Diagnosis and results of decompression. *J Bone Joint Surg [Br]* 1989; 71:131.

Thompson FM, Deland JT: Occurrence of two interdigital neuromas in one foot. *Foot Ankle* 1993; 14:15.

Chapter 128

TUMORS

Donna J. Astion

Tumors of the foot and ankle account for less than 5 percent of all musculoskeletal tumors diagnosed in the United States. Unfortunately, many of the malignant tumors of the foot are discovered in their late stages. The incidence of benign tumors in this area is difficult to estimate because most of these tumors are asymptomatic, found incidentally, and managed nonoperatively. Patients with a foot tumor most often complain of pain and functional impairment, with or without a palpable mass. As with other musculoskeletal tumors, the patient's age is an important part of the history and helps determine which tumors to include in the differential diagnosis. During the physical examination of the foot and ankle, areas of tenderness, masses, overlying skin changes, and adenopathy should be noted.

BONE FORMING TUMORS

BENIGN

Osteoid osteoma is a relatively common lesion which normally is painful, particularly at night. The pain is typically relieved with salicylates. This tumor presents more commonly in males and is most common in the second decade. Less than 1 percent of all osteoid osteomas occur in the foot. Radiographically the tumor has a central lucency (nidus) which is usually less than 1 cm, surrounded by a zone of sclerotic bone. While it is often difficult to visualize the tumor on plain radiography, a bone scan will show an area of increased uptake and a CT scan can be used to locate the nidus. In the foot, this tumor is most common in the tarsal bones. While the natural history of this lesion is often self-limiting, if the pain cannot be managed with salicylates, surgery is indicated to remove the nidus.

MALIGNANT

Osteosarcoma is a malignant tumor with bone-producing foci. This malignant tumor is more common in males and usually occurs in the second and third decades of life. While less than 1 percent of osteosarcomas are found in the foot, it is the second most common malignant primary bone tumor of the foot. Patients usually present with pain and swelling in the area of the lesion, and radiographs will demonstrate a destructive bone lesion of the cortex and medullary canal along with periosteal new bone formation. Surgical treatment of this malignant lesion of the foot usually involves foot or below-knee amputation with adjuvant chemotherapy.

CARTILAGE FORMING TUMORS

BENIGN

Enchondroma is a tumor of mature cartilage cells which form bone and is found within the medullary canal. These tumors occur most commonly in the second decade but can be seen in all age groups. This type of lesion can occur in isolation, be multiple (Ollier's disease), or can be associated with hemangiomas (Maffucci's syndrome). Enchondromas are the most common benign primary tumors of the foot and are most commonly found in the metatarsals and phalanges. While most often asymptomatic, they may become painful if a fracture occurs. Radiographically, the lesions are well-circumscribed radiolucent medullary defects with stippled calcification. They occur in the diaphysis or metaphysis, and on occasion, there is expansion of the overlying bone. When symptomatic, these lesions can be treated with curettage and bone grafting. Sarcomatous degeneration is associated with painful lesions which are increasing in size and radiographically demonstrate endosteal erosion and cortical destruction. These sarcomatous lesions are usually of very low grade and can be treated with local resection. However, if the lesion is more aggressive, amputation is necessary.

Osteochondromas are the most common benign lesions of bone. These lesions are developmental abnormalities of the growth plate and are found in the metaphyseal region of long tubular bones. Less than 1 percent of these lesions are found in the foot. Osteochondroma may occur as a single lesion or multiple lesions. These lesions usually present by the second decades of life as a painful mass. Radiographically, the lesions arise in the metaphyseal bone. There is continuity between the normal and lesional cortical and cancellous bone, and the stalk is either a sessile or pedunculated base, covered by a cartilaginous cap. If the lesion is symptomatic, it can be treated by excision of the bone, its cartilaginous cap, and the overlying bursa. The risk of malignant transformation is less than 1 percent in isolated lesions but increases to 10 percent in patients with multiple lesions.

Chondroblastoma is a very rare lesion and accounts for about 3 percent of benign bone tumors. It is more common in males, and the peak incidence is in the second and third decades. In the foot, this lesion is typically found in the calcaneus and the talus. A chondroblastoma usually presents with pain. Radiographically, the lesion appears within the medullary canal as a central area of lucency, often greater than 1.5 cm, surrounded by a margin of dense bone. Calcifications are sometimes seen within the lesion. If the chondroblastoma is symptomatic, it can be treated with curettage and bone grafting. Local recurrence is seen in about 10 percent of patients.

MALIGNANT

Chondrosarcoma is a slow-growing tumor which presents in adulthood between the fourth and sixth decades. It is the third most common primary malignant bone tumor but less than 1 percent of these lesions are in the foot. Chondrosarcoma of the foot usually presents with pain and swelling. Radiographs demonstrate a destructive expansile lesion of the bone, with a thickened cortex. In 65 percent of cases, areas of calcification are present. Often the lesion is expansile and the cortex is thickened. The tumor grade and adequacy of resection are prognostically significant. Low-grade lesions should be removed with wide margins while high-grade sarcomas are surgically treated with a foot or below-knee amputation. Patients should be followed closely for recurrence since recurrence have been reported as late as 10 years postresection.

FIBROUS TISSUE FORMING TUMORS

BENIGN

Plantar fibromatosis is a localized proliferation of fibrous tissue of the plantar aponeurosis which is analogous to Dupuytren's disease (palmer fibrosis) of the hand. This lesion is infiltrating and may involve the dermis as well as the underlying tendons. The disease is bilateral in 25 percent of cases and is more common in men than women. The incidence of plantar fibromatosis is higher in patients with seizures, diabetes, and a history of alcohol abuse. Patients usually present with a mass on the plantar aspect of the foot which may be painful with weightbearing activities. However, for many patients, these masses are asymptomatic. Nonoperative treatment with orthotics and shoe modifications often provide effective pain relief. Failing nonoperative treatment, a complete fascial excision is performed, as local excision is associated with a 57 percent recurrence.

MALIGNANT

Malignant fibrous histiocytoma comprises about 2 percent of foot tumors. This is a rapidly growing tumor which is often painful. Radiographically the lesion is radiolucent and destructive with poorly defined margins and minimal periosteal reaction. Treatment is adjuvant chemotherapy with either wide local resection or amputation.

ROUND CELL TUMORS (MALIGNANT)

Ewing's Sarcoma is a round cell tumor in the bone which has a 2 to 5 percent incidence in the foot. It is usually seen during adolescence but can be seen anytime before the 4th decade. Patients present with complaints of pain and swelling. They sometimes have constitutional symptoms such as fever, night sweats, and weight loss. Radiographically, the lesion is an aggressive, destructive, permeative, and lytic lesion of the bone, usually in the diaphysis of long bones. There is often extensive involvement of the bone and commonly an extraosseous mass. Infection should be in the differential diagnosis of this type of lesion. The most important prognostic indicator is the site of the lesion, as those of the distal appendicular skeleton have a better prognosis than lesions of the axial skeleton. In the distal appendicular skeleton, this type of tumor must be treated by amputation with adjuvant therapy.

GIANT CELL TUMORS

Giant cell tumors have a peak incidence between 20 and 40 years of age. When they occur, they are almost exclusively in the epiphysis of long bones and occur infrequently in the foot. Radiographically, the lesion is lytic and frequently violates the cortex and breaks out into the surrounding soft tissue. Surgical treatment includes curettage and bone grafting of the lesion or en-bloc resection and bone grafting. A recurrence rate as high as 50 percent has been reported.

VASCULAR TUMORS (BENIGN)

Glomus tumors are small, pea-sized vascular tumors found in subungual or subcutaneous locations. These tumors often cause significant pain and discomfort to the patient in the nail region. In most cases, simple excision affords great pain relief for the patient.

TUMOR-LIKE LESIONS

Simple (unicameral) bone cysts are common in the large tarsal bones and are often asymptomatic until a fracture occurs. These lesions typically present in children and adolescents. Radiographically, the lesion is radiolucent with well-defined borders and a thin adjacent cortex which is intact unless there has been a fracture. Simple bone cysts of the calcaneus are often asymptomatic. Treatment of asymptomatic lesions include observation or aspiration with steroid injection. For symptomatic lesions, curettage and bone grafting are advised.

Aneurysmal bone cysts occur in the foot in approximately 10 percent of the cases. This lesion is most commonly seen in the second and third decades and usually presents with pain, tenderness, and swelling at the site of the lesion. Radiographically, the lesion is expansile and eccentric with a thin, bulging cortex. Whenever this lesion is encountered, it is imperative to rule out another underlying primary tumor with aneurysmal bone cyst-like areas such as a giant cell tumor, osteoblastoma, chondroblastoma, osteosarcoma, or fibrous dysplasia. Surgically, as much of the lesion as possible should be removed and the area bone grafted as needed. However, there is a 19 percent recurrence rate of this lesion.

Ganglion cysts are well-encapsulated sacs filled with thickened synovial fluid which are connected with the underlying tendon or joint. These common benign tumors are usually associated with inflammatory or degenerative arthritis. They are most commonly found on the extensor surface of the foot. If the lesion is painful, it can be treated by aspiration. If this is not successful, surgical excision of the sac and its stalk is indicated.

Intraosseous ganglia are commonly found in the foot, particularly in the tarsal bones and the talus. Radiographically these lesions are well-circumscribed, round lucent defects in the subchondral bone. Patients usually present with complaints of pain and treatment consists of curettage and bone grafting of the lesion.

Nonossifying fibromas are reported to occur in up to 30 percent of children and adolescents with the peak incidence in the second decade. These lesions are usually asymptomatic except when associated with a pathologic fracture. Radiographically, these lesions appear in the metaphyseal area and have a sclerotic border. Over time, these lesions consolidate.

Subungual exostosis is a small osteochondroma or bone spur of the distal phalanx, below the nail. This condition is best treated by resection of the lesion.

METASTATIC BONE TUMORS

Metastatic bone disease is very rare in the foot. When it does occur, it is most commonly secondary to bronchiogenic carcinoma of the lung. Radiographically, theses metastatic lesions are lytic and produce a periosteal elevation. With any metastatic lesion, treatment is first directed toward the primary tumor and then toward the metastatic lesion.

MISCELLANEOUS MALIGNANCIES

Synovial cell sarcoma is the most common sarcoma of the foot and accounts for almost half of all foot sarcomas. *Clear cell sarcomas* can also be found in the foot. Both these sarcomas present as soft tissue masses which invade the surrounding tissue. These tumors have a high rate of metastasis and despite amputation, these tumors carry a very poor prognosis.

Malignant melanoma is frequently seen in the lower extremity and is most frequently found on the plantar surface of the foot. It is the most common malignant lesion of the foot. Women are affected almost twice as commonly as men, with a peak incidence in the fourth and fifth decades. The lesion should be differentiated from benign nevi. The depth of invasion of the lesion is the most important prognostic indicator. If the lesion is on the toe, an amputation is required, and when the lesion is in other areas of the foot, wide excision is recommended. Lymph node dissection is recommended for melanomas of intermediate thickness. Adjuvant therapy is used to treat the systemic spread of the tumor.

SUGGESTED READINGS

Enzinger FM, Weiss SW: *Soft Tissue Tumors*, 3d ed. St. Louis, MO: Mosby-Year Book; 1995.

Johnston JO: Tumors and metabolic diseases of the foot. In Mann RA, Coughlin MJ (eds): *Surgery of the Foot and Ankle*, vol 2, 6th ed. St. Louis, MO: CV Mosby; 1993:991.

Murari TM, Callaghan JJ, Berrey BH Jr, et al: Primary benign and malignant osseous neoplasms of the foot. *Foot Ankle* 1989; 10:68.

Chapter 129

THE DIABETIC FOOT

Donna J. Astion

The American Diabetic Association estimates there are 14,000,000 diabetics in the United States. It is also estimated that 20 to 25 percent of all hospital admissions of diabetic patients are foot-related problems and that 50 percent of all nontraumatic amputations in the United States (approximately 50,000 per year) are performed in patients with diabetes. Amputation in the diabetic population is performed for reasons such as multiple ulceration, neuropathy, infection, gangrene, and ischemia. Because diabetes affects many systems throughout the body, the diabetic patient often requires care by internists, endocrinologists, urologists, orthopaedic surgeons, vascular surgeons, and infectious disease doctors, as well as prosthetists, orthotists, and physical therapists. One of the most effective ways to lower the incidence of diabetic foot problems is to educate these patients at risk and provide them with resources to minimize their risk of developing foot problems. In short, treatment must be directed towards preventing and managing the complications of diabetes in the foot.

PATHOPHYSIOLOGY

PERIPHERAL NEUROPATHY

Peripheral neuropathy is the most common cause of diabetic foot and ankle pathology. It is estimated that 60 percent of the diabetic population has polyneuropathy, and this often coexists with peripheral vascular disease. Distal symmetric polyneuropathy is the most common. This neuropathy typically affects the lower extremities first and all components of the nerves (sensory, motor, and autonomic) are usually affected.

Sensory neuropathy is the primary cause of unrecognized injuries in the foot and ankle of diabetic patients. The signs and symptoms of sensory neuropathy are variable, but the earliest losses are usually vibratory sense and proprioception. Some patients may have numbness or paresthesias while other patients may experience burning or dysesthesia. Ulcerations on the plantar surfaces of the foot are caused by this sensory neuropathy, along with the repetitive trauma of standing and walking. These ulcerations usually occur in areas of high pressure concentration such as bony prominences or external points of pressure. Dorsal foot ulcerations are usually produced by external pressure, usually from a shoe.

Autonomic neuropathy is thought to be an important risk factor for the development of Charcot arthropathy in the diabetic foot. The autonomic system is responsible for the control of thermoregulation in the limbs, eccrine and apocrine gland function, and vascular control in the arteries. Patients with autonomic neuropathy have abnormal sweating in the extremities, loss of the normal hyperemic response, and loss of the limbs' thermoregulation.

Diabetic motor neuropathy can involve only a single nerve or multiple nerves. The common peroneal nerve is often involved and in the severe cases, the patients may develop a foot drop. Motor neuropathy which causes weakness of the intrinsic muscles of the foot can lead to clawtoe deformities, depression of the metatarsal heads, and increased pressure beneath the metatarsal heads. These areas of increased pressure can lead to skin ulcerations plantarly below the metatarsal heads or dorsally at the proximal interphalangeal (PIP) joints.

VASCULOPATHY

Vascular disease is about 30 times more common among diabetics when compared to the general population. In additon, atherosclerotic disease is more common, more diffuse, and more severe in the diabetic patient population. On radiographs, calcifications along the length of the arteries are often seen, and proximal large vessel occlusion often leads to distal ischemia. Endarterectomies and proximal bypasses are often helpful to assist in the salvage of ischemic foot lesions. Diabetic patients can also develop atherosclerotic disease at or distal to the popliteal trifurcation. In these cases, distal bypass or dilations are often helpful. Some authors discuss "microvascular disease" of diabetes while others contest existence of this entity. Many recent studies have not supported the presence of microvascular disease in the diabetic population.

EVALUATION

The orthopaedic evaluation of the foot and ankle in patients with diabetes should include a vascular examination. Each diabetic patient with a serious infection or ischemia of the foot requires a vascular evaluation to determine the adequacy of the local circulation. In the diabetic patient, the key to limb salvage is aggressive vascular reconstruction and a thorough and complete debridement of any infected and necrotic tissue in the foot. Limb salvage is important to maximizing the patient's function by minimizing the amount of work necessary to ambulate. As the level of amputation becomes more proximal, oxygen consumption during ambulation increases, and the associated morbidity and mortality of the patient also increases.

Any patient with nonhealing ulcers without palpable pulses requires a vascular evaluation. To heal a diabetic foot ulcer, a Doppler ratio of 0.45 or greater is necessary. It is important to remember that Doppler arterial pressure readings may be falsely elevated by arterial calcifications. The patients with an arterial brachial index > 1 will usually have an abnormally high Doppler arterial reading. Some recent studies have shown that absolute toe arterial pressures rather than ratios are more predictive of distal wound healing. A minimal toe pressure of 40 to 50mmHg is necessary for healing while lower pressures may warrant revascularization procedures.

Many anatomic changes seen radiographically due to diabetes can mimic other conditions. With this in mind it is important to clinically correlate any abnormality observed on imaging studies.

FOOT AND ANKLE ULCERS

On initial presentation, all diabetic foot ulcers need to be assessed for the depth of the ulcer and the presence of infection. The devitalized tissue should be debrided and radiographs should be obtained to detect foreign bodies, soft tissue gas, or bony abnormalities. The Wagner classification can be used to quantitate the depth of the diabetic foot ulcers (Fig. 129-1). In the grade 0 ulcer, the skin is intact. If a superficial ulceration with exposed subcutaneous tissue is present, then the ulcer is grade I. Grade II ulcers are those with exposed tendons and exposed deep structures, and grade III ulcers extend into deep tissues and include those with evidence of infection along the midfoot compartments, or osteomyelitis. With grade IV or V ulcers, the foot is devascular and gangrenous tissue is present. The depth and size of the ulceration, as well as anatomic location of the ulceration, affects the outcome. In general, forefoot lesions have a lower mortality rate and a greater incidence of limb salvage while more proximal lesions have a lower incidence of limb salvage.

Not all neuropathic foot ulcers become infected. Those that are infected usually present with local inflammation, purulent drainage, sinus tract formation or crepitus. Two-thirds of patients with limb-threatening infections do not have fevers, chills, or leukocytosis. Hyperglycemia is the most common sign of limb or life-threatening infections in the diabetic population. Erythema, swelling, and warmth in a nonulcerated foot may be due to infection or Charcot disease. While the presence of osteomyelitis can be determined by plain radiograph, MRI is the most sensitive and the most specific examination.

To effectively treat foot ulcers, pressure must be eliminated from the ulcer area. Plantar ulcers are ususally the result of abnormal weightbearing while dorsal ulcers are usually the result of ill-fitting shoes. Pressure relief on the ulcer area can often be accomplished with shoe modifications, orthotics, total contact casting, nonweightbearing, and bedrest. Diabetic ulcers which fail to heal due to excessive internal bony pressure may require excision of the bony prominence if external measures fail. Prior to undertaking any surgery, patients should undergo a vascular evaluation to determine the vascular supply of the foot. If a patient requires an amputation, the level of the amputation, the patient's nutritional status, and his or her abil-

ity to combat infection and to heal the wound postoperatively must be taken into account. Effective healing can be expected in patients with Doppler indices greater than 0.45 at the level of amputation.

Patients who have healed ulcers are at greater risk for repeated ulceration. These patients require education in lifelong footcare as well as prescription footwear and periodic callous and nailcare. Patients should be educated to avoid the preventable causes of ulceration and instructed to inspect their feet regularly. These patients should wear shoes which accommodate any deformity and provide cushioning at any point of contact between the foot and shoe. In addition, cushioned socks can aid in reducing pressure, and extra depth shoes with cushioned molded insoles or rigid rocker soles can be prescribed in appropriate cases.

NEUROPATHIC OR CHARCOT FRACTURES

Charcot joints are those joints destroyed from abnormalities extrinsic to the joint itself. It is estimated that Charcot fractures occur in 0.05 to 0.1 percent of diabetic patients. The etiology of Charcot joints in a patient with a sensory neuropathy may be due to fracture and destruction of the joint as the result of continued and unrecognized mechanical trauma. Others believe that the Charcot joint is due to resorption and, therefore, weakening of the bone from a neurally stimulated vascular reflux.

Charcot arthropathy can present as a slow gradual painful joint collapse with minimal or no swelling but, more commonly, patients experience the rapid onset of swelling and erythema, with mild pain. On physical examination, the foot is warm and swollen, and the pulses are intact. In the early stages of Charcot arthropathy, the radiographs may appear normal. In these cases, it is difficult to exclude gout and cellulitis from the differential diagnosis. Radiographic changes begin with osteopenia and progress to periarticular fragmentation of bone and joint dislocations (Fig. 129-2). It is often difficult to rule out osteomyelitis or septic arthritis in those cases where radiographs show mixed bony reactions of fragmentation with repair. One of the pathognomonic radiographic changes seen in a Charcot joint is bone particles embedded within the synovium. Often, combined technetium and indium scans are helpful in differentiating Charcot arthropathy from osteomyelitis or septic arthritis.

Charcot arthropathy can be seen in the midfoot, the hindfoot, or the ankle. Patients who have Charcot arthropathy in the midfoot often develop a rocker bottom deformity with severe midfoot valgus

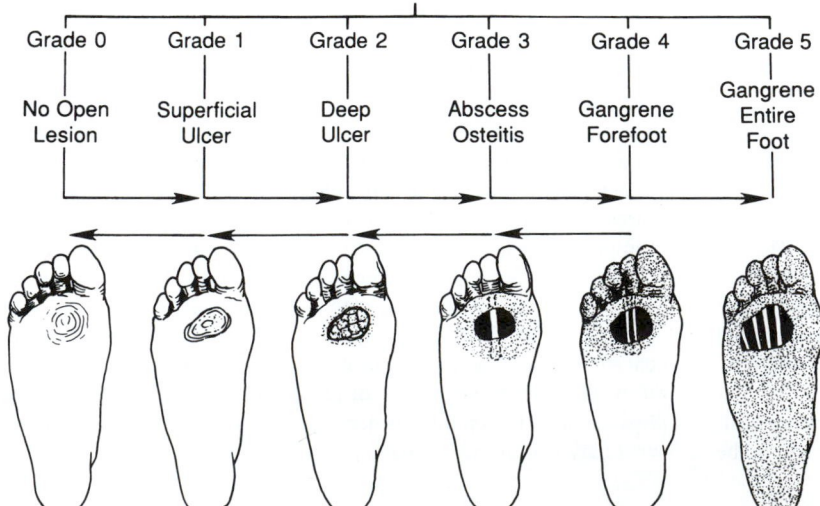

ORIGINAL RANCHO LOS AMIGOS HOSPITAL CLASSIFICATION

Grade 0	Grade 1	Grade 2	Grade 3	Grade 4	Grade 5
No Open Lesion	Superficial Ulcer	Deep Ulcer	Abscess Osteitis	Gangrene Forefoot	Gangrene Entire Foot

Figure 129-1
Wagner and Meggitt's original Ranchos Los Amigos classification of diabetic foot lesions. (Reproduced with permission from Brodsky JW: The diabetic foot. In: *Surgery of the Foot and Ankle.* St. Louis, MO: Mosby-Year Book; 1993:894.)

Figure 129-2
Lateral radiograph of a diabetic patient with a Charcot fracture of the midfoot.

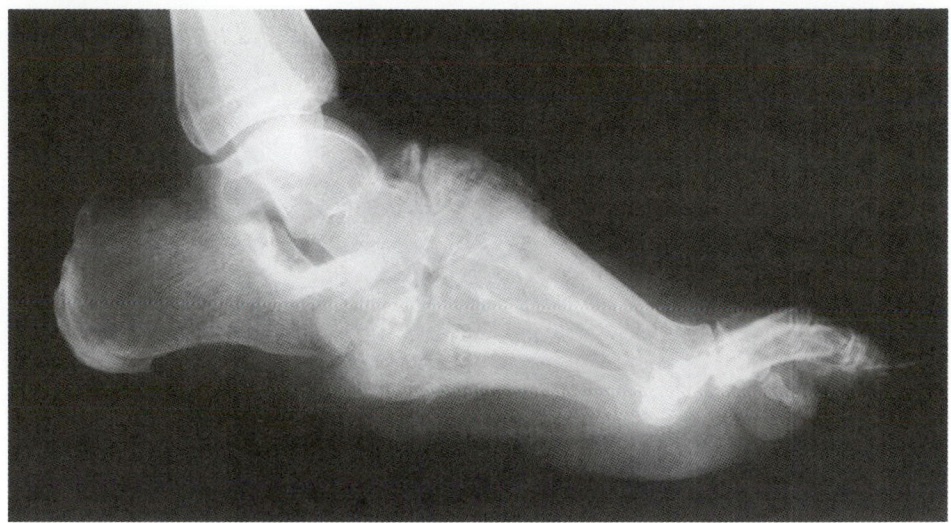

(Fig. 129-2). Bony prominences can cause increased pressure along the plantar aspect of the foot, and these patients frequently develop plantar ulcerations. Patients with hindfoot arthropathy may develop a progressive flat foot deformity. While patients with hindfoot arthropathy usually do not have problems with ulcerations, they often have difficulty fitting into normal shoes because of the persistent enlargement of the hindfoot after the fracture has healed. Patients with ankle arthropathy may develop a varus or valgus deformity of the ankle. These patients may have difficulty with ulcerations and joint stability.

In general, Charcot arthropathy can be treated nonoperatively with long periods of immobilization. Patients who present with a Charcot arthropathy should be treated first with elevation, restricted weight-bearing and casting. After the period of acute inflammation has subsided (about 8 weeks), patients may be allowed to bear weight on the limb in a brace or cast. Once the fracture has healed and the foot is stable, the patient may be advanced to a plastizote-lined ankle-foot orthosis or a custom-molded shoe with an insole. It may take 6 months to 2 years for the patient to advance to these less restrictive types of orthotic devices. While some authors advocate surgery to correct non-braceable deformities, complications and nonunion rates are extremely high in this patient population, and amputations are sometimes required. Charcot fractures occur in diabetic patients with peripheral neuropathy in the absence of overt trauma.

SUGGESTED READINGS

Brodsky JW: Outpatient diagnosis and care of the diabetic foot. In Heckman JD (ed): *Instructional Course Lectures.* Rosemont, IL: American Academy of Orthopaedic Surgeons; 1993; 42:121.

Caputo GM, Cavanagh PR, Ulbrecht JS, et al: Assessment and management of foot disease in patients with diabetes. *N Engl J Med* 1994; 331:854.

Clohisy DR, Thompson RC Jr: Fractures associated with neuropathic arthropathy in adults who have juvenile-onset diabetes. *J Bone Joint Surg [Am]* 1988; 70:1192.

Crandall RC, Wagner FW Jr: Partial and total calcanectomy: A review of thirty-one consecutive cases over a ten-year period. *J Bone Joint Surg [Am]* 1981; 63:152.

Duckworth T, Boulton AJ, Betts RP, et al: Plantar pressure measurements and the prevention of ulceration in the diabetic foot. *J Bone Joint Surg [Br]* 1985; 67:79.

Gould JS, Erickson SJ, Collier BD, et al: Surgical management of ulcers, soft-tissue infections, and osteomyelitis in the diabetic foot. In Heckman JD (ed): *Instructional Course Lectures.* Rosemont, IL: American Academy of Orthopaedic Surgeons; 1993; 42:147.

Harrelson JM: The diabetic foot: Charcot arthropathy. *Instructional Course Lectures* 1993: 42:141.

Larsson U, Andersson GBJ: Partial amputation of the foot for diabetic or arteriosclerotic gangrene: Results and factors of prognostic value. *J Bone Joint Surg [Br]* 1978; 60:126.

LoGerfo FW, Coffman JD: Current concepts: Vascular and microvascular disease of the foot in diabetes: Implications for foot care. *N Engl J Med* 1984; 311:1615.

McDermott JE: The diabetic foot: Diagnosis and prevention. In Heckman JD (ed): *Instructional Course Lectures.* Rosemont, IL: American Academy of Orthopaedic Surgeons; 1993; 42:117.

McDermott JE: The diabetic foot: Evolving techniques. In Heckman JD (ed): *Instructional Course Lectures.* Rosemont, IL: American Academy of Orthopaedic Surgeons; 1993; 42:169.

Papa J, Myerson M, Girard P: Salvage, with arthrodesis, in intractable diabetic neuropathic arthropathy of the foot and ankle. *J Bone Joint Surg [Am]* 1993; 75:1056.

Waters RL, Perry J, Antonelli DEE, et al: Energy cost of walking of amputees: The influence of level of amputation. *J Bone Joint Surg [Am]* 1976; 58:42.

Chapter 130

OSTEOCHONDROSIS

David S. Feldman

Osteochondrosis is classically defined as a disease of the growth or ossification centers in a child which begins as a degeneration or necrosis followed by regeneration or recalcification. There are a number of disease processes that fit this definition and they represent ailments of varied etiologies and clinical manifestations. The clinical problems occurring from osteochondrosis depend on whether the involved bone and cartilage is part of a joint, physis, or apophysis. Osteochondrosis of the femoral head (Legg-Calvés-Perthes Disease), proximal medial physis of the tibia (Blount's Disease), carpal lunate (Keinböck's disease), and spine (Scheuermann's disease) will be discussed in separate sections (Fig. 130-1).

OSGOOD-SCHLATTER DISEASE

Osgood-Schlatter disease is common and affects young adolescents between the ages of 10 and 15 years of age. It is a traction apophysitis of the tibial tubercle, caused either by multiple subacute fractures of the tibial tubercle or from inflammation at the tendon insertion. Pain in the knee is the presenting symptom, mainly after participating in sporting activities. Children may also complain of pain when ascending or descending stairs as well as on kneeling.

The physical exam is very specific. Point tenderness can be elicited over the tibial tubercle. There may or may not be a prominence of the tubercle. There should be no joint effusion or pain elsewhere in the knee, and the range of motion should be nearly full. Radiographs of the knee are the only imaging studies required and may demonstrate fragmentation of the apophysis as well as calcification in the insertion of the patella tendon.

Treatment consists of modification of activities. The children should decrease their jumping activities such as basketball and volleyball and place ice on the tubercle after sports. Quadriceps strengthening and stretching is helpful. There is no need for prolonged immobilization or steroid injections. Osgood-Schlatter is most often a self-limited disease that requires months or up to a year to resolve.

SINDING-LARSEN-JOHANSSON SYNDROME

Sinding-Larsen-Johansson syndrome (SLJ) is either an apophysitis of the distal pole of the patella or small repeated tears of the patella tendon attachment onto the distal pole of the patella with secondary calcification. SLJ presents with symptoms similar to that of adult jumper's knee and Osgood Schlatter disease. The children, usually young adolescents and usually between the ages of 10 and 15 years, present with knee pain after participating in sports and while stair climbing and kneeling.

On physical examination the children have tenderness over the distal pole of the patella and the proximal portion of the patella tendon. There should be no knee effusion. SLJ may coexist with Osgood-

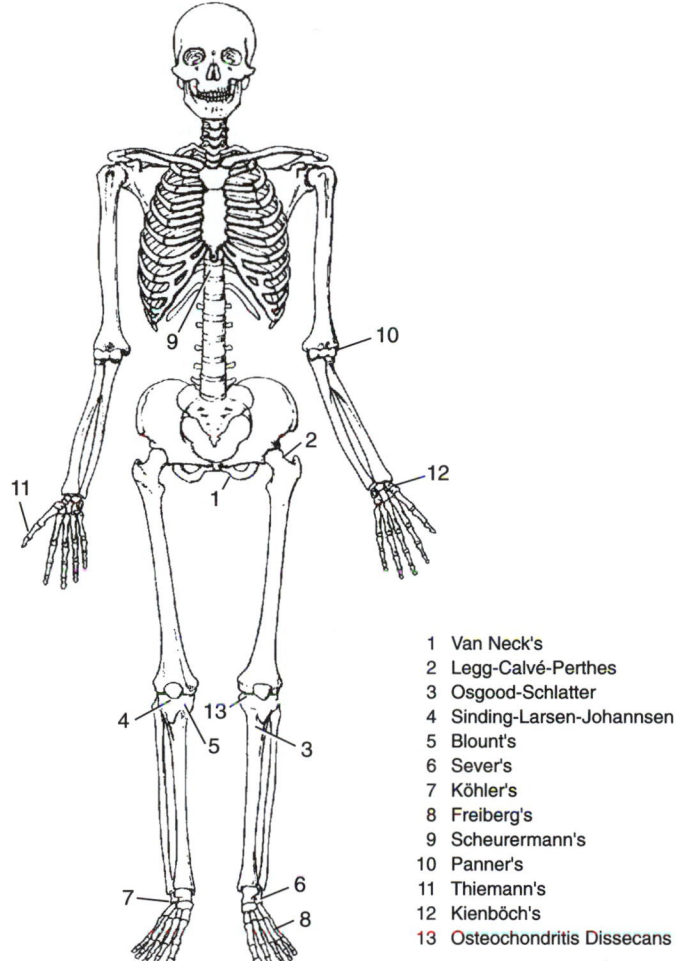

Figure 130-1
Common sites of osteochondrosis. (Reproduced and modified with permission from Miller MD: Basic sciences. In *Review of Orthopaedics.* Philadelphia: WB Saunders; 1992:71.)

1 Van Neck's
2 Legg-Calvé-Perthes
3 Osgood-Schlatter
4 Sinding-Larsen-Johannsen
5 Blount's
6 Sever's
7 Köhler's
8 Freiberg's
9 Scheurermann's
10 Panner's
11 Thiemann's
12 Kienböck's
13 Osteochondritis Dissecans

Schlatter disease but otherwise the rest of the knee should be asymptomatic. Treatment is the same as that for Osgood-Schlatter disease.

SEVER'S DISEASE

Sever's disease, or calcaneal apophysitis, is a traction apophysitis at the insertion of the achilles tendon. The patients present with heel pain, particularly with ambulation, and it occurs more often in children who are overweight. The diagnosis is made on clinical exam (i.e., tenderness directly over the posterior aspect of the calcaneus).

Radiographs are helpful only in ruling out other pathology of the heel (see below) such as a neoplasm. The calcaneal apophysis in most children not suffering from Sever's disease is irregular, fragmented, and sclerotic and therefore the diagnosis is not a radiographic one. Treatment consists of a heel lift and a soft heel cushion. This is a self-limited disease that resolves usually in a few months to a year after onset.

KÖHLER'S DISEASE

Köhler's disease or osteochondrosis of the tarsal navicular is a condition that affects young children, usually below the age of 6. The children may have an acute onset of pain in the medial aspect of the foot. There is point tenderness overlying the navicular. Radiographically, there is fragmentation of the navicular. Treatment consists of a short leg walking cast for 6 weeks, or in less severe cases a medial longitudinal arch may relieve symptoms. Köhler's disease is self-limited and may require 1 year until symptoms completely resolve. There are no long-term sequelae of this disease. Eventually, the navicular will reconstitute itself.

FREIBERG'S INFARCTION

Osteochondrosis of the second metatarsal head has been termed Freiberg's infarction. This disease presents as a painful forefoot in adolescence. There is tenderness directly over the second metatarsal head and limitation of motion of the metatarsal-phalangeal joint. Radiographs demonstrate an irregular, flattened, and large second metatarsal head and irregularity of the physis. Treatment consists of relieving the pressure on the second metatarsal head, as with casting or a metatarsal bar. Surgical intervention is reserved for those severe cases that have failed all nonoperative attempts at treatment. Surgery may range from re-establishing the contour of the second metatarsal head to excising the head or proximal phalanx.

OSTEOCHONDRITIS DISSECANS

Osteochondritis dissecans (OCD) affects many joints. It routinely affects the convex surface of the joint, such as the femoral condyle

of the knee (Fig. 130-2), dome of the talus in the ankle, and femoral head in the hip. Although called osteochondritis, inflammation is not involved in the pathologic process. OCD is characterized by avascular insufficiency of the subchondral bone. The etiology may be due to repetitive trauma; however, most are idiopathic. The signs and symptoms vary from mild aches to severe pain with a joint effusion and locking. The effect of the vascular compromise to the area has varied results on the overlying cartilage, ranging from mild softening to fibrillation to frank disruption of the articular fragment. Often treatment will depend on the status of the fragment (i.e., attached versus detached) as well as the age of the child on presentation.

OCD OF THE ELBOW: PANNER'S DISEASE

Panner's disease is an osteochondrosis of the capitellum that usually occurs in overhead throwing athletes. It presents with a painful elbow, particularly with throwing, and may be associated with swelling and locking of the elbow. The cause of the disorder is unknown, but it is associated with repetitive trauma. The age of presentation is the single most important factor in determining prognosis. Before the age of 10, although the capitellum may appear fragmented on plain radiographs, an osteochondral fracture or flap is very unlikely. In adolescents, however, fragmentation of the articular cartilage may occur and cause locking or early osteoarthritis. Therefore, in young children with this problem, restriction of overhead throwing and other forceful upper extremity activities, along with ice and anti-inflammatory medication, is the treatment of choice. The use of a sling in the acute phase maybe helpful as well.

The treatment of the older child and adolescent depends on the state of the articular cartilage. The cartilage can best be assessed with magnetic resonance imaging (MRI). The MRI can demonstrate a flap or a loose fragment in the joint. Elbow arthroscopy or arthrotomy are indicated if there is a loose fragment in the joint or if there is an os-

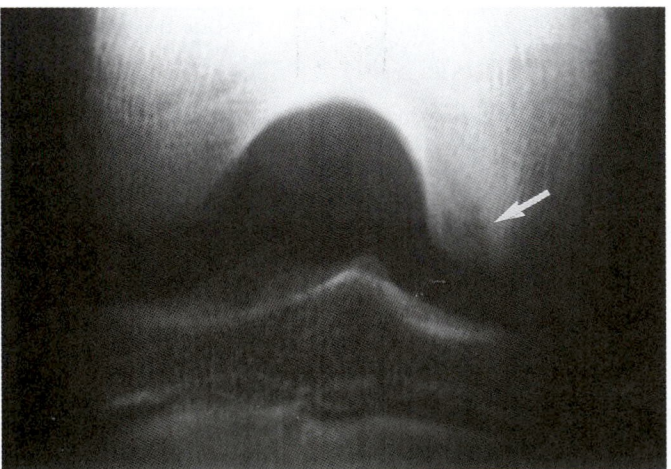

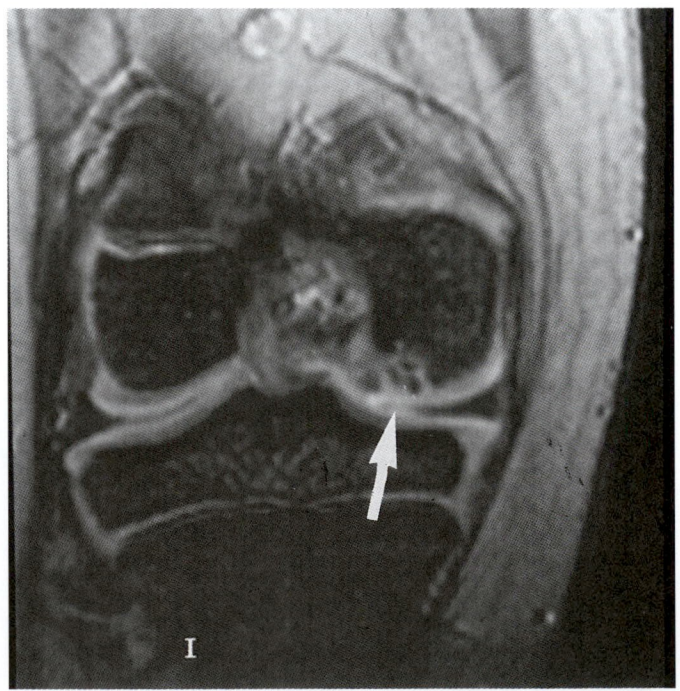

A

B

Figure 130-2
Osteochondrosis of the medial femoral condyle in 9-year-old child (*A*). MRI demonstrates intact articular cartilage with underlying osteochondrosis (*B*).

teochondral flap. The older child with this advanced stage of disease often cannot return to competitive athletics if it involves throwing. Prevention of this disorder is paramount. Training in the mechanics of throwing should be emphasized in young throwing athletes. Also, children and adolescents should be limited to only a few innings of pitching every week.

OCD OF THE KNEE

In the knee OCD most commonly affects the lateral portion of the medial femoral condyle, the posterior aspect of the lateral femoral condyle, and the patella. Care should be utilized in attributing the knee pain to the lesion seen on radiographs. Oftentimes, patients can have radiograph findings of OCD but be completely asymptomatic. The clinician should be alert for other pathology, such as in the hip, that is causing symptoms around the knee.

Evaluation with plain radiographs, including a tunnel view, is useful. MRI will demonstrate the state of the articular cartilage as well as the healing of the lesion.

Treatment of the disease depends on the age and skeletal maturity of the patient as well as the status of the fragment. Patients with intact overlying cartilage should be treated symptomatically with modification of activity, anti-inflammatory medication, and possibly a trial of short-term immobilization. A loose fragment or free fragment in the joint should be treated operatively and fixed in place if possible. Skeletally immature patients rarely require surgery for fragments that have not become loose, and have a good overall prognosis. Older patients with persistent pain without a loose fragment may benefit from in-situ pinning to aid revascularization or using bioresorbable pins such as polyactic acid (PLA). The older patients have a more guarded prognosis particularly with a free large fragment that cannot be fixed. These patients have a poor prognosis and some authors have recommended osteoarticular allografts for the treatment of these large symptomatic lesions or, if possible, the use of autologous osteochondral plugs from nonweightbearing areas of the knee. Long-term results of this treatment are not yet known.

OCD OF THE TALUS

OCD of the talus occurs usually either posteromedially or laterally. Nonoperative treatment consisting of limitation of activities, icing, and a trial of immobilization is the initial treatment of choice. If there is locking of the ankle or persistent pain with a cartilaginous flap demonstrated on MRI, then surgical intervention is necessary. Either arthroscopic pinning, if possible, or debridement of the lesion aiding revascularization are the treatments of choice.

SUGGESTED READINGS

Ogden JA, Southwick WO: Osgood-Schlatter's disease and tibial tuberosity development. *Clin Orthop* 1976; 116:180.

Ruch DS, Poehling GG: Arthroscopic treatment of Panner's disease. *Clin Sports Med* 1991; 10(3):629.

Siffert RS: Classification of the osteochondroses. *Clin Orthop* 1981; 158:10.

Woolfrey BF, Chandler EF: Manifestations of Osgood-Schlatter's disease in late teen age and early adulthood. *J Bone Joint Surg [Am]* 1960; 42:327.

Chapter 131

SKELETAL DYSPLASIAS

David S. Feldman

CLASSIFICATION

Skeletal dysplasias (chondrodysplasias) are a heterogeneous group of disorders that result in numerous orthopaedic abnormalities. The majority of the dysplasias, of which there are over 120 different types, result in dwarfism, in which the standing height is below the third percentile. In general, the hereditary intrinsic skeletal dysplasias cause *disproportionate* dwarfism, in which only the limbs or the trunk are shortened. In the types of dwarfism that primarily affect the limbs, the shortening may predominate in the proximal segments (rhizomelia), the middle segments (mesomelia), or the distal segments (acromelia). *Proportionate* dwarfism generally results from chromosomal, endocrine, nutritional, or nonosseous abnormalities.

Most cases of dwarfism are the result of a spontaneous mutation. Intelligence is normal in nearly all types of dwarfism. Exceptions include hypochondroplasia and the mucopolysaccharidoses.

ACHONDROPLASIA

Achondroplasia, which occurs in approximately 1 of 40,000 persons, is the most common and best-known type of dwarfism. It is transmitted by a single autosomal dominant gene, and results in abnormal endochondral bone formation. About 80 to 90 percent of cases are the result of a spontaneous mutation. The cause of achondroplasia is a point mutation in the gene coding for fibroblast growth factor receptor 3. This mutation causes a single amino acid change (arginine to glycine) in the transmembrane portion of this cell surface receptor, the function of which is not yet known. There has been an association identified with elevated paternal age (>36 years of age at time of conception).

CLINICAL FEATURES

The characteristic signs of achondroplasia are present at birth: disproportionate short stature, a normal to relatively long trunk, and rhizomelic shortening of the limbs. These patients have relatively large heads, with frontal and sometimes parietal bossing, a flat or depressed nasal bridge, and button noses (Fig. 131-1). Recurrent and chronic middle ear infections are common in infancy and early childhood and may lead to significant hearing loss.

Growth rate is normal in the first year of life, then drops to the third percentile. Adult height generally reaches anywhere from 42 to 52 in. Gross motor milestones are delayed, and patients should be evaluated against standards developed for children with achondroplasia. Motor skills are delayed because of hypotonia, ligamentous laxity, and the physical difficulties posed by a large head and short limbs. Cognitive skills are generally not delayed.

Initially, the legs appear straight but with ambulation may develop a bowleg deformity (genu varum) with or without back knee (genu recurvatum). The hands and feet may appear large in relation to the limbs, but the digits are short, broad, and stubby (brachydactyly). The short fingers are typically held in three groups, producing the classic trident hand. The arms are generally short, with the fingertips reaching only to the level of the trochanters. Elbow extension is restricted to 30 to 45 degrees, but this has little functional significance. The chest tends to be flat and broad and the abdomen and buttocks protuberant. Excessive lumbar lordosis and a tilted pelvis cause a waddling gait, and fixed flexion contractures of the hip appear early. In a sitting position, infants commonly exhibit thoracolumbar kyphosis. This kyphosis is related to a variety of factors, including ligamentous laxity and hypotonia. The kyphosis usually disappears once the child begins to walk.

Neurologic complications are common. The growth of the foramen magnum is severely impaired in the first year of life, resulting in compression of the medulla and cervical spinal cord. This can lead to apnea, paralysis of voluntary respiration, and compressive myelopathy at the level of the foramen magnum. Sudden infant death syndrome has been reported at an increased incidence. At older ages, stenosis of the lumbar spine, prolapse of intervertebral discs, osteophytes, and deformed vertebral bodies may also compress the spinal cord and/or nerve roots. Slowly progressive symptoms, such as paraesthesias, weakness, pain, and paraplegia, may develop by the teenage years. Muscle weakness and foot drop may also develop.

RADIOGRAPHIC FINDINGS

Although virtually all bones of the body are affected, the abnormal configuration of the skull, lumbar spine, and pelvis are hallmarks for this disease. The skull is large with a relatively small base. A diagnostic hallmark is a decrease of the interpedicular distance in a caudad direction in the lumbar spine (normally, the interpedicular distance increases in the caudad direction). A thoracolumbar kyphosis is present in infancy, and is replaced by an exaggerated lumbar lordosis with ambulation. The pelvis is short and broad with short, square iliac wings ("champagne glass" configuration). All tubular bones are short, with metaphyseal flaring. The distal femoral physis may look like an "inverted V".

TREATMENT

Nonoperative management consists of weight loss, which is a general problem for these patients, bracing for scoliosis, and exercises. Surgical management includes *spinal decompression,* which may be required at a young age, and fusion for kyphosis greater than 60 degrees; osteotomies and epiphysiodesis may also be needed to correct genu varum. Limb lengthening, which has been performed extensively in Italy and the former USSR, remains a controversial area.

HYPOCHONDROPLASIA

For many years, hypochondroplasia was considered a mild or atypical form of achondroplasia. It is also inherited as an autosomal dominant trait, with most cases appearing to be sporadic. About 10 percent of patients are mentally retarded.

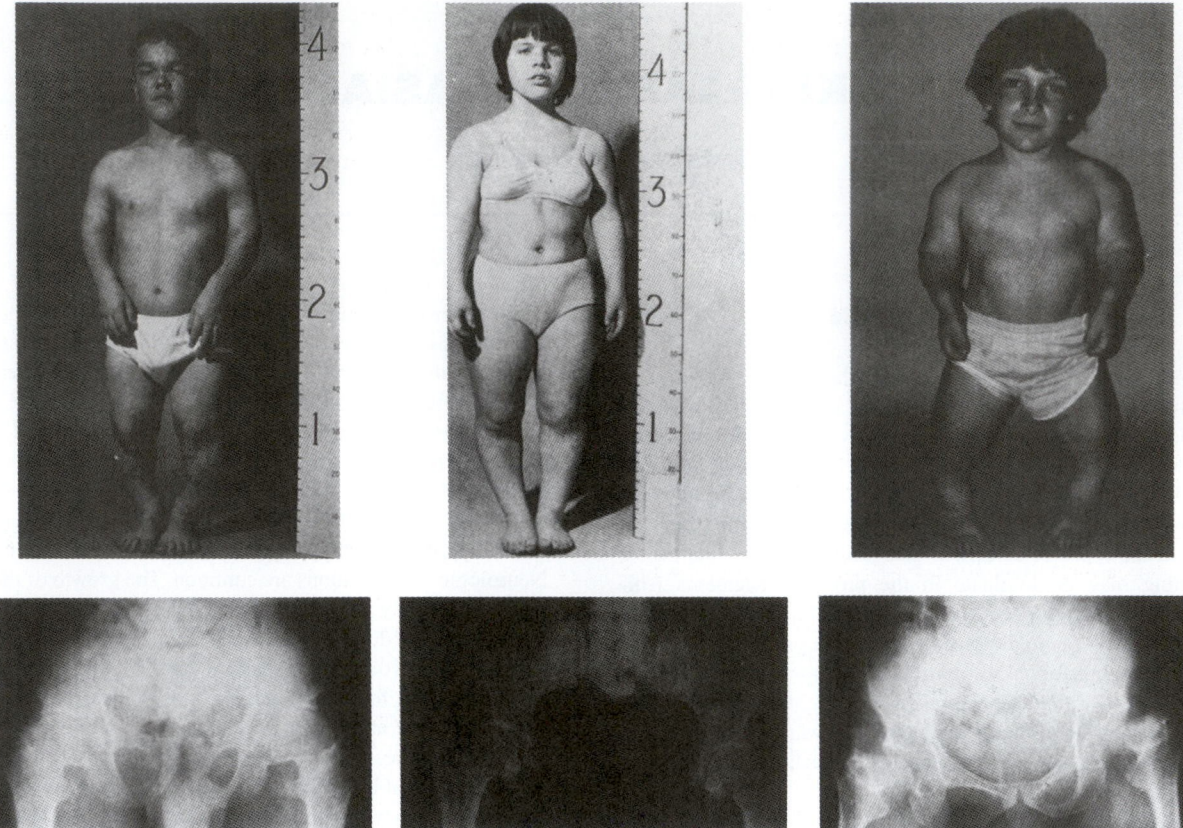

Figure 131-1

Clinical appearance and pelvic radiographs of patients with three related forms of skeletal dysplasia. *(Left)* Achondroplasia is characterized by rhizomelic short-limbed short stature, abnormal facies, short iliac wings, horizontal acetabula without early hip arthritis, and an adult height of 4 feet. *(Center)* Hypochondroplasia is characterized by an adult height of about 4.5 feet, normal facies, and minimal radiologic changes in the pelvis. *(Right)* Pseudoachondroplasia is characterized by short-limbed short stature with limb deformities, normal facies, and severe early dysplasia of the hips. (Reproduced by permission of Beals RK, Horton W: Skeletal dysplasias: An approach to diagnosis. *J Am Acad Orthop Surg* 1995; 3:175.)

CLINICAL FEATURES

Birth weight and length may be low normal. Head circumference is normal. The face, unlike that of achondroplasia, is normal with no midfacial hypoplasia or depression of the nasal bridge. The short stature may not be recognized until the patient is 2 or 3 years of age. In general, patients may achieve an adult height of 52 to 59 in. which is much taller than the achondroplast. The trunk is disproportionately long with relatively short limbs (Fig. 131-1). There may be some mild bowleg deformity that generally disappears with ambulation. Ligamentous laxity is mild, and the short fingers do not have a trident configuration as seen in achondroplasia.

The trunk shows a less exaggerated lumbar lordosis than in achondroplasia. Neurologic complications are much less frequent than in achondroplasia.

RADIOGRAPHIC FINDINGS

Thorough radiographic examination allows differentiation from achondroplasia. The skull is essentially normal, except for some mild bossing of the forehead. There is generalized shortening of the long bones with mild metaphyseal flaring. The femoral necks are short and broad, and the pelvis may be normal or mildly dysplastic. The vertebral bodies are of normal height (Fig. 131-1).

DIASTROPHIC DYSPLASIA

Diastrophic dysplasia is a rare short-limbed condition transmitted as an autosomal recessive trait. The disease is due to a defect in a gene on the long arm of chromosome 5, which codes for a novel sulfate transporter.

CLINICAL FEATURES

Like achondroplasia, this disorder is recognizable at birth. The head appears normal, but there is a characteristic circumoral fullness. The voice is typically soft. The nasal bridge is narrow, with broad, flared nostrils. More than 50 percent of patients have cleft or other abnormalities of the palate. In 80 percent of patients, the ear pinnae swell within the first six weeks after birth, with subsequent calcification and ossification, resulting in the so-called "cauliflower ear."

There is rhizomelic shortening of the limbs and flexion contractures of the joints. At least 20 percent of individuals have dislocated hips by adolescence. The "hitchhiker thumb" and ankylosis of the proximal interphalangeal joint (symphalangism) are hallmark hand deformities. Severe, rigid clubfoot is typically present at birth.

There is excessive lumbar lordosis early in life. Scoliosis becomes more severe with weightbearing and leads to trunk deformity and barrel chest. Spinal deformities include thoracolumbar kyphoscoliosis, severe cervical kyphosis, and odontoid hypoplasia with atlantoaxial instability.

RADIOGRAPHIC FINDINGS

The tubular bones are short and broad with flared metaphyses. Epiphyseal development is delayed, and this leads to joint deformities. The ulnas and fibulas are disproportionately short. The femoral heads have a saucer-shaped defect in the central weightbearing portion. Cervical spina bifida is uniformly present.

PSEUDOACHONDROPLASIA

Pseudoachondroplastic dysplasia was for many years confused with achondroplasia. It is also transmitted as an autosomal dominant disorder, but is not clinically apparent at birth. The cause of this disorder is a mutation in the calmodulinlike calcium-binding region of the gene coding for cartilage oligomeric matrix protein (COMP), which is present in the territorial matrix of cartilage.

CLINICAL FEATURES

Growth retardation is usually not apparent until the child is 2 or 3 years old. As the growth rate slows, the typical habitus of long trunk, lumbar lordosis, and rhizomelic shortening of the limbs develops (Fig. 131-1). Unlike achondroplasia, the cranium and face have a normal appearance.

Malalignment of the knees (varus, valgus, and windswept deformities), along with flexion contractures in the hips and knees, result in premature joint pain and osteoarthritis. The hands and feet are short and stubby, with marked ligamentous laxity. Pes planus also occurs. As in achondroplasia, there is limited extension of the elbow joint.

RADIOGRAPHIC FINDINGS

There are characteristic changes in the metaphyseal and epiphyseal regions of the long bones. In childhood, the small, irregular epiphyses of the femoral heads may become severely deformed and fragment by early adulthood. In the spine, there is moderate flattening of the vertebral bodies (platyspondyly) with central, anterior tonguelike projections. There is no narrowing of the interpedicular distances in the lumbar spine, as seen in achondroplasia. Odontoid hypoplasia with resultant atlantoaxial instability may be present.

SPONDYLOEPIPHYSEAL DYSPLASIA CONGENITA

Spondyloepiphyseal dysplasia congenita is an entity that results in short-limb disproportionate dwarfism. Although transmitted as an autosomal dominant trait, most cases are the result of a spontaneous mutation.

CLINICAL FEATURES

As infants, the head size is normal and the midface is flat. Cleft palate and wide-set eyes are other early signs. Myopia and retinal detachment occur in about 50 percent of patients, so periodic ophthalmologic examination is important. The limbs show rhizomelic and mesomelic shortening, with disproportionate shortening of the trunk and increased lumbar lordosis. Pectus carinatum, barrel chest, short neck, and scoliosis are also present.

As in achondroplasia, motor development is often delayed. In 50 percent of patients, there is hypotonia and ligamentous laxity. Odontoid hypoplasia results in atlantoaxial instability.

RADIOGRAPHIC FINDINGS

There is a generalized delay in the appearance of the primary ossification centers of the carpal and tarsal bones, as well as of the secondary ossification centers of the short and long tubular bones. The vertebral bodies become flattened and irregular with time, resulting in kyphoscoliosis. Coxa vara is common as well. Affected children are extremely susceptible to premature osteoarthritis of weightbearing joints.

SPONDYLOEPIPHYSEAL DYSPLASIA TARDA

Unlike spondyloepiphyseal dysplasia congenita, spondyloepiphyseal dysplasia tarda does not manifest until late childhood or adolescence. Many patients are initially referred for short stature, scoliosis, and hip pain. Some may be referred for what seems to be bilateral Legg-Calvé-Perthes disease. The mode of inheritance is most commonly X-linked recessive, although both autosomal dominant and autosomal recessive forms are known.

CLINICAL FEATURES

Many patients are above the third percentile for height and are thus not considered true dwarfs. The height reduction is primarily due to trunk shortening, secondary to mild platyspondyly or kyphoscoliosis, and associated exaggerated lumbar lordosis.

RADIOGRAPHIC FINDINGS

Epiphyseal involvement is observed generally in larger, more proximally located joints. As in the congenital form of the disease, there is delayed ossification of the epiphyses and a predisposition to early osteoarthritis. In the hips, coxa magna, flattening, and subluxation may resemble bilateral Legg-Calvé-Perthes' disease; however, the changes are symmetric bilaterally.

MULTIPLE EPIPHYSEAL DYSPLASIA

Multiple epiphyseal dysplasia is characterized by irregular and/or delayed ossification of multiple epiphyses. A severe form, the Fairbank type, has been distinguished from a milder form, the Ribbing type. Both are transmitted as an autosomal dominant trait, although autosomal recessive forms have been described.

CLINICAL FEATURES

The disease usually remains unrecognized until 5 to 10 years of age. Shortening of the limbs is variable, and the trunk is normal. Many patients are above the third percentile and are thus not considered truly dwarfed. Symptoms include morning stiffness, difficulty in running or climbing stairs, and a waddling gait. Valgus or varus deformities of the knees may occur. Osteoarthritis of the hips may become severe in older patients.

RADIOGRAPHIC FINDINGS

Diagnosis of the disease requires radiographs of the entire skeleton. Bilateral epiphyseal abnormalities in the hips, knees, and ankles are the chief manifestations. The ossification centers of the epiphyses appear late, and progressive joint deformities occur. The epiphyses of the femoral heads are symmetrically affected, which helps distinguish this disease from Legg-Calvé-Perthes disease.

METAPHYSEAL CHONDRODYSPLASIA

The metaphyseal chondrodysplasias are a heterogeneous group of disorders characterized by metaphyseal deformities of the tubular bones. The McKusick type and the Schmid type are the most common forms.

METAPHYSEAL CHONDRODYSPLASIA: McKUSICK TYPE

The McKusick type of this disorder is commonly known as cartilage-hair hypoplasia, as it is characterized by hypoplasia of the cartilage and small diameter of the hair shaft. It is transmitted as an autosomal recessive trait and is relatively common among the Old Order Amish population in Pennsylvania and in Finland.

CLINICAL FEATURES

At birth, weight is normal, but body length is reduced. The head and face are normal, although patients generally have sparse, light-colored hair which breaks easily. The elbows do not extend fully, but there is ligamentous laxity of the fingers and toes that permit hypermobility. There is fibular overgrowth distally, resulting in ankle deformity. Unilateral genu varum or genu valgum may be present as well. Atlantoaxial instability is common. About 10 percent of patients with the McKusick type of metaphyseal chondrodysplasia exhibit intestinal malabsorption and Hirschsprung's disease. Patients may also be unusually susceptible to chicken pox.

RADIOGRAPHIC FINDINGS

The metaphyses are widened and irregular, with sclerosis and cystic changes. The epiphyses appear normal.

METAPHYSEAL CHONDRODYSPLASIA: SCHMID TYPE

The Schmid type of disorder, described in 1949, is transmitted in an autosomal dominant fashion. The disease has been frequently confused with vitamin D-resistant rickets, because of similar clinical and radiographic findings. However, unlike vitamin-D resistant rickets, there are no changes in the serum calcium, phosphate, or alkaline phosphate, and there is no response to the administration of vitamin D.

CLINICAL FEATURES

The head and face are normal, and the short stature is not evident until 18 to 24 months of age. Bowleg is commonly the first sign and is evident when the child starts walking. The wrists are prominent and the fingers may not extend fully. The hands are otherwise normal. Poor alignment of the lower limbs can lead to symptomatic osteoarthritis in the hips and knees.

RADIOGRAPHIC FINDINGS

Metaphyseal abnormalities vary from mild scalloping to gross irregularities in the joints. These abnormalities appear to heal with bed rest, but recur once weightbearing is resumed. Epiphyseal lines are wide, but the ossification center appears normal.

CHONDRODYSPLASIA PUNCTATA: CONRADI-HÜNERMANN TYPE

The Conradi-Hünermann type of chondrodysplasia punctata is transmitted in an autosomal dominant manner, but there is variable clinical expression.

CLINICAL FEATURES

The disorder is evident at birth. The head is average size with a distinctively flat facies and relatively shortened neck. There is asymmetric shortening of the limbs. The hair is often coarse and sparse. Congenital cataracts are found in about 18 percent of patients. Scoliosis and joint contractures are common occurrences. The skin is dry and scaling, with linear striations.

RADIOGRAPHIC FINDINGS

Radiographs show punctate calcifications in the vertebral column and in the epiphyses of long bones, the tarsal and carpal bones, and the pelvic bones.

CHONDRODYSPLASIA PUNCTATA: X-LINKED DOMINANT TYPE

The X-linked dominant type of chondrodysplasia punctata contributes about 25 percent of the cases of chondrodysplasia punctata. It is an X-linked dominant trait that is usually fatal in males.

CLINICAL FEATURES

This disease shares many features with the Conradi-Hünermann type, but is distinguished by hypoplasia of the distal phalanges. There is severe shortening of the humerus, and sometimes of the femur, as well. Cataracts are much more common (72 percent as opposed to about 18 percent in Conradi-Hünermann).

RADIOGRAPHIC FINDINGS

A distinctive finding is very short, dumbbell-shaped humeri with punctate stippling. Otherwise, the disease shares the same radiographic features as the Conradi-Hünermann type.

CHONDRODYSPLASIA PUNCTATA: RHIZOMELIC TYPE

The rhizomelic type of chondrodysplasia punctata has an autosomal recessive inheritance and is considered the most severe of the three types of chondrodysplasia punctata described here.

CLINICAL FEATURES

Recurrent infections usually result in death in the first year. Survivors have a high incidence of neurologic abnormalities.

RADIOGRAPHIC FINDINGS

Calcification in and around the epiphyses are usually severe, although the vertebral column is spared. Lateral radiographs reveal clefts of the vertebral bodies. The humerus and femur show severe shortening and metaphyseal cupping.

CHONDROECTODERMAL DYSPLASIA (ELLIS-VAN CREVELD SYNDROME)

Chondroectodermal dysplasia is a very rare type of dwarfism transmitted in an autosomal recessive manner. It is common in the Old Order Amish of Lancaster County, Pennsylvania, where 13 percent of the population carries the gene.

CLINICAL FEATURES

Infants are of low-normal birth weight, and exhibit relatively large and long heads. There is a prominent forehead, flat face, and depressed nasal bridge, small mouth and jaw, and occasionally, wide set eyes and low-set ears. Cleft palate is commonly found. The tibias are shortened and bowed, and sometimes severely angulated to achieve a saber-shape. Resistant clubfoot is also common.

Associated abnormalities include congenital heart disease and hydronephrosis. Laryngotracheomalacia causes severe respiratory deficiency and usually results in death in the neonatal period.

RADIOGRAPHIC FINDINGS

There is a high incidence of congenital dislocation of the hip, and scoliosis or kyphoscoliosis. Hypoplastic scapulae are also a feature.

METATROPIC DYSPLASIA

Metatropic dysplasia is a rare disorder that is transmitted in an autosomal dominant manner, but an autosomal recessive form has been described. The name "metatropic" means changing, as the disease is characterized by changes in the body proportions with age.

CLINICAL FEATURES

At birth, patients have a normal face, short limbs, and a long, slender trunk. The trunk becomes increasingly shortened due to vertebral body flattening, kyphosis, and scoliosis. The expected life span is into early adulthood. Odontoid hypoplasia with atlantoaxial instability is a common problem.

RADIOGRAPHIC FINDINGS

Classic radiographic findings are dumbbell-shaped femurs and humeri, platyspondyly, and squared iliac crests.

MUCOPOLYSACCHARIDOSES

The mucopolysaccharidoses are a group of storage disorders caused by lysosomal enzyme defects and distinguished by the presence of complex sugars in the urine. There are seven types, which, with the exception of the X-linked recessive Hunter's syndrome (type II), are inherited as autosomal recessive traits. Hurler's, Hunter's, and Morquio's syndromes are all characterized by dwarfism.

HURLER'S SYNDROME

Hurler's syndrome (MPS 1-H) is transmitted as an autosomal recessive trait. Lab tests reveal a high concentration of dermatan sulfate and heparan sulfate in the urine.

CLINICAL FEATURES

Affected infants are large at birth, but growth slows down after the first few months. There is marked dwarfism and coarse facies, with a large tongue and lips. By 2 years of age, corneal clouding and motor and mental deterioration are seen. The abdomen is protuberant, partly due to hepatosplenomegaly. Umbilical hernias are common. Other associated complications include cardiac murmurs, respiratory difficulty, and deafness. Respiratory and cardiac problems are a usual cause of death by 10 years of age.

RADIOGRAPHIC FINDINGS

Findings are common to all the mucopolysaccharidoses. The sella turcica is enlarged, the ribs are splayed, and the lumbar vertebrae are beaked. Thoracolumbar kyphosis is generally seen early. The long bones are abnormally short and broad. Claw-hand deformity is also seen.

HUNTER'S SYNDROME

Hunter's syndrome (MPS II) has the same urinary laboratory findings as in Hurler's syndrome, but it has an X-linked recessive inheritance and milder clinical features.

CLINICAL FEATURES

Clinical signs are present only in males, and do not appear until after the age of 2 years. As in Hurler's syndrome, major features include coarse features, joint stiffness and contractures, claw-hand deformity, hepatosplenomegaly and umbilical hernia. However, corneal clouding is not as severe, mental deterioration is slower, and patients live to adulthood, reaching a height of 47 to 59 in.

RADIOGRAPHIC FINDINGS

Findings of an enlarged sella turcica, splayed ribs, beaking of the lumbar vertebrae, kyphosis, and shortening of the long bones are less pronounced than in Hurler's syndrome.

SANFILIPPO'S SYNDROME

Sanfilippo syndrome (MPS III-A, -B, and -C) has an autosomal recessive mode of inheritance, and is characterized by excessive amounts of heparin sulfate in the urine. The disease is characterized by CNS demyelination and may resemble cerebral palsy. The onset of disease characteristics is between the ages of 2 and 6 years and may present with hyperactivity, developmental delay, and hirsutism. Orthopaedically, short stature and mild joint stiffness are the only manifestations.

MORQUIO'S SYNDROME

Morquio's syndrome (MPS IV-A and -B) has an autosomal recessive inheritance. It is the most common of the mucopolysaccharidoses, and is characterized by the presence of keratan sulfate in the urine.

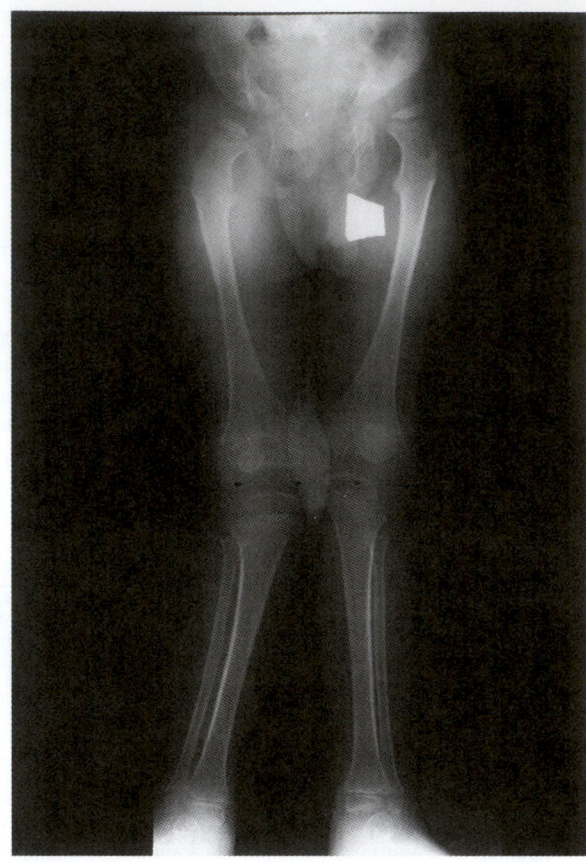

Figure 131-2
Three year-old male with typical findings of Morquio's syndrome, wide flat pelvis, unossified femoral heads, and genu valgum.

CLINICAL FEATURES

Patients present at about 2 years of age, when growth rate becomes stunted. Patients will have a waddling gait, severe knock-knee deformity, thoracic kyphosis, and pectus carinatum. The corneas become cloudy at 5 to 10 years of age, but less severely than in Hurler's syndrome. Unlike the other mucopolysaccharidoses, intelligence is normal. There is no organomegaly. Ligamentous laxity is severe and contributes to atlantoaxial instability. Patients can present with myelopathy requiring cervical decompression and fusion.

Patients live to adulthood. Growth generally stops at age 8 years, with average height ranging from 32 to 47 in.

RADIOGRAPHIC FINDINGS

There is thickening of the skull, odontoid aplasia or hypoplasia, wide ribs, anterior beaking of the vertebrae, wide flat pelvis, coxa vara, and unossified femoral heads. Metacarpals are bullet-shaped (Fig. 131-2).

SUGGESTED READINGS

Bassett GS: Orthopaedic aspects of skeletal dysplasias. In Green WB (ed): *Instr Course Lect.* Park Ridge, IL: American Academy of Orthopaedic Surgeons; 1990; 39:381.

Dietz FR: Genetic disorders and skeletal dysplasias. In Kasser JR (ed): *Orthopaedic Knowledge Update 5: Home Study Syllabus.* Rosemont, IL: American Academy of Orthopaedic Surgeons; 1996:181.

Beighton P, McKusick VA (eds): *McKusick's Heritable Disorders of Connective Tissue,* 5th ed. St. Louis: Mosby Year-Book; 1993.

Stefko RM, Wenger DR: Pediatric orthopaedics. In Miller MD (ed): *Review in Orthopaedics,* 2d ed. Philadelphia: WB Saunders; 1996:123.

Jones KL: *Smith's Recognizable Patterns of Human Malformation,* 4th ed. Philadelphia: WB Saunders; 1995.

Tolo V: Spinal disorders associated with skeletal and metabolic diseases. In Rothman RH, Simeone FA (eds.): *The Spine,* 3d ed. Philadelphia: WB Saunders; 1992:349.

Chapter 132

SYSTEMIC DISORDERS WITH ORTHOPAEDIC MANIFESTATIONS

David S. Feldman

There are numerous disorders, both genetic and acquired, that have orthopaedic manifestations. This chapter will divide these disorders into two categories, disorders of the hematopoietic system and genetic syndromes; discussion will be limited to orthopaedic manifestations of these diseases.

DISORDERS OF THE HEMATOPOIETIC SYSTEM

SICKLE CELL DISEASE

Sickle cell disease manifests a number of orthopaedic problems. First, children have increased susceptibility to osteomyelitis. Patients may develop pathologic fractures secondary to the osteomyelitis. This accounts for nearly half of the orthopaedic problems of these children. Second, patients develop aseptic necrosis of bone which, if articular, such as in the femoral head, may cause early osteoarthritis. Third, patients develop septic arthritis. Both *Staphylococcus aureus* and *Salmonella* have been commonly implicated as causative organisms for osteomyelitis. Patients present with a swollen and painful limb. Differentiation between a sickle crisis and osteomyelitis is best achieved with bone aspiration. Management includes intravenous antibiotics, debridement when necessary, and stabilization of the long bone to prevent pathologic fracture.

Osteonecrosis in sickle cell anemia is quite common, however, not all patients will be symptomatic. A number of patients with osteonecrosis of the femoral head or the humeral head have been known to become symptomatic, and may require late reconstructive procedures.

THALASSEMIA

Children with thalassemia have an increased incidence of fractures; approximately 15 percent of these may recur, that is, develop multiple fractures. If transfusion therapy is delayed, patients may also develop physeal arrests with asymmetric growth of both the proximal humerus and other long bones. The best orthopaedic outcome has been reported in children treated with transfusion therapy from a very young age.

FANCONI'S ANEMIA

In children with Fanconi's anemia, approximately one-third will have disorders of the hands with radial hemimelia, digital aplasia, or absence of the thumb. Patients may also have dislocations, as well as Klippel-Feil syndrome and Sprengel deformities.

GAUCHER'S DISEASE

Gaucher's disease is caused by a deficiency of the enzyme glucocerebrosidase. The disorder results in a number of orthopaedic manifestations. Gaucher's crisis, which like sickle cell disease causes a pseudoosteomyelitis, is quite common. True osteomyelitis in Gaucher's disease is uncommon. Patients also develop osteonecrosis of the femoral heads and sustain pathologic fractures of the long bones. Pathologic fractures have been known to demonstrate delayed union and nonunion, particularly those occurring in the femoral neck. Gaucher's disease is treated with alglucerase, an expensive enzyme replacement therapy. Alglucerase appears to have efficacy in preventing late orthopaedic complications, although this has not been fully elucidated.

HEMOPHILIA

Hemophilia is a disorder causing excessive bleeding in joints and hemarthrosis. Multiple episodes of bleeding into a joint will eventually result in stiffness, pain, and the development of early osteoarthritis. The goal of the orthopaedic surgeon in hemophilia is to prevent or minimize the hemarthroses. Synovectomy of joints is utilized in order to prevent recurrent bleeds. Maintaining motion of the knee with synovectomy is difficult; however, with intense physical therapy and continuous passive motion, it can be achieved. Many of the patients previously treated with Factor VIII or IX in the early 1980s are HIV-positive and this may play a role in the decision making for operative intervention. A total CD4 count is the most appropriate marker for tolerance of surgical intervention.

HISTIOCYTOSIS X

Histiocytosis X has differing modes of presentation, as an isolated lesion in bone as an eosinophilic granuloma, multiple osseous lesions, or multiple osseous lesions with visceral involvement. Orthopaedic intervention for this disease is two-fold: First is to arrive at the diagnosis and second is to treat the bony lesions in which a pathologic fracture may occur. Medical intervention with chemotherapy is utilized if there is visceral involvement, when the patient presents with diabetes insipidus, or when the multiple bony lesions are unremitting.

LEUKEMIA

Leukemia may present with primary complaints of bone and joint pain in approximately 20 percent of patients. These children have pain in their extremities and back, symptoms consistent with septic arthritis or osteomyelitis. Patients may also present with pathologic fractures. Radiologic findings include a metaphyseal band or lucency in up to 30 percent of patients. Diffuse osteopenia is found in approximately 25 percent of these patients and lytic or mixed sclerotic lesions in another 10 percent. Treatment of these lesions is medical. Pathologic fractures may require stabilization.

THROMBOCYTOPENIA-ABSENT RADIUS SYNDROME

Thrombocytopenia-absent radius syndrome is associated with bilateral absence of the radii with varying degrees of hypoplasia of the thumb. Lower extremity abnormalities include genu varum in approximately one-third of patients as well as other knee disorders in approximately another 20 percent including stiffness of the knee and patellar abnormalities. Patients may require surgery for the lower extremity including valgus osteotomies for the genu varum, as well as rotational osteotomies for internal tibial torsion. Stiffness of the knee is a common sequela of either surgery or nonoperative management of this disorder.

GENETIC SYNDROMES

DOWN'S SYNDROME (TRISOMY 21 SYNDROME)

Down's syndrome presents a number of problems to the treating orthopaedic surgeon. Cervical spine instability with myelopathy, hip dislocations, patellar instability, and calcaneovalgus instability of the foot represent the spectrum of associated orthopaedic disease. Surgical intervention is recommended in children with progressive atlanto-dens interval greater than 10 mm, as well as in patients with myelopathy, C1-2 fusion being the treatment of choice. Dislocation of hips often requires open reduction and femoral and/or pelvic osteotomies. The feet in Down's syndrome are frequently amenable to conservative measures; however, subtalar fusion or triple arthrodesis become necessary at times to stabilize the hind foot.

LARSEN'S SYNDROME

Larsen's syndrome is a autosomal dominant-transmitted disease that presents with a typical facies including hypertelorism, frontal bossing, and flattening of the midface. Orthopaedically, there may be dislocations of multiple joints including radial head dislocations associated with cubitus varus and knee and hip dislocations. Scoliosis and cervical kyphosis are quite common. Conservative treatment is usually ineffective in children with Larsen's syndrome, and knee dislocations need to be treated prior to undertaking either foot or hip surgery. Cervical spine kyphosis will often need to be addressed surgically.

NEUROFIBROMATOSIS

Neurofibromatosis is a neural crest disorder. It is an autosomal dominant disorder, with approximately one-half being spontaneous mutation. Type I neurofibromatosis has peripheral manifestations and type II is central, presenting with acoustic neuromas. Type I neurofibromatosis accounts for up to 90 percent of cases. A diagnosis of type I is made based on two or more of the following: (1) in children six café au lait spots larger than 5 mm; (2) two neurofibromas or one plexiform neurofibroma; (3) axillary or inguinal freckling; (4) two Lisch nodules; (5) a pseudoarthrosis; (6) optic glioma; and (7) a parent or sibling with neurofibromatosis type I. Orthopaedic manifestations include pseudoarthrosis, usually of the tibia with an anterolateral bow. This pseudoarthrosis can also affect other long bones such as the femur, ulna, radius, or clavicle.

Scoliosis is also a common problem in neurofibromatosis. The majority of curves resemble those found in idiopathic scoliosis. A dystrophic curve may also be present with scalloping of the vertebral body, as well as the adjacent rib. These curves are much more difficult to treat operatively and to achieve fusion. Anterior and posterior fusion with instrumentation is recommended; a vascular graft may be used anteriorly to improve the fusion rate. Macrodactyly and hemihypertrophy are also seen in neurofibromatosis. Children with neurofibromatosis have an increased incidence of malignancy with degeneration of the neurofibromas, as well as other neuronal tumors.

ARTHROGRYPOSIS MULTIPLEX CONGENITA

Arthrogryposis multiplex congenita is one of the contracture syndromes. The diagnosis is made by the position of the limbs and the type of contractures. Children usually have four-limb involvement. The lower extremities may be more involved than the upper extremities. Presentation of limb position is ordinarily with the shoulders adducted, elbows extended, and wrists flexed. There is decreased shoulder mass and decreased muscle mass throughout the upper and lower extremities. There may be hip-flexion contractures with either knee extension or flexion contractures. Affected children often have rigid clubfeet. Scoliosis is also a predominant feature in arthrogryposis.

Treatment should be for functional restoration and thought of in that fashion. Operative management may include surgery for knee hyperextension, clubfoot, and scoliosis. Surgery for dislocated hips is usually reserved for patients with unilateral dislocations. Treatment of bilateral dislocations is controversial.

Distal arthrogryposis is an autosomal dominant disorder involving only the hands and the feet; however, the foot deformity includes rigid clubfeet which, although attempts should be made at manipulative treatment, often requires surgical intervention.

The hand involvement is characteristic, with ulna deviation of the wrist and flexion deformities of the proximal interphalangeal and metacarpophalangeal joints. The thumb is ordinarily involved as well. Treatment includes serial manipulation and may require tendon lengthening. These patients usually achieve a good functional result due to the lack of involvement of the proximal musculature.

PTERYGIUM SYNDROME

Although there are a number of syndromes collected under the term, pterygium syndrome, these syndromes mainly involve the upper and lower extremity joints, as well as at times, the spine and the neck. The syndromes manifest with pterygium causing severe limitation of motion of the involved joints; scoliosis, as well as muscle weakness, may also be present. The extent of the involvement dictates the overall disability of the child. Surgery is quite difficult and there are times when amputation is required in order to treat severe fixed contractures.

PROTEUS SYNDROME

Proteus syndrome is a disorder that involves hemihypertrophy and macrodactyly and is thought to be an autosomal dominant disorder. Children may also present with a scoliosis and kyphosis, lower extremity deformity, and intraarticular problems such as acetabular dysplasia and genu valgum.

Proteus syndrome in children is notoriously difficult to treat, and the macrodactyly and hemihypertrophy cause great difficulty in surgical management. Each case needs to be treated in isolation with operative correction of deformities and either epiphysiodesis or limb lengthening used to correct leg length discrepancies. The macrodactyly of certain digits often requires amputation.

FREEMAN-SHELDON (WHISTLING FACE) SYNDROME

This is an arthrogryposis-like syndrome involving the hands and the feet. Patients have characteristic facies and may also have scoliosis. Surgical correction is usually required for the hand and foot deformities.

FAMILIAL DYSAUTONOMIA DISORDER

Familial dysautonomia is an autosomal recessive disorder that affects mostly Jews of Eastern European descent. Autonomic dysfunction causes wide swings in blood pressure, as well as aspiration pneumonia and difficulty in swallowing and eating. These children also suffer from congenital insensitivity to pain.

Orthopaedic manifestations include fractures secondary to insensitivity to pain, as well as Charcot joints. Children develop scoliosis in nearly all cases. This can be quite severe, and as soon as it demonstrates progression, surgical correction is indicated. These children also suffer from changes of osteochondritis desiccans in the knees, as well as osteonecrosis of the hip.

Operative management is quite difficult in these children, secondary to the autonomic dysfunction. Life expectancy is usually only into the teens.

TURNER'S SYNDROME

Children with Turner's syndrome are females who have short stature, a webbed neck, and also develop scoliosis, genu valgum, and cubitus valgus. Chromosomal anomalies include an XO sex chromosome constitution. Osteoporosis can also become a problem if the children are untreated. Children are usually managed with estrogen replacement and growth hormone during childhood, which allows for more normal development.

NOONAN'S SYNDROME

Noonan's syndrome presents with Turner-like features; however, patients have normal chromosomal analysis. Orthopaedic manifestations include short stature and cubitus valgus, with or without posterior dislocation of the radial head. Scoliosis is quite common in Noonan's syndrome and may be associated with congenital vertebral anomalies.

STICKLER SYNDROME

Stickler syndrome is an autosomal dominant disorder, a progressive arthroophthalmopathy characterized by a marfanoid appearance as well as ligamentous laxity. Children develop problems with their joints such as morning stiffness that may mimic juvenile idiopathic arthritis (JIA) [formerly termed juvenile rheumatoid arthritis (JRA)]. By adolescence, patients can have severe arthritis of multiple joints. These children may also have protrusio acetabula, coxa valga of the hips, and abnormal epiphyses throughout; ophthalmic disease may progress to blindness. Orthopaedically, children may develop loose bodies in their major joints, as well as degenerative spine disease and kyphosis. These conditions may require surgical treatment. Early joint arthroplasty is the treatment of choice due to early osteoarthritis in many of the large joints.

GOLDENHAR'S SYNDROME

Goldenhar's syndrome involves the eyes and ears, as well as the vertebrae. This syndrome is genetic, and its transmission is not well understood. Orthopaedically, the vertebral anomalies include congenital scoliosis, usually of the cervical or thoracic spine. If vertebral anomalies demonstrate progression, early fusion might be indicated. Children may also have Sprengel deformities and other rib deformities.

Nonorthopaedic manifestations include a characteristic facial appearance secondary to skin tags off of the ear, as well as a dermoid on the conjunctiva. These children may also have a hypoplastic mandible and cleft palate or cleft lips.

NAIL-PATELLA SYNDROME

Nail-patella syndrome is an autosomal dominant disorder. Children tend to have hypoplastic patellae which may be small or even absent. The patellae may also be congenitally dislocated or unstable. Children with nail-patella syndrome also demonstrate hypoplastic femoral condyles with deformities, both varus and valgus. Children may also have dislocated radial heads in the elbow. Hypoplastic condyles of the elbow mimic those of the knee. Children may also develop iliac horns which are found in the posterior aspect of the iliac wings; there is an exostosis in this area. In observing the hands of affected children, the nails are dystrophic; this feature may involve all or some of the nails, and is usually bilaterally symmetric.

Children may have a host of other orthopaedic problems such as foot deformities and joint contractures. Nonorthopaedic problems include kidney failure. Orthopaedic management is usually required for these children, and is very variable. Soft tissue releases or osteotomies are often required.

VATER SYNDROME

VATER is an acronym that describes an association of defects of the spine, GI tract, respiratory tract, and deformation of the upper extremity. The letters VATER stand for vertebral segmentation, anal atresia, tracheoesophageal fistula (with esophageal atresia), and radial aplasia and/or renal abnormalities. All or some of these problems may occur in children diagnosed with this syndrome. Patients often require extensive orthopaedic surgery of the upper and, at times, the lower extremity to improve function and cosmesis.

SUGGESTED READINGS

Cole WG: Genetics of connective tissue disease. *Med J Australia* 1993; 158:678.

Crawford AH Jr, Bagamery N: Osseous manifestations of neurofibromatosis in childhood. *J Pediatr Orthop* 1986; 6:72.

Diamond LS, Lynn P, Sigmen B: Orthopedic disorders in patients with Down's syndrome. *Orthop Clin North Am* 1981; 12:57.

Katz K, Horev G, Grunebaum M, et al: The natural history of osteonecrosis of the femoral head in children and adolescents who have Gaucher disease. *J Bone Joint Surg [Am]* 1996; 78:14.

Laville JM, Lakermance P, Limouzy F: Larsen's syndrome: Review of the literature and analysis of thirty-eight cases. *J Pediatr Orthop* 1994; 14:63.

Yoslow W, Becker MH, Bartels J, et al: Orthopedic defects in familial dysautonomia. A review of sixty-five cases. *J Bone Joint Surg [Am]* 1971; 53:1541.

Chapter 133

NEUROFIBROMATOSIS

Lynn J. Letko

Neurofibromatosis (NFM), a neurocristopathy or hamartomatous condition, is the most common single-gene disorder of the nervous system. This disorder was first described by Akenside in 1768. The term *neurofibroma* was coined by von Recklinghausen in 1882. Both the central nervous system and peripheral nervous system may be involved in this condition. NFM is probably of neural crest origin, but tissues of neuroectodermal, mesodermal, and endodermal origins may be involved in the disorder, from both neurologic and/or vascular anomalies.

CLASSIFICATION

Neurofibromatosis is classified into types 1 and 2.

NFM 1

NFM 1 has also been referred to as von Recklinghausen's disease or peripheral neurofibromatosis. The incidence is 1/4000 to 1/5000 live births. It is inherited in an autosomal dominant manner with a high penetrance rate but with variable expressivity. Up to half of all cases are the result of spontaneous mutation. Prenatal detection of the defect, which occurs on the long arm of chromosome 17, is not yet available. In 1987, the National Institutes of Health (NIH) Consensus Development Conference Statement put forth criteria of NFM 1. Two or more of the following are needed to make the diagnosis:

1. Six or more café-au-lait macules. These should measure more than 5 mm in prepubertal patients and more than 15 mm in postpubertal patients.
2. Two or more neurofibromas of any type or one plexiform neurofibroma. Various types of neurofibroma can occur. These include cutaneous, deep, and plexiform types. The plexiform type, or bag of worms, is often located in the head-and-neck, cervical, or lumbar regions, where it may compress the trachea, esophagus, or plexi.
3. Freckling in the axillary (Crowe's sign) or inguinal region.
4. Optic glioma.
5. Two or more Lisch nodules (iris hamartomas).
6. Distinctive osseous lesions such as sphenoid dysplasia or thinning of a long bone cortex with or without pseudarthrosis.
7. A first-degree relative with NFM 1.

NFM 2

NFM 2, or central neurofibromatosis, is characterized by bilateral acoustic neuromas. The incidence is 1/50,000 live births. It is inherited in an autosomal dominant fashion with 95 percent penetrance. The defect is on the distal long arm of chromosome 22. Criteria for diagnosis, as put forth by the NIH, include:

1. Bilateral cranial nerve (VIII) tumors
2. A first-degree relative with NFM 2 and either a unilateral cranial nerve VIII tumor or two or more of the following:
   A. Meningioma
   B. Ependymoma
   C. Neurofibroma
   D. Glioma
   E. Schwannoma (Fig. 133-1)
   F. Juvenile posterior subcapsular lenticular opacity (cataracts)

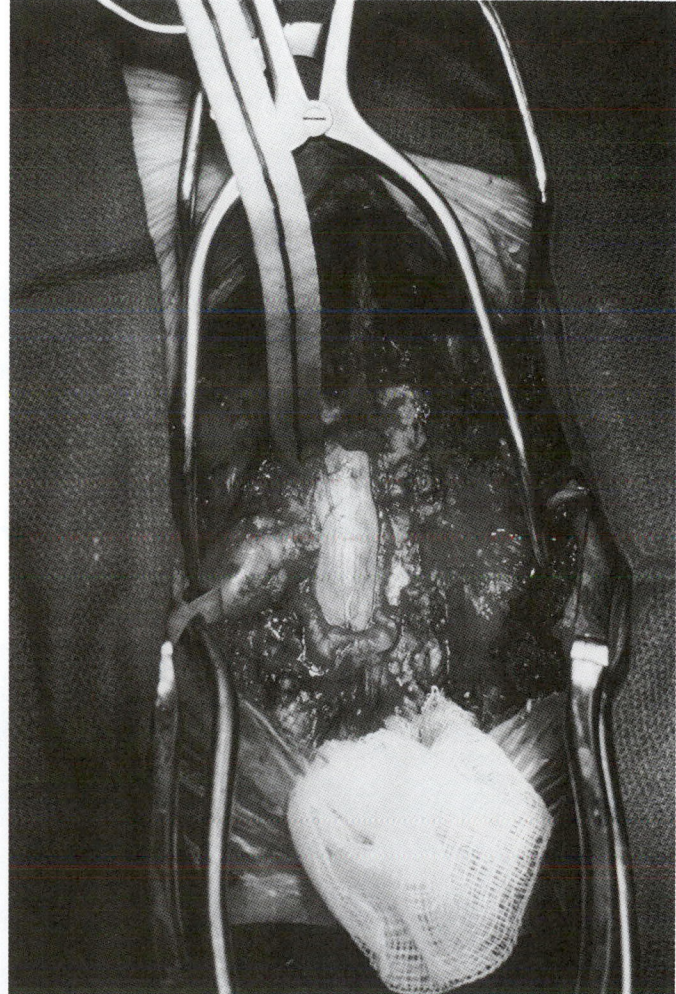

Figure 133-1
Dumbbell intradural and extradural spinal schwannoma.

NFM: OTHER MANIFESTATIONS

A variety of manifestations may be seen in NFM. Café-au-lait spots are common. Their border has been described as "coast of California" in contrast to the "coast of Maine," which has been used to describe those associated with Albright's syndrome. Sexual development may be either precocious or retarded. Malignant hypertension, secondary to renal artery stenosis, occurs in 1 to 2 percent of patients, whereas pheochromocytoma occurs in 0.5 percent. Elephantiasis neuromatosa or pachydermatocele occurs in 10 percent. Learning disabilities or mental retardation are frequent findings. Bantis syndrome, which is thrombocytopenia secondary to splenic obstruction by a fibroma, has been reported. Other associated anomalies include macrocephaly and short stature, as well as neurologic impairment. Neoplasms occur in approximately 5 percent of patients with NFM. The incidence of malignancy increases to greater than 20 percent in adults with NFM, with a higher incidence of malignant degeneration seen in more severely involved patients. Associated neoplasms include nonlymphocytic leukemia, Wilms' tumor, urogenital rhabdomyosarcoma, malignant peripheral nerve sheath tumors, optic glioma, astrocytoma, and acoustic neuroma (Fig. 133-2).

SKELETAL ABNORMALITIES

ANTEROLATERAL BOWING

Anterolateral bowing of the tibia is seen in 50 percent of patients with NFM 1, whereas 97 percent of patients with anterolateral bowing and congenital pseudarthrosis of the tibia are ultimately diagnosed with NFM. Bowing usually becomes evident within the first 2 years of life. The goal of treatment of anterolateral bowing is the prevention of fracture. The etiology of congenital pseudarthrosis of the tibia is uncertain. It may follow fracture or osteotomy, with the average age of fracture being 1.2 years.

Four radiographic presentations of anterolateral bowing and congenital pseudarthrosis of the tibia have been described. Type I is nondysplastic anterolateral bowing with a dense medullary canal. This type has the best prognosis, and patients may never suffer a fracture. Treatment involves follow-up without the use of an orthosis. Type II is dysplastic anterolateral bowing. Three subtypes have been described. Type IIA has an increase in medullary canal width and tubulation defect. Treatment involves protection with an orthosis and consideration of prophylactic intervention. Type IIB has a cystic postfracture lesion. Consideration should be given to early bone grafting, because these lesions have the tendency to fracture. Type IIC dysplastic lesions have the worst prognosis. Anterolateral bowing occurs with cysts, fracture, and frank pseudarthrosis.

Amputation should be considered early in the course of treatment if grafting procedures have been attempted without attainment of union, or if union is not obtained by age 7 years. The benefit of additional procedures should be questioned. Osteotomy should be avoided in these patients because of the increased risk of pseudarthrosis. When amputation is performed, it should be done at the ankle rather than through the pseudarthrosis site to allow better prosthetic biomechanical advantage and to avoid stump overgrowth.

OTHER SKELETAL ABNORMALITIES

Additional skeletal abnormalities seen with NFM include unilateral extremity shortening or lengthening, hypertrophy or giantism usually of one limb frequently associated with vascular lesions, cortical defects which may be erosive secondary to tumor, and spinal anomalies.

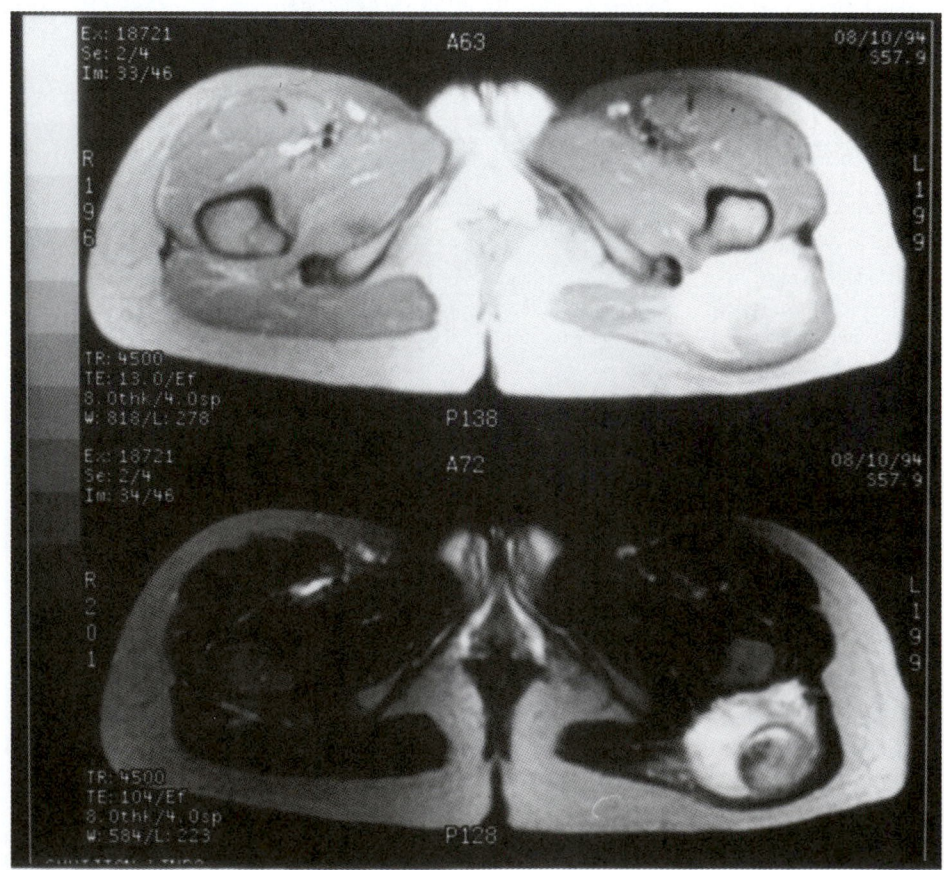

Figure 133-2
Computed tomography of malignant peripheral nerve sheath tumor of the buttock and thigh in a patient with previously undiagnosed neurofibromatosis

SPINAL ANOMALIES

SCOLIOSIS

Approximately 60 percent of patients with NFM 1 have some disorder of the spine. Scoliosis, which occurs in 10 to 60 percent of patients and is the most common osseous defect seen in NFM 1, is most often noted in the second decade of life and affects females slightly more frequently than males. Two types of scoliosis have been described: dystrophic and nondystrophic (Fig. 133-3). Dystrophic (dysplastic) scoliosis, which is believed to be developmental in nature, occurs approximately seven times more frequently than does nondystrophic scoliosis. It is more frequently located in the thoracic spines than in the thoracolumbar spines, and least frequently in the cervical spines. Progression may be aggressive or not occur at all. With anterior body kyphosis or scalloping, an increased risk of pseudarthrosis and progression exists. A recent classification system includes

- Type I: scoliosis with a normal sagittal curve
- Type II: scoliosis with thoracic lordoscoliosis
- Type III: kyphosing scoliosis with rotation such that the curve is evident only on the lateral radiograph
- Type IV: kyphoscoliosis in which an angular kyphosis predominates

Characteristics noted in dystrophic scoliosis include rotation, scalloping, and wedging of the vertebral bodies, short sharp curves (four to six segments), foraminal enlargement, penciling of the apical ribs, abnormal or absent pedicles, spindling of the transverse processes, and progression after puberty (Fig. 133-3).

Risk factors for progression of dystrophic curves include early age of onset, high Cobb angle at the time of presentation, vertebral scalloping, and severe apical rotation of more than 11 degrees. Additional risk factors for curve progression include the presence of an abnormal kyphosis, location of the curve apex at the middle or caudal thoracic spine, penciling of one or more ribs on the concavity of the curve, and penciling of 4 or more ribs.

Dystrophic curves frequently require treatment. Bracing is generally not effective. Treatment recommendations for curves of less than 20 degrees include observation at 6-month intervals. Posterior spinal fusion with segmental spinal instrumentation from neutral to neutral vertebra is recommended for curves of 20 to 40 degrees. Anterior and posterior spinal fusions are necessary to treat those curves that are greater than 80 degrees and to treat scoliosis with greater than 50 degrees of kyphosis.

Nondystrophic scoliosis seen in NFM patients is idiopathic in nature. The deformity should be observed closely because dystrophic changes may develop with growth. These patients have a higher pseudarthrosis rate when operated on (17 percent) than similar idiopathic curves. Specific treatment recommendations include observation of curves of less than 20 degrees, bracing for curves of up to 35 degrees, posterior spinal fusion with segmental spinal instrumentation for 35 to 45 degree curves, and anterior and posterior spinal fusion with segmental spinal instrumentation for curves of greater than 60 degrees.

KYPHOSIS

Kyphosis in NFM is a progressive deformity that is angular and has a high risk of paraplegia. Kyphosis of greater than 50 degrees should be treated by anterior spinal fusion with fibular strut grafting followed by posterior spinal fusion with segmental spinal instrumentation one to two segments past the end vertebra. Re-exploration of the fusion

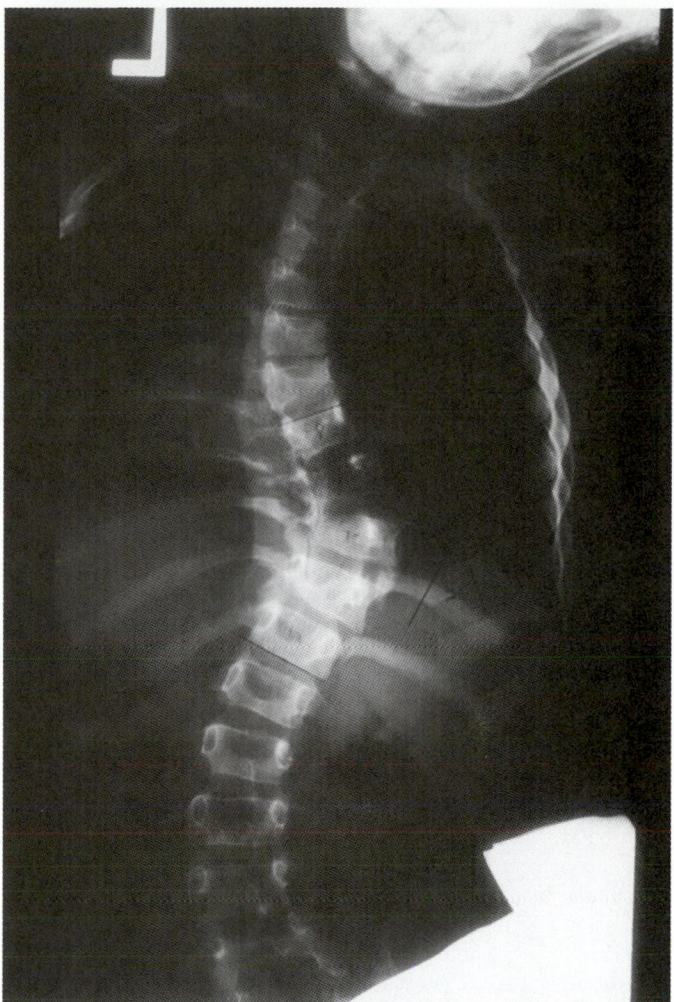

Figure 133-3
Dystrophic scoliosis secondary to neurofibromas.

mass and augmentation are recommended at 6 months if there is any concern regarding the fusion mass. Prior to undertaking surgical management, an intraspinal lesion must be ruled out. Laminectomy is contraindicated in the treatment of NFM kyphosis because it further destabilizes the spine.

THORACIC DISLOCATION

Two cases of thoracic dislocation have been reported in children with NFM. These cases occurred after minor trauma without neurologic impairment. Treatment included reduction, anterior spinal fusion, and posterior spinal fusion with segmental spinal instrumentation.

CERVICAL SPINE ABNORMALITIES

Cervical spine abnormalities have been reported to occur in up to 44 percent of NFM patients with short kyphotic or dystrophic thoracolumbar curves of greater than 65 degrees. These abnormalities include complete cervical dislocation, atlantoaxial rotatory subluxation, and atlantoaxial subluxation/dislocation. Cervical spine abnormalities are frequently asymptomatic in this population and may present as a neck mass, torticollis, or dysphagia. All patients with NFM should have cervical radiographs, including flexion and extension lateral films, prior to undergoing general anesthesia or application of traction for scoliosis. Indications for surgical treatment include neurologic impairment, progressive pain, and instability. Spinal fusion with segmental spinal instrumentation has been found to afford the best outcome in these patients and may need to be done both anteriorly and posteriorly. Patients should be forewarned preoperatively that they may require additional postoperative halo immobilization for adequate stabilization.

NEUROLOGIC COMPROMISE

Neurologic compromise may be secondary to intraspinal lesions such as pseudomeningoceles, dural ectasia, intraspinal neurofibromas, or malignant degeneration of existing neural tumors. Other causes of neurologic impairment include kyphosis or ribs entering the spinal canal, resulting in compression. Paraplegia without the presence of kyphosis is considered to be caused by an intraspinal lesion until proven otherwise. Work-up of such lesions should include magnetic resonance imaging and/or computed tomographic myelogram. Treatment of spinal compression depends on the location of the lesion and may include anterior excision, decompression and fusion, and/or posterior hemilaminectomy and tumor excision with posterior spinal fusion with segmental instrumentation and bone graft.

SPONDYLOLISTHESIS

Only nine cases of spondylolisthesis have been reported in patients with NFM. The incidence is less than 1 percent in this population versus 5 percent in the general population. When present, spondylolisthesis tends to progress secondary to dystrophic changes. Increasing size of the neuroforamina and elongation of the pedicles may result in pathologic spondylolisthesis. When progression is noted, surgical stabilization and fusion is indicated in these patients.

SURGICAL CONSIDERATIONS

When contemplating surgery for patients with NFM, several specific points should be considered. All patients with a diagnosis of NFM should have preoperative cervical spine radiographs. Patients with NFM tend to have poor bone quality. Patients should be forewarned that supplemental immobilization may be required. An increased rate of pseudarthrosis has been reported in the spine and tibia in this patient population and this alters treatment. In addition, blood loss may be significant. Wounds should be drained because bleeding tends to increase as patients become normotensive. An increased incidence of pheochromocytoma exists in this patient population. An appropriate workup for this should be done, if indicated. Lastly, tumors have a higher potential to undergo malignant degeneration in this population. Appropriate studies should be obtained for staging and the presence of metastasis.

SUGGESTED READING

Adkins JC, Ratvich MM: The operative management of von Recklinghausen's neurofibromatosis in children, with special reference to lesions of the head and neck. *Surgery* 1977; 82:342.

Betz RR, Iorio R, Lombardi AV, et al: Scoliosis surgery in neurofibromatosis. *Clin Orthop* 1989; 245:53–56.

Craig JB, Govender S: Neurofibromatosis of the cervical spine: A report of eight cases. *J Bone Joint Surg [Br]* 1992; 74:575–578.

Crawford AH: Neurofibromatosis in childhood. In Murray DG (ed): *Instructional Course Lectures.* Park Ridge, IL: American Academy of Orthopaedic Surgeons, 1981; 30:56–74.

Crawford AH: Neurofibromatosis. In Morrissy RT (ed): *Lovell and Winter's Pediatric Orthopaedics,* 3d ed. Philadelphia: JB Lippincott; 1990:175–201.

Crawford AH Jr, Bagamery N: Osseous manifestations in neurofibromatosis in childhood. *J Pediatr Orthop* 1986; 6:72–88.

Crawford AH, Gabriel KR: Dysplastic scoliosis: neurofibromatosis. In Bridwell KH, DeWald RL (eds): *The Textbook of Spinal Surgery,* 2d ed. Philadelphia: JB Lippincott; 1996:276.

Curtis BH, Fisher RL, Butterfield WL, et al: Neurofibromatosis with paraplegia: Report of eight cases. *J Bone Joint Surg [Am]* 1969; 51:843–861.

Funasaki H, Winter RB, Lonstein JB, et al: Pathophysiology of spinal deformities in neurofibromatosis: An analysis of seventy-one patients who had curves associated with dystrophic changes. *J Bone Joint Surg [Am]* 1994; 76:694–700.

Major MR, Huizenga BA: Spinal cord compression by displaced ribs in neurofibromatosis: A report of three cases. *J Bone Joint Surg [Am]* 1988; 70:1100.

National Institutes of Health Consensus Development Conference: Neurofibromatosis: Conference statement. *Arch Neurol* 1988; 45:575–578.

Rockower S, McKay D, Nason S: Dislocation of the spine in neurofibromatosis. A report of two cases. *J Bone Joint Surg [Am]* 1982; 64:1240–1242.

Roos KL, Dunn DW: Neurofibromatoses. *CA* 1992; 42:241–254.

Stone JW, Bridwell KH, Shackelford GD, et al: Dural ectasia associated with spontaneous dislocation of the upper part of the thoracic spine in neurofibromatosis: A case report and review of the literature. *J Bone Joint Surg [Am]* 1987; 69:1079–1083.

Tanno T, Moiriya ZH, Kitahara H, et al: Surgical treatment for cervical kyphosis in von Recklinghausen's disease. *Seikei Geka* 1990; 41:877–884.

Winter RB, Moe JH, Bradford DS, et al: Spine deformity in neurofibromatosis: A review of one hundred and two patients. *J Bone Joint Surg [Am]* 1979; 61:677–694.

Winter RB, Lonstein JE, Anderson M: Neurofibromatosis and hyperkyphosis: A review of 33 patients with kyphosis of 80 degrees or greater. *J Spine Disord* 1988; 1:39–49.

Yong-Hing K, Kalamchi A, MacEwen GD: Cervical spine abnormalities in neurofibromatosis. *J Bone Joint Surg [Am]* 1979; 61:695–699.

Chapter 134

NEUROMUSCULAR DISORDERS

Alfred D. Grant, Dan Atar, and Ellen S. Moran

BRACHIAL PLEXUS: BIRTH INJURIES (OBSTETRIC PALSY)

The incidence of brachial plexus birth injuries is 0.4 to 2.5 per 1000 live births. The etiology is generally traction during a traumatic delivery. Risk factors include high birth weight, breech presentation, and shoulder dystocia. Injury to the nerve roots vary from mild stretching to complete rupture of the trunks or avulsion of the roots from the spinal cord.

Ninety percent of the patients have upper arm paralysis of *ERB-Duchenne* in which the fifth and sixth cervical roots are damaged. The next most frequent type of injury is a complete lesion in which the whole plexus is involved (*whole limb* paralysis). Lower arm paralysis of *Klumpke* (C8, T1) is the least common.

The diagnosis is evident at birth. In the ERB-Duchenne type, the deltoid, supraspinatus, infraspinatus, teres minor, biceps brachi, brachialis, and the brachioradialis are paralyzed. The arm is positioned in internal rotation. Abduction is limited. Active elbow flexion may be absent. In the Klumpke type, the wrist flexors, the long flexors of the fingers, and the intrinsic muscles of the hand are affected. In entire limb paralysis, the whole limb is almost completely paralyzed.

Treatment of brachial plexus birth palsies consists of gentle passive exercises to maintain full range of motion of all joints. Splinting is discouraged by most authors. Recovery can be seen in 92 percent of patients within 3 months. Most authors recommend electromyography (EMG) and consideration of surgery if significant recovery is not evident by the age of 3 months. Surgery at this stage includes brachial plexus exploration and sural nerve interpositional graft for the damaged root. If the nerve roots are avulsed from the spinal cord neurotization may yield a worthwhile result.

In unresolved brachial plexus palsy, fixed deformities develop. They may require operative correction at a later stage, such as derotation osteotomy of the humerus for internal rotation and soft tissue and muscles transfer for fixed adduction and pronation.

MUSCULAR DYSTROPHIES

The muscular dystrophies are a group of disorders characterized by progressive muscle weakness and wasting without evidence of central or peripheral nervous system involvement. The pathology is in the muscle; innervation is normal. Age of onset, the muscle groups involved, and the rate of progression of the disorders may vary considerably. Current observations demonstrate that several childhood forms of muscular dystrophy including Duchenne, Becker, and the limb girdle muscular dystrophies share a common pathogenesis of muscle membrane instability. As such, there is marked elevation of serum enzymes, aldolase, and creatine kinase. Calcium levels in the muscle are elevated two to three times above normal. Affected mus-cles tend to be flaccid but not tender and there is no voluntary or percussion myotonia. The tendon reflexes may be depressed or absent. EMG changes reveal small action potentials of reduced amplitude and duration with an increase in the percentage of polyphasic potentials. Muscle biopsy demonstrates variation in muscle fiber size and fiber necrosis. As the disease progresses, muscle fibers are replaced by fat and connective tissue. The muscular dystrophies are all inherited.

DUCHENNE MUSCULAR DYSTROPHY

Duchenne muscular dystrophy (DMD) is an X-linked recessive disorder characterized by progressive and degenerative muscle wasting. The most common type of childhood dystrophy, DMD occurs primarily in males, with a population incidence of approximately 1/3500 live male births. Affected males have an unremarkable early childhood, with the first overt clinical symptoms appearing around 2 to 5 years of age. Most patients are confined to a wheelchair by age 10 and generally die by the end of the second or early third decade of life. DMD is caused by a defect in the gene which codes for the production of the protein, dystrophin. Dystrophin is a component of muscle tissue which supports the cytoskeleton of the muscle membrane complex. Absence of dystrophin disrupts the sarcolemma and leads to muscle fiber necrosis. Approximately 60 percent of males with DMD will show a molecular deletion of the gene localized to Xp21. Although most cases are transmitted via an unaffected, carrier mother, 30 percent of cases exhibit no previous family history and are considered de novo mutations. Approximately 25 percent of affected males will demonstrate an IQ of one standard deviation below the mean.

The onset of DMD may be vague but is usually recorded as being before the age of 5 years. Parents often report that their affected son never kept up with his peers in running and climbing. The child may be described as clumsy. There is a tendency for toe-walking secondary to muscle weakness and shortened achilles tendon, perhaps because of weakness to the anterior tibial muscles. Frequent falling is often a presenting feature. In the preclinical phase, the serum level of creatine kinase (CK) is highly elevated. Pelvic girdle weakness is usually more evident than shoulder girdle weakness in the early stages. Affected boys typically never learn to run normally and although they may be able to stand on one leg, they are unable to hop. Postural deformities produce a waddling gait and typical stance. There is marked lumbar lordosis and extension of the neck with a forward tilt of the pelvis. The feet may be in equinus. Pseudohypertrophy is observed in most patients at some stage of the disease and is most evident in the calf muscles, deltoids, and serratus anterior muscles.

The muscle weakness is steadily progressive and is particularly increased in the proximal musculature of the hip flexors and extensors, quadriceps, serratus anterior pectorals, biceps, and brachioradialis muscles. External ocular muscles are spared. The tendon reflexes are lost relatively early. As the muscle weakness progresses, difficulty rising from the floor and then from a low chair becomes obvious and the child begins to use his arms to help push his body off the floor with the legs extended, in order to stand.

Classic clinical signs present in the disease are the tendency of the patient to slide through the examiner's arms when an attempt is made to lift him (Meryon's sign) and climbing up his legs, pressing first on his knees, then the thighs to gain an erect posture (Gower's sign). These signs are a reflection of weakness in the pectoral and pelvic girdle musculature, respectively. Affected boys are usually confined to a wheelchair by age 11, at which time fixed contractures of the ankles, knees, and hips are likely to develop.

Kyphoscoliosis and diminished respiratory reserve are common features and cardiomyopathy is almost invariable. Death usually occurs in the early 20s due to respiratory infection or cardiac failure.

During the stage of independent ambulation no treatment is necessary. If a fracture occurs at this stage internal fixation is indicated to avoid prolonged recumbency. When the child ceases to ambulate independently (about age 10), releasing existing contractures and long leg braces are recommended to allow 2 to 3 more years of ambulation. In the wheelchair stage 25 percent of patients will develop significant scoliosis. Progressive curves over 25 degrees are considered for fusion if the patient's respiratory status allows.

BECKER MUSCULAR DYSTROPHY

This is an X-linked recessive form of muscular dystrophy characterized by proximal muscle weakness which is less severe than Duchenne.

The gene mutation is also localized to the Xp21 loci which codes for dystrophin. Dystrophin is present but is structurally abnormal or produced in decreased amounts. The distribution of muscle weakness is similar to the Duchenne type. Calf pseudohypertrophy, toe walking, and waddling gait are also similar features. CK levels are elevated. In Becker muscular dystrophy, however, there is a later age of onset (> 7 years) and the weakness progresses at a slower rate. Ambulation may be maintained until the second decade. The patients may live to their mid-40s. Early involvement of the myocardium is not a feature. Intelligence remains unaffected.

LIMB GIRDLE MUSCULAR DYSTROPHY

The limb girdle muscular dystrophies are a clinically heterogeneous group of disorders marked by proximal muscle weakness affecting predominantly the pelvic and shoulder girdle musculature. Age of onset may vary from the second year of life in the childhood forms to the second or third decade of life in the adult onset forms. The limb girdle muscular dystrophies are associated with abnormalities in the dystrophin associated protein complex known as the sarcoglycans. At least seven genetically distinct types of limb girdle muscular dystrophies have been discerned with both autosomal recessive and autosomal dominance reported. As such, both sexes may be equally affected. Muscle weakness and wasting may initially appear asymmetrical and the rate of progression is variable. Pseudohypertrophy of the calf muscles may occur and certain proximal muscles, particularly the biceps and periscapular muscles, may demonstrate atrophy. Cranial muscles are typically spared, but mild bilateral facial weakness may be present. Pelvic girdle weakness causes a waddling gait and difficulty in rising from the floor or a low chair. When the shoulder girdle is involved, the shoulders are hunched with difficulty in lifting the arms above the head. The tendon reflexes are usually present but may be difficult to elicit; the triceps reflex is usually relatively brisk. CK levels may be normal or moderately elevated, and dystrophin is normal. Disease progression is variable; however, by the fifth decade disability is usually marked. Treatment consists of physiotherapy, splinting to prevent contractures, and provision of aids for daily living.

The syndrome of limb girdle muscular dystrophy is used to refer to cases other than those in which there is a known metabolic or mitochondrial disorder. Diagnosis depends on the exclusion of other disorders, particularly disorders such as chronic spinal muscular atrophy and Becker muscular dystrophy.

FACIOSCAPULOHUMERAL MUSCULAR DYSTROPHY

Facioscapulohumeral muscular dystrophy (FSHMD) is an autosomal dominant, slowly progressive form of muscular dystrophy which affects both males and females with considerable variation. FSHMD has been found to be associated with a molecular deletion of genetic information mapped to chromosome 4. Age of onset is generally between the second and third decade of life, manifested by simultaneous weakness in the face and shoulder girdle musculature. Facial weakness is evident by inability to close the eyes properly, whistle, pout the lips, or wrinkle the brow.

Shoulder girdle weakness (scapulohumeral) includes atrophy of the trapezius, rhomboids, serratus anterior and posterior, biceps, and triceps (the forearm muscles are normal). The individual has difficulty abducting the arms with inability to stabilize the scapula (winging scapula). In the lower limb, the tibialis anterior and peronei are mainly affected. Foot drop may develop. Tendon reflexes are usually diminished early in the disease. Treatment includes ankle-foot orthoses to overcome the weakness of the foot extensors and scapular fixation for the scapular winging. Sensorineural deafness and/or retinal changes may be associated features of the disease.

CONGENITAL MUSCULAR DYSTROPHIES

The congenital muscular dystrophies are a group of disorders which present at birth or shortly thereafter. Patients may be classified into those with only skeletal muscle involvement and those with both central nervous system and skeletal muscle involvement. The muscle manifestations include hypotonia, proximal limb weakness, and joint contractures affecting the elbows, hips, knees, and ankles. The myopathic form of arthrogryposis multiplex congenita is considered a form of congenital muscular dystrophy. Congenital dislocation of the hip may be present. Weakness of facial muscles may occur, but other cranial nerve musculature is spared. The findings of full extraocular motility differentiates congenital muscular dystrophy from centronuclear myopathy. Tendon reflexes may be absent or depressed. EMG findings show a myopathic process. Muscle histology is characteristic of a dystrophy; serum enzymes are normal or elevated. A deficiency of the skeletal protein merosin has been demonstrated in a proportion of patients with congenital muscular dystrophy.

The severity of congenital muscular dystrophy varies greatly. Approximately one-half remain severely affected, never achieving the ability to stand independently. Rarely, patients die of respiratory insufficiency during the first few years of life. Conversely, one-half of patients exhibit delayed motor milestones but learn to walk, though difficulty in running and stair climbing persists. Treatment of deformity is conventional although there is high recurrence rate. Inheritance is autosomal recessive.

MYOTONIC DYSTROPHY

Myotonic dystrophy is an autosomal dominant, multisystem disorder which is the most common form of adult muscular dystrophy. Clinical manifestations of myotonic dystrophy include myotonia (delayed muscle relaxation), muscle wasting and weakness, cardiac conduction abnormalities, cataracts, and gonadal atrophy. There is a congenital form of myotonic dystrophy that is transmitted maternally and presents in the newborn period with nonspecific features of hypotonia, weakness, respiratory and feeding difficulties, and possibly arthrogryposis.

In the limbs, wasting may be prominent in distal muscles, especially forearm muscles and anterior tibia and calf muscles, but small hand muscles are usually spared until the late stages of the disease. The face appears expressionless. Myotonia is best demonstrated as a persistent dimpling after a sharp blow on a muscle belly of the thenar eminence, tongue, or deltoid. The course of the disorder is steadily progressive and usually leads to restricted ambulation within 15 to 20 years of the onset. However, there is considerable variation in the natural history of the disease. This is a reflection of the nature of the gene defect of myotonic dystrophy. The mutation is caused by an unstable, expanding DNA sequence of the myotonin protein kinase gene on chromosome 19. The size of the expanding sequence may vary between affected siblings and increase from generation to generation in parallel with increasing severity of the disorder.

NEUROPATHIES

SPINAL MUSCULAR ATROPHY

The childhood spinal muscular atrophies (SMAs) are a heterogenous group of disorders of unknown pathogenesis. They are characterized by idiopathic degeneration of anterior horn motor neurons in the spinal cord, medulla, and the mid-brain. Secondary denervation of voluntary muscle fibers results in progressive proximal muscle weakness, muscle wasting, fasciculation, and clinical paralysis. CK levels are generally normal or may be slightly elevated. EMG findings reveal characteristic denervation changes. Muscle biopsy will demonstrate denervated muscle fibers and grouped fiber atrophy.

Childhood SMA is divided into three categories according to severity and age of onset. Collectively, the SMAs of childhood comprise the second leading cause of mortality from a autosomal recessive genetic disorder. Approximately 95 percent of cases of SMA are associated with a deletion of the survival motor neuron (SMN) gene located on chromosome 5.

With type I or Werdnig-Hoffmann disease, the most severe form of spinal muscular atrophy, onset occurs within the first 6 months of life. In greater than 50 percent of cases, however, the disorder can be recognized at birth or in neonatal period. Clinically the patient will present with severe hypotonia and weakness. The child will lie with arms abducted and flexed at the elbows; the legs are abducted and flexed at the knees. Respirations are shallow and chest movements may be paradoxical. Swallowing and sucking are poor and there may be visible fasciculation of the tongue. Limb musculature may be difficult to assess because it is covered by adipose tissue, but atrophy may sometimes be recognized by palpation. The facial muscles are also involved in the denervation process; as such, the face appears expressionless and the child is unable to support its head. External ocular movements are normal. Startle and walking reflexes are difficult to elicit or absent; tendon reflexes are invariably absent. Between 10 to 25 percent of cases will present with congenital contractures or dislocation of hip. The disorder may present in a clinical picture similar to arthrogryposis congenita. A number of other disorders may also present in this manner, including infantile and neonatal myasthenia gravis, myotonic dystrophy, and certain congenital myopathies. However, when fasciculation of the tongue is noted, these other disorders may be excluded. The children generally succumb from pulmonary infection secondary to respiratory insufficiency and aspiration during feedings by age 3.

Intermediate, or type II, spinal muscular atrophy will present in infancy. Developmental milestones are normal the first few months of life with the child learning to sit independently. After 6 months of age, developmental milestones become delayed with the child never becoming able to achieve independent ambulation although standing may be observed in about 50 percent of patients. Fasciculation of other muscles is uncommon. Respiratory involvement is unusual in the early stages. The tendon reflexes are usually absent or diminished. There maybe a tremor of the outstretched fingers. Life expectancy is variable with the degree of respiratory muscle involvement the single most important factor. Many cases show little progression after presentation, with survival into adulthood common. In non-ambulatory patients a progressive coxa valga in the absence of actual motion and weight bearing may develop. Scoliosis is also a common orthopedic complication. In a curve of up to 20 degrees, bracing may be indicated. In a 40- to 60-degree curve surgery is recommended.

As fasciculation of limb muscles is rare in intermediate SMA, muscular dystrophy or other forms of infantile or childhood myopathy must be considered. Children with intermediate SMA, however, are often more severely disabled than children of the same age with muscular dystrophy, and muscular hypertrophy is uncommon in SMA. Fasciculation of the tongue is an important sign in differential diagnosis.

The mildest form of chronic childhood SMA, type III or Kugelberg Welander, generally presents after the age of 2 years but before adulthood. Typical age of onset occurs between 5 and 15 years. The first symptom is generally related to weakness of the thighs and hips. The child has difficulty getting up from the ground and climbing stairs. There is an associated waddling gait and in children with early onset there may be a delay in walking. Later, shoulder girdle weakness becomes evident causing weakness of the arm and winging of the scapulas. Paraspinal muscles may also be involved so that neck extensors and flexors become weak and lordosis may develop. Scoliosis may also occur. Weakness is usually proximal and symmetrical. Fasciculation may be found in limb muscles in about 50 percent of cases at some stage of the disease, usually in the early stage of the disease. Fasciculation of the tongue is uncommon. Hypertrophy of muscles, particularly of the calves, may also be observed. The tendon reflexes are diminished or absent. Survival into adulthood is a rule and many patients have a normal life span. Ambulation may be possible for many years.

Cases of Type III SMA may present similarly to limb girdle and facioscapulohumeral muscular dystrophy. Limb girdle muscular dystrophy in the juvenile age group is uncommon, whereas Kugelberg Welander accounts for the majority of patients presenting with proximal weakness at this age.

PERIPHERAL NEUROPATHIES

Hereditary motor and sensory neuropathy (HMSN I, II), peroneal muscular atrophy, and Charcot-Marie-Tooth (CMT) disease are synonymous.

The disease is characterized by slowly progressive distal wasting and weakness in the legs, predominantly affecting the anterior tibial and peroneal muscles. The patient complains about cramps in the legs and feet, difficulty in running, paresthesia in the legs. Nearly 60 percent of patients have depressed or absent ankle jerks. Cavus with clawing of the toes gradually develops. The deformity is present bilaterally. The peronei and intrinsic muscles of the foot are affected first. Later, the tibialis anterior and the toe extensors are weakened. As a result, foot drop develops. The upper limbs become involved at a later stage. Symmetric atrophy of the intrinsic muscles of the hand and forearm develops. Proprioceptive, light touch, and vibratory sensibilities in the feet are decreased.

Autosomal dominant type 1A (HMSN—demyelinating CMT) is the most common form of HMSN. Approximately 70 percent of cases will demonstrate a genetic duplication on chromosome 17. Motor nerve conduction velocity is delayed. Nerve biopsies show evidence of segmental demyelination, often accompanied by hypertrophic changes with "onion bulb" formation.

An autosomal recessive form of CMT 1B exists which is clinically similar to the dominant form although it appears to be more severe with earlier onset. Roussy-Lévy disease is a variant of HMSN type I with a clinical picture similar to the Charcot-Marie-Tooth but with associated tremor or ataxia. Neurophysiologic and pathologic features of the Roussy-Lévy syndrome and HMSN I are identical.

An X-linked dominant form of CMT exists which affects primarily males and is clinically similar to CMT 1. However, carrier females may be symptomatic.

The age of onset for type II (neuronal or axonal CMT) is generally later than type I, although the distribution and severity of muscle weakness are similar. Autosomal dominant and recessive forms have been reported as well as a severe autosomal recessive childhood form. Motor nerve conduction velocity may be normal or only slightly reduced. Nerve biopsy shows axonal degeneration.

HMSN type III, Déjèrine-Sottas disease or hypertrophic polyneuropathy, is an autosomal dominant disease. Symptoms are usually seen from infancy. The children have absent reflexes, walk late, and can become wheelchair bound in the second decade of life. There is marked sensory loss in all four extremities. Skeletal deformity, particularly scoliosis, is common and often severe. Ataxia is universal. Pathologic changes include hypomyelination as well as demyelination.

Refsum's disease (HMSN type IV) is an autosomal recessive disorder which manifests in childhood or at puberty. It is a hypertrophic neuropathy and is characterized chemically by excessive phytanic acid in the serum. It is accompanied by an atypical pigmentary degeneration of the retina, cerebellar limb ataxia, cardiomyopathy, and sensorineural deafness. There is a distal sensory and motor loss in the hands and the feet.

In the early stages of HMSN pes cavus can be corrected by serial casting and an orthosis. However, the deformity usually progresses. At this stage a plantar release is suggested. Once bony changes occur procedures such as wedge osteotomy or truncated osteotomy should be performed. In more than a 75 percent of cases, triple arthrodesis has a fair to poor result and is indicated only as a salvage procedure in patients with a severely rigid foot.

A recessively inherited disorder characterized by spinocerebellar degeneration and neuropathy, Freidreich's ataxia is associated with an unstable, expanding DNA sequence on chromosome 9. The clinical onset occurs between 6 to 20 years of age. Primary symptoms are an ataxic gait, pes cavus, clumsiness of the hands, dysarthria, and nystagmus. Seventy-five percent will have scoliosis and cardiomyopathy that often leads to death in the third to fourth decade of life. Most patients lose the ability to walk a few years after onset.

Scoliosis develops in 75 percent of patients with Friedreich's ataxia but rarely develops in patients with HMSN. Braces are poorly tolerated and progression often continues after maturity. In such cases spinal stabilization is indicated.

SPINA BIFIDA

Spina bifida is a congenital disorder characterized by a failure of fusion of the vertebral arch with or without dysplasia of the spinal cord and its membranes.

Isolated laminar defects are seen in 5 percent of lumbar spine x-rays. The incidence of myelomeningocele in the United States is 1 to 2 per 1000 live births. The incidence of spina bifida may vary by geographic location. Spina bifida is caused by multifactorial inheritance which is a genetic predisposition influenced by environmental factors such as nutritional (low intake of folic acid), drug induced (valproic acid), and maternal insulin-dependent diabetes.

The nervous system develops by the formation of the neural tube from deep ectoderm cells. After closure of this tube, superficial ectoderm fuses over it to close the back. Mesenchymal cells create the vertebral arch and the paraspinal muscles between the two layers of ectoderm. This process is completed by the fourth week of gestation. Spinal dysraphism (or myelodysplasia) is the generic term for defects in the fusion process.

Spina bifida occulta is the mildest form of dysraphism where the posterior bony arch of the vertebra is not fused. In some cases an associated skin dimple or tuft of hair can be seen. Intraspinal anomalies such as tethering or splitting of the cord (diastematomyelia) by a bony or cartilagenous bar may occur. In a meningocele, in addition to the unfused vertebral arch, there is a skin defect through which a meningeal sac is visible. This sac is filled with CSF and composed of dura or dura and arachnoid but no nerve tissue. Neurologic deficit is rare. In a myelomeningocele, the exposed meningeal sac contains part of the spinal cord and nerve roots. In the "closed" type the neural tube is fully formed and covered by membrane and skin. In the "open" type the cord may be in its primitive state, a neural plate that forms part of the sac. The spina bifida lesions are seen predominantly in the lumbosacral region, possibly due to rostral and caudal closure of the neural canal although they can occur at any level along the spine.

ASSOCIATED NEUROLOGIC CONDITIONS

Hydrocephalus

Among spina bifida patients, 80 to 90 percent have hydrocephalus that requires shunting. Hydrocephalus complicates 90 percent of cases of lumbosacral spina bifida.

Arnold-Chiari Malformation

Arnold-Chiari malformation is a caudal displacement of the posterior lobe of the cerebellum and is a common finding in patients with spina bifida. It represents a spectrum of anomalies involving caudal displacement and herniation of cerebellar structures. This results in weakness of the vocal cords and difficulties in feeding, crying, and breathing. In type 1 there is caudal displacement of the tonsils but not the brain stem, cerebellar vermis, or fourth ventricle and there is no kink in the cervicomedullary junction. Type II is associated with SB; the cerebellar vermis, the tonsils, and the medulla and/or fourth ventricle are displaced caudally. The upper cervical nerve roots tend to exit from the cord and run rostrally. The cervicomedullary junction is often kinked. Patients with either type may have syringomyelia and/or hydrocephalus.

Hydromyelia

Accumulation of fluid in the enlarged central spinal canal is frequent and may result in scoliosis.

Tethered Cord

Most patients have some tethering but only 20 percent will develop symptoms.

Urinary Problems

Ninety percent of cases will develop neurogenic bladder, either spastic or flaccid.

ASSOCIATED CONGENITAL ANOMALIES

Associated congenital anomalies can occur in 30 percent of cases. They include hip dislocation, clubfeet, and other anomalies of the spine and the genitourinary system. They may be primary or due to muscle imbalance or paralysis.

TREATMENT

Skin closure should be performed within 48 h. Careful dissection is needed.

Hydrocephalus develops within a few days of birth. Treatment should not be delayed. A ventriculoperitoneal shunt is usually inserted.

Children with Arnold-Chiari malformation have a high mortality rate (30 percent) and may need tracheotomy and cervical and posterior fossa decompression.

Urinary Problems: Ultrasound and intravenous pyelogram are used to detect anomalies. Intermittent catheterization is used for urinary incontinence. Urinary tract infections are common and management by a urologist familiar with spina bifida is essential.

PROGNOSTIC CLASSIFICATION OF SPINA BIFIDA PATIENTS (AMBULATION)

This classification is based on the level of the lesion.

Group I: High lumbar level or thoracic lesion. No quadriceps function and almost all patients are confined to wheelchair.

Group II: Low lumbar lesion with functioning quadriceps and medial hamstrings. Most require ankle-foot orthoses for support and crutches for trunk stability. About two-thirds of patients will use a wheelchair as an adult.

Group III: Sacral level lesion. Most children can walk without external support and may not require ankle-foot orthosis. The goal of the orthopedic treatment is to have these children walk with appropriate orthotic support by the age of eighteen months.

The care of each patient is individualized for thoracic and high lumbar levels. A frame for standing followed by parapodium supports over age 2 years, reciprocal gait orthosis (RGO), hip-knee-ankle-foot orthosis (HKAFO) for swing-through gait are used. For low lumbar and sacral level AFOs are used.

ORTHOPEDIC TREATMENT OF ASSOCIATED DEFORMITIES

Hip

Over 50 percent of children with sacral spina bifida have hip dislocation or subluxation. Treatment is by standard methods (e.g., Pavlik harness and traction). In low lumbar lesions hip dislocations are caused by imbalance. The extensors and abductors are weak and are overpowered by the flexors and adductors. Open reduction is indicated only in children with strong quadriceps muscles bilaterally, normal trunk balance, and normal upper extremities.

Ideally, treatment with muscle balancing will be performed prior to dislocation. In addition to the open reduction, muscle balancing procedures are suggested such as the transfer of the psoas tendon posterolaterally from the lesser to the greater trochanter through a large hole in the ileum (Sharrard) or laterally (Mustard). Hip dislocation in high-level lesions does not require open reduction. Only soft tissue contractures should be corrected. In older children it may be impossible to reduce a dislocation. Often it is best not to intervene.

Spine

Scoliosis is the most common deformity (100 percent in T12 lesions, 80 percent with L2 lesions, 70 percent with L3 lesions, 60 percent with L4, 25 percent with L5, and 5 percent with S1 lesions). Curves develop gradually until age 10 years and increase rapidly with the adolescent growth spurt. Braces may slow deterioration; however, when the child is old enough, operative correction and segmental stabilization are needed.

Kyphosis

Kyphosis occurs in 10 percent of patients. It usually presents at birth with the apex in the mid lumbar region. The deformity may exceed 90 degrees by 3 years of age. Braces have no place in the treatment of kyphosis. Surgery is indicated if patients develop recurrent skin breakdown with infection or are unable to sit upright without propping with their arms.

Foot

Thirty percent of spina bifida cases have clubfoot. It is rigid, and in most cases, not responsive to conservative treatment. Surgery is performed at 6 to 10 months (complete soft tissue releases). Patients may present with calcaneovalgus deformity (mainly L5-S1 lesions). Serial manipulation and casting followed by orthosis may be sufficient. In rigid cases, soft tissue release is indicated.

CEREBRAL PALSY

Cerebral palsy is a fixed nonprogressive brain lesion that occurs prenatally at birth or in the postnatal period (from birth until brain maturation at 2 years of age). The incidence of cerebral palsy is 2 in 1000 live births. The etiology includes prenatal, natal, and postnatal factors. Prenatal factors (30 percent of cases) include viral infection during early pregnancy, alcohol or drug use, diabetes mellitus, and thyroid abnormality. Natal factors include trauma, asphyxia during labor, and prematurity with intravascular hemorrhage. Postnatal factors include encephalitis, meningitis, trauma, and asphyxia.

There are four types of cerebral palsy described, based on the clinical presentation:

1. *Spastic* (60 percent of patients): These are generally the result of a cerebral cortex lesion.
2. *Dyskinetic* (25 percent of patients), including athetosis, dystonia, and rigidity: These cases result from mid-brain or base of brain lesions.
3. *Ataxic* (5 percent) cases have a cerebellar lesion.
4. *Mixed* (10 percent) have more widespread brain involvement.
   The distribution of the disability in cerebral palsy is as follows:

1. *Hemiplegic* (50 percent of cases): The patient has involvement predominantly on one side, arm, and leg. The arm is usually worse than the leg. These patients are usually spastic.
2. *Quadriplegic* (25 percent of cases): All four extremities are involved. The patients may be spastic or dyskinetic or a mixed type.

3. *Diplegic* (21 percent of cases): The lower extremities are predominantly involved, although there is some involvement of the upper extremities. Most patients are spastic.
4. *Triplegic* (3 percent of cases): Three or four extremities are affected. Most patients are spastic; they may be also dyskinetic.
5. *Monoplegic* (1 percent of cases). Only one extremity, either upper or lower, is affected.

About 80 percent of the cerebral palsy population have speech problems, 30 percent have visual defects, 20 percent are mentally retarded (especially those in the total body involvement), 15 percent have some deafness, 25 percent have seizures. About 50 percent have loss of sensation of two-point discrimination, stereognosis, and position sense.

TREATMENT

Any serious approach to treatment of cerebral palsy demands the multidisciplinary skills (teamwork) of the orthopaedic surgeon, neurologist, urologist, pediatrician, physiotherapist, occupational therapist, and speech therapist.

There is no cure for cerebral palsy. The goals of treatment are to increase the patient's physical independence and cognitive and speech abilities, and to create, as much as possible, a socioeconomic independence. Patients with cerebral palsy give the following order of preference in improving their quality of life: (1) education and communication, (2) activities of daily living, (3) mobility, and (4) ambulation.

The orthopaedic surgeon is seldom involved in the care of infants with cerebral palsy. An orthopaedist is consulted when abnormal posture or movement pattern appears, or if the child is unable to stand and walk. During this period intensive physiotherapy (there are some widely practiced methods) is begun. Physiotherapy continues through childhood and early adolescence. Splints are used to prevent fixed deformity, to facilitate improved patterns of movement, and to hold position after corrective surgery.

The indications for surgery in cerebral palsy are: (1) inability to control a spastic deformity by nonoperative measures; (2) to correct fixed deformity that interferes with function; and (3) to correct secondary bony deformities, hip dislocations, or joint instability.

The timing of surgery is important. Muscle releases before age 4 years have a high tendency to recur. If the contracture interferes with positioning, surgery should be performed even before this age. Preferably all surgical procedures should be performed in one session and be completed before school age (6 to 7 years).

Types of surgery include: (1) release of tight muscles; (2) tendon transfer to augment weak muscles; and (3) osteotomies or arthrodesis to correct fixed deformity.

Surgery for the Lower Limb

1. *Hip adduction deformity* results in "scissoring" gait or progressive hip subluxation. If passive abduction is less than 30 percent on each side, an adductor tenotomy is indicated. The adductor longus and gracilis in walkers, and the adductor brevis in nonambulators, is released. This may be combined with a neurotomy of the anterior branch of the obturator nerve.
2. *Hip flexion deformity* results in hyperlordosis. If flexion deformity is more than 30 degrees, iliopsoas recession or proximal rectus release are indicated.
3. *Hip internal rotation deformity* interferes with walking. In young children, up to age 6 years of age, muscle releases (adductors and

iliopsoas) are indicated. In the older child, derotation osteotomy of the femur is needed (intertrochanteric or supracondylar).
4. *Hip subluxation* results from a persistent flexion and adduction deformity. This leads to femoral anteversion, subluxation, and dislocation. Muscle release before age 6 may prevent the deformity. Older children need varus derotation osteotomy of the femur at times combined with acetabuloplasty.
5. *Knee flexion deformity* is due to tight hamstrings. It interferes with gait ability (measured by the popliteal angle). If the popliteal angle is greater than 60 degrees hamstring release is indicated.
6. *Knee extension deformity* results in "stiff knee" gait. Can be corrected by distal rectus release or transfer.
7. *Foot equinus* results in toe-toe gait. If fixed, tendoachilles lengthening is indicated.
8. *Varus foot* can be corrected by tibialis anterior and posterior split transfer.
9. Pronated foot may require arthrodesis.

A crouch gait can result from hip and knee flexion deformity and equinus. Before surgery is performed on one joint, other joints should be inspected carefully. Muscle releases should be done in all joints simultaneously.

Surgery for the Upper Limb

Surgery should be delayed till age 7 to 8 years.

1. Elbow flexion deformity: Usually no treatment is indicated.
2. Forearm pronation deformity: Pronator teres release may improve position. Also flexor carpi ulnaris (FCU) transfer to the extensor carpi radialis brevis and longus.
3. Wrist flexion deformity: FCU release and transfer are performed.
4. Flexion deformity of the fingers: Fractional lengthening of the flexors (sublimis and profundus may improve finger function) are performed.
5. Thumb in palm deformity: This can be improved by release of the thumb adductors.

Surgery of the Spine

Scoliosis is common in cerebral palsy. The curve is usually thoracolumbar; sometimes it is incorporated into the pelvis with obliquity. Surgery is indicated even in total body involvement to balance the trunk and to increase sitting ability.

In an effort to decrease spasticity by ablation of afferent impulses from the muscles, Peacock has suggested selective resection of the posterior rootlets in the L1-L5 vertebrae (selective posterior rhizotomy). Spasticity decreased remarkably in the operated cases. In some patients spasticity recurred in few months. Long-term results are still required to determine indications for this procedure.

SUGGESTED READINGS

BRACHIAL PLEXUS INJURIES

Gilbert A, Razaboni R, Amar-Khodja S. Indications and results of brachial plexus surgery in obstetrical palsy. *Orthop Clin North Am* 1988; 19:91.

Greenwald AG, Schute PC, Shiveley JL. Brachial plexus birth palsy: A 10-year report on the incident and prognosis. *J Pediatr Orthop* 1984; 4:689.

Tachdjian MO. Obstetrical brachial plexus palsy. In: *Pediatric Orthopaedics*, vol 3, 2d ed. Philadelphia: WB Saunders; 1990:2009.

DYSTROPHIES

Emery AEH, Rimoin DL. *Principles and Practice of Medical Genetics,* 2d ed. New York: Churchill Livingstone, 1990:539.

Hoffman EP, Kunkel KM. Dystrophin abnormalities in Duchenne/Becker muscular dystrophy. *Neuron* 1989; 2:1019.

Lee JH, Goto K, Matsuda C, Arahata K. Characterization of a tandemly repeated 3.3-kb KdnI unit in the facioscapulohumeral musclular dystrophy (FSHD) gene region on chromosome 4q35. *Muscle Nerve* 1995; (suppl 2):S6.

Mendell JR, Sahenk Z, Prior TW. The childhood muscular dystrophies: diseases sharing a common pathogenesis of membrane instability. *J Child Neurol* 1995; 10:2:150.

Roland EN. Neuromuscular disorders in childhood. *Curr Opin Pediatr* 1994; 6:636.

Sage PF. Muscular dystrophy. In: Crenshaw AH, ed. *Campbell's Operative Orthopaedics,* vol 5, 8th ed. St. Louis: Mosby-Year Book; 1992:2469.

Shapiro F, Bresnan MJ. Orthopaedic management of childhood neuromuscular disease. Part III: Diseases of muscle. *J Bone Joint Surg [Am]* 1982; 64:1102.

Swash M, Schwartz MS. Muscular dystrophies. In: Swash M, Schwartz MS, eds. *Neuromuscular Diseases: A Practical Approach to Diagnosis and Management,* 2d ed. New York: Springer-Verlag; 1988:163.

Tachdjian MO. Progressive muscular dystrophy. In: *Pediatric Orthopaedics,* vol 3, 2d ed. Philadelphia: WB Saunders; 1990:2126.

NEUROPATHIES

Emery AEH, Rimoin DL, eds. *Principles and Practices of Medical Genetics,* 2d ed. New York: Churchill Livingstone, 1990:565.

Filla A, De Michele G, Cavalcanti F, et al. The relationship between trinucleotide (GAA) repeat length and clinical features in Friedreich ataxia. *Am J Hum Genet* 1996; 59:554.

Kleyn PW, Gilliam TC. Progress toward cloning of the gene responsible for childhood spinal muscular atrophy. *Semin Neurol* 1993; 13:276.

Lefebvre S, Burglen L, et al. Identification and characterization of a spinal muscular atrophy-determining gene. *Cell* 1995; 80:155.

Miller G, Vannucci RC. Hereditary motor and sensory neuropathies. *Pediatr Ann* 1989; 18:428.

Roland EH. Neuromuscular disorders in childhood. *Curr Opin Pediatr* 1994; 6:636.

Schwentker EP, Gibson DA. The orthopaedic aspects of spinal muscular atrophy. *J Bone Joint Surg [Am]* 1976; 58:32.

Shapiro F, Bresnan MJ. Orthopaedic management of childhood muscular diseases. Part I: Spinal muscular atrophy. *J Bone Joint Surg [Am]* 1982; 64:785. Part II: Peripheral neuropathies. 1982; 64:949.

Swash M, Schwartz MS. Diseases of anterior horn cells. In: Swash M, Schwartz MS, eds. *Neuromuscular Diseases: A Practical Approach to Diagnosis and Management,* 2d ed. New York: Springer-Verlag; 1981:73–80.

Tachdjian MO. Hereditary motor and sensory neuropathies. In: *Pediatric Orthopaedics,* vol 3, 2d ed. Philadelphia: WB Saunders; 1990:1982.

SPINA BIFIDA

Asher M, Olson J. Factors affecting the ambulatory status of patients with spina bifida cystica. *J Bone Joint Surg [Am]* 1983; 65:350.

Beaty JH. Myelomeningocele. In: Crenshaw AH, ed. *Campbell's Operative Orthopaedics,* vol 3, 8th ed. St. Louis: Mosby-Year Book; 1992:2433.

Drennan JC, Banta JV, Bunch WH. Symposium: Current concepts in the management of myelomingocele. *Contemp Orthop* 1989; 19:63.

McLaughlin JF, Shurtleff DB, Lamers JY, et al. Influence of prognosis on decisions regarding the care of newborns with myelodysplasia. *N Engl J Med* 1985; 312:1589.

Samuelsson L, Skoog M. Ambulation in patients with myelomeningocele: A multivariate statistical analysis. J Ped Orthop 1988; 8:569.

Tachdjian MO. Myelomeningocele. In: Tachdjian MO, ed. *Pediatric Orthopaedics,* vol 3, 2d ed. Philadelphia: WB Saunders; 1990:1773.

CEREBRAL PALSY

Apley GA. Cerebral palsy. In: Apley GA, ed. *Apley's System of Orthopaedic and Fractures,* 7th ed. Oxford: Butterworth Heinemann; 1993:196.

Bleck EE. *Orthopaedic Management of Cerebral Palsy.* Philadelphia: WB Saunders; 1979.

Sage FP. Cerebral palsy. In: Crenshaw AD, ed. *Campbell's Operative Orthopaedics,* vol 4, 8th ed. Mosby-Year Book; 1992:2287.

Tachdjian MO. Cerebral palsy. In: Tachdjian MO, ed. *Pediatric Orthopaedics,* vol 3. Philadelphia: WB Saunders; 1990:1605.

Chapter 135

CONGENITAL LIMB MALFORMATIONS

Gail S. Chorney

This chapter will review congenital deformities of the lower extremities not covered in other chapters. The major anomalies involve bowing of the tibia and congenital absences of part or all of the tibia or fibula.

POSTEROMEDIAL BOWING OF THE TIBIA

The appearance of congenital posteromedial bowing of the tibia at birth can be quite frightening to the new parents and health care workers (Fig. 135-1). The natural history of this deformity and the subsequent treatment is benign, particularly when compared to anterolateral bowing. The typical appearance is of a shortened extremity below the knee with a severe calcaneovalgus foot. Except for its extreme position, the foot is normal with all rays present. Radiographs confirm that the entire tibia and fibula are also present. There is, however, significant bowing of the tibia with the fibula following in form. The apex of the curve is posteromedial. The angular deformity can be as high as 60 degrees.

The etiology of this angular deformity is unknown. The two theories are intrauterine positioning or prenatal injury to the physis with asymmetrical growth. It may be that both theories are correct with the latter accounting for the more severe deformities.

In the neonate period, treatment is education of the parents to the benign nature of the problem. It is not associated with other congenital anomalies. The major problem is an eventual leg length in-equality. The calcaneovalgus foot will usually resolve spontaneously. If it does not, manipulation and serial casting can be employed.

Even children with severe posteromedial bowing of the tibia begin independent ambulation on time. No orthotic intervention is necessary. These children do well despite the significant cosmetic deformity. As the children become older, a lift may be needed if the leg length discrepancy is greater than 2 cm.

The natural history is that the angular deformity decreases with growth. At skeletal maturity there is a leg length discrepancy and a small residual bowing. The leg length discrepancy averages 5 cm at maturity and may warrant lengthening. The residual bowing is approximately 6 degrees. This angular deformity can be corrected at time of lengthening. The bowing can be corrected acutely or gradually with the external fixator, depending on the surgeon's preference.

ANTEROLATERAL BOWING OF THE TIBIA

Anterolateral bowing of the tibia may not be as dramatic in appearance at birth as posteromedial bowing. In fact, the diagnosis may not be made at birth but during the first year of life. Its natural history, however, is not as benign and the treatment is far more complicated.

Anterolateral bowing of the tibia is a manifestation of congenital pseudoarthrosis of the tibia. The incidence is 1:140,000 live births. Approximately 50 percent of children with congenital pseudoarthrosis of the tibia have neurofibromatosis. Therefore, children with this

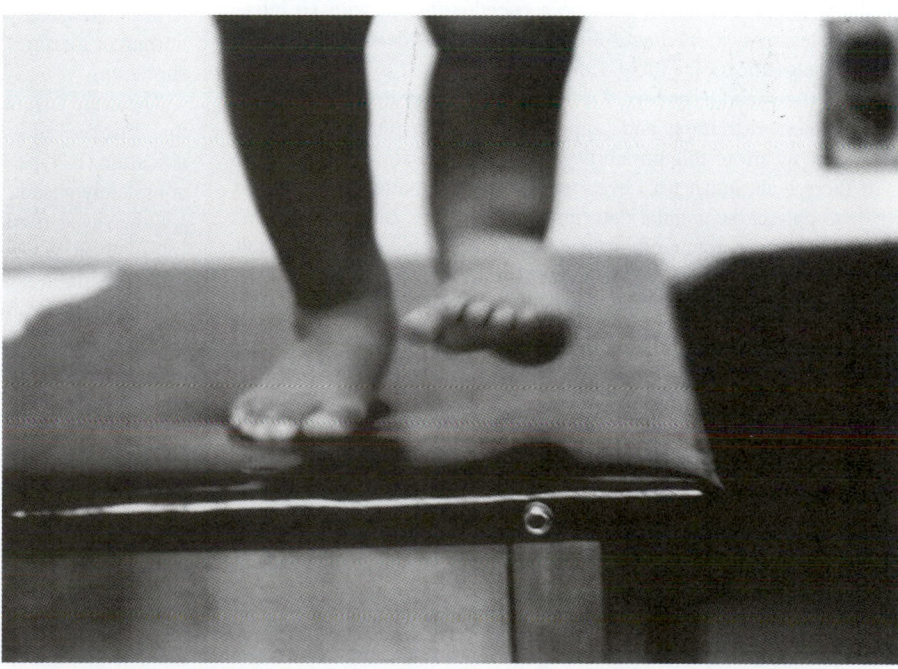

Figure 135-1
Child with posteromedial bowing of the tibia.

791

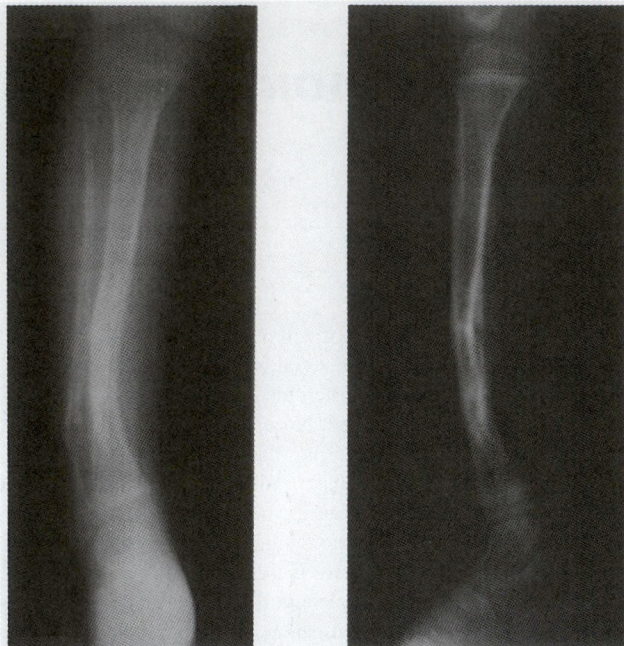

Figure 135-2
Radiographs of a tibia with congenital pseudoarthrosis with narrowing of the medullary canal and no fracture yet.

Table 135-1

Boyd Classification of Congenital Pseudoarthrosis of the Tibia

I	Tibia defect, bowing
II	Hourglass constriction in tibia, anterior bowing, associated with neurofibromatosis
III	Pseudoarthrosis through cystic lesion
IV	Pseudoarthrosis in sclerotic region of tibia, no narrowing of canal
V	Pseudoarthrosis, dysplastic fibula
VI	Pseudoarthrosis, intra-osseous neurofibroma

SOURCE: Modified and printed with permission from Beaty JH: Congenital anomalies of lower extremity. In Crenshaw AH (ed): *Campbell's Operative Orthopaedics,* 7th ed. St. Louis: CV Mosby; 1987; 2670–2671.

deformity should be checked regularly throughout their childhood for the other manifestations of neurofibromatosis. Often the other lesions do not become apparent until later in childhood. Conversely, only about 10 to 15 percent of individuals with neurofibromatosis have a congenital pseudoarthrosis of the tibia.

The radiographic presentation of pseudoarthrosis of the tibia falls into three major categories: (1) there may be an intact tibia with a sclerotic narrowing of the medullary canal; (2) bowing will be present (Fig. 135-2). Eventually, there will be a fracture through this narrowed area. There may be a pseudoarthrosis through a cystic lesion in the tibia; (3) there may also be a pseudoarthrosis with an intra-osseous lesion such as a neurofibroma. Boyd has developed a more detailed classification (Table 135-1). It is difficult to obtain fusion through the pseudoarthrosis. The patient may end up with a shortened useless extremity, and amputation may be required. Parents should be aware of this possibility early in the treatment plan.

If there is an intact tibia even with bowing, no attempt should be made to correct the angular deformity with surgery. An osteotomy invariably results in nonunion. Instead, the limb should be protected with a total contact orthosis. The natural history is that the tibia will fracture; at that time there will be ample opportunity to correct the deformity while attempting the difficult task of uniting the pseudoarthrosis. Refracture after union is also a frequent occurrence. There have been some case reports of spontaneous resolution of the bowing in an intact tibia. This should not be the expected outcome, however.

Multiple surgical procedures have been utilized to unite the congenital pseudoarthrosis of the tibia. The number of procedures is an indication of the poor results over the years. Treatment options include electrical stimulation, dual onlay bone grafting, intramedullary nailing with bone grafting, Ilizarov method of bone transport, and vascularized bone grafting. Complications of treatment include nonunion, stiff knee and ankle, and further growth arrest. The limb is already destined to be short and may need a lengthening. Often the

contralateral leg requires an epiphysiodesis in order to decrease the amount of lengthening needed. If there is a large limb length discrepancy and stiff joints at the end of treatment of the pseudoarthrosis, amputation and prosthetic fitting may still be the final option. Boyd Type II deformities are generally associated with the worst prognosis.

One of the goals of treatment should be to minimize the number of surgeries and emotional trauma to the child. Presently, it is common to start with intramedullary nailing and bone grafting as the first attempt to heal a pseudoarthrosis of the tibia. If this plan fails, a vascularized graft is the next option. Some surgeons proceed directly to the vascularized bone graft. If healing is achieved, the limb should still be protected with a total contact orthosis until skeletal maturity because of the risk of refracture.

FIBULAR HEMIMELIA

Fibular hemimelia is a limb deficiency that occurs spontaneously and is not associated with other congenital anomalies. The foot may be normal or missing several rays. Less obvious is an associated femoral shortening.

There are several classifications of fibular deficiency in the literature. The one most commonly used is the Achterman-Kalamachi classification. In type I, the fibula is present and in type II, the fibula is completely absent. Type I is further subdivided into A and B. In type IA, the distal fibular physis is at the same level as the tibial physis (normally it is more distal) (Fig. 135-3). In type IB, a large portion of the fibula is absent. The tibia itself is shorter than the contralateral side. In addition, there is usually anterior bowing of the tibia. The proportion of shortening of the tibia remains constant through life. The proportion is directly correlated with the amount of deformity. Type II deficiencies have the greatest amount of tibial shortening, often as much as 25 percent.

The foot may be normal in appearance or lacking one to two rays. It is always the lateral rays that are missing. The ankle is unstable because of the lack of lateral structures. Typically the ankle is in a valgus position. The femoral shortening will, of course, add to the overall limb length discrepancy.

When a child is born with complete absence of the fibula, amputation should be discussed with the parents. The shortening is severe enough to limit the potential of obtaining a satisfactory limb with

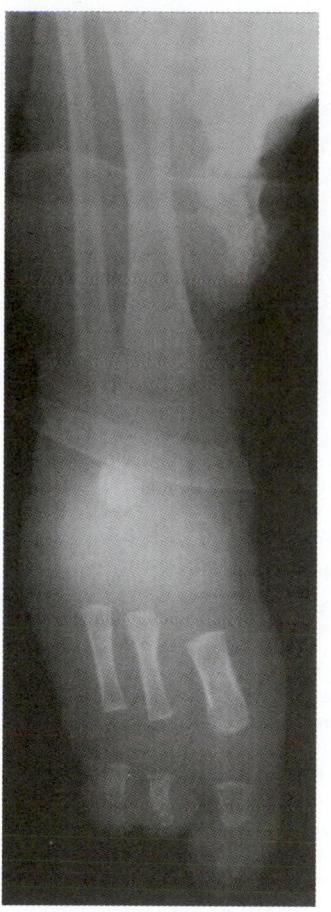
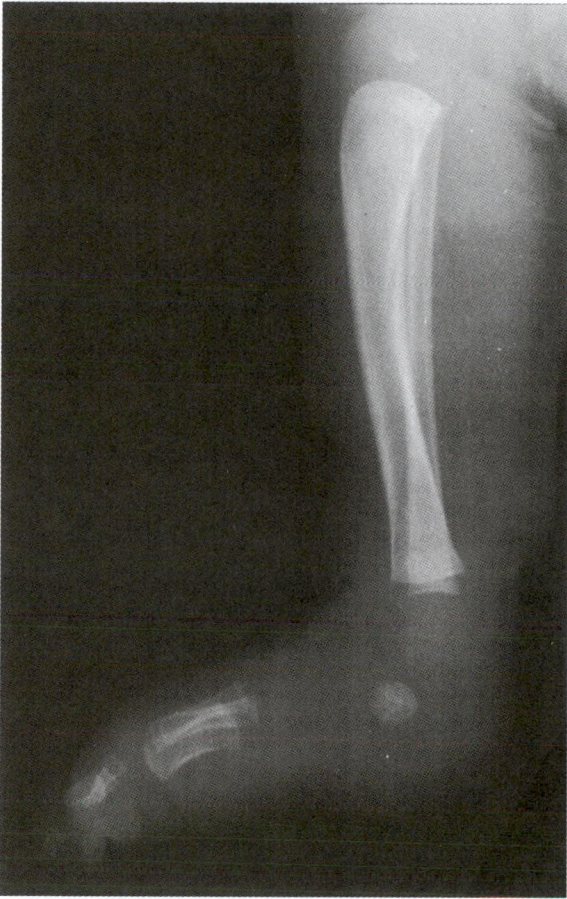
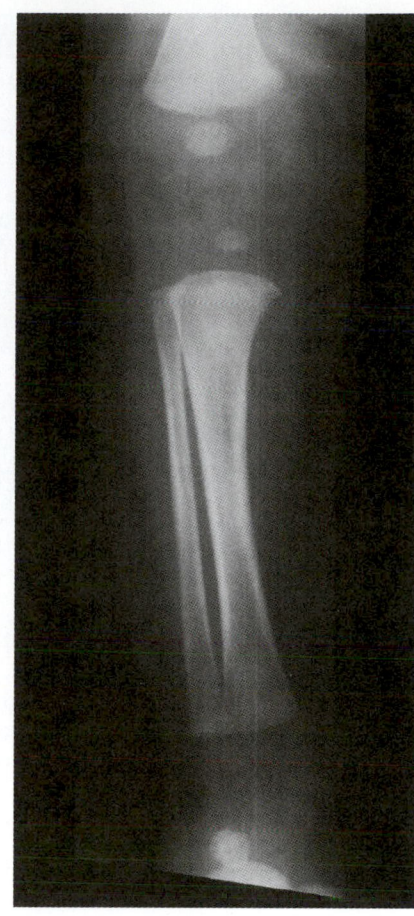

A   *B*   *C*

Figure 135-3
Radiographs of type IA fibular hemimelia.

multiple surgeries. The problem is particularly compounded if the foot is not normal. Since the goal is to normalize the child's function, the amputation should be preformed just before the child would start standing and ambulating. Therefore, the ideal timing would be just before the first birthday. The child would then learn to walk with the prosthetic limb. Function is excellent. More important, the psychological trauma is minimized.

A Symes amputation produces an excellent stump for prosthetic fitting. If there is sufficient bowing of the tibia to interfere with routine prosthetic fitting, a tibia osteotomy should be preformed at the time of the amputation.

If the fibula is partially present, treatment options depend on the foot and ankle anomalies and the amount of shortening predicted at skeletal maturity. If the foot is very deficient and the shortening is severe, the amputation still remains the best option. However, if there is a normal foot and ankle valgus is minimal, limb lengthening can yield a functional limb. The important factor is function of the limb. Preservation of a limb should not be the goal if function is sacrificed.

Symes amputation may be the ideal treatment for bilateral fibular hemimelia. Though the legs are the same length, they are disproportional to the remainder of the body. Bilateral prosthesis will offer a better cosmetic result as well as probably a more functional one. However, if the ankles and feet are very functional, bilateral lengthenings can be considered.

TIBIAL HEMIMELIA

Unlike fibular hemimelia, tibial hemimelia can be an inherited disorder and there is an association with other congenital problems. The inheritance may be autosomal dominant or autosomal recessive. The associated anomalies can include the upper extremity as well as the foot. In considering limb salvage versus amputation in treatment options, the knee as well as the ankle can be a problem.

The classification is by Jones. There are four types. In type I, the tibia is completely absent. In type II, the distal tibia is absent, while in type III, the proximal tibia is absent. In type IV, the distal tibial epiphysis lacks the joint surface at the ankle and the fibula and tibia diverge, leaving an unstable ankle. Type I is further subdivided into A and B based on the normalcy of the distal femoral epiphysis (Fig. 135-4).

In tibial hemimelia, the ankle joint is in varus. The articulation is abnormal. There may be tarsal coalitions. Shortening of the limb below the knee is significant.

Amputation remains the mainstay of treatment. It is almost impossible to achieve a good functional result with limb preservation if both the knee and ankle are abnormal. If the knee is normal and disarticulation of the ankle is the amputation of choice, a synostosis of the fibula and the tibia may have to be achieved first in order to provide a suitable stump.

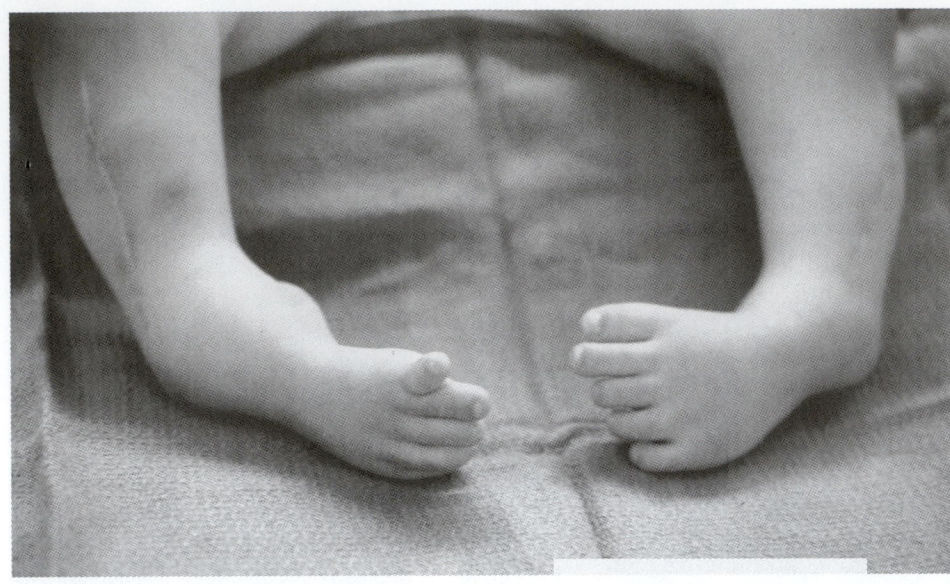

Figure 135-4
Child with tibial hemimelia. Note the extreme position of the foot.

In type IV, the talus can be fused to the distal tibia and a tibial lengthening can be preformed at a later date. This approach is to be considered if the predicted shortening is not that great. The foot must also be normal.

SUGGESTED READINGS

Bruce RW Jr: Torsional and angular deformities. *Pediatr Clin North Am* 1996; 43:867.

Fixsen JA: Major congenital shortening of the lower limb and congenital pseudarthrosis of the tibia [editorial]. *J Pediatr Orthop Part B* 1995; 4:142.

Gaine WJ, McCreath SW: Syme's amputation revisited: a review of 46 cases. *J Bone Joint Surg [Br]* 1996; 78:461.

Garg NK, Gaur S: Percutaneous autogenous bone-marrow grafting in congenital tibial pseudarthrosis. *J Bone Joint Surg [Br]* 1996; 77:830.

Gibbons PJ, Bradish CF: Fibular hemimelia: A preliminary report on management of the severe abnormality. *J Pediatr Ortho Part B* 1996; 5:20.

Gilbert A, Brockman R: Congenital pseudarthrosis of the tibia. Long-term followup of 29 cases treated by microvascular bone transfer. *Clin Orthop* 1995; 314:37.

Grill F: Treatment of congenital pseudarthrosis of tibia with the circular frame technique. *J Pediatr Orthop Part B* 1996; 5:6.

Huang SC, Yipp KM: Treatment of congenital pseudarthrosis of the tibia with the Ilizarov method. *J Formosan Med Assoc* 1997; 96:359.

Kanaya F, Tsai TM, Harkess J: Vascularized bone grafts for congenital pseudarthrosis of the tibia. *Microsurgery* 1996; 17:459.

Maffulli N, Fixsen JA: Management of forme fruste fibular hemimelia. *J Pediatr Orthop Part B* 1996; 5:17.

Naudie D, Hamdy RC, Fassier F, et al: Management of fibular hemimelia: Amputation of limb lengthening. *J Bone Joint Surg [Br]* 1997; 79:58.

Simmons ED Jr, Ginsburg GM, Hall JE: Brown's procedure for congenital absence of the tibia revisited. *J Pediatr Orthop* 1996; 16:85.

Turker R, Mendelson S, Ackman J, et al: Anatomic considerations of the foot and leg in tibial hemimelia. *J Pediatr Orthop* 1996; 16:445.

Chapter 136

HIP DISORDERS IN INFANCY AND EARLY CHILDHOOD

Dan Atar and Wallace B. Lehman

DEVELOPMENTAL DYSPLASIA OF THE HIP

INCIDENCE

The incidence of developmental dysplasia of the hip (DDH) is 1 per 1000 live births, with a female to male ratio of 5:1. The left side is affected three times as often as the right side. Twenty percent are bilateral.

HIGH RISK FACTORS

High risk factors include a positive family history, breech presentation, torticollis (20 percent of cases have DDH), metatarsus adductus (10 percent), calcaneovalgus (25 percent), and scoliosis (10 times more than normal children).

ETIOLOGY IS MULTIFACTORIAL

Genetic Factors

There is a familial tendency to dislocation associated with DDH. The chances of a second child being affected in a family with one DDH child is approximately 10 times the expected risk in the general population.

Ethnic Factors

DDH is significantly more common in Caucasian children than in African-American children. There is a high incidence among Navajo Indians and the Lapps who swaddle their babies and carry them with legs together fully extended, and a low incidence among the Chinese and African Negroes who carry their babies astride their backs with the legs widely abducted.

Mechanical Factors

There is greater incidence of hip dislocation in first-born children. This appears to be related to intrauterine malposture caused by conditions unique in the primigravida. Greater incidence is also related to oligohydramnios and breech presentation.

Hormonal Theory

High levels of maternal hormones in the last weeks of pregnancy increase joint laxity and allow dislocation of the hip during the neonatal period. DDH is rare in premature babies.

Pathology

The pathology depends on the type, grade, and age of dislocation. At birth, the hip, though unstable, is probably normal in shape. The capsule is often stretched and redundant. During infancy a number of changes develop, most of them due to adaptation to persistent instability. The femoral head dislocates posterolateral and then superolateral to the acetabulum. The ossific nucleus appears late. The acetabulum becomes shallow, a pad of fibrofatty tissue (pulvinar) lines its base. The transverse acetabular ligament, pulled by the stretched capsule, hypertrophies and blocks the lower part of the acetabulum. The ligamentum teres becomes elongated and hypertrophies. The labrum is pushed (inverted) by the dislocated head into the acetabulum. The proximal femur and the acetabulum are excessively anteverted. After weightbearing starts, the dislocated femoral head induces a false acetabulum to form above the shallow acetabulum. The capsule, squeezed between the iliopsoas muscle and acetabular edge, develops an hourglass deformity.

DIAGNOSIS

The diagnosis is made by clinical examination.

Up to age of 2 months: The Ortolani and the Barlow tests are reliable. The Ortolani test is performed by gently abducting and adducting the flexed hip to detect any reduction ("audible click") into or dislocation of the femoral head from the true acetabulum. The Barlow test is performed by direct pressure on the longitudinal axis of the femur while the hip is in adduction. If the femoral head can be made to slip in and out of the socket, the hip is "dislocatable" (Fig. 136–1).

Between age 2 months to walking age: The most reliable sign is a decrease in ability to abduct the dislocated hip because of a contracture of the adductors. The skin folds of the thigh and lateral creases become asymmetric with shortening of the affected side (Galeazzi sign). Twenty percent of normal children may have asymmetric folds.

At walking age: The child walks in a Trendelenburg gait ("waddling").

Imaging

Ultrasonography has replaced radiography for imaging hips in the newborn. Plain radiographs in the newborn may be misleading because the usual bony landmarks are not seen distinctly and lines are difficult to delineate accurately. (After age 4 to 6 months radiography is more reliable.) The most commonly used lines of references are the Perkin's vertical line and Hilgenreiner's horizontal line. Normally, the metaphyseal beak of the proximal femur will lie within the inner lower quadrant of these lines. Another line is the Shenton's line, which will be disrupted in the dislocated hip. The acetabular index indicates acetabular dysplasia and is generally 30 degrees or less (Figs. 136–2 and 136–3).

TREATMENT

Treatment is age related.

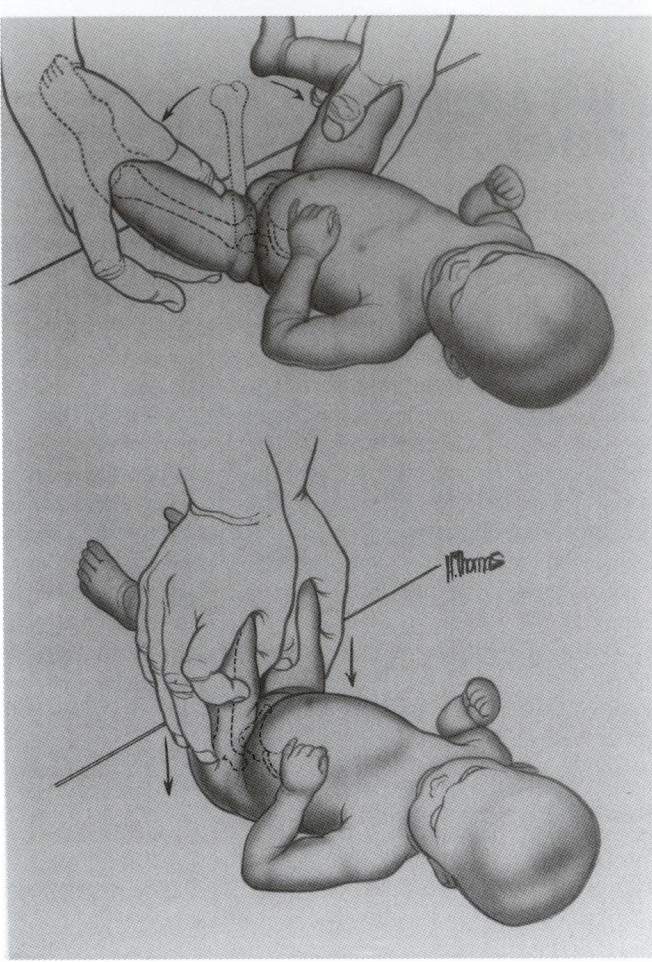

Figure 136-1
Ortolani test (*left*) Barlow test (*right*). See text for details.

Neonatal to Age 6 Months

Most of the dislocatable hips (Barlow positive) at birth will stabilize after 2 to 3 weeks. Hips that are dislocatable after 3 weeks or hips that are dislocated at the first examination (Ortolani positive) are placed in splints. The most popular are the Pavlik harness (Fig. 136–4), also in use are the Frejka splint, the von Rosen splint, or the Ilfeld splint. The object of the splint is to hold the hips in flexion and abduction. Extreme positions should be avoided to prevent avascular necrosis and the hips should be allowed some movement in the splints. Patients are maintained in the splints full time until the hips are clinically and radiographically stable. The rule of thumb to determine the treatment period is 2 months in splint for each month until treatment has begun. A success rate of 85 to 95 percent has been reported in children treated with splints during this period. If the dislocation persists after 4 weeks of splint treatment, it should be discontinued. Traction, closed or open reduction, are initiated.

Age 6 to 18 Months

Treatment at this age group includes preoperative traction for 2 to 3 weeks followed by an attempt of gentle closed reduction. If there is any tightness in the adductor muscles, adductor tenotomy may be required. The hip is then placed in a spica cast in the "human" position (90 degrees flexion, 60 degrees abduction). If gentle closed reduction cannot be achieved, an arthrogram is indicated. This will usually identify soft tissue obstruction and suggest the necessity of open reduction.

Age 18 Months to 3 Years

The treatment of choice for this age group is open reduction, with varus derotation osteotomy of the proximal femur. The acetabulum has remarkable remodeling ability up to age 4 years. Thus, pelvic osteotomy may not be needed after the femoral head has been concentrically seated in the dysplastic acetabulum.

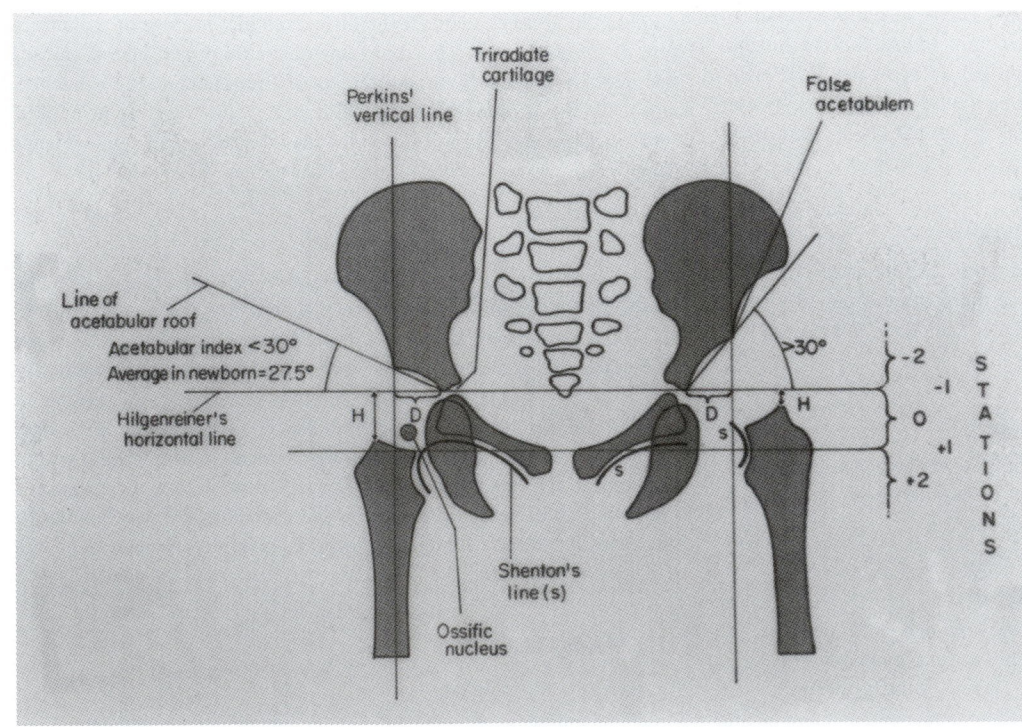

Figure 136-2
Roentgenographic lines of references for developmental hip dysplasia.

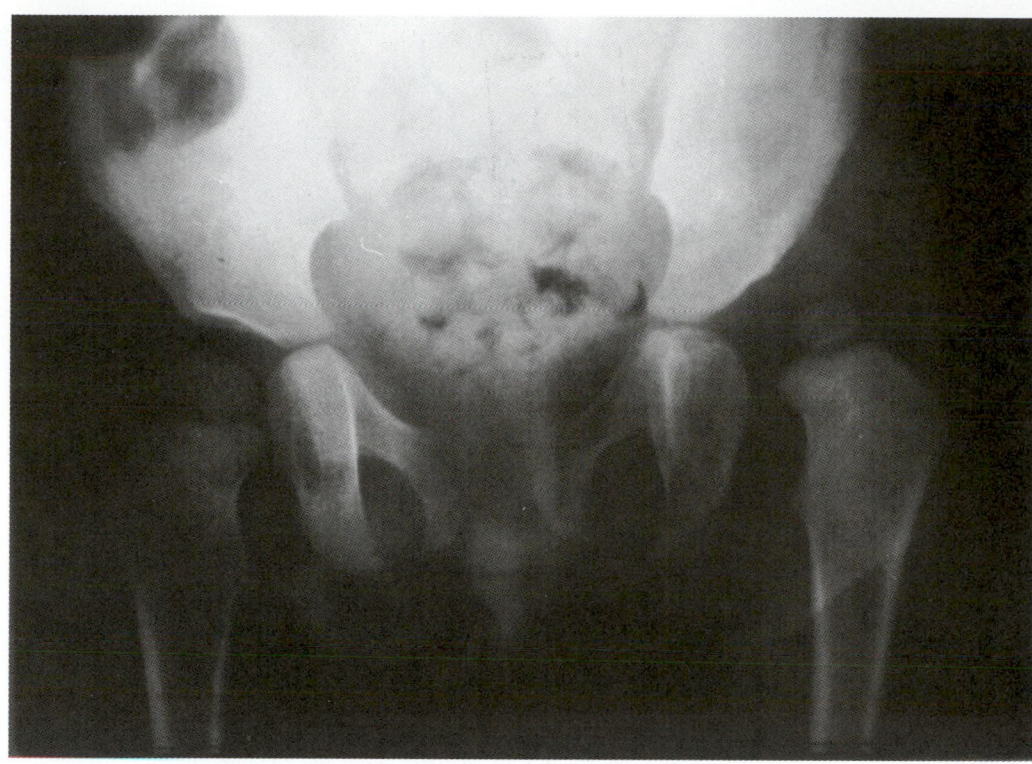

Figure 136-3
Dislocated left hip in 6 month old.

Age 3 to 8 Years

In uni- or bilateral cases, the treatment should be combined hip surgery to include open reduction, femoral shortening, and varus derotation osteotomy combined with pelvic osteotomy (Salter, 1974; Chiari, 1974) (Fig. 136–5).

Age over 8 Years

Bilateral dislocations in this age group should be left unreduced; joint replacement may be carried out during adulthood. In unilateral dislocation, the hip is mobile; the patient limps but has little pain until middle life. Many authors consider it as a justification for noninter-

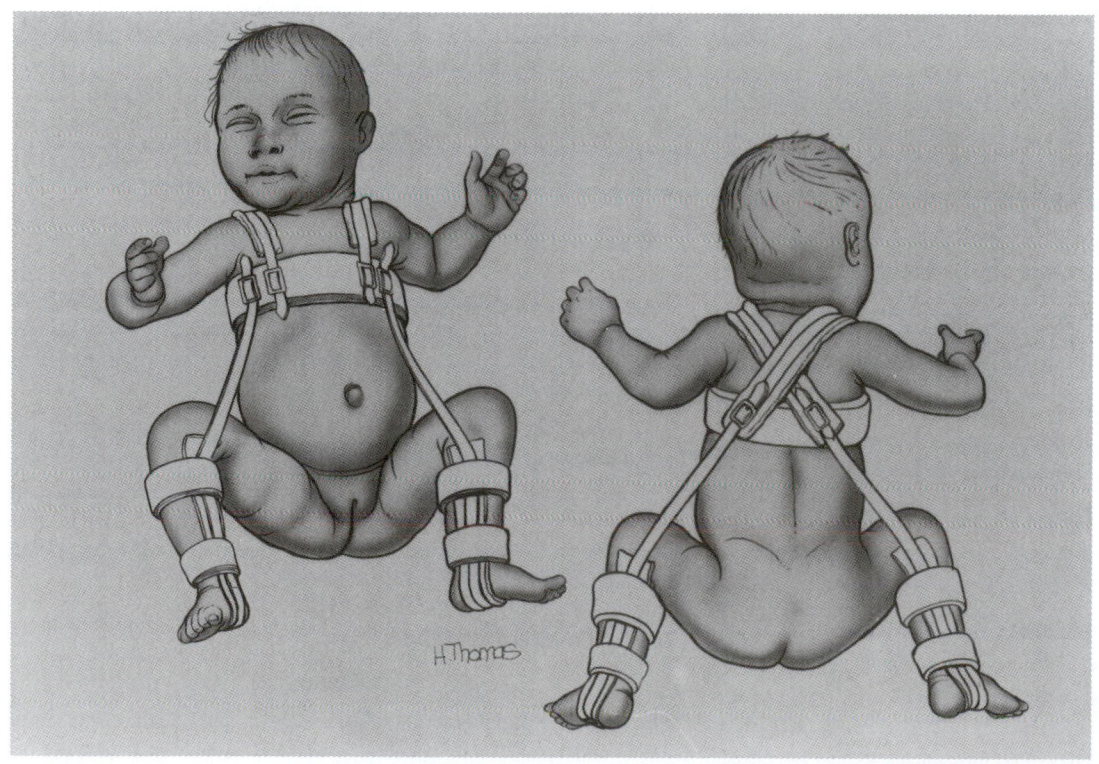

Figure 136-4
The Pavlik harness.

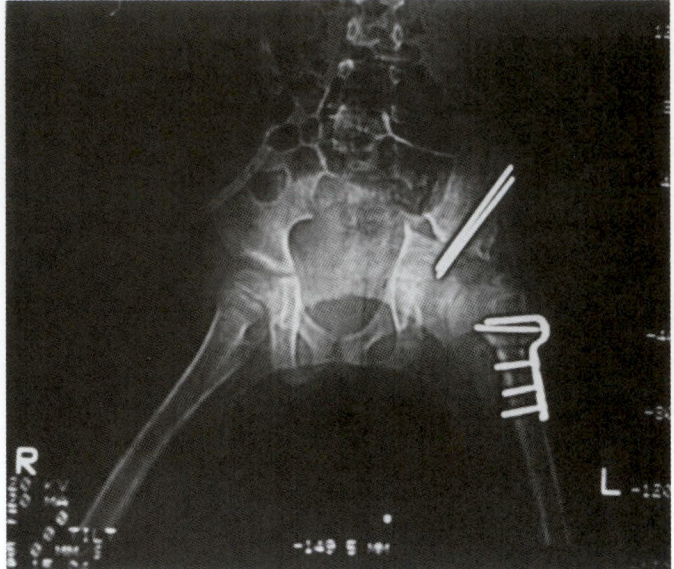

Figure 136-5
Combined hip surgery in 6 year old: open reduction, VDO, Chiari osteotomy.

vention. Some authors recommend shelf procedures or combined hip surgery. Persistent subluxation, however, may be improved by a Chiari or triple osteotomy (Steel, 1973; Ganz, 1988; Töonis, 1981) or by shelf procedure (Staheli, 1981).

COMPLICATIONS

Avascular Necrosis

Avascular necrosis (AVN) is the most serious complication associated with DDH treatment. It may occur also in the normal head as the result of positioning in spica cast. Sequelae of AVN include femoral head deformity, overgrowth of the greater trochanter, leg length discrepancy, and late osteoarthrosis. Kalamchi and MacEwen have proposed an AVN classification system of four types based on morphologic changes in the capital femoral epiphysis, metaphysis, and physis (Table 136–1 and Fig. 136–6). The classification should be iden-

---
Table 136-1

Avascular Necrosis Classification System[a]

Group I:	Delayed appearance of ossific nucleus. Flattening and fragmentation with revascularization. Excellent outcome.
Group II:	Premature lateral epiphysiodesis occurs with valgus tilt of the head.
Group III:	Central damage to the growth plate. Relative overgrowth of the great trochanter occurs with leg discrepancies.
Grop IV:	Total damage to the head and physis with irregularity and flattening of the head. Widening and shortening of the metaphysis.

[a]See Kalamchi A. and MacEwen GD (1980) for complete details associated with each type.

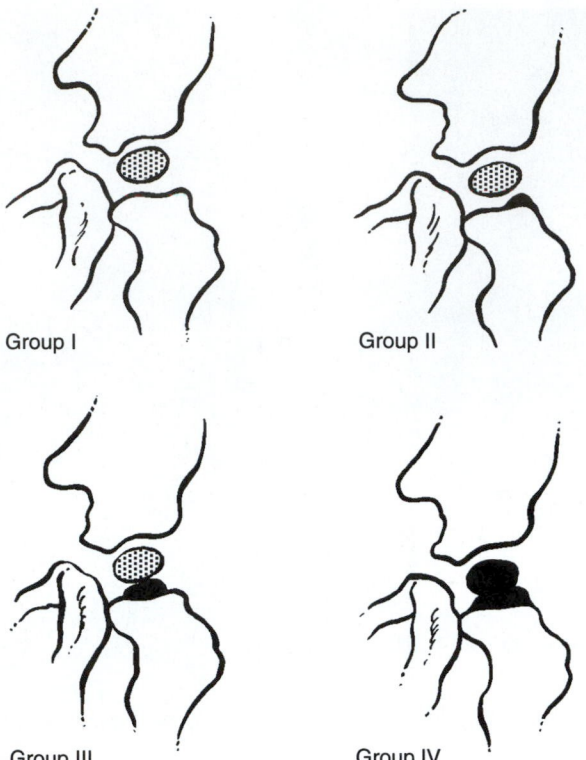

Group I   Group II

Group III   Group IV

Figure 136-6
Classification of avascular necrosis. Group I: Localized involvement of femoral head. Group II: Lateral epiphyseal involvement. Group III: Central epiphyseal involvement. Group IV: Total involvement of head and epiphysis. (Reproduced with permission from Kalamchi A, MacEwen D: Avascular necrosis following treatment of congenital dislocation of the hip. *J Bone Joint Surg [Am]* 1980; 62:885.)

tifiable on x-rays within 2 years of treatment and confirmed by the age of 6 years. Many patients will not require treatment. Some, however, will require limb lengthening, advancement of the greater trochanter or femoral, and pelvic osteotomies.

COXA VARA

TYPES OF COXA VARA

There are three types of coxa vara

Congenital: The congenital type is very rare. It presents at birth and is often associated with congenital anomalies such as: proximal focal deficiency, cleidocranial synostosis, and multiple epiphyseal dysplasia.

Developmental: The developmental type is not distinguished until walking. It is not associated with other anomalies.

Acquired: The acquired type occurs in children after rickets, and possibly Legg-Calvé-Perthes and fibrous dysplasia. In adults it occurs with osteomalacia or Paget's disease, or after pyogenic infection or fracture.

DEVELOPMENTAL COXA VARA

Incidence

The incidence of developmental coxa vara is 1 in 25,000 births. Both males and females are affected. Unilateral involvement is twice as common as bilateral.

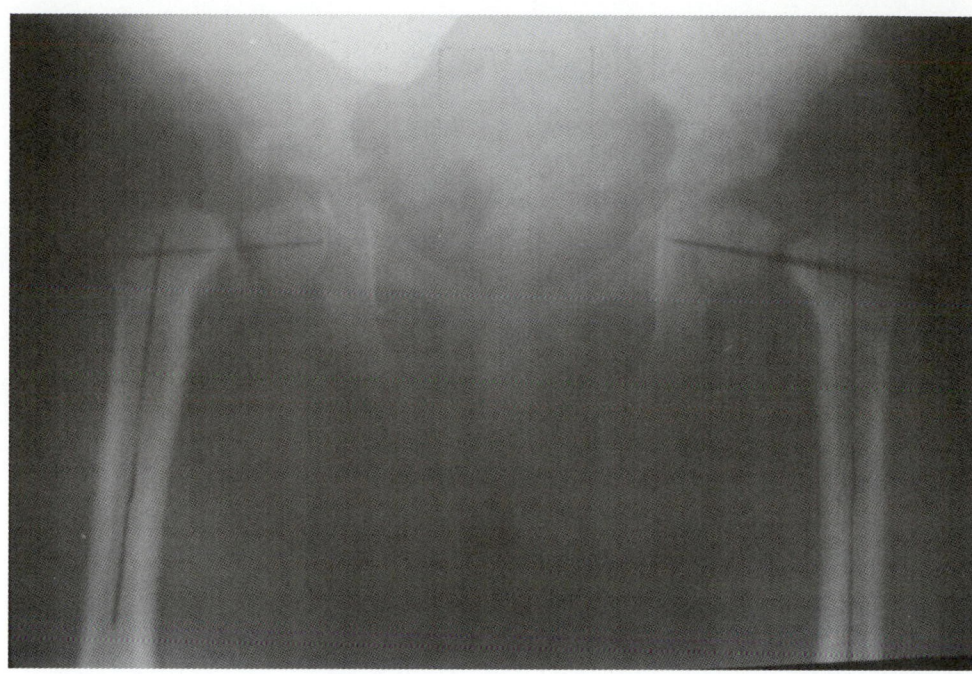

Figure 136-7
Coxa vara in 4-year-old child. Neck shaft angle of 100 degrees.

Etiology

The etiology is unknown; heredity seems to play a role.

Pathology

The pathology is the result of a defect of enchondral ossification in the medial part of the femoral neck. The neck is weakened mechanically and passively deformed into varus under the stress of body weight.

Clinical Symptoms

The condition is diagnosed when the child starts to walk. The child walks in a painless lurching limp when one hip is involved or in "waddling" gait when both hips are involved. Patients are short and sometimes have lumbar hyperlordosis, especially if the deformity is bilateral. Abduction and internal rotation are limited. Pelvic radiographs reveal a decreased neck shaft angle (normally, 150 degrees at 1 year of age and decreasing to 125 degrees in adult life), an almost vertical physeal line, and a separate triangle of bone in the inferior portion of the metaphysis (Fig. 136–7).

TREATMENT

The treatment of choice is inter- or subtrochanteric valgus osteotomy (Fig. 136–8). Surgery is indicated when the neck shaft angle is 110 degrees or less. If the operation is preformed after age 8 years, the prognosis for providing a normal hip rapidly diminishes. The deformity can recur. Children should be examined periodically until maturity. If the deformity recurs, the operation is repeated.

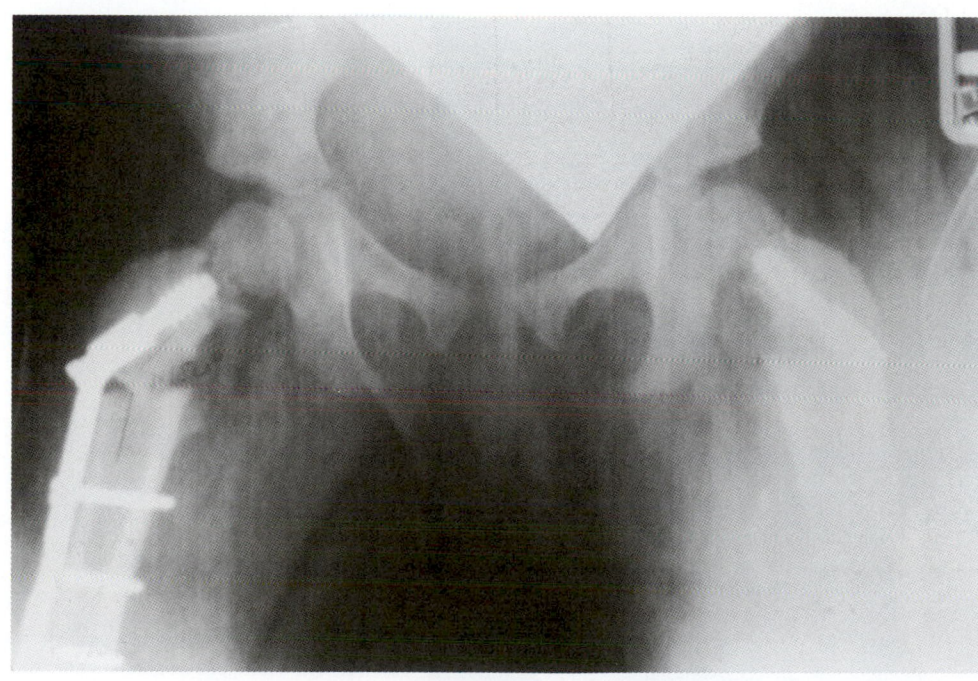

Figure 136-8
Same patient in Fig. 136-7 after bilateral subtrochanteric osteotomies.

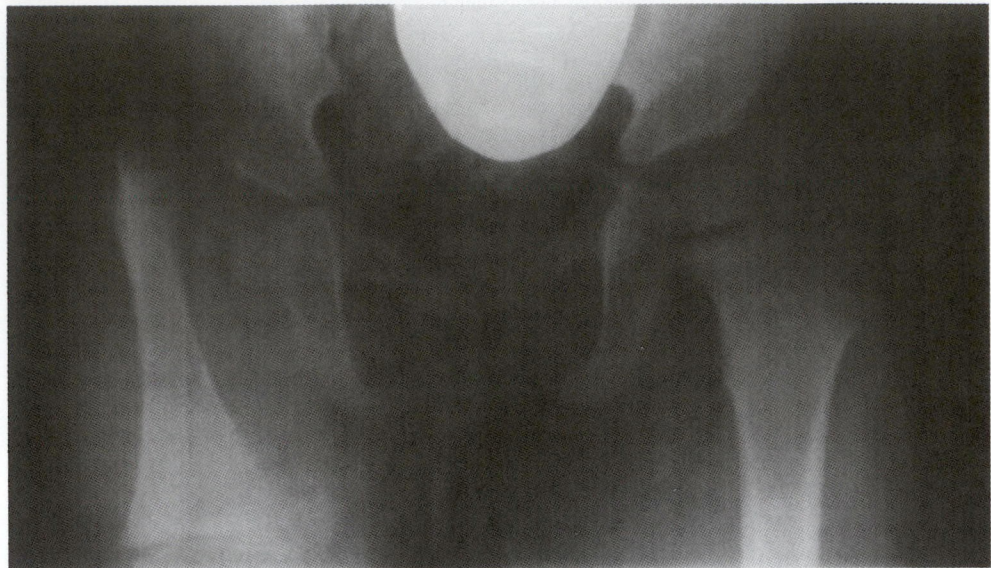

Figure 136-9
PFFD of left hip. Aitken class A. One-year-old child.

PROXIMAL FEMORAL FOCAL DEFICIENCY

INCIDENCE

The incidence of proximal femoral focal deficiency (PFFD) is 1 in 50,000 live births.

PATHOLOGY

The ileum and the proximal end of the femur develop from a common cartilaginous anlage. The hip joint is created by the formation of a cleft in the anlage. By the ninth week of fetal life the hip joint resembles the adult hip. In fetuses in which there is no acetabulum, no femoral head develops. During this period of fetal life, teratogenic agents may produce PFFD. These agents can include irradiation, anoxia, ischemia, bacterial toxins, viral infection, or drugs. Most patients with PFFD have a high incidence of associated anomalies.

CLASSIFICATION

Pappas

The Pappas (1983) classification consists of nine categories, five of which include patients with (1) hypoplastic normal femur; (2) congenital absence of femora; (3) short femora and coxa valga; (4) short femur and coxa vara; and (5) irregular distal femur. The remaining four groups almost match those in the Aitken classification, which have gained the widest acceptance.

Aitken Classification

The Aitken (1969) classification consists of the following four classes:

Class A: There is a normal acetabulum and femoral head, with shortening of the femur and absence of the femoral neck (Fig. 136–9). With age the cartilaginous neck ossifies, but a pseudarthrosis is present. This latter may heal, but the usual radiographs show severe coxa vara with significant shortening of the limb (Fig. 136–10).

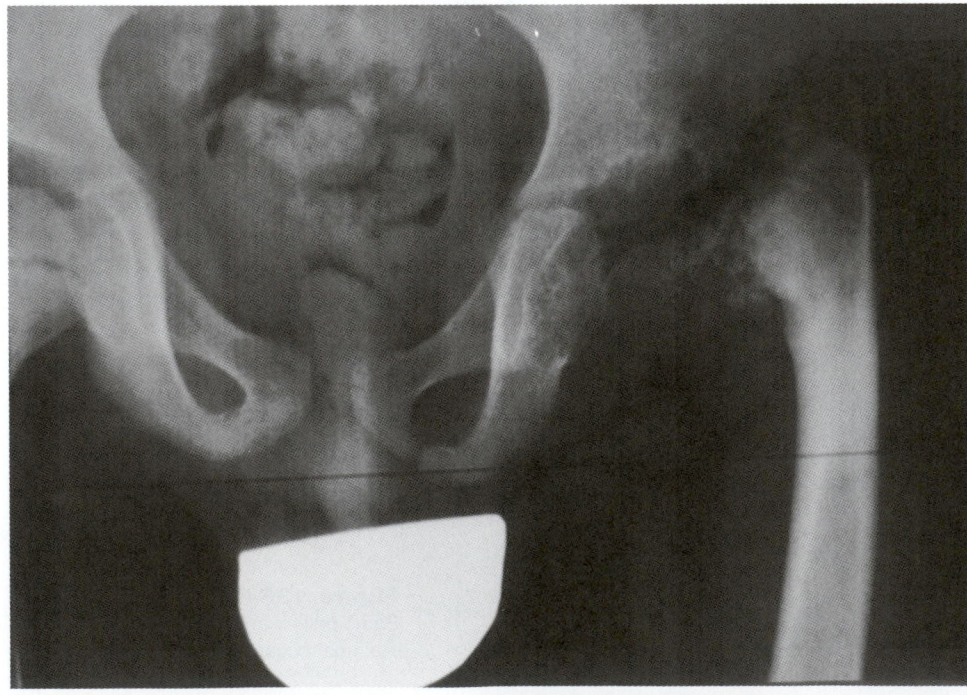

Figure 136-10
Same patient in Fig. 136-9 at 3 years old. Femoral neck ossified in severe coxa vara.

Class B: The acetabulum and femoral head are present. The femoral head is rudimentary. The femur is short. There is a small bone tuft in the proximal end of the femur. At skeletal maturity, there is no connection between the femoral head and the proximal end of the femur.

Class C: Anomalies include a dysplastic acetabulum, no femoral head, a short femur, and an ossified tuft at the proximal end of the shaft (Fig. 136–11).

Class D: The acetabulum and the femoral head are absent. The markedly short femur is not associated with a proximal tuft (Fig. 136–12).

CLINICAL PRESENTATION

The affected thigh is short and bulky (Fig. 136–13). The extremity is abducted, flexed, and externally rotated. Often the extremity is so short that the ankle on the affected side is level with the contralateral knee. Examination of the hip is not diagnostic; in about 50 percent of the cases, the ipsilateral fibula is absent and the tibia is shortened. The patella may be absent or hypoplastic and riding high and laterally. Absence of lateral rays of the foot may be present as other anomalies in other parts of the body.

TREATMENT

Bilateral Involvement

Most authors agree that bilateral PFFD is best treated without surgery. These patients can walk on their natural feet, but for social or cosmetic reasons, extension prostheses may be provided.

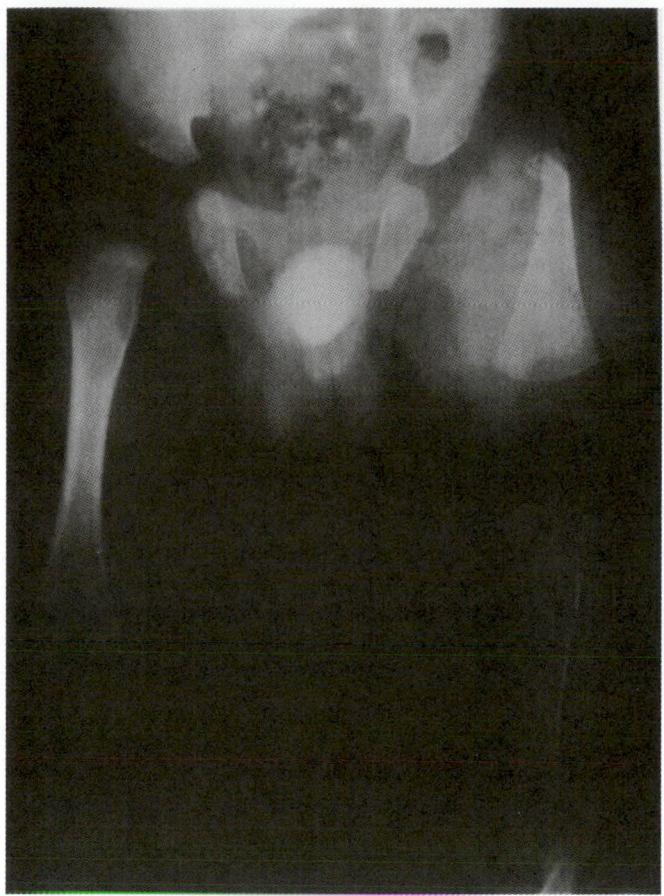

Figure 136-11
PFFD Aitken class C (see text for details).

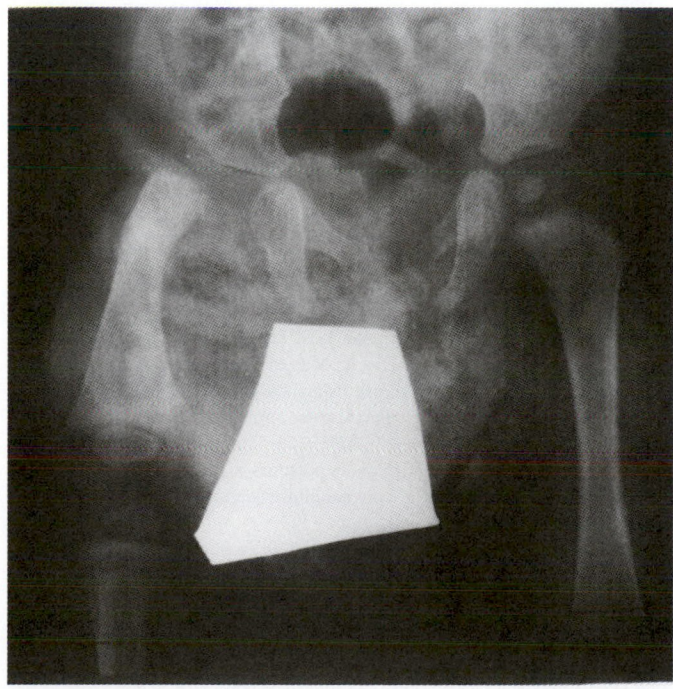

Figure 136-12
PFFD Aitken class D (see text for details).

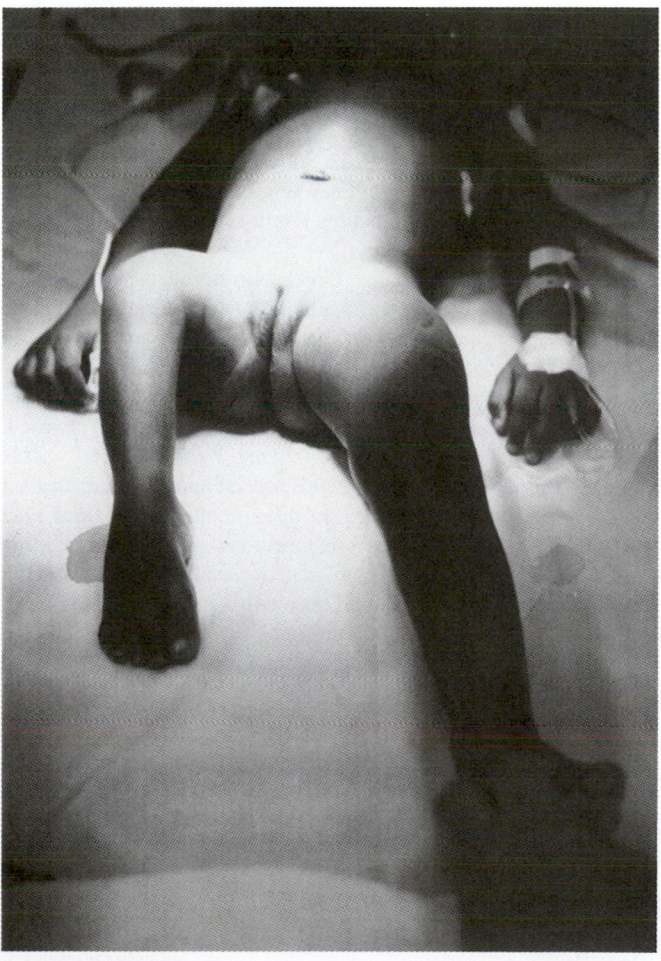

Figure 136-13
PFFD: The right thigh is short and bulky.

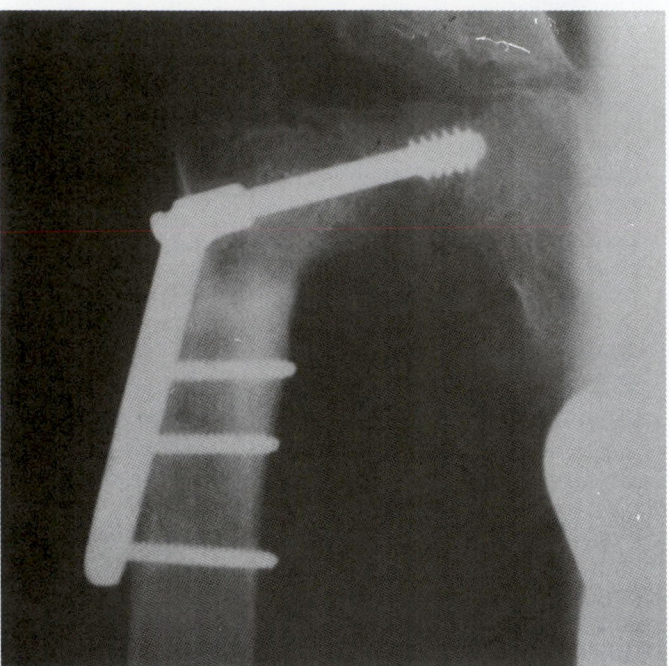

Figure 136-14
Same patient in Fig. 136-10 after subtrochanteric osteotomy.

Unilateral Involvement

Hip Stability With Aitken classes C and D most authors recommend that no attempt be made at hip reconstruction (although some authors describe fusion of the femoral remnant to the ileum, allowing the knee joint to assume the function of the hip joint). In Aitken classes A and B an arthrogram may be helpful to evaluate the unossified neck. Subtrochanteric osteotomy, internal fixation, and bone grafting were recommended (Fig. 136–14). Some authors found that patients in classes A and B who have not had surgical intervention have painless hips with good range of motion. For this reason they do not advocate surgery for these cases.

Limb lengthening is difficult in PFFD patients with unstable hips and knees. The preferred treatment in significant limb length discrepancy rather than lengthening is knee arthrodesis and foot amputation. The foot amputation should be performed between 1 to 2 years of age, before the child and parents become psychologically attached to the concept of having a foot. After foot ablation, an above the knee prosthetic socket that includes the entire femur is fitted. Knee arthrodesis can be done later. It is possible to fuse the knee over an intramedullary nail and still allow longitudinal growth of the distal femur and proximal tibial epiphyses. An alternate approach is to use the prosthesis to mold the foot into equinus so that it fits into an above knee prosthetic socket.

Another alternative is the Van Ness rotation plasty which combines arthrodesis of the knee with rotation of the distal tibia 180 degrees externally so that the ankle joint becomes a functional knee joint. The procedure should be deferred until the patient is 9 to 12 years of age.

TRANSIENT SYNOVITIS

Transient synovitis is the most common cause of hip pain in children.

INCIDENCE

The incidence of transient synovitis is 3 percent; the age group range is 3 to 12 years of age. The boys-to-girls ratio is 2:1.

ETIOLOGY

The etiology is unknown. Trauma, bacterial or viral infection, and allergy have been suggested.

CLINICAL SYMPTOMS

There may be pain at the groin, thigh, or knee, along with a limp. Limitation of the hip is mainly internal rotation, extension, and abduction. Temperature is normal to slightly elevated (rarely over 100°F). Sedimentation rate and WBC are normal or mildly elevated.

Joint aspiration will yield clear and sterile fluid.

Radiographs are normal. (There may be some widening of the medial joint space, mostly due to the hip position.)

Bone scans are normal. Ultrasonography can assess the joint effusion.

DIAGNOSIS

Diagnosis of transient synovitis is by exclusion (differential diagnosis: septic arthritis, Perthes disease, rheumatic fever, juvenile rheumatoid arthritis, and slipped epiphysis).

TREATMENT

Treatment consists of bed rest at home. The hip should be kept flexed and in some external rotation. (This posture decreases the pressure inside the hip joint.) Resolution of symptoms is expected within several days. Two-and-a-half to 10 percent of the cases will develop Perthes disease in 2 to 6 months after an episode of transient synovitis. Obtaining a pelvic x-ray is recommended 4 to 6 months after this episode.

SUGGESTED READINGS

DEVELOPMENTAL DYSPLASIA OF THE HIP

Atar D, Lehman WB: Pavlik harness vs Frejka splint in treatment of developmental dysplasia of the hip: Bicenter study. *J Pediatr Orthop* 1993; 13:311.

Bennett JD, MacEwen GD: Congenital dislocation of the hip. Recent advances and current problems. *Clin Orthop* 1989; 247:15.

Chiari K: Medial displacement osteotomy of the pelvis. *Clin Orthop* 1974; 98:55.

Ganz R, Klaue K. Vinh TS, et al: A new periacetabular osteotomy for the treatment of hip dysplasias. *Clin Orthop* 1988; 232:26.

Graf R: Fundamentals of sonographic diagnosis of infant hip dysplasia. *J Pediatr Orthop* 1984; 4:735.

Ilfeld FW, Westin GW, Makin M. Missed or developmental dislocation of the hip. *Clin Orthop* 1986; 203:276.

Kalamchi A, MacEwen GB: Avascular necrosis following treatment of congenital dislocation of the hip. *J Bone Joint Surg [Am]* 1980; 62:876.

Kastenbaum DM, Avella BG, Lehman WB: Infantile hip dysplasia (congenital dislocation of the hip). In Dee R, Mango E, Hurst LC (eds): *Principles of Orthopedic Practice.* New York: McGraw-Hill; 1989:1085.

Lehman WB, Atar D, Grant AD: Pelvic osteotomies in children. *Bull NY Acad Med* 1992; 68:483.

Salter RB, Dubos JP: The first 15 years personal experience with innominate osteotomy in the treatment of congenital dislocation and subluxation of the hip. *Clin Orthop* 1974; 98:72.

Staheli LT: Slotted acetabular augmentation. *J Pediatr Orthop* 1981; 1:321.

Steel HH: Triple osteotomy of the innominate bone. *J Bone Joint Surg [Am]* 1973; 55:343.

Tachdjian MO: Congenital dysplasia of the hip. In: *Pediatric Orthopedics*, 2d ed. Philadelphia: WB Saunders; 1990:297.

Toonis D, Behrens K, Tscharani F: A modified technique of the triple pelvic osteotomy. *J Pediatr Orthop* 1981; 1:241.

COXA VARA

Schmidt TL, Kalamchi A: The fate of the capital femoral physis and acetabular development in developmental coxa vara. *J Pediatr Orthop* 1982; 2:534.

Stevens PM, Coleman SS: Coxa breva: Its pathogenesis and a rationale for its management. *J Pediatr Orthop* 1985; 5:515.

Tachdjian MO: Developmental coxa vara. In: *Pediatric Orthopedics*, 2d ed. Philadelphia: WB Sanders; 1990:583.

Weinstein JN, Kuo KN, Millar EA: Congenital coxa vara. A retrospective review. *J Pediatr Orthop* 1984; 4:70.

PROXIMAL FEMORAL FOCAL DEFICIENCY

Aitken GT: Proximal femoral focal deficiency: definition, classification and management. In Aitken GT (ed): *Proximal Femoral Focal Deficiency:A Congenital Anomaly*. Washington, DC: National Academy of Science; 1969:1.

Epps CH: Proximal femoral focal deficiency. *J Bone Joint Surg [Am]* 1983; 65:867.

Koman LA, Meyer LC: Proximal femoral focal deficiency: A 50 year experience. *Dev Med Child Neurol* 1982; 24:344.

Pappas AN: Congenital abnormalities of the femur and related lower extremity malformations: Classifications and treatment. *J Pediatr Orthop* 1983; 3:45.

Tachdjian MO: Congenital longitudinal deficiency of the femur. In: *Pediatric Orthopedics*, 2d ed. Philadelphia: WB Saunders; 1990:553.

Westin GW: Proximal femoral focal deficiency. A review of treatment experience. In Aitken GT (ed): *Proximal Femoral Focal Deficiency: A Congenital Anomaly*. Washington, DC: National Academy of Science; 1969:100.

TRANSIENT SYNOVITIS

Hardinge K: The etiology of transient synovitis of the hip in childhood. *J Bone Joint Surg [Br]* 1970; 52:101.

Illingworth CM: Recurrences of transient synovitis of the hip. *Arch Dis Child* 1983; 58:620.

Jacobs BW: Synovitis of the hip in childhood and its significance. *Pediatrics* 1974; 47:558.

Landin LA, Danielsson LG, Wattsgard C: Transient synovitis of the hip. *J Bone Joint Surg [Br]* 1987; 69:238.

Vegter J: The influence of joint posture on intra-articular pressure. A study of transient synovitis and Perthes disease. *J Bone Joint Surg [Br]* 1987; 69:71.

Chapter 137

HIP DISORDERS IN ADOLESCENCE

Dan Atar and Wallace B. Lehman

SLIPPED CAPITAL FEMORAL EPIPHYSIS

The *incidence* of slipped caital femoral epiphysis (SCFE) is 1 to 3:100,000 in the Caucasian and 7:100,000 in the black population. The male–female ratio is 2 to 5:1, and the age of onset for males is 13 to 15 years and for females is 11 to 13 years. Bilateral involvement is found in 25 percent of the cases.

ETIOLOGY

The immediate cause of slipping is mechanical. The growth plate's stability is provided mainly by the perichondral ring and the transepiphyseal collagen fibers. During adolescent rapid growth spurts, the ability of these structures to hold the femoral head is decreased. Hence, overloading the growth plate at this age abruptly (40 percent of the cases give a history of trauma) or slowly (as in obese patients, as seen commonly in SCFE) results in slipping of the femoral head.

Hormonal imbalance has also been suggested as a cause for further weakening of these structures. Deficiency of sex hormone (large, obese adolescents) or excess of growth hormone (tall, thin children) was reported in adolescents with SCFE, as well as hypoparathyroidism, hypopituitarism, and hypothyroidism. The majority of cases occur sporadically. However, there is some hereditary predisposition to this disease.

PATHOLOGY

The physis is widened and may be twice its normal width. The hypertrophic zone may constitute 60 to 80 percent of the growth plate (normally 30 percent) and has an abnormal matrix. The plane of the slip passes through the different zones of the physis, extending toward the germinal zone or into the metaphysis. This line of separation is due to the irregularity of the contour of the physis in this age group. The physeal disruption leads to premature fusion of the physis, usually in 1 to 2 years. The displacement of the epiphysis is almost always posterior and inferior. Occasionally, the femoral head is displaced laterally (superiorly) and posteriorly (valgus slip). Very occasionally in traumatic slip, the femoral head may be displaced anteriorly.

CLINICAL SYMPTOMS

The clinical presentation varies according to the type of slip:

Preslip (6 percent of cases). Some groin and thigh pain, and limitation of internal rotation.

Acute slip (11 percent of cases). Pain and inability to bear weight on the affected leg for less than 2 weeks.

Chronic slip (60 percent of cases). Intermittent groin and thigh pain or knee pain of several weeks, with limitation of flexion, internal rotation, and abduction. The leg is sometimes laterally rotated.

Acute on chronic slip (23 percent of cases). After several weeks or months of hip–thigh–knee pain, the pain is suddenly exacerbated.

RADIOLOGIC ASSESSMENT

Anteroposterior (AP) and lateral (frog position) views of the pelvis are imperative. On AP view, in a slip, a line drawn along the superior border of the neck remains superior to the head instead of passing through it (Trethowan's sign in the English literature or Klein's or Rennies' line in the American literature). Also, in a slip, the physis looks wider and irregular. In the lateral view, the angle between the femoral neck to the epiphyseal base is normally 90 degrees. In a slip, this angle decreases.

The degree of slipping is generally graded as to the amount of head displaced in proportion to the width of the femoral neck on AP radiographs (Fig. 137-1):

Preslip (grade I). There is widening and rarefaction of the physis without displacement.

Mild slip (grade II). The displacement is up to one-third of the femoral neck on AP radiographs and less than a 20-degree tilt on lateral radiographs.

Moderate slip (grade III). Displacement is 30 to 50 percent (a 20 to 40 degree tilt on the lateral view).

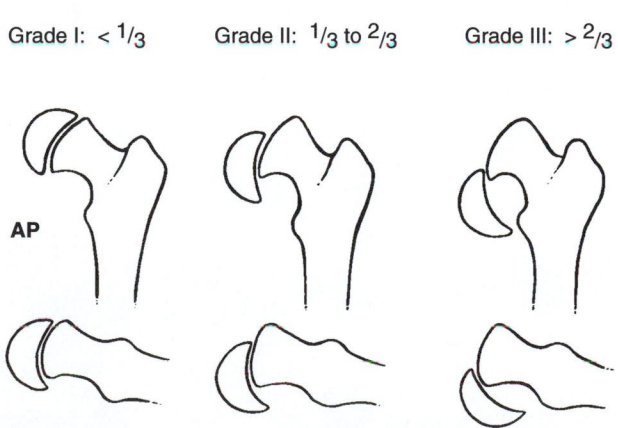

Grade I: < 1/3   Grade II: 1/3 to 2/3   Grade III: > 2/3

AP

L

Figure 137-1
Slipped capital femoral epiphysis: schematic drawings of anteroposterior and lateral views of the femoral head and neck (grade I, mild slip; grade II, moderate slip; and grade III, severe slip).

Severe slip (grade IV). Displacement of over 50 percent (more than a 40-degree tilt on the lateral view) (Fig. 137-2). Southwick (1967) recommends measurement of the head-shaft angle in the frog position to record the amount of slipping.

TREATMENT

Minor slip (grades I–II). Pinning in situ with 1 to 2 cannulated pins (Fig. 137-3).

Moderate slip. Pinning in situ. One to two years later, if there is any noticeable deformity, corrective intertrochanteric osteotomy is indicated.

Severe slip. Closed reduction by manipulation is dangerous (avascular necrosis). Some recommend traction to obtain a slow reduction and then pinning. Others recommend femoral neck osteotomy (cuneiform) with a high risk of avascular necrosis. Most authors advocate pinning in situ (pins should be inserted from the anterior portion of the femoral neck). As soon as fusion is complete, compensatory triplane intertrochanteric osteotomy is performed (as described by Southwick).

Valgus slip. This is rare and associated with coxa vara. Patients are tall. There is limitation of adduction and flexion. AP radiographs show superior displacement of the femoral head, and lateral radiographs show posterior displacement. Pinning in situ is difficult, especially in severe valgus. In such cases, open epiphysiodesis is a safer treatment.

Anterior slip. This is very rare, with only two cases reported. Hip motion in these cases was limited in lateral rotation and abduction, and the hips were in flexion deformity. Treatment was femoral neck osteotomy and pin fixation.

COMPLICATIONS

The incidence of *avascular necrosis* is 10 to 15 percent of cases, which are mainly iatrogenic. Complications can also follow forceful manipulation or femoral neck osteotomy. *Chondrolysis* occurs in 1 to 40 percent of cases. Complications occur in 36 percent of surgically treated patients (pin penetration) and in 6 to 30 percent of patients

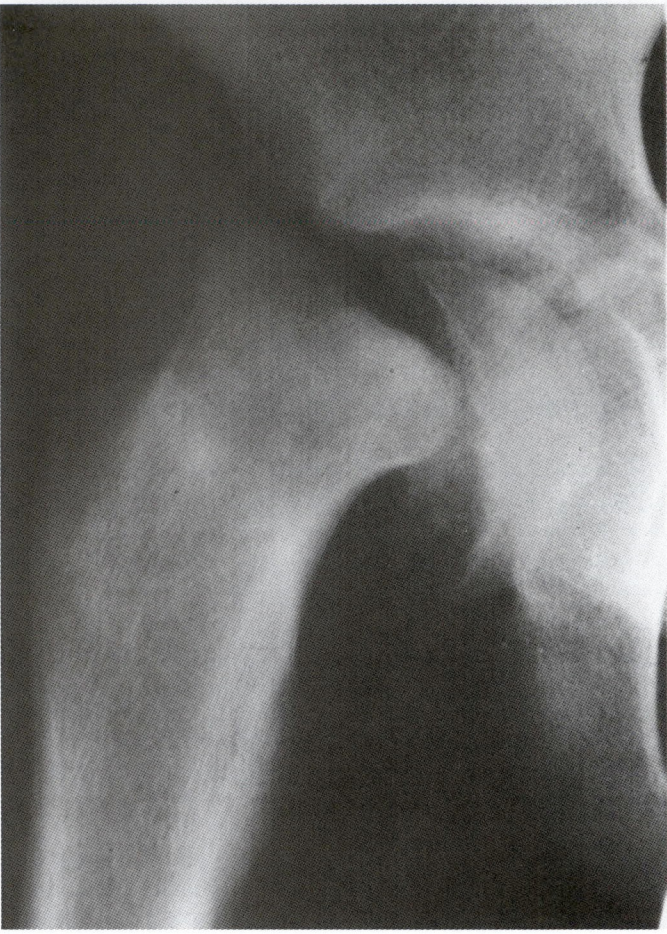

Figure 137-2
Anteroposterior view of severe slip.

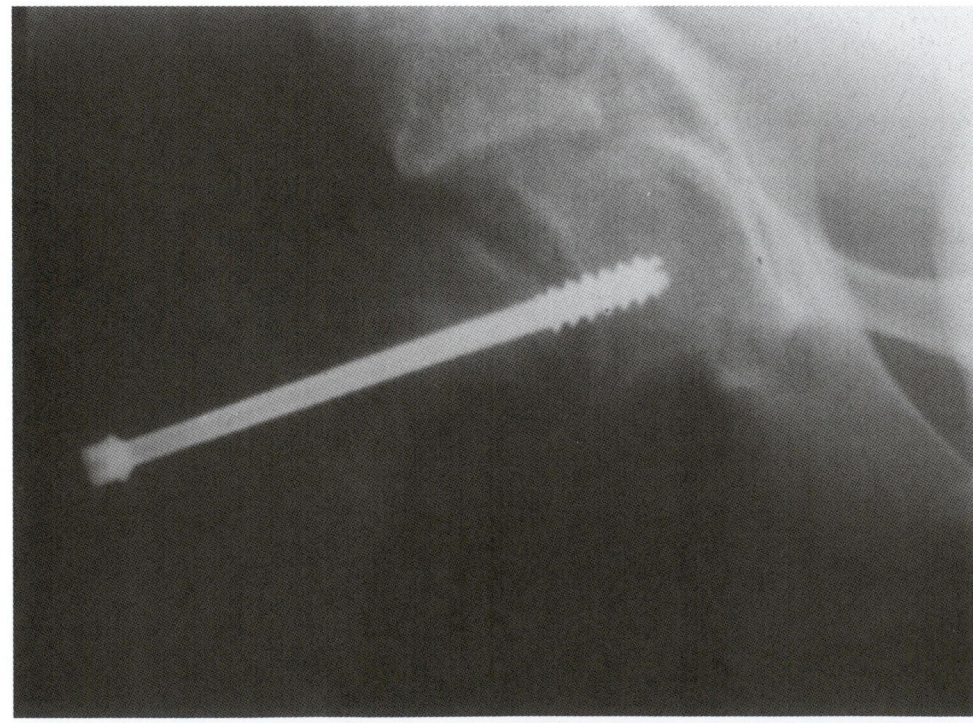

Figure 137-3
Pinning in situ of a chronic minor slip with a cannulated screw.

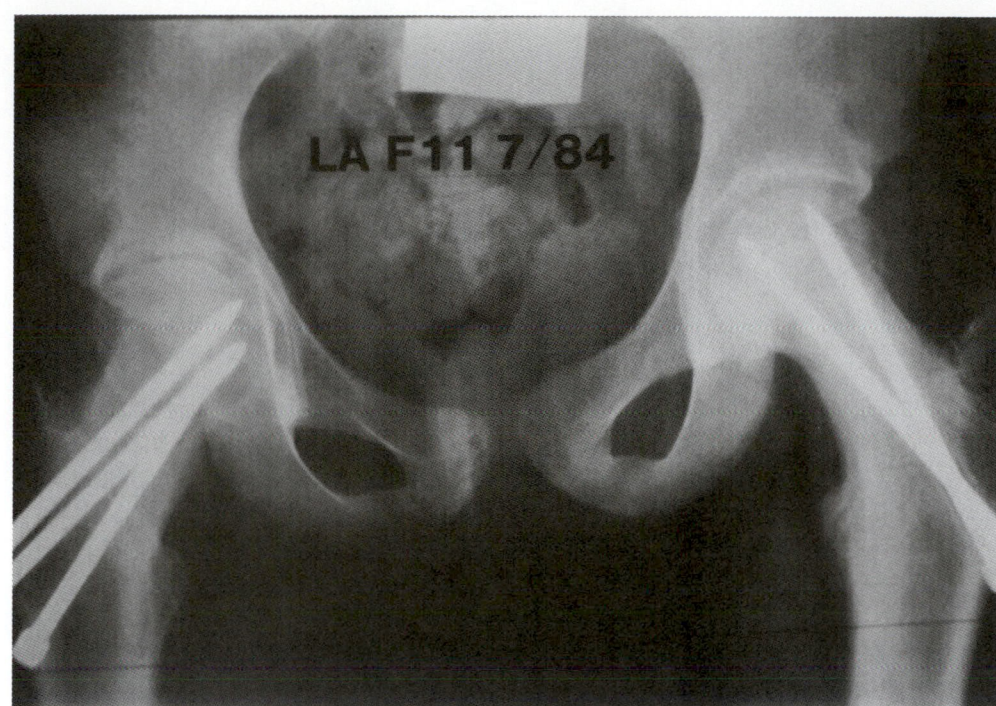

Figure 137-4
Radiograph of bilateral slipped capital femoral epiphysis treated with in situ pinning. Note the chondrolysis of the right hip joint.

who have not undergone surgery. Cartilage is destroyed, which may be related to an autoimmune response?) and joint space is progressively narrowed (Fig. 137-4). In severe cases, ankylosis may develop. About one-third of the cases may resolve spontaneously.

LEGG-CALVÉ-PERTHES DISEASE

The condition Legg-Calvé-Perthes disease (LCPD) was described independently, in 1910, by Legg in Boston, Calvé in France, and Perthes in Germany. Its *incidence* is 1:10,000, with 10 percent of cases bilateral. The affected age group range is 2 to 13 years, and the boy–girl ratio is 4:1.

ETIOLOGY

The etiology is ischemia of the femoral head for unknown reasons. Several theories have been suggested: increased intraarticular pressure preceding episodes of transient synovitis hereditary factors and constitutional factors (short stature).

PATHOLOGY

The disease is self-limited, with the pathologic process taking 2 to 4 years to complete and passing through three stages:

Initial stage. All or part of the bony aspect of the head is dead. Trabecular fractures occur and create the crescent sign, as described by Salter. The cartilaginous part (nourished by the synovial fluid) becomes thicker than normal.

Resorption stage. Within weeks of infarction, the femoral head is revitalized by "creeping substitution." The new lamellae laid down on the dead trabeculae produce increased density on radiographs. Some dead trabeculae are replaced by fibrous tissue. Alternating areas of sclerosis and fibrosis appear as "fragmentation" on radiographs. In the metaphysis and acetabulum, cysts may appear. This stage lasts 1 to 3 years.

Reparative stage. Normal bony architecture replaces the diseased bone, and the femoral head continues to remodel until patients reach maturity.

Waldenstrom divided the natural history of the disease into four stages according to radiographic changes: (1) the incipient stage (with no radiographic changes), (2) the necrotic stage (equivalent to the initial stage), (3) the fragmentation (Fig. 137-5) and reossification stage (resorption stage), and (4) the remodeling stage (reparative stage) (Fig. 137-6).

Catterall (1989) described four groups based on the radiographic appearance (AP and lateral) of the femoral head: group I, less than half of the epiphysis is sclerotic with no collapse; group II, half of the epiphysis is involved with some collapse; group III, the lateral half of the epiphysis is collapsed with some metaphyseal changes; and group IV, the whole head is involved with metaphyseal cysts (Fig. 137-7).

Salter and Thompson (1984) described a simpler classification, which they based on the subchondral crescent-shaped radiolucent line that appears early in the disease. In group A, the extent of the subchondral fracture is less than half of the femoral head (Catterall I and II) and, in group B, more than half the head is involved (Catterall III and IV). A lateral pillar classification that was suggested recently by Herring (1992) but remains controversial, includes three groups based on radiolucency of the lateral pillar of the femoral head during the fragmentation stage (the lateral pillar comprises 15 to 30 percent of the femoral head on AP radiographs) (Table 137-1).

CLINICAL SYMPTOMS

The presenting symptoms are a limp and pain. The pain is in the groin or referred to the thigh or the knee. The child appears to be well, but hip motion is limited and painful especially in internal rotation and abduction. The results of all blood tests are normal.

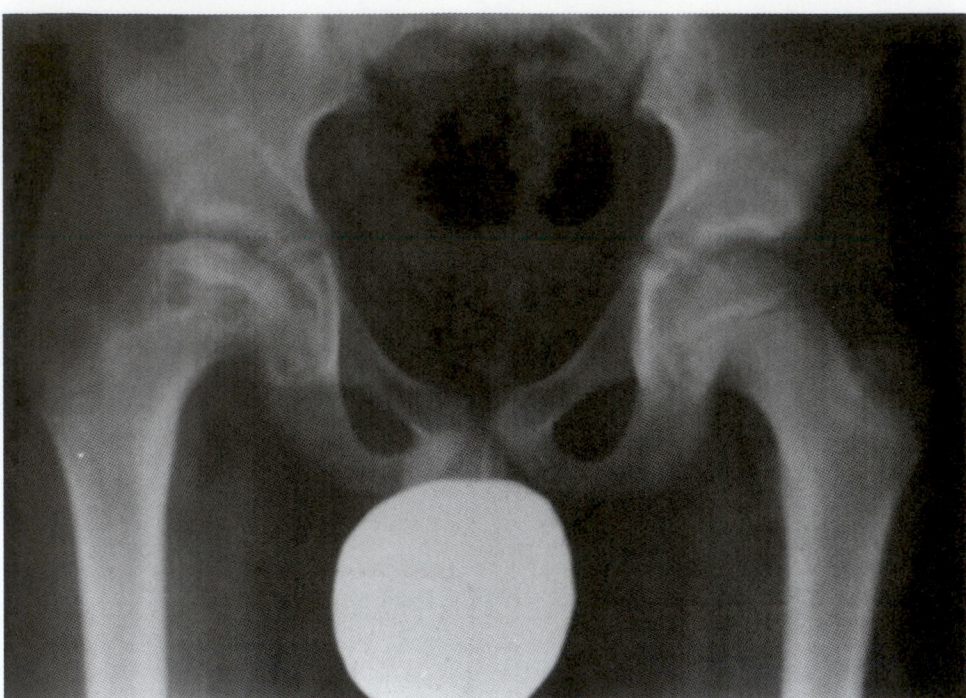

Figure 137-6
Waldenstrom remodeling stage
(see the text).

DIFFERENTIAL DIAGNOSIS

This includes transient synovitis, infection, rheumatic fever, early-onset rheumatoid arthritis, [juvenile rheumatoid arthritis], Gaucher's disease, sickle cell disease, and multiple epiphyseal dysplasia or hypoparathyroidism in bilateral hip involvement.

PROGNOSIS

The two prognostic factors are femoral head involvement and age. The greater the degree of femoral head involvement, the worse is the outcome. The "head at risk" signs that are also an indicator of poor prognosis include: (1) calcification lateral to the epiphysis, (2) diffuse metaphyseal rarefaction, (3) lateral extrusion of the femoral head, (4) growth disturbance of the physis, and (5) rarefaction in lateral part of the epiphysis and subjacent metaphysis (Gage's sign).

The age remains the strongest prognostic factor. In children younger than the age of 6 years, the outcome is almost always good, whereas those older than 9 years have a poor prognosis.

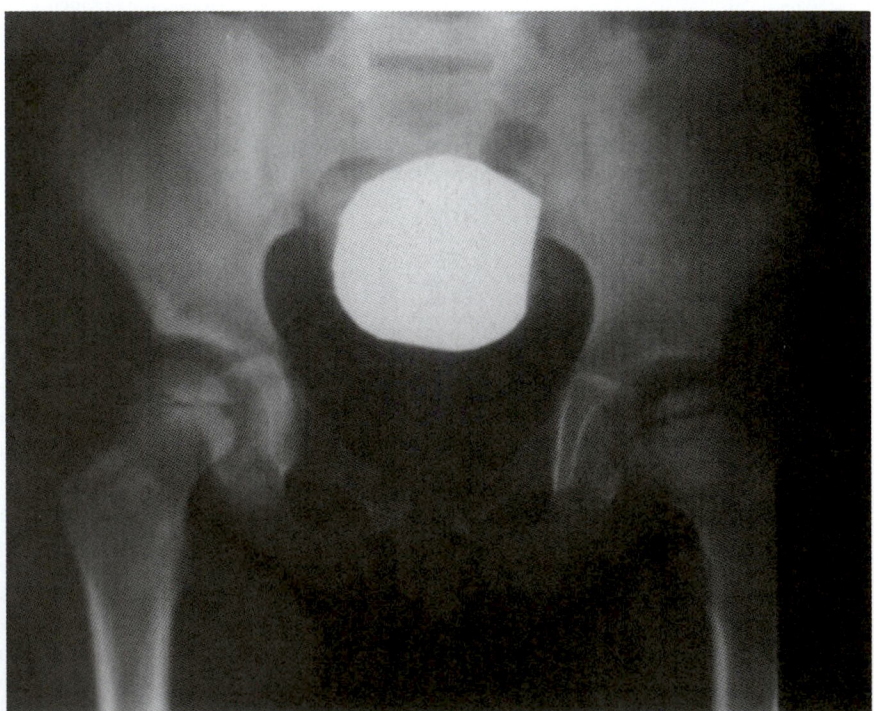

Figure 137-5
Waldenstrom fragmentation stage
(see the text).

Table 137-1

Lateral Pillar Classification[a] Based on Radiolucency		
Group A	No involvement of the lateral pillar (good outcome)	
Group B	More than 50% of the lateral pillar height is maintained (good prognosis for patients younger than 9 years of age)	
Group C	Less than 50% of the lateral pillar height is maintained (bad prognosis)	

[a]See the text.

SOURCE: Modified from Herring et al (1992), with permission.

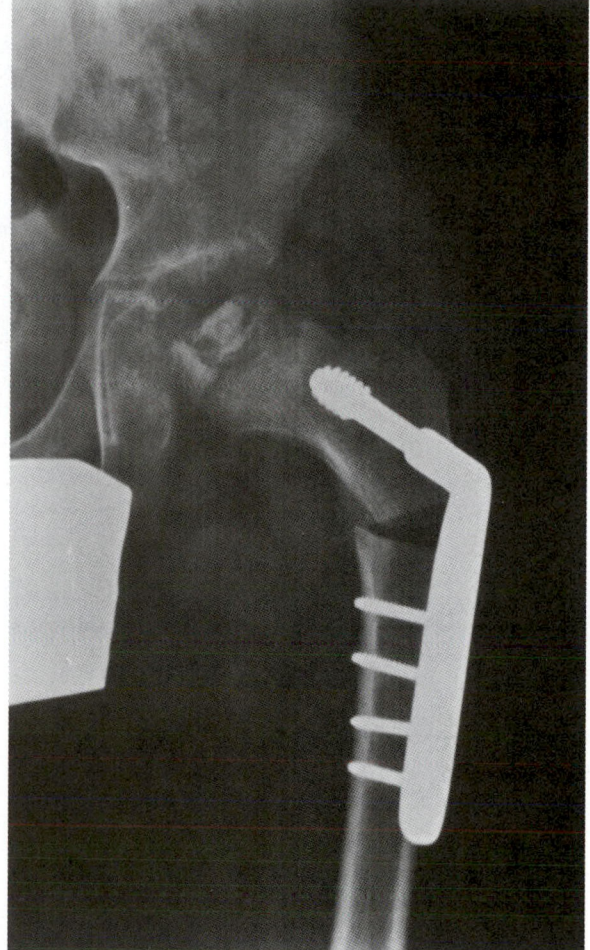

Figure 137-8

Containment with femoral varus osteotomy. Catterall group IV, Salter group B.

CURRENT CONCEPT OF TREATMENT

The goal of treatment is the prevention of deformity of the femoral head, mainly by containment of the femoral head and restoration of the hip motion.

Patients who are less than six years old. There is no evidence that any form of treatment alters the outcome. Most patients have good results. Treatment is to alleviate symptoms only and includes traction, nonweightbearing, and nonsteroidal anti-inflammatory drugs.

Patients 6 to 8 years old. These patients have a better outcome when managed with containment methods. There is no difference between the various methods of containment: brace, femoral osteotomy (Fig. 137-8), or innominate osteotomy.

Patients over 9 years old. These patients usually refuse braces. Operation is the treatment of choice.

Restoration of hip range of motion is necessary before and after any treatment. This is done by physical therapy, traction, Petrie plaster casts, and sometimes muscle releases.

SUGGESTED READINGS

SLIPPED CAPITAL FEMORAL EPIPHYSIS

Canale ST: Problems and complications of slipped capital femoral epiphysis. In Barr JS Jr (ed): *Instructional Course Lectures,* vol 38. Park Ridge, IL: American Academy of Orthopaedic Surgeons; 1989:281.

Kelsey J, Southwick WO: Etiology, mechanism and incidence of slipped capital femoral epiphysis. In *Instructional Course Lectures (AAOS),* vol 21. St. Louis: CV Mosby; 1972:182.

Lehman WB, Grant A, Rose D, Pugh J, Norman A: A method of evaluating possible pin penetration in slipped capital femoral epiphysis using a cannulated internal fixation device. *Clin Orthop* 1984; 186:65.

Morrissy RT: Principles of *in situ* fixation in chronic slipped capital femoral epiphysis. In Barr JS Jr (ed): *Instructional Course Lectures,* vol 38. Park Ridge, IL: American Academy of Orthopaedic Surgeons; 1989:257.

Southwick WO: Osteotomy through the lesser trochanter for slipped capital femoral epiphysis. *J Bone Joint Surg [Am]* 1967; 49:807.

Tachdjian MO: Slipped capital femoral epiphysis. In *Pediatric Orthopedics,* vol 2, 2d ed. Philadelphia, WB Saunders, 1990:1016.

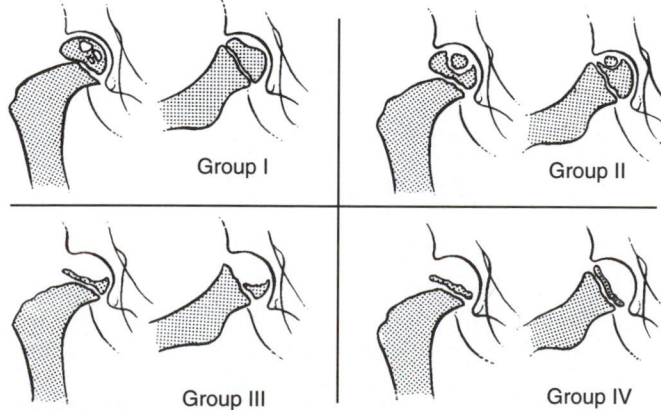

Figure 137-7

Catterall classification: group I, *top left;* group II, *top right;* group III, *bottom left;* and group IV, *bottom right.*

LEGG-CALVÉ-PERTHES DISEASE

Beaty JH: Legg-Calvé-Perthes disease: Diagnostic and prognostic techniques. In Barr JS Jr (ed): *Instructional Course Lectures,* vol 38. Park Ridge, IL: American Academy of Orthopaedic Surgeons; 1989:291.

Catterall A: Legg-Calvé-Perthes disease. In Barr JS Jr (ed): *Instructional Course Lectures,* vol 38. Park Ridge, IL: American Academy of Orthopaedic Surgeons; 1989:297.

Fackler CD: Non-surgical treatment of Legg-Calvé-Perthes disease. In Barr JS Jr (ed): *Instructional Course Lectures,* vol 38. Park Ridge, IL: American Academy of Orthopaedic Surgeons; 1989:305.

Herring JA: The treatment of Legg-Calvé-Perthes disease. *J Bone Joint Surg [Am]* 1994; 76:448.

Herring JA, Neustadt JB, Williams JJ, et al: The lateral pillar classification of Legg-Calvé-Perthes disease. *J Pediatr Orthop* 1992; 12:143.

Salter RB, Thompson GH: Legg-Calvé-Perthes disease: The prognostic significance of the subchondral fracture and a two-group classification of the femoral head involvement. *J Bone Joint Surg [Am]* 1984; 66:479.

Tachdjian MO: Legg-Calvé-Perthes disease. In *Pediatric Orthopedics,* vol 2, 2d ed. Philadelphia: WB Saunders; 1990:933.

Waldenstrom H: The first stages of coxa plana. *J Bone Joint Surg [Am]* 1938; 20:559.

Chapter 138

LIMB LENGTH INEQUALITY

Gail S. Chorney

The clinical approach to limb length inequality requires understanding the etiology of the inequality, the natural history of that etiology, the child's potential height, and the family's expectations. The treatment options range from no intervention to amputation. The major focus is on the lower extremities because of the obvious need for both feet to touch the ground for ease of ambulation. A significant leg length discrepancy increases the amount of energy expenditure in gait. There is no conclusive evidence that a leg length inequality contributes to low back pain. Smaller discrepancies in the upper extremities are usually less of a clinical problem. However, individuals with large discrepancies in the length of the humeri may present for a lengthening procedure.

ETIOLOGIES

The possible etiologies of a limb length inequality are extensive. Establishing the origin of the problem allows an understanding of the natural history and a knowledge of whether the inequality will increase, decrease, or remain static. Knowing whether the long leg is the normal leg or the pathologic one is also important.

A major cause of limb length inequality is infection. Multifocal neonatal osteomyelitis can lead to significant limb deformity. The origin of the discrepancy may be the result of damage to one or more of the physes in the lower extremities. There may also be significant hip dysplasia or angular deformity secondary to asymmetrical growth arrest. These deformities would have to be addressed at the same time or prior to surgical intervention for the limb length inequality. Osteomyelitis in later childhood, if not diagnosed and treated early, can lead to premature closure of the physis. Although the consequences of this infection may not be as devastating as multifocal neonatal osteomyelitis, there may still be enough of a problem to warrant intervention.

Trauma is another leading cause of limb length inequality. A mid-shaft femur fracture between the ages of 2 and 10 years may lead to overgrowth of the injured limb. When treating these fractures with traction and spica casts, the fractured ends are purposely overlapped to avoid this problem. However, there may still be enough of a discrepancy to again demand intervention. More obvious are the problems of premature growth arrest secondary to a fracture through the growth plate. Salter-Harris type I and II fractures are rarely associated with a growth arrest. The exception is a fracture through the distal femoral physis. Because of the undulating nature of this physis, Salter-Harris I and II fractures will damage the upper layers of the proliferative zone and result in premature closure. Because of the large amount of growth from this physis, the consequences can be considerable. Salter-Harris type IV and V fractures have a high incidence of premature closure even with anatomic reduction. Patients with fractures that may be asso-

ciated with growth disturbances should be followed for 2 years post injury in order to diagnose the problem and provide timely treatment.

Neoplasm may cause a growth disturbance primarily or the treatment of the tumor may result in a leg length inequality. Radiation therapy for a malignancy may destroy a physis. Ollier's disease (multiple enchondromatosis) is associated with deformity as well as limb length inequality.

Congenital malformations may result in some of the more severe leg length discrepancies. Unilateral fibular or tibial hemimelia can lead to a degree of discrepancy that will have a significant impact on the overall treatment plan. Posterior medial bowing of the tibia may spontaneously resolve with time, but there is usually a residual leg length discrepancy. Anterior lateral bowing resulting from pseudoarthrosis of the tibia presents the treating physician with not only the problem of how to heal the pseudoarthrosis but of how to deal with the growth disturbance. Proximal femoral focal deficiency (PFFD) is another treatment challenge because of the degree of shortening that may be seen.

Paralysis, complete or partial, of a single extremity can also result in a significant limb length discrepancy. Before the advent of the polio vaccine, paralysis secondary to poliomyelitis was a common occurrence. Today, paralysis secondary to asymmetric neurologic defect in a child with myelodysplasia is the more common etiology.

Avascular necrosis of the femoral head due to Legg-Perthes Disease or as a complication of a slipped femoral capital epiphysis may result in a leg length discrepancy, although not usually one of a large extent. This is because the femoral capital epiphysis contributes only about 15 percent of the total length of the leg. However, if the avascular event involved the entire epiphysis or occurred when the child was very young, there might be enough of a difference to require intervention.

Certain conditions actually result in stimulation of growth causing the pathologic leg to be the longer one. The most common disorder in which this occurs is juvenile rheumatoid arthritis. Other disorders which involve increased vascularity to a limb and therefore result in overgrowth are Klippel-Weber-Trenaunay and hemophilia.

PREDICTION OF GROWTH

Information on the growth of the legs is a result of the work done by Green and Anderson (1963). The length of legs in boys and girls at various ages was recorded, as well as sequential studies of growth in the same children. Growth was related to skeletal age. Although the children in these studies did not represent a diversity in race or ethnicity, the Green-Anderson charts are still widely used.

Sixty-five percent of the growth of the leg occurs at the distal femoral and proximal tibial physes. Therefore, any damage to these physes results in significant alteration in growth. The distal femoral physis contributes 37 percent while 28 percent is from the proximal tibia. Another method of stating the growth potential from these physes is knowing in actual amounts how much growth per year is obtained:

distal femur	10 mm = 3/8 in./year
proximal tibia	6 mm = 1/4 in./year

Clinically, leg lengths are measured from the anterior superior iliac spine to the medial malleolus. To determine treatment, the leg lengths should be measured radiographically. There are several radiographic methods available. In order not to be comparing apples to oranges, the same method should be used for each individual patient. Scanograms do not need to be obtained until the patient reaches 5 years of age. The various graphs for determining the final discrepancy have their first point at this age. In addition, it is unlikely that epiphysiodesis or lengthening will be performed before this age. Usually, scanograms are obtained yearly. However, if the patient presented late for treatment, scanograms will need to be obtained more frequently in order to obtain enough data for decision making.

The orthoroentgenogram is done with the patient supine on the x-ray table. The beam is taken from 6 feet away. Three exposures are taken; one each over the hip, knee, and ankle. This technique eliminates the problem of magnification. This results in one long film with the entire leg visible. The advantage is that pathology or angular deformities are visible.

The scanogram is taken in a similar way with the three exposures and a ruler along side the patient. The film is moved down the leg for each exposure. The advantages are again the elimination of magnification and a smaller film to deal with.

The state of the art technique utilized today is the CT scanogram. The amount of radiation is smaller than with the other techniques and the accuracy is greater (Fig. 138-1).

The amount of discrepancy predicted to be present at the time of skeletal maturity is the number needed to make a good clinical deci-

sion regarding treatment course. There are three methods used to determine the final discrepancy.

The simplest method is the Menelaus or White method. This method involves calculating the discrepancy by utilizing the amount of growth per year in the physes about the knee. In addition to those assumptions, this method also assumes that girls stop growing at 14 and boys at 16 years. The discrepancy is felt to increase at the rate of 3 mm (1/8 in.) per year. The simplicity of the method is obvious. There are disadvantages. The method is inaccurate if the child is very young because the rate of growth is different. The assumptions of rate of growth are reasonable only in the last few years of growth. In addition, only the chronologic age is used. The maturity of various children of the same chronologic age can differ significantly. This method can still be very useful, though, in determining the timing of epiphysiodesis in patients with relatively small discrepancies (2 to 4 cm).

The Green-Anderson method is the more complicated tool. Multiple graphs are needed. The final growth of both legs is determined from the Green-Anderson charts for leg length plotted against skeletal age. The inhibition of growth factor is calculated from the following formula:

$$\frac{\text{growth* of long leg} - \text{growth of short leg}}{\text{growth of long leg}}$$

*growth = present length − first length

The timing of epiphysiodesis can be determined from a second growth remaining chart.

The Green-Anderson data has been compiled into the Mosley straight line graph. This graph and its instructional use are available in every pediatric orthopaedic textbook. It is now available on computer (Fig. 138-2).

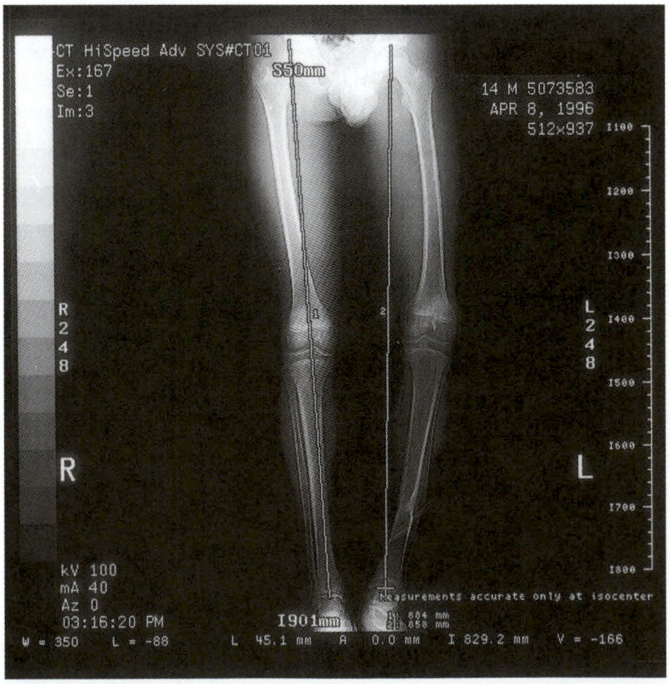

TREATMENT

Treatment options consist of no intervention, shoe lift, epiphysiodesis, shortening the long leg, lengthening the short leg, and amputation. Children usually tolerate a discrepancy of <2 cm without requiring a lift. While awaiting definite treatment for larger discrepancies, lifts that are less than the actual difference may be prescribed.

The current recommendations for treatment for various differences are as follows:

<2 cm	No treatment
2 to 6 cm	Shoe lift, epiphysiodesis
6 to 15 or 20 cm	Lengthening
>20 cm	Amputation

These recommendations may be modified based on each individual patient's needs. For instance, a child with a predicted discrepancy of 6 cm but with a predicted total height at skeletal maturity of only 5 feet would be better served by a lengthening rather than an epiphysiodesis with its loss of total final height. Lengthening of large discrepancies may be made simpler by combining with an epiphysiodesis.

When the predicted leg length discrepancy is going to be over 15 cm amputation is often advised. In more recent years, the amount of lengthening may be as high as 20 cm. This amount is usually achieved by staged lengthening. A goal of 15 percent of the total length of the bone is still the best guideline for successful lengthening. Other issues to consider in deciding whether to amputate or lengthen are normalcy of the foot, a patient's tolerance for multiple surgeries, and condition of the hip and knee.

Figure 138-1
CT scanogram for measuring leg lengths.

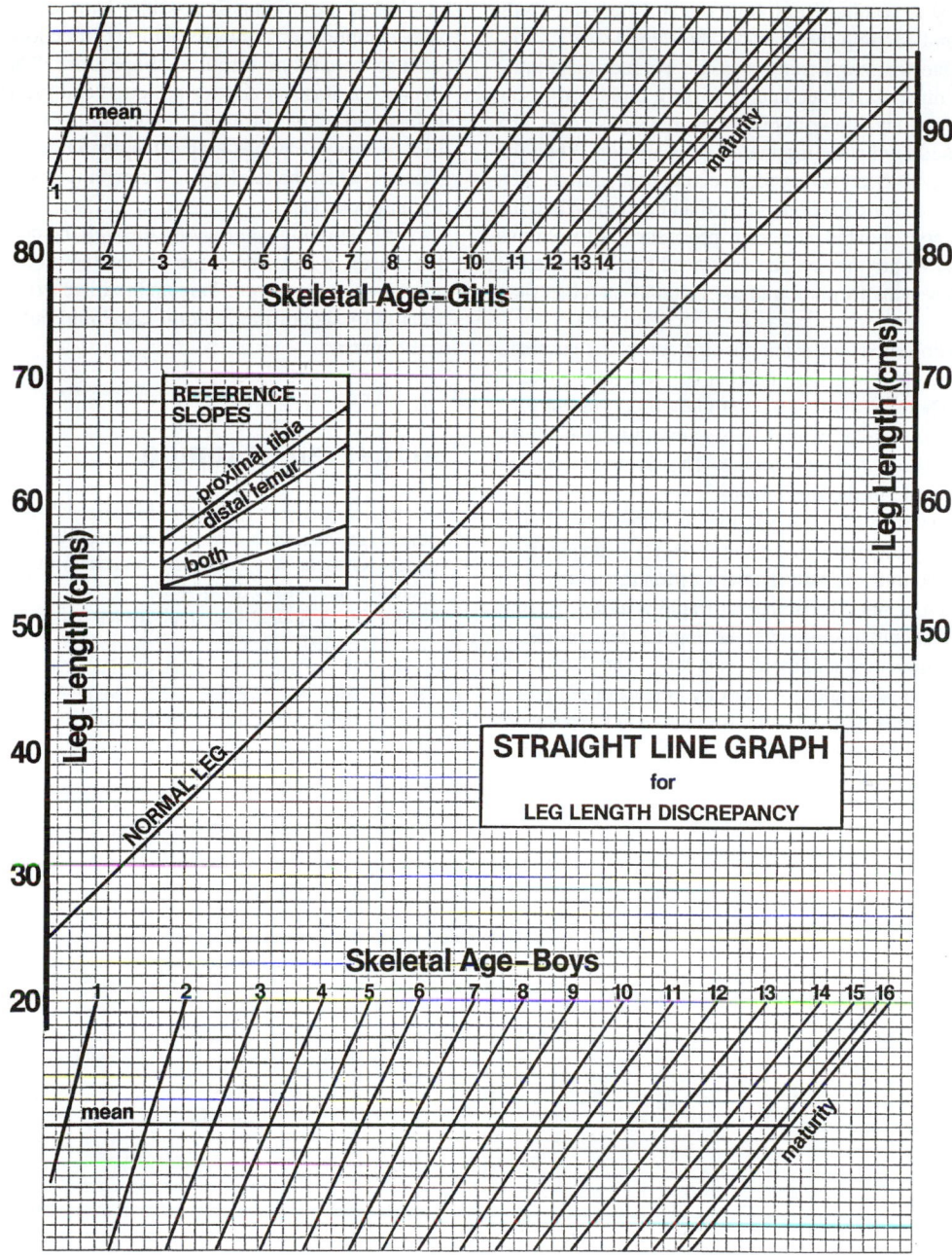

Figure 138-2
The Moseley straight line graph for determining final discrepancies. (Reproduced with permission by Moseley CF: A straight-line graph for leg-length discrepancies. *J Bone Joint Surg [Am]* 1977; 59:176.)

Epiphysiodesis is more correctly called physiodesis since it involves a destruction of the growth plate in order to stop the growth in the long leg and allow the short limb to catch up. Epiphysiodesis, however, has remained in the literature. There are three methods of epiphysiodesis.

The modified Phemister method involves removing a rectangular block of bone around the physis from both lateral and medial sides and then curetting the physis from each side. The block is fashioned by having two-thirds of the block on the metaphyseal side and one-third on the epiphyseal side. The block is replaced after rotating it 180 degrees. In the original description, only the block was rotated. This method resulted in a high number of failures, however, so that actual destruction of the growth plate was added.

Epiphysiodesis has been further sampled by performing it percutaneously. The physis is drilled from lateral and medial sides under the guidance of the image intensifier. The advantage is a quicker recovery.

Blount stapling is performed by placing three staples over the physis, both lateral and medial. The advantage is that the staples can be removed and growth resumed if the timing was inaccurate. Resumption of growth, however, was not always predictable. Blount stapling is used more routinely now for angular deformities.

Each technique is relatively easy. Determining the timing of the procedure is the more difficult task. The timing can be determined by any of the methods mentioned. Whether a distal femoral or proximal tibial closure, or both, are required is determined by knowing where the discrepancy is coming from, how much difference needs to be corrected for, and keeping the knees at the same level.

The initial technique for lengthening was the Wagner technique. By definition, it is a three-staged technique. First, a unilateral external fixator is applied and an osteotomy in the diaphysis is done. The bone is then lengthened by distracting the external fixator. When the amount of lengthening has been achieved, a second procedure is then performed. The lengthened area is bone grafted and plated. When the graft has been fully consolidated, the third procedure is to remove the plate. The Wagner technique has been replaced by the new techniques that rely on new bone formation in the metaphysis rather than bone grafting.

Distraction epiphysiolysis involves lengthening across the physis itself. This technique resulted in a high number of premature closures of the growth plate. Therefore, it is not commonly used presently.

Callostasis utilizing a circular or unilateral external fixator are the currently accepted methods for lengthening. The fixator is applied and an osteotomy is made in the metaphysis.

The lengthening is started after 1 week, thus it is the callus that is being lengthening. The principle is that osteogenesis has already been established and is just being elongated. The distraction rate empirically is 1 mm/day in four segments. The unilateral frame is easier to apply but the circular frame allows for correction of angular deformities.

The list of complications for lengthenings is long. The family and physician must be prepared to address them by performing a procedure. The patient must start with a stable hip and knee because dis-location of these joints is possible with a femoral lengthening. The other complications involve pin tract infections and neurologic compromise, as well as vascular compromise. The latter two complications necessitate an end to the lengthenings. The complications can be lessened by performing a lengthening of only 5 cm at a time. The tibia probably tolerates longer lengthenings better than the femur. In addition, when the etiology is a congenital issue there is a higher rate of complications.

Post fixator removal fracture through the new bone is common. For this reason, a new technique of lengthening over an intramedullary rod has been employed. This method is useful only in the older child because of size of the femoral canal and not wanting to do damage to the physis.

SUGGESTED READINGS

Anderson M, Green WT, Messner MB: Growth and predictions of growth in the lower extremities. *J Bone Joint Surg [Am]* 1963; 45:1.

Guidera KJ, Helal AA, Zuern KA: Management of pediatric limb length inequality. *Adv Pediatr* 1995; 42:501.

Moseley CF: A straight-line graph for leg-length discrepancies. *J Bone Joint Surg [Am]* 1977; 59:174.

Moseley CF: Leg length discrepancy and angular deformity of the lower limbs. In Morrissy RT, Weinstein SL (eds): *Lovell and Winter's Pediatric Orthopaedics*, vol 2, 4th ed. Philadelphia: Lippincott; 1996:chap 22.

Chapter 139

LOWER LIMB DISORDERS

David S. Feldman

In order to understand the various pathologic entities that affect the lower extremities from infancy through adolescence, one must understand the normal angular and rotational development of the growing child. In each category of disease the normal spectrum of lower extremity alignment will be discussed.

INTOEING

Intoeing is one of the most common complaints brought by the parents to their physician. In an otherwise normal child intoeing occurs for one of three reasons. These include excessive femoral anteversion, internal tibial torsion, and metatarsus adductus. Some patients may have a combination of one or more of these entities. This chapter will discuss excessive femoral anteversion and internal tibial torsion. Metatarsus adductus is reviewed in Chap. 140.

EXCESSIVE FEMORAL ANTEVERSION

The infant and child undergo significant rotational changes of the lower extremity with growth. The newborn can have up to 40 degrees of femoral anteversion, which over the first decade will derotate to the final 10 to 15 degrees of anteversion. The manifestation of intoeing or excessive internal rotation of the hip from increased femoral anteversion does not occur until the second or third year of the child's life.

In an otherwise healthy child excessive femoral anteversion (>25 degrees) presents with intoeing, and, at times, medial rotation of the patella with ambulation. On examination, there is an increased internal rotation of the hip with relatively less external rotation. In order to gauge the amount of femoral anteversion, one can place the child prone on the examining table and palpate the ipsilateral greater trochanter while rotating the leg. The angle that the leg makes with the table when the trochanter is in mid-position parallel with the table is the amount of femoral anteversion.

Before the age of 8 years this is a normal developmental finding and should not be treated. Some physicians recommend avoiding the "W" position when a child is seated so as not to stretch the anterior hip capsule. Any other intervention in this age group is not indicated. Mild residual femoral anteversion with some intoeing is actually a mechanical advantage for running, and many sprinters and professional athletes have mild intoeing.

There is a rare subgroup of children who have residual excessive femoral anteversion into adolescence. If the condition becomes either *functionally* or cosmetically unacceptable, then a femoral derotational osteotomy can be performed near skeletal maturity. The CT scan is the most accurate measure of femoral anteversion, and should be utilized prior to undertaking any surgical procedure. Children may also develop compensatory external tibial torsion; therefore, although they have excessive femoral anteversion, their foot progression angle is normal. When children or adolescents walk, their patellas may face slightly inward. In most patients, this combination of findings is benign, but in a small percentage of patients patella-femoral symptoms can become problematic. There is no proof that osteoarthritis is a sequela of excessive femoral anteversion.

TIBIAL TORSION

Tibial torsion is a common finding in children up to the age of 3 years. Internal tibial torsion (more common) and external tibial torsion may be thought of as normal developmental variants in an otherwise uninvolved child. The normal thigh-foot angle is between 0 and 20 degrees; measurements which are slightly more or less than these numbers are not necessarily pathologic.

Tibial torsion presents clinically as either intoeing (internal tibial torsion) or outtoeing (external tibial torsion). The etiology and exact location of the twisting is unclear. Children usually present with intoeing during the second year of life. The parents have usually noticed the problem since their children began to walk and that they tripped over their feet when attempting to run. Most pediatric orthopedic surgeons view internal tibial torsion as a normal developmental variant that usually corrects itself by age 3. The use of nighttime Dennis Browne bars or other such devices is controversial and is usually reserved for children who do not self correct—even then use of these applications and their efficacy is questionable. The need for supramalleolar osteotomies is exceedingly rare and is reserved for the older child whose persistent torsion is either cosmetically or functionally unacceptable.

OUTTOEING

Persistent outtoeing is a less frequent complaint than intoeing. During infancy the feet of many children will appear to be externally rotated from external rotation hip contractures because of fetal positioning. This condition usually resolves in the first 18 months of life. Persistent outtoeing in an adolescent may be secondary to external tibial torsion or less commonly to femoral retroversion. If this is cosmetically or functionally unacceptable, then an osteotomy can be performed.

KNEE DEVELOPMENT (VARUS AND VALGUS)

When children are born, the mechanical axis of their lower extremities is in maximal varus. Gradually, over the first two years of life this physiologic varus should resolve; by the age of 3 to 4 years there is a physiologic valgus of seven to ten degrees. This resolves by the age of 7 to 8 years to the normal 3 to 7 degrees of valgus.

During these various normal developmental milestones, the child may have an increase of the normal varus and valgus. This may or may not represent a pathologic process. For instance, a 1-year-old child may have a 20-degree varus deformity of the knees. If observed and improvement is noted over the next 6 months, then this represents a normal variant. There are certain physical signs that distinguish the physiologic varus from a pathologic process. First, the child's overall height should be monitored and charted. If the child is consistently below the fifth percentile, evaluation for a skeletal dysplasia or rickets should be performed. A lateral thrust with ambulation or varus instability on examination is a pathologic finding. If the child is above the age for physiologic varus or demonstrates pathologic findings on physical examination, then a lower extremity radiograph is indicated. This will aid the physician in diagnosing a skeletal dysplasia versus metabolic bone disease (rickets) versus physiologic varus.

BLOUNT'S DISEASE

Tibia vara, or Blount's disease, has three forms: infantile, juvenile, and adolescent.

Infantile Blount's disease is a disorganization of the medial growth plate of the proximal tibia causing an asymmetric growth and leading to a progressive varus deformity of the knee.

Children with Blount's disease ordinarily present after the age of 2 years with a progressive varus deformity. A number of methods are utilized to distinguish physiologic varus. The first and simplest method is asking the parents if this deformity is worsening or improving. After the age of 2 years, a physiologic varus should be improving. Second, on physical examination, the presence of a lateral thrust with ambulation and persistent internal tibial torsion may represent Blount's disease. Third, a lower-extremity radiograph with demonstration of medial beaking of the proximal tibia and a metaphyseal-diaphyseal angle greater than 16 degrees is diagnostic for Blount's disease (Fig. 139-1).

The etiology of Blount's disease is unknown. It is thought to be due to excessive force on the medial tibial physis. This may occur in children who are obese or who walk early. Genetic predisposition may play a factor as certain races, such as African-American, are more commonly affected.

Once the diagnosis of Blount's disease is made, classification (staging) of the disease is of utmost importance. Langeskjold classified the disease into six stages (Fig. 139-2). As the medial plateau dips and the medial epiphysis follows, this represents stage IV and the growth plate is thought to be irreversibly damaged (Fig. 139-3). If possible, treatment should be administered prior to this stage. Some authors have advocated bracing at stage I and II of the disease. A knee-ankle-foot orthosis (KAFO) is utilized to restore the mechanical axis. The brace must be worn 23 h a day until the mechanical axis has returned to normal. Resolution to a normal axis may take more than 1 year. Surgery is indicated if the varus is progressive or if the child reaches stage III. A tibia and fibula osteotomy, which restores

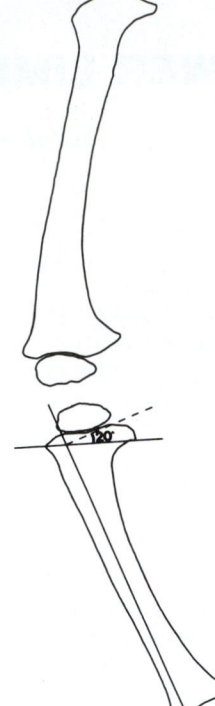

Figure 139-1
The metaphyseal angle is determined by first drawing a line perpendicular to the longitudinal axis of the tibia (dotted line). A second line is drawn through the two beaks of the metaphysis to determine the transverse axis of the tibial metaphysis. (Reproduced and modified with permission from Levine AM, Drennan JC: Physiologic bowing and tibia vara. *J Bone Joint Surg [Am]* 1982; 64: 1159.)

the normal mechanical axis, is the standard treatment. If the child has reached stage IV prior to treatment, then the deformity will recur and sequential osteotomies will need to be performed until the child is of adequate height to undergo an epiphysiodesis.

ADOLESCENT BLOUNT'S DISEASE

Adolescent Blount's disease is thought to occur secondary to trauma. The proximal medial tibial physis is affected, and a progressive varus deformity develops. This disease is most often unilateral and affects males more commonly than females. Treatment is always surgical.

If the child has greater than 1 year of growth remaining, then a hemiepiphysiodesis may be indicated with approximately 7 degrees of angular correction expected per year of growth. Care must be taken not to overcorrect. Tibia and fibula osteotomy below the tibial tubercle is the treatment of choice for children with insufficient growth remaining or significant concomitant internal tibial torsion. Adolescents

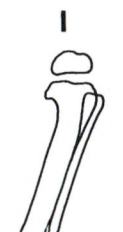 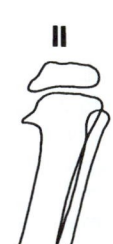 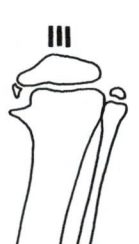 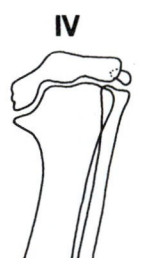 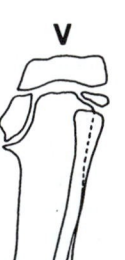 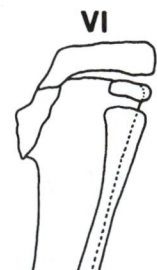

I   II   III   IV   V   VI

Figure 139-2
Blount's disease: Infantile tibia vara. Six stages of the disease. [Reproduced with permission from Resnick D: Osteochondroses. In Resnick D (ed): *Diagnosis of Bone and Joint Disorders,* 3d ed. Saunders; 1995; vol 5:3591.]

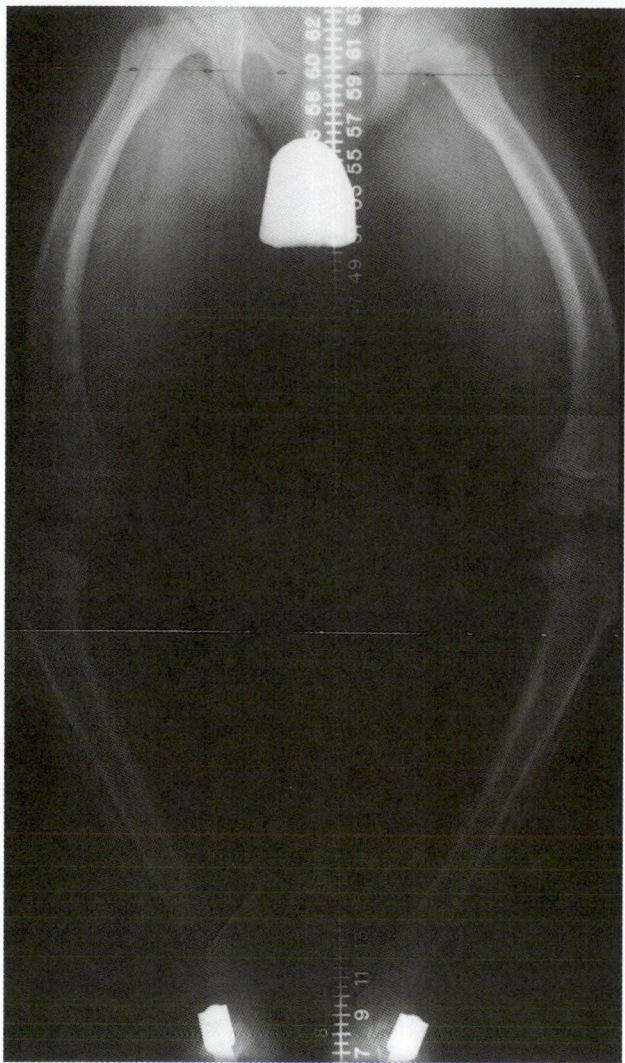

A

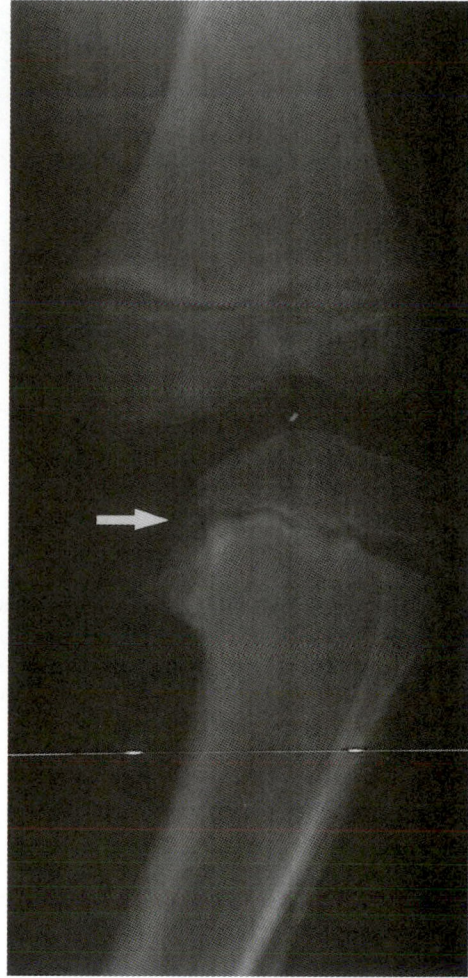

B

Figure 139-3
A. Stage IV infantile Blount's disease demonstrating severe varus and knee subluxation. *B*. Epiphysis dipping into metaphyseal defect (*arrow*).

are often very large, and fixation of the osteotomy has been a problem in the past, as well as delayed union, compartment syndromes, and peroneal nerve palsies. External fixation is commonly employed today, and the newer devices have been quite versatile, obviating the need for casting and decreasing complications.

GENU VALGUM

Genu valgum is a normal physiologic entity in children between the ages of 3 and 8 years. After 8 years of age, pathologic genu valgum in children is uncommon and difficult to treat. In a young child with severe genu valgum the physician should consider a skeletal dysplasia diagnosis such as Morquio's syndrome.

If the disorder is idiopathic, treatment is based on the age of the patient and location of the valgus. The valgus is most commonly seen at the distal femur; however, it may be present in the proximal tibia or distal tibia as well. Rarely, a diaphyseal deformity is seen.

In the common location of distal femoral valgus, treatment could

consist of a KAFO with a varus moment in a young child 2 to 6 years of age to a hemiephysiodesis of the medial distal femoral physis in a child 6 to 10 years of age to a distal femoral osteotomy in an adolescent.

SUGGESTED READINGS

Bowen JR, Leahey JL, Zhang ZH, et al: Partial epiphysiodesis at the knee and correct angular deformity. *Clin Orthop* 1985; 198:184.

Feldman MD, Shoenecker PC: Use of metaphyseal-diaphyseal angle in the evaluation of bowed leg. *J Bone Joint Surg [Am]* 1993; 75:1602.

Heath CH, Staehli LT: Normal limits of knee angle in white children—genu varum and genu valgum. *J Pediatr Orthop* 1993; 13:259.

Paley D, Tetsworth K: Mechanical axis deviation of the lower limbs. Preoperative planning of uniapical angular deformities of the tibia or femur. *Clin Orthop* 1992; 280:65.

Staheli LT, Corbett M, Wyss C, et al: Lower extremity rotational problems in children. Normal values to guide management. *J Bone Joint Surg [Am]* 1985; 67:39.

Chapter 140

FOOT DISORDERS IN INFANCY

Wallace B. Lehman
Dan Atar

CONGENITAL CLUBFOOT (TALIPES EQUINOVARUS)

The *incidence* of congenital clubfoot is 1:1000 live births. Bilateral feet are involved in 50 percent of cases, the right side is affected more than the left, and males are affected twice as often as females. The *heredity* is of a polygenic pattern. If a first-born male is affected, there is nearly a 40 times increased incidence of another male being affected.

ETIOLOGY

The etiology is unknown, but a few theories have been suggested: In the *mechanical theory,* the foot is forced into the deformed posture in the uterus; in the *neuromuscular theory,* the deformity is the sequelae of neuromuscular imbalance and the talar deformity is secondary; and in the *germ plasm defect theory,* the talus never develops into a normal size and shape. All other deformities are seen as secondary to the primary talar deformity.

PATHOLOGIC ANATOMY

The ankle is in equinus, the heel is inverted, and the forefoot is adducted and supinated (Fig. 140-1). There is obvious atrophy of the calf muscles, and the affected foot is smaller. Turco (1979) attributed the deformity to the medial displacement of the navicular and calcaneus around the talus. The talus is forced into equinus. The head and neck of the talus are deviated medially. The calcaneus is inverted under the talus. McKay (1982) described abnormal rotation in sagittal, coronal, and horizontal planes of the talocalcaneal joint. The talonavicular joint is in an extreme position of inversion as the navicular moves around the head of the talus. Contracture of soft tissues exerts further deforming forces and resists realignment of the joints.

RADIOGRAPHY

In the anteroposterior (AP) radiographs, lines through the long axis of the talus and calcaneus cross at an angle of 20 to 40 degrees. In clubfoot, the two lines may be almost parallel (Fig. 140-2). In the lateral radiographs, the lines through the longitudinal axis of the talus and calcaneus cross also at an angle of 20 to 40 degrees. In clubfoot, the angle is less than 20 degrees (Fig. 140-3).

TREATMENT

Treatment consists of weekly serial manipulation and casting. The correction of the forefoot adduction should be first, followed by correction of the heel varus, and, finally, the correction of the hindfoot equinus. If correction of the equinus is done earlier, rocker-

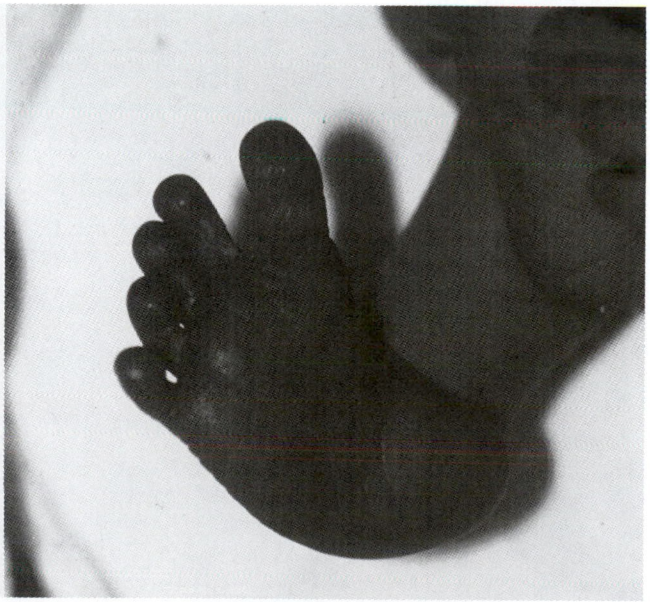

Figure 140-1
Club foot. Note the three components: midfoot adduction, heel varus, heel equinus.

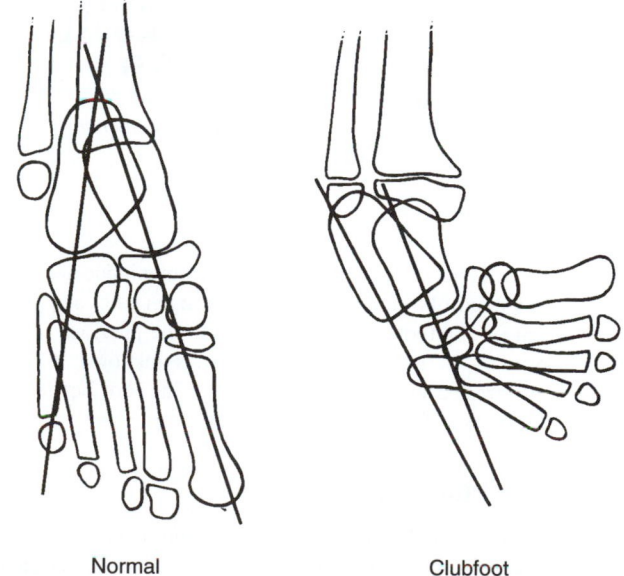

Normal   Clubfoot

Figure 140-2
Schematic drawing of lines through the long axis of the talus and calcaneus in anteroposterior view of a normal foot (*left*) and clubfoot (*right*).

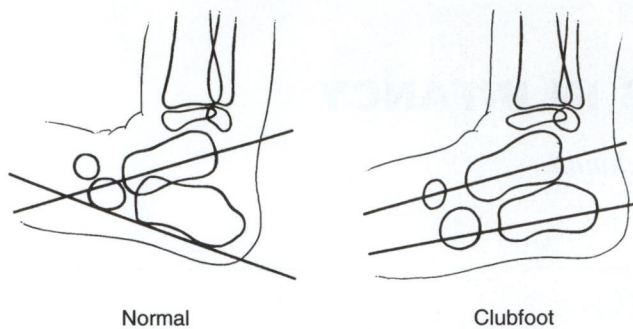

Normal   Clubfoot

Figure 140-3
Schematic drawing of lines through the long axis of the talus and calcaneus in lateral view of a normal foot (*left*) and clubfoot (*right*).

bottom deformity may be created. In most cases (75 to 80 percent),
correction can be achieved in 2 to 3 months. The feet should be held
in cast for a further 4 weeks, followed by wearing of outflare shoes
for a year. Parents are taught daily manipulative exercises for their
children. In the feet with the persisting deformity, surgery is indicated. The recommended age for surgical intervention is 3 to 6
months. Surgery should include complete soft tissue release done systematically. Surgery includes Z-plasty of the Achilles tendon; fractional lengthening of the flexor digitorum and flexor hallucis longus;
section of the tibialis posterior (up to age 2 years) and the abductor
hallucis; capsulotomies of the posterior tibiotalar joint, talocalcaneal
joint, and talonavicular joint; and section of the fibulocalcaneal ligament. The talonavicular joint and calcaneus are realigned and held in
plaster casts for 6 weeks, followed by outflare shoes and manipulations for a year after surgery.

Among these patients, 15 to 50 percent may relapse after surgery.
The revision clubfoot surgery should be carefully planned according
to the algorithm outlined by Atar and colleagues (1991). Redo soft
tissue release, calcaneocuboid fusion, cuboid decancellization, wedge
tarsectomy, metatarsal osteotomy, and triple arthrodesis are all used
for recurrent clubfoot salvage procedures.

CONGENITAL VERTICAL TALUS
(CONGENITAL CONVEX PES PLANOVALGUS)
(ROCKER-BOTTOM FOOT)

Congenital vertical talus deformity is very rare (*incidence,* 1:10,000
births), sex distribution is equal, and involvement may be bilateral.

ETIOLOGY

Vertical talus can be in association with myelomeningocele, arthrogryposis, and neurofibromatosis. It can be iatrogenically acquired in
the treatment of clubfoot (as was described in the previous section)
or can be primary. In the latter case, the cause is unknown. It may be
the result of arrested prenatal development of the foot between the
7th and 12th weeks of pregnancy.

CLINICAL APPEARANCE

The hindfoot is in fixed equinus, and the forefoot is dorsiflexed and
pronated. The sole of the foot is convex and has a rocker-bottom appearance. The head of the talus is prominent on the medial and plantar aspect of the foot. There are deep creases on the dorsolateral aspect of the foot anterior and inferior to the lateral malleolus (Figs.
140-4 and 140-5). The deformity is rigid. When weightbearing is be-

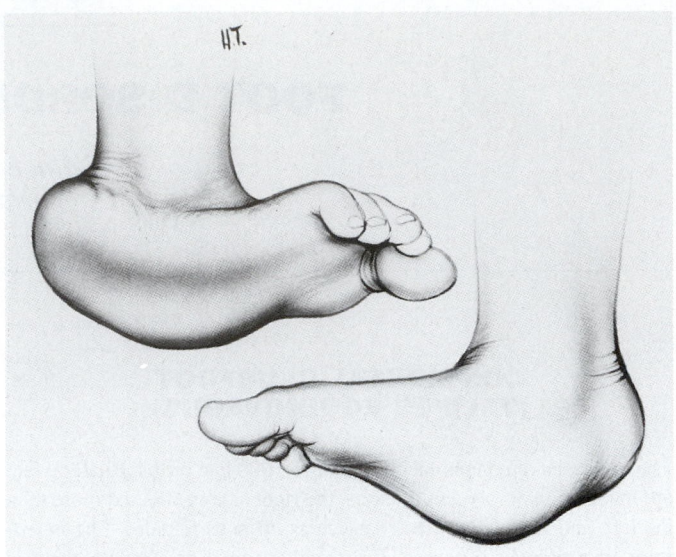

Figure 140-4
The rocker-bottom foot.

gun, adaptive changes occur in the bones and soft tissue. Congenital
vertical talus may be difficult to distinguish from congenital calcaneovalgus (here the calcaneus is not in equinus and the deformity is
quite flexible) or from oblique talus. In older children, oblique talus
is often associated with pes planus. In severe cases, the diagnosis is
made by radiography: Standing AP and lateral views are required with
lateral forced plantar flexion and dorsiflexion views. Forced dorsiflexion will demonstrate the navicular located over the dorsal surface
of the neck of the talus. In an unossified navicular (it ossifies by
3 years of age), the long axis of the first metatarsal will point dorsally to the head of the talus (Fig. 140-6). (In normal foot, it bisects
the head of the talus.) In oblique talus, the navicular remains articu-

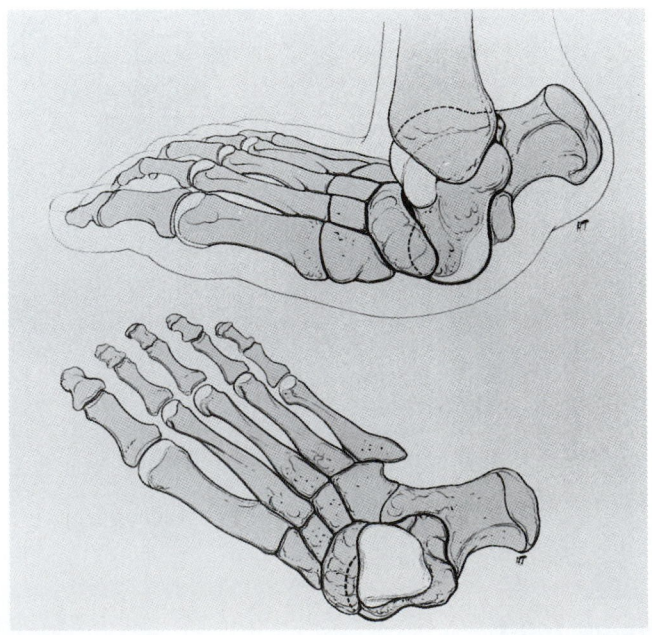

Figure 140-5
Schematic drawings of the talo-calcaneus-navicular. Relationship in the
rocker-bottom foot (anteroposterior, *bottom*; and lateral, *top*).

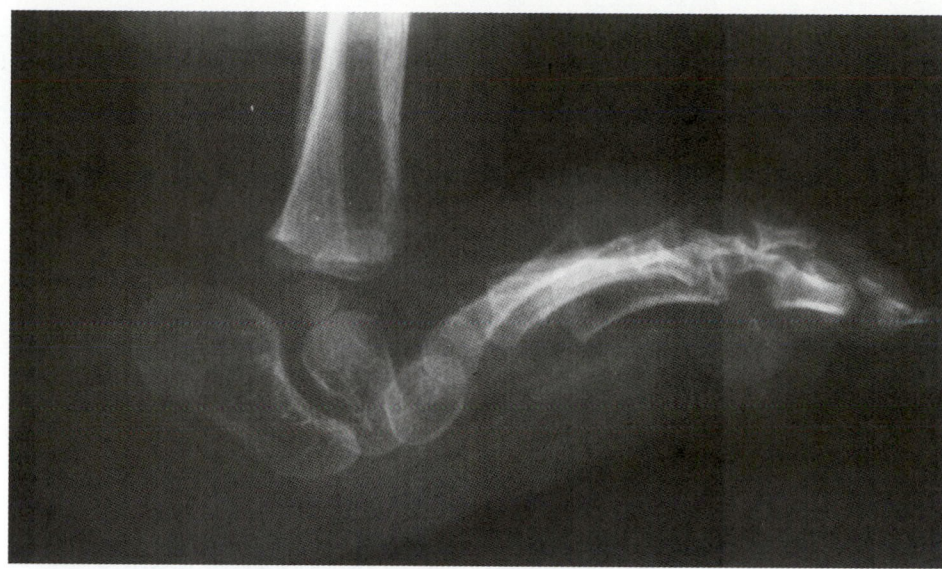

Figure 140-6
Lateral radiograph of vertical talus. The navicular is unossified.

lated with the upper part of the talar head even when the foot is forcibly dorsiflexed. Plantar flexion will correct any subluxation of the talonavicular joint in oblique talus whereas, in vertical talus, the talonavicular dislocation will not be corrected.

TREATMENT

At birth, gentle manipulation and serial casting are beneficial to stretch the soft tissues, but the reduction of the talonavicular joint almost always requires surgical intervention. The procedure should include complete soft tissue release as for clubfoot, plus lengthening of the extensors and the peronei. In children over 6 years of age, it is best to wait until age 10 and perform triple arthrodesis.

PES CALCANEOVALGUS

Pes calcaneovalgus is the most common foot deformity seen at birth (30 to 50 percent of live births). Its incidence is higher in firstborns.

ETIOLOGY

The etiology is postural dorsal compression of the feet, particularly in primigravida.

CLINICAL APPEARANCE

The entire foot is dorsiflexed and everted. In severe cases, the foot may touch the anterior aspect of the tibia. Neuromuscular diseases and congenital convex pes planovalgus (rocker bottom) foot should be excluded.

TREATMENT

In most cases, passive stretching exercises at the time of diaper changes are sufficient. Severe cases or, in persistent cases, manipulation and serial casting are needed.

FLEXIBLE FLATFOOT (PES PLANUS)

Flexible flatfoot refers to a foot that, on weightbearing, the medial border is in contact with the ground. When weightbearing is removed,

an apparent longitudinal arch reappears. The longitudinal arch is maintained only by the configuration of the tarsal bones and joints and the strength of the ligaments that bind them together. Flatfeet result from excessive ligamentous laxity, the exact cause of which is unknown. There is a common familial incidence to this condition.

RADIOGRAPHIC APPEARANCE

In standing radiographs of a normal foot, the longitudinal axis of the talus, navicular, medial cuneiform, and the first metatarsal forms a straight line. In a flexible flatfoot, this line is broken, and there is a sag at the talonavicular joint or the naviculocuneiform joint. Footprints can also demonstrate the degree of the deformity.

CLINICAL SYMPTOMS

Flexible flatfeet are asymptomatic. Children seldom complain about their feet, and their parents are usually concerned about the appearance of the child's feet (Fig. 140-7) or the shoe wear. A child's complaint

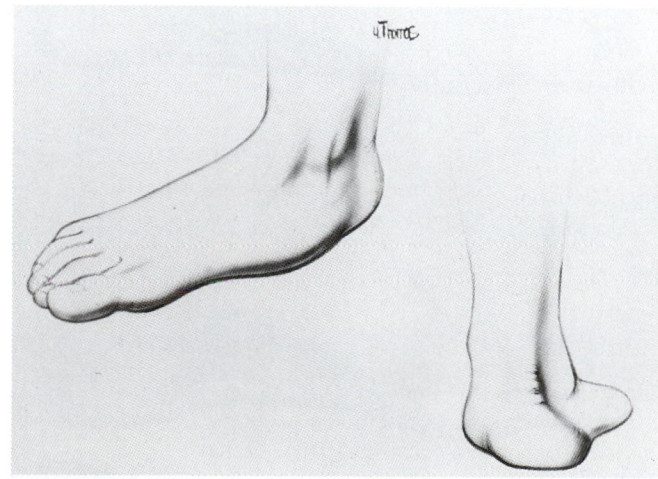

Figure 140-7
Severe flatfoot.

about foot pain might be related to contracture of the gastrocnemius, tarsal coalition, or inflammatory process involving the subtalar and midtarsal joints. In adults, the deformity may become progressively rigid, and they may complain about pain because of foot strain.

TREATMENT

Most cases of flexible flatfoot do not need treatment. In symptomatic cases, muscle-stretching exercises and arch supports may be indicated. In severe symptomatic flatfeet, heel cups are indicated. Surgery is reserved for a small percentage of patients who failed to respond to conservative treatment. Surgery may include soft tissue procedures (ligamentous tightening or tendon transfer), bony procedures (arthrodesis of tarsal joints, osteotomy of tarsal bones, or a combined procedure), or artificial subtalar implants.

PES CAVUS

Pes cavus, which is a foot with an abnormally high arch often associated with clawing of the toes (Fig. 140-8), is a manifestation of neuromuscular disease unless proven otherwise. In about 80 percent of cases, a careful, detailed medical history, neurologic evaluation, radiography of the entire spine, magnetic resonance imaging, electromyography, and nerve conduction tests can reveal neuromuscular disease such as Charcot-Marie-Tooth disease, poliomyelitis, spinal dysraphism, cerebellar disease, or arthrogryposis. Traumatic pes cavus can also occur after fracture of the tibia or fibula and after pos-

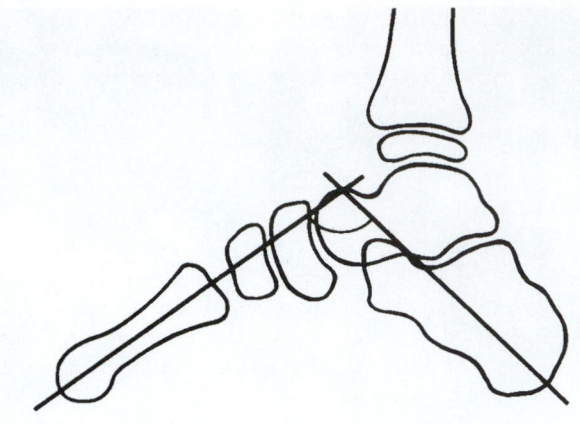

Figure 140-9
Schematic drawing of the bony relationship in the pes cavus (see the text).

terior compartment syndrome that cause muscle fibrosis of some of the calf muscles or the intrinsic muscles of the foot and progress gradually to a cavovarus foot with clawtoes. In some cases, no definite cause is discovered.

CLINICAL SYMPTOMS

Patients usually present at age 8 years. The deformity can be noticed before there are any symptoms. Pain may be felt under the metatarsal heads with callosities. In standing radiographs of a normal foot, the

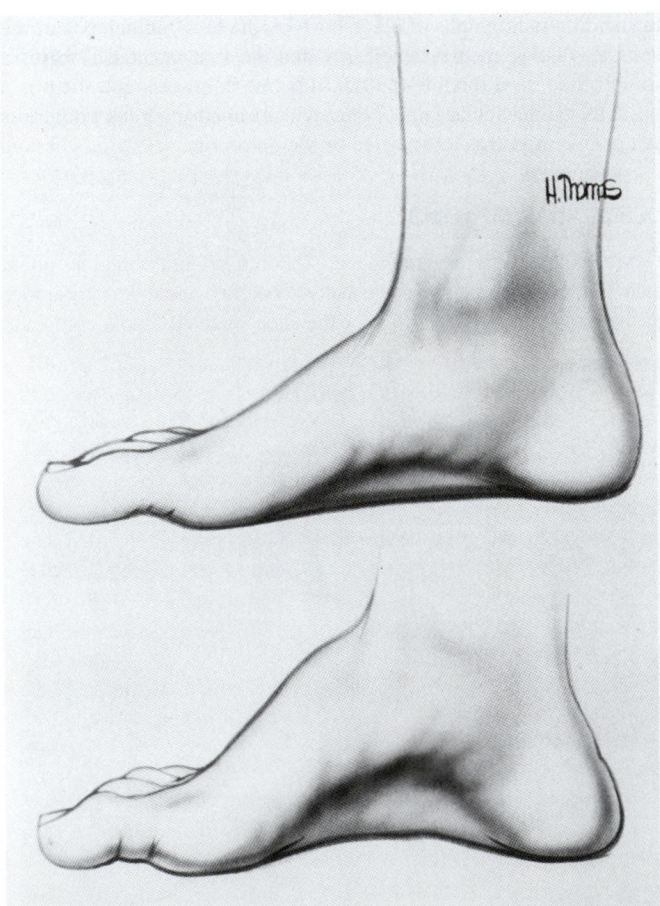

Figure 140-8
Top, normal arch; and *bottom,* pes cavus.

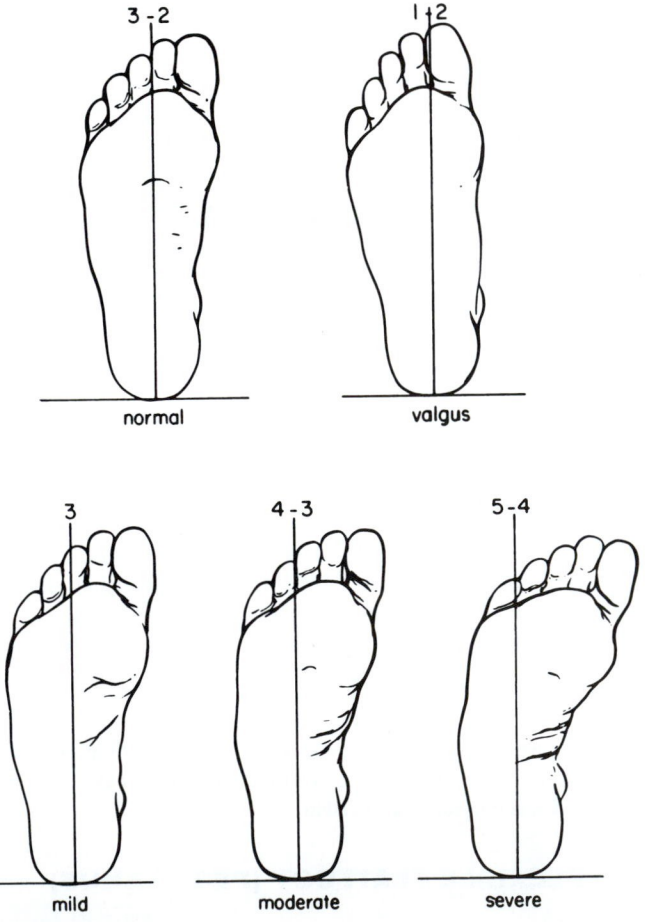

Figure 140-10
Mild, moderate, and severe metatarsus adductus.

longitudinal axis of the talus is parallel with that of the first metatarsal. In pes cavus, an angle forms between the lines. An alternative measurement can be the angle between the longitudinal axis of the calcaneus and talus. An angle of more than 140 degrees suggests pes cavus (Fig. 140-9).

TREATMENT

Symptomatic patients can be relieved by a combination of arch support and specially made shoes. When conservative measures fail, surgery is indicated, but should be delayed until progressive neuromuscular deficit has been ruled out. Surgery should first include release of the plantar fascia, short plantar muscles, and long flexor tendons, followed by bony osteotomies.

METATARSUS ADDUCTUS

Metatarsus adductus and metatarsus varus are sometimes considered to be synonyms. Some authors differentiate between the two, observing that in metatarsus adductus the forefoot deviates toward the midline and in metatarsus varus the forefoot is also inverted, the medial border is concave, the lateral border is convex, and the prominence on this border consists of the subluxing second and third cuneiform (Fig. 140-10).

ETIOLOGY

The etiology has been considered as malposition in utero. Up to 10 percent of cases may also have developmental dysplasia of the hip.

TREATMENT

Most of the metatarsus adductus will resolve spontaneously. Moderate to severe forms require serial manipulation and casting. The metatarsus varus feet increase with severity if left untreated. They require early manipulation and serial casting (Fig. 140-11). During manipu-

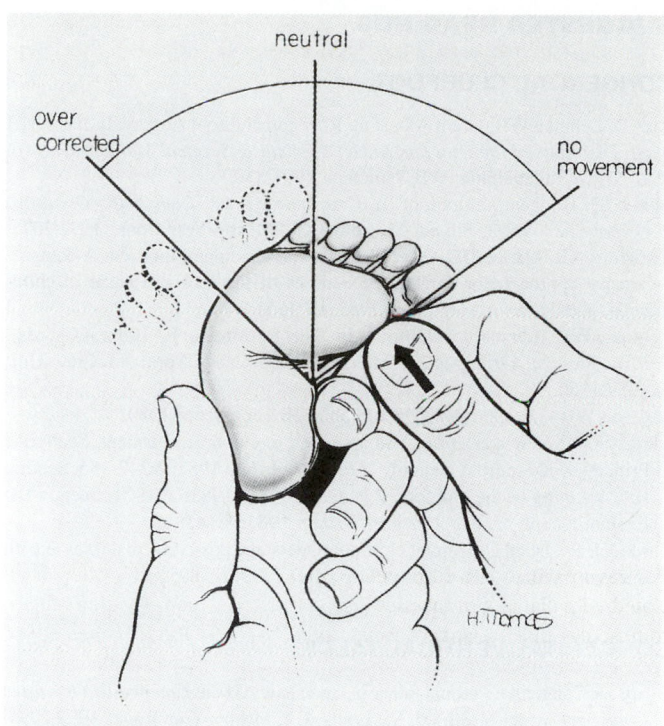

Figure 140-11
Manipulation of the metatarsus varus.

lations, the calcaneus should be held in a neutral position. For children with residual deformity (about 10 percent of the cases), surgery is indicated. Tarsometatarsal capsulotomies (Heyman-Herndon) have been suggested for children younger than age 5, although in recent reports about a 41 percent failure rate was reported. For children older than age 5, metatarsal osteotomy is the procedure of choice (Fig. 140-12).

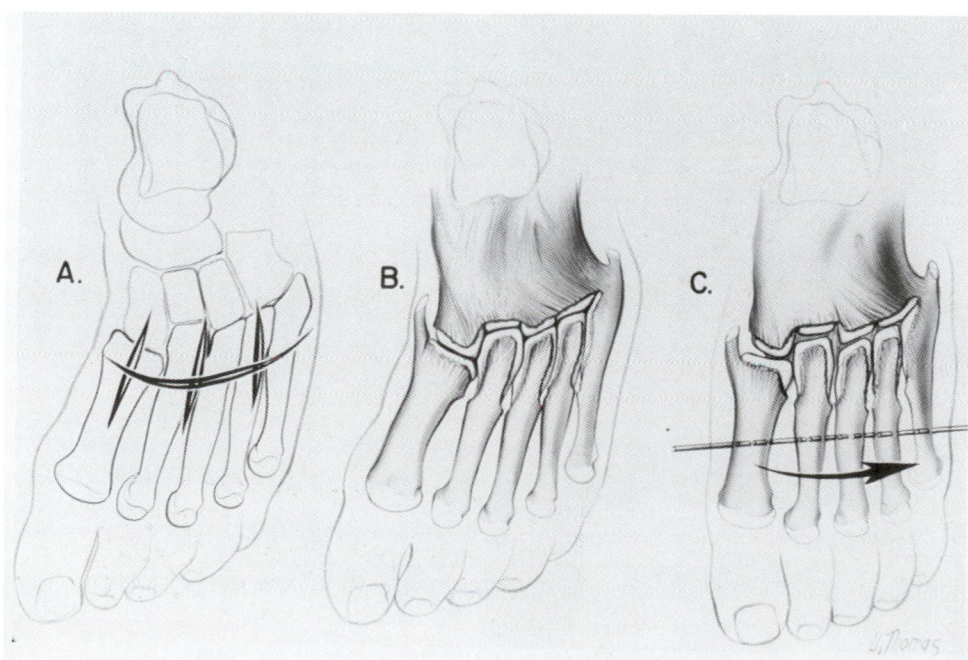

Figure 140-12
Metatarsus osteotomies for persistent forefoot adduction.

SUGGESTED READINGS

CONGENITAL CLUBFOOT

Atar D, Lehman WB, Grant AD, et al. Revision clubfoot surgery. In Jahss MH ed: *Disorders of the Foot and Ankle: Medical & Surgical Management,* vol 1, 2d ed. Philadelphia: WB Saunders; 1991:830.

Beaty JH: Congenital clubfoot. In Crenshaw AH ed: *Campbell's Operative Orthopedics,* vol 3, 8th ed. St. Louis: CV Mosby-Year Book; 1992:2075.

Crawford AH, Marxen JL, Osterfeld DL: The Cincinnati incision: A comprehensive approach for surgical procedures of the foot and ankle in childhood. *J Bone Joint Surg [Am]* 1982; 64:1355.

Lehman WB: Idiopathic clubfoot. In Dee R, Mango E, Hurst LC (eds): *Principles of Orthopedic Practice,* vol 2. New York: McGraw-Hill; 1989:1150.

Lehman WB: *The Clubfoot.* Philadelphia: JB Lippincott; 1980.

McKay DW: New concept of and approach to clubfoot treatment. Section I: Principles and morbid anatomy. *J Pediatr Orthop* 1982; 2:347-356. Section II: Correction of the clubfoot. *J Pediatr Orthop* 1983; 3:10-21. Section III: Evaluation and results. *J Pediatr Orthop* 1983; 3:141.

Turco VJ: Resistant congenital clubfoot: One-stage posteromedial release with internal fixation. *J Bone Joint Surg [Am]* 1979; 61:805.

CONGENITAL VERTICAL TALUS

Beaty JJ: Congenital vertical talus. In Crenshaw AH ed: *Campbell's Operative Orthopedics,* vol 3, 8th ed. St. Louis, CV Mosby-Year Book; 1992:2091.

Jacobsen ST, Crawford AH: Congenital vertical talus. *J Pediatr Orthop* 1983; 3:306.

Kumar SJ, Cowell HR, Ramsey PL: Foot problems in children. Part I: Vertical and oblique talus. In Frankel VH (ed): *Instructional Course Lectures,* vol 31. Park Ridge, IL: American Academy of Orthopaedic Surgeons; 1982:235.

Tachdjian MO: Congenital convex pes valgus. In Tachdjian MO ed: *Pediatric Orthopedics,* vol 4, 2d ed. Philadelphia: WB Saunders; 1990:2557.

PES CALCANEOVALGUS

Edwards ER, Menelaus MB: Reverse clubfoot: Rigid and recalcitrant talipes calcaneovalgus. *J Bone Joint Surg [Br]* 1987; 69:330.

Tachdjian MO: Talipes calcaneovalgus. In *Pediatric Orthopedics,* vol 4, 2d ed. Philadelphia: WB Saunders; 1990:2423.

FLEXIBLE FLATFOOT

Barry RJ, Scranton PE, Jr: Flatfeet in children. *Clin Orthop* 1983; 181:68.

Richardson GE: Flexible pes planus. In Crenshaw AH ed: *Campbell's Operative Orthopedics,* vol 4, 8th ed. St. Louis: CV Mosby-Year Book; 1992:2693.

Staheli LT, Chew DE, Corbett M: The longitudinal arch: A survey of eight hundred and eighty-two feet in normal children and adults. *J Bone Joint Surg [Am]* 1987; 69:426.

Tachdjian MO: Flexible pes planovalgus. In *Pediatric Orthopedics,* vol 4, 2d ed. Philadelphia: WB Saunders; 1990:2717.

Wenger DR, Mauldin D, Speck G, et al: Corrective shoes and inserts as treatment for flexible flatfoot in infants and children. *J Bone Joint Surg [Am]* 1989; 71:800.

PES CAVUS

Jahss MH: Evaluation of the cavus foot for orthopedic treatment. *Clin Orthop* 1983; 181:52.

McCluskey WP, Lovell WW, Cummings RJ: The cavovarus foot deformity: Etiology and management. *Clin Orthop* 1989; 247:27.

Richardson GE: Cavus foot. In Crenshaw AH ed: Campbell's *Operative Orthopedics.* St. Louis: CV Mosby-Year Book; 1992:2792.

Tachdjian MO: Pes cavus. In *Pediatric Orthopedics,* vol 4, 2d ed. Philadelphia: WB Saunders; 1990:2671.

METATARSUS ADDUCTUS

Bleck EE: Metatarsus adductus classification and relationship to outcomes of treatment. *J Pediatr Orthop* 1983; 3:2.

Gruber MA, Dee R: Congenital metatarsus varus. In Dee R, Mango E, Hurst LC eds: *Principles of Orthopedic Practice,* vol 2. New York: McGraw-Hill; 1989:1148.

Stark JG, Johnson JG, Winter RB: The Heyman–Herndon tarseometatarsal capsulotomy for metatarsus adductus: Results in 48 feet. *J Pediatr Orthop* 1987; 7:305.

Tachdjian MO: Congenital metatarsus varus. In *Pediatric Orthopedics,* vol 4, 2d ed. Philadelphia: WB Saunders; 1990:2612.

Chapter 141

FOOT DISORDERS IN EARLY CHILDHOOD AND ADOLESCENCE

Wallace B. Lehman and Dan Atar

TARSAL COALITION

Tarsal coalition, rigid pes planus, and peroneal spastic foot are synonyms. Coalition of the tarsal bone may be *congenital* (due to a failure of segmentation of the primitive mesenchyme) or *acquired* after trauma or inflammation. Its *incidence* is 1 percent, and it can occur bilaterally in about 50 percent of cases. The most common type is calcaneonavicular, followed by the talocalcaneal.

CLINICAL SYMPTOMS

Some coalitions never become symptomatic and are accidental findings on radiographs. All coalitions are cartilaginous at birth and may allow motion. When they ossify, they restrict motion. The age for clinical presentation varies for the different types of coalition and correlates with the age at which each type ossifies. The talonavicular ossifies between 3 and 5 years of age. Symptoms may present at 8 years of age. Calcaneonavicular ossifies at age 8 to 12 with symptoms at age 16. Talocalcaneal coalition ossifies at age 12 to 16 with symptoms at age 18. Pain is the presenting symptom. The foot is rigid, flat, and everted. The peroneal and sometimes the extensors are spastic. Ankle motion is normal, but subtalar motion is restricted and painful. Midtarsal movements also are restricted. Talonavicular bars are readily diagnosed on lateral radiographs. Oblique radiographs may demonstrate the calcaneonavicular bar (Fig. 141-1). The Harris and Beath view (a tangential radiograph of the subtalar joint) can demonstrate the talocalcaneal bar. (Sometimes, secondary signs such as talar beaking are helpful.) Computed tomographic scan is the best modality and can provide detailed knowledge of the bar anatomy (Fig. 141-2).

TREATMENT

Conservative treatment is initially indicated: cast immobilization, special shoes, and orthosis. When the pain persists, surgery is indicated. Resection of the bars with fat interposition is usually recommended. Arthrodesis is performed when degenerative changes occur.

JUVENILE/ADOLESCENT BUNIONS

Varus of the first metatarsal with a widened first to second intermetatarsal angle (more than 10 degrees) is almost always present. Because of the soft tissue attachments (adductor halluces) to the proximal phalanx of the great toe, the proximal and distal phalanxes of

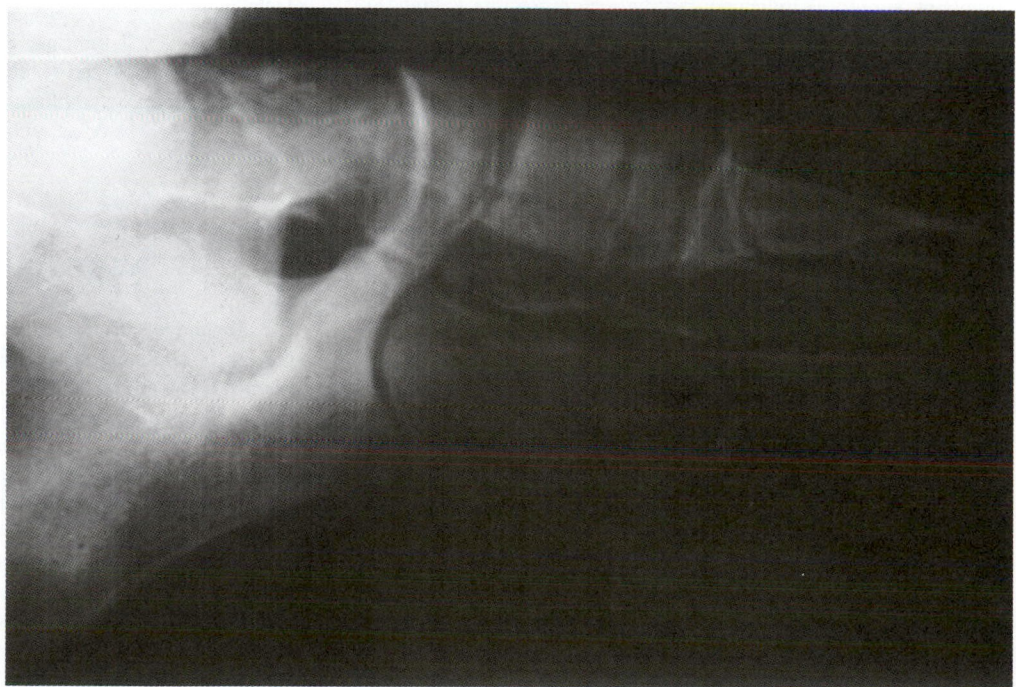

Figure 141-1
Oblique radiograph demonstrates a calcaneonavicular bar.

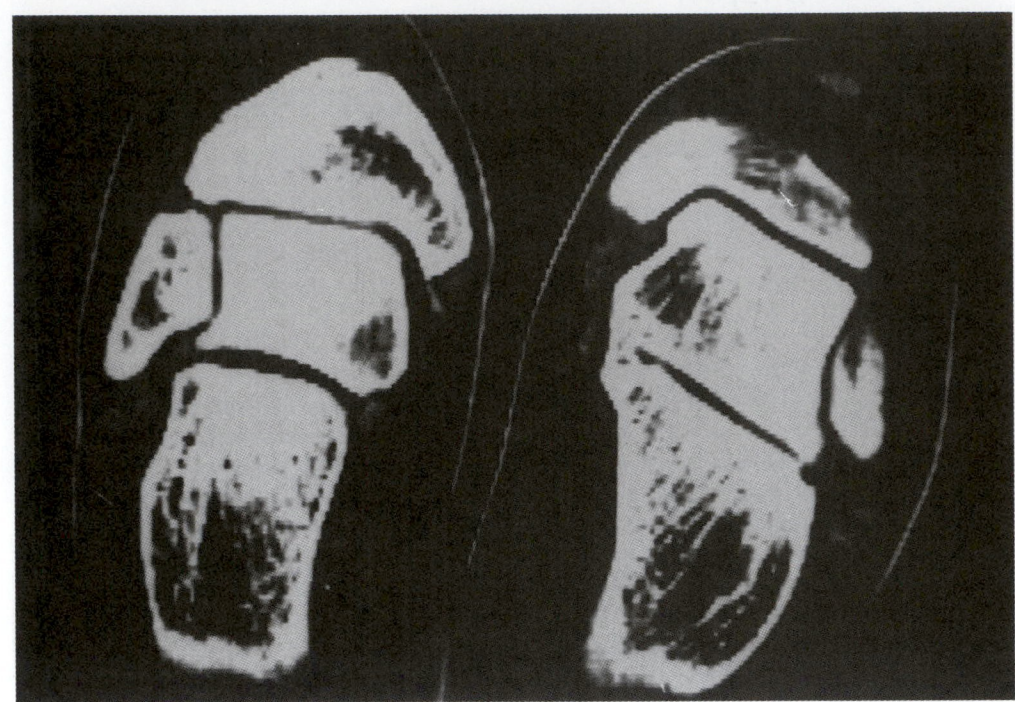

Figure 141-2
Computed tomographic scan demonstrates the talocalcaneal bar (medial facet) of the left foot.

the great toe deviate laterally, producing hallux valgus. A bunion of the head of the 1st metatarsal is a major part of the deformity. Hypermobile pronated flatfoot is frequently associated. A positive family history is to be expected. Patients present for treatment at age 10 to 14. Cosmesis for unattractive feet, rather than pain, is the primary complaint (Fig. 141-3). The initial treatment should be conservative. Patients should be advised to change shoes. For a persistent complaint, surgery is indicated, but the recurrence rate is high. Soft tissue procedures alone are unlikely to result in permanent correction. They should be combined with metatarsal osteotomy (proximal or distal) to realign the first metatarsal.

KÖHLER DISEASE

Osteochondrosis of the tarsal navicular, which was originally described by Köhler in 1908, occurs more in males (80 percent of cases). The average age is 5 years for males and 4 years for females.

ETIOLOGY

The navicular bone ossifies in boys at age 3 and girls at age 2. It is located at the apex of the longitudinal arch of the foot and is subjected to constant stress during walking. An ischemia of unknown origin associated with stress on an unossified bone has been proposed as an etiology.

CLINICAL SYMPTOMS

The child presents with a limp and pain localized over the navicular. Radiographs reveal irregular rarefaction, sclerosis, and flattening of

the navicular. In 20 percent of cases, both feet have the same changes although one foot may be asymptomatic. Irregular ossification of the navicular is seen without symptoms in 30 percent of boys and 20 percent of girls.

TREATMENT

The disease is self-limiting. The navicular reconstitutes itself in 1 to 3 years, and usually no residual deformity or disability will be left. When the feet are symptomatic, some recommend using a walking cast for few weeks or an arch support for a few months.

ACCESSORY NAVICULAR

Other synonyms are prehallux or tibialis externum. It presents in 10 percent of children's feet. However, it persists as a separate ossicle in only 2 percent of adult feet. It is often bilateral and is located at the medial end of the navicular (Fig. 141-4). The tibialis posterior tendon is attached to it. Kidner in 1929 stated that the support to the longitudinal arch was compromised by the abnormal insertion of the tibialis posterior. This is as yet unproven, since many people with an accessory navicular have a normal longitudinal arch. The presenting symptoms are localized pain and planovalgus deformity of the foot. Initial treatment includes arch support, hydrocortisone injection, and plaster cast. If symptoms persist, surgical excision of the accessory navicular with rerouting of the tibialis posterior tendon (Kidner, 1929) are indicated.

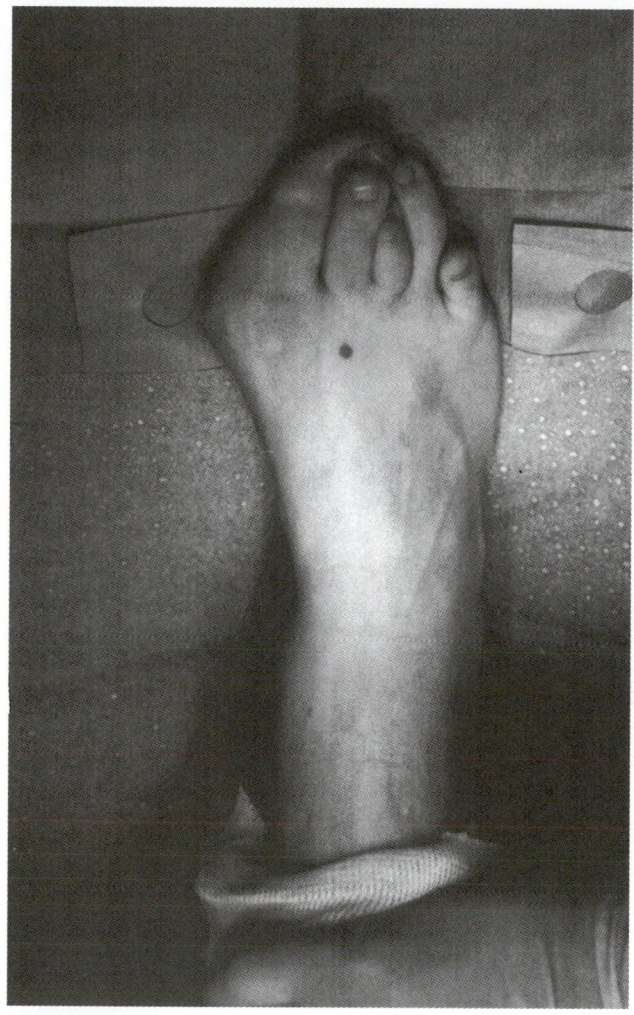

Figure 141-3
Adolescent bunion.

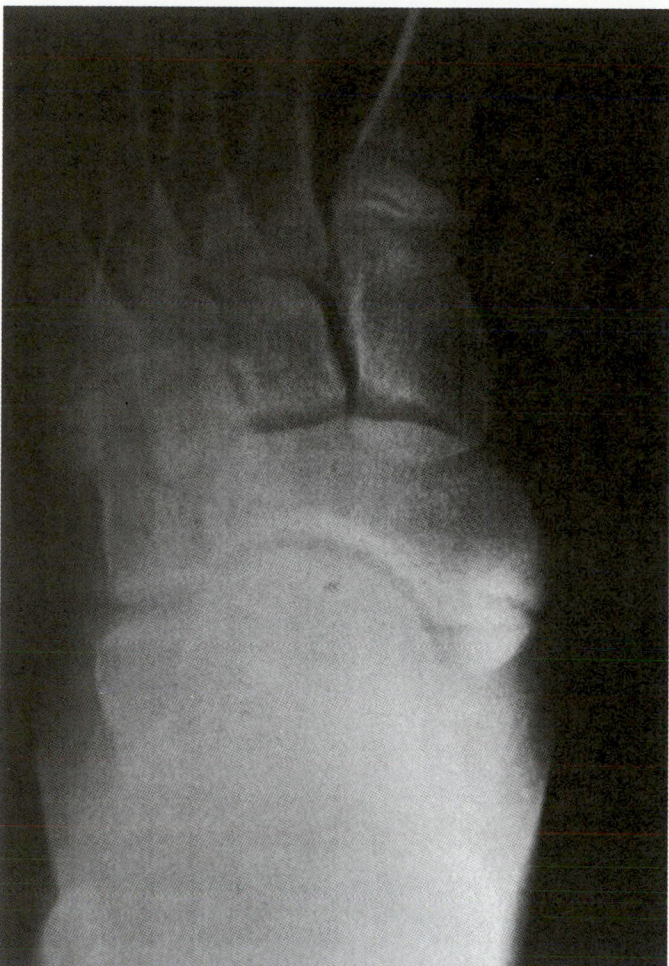

Figure 141-4
Radiograph of a foot with accessory navicular.

SUGGESTED READINGS

TARSAL COALITION

Jayakuma S, Cowell HR: Rigid flatfoot. *Clin Orthop* 1977; 122:77.

Mosier KM, Asher M: Tarsal coalitions and peroneal spastic flat foot: A review. *J Bone Joint Surg [Am]* 1984; 66:976.

Richardson EG: Tarsal coalition. In Canale ST (ed): *Campbell's Operative Orthopedics,* vol 2, 9th ed. St. Louis, Mosby; 1998:1732.

Swiontkowski MF, Scranton PE, Hansen S: Tarsal coalition long-term results of surgical treatment. *J Pediatr Orthop* 1983; 3:287.

Tachdjian MO: Tarsal coalition. In Tachdjian MO (ed): *Pediatric Orthopedics,* vol 4, 2d ed. Philadelphia, WB Saunders; 1990:2578.

Wilkins KE: The painful foot in the child. In Bassett FH III (ed): *Instructional Course Lectures,* vol 37. Park Ridge, IL, American Academy of Orthopaedic Surgeons; 1988:77.

JUVENILE/ADOLESCENT BUNIONS

Coughlin MJ, Mann RA: The pathophysiology of the juvenile bunion. In Griffin PP (ed): *Instructional Course Lectures,* vol 36. Park Ridge, IL, American Academy of Orthopaedic Surgeons; 1987:123.

Helal B: Surgery for adolescent hallux valgus. *Clin Orthop* 1981; 157:50.

Mann RA: Decision-making in bunion surgery. In Greene WB (ed): *Instructional Course Lectures.* Park Ridge, IL, American Academy of Orthopaedic Surgeons; 1990; 39:3.

Scranton PE, Zuckerman JD: Bunion surgery in adolescents: Results of surgical treatment. *J Pediatr Orthop* 1984; 4:39.

Tachdjian MO: Congenital metatarsus primus varus and hallux valgus. In Tachdjian MO (ed): *Pediatric Orthopedics,* vol 4, 2d ed. Philadelphia, WB Saunders; 1990:2626.

Richardson EG: Disorders of the hallux. In Canale ST (ed): *Campbell's Operative Orthopedics,* 9th ed, vol 2. St. Louis, Mosby; 1998:1621.

KÖHLER DISEASE

Tachdjian MO: Köhler disease of the tarsal navicular. In Tachdjian MO (ed): *Pediatric Orthopedics,* vol 2, 2d ed. Philadelphia, WB Saunders; 1990:1003.

Williams GA, Cowell HR: Köhler disease of the tarsal navicular. *Clin Orthop* 1981; 158:53.

ACCESSORY NAVICULAR

Kidner FC: The prehallux (accessory scaphoid) in its relation to flatfoot. *J Bone Joint Surg* 1929; 11:831.

MacNicol MF, Voutsinas S: Surgical treatment of symptomatic accessory navicular. *J Bone Joint Surg [Br]* 1984; 66:218.

Richardson EG. Accessory navicular. In Canale ST (ed): *Campbell's Operative Orthopedics,* 9th ed, vol 2. St. Louis, Mosby, 1998:1725.

Tachdjian MO: Accessory tarsal navicular. In Tachdjian MO (ed): *Pediatric Orthopedics,* vol 4, 2d ed. Philadelphia, WB Saunders, 1990:2412.

Chapter 142

INFECTIONS

David S. Feldman

Infections of bone (osteomyelitis) and joints (septic arthritis) are of great concern to the orthopaedic surgeon. Delay in diagnosis and management can have severe deleterious effects on the long-term outcome. Destruction of the articular cartilage by lysosomal enzymes starts within hours after the initiation of the septic arthritis, and destruction of the growth plate may be the inevitable sequelae of metaphyseal osteomyelitis. Careful physical examination, timely and appropriate diagnostic tests, and early medical, and—when appropriate—surgical intervention can often prevent many of the long-term sequelae of these diseases, including joint stiffness, arthritis, and physeal arrest.

Osteomyelitis has two general forms: hematogenous and post-traumatic (direct inoculation). Children are more susceptible to hematogenous metaphyseal osteomyelitis due to the metaphyseal end arterioles at the level of the physis. This decreases the rate of blood return from this region of bone, and therefore bacterial seeding is likely in this area. In the neonatal period and up to 6 months of age, the children have transphyseal vessels, and therefore metaphyseal osteomyelitis is associated with septic arthritis. The knee and the hip are the most common locations for osteomyelitis and septic arthritis. Trauma is thought to precede osteomyelitis, perhaps by making the area more susceptible to infection.

Septic arthritis may affect any joint but most commonly affects the hip or knee of the child. Septic arthritis may be caused by hematogenous spread or by osteomyelitis from transphyseal vessels in young children. It can also occur secondary to a direct inoculation.

CLINICAL PRESENTATION

Children at different ages and with various preexisting underlying diseases may present with a broad range of symptoms. In the neonatal period, infants with either septic arthritis or osteomyelitis may have pseudo-paralysis of the affected limb and may lack the usual symptoms of fever and swelling. The older child will often stop walking, hold the hip or knee in a flexed position, and often have a high fever. Adolescents will present with severe pain and limitation of motion of the affected joint and may not have a high fever.

Osteomyelitis usually presents with swelling and erythema, as well as bony tenderness. Septic arthritis will present with swelling if the joint is not covered by muscle, such as the knee and elbow. However, a shoulder or hip septic arthritis may not demonstrate discernible swelling on the surface of the limb. A painful joint effusion is the rule in septic arthritis while in osteomyelitis, although an effusion may be present, it is not associated with severe restricted or painful motion.

LABORATORY STUDIES

Increased erythrocyte sedimentation rate (ESR) and an elevated white blood cell count (WBC) with a shift to the left is present in up to 90 percent of the cases, but their absence does not exclude the disease. C-reactive protein (CRP) is a sensitive marker for infection, but often is valuable only in determining the effects of treatment and not in the initial evaluation. Neonates and adolescents may lack some or all of these markers, and the cessation of movement in a limb in neonates or the severe pain in the adolescent may be the only clue to the disease. Blood cultures (positive in up to 50 percent of cases of septic arthritis), joint aspiration (positive in approximately 50 percent of cases of osteomyelitis or septic arthritis), and bone/joint aspiration are essential in the evaluation and treatment of osteomyelitis and septic arthritis. Synovial fluid analysis is often helpful in diagnosing septic arthritis. A joint fluid white cell count over 80,000 μL with 75 percent polymorphonuclear leukocytes is consistent with infection. This number may overlap and be confused with juvenile idiopathic arthritis (formerly termed juvenile rheumatoid arthritis); however, all other entities, such as synovitis ($<$15,000 μL) or trauma ($<$5000 μL), are easily differentiated by a synovial fluid cell count. This count is only true in otherwise healthy children; it may not be elevated in immunosuppressed children, such as those children receiving chemotherapy.

IMAGING STUDIES

Plain radiographs are of some value in the initial workup of both septic arthritis and osteomyelitis. First, they rule out other possibilities such as a fracture or neoplasm mimicking a septic process. Second, although the radiographic changes in bone, such as periosteal reaction and bone resorption, do not occur until 7 to 10 days after the onset of the disease, soft tissue swelling and loss of normal fat planes in the affected extremity may be seen. This is much less specific in joints like the hip and shoulder which are covered with muscle. Widening of the joint space, such as in the pediatric infected hip, is a finding that may be present, but its absence does not preclude infection.

A bone scan (technetium-99m), particularly in the third phase, is a useful tool to demonstrate bone turnover. It can demonstrate the area of the problem, but it cannot be used to differentiate septic arthritis from osteomyelitis. Bone scan should be utilized when there is a question regarding the location of the pathology. It is not necessary if the location and nature of the disease is obvious.

Magnetic resonance imaging (MRI) is an excellent technique in evaluating osteomyelitis, particularly if anatomic detail is needed for

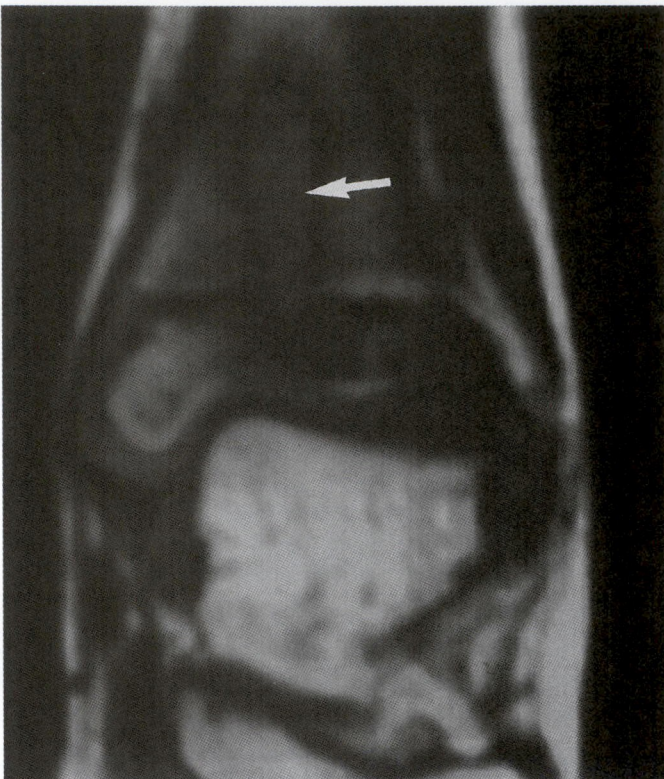

Figure 142-1
MRI demonstrating subacute osteomyelitis in distal tibia of 11-year-old child.

aspiration or treatment (Fig. 142-1). It is also useful if the clinician needs to differentiate neoplasm from infection. The high cost and need for heavy sedation in children precludes its routine use in osteomyelitis.

Computed tomographic scanning is reserved for those cases in which anatomic detail for biopsy is needed. It may be useful as a guide to performing an aspirate of a spine or pelvic osteomyelitis.

Ultrasound is a useful tool in demonstrating fluid. It has been used in determining if the hip joint has an effusion. It still cannot accurately differentiate a synovitis from an infection if fluid is present. Sonography is commonly being used in osteomyelitis to demonstrate the presence of an abscess or in diagnosis by soft tissue or periosteal changes. The accuracy of ultrasound, in this setting, is dependent on the experience of the sonographer, and its sensitivity and specificity have yet to be determined.

DIFFERENTIAL DIAGNOSIS

Clinically, osteomyelitis may mimic a number of disorders. First, trauma can often present like osteomyelitis, as it can cause pain and swelling in the affected extremity. Often plain radiographs as well as a complete blood count (CBC) and ESR will differentiate the two entities. Neoplasm, such as leukemia, Ewing's sarcoma, and histiocytosis X, may mimic osteomyelitis. In these cases where changes are noted on plain film, a formal biopsy may be required in order to make a diagnosis. Leukemia is the most difficult of these as children may present with normal or low white counts and minimal changes on radiographs. The clinician should be suspicious of leukemia if the child has multiple bone pain, a low or high WBC, low platelets, fatigue, or easy bruisability. Avascular necrosis associated with bone crisis in

children with sickle cell anemia or Gaucher's disease is easily confused with osteomyelitis, because these children have fever, and an increased WBC and ESR. This differential can be resolved only with a bone aspirate.

The differential diagnosis for septic arthritis is more difficult and extensive than that of osteomyelitis. Juvenile idiopathic arthritis (particularly Still's disease) can mimic all the signs and symptoms of septic arthritis. Severe toxic synovitis, Lyme disease, rheumatic fever, Henoch-Schönlein purpura, enteroarthritis (Salmonella or Yersinia), Kawasaki disease, and discitis may all present with similar symptoms. The clinician must be familiar with the presenting signs and symptoms of each of these diseases. In many of these diseases, there is no significant articular pain, (i.e., the child continues to walk, as in toxic synovitis and juvenile idiopathic arthritis). However, in cases where a joint effusion is present and the clinical picture resembles septic arthritis, a joint aspirate should be performed for diagnostic purposes.

INITIAL EVALUATION

The initial workup of a child with suspected osteomyelitis or septic arthritis is to obtain a CBC, ESR, CRP, and blood cultures. The results of these tests are not necessary to institute treatment. The diagnosis must be made on clinical grounds with diffuse swelling and pain over the metaphyseal region of the bone in osteomyelitis, and limitation of joint motion with pain in septic arthritis. Plain radiographs of the affected area should be performed. Joint aspirate for septic arthritis and bone aspirate for osteomyelitis is essential in the initial evaluation. The bone aspirate should be performed at the level of the periosteum and, if no pus is present, inside the metaphyseal bone. The aspirate, even if it is bloody, should be sent for gram stain and cultures. Aspiration of certain relatively inaccessible joints such as the hip may be performed in the operating theater. If no fluid is aspirated, an arthrogram is performed to be certain the needle is located in the joint. One should make all attempts not to aspirate a joint through an area of cellulitis, in order to avoid inoculating the joint and causing a septic arthritis.

MICROBIOLOGY

In children of all ages, with or without an underlying illness, *Staphylococcus aureus* is the most common causative organism (up to 80 percent). *Haemophilus influenzae* type B is becoming more common and may be seen in children below the age of 3 years. Salmonella is not uncommon in children with sickle cell anemia, and *Pseudomonas aeruginosa* is often found in the heel from direct inoculation through the shoe.

Septic arthritis is also caused most commonly by *Staphylococcus aureus*. However, *Haemophilus influenzae* type B is a common organism in children below the age of 3 years. Neonates may be infected by Group B streptococcus. Therefore, although *Staphylococcus aureus* is the most common organism, the age of the child must determine which antibiotic is given while awaiting cultures.

TREATMENT

HEMATOGENOUS OSTEOMYELITIS

After the initial evaluation has been performed as described above, empirical antibiotic therapy should commence. Treatment should consist of cefotaxime (third generation cephalosporin) in neonates, cefuroxime (second generation cephalosporin) in children 6 months to 4 years, and a first generation cephalosporin in older children.

Antibiotics should then be changed depending on the sensitivity of the organism cultured.

In hematogenous osteomyelitis, surgery is reserved for patients with soft-tissue abscesses or for those with a poor response to antibiotics after 48 h. The presence of a sequestrum is not, by itself an indication for surgery. The surgery is tailored specifically to treat the soft-tissue abscess and possibly to drill holes in the bone, in order to decompress an intraosseous abscess and remove any grossly necrotic tissue. Bone should not be routinely excised.

The duration of the intravenous antibiotics should depend on the organism cultured and on the patient's clinical response. Prior to switching to oral antibiotics, one should see a good clinical response, (i.e., decreasing pain and swelling, as well as a CRP that is returning to normal). Also, the organism cultured must be sensitive to an oral antibiotic. The duration of antibiotic treatment is usually 4 to 6 weeks and the ESR should have returned to normal.

SEPTIC ARTHRITIS

The treatment of septic arthritis is either serial arthrocentesis or incision, drainage, irrigation, and debridement of the joint. Large joints, such as the hip and shoulder, require surgical intervention due to the difficulty in performing serial aspirates. Serial aspirates may be inadequate in removing necrotic tissue, particularly in a joint where loculations are present, such as the knee. In addition, children do not tolerate serial aspirations well. Urgently performing either a small arthrotomy or an arthroscopy of a large joint may be the treatment of choice. Septic arthritis of the ankle, wrist, and finger may be treated with aspiration and antibiotics.

The choice of empirical antibiotic coverage is the same as that described for osteomyelitis. The principles regarding the duration of antibiotic treatment is similar to that of osteomyelitis, although, often, the response is faster and therefore the duration of treatment is shorter.

PUNCTURE WOUNDS OF THE FOOT

Direct inoculation of microorganisms into bone from the outside environment may occur from open fractures or puncture wounds; both must be treated surgically. Open fractures, similar to those of adults, must be irrigated and debrided with removal of the bone, devoid of soft tissue attachments. Heel puncture wounds through running shoes may lead to an osteomyelitis of the calcaneus due to *Pseudomonas aeruginosa.* Deep puncture wounds of the heel should be surgically debrided. Tetanus prophylaxis should be administered, and if a cellulitis develops antibiotics alone with local wound care is sufficient. If osteomyelitis develops, then the treatment of choice is surgical debridement of the calcaneus as well as administering the appropriate antibiotics; these should include a third generation cephalosporin such as ceftazidime, as well as coverage for *Staphylococcus aureus,* such as nafcillin. It may be difficult to clinically differentiate cellulitis from osteomyelitis. An MRI will often distinguish between the two.

UNUSUAL INFECTIONS OF BONE AND JOINTS

GONOCOCCAL ARTHRITIS

Septic arthritis in adolescent patients may be gonococcal arthritis, a sexually transmitted disease, caused by *Neisseria gonorrhoea.* Less commonly, this disease is seen in neonates and is contracted from passage through the birth canal of an infected mother. Any child or

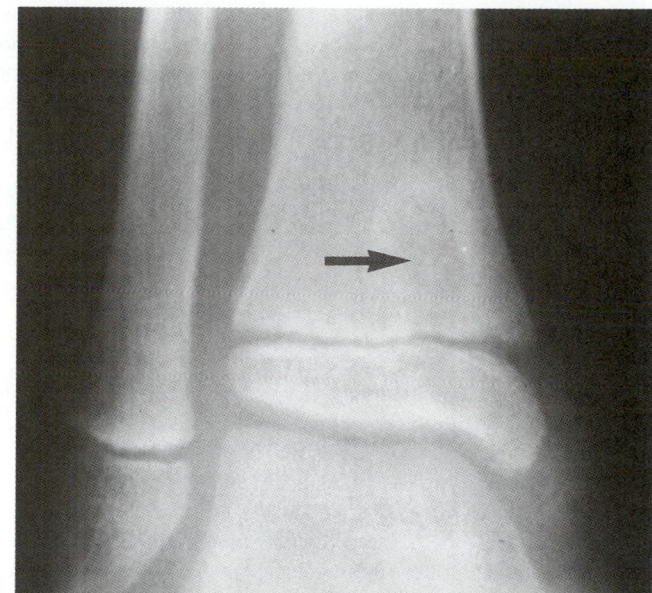

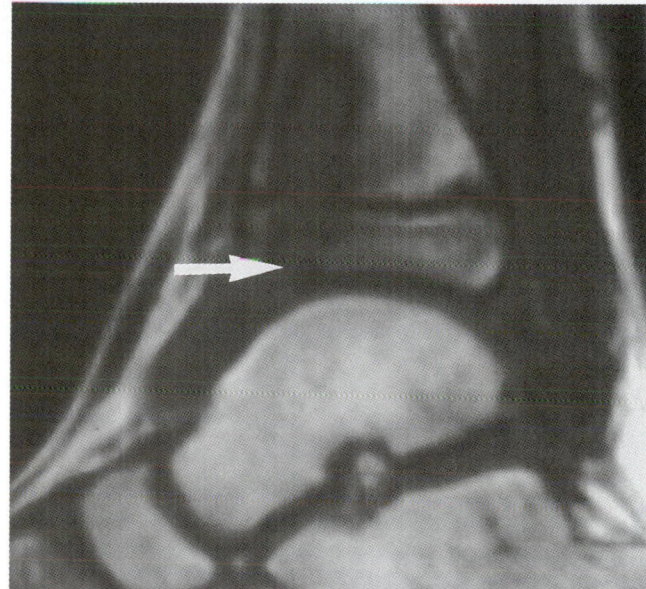

Figure 142-2
Subacute osteomyelitis of the distal tibia (*A*). MRI demonstrating invasion into the ankle joint (*B*).

adolescent presenting with gonococcal arthritis should be evaluated for child abuse. Presenting symptoms include a maculopapular rash, low-grade fever, chills, and a migratory polyarthritis (or arthralgia). Cultures are often difficult with the best results obtained from the genitourinary tract. Unless the arthritis involves the hip joint, the treatment of choice is aspiration of the effected joint and administration of ceftriaxone intravenously for at least 7 days.

SUBACUTE OSTEOMYELITIS

Subacute osteomyelitis is an infection of bone without the acute phase of the disease (Fig. 142-2). Patients had no acute symptoms and were not treated with antibiotics. The presenting symptom is usually that of pain. The initial radiographs often demonstrate a metaphyseal or epiphyseal cavitary lesion with or without periosteal reaction. The lesion often has to be differentiated from a giant cell tumor, osteoblastoma, chondroblastoma, eosinophilic granuloma, enchondroma, and chondromyxoid fibroma. If there has been bone erosion in the metaphysis, then osteosarcoma must be ruled out. Blood markers for infection, such as elevated WBC or ESR, are inconsistent.

Treatment of subacute osteomyelitis is antibiotics, initially intravenously, and then orally, for a total of 6 weeks. If the lesion is aggressive, then open biopsy and curettage (if osteomyelitis is confirmed) is indicated.

LYME ARTHRITIS

Lyme disease is transmitted via a tick (*Ixodes*) bite; this parasitic insect is often carried by deer and rodents. The disease may start as a rash, erythema migrans, as well as flulike symptoms. Children often skip this stage and present with monoarticular or polyarticular arthritis. The large joints are most commonly affected and often are not as acutely painful as those seen with septic arthritis from a bacterial etiology. Children will often walk with an antalgic gait, while with septic arthritis they will almost uniformly cease walking. This disease is more likely to be confused with juvenile idiopathic arthritis (formerly JRA).

Lyme disease is caused by a spirochete, *Borrelia burgdorferi*. Diagnosis is confirmed by enzyme-linked immunosorbent assay (ELISA). Anti-nuclear antibody (ANA) titers may also be positive.

The treatment of the arthritis is oral amoxicillin for one month. For later stages of the disease, intravenous penicillin is indicated. Nonresponders, which is very unlikely in children, should be treated with ceftriaxone intravenously. The overwhelming majority of children will be cured without sequelae using this regimen.

SUGGESTED READINGS

Green NE, Edwards K: Bone and joint infection in children. *Orthop Clin North Am* 1987; 18:555.

Hamdy RC, Lawton L, Cary T, et al: Subacute hematogenous osteomyelitis: Are biopsy and surgery always indicated? *J Pediatr Orthop* 1996; 16:220.

Betz RR, Cooperman DR, Wopperer, et al: Late sequelae of septic arthritis of the hip in infancy and childhood. *J Pediatr Orthop* 1990; 10:365.

Lauschke FH, Frey CT: Hematogenous osteomyelitis in infants and children in the northwestern region of Namibia. Management and two-year results. *J Bone Joint Surg [Am]* 1994; 76:502.

Mazur JM, Ross G, Cummings J, et al: Usefulness of magnetic resonance imaging for the diagnosis of acute musculoskeletal infections in children. *J Pediatr Orthop* 1995; 15:144.

Chapter 143

AMPUTATIONS

John W. Michael

LOWER-LIMB AMPUTATIONS

INDICATIONS

The most common cause of lower-limb amputation in North America is now peripheral vascular disease. As a result, the "typical" new amputee is an adult aged 50 to 70 years, often with diabetes mellitus or other medical conditions in addition to the precipitating cause for the amputation. Limb loss due to trauma does still occur in industrial and transportation accidents, but with less frequency each decade, as safer equipment and operating conditions proliferate in combination with better limb salvage techniques. Congenital absences and malformations affect a small percentage of the population each year, as do malignant tumors. Due to steady improvements in medical therapies and surgical solutions, limb loss due to cancer is less common than in previous decades.

Limb ablation is now widely acknowledged as an important reconstructive surgical procedure. When performed properly, amputation not only eliminates the diseased or damaged segment but also creates a residual limb surgically optimized for controlling a prosthesis. When prosthetic fitting is provided as soon after surgery as is practical, rehabilitation success increases and most individuals return to within one level of their preamputation functional ability. Meticulous amputation technique and early experience with a preparatory prosthesis are the keystones of modern rehabilitation practice.

LEVEL SELECTION AND SURGICAL PRINCIPLES

Many factors influence the level of amputation selected. In the case of trauma or dysvascularity, viability of the tissue is a major concern. Although a number of objective tests that help predict healing rates, including segmental laser Doppler studies and transcutaneous oxygen measurements, have been investigated, at present there is no universally acknowledged "gold standard" which will guarantee a good outcome. In general, the surgeon must combine clinical judgment based on experience with available objective data when determining specific amputation levels.

Retrospective studies have shown clearly that the lower the level of amputation, the higher the level of community independence following rehabilitation. Preservation of a *functional* knee joint, in particular, has been demonstrated to significantly reduce the energy required to walk with a prosthesis. In general, medium to long diaphyseal amputations offer leverage advantages when controlling a prosthesis, as compared to short or very short levels. Ankle (Syme) and knee disarticulations remain controversial levels for adults due to the limitation in prosthetic components and unnatural appearance that results from these bulbous residual limbs. However, disarticulations also offer functional advantages such as end weightbearing and full-length musculature, and are the preferred technique *for growing*

children to avoid the risk of bony overgrowth which often occurs following a pediatric diaphyseal ablation.

Although earlier works tried to define an "ideal" amputation level, present consensus is to preserve all prosthetically useful length, which varies with each individual case. Important surgical principles include:

1. Careful rounding and smoothing of all bony terminations
2. Gentle handling of all tissues, particularly dysvascular ones
3. Stabilization of transected muscles in a normal, nonretracted position via *myoplasty* (suture to fascia of antagonist muscles) or *myodesis* (suture to bone ends via small drill holes)
4. Careful tailoring of skin flaps to create mobile, nonadherent scars
5. Placement of cut nerve ends well away from bony or pressure areas, by transection while under *slight* tension

SPECIFIC AMPUTATION LEVELS

In 1990, a number of leading surgeons, engineers, and prosthetists from around the world met at the University of Strathclyde in Scotland, having reviewed all available literature on amputation published in the English language over the past 50 years. The International Society for Prosthetics & Orthotics published the results of their deliberations, which form the basis for the recommendations regarding specific amputation levels that follow in this chapter. Common levels of amputation are illustrated in Fig. 143-1.

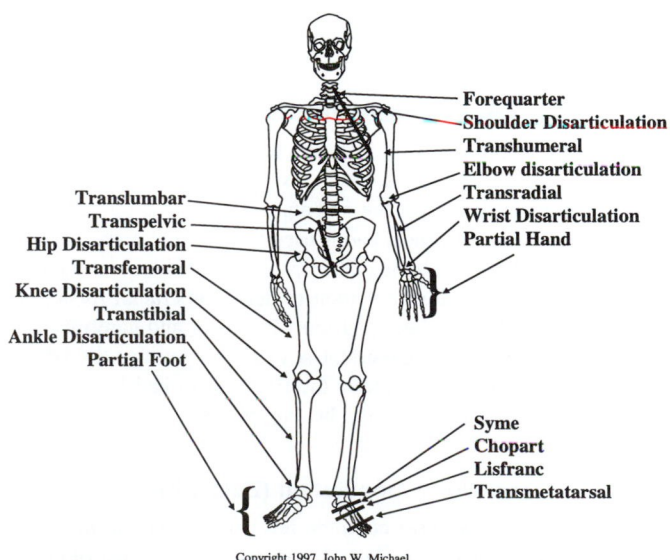

Copyright 1997, John W. Michael

Figure 143-1

This graphic represents common anatomic levels for elective amputation.

Partial Foot Amputation

Many variations in partial foot ablations have been reported, with widely varying results. In general, the more proximal the amputation, the more controversial is the long-term outcome: this is a result of the reduction in plantar surface area for weightbearing and the progressive muscle imbalance from unopposed gastroc-soleus musculature. The presence of scarred skin in weightbearing areas is almost always troublesome, particularly when adherent.

With the exception of skeletally immature pediatric cases, hindfoot and midfoot levels of amputation such as Boyd, Pirigoff, Chopart, and Lisfranc are not routinely performed although they frequently result following trauma. Whenever such procedures are elected, tibialis anterior transfer combined with tendo-Achilles lengthening is recommended to reduce the risk of progressive equinovarus deformity. The Boyd procedure, where the talus is removed (along with the metatarsal-phalanges) and replaced by the remaining aspect of the calcaneous, is sometimes used in the case of toddlers or young children. Advocates point out that it results in a weightbearing hindfoot residuum with both the proximal and distal tibial growth plates undisturbed. Others argue that a Syme-type ankle disarticulation is equally effective while the greater limb shortening permits more prosthetic ankle options.

Transmetatarsal amputation, particularly just proximal to the heads, can offer good results so long as the amputee realizes that strenuous activities such as running and competitive sports are virtually impossible without an intact first ray. Beveling the distal ends of the cut bones into a rocker contour will significantly improve comfort during roll-over and permit a more normal stride length. Limited ambulators, who can walk only short distances due to cardiopulmonary restrictions, may do quite well with simple shoe modifications or a weight-transferring foot orthosis following transmetatarsal ablation.

Toe disarticulations are generally useful, as are partial toe amputations. When intermediate toes must be removed (2, 3, or 4), it is usually best to remove the entire ray and create a narrower foot. Otherwise, over time, the adjacent toes will drift into varus deformity due to the gap between the toes.

Ray amputations of up to three lateral rays can also result in a stable foot remnant which can be managed with prosthetic-orthotic supports and shoe modifications. As much of the first ray should be preserved as possible, since it aids both balance and push off.

Ankle Disarticulation (Syme)

The preferred technique of ankle disarticulation is described by James Syme in 1843, which creates a bulbous, end weightbearing residual limb suitable for short-distance ambulation without a prosthesis. In this technique, the intact heel pad is used to cover the bony resection done transversely through the distal tips of both malleoli at the level of the plafond. Meticulous attention to details is crucial for a good result. In particular, the heel pad must be intact and carefully centered beneath the remaining bones. Use of a postoperative rigid dressing has been suggested to protect the fragile heel pad from rupture or displacement during the initial healing phase.

Trans-Tibial Amputation (Below Knee)

Below the knee is the most common level of amputation in the developed world. Almost all unilateral amputees and the majority of bilateral amputees with this level of loss are able to ambulate with a near-normal gait, although some elderly individuals will use one or two canes for balance.

The shortest limb remnant that can power a prosthesis terminates at the tibial tubercle level; longer lengths are preferred and increase the amputee's leverage and functional abilities. Some studies suggest a lower energy cost for the longer-level amputations. Whenever possible, myodesis of the muscles should be performed to improve the amputee's proprioception and control of the prosthesis. Although early authors recommended transecting the fibula quite proximal to the tibia to create a conical residual limb, modern total-contact prostheses can take advantage of the contours of a more cylindrical residuum. The fibula should be cut just proximal to the tibial (< 1 cm) so that its maximum length is available to provide lateral stability in the prosthesis.

The long posterior flap, popularized by Burgess, works quite well. There is ample evidence, however, that a variety of skin flaps can be equally successful. Trauma and dysvascularity often dictate the available skin for closure, so the creative surgeon can create "skew" flaps as necessary to preserve as much bony length as is practical.

The practical goal of trans-tibial surgery is to create a "non-tender stump covered with mobile, durable, and sensate skin and powered by muscles about the knee with full range of motion and normal strength." The better the amputation technique, the greater the quality of life, comfort, and activity level for the amputee.

Knee Disarticulation

Knee disarticulation remains an uncommon level worldwide, despite having strong proponents who note the functional advantages of the bulbous, end weightbearing residual limb that results. It is most often performed when the knee joint is ankylosed, painful, or severely contracted yet the surrounding skin is intact.

Suturing of the patellar ligament and hamstrings to the stumps of the cruciate ligaments is recommended to preserve normal muscle tension. It is not necessary to remove the patella unless it was painful prior to amputation. So long as it is mobile, the scar can be placed anywhere except directly under the condyles. Most often, sagittal flaps are used so the scar rests within the intercondylar notch.

Trans-Femoral Amputation (Above Knee)

Amputation through the femoral diaphysis markedly increases the energy requirements for walking. Particularly for the debilitated elderly individual, this can significantly reduce the amputee's functional capabilities. Meticulous surgical technique to preserve as much bony leverage and muscle power as is practical, advocated by Gottschalk, can significantly improve the trans-femoral amputee's quality of life.

Transecting the femur 7.5 to 10 cm proximal to the joint space (in the adult) will preserve most of the proximal adductor magnus attachment, preventing the muscle from retracting. The distal insertion of the magnus may then be wrapped over the smoothed end of the bone and sutured through drill holes in the lateral femur. With the hip in full extension (to avoid creating an iatrogenic hip flexion contracture), the quadriceps may be sutured to posterior drill holes, and the hamstrings anchored to the posterior aspect of the adductor magnus. Gentle closure of the fascia and later approximation of the skin edges with widely spaced sutures completes the procedure.

Roentgenographic studies have shown than when trans-femoral amputation is performed in this manner, normal skeletal adduction is maintained on the amputated side. With the muscles anchored near their resting length, maximum available strength is preserved and prosthetic rehabilitation is enhanced.

Hip Disarticulation and Trans-Pelvic Amputation (Hemipelvectomy)

High level amputations at the hip and pelvis are relatively rare, most often becoming necessary due to the presence of malignant tumor or extensive trauma. The specific techniques are well described in available texts and will not be described here. As with lesser procedures, the goal is to create a comfortable, painless residuum with sensate, nonadherent skin coverage that will tolerate the stresses of prosthetic use.

Although the energy consumption to use a prosthesis for this level of loss has been measured at more than 200 percent that of the nonamputee, a significant number of individuals who are otherwise in good health and have sufficient energy reserves will be able to use an artificial limb. Those who develop sufficient balance and skill to ambulate without external aids, or with only one cane, often continue using the prosthesis long term.

UPPER-LIMB AMPUTATIONS

GENERAL PRINCIPLES

In the developed world, upper-limb amputation most commonly follows traumatic injury, and the degree of injury or infection often dictates the level of amputation that is possible. In unilateral cases, where the contralateral limb is fully functional, the amputated side inevitably becomes the nondominant, assistive extremity. The surgical goals are primarily the creation of a pain-free, mobile, and sensate residual limb that is suitable for prosthetic fitting. As present technology cannot restore the intricacies of human hand function, and only offers gross grasp and release capabilities, a significant number of upper-limb amputees choose not to wear a prosthetic device. This is particularly true when higher-level amputation is necessary. Those who do use prostheses may require more than one device, as no presently available prostheses can simultaneously maximize cosmetic appearance with functional grasp.

The bilateral amputee, or the individual with limited function in the contralateral limb, presents a special challenge. In many cases, they will become very adept prosthetic users from necessity. In this group, functional capabilities are usually of paramount importance, and heroic efforts to preserve small degrees of voluntary movement or residual limb length may sometimes be justified.

SPECIFIC AMPUTATION LEVELS

Partial Hand Amputation

Partial hand amputation is a very complex and challenging area, increasingly managed by the hand specialist. Mechanical prosthetic devices are almost always rejected as too cumbersome, although many individuals can benefit from a passive, cosmetic restoration to partially disguise the disfigured hand remnant. Psychological trauma associated with hand disfigurement is quite common, and is only partially addressed by prosthetic devices. From a functional standpoint, the hand which retains sensate, voluntary opposition of any digit with the thumb has more inherent usefulness than any modern prosthesis.

Wrist Disarticulation

As is the case in the lower limb, disarticulations are uncommon and tend to be controversial—except in the case of the skeletally immature child, with whom they are the procedure of choice to avoid bony overgrowth. The functional advantages of disarticulations, such as improved rotational control and suspension of the prosthesis, must be weighed against the disadvantages of limited component options and an abnormal appearance in the finished prosthesis due to the length and girth of the disarticulated limb.

For the individual with bilateral upper-limb loss or limitations, and anyone whose primary motivation is to maximize function, even at the expense of appearance, the wrist disarticulation can offer advantages. Most importantly, so long as the interosseous membrane is undamaged, wrist disarticulation should preserve nearly the full range of voluntary pronation and supination.

Trans-Radial Amputation (below Elbow)

Except for the distal 2 to 3 cm, which can interfere with prosthetic component placement, it is useful to preserve all available bony length that can be covered with good skin. This increases the amputee's comfort and improves control of the artificial limb. As in the lower limb, it is important to smooth the bone ends carefully and treat the soft tissues gently. Myodesis or myoplasty is strongly recommended to stabilize the muscle mass, and can enhance stability of the EMG signals that may be used for control of a myoelectric device.

Even very short trans-radial residual limbs can be successfully fitted with a modern prosthesis, although tolerance for weight obviously diminishes with reduced length. So long as some forearm remnant protrudes anterior to the cubital fold with the elbow flexed to 90 degrees, fitting may be possible.

Elbow Disarticulation

Amputation at the elbow disarticulation level is common only for growing children. It has much the same advantages and disadvantages as the wrist disarticulation level, as noted previously.

Trans-Humeral Amputation (above Elbow)

Trans-humeral amputation is somewhat analogous to the transfemoral level in the lower limb: prosthetic use becomes notably more difficult due to the number of limb functions that have been lost. Meticulous surgical technique and careful myodesis to restore the resting length of the transected muscles can be very useful, especially in very short residual limbs. Overzealous preservation of soft tissues that results in a bulbous or redundant, flabby residual limb is an impediment to prosthetic use. The ideal residuum will have firm, stable musculature covered by mobile, sensate skin and will terminate at 5 to 6 cm proximal to the elbow joint to allow consideration of the full range of prosthetic component options.

Shoulder Disarticulation and Forequarter Amputation

These rare, high-level ablations are usually due to the presence of a malignant tumor or very severe trauma. Use of a functional prosthesis is difficult but not impossible, provided the amputee will tolerate the rather large torso socket that is required to stabilize the artificial limb. Often, a lightweight, passive device that primarily improves the appearance is more successful. Myoplasty to anchor the deltoid remnants securely, in the case of the shoulder disarticulation, can significantly improve the chances for practical use of a myolelectrically controlled device.

SUGGESTED READINGS

Bowker JH, Michael JW (eds): *Atlas of Limb Prosthetics: Surgical, Prosthetic, and Rehabilitation Principles,* 2d ed. St. Louis: Mosby-Year Book; 1992.

Murdoch G, Jacobs NA, Wilson AB, (eds): Report of International Society of Prosthetics and Orthotics (ISPO) Consensus Conference on Amputation Surgery; Copenhagen; 1992.

Murdoch G, Wilson AB (eds): *Amputation: Surgical Practice and Patient Management.* Oxford: Butterworth Heineman; 1996.

Chapter 144

OVERVIEW OF PROSTHESES

John W. Michael

LOWER-LIMB PROSTHESES

The quality and usefulness of prosthetic devices have improved significantly, particularly within the past decade. Reliability, durability, and functional capabilities have all increased. Modern components are made from composite plastics and lightweight metal alloys, with microprocessor controls for selected upper-limb and lower-limb devices now available. Socket design often includes flexible materials which allow improved comfort and suspension, even for very intimately fitted interfaces.

At the same time, the increasing percentage of debilitated, elderly amputees has increased the difficulty of prosthetic rehabilitation and emphasized the importance of early mobilization of the new amputee. At present, there are four types of prosthetic devices which can be combined to create a comprehensive rehabilitation program.

1. *Immediate Postoperative Prostheses* are applied in the operating theater, so the patient awakens following elective amputation with the first prosthetic device already in place. This is a very positive approach from a psychological standpoint and may be of particular importance when multiple amputations are anticipated.

   Although technically possible in almost any case, *immediate* fittings are currently offered selectively: primarily to younger, healthier persons with excellent vascularity and who are undergoing trans-tibial or trans-radial amputations where the risk of complications is considered low. A plaster or synthetic cast which immobilizes the joint proximal to the amputation site typically serves as the foundation for attachment of a foot or upper limb terminal device. Due to rapid atrophy of the residual limb, the *immediate* prosthesis must be reapplied within a week to 10 days.

   For a variety of reasons, many centers no longer attach the prosthetic components but continue to apply a cast postoperatively. This *rigid dressing* technique offers many of the benefits of the original immediate fitting, including protection and support of the healing tissues, without all the costs and risks associated with full prosthetic mobilization.

2. *Early Prostheses* are, by definition, applied soon after surgery while the sutures are still present and the wound is not yet healed. They use techniques similar to the *immediate* prosthesis, and were originally developed for application in secondary hospitals that received the amputees within a few days following surgery. In most cases, the *early* prostheses are removable to allow inspection of the wound. As was the case with *immediate* devices, many centers no longer apply the prosthetic components but continue with the *removable rigid dressing (RRD),* due to its well-documented advantages in promoting wound healing and accelerating rehabilitation.

3. *Preparatory Prostheses* are almost always prescribed within the first 30 days following amputation, and allow the new amputee to begin active rehabilitation with a well-fitted and functional device. Originally, the *preparatory prosthesis* was a crude plaster socket attached to a broomstick pylon, and later a prefabricated socket shape attached to simplified components—to determine if the amputee was capable of using a more sophisticated device. Although this was perhaps useful in the era of young, vigorous postwar amputees, such crude devices are not useful in predicting the capabilities of the debilitated elderly person with limited energy reserves. As a result, today's *preparatory prosthesis* usually includes a very well-fitted custom-made socket and functional components appropriate to the amputee's goals. Structural reinforcements and external finishing are usually omitted to reduce the cost and facilitate the frequent adjustments and modifications that are necessary as the configuration of the residual limb gradually matures.

4. *Definitive Prostheses* are, by definition, completely finished devices which not only fit and function optimally but also have a protective outer covering which imparts a lifelike appearance to the device. The earlier term, *permanent,* is now considered misleading, since no prosthesis is ever suitable for a lifetime of use. Like all mechanical devices, prostheses need periodic maintenance or repairs, and will eventually need replacement. For the adult amputee with a mature residual limb, the *definitive prosthesis* usually fits comfortably and performs reliably for 3 to 5 years—although the first *definitive prosthesis* may need replacement more quickly due to residual limb atrophy.

Although it may be ideal for the amputee to progress through all four stages of prosthetic management, from the *immediate* fitting all the way to the *definitive,* very few centers offer this option. In most cases, practical considerations dictate when prosthetic rehabilitation begins and the amputee starts the process at that time in the recovery process. For example, the amputee who is transferred to the rehabilitation setting within 14 days of surgery may begin with a RRD and progress to a *preparatory* and then *definitive prosthesis.* The patient who arrives two months or more after amputation will more commonly begin directly with the *preparatory* device.

ENDOSKELETAL VERSUS EXOSKELETAL DESIGN

Prior to the 1960s, almost all prostheses worldwide were constructed of wood, hollowed out to a thin-wall structure, and reinforced with an outer "skin" of rawhide and later plastic laminate. Forces transmitted to the socket during weightbearing traveled through the rigid outer shell to the floor, as is the case with crabs, lobsters, and other crustaceans. This form of construction is termed "exoskeletal" since the rigid members are external.

OVERVIEW OF TRANSTIBIAL SUSPENSION

GENERIC CLASS	EXAMPLES	PRIMARY INDICATION	ADVANTAGES	DISADVANTAGES
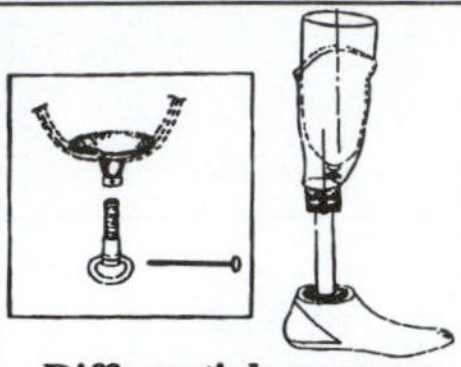 Differential pressure	Suction" via valve; "wet fit" with lotion ************** Elastomer sleeves; 3S/ICEROSS; Hypobaric seals in textile socks	Whenever feasible	Most secure suspension + best proprioception + greatest range of motion	Stable limb volume + good skin required ************** Precise fit; exact donning necessary
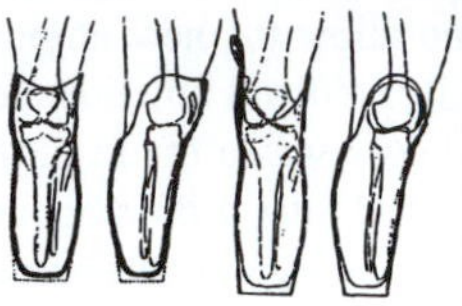 Anatomic	Supracondylar wedge with or without Suprapatellar extension	Added knee stability, such as for short residual limb; When differential pressure is not feasible	Easy to don and doff, even with limited hand function + Adds stability: SC = ML SP = AP	Restricts full knee flexion + localized pressure over condyles
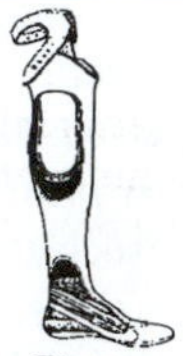 Straps	Cuff Cuff + waist belt Fork strap + belt	Volume changes anticipated	Easy to adjust + Good auxiliary suspension	Slight pistoning Belt uncomfortable Effect on circulation?
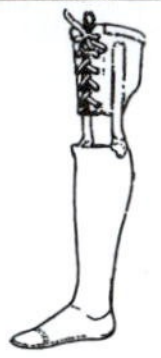 Hinged	Thigh corset ["Joints & Lacer"]	Damaged knee or residual limb	Maximum ML/AP support + Partial unloading of residual limb	Heavy, bulky, pistoning, donning properly takes skill

A

FIGURE 144-1
This matrix summarizes transtibial (*A*) and transfemoral (*B*) suspension options. COPYRIGHT 1997, JOHN W. MICHAEL, MED, CPO.

Since 1970, with the advent of high-quality miniaturized components made of lightweight plastic and metal alloys, "endoskeletal" construction has become increasingly popular. Analogous to the human skeleton, weightbearing forces are transmitted through the strong inner structures in endoskeletal prostheses. The outer covering can then be made of soft materials and sculpted to match the contralateral limb contours, since it serves primarily to protect the internal parts from damage.

Some endoskeletal components offer an additional advantage: multiplanar adjustability, even in the finished prosthesis. Such specially designed components permit the prosthetist to economically "fine tune" the alignment of the device as the amputee's needs or abilities change over time. This has proved to be such a benefit to today's elderly amputees, who often require many months to fully recover their preamputation capabilities, that realignable endoskeletal construction is now the norm in the developed world.

Exoskeletal construction is usually reserved for individuals whose work or hobbies demand a durable outer shell, and for very large or unusually active individuals who need a very heavy duty limb. Garage mechanics, construction laborers, and active children who play in sand and mud are all examples of individuals for whom exoskeletal construction is still commonly provided.

SUSPENSION

Suspension of the prosthetic device is one of the critical variables that influences both function and acceptance. As a general rule, the most secure suspension that the amputee can manage will give the best results. *Differential pressure suspension* is by far the most powerful type of suspension, since it uses atmospheric pressure (vacuum) to hold the artificial limb onto the residuum. Originally, the only known method of differential pressure suspension was to create a very snugly fitted socket which was in direct contact with the skin. Although quite effective when the limb volume is stable, such "suction sockets" have practical limitations for many individuals, particularly if scarring or skin grafting is present.

Over the past decade, many additional methods of securing differential pressure suspension have been developed which accommodate moderate volume changes and may be feasible even for amputees with less-than-perfect skin coverage. One of the most common methods is to apply an elastic sleeve of silicone or urethane rubber over the residual limb and anchor the socket to it distally with a locking mechanism or hook-and-loop strap arrangement. Atrophy of the residual limb is easily compensated by adding limb socks between the silicone suction sleeve and the socket interface.

OVERVIEW OF TRANSFEMORAL SUSPENSION

GENERIC CLASS	EXAMPLES	PRIMARY INDICATION	ADVANTAGES	DISADVANTAGES
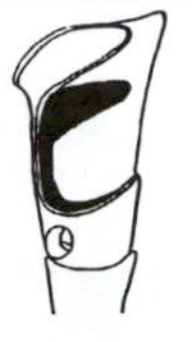 Differential pressure	Suction" via valve; "wet fit" with lotion ************** 3S/ICEROSS; Hypobaric seals in textile socks	Whenever feasible	Most secure suspension + best proprioception + greatest range of motion	Stable limb volume + good skin required **************** Precise fit; exact donning necessary
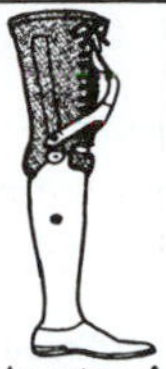 Anatomic	Supracondylar wedge for knee disarticulation	Knee disarticulation or congenital malformations only	Good suspension	Localized pressure over suspension areas
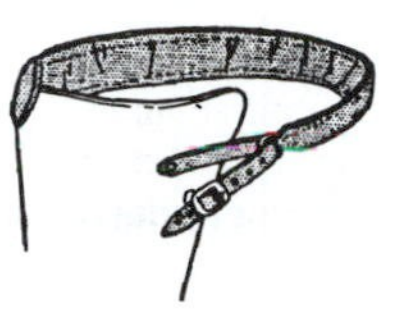 Straps	Silesian belt varients T.E.S. belt	Volume changes anticipated or differential pressure not feasible	Easy to adjust + Good auxiliary suspension + Controls rotation	Slight pistoning; Belt uncomfortable; Donning properly takes skill
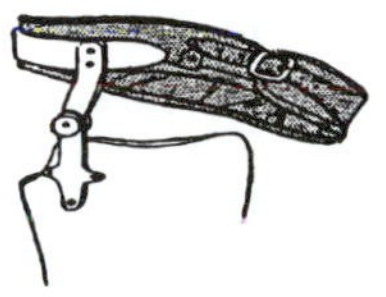 Hinged	Pelvic joint & belt	Short, weak, or flabby residual limb	Maximum ML support + Partial rotational control	Heavy, bulky, pistoning; Donning properly takes skill

B

FIGURE 144-1 (*Continued*) COPYRIGHT 1997, JOHN W. MICHAEL, MED, CPO.

Another variant involves the use of "hypobaric" limb socks which have a band of silicone rubber molded into an otherwise conventional textile limb sock. The silicone serves as a gasket and creates a suction seal which aids retention of the socket, while the textile fibers provide cushioning and help wick perspiration away from the skin.

The simplest method is to use a rubberized knee sleeve which seals against the proximal thigh and the outer surface of the prosthesis. So long as the sleeve remains intact, the resulting vacuum seal will suspend the prosthesis. One advantage of this approach is that the amputee can wear conventional limb socks under the sleeve suspension, to manage volume changes by adding or subtracting sock plies. The knee sleeve is also commonly provided as auxiliary suspension to augment another type of suspension.

Anatomic suspension is the second most desirable option. In many cases, careful contouring of the proximal socket walls can create a prosthesis that "clips on" just above the epicondyles. Particularly for individuals with shorter residual limbs, such "supracondylar" suspension will also add to the mediolateral stability of the socket/amputee connection. The two primary limitations to anatomic suspension are the localized pressure as compared to differential pressure and the inevitable restriction in full flexion of the joint that results. For most unilateral amputees, and many bilaterals as well, the advantages outweigh the limitations and "supracondylar" suspension is well accepted.

When the first two choices are not feasible, then *strap suspension* is selected. Its virtues are easy adjustability by the amputee to accommodate volume changes, so a strap or hook and loop closure is often used for new amputees and for those who live in remote areas. The chief disadvantage is that, even if a waist belt is added, strap suspensions inevitably permit some pistoning of the socket on the residual limb.

The final suspension option involves the use of a *mechanical hinge* for suspension. Originally the only suspension technique known, such bulky and cumbersome solutions are rarely needed in the modern world. One of the byproducts of using a mechanical hinge to suspend the prosthesis is added mediolateral stability and—in the case of transtibial joints attached to a leather thigh corset—partial unloading of the residual limb. This may be useful if the skin or knee joint have been damaged.

Figure 144-1 presents a detailed summary of trans-tibial and transfemoral suspension options.

OVERVIEW OF PROSTHETIC FEET/ANKLES

GENERIC CLASS	BASIC FUNCTION	GENERAL INDICATION	EXAMPLES	ADVANTAGES	DISADVANTAGES	ANALOGY
S.A.C.H. 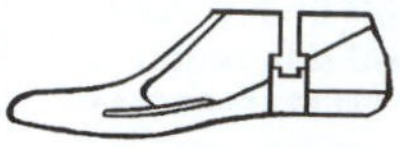	Simplicity	Limited ambulation	Otto Bock, Kingsley, USMC, et cetera	Inexpensive and durable	Rigid forefoot Energy consuming?	Bicycle
Single Axis 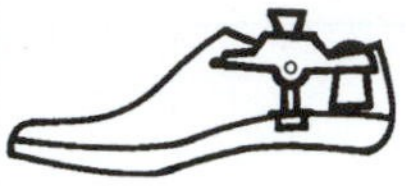	Rapid footflat	To enhance knee stability	Various, as above	Stability in early stance phase	Abrupt dorsiflexion stop; increased weight, cost, maintenance	Tricycle
Multiple Axis 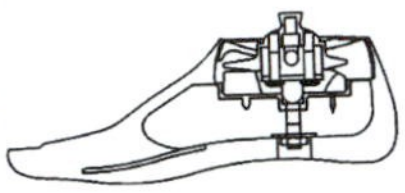	Hindfoot in/eversion + Int/external rotation	To accommodate uneven surfaces	Otto Bock "Greissinger", Endolite "Multiflex", et cetera	Relieves stress on skin and prosthesis	Increased weight, cost, maintenance	Offroad vehicle
Elastic Keel 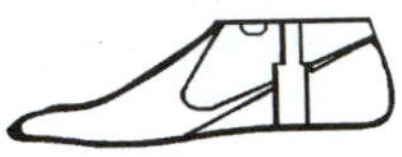	Smooth, easy rollover	Easier ambulation	Otto Bock "Dynamic", S.A.F.E. II, et cetera	Comfortable, reliable	Limited pushoff, increased cost	4 cylinder sedan
Dynamic Response 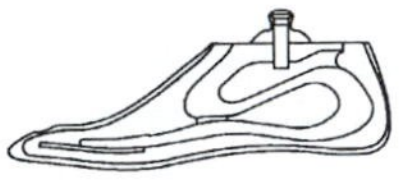	Active pushoff	To increase activity level	Carbon Copy, Seattle, Flex-Walk, Flex-Foot, et cetera	Responsiveness	Increased cost	V-6 sedan

FIGURE 144-2

This matrix summarizes basic prosthetic foot options. COPYRIGHT 1997, JOHN W. MICHAEL, MED, CPO.

SOCKET LINERS

Socket liners are useful to cushion and protect the more fragile residual limbs. Some may also provide suspension (silicone suction suspension or supracondylar suspension with the wedge built into the liner). A variety of cushioning materials are now available, including silicone and urethane elastomers. The most common material for the liner is an expanded polyethylene foam, which is very lightweight and easy to mold yet reasonably durable. For special cases, including severe burn scarring, very soft gel liners and similar special materials may be necessary.

ANKLE/FOOT COMPONENTS

For the partial-foot amputee, space constraints require individualized foot restorations which offer only limited functional capabilities. Construction of a one-piece socket plus toe filler of silicone elastomer is increasingly popular. All higher-level amputees can use a commercially manufactured foot which offers much higher levels of function and durability than hand-made devices.

Although there are presently more than 100 commercially available prosthetic feet, they can all be described generically as belonging to one or more of five functional groups (Fig. 144-2).

1. *Solid Ankle Cushion Heel (SACH)* feet were developed in the 1950s and remain the simplest designs, and therefore, the least expensive and most reliable foot components that are clinically acceptable. The heel of the foot, made of a foam rubber, compresses in early stance and simulates plantar-flexion rather well—even though the ankle is rigidly attached to the prosthesis. At midstance, the rigid hardwood keel inside the foot provides reasonable stability. With sufficient momentum, the amputee is able to roll over the rigid keel in late stance as the heel rises from the floor and the flexible toe bends at the metatarsal head region.

   The availability of more sophisticated prosthetic feet has progressively decreased the use of SACH designs. They are now commonly prescribed only for limited household ambulators and for small children: applications where simplicity and low cost are paramount.

2. *Single-Axis* feet have been available for centuries, and suffer from the twin deficits of added weight and the need for periodic maintenance. Based on extensive studies performed in the 1970s, it is now clear that the single-axis foot performs much like the SACH foot in most respects. It is, therefore, seldom prescribed if a SACH would be suitable.

The one benefit of the single-axis foot is that it can achieve foot flat more quickly than any other foot available to date. When knee stability is the primary concern, this characteristic makes the single-axis foot preferable, and is the major indication for prescribing it. The more quickly the foot is fully in contact with the ground, the more stable the prosthetic knee, and indeed, the entire prosthesis. So, despite the added weight and need for periodic servicing, the single-axis foot is often recommended for above-knee amputees who have difficulty managing the prosthetic knee.

3. The *Multiaxial* foot adds inversion-eversion and transverse rotation capabilities to the functions of the single-axis foot, and is often recommended to accommodate uneven terrain. Golfers, hikers, surveyors, fisherman, and others who work or play outdoors often choose this type of foot. The weight and maintenance requirements are similar to the single-axis foot, so most prescribers feel the added functions make the multiaxial foot preferable for moderately active individuals.

4. In 1980, the first *Elastic Keel* foot became commercially available. Called the Stationary Ankle Flexible Endoskeleton foot [quickly shortened to SAFE], it demonstrated that the flexible rubber keel allowed a smoother rollover and was preferred over the rigid keel of the SACH by most amputees. This type of foot is now widely accepted, and is suitable for most amputees who can load the forefoot of the prosthesis.

5. Just a few years later, the "Seattle" foot and "Flex-Foot" demonstrated the advantages of using a plastic spring in the keel of the prosthesis. The original term "energy storing" has fallen into disfavor since it may mislead amputees into believing the foot will *conserve* energy; such mechanisms are now called *Dynamic Response* feet. Despite tremendous amputee acceptance worldwide, researchers have failed to determine precisely why almost all amputees do very well with such feet, and no significant reduction in energy expenditure has been demonstrated provided the amputee is walking on level ground at a normal speed. For more vigorous activities, such as running or walking uphill, dynamic response feet are clearly more efficient than alternatives and they are now the component of choice for most recreational and competitive athletes. At present, they remain clinically suitable for amputees who can load the forefoot and wish to increase their activity level—a very broad indication.

The most recent trend in prosthetic component development has been to create designs that combine functions of two or more generic groups. For example, the use of feet having a multiaxial ankle mechanism combined with a dynamic response keel is growing rapidly, based on strong subjective preferences expressed by many amputees who have tried such "hybrid" functional prosthetic feet. As a result, the development of additional "multifunctional" feet is expected in the coming decade.

KNEE COMPONENTS

As is the case with prosthetic feet noted above, the plethora of prosthetic knees available can be categorized as offering one of five generic functions (Fig. 144-3).

1. The *Single-Axis* knee offers the simplest function: a simple hinge, usually with adjustable friction for swing phase damping. Like the SACH foot, the simplicity of these mechanisms makes the single axis knee the least expensive and most reliable alternative available, making it particularly suitable for individuals who live in a remote area. They are also commonly prescribed for small children.

This knee has two major limitations: The amputee must walk at only one speed, and must use voluntary muscle control to keep the knee stable. As a result, it is not commonly prescribed when more sophisticated alternatives are appropriate.

2. To address the need for more stance stability, the *Stance Control* knee was developed. Most present designs use a weight-activated brake which adds friction to the knee axis and prevents it from bending under weightbearing. This can be useful in early gait training and in the event of an inadvertent misstep, or to supplement the efforts of a debilitated geriatric amputee.

There are two limitations to this category of knees: the brake wears overtime and loses its effectiveness, and the knee cannot be flexed under weightbearing conditions—even where this is desirable such as when descending stairs. The first limitation makes the friction brake stance control inappropriate for amputees who have zero ability to voluntarily control the knee; the second makes it less than optimal for amputees capable of initiating swing phase, since it will delay the onset of knee flexion until all weight is transferred to the leading leg. Both groups are often better served by the next group of knee mechanisms.

3. *Polycentric* knees can be recognized by their multiple centers of rotation, which provide a number of unique functional capabilities. Modern examples are both reliable and easily adjusted, which has increased their frequency of clinical application over the past decade or so.

Many polycentric knees are designed to offer enhanced knee stability early in stance phase, combined with the ability to flex under weightbearing just prior to swing phase. This combination of characteristics makes these mechanisms preferable for moderately to highly active amputees, particularly those who will be walking on uneven terrain at times.

A special subgroup of polycentric knees is designed specifically for the amputee with a very long trans-femoral or knee disarticulation residual limb. Long linkage bars move the shin posterior on the thigh when flexed to 90 degrees, thus minimizing the protrusion beyond the anatomic knee center. Such "cosmetic four-bar knees" may or may not provide added stance stability, depending on their specific mechanical construction.

4. *Manual Locking* knees are considered knees of last resort, to be used only when no other alternative is feasible. The stiff-legged gait that results from having a locked knee disrupts swing phase and forces the amputee to "pole vault" over the prosthesis. It is best to use locked knees only temporarily, such as when hiking on very rough terrain, to avoid developing such gait deviations as circumduction or an abducted swing phase. It should be noted that to provide ground clearance at midswing, any prosthesis with a locked knee must be at least 1 cm shorter than the contralateral side.

5. *Fluid Controlled* knees use a chamber filled with either gases such as air (pneumatic) or oils such as silicone (hydraulic) to permit a variable speed swing phase. Due to the properties of a fluid-filled cylinder, the amputee is able to increase or decrease walking cadence, and the knee automatically compensates. As a general rule, pneumatic control units are for moderate cadences and hydraulic control units are for moderate to higher cadences.

PROSTHETIC KNEE MECHANISMS

ICON + ABBREVIATION	FUNCTIONAL CLASS	GENERAL INDICATIONS	ADVANTAGES	DISADVANTAGES
SA	SINGLE AXIS ["Constant Friction"]	Single speed walking on level surfaces, ONLY if hip control is good or better	Simple Inexpensive Reliable	Fixed cadence Low stability
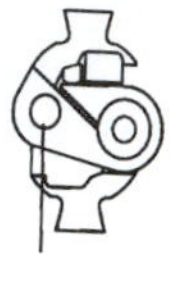 SC	STANCE CONTROL ["Safety"]	Initial prosthesis; General debility; Poor hip control; [Uneven terrain]	Improved knee stability	Delayed swing phase; Must unload FULLY to flex and sit; Bilateral = risk in falling
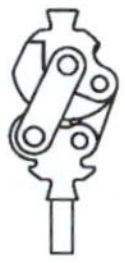 PC1 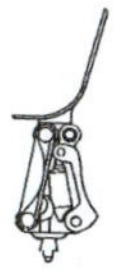 PC2	POLYCENTRIC ["4 Bar"] 1. Positive stability -------------------------- 2. Sitting cosmesis	1. Same as Stance Control -------------------------- 2. Knee disartic or very long transfemoral	1. Excellent knee stability -------------------------- 2. Improved cosmesis for long amputations	1&2. Added weight and cost -------------------------- 2. NOT heavy duty
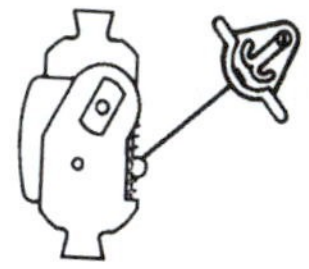 ML	MANUAL LOCKING ["Lock"]	Knee of last resort	Ultimate knee stability	Abnormal gait Awkward sitting Bilateral - risk in falling
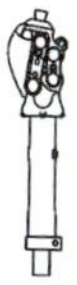 FC1 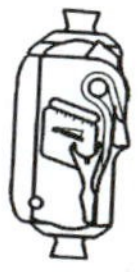 FC2	FLUID CONTROLLED 1. Pneumatic = gas [air] 2. Hydraulic = liquid [oil]	Able to vary walking speed	Variable cadence; Smoothest, most natural gait; Sophisticated stability [SNS ONLY]	Greater weight, cost, maintenance
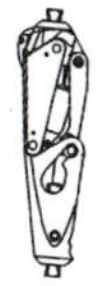 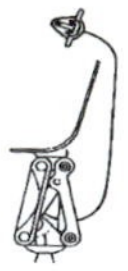 HYB	HYBRID	For combined functions from two or more classes	One knee allows multiple functions	Greater cost and complexity

FIGURE 144-3

This matrix summarizes basic prosthetic knee options. COPYRIGHT 1997, JOHN W. MICHAEL, MED, CPO.

The most advanced designs now offer sophisticated hydraulic stance phase stability in addition to swing phase responsiveness. Such devices are often termed "SNS units" in homage to the Mauch "S-N-S" knee, the first to provide hydraulic stance and swing controls.

As was the case with prosthetic feet, there have been a number of developments combining functions of two or more of these generic groups. Such hybrid knees offer the broadest range of function for the amputee and are increasingly popular. One common strategy is to combine the stability of a polycentric knee with the responsiveness of a fluid-controlled cylinder. The addition of mi-

croprocessor control to prosthetic knees is just beginning to be explored clinically.

SPECIAL COMPONENTS

There are presently two specialty components that may be added to lower limb prostheses in addition to the devices previously discussed, to add additional transverse plane functions. The *Torque Absorber* (or *Torsion Adapter*) allows the leg to rotate with reference to the socket during stance phase, automatically returning the leg to the normal position during swing phase. Although such components are suitable for any amputee, they are particularly appreciated by those who engage in activities where rotation is prevalent: golfing, bowling, dancing, and so on. The higher the level of amputation, the greater the loss of the body's natural torsional capabilities and the more crucial prescription of a torsion adapter is likely to be.

The second item is a *Locking Transverse Rotation Unit,* usually placed just above the prosthetic knee. When the amputee is seated, the locking transverse rotation unit can be unlocked by pressing a button, and the entire knee-shin-foot assembly can be rotated more than 90 degrees. This device makes tying shoelaces and entering confined spaces such as automobiles or restaurant booths much easier. Suitable for all amputees, the locking transverse rotation unit is particularly helpful to individuals with long legs or high-level amputations; these individuals often have a difficult time with these tasks.

SOCKET CONFIGURATIONS

Designing and fitting a prosthetic socket that is comfortable and suspends securely throughout a broad range of activities is the essence of the prosthetic art. Although certain fundamental principles can be identified, this remains an empirical skill which develops only with experience. As a general rule, so that the prosthetist may be fully accountable for the final result, it is also critical that he or she have as much latitude as possible in creating a clinically effective socket. The physician usually offers only broad guidelines to communicate clearly the desired suspension and weightbearing characteristics.

Suspension characteristics are determined as noted above. Weightbearing possibilities are largely determined by the level of amputation and the quality of the surgery. For each major level of amputation, characteristic socket designs have evolved which have proved successful over time.

Partial Foot

Due to the complexity of the ankle-foot complex and the infinite permutations of partial foot amputation, numerous socket designs are required to meet the needs of this challenging group of amputees. Generally, the higher the desired activity level or the more proximal the amputation level, the more complex (and costly) the required prosthesis.

At the transmetatarsal level, very limited ambulators require only a simple toe filler to keep the shoe from collapsing. Those who walk a bit more will benefit from a steel shank inserted into the sole of the shoe and often a mild rocker sole to prevent the bending of the shoe during rollover from ulcerating the distal end of the residual foot. Better ambulators may need an additional special orthosis to redistribute the forces away from the cut bones. Unlimited community and household ambulators usually require a prosthesis per se, which combines the biomechanical effects of all the previous shoe modifications and orthotic support into one comprehensive device that can be used with a variety of shoes.

Flexible elastomer "slipper" prostheses, terminating just above or below the malleoli, have proved very effective for many mid- and forefoot amputations. Suction suspension is sometimes possible or Velcro tapes are used for closure. Custom sculpted variants—although somewhat costly—can offer surprisingly good cosmesis, as well as good protection for the foot remnant.

Highly active individuals, particularly those with mid- and hindfoot amputations, are often unable to tolerate full weightbearing on the limited amount of plantar skin remaining. Such cases typically require a rigid, high-profile prosthesis which fully encases the leg to at least the patellar tendon level and that is carefully designed to transfer weightbearing stresses to the shin as much as possible. Unfortunately, the necessary bivalve construction results in a struc-

ture that is bulky and somewhat fragile, since the rigid socket is split into anterior and posterior sections. Modified thermoplastic ankle-foot orthoses of various types have also been used successfully, primarily for mid-foot amputees with low activity levels who can tolerate full plantar-surface weightbearing.

Ankle Disarticulation (Syme)

So long as meticulous surgery results in a Syme disarticulation with full end weightbearing, this level offers functional advantages over higher levels, including requiring lower energy consumption to cover a given distance. The rigid socket usually suspends anatomically via intimate contours just proximal to the malleoli. Careful planning is necessary to create an opening sufficient to allow the bulbous distal end to enter the socket, yet not weaken the structure excessively. Most commonly located medially, the opening may be placed anywhere on the socket that unusual residual limb contours dictate. A soft liner, precisely molded so the inner contours fit the residual limb irregularities, is sometimes used for suspension. When a cylindrical "stovepipe" socket is applied over the liner, durability is markedly increased since no opening in the rigid socket is necessary.

Transtibial (below Knee)

Although the original term "patellar tendon bearing" is often still used colloquially, it is now widely recognized that "total surface bearing" is a more accurate description of the modern, total contact transtibial socket. Every square millimeter of the residual limb may be in contact with the socket at some time during the gait cycle, and therefore, each area can contribute to weightbearing, proprioception, and control of the prosthesis. In designing the individual socket, the prosthetist varies the forces applied to the skin very carefully, in accordance with the pressure and stress-tolerance of particular tissues.

It is now well documented that unsupported distal end tissues are at risk for chronic edema syndromes, such as verrucous hyperplasia. This makes total contact essential for all modern lower limb sockets. Depending on the quality of the surgical result, this may be accomplished with a "hard socket" of rigid plastic or with a softer foam elastomer end pad.

The rigid plastic socket, particularly when laminated with thermoset resin, is clearly the most durable material choice. Use of thermoplastic materials, which can be locally remolded to accommodate bony prominences, is rapidly increasing. Due to increased comfort for the amputee, the use of flexible inner sockets is also increasingly common. Soft liners, to further protect the residual limb, are added as necessary.

Suspension alternatives have been previously reviewed, and may often be incorporated within the socket liner. To provide added knee control for the individual with a very short residual limb, one common design is to incorporate a supracondylar wedge for suspension within a soft polyethylene foam insert. Even with limited hand function, the amputee can easily push the residual limb into the soft liner. The liner-covered limb is then placed in the socket inlet, and by standing up, the individual's body weight completes the donning of such a self-suspending socket.

Knee Disarticulation

Very much analogous to the Syme alternatives, so long as comfortable end weightbearing is possible, the chief variable in knee disarticulation socket design is the placement of the opening. A medial "door" is typical but can be varied as necessary. Another common design uses an anterior closure with laces or hook-and-loop tape to don the socket. When weightbearing capacity is limited, due to high activity levels or a poor residual limb, proximal weightbearing features similar to those required for trans-femoral amputation must be added. Particularly for bony, elderly individuals, a soft insert may be helpful.

Transfemoral (above Knee)

As noted earlier, the greatest liability at the above level of loss is the marked increase in effort required to walk, even on level surfaces at a slow speed. As a result, careful fitting of the socket, meticulous alignment of the proper components, and secure suspension choices are particularly critical in trans-femoral prostheses.

Although the ischial-weightbearing "quadrilateral" socket probably remains the most widely available design worldwide, it is rapidly being supplanted by the more global-weightbearing "ischial containment" socket. With numerous variants designated by a variety of acronyms, the ischial containment socket style is particularly preferred for more active individuals and for those with shorter residual limbs: the much more proximal trimlines increase the area of the pelvis used for weightbearing, and thereby reduce the pressure per unit area. A general trend to reserve the quadrilateral for satisfied previous wearers and limited ambulators has been noted. The conclusion of an international consensus conference, that "there is no absolute contraindication for any socket style," remains valid. The specifics are a complicated, empirical choice which requires careful consideration of the prosthetist's recommendations for each individual.

Suspension alternatives have already been discussed. Suction suspension is preferred but not always feasible, and may need to be supplemented with a fabric strap such as the "Silesian belt." The rigid pelvic joint and belt combination is usually reserved for situations where additional external support at the hip is required, such as a very short amputation level. Because it encumbers the amputee, and can make access to confined spaces such as automobiles more difficult, use of the pelvic joint is decreasing as alternative suspension techniques are developed.

Hip Disarticulation and Transpelvic

Specialized designs for hip and transpelvic amputation must be individualized for each amputee, although both can be described as a "pelvic girdle." Due to the loss of bony weightbearing structure, the socket for the transpelvic amputee must fully contain the soft tissues to allow hydrostatic support of the body weight. This sometimes requires extension of the proximal socket higher onto the torso, particularly for obese individuals.

Although an anterior or lateral opening is most common, it can be located virtually anywhere on the socket according to the individual's needs. Many materials have been used successfully. As is the case in other levels, a general trend toward the use of thermoplastics and other flexible materials has been noted.

Suspension is almost always based on intimate contouring just proximal to the iliac crests bilaterally. In the case of the trans-pelvic amputee, and extremely obese individuals, it may be necessary to add a bandoleer strap or similar auxiliary suspension.

Prescription Criteria

Prescription of specific prosthetic components and designs is presently an empirical decision, based primarily on experience with previously successful applications. As a result, more often than not there are several plausible prosthetic alternatives for a given individual.

The basic information previously reviewed should help the clinic team to quickly rule out inappropriate choices based on the amputee's stance and swing phase needs, and to generate a generic prescription based on the desired functions, such as "transfemoral ischial containment prosthesis, endoskeletal construction, suction suspension,

stable polycentric knee with fluid swing phase control, and dynamic response foot." The Certified Prosthetist must then select specific components and materials that fall within these guidelines, based on the present clinical consensus regarding their efficacy and durability, trying to minimize overall cost and weight as much as possible.

COMMON PROBLEMS

Shoes with Differing Heel Heights

Perhaps the most common early complication seen in prosthetic clinics is the amputee who complains that the prosthesis no longer "walks" as it previously did. In many cases, the problem can be directly traced to the purchase of new footwear which appeared similar but differed in heel height from the original shoes. A lower heel will create a hyperextension moment at the knee as the foot tries to "rock backwards" until the heel contacts the ground. A higher heel height will push the shin forward and increase the knee flexion moment at midstance. Most instances of what at first appears to be gross anteroposterior misalignment can be corrected by changing the heel height of the shoes appropriately. As a general rule, the lower-limb amputee can wear many different *styles* of shoes so long as they have approximately the same heel height.

Volume Fluctuation

Perhaps even more common than a change in footwear is the amputee complaint that "my socket no longer fits right." Since the prosthesis has a fixed size, a change in the volume of the residual limb is virtually always the cause. Increased volume due to edema or weight gain causes the residual limb to be excessively compressed at first and then "lifted" out of the prosthetic socket, making the leg appear "too long." Decreased volume causes the residuum to sink into the socket, usually causing discomfort, and makes the leg appear "too short." Permanent changes can often be accommodated by socket modifications such as adding linings; temporary changes such as edema are better addressed by compression bandaging or the use of diuretics, or simply changing the ply of limb socks to compensate.

Inadequate Suspension

Inadequate suspension results in swing-phase pistoning: displacement of the prosthesis on the residual limb. In effect, the prosthesis appears to be "too long" in swing phase, and toe clearance problems may arise. Readjustment of the suspension mechanism is usually sufficient; additional training in applying the limb properly is also helpful. In recalcitrant cases, additional auxiliary suspension may be added.

Incorrect Knee Adjustments

Particularly when the amputee's cadence increases as confidence in the prosthesis develops, it may be necessary to readjust the knee resistance. A knee with too much friction will cause a stiff-legged gait and may give rise to such deviations as circumduction, abducted swing phase, or vaulting on the contralateral side. Such gait deviations are often strategies to clear a limb which is functionally "too long."

A knee with insufficient swing-phase resistance will allow excessive heel rise, and as a result, the shin will fail to swing through quickly enough for a smooth gait. Adding mechanical friction or changing to a fluid-controlled knee are the preferred solutions, as opposed to forcing the amputee to slow down to compensate for the components' limitations.

Alignment Errors

Alignment errors are very difficult to identify and are, fortunately, no longer very common. Today's readjustable endoskeletal systems allow the prosthetist to refine the alignment continuously, as the amputee's gait pattern changes. Before making any determinations about the alignment of the prosthesis, it is important to look for changes or inconsistencies in the amputee's gait.

For example, what at first appears to be malalignment causing the amputee to walk on the medial border of the foot is often a result of the patient increasing the distance between the feet for increased balance. Additional practice, and cueing to bring the feet closer together, usually eliminates this problem. Persistence of an abducted gait despite a normal walking base may require realignment.

Intermittent occurrences of "stubbing the toe" during swing are most often the result of poor gait timing, improperly applied suspension, or weight gain. Only when these variables have been conclusively ruled out is it necessary to shorten the prosthesis further. Erratic episodes of "knee buckle" more often than not indicate inconsistent hip control and are best addressed with more intensive gait training. Making the prosthetic alignment more stable is only appropriate as a last resort.

The best general guideline is that prosthetic alignment errors almost always result in consistent problems, apparent in the majority of steps. Inconsistent problems are most often caused by erratic walking by the amputee, symptomatic of the need for more gait training or more time to regain full strength and control over the prosthesis. Problems which do not diminish over time can sometimes be overcome by compensating with alignment changes. For example, the amputee who tends to "forget" to make the knee stable may ultimately benefit from very slight plantarflexion of the foot, as the resultant floor reaction hyperextension moment will increase knee stability.

PEDIATRIC PROSTHESES

Although the components and other elements are simply miniature versions of adult prostheses, the rationale for children's devices is somewhat different. Unlike the adult, the child typically has exuberant healing capabilities, unlimited energy, and an inherent drive to overcome new challenges. Even more importantly, the complexity of the prosthesis must be limited in accord with the child's developmental abilities and adjusted regularly for growth.

There is no absolute age requirement to begin prosthetic fitting, but most authorities suggest that the initial upper-limb device be offered just as the child is mastering sitting balance: at about three months of age. Lower-limb devices are usually deferred until the unilateral child begins to pull-to-stand, at 6 to 10 months; for bilateral lower limb loss, fitting may be delayed even longer. In general, the initial prostheses are simplified versions with limited capabilities. The knee is often omitted until the child is able to begin walking with a free knee, which can vary from age two and older. The initial upper-limb device may be passive, or an active device without harnessing, with some centers reporting good long-term results with fitting a simplified myoelectric limb as the initial prosthesis.

As the child grows older, options are gradually added to the prosthesis until the prostheses are essentially adult devices by the teen years. Often, simplicity and durability in the sandbox are important criteria initially, with a pleasing appearance gradually becoming important as the child matures. Many children are active in sports activities and benefit greatly from specialty upper- and lower-limb devices to encourage an active lifestyle.

Planning ahead for increases in circumferential and linear growth usually results in a useful life span of at least one year for the prosthesis, although modifications and adjustments every 3 to 4 months are typical when the child is actively growing.

Acceptance of lower-limb prostheses is high due to the increase in mobility that results. The rejection rate for upper-limb devices is considerably higher, with many choosing not to use an upper-limb prosthesis. Fitting children with congenital absence of a limb has been challenged by some since the child has been born with a "difference" rather than a loss. Most clinics offer a prosthesis as one possible option, but encourage the child and family to decide if the value is sufficient to continue use in the long term.

UPPER-LIMB PROSTHESES

Many of the same principles and guidelines already discussed apply to the upper-limb prosthesis as well. The choice of materials, suspension, construction, and types of prosthesis are essentially the same. This segment will highlight only the major differences.

The most important difference is that the upper limb is not a weight-bearing organ but rather a prehensile member. The focus in upper-limb prosthetic design is on the ability to place the arm in space and operate the grasping device effortlessly. Rather than being concerned with knee and ankle/foot components, upper-limb design focuses on the terminal device and control strategy selected.

TERMINAL DEVICES

The termination of an upper limb prosthesis can be broadly divided into "passive" and "active" devices (Fig. 144-4). As the name implies, passive devices are fixed and cannot be moved by the amputee. As a rule, they are simple, lightweight, and less costly than mechanical alternatives. *Aesthetic* devices can be quite lifelike in appearance and serve primarily to restore a balanced appearance and body image. Psychological benefits from such a device can be tremendous, and passive functions are offered as well (such as stabilizing paper on the desk while the contralateral hand writes). *Sports adaptations* are available in numerous configurations and are useful in permitting the amputee to safely participate in recreational and competitive activities.

Active terminal devices are first subdivided by the method of control. Those using a series of straps and cables to transmit shoulder motions are termed *body powered* while those that operate electrically are considered *externally powered*. As a general rule, the *body powered* devices are lighter, simpler, less costly, and more rugged, and the harness offers gross proprioception about how much force is being exerted to operate the terminal device. Externally powered devices typically offer a more powerful grip with minimal effort, and are frequently necessary if higher-level amputees are to be fitted with active devices.

Terminal devices can be further grouped into those which appear "hooklike" and those which appear "handlike." As a rule, the "hooklike" devices are functional tools—similar to a Swiss army knife—offering a variety of gripping options in one multipurpose package. These are among the simplest, lightest, and most reliable alternatives—and most have a very low cost as well. Their chief liability is the unnatural appearance, which makes them absolutely unacceptable for many amputees and cultures despite their practical usefulness. The "handlike" devices, in contrast, offer a much more lifelike appearance when covered with a flexible plastic glove but offer only spherical and palmar grasp patterns. The glove makes them fragile, and it must be replaced every few months due to soiling and tearing from everyday activities.

One final distinction with body-powered devices is that most open when the amputee activates the cable (voluntary opening or VO) and close from spring or rubber band tension when the cable is relaxed.

OVERVIEW OF UPPER LIMB TERMINAL DEVICES - I

PREHENSION TYPE	GENERIC CLASS	EXAMPLES	ADVANTAGES	DISADVANTAGES
PASSIVE	Cosmetic restoration	Cosmetic hand 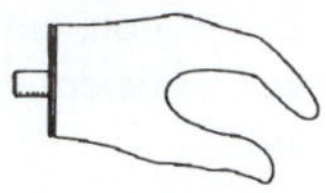	Light & cosmetic; Silicone is durable	Passive grip; Custom-sculpted are costly
PASSIVE	Special adaptations	Sports mitt 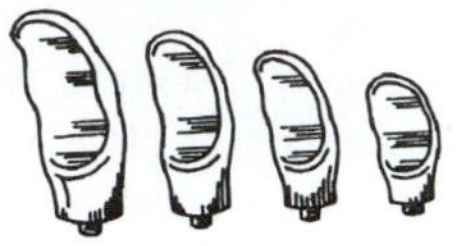	Useful for tasks	Limited purpose
ACTIVE	Externally Powered	Electronic hand 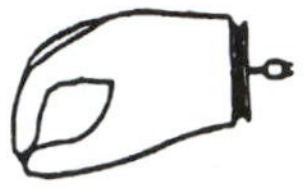	Easy to use; Good appearance; Powerful grip	Weight, cost
ACTIVE	Externally Powered	Electronic hook 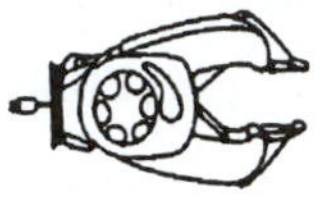	Easy to use; Powerful grip; Precise grasp	Cost
ACTIVE	Externally Powered	Prehension Actuator 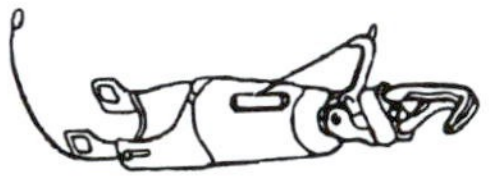	Easy operation	Limited pinch force [VO TD's only]

A

FIGURE 144-4
These matrices (*A* and *B*) summarize common upper-limb terminal device alternatives. COPYRIGHT 1997, JOHN W. MICHAEL, MED, CPO.

Although it takes effort to open such a device, once the grip is secure it can be maintained automatically by the closing mechanism and the amputee can relax. This ease of operation is probably why VO devices are particularly well accepted by adults with an acquired amputation.

The other group of body-powered devices closes when the cable is activated and is therefore termed voluntary closing (VC). This control scheme allows the amputee to easily control the force at the terminal device, since the more vigorously the shoulders are moved, the more powerful the grip exerted. This "graded prehension" can be an advantage, particularly for active amputees with a long trans-radial or wrist disarticulation amputation. The downside is that the amputee must maintain tension of the cable to continue holding an object, and some find the required concentration too difficult. Although suitable for most amputees, VC devices have been particularly well accepted by child amputees and those with vigorous vocations or avocations.

In North America, the most commonly prescribed terminal device is one of the many VO hooks. Although new amputees often request and wear a mechanical hand from time to time in the early period following limb loss, most ultimately reject mechanical hands due to their limited grasp capabilities. In contrast, the externally powered hand, particularly if myoelectrically controlled, enjoys a very high rate of acceptance. This is believed to be due, at least in part, to the powerful grasp capabilities of the motorized device and the ease of

control—which are far superior to the mechanical body-powered hand. A limited number of externally powered hooks are now available and have also been well accepted by those who do not demand a handlike appearance for the terminal device.

WRIST COMPONENTS

The great majority of amputees use the "constant friction" wrist which allows passive pronation and supination of the terminal device. Those who interchange different terminal devices may prefer a "quick disconnect" style. Bilateral users, and selected unilateral users, often benefit from the use of a wrist that adds flexion of the terminal device as well. This is particularly helpful in midline activities such as eating and toileting. Externally powered wrist rotators are available and have been well accepted, particularly when applied on the dominant side for bilateral upper-limb amputees.

ELBOW COMPONENTS

For the trans-radial amputee, flexible textile hinges are preferred to allow maximum voluntary pronation and supination. To protect selected short residual limbs against torque loads, rigid metal single axis or polycentric hinges may be used. The latter improve the range

OVERVIEW OF UPPER LIMB TERMINAL DEVICES - II

PREHENSION TYPE	GENERIC CLASS	EXAMPLES	ADVANTAGES	DISADVANTAGES
ACTIVE	Body Powered	VO hook: 5XA 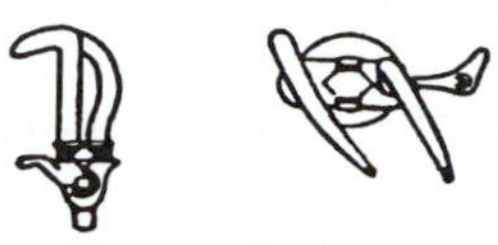	Light, versatile, inexpensive, easy to use	Limited pinch force + mechanical appearance
ACTIVE	Body Powered	VO hook: #7 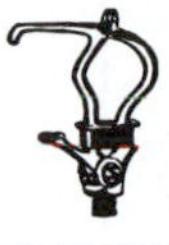	Rugged, versatile, inexpensive	Limited pinch force + mechanical appearance
ACTIVE	Body Powered	VC hook: GRIP 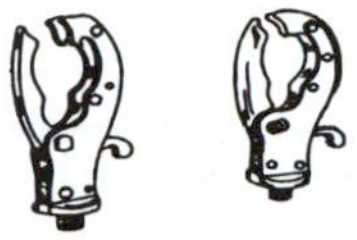	Rugged, powerful grip, graded prehension	Requires constant force to maintain grip
ACTIVE	Body Powered	VO Mechanical Hand 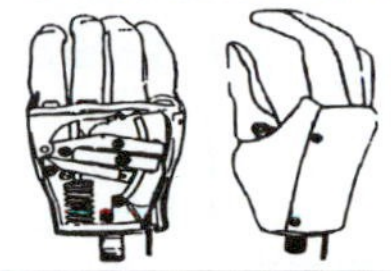	Pleasing appearance	Limited grip force and versatility
ACTIVE	Body Powered	VC Mechanical Hand 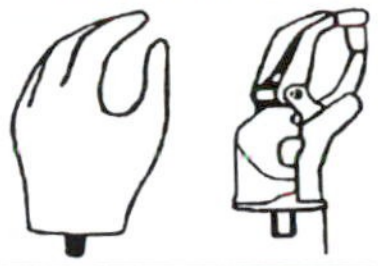	Pleasing appearance + graded prehension	Limited grip versatility

B

FIGURE 144-4 (*Continued*) COPYRIGHT 1997, JOHN W. MICHAEL, MED, CPO.

of elbow flexion, which is important mostly for bilateral amputees. Highly specialized hinges which control forearm movements independently from the residual limb motion are used sparingly. Usually reserved only for those with the very shortest residual limbs, such "step-up" hinges or "stump-activated locking" hinges can help the bilateral upper-limb amputee remain independent.

For the transhumeral and higher-level amputee, a body-powered "internal locking" elbow is commonly prescribed. Mastery of the required body movements allows the adept user to pre-position the forearm almost anywhere in space. An externally powered elbow is also available from several manufacturers, and is often used for those with very high levels of limb loss.

SHOULDER COMPONENTS

Due to the difficulty in successfully operating such a high-level prosthesis over time, many of these amputees do not wear an artificial limb. Those that do choose to try an active prosthesis may prefer that the humeral sections simply be sculpted to flow directly into the torso jacket portion of the socket, and avoid the need for any mechanism. To allow limited pre-positioning of the arm, several permutations of a friction-stabilized shoulder joint are available.

HARNESSING

Harnessing may be used to provide suspension and to operate body-powered components (Fig. 144-5). The most common configuration has a loop which encircles the contralateral shoulder, an anterior strap to suspend the prosthesis, and a posterior strap which connects to the control cable. Viewed from the back, this harness looks like the numeral "8", rotated 90 degrees: hence the name, "figure of eight" harness. This is the most common strap arrangement for body-powered prostheses for amputations below the axilla level.

If the amputee uses a self-suspending socket (e.g., suction or anatomic suspension), the anterior suspensor is deleted and it is termed a "figure of nine" harness. Some persons have difficulty tolerating the pressure generated by the axilla loop of these harnesses, and some will complain of discomfort, numbness, or color change of the contralateral hand.

An alternative harness, which shifts the forces to the chest wall, uses a wide strap crossing the chest inferior to the clavicle. Termed a "chest strap" or "shoulder saddle" harness, it is most commonly prescribed for laborers who lift heavy axial loads with the prosthesis. Because it crosses the upper chest, this style is often objectionable to individuals who wish to wear an open collar shirt or blouse.

Basic Upper Limb Harnessing Variants

Type	Application	Advantages	Disadvantages
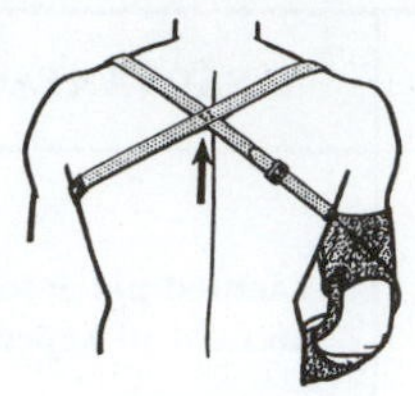 **Figure of Eight**	Transradial (BE) Elbow Disarticulation (ED) Transhumeral (AE)	Easy to don and doff Provides both suspension and control Chest is uncovered	Encumbers contralateral shoulder Creates axillary pressures
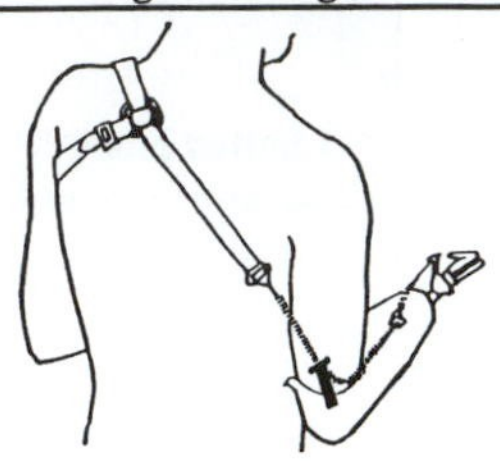 **Figure of Nine**	Transradial (BE) Elbow Disarticulation (ED) Transhumeral (AE)	Easiest to don and doff Provides good control Chest is uncovered	Requires self-suspending socket Encumber contralateral shoulder Creates axillary pressures
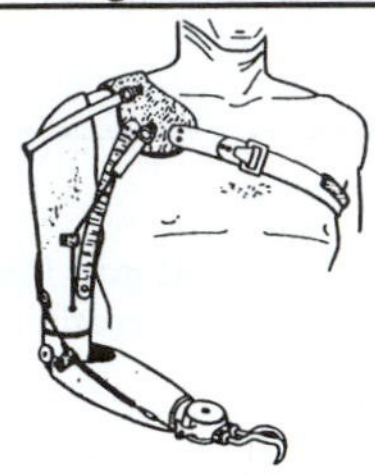 **Shoulder Saddle with Chest Strap**	Transradial (BE) Elbow Disarticulation (ED) Transhumeral (AE) Chest Strap Only = Shoulder Disarticulation (SD) & Interscapular Thoracic	Eliminates axilla pressures Frees contralateral shoulder Shoulder saddle supports heavy axial loads	Slightly more difficult to don Strap crosses chest = reduced cosmesis

A

Basic Upper Limb Control Motions - 1

Type	Application	Advantages	Disadvantages
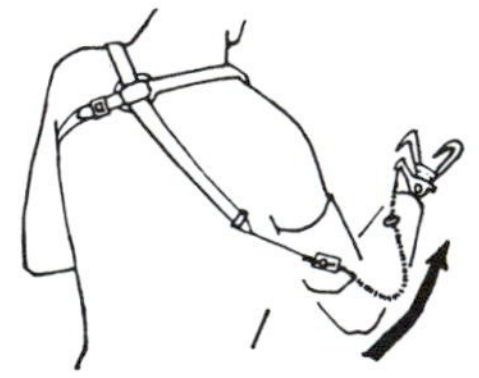 **Glenohumeral Forward Flexion**	Terminal Device [TD] operation OPTIONAL: Elbow flexion/extension [Requires split cable housing + locking elbow mechanism]	Natural movement Generates excellent power Excellent excursion available Good proprioceptive feedback through harness	TD moves while opening/closing
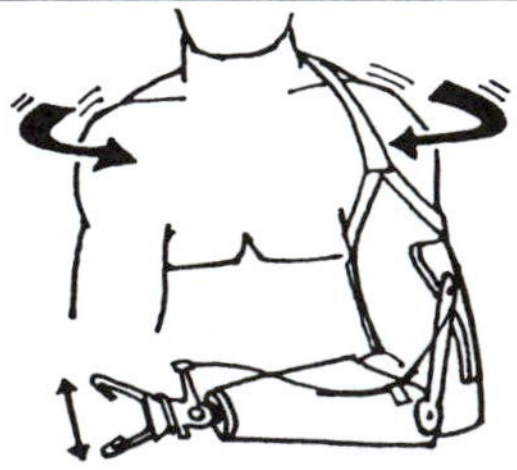 **Biscapular ABduction**	Terminal Device [TD] operation	TD is stationary during opening/closing	Somewhat awkward motion Generates less force and excursion
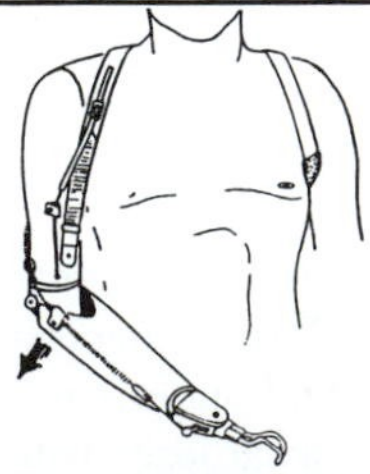 **G-h Depression, Ext, ABduction**	Reciprocal Elbow lock-unlock	Does not interfere with TD operation motions	Unnatural movement Somewhat difficult to master

B

Basic Upper Limb Control Motions - 2

Type	Application	Advantages	Disadvantages
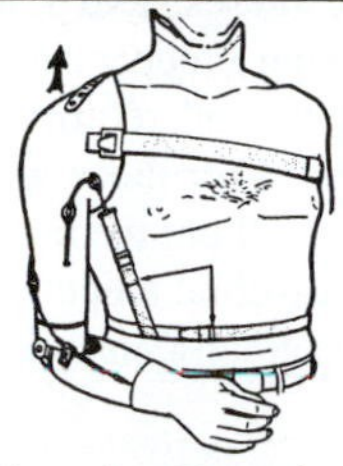 Scapular Elevation	Reciprocal Elbow lock-unlock	Simple to master	Requires waist belt or attachment to slacks
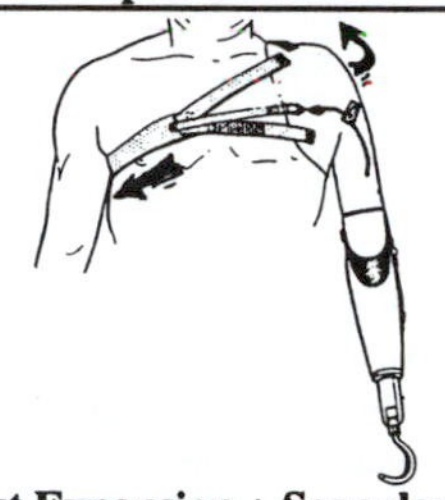 Chest Expansion + Scapular ADd	Reciprocal Elbow lock-unlock	Does not interfere with TD operation motions	Somewhat awkward motion
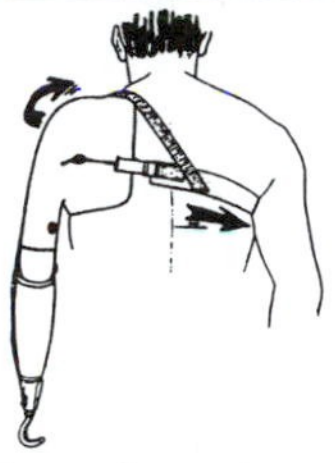 Chest Expansion + Scapular ABd	TD operation OPTIONAL: Elbow flexion/extension [Requires locking elbow]	Does not interfere with TD operation motions	Somewhat awkward motion Generates limited force and excursion

C

FIGURE 144-5
This matrix summarizes (A) upper limb harnessing alternatives and (B, C) body-powered control motions. COPYRIGHT 1997, JOHN W. MICHAEL, MED, CPO.

PRESCRIPTION

There are three prerequisites for upper-limb function: proximal stability, placement in space, and grasp/release control. Sensory or proprioceptive feedback is also highly desirable. Prosthetic prescription is simplified if these fundamentals are considered for each amputation level, along with the amputee's vocational and avocational needs. Selecting the terminal device first, and then determining the more proximal components, is suggested.

SPECIFIC UPPER-LIMB PROSTHESES

For the wrist disarticulation amputee, the distal styloids are commonly used for anatomical suspension of the socket, while flexible elbow hinges permit full use of residual voluntary pronation and supination. Terminal device options are determined primarily by the tasks the amputee wishes to undertake. For example, a motor mechanic will most likely benefit from a body-powered VO hooklike device, due to the grease and oil encountered daily. The housewife or teacher may be just as happy with a myoelectric prosthesis, due to the freedom from a harness and the effortless grasp.

Although the majority of transradial (below elbow) prostheses are body powered, a rapidly growing percentage of amputees worldwide use myoelectric controls. Self-suspending sockets can be used to minimize the need for harnessing or to delete the harness entirely. Flexible

socket designs and the use of thermoplastic materials are increasing, as is the use of silicone elastomeric products for suspension. Since the major deficit is loss of grasp and release, selection of an optimal terminal device is the primary decision facing the clinic team.

As with other disarticulation levels, the choice of elbow function for the elbow disarticulation amputee is limited primarily to external locking hinges, which are moderate-duty at best and increase the bulk of an already uncosmetic prosthesis. Occasionally, usually when fitting very small children, the hinges are omitted to save weight. This significantly restricts placement in space, however, and is therefore an option only for unilateral amputees. Terminal device choices, to restore grasp functions, are the same as for other levels.

For the transhumeral (above elbow) amputee, use of an internal locking mechanical elbow is preferred for those who can generate sufficient range of motion to operate this component. Terminal device choices are made in the same manner as for all other levels. When a body-powered elbow is not suitable, particularly for higher-level amputees or those with brachial plexus injury or other complicating factors, an externally powered elbow is a very useful choice. Occasionally, for pediatric or passive prostheses, a friction elbow that may be passively pre-positioned is used. As is the case in the lower limb as well, the higher the amputation level, the more difficult the prosthetic challenge and the lower the long-term use rate of the prosthesis.

Only a small percentage of highly motivated individuals who have sustained a shoulder disarticulation or forequarter amputation will use an active prosthesis long-term. The loss of the shoulder joint severely restricts the ability of the amputee to place the prosthesis in space, and a rather bulky socket is required to stabilize the prosthesis on the remaining torso. Use of externally powered components, in whole or in part, is typically required. A somewhat larger percentage will wear a lightweight passive prosthesis, usually of endoskeletal construction. Most forequarter amputees prefer a very lightweight and simple cosmetic shoulder restoration, without the arm segments attached, to restore torso symmetry and make wearing conventional shirts and jackets more comfortable.

BILATERAL UPPER LIMB LOSS

The individual who has suffered bilateral upper limb loss is often best managed by referral to an experienced specialty center for rehabilitation. In this circumstance, the prostheses serve as tools for survival and independence rather than gross assistance to the remaining hand. Meticulous fitting, extended trials with a variety of component options, and specialized use training are generally necessary for an optimal result. Even small changes in the alignment or construction of the artificial arms can enhance the usefulness of the devices.

Perhaps as a result of necessity, the bilateral user quickly becomes expertly proficient in the use of prostheses, and many users can demonstrate remarkable dexterity. Living independently, driving an automobile with minimal modifications, and returning to full-time employment are tasks which are practical for those with lower-level bilateral loss and possible for some with all but the highest level loss. Analogous to the situation with the trans-tibial amputee, preservation of at least one functioning elbow joint greatly enhances the individual's independence.

SUGGESTED READINGS

Atkins DJ, Meier RH (eds): *Comprehensive Management of the Upper-Limb Amputee.* New York: Springer-Verlag; 1989.

Bowker JH, Michael JW (eds): *Atlas of Limb Prosthetics: Surgical, Prosthetic, and Rehabilitation Principles,* 2d ed. St. Louis: Mosby-Year Book; 1992.

Murdoch G, Wilson AB (eds): *Amputation: Surgical Practice and Patient Management.* Oxford: Butterworth Heineman; 1996.

Chapter 145

OVERVIEW OF ORTHOSES

John W. Michael

Many devices meet the simplest definition of an orthosis: "An external device that applies biomechanical forces to the body." Plaster or synthetic casts, off-the-shelf supports, modular devices assembled from prefabricated elements, and custom-made thermoplastic devices vacuum-molded over a rectified positive model of the affected body part can all be considered "orthoses."

The International Standards Organization has now officially adopted the proposal, originated by a group of U.S. physicians, engineers, and orthotists in the 1970s, that all orthoses be described by the segment of the body encompassed by the device and the biomechanical controls desired. Colloquial names and eponyms honoring the inventor or popularizer may be used locally but do little to clarify international communication. As a matter of convenience, the acronym formed by the first letter of each body segment is the accepted abbreviation: For example, an orthosis beginning at the toes, crossing the ankle, and terminating on the calf is referred to worldwide as an "Ankle-Foot Orthosis" or "AFO."

Each orthosis is further described by the type of biomechanical control it offers each anatomic joint. Listed from the least to the most restrictive, there are five joint controls possible:

1. *Free:* unrestricted motion in the stated plane
2. *Assist:* external force applied to increase the range, force, or velocity of a desirable motion
3. *Resist:* the reverse of previous control, to influence undesired motion
4. *Stop:* prevents motion in one direction
5. *Hold:* immobilizes the body segment in all planes

Four additional descriptors may be used, if desired, to specify the orthosis even more explicitly:

1. *Lock:* describes a "removable Hold," as might be used at the knee joint
2. *Degree:* indicates the range end points for a Stop to limit motion
3. *Variable:* specifies an adjustable Stop which can be easily varied
4. *Axial Unloading:* a special circumstance where distal unloading is desirable

Together, these descriptors allow complete specification of the functional outcome desired for a specific orthosis. Using these goals as a guideline, the Certified Orthotist can then evaluate the patient and select the most effective combination of materials and available components to solve a particular problem.

Successful orthotic devices offer one or more of the following benefits to the patient:

1. *Control of Motion*
   A. Prevent motion (immobilize)
   B. Limit motion (to a certain range)
   C. Delay/prevent deformity (recurrence or initial development)
2. *Correction of Deformity*
3. *Compensation for Weakness*
4. *Partial Axial Unloading*

The prescriber should take care to insure that all recommended orthoses are expected to offer at least one of the above advantages to the recipient.

UPPER-LIMB ORTHOSES

It must be clearly emphasized that orthoses are not diagnosis-specific. They are prescribed based on the functional deficits present regardless of the underlying cause. Therefore, the concept of a "polio splint" is obsolete, as an identical device may be properly prescribed for patients with varying pathologies so long as the functional deficits are comparable.

Treatment of the spinal cord injury survivor is individualized based on the remaining functioning musculature. Particularly for those with low cervical level injuries, a well-fitted Wrist-Hand Orthosis (WHO) can become a lifetime assist in restoring grasp. If sufficient voluntary wrist extension is present, it can be harnessed with a linkage bar to create a tenodesis grasp. (Fig. 145-1). Since wrist extensor muscles are innervated by C6 roots, this level must

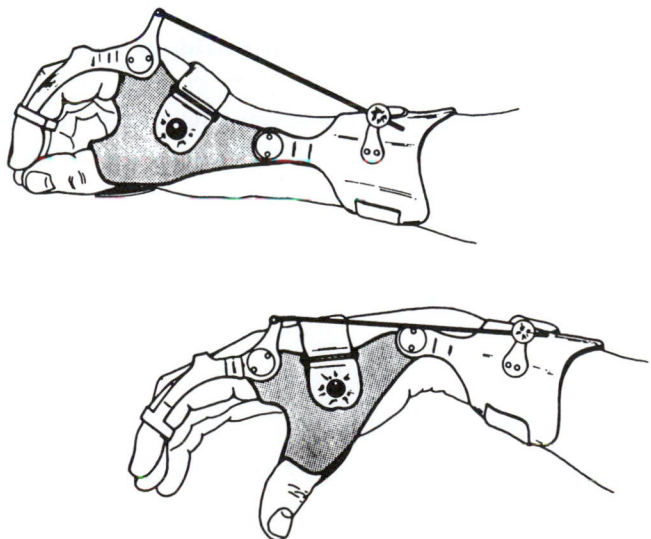

Figure 145-1
Tenodesis wrist-hand orthosis (WHO) uses residual wrist extension to provide grasp and release despite complete hand paralysis. [Reproduced with permission from Michael JW: Orthotic treatment of neurological deficits. In Good DC, Couch JR (eds): *Handbook of Neurorehabilitation.* New York: Marcel Dekker; 1994:271.]

be intact for such an orthosis to succeed. Higher-level lesions may require the addition of external power in the form of a miniature electronically controlled motor. Although the strongest side is usually fitted initially, some patients can master the use of bilateral WHOs. Due to the lack of protective sensation, the fit of such devices must be very precise.

Placement in space is the second requirement for functional prehension. For those patients who lack sufficient strength to overcome the force of gravity, a special Shoulder-Elbow-Wrist-Hand Orthosis (SEWHO) may be helpful. Colloquially termed the "balanced forearm orthosis," this wheelchair-mounted device is adjusted to counterbalance the paralyzed arm and hand, allowing the patient to use trace muscles and "body English" to move the arms voluntarily.

The final prerequisite for prehension is proximal stability. For those with lower thoracic lesions, the trunk muscles may be sufficient. If not, special customized seating modules can be designed to cradle the torso in an upright position.

Brachial plexus injuries are complex and result in varying long-term deficits. One subset that responds well to orthotic intervention leaves the patient with a fully functioning hand attached to a completely flail arm. If the hand has sensation, provision of an elbow orthosis with a locking elbow joint can position the hand at desktop level for functional tasks.

Completely flail arms have been managed with full-arm orthoses but without consistent results. One British surgeon has claimed a 70 percent long-term use rate based on multiple-year follow-up of several hundred brachial plexus injury cases fitted with functional SEWHOs.

Stroke, traumatic brain injury, and similar insults can result in a spastic, nonfunctioning upper limb. Although functional orthoses have shown little success for such severe deficits, selective treatment to reduce residual marked spasticity has been useful. An orthosis to hold the hand and wrist in a relaxed position, with or without gentle traction on contracted fingers, may sometimes increase the flexibility of the hand and make hygiene easier than with a clenched fist.

Many peripheral nerve palsies are temporary and may therefore be treated with an appropriate prefabricated hand orthosis. When the orthosis serves primarily as an adjunct to hand therapy, low temperature thermoplastic splints fabricated by the occupational therapist are usually provided. Low-temperature plastics can be readily modified, making them particularly useful for postoperative applications as well. Specific designs depend on the nature of the injury or surgery and are often intended to support the wrist, hand, or fingers in a functional position while healing occurs. For example, an isolated radial nerve injury at the cubital fold would cause loss of extensor function and therefore requires an orthosis which supports the hand and holds the wrist in moderate extension, to overcome gravity and prevent the development of contracture due to the unopposed muscles.

SPINAL ORTHOSES

Cervical orthoses (COs) serve as a reminder to the patient and limit cervical spine motion to varying degrees (Table 145-1). Soft foam collars may warm the muscles and cue the wearer to keep the head still but demonstrate little limitation of neck movement. Prefabricated COs are indicated only for clinically stable applications. Only the halo-vest apparatus, with skeletal fixation from skull pins, provides marked restriction of cervical motion. The halo is also the only device capable of limiting upper spine motion at the C2-Occiput level. Despite fixation at the head and from the trunk vest, significant translatory movement of the cervical spine can occur while wearing the halo. This motion has been documented radiographically when moving from the supine to upright position, and increases when the trauma has disrupted the ligamentous and bony structures of the spine.

Cervico-Thoracic Orthoses (CTOs) cover more of the torso than collars and improve the immobilization provided, but are less accepted by the patients. Finding the optimum compromise between comfortable but ineffective devices and more rigid ones that are not as well tolerated by the wearer is the challenge of COs. One variant,

---

Table 145-1

Percentage of Residual Motion Permitted by Typical Cervical Orthoses

MOTION ALLOWED FROM THE OCCIPUT TO THE FIRST THORACIC VERTEBRA WITH VARIOUS ORTHOSES

Test Situation	No. of Subjects	Mean Age (yr)	Flexion-Extension	Rotation	Lateral Bending
Normal unrestricted (all subjects)	44	25.8	100	100	100
Soft collar	20	26.2	74.2	82.6	92.3
Philadelphia collar	17	25.8	28.9	43.7	66.4
Four-poster brace	27	25.9	20.6	27.1	45.9
Cervicothoracic brace	27	25.9	12.8	18.2	50.5
Halo with plastic body vest	7	40.0	4	1	4

NOTE: The mean of normal motion allowed fell in the range ±10% of indicated values.

SOURCE: Reproduced with permission from Michael JW: Orthotic treatment of neurological deficits. In Good DC, Couch JR (eds): *Handbook of Neurorehabilitation*. New York: Marcel Dekker; 1994:261–315 (based on the original from Johnson RM, Hart DL, Simmons EF, et al: Cervical Orthoses. *J Bone Joint Surg [Am]* 1977; 59:334.)

the sternal occipital mandibular immobilizer (SOMI), has been shown to offer nearly as much immobilization as four-post CTOs, yet it is tolerable for most patients. It can also be fitted to the patient who is supine in bed. Custom CTOs are reserved for special cases not amenable to management with prefabricated orthoses.

Cervico-Thoracic-Lumbo-Sacral Orthoses (CTLOs) offer greater immobilization yet and are reserved for more involved injuries. As noted previously, the halo-vest apparatus offers the greatest immobilization of any available cervical device. Although the cranial attachment of the halo is quite secure, some motion of the vest on the torso is inevitable. Prefabricated vest systems, when carefully fitted, have been shown to provide approximately 95 percent immobilization of the cervical spine. For added stability, or to accommodate unusual torso contours such as those associated with achondroplastic dwarfism, a custom-made Thoraco-Lumbo-Sacral-Orthoses (TLSO) "body jacket" may be added to the commercial halo superstructure. Alternatives to the halo include casts such as the Minnerva, but these devices are not as well tolerated by most patients.

Numerous complications have been reported from improper use of the halo ring and skull pins, including pin site infections, pin loosening, skull penetration, and injury to the supraoccular structures. Meticulous hygiene, careful application of the pins in accordance with the manufacturer's instructions, and regular follow-up will prevent or mitigate most difficulties. Widespread availability of new materials compatible with magnetic resonance imaging (MRI) allows immediate application of the halo CTLSO in the emergency room without fear of interfering with later diagnostic studies.

Muscle atrophy is a normal result of prolonged halo-vest immobilization. It is useful to provide a semirigid CO such as a Philadelphia collar to be worn for a few days after halo removal until head control improves.

Although the thoracolumbar spine may be viewed as a semiflexible rod, it is virtually impossible to press directly upon it. As a result, spinal orthoses can only be expected to manage fractures or lesions that have some intrinsic stability.

Postoperative application of the TLSO (plastic body jacket) is well accepted, but specific applications remain controversial and practice varies widely from center to center. In general, the more stable the internal construct provided, the less the need for external support.

Rigid metal orthoses are much less commonly prescribed than in the past, having been displaced in large measure by total-contact plastic devices when immobilization is desired and by fabric supports when immobilization is unnecessary. An almost infinite array of traditional metal orthoses can be constructed by combining various elements such as pelvic and thoracic bands, vertical uprights, and a canvas anterior panel. The more of the torso covered, the greater the restriction in motion. Recent research suggests that when treating chronic low back pain, a "diagnostic orthosis" which varies the amount of lumbar lordosis can be used to specify the contours of the definitive device and to predict when pain reduction will result.

A prefabricated metal orthosis is still frequently prescribed following spinal compression fractures, to apply a hyperextension force to the trunk, thereby unloading the anterior vertebral bodies until healing occurs. For example, the Jewett hyperextension TLSO creates a three-point pressure system with posteriorly directed forces at the sternum and suprapubic area and an anteriorly directed force in the lower thoracic area. Orthoses are least effective biomechanically at their margins, so these devices work best to prevent flexion at the lower thoracic and thoracolumbar regions.

Like all spinal supports, such devices also require a compliant patient who will wear the orthosis faithfully and correctly for any benefit to occur. Orthoses are generally ineffective when offered to confused, irrational, or uncooperative individuals.

The soft lumbar corset is believed to be the most commonly prescribed spinal orthosis in the United States, in part because it is so well tolerated by most patients. Although such cloth garments offer only limited biomechanical control, many patients have reported a reduction in low back pain when the corset is used as a short-term treatment. Non-elastic fabric corsets may function by one or more of the following mechanisms:

1. Increasing intracavitary pressure by compressing the abdomen, which has been shown experimentally to decrease loading on the lumbar spine
2. Providing a kinesthetic reminder to withdraw, encouraging upright posture
3. Providing a psychological reassurance that "something" is being offered

Elastic garments move and expand with the body, thereby reducing or eliminating the first two benefits. Both LSO and TLSO corsets are available. It is generally recommended that corsets only be used as short-term measures, due to their tendency to encourage disuse atrophy of the abdominal muscles.

Custom-molded plastic orthoses are widely acknowledged as providing the most effective overall thoracolumbar spinal control available. Both LSO and TLSO body jackets may be custom-made from a plaster cast or custom-fitted from a module based on measurements. Computer-assisted manufacturing is just becoming available, allowing creation of a plastic orthosis based on data from optical scans of the torso.

In addition to postoperative and posttrauma applications, plastic TLSOs are the treatment of choice for selected cases of idiopathic scoliosis. Curves less than 20 degrees are now known to have little risk of progression and are simply monitored at regular intervals to watch for progression. Most curves less than 30 degrees do not require orthotic treatment, but larger curves and those with documented progression are often appropriate for brace fitting. Patients with curves greater than 40 to 45 degrees seldom respond well to bracing and are typically surgical candidates. The present window for brace management is therefore curves between 25 to 40 degrees with documented progression in a skeletally immature child. The more years of skeletal growth remaining (Risser 0 or 1), the greater the risk of progression even with the smaller curves.

For many decades, the Milwaukee CTLSO was the only available nonoperative treatment for idiopathic scoliosis, and it remains the orthosis of choice for all higher-level curves (generally with apices above T8). The Milwaukee also has the greatest volume of studies documenting a favorable outcome in limiting curve progression. For Scheuermann's juvenile kyphosis, a modified Milwaukee brace has been shown not only to arrest curve progression but often to correct the deformity within 6 to 12 months as the child's spine grows.

Concerns over the psycho-social impact of having adolescents wear a brace with a visible cervical component, combined with new evidence of a much lower compliance rate in this population than originally assumed, led to the development of numerous TLSO jackets as alternatives to treat lower curves from idiopathic scoliosis and Scheuermann's kyphosis. The best known of such "underarm" devices is the Boston Brace. It appears that for curves below T7, properly designed and fitted TLSOs are equal in effectiveness to the Milwaukee CTLSO. Some physicians will always begin brace treatment with a TLSO, adding the Milwaukee superstructure whenever radiographic evidence shows that the plastic jacket alone is insufficient to prevent progression.

Many other treatments have been tried over the years, including exercise programs, neuromuscular electrical stimulation, and nocturnal orthoses which overcorrect the curves while sleeping (such as the Charleston bending brace). Unfortunately, outcome studies to date suggest that none of these alternatives can equal the success rate of the Boston or Milwaukee orthoses.

Regardless of the particular TLSO or CTLSO style chosen, the child must wear the orthosis 16 to 23 h daily until skeletal maturity, when gradual weaning from the brace can occur safely. Initial correction of flexible curves may be 50 percent or more, but long-term studies suggest a gradual return over many years to the original presenting curve at initiation of the orthosis. In essence, successful brace treatment seems to halt further progression of idiopathic scoliotic curves rather than providing long-term correction. Where brace management is unsuccessful for whatever reason, surgical stabilization is generally recommended.

Both prefabricated and custom-molded TLSOs are available. Grossly abnormal torso contours generally require that the device be custom made. The prescription should describe the type and style of orthosis recommended and clearly indicate the levels and magnitudes of all curve segments. Corrective pads are placed at or just inferior to the apices of the major curves, and the result is checked with an in-brace standing radiograph to measure the initial correction. For best results, the orthotist should have access to a pre-brace standing x-ray to assist in visualizing the curves and in specific pad placement.

Plastic TLSOs may also be used for a variety of other applications, including reduction of excessive lumbar lordosis due to spondylolisthesis or postural deficits. When hip flexor tightness is present, a properly fitted TLSO will prevent compensatory lordosis and force the patient to assume a "bent knee" stance since the hips are flexed. Over time, the normal righting reflex will cause the patient to gradually stretch out the contractures and normal upright stance is then possible.

One caveat applies to all orthoses: Their efficacy diminishes at the margins and is most effective at the midpoint. Norton and Brown demonstrated many years ago that a rigid spinal orthosis may actually *increase* motion at the lumbosacral junction. Effective immobilization at this level requires a rigid extension to immobilize at least one thigh, analogous to a hip spica cast.

LOWER-LIMB ORTHOSES

The clinical preponderance of lower-limb orthoses reflects both the strong desire to walk (or at least stand) by most individuals with a disability and the fact that present orthotic technology is reasonably effective at restoring gross physical functions, such as walking and standing. In addition, for the extremely active competitive athlete, rather subtle interventions with foot orthoses can sometimes overcome small physiological deficits that would otherwise limit performance. Lower-limb orthoses are therefore applicable to enhance function for many deficits, large and small.

Custom footwear and modifications to commercial footwear are extremely important aspects of both orthotic and pedorthic practices. Not only can shoe adaptations successfully treat many simpler problems, they can also significantly enhance the effectiveness of orthotic management when more proximal devices are required. Common examples would include prescribing a shoe with a deep toe box to accommodate hammer toes, adding a rocker sole to partially compensate for limited ankle dorsiflexion, and specifying hook-and-loop closures due to upper limb impairment.

FOOT ORTHOSES

Foot orthoses (FOs), are the foundation for lower-limb management. Not only are they suitable for managing many of the basic problems encountered in daily practice, it should also be noted that each and every more proximal orthosis (e.g., AFO, KAFO, and HKAFO) is first and foremost an FO. In general, the FO portion should be used to manage as many deficits as possible, relying on more proximal designs *only* when an FO alone will be insufficient. This is the most cost-effective approach, enhancing patient acceptance since most FOs are "invisibly" contained within the footwear.

Conceptually, FOs are usually divided into three broad categories:

1. Accommodative or soft devices
2. Intermediate or semi-rigid devices
3. Corrective or rigid devices

Accommodative FOs are typically used to "cradle" and protect rigidly deformed or dysvascular feet, and are constructed from a variety of soft or flexible materials. Very minor problems such as mild metatarsal pain may respond to "over-the-counter" (OTC) or prefabricated "inserts" of resilient materials. Such limited function devices are often worth a trial when treating minor complaints.

Corrective FOs made of rigid materials can be extremely difficult to fit successfully, as they require meticulous attention to detail as well as a weaning period of several weeks to insure successful patient acceptance. Most practitioners reserve such rigid materials for easily correctable, flexible deformities such as mild ankle valgus or for subtle control of a nearly normal foot with slight biomechanical deficits, such as the Olympic-level sprinter with a few degrees of excess pronation. In general, the more pronounced the flexible deformity, the more extensive the design and trimlines of the orthosis must be.

Intermediate FOs made of semi-rigid materials are very popular clinically, as they may be fabricated from multiple layers of slightly different densities to provide graduated degrees of control, thereby enhancing patient acceptance. As noted before, mild problems such as plantar pain without ulceration may respond to OTC, prefabricated, or modular intermediate FOs. Some clinicians use such devices for a field trial to verify the effectiveness of orthotic management in a given case prior to creating a custom orthosis. Chronic conditions, as well as moderate and severe biomechanical deficits, typically require custom-molded devices to insure the best result. Carefully designed and meticulously fitted custom devices are virtually mandatory for all feet with a history of ulceration or sensory limitation, due to the risk of injury from the orthosis itself when protective sensation is absent or impaired.

Most foot orthoses are based on one or more of the following principles:

1. Total surface contact
2. Support of the foot in a biomechanically corrected position
3. Limitation of excessive motion
4. Compensation for restricted motion or fixed deformity
5. Attenuation of impact

Total surface contact is inherent in all custom-molded FOs. By spreading the weightbearing load across the entire plantar surface of the foot, the pressure under any specific area is decreased. This is an excellent application of the classic equation from basic physics: $P = F/A$, where P = pressure; F = force; A = area. Many insensate feet, whether diabetic or dysvascular or both, respond well to total surface contact—particularly when combined with a self-relieving material such as Plastazote which also attenuates impact forces.

Principle 2 is the primary technique to manage flexible, fully correctable deformities. For example, a talus may be held in neutral with only mild pressure from the orthosis. On the other hand, if the talus remains positioned in even slight varus, the ground reaction forces of walking will increase the pressure against the orthosis tremendously.

Hypermobility at any joint can often be reduced by the application of a supportive orthosis. The most common example in sports medicine is the provision of support along the medial longitudinal arch to diminish excessive pronation. Fixed deformities, by definition, can only be managed by accommodation with an orthosis (or surgical correction). In this context, the orthosis can be viewed as a shim between the rigidly deformed foot and the floor.

It must always be remembered that the foot is a dynamically changing organ during the gait cycle while the FO is a static device. A thorough understanding of the foot and ankle biomechanics, in addition to careful follow-up and adjustments, is essential for long-term success with this treatment modality.

ANKLE-FOOT ORTHOSES

AFOs can be designed with sufficient lever arms to fully control the ankle complex and to indirectly influence the knee joint, making AFOs applicable for more extensive disabilities than FOs. At present, AFOs based on electrical stimulation of paraplegic muscles are primarily research applications in North America. If they prove economical and reliable, we may see them as clinically available devices in the very near future.

For now, the clinician must choose between metal alloy-based devices, plastic-based devices, and a hybrid assembly incorporating both materials. In most cases, the orthotist and patient spend time discussing the various advantages and disadvantages to each approach and arrive at a final choice. In general, plastic or hybrid plastic-metal systems predominate in North America due to the greater degree of patient acceptance and circumferential control they offer.

The older-style metal and leather orthoses are usually reserved for selected applications such as satisfied previous wearers, unusually large or heavy individuals, and conditions where minimal contact with the leg is desirable, such as persons with fluctuating edema and heat-sensitive individuals who cannot tolerate the more intimately fitting plastic contours. Some clinicians prefer metal systems for growing children due to their adjustability for growth, but many others feel that plastic or hybrid devices are just as versatile in this regard. One of the most critical factors is patient (or parental) preference, which largely determines acceptance and should play a significant role in the final decision.

As has been noted earlier, all orthotic devices, including AFOs, must fulfill one of the following fundamental goals:

1. Control of motion
2. Correction of deformity
3. Compensation for weakness
4. Partial axial unloading

One common application of control of motion would be a rigid, plastic AFO with the ankle locked in slight dorsiflexion and a well-padded anterior proximal segment to stabilize the tibia. This design, first reported in 1969 by an Israeli orthotist, Jimmy Saltiel, is often colloquially termed a "floor reaction" AFO since the extended, rigid forefoot section accentuates the knee *extension* moment at midstance and thereby prevents tibial collapse due to weak or absent gastroc-soleus musculature. This illustrates one of the critical treatment principles of orthotic management: The orthosis may indirectly affect remote body segments, and this characteristic can be used therapeutically.

Orthoses may be rationally prescribed based on the biomechanical function desired. The plastic "floor reaction" AFO, with the ankle locked in slight dorsiflexion, is usually applicable when the patient has a paralyzed ankle-foot complex but good or better quadriceps and balance. Examples of pathologies that could give rise to this clinical picture would include myelodysplasia, incomplete spinal cord injury, peripheral nerve injury, poliomyelitis, and gastroc-soleus trauma.

One of the most common lower-limb deficits is a flaccid equinus, which may result from many etiologies including Charcot-Marie-Tooth disease, mild cerebral vascular accidents, and muscular dystrophy, as well as peroneal palsies of various types. The orthotic options to definitively compensate for pretibial compartment weakness or paralysis, shown in Fig. 145-2, include: (1) bilateral 2-in. heel lifts; (2) spring wire AFO; (3) Klenzak style AFO; (4) flexible plastic AFO; (5) and peroneal function electrical stimulation (FES).

A functionally based prescription, such as "Orthosis to compensate for weakened pretibial musculature" will insure that the Certified Orthotist considers all available alternatives before selecting the optimum solution for a particular patient. A more specific prescription, such as "Prefabricated plastic AFO to provide dorsiflexion assist" is appropriate only if that is indeed the *sole* desirable solution, and all others are to be automatically ruled out. In general, only the physician with special training and experience in rehabilitation will be able to write such specific prescription instructions. The alternative—"Evaluate for orthosis to . . . . and call to discuss prescription"—is more practical in most circumstances.

The first alternative, which may be supplied by the two inch heels inherent in cowboy footwear, will prevent the plantarflexed forefoot from dragging in swing phase—because the boot stabilizes the flaccid foot, and the heel height lengthens both legs sufficiently for clearance of a plantarflexed extremity. This is obviously the least expensive option, and may be acceptable in some geographic locations.

The next two choices are essentially spring-loaded metal systems attached to the patients' shoes. Use of a caliper box and removable stirrups with the Klenzak AFO would allow shoe interchange, but the cost and inconvenience of modifying all shoes for compatibility with the orthosis should not be underestimated. The chief advantage of the metal systems is the limited contact with the leg, which must be balanced against the bulk, weight, and maintenance required for such devices.

The fourth option may be either prefabricated or custom-molded. In general, prefabricated solutions are applicable for short-term use with sensate extremities (such as a mild iatrogenic palsy from cast application) so long as the limb contours are within normal limits. Deformed limbs, insensate limbs, and definitive applications generally require custom-made devices to insure long-term comfort and success.

As noted previously, the fifth option (FES) is presently considered experimental. Various elastic "slings" available for temporary management of flaccid equinus have been omitted from the discussion since such OTC items are intended as "therapy gym equipment" to facilitate gait retraining, and are usually inappropriate for long-term, outpatient use. The discussion has also excluded the compensatory "steppage gait" characterized by excess hip flexion, which is a common *adaptation* to untreated flaccid equinus.

All the devices discussed in this segment offer the same biomechanical function: compensation for pretibial muscle weakness. The particular orthosis selected for an individual patient must take into

ORTHOTIC SOLUTIONS FOR FLACCID EQUINUS

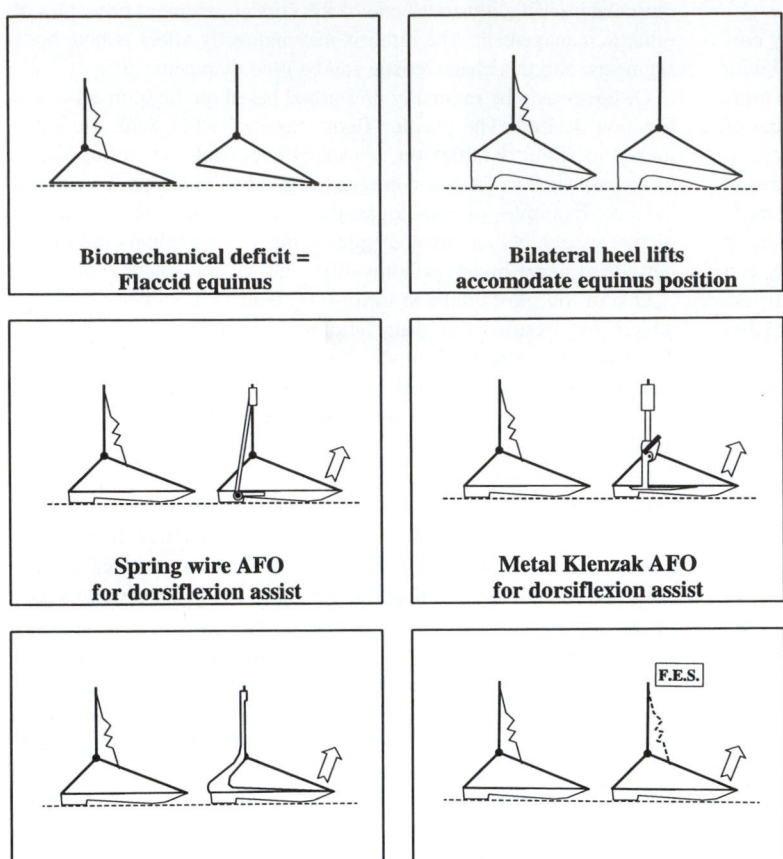

Figure 145-2

Matrix summarizing functional orthotic alternatives to manage flaccid equinus. [Reproduced with permission from Michael JW: Lower limb orthoses: Overview of principles, materials and components. In Goldberg B, Hsu J (eds): *Atlas of Orthoses and Assistive Devices,* 3d ed. Philadelphia: Mosby-Year Book; 1997:211.]

consideration of a variety of additional criteria beyond the simple diagnosis and gross functional deficit, including such additional clinical data as ease of donning, weight, cost, patient acceptance, and durability.

Correction of *flexible* deformities is so common in lower-limb orthotic management that it has become a *sine qua non* for modern treatment: reduce all flexible deformities to a neutral or balanced position. Such careful alignment markedly reduces the floor reaction moments trying to further collapse the limb segment, lowers the magnitude of stabilizing force necessary, and results in a more comfortable orthosis thus enhancing long-term acceptance.

Correction of more *rigid* deformities is feasible only in carefully selected cases. Children can sometimes be braced sufficiently to "grow out of the deformity," as is the case with tibial bowing due to Blount's disease. In adults, correction with orthotic management is feasible only where the cause is short-term and primarily soft-tissue related. Figure 145-3 illustrates bilateral hybrid AFOs designed to allow ambulation, as well as to help reduce the plantarflexion contractures due to a hypertonic gastrocnemius following a transamatic brain injury.

Initially, the ankle joints were set to accommodate the full contracture and the plastic foot and tibial shells held the limb securely, eliminating clonus. External wedges of a lightweight material were

added to the plantar surface of the orthosis so that the tibia-to-floor angle simulated slight dorsiflexion, which allowed ambulation without the painful hyperextension moment at the knee that occurred during barefoot walking. Over time, in response to antispasticity medication and physical therapy mobilization, the contracture began to become slightly more flexible. By incrementally readjusting the ankle joints, the orthosis was then used to maintain the limb in a less deformed attitude, 24 h per day, to consolidate the gains made during daily treatments. As the contracture diminished, slices of the wedge material were removed to restore the proper tibia-to-floor attitude as the ankle attitude approached neutral. Ultimately, the patient was discharged as a community ambulator with her ankles held in slight dorsiflexion by the orthoses, which now fit comfortably inside conventional athletic footwear.

This case example illustrates two important additional orthotic treatment principles:

1. Application of low-level, tolerable forces over an extended period may result in significant changes to the musculoskeletal anatomy
2. The tibia-to-floor angle may be varied *independently* of the ankle-foot attitude, to facilitate a reasonable gait despite lower-limb abnormalities.

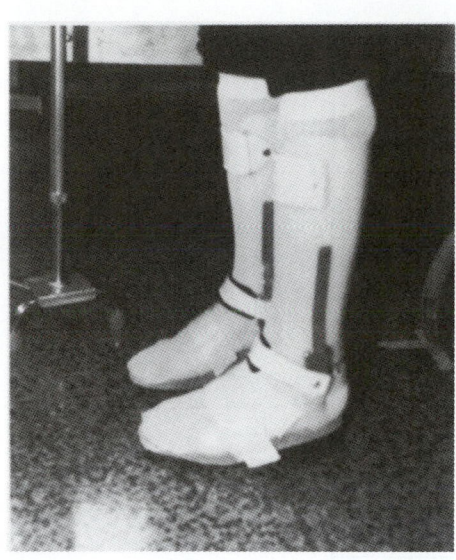

A

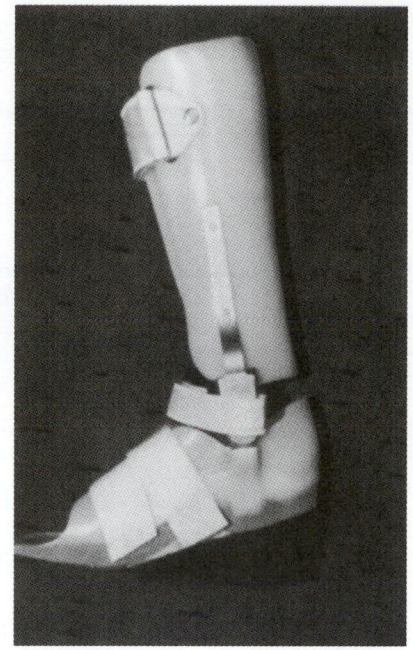

B

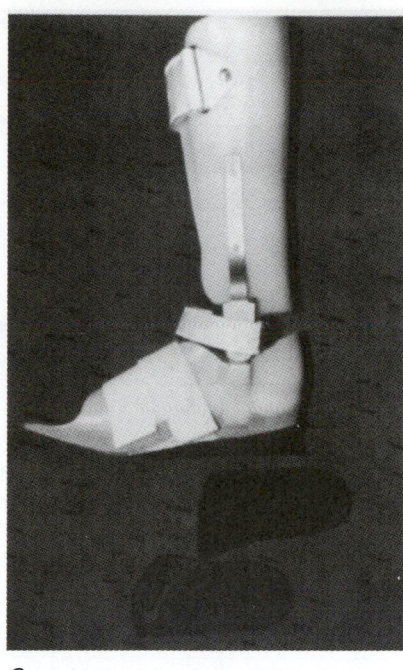

C

Figure 145-3

These hybrid metal and plastic orthoses allowed early ambulation despite significant soft-tissue contractures at the ankles secondary to spasticity (*A*). As the contractures resolved, the ankle position and compensatory sole wedging was adjusted (*B, C*) until a plantigrade attitude was achieved. [Reproduced with permission from Michael JW: Lower limb orthoses: Overview of principles, materials and components. In Goldberg B, Hsu J (eds): *Atlas of Orthoses and Assistive Devices,* 3d ed. Philadelphia: Mosby-Year Book; 1997:211.]

The matrix in Fig. 145-4 summarizes the motion control options available at the ankle, and provides examples of both metal and plastic AFOs that offer such function. This graphic summary helps in visualizing the available options. Much like the ingredients in a recipe, these simple prescription options, when properly and creatively combined, achieve a clinical result that is more effective than just the sum of the individual parts.

On rare occasions, orthoses may be prescribed to offer an additional function: *partial* axial unweighting of more distal limb segments. Such orthoses are sometimes used to protect hindfoot fractures, recalcitrant heel ulcerations, and similar pathologies or to reduce the risk of bony collapse during the consolidation phase of neuropathic (Charcot) arthropathy. Although the original unweighting orthoses incorporated quadrilateral and patellar tendon bearing shapes from prosthetic experience, the present trend is to emphasize circumferential soft-tissue containment using total contact designs. Since the thigh and distal calf have a contour similar to an inverted cone, when such an orthosis is cinched snugly against the skin and underlying muscles, the soft tissues can accept a portion of the vertical loading of the body, thereby reducing the load on the more distal skeletal structures.

KNEE-ANKLE-FOOT ORTHOSES

As noted previously, simpler orthoses enjoy a much higher long-term acceptance rate than more complex devices. Therefore, a Knee-Ankle-Foot-Orthoses (KAFO) should not be prescribed unless there is a compelling reason to do so.

The most common justification for a KAFO is the need for direct control of the knee complex, which cannot be accomplished in another fashion, *in addition to a need for ankle/foot control or suspen-*sion. Obviously, if knee control alone is the objective, the simple knee orthosis (to be discussed next) will suffice.

Figure 145-5 depicts the range of controls possible at the knee joint, and examples of plastic and metal devices that offer such functions. When combined with the plethora of ankle controls available, literally scores of orthoses can be constructed. Prescribing orthotic management on a functional basis allows the physician to direct the team's efforts, while simultaneously allowing the knowledgeable Certified Orthotist to consider all available permutations before selecting the preferred approach.

Figure 145-6 presents a metal KAFO designed for a polio survivor with a flail leg from the hip distally. The offset knee joints are held in extension during stance by loading on the anterior proximal thigh band. The patient's knee is allowed to go into very slight recurvatum, sufficient to stabilize it via floor reaction forces, which occur when the dorsiflexion stop inside the orthotic ankle joint applies force to the extended steel shank placed inside the sole of the shoe.

The biomechanics at heel strike are also crucial. The counterforces from a mild plantarflexion resist spring in the ankle allows the foot to descend to the floor in a controlled manner, replacing the function of the pretibial muscles. If a rigid plantarflexion stop had been provided instead, the resultant knee-flexion moment could cause the orthotic knee joint to flex prior to foot flat and the patient might fall.

It is important to carefully analyze the resultant forces throughout the device to anticipate and deal with their effect. If a rigid ankle device were prescribed in this situation, then a locked knee mechanism would also be required for the same biomechanical reason. Particularly for patients with good proprioception as in this case, locking the knee joint is undesirable since it disrupts the gait mechanics and may increase the effort required to ambulate.

Orthotic Ankle Control Options

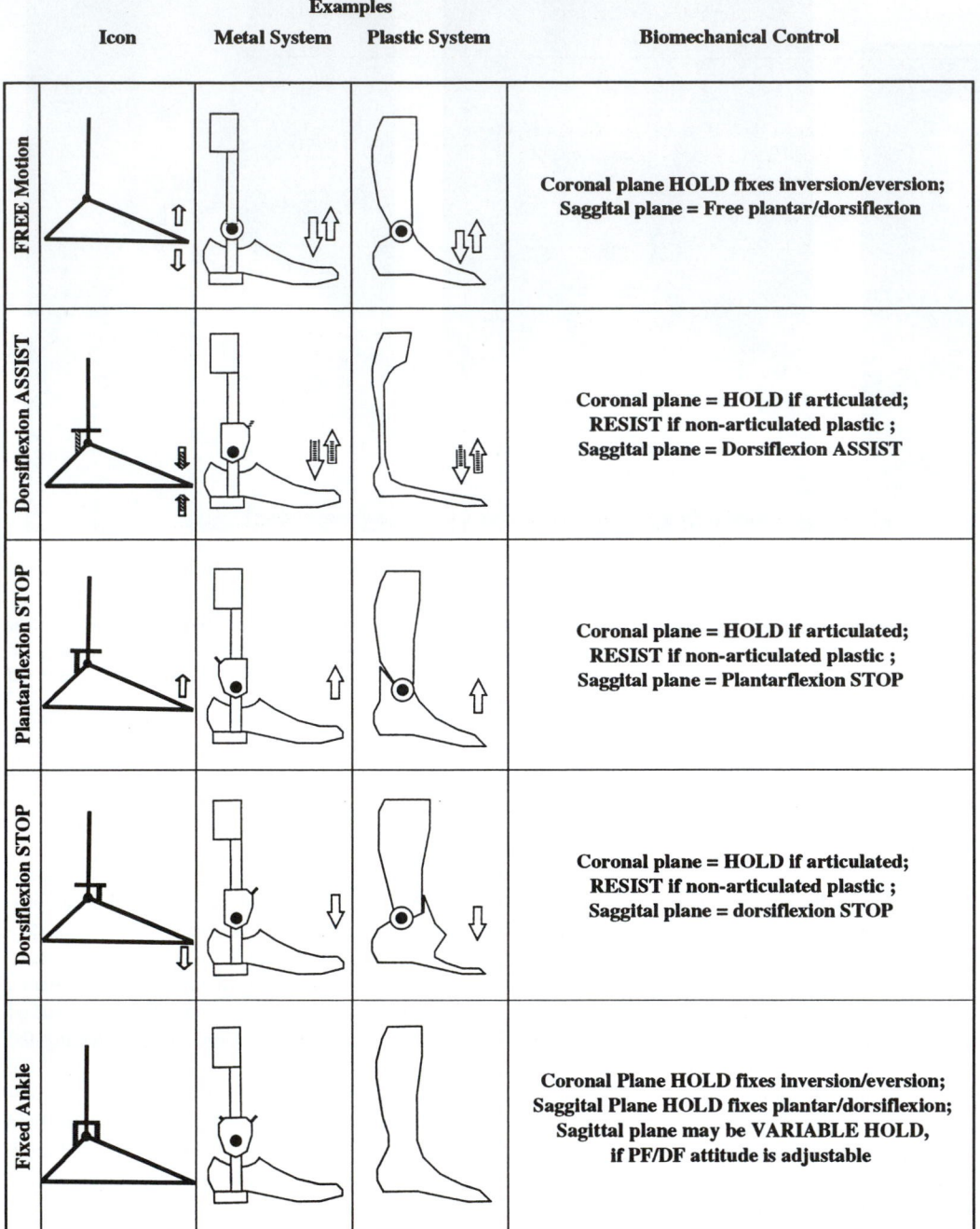

	Examples			
	Icon	Metal System	Plastic System	Biomechanical Control
FREE Motion				Coronal plane HOLD fixes inversion/eversion; Saggital plane = Free plantar/dorsiflexion
Dorsiflexion ASSIST				Coronal plane = HOLD if articulated; RESIST if non-articulated plastic; Saggital plane = Dorsiflexion ASSIST
Plantarflexion STOP				Coronal plane = HOLD if articulated; RESIST if non-articulated plastic; Saggital plane = Plantarflexion STOP
Dorsiflexion STOP				Coronal plane = HOLD if articulated; RESIST if non-articulated plastic; Saggital plane = dorsiflexion STOP
Fixed Ankle				Coronal Plane HOLD fixes inversion/eversion; Saggital Plane HOLD fixes plantar/dorsiflexion; Sagittal plane may be VARIABLE HOLD, if PF/DF attitude is adjustable

Figure 145-4

Matrix summarizing the biomechanical control available from various orthotic ankle mechanisms. [Reproduced with permission from Michael JW: Lower limb orthoses: Overview of principles, materials and components. In Goldberg B, Hsu J (eds): *Atlas of Orthoses and Assistive Devices,* 3d ed. Philadelphia: Mosby-Year Book; 1997:214.]

The variety of knee lock mechanisms available suggests how often pathologic conditions require this level of security, despite the obvious gait deviation that results. Recent experimental results have shown that a joint which electromagnetically unlocks for swing phase would be more energy efficient, but no such device is presently commercially available. Perhaps the most common application of knee locks is for paraplegia, which may result from a variety of neuromuscular diseases, as well as many traumatic causes including sinal cord injury.

Figure 145-7 illustrates one of the simplest approaches permitting limited ambulation, using forearm crutches, despite full paralysis of the lower limbs. The fixed ankle with adjustable joints, combined with specially reinforced shoes, provide a solid base of support. Careful adjustment into a slightly dorsiflexed attitude, combined with the locked-knee mechanisms and therapy training to teach the patient to extend the hips and "hang" on the hip ligaments, results in hands-free balance. Ambulation for limited distances is possible using crutches, at least for the young or vigorous individual. This type of

Orthotic Knee Joint Options

	Examples	Biomechanical Control	Typical Application
Single Axis	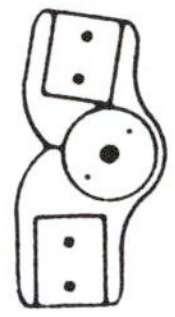	Coronal plane HOLD fixes genu varum-valgum; Saggital plane = Free flexion-extension; integral hyperextension stop	Mild to moderate genu varum or valgum
Offset	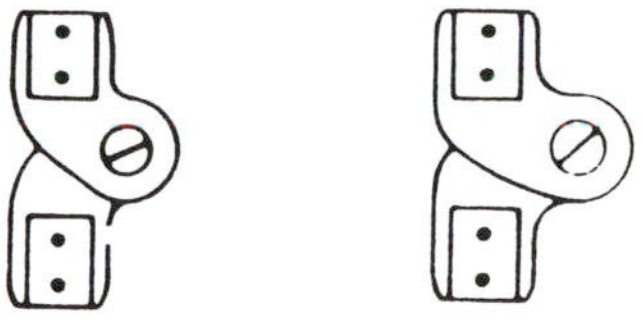	Coronal plane HOLD fixes genu varum-valgum; Saggital plane = Free flexion-extension; integral hyperextension stop	Moderate genu recurvatum
Polycentric	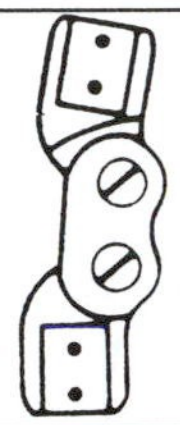	Coronal plane HOLD fixes genu varum-valgum; Saggital plane = Free flexion-extension; integral hyperextension stop	Usually, self-suspending orthoses - to track the knee axis more closely
Lock	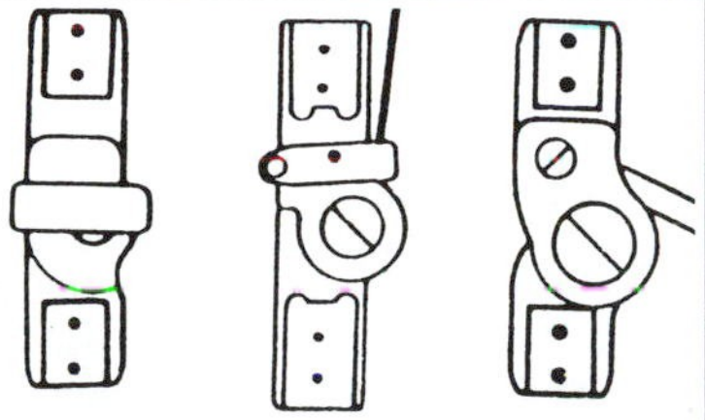 Droplock Wedge Lock Bail Lock	Coronal Plane HOLD fixes genu varum-valgum; Saggital Plane = removable LOCK in full extension	Paralysis, severe paresis, severe genu varum/valgum or recurvatum
Lock + Variable Flexion	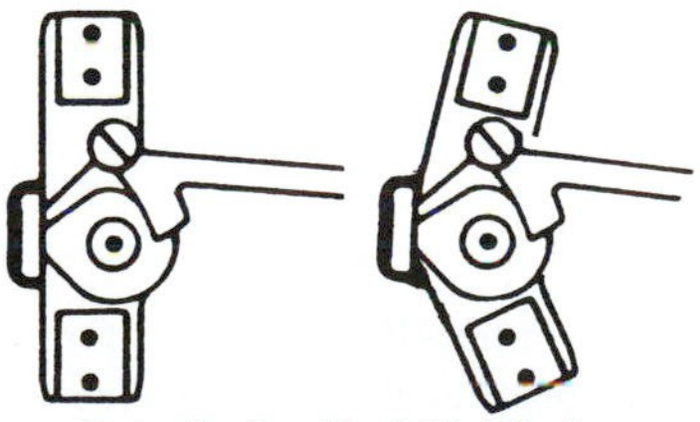 Swiss Lock + Variable Flexion	Coronal Plane HOLD fixes genu varum-valgum; Saggital Plane = removable LOCK, in variable degrees of flexion	Usually, spastic paralysis with reducible knee flexion contractures

Figure 145-5
Matrix summarizing available orthotic knee joint alternatives. [Reproduced with permission from Michael JW: Lower limb orthoses: Overview of principles, materials and components. In Goldberg B, Hsu J (eds): *Atlas of Orthoses and Assistive Devices,* 3d ed. Philadelphia: Mosby-Year Book; 1997:217.]

KAFO bears the eponym "Scott Craig" after the Colorado rehabilitation hospital that popularized its application for persons with paraplegia following lumbar or low thoracic spinal cord injury.

KNEE ORTHOSES

Knee orthoses (KOs) were originally rarely prescribed, with their application limited to isolated knee pathologies—typically varus or valgus angulation secondary to advanced arthritic destruction on the condylar area. To unload the painful condyle, as well as to prevent further progression, extensive bracing with long moment arms was required. The need for self-suspension was met by careful contouring to the deformed limb, supplemented with a supracondylar contour similar to the prosthetic suspension technique.

The Lenox Hill brace was first developed about two decades ago, gradually becoming the first widely accepted knee orthosis for sports applications. Over the ensuing years, literally hundreds of imitators have developed slight variations on the theme of a self-suspending KO with dual freely moving knee hinges. The original custom-molded designs have gradually been supplanted in many cases with prefabricated and even OTC variants. Many have only superficial differences; others are made of poor-quality materials; none has been convincingly demonstrated to be generally "superior" to any other variant.

Indications for sports-knee orthoses remain equivocal, other than for nonoperative applications where surgery has been refused or is not feasible. Postoperative use is largely subjective and probably prevents litigation as much as re-injury. Prophylactic application to pre-

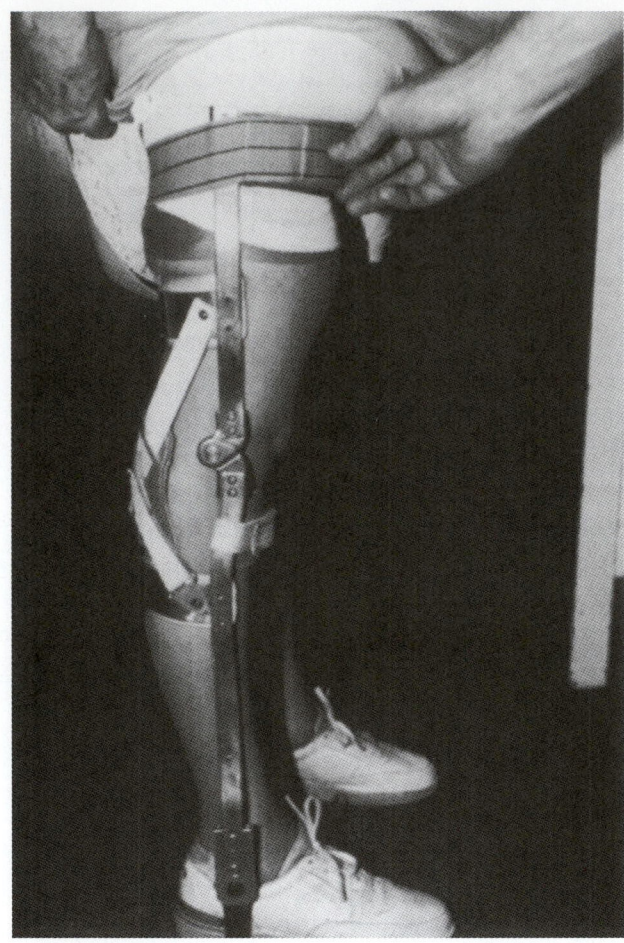

Figure 145-6
This knee-ankle-foot-orthosis (KAFO) with free motion, offset knee joints allows sufficient genu recurvatum for the ground reaction force to stabilize the flail knee in stance, and yet allow free swing phase motion. This approach is clinically most successful when the individual has residual sensation in the paralyzed limb as is the case with this polio survivor. [Reproduced with permission from Michael JW: Lower limb orthoses: Overview of principles, materials and components. In Goldberg B, Hsu J (eds): *Atlas of Orthoses and Assistive Devices,* 3d ed. Philadelphia: Mosby-Year Book; 1997:218.]

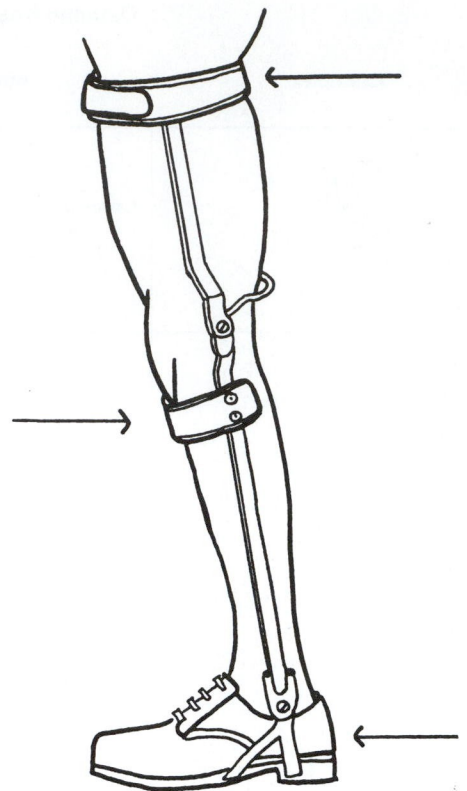

Figure 145-7
Orthosis with locked knees and adjustable ankle stops are sometimes used to allow persons with acquired paraplegia to ambulate with crutches using a swing-through gait. Arrows indicate the stabilizing forces during static standing. Due to the energy required to walk in this fashion, few persons continue with this mode of mobility more than a year or so. [Reproduced with permission from Michael JW: Lower limb orthoses: Overview of principles, materials and components. In Goldberg B, Hsu J (eds): *Atlas of Orthoses and Assistive Devices,* 3d ed. Philadelphia: Mosby-Year Book; 1997:219.]

vent injuries has never been shown definitively to be effective, and such bracing may increase the risk of "transfer injuries" to adjacent unprotected joints.

HIP ORTHOSES

Hip orthoses (HOs) are indicated for isolated problems in the acetabular region, which may be the result of: dysplastic disorders; traumatic injury; and surgical procedures (total hip replacement).

A variety of devices are available to treat infantile developmentally dysplastic hips (DDH), with generally good results. The prefabricated Pavlik harness is one of the most common. A variety of custom-made HOs have been used to treat Legg-Calvé-Perthes disease in adolescents, based on the containment theory which states that if the femoral head is maintained in the acetabulum during the active phase of the disorder, a more congruent head will result. The scientific evidence to support the containment theory is equivocal, and such treatment is now being challenged.

The most common application for the HO in adults is for postoperative protection after total hip replacement, especially after revision surgery. In general, those devices which incorporate an extensive hemi-shell at the hip, as well as an extension to the distal thigh—and are therefore technically called LSHOs—provide the most effective biomechanical control. It should be noted that no orthosis has yet been developed that can fully "protect" the at-risk hip, particularly with an uncooperative or incoherent patient. A well-designed and well-fitted HO may decrease the risk of dislocation but no orthosis can eliminate the possibility.

Definitive HO applications are rare. A young man with total loss of adductor power, secondary to one of the muscular dystrophies, complained of progressive abduction as he walked, which ultimately prevented further progress when his legs became maximally abducted. A lightweight, custom-made HO that held his hips in normal abduction, while allowing free sagittal plane motion, restored him to community ambulator status.

HIP-KNEE-ANKLE-FOOT ORTHOSES

Hip-knee-ankle-foot orthoses (HKAFOs) are most commonly prescribed for pediatric patients, who do remarkably well even with such complex devices. They are selectively recommended for adults, who

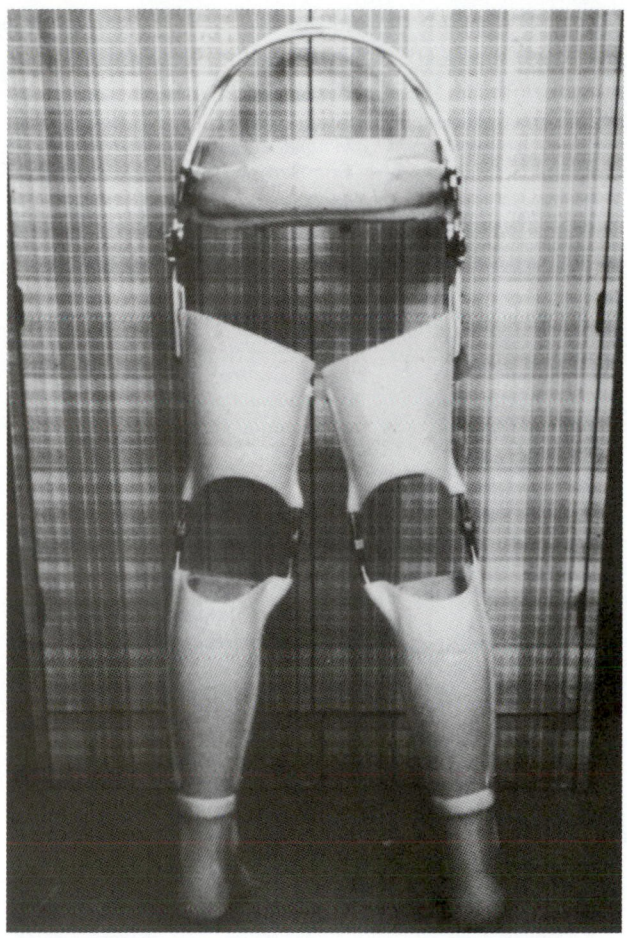

Figure 145-8
This reciprocating gait orthosis (RGO) links flexion of one hip with extension of the other, allowing the paraplegic to walk with a foot-after-foot gait. This has been shown to be a slower but more energy efficient gait than previous orthoses permitted. To move more quickly, a swing-through gait may be used as well. [Reproduced with permission from Michael JW: Orthotic treatment of neurological deficits. In Good DC, Couch JR (eds): *Handbook of Neurorehabilitation.* New York: Marcel Dekker; 1994:309.]

tend to abandon more involved orthoses after the first year or so due to the tremendous energy consumption required to use bilateral devices that cross the knee. Unilateral applications are rare.

One of the most common HKAFO uses is as a mechanical linkage to couple flexion of one hip with extension of the other. Such mechanisms allow the option of a reciprocal step-over-step gait, which has been shown to be more energy efficient, albeit slower, than the traditional swing-through gait. One example of such an HKAFO is illustrated in Fig. 145-8. Colloquially referred to as reciprocating gait orthoses or RGOs, these HKAFOs are used for a variety of pathologies that result in paraplegia, including spinal cord injury and myelodysplasia.

COMPOUND ORTHOSES

Devices which cross more than five body segments may be considered "compound" orthoses, composed of two or more less complex devices. The terminology reflects this perspective as two or more individual orthoses, with the device pictured in Fig. 145-9 described as a TLSO + HKAFOs. Such extensive bracing is occasionally successful with young adults who are extremely motivated.

Children, on the other hand, typically do very well with such complexity. Even if a TLSO is required full-time for scoliosis management, and superincumbent HKAFOs are used daily for ambulation, youngsters with paraplegia often wear such compound orthoses without complaint and ambulate reasonably well with a reversed walker until their teen years, when the increase in their height and body weight make such ambulation too difficult to sustain for almost all individuals with higher-level lesions. At that point wheelchair use, previously reserved for covering longer distances, becomes the primary source of mobility.

SEATING AND MOBILITY SYSTEMS

Medical advances have resulted, in recent decades, in the long-term survival of large numbers of people with marked mobility impairments. Whether the underlying pathology is severe cerebral palsy, sinal cord injury, or a progressive neuromuscular disorder, it is now recognized that all persons who spend substantial time in an upright, immobile position should receive a thorough evaluation of their seating and mobility needs.

The ubiquitous "hospital wheelchair" is inappropriate for long-term use, although it functions well for temporary use while recovering

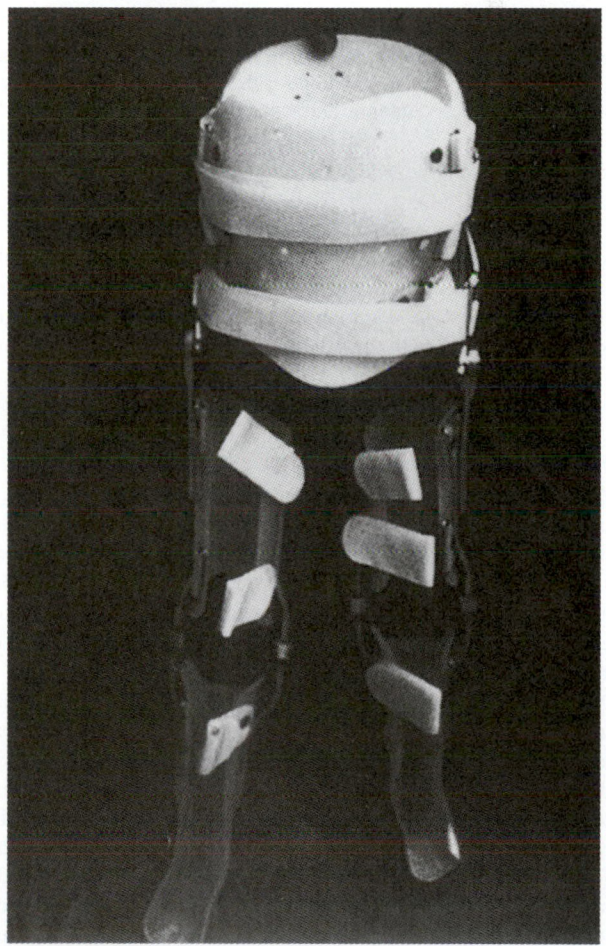

Figure 145-9
Compound orthosis providing trunk support as well as full lower limb bracing. [Reproduced with permission from Michael JW: Orthotic treatment of neurological deficits. In Good DC, Couch JR (eds): *Handbook of Neurorehabilitation.* New York: Marcel Dekker; 1994:310.]

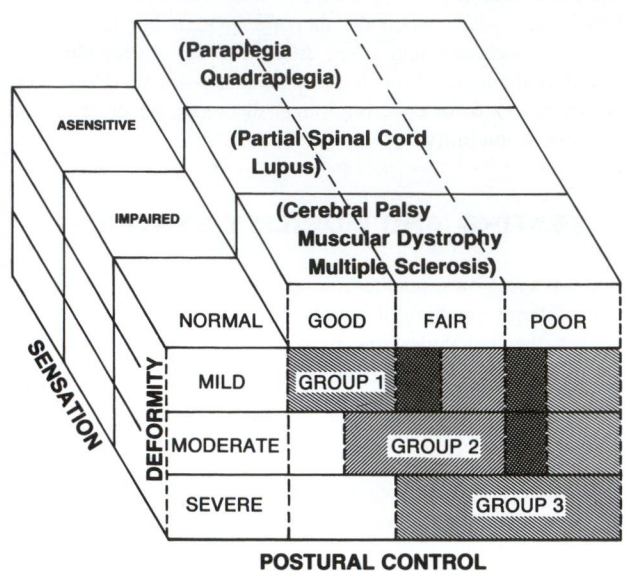

	Generic Seating Devices		Needs Group
Type I	Noncontoured	*(Simple foam and plywood)*	Group I
Type II	Precontoured Modules	*(MPI, Pin Dot Modular System, Otto Bock MOSS)*	Group II
Type III	Multiadjustable	*(Mullholland, E & J Postural)*	Groups I & II
Type IV	Custom Contoured		Groups II & III
a.	Complex Foam & Plywood	*(Custom contoured foam cutouts)*	
b.	Traditional Orthotic Approach	*(Plaster positive complete with plastic body jacket)*	
c.	Vacuum Consolidation (1 & 2 step)	*(Bead Seat, Gillette Spinal Support, and DESMO)*	
d.	Foaming (1 & 2 step)	*(Foam-in-Place, Contour-U, Canadian Posture)*	
e.	Shapable Matrices	*(Clinical Engineering Design, London, England MERU-UBC)*	

A

B

Figure 145-10

Matrix summarizing the key intrinsic factors (*A*) that suggest specific seating system approaches (*B*) for various pathologies. (Reproduced with permission from Hobson DA: Research and development considerations and engineering perspective. *Clin Prosthet Orthot* 1986; 10(4):124, 127.)

from various surgical or medical procedures. In most cases, a lighter and more stable wheelchair with appropriate accessories is necessary for full-time users. One common prescription would be for a lightweight, folding, manually-propelled chair with removable, swing-away leg rests. When chair-to-bed transfers are anticipated, removable desk arms should also be specified. For optimum results it is crucial that the chair be sized according to the physiology and needs of the individual user.

Modifications for amputee use could include elevating leg rests to reduce the risk of knee-flexion contracture immediately following trans-tibial amputation, and a posteriorly offset axle to compensate for the shift in the anatomic center of gravity due to lower-limb loss. Axle placement is particularly important for bilateral lower-limb amputees as they are at significant risk of having a standard chair tip over backwards on a small incline or uneven surface.

Other mobility modifications are based on the neuromuscular deficit present. Following stroke or other pathologies that impair upper-limb function, a "one hand drive" wheelchair can be considered. Anti-tipping bars are commonly prescribed to increase the users' safety. When necessary, various battery-powered chairs are available using a wide range of control inputs, including joystick or "sip-and-puff" breath-activation. Designs with oversized tires or "tank treads" are available for outdoors use. Numerous specialty mobility devices are now readily available, such as pediatric strollers and electrically operated "standing frames."

The standard hospital sling seat is also adequate only for *temporary* use. Whenever a mobility aid is necessary for long-term mobility, some seating adaptation is required. As an overall guideline, the complexity of the seating system should be proportional to the de-

gree of deformity or paralysis present. Figure 145-10 presents a selection matrix to help determine the general type of seating system required for a given level of deformity. Elderly persons with protective sensation and good trunk balance may only need a solid drop seat and basic OTC foam cushion to insure comfort and a stable posture. When trunk balance is limited or absent, a back support must also be created, perhaps with added lateral support features.

Certain forms of spasticity are aggravated by particular postures. Careful positioning in a well-designed seating system can markedly improve both sitting balance and upper limb functioning in such cases. Moderate spasticity is often amenable to management with a modular seating system assembled from prefabricated elements. Custom-made plywood and foam devices offer additional possibilities. More severely involved individuals, particularly when fixed deformities are also present, may need an intimately fitted, custom-molded seating system.

Fabrication of a custom-molded seating system generally begins from either a plaster-of-Paris negative impression or electronic digitization of the client, to produce the positive plaster model of the affected individual's torso and legs. After the positive model has been rectified to optimize the alignment and pressure distribution, the back and seat portions of the system are fabricated. For optimal results, the back and seat must be attached to the mobility base in a manner that maximizes the user's independence. For example, if the seat is mounted too high in the frame, this prevents individuals from using their legs for transfers or propulsion. Accessories such as arm-support troughs and head rests must also be added, as necessary. Leg and foot rests must be correctly oriented to support and stabilize the lower limbs, particularly when deformities are present.

Although most seating systems are an integral part of the mobility base, some—notably, the Gillette spinal seating orthosis—are specially designed to function independently as well. Particularly for pediatric patients, this approach permits proper positioning in the classroom, home environment, automobile, and school bus, without the person being confined to the same wheelchair during all waking hours.

[NOTE: The segment on Overview of Orthoses is adapted in part from Michael JW, "Orthotic Treatment of Neurological Deficits" in Good DC and Couch JR, *Handbook of Neurorehabilitation,* Marcel Decker, Inc; NY, 1994 and Michael JW, "Lower Limb Orthoses: Overview of Principles, Materials, & Components" in Goldberg B and Hsu J, *Atlas of Orthoses and Assistive Devices: Third Edition*, Mosby, Philadelphia 1997 - with permission.]

SUGGESTED READINGS

Bergen AF, Presperin J, Tallman T: *Positioning for Function: Wheelchairs and Other Assistive Technologies.* Valhalla, NY: Valhalla Rehabilitation Publications, Ltd.; 1990.

Bowker P, Condie DN, Bader DL, Pratt DJ: *Biomechanical Basis of Orthotic Management.* Oxford: Butterworth Heinemann; 1993.

Bunch WH, Patwardhan AG: *Scoliosis: Making Clinical Decisions.* St. Louis: Mosby; 1989.

Cooper PR, (ed): *Management of Posttraumatic Spinal Instability.* Park Ridge, IL: American Association of Neurological Surgeons; 1990.

Goldberg B, Hsu JD (eds): *Atlas of Orthoses and Assistive Devices,* 3d ed. St. Louis: Mosby; 1997.

Yarkony GM, (ed): *Spinal Cord Injury: Medical Management and Rehabilitation.* Gaithersburg, MD: Aspen Publishers; 1994.

Chapter 146

PEDIATRIC RHEUMATOLOGY

Kathleen A. Haines

JUVENILE IDIOPATHIC ARTHRITIS

It has long been recognized that juvenile rheumatoid arthritis (JRA), also known as juvenile idiopathic arthritis (JIA), is markedly different from adult rheumatoid arthritis in presentation. Moreover, this ostensibly single diagnosis has several distinct subtypes, each of which also differ by age of onset, clinical presentation, and typical outcome. In addition, these same conditions have been given different names in various parts of the world. To distinguish these distinct syndromes better, the International League Against Rheumatism (ILAR), in 1994, organized a task force to classify the juvenile arthritides. Although the reclassification system proposed (Fink and Fernandez-Vina, 1995) will not be adopted until it has been validated against the current ARA (now American College of Rheumatology) and EULAR (European League Against Rheumatism) criteria, it is clear that the term JRA will be abandoned in the near future. This chapter, therefore, will avoid the term "rheumatoid" except as it implies a parallel with adult-type RA, but will continue to follow the currently used classifications.

CRITERIA FOR CLASSIFICATION

JIA is first and foremost a diagnosis of exclusion. All other potential causes must be first ruled out before idiopathic arthritis can be entertained. JIA is defined as follows: (1) onset before age 16; (2) manifest by arthritis (joint swelling, tenderness, and/or loss of motion not due to mechanical derangement) in at least one joint; and (3) persis-

tent for 6 weeks or more. Currently recognized classifications of JIA include systemic onset, polyarticular arthritis-rheumatoid factor (RF) negative, polyarticular arthritis-RF positive, oligoarticular arthritis, and the seronegative arthritis with enthesitis (SEA) syndromes, including juvenile spondyloarthritis, inflammatory bowel disease, Reiter's syndrome, and psoriatic arthritis (Table 146-1).

ETIOLOGY

As with most of the rheumatologic diseases, the etiology of JIA is unknown. Historically, these arthritides were believed to be a chronic infection, with organisms such as *Mycoplasma pneumoniae* and *M. tuberculosis* as leading candidates, and led to the use of such agents as injectable gold salts, antibiotics, and antimalarial drugs as treatment for arthritis. All of these drugs have some efficacy; however, their anti-arthritic effects most likely derive from additional anti-inflammatory properties rather than microbicidal ones.

With the growth of immunology, the juvenile arthritides were next believed to be a pure autoimmune response; that is, the immune system had a genetically coded "programming error" that caused the immune system to attack the joints. This hypothesis was supported by the discovery that susceptibility to the various types of juvenile arthritides is linked to different HLA molecules, known at the time as "transplantation antigens." Family studies, including those of identical twins, simultaneously supported and negated this hypothesis: although concordance for arthritis is, at best, 50 percent in twin pairs and siblings sharing HLA alleles, this figure is far greater than the

---

Table 146-1

Selected Clinical and Laboratory Manifestations of the Juvenile Arthritides

Disease	Female to Male Ratio	Age at Onset	Fever	Arthritis	WBC	ESR	RF	ANA
Systemic Onset	1:1	All ages	+++	May be late	+++	+++	Negative	<10%
Polyarticular								
-RF-negative	3:1	Often <5y	− to ++	At onset	++	++	Negative	25–50%
-RF-positive	5:1	Often >10y	− to +	At onset/erosive	++	++	Positive	50–75%
Oligoarticular	4:1	1–5 yrs.	−	At onset	Normal	Normal	Negative	50–75%
SEA syndromes	1:5	>6 yrs.	− to ++	Insidious onset	nl to ++	nl to ++	Negative	Negative
Psoriatic arthritis	1.5:1	All ages	−	Insidious onset	Normal	nl to +	Negative	15–25%

NOTE: −, absent; +, mild; ++, moderate; +++, high.

incidence in the general population. Thus, genetic susceptibility is necessary but not sufficient for the development of the arthritides; what is required are "genes and something else."

Over the last 10 years, we have learned much about the genes of autoimmunity. The proteins encoded by the HLA genes are uniquely involved in activating immune effector cells and define what antigens to which one can respond. However, the "something else" of autoimmunity remains open to question. Three potential models for arthritis follow. Evidence for JIA as a chronic infection remains scattered through the literature, with Lyme arthritis as the prototypical example. In this model, the affected host is genetically less able to clear the infecting agent than the general population. Hence, the intraarticular infection and resultant arthritis persist. The second model proposes that JIA is triggered by infection with an agent that displays antigens which are cross-reactive with joint tissue, most recently exemplified by heat-shock proteins. In this model, the affected host produces a vigorous immune response to these antigens and, whereas the infection is cleared, the immune response persists and the arthritis becomes chronic. A third model has been entertained whereby a bacterial toxin (superantigen) or local trauma acts as a nonspecific immune adjuvant. In genetically susceptible individuals, immune tolerance to joint antigens is thus broken and arthritis results. Whether any or all of these models trigger immune arthritis remains to be determined.

SYSTEMIC ONSET ARTHRITIS (SYSTEMIC ARTHRITIS)

Clinical Features

Systemic onset arthritis, or Still's disease, can present at any time from infancy through adolescence. It affects males and females in an equal ratio. Systemic onset arthritis is marked by fevers to 39° C or more, which typically peak once or twice daily and rapidly return to normal (quotidian fevers). Classically, a macular, erythematous, or salmon-colored rash distributed on the trunk and proximal extremities appears during the fever spikes. Hepatosplenomegaly, carditis, and/or serositis may occur. The arthritis may not be evident at the onset of Still's disease; it often presents weeks to months afterward and more rarely commences a year or more after systemic symptoms have begun. Associated inflammatory uveitis is extremely rare in systemic onset arthritis (see Table 146-1).

Laboratory Findings

Typical laboratory features in children with systemic onset arthritis include anemia (hemoglobin 10 mg/dl or less), an elevated white blood cell count (15 to >20,000/mm³) with the increase primarily in polymorphonuclear leukocytes, and a marked thrombocytosis. All acute phase indicators—erythrocyte sedimentation rate, C-reactive protein, the complement components C3 and C4, as well as others—are extremely elevated. RF is negative; anti-nuclear antibody is usually negative or in low titer. Arthrocentesis usually reveals inflammatory joint fluid with a cell count that may be as high as 25,000/mm³, principally neutrophils.

Other Diseases

As a monoarticular arthritis presenting within days of the onset of other systemic symptoms, systemic onset arthritis may be extremely difficult to distinguish from septic arthritis or osteomyelitis with effusion. Negative cultures of joint fluid and blood coupled with a lack of response to antibiotics may be required to differentiate between these diseases. Acute leukemias can mimic systemic onset arthritis

with no distinguishing laboratory features. Serum-sickness, like drug reactions, can mimic systemic arthritis; however, these are frequently accompanied by a rash that is not typical for systemic onset arthritis. Systemic lupus erythematosus and dermatomyositis can appear as a polyarthritis with systemic symptoms, but usually can be distinguished by their blood chemistries and unique serologies. Absent arthritis in systemic onset disease, a vigorous search for occult infection must be made.

POLYARTICULAR JUVENILE IDIOPATHIC ARTHRITIS, RHEUMATOID FACTOR (RF) NEGATIVE

Clinical Features

Polyarticular JIA-RF− has its peak incidence between ages 1 and 3, but is not rare throughout childhood. There is an increased incidence in females, with a ratio of approximately 3:1. Polyarticular juvenile arthritis, which is defined as a chronic arthritis involving five joints or more, is a relatively symmetric arthritis involving both large and small joints. Knees, ankles, wrists, metacarpophalangeal joints, proximal interphalangeal (PIP) joints of the hands, and cervical spine are often involved early on. Involvement of the temporomandibular joint is also frequent and results in the micrognathia typical of the facies of JIA. Children with polyarticular arthritis may have systemic features with fever, weight loss, and occasional organomegaly, but are not as toxic-appearing as those with systemic onset. The typical history, common to all inflammatory arthritides, is of stiffness after morning awakening which recurs after periods of inactivity such as sitting at a desk or napping at midday. Approximately 5 percent of these patients may develop a chronic, painless uveitis with a significant risk for loss of vision.

Laboratory Findings

Children with polyarticular JIA have anemia, a normal to somewhat increased white blood cell count, and usually a thrombocytosis. They have increased acute-phase indicators such as sedimentation rate, C-reactive protein, and complement components. RF is negative; antinuclear antibodies may be positive in 25 percent or more. Quantitative immunoglobulins are often high and can be a good indicator of disease progression or remission.

Other Diseases

Lyme arthritis can present as a chronic, polyarticular arthritis, although it is more commonly a pauciarticular disease. Viral diseases such as rubella, parvovirus B19, and hepatitis, among others, can present as a polyarthritis. Acute leukemias can mimic polyarticular arthritis. Most often, the differential diagnosis includes other rheumatologic disorders such as systemic lupus erythematosus, dermatomyositis, SEA syndromes, or sarcoidosis. These can be distinguished by appropriate serum chemistry and serologic tests.

POLYARTICULAR JUVENILE IDIOPATHIC ARTHRITIS, RHEUMATOID FACTOR (RF) POSITIVE

Clinical Features

Polyarticular JIA-RF+ is the expression of classic rheumatoid arthritis in childhood. This condition is most common in females with an increasing incidence from late childhood through adolescence. Their history is one of an inflammatory arthritis as just described; the arthritis itself is symmetric, involving both large and small joints.

Rheumatoid nodules can be present; the arthritis can be either insidious in onset or quite rapidly erosive.

Laboratory Findings

A positive test for RF is required for diagnosis. Other laboratory findings are similar to those for RF-negative disease.

Other Diseases

As with RF-negative arthritis, the primary diagnoses are aforementioned rheumatologic disorders. In adolescents, however, gonococcal arthritis can present in this manner. Subacute bacterial endocarditis can also present with fever, positive RF, and arthritis and must always be considered in the differential diagnosis.

PAUCIARTICULAR JUVENILE IDIOPATHIC ARTHRITIS (OLIGOARTHRITIS)

Clinical Features

Pauciarticular JIA is the most common form of the idiopathic childhood arthritides, accounting for approximately 50 percent of the cases. It has a peak incidence at 2 years of age and females outnumber males by approximately 4:1. Pauciarticular arthritis, which is defined as four or fewer involved joints, is often monoarticular, with the knee as the joint most commonly affected. Approximately 20 percent of children with pauciarticular arthritis develop the chronic painless uveitis that puts their vision at risk. The uveitis usually develops within the first 5 years of the disease, but may either antecede the arthritis or develop years later.

Laboratory Findings

Most of these children have no laboratory abnormalities indicative of inflammatory disease. However, anti-nuclear antibodies may be positive in over 50 percent; this subgroup is at highest risk for development of uveitis.

Other Diseases

Lyme arthritis, septic arthritis, osteomyelitis with effusion, as well as tumors can present as monoarticular arthritis and must be considered in the differential diagnosis. Serologic studies, blood and joint cultures, and imaging studies should distinguish these diseases.

SERONEGATIVE ENTHESITIS WITH ARTHRITIS (SEA) SYNDROMES

The SEA syndromes—which include reactive arthritis, Reiter's disease, psoriatic arthritis, inflammatory bowel disease, and juvenile spondyloarthritis—are a group of diseases that present with similar oligoarticular findings, but appear to have distinct etiologies.

Clinical Features

These arthritides present as asymmetric large and small joint involvement, primarily of the lower extremities, and may include the axial skeleton. Inflammation at the entheses, particularly at the insertions of the Achilles tendon and the plantar fascia, is a hallmark of these diseases. Other than psoriatic arthritis, the SEA syndromes are more common in males, with a male–female ratio of approximately 5:1; they typically appear in children older than age 6. Reactive arthritis and Reiter's disease (conjunctivitis, urethritis, and arthritis)

may appear within weeks following a bout of infectious diarrhea. These are both often self-limited syndromes; Reiter's, however, can be an idiopathic, chronic arthropathy. Psoriatic arthritis may frequently appear before the skin manifestations and is diagnosed by identifying nail changes such as pitting and onycholysis along with a family history of psoriasis. Inflammatory bowel disease may be an occult finding with arthritis, systemic symptoms (weight loss, fever, and anemia), and erythema nodosum as a clinical presentation. Juvenile ankylosing spondylitis may be indistinguishable clinically from pauciarticular arthritis except the sex and age are atypical. Sacroiliac involvement is a distinguishing characteristic, but often appears later in the disease. All of these diseases may have associated acute or chronic inflammatory uveitis.

Laboratory Findings

The indices of acute inflammation are elevated: mild thrombocytosis, increased erythrocyte sedimentation rate, increased C-reactive protein, and complement components as examples. RF and antinuclear antibodies are usually negative.

TREATMENT

Anti-inflammatory (rather than analgesic) doses of nonsteroidal anti-inflammatory agents are used as first-line therapy in all these disorders. These drugs may require 6 weeks of use before maximal efficacy may be achieved. Second-line agents include hydroxychloroquine, sulfasalazine, and methotrexate. Oral prednisone should be reserved for unremitting symptoms of systemic JIA and rarely as a stopgap measure while waiting for other slower-acting drugs to take effect.

ACUTE RHEUMATIC FEVER

ETIOLOGY

Despite the knowledge since the 1930s that acute rheumatic fever (ARF) is a sequelae of infection with *Streptococcus pyogenes*, or group A beta-hemolytic streptococci, its molecular pathogenesis remains a mystery. Twin studies, HLA associations, and B-cell antigen associations have confirmed a genetic predisposition. Moreover, patients with rheumatic fever make much higher antibody titers to streptococcal antigens than do unaffected individuals. In addition, antibodies to streptococcal proteins bind to heart and areas of the central nervous system. However, none of these antibodies are cytotoxic; thus, their causality is unlikely. In sum, whereas the etiologic agent is clear, the mechanism of disease is not.

CLINICAL FEATURES

Acute rheumatic fever typically affects children between the ages of 5 and 12 years; it is extremely rare in children younger than age 3. A streptococcal pharyngitis antecedes the disease by 2 to 5 weeks, although this often is a subclinical infection. ARF presents as a migratory, painful arthritis primarily affecting the large joints, typically knees, ankles, elbows, and wrists, although small joints of the hands and feet are often involved as well. Children with ARF are frequently quite ill with high fever and malaise. Associated carditis can be life-threatening. ARF has an associated macular rash with well-defined, "snake-like" borders known as erythema marginatum. This rash appears primarily on the trunk and proximal extremities. Like the arthritis, it is migratory and often quite transient. Diagnosis of definite ARF

Table 146-2

Jones Criteria (Revised) for the Diagnosis of Acute Rheumatic Fever[a]

I. Major Criteria
   A. Carditis
   B. Polyarthritis
   C. Chorea
   D. Erythema marginatum
   E. Subcutaneous nodules

II. Minor Criteria
   A. Fever
   B. Arthralgia
   C. Previous ARF or rheumatic heart disease
   D. Elevated ESR or positive CRP
   E. Prolonged P-R interval

---

[a]Plus evidence of preceding streptococcal infection: positive throat culture, increased antistreptococcal antibody titer, recent scarlet fever.

is made by use of the modified Jones criteria (Table 146-2), requiring evidence of a streptococcal infection *and* the presence of two major criteria or one major criterion and two minor criteria.

LABORATORY FINDINGS

In ARF, the indices of acute inflammation are quite elevated. As children often have a chronically elevated titer of anti-strep antibodies, a modest elevation in these enzymes is not helpful. Therefore, antistreptolysin O (or other strep-related antibodies such as anti-DNase B or antihyaluronidase) should be very high or demonstrate a significant change in titer (either increase or decrease) that will indicate a recent infection. Throat cultures may be positive for strep.

OTHER DISEASES

Systemic JIA, septic arthritis, or viral arthritis may be confused with ARF, but the migratory nature of the arthritis, after a period of observation, should distinguish ARF from these disorders. Bacterial endocarditis must be considered, but should reveal itself with positive blood cultures.

TREATMENT

Salicylates at anti-inflammatory doses are the drug of choice for treatment of ARF and should be continued until the C-reactive protein is normal. The presumed streptococcal infection should be treated with 10 days of oral penicillin or a depot injection. Prophylaxis of 1.2 million units of benzathine penicillin G administered intramuscularly should be given monthly to prevent recurrences. Oral prophylaxis with sulfadiazine or penicillin can be used successfully as well. If carditis was not a feature of the disease, most authors agree that prophylaxis can be stopped by age 18. However, if carditis was present, injections are recommended every 3 weeks, and the duration of the prophylaxis has been recommended for life by some authors and through the fourth decade by others.

SUGGESTED READINGS

Amigo M-C, Martinez-Lavin M, Reyes PA: Acute rheumatic fever. *Rheum Dis Clin North Am* 1993; 19:333.

Anonymous [Committee on Rheumatic Fever, Endocarditis and Kawasaki Disease of the Council on Cardiovascular Disease in the Young of the American Heart Association]: Guidelines for the diagnosis of rheumatic fever: Jones criteria, 1992 update. *JAMA* 1992; 268:2069 Erratum: *JAMA* 1993; 27:2084].

Anonymous [Criteria Subcommittee of the Diagnostic and Therapeutic Criterial Committee of the American Rheumatism Association Section of the Arthritis Foundation]: Current proposed revision of JRA criteria. *Arthritis Rheum* 1977; 20:195.

Bisno AL: Acute rheumatic fever: A present-day perspective. *Medicine* 1993; 72:278.

Boog CJ, de Graeff-Meeder ER, Lucassen MA, et al: Two monoclonal antibodies generated against human hsp60 show reactivity with synovial membranes of patients with juvenile chronic arthritis. *J Exp Med* 1992; 175:1805.

Clemens LE, Albert E, Ansell BM: Sibling pairs affected by chronic arthritis of childhood: Evidence for a genetic predisposition. *J Rheumatol* 1985; 12:108.

De Graeff-Meeder ER, van der Zee R, Rijkers GT, et al: Recognition of human 60kD heat shock protein by mononuclear cells from patients with juvenile chronic arthritis. *Lancet* 1991; 337:1368.

De Inocencio J, Giannini EH, Glass DN: Can genetic markers contribute to the classification of juvenile rheumatoid arthritis? *J Rheum* 1993; 20 (suppl 40):12.

Dresner E: Aetiology and pathogenesis of rheumatoid arthritis. *Am J Med* 1955; 18:74.

Fink CW, Fernandez-Vina M: The genetics of juvenile rheumatoid arthritis. *Bull Rheum* Dis 1995; 44:5.

Friedman SM, Tumang JR, Crow MK: Microbial superantigens as etiopathogenic agents in autoimmunity. *Rheum Dis Clin North Am* 1993; 19:207.

McCarty M: Evidence for the relationship of group A streptococcal infections to rheumatic fever. In Cruickshank R, Glynn A, eds. *Rheumatic Fever Epidemiology and Prevention.* Oxford: Blackwell; 1959:65.

Ostrov BE, Goldsmith DP, Athreya BH: Differentiation of systemic juvenile rheumatoid arthritis from acute leukemia near the onset of disease. *J Pediatr* 1993; 122:595.

Rose CD, Doughty RA: Pharmacological management of juvenile rheumatoid arthritis. *Drugs* 1992; 43:849.

Rosenberg AM, Petty RE: A syndrome of seronegative enthesopathy and arthropathy in children. *Arthritis Rheum* 1982; 25:1041.

Steere AC, Malawista SE, Snydman DR, et al: Lyme arthritis: An epidemic of oligoarticular arthritis in children and adults in three Connecticut communities. *Arthritis Rheum* 1977; 20:7.

Chapter 147

ADULT RHEUMATOLOGY

Paula J. Rackoff

A patient's joint complaints may arise from the joint itself, from the periarticular area, or from elsewhere in the musculoskeletal system. The first step in assessing whether arthritis is the source of a patient's complaints is to determine if there is pain, swelling, and/or tenderness localized to the joint and whether there is decreased range of motion and/or deformity of the joint. Once arthritis is determined to be present in a particular joint, the remainder of the musculoskeletal system should be examined to determine (a) if this is a monoarticular, pauciarticular (one to four joints), or polyarticular process, and (b) if this is an inflammatory or noninflammatory arthritis. A careful physical exam, data obtained from laboratory analysis of blood and synovial fluid, plain radiographs, high resolution imaging techniques, and even immunogenetic analysis can be employed to make a specific diagnosis.

The most common causes of monoarthritides are relatively limited and treatable. In the adult this usually falls into one of the following categories: trauma, infection, crystal induced, or an initial presentation of a polyarticular disease. Unless it is certain that a patient's complaints are secondary to a polyarticular process, arthrocentesis should be performed, as synovial fluid analysis can be helpful and at times diagnostic. Microscopic findings can be specific for gout (monosodium urate crystals), pseudogout (calcium pyrophosphate crystals), infectious arthritis (positive gram stain for bacteria), and trauma (grossly bloody fluid).

The appearance of synovial fluid and the cell count are helpful in distinguishing different arthritides but are rarely diagnostic (Table 147-1). The synovial fluid of a normal joint is clear and has a white blood cell count of less than 200 WBC/mm^3. Clear fluid is commonly seen in osteoarthritis, cloudy fluid in inflammatory arthritis, and pu-

rulent fluid in infection. A high cell count (>50,000 with a predominance of polymorphs) is indicative of crystal-induced synovitis or infection. Infection can only be excluded by Gram's stain and culture of the aspirated fluid. Infection may accompany crystal induced arthritis, inflammatory arthritis, and traumatic arthritis. When the history and physical exam even suggest the possibility of infection, the patient should be treated for such until cultures are known.

A persistent monoarthritis without evidence of infection, crystals, trauma, or polyarthritis requires evaluation by MRI or CT scan and possibly synovial biopsy. The differential diagnosis for such a clinical situation includes pigmented villonodular synovitis, infiltrative diseases (amyloidosis), granulomatous diseases, and synovial malignancy.

Polyarthritis can be separated into noninflammatory, inflammatory, and metabolic causes. The history, physical exam, and certain laboratory tests are necessary to arrive at a diagnosis.

NONINFLAMMATORY ARTHRITIDES

This group of arthritides includes the general category of osteoarthritis (OA) and the diseases that can be associated with OA (acromegaly, Gaucher's, Wilson's, hemochromatosis, ochronosis), neuropathic arthropathy, acute rheumatic fever, and local joint disturbances (aseptic necrosis, osteochondromatosis).

OSTEOARTHRITIS

Osteoarthritis (OA) is the most common musculoskeletal problem in people over 50 years of age. Patients typically complain of pain, stiff-

---

Table 147-1

Synovial Fluid Analysis

Classification	Disease	Color	WBC/mm^3	%Polys
Normal	Normal	Yellow	<200	<25
Noninflammatory	OA	Yellow	<2000	<2.5
	Trauma	Pink/red	<2000	<25
Inflammatory	SLE	Yellow	0–9000	<25
	Acute rheumatic fever	Yellow	0–60,000	25–50
	Pseudogout	White/yellow	50,000–75,000	90
	Gout	White/yellow	100,000–160,000	90
	RA	Yellow/purulent	3000–50,000	50–75
Infectious	TB	Purulent	2500–100,000	50
	Bacterial	Purulent	50,000–300,000	>90

ness, joint enlargement or deformity, decreased range of motion, and palpable grating of the joint (i.e., crepitus). The two major clinical subsets of the disease are primary osteoarthritis and secondary osteoarthritis. In both forms of OA, the initial insult begins in the articular cartilage. Focal areas of damage lead to articular cartilage softening, vertical clefts, and ulcerations of the articular cartilage. This leads to histologic changes of sclerosis, cyst formation, bone thickening, and neoformation of bone and cartilage.

In addition to fibrillation described above, histologic changes in progressive OA include loss of proteoglycan staining and clumping of chondrocytes into clones. Eventually, there is destruction of the collagen network with exposure of underlying bone. Destruction of the matrix is mediated by metalloproteinases (collagenase, gelatinase, and stomelysin) and cysteine proteinases (cathepsins L, B, and N). When cartilage damage extends to the subchondral bone, attempts at repair do take place with the formation of fibrocartilage in the place of the prior articular cartilage.

There are several factors that contribute to the development of OA:

1. Mechanical factors: Secondary to wear and tear from repetitive microtrauma or congenital/developmental abnormalities in joint shape (Legg-Calvé-Perthes, slipped capital epiphysis).
2. Genetic factors: Particularly Heberden's nodes in women (associated with HLA A1-B8) and with monozygotic alpha 1 antitrypsin phenotypes.
3. Age: The prevalence of osteoarthritis increases with age in all populations studied. Alterations in proteoglycans have been noted with decreased chondroitin sulfate to keratin sulfate ratio.
4. Biochemical factors: In the early stages of OA, cartilage is thicker than normal with an increased net synthesis of proteoglycans; as the disease progresses the cartilage becomes thinner and the concentration of proteoglycans decrease ultimately leading to softer cartilage.

SECONDARY OSTEOARTHRITIS

Secondary osteoarthritis stems from disorders that damage joint surfaces: prior trauma, prior inflammatory disease, prior bone disease (such as Paget's or avascular necrosis), bleeding dyscrasias, endocrinopathies, crystal diseases, ochronosis, Wilson's disease, and hemochromatosis.

BLEEDING DYSCRASIAS

Bleeding dyscrasias such as hemophilia leads to hemarthrosis in 90 percent of those with the disease, most commonly in the knee, ankle, and elbow. With recurrent bleeding into the joint, a proliferative synovitis develops. Radiologic changes include widening of the femoral intercondylar notch, squaring of the inferior patella, joint space narrowing, and large subchondral cyst formation. Skeletal manifestations of sickle cell disease are more commonly bone and periarticular pain from infarction, rather than a true arthropathy. Radiologic changes seen are secondary to hyperactive bone marrow: widening of the medullary cavity, thin cortex, and cupping of vertebrae.

ENDOCRINE DISEASES

Endocrine diseases have a myriad of musculoskeletal manifestations. Table 147-2 indicates the major rheumatic symptoms of the most common endocrinopathies.

NEUROPATHIC ARTHROPATHY

Neuropathic arthropathy has characteristic clinical and radiologic features. Neurologic disease of the spinal cord or peripheral nerves can lead to a neurologic deficit in the area of a particular joint. The affected joint is characterized by soft tissue swelling, joint laxity, and instability, all of which are painless. Radiograph examination reveals joint destruction with osteopenia, and both bone resorption and proliferation leading to the appearance of a "disorganized joint." The joint(s) affected depend on the underlying neuropathy. Diabetes most commonly affects the foot, syringomyelia the large joints of the upper limbs, and tabes dorsalis the large joints of the lower limbs.

The treatment options for a neuropathic joint are very limited. Treatment of the neurologic disease is indicated but has no effect on the arthropathy already present. Joint replacements are generally contraindicated because of the poor quality of the bone. Joint protection is mandatory. Immobilization of the joint with braces or external supports should be done as soon as possible. If after conservative treatment with nonweightbearing a joint is still unstable, arthrodesis can be considered. However, joint fusions of a neuropathic joint may fail because of nonunion.

OCHRONOSIS

Ochronosis is a rare autosomal recessive disorder resulting from a lack of homogentisic acid oxidase and the subsequent accumulation of its substrate in cartilage, skin, and sclera. The earliest symptoms of ochronotic arthritis is limitation of movement of the hips, knees, or shoulders with episodes of acute inflammation. Joint space narrowing, marked subchondral sclerosis, osteophytes, and loose bodies are commonly seen on radiograph. In late ochronosis there is marked limitation of movement of the spine with typical wafer-like calcifications in the intervertebral discs.

WILSON'S DISEASE

Wilson's disease (disorder of copper metabolism) manifests in the musculoskeletal system as premature osteoarthritis, pseudogout, and chondromalacia.

OSTEONECROSIS

Osteonecrosis (ON) is the term used to describe the final common pathway of a number of conditions which lead to ischemia of bone. Although this impairment of blood supply can happen in any bone, the femoral head and condyles are the most common and severe locations of osteonecrosis. Anatomic, inflammatory, and metabolic diseases can lead to necrosis. Revascularization leads to resorption of dead bone, diminished bone stock, and eventual bony collapse. Conditions associated with osteonecrosis are listed in Table 147-3.

Stages of the disease have radiologic and clinical characteristics which parallel one another.

Stage 0: Asymptomatic patient; plain film, bone scan, MRI all normal, but osteonecrosis seen histologically.
Stage 1: Asymptomatic patient with normal plain films, but cold spot seen on radionuclide bone scan or double band on T2-weighted MRI.
Stage 2: Mild pain; radiographs reveal sclerosis, cysts, osteopenia without collapse.
Stage 3: Moderate pain; radiographic "crescent sign" signifying osteochondral fractures and collapse.
Stage 4: Severe pain; advanced subchondral collapse and joint destruction.

Medical treatment of ON is limited to reducing activity, encouraging nonweightbearing, and maintaining range of motion, all of which can help patients with stage 1 disease, and sometimes those with stage 2 disease. Core decompression is advocated in some institutions for stages 1 and 2, but is not universally accepted. In late stages with evidence of collapse, total hip replacement is recommended. Bone graft or osteotomy is recommended in intermediate stages, particularly in unilateral cases with controlled and treated causative factors.

OSTEOCHONDROMATOSIS

Osteochondromatosis is a rare disorder presenting as monoarticular arthritis. For reasons that are unclear, cartilage formation occurs within the synovium. Primary osteochondromatosis is thought to reflect metaplastic changes of fibroblasts into cartilage-making cells. Secondary osteochondromatosis can result from trauma and osteoarthritis. Radiologically, the two forms are identical with multiple loose bodies seen within joint cavities. The knee is the most com-

Table 147-2

Major Rheumatic Symptoms of Common Endocrinopathies

Endocrinopathy	Rheumatic Manifestation
Hyperthyroidism[a]	Muscle weakness with normal CPK; thyroid acropachy: periostitis of the metacarpals causing diffusely swollen hands
Hypothyroidism[a]	Muscle weakness with increased CPK Symmetric joint swelling mimicking rheumatoid arthritis Hyperuricemia Calcium pyrophosphate deposition
Hyperparathyroidism	Diffuse arthralgias and stiffness Subperiosteal bone resorption Hyperuricemia Calcium pyrophosphate deposition Osteitis fibrosa cystica
Hypoparathyroidism	Short metacarpals/metatarsals
Hyperpituitarism (acromegaly)	Increased muscle mass leading to myopathy Cartilage hypertrophy leading to joint space narrowing Hypermobility
Hypopituitarism	Short stature
Hyperadrenalism	Osteoporosis Avascular necrosis Proximal muscle weakness with normal CPK
Hypoadrenalism	Severe muscle cramps
Diabetes	Charcot joints Dupuytren's contracture Palmar fasciitis Cheiroarthropathy Decreased joint mobility
Hemochromatosis	Calcium pyrophosphate deposition "Hooks" on 2d and 3d metacarpophalangeal joints

[a]Note that with treatment of hypo- or hyperthyroid states, mild to moderate myalgias and arthralgias are common.

NOTE: CPK, creatine kinase.

Table 147-3

Diseases Associated with Osteonecrosis

Trauma

Alcoholism

Congenital malformations

Hemoglobinopathies

Vasculitis/Vasculopathy

Corticosteroids

Cushing's syndrome

Caisson's disease

Infiltrative bone marrow diseases (e.g., Gaucher's)

Arteriosclerosis

Pregnancy

Hypercoagulable states

Fat embolism

Diabetes

---

monly affected joint, followed by the hip and elbow. Treatment options depend on the extent of the disease and disability of the patient; they range from observation to complete removal of the loose bodies and synovectomy.

INFLAMMATORY ARTHRITIDES

CRYSTAL-INDUCED DISEASE

Crystal-induced disease can cause both monoarticular and polyarticular arthropathies. Uric acid, calcium pyrophosphate, and calcium hydroxyapatite are the most common crystals which lead to arthritis (Fig. 147-1).

Hyperuricemia results from a disorder of purine metabolism or from abnormal excretion of uric acid. Primary gout refers to cases that appear to be inborn or not secondary to another acquired disease. In only 1 percent of primary gout patients enzyme deficiencies are found (deficiency of hypoxanthine-guanine phosphoribosyl transferase or increased activity of phosphoribosylpyrophosphate synthetase). Both enzyme deficiencies are X-linked and present in early adulthood with an increased incidence of kidney stones. Most primary gout patients fall into the idiopathic category as no precise metabolic defect can be isolated. Secondary gout refers to those cases which develop in the course of another disease or secondary to drugs (Table 147-4).

The diagnosis of gout can be made by history, physical examination (Fig. 147-2), and most importantly, examination of the synovial fluid by compensated polarized microscopy. If carefully sought, uric acid crystals can be found in 85 percent of acute gout patients. Under polarized light urate crystals appear yellow when parallel to the axis of the red compensator and blue when perpendicular to the axis. The urate crystals are slender and needle shaped. Although serum uric acid level is usually elevated, it is normal in about 10 percent of patients and therefore cannot be used to make a definitive diagnosis of gout.

The differential diagnosis to be considered in suspected gouty arthritis includes a septic arthritis, trauma, pseudogout, and atypical rheumatoid arthritis. Gout and pseudogout can occur together in the same joint.

The response to treatment of gout is usually quite dramatic. For most patients nonsteroidal anti-inflammatory agents (NSAIDs) are the drugs of choice. Although indomethacin is the NSAID most commonly used, all the other NSAIDs have successfully been used as alternative agents provided they are used in appropriate doses. Indomethacin, however, is also available in suppository form for those patients unable to tolerate the oral form. Generally, 50 mg of indomethacin four times per day is an effective dose for an acute attack with a tapering schedule as the attack abates.

Oral colchicine is still used for an acute attack of gout; however, it often causes diarrhea at the doses needed to control an acute attack. Intravenous colchicine is recommended in those patients with peptic ulcer disease and in those in whom the salt-retaining effects of NSAIDs should be avoided. While intravenous colchicine is efficacious, it should be used with caution as its potential side effects are serious: local extravasation leading to necrosis, bone marrow toxicity, myopathy, and neuropathy.

Glucocorticoids can be injected intraarticularly into the involved joint. Pain relief is usually quite prompt, but concomitant treatment with an NSAID or colchicine is usually necessary. Patients who have failed to respond to colchicine or NSAIDs, or when these medications are contraindicated, may be treated with systemic steroids in the form of intramuscular corticotrophin (recommended dosage of 40 to 80 IU in a single IM injection) or oral corticosteroids (recommended dosage of oral prednisone is 40 mg/day initially for 3 to 5 days followed by a slow taper by 5 mg decreases over 10 to 14 days).

Prophylactic therapy is aimed at the prevention of recurrent attacks. Although colchicine is highly effective in reducing the frequency of attacks, only correction of the underlying hyperuricemia can alter the tendency to gouty attacks. The drugs used to correct hyperuricemia act either by promoting renal excretion of urate (uricosuric drugs) or by inhibiting xanthine oxidase and thereby decreasing urate production (allopurinol). Although underexcretion of uric acid is much more common than overproduction, many patients show features of both processes. The xanthine oxidase inhibitor allopurinol may be used in most situations to lower uric acid even when there is urate underexcretion. Uricosuric agents (probenecid, sulfinpyrazone) should be avoided in renal insufficiency, renal colic, and if there is an inadequate urine volume. The uricosurics are most commonly used when there is an allergy to allopurinol.

Asymptomatic hyperuricemia has not been shown to lead to renal disease or joint deformity. Therefore, long-term urate-lowering drug therapy is not recommended.

In tophaceous gout, the principle of treatment is to lower the plasma urate concentration so that urate is resorbed from the surface of the tophi. Surgery is rarely indicated for tophi except in the unusual situations where they become infected, interfere with joint function, or exert pressure on an important structure (e.g., the spinal cord).

PSEUDOGOUT

Pseudogout is an inflammatory arthropathy caused by deposition of calcium pyrophosphate dihydrate (CPPD). The CPPD crystals are shed into the joint, phagocytized by leukocytes which release lysosomal enzymes, resulting in an acute inflammatory response. The classic acute synovitis of pseudogout is the most common cause of monoarthritis in adults. Although any joint may be involved, the knee is the most common site. A chronic pyrophosphate arthropathy is also commonly seen in the elderly population. Joint examination generally reveals signs of osteoarthritis with superimposed synovitis most evident clinically at the knees, wrists, and shoulders.

Diseases associated with CPPD include hyperparathyroidism, hypothyroidism, hemochromatosis, hypophosphatasia, hypomagnesemia, gout, osteoarthritis, Wilson's disease, and neuropathic arthropathy.

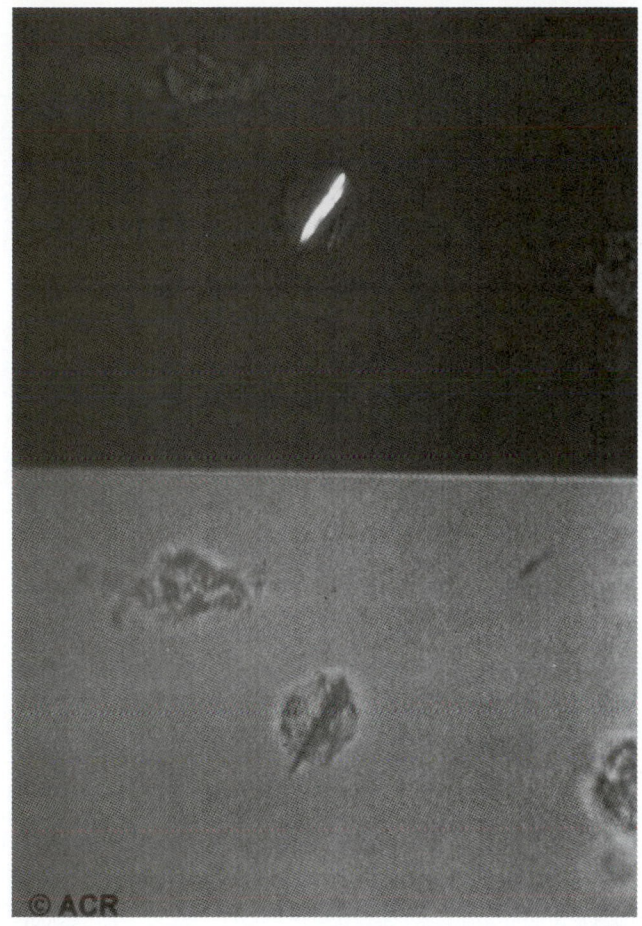

A © ACR

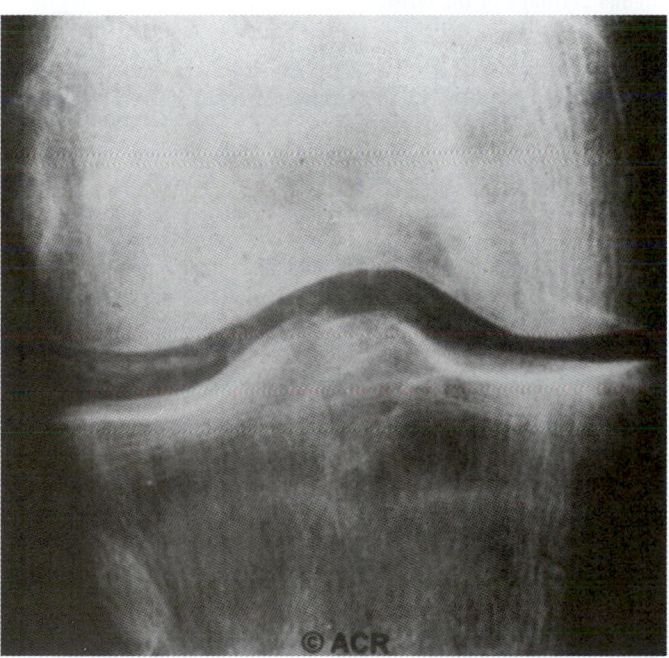

C © ACR

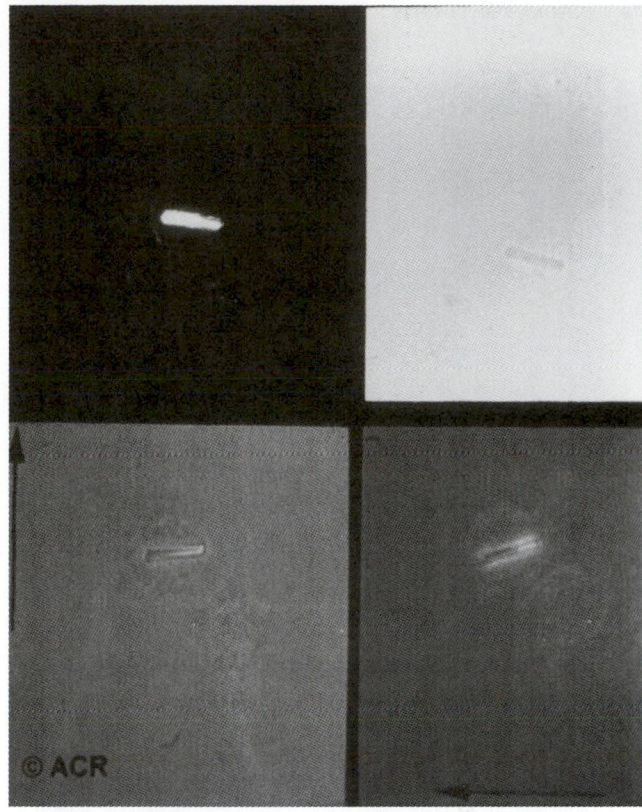

B © ACR

Figure 147-1

A. Gout: Phagocytosed urate crystals (polarized and ordinary light microscopy). *Top,* Compensated polarized light clearly demonstrates two longer crystals (approximately 13 μm) and one shorter crystal (approximately 9 μm). *Bottom,* In the same field under ordinary light, only one of the longer crystals is identifiable. These monosodium urate monohydrate crystals have been phagocytosed by a polymorphonuclear leukocyte in the joint fluid during an acute attack of gout. This image demonstrates the superiority of compensated polarized light over ordinary light microscopy when evaluating joint fluid for crystals. (Reprinted from the Clinical Slide Collection on the Rheumatic Diseases, copyright © 1991, 1995, 1997. Used by permission of the American College of Rheumatology.) *B.* Chondrocalcinosis: Calcium pyrophosphate crystals (ordinary, polarized, and compensated polarized light microscopy). This calcium pyrophosphate dihydrate crystal from synovial fluid is being engulfed by a leukocyte. The crystal is shown with regular light microscopy in the upper left view and with the addition of polarized lenses in the upper right panel. In the two lower panels, compensated polarized light microscopy is used with the crystal parallel to the plane of the compensator (*arrow*) on the left and perpendicular on the right. The crystal has weakly positive birefringence. (Reproduced with permission from the American College of Physicians *Self Learning Series*, 1978, Philadelphia.) *C.* Chondrocalcinosis: Knee (roentgenogram). This posteroanterior projection of the knee demonstrates calcification of the menisci and articular cartilage that is typical of chondrocalcinosis. The calcification is due to focal deposits of calcium pyrophosphate dihydrate crystals in articular cartilage. In this view, the deposits are more marked in the lateral compartment of the joint. Classically, both knees are involved and the calcifications, although linear, are not smooth and continuous but are interrupted by multiple focal deposits, as seen here. Statistically, the knee is the most frequent site of such calcifications and attacks of pseudogout. However, other joints may be involved. Many patients with chondrocalcinosis on roentgenogram have not had clinical attacks of pseudogout, and some patients with proven attacks of pseudogout do not have radiographic evidence of chondrocalcinosis on routine roentgenograms. (Reprinted from the Clinical Slide Collection on the Rheumatic Diseases, copyright © 1991, 1995, 1997. Used by permission of the American College of Rheumatology.)

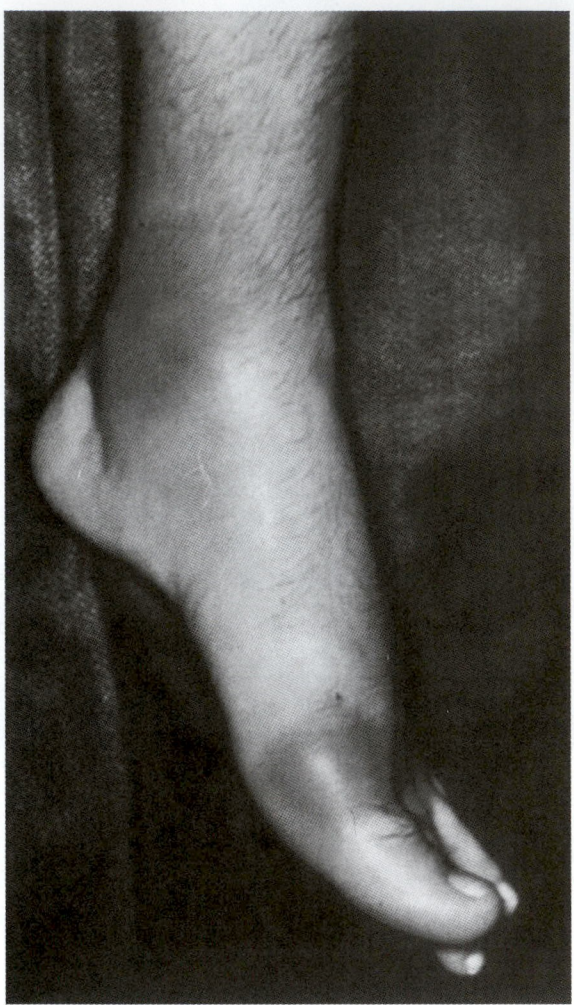

A

Table 147-4
Classification of Hyperuricemia
Overproduction of uric acid
Primary gout
Myeloproliferative disorders
Psoriasis
Chemotherapy
Hemolysis
Underexcretion of uric acid
Chronic renal failure
Drugs: Low-dose aspirin, diuretics
Lactic acidosis and ketosis
Hyperparathyroidism

CPPD crystals can be seen by compensated polarized microscopy as rhomboid shaped with weak positive birefringence. Linear or punctate radiodensities within cartilage can be identified in approximately 75 percent of patients on plain films. Sites most likely to identify the calcifications include the symphysis pubis, knee menisci, and the triangular cartilage of the wrist.

Treatment of pseudogout attacks is similar to that described above for gouty attacks. Any associated diseases such as hemochromatosis, hypothyroidism, or hyperparathyroidism should be managed, but treatment of the underlying disease may not prevent recurrent arthritis.

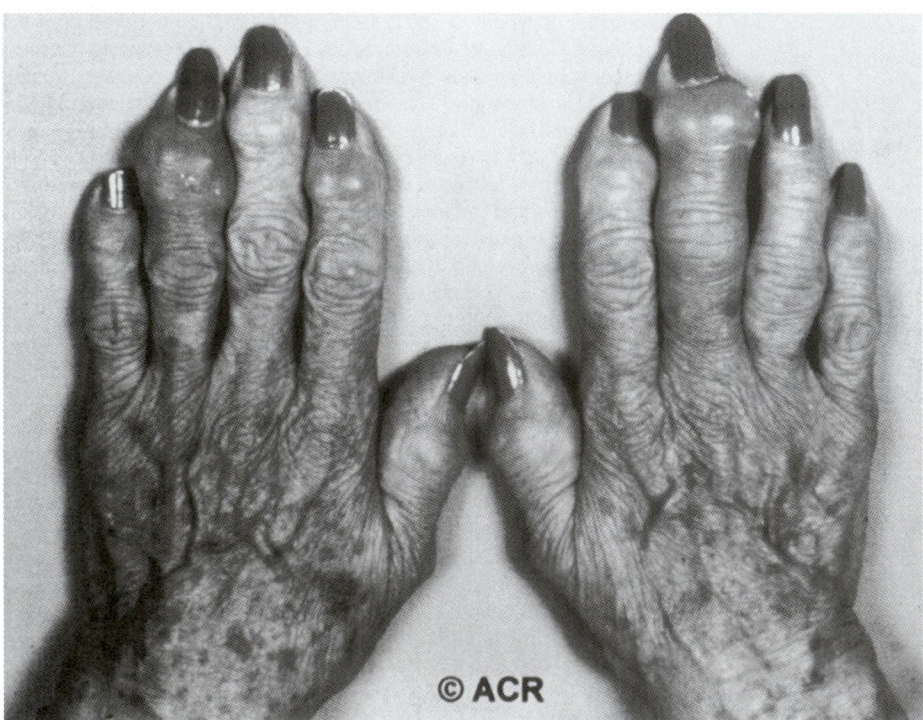

© ACR

B

Figure 147-2

A. Gout: Podagra. The base of the big toe and ankle are red, swollen, and extremely painful due to an acute attack of gout. As the attack subsides, the superficial skin may peel. Clinical findings of acute gout may be indistinguishable from acute cellulitis. *B.* Gout of distal interphalangeal joints simulating osteoarthritis. Tophaceous enlargement and erythema of the right third and left fourth distal interphalangeal joints are present. These findings may simulate and/or coexist with Heberden nodes, as is seen in the second left distal interphalangeal joint. (Reprinted from the Clinical Slide Collection on the Rheumatic Diseases, copyright © 1991, 1995, 1997. Used by permission of the American College of Rheumatology.)

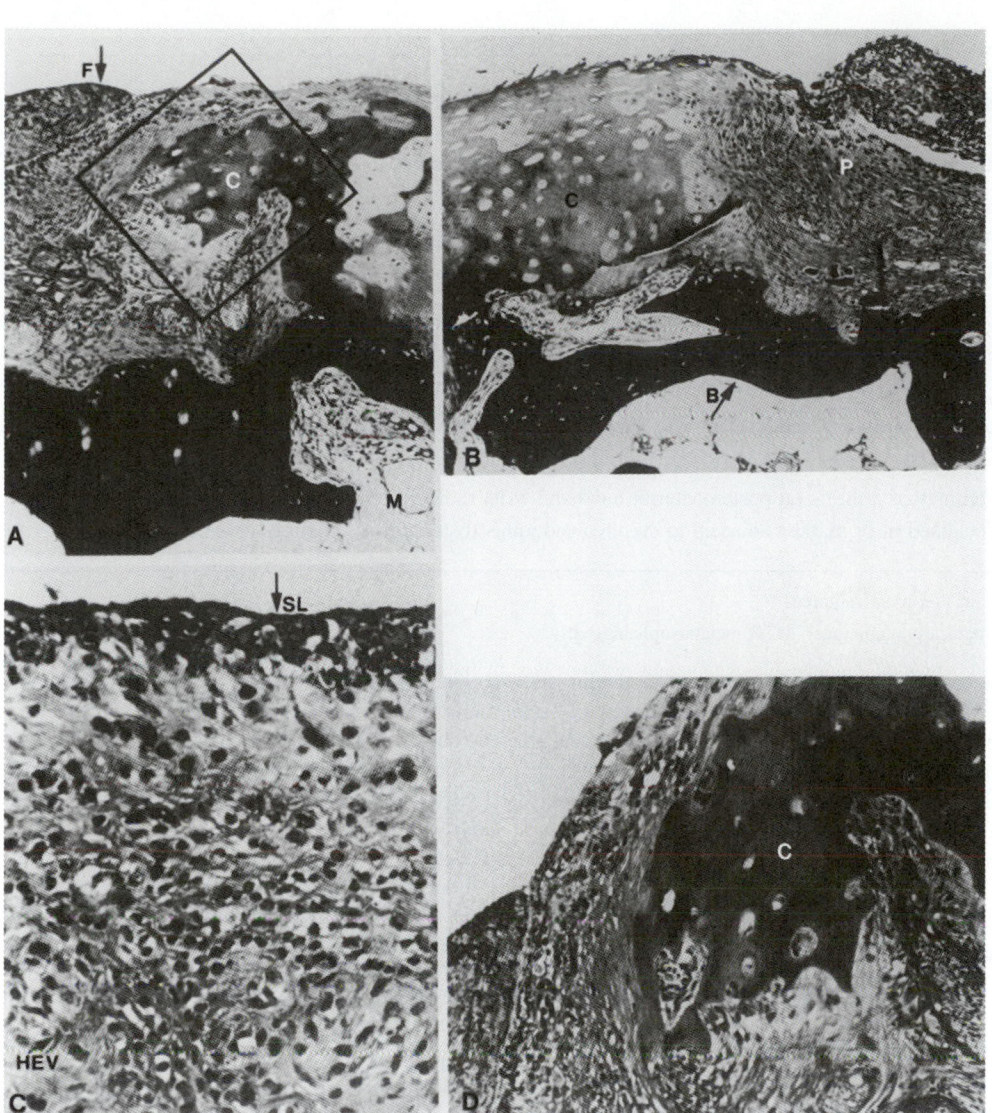

Figure 147-3
Four microscopic views of a rheumatoid metatarsal head. In *A* and *B*, the black areas represent subchondral bone (M, marrow; P, pannus; C, cartilage; the area in detail is shown in panel *D*). *A*. The heterogeneity of the invasive pannus is shown here. Whorls of proliferative synovial tissue become relatively avascular as they abut against the remaining cartilage, destroying it by proteases. *B*. A similar picture to *A*. In the ivasive pannus, there are numerous lymphocytes; individual chondrocytes that have been activated to produce proteases by cytokines. *C*. A section through synovial tissue near the invasive front. The synovial cells on the surface (*SL*), in continuity with synovial fluid, always develop a distinct morphology from sub-lining cells, even though they are, presumably, the same cell (macrophage or fibroblast). One small capillary, *eV*, shows plump, tall endothelium. *D*. Different patterns of cells surrounding cartilage being destroyed. [Reproduced with permission from Harris ED Jr: Etiology and pathogenesis of rheumatoid arthritis. In Kelley WN, Harris ED Jr, Ruddy S, et al (eds): *Textbook of Rheumatology*, 4th ed. Philadelphia: WB Saunders; 1993:863. Copyright © 1993 Edward D. Harris, Jr., M.D.]

RHEUMATOID ARTHRITIS

Rheumatoid arthritis (RA) is a chronic inflammatory disease in which an erosive, symmetrical polyarthritis leads to progressive disability and mortality. Constitutional symptoms and extraarticular manifestations add to the morbidity of the disease. The diagnosis of RA may not always be obvious as the signs and symptoms of the disease range from very mild, vague symptoms early on to severe, deforming manifestations in later years.

Although women are affected two to three times more than men, recent studies have suggested that the incidence in women may be decreasing, possibly secondary to the use of oral contraceptives and postmenopausal estrogens. RA increases in prevalence with age; the prevalence of RA is said to approximate 1 percent in the United States and Canada.

Early pathologic observations of a joint affected by RA show infiltration of the synovium with lymphocytes (primarily CD4 helper/inducer cells), plasma cells, and mononuclear cells (Fig. 147-3). The synovial tissue becomes increasingly thickened leading to granulation tissue, i.e., pannus. The pannus can erode into the bone at the joint margin, causing fibrous adhesions and occasionally bony ankylosis. These pathologic observations, along with the finding of rheumatoid factors (antibodies directed at the Fc fragment of IgG), immune complexes, an increased production of various cytokines, and the association with HLA-DR4 in white patients, suggest that immune mechanisms are important in any explanation of the pathogenesis of RA. The nature of the causative agent(s) of RA has not yet been found.

Clinical Features

In 1987, the American College of Rheumatology revised the criteria for the classification of RA (Table 147-5). The criteria emphasize that the diagnosis of RA remains a clinical diagnosis.

The onset of RA is characteristically insidious with prodromal symptoms of fatigue, weight loss, joint pain, and joint swelling. RA can, however, present acutely with an explosive arthritis developing in one or many joints. Stiffness is a prominent symptom. It can last for hours and may involve the entire body rather than just the involved joints. The duration of morning stiffness is often used by clinicians to assess both the degree of activity of the disease and the clinical response to therapy.

Less than 10 percent of RA patients ever go into a prolonged remission. There may, however, be intervals of almost complete freedom from pain between attacks of inflammation before the disease becomes established in a joint. The best laboratory indicator of prognosis is the serum rheumatoid factor. High titers of rheumatoid factor (i.e., seropositivity) are associated with extraarticular manifes-

---

Table 147-5

American College of Rheumatology Criteria for the Classification of Rheumatoid Arthritis 1987[a]

1. Morning stiffness in and around the joints, lasting at least 1 h before maximal improvement.

2. At least three joints simultaneously have had soft tissue swelling or fluid (not bony overgrowth alone) observed by physician. The 14 possible areas are right or left PIP, MP, wrist, elbow, knee, ankle, and MTP joints.

3. At least one area swollen (as defined above) in a wrist, MP, or PIP joint.

4. Simultaneous involvement of the same joint areas (as defined in two) on both sides of the body (bilateral involvement of PIPs, MPs, or MTPs is acceptable without absolute symmetry).

5. Subcutaneous nodules over bony prominences, extensor surfaces, or in juxtaarticular regions observed by a physician.

6. Demonstration of abnormal amounts of serum rheumatoid factor by any method for which the result has been positive in less than 5 percent of normal control subjects.

7. Radiographic changes typical of rheumatoid arthritis on posteroanterior hand and wrist radiographs, which must include erosions or unequivocal bony decalcification localized in or marked adjacent to the involved joints (osteoarthritis changes alone do not qualify).

[a]For the diagnosis of RA, four of the seven critieria are required.

NOTE: PIP, proximal interphalangeal; MP, metacarpophalangeal; MTP, metatarsophalangeal.

---

tations of RA such as nodules and rheumatoid vasculitis. Patients with seropositive disease often have more erosive disease than those with seronegative disease, although there are exceptions. HLA-DR4 has been found in greater frequency in seropositive patients and in those seronegative patients with erosive disease. A recent study reported that heterozygosity for DR4DW4 was associated with rheumatoid nodules, vasculitic skin ulcers, neuropathy, and lung disease.

Physical Examination

In early RA, one or a few isolated joints may be involved; but as the disease progresses, joint involvement tends to be bilaterally symmetrical. Joint findings on one side of the body should always be compared to findings on the opposite side. Swelling, tenderness, heat deformity, range of motion, muscle changes, crepitus, and the presence of nodules should all be documented. Subcutaneous nodules are not specific for RA; they can also be seen in gout, pseudogout, rheumatic fever, sarcoid, panniculitis, vasculitis, type II hyperlipoproteinemia, and SLE. In adults, joint symptoms frequently originate symmetrically in the proximal interphalangeal and metacarpophalangeal joints of the hands and the metatarsophalangeal joints of the feet. MCP involvement with eventual volar subluxation and ulnar drift is a typical deformity of RA. Synovitis in the proximal interphalangeal (PIP) joint produce three characteristic deformities due to lack of collateral ligament support: the boutonniere, the Swanneck, and the unstable PIP joint. However, all other joints may be involved eventually.

Laboratory Tests

There is no specific diagnostic test for rheumatoid arthritis. A positive blood test for rheumatoid factor (RF) fulfills only one of the four to seven necessary criteria for RA, emphasizing again that RA is a clinical diagnosis. The latex fixation test for RF is positive in approximately 85 percent of RA patients. However, RF is also found in almost 20 percent of patients with systemic lupus erythematosus, in a smaller percentage of patients with other rheumatic conditions, and in patients with chronic infections. Rheumatoid factor is not a measure of inflammation; therefore, serial changes in serum titer do not occur as the level of clinical RA changes. However, seropositive patients with high titers tend to have more serious articular and ex-

traarticular disease. The erythrocyte sedimentation rate (ESR) is a measure of inflammation. Red blood cells in inflammatory disorders tend to form stacks (rouleaux) that partly result from increased levels of fibrinogen and thus sediment more rapidly. Although the ESR is usually increased in rheumatoid arthritis, it may not always correlate with disease activity.

Synovial fluid analysis can be of help in the diagnosis of rheumatic conditions; however, a normal cell count or negative findings on examination do not exclude a diagnosis. In inflammatory arthritides such as RA, the synovial fluid is usually cloudy, the white blood cell count elevated (15,000 to 25,000 WBC/mm^3) with 60 to 70 percent neutrophils.

Radiologic Examination

Radiographic findings may aid in the diagnosis of RA and are useful as a means of following the progression of a patient's disease. Soft-tissue swelling, juxtaarticular osteoporosis, and erosive changes are evident in most RA patients within the first two years of diagnosis. The earliest radiologic changes are more likely to be found in radiographs of the hands and feet. With advanced disease, joint spaces narrow, often with ankylosis and/or subluxation. There is a strong correlation between erosive changes on radiographic and clinical symptoms of morning stiffness, synovitis, and elevated ESR. In autopsy studies, up to 50 percent of RA patients show some cervical involvement. RA patients are at risk for atlantoaxial subluxation, atlantoaxial impaction, subaxial subluxation, and lateral mass collapse. Clinically, this manifests as neck and shoulder girdle pain, head tilts, and when severe, a myelopathy. The presence of progressive neurologic changes, severe pain, severe atlantoaxial and subaxial subluxation, and atlantoaxial impaction are indications for surgical fixation. Flexion/extension MRI has become the procedure of choice for evaluation of cervical disease in rheumatoid arthritis.

Extraarticular Manifestations

Although much of the diagnosis and treatment of RA is focused on joint symptoms, RA is a systemic disease, particularly in seropositive patients with high RF titers. As discussed below, some of these manifestations may only become evident on preoperative screening; they may also make postoperative recovery more complicated.

Up to 40 percent of RA patients have pleural involvement (pleural effusions) at the time of autopsy. Clinically, however, this may go unnoticed until a chest radiograph (CXR) is ordered. Other pulmonary manifestations include interstitial fibrosis, nodules, and lymphoid hyperplasia. Of significance is that the severity of the lung disease does not correlate with the duration or the severity of the arthritis.

Cardiac manifestations are rare, but include pericardial disease, coronary arteritis, and valvular dysfunction secondary to rheumatoid nodules.

Secondary Sjögren's syndrome with the sicca syndrome (dry eyes and dry mouth) is common in RA and requires local attention in the perioperative and postoperative period, particularly when anesthesia requires intubation.

The anemia of RA is multifactorial. Iron utilization is impaired, erythropoietin levels are decreased, and the marrow response to erythropoiesis is depressed. The degree of anemia usually correlates with the activity of the arthritis. Unless complicated by blood loss, poor nutrition, hemolysis, or marrow suppression from medications, the anemia of RA is commonly normocytic, normochromic. Repletion of iron in iron deficiency may be difficult in an inflammatory state such as RA since part of the anemia is due to inhibition of hemoglobin synthesis caused by inflammation.

Thrombocytosis is a frequent abnormality in active disease and correlates with the degree of inflammation. The thrombocytosis does not predispose to thrombotic events and does not represent marrow neoplasia.

Felty's syndrome consists of RA, splenomegaly, and granulocytopenia. It characteristically occurs in patients with long-standing seropositive, nodular, deforming RA. Recurrent bacterial infections and leg ulcers are common complications.

More rarely, systemic vasculitis is observed in RA manifesting as palpable purpura, cutaneous ulcers, and mononeuritis multiplex, all of which may complicate surgical procedures. Ulcers can be sources of infection. Positioning patients with neuropathies during surgical procedures takes care, as prolonged compression of an already ischemic nerve can lead to unexpected paralysis. The medications needed to treat vasculitis (e.g., as prednisone, methotrexate, cyclophosphamide) can complicate wound healing and increase the risk of infections.

Treatment

The three main objectives in the management of RA are decreased pain and swelling, optimal range of motion of individual joints, and minimal drug toxicity. Exercise, rest, physical therapy, occupational therapy, medications, and surgical intervention are all part of the required multidisciplinary approach to rheumatoid arthritis. The role of surgery may be prophylactic, reconstructive, or palliative.

Medical therapy is aimed at suppression of synovial inflammation and disease remission. Complete success in this regard without any drug therapy is, unfortunately, quite uncommon. The three major classes of medications used are NSAIDs, corticosteroids, and disease-modifying antirheumatic drugs (DMARDs). There has been a strong trend over the past several years to use DMARDs early in the course of RA before bony destruction is established.

NSAIDs have taken the place of aspirin, as they have a less frequent dosing regimen and are generally better tolerated. NSAIDs decrease inflammation via inhibition of cyclooxygenase, lipoxygenase, and free radicals. NSAIDs also suppress fever; both aspirin and NSAIDs inhibit platelet cyclooxygenase and decrease platelet aggregation. The effect of NSAIDs on platelets is only temporary, the duration of which depends on the individual drug's half-life. The effect of aspirin on platelets is irreversible for the life span of the platelet.

Although almost ubiquitous in use, NSAIDs have considerable morbidity and even mortality. In the United States, NSAID-induced gastrointestinal complications account for at least 2000 deaths and 20,000 hospitalizations per year for RA patients alone. The most common adverse reactions of NSAIDs include gastrointestinal upset, which ranges from dyspepsia to major gastrointestinal hemorrhage.

There are medications available for the prophylaxis and/or treatment of NSAID-induced gastroduodenal disease. Misoprostol has been shown to heal NSAID-induced gastroduodenal erosive disease and prevents NSAID-induced duodenal disease. It does not, however, relieve dyspeptic symptoms. H2 antagonists can heal and prevent duodenal lesions; they can heal NSAID-induced gastric lesions, but have little effect in the prevention of gastric lesions. The H2 antagonists do help to improve dyspeptic symptoms. Sucralfate has not been shown to prevent or heal gastric ulcers. Antacids need to be taken in extremely high doses to be useful.

Hepatotoxicity, including hepatic failure, has been seen, particularly with diclofenac. Central nervous system side effects such as headaches, confusion, dizziness, and depersonalization reactions have been seen with all the NSAIDs and occur more commonly with increasing age. Aseptic meningitis has been reported with ibuprofen.

NSAIDs should be avoided in persons with chronic renal disease and severe congestive heart failure as inhibition of prostaglandin synthase leads to imbalance in vasoconstrictors and vasodilators and can exacerbate each condition.

Corticosteroids are potent anti-inflammatory and immunosuppressive agents. They have important effects on the cellular components of the immune system. T lymphocytes are more sensitive to the immunosuppressive effects of corticosteroids than B lymphocytes. The combined effect of steroids on monocytes, macrophages, and T lymphocytes often leads to anergy. In chronic inflammatory diseases, corticosteroids should ideally be used as temporary "therapeutic bridges" between the onset of severe pain/swelling and the time when remittive agents take effect. Unfortunately, many clinical situations such as refractory inflammatory arthritis, vasculitis, and other severe forms of connective tissue diseases warrant their long-term use in high doses. Divided doses of steroids suppress the pituitary-adrenal axis more than single dosing, but are often required for the initial treatment of severe inflammatory disease. Single morning dosing is usually all that is required for moderate conditions. Alternate day dosing is associated with less interruption of the pituitary-adrenal axis. Although glucocorticoids can be life-saving, their side effects contribute to significant morbidity and mortality (Table 147-6).

The clinical response to intraarticular corticosteroids correlate with a decrease in synovial inflammation and a decrease in gene expression for collagenase, metalloproteinases, C2, and human leukocyte antigen HLA DR antigens.

Surgical management of patients on corticosteroids requires careful attention. Due to the immunosuppressive effects of corticosteroids on pituitary-adrenal function, patients who are on corticosteroids or who have received them in large doses or for prolonged periods of time within the past year should be treated for pituitary-adrenal axis suppression. Because there is great variation from patient to patient, it is not possible to definitively anticipate the shortest interval for the smallest dose of steroids at which suppression may occur. In general, the stress from general anesthesia and surgery is not hazardous to patients who have only received early morning replacement doses (no more than 25 mg of hydrocortisone, 5 mg of prednisone, 4 mg of triamcinolone, or 0.75 mg of dexamethasone). Evening doses inhibit the diurnal release of ACTH. When adrenal suppression is suspected, one may perform a Cortrosyn stimulation test or one may treat the patient as though adrenocortical insufficiency were present. Basal plasma cortisol levels are poor predictors of pituitary-adrenal axis function.

Table 147-6

Glucocorticoid Toxicities

Ophthalmic	Cataracts, increased intraocular pressure
Cardiovascular	Hypertension, fluid retention
Gastrointestinal	Peptic ulcer disease, pancreatitis
Endocrine	Truncal obesity, moon facies, acne, hirsutism, hyperglycemia, increased appetite
Musculoskeletal	Myopathy, osteoporosis,[a] avascular necrosis
Neuropsychiatric	Seizures, pseudotumor cerebri, moodswings
Dermatologic	Facial erythema, fragile skin, striae, impaired wound healing
Immunologic	Suppression of delayed hypersensitivity, neutrophilia, monocytopenia, lymphopenia, increased susceptibility to infection

[a]Of note is that bone loss is greatest in the first 6 months of steroid treatment. Trabecular bone, which is proportionately greater in the spine and in the distal radius, is lost to a greater extent than cortical bone. Men are just as sensitive to the bone loss induced by steroids as are women.

DMARDs constitute a large number of drugs used in the management of chronic inflammatory rheumatic diseases. DMARDs are believed to significantly alter the inflammatory process. Rheumatologists commonly use DMARDs in the early stages of inflammatory arthritis before the onset of erosions and deformities.

Azathioprine is a derivative of 6-mercaptopurine. Both drugs inhibit cell-mediated and humoral immunity. Azathioprine and 6-mercaptopurine are generally administered in doses of 2 mg/kg per day. One of the pathways for the metabolism of both drugs is by the enzyme xanthine oxidase. In patients taking allopurinol, the usual dose of azathioprine must be reduced to one-third the previous dose, as allopurinol is a xanthine oxidase inhibitor. Major side effects of azathioprine that limit treatment are gastrointestinal tolerance, marrow toxicity, infection, and hepatitis. There is also an increased incidence of lymphoma in azathioprine-treated patients. In renal transplant patients taking azathioprine, the increased incidence is 60-fold; one similar study in rheumatoid arthritis patients reported a 13-fold increase.

Gold compounds may be used orally or intramuscularly and are mainly used in both juvenile idiopathic arthritis (JIA; formerly called juvenile rheumatoid arthritis or JRA) and adult RA. Gold treatment is most effective in early active synovitis; it is not indicated for advanced RA. Gold has been shown to inhibit the function of macrophages and neutrophils, to decrease antibody production, and to have a weak antibacterial effect. Oral gold is, in general, not as effective as IM gold, but has fewer side effects than that seen with the parenteral preparations. Few patients are on gold for more than 5 years secondary to loss of efficacy or adverse reactions. The toxicity of parenteral gold falls into three major areas: dermatologic (various types of rashes), hematologic (anemia, leukopenia, and thrombocytopenia), and renal (proteinuria and membranous glomerulonephritis). Oral gold's most common side effect is diarrhea, but effects on the marrow, kidney, and skin can also be seen. Although gold has generally been supplanted by the use of methotrexate, it had been used for decades by rheumatologists when NSAIDs were not fully effective.

Hydroxychloroquine and chloroquine are used in the treatment of inflammatory arthritis, systemic lupus erythematosus, and autoimmune skin diseases. Among other anti-inflammatory effects, these antimalarial agents interfere with lysosomal enzyme release, interfere with antigen processing, and inhibit interleukin secretion by monocytes. They are commonly used in the treatment of mild-to-moderate inflammatory arthritis either alone or in combination with NSAIDs. The most serious potential side effects are related to the eyes, where antimalarials can cause corneal and retinal deposits. Although this rarely occurs, biannual eye exams are required.

Sulfasalazine is an oral anti-inflammatory agent in which gastrointestinal bacterial enzymes cleave the drug in the large intestine into sulfapyridine and 5-aminosalicylic acid. Sulfapyridine is the main compound absorbed. Certain effects like prostaglandin inhibition are unique to the whole molecule; inhibition of killer cell activity is an effect of the sulfapyridine moiety. Liver function tests and blood counts need monitoring; hematologic side effects that are serious include leukocytopenia, agranulocytosis, and thrombocytopenia. Sulfasalazine in high doses can inhibit folate absorption resulting in abnormal erythrocyte morphology.

Methotrexate, an analogue of folic acid, inhibits the enzyme dihydrofolate reductase, thereby impairing DNA synthesis. It is a potent anti-inflammatory agent and is widely used in the treatment of rheumatoid arthritis, vasculitis, and other autoimmune diseases where it is prescribed orally or parenterally once per week. Although rare, long-term administration may be associated with hepatic fibrosis, including cirrhosis. Patients at increased risk for liver complications are those with preexisting liver disease, diabetes mellitus, renal disease, excess alcohol intake, psoriasis, and older age. A rare, but potentially lethal, complication is acute hypersensitivity pulmonary injury. Anemia, leukopenia, and thrombocytopenia are other possible side effects. The risk of malignancy in patients taking methotrexate is not increased, but there have been case reports of temporally associated cancers.

D-penicillamine is another antirheumatic agent that is used in seropositive RA patients with high rheumatoid factor titers. Its use demands particular care because of its toxicity. Marrow suppression can be severe. Twenty percent of patients get proteinuria, and it has a unique ability to induce autoimmune diseases including SLE, Goodpasture's syndrome, myasthenia gravis, polymyositis, and Sjögren's syndrome.

Cyclophosphamide is a nitrogen mustard alkylating agent used in autoimmune diseases in which there is serious risk of vital organ damage, or in patients who require long-term high doses of steroids for disease control. Intravenous boluses of Cytoxan have been shown to decrease the risk of end-stage renal failure in patients with lupus nephritis. Cytoxan has also dramatically decreased the morbidity and mortality of Wegener's granulomatosis, systemic vasculitis, and transverse myelitis.

Other approaches to immunosuppression in active rheumatic diseases include using monoclonal antibodies directed against molecules on the surface of T cells and anti-interleukin-2 receptor antibodies. These have been used with limited success in a small number of patients with RA. It is likely that other cytokines and adhesion molecules will be targets in the future.

SYSTEMIC LUPUS ERYTHEMATOSUS

Systemic lupus erythematosus (SLE) is the prototypic autoimmune disease with a wide spectrum of clinical manifestations. The major target organs of the disease are the skin, joints, serous membranes, marrow, kidneys, and brain. SLE is characterized by both humoral and cellular immunologic abnormalities, including multiple autoantibodies that may participate in tissue injury.

Epidemiology

Most series of adult patients recognize a female:male ratio of 9:1. This ratio is less striking in childhood and in the elderly. Symptoms usually first occur in the reproductive years, in the second through fourth decades of life. Although lupus occurs in all races, it is more common in blacks and Asians than whites. SLE is associated with HLA class II antigens HLA-DR2, HLA-DR3, and most probably HLA-DQw1. It is estimated that 5 to 12 percent of relatives of patients with SLE go on to develop SLE.

Pathogenesis

Although there is no histologic feature which is pathognomonic for SLE, several pathologic findings have been considered characteristic of SLE: (1) the hematoxylin body, which contains aggregates of chromatin and immunoglobulins; engulfment of hematoxylin bodies by phagocytes produces the characteristic LE cell; (2) "onion skin" thickening of the arterioles of the spleen; and (3) fibrinoid necrosis of blood vessels and connective tissue.

Synovial biopsies often show fibrinous villous synovitis. The presence of pannus formation or bony erosions, however, is rare, and is a distinguishing feature from rheumatoid arthritis. The kidney has been the most intensively studied organ in SLE. The entire range of glomerulonephritis is seen: membranous, mesangial, proliferative, and membranoproliferative. Findings in skin, muscle, nerves, and other viscera range from a nonspecific perivascular neutrophilic infiltrate to frank vasculitis. As is typical of immune complex-mediated disease, immunofluorescence studies show deposits of immunoglobulins and complement in tissues; this has been best studied in the skin at the dermal-epidermal junction and in the glomerulus.

Immunology

Cellular and humoral immunity is dysregulated in SLE. Anergy is common as is lymphopenia. Interleukin-2 production, a T-cell derived cytokine that plays a key role in immune responses, is deficient. Overactivity of the humoral component is manifested by autoantibodies, hypergammaglobulinemia, and circulating immune complexes. Among the autoantibodies the anti-nuclear antibodies (ANAs) are the most characteristic, and are found in 95 percent of SLE patients. ANAs can be directed against DNA and RNA, as well as any of the other nuclear protein complexes. In addition, cytoplasmic proteins associated with RNA can be targets of autoantibodies (Table 147-7). It has been shown that certain autoantibodies contribute directly to tissue in-

Table 147-7

Autoantibodies in Systemic Lupus Erythematosus

Target	Clinical Significance
dsDNA	Highly specific for SLE Correlates with disease, especially renal disease
ssDNA	Low diagnostic specificity
Sm (Smith)	Highly specific for SLE
U1 RNP	Mixed connective tissue disease
Histones	SLE and drug-induced lupus
ro and la	Sjögren's syndrome Photosensitivity Subacute cutaneous lupus Neonatal lupus
Phospholipids	Thrombosis Recurrent abortion Inhibition of laboratory coagulation tests Thrombocytopenia Stroke

Table 147-8

Revised ACR Criteria for Classification of SLE

Criteria	Definition
Malar rash	Fixed erythema over the malar eminences
Discoid rash	Erythematous raised patches with scaling and plugging
Photosensitivity	Skin rash as a result of unusual reaction to sunlight
Oral ulcers	Usually painless, must be observed by a doctor
Arthritis	Nonerosive arthritis involving two or more joints
Serositis	Pleuritis or pericarditis
Renal disorder	Persistent proteinuria >0.5 g/day or cellular tests
Neurologic disorder	Seizures or psychosis
Hematologic disorder	Hemolytic anemia or Leukopenia <4000/mm^3 total or Lymphopenia <1500/mm^3 or Thrombocytopenia <100,000/mm^3
Immunologic disorder	Positive LE cell prep or Anti-DNA antibody or Anti-Sm antibody or False positive VDRL
Antinuclear antibody	An abnormal titer of ANA

NOTE: ANA, antinuclear antibody; VDRL, Venereal Disease Research Laboratories.

jury. Anti-DNA antibodies have been found in renal glomerular lesions of SLE patients. Although the titer of antinuclear antibodies usually does not correlate with disease activity, the level of anti-DNA antibodies often does vary with the severity of renal disease.

Clinical Features

SLE is a multisystem disease with a myriad of presenting symptoms and signs. No single finding makes the diagnosis. Criteria for diagnosis have been devised by the American College of Rheumatology to ensure uniformity for disease classification in clinical studies (Table 147-8).

The presence of four criteria is required to classify a patient with SLE, although in clinical practice it is understood that certain findings, such as antibodies to double-stranded DNA, anti-Sm antibodies, and malar rash, are more suggestive than others. A positive antinuclear antibody is a signal to consider the diagnosis of SLE further.

Arthritis and/or arthralgias are the most common presenting manifestation of SLE. The arthritis of SLE can affect both small and large joints, usually in a symmetric distribution. Unlike RA, the arthritis of SLE does not typically cause bony erosions. Synovial thickening is common over proximal interphalangeal joints and tendon sheaths, leading to ulnar deviation of the fingers and subluxations and contractures. Tendon ruptures may occur. The pattern of nonerosive but deforming disease in the hand is termed Jacoud's arthropathy. Septic arthritis and osteonecrosis are more common in SLE and can mimic an acute synovitis. Osteonecrosis may be from underlying lupus or secondary to steroid intake. The same surgical and anesthetic precautions described for RA patients taking corticosteroids apply to SLE patients.

Treatment

The development of more sensitive immunologic testing for autoantibodies has facilitated the diagnosis of milder forms of SLE. Treatment must therefore be individualized to consider the distribution and severity of organ systems involved. General measures include rest, avoidance of stress, and avoidance of ultraviolet light exposure. Aspirin and NSAIDs are used for the treatment of fevers and arthritis. Antimalarials are used for constitutional symptoms, cutaneous diseases, and arthralgias and arthritis. Oral corticosteroids are reserved for serious end-organ disease manifesting as pneumonitis, hemolytic anemia and thrombocytopenia, vasculitis, neurologic disease, renal disease, or arthritis unresponsive to NSAIDs and antimalarials. Cytotoxic therapy (cyclophosphamide, azathioprine) is indicated in patients with serious major organ involvement, particularly nephritis, or in patients requiring high doses of corticosteroids. Low-dose methotrexate has also been used in the treatment of end-organ disease.

SCLERODERMA

Scleroderma is a syndrome characterized by microvascular abnormalities and excessive synthesis of collagen in multiple organs, including the skin, lung, kidney, vasculature, and gastrointestinal tract. Patients with scleroderma are divided into two subsets: a limited type, termed CREST (calcinosis, Raynaud's phenomenon, esophageal dysfunction, sclerodactyly, telangiectasis) and a diffuse cutaneous type. Approximately 90 percent of patients have detectable antinuclear antibodies. Antibodies to the centromere can be identified in most patients with limited scleroderma and antibodies to topoisomerase 1 (Scl 70) are seen in 30 percent of patients with diffuse scleroderma.

Endothelial cell injury and an increase in local growth factors and cytokines (transforming growth factor-B, epidermal growth factor, platelet-derived growth factor) have been implicated as causes of the excessive synthesis of collagen by fibroblasts.

Pulmonary hypertension in both the limited and diffuse types, and renal involvement in the diffuse type are the major causes of morbidity and mortality. Musculoskeletal symptoms include arthralgias and morning stiffness. Loss of hand function is a significant problem for many patients but is more likely secondary to tethering effects of skin thickening than to pathologic joint involvement. Physical examination often reveals tendon friction rubs over the wrists, ankles, and knees. Bony erosions are seen radiographically in 20 to 30 percent of patients. Radiographs may reveal resorption of the tufts of the terminal phalanges secondary to chronic digital ischemia. Subcutaneous calcinosis occurs in 50 percent of patients with CREST and in 10 percent of patients with diffuse scleroderma. They can get intermittently inflamed and infected. Like subcutaneous rheumatoid nodules, surgical resection is done as a last resort, as they recur. Due to the microvascular abnormalities, wound healing can be delayed and complicated. A myopathy can also be seen in scleroderma secondary to disuse atrophy and muscle fiber fibrosis.

SARCOIDOSIS

Sarcoidosis is a noncaseating granulomatous disease affecting bone, muscles, and synovium. Nonmusculoskeletal manifestations include bilateral hilar adenopathy, pulmonary infiltrates, uveitis, and erythema nodosum skin lesions. The most common arthropathy is acute or chronic polyarthritis of the knees and ankles, although any joint can be involved. Cystic bone lesions may cause dactylitis of the affected digit. Rarely, resorption of distal digits can occur. Granulomata can be found in tendon sheaths, vertebrae, ribs, the pelvic bones, and the skull. Most patients with sarcoid arthropathy respond to NSAIDs; the chronic, persistent forms of arthritis are often associated with more severe forms of sarcoidosis where corticosteroids are required.

INFECTIOUS ARTHRITIS

Infectious arthritis may be caused by bacteria, spirochetes, viruses, rickettsia, fungi, and parasites. The latter three infections do not lead to polyarticular disease as often as the former three organisms.

Disseminated gonococcal infection is a very common cause of inflammatory arthritis in sexually active individuals. Three-quarters of patients present with a migratory polyarthritis. Most patients do not have symptoms of genitourinary infection. Classic findings include vesicular and pustular dermatitis and tenosynovitis (usually involving the hands/wrists or ankles/feet) (Fig. 147-4). In almost all cases of gonococcal arthritis successful treatment can be accomplished by appropriate antibiotics and daily needle aspiration. Surgical drainage is rarely required unless the hip is involved. The current treatment recommendation of the Centers for Disease Control and Prevention is: (1) ceftriaxone, intravenously, 1 g daily for 7 to 10 days, or (2) ceftizoxime or cefotaxime, intravenously, 1 g every 8 h until 2 or 3 days or clinical improvement; then cefixime, orally, 400 mg twice daily, or ciprofloxacin, orally, 500 mg twice daily to complete 7 to 10 days of therapy. However, if the infecting strain is known to be sensitive to penicillin or tetracycline, therapy should be changed accordingly.

RHEUMATIC FEVER

Rheumatic fever seems to be increasing in frequency among adult populations. Clinically, patients present with fever, history of pharyngitis (this may be subclinical), and pain and swelling of the large joints of the lower extremities.

The migratory pattern of arthritis commonly seen in children is not characteristic of rheumatic fever in adults. Carditis is uncommon, and chorea and subcutaneous nodules are rare. Diagnosis is made by throat culture (however, cultures can be negative), and rising antistreptolysin and anti-DNase B antibodies. Treatment of the primary pharyngitis is required with at least 10 days of antibiotics. Prophylactic antibiotic treatment of 5 years is recommended for those

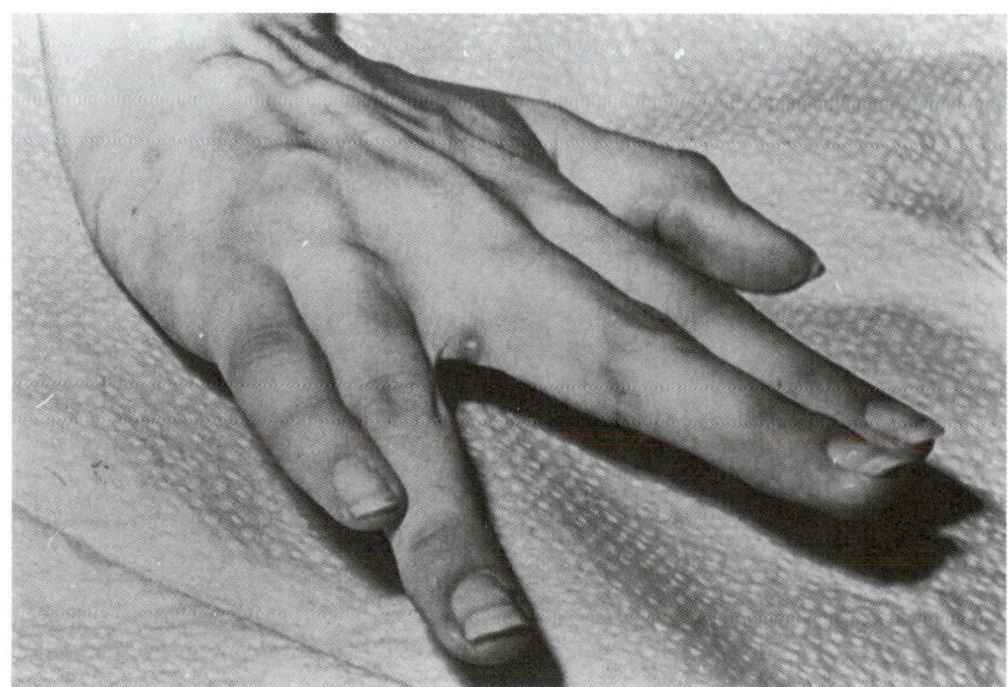

Figure 147-4
Vesiculopustular skin lesion on hand of patient with gonococcal arthritis. (Reproduced with permission from Healy LA: Gonococcal urethritis: No longer a rarity. *Res Staff Phys* 1978; 24:66.)

adults who get rheumatic fever in an epidemic setting and those adults who also get carditis. Uncomplicated poststreptococcal reactive arthritis unassociated with high antibody titers does not require prolonged treatment with antibiotics.

LYME DISEASE

Lyme disease is caused by the spirochete *Borrelia burgdorferi*. Diagnosis is based on geographic, seasonal, clinical, and laboratory features. Early Lyme disease can be subclinical, but frequent manifestations include malaise, fever, headache, migratory arthralgias, and the characteristic rash of erythema chronica migrans. Less common features include meningoencephalitis, neuropathy (particularly Bell's palsy), radiculopathy, and carditis. Onset usually corresponds to the nymph stage of the infected tick infecting the arthropod vector from late spring through early fall. The enzyme-linked immunosorbent assay (ELISA) test may be negative early in infection, as the immunoglobulin (IgM) response develops 4 to 6 weeks after the acute infection. Chronic disease is more typically characterized by frank arthritis (usually oligoarthritis); 60 percent of untreated patients develop arthritis of large joints months following the infection. Very rarely, Lyme arthritis can present symmetrically and mimic RA. However, it rarely produces erosions or joint deformities. Neurologic symptoms of encephalopathy and radiculopathy may also be delayed by months. Testing for Lyme disease has not been completely standardized, but in reputable laboratories it is reliable. Routine testing involves the ELISA test; Western blot analysis is helpful when clinical suspicion is low and the ELISA is equivocal. In difficult clinical situations, the polymerase chain reaction technique can be used to detect spirochetal DNA. Treatment for early Lyme disease is with doxycycline (100 mg b.i.d. for 14 to 21 days), Amoxicillin (500 mg t.i.d. for 14 to 21 days), or erythromycin 250 mg (q.i.d. for 14 to 21 days). Bell's palsy and uncomplicated Lyme arthritis can be treated with oral antibiotics for 30 days. Meningitis, neuropathies, carditis, and refractory arthritis require intravenous antibiotics.

The most common viral-related polyarthritis is associated with hepatitis B. In the prodromal, preicteric phase transient arthritis occurs, usually involving the small joints, in association with an urticarial or purpuric rash. As the patient becomes icteric, the arthritis begins to clear. Rubella, rubella immunization, mumps, and infectious mononucleosis can all be associated with transient polyarthritis. Human B19 parvovirus can cause an arthropathy in both children and adults. Arthropathy occurs in up to 5 percent of infected children, usually in association with a "slapped cheek" appearance. Parvovirus can cause both a transient and permanent symmetric polyarthritis in adults.

SERONEGATIVE ARTHRITIS

Several syndromes exist in which entheses, peripheral joints, and the axial skeleton are susceptible to inflammation. This type of inflammation is much more common in patients who are HLA-B27 positive. Environmental triggers and possibly other genetic factors put HLA-B27 patients at risk for this type of arthropathy. Of significance, however, is that less than 10 percent of people with B27 develop any form of arthritis.

ANKYLOSING SPONDYLITIS

Ankylosing spondylitis (AS) primarily affects the spine, the sacroiliac joints, and the large proximal joints. The prevalence rate in white populations is between 0.1 to 1.0 percent. In African-Americans the prevalence is one-quarter that of whites. The earliest radio-

graphic findings are seen in the sacroiliac joints as erosions, pseudo-widening and eventual sclerosis. As the disease progresses spinal motion is lost due to the distinctive tendency of the disease toward fibrosis with secondary ossification ("marginal" syndesmophytes) and ankylosis of involved joints. Other radiographic changes include squaring of vertebral bodies, symmetric syndesmophytes, and the eventual appearance of the bamboo spine.

The classic patient with AS is a young white man between 15 and 40 years of age with the insidious onset of low back pain and stiffness which is worse in the early morning hours and improves with physical activity. Peripheral arthritis occurs in 50 percent of patients, usually involving the hip, shoulder, or knee. Chest wall pain is common and is due to enthesitis of the costovertebral and sternocostal junctions. Late complications of spinal arthritis include atlantoaxial subluxation and spinal stenosis. The rigid spine is also prone to fracture. Extraarticular manifestations of AS include uveitis (25 percent of patients), aortic insufficiency, conduction defects (5 percent of patients), and apical lobe fibrosis in long-standing disease (less than 1 percent of patients).

There are no pathognomonic tests for ankylosing spondylitis. HLA-B27 is ordered only when the clinical or radiographic picture is uncertain.

Medical treatment may relieve pain but does not slow the progression of disease. NSAIDs and sulfasalazine are used to treat the inflammation. Intraarticular steroids can be used to treat episodes of peripheral arthritis. Aggressive physical therapy, particularly swimming, is critical to help patients maintain erect posture and range of movement of joints. Surgical procedures are done in patients with deformities causing severe pain and/or loss of function. Total hip replacement is the most common operation performed in AS patients. Other common surgical procedures are knee replacement, cervical an lumbar osteotomies to correct spinal kyphosis, stabilization of atlantoaxial subluxation, and condylar resections of ankylosed temporomandibular joints. Ectopic calcification and prolonged bed rest postoperatively put many patients at risk for reankylosis.

REITER'S SYNDROME

Reiter's syndrome is classically defined as the triad of arthritis, urethritis, and conjunctivitis. The diagnosis of Reiter's, or "reactive arthritis" is usually diagnosed clinically, but in uncertain cases a positive test for HLA-B27 is helpful. The typical presentation is of an asymmetric oligoarthritis (most commonly the knee) with inflammation of an adjacent enthesis (such as a sausage toe). The appearance of symptoms may follow a genitourinary infection with *Chlamydia* or *Mycoplasma*, or a gastrointestinal infection with *Shigella*, *Salmonella*, or *Yersinia*. Radiographs may show periosteal proliferation near involved joints; sacroiliitis is seen in up to 80 percent of patients with chronic disease. Laboratory tests reveal an elevated erythrocyte sedimentation rate, often greater than 100 mm/h in acute attacks. Pyuria and hematuria are common.

Treatment is with NSAIDs and in the past, with phenylbutazone. Tetracyclines have been used to shorten the duration of reactive arthritis due to venereal disease.

PSORIATIC ARTHRITIS

Psoriatic arthritis affects 5 percent of patients with psoriasis. Five presentations are described: (1) oligoarthritis affecting a few distal interphalangeal, proximal interphalangeal, and metacarpophalangeal joins with diffuse swelling characteristic of a "sausage toe or finger" (70 percent of patients); (2) distal interphalangeal joint involvement

---

Table 147-9

Rheumatic Syndromes Associated with Inflammatory Bowel Disease

Features	Spondylitis	Peripheral arthritis
HLA-B27	Yes	No
Sex incidence	Male	Equal
Onset before IBD	Yes	No
Parallels activity of colitis	No	Yes
Predominant IBD	Ulcerative colitis	Crohn's disease

---

with nail changes (10 percent); (3) arthritis mutilans with severe deformities characterized by flail hands secondary to osteolysis of the affected joints (5 percent); (4) symmetric polyarthritis mimicking rheumatoid arthritis (15 percent); (5) spondyloarthritis presenting as sacroiliitis and/or spondylitis (5 percent).

There are a myriad of characteristic radiographic changes: erosions of the distal interphalangeal joints of the fingers and interphalangeal joints of the toes, periostitis, "pencil-in-cup" appearance of DIP joints, asymmetric sacroiliitis, and asymmetric syndesmophytes on the spine.

Treatment options are similar to rheumatoid arthritis: physical therapy, NSAIDs, and immunosuppressive therapy. Methotrexate is used in patients with severe disease and has the additional benefit of suppressing the skin manifestations of the disease. Hepatotoxicity appears to be a greater problem in psoriatic patients than in rheumatoid patients. Gold injections and antimalarial therapy is also used. An increased incidence of exfoliative skin reactions have been seen with antimalarials. Reconstructive surgery is recommended for patients with end-stage joint destruction.

INFLAMMATORY BOWEL DISEASE

Inflammatory bowel disease (IBD) is associated with two distinct forms of arthritis: spondyloarthritis and peripheral arthritis. Spondyloarthritis is seen in approximately 10 percent of patients with inflammatory bowel disease; 50 to 75 percent are HLA-B27 positive. The typical patient is a man with back pain and enthesitis; particularly of the heels, hip, and/or knee. Peripheral arthritis occurs in 20 percent of patients with IBD and most often affects the knee and ankle. Features specific to Crohn's disease and ulcerative colitis are described in Table 147-9.

Although the disease classifications in this chapter facilitate the understanding of the pathophysiology and treatment of arthropathies, it is clear that there is often great overlap among the diseases in cellular mechanisms and in clinical practice. Laboratory advances in the immunogenetics of diseases and serologic and immunologic analysis will likely provide new insights into rheumatic diseases in the near future.

SUGGESTED READINGS

Arnett FC, Edworthy SM, Block DA, et al: The American Rheumatism Association 1987 criteria for the classification of rheumatoid arthritis. *Arthritis Rheum* 1988; 31:315.

Dieppe P, Cushnaghan J: The natural course and prognosis of osteoarthritis. In Moskowitz RW, Howell DS, Goldberg VM, et al (eds): *Osteoarthritis: Diagnosis and Management*, 2d ed. Philadelphia: WB Saunders; 1992:399.

Dluhy RG, Newmark SR, Lauler DP, et al: Pharmacology and chemistry of adrenal glucocorticoids. In Azarnoff DL (ed): *Steroid Therapy*. Philadelphia: WB Saunders; 1975:1.

Hochberg MC: Systemic lupus erythematosus. *Rheum Dis Clin North Am* 1990; 16:617.

Khan MA, Van der Linden SM: A wider spectrum of spondyloarthropathies. *Sem Arthritis Rheum* 1990; 20:107.

Roubenoff R: Gout and hyperuricemia. *Rheum Dis Clin North Am* 1990; 16:539.

Schwarzer AC, Arnold MH, Brooks PM: Combination therapy in rheumatoid arthritis. *Baillieres Clin Rheum* 1990; 4:663.

Steere AC, Bartenhagen NH, Craft JE, et al: The early clinical manifestations of Lyme disease. *Ann Intern Med* 1983; 99:76.

Chapter 148

METABOLIC BONE DISEASES

Stanley Wallach

The skeleton comprises approximately 8 percent of body weight, and is a complex, metabolically active tissue containing 35 percent organic and 65 percent inorganic fractions. The organic component is predominantly type I collagen, but a large number of noncollagenous proteins are present in trace amounts whose functions are only currently being explored. Examples of noncollagenous proteins are the glycosaminoglycans, proteoglycans, osteocalcin, osteonectin, and osteopontin. The inorganic fraction is a crystalline calcium phosphate salt known as hydroxyapatite, which has the stoichiometric formula of $Ca_{10}(PO_4)_6(OH)_2$. The hydroxyapatite crystals are highly organized but imperfect in that several lattice positions for each of the elements involved are empty or substituted by other cationic or anionic species. The hydroxyapatite is deposited in a highly structured manner within the interstices of the type I collagen molecules.

In young adults, the skeleton turns over at an overall rate of approximately 8 percent per year. However, cortical (or compact) bone is relatively inert and remodels less rapidly, approximately 4 percent per year. In contrast, trabecular bone, in part because of its high surface area, remodels at a rate closer to 25 percent per year. These rates diminish with increasing age. The first step in the remodeling process is bone resorption, which occurs by the recruitment of osteoclasts to sites of defunct bone that has suffered strain and microfractures from stress. Mature osteoclasts evolve from precursor stem cells of the macrophage/monocytic series present in the bone marrow; they first proliferate, then fuse, and finally differentiate into multinucleate cells capable of bone resorption. Bone resorption is then accomplished by attachment of a cytoplasmic collar around the area to be resorbed, followed by the secretion of acid hydrolytic enzymes and protons into the sequestered area so that bone mineral and matrix are resorbed simultaneously. The products of resorption pass through the cytoplasm of the osteoclast, and are then extruded and removed by the marrow circulation.

Once resorption has occurred, a quiescent phase is followed by a phase of new bone formation to replace the lost bone. Osteoblast precursor cells, related to marrow stromal cells, undergo proliferation and then differentiate into mature osteoblasts, which produce new bone matrix sufficient to fill the defect created by the resorbing osteoclasts. As new bone matrix appears, it is mineralized by the deposition of an amorphous calcium phosphate salt, which then converts to hydroxyapatite crystals. In young adults, the replacement process is closely coupled to the bone resorption process, both qualitatively and quantitatively, so that there is neither gain nor loss of bone. The net result is the replacement of structurally inadequate bone with new bone that maintains the vitality of the skeleton and its ability to withstand stress.

The entire process is orchestrated by a combination of hormones and by local factors that are either growth-stimulating or resorption-stimulating cytokines. There is also modulation by other influences to include heredity, environment, life style, and other "risk factors" (Table 148-1). The local factors involved are in part self-regulating, in part under hormonal control, and in part responsive to modulating factors. As such, they are the moieties that directly influence osteoclastic and osteoblastic activity, and the balance between them.

The term *metabolic bone disease* refers to a large number of skeletal afflictions that arise from disturbances in the orderly sequence of skeletal modeling during growth and development, and *with* skeletal turnover in *adults*. Many rare examples have their basis in genetic mutations affecting the controlling hormones or their receptors, local factors and their receptors, or the assembly of the type I collagen molecules during bone matrix formation. Examples of diseases arising from these defects are presented in Table 148-2. The most common metabolic bone diseases—osteoporosis, Paget's disease of bone, osteomalacia, and renal osteodystrophy—in many cases have an element of genetic predisposition. However, evolving knowledge of the causes of these conditions indicates that an interplay of inherent and "environmental" factors is operative. Therefore, both preventive and interventional actions can be taken to limit the impact of these impinging factors, and their eventual expression as a metabolic bone disease.

Table 148-1

Risk Factors For Bone Loss

Genetic	Female sex
	Caucasian/Asian ethnicity
	Family history of osteoporosis
Life Style	Low calcium intake
	Excessive alcohol use
	Cigarette smoking
	Excessive caffeine use
	Extreme or insufficient athlecity
	Excessive acid ash diet (high protein/soft drink intakes)
Medical	Early menopause
	Gonadal hormone deficiency states
	Eating disorders
	Chronic liver/kidney disease
	Malabsorption syndromes
Iatrogenic	Corticosteroids
	Excessive thyroid hormone
	Chronic heparin therapy
	Radiotherapy to skeleton
	Long-term anticonvulsants
	Loop diuretics

Table 148-2

Examples of Genetic Mutations Contributing to Metabolic Bone Diseases

Enzyme defects
  Carbonic anhydrase II: Osteopetrosis
  1-Hydroxylase (25-OH-D): Vitamin D dependent rickets
Receptor defects
  PTH-PTH related protein receptor: Jensen's metaphyseal chondrodysplasia
  Fibroblast growth factor 3 receptor: Achondroplasia
  Calcium sensing receptor: Familial hypocalciuric hypercalcemia (inactivating)
  Calcium sensing receptor: Autosomal dominant hypoparathyroidism (activating)
  Vitamin D receptor: Vitamin D resistance syndromes
Signaling mechanism defects
  Gs protein excess: McCune-Albright syndrome
  Gs protein deficiency: Pseudohypoparathyroidism
Structural gene defects
  Type I collagen genes: Osteogenesis imperfecta
  Bone morphogenetic protein 4: Fibrodysplasia ossificans progressiva (activating)

Table 148-3

General Factors Predictive of Osteoporosis

Peak bone mass at maturity
  Genetic/familial
  Nutritional
  Physical (activity status, exercise, etc.)
  Life style (alcohol, cigarettes, caffeine)
  Medical (chronic diseases, hypogonadal states, etc.)
  Iatrogenic (corticosteroids, anticonvulsants, etc.)
Postmenopausal bone loss
  Accelerated trabecular bone loss for 3 to 10 years postmenopausally
  Due to increased bone resorption secondary to estrogen loss
  Loss normally 1 to 2% per year to a maximum of 10%
Age-related (involutional) bone loss
  Starts at age 35 to 40 years in both sexes, continues for 30 to 40 years
  Subtle uncoupling of rates of bone formation and resorption
  Both cortical and trabecular bone affected
  Loss normally less than 0.5% per year to a maximum of 20%
Risk factors (see Table 148-1)

OSTEOPOROSIS

EPIDEMIOLOGY

Osteoporosis is defined as a state of severe bone loss and microarchitectural disturbance of the skeleton that renders *bone* susceptible to fracture with minimal trauma. It is a major health problem in many parts of the world, especially among Caucasian and Oriental females. Of *women* who survive to age 80, *35 to 50 percent* will have sustained at least one major osteoporotic fracture. Men are not immune, especially aged men, and approximately 15 percent will eventually develop osteoporotic fractures. The annual cost of health care of osteoporotic fractures currently exceeds 10 billion dollars, and will probably increase four-fold over the next 50 years, if no preemptive actions are taken to limit the disease. These figures do not include the costs of osteoporosis treatment itself. The ideal treatment of osteoporosis is preventive. The outlook for prevention has improved greatly due to better understanding of the multifactorial causes of osteoporosis, the availability of predictive measurements for fracture, and an increasing number of bone-active therapeutic agents under study.

CAUSATIVE FACTORS

Four sets of factors have been identified as playing a role in the genesis of osteoporosis (Table 148-3). Many patients who manifest osteoporosis in later life have failed to achieve optimal bone mass during growth and development, and enter their mature years with suboptimal bone mass. In many instances, a hereditary component mandating low bone mass is present, but, in addition, many patients lack adequate calcium intake during their early years, and also lack physical conditioning. The early use of alcohol, tobacco products, and excessive caffeine also contributes to bone loss. In some instances, the intercession of chronic diseases, especially if they are endocrine and associated with hypogonadism, plays a role. Finally, the use of certain drugs that predispose one to diminished bone accretion during growth may add to the problem.

The loss of estrogen secretion during menopause contributes significantly to later bone loss, working through activation of resorption-stimulating cytokines such as interleukins 6 and 1, and inhibition of growth factors such as insulin-like growth factor 1 (somatomedin or IGF-1). Bone turnover accelerates during the perimenopausal period and for several years thereafter. Unfortunately, the bone resorption rate exceeds the formation rate, and bone is lost; sometimes excessively for an unduly long period. Normally, postmenopausal bone loss averages 1 to 2 percent per year for 3 to 10 years; the total loss sustained through estrogen deficiency should not exceed 10 percent of the skeleton. Because of its greater surface area and metabolic activity, this overall loss can translate into a loss of trabecular bone of approximately 30 percent, whereas cortical bone loss may be as little as 5 percent.

A third component contributing to bone loss in osteoporosis is age-related (involutional) bone loss, which occurs with normal or even low bone turnover. It represents a subtle uncoupling of the rates of bone resorption and formation and begins at approximately age 35 to 40, continuing thereafter for approximately 40 years. Normally, the uncoupling does not cause bone loss greater than 0.5 percent per year and a cumulative lifetime loss of 20 percent. Cortical and trabecular bone are affected, but the latter more so. The rate of loss tends to be slower in men than in women. The cause(s) of age-related bone loss are unknown, and are therefore not directly accessible to treatment.

It has been speculated that exaggerated age-related bone loss may depend on disturbed local factor function and that, once the operative factor(s) can be identified, appropriate intervention will be possible. This is especially desirable since this component is quantitatively the greatest loss that occurs over the lifetime, and may be specifically involved in hip fractures.

The fourth set of general factors in bone loss underlying osteoporosis are the so-called risk factors, which represent a miscellaneous group of hereditary, environmental, life-style, medical, and iatrogenic factors, as indicated by the extensive list in Table 148-1. Of the multiple risk factors cited, inadequate calcium intake, inadequate physical conditioning, and the excessive use of alcohol, tobacco, and caffeine are probably most important. Patients with hypothyroidism, who are being treated with excessive doses of thyroxin, and patients who require pharmacologic doses of corticosteroids are at particular risk. Risk factor reduction, if applied early, will also optimize skeletal mass during growth and development. Early attention to risk factors and postmenopausal bone loss (by hormone replacement treatment) should reduce the incidence of osteoporosis by more than 50 percent, even though our ability to manage age-related bone loss is limited.

The net result of the interplay among the factors promoting bone loss is the development of a fragile skeleton with an overall loss greater than 30 percent, but with predominant trabecular bone loss. Until back pain or peripheral fractures appear, the condition is usually silent and patients are not aware of the progressing osteopenia. Once the amount of bone loss exceeds a hypothetical fracture threshold, however, patients become increasingly at risk for fractures following minor trauma, or even from the stress placed on the skeleton by everyday activities. Eventually, clinical manifestations of osteoporosis develop that are characterized by chronic or intermittent back pain, and punctuated by episodes of severe back pain as overt vertebral compression fractures occur. Patients may also sustain peripheral fractures, predominantly at sites that depend on trabecular bone for structural support; that is, the ends of the long bones such as the upper femur, distal radius, and upper humerus, the pubic rami, and ribs. The degree of pain and disability is variable, as is the rate of progression. Vertebral compression fractures cause loss of stature with the development of kyphosis, and eventually the abutment of the lower rib margins on the iliac crests. In some cases, either before or after vertebral compression, an additional component of scoliosis is present, further adding to deformity, height loss, pain, and disability.

BONE DENSITOMETRY

Both early and late radiographic changes accompany this process (Table 148-4), but the so-called early changes indicate significant microfracturing of trabecular bone in the vertebral bodies, and imminence of overt compression fractures. Biochemical abnormalities are generally absent, except for an occasional transient elevation of the serum total and bone-specific alkaline phosphatase levels, secondary to recent fractures. The presence of persistent biochemical abnormalities should alert physicians to the possibility of another disease condition either complicating osteoporosis or causing the bony fragility. Bone scans often show focal abnormalities at the site of previous fractures; these abnormalities may persist for a prolonged period after a previous fracture and may be misread as indicative of metastatic disease. In general, bone scans should not be done in suspected osteoporosis unless a different skeletal diagnosis is being seriously entertained.

An essential component of the clinical evaluation of patients with evolving or established osteoporosis is the quantitation of bone mineral density (BMD). This can be accomplished by one of three methodologies: dual x-ray absorptiometry (DXA) of the lumbar spine

and upper hips, quantitative computed tomographic scanning of the lumbar spine, and bone histomorphometry of a transiliac bone biopsy. Of the three methods, DXA is the method of choice based on its noninvasive character, ease of performance, low radiation exposure, and cost. It is also the most widely available, especially in urban communities. DXA is based on the differential absorption by bone and surrounding soft tissues of two low energy (40 keV and 100 keV) x-ray beams that are emitted by a filtered x-ray source contained within the instrument. This x-ray source scans the areas of interest rectilinearly and is tracked by a highly collimated detector that quantifies the attenuation of the x-ray beams, corrects for soft tissue absorption, and compares them to standards based on young adults and normal subjects of similar age. The output yields the BMD of lumbar vertebrae separately, and as an average. Various sites in the upper femur are also quantitated and, with some instruments, an average for the entire upper femur is displayed. The outputs of the various DXA instruments on the market vary and are not directly intercomparable. To help obviate this problem, DXA data are most conveniently evaluated as the number of standard deviations below the mean for an appropriate comparison population (T or Z score). Most experts feel that comparisons with young adults are most meaningful (T score), and base their treatment recommendations on the T score (Table 148-5). Whenever possible, follow-up DXA studies should be done on the same instrument and at the same location as the baseline DXA study.

Table 148-4

Radiologic Changes in Osteoporosis

"Early"
- Increased width of intervertebral spaces
- Schmorl's nodes
- Relative accentuation of cortical plates
- Visible vertical striations of vertebral bodies

Late
- Vertebral compression
- Cortical plate fractures
- Crush fractures
- Wedged vertebrae
- Peripheral fractures at ends of long bones (femoral neck, proximal humerus, distal radius, etc.)

Table 148-5

Representative Scheme for Interpreting DXA Generated Bone Density Data

T Score (No. of SD below mean of young adults)	Degree of bone loss	Risk of fracture
0 to −1	None	None
−1 to −2	Moderate	Small
−2 to −3	Severe	Moderate
Below −3	Very severe	Severe

Table 148-6

Goals of Osteoporosis Prevention

Optimizing skeletal development (see Table 148-3)
  Nutrition
  Physical activity
  Life style changes
  Minimize medical/iatrogenic factors
Minimize postmenopausal bone loss
  Early identification of patients at risk
  Reduce risk factors (see Table 148-1)
  Hormone replacement therapy (HRT)
  Other agents preemptively if HRT contraindicated
  raloxifene, alendronate
Minimize age-related bone loss
  Identification of patients at risk
  Reduce risk factors (see Table 148-1)
  Full prevention and exercise programs (physical therapy)

PREVENTIVE TREATMENT

Preventive treatment involves both primary and secondary methodologies. Measures that can be applied population-wide and can be started at an early age involve the avoidance of the aforementioned risk factors that are relevant to the entire population (Table 148-1). Secondary prevention procedures are similar to those for primary prevention, but may also include the prescription of a bone-active agent, such as hormone replacement treatment, in postmenopausal women who have lost significant bone mass but have not yet had a fracture. Goals and procedures that are used in a prevention program are listed in Tables 148-6 and 148-7.

TREATMENT OF ESTABLISHED OSTEOPOROSIS

The treatment of established osteoporosis involves both general management and drug therapy. Attention to proper diet, encouragement of

---
Table 148-7

Elements of Osteoporosis Prevention

Reduce risk factors (see Table 148-1)
  Appropriate diet: 1 to 1.5 g of calcium per day from
                        all sources
                        600- to 800-IU vitamin D per day
                        Delete sources of excessive protein
                        and phosphorus
  Appropriate exercise program
  Adjustment of life style   Avoid alcohol/cigarettes
                               Reduce caffeine intake
  Treat predisposing medical conditions
  Minimize iatrogenic factors (see Table 148-1)
Baseline measurements of DXA generated bone density
  Periodic remeasurements if indicated
Prophylactic drug therapy when indicated (HRT, raloxifene, alendronate)

maximum mobility, rehabilitation therapy when necessary, and risk factor reduction are important. Most devastating osteoporotic fractures occur after a fall, and proper rehabilitation should instruct patients on how to reduce falls. Physical barriers and hazards in a patient's home and other living areas should be eliminated. Psychotropic drugs should be prescribed sparingly because they reduce a patient's awareness of hazards. It is necessary to provide reasonable analgesia for back and other musculoskeletal pain, but not at the expense of reducing awareness and mobility. Judicious use of weak narcotics, such as propoxyphene and oxycodone combined with either salicylates or acetaminophen, is usually sufficient. In some patients, the addition of nonsteroidal anti-inflammatory drug (NSAID) may be advisable.

Four classes of drugs have been used to treat established osteoporosis in an attempt to augment bone density or stabilize the skeleton so that no further loss occurs (Table 148-8). In many patients, these agents can increase bone density by 3 to 10 percent, and theoretically reduce risk of subsequent fracture by 20 to 50 percent. Three are approved by the Food and Drug Administration (FDA): hormone replacement treatment (HRT), synthetic salmon calcitonin (SCT), and bisphosphonates. Sodium fluoride (NaF) is no longer used because of concerns, not convincingly proven, that it may adversely affect cortical bone and predispose individuals to peripheral fractures despite its ability to stimulate trabecular bone formation and increase vertebral trabecular bone mass. A slow-release form of NaF that is before the FDA for licensing does not appear to have these complications. Raloxifene is FDA approved for prevetion only.

Hormone Replacement

HRT is considered to be the "gold standard" of the present-day drug treatment of osteoporosis. It has had widespread use over the past 50 years for both secondary prevention in patients with decreased bone mass but no fractures and in patients after fracture. Although there are a number of contraindications, both absolute and relative, as well as annoying side effects that are usually transient, the large majority of women can take HRT with good benefit, not only to their skeleton, but also as a cardioprotective agent to prevent coronary artery disease. HRT requires careful monitoring by a generalist, endocrinologist, or gynecologist, with at least yearly breast and pelvic examinations, Pap smear, and mammogram. Despite advocacy for HRT on the part of most knowledgeable practitioners, there is widespread concern among patients as to safety, with the predominant concern being carcinoma of the breast. This is a controversial issue, and it is unclear whether there is a small increase in risk with HRT. In view of the cardioprotective effect of HRT, however, there is an overall benefit to patients. It has been estimated that only 50 percent of women who should be taking HRT for either secondary prevention or for treatment for established osteoporosis are willing to start treatment, and only half of these will continue treatment beyond 6 months.

Table 148-8

Therapeutic Agents in Osteoporosis

Hormone replacement therapy (estrogen/progesterone)
Sodium fluoride, sustained release fluoride preparations
Calcitonin (salmon)
Bisphosphonates (etidronate, alendronate, higher generation
  bisphosphonates)
Selective estrogen receptor modulators (reloxifene)

In an attempt to overcome this problem, "designer estrogens," known as selective estrogen receptor modulators (SERMs) have been developed and one, raloxifene (an analog of tamoxifen), is now FDA approved for the prevention of osteoporosis. The SERMs have properties similar to estrogens with regard to skeletal actions and cardioprotection, but do not stimulate the breast or uterus. Therefore, they can be used in place of HRT with greater safety and less monitoring.

Calcitonin

SCT is a nongonadal, bone-active hormone with few of the problems associated with HRT. In approximately 70 percent of treated patients, SCT will not only accomplish the same results as HRT, but has a greater effect in reducing bone pain. However, there are other problems with its use as an injectable, including early side effects, such as nausea and facial flushing, which are a relatively short-term nuisance but often influence patients not to continue treatment. The need to self-inject daily or every other day and the drug's cost are also concerns. SCT is not generally used for secondary prevention, but is highly effective in established osteoporosis. For this indication, it has an additional benefit as a "bone analgesic" with a noticeable reduction in bone pain gradually over the first few months of treatment. SCT is a foreign protein, and secondary resistance will occur after prolonged treatment in a small percentage of patients. Secondary resistance in osteoporosis is manifested by a resumption of bone pain and a loss of the stabilizing or augmenting effect of SCT on bone density, as measured by DXA.

To obviate compliance problems associated with side effects and the need for injections, a nasal preparation of SCT, already available in many countries, is now licensed by the FDA for use in the United States. Nasal calcitonin retains the positive features of calcitonin use. Further, the cost has been curtailed to widen possible indications for use. Nasal SCT has largely supplanted injectable SCT and appears to be as effective.

Bisphosphonates

The bisphosphonates are analogs of pyrophosphate, a natural inhibitor of bone metabolism. They are immune to degradation by alkaline phosphatase and, although poorly absorbed, have a prolonged action once deposited in the skeleton. The first-generation bisphosphonate, disodium etidronate, has had extensive clinical trials as a treatment for osteoporosis over the past decade and, when given cyclically, can produce approximately a 5 percent increase in lumbar BMD in many patients. Thus far, architectural deterioration of the spine, as might occur if the agent's anti-mineralization effect caused defective hydroxyapatite deposition, has not been observed. Etidronate has failed to receive FDA approval because it is still unclear whether its use reduces fracture incidence. A newer bisphosphonate, alendronate, has received FDA approval. In established osteoporosis, a decrease in biochemical markers of bone resorption is noted, and a consistent increase in BMD of 5 to 8 percent occurs in both the lumbar spine and upper femur. Prevention of postmenopausal bone loss and decreased fracture rates have also been reported. Alendronate has come into widespread use since its introduction.

Dose and Duration

The duration of drug treatment for osteoporosis obviously depends on the agent. HRT will have beneficial effects on bone density for as long as it is administered, since "catch-up" bone loss can occur after its discontinuation. It is generally believed that HRT, once started, should not be discontinued, but should be taken for as long as the patient is able. Recent studies suggest that if the total duration of treatment is less than 5 years, no long-term benefit is likely. Once HRT is well established, it generally provides few problems thereafter, so long as proper monitoring is maintained. Many women are capable of taking this form of treatment beyond age 75 with few problems. Bone density should be measured by DXA yearly to monitor the effects of treatment.

The recommended durations of SCT and alendronate have not been determined; nor have the doses or frequency of administration. The therapeutic range for injectable SCT is from 50 IU three times a week to 100 IU daily and, for nasal SCT, 200 IU per day, alternating nostrils. Some physicians advocate intermittent treatment for SCT, although there is, as yet, no definitive scientific data to support intermittent programs of treatment. One possible concern with intermittent programs is promotion of secondary resistance. Alendronate is usually given daily in a dose of 10 mg, not cyclically, and must be taken on an empty stomach with no food, beverages, or other drugs for approximately 1 h. Patients should use a full glass of water to swallow the pill, and remain in the upright position for 1 h to prevent lower esophageal side effects. In these treatment programs, bone density should also be measured yearly by DXA to determine the progress of treatment. More recently, a 5 mg dose size of alendronate has received FDA approval for the prevention of postmenopausal bone loss.

PAGET'S DISEASE OF BONE

EPIDEMIOLOGY

Paget's disease (osteitis deformans) is an inflammatory condition characterized by painful, deformed bones that limit mobility and fracture easily. The disease varies in severity, from no symptoms with few bones involved to a highly disabling and sometimes fatal form. Paget's disease is a focal disease, both demographically and anatomically. In the United Kingdom, 4 to 6 percent of the Caucasian population over the age of 50 are affected. Paget's disease has spread to other areas settled by the English, and its frequency in Australia and New Zealand is also high. In France, Germany, the United States, and certain parts of Italy, a frequency of 3 percent of the Caucasian population over the age of 50 is affected. Paget's disease is uncommon in Scandinavia, as well as in African-Americans and Asians.

There is a marked familial incidence of Paget's disease, and the parents and siblings of index cases have a sevenfold to tenfold greater frequency of the disease than the first-order relatives of their spouse, if radiographs and biochemical studies are included to detect patients who are asymptomatic. Patient awareness is estimated to be approximately 15 percent. In severe cases, a careful documentation of the medical history may disclose early symptoms dating from the third to fourth decades of life. There are approximately one million cases in the United States.

ETIOLOGY

The etiology of Paget's disease remains unknown. Hereditary factors are operative, but the interaction is unclear. Recent studies suggest precise genetic loci may be involved. Hormonal abnormalities are considered to be secondary effects. The most prevalent etiologic theory is that Paget's disease represents a slow virus infection of the afflicted bones. The major evidence consists of the ubiquitous finding of "nucleocapsid-like" inclusion bodies in the nuclei and cytoplasm of pagetic osteoclasts, suggesting paramyxoviral infection. Although there is supporting cytoimmunochemical and *in situ* hybridization evidence, there is no agreement as to the identity of the putative virus, with measles, respiratory syncytial virus (RSV), parainfluenza 3 virus, and the canine distemper virus (CDV)—all potential candidates. Until viral rescue from pathologic lesions is accomplished, the slow-virus theory remains unproven.

Osteoclasts are activated during the pathogenesis of the condition to proliferate wildly with the development of bizarre osteoclasts that may contain up to 100 nuclei. In response to intense, chaotic, but focal osteolysis, osteoblasts are recruited and, in an equally chaotic and unregulated fashion, they attempt to repair the osteolytic damage. This sequential process can move across an area of involved pagetic bone several times. Eventually, bone formation exceeds resorption, and an excessive amount of poorly organized, structurally deficient, under-mineralized bone appears, the so-called sclerotic phase. Radiographically, this sequential process can be recognized as a front of resorptive activity that moves across an involved bone, followed behind by thickened areas of sclerotic bone.

CLINICAL FEATURES

The cardinal clinical features are pain, deformities, and fractures (Table 148-9). Direct skeletal pain is due to periosteal irritation, deep and boring, and worse at night. The pain lessens but does not disappear during physical activity. In some patients, this pain is referred to the joints or muscles, but may also be due to the secondary osteoarthritis that commonly occurs. Deformed pagetic bone may also cause intervening joints to operate at a mechanical disadvantage, causing muscular pain. Impingement on exiting cranial and spinal nerves may produce radiculo-neuropathic pain. Patients with extensive Paget's disease of the skull commonly complain of headaches.

The structurally abnormal bone deforms under stress, causing bowing of thickened long bones, or flattening of the skull, which leads

---

Table 148-9

Skeletal Features of Paget's Disease

Pain
  Skeletal
  Osteoarthritic
  Muscular
  Radicular
  Headache
Deformities
  Thickening/bowing
  Head enlargement, platybasia
  Kyphoscoliosis
  Acetabular protrusion
Fractures
  Complete fractures
  Fissure fractures
  Vertebral compression and collapse
Miscellaneous
  Malignant conversion
  Giant cell tumor
  Osteoporosis circumscripta
  Osteoarthritis
  Increased vascularity (increased skin temperature)
  Immobilization hypercalcemia

---

to a condition known as platybasia or basilar invagination. Pagetic vertebrae commonly compress. Weakened acetabula may cause acetabular protrusion. Fractures occur with minimal trauma and may be complete fractures or incomplete fractures; the latter are known as fissure fractures through the cortex of long bones along the convex side of deformities. Fissure fractures may later become complete horizontal fractures.

Miscellaneous skeletal abnormalities can include a fan-like wave of bone resorption in the calvarium known as osteoporosis circumscripta cranii, which is later replaced by more characteristic "cotton-ball" sclerotic lesions. Pagetic bone is highly vascular and has a large, low-pressure, high cross-section capillary bed. When 30 percent or more of the skeleton is involved, an increased cardiac output is required for adequate perfusion of the skeleton. Increased bone vascularity is palpable as an increase in skin temperature.

An unusual neoplastic complication is the development of benign giant cell tumors, which consist of neoplastic osteoclast-like cells in a fibrous background. These benign tumors are resistant to extirpative therapy, but there are some reports of regression with corticosteroid therapy. A more serious neoplastic complication is conversion into a mesenchymal malignancy, such as osteogenic sarcoma, fibrosarcoma, chondrosarcoma, or other variants. These sarcomas are highly malignant and particularly resistant to both surgical and nonsurgical forms of palliation. Death usually occurs within 2 years, but scattered reports of long survival after high-dose x-ray radiation treatment have appeared.

Neurologic symptoms and findings can accompany Paget's disease of the skull and spinal column by direct impingement or ischemia due to a "pagetic steal syndrome." Typical neurologic deficits are listed in Table 148-10. The most common deficit is sensorineural hearing loss. Optic nerve involvement can cause focal visual defects. Paget's disease of the posterior skull may affect the lower cranial nerves, medulla, and cerebellum. Partial obstruction in the aqueductal region may cause Valsalva-induced cranial pain. In the spinal cord, a combination of myelopathy and radiculoneuropathy can occur.

Two retinal lesions, angioid streaks and mottled retinal degeneration, which are not directly neurologic in origin, can cause serious visual impairment. In the cardiovascular system, medial calcinosis and intimal atherosclerosis occur commonly. Renal calculi may be composed of either uric acid or calcium salts.

Excessive osteoclastic activity can be monitored by increased urinary excretion of pyridinium collagen cross-links or the N-telopeptide, which represent degraded and nonreutilized portions of the bone collagen molecule. Serum tartrate-resistant acid phosphatase (TRAP), a constituent of osteoclasts, is also increased. Osteoblastic activity is indicated by total serum alkaline phosphatase (if liver disease is absent), bone-specific alkaline phosphatase, and serum osteocalcin levels. Another osteoblast marker are the procollagen extension peptides, which are nonutilized terminal peptides released during assembly of the collagen molecule.

Radiographs show an irregular pattern of alternating bone formation and resorption in enlarged, deformed bones. Resorptive fronts at the advancing edge of the disease process is an early finding. There is intense uptake of radiotechnetium in affected bones on bone scans. Bone scans define the full extent of the disease so that x-rays can be directed at determining essential anatomic features. Computed tomography and magnetic resonance imaging of pagetic lesions are rarely needed, but can demonstrate extra-bony extension when sarcomatous change is suspected. Bone biopsy should be done only if there is confusion regarding diagnosis or suspicion of a sarcomatous complication. Differential diagnostic considerations are usually minimal since it is usually easy to distinguish Paget's disease from polyos-

---
Table 148-10

Neurologic Features of Paget's Disease

CRANIAL NERVE

I:	Anosmia
II:	Optic atrophy, field defects, papilledema, proptosis, angioid streaks, mottled retinal degeneration
III, IV, VI:	Oculomotor palsies, diplopia, ptosis
V:	Trigeminal neuralgia and sensory deficits
VII:	Hemifacial spasm, Bell's palsy
VIII:	Deafness, tinnitus, vestibular dysfunction
IX, XI, XII:	Dysphagia, dysarthria, pharyngeal, lingual, and shoulder muscle weakness

MEDULLA AND CEREBELLUM

Pyramidal tract signs, Valsalva induced headaches, ataxia, cerebellar dysfunction, hydrocephalus-dementia syndrome

SPINAL CORD AND NERVES

Myelopathy, neuroradiculopathy, spinal stenosis, cauda equina syndrome.

MISCELLANEOUS

Pagetic "steal syndromes", peripheral nerve entrapment, carpal and tarsal tunnel syndromes

---
Table 148-11

Indications for Treatment of Paget's Disease

Pain (moderate to severe), not relieved by NSAIDs
Progressive skeletal involvement[a]
    Fractures, progressing deformities, platybasia, vertebral compression, acetabular protrusion
Predominant resorptive features[a]
    Osteoporosis circumscripta, resorptive fronts, lenticular-shaped resorptive foci, fissure fractures
Neurologic deficits
    All types, progressive auditory and/or visual loss.
Preparation for orthopaedic surgery[a]
Prolonged immobilization: post-fracture/surgery.[a]
Cardiovascular complications (secondary to increased cardiac output)
Preemptive treatment (for extreme biochemical abnormalities)

[a]See under Paget's Disease, Treatment.

---

totic fibrous dysplasia, primary bone neoplasm, mixed osteolytic–osteoblastic metastases, or skeletal hyperparathyroidism.

TREATMENT

Indications for treating Paget's disease are presented in Table 148-11. Minimal pain is best relieved by NSAIDs, but more severe pain requires specific treatment. Progressive skeletal involvement with loss of structural integrity, such as with fractures, progressing deformities (including platybasia of the skull), vertebral compression, and acetabular protrusion, should always be treated, as should extensive resorptive features noted on bone radiographs. Neurologic deficits may be partially or completely reversed except for hearing and visual changes, which will remain static and hopefully not progress. Orthopaedic surgery can cause bleeding because of excessive vascularity of pagetic bone, whereas softening or hardening of pagetic bone may cause problems with prostheses. Specific suppressive treatment reduces vascularity within days, but other problems may require up to 6 months of such prior treatment.

Four classes of drugs (Table 148-12) are available to treat Paget's disease: the calcitonins, the bisphosphonates, plicamycin, and gallium nitrate. NSAIDs should also be included to treat minor pain and secondary osteoarthritis. The calcitonins have the longest track record of efficacy, with positive subjective and objective responses in 85 percent of treated patients. Biochemical parameters of disease activity decrease 50 to 70 percent. Radiographs show gradual filling in of lytic lesions, but sclerotic lesions do not change nor is there a correction of previous deformities. Sequential bone biopsies show a partial reversal of the abnormal histology typical of the disease. Bone vascularity decreases. Injectable SCT, 50 IU three times a week, is the preferred calcitonin, and should be given for 12 to 18 months. In approximately 20 percent of initially responsive patients, secondary resistance will eventually occur, and can be reversed by switching to a bisphosphonate. A prolonged clinical response is often seen after the cessation of treatment, but there is eventually a return of biochemical parameters to baseline and a resumption of symptomatology. Nasal SCT does not carry an FDA-approved indication for Paget's disease, but is often effective, and can be used to replace injectable SCT using the 200 IU dose, as in osteoporosis. It is unclear whether daily to every-other-day treatment will suffice.

Disodium etidronate, mentioned previously as a non-FDA-approved treatment for osteoporosis, is FDA-approved for Paget's disease. It is usually administered on an empty stomach in a dose of 400 mg daily, in 6-month courses, with 3- to 6-month rest periods between courses. In most patients in need of treatment, etidronate accomplishes the same result as SCT. However, there are some indications for treatment (footnote in Table 148-11) where SCT is probably preferable, because it does not have an inhibitory effect on osteoblastic action or mineralization. This is undesirable in patients with rapidly progressive bone changes, or radiologic evidence of predominant resorptive

---
Table 148-12

Therapeutic Agents for Paget's Disease

Calcitonins: salmon, eel
Bisphosphonates: etidronate, pamidronate, alendronate, teludronate, residronate.
Plicamycin
Gallium nitrate
NSAIDs

---

disease, and in individuals who have recently incurred fractures or undergone orthopaedic surgery. With these exceptions, etidronate is a reasonable alternative to SCT. It has the advantage of oral administration (on an empty stomach), but is no less expensive than SCT. Nasal SCT, although not specifically licensed for Paget's disease, is also an option.

Both an intravenous bisphosphonate (pamidronate) and three newer oral bisphosphonates (alendronate, teludronate, and risedronate) are now licensed for use in Paget's disease. Pamidronate requires sequential intravenous infusions either in the hospital or at an infusion center and is expensive. It is not being used as first-line treatment in the United States although it is the preferred treatment in other countries. Pamidronate is reasonably well tolerated with relatively few, transient, side effects. It is preferred in patients who have become resistant or intolerant of either SCT or etidronate. It does not have the antimineralization qualities that can sometimes be a problem with etidronate.

Alendronate, in a daily dose of 40 mg (higher than the 5- and 10-mg doses in osteoporosis), is also an effective treatment for Paget's disease, and has the advantage over pamidronate of the oral route. The same precautions as for osteoporosis treatment should be followed. Also, like pamidronate, it does not have antimineralization properties, and can be used for the footnoted indications in Table 148-11. Similarly, teludronate in a daily dose of 400 mg and risedronate in a daily dose of 30 mg are effective treatment. These newer bisphosphonates are usually given in courses, 6 months for alendronate, 3 months for teludronate, and 2 months for residronate.

Plicamycin has been used to treat resistant Paget's disease for over two decades and is as effective as any of the agents that are in more common use. Its major drawback is that it requires administration in either an infusion center or a hospital. In addition, it has many serious side effects, including gastrointestinal (GI) side effects, hematologic abnormalities (especially thrombocytopenia), and hepatic and renal dysfunction. In most patients, these side effects are transient, but must be monitored carefully. Patients with preexistent hematologic, GI, hepatic, and/or renal problems (especially a history of prior upper GI bleeding) should not be treated with plicamycin. Gallium nitrate is the most recent form of treatment to be advocated for Paget's disease and also is not FDA-approved for this indication. There is insufficient experience to indicate whether it is as effective as other agents, but the extant data suggest that it is. Like pamidronate, it must be given intravenously in an infusion center or hospital, and has relatively few and acceptable side effects, but is also expensive. It is an option for treatment when other agents are either ineffective or cannot be used.

With all forms of treatment, the cases of patients should be followed at approximately 2- to 3-month intervals with either total serum or bone-specific alkaline phosphatase measurements to indicate the progress of treatment. Testing after a completed course of treatment will determine whether clinical improvement is being maintained or relapse is imminent. All classes of drugs are capable of inducing relatively prolonged remissions of 6 months or longer after treatment is complete. Recurrence will usually be sooner with SCT than with the other agents.

In addition to specific antipagetic treatment, as just outlined, many patients will require concomitant treatment with a NSAID, because a significant amount of their symptomatology relates to the secondary osteoarthritis that so commonly accompanies Paget's disease. Continued pain in the presence of a declining alkaline phosphatase level (which indicates that specific treatment is effective) is a prime indication for NSAID use. In 10 to 15 percent of patients, the antimineralizing property of etidronate causes increased rather than decreased bone pain at the site of pagetic lesions. In these patients, the drug must be discontinued and an alternate form of treatment sought.

SKELETAL HYPERPARATHYROIDISM

Parathyroid hormone has complex effects on the skeleton, depending on the degree, duration, and cyclicity of parathyroid gland secretion. Under physiologic conditions, it will promote cortical bone resorption via osteoclast stimulation, but at the same time can facilitate trabecular bone formation via osteoblast stimulation. When hypersecreted in large amounts over a prolonged period, a situation rarely encountered today as a primary abnormality, significant bone loss can occur characterized by subperiosteal cortical bone resorption and "tunneling"; that is, excavation of osteons within the interior of the cortices. Typical radiographic and histologic patterns consist of scalloping and porotic cavities within bone, with intense osteoclastic and osteoblastic reactions within a fibrous matrix. Although primary hyperparathyroidism is a relatively common condition, especially in older patients, it rarely causes this severe skeletal dysfunction. More commonly, skeletal architecture and mass are preserved, or bone loss resembling osteoporosis occurs. However, cortical bone is more severely affected than in osteoporosis. Any degree of skeletal loss in primary hyperparathyroidism is considered an indication for parathyroid exploration with removal of an offending parathyroid adenoma or subtotal resection of diffuse parathyroid hyperplasia.

OSTEOMALACIA

Unlike osteoporosis, Paget's disease, and skeletal hyperparathyroidism, in which there are profound disturbances in bone formation and resorption, the osteomalacic syndromes that have been recognized (Table 148-13) arise primarily from a deficit in the mineralization of bone matrix. Mineralization requires osteoblastic intervention, adequate provision of the minerals to be deposited (calcium, phosphorus, and hydroxyl ions), and provision of active vitamin D metabolites such as calcitriol (1,25-dihydroxy-vitamin D). Clinically, osteomalacia may mimic osteoporosis and must be ruled out before initiating treatment for osteoporosis. The clinical features that can distinguish osteomalacia from osteoporosis are outlined in Table 148-14. Pseudofractures are serpentine, and are often symmetric defects at sites in the bone cortex where muscular arteries wrap around

---

Table 148-13

Causes of Osteomalacia

Vitamin D deficiency: nutritional, secondary to Billroth II gastrectomy

Malabsorption syndromes

Vitamin D dependent rickets (1-alpha hydroxylation defect)

Familial hypophosphatemic rickets (vitamin D "resistant")

Vitamin D receptor defects

Chronic renal disease (tubular, occasionally glomerular)

Oncogenic osteomalacia (mesenchymal tumors)

Hypophosphatasia

Drugs/toxic agents

    Anticonvulsants, phosphate binders (mega doses), etidronate, aluminum, cadmium, fluoride, iron

---

Table 148-14

Distinguishing Clinical Features of Osteomalacia

Diffuse musculoskeletal pain
Muscle weakness, waddling gait
Deformities characteristic of childhood rickets
Pseudofractures
Increased total and bone specific alkaline phosphate levels
Decreased serum Ca × P product
Bone biopsy showing increased osteoid and decreased mineralization rate

---

Table 148-16

Treatment of Renal Osteodystrophy

Optimize renal function and dialysis procedures, consider renal transplantation
Remove excess skeletal aluminum and iron, if present (chelators such as desferrioxamine)
Calcium supplements (as phosphate binders)
Reduced phosphorus, magnesium, protein, acid ash in diet
Calcitriol (to tolerance)
Parathyroid ablation (in selected cases)
Calcitonin

---

bone or enter bone cortex as a nutrient artery. Pseudofractures can evolve into complete fractures at any site in the skeleton. If pseudofractures are not present, the diagnosis of osteomalacia requires a nondecalcified transilial bone biopsy subjected to quantitative histomorphometric techniques including prelabeling with tetracycline. The treatment of osteomalacia requires correcting the cause (if known and treatable) and the provision of mineral supplements and appropriate vitamin D analogs (Table 148-15).

RENAL OSTEODYSTROPHY

Renal osteodystrophy is a nonspecific term used to describe the complex skeletal changes that occur during long-standing, end-stage glomerular failure, which is usually under treatment with hemodialysis or peritoneal dialysis. The major component is skeletal hyperparathyroidism, secondary to parathyroid hyperplasia; but in many patients there is also a component of osteomalacia, most often due to aluminum accumulation from the use of aluminum-containing phosphate binders. Generalized osteoporotic changes are also present. A curious fourth component, osteosclerosis, is sometimes present. Many theories have been advanced to account for the osteosclerosis, but none is generally accepted. The clinical consequences of renal osteodystrophy can be serious, and they cause more disability than the underlying renal failure. Treatment is complex, difficult, and not always effective (Table 148-16).

Table 148-15

Treatment of Osteomalacia

Nutritional: calcium, vitamin D supplements
Malabsorption: gluten-free diet, pancreatic enzymes, calcium, vitamin D supplements
Vitamin D dependent rickets: calcium, calcitriol
Familial hypophosphatemic rickets: phosphate, vitamin D supplements, calcitriol
Chronic renal disease: calcium, calcitriol
Oncogenic osteomalacia: locate and excise mesenchymal tumor

NEOPLASTIC INVASION OF THE SKELETON

A number of malignant neoplasms can affect skeletal metabolism, by virtue of the ability of their skeletal metastases or deposits to secrete cytokines and growth factors capable of stimulating osteoclasts and osteoblasts. In solid tumors, parathyroid hormone-related protein (PTHRP) secreted by the tumor and/or its skeletal deposits is the most common inciting factor, and may even cause systemic hypercalcemia. In most instances, the lytic and/or blastic lesions that occur are discrete and readily identified. On rare occasions, the neoplasm-related bone resorption may be diffuse, without hypercalcemia, and mimic osteoporosis. In the case of multiple myeloma and other hematologic neoplasms, cytokines rather than PTH-RP are responsible. The lytic skeletal changes are diffuse as often as they are discrete, and a misdiagnosis of osteoporosis is often made. Proper diagnosis of neoplastic invasion sometimes requires histologic identification of the neoplastic cells in a bone marrow aspiration or biopsy. A bone biopsy may be needed. Treatment involves appropriate chemotherapy and radiotherapy in sensitive tumors and treatment of hypercalcemia, if present. Recently, palliation of the responsible tumor has been reported in research studies involving calcitonin and higher-generation bisphosphonates, based on their ability to oppose cytokine-induced bone resorption. Pamidronate is now FDA-approved for certain skeletal malignancies.

ORTHOPAEDIC ASPECTS

The majority of the metabolic bone diseases discussed have endocrine/rheumatologic treatments that will generally result in significant improvement. Orthopaedic surgeons are also interested in these conditions, and may play a nonoperative therapeutic role. With regard to operative intervention, surgery is most commonly needed as a result of fragility fractures that require closed or open reduction/stabilization. Other procedures that may be required in this patient group include osteotomy to correct deformities, total joint replacement, scoliosis stabilization, and bone biopsy.

Except for acute fracture intervention, operative procedures should not be undertaken until available treatment for the underlying metabolic bone disease has been instituted and the desired effect achieved. As an example, elective osteotomies and joint replacements in Paget's disease should be delayed as long as possible to allow the markedly increased blood flow through pagetic bone to decrease and for the quality of the bone to improve maximally. Osteomalacic bone heals particularly poorly, and appropriate nonoperative treatment should be instituted first to maximize postoperative healing. A major exception is osteoporotic bone that heals normally after orthopaedic surgery and is not enhanced by treatment intended to increase bone density. The drugs used to treat metabolic bone diseases do not, in general, have an adverse effect on bone healing, except when they have an anti-mineralization action at therapeutic doses, such as the first-generation bisphosphonate, disodium etidronate, and high doses of sodium fluoride that are not prepared specially for slow release. When bone exposed to these latter agents requires an orthopaedic procedure, including open fracture reduction, precautions should be taken to ensure optimal fixation and apposition of the bone fragments.

Bone biopsies are seldom required to diagnosis metabolic bone diseases, but when necessary, every attempt should be made to use the ilial bone, which is nonweightbearing. However, conditions that require diagnosis are often focal, and strategic bones may have to be biopsied with some risk of later fracture through the biopsy site. In such cases, the biopsy should be as small as possible. If an unequivocal histologic picture characterizes the condition to be diagnosed, biopsy can be performed without pretreatment with bone turnover markers such as the tetracyclines, which absorb to mineralizing surfaces. Such simple biopsies should be handled by both decalcified and nondecalcified techniques, the latter to assess the amount of unmineralized bone present. When knowledge of the state of skeletal turnover and bone mineralization rate is important, the nondecalcified technique should be employed with two prior pulse tetracycline administrations at 12-day intervals to enable double labeling and estimation of the bone mineralization rate. An attempt at double labeling should always be made when osteoporotic or osteomalacic patients are being evaluated by bone biopsy. To maximize the accuracy of reading such biopsies, a 6- to 8-mm trephine or bone biopsy needle should be employed and a "through-and-through" biopsy taken of the ilial plate, 2 cm below and 2 cm behind the superior anterior iliac spine. The actual technique of the biopsy and of preparing and reading the biopsy slides is beyond the scope of this discussion.

SUGGESTED READINGS

OSTEOPOROSIS

Christiansen C: What should be done at the time of menopause? *Am J Med* 1995; 98(2A):56S.

Kanis JA: Treatment of osteoporosis in elderly women. *Am J Med* 1995; 98(2A):60S.

Kaplan FS: Prevention and management of osteoporosis. *Clin Symp* 1995; 47:2.

Kelepouris N, Harper KD, Gannon F, et al: Severe osteoporosis in men. *Ann Intern Med* 1995; 123:452.

Lobo RA: Benefits and risks of estrogen replacement therapy. *Am J Obstet Gynecol* 1995; 173(3, Pt 2):982.

Palmieri GM: Calcium, why and how much? *Miner Electrolyte Metab* 1995; 21(1–3):236.

Prestwood KM, Pilbeam CC, Raisz LG: Treatment of osteoporosis. *Annu Rev Med* 1995; 46:249.

Seeman E: The dilemma of osteoporosis in men. *Am J Med* 1995; 98(2A): 76S.

Ziegler R, Scheidt-Nave C, Scharla S: Pathophysiology of osteoporosis: Unresolved problems and new insights. *J Nutr* 1995; 125 (suppl 7):2033S.

PAGET'S DISEASE

Bockman RS, Wilhelm F, Siris E, et al: A multicenter trial of low dose gallium nitrate in patients with advanced Paget's disease of bone. *J Clin Endocrinol Metab* 1995; 80:585.

Greenspan A: A review of Paget's disease: Radiologic imaging, differential diagnosis and treatment. *Bull Hosp Jt Dis Orthop Inst* 1991; 51:22.

Hadjipavlou A, Lander P, Srolovitz H, et al: Malignant transformation in Paget disease of bone. *Cancer* 1992; 70:2802.

Hamdy RC: Clinical features and pharmacologic treatment of Paget's disease. *Endocrinol Metab Clin North Am* 1995; 24:421.

Klein RM, Norman A: Diagnostic procedures for Paget's disease: Radiologic, pathologic and laboratory testing. *Endocrinol Metab Clin North Am* 1995; 24:437.

Morales-Piga AA, Rey-Rey JS, Corres-Gonzalez J, et al: Frequency and characteristics of familial aggregation of Paget's disease of bone. *J Bone Miner Res* 1995; 10:663.

Singer FR, Minoofer PN: Bisphosphonates in the treatment of disorders of mineral metabolism. *Adv Endocrinol Metab* 1995; 6:259.

Chapter 149

ORTHOPAEDIC ANESTHESIA

Ralph L. Bernstein and Andrew D. Rosenberg

MANAGEMENT OF THE AIRWAY IN ORTHOPAEDIC SURGERY

Obtaining and maintaining an airway for oxygen exchange and ventilation is crucial in caring for injured patients requiring emergency intubation as well as in patients undergoing elective surgery who have anatomic alterations of their airway. Orthopaedic patients present a unique population with special airway considerations.

MANAGEMENT OF PATIENTS WITH ACUTE CERVICAL SPINE INJURY

Patients presenting with spinal cord injury are usually young males in the 15- to 35-year age group. Spinal cord injuries are commonly caused by motor vehicle accidents, falls, or trauma during sports. Cervical spine injuries may be associated with head injury, fracture of the skull, facial injury, tracheal injury, and esophageal perforation. Obtaining an airway is one of the major concerns in caring for patients with cervical spine injury. Neurologic damage at a high cervical level may preclude adequate respiratory function and require emergent intubation. In addition, the usual maneuvers used to obtain an airway may result in additional neurologic damage.

Securing and Maintaining the Airway in Patients with Cervical Spine Injury

The indications for tracheal intubation in patients with cervical spine injury are

1. Relief of airway obstruction
2. Treatment of ventilatory failure
3. Facilitation of pulmonary toilet
4. Prevention of aspiration of gastric contents
5. Hyperventilation to treat elevated intracranial pressure
6. Securing of an airway for surgery

Awake Patients

In awake patients with a complaint of neck pain, movement of the neck should be avoided while obtaining an airway. In awake but uncooperative patients who may be thrashing about, a rapid sequence technique for endotracheal intubation is used. Thiopental (350 to 400 mg) is administered intravenously, followed by succinylcholine (100 mg) to provide muscle relaxation while cricoid pressure is applied by an assistant. This is done by placing two fingers on the cricoid cartilage and pressing down to occlude the esophagus against the spine to prevent regurgitation and aspiration of gastric contents.

Succinylcholine, which may cause the release of potassium in patients with a spinal cord injury, can be safely used for up to 24 h after spinal injury. The use of cricoid pressure does not appear to exacerbate cervical spine injury.

Unconscious Patients

Manipulation of the neck is avoided in unconscious patients. Ventilation is provided with a bag and mask to ensure adequate oxygenation before attempting intubation of the trachea. Blind nasotracheal intubation must not be used if a patient has fractures of the face or if a basilar skull fracture is suspected; an airway or endotracheal tube can enter the brain. If ventilation by bag or mask does not result in expansion of the lungs, injury to the soft tissues of the pharynx may be present. It is important to examine the lateral radiograph of the cervical spine to determine whether the normal soft tissue contours are disrupted. In this situation, endotracheal intubation even with fiberoptic assistance may not be possible since the obstruction is below the vocal cords, and a tracheotomy may be necessary to secure the airway. Techniques to secure an airway in the unconscious patient include

1. Orotracheal intubation while a qualified physician stabilizes the head and neck.
2. Oral fiberoptic intubation using a mask to ventilate the patient that permits the passage of a fiberoptic bronchoscope.
3. The use of transtracheal jet ventilation to maintain oxygenation while an airway is being secured.
4. Retrograde intubation of the trachea in which a wire is passed through a needle inserted through the cricothyroid membrane and passed up into the mouth. An endotracheal tube can be passed over the wire and into the larynx. Alternatively, the end of the wire can be inserted into a fiberoptic bronchoscope that is "loaded" with an endotracheal tube. The fiberoptic bronchoscope is guided into the larynx by means of the wire, and the endotracheal tube can then be passed into the larynx.
5. A cricothyroidotomy or tracheotomy is performed if endotracheal intubation cannot be accomplished using the foregoing techniques.

Use of Jet Ventilation

Jet ventilation can be used to provide oxygenation if there is difficulty in establishing an airway. A large-bore intravenous catheter is placed into the trachea through the cricothyroid membrane and held in place so that kinking does not occur. The catheter must also not migrate out of the trachea into the subcutaneous tissues, because subcutaneous emphysema will occur. Upper airway obstruction will hinder the escape of expired air and can result in a tension pneumothorax. Therefore, upper airway obstruction must not be present during jet ventilation. This technique can provide oxygenation until a definitive airway is established.

MANAGEMENT OF THE AIRWAY IN PATIENTS WITH RHEUMATOID ARTHRITIS

Securing an airway in patients with rheumatoid arthritis may be difficult because of the destructive changes that can occur in the jaw, larynx, and cervical spine. A neurologic examination and appropriate radiologic procedures will aid in determining the presence and extent of encroachment on the cervical spinal cord with any attendant changes, such as myelopathy.

Ankylosis of the Temporomandibular Joint

Ankylosis of the temporomandibular joint leads to decreased mouth opening. If the distance between the upper and lower teeth is less than 5 cm with the mouth fully open, there may be difficulty in intubation.

Receding Chin

A patient may have a receding chin with a hypoplastic mandible, which can be detected by examining the patient from the side. An overbite may be present with the upper teeth extending beyond the lower teeth when the mouth is closed.

Cricoarytenoid Arthritis

The cricoarytenoid joint of the larynx can become involved during acute exacerbations of the disease. In this situation, patients have acute inflammation of the joint with pain on swallowing, accompanied by a feeling of fullness in the throat with radiation of pain to the ears. Hoarseness and stridor may be present because of swelling and fixation of the cords. With exacerbations and remissions of the disease, fixation of the vocal cords may result in stridor during sleep. There may be occasional hoarseness or mild respiratory distress. The effects of cricoarytenoid arthritis may not become obvious because the general condition of the patient does not lead to a great deal of stressful activity requiring rapid, deep breathing. If patients complain of "asthma," difficulty in swallowing, laryngeal tenderness, or hoarseness or snoring at night, the presence of cricoarytenoid arthritis should be considered. Problems may not occur until the postoperative period, when stridor may develop. The difficulty in breathing attendant to this problem may be diagnosed as asthma, but cricoarytenoid arthritis must be considered. If this occurs, steroids should be administered.

Cervical Spine Involvement

Instability of the cervical spine caused by destruction of supporting ligamentous structures may lead to atlantoaxial subluxation, subaxial subluxation, and superior migration of the odontoid process. Destruction of the transverse axial ligament and alar ligaments may lead to atlantoaxial subluxation. All patients with rheumatoid arthritis should have lateral cervical spine films in flexion and extension to delineate the extent of atlantoaxial subluxation, if present. To avoid compression of the cervical spinal cord, the neck should be kept in extension, which reduces the subluxation. If the atlas–dens interval is greater than 3 to 4 mm in flexion, the patient may exhibit neurologic findings. If subaxial subluxation and upward migration of the odontoid are present, there may be spinal cord damage with myelopathy, which can be affected by manipulation of the neck.

If general anesthesia is required in patients with rheumatoid arthritis and cervical spine involvement with encroachment on the spinal cord, an awake fiberoptic intubation under topical anesthesia should be performed to secure the airway. In those procedures in which patients have to be placed into the prone or lateral position, intubation should be performed with the patients awake. The patients can then be positioned awake and evaluated neurologically so that any neurologic changes resulting from positioning, such as weakness or tingling, would be noted. After positioning and assessing neurologic function, general anesthesia can be instituted.

Upward migration of the odontoid process into the foramen magnum leads to encroachment on the spinal cord, leading to compression with myelopathy. Awake fiberoptic endotracheal intubation provides a method of securing the airway without manipulation of the neck with possible spinal cord injury.

The architecture of the larynx and trachea is affected by the changes in the cervical spine in rheumatoid arthritis. As changes in the cervical vertebrae occur with resultant shortening of the cervical spine, the semirigid trachea and larynx may become twisted, which leads to a predictable rotation of the trachea and larynx because of the tethering effect of the arch of the aorta as it passes over the left mainstem bronchus.

Ankylosing Spondylitis

Patients with ankylosing spondylitis are frequently difficult to intubate and at risk for neurologic damage if the neck is forced into extension. In addition, arthritis of the temporomandibular joint may restrict mouth opening. Cricoarytenoid arthritis with pain on swallowing, hoarseness, stridor, and snoring may also be noted.

Ankylosing spondylitis involves the spine in the lumbar, thoracic, and cervical areas, with fixation of the spine and limitation of motion. Ankylosis of the cervical spine frequently leads to problems in endotracheal intubation. Extension of the neck to achieve proper position for intubation may lead to fractures. In patients who have atlanto-occipital fusion, fractures of the dens can occur. The cervical spine may be fixed in flexion or in neutral. A neck that is fixed in the neutral position may be rigid and present a problem in intubation. To determine the degree of difficulty involved in securing an airway, patients should be evaluated to determine whether there is any difficulty in opening the mouth and the degree of flexion and extension of the neck. If there is any question, a fiberoptic endotracheal intubation should be planned. When a patient is placed on the operating table, adequate support to the neck and upper thoracic area must be provided, because fractures of the spine can occur if proper positioning and padding are not provided in those patients with cervical and thoracic spine deformities. Awake fiberoptic intubation after anesthesia of the airway is the method of choice in securing an airway. General anesthesia is induced after the airway is secured. Patients are then positioned with proper padding so that injury to the spine is avoided.

Problems in Ventilation

Fixation of the thoracic vertebrae and the costovertebral, costochondral, and manubriosternal joints leads to limited expansion of the lungs, resulting in a restrictive pattern of respiration. If the restriction is significant, patients may hyperventilate with a rapid, shallow breathing pattern dependent on diaphragmatic activity. A decreased $PaCO_2$ on an arterial blood gas is indicative of hyperventilation. Encroachment on the vertebral arteries may result in vertebrobasilar insufficiency. Spinal stenosis may lead to a cauda equina syndrome. A hypochromic microcytic anemia as a result of occult gastrointestinal bleeding from anti-inflammatory agents or from the disease itself may be present. The anti-inflammatory agents may affect renal function.

Table 149-1

Conditions Associated with Neck/Cervical Spine Problems of Note to Anesthesiologists

Congenital muscular torticollis

Klippel-Feil syndrome

Morquio syndrome

Down syndrome

Congenital scoliosis

Osteogenesis imperfecta

Neurofibromatosis

Abnormalities of the odontoid process
Congenital separation: *Os odontoideum*
Congenital absence
Hypoplasia
Infection of the retropharyngeal space: Grisel's syndrome
Trauma: absorption of the odontoid process after fracture

Performance of spinal or epidural anesthesia may be difficult because of the alterations in the spine. If the sacral hiatus is open, caudal anesthesia may be possible.

Other conditions with associated neck/cervical spine problems of importance to anesthesiologists are noted in Table 149-1.

RHEUMATOLOGIC CONDITIONS OTHER THAN RHEUMATOID ARTHRITIS

Systemic Lupus Erythematosus

Systemic lupus erythematosus is a condition involving multiple organ systems. There can be cardiac involvement with possible myocarditis, cardiomegaly, congestive heart failure, pericarditis, and endocarditis of the mitral valve. There may be pleural effusion, pneumonia, and pulmonary infiltrates with fibrosis. Nervous system involvement can lead to cerebrovascular accidents and psychiatric disorders. There may be psychosis with a schizophrenic type of reaction. Migraine headaches may occur, and transverse myelopathy, cranial nerve palsies, and peripheral neuropathy may be seen. Anemia, leukopenia, and thrombocytopenia with coagulation disorders may be present. One of the major problems in patients with lupus erythematosus is renal involvement leading to renal insufficiency. Crossmatching may be a problem if antibodies to red blood cells are present.

Anesthetic Considerations Preoperative evaluation of the airway must be carried out since many of these patients have changes in the oral and nasal mucosa that may lead to problems with endotracheal intubation.

Pulmonary System Chest radiographs, arterial blood gases, and pulmonary function tests may aid in determining the extent of pulmonary involvement. Pleural effusions or pneumonia should be treated prior to embarking on elective surgery. If pulmonary disease is extensive, determine whether postoperative ventilation is indicated.

Cardiac System Congestive heart failure should be treated, and arrhythmias should be controlled. If valvular lesions are present, antibiotic prophylaxis must be considered. In developing an anesthetic plan, agents that are known to cause myocardial depression should be avoided. Judicious use of fluids is indicated to prevent cardiac failure.

Renal System If a significant degree of renal insufficiency is present, agents that depress kidney function and those that depend on renal excretion should be avoided. Maintain adequate blood pressure to ensure renal perfusion.

Crossmatching of Blood

Some patients may exhibit antibodies to red blood cells, making crossmatching of blood a problem. It may be wise to investigate this matter as soon as surgery is contemplated.

MEDICAL CONDITIONS OTHER THAN RHEUMATOID ARTHRITIS

Acromegaly

Securing and maintaining an airway may be difficult in patients with acromegaly because of the enlarged mandible. Upper airway obstruction may result from an enlarged tongue and epiglottis. Fiberoptic intubation may be necessary to secure the airway. Cardiovascular involvement includes hypertension, arrhythmias, and conduction defects. There may be left ventricular hypertrophy and heart failure.

Echocardiography may reveal an increased size of wall chambers with a cardiomyopathy. Diabetes and hypertension may be present.

Osteitis Deformans (Paget's Disease of Bone)

There is intense resorption of bone with osteitis deformans followed by the deposition of new abnormal bone. Because of the increased vascularity accompanying the resorption and replacement of bone, extensive arteriovenous fistulae may be present with increased perfusion leading to a high cardiac output. The increased heart rate should not be slowed with beta blockers, because the tachycardia is a result of a high cardiac output state.

Cardiac changes include calcification of the aortic valve and of the interventricular system, as well as conduction abnormalities. Spinal involvement may lead to neural compression with radicular pain. This should be considered if spinal anesthesia is contemplated. Since the bone is not properly calcified fractures may occur during positioning of the patient.

Progressive Systemic Sclerosis (Scleroderma)

Scleroderma is more prevalent in women aged 40 to 50 years and involves not only the skin and joints but internal organs as well. Because of the skin tightness, mouth opening may be limited. Strictures of the esophagus with decreased motility and peristalsis can result in inability to swallow food that may become lodged in the esophagus, leading to regurgitation under anesthesia. Pulmonary fibrosis and pulmonary hypertension can occur. Pulmonary function testing can demonstrate decreased vital capacity, decreased lung volumes, and decreased diffusing capacity. Tightness of the skin of the chest can further decrease compliance. Cardiac involvement leads to myocardial fibrosis, left ventricular hypertrophy with arrhythmias, and conduction defects. Renal insufficiency can occur as a result of kidney involvement.

Anesthetic Considerations   Securing of the airway may be difficult because of decreased mouth opening. Endotracheal intubation by means of fiberoptic bronchoscopy with patients in the head-up position to avoid regurgitation because of esophageal involvement is the method of choice in securing the airway.

If possible, anesthesiologists should avoid arterial punctures, because there may be interference with adequate perfusion following this procedure. Undue pressure should be avoided on delicate skin. If a pulse oximeter is used, change fingers frequently to decrease the effect of the heat or pressure from the sensor on any one finger.

If regional anesthesia is used, epinephrine should be avoided in peripheral nerve blocks because its use may cause problems of circulation to the extremities.

If surgery is performed under regional anesthesia, deep sedation should be avoided, and patients should be kept in the head-up position to avoid regurgitation and aspiration.

Postoperative care of patients with progressive systemic sclerosis may involve the maintenance of ventilatory support because of the poor lung and chest wall compliance. The patients should not be extubated until completely awake and able to breathe adequately and maintain upper airway reflexes.

Marfan's Syndrome

The basic defect in Marfan's syndrome is the inability to manufacture normal elastin fibers of collagen, leading to changes in the connective tissue throughout the body. Changes in Marfan's syndrome that affect anesthesia are the prognathism and the high arched palate that can lead to difficulties in endotracheal intubation. Patients should be examined to determine whether fiberoptic intubation is necessary. Aortic valve insufficiency and dilatation of the ascending aorta as well as mitral insufficiency may be present. Weakness of the wall of the ascending aorta may lead to dissecting aortic aneurysm. To decrease the heart rate and the force of ejection of blood against the wall of the aorta, patients are maintained on beta blockers.

Mitral valve prolapse may be present, and antibiotic prophylaxis may be necessary. The anesthetic technique should be designed so that the velocity of left ventricular contraction is controlled to avoid high ejection pressures on the wall of the ascending aorta. Vasodilators should be used in conjunction with beta blockers in controlling blood pressure to control the left ventricular ejection velocity. Inhalation anesthetic agents can aid in decreasing the force of myocardial contractility. During positioning of patients, care should be taken to avoid joint dislocation.

Neurofibromatosis

In neurofibromatosis there are abnormal growths of neural tissue throughout the body. Neurofibromas in the airway may result in possible respiratory obstruction. There may be cervical spine involvement with atlantoaxial instability. Hypertension in this disease may be associated with pheochromocytoma, which must be treated prior to surgery when present. Severe kyphosis may be associated with pulmonary dysfunction.

Sickle Cell Disease

In patients with sickle cell disease, treatment is directed to decrease the level of hemoglobin S, which is best accomplished under the direction of a hematologist. Infection should be treated and brought under control. Patients should be adequately hydrated. The aim of anesthesiologists is to avoid all situations that may induce sickling. These include hypotension, hypercarbia, hypoxia, hypothermia, and hypovolemia.

Anesthetic Considerations   The blood pressure should be maintained in a normal range. Adequate ventilation should be provided to prevent hypoxia and hypercarbia, with pulse oximetry and end-tidal carbon dioxide monitoring. Hypothermia should be avoided by warming the patient, the operating room, and the intravenous fluids. Hypovolemia is avoided by maintaining adequate hydration and blood replacement.

The use of tourniquets should be avoided, if possible. If exsanguination of the limb is not complete, trapped red blood cells may sickle. On release of the tourniquet, acid products enter the circulation, which may also cause sickling. In the immediate postoperative period, patients should receive oxygen for 48 h. Narcotics and sedatives should be administered judiciously to prevent hypoventilation with hypoxia and hypercarbia; they should not be withheld, however, because the postoperative stress response may result in sickling. Monitor oxygen saturation with a pulse oximeter. Maintain adequate hydration; avoid hypothermia and shivering.

Sickle Cell Trait

Under stressful conditions, patients with sickle cell trait may develop complications. Anesthetic management includes the avoidance of hypoxia, hypotension, hypovolemia, hypocarbia, and hypothermia. An increased inspired oxygen concentration should be administered during anesthesia and in the early postoperative period.

PEDIATRIC ORTHOPAEDICS

Latex Allergy and Anaphylactic Reactions

Anaphylactic reactions to latex have been reported in patients with myelodysplasia. A number of these patients undergo orthopaedic surgical procedures. Patients with myelodysplasia are frequently exposed to materials containing latex, such as gloves and catheters, and this frequent exposure may predispose them to anaphylaxis. Allergic reactions to latex are mediated through immunoglobulin E. The allergic reaction can be manifested by rash, urticaria, wheezing, and hypotension.

Patients who are suspected of being allergic to latex should be questioned about this condition. If an allergic history to latex is present, the following preparations should be made:

1. Allergic patients should receive medications to prevent allergic reactions 24 h prior to surgery and 24 h following surgery. These medications are
   Diphenhydramine, 1 mg/kg every 6 h with a maximum dose of 50 mg.
   Methylprednisolone, 1 mg/kg every 6 h with a maximum dose of 125 mg.
   Cimetidine, 5 mg/kg every 6 h with a maximum dose of 300 mg.
2. A latex-free environment should be created for patients during their stay in the hospital.

Management of these patients during surgery includes

1. Advise all operating-room personnel of the allergic history of these patients.
2. A sign stating "Latex-free Environment" should be posted on the doors to the operating room.
3. All personnel should wear nonlatex gloves.
4. The anesthesiologist should not apply a rubber face mask.
5. Intravenous tubing with rubber injection ports should not be used. Do not use the rubber port in an intravenous bag. To gain

access three-way stopcocks should be employed.

6. All drugs should be drawn up using filtered needles.
7. Padding should be placed under any areas that may be exposed to a rubber-containing item, such as a blood pressure cuff.
8. Urinary catheters should be latex free.
9. The anesthesiologist must be on the alert for any signs of allergy to latex such as hypotension or wheezing.
10. An epinephrine infusion should be prepared and ready for use.

Arthrogryposis

Intravenous access in arthrogryposis patients is usually very difficult because of the alterations in the joints and abnormalities in the soft tissues. Intubation may be difficult if mandibular hypoplasia is present.

Achondroplasia

The head may be enlarged in achondroplasia, possibly as a result of hydrocephalus. A small foramen magnum and abnormalities of the odontoid process may lead to encroachment on the spinal cord with pressure. A prominent mandible and a short maxilla may be present, which may lead to problems with endotracheal intubation. Abnormality of the development of the chest may lead to deformity. During intubation and positioning, the cervical spine should not be hyperextended or hyperflexed.

Osteogenesis Imperfecta

There is poor bone formation in osteogenesis imperfecta, that is a result of abnormalities in the synthesis of collagen. Abnormalities of the odontoid process and atlantoaxial instability may be present. Radiographs in flexion and extension should be obtained prior to surgery to determine the extent of any abnormalities. Scoliosis may be present, leading to poor pulmonary compliance. Brittle teeth make endotracheal intubation a problem. There may be aortic and mitral regurgitation and medial necrosis of the wall of the aorta. Metabolic abnormalities include increased sweating, heat intolerance, increased body temperature, tachycardia, and tachypnea. An elevated body temperature during anesthesia may not be a manifestation of malignant hyperthermia. Although malignant hyperthermia may occur in patients with osteogenesis imperfecta, there is not an increased risk in these patients. Platelet function may be defective, with problems in adhesion of platelets and clot retraction. Deafness may make communication with patients difficult. Manipulation in these patients can lead to fractures, so care must be used when applying blood pressure cuffs and tourniquets.

Muscular Dystrophy

In the muscular dystrophies, anesthesiologists are mainly concerned with cardiac involvement, pulmonary function, and weakened musculature.

Duchenne Muscular Dystrophy

There is the possibility of aspiration in Duchenne dystrophy because of decreased laryngeal and pharyngeal reflexes and a weak cough. Patients should be kept NPO for at least 8 h. If decreased gastric motility or gastric dilatation is suspected, a nasogastric tube should be inserted. The cardiac status must be evaluated by means of an electrocardiogram and echocardiogram. Pulmonary status should be evaluated by preoperative pulmonary function tests. Inhalation anesthetic agents should be avoided, because they may cause cardiac depression. Postoperative pulmonary ventilation may be necessary in patients who have a decreased vital capacity.

Since patients with Duchenne's muscular dystrophy are at high risk for developing malignant hyperthermia, anesthetic management should consist of nontriggering agents, including narcotics, nitrous oxide, oxygen, and acceptable muscle relaxants. Succinylcholine should not be used in these patients, because they may develop hyperkalemia and rhabdomyolysis after its administration.

In the immediate postoperative period, assisted or controlled ventilation should be maintained if there is evidence of inadequate ventilation. Patients should be observed for the development of malignant hyperthermia. Procedures to prevent postoperative pulmonary infection should be instituted. The patients should be weaned from the ventilator as soon as possible to avoid loss of muscle mass.

ELDERLY PATIENTS WITH FRACTURED HIP

The management of the patient with a fractured hip requires the combined efforts of the orthopaedic surgeon, internist, anesthesiologist, and the intensivist. Patients scheduled for surgical repair of a fractured hip frequently suffer from several other medical conditions or comorbidities. These associated illnesses include cardiac problems, elevated blood pressure, pulmonary dysfunction, metabolic disorders such as diabetes, neurologic problems such as parkinsonism and dementia, as well as renal or gastrointestinal disorders.

THE EFFECT OF COMORBIDITY ON OUTCOME

The number of concurrent medical problems or comorbidities, and their significance, is an important indication of outcome in patients with a hip fracture. Kenzora and colleagues (1984) found that an increased mortality rate was noted if there were four to six comorbidities. Davis (1987) noted that increased age and concurrent medical problems increased the mortality in geriatric patients with fractured hips.

White (1987) found increased morbidity with higher American Society of Anesthesiologists (ASA) classifications. In fact, healthy patients with hip fractures did not have a higher mortality rate than matched controls, whereas ASA III and IV classification patients did have a higher mortality rate than matched controls.

It appears that high ASA classification, concurrent medical problems, and increased age are the risk factors associated with a higher mortality in patients with fracture of the hip.

OPTIMAL TIMING FOR REPAIR OF FRACTURED HIPS

While the patient with a fractured hip benefits from having surgery performed as soon as possible, there are medical considerations that necessitate treatment prior to surgery.

Schultz and coworkers (1985) demonstrated a decrease in the mortality rate from 29 to 2.9 percent in patients who benefited from intense preoperative treatment and correction of their altered physiologic state. Kenzora and colleagues (1984) documented a higher mortality rate in those patients in whom surgery was performed within the first 24 h in comparison to patients who were properly prepared and then operated on, even if a few days were necessary.

In general, if the patients are healthy, early surgery is beneficial, whereas correction of medical conditions and surgical delay is better for the sicker patients.

ANESTHETIC MANAGEMENT

Many physicians consider regional anesthesia as the safer technique for patients with a hip fracture. However, in studies to determine whether regional or general anesthesia is superior, Valentin (1986)

Table 149-2

Practical Considerations in Choosing an Anesthetic Technique

Anesthesia	Pros	Cons
Regional	Avoids pulmonary irritation in patients with chronic obstructive pulmonary disease Decreases stress response Patients with history of congestive heart failure tolerate it well Decreases afterload Patients are more awake postoperatively May prevent thromboembolism	May require additional sedation, causing respiratory depression Bad for hypovolemic patients Bradycardia Time factor Not for patients with moderate to severe aortic stenosis Not for very confused or disoriented patients Not for patients with uncorrected coagulopathy
General	Ease of administration Patient comfort Higher F_IO_2, if necessary	Myocardial depression Not protective against thromboembolism Airway manipulation necessary Prolonged effects of medications (narcotics, muscle relaxants, inhalation agents)

SOURCE: Reproduced with permission from Bernstein RL, Rosenberg AD: The fractured hip. In *Manual of Orthopedic Anesthesia and Related Pain Syndromes*. New York: Churchill Livingstone; 1993:105.

---

and Davis were unable to find any significant difference in short-term or long-term mortality based on anesthetic technique. Davis also noted that there was an increased mortality in those patients who had been suffering from dementia.

In a study of 622 patients at the Hospital for Joint Diseases (Koval and coworkers, 1999), we noted that in patients with ASA classification III or IV there was no statistically significant difference in in-hospital mortality rates for those who received general or regional anesthesia. For practical considerations in choosing an anesthetic technique, see Table 149-2.

If general anesthesia is chosen, there is ease of administration and increased patient comfort, and a high concentration of oxygen can be administered. The disadvantages of a general anesthetic technique include possible myocardial depression and prolonged effects of the medications used (e.g., muscle relaxants and inhalation agents).

The advantages of a regional anesthetic technique are that the stress response may be decreased and the technique may prevent thromboembolism. Patients appear to be more alert and awake after regional techniques. Pulmonary irritation may be avoided in those patients with chronic lung disease and asthma. Regional anesthesia decreases afterload on the heart and is beneficial for patients who may have a history of congestive heart failure.

By decreasing sympathetic tone, regional anesthesia techniques can decrease blood pressure. However, it must be remembered that if the blood pressure falls following the administration of spinal anesthesia, it is better to treat patients with a vasopressor and not with large amounts of fluid. At the end of the procedure when the spinal recedes, the fluid may then cause congestive heart failure and pulmonary edema.

The problems with spinal anesthesia are that patients may become unruly and require large amounts of sedation, which may lead to respiratory depression and hypoxemia. Spinal anesthesia may lead to significant drops in blood pressure in hypovolemic patients.

Therefore, adequate intravascular volume should be present prior to initiating spinal anesthesia. Patients with a history of congestive heart failure who have a hip fracture may be hypovolemic from the loss of blood into the thigh, and administration of diuretics to maintain these patients "dry." The onset of a spinal anesthetic in patients may result in profound hypotension. Spinal anesthesia is contraindicated in patients with severe aortic stenosis. Regional anesthesia is to be avoided in patients with a coagulopathy.

Spinal anesthesia may also have a time factor consideration based on the local anesthetic and may wear off before the surgical procedure is finished.

NERVE BLOCKS IN ORTHOPAEDIC SURGERY

A nerve or group of nerves to be blocked can be located by eliciting a paresthesia or with the use of the nerve stimulator. Use of a paresthesia requires the cooperation of patients, which precludes the use of sedation.

The use of a nerve stimulator is an effective aid in blocking peripheral nerves. A peripheral nerve stimulator can be used to locate any nerve that has a motor component. The advantage of using a nerve stimulator is that the cooperation of patients is not necessary as it is when trying to elicit a paresthesia. In addition, less current is needed to stimulate the motor component of a mixed motor and sensory nerve than to stimulate the sensory or pain fibers. The endpoint of the nerve stimulator techniques is to obtain the maximal twitch response at the lowest milliamperage possible. This ensures that the needle is in very close proximity to the nerve. Currents of 0.1 to 0.3 mA provide the greatest success. It is important to choose the correct block for upper extremity surgery so the appropriate area is anesthetized (Table 149-3).

Table 149-3

Choice of Blocks for Upper Extremity Surgical Procedures[a]

	Interscalene	Infraclavicular	Axillary
Arthroscopy of shoulder	√		
Closed reduction, dislocation of shoulder	√		
Total shoulder replacement	√		
Resection, distal end of clavicle	√		
Arthroplasty of shoulder for chronic dislocation	√		
Elbow surgery		√	√
Ulnar nerve transposition		√	√
Open reduction, internal fixation of olecranon		√	√
Procedure on 4th and 5th digits		√	√
Excision, distal end of ulna		√	√
Carpal tunnel release	√	√	√
de Quervain's release	√	√	
Volar ganglion resection	√	√	√
Dupuytren's contracture			√
Excision of ganglion, dorsum of wrist		√	
Radial collateral ligament repair	√	√	
Arthroplasty of thumb	√	√	
Open reduction, internal fixation of fracture radius	√	√	
Excision, distal radius	√	√	
Procedures on digits		√	

[a] Ask surgeon where incision is going to be.
SOURCE: Reproduced and modified with permission from Bernstein RL, Rosenberg AD: Regional anesthesia. In *Manual of Orthopedic Anesthesia* and *Related Pain Syndromes.* New York: Churchill Livingstone; 1993:177.

UPPER EXTREMITY BLOCKS

Regional Anesthesia for Surgery of the Shoulder

An interscalene brachial plexus block is the method of choice for shoulder surgery under regional anesthesia.

Technique   The nerves are blocked in the groove between the anterior and medial scalene muscles as they exit from the spinal column. The patient is placed on the operating-room table in the supine position with the head turned to the side. The anesthesiologist palpates the sternal head and clavicular head of the sternocleidomastoid muscle and slides off laterally until the anterior scalene muscle is encountered. The insulated needle is then inserted in the groove between the anterior and medial scalene muscles (Fig. 149-1).

Once twitches are obtained at the lowest milliamperage possible within the distribution of the nerves innervated by the brachial plexus, the anesthetic agent is injected after aspiration to make certain that the needle is not intravascular. Hemidiaphragmatic paralysis on the side of the block frequently results. This is important in patients who have a history of pulmonary disease where diaphragmatic paralysis may be dangerous. A large number of patients develop Horner's syndrome on the side of the block. This possibility should be considered when an interscalene block is performed in patients who are suspected

of having head injury. The interscalene block does not provide anesthesia in the medial aspect of the forearm and hand.

Upper Extremity Surgery Below the Shoulder

Infraclavicular Brachial Plexus Block   This block provides anesthesia from the hand up to, but not including, the shoulder, allowing all operations on the upper extremity to be performed under this block except shoulder surgery.

Infraclavicular brachial plexus block provides anesthesia of the cords and branches of the brachial plexus, including the musculocutaneous and axillary nerves. The medial cord is blocked, providing anesthesia of the ulnar nerve.

The infraclavicular brachial plexus block is our choice for upper extremity surgery since the interscalene block does not block the ulnar area and the axillary brachial plexus block may not block the distribution of the musculocutaneous nerve, leaving the lateral aspect of the hand and forearm unblocked (Fig. 149-2).

Position   The patient is placed on the operating-room table in the supine position. The head is turned away from the extremity to be blocked. The anesthesiologist stands on the side opposite the side to be blocked. A skin wheal is raised 1 inch below the midpoint of the

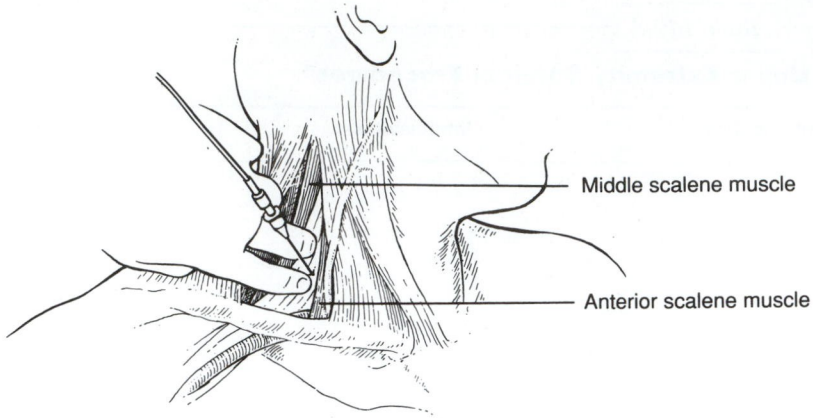

Figure 149-1
Interscalene brachial plexus block. The needle is inserted between anterior and middle scalene muscles and is directed caudad, mesiad, and posterior. *[From Rosenberg and Bernstein (1993:182), with permission.]*

clavicle. This block requires the use of a nerve stimulator. A sheathed needle is inserted at a 45 degree angle with the chest wall and directed toward the pulsations of the axillary artery in the axilla. Although it appears that a pneumothorax can occur because of the position, the entire procedure is extrathoracic, and the chance of pneumothorax is exceedingly rare. To achieve a solid block, twitches are sought in the muscles below the elbow.

LOWER EXTREMITY BLOCKS

Femoral Nerve Block

Femoral nerve blocks are useful in providing pain relief for patients who have fractures of the hip or fractures of the shaft of the femur. This block, when combined with a lateral femoral cutaneous nerve block, can provide anesthesia for some fractures of the hip requiring transcervical pinning.

In a patient with a femoral shaft fracture, a femoral nerve block can provide pain relief while the patient is being observed and when the patient is being transferred from the bed to the operating table. This block will also decrease the need for deep anesthesia and probably provide some pain relief in the immediate postoperative period.

The femoral nerve is blocked 1 inch below the inguinal ligament lateral to the pulsations of the femoral artery.

Lateral Femoral Cutaneous Nerve Block

Lateral femoral cutaneous nerve blocks are useful for surgical anesthesia in the lateral aspect of the thigh in combination with a femoral nerve block for repair of fracture of the hip. It is also useful in the

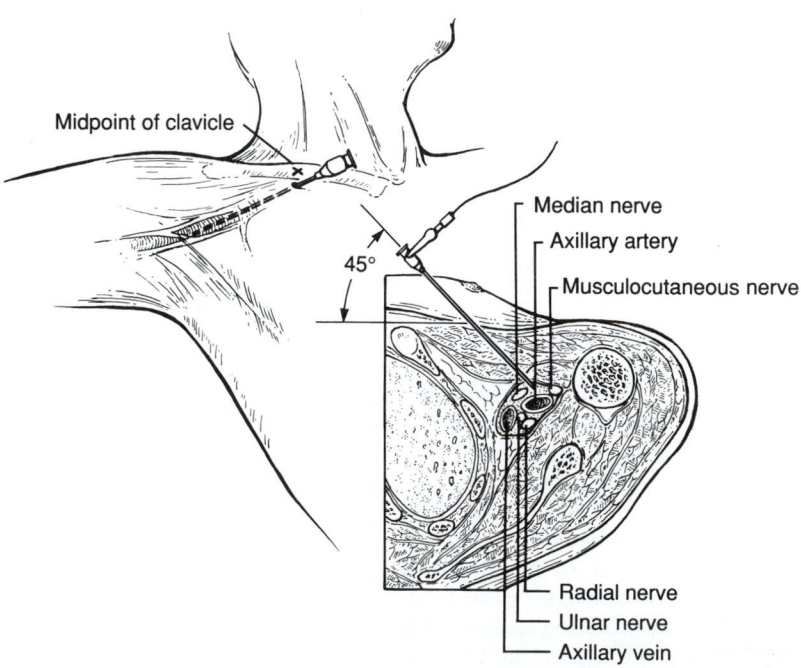

Figure 149-2
Infraclavicular brachial plexus block. The operator stands on the side opposite to the one to be blocked. The needle is inserted 1 inch below the midpoint of the clavicle at a 45 degree angle and directed toward pulsations of the axillary artery. *[From Rosenberg and Bernstein (1993:184), with permission.]*

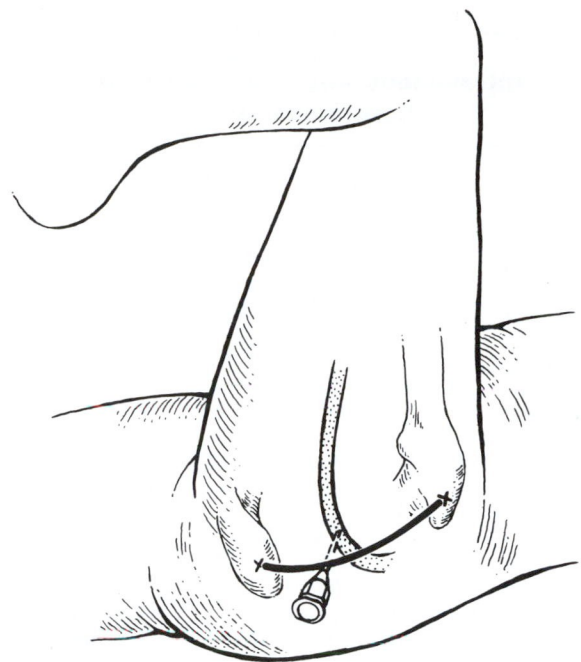

Figure 149-3
Supine approach to sciatic nerve block. The needle, which is kept parallel to table, is inserted between the ischial tuberosity and the greater trochanter and advanced. *[From Rosenberg and Bernstein (1993:213), with permission.]*

treatment of *meralgia paresthetica* and for anesthesia for muscle biopsy. This is a sensory nerve that arises from the lumbar plexus and passes through the fascia lata below the inguinal ligament.

Technique   The nerve is blocked by inserting a needle at a point 1 inch medial and 1 inch inferior to the anterior superior iliac spine. Anesthetic solution is infiltrated in a fanwise direction from medial to lateral.

Sciatic Nerve Block

Posterior Approach of Labat   The patient is placed on the operating table in the Sims position. A line is drawn from the posterior superior iliac spine to the greater trochanter. Another line is drawn from the tip of the coccyx to the greater trochanter. A perpendicular line connecting the midpoint of the first line overlies the sciatic nerve at the intersection of the second line. At this point, the needle is passed perpendicular to the skin and, with the use of the nerve stimulator, muscle twitches are sought in the distribution of the sciatic nerve.

Supine Approach to the Sciatic Nerve   The patient is placed on the operating table in the supine position. The hip and knee are flexed at 90 degrees. A line is drawn between the ischial tuberosity and the greater trochanter. At approximately the midpoint of this line with the needle parallel to the table, the needle is passed until twitches are noted in the distribution of the sciatic nerve. Local anesthetic is administered (Fig. 149-3).

Anterior Approach to the Sciatic Nerve   This approach can be used when the lower extremity cannot be moved, and the patient cannot be placed into the Sims position. The patient is placed on the operating table in the supine position. A line is drawn from the anterior superior iliac spine to the pubic tubercle. A line parallel to this line is drawn at the level of the greater trochanter. A line from the junction of the medial one-third and middle one third of the first line, which represents the inguinal ligament is drawn perpendicular to the second line. At the intersection of this perpendicular line with the line through the greater trochanter a skin wheal is raised, and the needle is passed perpendicular to the skin. A nerve stimulator is used to seek paresthesias in the distribution of the sciatic nerve (Fig. 149-4).

Lateral Approach to the Sciatic Nerve   The patient is placed on the operating table in the supine position. A small pillow is placed behind the knee. The posterior border of the greater trochanter is palpated. A skin wheal is raised 1 inch posterior to the greater trochanter and through this wheal a needle is inserted perpendicular to the skin and directed medially and slightly anteriorly. With the use of the nerve stimulator, twitches in the distribution of the sciatic nerve are sought.

INTRAVENOUS REGIONAL ANESTHESIA

In intravenous regional anesthesia, local anesthetic is injected into an extremity that has been exsanguinated and has the arterial supply occluded by a tourniquet. Anesthesia is obtained up to the area of the tourniquet. Contraindications to the use of intravenous regional anesthesia are listed in Table 149-4.

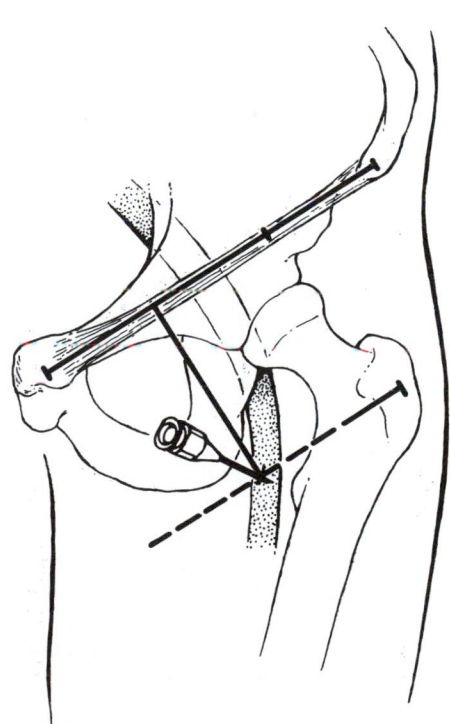

Figure 149-4
Anterior approach to sciatic nerve block. A line is drawn from the anterior superior iliac spine to the pubic tubercle. A second line is drawn parallel to this line from the greater trochanter. A perpendicular line is dropped from the inner one-third of the first line to the second line. At the point of intersection, the needle is inserted perpendicularly. *[From Rosenberg and Bernstein (1993:214), with permission.]*

Technique

A double tourniquet with a proximal and distal chamber that can be inflated separately is placed on the padded arm. A 20-gauge cannulae with an appropriate-sized stylet is inserted into a vein on the hand. The extremity to be blocked is raised and is exsanguinated by means of an Esmarch's bandage. The proximal tourniquet is inflated. Local anesthetic solution consisting of 3 mg/kg of 0.5 % preservative-free, epinephrine-free lidocaine up to 40 ml is injected slowly to prevent injection underneath the inflated tourniquet. The local anesthetic solution is especially made for intravenous regional use and does not contain any preservatives or epinephrine. Onset of anesthesia is usually within 5 min. If surgery is to be performed on the hand, the first one-third of the solution is injected while a separate tourniquet is placed on the distal forearm to force the anesthetic to stay in the hand for a more immediate, intense block.

After 20 min, the distal tourniquet should be inflated and the proximal tourniquet should be deflated. This will provide anesthesia under the tourniquet for the remainder of the operation. When using intravenous regional anesthesia, it is recommended that the tourniquet not be let down until at least 20 min have elapsed, because this is the time necessary for the local anesthetic agent to be fixed to the tissues. Deflation of the tourniquet sooner than this may cause local anesthetic solution to be released into the circulation, with the possibility of a resultant toxic effect.

Release of the tourniquet may lead to signs of local anesthetic toxicity, such as ringing in the ears, numbness of the lips, or metallic taste in the mouth. In severe cases, a seizure can occur. If toxic effects of local anesthesia are manifested, treatment with benzodiazepine intravenously may be useful. Seizures may need to be treated with a barbiturate or propofol.

Warning: Do not use bupivacaine for intravenous regional anesthesia, because the release of bupivacaine may cause severe toxicity to the myocardium, with possible cardiac arrest.

Intravenous Regional Anesthesia with Forearm Tourniquets

From time to time, surgeons require that patients move the fingers during surgery. To achieve this a tourniquet is placed on the forearm a few centimeters below the elbow, and the procedure is carried out as above. The dosage recommended is 2 mg/kg of 0.5 % preservative-free, epinephrine-free lidocaine. The injection must be carried out slowly to avoid overcoming the tourniquet's occlusion pressure. Leakage, however, may occur. Proper occlusion may not be achieved because blood vessels run along the interosseous membrane between the radius and ulnar and preclude the possibility of complete arterial occlusion.

Intravenous Regional Anesthesia in the Lower Extremity

A double tourniquet made for lower extremity use is applied over Webril padding on the thigh, and 100 ml of preservative-free, epinephrine-free lidocaine 0.3 % manufactured for intravenous regional use only is used. The 100 ml of 0.3 % solution is made by adding 40 ml of normal saline to 60 ml of 0.5 % solution. The normal saline should be without preservative. In the lower extremity, do not use any solutions containing epinephrine or preservatives.

MALIGNANT HYPERTHERMIA

In 1960, Denborough and Lovell described a 21-year-old Australian man with an open leg fracture who was more anxious about anesthesia than about surgery, because ten of his relatives had died during or after anesthesia. The patient underwent the surgical procedure

---

> *Table 149-4*
>
> ### Intravenous Regional Anesthesia: Contraindications
>
> Infection
>
> Allergy to local anesthetics
>
> Scleroderma
>
> Sickle cell disease
>
> Raynaud's disease
>
> Malignancy
>
> Thrombophlebitis, deep vein thrombosis
>
> Vascular insufficiency

under general anesthesia during which he developed malignant hyperthermia (MH) but survived. This is one of the earliest reported cases of MH. It is of interest that it occurred in a patient requiring treatment of a fracture.

MH is a syndrome in which there is a rapidly rising body temperature that occurs during general anesthesia. Individuals susceptible to MH have an autosomal dominant disorder in which there is an alteration in calcium metabolism in muscle. This usually occurs following exposure of the individual to potent inhalation anesthetic agents when associated with the use of succinylcholine or following the use of succinylcholine alone. When agents such as volatile anesthetics, succinylcholine, or potassium salts are given to a susceptible individual resulting in development of MH, it is known as *anesthetic triggering*. Although the onset of MH usually occurs immediately following the administration of triggering agents, it can be delayed and may not become manifest until the patient is in the recovery room.

To determine which patients may be susceptible, a history of prior experiences may be helpful. Suspicion is raised if a patient has had muscle rigidity or a high fever of unknown etiology during a previous anesthetic. Suspicion is raised also if direct blood relatives had MH, or died unexpectedly during or after anesthesia or if the patient has abnormal temperature responses to minor stress, or myopathic or neuropathic disorder which may be associated with MH. To determine whether a patient is susceptible, a muscle biopsy with contracture responses to caffeine or halothane is necessary.

If a patient presents with the foregoing history, the surgical procedure can be carried out if precautions are taken. The anesthesia machine is prepared by removing the vaporizer containing volatile anesthetic agents, changing the soda lime, using new tubing, and flushing the machine with oxygen for about 5 min. Nontriggering agents should be used for induction and maintenance of anesthesia. The patient should be observed postoperatively for any signs of MH.

MASSETER MUSCLE RIGIDITY

Masseter muscle rigidity (MMR) may precede MH in some instances, although a normal increase in jaw muscle tone may occur in some patients who do not have MH. Among patients with MMR, 50 to 55 percent are positive for MH.

If MMR occurs and the anesthetic is converted to a nontriggering type, the procedure may continue. Dantrolene should be available, and the team should be experienced in managing MH.

In MH, there is a problem of calcium metabolism in muscle. There appears to be an inability of the muscle to return calcium to the sar-

---

Table 149-5

Contents of Malignant Hyperthermia (MH) Cart

MHAUS Emergency Hotline (800) 644-9737 (prominently displayed on cart)

1. Dantrolene sodium: supplied in 70-ml bottles containing 20 mg of drug; keep at least 36 bottles immediately available in cart; have access to at least 72 bottles
2. Bottles of sterile water needed to reconstitute dantrolene, not normal saline
3. Emergency drugs
   a. Sodium bicarbonate: 12 ampules
   b. Furosemide: four 100-mg ampules
   c. Regular insulin: one 100-unit ampule
   d. Dextrose 50% in water: one 50-ml ampule
   e. Mannitol 25%: four 12.5-g ampules
   f. Procainamide: one 1-g ampule
4. Refrigerated intravenous fluids: 5 liters
5. Ice: make certain supply readily available
6. Nasogastric tube
7. Urinary catheter
8. Syringes, needles
9. Blood gas kits

NOTE: Acknowledgment to Malignant Hypothermia Association of the United States (MHAUS), Sherburne, NY.

---

coplasmic membrane after contraction. The excess calcium in the sarcoplasm causes activation of ATPase, with hydrolysis of ATP and depletion of ATP and creatine phosphate. There may also be an uncoupling of oxidative phosphorylation. This results in a hypermetabolic state with an excessive production of carbon dioxide, an elevated body temperature, skeletal muscle rigidity, and acidosis. The hypermetabolic state and hypercarbia lead to sympathetic nervous system stimulation with tachycardia and tachypnea, which *may be the first signs noted*. If the patient under general anesthesia received muscle relaxant and is paralyzed, the tachypnea may not be manifest. There may be increased blood pressure, ventricular arrhythmias, muscle rigidity, and evidence of desaturation of the blood, with a continued rise in the body temperature. The anesthesiologist may note that the carbon dioxide absorber becomes warm because of the excess carbon dioxide being neutralized by the soda lime, which is an exothermic reaction. Hyperkalemia, hypercalcemia, and myoglobinuria occur. There will be a rise in the creatinine phosphokinase. Disseminated intravascular coagulation may occur as well.

TREATMENT

As soon as the diagnosis is suspected, the surgeon should stop the operation and the anesthesiologist should discontinue the anesthetic (Tables 149-5 and 149-6). Dantrolene sodium is mixed in sterile water (not normal saline) and given to the patient intravenously. The initial dose is 2.5 mg/kg every 5 min, which can be increased up to 10 mg/kg or even higher if needed. Dantrolene sodium may be difficult to dissolve, so it should be heated to get it into solution, if necessary.

Table 149-6

Treatment of Malignant Hyperthermia

1. Stop surgery
2. Discontinue anesthetic
3. Assistant mixes dantrolene
   Use sterile distilled water
   Heat bottle of dantrolene in hot water to aid solution
4. Administer *2.5 mg/kg dantrolene every 5 min*
   Use up to 10 mg/kg and more if needed as determined by clinical situation
   Each bottle contains 20 mg of dantrolene
   Initial treatment for a 70 kg patient: $70 \times 2.5 = 175$ mg
   Use 9 vials ($9 \times 20 = 180$)
5. Administer 2 to 4 mg/kg bicarbonate; follow with blood gases
6. Hyperventilate with 100% oxygen
7. Lower body temperature
8. Monitor urinary output

NOTE: Acknowledgment to Malignant Hypothermia Association of the United States (MHAUS), Sherburne, NY.

Refrigerated intravenous fluids should be administered and exposed areas such as the axilla and groin packed in ice. If a body cavity is open iced, sterile saline can be placed into it. Sodium bicarbonate can be used to correct the metabolic acidosis. Use blood gases to monitor treatment. Hyperventilation of the patient should be carried out. Furosemide, intravenously, will increase urine output. All of these treatments are secondary and should not take precedence over the administration of the dantrolene sodium. If hyperkalemia is present, dextrose plus insulin can be used to drive the potassium intracellularly. A nasogastric tube can be inserted through which iced normal saline can be introduced into the stomach.

A urinary catheter is inserted to monitor urine output. The urinary catheter can also be used to introduce iced saline for bladder irrigation to help lower body temperature. Myoglobinuria may result from muscle damage (Table 149-6).

POSTOPERATIVE MANAGEMENT

Patients should be placed in the intensive care unit and monitored for at least 24 h. Dantrolene sodium intravenously in a dose of 1 mg/kg should be given every 6 h. The intravenous dantrolene can be discontinued if there are no signs of recurrence of the MH. After patients are stable, 1 mg/kg oral dantrolene is administered every 6 h for 24 to 48 h.

Management of Patients Who Have Suffered an Attack of Malignant Hyperthermia and Now Present for Surgery

Anesthesia should be maintained with safe nontriggering agents, and all preparations to treat MH should be present. Volatile anesthetics and succinylcholine should not be used. Safe agents include

1. Barbiturates
2. Benzodiazepines
3. Droperidol
4. Etomidate
5. Ketamine
6. Narcotics
7. Nitrous oxide
8. Non-depolarizing muscle relaxants
9. Propofol

Spinal anesthesia, epidural anesthesia, regional blocks, and local anesthesia can be safely used. Patients should be observed following surgery for any signs of MH.

SUGGESTED READINGS

Davis FM, Woolner DF, Frampton C, et al: Prospective, multi-centre trial of mortality following general or spinal anesthesia for hip fracture surgery in the elderly. *Br J Anaesth* 1987; 59:1080.

Donlon JV: Ear, nose and throat diseases. In Katz J, Beneumof JL, Kadis LB (eds): *Anesthesia and Uncommon Diseases,* 3d ed. Philadelphia, WB Saunders, 1990:293.

Eisele JH Jr: Connective tissue diseases. In Katz J, Beneumof JL, Kadis LB (eds): *Anesthesia and Uncommon Diseases,* 3d ed. Philadelphia, WB Saunders, 1990:645.

Gronert GA, Schulman SR, Mott J: Malignant hyperthermia. In Miller RD (ed): *Anesthesia,* 3d ed. New York, Churchill Livingstone, 1990:935.

Keenan MA, Stiles CM, Kaufman RL: Acquired laryngeal deviation associated with cervical spine disease in erosive polyarticular arthritis. *Anesthesiology* 1983; 58:441.

Kelly K, Setlock M, Davis JP: Anaphylactic reactions during general anesthesia among pediatric patients: United States, January 1990–January 1991. *MMWR* 1991; 40:437.

Kenzora JE, McCarthy RE, Lowell JD, et al: Hip fracture mortality: Relation to age, treatment, preoperative illness, time of surgery and complications. *Clin Orthop* 1984; 186:45.

Koval KS, Aharonoff GB, Rosenberg AD, et al: Hip fracture in the elderly: The effect of anesthetic technique. *Orthopaedics* 1999; 22:31.

Meeropol E, Frost J, Pugh L, et al: Latex allergy in children with myelodysplasia: A survey of Shriners hospitals. *J Pediatr Orthop* 1993; 13:1.

Miller JD, Lee C: Muscle diseases. In Katz J, Beneumof JL, Kadis LB (eds): *Anesthesia and Uncommon Diseases,* 3d ed. Philadelphia, WB Saunders, 1990:590.

Pavlin EG: Respiratory diseases. In Katz J, Beneumof JL, Kadis LB (eds): *Anesthesia and Uncommon Diseases,* 3d ed. Philadelphia, WB Saunders, 1990:chap 7.

Raj PP, Parks RI, Watson TD, et al: A new single-position supine approach to sciatic–femoral nerve block. *Anesth Analg* 1975; 54:489.

Rodman GR, Schumacher R (eds): *Primer on Rheumatic Diseases,* 8th ed. Atlanta, Atlanta Arthritis Foundation, 1983.

Rosenberg AD, Bernstein RL. Regional anesthesia. In *Manual of Orthopedic Anesthesia and Related Pain Syndromes.* New York, Churchill Livingstone, 1993.

Rosenberg H, Fletcher J, Seitman D: Pharmacogenetics. In Barash PG, Cullen BF, Stoelting RK (eds): *Clinical Anesthesia,* 2d ed. Philadelphia, JB Lippincott, 1992:589.

Salem MR, Klowden AJ: Anesthesia for orthopedic surgery. In Gregory GA (ed): *Pediatric Anesthesia,* 3d ed. New York, Churchill Livingstone, 1994:607.

Schultz RJ, Whitfield GF, LaMura JS, et al: The role of physiologic monitoring in patients with fractures of the hip. *J Trauma* 1985; 25:309.

Steen VD: Systemic sclerosis in rheumatic diseases. *Rheum Dis Clin North Am* 1990; 16:641.

Tachdjian MO: Congenital deformities. In Tachdjian MO (ed): *Pediatric Orthopedics,* 2d ed. Philadelphia, WB Saunders, 1990:104.

Urmey WF, Talts KH, Sharrock NE: One hundred percent incidence of hemidiaphragmatic paresis associated with interscalene brachial plexus anesthesia as diagnosed by ultrasonograph. *Anesth Analg* 1991; 72:498.

Valentin N, Lomholt B, Jensen JS, et al: Spinal or general anesthesia for surgery of the fractured hip? A prospective study of mortality in 578 patients. *Br J Anesth* 1986; 58:284.

White BL, Fisher WD, Laurin CA: Rate of mortality for elderly patients after fracture of the hip in the 1980s. *J Bone Joint Surg [Am]* 1987; 69:1335.

Winnie AP: Interscalene brachial plexus block. *Anesth Analg* 1970; 49:455.

Chapter 150

TRANSFUSION CONSIDERATIONS

Andrew D. Rosenberg

Ralph L. Bernstein

Linda Stehling

Concern about transmission of infectious diseases, such as hepatitis or AIDS, from allogeneic (homologous) blood transfusions has revolutionized the approach of many physicians regarding when to transfuse patients. Orthopaedic surgeons have been leaders in instituting methods to avoid allogeneic blood transfusions. This has been accomplished by instituting predonation programs, by perioperative blood salvage techniques, and by accepting lower hemoglobin (Hb) and hematocrit (Hct) levels than in the past, prior to ordering a transfusion. In the 1970s and early 1980s, many patients were transfused when the Hb and Hct levels decreased below 10 g/dl and 30 percent, respectively. Thus, 10/30 became the transfusion trigger below which many patients received allogeneic blood. In retrospect, many people may have been overtransfused because of this concept. The current state of the art in transfusion medicine is not to transfuse at any given number or "transfusion trigger," but to administer red blood cells (RBCs) on an individual basis in order to improve oxygen-carrying capacity to the patient. This requires an understanding of the physiologic basis for transfusion.

WHEN TO TRANSFUSE?

A number of factors are considered important when determining the need for transfusion. To tolerate a low Hb, patients must be able to compensate for diminished oxygen-carrying capacity. This can be accomplished by many healthy patients without problem, but patients with medical conditions including cardiac, respiratory, or cerebrovascular disease may not be able to compensate when confronted with decreased oxygen-carrying capacity. If cardiac or respiratory disease exists, increases in cardiac output or respiratory function may be insufficient to meet cellular oxygen requirements. The etiology and chronicity of the anemia are also important. Long-standing anemia, such as that occurring in patients with rheumatoid arthritis and even to a larger extent in patients with chronic renal disease, is frequently better tolerated than in age-matched controls. These patients have adapted to lower Hb levels, compensated physiologically, and do not need transfusions unless they lose blood. By comparison, rapid blood loss in patients with a baseline normal Hb and Hct but who suffer from cardiac disease, may require early transfusion. Even in healthy patients, a transfusion must be considered once enough blood is lost such that the patient will not be able to compensate for diminished oxygen-carrying capacity. Oxygen utilization by vital organs such as the brain, heart, and kidney must be evaluated when making a determination as to the minimal acceptable Hb and Hct. Since patients are transfused to increase oxygen-carrying capacity, blood transfusion should be reserved only for this purpose and not to increase intravascular volume in hypovolemic patients. Crystalloid or other intravascular volume expanders, and not blood, are indicated for volume expansion.

Two major factors, oxygen delivery and tissue oxygen consumption, are considered important when deciding to transfuse RBCs. Oxygen delivery (D_{O2}) is a function of arterial oxygen concentration (Ca_{O2}) and cardiac output. $Ca_{O2} = \% \ O_2$ saturation $\times (1.34 \times Hb) + (0.0031 \times Pa_{O2})$. The formula indicates that a patient's Hb level is very important in oxygen delivery. The other component of oxygen delivery, cardiac output, reflects a patient's ability to increase the heart rate and stroke volume in response to anemia. Healthy patients can easily increase their cardiac output, but patients with myocardial dysfunction or pulmonary disease usually cannot adequately compensate and fail under the stress of increased cardiac output requirement. Additional patients who may not be able to compensate adequately include those who are pharmacologically prevented from increasing their heart rate, such as patients receiving beta-blockade medication.

Analysis of the available data concerning at which point patients require transfusions indicates that most patients with Hb levels <10 g/dl do not usually need a transfusion. A difficult question to answer is how low the Hb can fall without placing patients at significant danger for suffering a complication. Although many patients with Hb levels of >10 g/dl will not require a transfusion, most patients will require a transfusion if they have <6 g/dl Hb concentration. Observations in the Jehovah's Witness patient population have revealed that patients can tolerate Hb levels much lower than we had expected or allowed in the past. In one study of patients who refused blood transfusion and underwent surgery, mortality was only 7 percent when Hb levels were >10 g/dl, but increased to 62 percent when Hb levels dropped to <6 g/dl. An analysis involving patients from 1970 to 1993 demonstrated that, with the exception of patients (three) who died after cardiac surgery, all patients who died secondary to anemia had Hb levels of ≤5 g/dl. Many studies have documented that Hb levels of >6 g/dl are well tolerated. In a study of patients undergoing primary total hip replacement, no correlation could be drawn between the Hb level at discharge, the preoperative Hb, or decrease in Hb concentration and the number of days to discharge from the hospital. At discharge time, Hb levels were in the 9 to 12 g/dl range.

Concern exists that, as a result of withholding a transfusion, a patient may suffer a complication such as a myocardial infarction, arrhythmia, or cerebrovascular accident. This concern was addressed in one study that involved perioperative electrocardiographic monitoring of patients undergoing infrainguinal arterial bypass. A total of 27 high-risk patients were studied. Of 13 patients with Hct levels of <28 percent, ten developed postoperative myocardial ischemia, six of whom developed either unstable angina or myocardial infarction, or died of cardiac disease or pulmonary edema secondary to ischemia. In patients with Hct levels of >28 percent, only two developed myocardial ischemia and there were no incidents of death or of pulmonary edema. Significance was noted between anemia on day 1 postoperatively and postoperative myocardial ischemia and cardiac death.

The degree of coronary disease and accompanying left ventricular dysfunction is an important determinant in outcome as it relates to Hb level. In a series of patients who underwent cardiac revascularization, patients with postoperative Hb levels of >12.1 g/dl had better myocardial metabolism than did patients with Hb levels of 8.0 g/dl. Of particular interest is that patients with coronary artery disease and Hb levels <9.6 g/dl combined with left ventricular dysfunction did worse than patients who had no ventricular dysfunction.

Thus, when evaluating each patient as to when he or she should receive a transfusion, one must consider each patient's underlying medical condition, their ability to compensate for lower Hb and Hct levels, the actual blood loss, anticipated blood loss for the remainder of the operation, and whether any particular organs are at risk.

ADVERSE EFFECTS OF ALLOGENEIC TRANSFUSIONS

Transfusions have decreased for fear of transmitting human immunodeficiency virus (HIV) and hepatitis to recipients. Although blood is tested, one concern is that the donor will be in the "window period" for determining infectivity. This means that the blood donor may be infected with the disease and be capable of transmitting the disease, but not have had sufficient time to develop antibodies to the virus. Testing for the HIV antigen will avoid this problem, and some centers are currently doing this. However, the antibody test is currently used in most centers to determine seropositivity. Thus, if no antibodies exist, the blood is considered free of disease when in fact this may not be true. Because of the "window period," patients can become infected with blood that tests negative for the antibody to HIV but is actually infected. Currently, the "window period" is approximately 22 days. In one review, 39 patients became seropositive from 182 previously seronegative donors who subsequently tested positive. It is believed that these donors were actually infected with the HIV virus, but had not developed antibodies at the time of donation.

In addition to transmission of HIV, concern exists about transmission of hepatitis B, hepatitis C, and cytomegalovirus (CMV). CMV is present in much of the blood that is transfused. In immunosuppressed patients, special care must be taken to ensure that CMV is not present in transfused blood. Reports of transmission of bacterial and parasitic infections also exist. Other complications associated with transfusions include allergic reactions, hemolytic transfusion reactions, and volume overload.

There is some concern that transfusions can also result in immunosuppression or immunomodulation of recipients. It was noted that renal transplant patients had lower allograft rejection rates and improved allograft survival times if patients received transfusions of allogeneic blood prior to receiving their allograft. In the 1970s, some institutions actually required patients receiving cadaveric renal transplants to receive transfusions prior to renal transplant. Prior transfusion with whole blood was a stronger enhancer of allograft survival than was packed RBCs. It was believed that the transfusion induced an immunosuppressive effect on patients and therefore, when patients received the renal transplant, rejection did not occur. Cyclosporin A, an immunosuppressive agent, has supplanted the role of transfusion in inducing an immunosuppressive effect in the host.

Cancer patients who receive allogeneic transfusions at the time of surgery have lower survival rates and an increased incidence of re-

currence. Recent meta-analysis studies have demonstrated this to be true in both head-and-neck and colorectal cancer patient populations. Patients with osteosarcoma who receive perioperative blood transfusions have an increased incidence of metastases and shorter survival compared with those patients who did not receive blood.

There is an altered immunological status as a result of receiving a blood transfusion. Cell-mediated immunity, macrophage migration, and natural killer cell activity decrease. Other effects of allogeneic transfusion include decreases in T helper cells, the cells that incite B lymphocytes to differentiate and produce antibodies. These alterations result in an immunosuppressive effect and are thought to be secondary to either antigen excess, a graft-versus-host phenomenon, a reactivation of immunosuppressive viruses, or a result of transfused white blood cells that are administered along with RBCs.

Interestingly, allogeneic blood transfusions have also been implicated in causing postoperative infections. This has been studied in the orthopaedic patient population. Murphy and colleagues (1991) and Triulzi and coworkers (1992), in separate studies, demonstrated the predictive effect of allogeneic blood transfusions in producing a postoperative infection. In patients who received an allogeneic blood transfusion during either total hip or spine surgery, there was a significant increase in postoperative infection rates compared with those who did not. In the Triulzi study of 102 patients undergoing 109 spinal fusions, there was an infection rate of 20.8 percent in those who received allogeneic blood. Patients who did not receive allogeneic blood had an infection rate of only 3.5 percent. Triulzi and colleagues (1992) also studied natural killer cell activity, an indicator of immunological function, and demonstrated that the patients who received allogeneic blood developed immunomodulation and their natural killer cell activity decreased. A specific dose–response curve from transfusions demonstrated that patients who received two transfusions had a higher infection rate than did patients who received either one or no transfusions. In another study, Fernandez and coworkers (1992) demonstrated that only patients who received homologous whole blood had a higher incidence (20 percent) of infection compared to the overall (6.1 percent) infection rate for all the patients in the study. Agarwal (1993) demonstrated that patients who had suffered from trauma had a higher incidence of infection after receiving a transfusion when controlling for variables such as age, sex, and mechanism of injury. At the Hospital for Joint Diseases (1997), we demonstrated that patients who underwent hip surgery to repair a fracture and received a blood transfusion had a significantly higher incidence of infection, when compared with those patients who did not receive an allogeneic transfusion.

Not all studies indicate that transfusion in orthopaedic patients is associated with a higher incidence of infection. A meta-analysis by Vamvakas and coworkers (1995) was unable to demonstrate a clear relationship between transfusion and infection. However, their study criteria defined a significant relationship between transfusion and infection as one that would result in an infection rate greater than double the baseline occurrence rate.

AVOIDING TRANSFUSION IN THE PERIOPERATIVE PERIOD

A number of methods exist for decreasing transfusion requirements in the perioperative period. These include autologous donation, normovolemic hemodilution, intraoperative cell salvage, postoperative salvage and reinfusion, pharmacologic methods, patient positioning, hypotensive anesthesia, and surgical technique. The techniques involving blood are addressed in this section.

PREDONATION

Predonation of blood prior to the surgical procedures appears to be very effective in decreasing the requirements for allogeneic transfusion. Criteria for predonation include Hb level of 11 g/dl. In addition, although many patients, including pregnant patients, can and do predonate, certain patients, such as those with unstable angina or severe aortic stenosis, should not predonate. Initially, it was believed that the patient population that predonated might not be as healthy as the allogeneic donation population and therefore would develop more complications while donating. Studies have demonstrated that preoperative donation poses no greater risk to presurgical patients than to patients who give regular allogeneic donations to the blood bank. Interestingly, elderly patients have a lower incidence of reactions than do younger patients. Overall, complications of predonation include a 3 percent incidence in light-headedness, 0.3 percent incidence in loss of consciousness that is transient, and a 0.03 percent incidence in seizures that are of self-limited duration. The populations considered at increased risk for complications are patients who have had a previous problem with donation, patients with low body weight, and first-time donors. To determine the incidence of complications in autologous donators when compared with allogeneic donators, a study was performed in which 10,299 predonators were compared with 219,307 allogeneic donors. The data demonstrated that there was no significant difference in reactions between the groups.

At the time of predonation, patients should be placed on iron supplementation. Genetically engineered erythropoietin (EPO) is used in specific circumstances to increase endogenous RBC production. Patients who received EPO and iron were able to predonate more units of blood than controls. However, it appears that EPO should be reserved for those situations in which patients are severely anemic, or need to produce extraordinary amounts of RBCs.

Body weight of <50 kg is a criterion described by some as a cutoff for predonation. In this situation, however, there are methods for predonating partial units based on body weight. This has been used successfully in scoliosis patients. Of 100 patients, 63 percent were able to avoid allogeneic transfusions by predonating 2 or more partial units.

In general, at the Hospital for Joint Diseases, patients undergoing elective total hip surgery are advised to predonate 2 units of blood. With the combination of predonation, intraoperative cell salvage, and postoperative reinfusion, the patients undergoing total hip replacement have been able to decrease their risk of requiring an allogeneic transfusion to only 4 percent.

ACUTE NORMOVOLEMIC HEMODILUTION (ANH)

This technique involves the rapid withdrawal of the patient's blood while maintaining intravascular volume by reinfusion of colloid or crystalloid. With this method, patients are maintained in a normovolemic but relatively anemic condition. Thus, intraoperatively, a patient loses blood at a lower Hct level and, at the conclusion of the procedure, the patient's blood that was withdrawn at the beginning of the procedure can be reinfused. A patient who arrives in the operating room with a preoperative Hct of 45 percent can be hemodiluted to an Hct of 25 percent. If the patient now loses 1 liter of blood, he or she has lost only 250 ml of RBC, as compared with the 450 ml that would have been lost had all the bleeding occurred at the admission Hct. When the RBCs are reinfused, the patient is receiving blood with an Hct of 45 percent as well as fresh clotting factors and platelets.

It appears that healthy patients tend to tolerate hemodilution and can increase and maintain their cardiac output and coronary blood flow for extended periods of hemodilution. In patients with coronary artery disease, however, one must be very careful about hemodilution techniques. Studies in canine models with stenosed left anterior descending arteries have demonstrated myocardial dysfunction at Hcts of 35 percent. More recent studies have indicated that some canine models can maintain adequate contractility at Hb levels of 7.5 g/dl. In this model, when contractile function deteriorated, it was improved by slightly increasing the Hb and Hct levels.

The anesthesiologist and surgeon must consider a patient's coronary artery disease prior to the institution of hemodilution. Increases in cardiac output and thus in heart rate may not be well tolerated and the patient may develop ischemia. To determine the amount of blood that can be withdrawn, the formula

$$\frac{EBV\ (H_o - H_t)}{\left(\frac{H_o + H_t}{2}\right)}$$

is used, where EBV = estimated blood volume and is calculated as weight in kilograms $\times$ 70 ml/kg. H_o is the starting Hct, and H_t is the final or target Hct. Donation bags already prepared with anticoagulants exist to collect 450 ml of blood. The blood can be withdrawn through a large-bore intravenous, central line, or arterial line by gravity drainage. Normovolemia is maintained by crystalloid 3:1 or colloid 2:1 replacement. Properly label the blood and store appropriately until use.

Hypotensive anesthetic techniques and hemodilution should not be combined.

INTRAOPERATIVE CELL SALVAGE

Intraoperatively, blood that is lost from the wound and usually suctioned into canisters and discarded can now be collected, washed, and reinfused into the patient. This requires removal of debris, bone chips, anticoagulant, and hemolyzed RBCs. Many patients are candidates for use of intraoperative cell salvage, but infection or malignancy at the operative site are considered contraindications by many. Blood is initially collected in a heparinized solution. It is then spun in a centrifuge bowl where supernatant waste, free Hb, anticoagulant, and surgical debris are washed from the RBCs as the centrifuge is spun. Saline is added to the solution to further wash the debris from the RBCs. As RBCs settle to the bottom of the centrifuge and the debris is washed from the top, the Hct level continues to rise until it reaches a level of about 50 to 60 percent. Once the blood is well washed, it is pumped into a blood delivery bag and reinfused. Insufficient washing has been noted to result in patients receiving free Hb, fat, and bone marrow debris or excess anticoagulant. Free Hb can cause renal damage. There were some early reports of air embolism as a result of incorrectly connecting tubing, but this problem appears to have been corrected in newer cell salvage models. Disseminated intravascular coagulation has been reported. Both patients in the report appear to have received blood that had been collected with the suction apparatus at too high a level, and the reinfused blood was not adequately washed. Because of the presence of bone, fat, and surgical debris, it is generally recommended that blood salvaged from orthopaedic procedures be washed more rigorously.

POSTOPERATIVE SALVAGE DEVICE

Blood that drains into a wound drainage apparatus in the postoperative care unit can now be collected and reinfused into patients. By sterile technique, the wound drainage is passed through a 265 μm filter as it is collected and then reinfused through a 40 μm filter. The reinfused fluid has an Hct level slightly lower than that of the patient's current intravascular Hct. It also contains low platelet counts, increased fibrin degradation products, and an elevated prothrombin (PT) and partial thromboplastin time (PTT). Additionally, free Hb is present. In our institution, because of the elevated PT and PTT, additional anticoagulant is not added to the collection apparatus.

Concerns with reinfusion of postoperative salvaged blood include renal damage from free Hb, reinfusion of anticoagulants, adult respiratory distress syndrome (ARDS), disseminated intravascular coagulation, and complement activation. One report describes a patient who developed acute upper airway edema following administration of wound drainage. Some physicians suggest washing wound drainage blood prior to reinfusion. In our institution, however, we have reinfused unwashed drainage into many patients without serious sequelae.

CONCLUSION

Many methods exist to decrease the chance of patients requiring an allogeneic transfusion. For elective surgical patients, a plan can be outlined to minimize the chances of a patient requiring bank blood. In addition to this, patients should be transfused when they actually need the blood based on physiologic requirements to improve oxygen-carrying capacity.

SUGGESTED READINGS

Agarwal N, Murphy JG, Cayten CG, et al: Blood transfusion increases the risk of infection after trauma. *Arch Surg* 1993; 128:171–177.

Birgegard G, Danersund A, Hogman C, et al: Physiological response to phlebotomies for autologous transfusion at elective hip–joint surgery. *Eur J Haematol* 1991; 46:136.

Faris PM, Ritter MA, Keating EM, et al: Unwashed filtered shed blood collected after knee and hip arthroplasties: A source of autologous red blood cells. *J Bone Joint Surg [Am]* 1991; 73:1169.

Fernandez MC, Gottlieb M, Menitove JE: Blood transfusion and postoperative infection in orthopedic patients. *Transfusion* 1992; 32:318.

Goodnough LT, Rudnick S, Price TH, et al: Increased preoperative collection of autologous blood with recombinant human erythropoietin therapy. *N Engl J Med* 1989; 321:1163.

Koval KJ, Rosenberg AD, Zuckerman JD, et al: Does blood transfusion increase the risk of infection after hip fracture? *J Orthopaedic Trauma* 1997; 11:260–265.

Landers DF, Hill GE, Wong KC, et al: Blood transfusion-induced immunomodulation. *Anesth Analg* 1996; 82:187.

MacEwen GD, Bennett E, Guille JT: Autologous blood transfusions in children and young adults with low body weight undergoing spinal surgery. *J Pediatr Orthop* 1990; 10:750.

Mann DC, Wilham MR, Brower EM, et al: Decreasing homologous blood transfusion in spinal surgery by use of the cell saver and predeposited blood. *Spine* 1989; 14:1296.

McVay PA, Andrews A, Hoag MS, et al: Moderate and severe reactions during autologous blood donations are no more frequent than during homologous blood donations. *Vox Sang* 1990; 59:70.

Murphy P, Heal JM, Blumberg N: Infection or suspected infection after hip replacement surgery with autologous or homologous blood transfusions. *Transfusion* 1991; 31:212.

Murray DJ, Gress K, Weinstein SL: Coagulopathy after reinfusion of autologous scavenged red blood cells. *Anesth Analg* 1992; 75:125.

Nelson AH, Fleisher LA, Rosenbaum SH: Relationship between postoperative anemia and cardiac morbidity in high-risk vascular patients in the intensive care unit. *Crit Care Med* 1993; 21:860.

Seltzer DG, Brown MD, Tompkins JS, et al: Toward the elimination of homologous blood use in elective lumbar spine surgery. *J Spinal Disord* 1993; 6:412.

Stehling L, Simon TL: The red blood cell transfusion trigger: Physiology and clinical studies. *Arch Pathol Lab Med* 1994; 118:429.

Stehling L: Perioperative mortality in anemic patients. *Transfusion* 1989; 29:37S.

Toy P: Autologous transfusion. *Anesthesiol Clin North Am* 1990; 8:533.

Triulzi DJ, Vanek K, Ryan DH, et al: A clinical and immunologic study of blood transfusion and postoperative bacterial infection in spinal surgery. *Transfusion* 1992; 32:517.

Vamvakas EC, Moore SB, Cabanela M: Blood transfusion and septic complications after hip replacement surgery. *Transfusion* 1995; 35:150.

Zauder HL: Preoperative hemoglobin requirements. *Anesthesiol Clin North Am* 1990; 8:471.

Chapter 151

ANTIBIOTICS IN ORTHOPAEDICS

Christina M. Hift

ROLE OF ANTIBIOTICS IN ORTHOPAEDIC INFECTIONS

Antibiotics have markedly changed the outcome of orthopaedic infections over the years. Today there is a wide range of antibiotics with different spectra, different half-lives, and different toxicities. To make the most appropriate choice, a precise microbiologic diagnosis is required.

Antibiotics alone are often not sufficient in the treatment of orthopaedic infections. Adequate debridement of necrotic tissue is always necessary, as well as drainage of any abscess. For this reason, the orthopaedist and the infectious disease specialist must work closely together to determine the optimum treatment plan for each patient.

THE MAJOR ORGANISMS

Orthopaedic infections are usually caused by a small number of different organisms. The majority are caused by staphylococci, streptococci, and a few gram-negative rods such as *Escherichia coli, Proteus,* and *Pseudomonas.* Of course, we have seen single infections caused by a vast variety of unusual organisms. Table 151-1 lists the major pathogens in orthopaedic infections, with their particular characteristics.

CHOICE OF INITIAL ANTIBIOTIC THERAPY

In the ideal situation, when a patient presents with an orthopaedic infection, a culture is obtained and the initial therapy is tailored to the gram stain results. Table 151-2 outlines this decision making.

When the gram stain is negative and no culture is yet available, the choice of therapy is based on many factors. Considerations include the most likely organism according to the patient's risk factors and exposures, the rate of progressions of the infection, the response to prior antibiotics, and the severity of the symptoms. When choosing initial antibiotic therapy, in particular when there is a possibility of a negative or no culture, an antibiotic with the narrowest spectrum, often ideally with an oral equivalent and the least toxicity, should be chosen. Initial antibiotic therapy is also very much influenced by the severity of the infection. When faced with a toxic, severely ill patient, broad-spectrum coverage is always recommended until culture results are available. Table 151-3 outlines suggestions for empiric therapy to be used when faced with a negative gram stain and negative culture results.

SENSITIVITIES OF COMMONLY USED ANTIBIOTICS

Table 151-4 is to be used only as a guideline to choosing antibiotics pending the availability of the final sensitivities. A plus sign indicates that most bacteria are sensitive to a given antibiotic and a minus sign that most are resistant. The sensitivity patterns of bacteria in a given geographic area or hospital should also be taken into consideration.

FINAL CHOICE OF ANTIBIOTICS

GENERAL CONSIDERATIONS

The final choice of antibiotics is based on multiple considerations. Antibiotics should have the narrowest spectra, least toxicity, lowest

---

Table 151-1

Major Pathogens	Gram Stain	Lab/Clinical Characteristics
Staphylococcus aureus	Gram-positive cocci	Purulent discharge
Staphylococcus epidermidis	Gram-positive cocci	Discharge variable
Streptococci groups A & B	Gram-positive cocci, often in chains	Rapidly spreading infection
Gram-negative bacilli	Gram-negative rods	Greenish discharge (often pseudomonas)
Anaerobic bacteria	Gram-positive rods, gram-negative cocci and rods	Foul-smelling
Haemophilus influenzae	Gram-variable rods	Must grow on chocolate agar, blood cultures often not cloudy—must be smeared
Neisseria	Gram-negative rods	Grow on Thayer-Martin media

Table 151-2

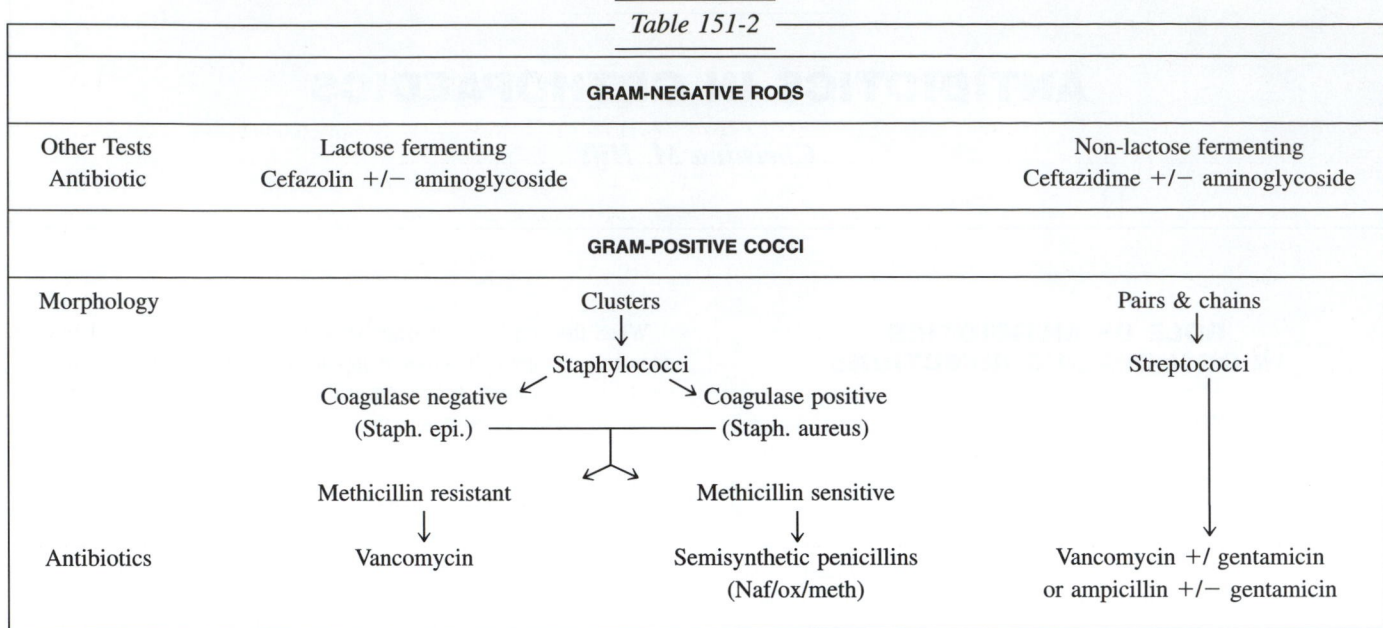

GRAM-NEGATIVE RODS

Other Tests	Lactose fermenting	Non-lactose fermenting
Antibiotic	Cefazolin +/− aminoglycoside	Ceftazidime +/− aminoglycoside

GRAM-POSITIVE COCCI

Morphology — Clusters → Staphylococci → Coagulase negative (Staph. epi.) / Coagulase positive (Staph. aureus) → Methicillin resistant / Methicillin sensitive — Pairs & chains → Streptococci

Antibiotics — Vancomycin — Semisynthetic penicillins (Naf/ox/meth) — Vancomycin +/ gentamicin or ampicillin +/− gentamicin

Table 151-3

Type of Infection	Suspected Organism	Empiric Therapy
INFECTED JOINT REPLACEMENT		
Early Infection	*Staphylococcus aureus*	Nafcillin
Revision/late infection	*Staphylococcus aureus/* Streptococcus (including Enterococcus)	Vancomycin and Gentamycin[a]
SEPTIC ARTHRITIS IN CHILDREN		
Less than six years of age	*Staphylococcus aureus/*Group A Streptococci/ *Haemophilus influenzae*	Cefuroxime
Greater than six years of age	*Staphylococcus aureus/*Group A Streptococci	Nafcillin
Young adult	*Neisseria gonorrhoeae/ Staphylococcus aureus*	Nafcillin and Ceftriaxone
Older adult	*Staphylococcus aureus/*Enteric gram-negative rods	Nafcillin and Ceftazidime
OSTEOMYELITIS		
Less than six years of age	*Staphylococcus aureus/ Haemophilus influenzae*	Cefuroxime
Greater than six years of age	*Staphylococcus aureus*	Nafcillin
Infection of the diabetic foot	Enteric gram-negative rods (including Pseudomonas)/ *Staphylococcus aureus/*Anaerobes	Ticarcillin/Clavulanate potassium and Tobramycin

[a] Consider adding rifampin if there is poor progression of laboratory results and if further surgical debridement is not indicated.

Table 151-4

	Staph		Strep	Gram-negative rods		Enterococcus	Anaerobes
	MR	MS		LF	NLF		
Penicillin	−	−	+	−	−	+	+/−
Cefazolin	−	+	+	+	−	−	−
Semisynthetic penicillins	−	+	−	−	−	−	−
Aminoglycosides	+	+	+	+	+	+	−
Clindamycin	−	+	+	−	−	−	+
Metronidazole	−	−	−	−	−	−	+
Timentin	−	+	+	+	+	−	+
Ampicillin/sulbactam	−	+	+	+	−	+	+
Ceftazidime	−	−	−	+	+	−	−
Ciprofloxacin	+/−	+	−	+	+	−	−
Vancomycin	+	+	+	−	−	+	−

cost, and greatest convenience for administration in particular when home intravenous therapy is desired. Ideally, they should also have the fewest side effects.

INTERPRETATION OF CULTURE RESULTS

Interpretation of the culture results and antibiotic sensitivities is usually fairly straightforward. A few special circumstances should be mentioned. A common problem occurs when an organism grows in culture, often after several days and only on the thioglycollate liquid media. This usually is indicative of a possible contaminant and not a meaningful culture for the patient. Another problem occurs when the culture is taken from a normally nonsterile site and represents colonization rather than infection. The absence of white blood cells is further evidence for this interpretation.

There are a few situations in which the culture report will indicate that the organism is sensitive although it has been shown not to be effective in vitro. The most common example involves methicillin-resistant *Staphylococcus aureus* (MRSA). The organism may be sensitive to cefazolin in the laboratory. A cephalosporin should not be used, however, when a *S. aureus* is shown to be methicillin resistant.

Another confusing situation arises when a *S. aureus* is shown to be sensitive to penicillin. This has of course become increasingly rare. When this does occur, however, these staphylococci are usually very sensitive to penicillin and this is the drug of choice over the semisynthetic penicillins (oxacillin, nafcillin, and methicillin).

In contrast to MRSA, certain antibiotics are effective against *Enterococcus* although it is reported as showing intermediate resistance. Further complicating the situation is the fact that *Enterococcus* has recently acquired increased resistance to certain antibiotics. This has mandated that laboratories test the sensitivity of *Enterococcus* to penicillins, vancomycin, and the aminoglycosides. To choose the appropriate antibiotics, the mechanisms of resistance must be determined. Table 151-5 demonstrates the different mechanisms.

Since penicillins are not normally bactericidal for *Enterococcus*, synergy with aminoglycosides is required in cases of serious infections. If the *Enterococcus* produces altered penicillin-binding proteins, however, the synergy will not be effective. If the resistance is secondary to production of beta-lactamases, then amoxicillin plus clavulanic acid, imipenem, or ampicillin plus sulbactam would be effective.

Table 151-5

Mechanisms of Resistance of Enterococcus

1. Penicillins
   Beta lactamase production
   Penicillin-binding proteins
2. Aminoglycosides
   Aminoglycoside modifying enzymes
3. Vancomycin
   Three different levels of resistance

If the *Enterococcus* produces aminoglycoside-modifying enzymes, then aminoglycoside antibiotics will not be effective. This can be determined by measuring the minimum inhibitory concentration (MIC). If the MIC is between 8 and 256, resistance can be overcome by combination therapy. If the MIC is greater than 500 mg/ml, aminoglycosides will not be effective even in combination with another antibiotic.

Resistance to vancomycin can be divided into three levels according to the MIC values that correspond to the genetic characteristics of the *Enterococcus*. Usually only at the lowest level of resistance—that is, an MIC of less than 32—will the drug remain effective.

MECHANISM OF ACTION AND TOXICITY OF ANTIBIOTICS

The antibiotics most commonly used in orthopaedic infections are reviewed in Table 151-6.

DOSES OF MOST COMMONLY USED ANTIBIOTICS

Table 151-7 contains the doses of antibiotics for patients with normal renal and hepatic function.

Table 151-6

Most Commonly Used Antibiotics in Orthopaedic Infections

Antibiotic	Mechanism of Action	Toxicity
Penicillin	Cell wall inhibitor	Allergic reactions
Nafcillin	Cell wall inhibitor	Neutropenia
Oxacillin	Cell wall inhibitor	Liver function abnormalities
Methicillin	Cell wall inhibitor	Nephritis
Cephalosporins	Cell wall inhibitors	Rare
Aminoglycosides	Inhibit bacterial protein synthesis	Renal Ototoxic
Quinolones	DNA gyrase inhibitors	Central nervous system
Vancomycin	Cell wall inhibitor	Eighth nerve (mainly hearing) Renal
Clindamycin	Bacterial protein synthesis inhibitor	Pseudomembranous colitis

---

Table 151-7

Doses of Most Commonly Used Antibiotics for Patients with Normal

Renal and Hepatic Function

Parenteral Antibiotics	Adult Dose	Pediatric Dose (Never exceed adult dose)
Penicillin G	12–24 million units/day divided q4–6h	100,000–250,000 units/kg/day divided q4–6h
Cefazolin	3–6 g/day divided q8h	50–100 mg/kg/day divided q8h
Oxacillin	8–12 g/day divided q6h	100–200 mg/kg/day divided q6h
Nafcillin	8 g/day divided q6h	100–200 mg/kg/day divided q6h
Methicillin	8–12 g/day divided q6h	100–200 mg/kg/day divided q6h
Ciprofloxacin	400 mg q12h	Not approved
Clindamycin	800 mg q8h	40 mg/kg/day divided q6h
Vancomycin	2 g/day divided 6–12h	40 mg/kg/day divided q6h
Gentamicin	3–5 mg/kg/day divided q8h	7.5 mg/kg/day divided q8h
Tobramycin	3–5 mg/kg/day divided q8h	7.5 mg/kg/day divided q8h
Amikacin	15 mg/kg/day divided q8–12h	15 mg/kg/day divided q8–12h
Ceftriaxone	2 g q24h	50 mg/kg q24h
Cefuroxime	2 g q8h	150 mg/kg/day divided q8h
Once daily dosing for aminoglycosides[a]		**Desired peak**
Gentamicin	4–7 mg/kg	10–20 μg/ml
Tobramycin	4–7 mg/kg	10–20 μg/ml
Amikacin	15 mg/kg	54 μg/ml
Oral Antibiotics		
Ciprofloxacin	250–750 mg bid	Not approved
Rifampin	300 mg bid or tid	20 mg/kg/day divided bid
Amoxicillin/Clavulanic acid	500 mg tid	40 mg/kg/day divided tid
Cephalexin	250–500 mg qid	50 mg/kg/day divided qid

[a]*Recommended curently only for nonneutropenic patients with normal renal function infected with gram-negative organisms excluding *Pseudomonas aeruginosa*.

EVALUATION OF TREATMENT

Orthopaedic infections present certain unique problems in monitoring their progress. Often there is nothing visible that can be followed by physical examination. One must therefore rely heavily on laboratory results. We have found the C-reactive protein (CRP) to be the most helpful laboratory test. CRP is produced by the liver in response to infection and inflammation. Laboratory tests such as the white cell count and sedimentation rate may be only minimally altered by infection. Conversely, the sedimentation rate may become markedly elevated and decrease only slowly with resolution of the infection.

We have followed the CRP in a wide range of orthopaedic patients. Although the rate of decline varies slightly from patient to patient, it appears to correlate well with the resolution of infection.

The CRP has been particularly useful in helping us decide which patients need a change of antibiotics or orthopaedic intervention, usually in the form of further debridement. We also find the CRP a useful guide in determining the length of treatment with antibiotics for a given patient. A negative CRP for at least 2 weeks' while on a full course of antibiotics appears to be predictive of adequate treatment. The CRP can also be used to monitor patients on prolonged oral treatment after a course of intravenous antibiotics. The CRP has also been useful in following the cases of patients after the end of their antibiotic treatment in order to detect early relapses.

CONVERSION OF INTRAVENOUS TO ORAL ANTIBIOTIC TREAMENT

Table 151-8 lists intravenous antibiotics and their oral equivalents.

Multiple factors must be considered when choosing an oral antibiotic. The major consideration is tolerance by the patient. It should also be noted that certain intravenous antibiotics have no oral counterparts. Table 151-9 lists organisms for which oral antibiotics are currently unavailable.

ORAL TREATMENT

Orthopaedic infections can often be treated orally. However, certain criteria need to be fulfilled. The ideal situation is an orthopaedic in-

Table 151-9
Organisms Often Not Covered by Oral Antibiotics

Staphylococcus aureus (methicillin resistant/ciprofloxacin resistant)
Enterococcus (penicillin resistant)
Pseudomonas (ciprofloxacin resistant)
Enterobacter (ciprofloxacin resistant)
Serratia (ciprofloxacin resistant)

fection that has resulted from a hematogenous source such as in the case of pediatric osteomyelitis. This ensures that high levels of antibiotic will reach the source of the infection. Patient reliability and tolerance of the oral antibiotic are also important.

The organism must be isolated and shown to be sensitive to an oral antibiotic. Ideally, one would also like to have the organism available so that a Schlichter test can be performed. Extrapolating from the endocarditis literature, a Schlichter test with a bactericidal level of 1:8 at the peak of the antibiotic is considered ideal. One study found a serum bactericidal level of 1:2 or greater to be adequate. The Schlichter test measures bactericidal and bacteriostatic levels at the peak and trough of the antibiotic. The levels represent the maximal dilution of the patient's serum that will kill or inhibit 99.9 percent of the infecting organism in vitro.

We have also found that persistence of a negative CRP ensures that the treatment is adequate. However, a satisfactory response must also be documented to intravenous antibiotics before switching to oral antibiotics.

PROPHYLAXIS FOR ORTHOPAEDIC PROCEDURES

It is standard practice to prophylax orthopaedic procedures that involve placement of prostheses or placement of hardware to achieve internal fixation.

The choice of antibiotics should be based on the sensitivities of the organisms in a given hospital. For instance, in a hospital with many methicillin-resistant organisms, vancomycin would be the appropriate antibiotic. Otherwise, cefazolin is usually used because of its long half-life and low toxicity.

Several studies have tried to compare different treatment schedules. It remains unclear whether one perioperative burst may not be as effective as 48 h of antibiotics. There is definite concern that prolonged use of prophylactic antibiotics may select out for resistant organisms. No definite conclusions can be drawn from the literature. It appears that most orthopaedists use the 48 h schedule.

PROPHYLAXIS FOR DENTAL, GENITOURINARY, AND GASTROINTESTINAL PROCEDURES FOR PATIENTS WITH JOINT REPLACEMENTS

Joint replacements can be infected by hematogenous spread. Therefore, any procedures that can cause a bacteremia have the potential of infecting a joint replacement. In selecting an antibiotic for prophylaxis, it is logical to consider the most likely organism from the given anatomic site. One cannot cover all possible organisms. In

Table 151-8
Antibiotics

Intravenous	Oral
Penicillin G	Penicillin VK
Oxacillin	Dicloxacillin
Methicillin	Dicloxacillin
Ampicillin/sulbactam	Amoxicillin/clavulanic acid
Cefazolin	Cephalexin
Ciprofloxacin	Ciprofloxacin
Vancomycin	No oral equivalent, oral vancomycin not absorbed
Ticarcillin/clavulanate potassium	No oral equivalent
Ceftazidime	No oral equivalent
Gentamicin	No oral equivalent
Tobramycin	No oral equivalent
Amikacin	No oral equivalent

Table 151-10

Recommendations For Prophylaxis

Dental and Upper Respiratory Procedures

Amoxicillin	3 g 1 h before procedure and 1.5 g 6 h later
Penicillin allergy: Erythromycin	1 g 1 h before procedure and 500 mg 6 h later

GASTROINTESTINAL AND GENITOURINARY PROCEDURES

Amoxicillin	3 g 1 h before procedure and 1.5 g 6 h later
Penicillin allergy	No oral prophylaxis available Vancomycin 1 g IV 1 h before procedure given over 1 h plus Gentamycin 1.5 mg/kg IV 30 min before procedure

the case of orthopaedic infections, there is a further dilemma because the majority are caused by staphylococci that are not often found in dental, genitourinary, and gastrointestinal sites.

The studies remain inconclusive and, at the present time, most orthopaedists appear to be using modifications of the recommendations of the American Heart Association for the prevention of endocarditis (see Table 151-10).

SPECIAL ISSUES IN PEDIATRIC ORTHOPAEDIC INFECTIONS

The selection of antibiotics for children differs from that for adults in several respects. Children have a much higher incidence of meningitis, and this influences the diagnostic workup and the initial choice of antibiotics. The highest incidence of meningitis occurs in children younger than 1 year of age. Children also are at an increased risk for bacteremia between 6 months and 2 years of age. The bacteremia can lead to meningitis and orthopaedic infections, as well as to epiglottitis or sinusitis. For this reason, blood cultures are standard practice in pediatric evaluations, and treatment is often started prior to the availability of culture results.

Children are also at risk for slightly different pathogens than adults, and this should be considered when choosing their initial treatment. In infants, the incidence of group B streptococci is much higher than in other age groups. Similarly, the incidence of *Haemophilus influenzae* is higher in children younger than age 6.

This may change in the near future, since there is now a vaccine for *H. influenzae*.

Because of the hematogenous source of many pediatric infections, oral antibiotics are particularly appropriate for these patients. Also, the smaller size of pediatric patients and their generally good gastrointestinal absorption make them good candidates. Probenecid can also be used to increase the blood levels of certain antibiotics such as penicillin, ampicillin, and the semisynthetic penicillins. Oral treatment should be considered when treating pediatric patients if the social situation appears to be reliable.

SUGGESTED READING

Ahlberg A, Carlsson AS, Lindberg L: Hematogenous infections in total joint replacement. *Clin Orthop* 1978; 137:69.

Brause BD: Infections associated with prosthetic joints. *Clin Rheum Dis* 1986; 12:523.

Cunha BA (ed): Antimicrobial therapy. *Med Clin North Am* 1982; 66(1):313.

Dirschl DR: Acute pyogenic osteomyelitis in children. *Orthop Rev* 1994; 23:305.

Goldenberg DL, Reed JI: Bacterial arthritis. *N Engl J Med* 1985; 312:764.

Hill C, Flamant R, Mazas F, et al: Prophylactic cefazolin versus placebo in total hip replacement. Report of a multicentre double-blind randomized trial. *Lancet* 1981; 1:795.

Larsson S, Thelander U, Friberg S: C-reactive protein (CRP) levels after elective orthopedic surgery. *Clin Orthop* 1992; 275:237.

Marks KE, Nelson CL, Lautenschlayer EP: Antibiotic-impregnated acrylic bone cement. *J Bone Joint Surg [Am]* 1976; 58:358.

Nasser S: Prevention and treatment of sepsis in total hip replacement surgery. *Orthop Clin North Am* 1992; 23:265.

Nelson JD, Norden C, Mader JT, et al: Evaluation of new anti-infective drugs for the treatment of acute hematogenous osteomyelitis in children: Infectious Diseases Society of America and the Food and Drug Administration. *Clin Infect Dis* 1992; 15(suppl):S162.

Norden CW: Antibiotic prophylaxis in orthopedic surgery. *Rev Infect Dis* 1991; 13(suppl 10):S842.

Patzakis MJ (ed): Antibiotics in orthopaedics. *Clin Orthop* 1984; 190:2.

Pollard JP, Hughes SPF, Scott JE, et al: Antibiotic prophylaxis in total hip replacement. *BMJ* 1979; 1:707.

Roine I, Faingezicht I, Arguedas A, et al: Serial serum C-reactive protein to monitor recovery from acute hematogenous osteomyelitis in children. *Pediatr Infect Dis J* 1995; 14:40.

Stambough JL, Beringer D: Postoperative wound infections complicating adult spine surgery. *J Spinal Disord* 1992; 5:277.

Ullman RF, Cunha BA: Antibiotic selection in the penicillin allergic patient. *Intern Med* 1986; 7:100.

Wahl MJ: Clinical issues in the prevention of dental-induced endocarditis and prosthetic joint infection. *Pract Periodontics Aesthetic Dent* 1994; 6:25.

Williams DN, Gustilo RB. The use of preventive antibiotics in orthopaedic surgery. *Clin Orthop* 1984; 190:83.

Yentis SM, Soni N, Sheldon J: C-reactive protein as an indicator of resolution of sepsis in the intensive care unit. *Intensive Care Med* 1995; 21:602.

Chapter 152

THROMBOEMBOLIC COMPLICATIONS

David J. Steiger, William N. Rom, Omar E. Burschtin

Venous thromboembolism is a major cause of morbidity and mortality in hospitalized patients. It causes in-hospital death in more than 100,000 patients each year in the United States and contributes to death in another 100,000. The disease is often clinically silent, and pulmonary embolism (PE) is unsuspected in 70 to 80 percent of patients whose condition are diagnosed at autopsy. Fatal PE may be the most common preventable cause of hospital death.

Although the frequency of deep venous thrombosis (DVT) has been well documented in surgical patients, the rate of DVT in medical patients has not often been evaluated. A recent study described a high rate of DVT (33 percent) in a medical ICU; 48 percent were proximal DVTs (15 percent were upper extremity), despite the use of prophylaxis in 61 percent of patients. This study underscores the prevalence of DVTs in this high-risk population.

Routine DVT prophylaxis is notoriously under-used despite overwhelming evidence on the efficacy of a wide variety of prophylactic agents. The application of effective prophylaxis depends on the knowledge of specific clinical risk factors in individual patients. Congenital and acquired hypercoagulable states assume greater importance in hospitalized patients. In many patients, multiple risk factors are present, and risks are cumulative.

CAUSES OF VENOUS THROMBOEMBOLISM

At least 90 percent of clinically important PE results from lower extremity DVT. Virchow's triad describes three factors responsible for thrombus formation: (1) stasis of blood flow, (2) intimal injury, and (3) hypercoagulability. The risk of thromboembolism increases in proportion to the number of specific predisposing factors (Table 152–1). In many patients, multiple risk factors may be present.

THE ORTHOPAEDIC PATIENT

PATIENTS UNDERGOING MAJOR ORTHOPAEDIC SURGERY OF THE LOWER LIMB

These patients are at high risk for postoperative venous thromboembolism (Table 152–2), despite modern surgical techniques and early patient immobilization.

MULTIPLE TRAUMA

A recent large study established that major trauma patients have an extremely high risk of venous thromboembolism, with an incidence of 58 percent. There was, as expected, a high rate of DVT in patients with lower extremity fractures (69 percent) and spinal cord injury (62 percent), but there was also a high rate of DVT following facial, chest, and abdominal trauma.

HEMATOLOGIC RISK FACTORS

Risk factors related to abnormal clotting mechanisms include lupus anticoagulant, proteins C and S deficiency, antithrombin III deficiency, and reduced fibrinolytic activity. Recently, Dahlback (1993) demonstrated an inherited resistance to the anticoagulant effect of activated protein C. The estimated prevalence of activated protein C resistance in patients with thromboembolic disease is 21 to 52 percent. The prevalence in the normal population is approximately 5 percent. It is the most common inherited thrombophilic disorder. The molecular basis for the disease is secondary to a point mutation in the gene encoding for Factor V, commonly known as the Factor V Lieden mutation. Persons heterozygous for the mutation have a mild (8- to 10-fold) increased risk of venous thrombosis; the homozygous state confers a high (80-fold) risk of thrombosis. Recent studies have identified hyperhomocystinemia to be a risk factor for recurrent thrombosis in patients between ages 20 to 70 years compared to the general population.

CLINICAL FEATURES AND NATURAL HISTORY OF DVT AND PE

DVT may be silent and is often undetectable at the bedside. Edema, distended veins, localized areas of discoloration, and increased heat and tenderness are signs which should raise the spectre of a DVT diagnosis.

Table 152-1

Specific Risk Factors

Age >40 years
Obesity
History of venous thromboembolism
Cancer
Bed rest >5 days
Major surgery
Congestive heart failure
Lower extremity fracture
Stroke
Immobility
Multiple trauma
Childbirth
Myocardial infarction
Hypercoagulable state

Table 152-2

Venous Thromboembolism Prevalence following Major Orthopaedic Surgery of the Leg

Procedure	DVT (%)*a*		PE(%)	
	Total	Proximal	Total	Fatal
THR	45–57	23–36	6–30	3.4–6
TKR	40–84	9–20	1.8–7	0.7
Hip fracture surgery	36–60	17–36	4.3–24	3.6–12.9

*a*Data based on post-operative venography from recent placebo controlled, randomized trials.

NOTE: THR, total hip replacement; TKR, total knee replacement

Thrombi limited to the calf veins are rarely associated with PE. Popliteal and more proximal venous thrombi carry a high embolic risk. However, most above-knee DVTs represent extension of thrombus from calf vein DVTs. Approximately 15 percent of calf vein thrombi extend proximally.

DVT and PE represent parts of a continuum in the spectrum of thromboembolic disease. Greater than 50 percent of patients with PE have a proximal DVT, and greater than 50 percent of patients with symptomatic DVT have asymptomatic PE.

CLINICAL FEATURES OF PE

Of patients with a PE, 40 to 60 percent are asymptomatic. The most common symptoms include apprehension, breathlessness, and palpitations. Pleuritic chest pain and hemoptysis are rare and more likely to accompany pulmonary infarction. This entity occurs in patients with a large PE, or in those patients with a smaller PE but with impaired cardiopulmonary reserve. Syncope is rare and is a manifestation of a massive PE.

The most common sign of PE is tachycardia. Evidence of right-sided heart strain and hypotension are rare, and signify a hemodynamically significant PE. A pleural rub occurs with pulmonary infarction.

LABORATORY FINDINGS

Hypoxia, respiratory alkalosis, and an increased alveolar-arterial (A-a) oxygen difference are seen in PE, but a normal (A-a) difference does not exclude a PE. The hypoxia is secondary to ventilation-perfusion mismatch, increased dead space ventilation from decreased alveoli perfusion, decreased surfactant, and an intracardiac shunt in massive PE with pulmonary hypertension, in patients with a patent foramen ovale.

ECG findings are usually nonspecific, with sinus tachycardia being the most common abnormality.

THE DIAGNOSTIC APPROACH TO THROMBOEMBOLIC DISEASE

DIAGNOSIS OF DVT

Since symptoms and the clinical exam for the diagnosis of DVT are notoriously unreliable, a reliable objective test is required to provide guidance in the critical decision of whom to treat, because of the potentially dire consequences of delayed diagnosis and treatment.

Contrast venography is the acknowledged gold standard, but the procedure is invasive and not without risk.

Impedance plethysmography was favored due to its low cost, relative accuracy, and ease of use on serial testing; it was associated with a diagnostic accuracy of over 90 percent. However, the test's inability to distinguish extravascular from intravascular compression has led to questioning of the test's high sensitivity.

Duplex ultrasonography has become the primary screening test for evaluation of DVT. Its accuracy of diagnosis is measured against venography and by longitudinal analysis which assesses the consequences of clinical decisions based on ultrasound test results. Duplex ultrasonography has a sensitivity and specificity of approximately 95 percent for symptomatic femoral and popliteal DVT, but is less accurate in detecting calf and pelvic DVTs. Sonography is operator dependent, may not be specific in cases of recurrent DVT, and has a sensitivity of approximately 66 percent for asymptomatic DVTs.

MRI has become a valuable tool in the accurate diagnosis of DVT. Venous thrombi can be seen with conventional spin echo techniques. Normal flowing blood has a low signal intensity (i.e., its image is dark); thrombus has a higher intensity. Gradient echo technique (normal flowing blood has high intensity, white on the images; thrombus has a low intensity) has a higher specificity for DVT (100 versus 75 percent for spin echo), but the sensitivities for the two techniques are similar.

In a prospective study of 61 patients, the diagnostic performance of MRI was better than that of venography in the pelvis, the same as venography in the thigh, and a worse diagnostic tool in the calf.

Summary of Recommended Diagnostic Tests for Thromboembolic Diseases

The choice of diagnostic test depends on the signs, symptoms, clinical risk, availability of different imaging tools, and clinical expertise of the practitioners performing and interpreting the studies. Guidelines include

1. Rule out symptomatic DVT of the thigh or popliteal vein: ultrasonography
2. High-risk patient with possible asymptomatic DVT: MRI
3. Bilateral lower extremity signs or symptoms: ultrasonography should be the initial screening test; consider MRI due to greater likelihood of pelvic and abdominal extension
4. Prior history of DVT: baseline follow-up ultrasound; if this is not available, perform MRI or venography to distinguish acute from chronic DVTs

5. Rule out extravascular pathology: MRI
6. Rule out calf DVT (< 20 percent calf DVTs extend to the upper thigh or popliteal vein): if ultrasonography of the thigh is negative, perform serial studies to rule out extension; one can perform venography/MRI to evaluate the calf veins directly

THE DIAGNOSIS OF PULMONARY EMBOLI

Ventilation/Perfusion (V/Q) Scans

In many patients with suspected PE, the V/Q scan is nondiagnostic. Studies have shown that a PE can be ruled out on the basis of a normal scan, and there is a 4 percent prevalence for PE if the scan is low probability and the clinical suspicion is low. Of patients with a high probability scan 87 percent had a positive angiogram. However, in patients with pulmonary angiographic evidence for PE, only 41 percent of patients had a high probability scan, and 42 percent had an intermediate probability scan. Fifteen percent of patients with a low probability scan had a positive angiogram.

CT Scan in the Diagnosis of Pulmonary Emboli

Early reports have documented the ability of CT to demonstrate clots in the central pulmonary artery, with a sensitivity of 100 percent and specificity of 96 percent. In addition, the detection of proximal clots on CT scan among patients with clinically unsuspected PE has been shown. Helical CT and electron-beam CT have improved visualization of the pulmonary arterial tree. A recent study documented emboli as distal as segmental vessels. CT and angiographic findings correlated well with respect to the location of emboli. The CT is superior to V/Q scanning, but less accurate than conventional angiography.

MRI in the Diagnosis of Pulmonary Embolus

MRI is evolving as a potential noninvasive means of directly depicting pulmonary artery clots. The distinct advantages of MRI over CT scans include: (1) no requirement of iodinated contrast material and (2) pulmonary vascular imaging may be combined with MR venography of the legs and pelvis for evaluation of DVT. Technical advances have enabled visualization of intraparenchymal pulmonary vasculature, as well as central vessels. While it is possible to visualize vessels down to the seventh generation, the ability to detect emboli is limited.

Summary/Diagnostic Algorithm in Diagnosis of Possible PE

The precise role of CT and MRI within the diagnostic work-up of patients suspected of acute PE is not well defined.

Possible indicators are

1. CT scan: for intermediate V/Q and negative DVT studies; if the patient is unstable, perform angiogram to facilitate clot extraction/lysis/IVC filter placement (see below)
2. Combined MR angiogram and MR venography of lower extremities and pelvis: this requires further improvement in the accuracy of MRI pulmonary angiography for detection of smaller pulmonary artery clots

PROPHYLAXIS OF VENOUS THROMBOEMBOLISM

The rationale for prophylaxis of venous thrombosis is based on the clinically silent nature of the disease. Both DVT and PE manifest few specific symptoms, and the clinical diagnosis is insensitive and unreliable. Morgenthaler (1995) noted that the classical symptoms of PE were frequently absent in patients who died of PE. Most patients who die of PE, do so in the first 30 min of the acute event. Therefore, DVT prophylaxis should be the cornerstone of management of thromboembolic disease. The intensity of prophylaxis should match the magnitude of risk, using physical and chemical methods of prophylaxis.

PROPHYLACTIC MEASURES

Physical Methods

Elastic Stockings   Elastic stockings are inexpensive and simple to use and to combine with other prophylactic measures.

Intermittent Compression Devices   Intermittent compression devices increase blood flow to the femoral veins and exert fibrinolytic activity. They are uniquely beneficial in patients for whom anticoagulation is contraindicated.

Pharmacologic Methods

Coumadin   Coumadin has not gained wider acceptance due to fear of bleeding complications, the need for frequent laboratory monitoring, and the delay of 3 to 4 days after initiating therapy before therapeutic effects are manifest.

Low-Molecular-Weight Heparins   Low-molecular-weight heparins (LMWHs) represent an exciting advance in the prophylaxis and treatment of venous thromboembolism. The LMWH preparations are currently only approved for use in the United States for total knee and total hip replacement DVT prophylaxis, but their use may expand to include treatment of established DVT. LMWH is prepared from unfractionated heparin (UFH) by chemical and enzymatic depolymerization. Its different anticoagulation profile to UFH is secondary to its difference in size. Only one-third of the LMWH molecules contain the pentasaccharide required for anti-thrombin III binding (which accelerates the inactivation of thrombin, factor IXa, and factor Xa in a ternary complex). Inactivation of Xa by heparin/anti-thrombin III requires only binding to antithrombin III, and does not require a ternary complex with thrombin. Heparin molecules smaller than 18 saccharide units are unable to bind thrombin and anti-thrombin III, but retain their ability to catalyze the inhibition of Xa by anti-thrombin III. Therefore, the LMWH fractions have relatively more anti-Xa than thrombin (IIa) activity. LMWH's reduced nonspecific binding to endothelial cells and plasma proteins contributes to its superior bioavailability, and to a plasma half-life four times longer than UFH. There is less platelet inhibition and decreased microvascular bleeding from LMWH compared to UFH. Metaanalyses and clinical trials have demonstrated the superiority of LMWH compared to UFH in preventing DVT after general orthopaedic surgery, specifically after total hip and total knee replacement (see below), in patients with acute ischemic stoke, and after major trauma.

Dextran   Dextran, a colloid, reduces plasma viscosity, alters platelet function, and reduces fibrin polymerization. Major complications of dextran include fluid overload, anaphylaxis, and renal toxicity.

SPECIFIC RECOMMENDATIONS FOR ORTHOPAEDIC SURGERY

Elective Hip Replacement

LMWHs and coumadin are effective, reducing venous thromboembolism risk by 60 to 70 percent. Although more expensive than other

Table 152-3

DVT Prevention following Total Hip Replacement[a]

Regimen	No. of Patients	Incidence (%)	Relative Risk Reduction (%)
Controls	655	51	—
L.M.W.H.	2571	15	71
Low intensity coumadin	637	20	61
Aspirin	357	56	—
Dextran 70	229	30	41
Pneumatic stockings	359	22	57
Elastic stockings	137	38	25

[a]Pooled data from trials requiring venography.

agents, LMWHs are becoming the prophylactic agent of choice because of their efficacy, lack of need for laboratory monitoring, ease of administration, and relatively low risk of bleeding (Table 152–3).

Elective Knee Replacement (see Table 152–4)

Both LMWHs and pneumatic stockings are highly effective in reducing the incidence of venous thromboembolism following knee replacement, with an approximate risk reduction of 60 percent.

DVT Prophylaxis following Hip Fracture Surgery

Prophylaxis of hip fracture surgery is a major challenge due to the risk of bleeding in these typically elderly patients with recent trauma. Five studies each of LMWH and low intensity coumadin show similar and substantial reductions in relative risk of approximately 50 percent compared to placebo. Bleeding complications were similar, although there are differences in the reporting of this complication. Either agent can be used, and treatment should be initiated preoperatively, when the patient is clinically stable.

Controversies in Thromboembolism Prevention

There are a number of unresolved controversies in venous thromboembolism prevention.

The optimal duration of DVT prophylaxis administration in patients requiring surgery remains unclear. With decreasing lengths of acute hospitalization, it is possible that an increasing proportion of venous thromboembolism is occurring in the out-patient setting. Consensus statements recommend that prophylaxis continue until the patient is ambulatory—which may be delayed in orthopaedic patients.

In a study by Bergquist (1996), 262 patients undergoing total hip replacement received LMWH during hospitalization (mean stay, 11 days), and then randomized to LMWH or placebo injection as outpatient therapy after a baseline normal venogram was obtained. There was a significant reduction in venographically documented DVT and incidence of PE in the LMWH group compared to the UFH group. However, the optimal duration of prolonged DVT prophylaxis remains unclear.

Inferior vena cava filters have been inserted as primary prophylaxis in patients at high risk for thromboembolism in whom a PE would be fatal, such as in patients with poor cardiopulmonary reserve. In addition, their use has extended to include patients with multiple injuries including patients with acute intracranial pathology, who would be intolerant of anticoagulation, or where physical methods of prophylaxis would not be possible. In view of the multiple potential complications associated with the insertion of IVC filters, their use as primary prophylaxis should still be considered experimental.

TREATMENT OF THROMBOEMBOLIC DISEASE

Patients with a DVT or PE should be treated with IV heparin sufficient to prolong the PTT to 1.5 x control. Heparin may be bolused by loading with 80 U/kg per h and giving a maintenance dose of 18 U/kg per h. Heparin should be continued for 5 to 10 days, and oral anticoagulation should be overlapped with heparin therapy for 4 to 5 days. For a massive PE or ileo-femoral vein thrombosis, prolonged IV heparin may be required. Long-term anticoagulation should

Table 152-4

DVT Prevention following Total Knee Replacement[a]

Regimen	No. of Patients	Incidence (%)	Relative Risk Reduction (%)
Controls	116	61	—
L.M.W.H.	1354	30	51
Low Intensity Coumadin	1033	47	23
Aspirin	27	79	—
Dextran 70	229	30	41
Pneumatic Stockings	366	11	82

[a]Pooled data from trials requiring venography.

be continued for at least 3 months, aiming for an International Normalized Ratio (INR) of 2.0 to 3.0. Patients with recurrent venous thrombosis, a continuing risk factor, or a hypercoagulable state should be treated indefinitely.

LMWH has been compared with continuous UFH for the treatment of established DVT in a number of clinical trials, using repeat venography as the clinical endpoint. When comparing published trials, it is important to note that the LMWH preparations and timing of coumadin administration were variable; the LMWH doses were adjusted for weight of patient or based on anti-factor Xa activity. In a prospective, randomized, multicenter European trial, there was a statistically significant improvement in quantitative venography score at 10 days in the LMWH group. A more recent trial revealed superior venographic results at day 10, and a decreased incidence of recurrent thromboembolic events. Several large clinical trials of LMWH versus UFH for venous thromboembolism are in progress. Clinical outcome and objective parameters (venography and angiography) will be used.

The longer half-life, better bioavailability, and more predictable anticoagulation response of LMWHs compared to UFH, make them attractive for home use. Two recent trials compared standard heparin administered in hospital with LMWH (subcutaneous, weight-adjusted, twice a day). In both studies, a significant proportion of patients were excluded for reasons such as coexisting conditions, potential noncompliance, and risks of bleeding. However, both studies demonstrated that LMWH was as efficacious as VFH, with a similar rate of bleeding complications and comparable rates of anticoagulation failure.

Heparin-induced thrombocytopenia (HIT) is a relatively common complication of heparin use, and is associated with the development of thromboembolic disease, disseminated intravascular coagulation (DIC), PE, and ischemia to the extremities. It is caused by heparin-dependent IgG antibodies that activate platelets through their Fc receptor. In a prospective, controlled study in patients receiving DVT prophylaxis after hip surgery, none of 332 patients treated with LMWH had heparin-induced thrombocytopenia, 9 of 332 patients treated with UFH had HIT, and 8 developed thromboembolism. Heparin-associated antibodies developed in 8 percent in the UFH group and in 2.2 percent in the LMWH group. The explanation for these findings could be secondary to LMWH being less capable of activating resting platelets.

In a patient who develops HIT, LMWH should not be used. Alternative prophylactic agents include danaproid and hirudin. Danaproid is a heparinoid with a mean molecular weight of 5500 daltons. It has low cross reactivity with heparin-induced antibodies. It has been demonstrated to be an effective prophylactic agent for hip surgery. Hirudin is a direct thrombin inhibitor that has better biophysical properties than UFH or LMWH. It is a direct thrombin inhibitor since it can access and inactivate fibrin-bound thrombin, unlike the heparin/antithrombin III complex. Like LMWH, its superior pharmacokinetic profile compared to UFH is secondary to less nonspecific binding to protein and cell surfaces. It is not known to be associated with HIT. It has been shown to be a more effective agent than UFH for DVT prophylaxis in patients undergoing total hip replacement. It has not been compared with LMWH or coumadin.

MASSIVE PULMONARY EMBOLISM

Most patients with an acute PE do not succumb to the initial insult because the pulmonary circulation has a tremendous reserve. Normally, at rest much of the pulmonary vasculature is nonperfused, but can accommodate increased flow when cardiac output increases or when there is a small blood clot, without a change in V/Q matching, right ventricular (RV) function, and pulmonary vascular resistance (PVR). When the clot obliterates more than 50 percent of the vascular bed, however, there is worsening V/Q matching secondary to increased dead space, profound hypoxemia, and increased PVR with RV strain and failure.

In a patient with normal cardiopulmonary reserve, hypoxia suggests a large clot burden. The patient may present with unexplained tachycardia, hemodynamic instability, syncope, or shock. If the patient is too unstable for noninvasive diagnostic work-up, a bed-side echocardiogram demonstrating a volume-overloaded dyskinetic RV in the appropriate clinical context is sufficient to make the diagnosis.

Treatment of massive PE involves management of the hemodynamic abnormalities and anatomic treatment of the clot. Increasing the intravascular volume increases the preload of the RV to overcome the high PVR. A CVP = 15 mmHg is used as a goal. However, RV ischemia may be magnified by excessive increases in RV preload.

Inotropic agents are used to increase RV contractility. These include dobutamine and dopamine.

Interest in thrombolytic therapy increased when it was shown to improve survival in patients with an acute myocardial infarction (MI). However, the role of thrombolytic therapy remains unclear. Thrombolytic therapy has been shown to improve pulmonary arterial hemodynamics, normalize RV function, and improve V/Q scan and pulmonary arteriographic abnormalities earlier than IV heparin. Despite this, there has been no demonstrable improvement in patient outcome. A National Institutes of Health consensus recommended thrombolytic therapy when at least 40 percent of the pulmonary vascular bed is obliterated, for severe RV strain and for significant hypoxia.

Three thrombolytic agents are available for treating PE: streptokinase, urokinase, and tissue plasminogen activator (tPA). The choice of agent is based on cost and necessity for rapid clot dissolution. tPA is recommended for patients in shock, where rapid clot lysis is warranted. Thrombolytic therapy can be given peripherally. Bleeding is the most serious complication of therapy. Intracranial bleeding has been observed in 0.15 to 0.6 percent in patients treated for an acute MI.

To prevent clot migration, an inferior vena cava (IVC) filter can be used. It is commonly inserted when there are contraindications to, or failure of, anticoagulation and for massive PE to prevent death from a further DVT. The filter can be inserted through the same venous access route following pulmonary angiography. Complications of IVC filter placement include (1) recurrent PE (2 percent), (2) migration of the filter, (3) penetration of the IVC, and (4) IVC obstruction (8 to 33 percent after 55 months) and venous insufficiency.

Physical removal of the pulmonary clot is another treatment strategy in the patient with a massive PE. Open surgical embolectomy should be considered when other modalities have failed, for refractory hypotension, and where thrombolytic therapy is contraindicated. The mortality rates for surgical embolectomy range from 11 to 64 percent, depending on the absence or presence of preceding cardiac arrest. There is unlikely to be a trial comparing thrombolytic therapy with surgical embolectomy, since thrombolytic therapy is easier to undertake immediately, obviating the need for highly expert personnel to perform cardiopulmonary bypass.

Percutaneous catheter embolectomy has been used to reduce clot burden in patients with massive PE, although no trials have compared it with other forms of therapy in controlled studies with a large number of patients.

A few case reports have described the successful use of percutaneous catheter fragmentation, sometimes with concurrent thrombolytic administration.

Before attempting any of the clot removal procedures, an IVC filter should be placed.

SUGGESTED READINGS

4th American College of Chest Physicians Consensus Conference on Antithrombotic Therapy; ACCP Proceedings, Tucson, AZ, April, 1995. *Chest* 1995; 108(4 Suppl):225S.

Bergqvist D, Benoni G, Bjorgell O, et al: Low-molecular-weight heparin (enoxaparin) as prophylaxis against venous thromboembolism after total hip replacement. *N Engl J Med* 1996; 335:696.

Dahlback B, Carlsson M: Familial thrombophilia due to a previously unrecognized mechanism characterized by poor anticoagulant response to activated protein C: Prediction of a cofactor to activated protein. *Proc Natl Acad Sci USA* 1993; 90:1004.

Dalen JE, Alpert JS: Natural history of pulmonary embolism. *Prog Cardiovasc Dis* 1975; 17:257.

den Heijer M, Koster T, Blom HJ, et al: Hyperhomocysteinemia as a risk factor for deep vein thrombosis. *N Engl J Med* 1996; 334:759.

Erdman WA, Peshock RM, Redman HC, et al: Pulmonary embolism: Comparison of MR images with radionuclide and angiographic studies. *Radiology* 1994; 190:499.

Eriksson BI, Ekman S, Kälebo P, et al: Prevention of deep-vein thrombosis after total hip replacement: Direct thrombin inhibition with recombinant hirudin. *Lancet* 1996; 347:635.

Evans A, Beam C: Detection of deep venous thrombosis DVT: Prospective comparison of MR imaging with contrast venography. *Am J Roentgenol* 1993; 161:131.

Geerts WH, Jay RM, Code KI, et al: A comparison of low-dose heparin with low-molecular-weight heparin as prophylaxis against venous thromboembolism after major trauma. *N Engl J Med* 1996; 335:701.

Goldhaber SZ, Savage DD, Garrison RJ, et al: Risk factors for pulmonary embolism. The Framingham study. *Am J Med* 1983; 74:1023.

Hirsch DR, Ingenito EP, Goldhaber SZ: Prevalence of deep venous thrombosis among patients in medical intensive care. *JAMA* 1995; 274:335.

Imperiale TF, Speroff T: A meta-analysis of methods to prevent venous thromboembolism following total hip replacement. *JAMA* 1994; 271:1780.

Koopman MM, Prandoni P, Piovella F, et al: Treatment of venous thrombosis with intravenous unfractionated heparin administered in the hospital as compared with subcutaneous low-molecular-weight heparin administered at home. The Tasman Study Group. *N Engl J Med* 1996; 334:682.

Levine M, Gent M, Hirsh J, et al: A comparison of low-molecular-weight heparin administrated primarily at home with unfractionated heparin administered in the hospital for proximal deep-vein thrombosis. *N Engl J Med* 1996; 334:677.

Morgenthaler TI, Ryu JH: Clinical characteristics of fatal pulmonary embolism in a referral hospital. *Mayo Clin Proc* 1995; 70:417.

Moser KM, Fedullo PF, Little John JK, et al: Frequent asymptomatic pulmonary embolism in patients with deep venous thrombosis. *JAMA* 1994; 271:223 [published erratum *JAMA* 1994; 271:1908].

The PIOPED Investigators: Value of the ventilation/perfusion scan in acute pulmonary embolism. Results of the prospective investigation of pulmonary embolism diagnosis (PIOPED). *JAMA* 1990; 263:2753.

Tapson VF, Hull RD: Management of venous thromboembolic disease. The impact of low-molecular-weight heparin. *Clin Chest Med* 1995; 16:281.

Teigen CL, Maus TP, Sheedy PF II, et al: Pulmonary embolism: Diagnosis with contrast-enhanced electron beam CT and comparison with pulmonary angiography. *Radiology* 1995; 194:313.

Wells PS, Lensing AW, Davidson BL, et al: Acccuracy of ultrasound for the diagnosis of deep venous thrombosis in asymptomatic patients after orthopedic surgery: A meta-analysis. *Ann Intern Med* 1995; 122:47.

Chapter 153

FAT EMBOLISM SYNDROME AND THE ACUTE RESPIRATORY DISTRESS SYNDROME

Mark F. Sloane

THE ACUTE RESPIRATORY DISTRESS SYNDROME: OVERVIEW

In 1967, Ashbaugh and colleagues described a syndrome of acute respiratory failure in association with a variety of clinical conditions. Today, the acute (or adult) respiratory distress syndrome (ARDS) is a syndrome of respiratory dysfunction due to a spectrum of processes which cause lung injury. This injury is generally thought to be due to inciting events which activate cellular elements and coagulation factors leading to the release of direct toxins, chemotactic factors, and mediators of injury. The common endpoint is the development of abnormal alveolar-capillary permeability and the development of a noncardiogenic pulmonary edema. Abnormal lung compliance and gas exchange derangements ensue. Ventilation-perfusion mismatch occurs with the generation of an intrapulmonic shunt. Chest radiograph reveals bilateral alveolo-reticular infiltrates. The pulmonary capillary wedge pressure classically is not elevated, supporting the noncardiac etiology of this pulmonary edema. A variety of etiologies of ARDS have been described, including the sepsis syndrome or systemic inflammatory response syndrome, trauma, gastric aspiration, smoke inhalation, fat embolism, burns, near drowning, pancreatitis, toxic inhalations, lung contusions, cardiopulmonary bypass, pulmonary infections, blood product transfusions, and possibly air emboli and amniotic fluid emboli.

The treatment of ARDS is generally supportive and additionally concentrates on the treatment of the underlying disease process. For example, in ARDS associated with sepsis, therapy directed against the infectious pathogen and aggressive management of the sepsis syndrome are pursued. In addition to significant advancements in supportive care, including ventilatory management and hemodynamic support, various therapeutic modalities recently have been studied. These include the use of *N*-acetylcysteine as a free radical scavenger, inhaled nitric oxide as a selective pulmonary vasodilator and bronchodilator, anti-inflammatory agents, alveolar surfactant administration, and immunologic therapy. Aggressive methods of supportive care have been evaluated, including extracorporeal membrane oxygenation.

Just as the etiology of ARDS is varied, its prognosis differs as well. For example, while ARDS following sepsis is associated with a 90 percent mortality, ARDS caused by fat embolism is associated with greater than 90 percent survival. It is clear that orthopaedists may encounter a variety of clinical syndromes associated with ARDS; however, an in-depth understanding of the fat embolism syndrome is of paramount importance to orthopaedic surgeons.

THE FAT EMBOLISM SYNDROME

Fat embolism syndrome (FES) is a well-recognized phenomenon associated with orthopaedic trauma as well as long-bone fracture stabilization and repair. FES has been surrounded by marked debate as to its etiology, incidence, pathogenesis, and treatment. Fat embolism was first reported by Zenker in 1862 when he found fat globules during the autopsy of a railroad worker who had sustained a fatal thoracoabdominal crush injury. The clinical syndrome was first described in 1873 by von Bergmann in a patient with a femur fracture in whom fat embolism was confirmed at autopsy. It may be helpful to view fat embolism as a continuum of disease—from the embolization of fat which may asymptomatically occur to a syndrome of systemic derangement which may itself be either mild or severe.

The reported incidence of FES after long-bone fractures varies from 1 to 20 percent. This variability in the reported incidence is, in large part, due to difficulty in accurately defining the clinical diagnostic criteria for FES. It has been reported that up to 90 percent of patients who sustain long-bone or pelvic fractures have hematogenous fat identified. Furthermore, it has been observed that during insertion of the prosthetic device in total hip replacement, all patients have fat globules released into the venous circulation. FES in its most rigorous definition is associated with respiratory insufficiency and hypoxemia, central neurologic deficits, and petechiae. In a study of trauma patients, the incidence of a substantial presentation of FES was 1.4 percent while a milder form was noted in 9 percent. If mild forms of FES may be identified by an abnormal alveolar-arterial oxygen gradient, the incidence may be as high as 11 percent. Earlier literature reported mortality in FES between 10 and 20 percent. Recent experience, however, suggests a lower mortality rate was likely due to advancements in supportive care. FES classically occurs in settings of multiple trauma, typically with fractures of the long bones or pelvis. Additionally, a variety of nontraumatic clinical conditions may be associated with FES. These include nontraumatic orthopaedic procedures, soft tissue injuries, cardiac massage, bone marrow transplantation and harvesting, osteomyelitis, liposuction, fatty liver, lipid hyperalimentation, pancreatitis, burns, renal transplant, sickle cell disease, steroid therapy, cisplatinum chemotherapy and bone tumor lysis, altitude decompression, diabetes mellitus, cyclosporin-A solvent, and carbon tetrachloride poisoning.

In the classic presentation of FES, symptoms generally occur 24 to 72 h after the inciting event, which is generally trauma to long bones or the pelvis. These symptoms classically include respiratory insufficiency, central neurologic abnormalities, and petechiae. If massive embolism of fat and marrow contents occurs during trauma or orthopaedic manipulation, sudden death may ensue quite rapidly. Significant elevations of pulmonary artery pressures have been demonstrated in both humans and experimental animal models with acute fat embolism. The cause of death in this acute massive fat embolism is felt to be due to acute pulmonary hypertension and resultant right heart failure. In a majority of cases of fat embolism, a lesser degree of pulmonary circulatory obstruction occurs. These events are generally acutely well tolerated, likely due to autoregulatory factors as well as the high compliant nature of the pulmonary vasculature. A delayed or biochemical phase occurs after fat embolization which, most commonly, is seen in patients with FES. This phase is associated with arterial hypoxemia which is thought to be due to the development of a ventilation-perfusion shunt. Endothelial cells in the alveolar capillaries secrete lipoprotein lipase which hydrolyses neutral fats and triglycerides into free fatty acids (FFAs) and glycerol. FFAs are toxic to lung parenchyma, causing toxicity to alveolar capillary endothelium, reduced surfactant production, interstitial hemorrhage, and pulmonary edema. Moylan and Everson suggested in 1977 that catabolism associated with trauma increases unbound FFA. This may help to explain the suggested correlation between FES and severity of trauma. Additionally, after fat embolization, aggregates of fat, platelets, fibrin, and leukocytes are found in the pulmonary microcirculation. Breakdown of cellular components is associated with further tissue insult and disruption of gas exchange. Platelet destruction may cause the release of serotonin which causes vascular congestion. In addition, platelet-derived vasoactive amines and prostaglandins serve as chemotactic factors which attract granulocytes. Granulocytes, in turn, release proteases, leukotrienes, and oxygen radicals which cause pulmonary parenchymal injury. Additionally, mast cell release of histamine causes airway constriction and inflammation. The time lag between the initial embolic events and onset of systemic derangements in FES may be explained by the time necessary for lipoprotein lipase to convert the embolized neutral fat to FFA, as well as the development of the cellular inflammatory response, as described.

CLINICAL PRESENTATION

FES presents primarily with neurologic, pulmonary, and cutaneous abnormalities classically after long-bone or pelvic trauma. Although symptoms may appear rapidly as in cases with massive emboli, generally there is a 12- to 24-h latent period between inciting event and the onset of the clinical syndrome. Symptoms develop in 60 percent of patients within 24 h and in 85 percent of patients within 48 h. Neurologic abnormalities occur in up to 86 percent of patients. Affected patients generally develop alterations in mental status ranging from mild disorientation to the onset of an acute confusional state which may progress to stupor and coma. Focal or generalized seizures may occur. Less frequently, focal neurologic defects may be encountered, including anisocoria, hemiplegia, scotomata, apraxia, aphasia, and conjugate eye deviation. These findings, when present, usually follow the alterations in cognition. The etiology of neurologic dysfunction is thought to be embolization of arterial fat via a patent foramen ovale and pulmonary arteriovenous shunts. Pathologically, diffuse petechial hemorrhage associated with the presence of microvascular fat globules may be seen involving predominantly the cerebral white matter. Computerized tomographic (CT) scan and magnetic resonance imaging (MRI) of the brain have variable yield. Although permanent focal injuries such as pontine hemorrhage may be seen, neurologic recovery usually occurs.

Pulmonary dysfunction is a common and, at times, a life-threatening manifestation of FES. Although at times clinically inapparent, hypoxemia is nearly universal when measured. Of patients, 75 percent develop respiratory insufficiency. Of those patients, 10 percent will progress to respiratory failure. Clinically, patients may experience dyspnea and develop tachypnea. Physical exam may reveal diffuse fine inspiratory rales. Arterial blood gas analysis demonstrates a respiratory alkalosis and decreased arterial oxygen tension, usually less than 60 mmHg. The chest radiograph may reveal bilateral alveolar or reticular infiltrates in 30 to 60 percent of patients. Of note, there is a delay in onset of radiographic abnormalities. This time lag from injury to radiographic manifestation may be of diagnostic value in that other pulmonary injuries such as aspirations, toxic or thermal injuries, other forms of adult respiratory distress syndrome, or pulmonary contusions reveal earlier radiographic abnormalities. Even when chest radiographs are normal, a ventilation and perfusion scan may demonstrate a mottled pattern of subsegmental perfusion defects with normal ventilation. Although this pattern is nonspecific, this observation may be of clinical value. The pathophysiology of pulmonary parenchymal injuries is associated with intravascular fibrin clot, hemorrhagic interstitial and alveolar edema due to toxicity of FFAs, and the inflammatory cellular response as described previously.

Petechiae are present in 20 to 50 percent of patients with FES and occur 48 to 72 h after injury. A petechial rash is an uncommon finding in patients with respiratory failure and neurologic dysfunction and, therefore, when present in the appropriate setting, supports the diagnosis of FES. Petechiae typically occur in the nondependent areas of skin such as the neck, anterior thorax, and axillae, as well as conjunctivae. Originally, this characteristic rash was thought to be due to thrombocytopenia associated with FES. However, skin biopsies have revealed the presence of fat globules in the dermal capillaries with vascular damage and local hemorrhage. The presence of petechiae in nondependent areas may be explained by the observation that these regions derive their blood supply from proximal branches of the aorta. Fat globules may rise to the surface of the blood column and be "skimmed off" into the vessels.

Additional clinical signs associated with FES include tachycardia and fever, and funduscopic exam may reveal fat emboli, hemorrhage, fluffy exudates, and macular edema. The electrocardiogram may show tachycardia, ST-segment changes, and signs of right heart strain. While renal insufficiency is rare, lipuria is common. Hematologic abnormalities are common. Thrombocytopenia and a sudden decrease in the hematocrit may be seen. Prolongations of the protime and prothrombin time may be noted if disseminated intravascular coagulation occurs. An increase in the erythrocyte sedimentation rate and C-reactive protein has been observed as well. Hypocalcemia may occur, thought due to the binding of calcium to FFA.

DIAGNOSIS

The clinical diagnosis of FES is made by a constellation of clinical findings, which include tachypnea, dyspnea, hypoxemia, respiratory alkalosis, and radiographic pulmonary infiltrates, as well as cerebral dysfunction and a petechial rash. Additional findings include tachycardia, fever, and thrombocytopenia. These abnormalities in the setting of long-bone or pelvic fracture support the diagnosis of FES. Several authors have proposed formal diagnostic criteria and scoring indices to increase diagnostic certainty. Masson and Ruggieri (1985) suggested the use of a pulmonary artery catheter to sample pulmonary capillary blood to determine fat content. Bronchoalveolar lavage has been used to demonstrate intrapulmonary fat as well. While a high percentage of bronchoalveolar cells exhibiting intracellular fat (greater than or equal to 5 percent) is supportive for the diagnosis of FES, the presence of fat in the cells is nonspecific. Recently, transesophageal echocardiography has been used to monitor the amount of emboli released during repair of long-bone fractures. The use of ventilation-perfusion lung scanning and head CT and MRIs, as discussed, may be useful and offer the added benefit of ruling out alternate etiologies for pulmonary and cerebral dysfunction.

TREATMENT

Management of patients at risk for the development of FES is primarily preventive, while the treatment of patients who have developed signs and symptoms of FES is essentially supportive in nature. In the early management of trauma patients, there are measures which must be undertaken to decrease the incidence and severity of FES. Long-bone fractures need to be stabilized as early and effectively as possible by the use of air splints and careful patient handling at the scene of the accident. After arrival at the hospital, early immobilization of fractures, including balanced traction, casting, or open reduction and internal fixation of long-bone fractures, is crucial. Additionally, treatment or prevention of hypovolemic shock is indicated by maintaining intravascular volume by using colloids, crystalloids, and/or blood transfusions. Of interest, in the animal model, the presence of shock has been reported to increase the incidence of fat embolism. After resuscitative measures have been undertaken, supportive management largely surrounds the pulmonary manifestations of FES.

Detection and treatment of hypoxemia is paramount. Supplementary oxygenation via nasal cannula or face mask is appropriate for mild hypoxemia. Endotracheal intubation and mechanical ventilation is necessary for severe hypoxic respiratory failure, or for airway protection in the case of severe cerebral dysfunction. Methylprednisolone has been used in the treatment and prophylaxis of FES. Ashbaugh and colleagues suggested its use after apparent effectiveness in two treated patients. Subsequently, numerous studies have suggested a benefit when corticosteroids are used prophylactically. Increased risk for infection associated with steroids is well known and should temper the aggressive use of prophylactic steroids in patients with long-bone fractures. In one study, while steroids appeared effective in reducing the incidence of FES, the only death which occurred was in a steroid-treated patient who died of infection. At present, methylprednisolone appears to be beneficial in reducing the incidence of FES when used prophylactically. Its use should be tempered by awareness of increased infection risk. Finally, the use of steroids in the treatment of established FES has not been studied in humans. Other therapeutic interventions in the treatment of FES have been postulated, including intravenous heparin, ethanol, low molecular weight dextran, clofibrate, protease inhibitors, nonsteroidals, and infusions of glucose and insulin. The usefulness of these treatments has not been supported in the literature. The use of albumin may have a role in the treatment of FES. FFAs, when complexed to albumin, do not produce the toxic effects seen with unbound FFA in vitro. Preliminary studies suggest the possible, although yet unproven, role for albumin administration in the treatment of FES. At present, accurate diagnosis, early immobilization and surgical intervention, and supportive care are the standard of care in the treatment of FES. Methylprednisolone may have a prophylactic role in patients at high risk for developing FES. The role of other treatments has yet to be supported in the literature. FES generally resolves in 3 to 7 days. The long-term prognosis overall is generally good for those who survive the initial trauma and pulmonary injury. Both respiratory and neurologic manifestations generally resolve, although permanent sequelae may occur. Prognosis may be more related to the severity of the initial injury than to FES itself.

In summary, FES is a relatively uncommon complication of long-bone fractures and orthopaedic trauma. The pathophysiology and incidence have been avidly debated and discussed. This syndrome's primary presentation is one of respiratory insufficiency, cerebral dysfunction, and a petechial rash. Although a variety of objective diagnostic tests have been sought, the diagnosis of FES remains a clinical one based on a constellation of signs and symptoms in the appropriate clinical setting. Effective treatment depends on early diagnosis of respiratory or neurologic impairment and is primarily supportive in nature. Early immobilization and operative intervention for long-bone fractures are indicated to decrease the incidence and severity of FES. The potential role of prophylactic steroids has been addressed. The long-term prognosis for patients suffering from FES is generally good for those who survive the initial injuries and respiratory dysfunction. While much is understood, clearly further research is warranted to unravel further the pathophysiology leading to FES. With a more complete understanding of the molecular and cellular processes producing the syndrome, further therapies will likely become available.

SUGGESTED READINGS

Ashbaugh DG, Bigelow DB, Petty TL, et al: Acute respiratory distress in adults. *Lancet* 1967; 2:319.

Cunningham AJ: Acute respiratory distress syndrome: Two decades later. *Yale J Biol and Med* 1991; 64:387.

Dines DE, Linscheid RL, Didier EP: Fat embolism syndrome. *Mayo Clin Proc* 1972; 47:237.

Evarts CM: The fat embolism syndrome: a review. *Surg Clin North Am* 1970; 50:493.

Fischer JE, Roderick H, Turner RH, et al: Massive steroid therapy in severe fat embolism. *Surg Gynecol Obstet* 1971; 132:667.

Gossling HR, Pellegrini VD Jr: Fat embolism syndrome: A review of the pathophysiology and physiological basis of treatment. *Clin Orthop* 1982; 165:68.

Hulman G: Pathogenesis of nontraumatic fat embolism. *Lancet* 1988; 1:1366.

Hulman G: Pathogenesis of fat embolism. *J Pathol* 1995; 176:3.

Masson RG, Ruggieri J: Pulmonary microvascular cytology: A new diagnostic application of the pulmonary artery catheter. *Chest* 1985; 88:908.

Matthay MA: The adult respiratory distress syndrome: Definition and prognosis. *Clin Chest Med* 1990; 11:575.

Moreau JP: Fat embolism: A review and report of 100 cases. *Can J Surg* 1974; 17:196.

Moylan JA, Everson MA: Diagnosis and treatment of fat embolism. *Annu Rev Med* 1977; 28:85.

Niden AH, Aviado DM: Effects of pulmonary embolism on the pulmonary circulation with special reference to arteriovenous shunts in the lung. *Circ Res* 1956; 4:67.

Oh WH, Mital MA: Fat embolism: Current concepts of pathogenesis, diagnosis and treatment. *Orthop Clin North Am* 1978; 9:769.

Peltier LF: The diagnosis of fat embolism. *Surg Gynecol Obstet* 1965; 121:371.

Riska EB, Myllynen P: Fat embolism in patients with multiple injuries. *J Trauma* 1982; 22:891.

Riska EB, von Bonsdorff H, Hakkinen S, et al: Prevention of fat embolism by early internal fixation of fractures in patients with multiple injuries. *Injury* 1976; 8:110.

Robert JH, Hoffmeyer P, Broquet PE, et al: Fat embolism syndrome. *Orthop Rev* 1993; 22:567.

Schonfeld SA, Ploysongsang Y, DiLisio R, et al: Fat embolism prophylaxis with corticosteroids: A prospective study in high-risk patients. *Ann Intern Med* 1983; 99:438.

Shier MR, Wilson RF, James RE, et al: Fat embolism prophylaxis: A study of four treatment modalities. *J Trauma* 1977; 17:621.

von Bergmann EB (1873). Cited as Bergmann EB von by: Peltier LF: The diagnosis of fat embolism. *Surg Gynecol Obstet* 1965; 121:371.

Wenda K, Degreif J, Runkel M, et al: Pathogenesis and prophylaxis of circulatory reactions during total hip replacement. *Arch Orthop Trauma Surg* 1993; 112:260.

Zenker FA (1862). Cited by: Peltier LF: The diagnosis of fat embolism. *Surg Gynecol Obstet* 1965; 121:371.

Chapter 154

MEDICAL COMPLICATIONS

Omar E. Burschtin, William N. Rom, and David J. Steiger

COMPLICATIONS OF BLOOD TRANSFUSIONS

Orthopaedic patients frequently need transfusions of blood products due to blood loss from bone fractures, surgery-related blood loss, perioperative complications (including upper gastrointestinal bleeding), or correction of chronic anemia. When planning elective surgery, one has the advantage of obtaining autologous blood, to be used during and/or after surgical procedures. The benefits are both decreased complications and disease transmission hazards (see below).

Transfusion reactions can be divided into immediate and delayed reactions.

RED CELL–RELATED COMPLICATIONS

Immediate Transfusion Reactions

Hemolytic transfusion reactions result from antibodies in the recipient's plasma reacting with donor red cells. The reaction can cause intravascular or extravascular hemolysis.

Intravascular Hemolysis   This condition occurs if the antibody is an IgG or IgM type that activates complement. Intravascular hemolysis is rapid, occurring after transfusion of a few cubic centimeters of blood. The patient presents with fever, shaking chills, headache, urticaria, hypotension, bronchospasm, and a burning sensation at venous access sites, chest pain, back pain, and facial flushing. The patient develops hemoglobinemia, hemoglobinuria, hyperbilirubinemia, and a decreased haptoglobin and disseminated intravascular coagulation (DIC).

Treatment   Discontinuation of the transfusion is mandatory and infusion with normal saline should be performed through new IV tubing, maintaining a minimum of 30 ml/h. of urine output. The blood pressure should be monitored and stabilized if hypotension is present. The blood bank must be notified immediately, and labels on the donated blood checked with patient identification. Laboratory studies to be sent include: BUN, Cr, electrolytes, prothrombin (PT), partial prothromboplastin (PTT), fibrinogen, platelet count, fibrinogen degradation products, hemoglobin, urine hemoglobin, serum or plasma hemoglobin and haptoglobin, and serum bilirubin. Urgent hematology consultation must be done as well as possible therapeutic interventions which include whole blood or plasma exchange, heparin infusion, and/or hemodialysis, depending on the diagnostic workup.

Extravascular Hemolysis   This occurs with IgG or IgM antibodies that do not bind complement, or only partially bind and activate complement. The reaction is usually mild, and the patient may develop fevers and chills. Treatment is supportive. The hemoglobin should be monitored, and the patient well hydrated.

Delayed Hemolytic Transfusion Reaction

A recipient may take hours to weeks to develop antibodies to a specific antigen. Extravascular hemolysis occurs, resulting in anemia and increased bilirubin. The patient will require a blood bank workup for a confirmatory diagnosis. Occasionally, the rare complication intravascular hemolysis will occur with potentially lethal consequences.

PLASMA-RELATED COMPLICATIONS

Allergic reactions can be mild or severe (anaphylactic). Mild reactions occur secondary to allergy to a substance in the donor plasma. Treatment with an antihistamine is usually effective and the transfusion can be continued. Occasionally, asthma or glottal edema occurs, mandating more aggressive therapy with epinephrine and steroids.

An anaphylactic reaction is seen during the first 10 ml of blood transfusion, more commonly observed among IgA-deficient patients receiving blood or plasma containing IgA from a donor. Anaphylaxis is due to the binding of high titers of complement-binding anti-IgA antibodies (developed from a previous transfusion) to IgA transfused in the blood products. The patient manifests bronchospasm, hypotension, abdominal cramps, and shock. Urgent treatment includes 10 ml of intravenous epinephrine in a 1:10,000 solution, 50 mg of intravenous diphenhydramine, and intravenous steroids. Subsequently, patients should be transfused either with red cells washed repeatedly, depleting IgA, or autologous blood or blood from IgA-deficient donors.

WHITE CELL–RELATED COMPLICATIONS

A febrile reaction is the most common transfusion complication and is characterized by fever and chills, and rarely hypotension. Such reactions are mainly due to antiplatelet and antileukocyte antibodies. Transfusion must be terminated and an evaluation for a hemolytic process needs to be initiated. Prophylactically, a patient with history of febrile reaction should be transfused with leukocyte-depleted blood.

COMPLICATIONS OF MASSIVE BLOOD TRANSFUSION

Massive transfusion means transfusion within a 24-h period that approximates a patient's total blood volume. The complications, a list of which follows, of massive transfusion are secondary to the effects of shelf storage and the dilutional effects on platelets and clotting factors.

1. *Hypocalcemia* is due to citrate (the anticoagulant in blood) binding to the patient's ionized calcium. Serum and ionized calcium should be followed.
2. *Hyperkalemia* may occur after multiple transfusions, from high concentrations of K^+ in stored blood. This is compounded by the presence of acidosis, renal insufficiency, and shock. Hypokalemia may result from the metabolism of citrate to bicarbonate, causing a metabolic alkalosis.

3. *Hypothermia* can occur after multiple transfusions of blood stored at 40°C. An external blood warmer should be used during massive transfusion.
4. *Lactic acidosis* increases during prolonged blood storage, leading to decreased glycolysis, and thus to decreased 2,3-DPG production. Since 2,3-DPG competes with hemoglobin for oxygen association, there is an increased binding of oxygen to hemoglobin and therefore decreased oxygen delivery. The increased cardiac output resulting from the transfusion and the rapid regeneration of 2,3-DPG in vivo can compensate for this decrease.
5. *Coagulopathy* occurs after massive transfusion because functional platelets are depleted in stored blood, and coagulation factors V and VIII deteriorate with storage. Management is guided by the results of platelet counts, fibrinogen, PT, and PTT, as well as the presence or absence of clinical bleeding.

UPPER AIRWAY OBSTRUCTION

Acute upper airway obstruction (UAO) is a serious, potentially fatal condition that requires immediate medical intervention. Airway resistance is inversely related to the fourth power of the radius. Therefore small changes in the cross-sectional diameter of the airways will cause proportionally greater decreases in air conductance and increases in the resistive load, with risk of asphyxiation.

CAUSES OF UPPER AIRWAY OBSTRUCTION

The causes of UAO follow:

Foreign bodies (the most common)

Traumatic (laryngeal injury and stenosis, airway burn)

Infections (epiglottitis, laryngitis, tonsillitis)

Tumors (laryngeal tumors)

Angioedema (ACE inhibitors, C1 inhibitor deficiency and anaphylaxis)

Vocal cord paralysis

Endotracheal tube trauma

CLINICAL FEATURES

Signs and symptoms include respiratory distress, cyanosis, stridor, and absent air movement. As asphyxiation continues, bradycardia, hypotension, and death occur. Unlike an acute asthma attack, the obstructive noises in UAO are intensified on inspiration and are localized to the upper airway.

SELECTED CAUSES OF UPPER AIRWAY OBSTRUCTION

Facial Trauma

Facial trauma after a motor vehicle accident that includes maxillary and mandibular fractures can cause UAO. Establishing an airway is a priority. If the cervical spine is unstable, fiberoptic intubation is preferred.

Laryngeal Stenosis

Airway injury during tracheal intubation, prolonged endotracheal intubation, and extubation injury are iatrogenic complications that can affect the glottis, subglottis, and trachea. Damage ranges from self-limited vocal cord edema and ulceration and granuloma to more severe laryngeal stenosis. Special attention is required in patients with a tracheostomy due to frequent scarring and subsequent stomal stenosis; after decanulation of the tracheostomy tube the patient may develop respiratory distress due to scarring and also to vocal cord abduction. Chronic UAO in a stable patient should be evaluated by pulmonary function test, plain radiography of the chest and neck, simple tomography, spatial computed tomography of the airways with contrast, or magnetic resonance imaging.

Laryngospasm

Spasm may be precipitated by a variety of laryngeal stimuli, including blood, mucus, and direct contact during intubation or after extubation. A short-acting paralyzing agent may be required followed by bag-mask ventilation (until the spasm has resolved) or translaryngeal intubation.

MANAGEMENT STRATEGIES APPLICABLE TO ALL FORMS OF UPPER AIRWAY OBSTRUCTION

Securing and maintaining a patent airway, whether by mechanical, chemical, physical, or surgical means, is of paramount importance. Simple nasopharyngeal or oropharyngeal airways may be enough for supraglottic soft tissue collapse. Transnasal or transoral endotracheal intubation, intubation over a fiberoptic bronchoscope, and tracheotomy not only secure but also maintain airway patency. Racemic epinephrine decreases the laryngeal mucosal edema but may be deleterious in cases of epiglottitis; it can be used either alone or in combination with dexamethasone. Dexamethasone is very effective in cases of postextubation laryngeal edema but has no role as a prophylactic agent. Steroids are also contraindicated in cases of epiglottitis. Heliox, a helium-oxygen mixture, has physical characteristics that are responsible for its benefit in acute UAO. The low density of the gas mixture reduces the flow-resistant forces, increases air conductance, and transforms turbulent flow to laminar flow, decreasing the work of breathing. It can be used as a temporizing measure until edema or an anatomical defect is corrected. Chronic subglottic laryngeal and tracheal stenosis can be treated by bronchoscopic dilatation, laser therapy, stent placement, and tracheal or laryngeal resection and reconstruction according to the etiology and expected prognosis.

ADDISONIAN CRISIS

Causes of adrenal cortical hypofunction can be primary or secondary.

PRIMARY ADRENAL HYPOFUNCTION

1. *Autoimmune adrenalitis*, the most common cause of primary adrenal hypofunction, is due to circulating antiadrenal antibodies which can coexist with other endocrine-deficient syndromes from polyglandular autoimmune diseases, and affect the pancreas, gonads, thyroid, and parathyroids.
2. *Infiltrative diseases* that can cause primary adrenal hypofunction include sarcoidosis, hemochromatosis, tuberculosis, fungal diseases, malignant transformation, hemorrhage from anticoagulation therapy, pseudomonas sepsis, or meningococcemia.

SECONDARY ADRENAL INSUFFICIENCY

Causes of secondary adrenal insufficiency include:

1. Hypothalamic and/or pituitary dysfunction due to intrinsic disease.
2. Long-term glucocorticoid therapy (with secondary suppression of ACTH) and the sudden discontinuation of the steroid formulation, or secondary to acute physiologic stress, such as a surgical procedure, in the steroid-dependent patient.

CLINICAL FEATURES AND LABORATORY ABNORMALITIES

Primary Addison's disease is manifested by darkening of the skin, nausea, weight loss, and weakness. Postural hypotension, hyponatremia, and hyperkalemia occur secondary to loss of adrenal mineralocorticoid function. Secondary adrenal insufficiency does not present with skin darkness, hyperkalemia, or sodium loss due to intact aldosterone function. Hyponatremia may result from water retention. Laboratory abnormalities show hyperkalemia (due to aldosterone deficiency), hyponatremia, pre-renal azotemia, and mild acidosis. Acute adrenal insufficiency (adrenal crisis) is the most serious manifestation of adrenal insufficiency and may present as an exacerbation of chronic adrenal insufficiency. It presents as severe hypotension with hypovolemic vascular shock, fever, abdominal pain, nausea, vomiting, and lethargy.

DIAGNOSIS OF ADRENAL INSUFFICIENCY

The diagnosis is made by an ACTH stimulation test. In the clinically obvious case, a low morning serum cortisol may be sufficient to confirm the diagnosis. In an Addisonian crisis, treatment should be initiated immediately by glucocorticoid replacement (100 mg of I.V. cortisol, repeated every 6 h), or a continuous infusion of 10 mg/h of cortisol, electrolyte, and volume correction. Recommended therapy includes 5% glucose in normal saline. Transient use of vasopressors may be needed until volume replacement and hypotension is corrected. After stabilization and improvement, a steroid taper can be initiated.

Patients with a history of adrenal insufficiency or patients on long-term steroid therapy scheduled for elective surgery should receive adequate cortisol supplementation one day before surgery, the day of surgery and subsequent postoperative days with a tapering schedule. The duration of the steroid taper should be individualized, based on the presence of severe pain or the development of medical complications.

COMPARTMENT SYNDROME AND RHABDOMYOLYSIS

COMPARTMENT SYNDROME

Compartment syndrome (CS) is defined as an elevation of the interstitial pressure in a closed osseofascial compartment, resulting in microvascular compromise. The mechanism of injury is obstruction of the circulation due to post-injury swelling causing tissue hypoxia, anoxia, and necrosis. The most common causes of CS include: massive soft-tissue trauma, crush injuries, prolonged limb compression, long bone fracture, and complications following revascularization of an ischemic limb. Within the orthopaedic population, a bone fracture is the most frequent cause of CS either before or after surgical correction or casting. It is most commonly seen in the leg and forearm but is also observed in the thigh, foot, and hand. In the lower extremity, the anterior compartment can be involved due to tibial fractures. The anterior tibial muscle is nourished only by the anterior tibial artery with no alternate blood supply. The deep posterior compartment of the lower extremity is affected by fracture of the tibia and fibula. The lower extremity may manifest chronic presentations of CS, with milder symptoms that are usually exacerbated after exercise.

Clinical Presentation

There are signs and symptoms of muscle ischemia (pain, pallor), vascular deficiency (absent or decreased pulse), and neurologic abnormalities (paresthesias, weakness, and paralysis). The area with CS manifests swelling and tenderness on physical examination; the cardinal sign is severe pain during passive stretching. If the patient is unconscious, measurement of the intracompartmental pressure can be performed. Diagnostic tools include Doppler ultrasound and Tc-99 scintigraphy, which can demonstrate focal areas of muscle necrosis. Compartmental pressure can be measured directly by catheter manometry. When the pressure exceeds systemic diastolic pressure, emergency fasciotomy is indicated.

The most significant medical complication of CS is the development of renal insufficiency due to myoglobinuria, hyperkalemia, hyperphosphatemia, hypocalcemia, DIC, metabolic acidosis, and irreversible damage of the nerves and muscles involved.

Treatment of an Acute Compartment Syndrome

Fasciotomy should be performed shortly after the diagnosis is made, as better results are obtained if surgery occurs within the first 8 h of the onset of CS. After 8 h, if untreated, the damage is irreversible and the limb progresses to a chronic ischemic fibrotic contraction (Volkmann's ischemic contraction) resulting in paralysis of the extremity. Medical management of the complications of CS is focused on correction of the metabolic acidosis and electrolyte abnormalities, the prevention and treatment of hypotension, obtaining an adequate urine output, and the management of myoglobinuria and renal insufficiency (see below). Finally, treatment should address the coagulopathy and the management of possible infection.

RHABDOMYOLYSIS

Skeletal muscle can be injured by numerous causes. When the insult produces a disruption of the sarcolemma, the release of muscle cell contents into the circulation is responsible for the rhabdomyolysis syndrome.

Causes of Rhabdomyolysis

The causes of rhabdomyolysis include:

Trauma

Compartment syndrome

Burns

Tissue hypoxia

Metabolic abnormalities (DKA, hypokalemia, hypophosphatemia, hyponatremia)

Genetic disorders of the carbohydrate and lipid metabolism

Drugs (aspirin, cocaine, heroine, codeine, succinylcholine)

Miscellaneous causes: toxins, infections, hypothermia, and hyperthermia

Clinical Features/Metabolic Abnormalities

The disruption of the cell membrane allows intracellular K^+, intracellular PO_4, and myoglobin to exit the cell to the extracellular spaces and intravascular compartment with subsequent development of hyperkalemia, hyperphosphatemia, and myoglobinemia. Calcium influx to the cell increases and hypocalcemia develops. Acute renal failure is the most important complication of rhabdomyolysis, commonly due to acute tubular necrosis as a result of myoglobin nephrotoxicity. Contributory factors are hypovolemia, hypotension, and high uric acid accumulation in the renal tubules (worsening the obstruction to the urinary flow).

Clinical Manifestations   Presentation depends on the underlying disease process. The medical history and the physical examination may only give limited information. Swelling, weakness, and muscle tenderness are rarely seen.

Laboratory Diagnosis

CK levels five times normal or greater indicate the presence of rhabdomyolysis. Serum CK elevation is seen immediately after muscle damage and peaks within 24 to 36 h. Ongoing muscle injury must be suspected if CK level fails to decrease. Myoglobin level in serum is not a reliable marker due to its very short half-life. Urine myoglobin can be measured by radioimmunoassay and dipstick test. The dipstick test can not distinguish myoglobin from hemoglobin, but a positive dipstick test combined with the absence of RBCs in the urinalysis can be indicative of the presence of rhabdomyolysis. One should be aware, however, that myoglobinuria can only be seen after rhabdomyolysis, while rhabdomyolysis can exist in the absence of myoglobinuria due to variability in glomerular filtration rate from one patient to another. The most lethal complication of rhabdomyolysis is acute renal failure. Laboratory values found in acute renal failure and acute tubular necrosis include a specific gravity less than 1.015, urine osmolarity of less than 350 mOsm/L, dirty brown casts, urine sodium greater than 20 to 40 mEq/L, and fractional excretion of sodium over 1 to 2%.

Treatment

Treatment should focus on the original insult, stabilization of the airway, ventilation and circulation, correction of metabolic disorders, monitoring of coagulation profiles and correction of coagulopathy if present, prevention of compartment syndrome with frequent measurement of compartmental pressures, and prevention and treatment of renal insufficiency. The most important therapeutic intervention to prevent renal failure is the administration of an adequate volume of normal saline in order to obtain an ideal tubular flow and avoiding renal tubular obstruction and accumulation of nephrotoxic waste released from the injured muscle cell. Urine output must remain in the 200 to 300 cc/h rate; over 20 L of fluid may be required in the first 24-h period. Patients with a history of fluid retention, congestive heart failure, and hypertension need special close monitoring and adjustment of their fluid balance. There is controversy regarding the use of sodium bicarbonate as a tool for urine alkalinization. The rationale is that myoglobin and uric acid are both more toxic in acid urine, but large prospective randomized double blind control trials are lacking. In the presence of adequate saline infusion but a poor urine output response, furosemide or mannitol can be used; in the absence of appropriate urine output, dialysis is indicated.

FLUID OVERLOAD

Fluid overload is a common complication in hospitalized patients and is the result of an imbalance between intake and output. It is mainly due to a disproportionate intravenous fluid and/or blood products administration, but also due to mobilization of sequestered "third space" fluid seen after complications such as sepsis or hypoalbuminemia.

Intravascular hypervolemia results when the input of sodium and water (or blood) exceeds their loss, and implies a deficit in renal elimination, either intrinsic or due to poor cardiac output. The most remarkable clinical presentation of fluid overload is pulmonary edema with hypoxic respiratory failure. The patient increases the work of breathing, and exhaustion may occur with subsequent hypercapnic respiratory failure. The most common presentation of fluid overload in hospitalized patients manifests with hypoosmolarity and congestive heart failure (CHF) due to excessive retention of free water and/or iatrogenic fluid administration with isotonic or hypotonic solutions. Free water renal excretion requires optimal renal, adrenal, and thyroid function. A patient with fluid overload and CHF must have a complete evaluation for acute or chronic coronary insufficiency, cardiomyopathy, and valvular dysfunction. Excessive water retention can be seen in the postoperative orthopaedic patient due to ADH release secondary to pain, nausea, and morphine administration. However, this state of inappropiate ADH secretion presents as a euvolemic state. Treatment of fluid overload needs to be individualized to each particular case according to the pathophysiological mechanisms implicated in the defect. The main goals of therapy are to stabilize the hemodynamic state, optimize the cardiac index and the oxygen delivery, establish optimal diuresis, normalize electrolyte values, and achieve volume homeostasis.

BLOOD LOSS

The skeleton has a very rich blood supply and patients with bone fractures may present with significant blood loss, shock, and risk of death. Vascular injuries are particularly associated with certain fractures. In adults, a pelvic fracture may lose between 1500 to 3000 ml of blood, a femoral fracture averages 1000 ml of blood loss, and a radius and ulnar fracture between 150 to 250 ml. Patients undergoing surgical procedures have an increased risk of hemorrhage during surgery and immediately post-op.

PERIOPERATIVE CAUSES OF BLOOD LOSS

These include:

1. *Disseminated intravascular coagulation* can be due to fat embolism, hemolysis, tissue damage (burns, frostbite, head injury) and bacterial, viral, or parasitic infections.
2. *Gastrointestinal bleeding*, retroperitoneal or intraabdominal bleeding, hemorrhagic pleural effusion, hematuria, hemoptysis
3. *Anticoagulation therapy* is usually given to prevent or treat thromboembolic diseases.

CLINICAL MANIFESTATIONS OF HEMORRHAGE

The clinical features of hemorrhage depend on the rate and extent of the blood loss and the patient's age and medical comorbidities. Rapid blood loss produces orthostatic hypotension, decreased venous return to the heart, decreased cardiac output, reactive vasoconstriction, and decreased urine output. The patient may present with syncope, nausea, and thirst. Other manifestations may represent end organ claudication secondary to anemia, such as chest pain, dyspnea, or headache. Physical examination reveals tachycardia, hypotension, pallor, and cold skin. When 40 percent of the blood volume is lost, shock is imminent and urgent volume resuscitation must ensue.

Laboratory findings include mild leukocytosis and an increased number of platelets. A normal or mildly low hematocrit does not reflect the acute amount of blood loss. The true magnitude of the anemia is apparent after equilibration occurs with the extravascular fluid.

DIAGNOSTIC APPROACH TO HEMORRHAGE

1. *Baseline studies*: Studies must include hemoglobin, red cell morphology characteristics [mean cell volume (MCV), mean cell hemoglobin (MCH), red cell distribution width (RDW)] prothrombin time (PT), partial thromboplastin time (PTT), and clotting factors when appropiate.
2. *Vascular injury*: If vascular injury is suspected by the absence of pulses and/or poor capillary filling, arterial Doppler or arteriography should be performed.
3. *Hemolysis*: Routine blood film, reticulocyte count and marrow examination should be performed; serum bilirubin, haptoglobin, plasma hemoglobin, lactate dehydrogenase, and methemalbumin need to be evaluated; in urine, bilirubin, urobilinogen, hemosiderin, and hemoglobin must be measured. Hemolysis can be due to sequestration, in the spleen with hypersplenism. Hemolysis may be auto-immune, due to antibodies (idiopathic, lymphomas, SLE, drugs, mycoplasma infection, infectious mononucleosis, and paroxysmal hemoglobinuria).
4. *DIC*: Observe thrombocytopenia; schistocytes (fragmented red cells); elevated PT, PTT, and thrombin time; reduced fibrinogen level; and elevated fibrinogen degradation products.

If ascites or a pleural effusion is present, a paracentesis and thoracentesis may need to be done (in the absence of chest tube or abdominal drainage) to confirm a hemothorax or an intraabdominal bleed.

TREATMENT OF BLOOD LOSS

The first priority is to correct the blood volume in order to avoid organ hypoperfusion, ensuring adequate circulation and oxygen delivery. Then, the values of red cells and platelets must be corrected to desirable levels, avoiding complications such as fluid overload, dilutional coagulopathy, and electrolyte imbalance. Patients with massive blood loss with shock require airway and breathing evaluation to monitor the need for airway intubation and mechanical ventilation. Hypoxemia, an elevated and rising PCO_2, and a decreasing arterial pH establishes the diagnosis of respiratory failure. Patients with ventilatory failure may be more acidotic at the tissue level with high mixed venous PCO_2 level and high arterial-venous CO_2 difference.

Initial therapy includes leg elevation, obtaining venous access with large bore catheters, and infusion of normal saline and blood components. These methods should be continued until blood pressure normalizes. Before adequate volume repletion is achieved, one may start a dopamine infusion, increasing the dose from 1 to 20 µg/kg per minute. If higher doses are needed, norepinephrine from 2 to 30 µg/min should be added. These drugs must be stopped as soon as volume status and hemostasis are stabilized.

SUGGESTED READINGS

Demuynck K, Van Calenbergh F, Goffin J, et al: Upper airway obstruction caused by a cervical osteophyte. *Chest* 1995; 108:283.

Dodd FM, Simon E, McKeown D, et al: The effect of a cervical collar on the tidal volume of anesthestized adult patients. *Anaesthesia* 1995; 50:961.

Ferreira TA, Pensado A, Dominguez L, et al: Compartment syndrome with severe rhabdomyolysis in the postoperative period following major vascular surgery. *Anaesthesia* 1996; 51:692.

Hall JB, Schmidt GA, Wood LDH: *Principles of Critical Care*. New York: McGraw-Hill; 1992:1710–1718, 1913–1919, 1977–1984.

Jeter EK, Spivey MA: Noninfectious complications of blood transfusion. *Hematol Oncol Clin North Am* 1995; 9(1):187.

Norfolk DR, Williamson LM: Leukodepletion of blood products by filtration. *Blood Rev* 1995; 9:7.

Perkins H: Transfusion reactions: The changing priorities. *Immunol Invest* 1995; 24(1–2):289.

Practice guidelines for blood component therapy: A report by the American Society of Anesthesiologists Task Force on blood component therapy. *Anesthesiology* 1996; 84:732.

Schepsis AA, Lynch G: Exertional compartment syndromes of the lower extremity. *Curr Opin Rheumatol* 1996; 8:143.

Schneider JM, Roger DJ, Uhl RL: Bilateral forearm compartment syndromes resulting from neuroleptic malignant syndrome. *J Hand Surg [Am]* 1996; 21:287.

Turnipseed WD, Hurschler C, Vanderby R Jr: The effects of elevated compartment pressure on tibial arteriovenous flow and relationship of mechanical and biochemical characteristics of fascia to genesis of chronic anterior compartment syndrome. *J Vasc Surg* 1995; 21:810 (discussion, 816).

Chapter 155

NONSURGICAL PAIN MANAGEMENT

Paul Gusmorino

A good understanding of pain, pain mechanisms, and pain management is essential for the proper care of orthopaedic patients. No matter how skillful the surgeon or how successful the surgery, without proper management of pain it usually becomes a significant element of most orthopaedic procedures. Postoperative pain can be managed effectively through relatively simple means in most patients, although unfortunately, postoperative pain is frequently undertreated. This chapter focuses on pain mechanisms and pathways, practical approaches to acute pain management, and a brief discussion of chronic pain—how it differs from acute pain, and how the approach to chronic pain should be primarily different from the approach to acute pain.

DEFINITION OF PAIN

Pain, as defined by the International Society for the Study of Pain, is an unpleasant sensory and emotional experience defined in terms of tissue damage or potential tissue damage. It is clear from this definition that pain is a subjective experience and that the only instruments we have for clinical evaluation depend on patients' reports. Clearly, this makes pain evaluation somewhat difficult when we have a patient with whom communication is a problem. While it is true that with acute pain there are often clear signs of autonomic arousal, including elevated pulse rate and blood pressure, these are not unique to the experience of pain, but rather general indicators of distress and often absent in patients with more chronic pain.

PAIN MECHANISMS

Although pain is clearly a whole human experience and any attempt to look at it with a mind-body dualism is fraught with problems, it is important to have an understanding about the physiologic mechanisms involved in pain and its transmission to best understand a rational approach to prevention and management. Pain perception is mediated by all of the neural processes that modulate perception. It is composed of both a somatic signal that something is wrong with the body and a message or interpretation of that signal involving attentional, cognitive, affective, and social factors. Higher brain centers provide means of modulating pain signals, either amplifying them through excessive attention or minimizing them through denial, inattention, relaxation, or attention-control techniques. (This helps to explain how athletes are able to sustain serious injury in the height of sport and not be aware of pain until the injury is brought to their attention.) It is known that the meaning attributed to pain by the individual may influence the intensity of pain. In a classic study, Beecher (1956) noted how soldiers injured in combat seemed to require relatively little in the way of analgesic medication. He compared these soldiers to a set of civilian surgical patients with equivalent surgically-induced wounds. The surgical patients demanded much more analgesic medication than the soldiers injured in combat. Beecher explained this discrepancy based on a difference in the meaning of pain. While to the surgical patients pain signified a potential problem with their surgery and threat to their health, to the soldiers the meaning of pain was that they were alive and likely to return home and no longer face combat.

Complex interactions of many different peripheral and central nervous system structures, from the skin surface to the cerebral cortex, are known to be involved in the processing of pain. At any level, blockade of these pathways may be considered to treat pain. When a potentially damaging stimulus is applied to a sensitive area of the body such as the skin, a chain of signals is initiated that results in the identification of the stimulus as painful.

Nociceptors are specific primary afferent nerves for signaling noxious stimulation. After a noxious stimulus has been detected by a nociceptor, the resultant impulse travels away from the point of origin via the primary afferent nerve. The primary afferent nerves that carry pain impulses are almost exclusively unmyelinated C fibers and finely myelinated A delta (Aδ) fibers. Most C fiber afferents originate from polymodal nociceptors that are activated by mechanical, chemical, and thermal noxious stimuli. The conduction velocity of these C fibers is approximately 1 m/s, which likely explains the "slow pain" felt 1 to 2 s after the application of a noxious stimulus. The finely myelinated Aδ fibers also transmit pain impulses, but the conduction velocity of these neurons is much faster (12 to 30 m/s). Aδ fibers are particularly sensitive to stimulation with sharp instruments. About 20 to 50 percent of the Aδ fibers respond to heat as well as mechanical stimulation. These primary afferent nociceptors make up the majority of fibers in any peripheral nerve. The cell bodies of all somatic primary afferent fibers are in the dorsal root ganglia adjacent to the spinal cord. Fibers from the dorsal root are organized within the root according to diameter. The large-diameter afferents enter the spinal cord in the dorsal region of the entry zone, whereas the small-diameter afferents enter into the lateral region of the cord. In the spinal cord, the primary afferent fibers (Aδ and C) bifurcate into both cephalad and caudad projecting branches as part of the dorsolateral tract. Most of these fibers terminate in the ipsilateral dorsal gray matter, but a small number will cross behind the central canal to terminate in the dorsal gray matter of the contralateral side. These neurons then project to one of several areas: the thalamus by way of the contralateral spinothalamic tracts, the ipsilateral dorsal white matter, or the ipsilateral dorsal gray matter for an area of several segments.

The spinothalamic and spinoreticular systems represent the most important tracts associated with pain transmission. The fibers from these tracts make up the anterolateral funiculus. Several nuclear groups of the thalamus are associated with the relay of nociceptive afferent impulses. In the thalamus, spinothalamic neurons terminate largely on the ventroposterolateral and the centromedian nuclei. The centromedian nucleus is involved in the qualitative aspects of pain perception in that stimulation of this region triggers the unpleasantness associated with tissue damage (Besson and Chaouch, 1987). The somatosensory cortex receives processed input from spinothalamic, spinoreticular, and dorsal column systems. Understanding descending modulation is critical to pain management. Modulation of pain stimuli can occur at virtually every pathway carrying nociceptive information, including the spinothalamic and spinoreticular tracts, which are under modulatory control from supraspinal systems.

ACUTE PAIN MANAGEMENT

Pain management strategy should begin prior to surgery, because an assessment of the patients' previous experience with pain or operative procedures is most helpful in alleviating patients' fears, understanding their preferences, and preparing them for their postoperative experiences, thus giving them the best chance at feeling in control and confident. Patients' perceptions vary greatly: from the one extreme of expecting that severe postoperative pain is inevitable and their determination (to their detriment) to endure this quietly, to the other extreme of patients who interpret any pain postoperatively as an indication of a severe complication of the surgery and a grave threat to well-being. Naturally, most patients fall somewhere in the middle. It is extremely helpful to patients to approach surgery with a realistic understanding of what to expect and what options they have to manage the pain. While behavioral techniques, physical modalities, and nonsteroidal anti-inflammatory drugs (NSAIDs) all have a role to play for the vast majority of orthopaedic cases, the opioids are clearly the drugs of choice for postoperative pain management. Opioids are effective, inexpensive, easily titrated, have a favorable benefit-to-risk ratio, and usually work quickly.

Patients and, too often, medical professionals tend to have exaggerated fears of opioid analgesics, based on misinformation. The most common misperceptions have to do with fear of a very narrow range between a therapeutic and lethal dose range and with the fear of drug addiction. It is well understood that pain is easier to prevent than to relieve once it has become severe. Maintaining a fairly stable blood level of the analgesic is important. There are different routes of administration of drugs to be considered. This chapter is limited to those of parenteral and oral administration, which are the most common, readily available in all settings, and generally quite effective. The goal with good pain control is maintaining a fairly consistent level of analgesic blood level and enabling patients to maintain control over this process.

PATIENT-CONTROLLED ANALGESIA

In the immediate postoperative period, patient-controlled analgesia (PCA) is often the best choice. This is a system where a patient has the ability to self-administer an opioid analgesic (usually morphine) intravenously at a dosage and time interval predetermined by the physician. The system can be set so that a predetermined dose is delivered at a predetermined interval without the patient's initiative or is exclusively triggered by the patient's action. A clear benefit of this is that the patient has a sense of mastery and control and can often fine-tune the medication level to his or her need. Most patients find that this system works well for them, and studies of its use have demonstrated good patient satisfaction, shorter recovery times, and use of less opioids than with traditional intramuscular p.r.n. scheduling.

Difficulties with PCA may be related to intrinsic properties of the opioids such as excessive sedation, nausea, ileus, or pruritus and not the PCA system. Some patients have difficulty with the PCA system because of their poor understanding of it and ineffective use. There are patients who make as many as 100 attempts in 1 h and end up receiving far less medication than what has been allowed had they used the system effectively. Understandably, these patients, in addition to suffering pain, end up frustrated and demoralized. Another problem with PCA is the difficulty that patients have in maintaining comfort during the night if they are able to sleep and are not actively pressing for medication at regular intervals. Apparently, their blood level falls to a point where they need to be up and pressing for some continuous intervals to regain comfort and then repeat this cycle again when they fall back asleep. Incidents of mechanical failure can result in patients not receiving their medication, with subsequent poor pain control as a result of this. Mechanical tampering with the PCA machine by patients with histories of drug abuse has also been reported.

In the immediate postoperative period, if patients are unable to take oral medications and PCA is unavailable, the intravenous route is preferable to intramuscular, and patients' opioid levels can be maintained either by continuous infusion or a regular bolus injection every 2 to 3 h, depending on the drug chosen and patient response. Because continuous infusion involves the greatest risk of overdosage and allows less for patient modulation, it is rarely the treatment of choice. When the decision is made for parenteral periodic bolus injections, it as important to recognize that the active period of analgesia with opioids given this way is approximately 3 h to administer medications at an effective interval and dosage to maintain comfort—without subjecting patients to periods of oversedation—alternating with periods of poor pain relief. With intramuscular injections, absorption can vary significantly. There is quicker onset of action and more consistency if injections can be given intravenously. Opioids can also be given rectally, and hydromorphone comes in a suppository formulation.

ORAL OPIOIDS

As soon as oral opioids can be tolerated, patients should be switched from PCA and other forms of parenteral opioid administration. The effective parenteral dose of morphine can easily be converted to an equianalgesic dose of oral morphine and given on an every 4-h around-the-clock schedule. Hydroxyzine (Vistaril) 25 mg can be added, as it has benefits of counteracting the nausea and pruritus side effects of opioids and can enhance the analgesic effect. Although maintaining a steady level is important, it is equally important to allow for a rescue dose (usually about 30 percent of the every-4-h dose) should patients experience an increase in pain, possibly due to activity or dressing changes. What cannot be emphasized enough is the importance of reassessing the patient's comfort and level of sedation at regular intervals with the intention of adjusting medication dosage and schedule as needed. The patient's respiratory rate should be monitored and the opioid withheld if respirations are fewer than 10/min. Adding a stool softener like docusate sodium (Colace)100 mg three times a day is important to prevent difficulty with constipation. When patients are doing well, their medication can generally be decreased by 20 to 30 percent on a daily basis, still maintaining the every-4-h dose schedule. When asleep during the night, most patients prefer to be awakened and given their scheduled pain medication as it is due, which they find preferable to awakening on their own, 1 or 2 h in pain, and having more difficulty reestablishing comfort. Generally, patients are encouraged to continue on an around-the-clock schedule with reducing doses as they recover and, only when they are on an opioid equivalent of about 10 mg morphine orally, switch to an as-needed schedule. If patients are to be discharged from the hospital while still on opioid pain medications, it is important to give them written instructions of the medication reduction schedule and specify when they are expected to stop using the opioid analgesics. The equianalgesic doses, oral and parenteral, of the more commonly used opioid analgesics are identified in Table 155-1.

When using opioid analgesics for pain control, it is important to be aware of some of the potential problems associated with their use. Opioids slow gut motility, and this can easily be a problem resulting

---

Table 155-1

Dosing Data for Opioid Analgesics

DRUGS			RECOMMENDED STARTING DOSE (ADULTS MORE THAN 50KG BODY WEIGHT)	
Opioid Agonist	Approximate equianalgesic oral dose	Approximate equianalgesic parenteral dose	Oral	Parenteral
Morphine	30 mg q3–4h (around the clock dosing) 60 mg q3–4h (single dose or intermittent dosing)	10 mg q3–4h	30 mg q3–4h	10 mg q3–4h
Codeine	130 mg q3–4h	75 mg q3–4h	60 mg q3–4h	60 mg q2h (intramuscular/subcutaneous)
Hydromorphone (Dilaudid)	7.5 mg q3–4h	1.5 mg q3–4h	6 mg q3–4h	1.5 mg q3–4h
Hydrocodone (in Lorcet, Lortab, Vicodin, others)	30 mg q3–4h	Not available	10 mg q3–4h	Not available
Levorphanol (Levo-Dromoran)	4 mg q6–8h	2 mg q6–8h	4 mg q6–8h	2 mg q6–8h
Meperidine (Demerol)	300 mg q2–3h	100 mg q3h	Not recommended	100 mg q3h
Methadone (Dolophine, others)	20 mg q6–8h	10 mg q6–8h	20 mg q6–8h	10 mg q6–8h
Oxycodone (Roxicodone, also in Percocet, Percodan, Tylox, others)	30 mg q3–4h	Not available	10 mg q3–4h	Not available
Oxymorphone (Numorphan)	Not available	1 mg q3–4h	Not available	1 mg q3–4h

---

in ileus in a postoperative patient whose bowel is inactive from surgery and anesthesia. The effect of slowing bowel motility is a central effect, so parenteral administration is not the solution, and sometimes all opioids need to be held until bowel function is reestablished. In this situation, the use of a parenteral NSAID, ketorolac (Toradol), which does not affect bowel motility, can often be effective. Given 30 mg IM every 6 h, it has demonstrated analgesia roughly equivalent to parenteral morphine 10 mg. As with most NSAIDs, it also affects platelet aggregation and, if bleeding is a concern, this needs to be taken into account with its use. Another potential problem with opioids is their sedating effects, which are not well tolerated by some patients. Sometimes, backing down slightly on the opioid dose will improve this, but some patients experience acceptable pain relief only at a dose that they find too sedating. This can often be resolved by switching to another opioid at a roughly equianalgesic dose, such as switching patients to hydromorphone when morphine is oversedating. Another possible intervention is reducing the opioid dose and adding another nonopioid analgesic, usually a NSAID. Here again, ketorolac (Toradol) 30 mg IM q6h can often be quite effective for a brief period until the patient's pain improves and can be well controlled on a lower opioid dose. Nausea, which is a fairly common side effect of opioids, can usually be managed with standard antiemetics like prochlorperazine (Compazine). The addition of hydroxyzine to the opioid dose is also often effective in controlling nausea, as well as enhancing the analgesic effect.

While the proper use of opioid analgesics is the mainstay of pain control for the majority of orthopaedic patients, there is a clear role for other medications and interventions for many patients. NSAIDs are effective analgesics for mild to moderate pain and can often be given in conjunction with opioid analgesics. The combination of NSAIDs and opioids can be "opioid sparing," allowing for a lower opioid dose. NSAIDs have a ceiling effect, which means that increasing the dosage after a certain point will not increase the analgesic effect, but only the side-effect profile. With the exception of choline magnesium trisalicylate (Trilisate), NSAIDs have significant antiplatelet activity and are relatively contraindicated in patients with renal and hepatic disease and risk of, or actual, coagulopathy. See Table 155-2 for dosing data for NSAIDs.

With many orthopaedic procedures, severe muscle spasm in the postoperative period is often a problem; however, it can usually be helped with diazepam (Valium) 5 to 10 mg PO q6h.

In addition to pharmacologic treatments, there are a number of nonpharmacologic interventions from simple relaxation training to the use of transcutaneous nerve stimulation (TENS). There is good evidence to support that a simple discussion with patients of what to expect after surgery and what options are available for managing pain has a positive effect on patients' postoperative pain. Patients can easily be instructed in using relaxation exercises as simple as clenching their fists, breathing in deeply, holding it a minute, then breathing out slowly, and relaxing their hand. Slow rhythmic breathing exercises,

---
Table 155-2

Dosing Data for Acetaminophen and NSAIDs

Drug	Usual adult dose	Comments
Acetaminophen	650–975 mg q4h	Acetaminophen lacks the peripheral anti-inflammatory activity of other NSAIDs
Aspirin	650–975 mg q4h	The standard against which other NSAIDs are compared. Inhibits platelet aggregation; may cause postoperative bleeding
Choline magnesium trisalicylate (Trilisate)	1000–1500 mg bid	May have minimal antiplatelet activity; also available as oral liquid
Diflunisal (Dolobid)	1000 mg initial dose followed by 500 mg q12h	
Etodolac (Lodine)	200–400 mg q6–8h	
Fenoprofen calcium (Nalfon)	200 mg q4–6h	
Ibuprofen (Motrin, others)	400 mg q4–6h	Available as several brand names and as generic; also available as oral suspension
Ketoprofen (Orudis)	25–75 mg q6–8h	
Magnesium salicylate	650 mg q4h	Many brands and generic forms available
Meclofenamate sodium (Meclomen)	50 mg q4–6h	
Mefenamic acid (Ponstel)	250 mg q6h	
Naproxen (Naprosyn)	500 mg initial dose followed by 250 mg q6–8h	Also available as oral liquid
Naproxen sodium (Anaprox)	550 mg initial dose followed by 275 mg q6–8h	
Salsalate (Disalcid, others)	500 mg q4h	May have minimal antiplatelet activity
Sodium salicylate	325–650 mg q3–4h	Available in generic form from several distributors
Parenteral NSAID		
Ketorolac (Toradol)	30 or 60 mg initial dose followed by 15 or 30 mg q6h Oral dose following IM dosage 10 mg q6–8h	Intramuscular dose not to exceed 5 days

as well as simple imagery, are also easy to instruct patients in and often effective. Patients can be told to bring a tape or compact disc player with them, because listening to music can be effective in reducing mild to moderate pain.

PAIN MANAGEMENT IN TEN BASIC STEPS

1. Explain to patients that, while some pain is to be expected and is not an indication of anything wrong, severe pain can usually be well controlled by taking medications on a regular basis.
2. Find out what has worked well for patients in the past, and if it is reasonable, use it.
3. When patients are unable to take oral medications, usually in the immediate postoperative interval, intravenous opioids are better than intramuscular, and PCA is a good means of administration.
4. When patients can take oral medication, it is usually the best strategy, easy to administer, and inexpensive. Morphine and hydromorphone (Dilaudid) are standards and usually work well given every 4 h around the clock. Allow for a rescue dose, about 30 percent of the regular dose, and if the patient is using the rescue dose consistently, it often means that the standing dose needs to be increased.
5. Be prepared for the common opioid side effects—nausea, constipation, and sedation—and treat them actively.
6. Frequent assessment of pain and pain relief, with adjustment of dosage to the individual's needs, is critical (15 to 30 min after parenteral drug therapy and 1 h after oral administration).
7. Know the equianalgesic doses of the drugs used.
8. When patients are doing well and recovering, begin to reduce the dosage rather than lengthen time intervals.
9. Use other modalities (behavioral strategies, physical modalities, or NSAIDs) to supplement pain relief, and reduce opioid dosage when possible.
10. If patients are ready for discharge from the hospital and still using pain medications, give clear instructions for continued use at home with a written schedule for decreasing dose and discontinuing medication.

CHRONIC PAIN

Unfortunately, a number of patients continue to report significant difficulty with pain that goes well beyond the postoperative healing phase and appears to be out of proportion to any objective findings of ongoing tissue damage that can explain this pain. For many of these patients, their struggle to relieve this pain has taken over their lives and leads to a series of treatment failures as they continue to pursue treatments appropriate for acute pain. Often these patients seek surgical solutions for their difficulty, which has become much more complicated than could ever be corrected by a simple approach at relieving a source of nociception, and their chances for success with successive operations rapidly declines. The major pitfall for or-

thopaedic surgeons in wanting to help these unfortunate and often very suffering individuals is focusing on the acute nociceptive model and failing to realize the extent to which the patients' pain and suffering is being maintained by multiple other elements in the patients' life situation. These patients need to be evaluated and treated by specially trained multidisciplinary pain centers where the emphasis is on rehabilitation with a balance between physical and behavioral rehabilitation. Many of these patients suffer with degrees of depression that vary from moderate to severe. This must be addressed with both psychotherapy and appropriate use of antidepressant medications. Often the family system is severely disrupted by a patient's continued difficulty with pain and, at the same time, this family stress exacerbates difficulty with pain and suffering. Clearly, these circumstances need experienced family therapy intervention.

The vast majority of the chronic pain population has become significantly physically deconditioned and needs an active physical therapy program to address this decline. Patients also need to be educated that using pain as a guide to activity is not likely to be a successful strategy and to learn to organize preplanned structured activities independent of pain.

In brief, the key is in recognizing that acute and chronic pain approaches need to be different. Acute pain strategies that focus on looking for sources of nociception, prescribing rest, using pain as a guide to activity, and increasing dosage of analgesic medications to relieve pain are generally not effective strategies for chronic pain patients.

SUGGESTED READINGS

Acute Pain Management Guideline Panel: Acute pain management: operative or medical procedures and trauma. *Clinical Practice Guideline.* AHCPR Pub 192-0032. Rockville, MD, Agency for Health Care Policy and Research, Public Health Service, 1992 (Feb); US Department of Health and Human Services.

American Pain Society: *Principles of Analgesic Use in the Treatment of Acute Pain and Chronic Cancer Pain: A Concise Guide to Medical Practice.* Skokie, IL: American Pain Society; 1992.

Beecher HK: Relationship of significance of wound to pain experienced. *JAMA* 1956; 161:1609.

Besson JM, Chaouch A: Peripheral and spinal mechanisms of nociception. *Physiol Rev* 1987; 67:67.

Blumer D, Heilbronn M: Chronic pains as a variant of depressive disease: The pain-prone disorder. *J Nerv Ment Dis* 1982; 170:381.

Bonica JJ: Evolution and current status of pain programs. *J Pain Symptom Manage* 1990; 5:368.

Dworkin SF, Von Korff M, LeResche L: Multiple pains and psychiatric disturbance: An epidemiological investigation. *Arch Gen Psychiatry* 1990; 47:239.

Katon W, Egan K, Miller D: Chronic pain: Lifetime psychiatric diagnosis and family history. *Am J Psychiatry* 1985; 142(10, Pt 2):1156.

Pilowski I, Chapman CR, Bonica JJ: Pain, depression and illness behavior in a pain clinic population. *Pain* 1977; 4:183.

Willis WD: Thalamocortical mechanisms of pain. In Fields H, Dubner R, Cervero F (eds): *Advances in Pain Research and Therapy,* vol 9. New York, Raven; 1985.

Chapter 156

NEUROSURGICAL MANAGEMENT OF CHRONIC PAIN

Werner K. Doyle

Criteria for surgical management of intractable pain is met when all attempts at conservative management have failed to provide adequate relief, and a thorough investigation eliminating possible correctable etiologies of the pain has been performed. For example, low back pain from instability would require that spinal fusion be considered first rather than surgery directed toward the symptom of chronic pain. Chronic pain is different than acute pain, in that the former is persistent and without anticipated resolution. Psychological contraindications should also be ruled out prior to surgery directed at pain control. Psychological, social, and other environmental factors may play an important role in the setting of chronic pain of benign etiology. A successful outcome may be compromised if they are overlooked.

Location and mechanism of pathophysiologic pain determine the particular surgical procedure chosen to manage chronic intractable pain. The two pathophysiologic categories of pain are nociceptive pain and deafferentation pain. Nociceptive pain, sometimes referred to as somatic pain, is associated with ongoing tissue injury. Examples of this include cancer invading bone or malignancy involving viscera. In this pain category, the sensory nerve receptors are initiating the pain sensation, which is transmitted via the usual neural routes to the central nervous system to be perceived appropriately as pain. Deafferentation, or neurogenic, pain is the result of injury to the peripheral or central nervous system. In this case, the pain signal originates within pain pathways. Actual ongoing tissue damage is absent. This abnormal sensation is due to dysfunction of the nervous system. Examples of this include phantom limb pain and arachnoiditis.

Nociceptive pain is usually well localized, sharp, stabbing, or aching. In addition to tissue injury, inflammation or nerve compression can produce this. Nociceptive pain will typically respond to interruption of the nociceptive pathway, but this may compromise normal function or may even result in a deafferentation pain syndrome. The management of choice for nociceptive pain is treating the underlying pathology whenever possible. Deafferentation pain, in contrast, is poorly localized, described as crushing, or tearing, and often accompanied by paresthesias. Classically, its quality is burning with dysesthetic numbness. It can often be lancinating. Deafferentation pain will initially respond to interrupting the pain pathway proximal to the pathology, but has a high likelihood of recurring with even worse manifestations with this form of surgical treatment. Sympathetically mediated pain such as causalgia and reflex sympathetic dystrophy (RSD) is considered by some as a separate pain category, but we will consider it as a subtype of neurogenic (deafferentation) pain. The medical history and physical examination are essential to distinguishing the pain syndrome. It is also possible to have more than one kind of coexistent pain.

There is little consensus about which procedure is the most beneficial for treatment of a particular pain type (Table 156-1). In fact, similar results have been reported using various modalities to treat the same pain situations. In many cases, the setting in which the pain occurs can be more important than the type of pain when selecting the most appropriate management modality for a given patient. For example, pain used by a patient to avoid work, or pain used as the patient's foundation for litigation, is a possible contraindication for surgical management. A description of surgical procedures will be reviewed. Though a clear consensus may not always exist with respect to treating a particular pain syndrome, chronic pain examples that have been successfully treated by each modality are listed.

Table 156-1

Surgical Procedures

Though a clear consensus may not always exist with respect to treating a particular pain syndrome, the following is a guideline supported by the referenced literature.

Electrical stimulation
  Spinal column stimulation
    Indication: benign deafferentation pain, reflex sympathetic dystrophy, failed back, nerve-root injury, causalgia, intercostal neuralgia, postherpetic neuralgia, arachnoiditis, and ischemic and vasculopathic pain
    Contraindication: nociceptive pain
  Deep brain stimulation
    Indication: similar to spinal cord stimulation (arachnoiditis and peripheral neuropathies) and nociceptive pain[a]

Intraspinal drug administration
  Intrathecal morphine
    Indication: malignant nociceptive pain (cancer pain)
    Contraindication: neurogenic pain (recent data suggest that chronic nonmalignant pain may no longer be a contraindication)

Intracranial ablative procedures
  Cingulotomy, mesencephalic tractotomy, and thalamotomy
    Indication: face, ear, oropharynx, and neck shoulder pain

Spinal ablative procedures
  Cordotomy
    Indication: unilateral malignant cancer nociceptive pain in patients with short life expectancy
    Contraindication: ipsilateral respiratory compromise

[a]No current FDA approval.

(continued)

Table 156-1 (Continued)

Surgical Procedures

Commissural myelotomy
  Indication: multisegmental somatic or deafferentation
    pain, lower abdominal, pelvic, perineum, and lower
    extremity cancer pain
  Contraindication: intact motor function below lesion,
    since the lesion will produce deficits

Dorsal root entry zone (DREZ) lesion
  Indication: deafferentation syndromes such as
    postherpetic neuralgia, traumatic brachial or
    lumbosacral root avulsion, phantom limb pain, and
    spinal cord injury pain
  Contraindication: diffuse nondermatomal, constant,
    burning, nonparoxysmal variety of spinal cord injury
    pain

ELECTRICAL STIMULATION

Spinal cord stimulation (SCS) or dorsal column stimulation is accomplished by placing an electrode array, either percutaneously or via an open laminotomy, into the dorsal epidural space of the spinal cord (Fig. 156-1). The electrodes deliver an electrical signal of differing pulse widths, frequency, and amplitudes to the spinal cord over an area several segments rostral to the segmental level of the pain. The electrodes are usually implanted as a trial, leaving the wire leads externalized and giving patients the opportunity to test various settings and electrode combinations before permanent implantation of the programmable pulse generator. The electrodes are placed in patients while they are awake, and the electrodes repositioned to superimpose the stimulator-induced paresthesias over the area of pain. In the case of deafferentation pain involving a large area, two multicontact electrodes have been advocated. Pain control persists beyond the stimulation time and is not reversed by naloxone. The mechanism of action is unknown.

There is no agreement as to specific indications for SCS, but chronic pain from failed back surgery is probably the most common reason SCS is performed. Axial low back pain may be mechanical and nociceptive and therefore may not respond to SCS as well as pain associated with nerve injury or deafferentation. More recent data suggest a better outcome with SCS in patients with unilateral lower extremity pain following low back surgery since this probably represents nerve-root injury.

Other indications for SCS include RSD, causalgia, intercostal neuralgia, and multiple sclerosis. SCS has also been shown to benefit patients with postherpetic neuralgia and ischemic and vasculopathic pain. It is not effective for treatment of nociceptive pain. The general success rate is 50 percent improvement in 50 percent of patients selected by a multidisciplinary team. Poor results have been reported in pain from spinal cord injury, lesions proximal to the ganglion (e.g., root avulsion), failed back syndrome with back pain as the primary complaint rather than leg pain, and in patients with coexisting significant psychological factors. SCS is nondestructive and reversible, making it more attractive than ablative procedures. Surgical options for SCS include percutaneous versus open electrode implantation, single-stage versus two-stage surgery involving a stimulation trial, mul-

tiple versus single electrode arrays, and internal versus external generator designs.

Deep brain stimulation (DBS) is similar to SCS except that the stimulation involves ascending or descending brain tracks that play a role in modulating pain. The pain systems involved include the descending endorphin pathways and the ascending lemniscal system. In a multicenter study, DBS was shown to be effective in 40 percent of patients with deafferentation pain (arachnoiditis and peripheral neuropathies) and in 60 percent of patients with nociceptive cancer and "failed back" pain. Periventricular and periaqueductal gray-area stimulation was useful for nociceptive pain, whereas thalamic (ventralis posteromedial–ventralis posterolateral somatosensory thalamic nucleus) and capsular (posterior limb of internal capsule) stimulation were more efficacious in deafferentation pain. The electrodes are inserted into the brain by using stereotactic neurosurgical methods, and intraoperative stimulation is used for finer physiologic localization. Though DBS electrical stimulators are FDA approved for other neurological problems such as tumor, they are not FDA approved for pain—limiting their availability to centers conducting experimental trials.

INTRASPINAL DRUG ADMINISTRATION: INTRATHECAL MORPHINE

The main advantage of direct intrathecal administration of morphine is pain control without systemic side effects such as sedation, confusion, decreased gastrointestinal motility, and nausea. The doses of intrathecal morphine are very small. This method probably works by morphine binding to receptor sites in the superficial parts of the posterior horns of the spinal gray matter, in the nucleus caudalis, and in brainstem sites. Up to 80 percent of patients may receive significant short-term relief. Because it was believed that long-term efficacy was significantly reduced, direct intrathecal morphine was generally not indicated for chronic benign pain. Recent reports of long-term success have broadened its indication to the failed back syndrome and

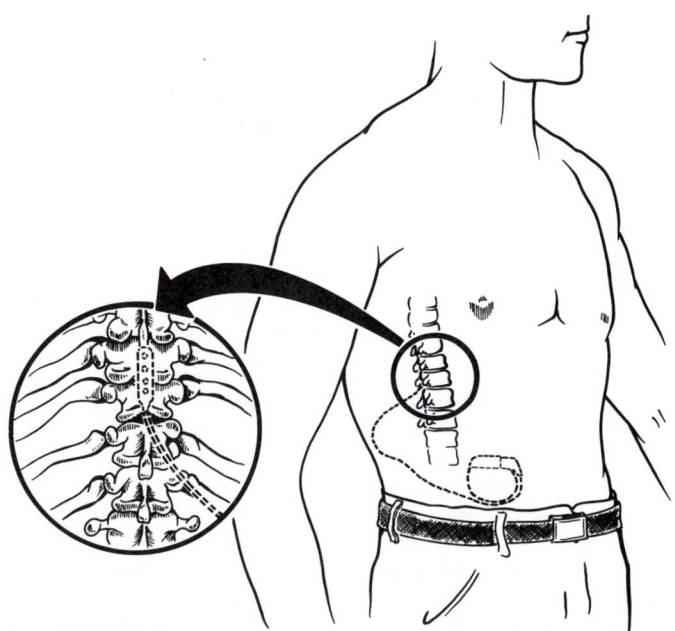

Figure 156-1
Placement of epidural electrode and subcutaneous generator of a spinal cord stimulator system. *(Courtesy of Medtronic, Inc., Minneapolis, Minnesota.)*

Figure 156-2
Typical placement of a continuous infusion intrathecal morphine pump. *(Courtesy of Medtronic, Inc., Minneapolis, Minnesota.)*

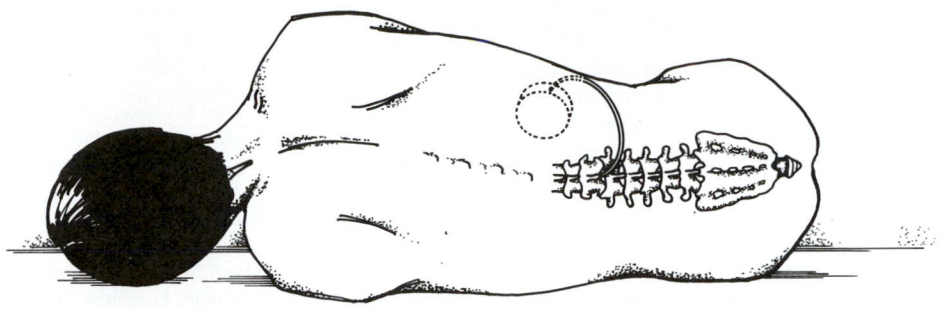

other nonmalignant pain. Urinary retention, pruritus, confusion, dysphoria, hallucinations, nausea, and emesis may occur. Respiratory depression is not usual. Similar to SCS, a test trial is recommended, though there may not be direct correlation between trial and long-term efficacy. Intrathecal morphine via lumbar puncture is administered prior to permanent implantation of a bolus reservoir system or of a continuous infusion pump (Fig. 156-2). Continuous infusion has been shown to be superior to bolus administration. The addition of bupivacaine has increased the efficacy of this treatment in patients whose initial success went on to fail.

INTRACRANIAL ABLATIVE PROCEDURES: CINGULOTOMY, MESENCEPHALIC TRACTOTOMY, AND THALAMOTOMY

Cingulotomy is a frontolimbic disconnection procedure that significantly reduces the intense anxiety associated with chronic pain. Stereotactically guided lesions placed bilaterally in the cingulate gyrus does not eliminate the pain or alter pain threshold, but it will reduce the unpleasant affect of pain. Good results are achieved in up to 80 percent of properly selected patients over the course of their malignant disease without deterioration in their intellectual abilities or changes in their personality.

Two other important intracranial ablative procedures are mesencephalic tractotomy and thalamotomy. Stereotactic mesencephalic tractotomy is effective in eliminating face, ear, oropharynx, neck, and shoulder pain. Lesions of the centromedian nucleus of the thalamus have limited success for nociceptive, cancer, or deafferentation pain, with aphasia and hemiparesis as important complications.

SPINAL ABLATIVE PROCEDURES

Intrathecal alcohol has been advocated for treatment of pain isolated to one or two unilateral spinal segments. This modality may last up to 6 months, at which time it must be repeated.

CORDOTOMY

For pain relief in the contralateral lower extremity or torso, due to cancer, lateral spinothalamic tract transection has been performed. Radio-frequency ablation via a percutaneous route in the high cervical region offers effective control of unilateral multisegmental malignant pain at segmental levels C5 and below. Direct transection of the lateral spinothalamic tract with a knife at a high thoracic area provides pain relief to segments T8 and lower. Deafferentation pain and bilateral pain are contraindications to performing this procedure. Cordotomy in the setting of deafferentation pain risks exacerbation of the pain with the production of dysesthesias in areas of neurologic deficit. Respiratory compromise from damage to the involuntary respiratory pathways located in the anterolateral quadrant of the spinal cord limits cervical cordotomy on the side contralateral to any pulmonary dysfunction. Fatal sleep apnea would result if cordotomy injured the respiratory pathway in a patient without an intact contralateral pathway or without intact contralateral pulmonary function. Similarly, bladder dysfunction may result with bilateral cordotomy below the cervical region. Cervical cordotomy is 60 to 80 percent successful at 1 year, but this falls to 40 percent by 2 years. When reserved for patients with a limited life expectancy, this procedure can be very satisfactory for unilateral refractory nociceptive cancer pain. If the patient has bilateral pain and the procedure is performed on the side of the most severe pain, the contralateral pain will often become magnified, leading to failure. For cervical cordotomy, the preoperative evaluation includes pulmonary function tests. Complications include ataxia, ipsilateral paresis, bladder dysfunction, dysesthesia, sleep apnea, and death, usually due to respiratory failure.

COMMISSURAL MYELOTOMY

For limited multisegmental somatic or deafferentation pain, single-stage commissural myelotomy may be appropriate. The procedure entails a midsagittal longitudinal incision in all spinal cord segments involved in the symptomatic pain transmission. To assure success, the laminectomy must extend at least three levels above the highest dermatome involved with pain. It is used commonly for lower abdominal, pelvic, perineum, and lower extremity cancer pain. Bladder dysfunction, motor loss, and dysesthesias complicate this procedure, which has a 60 percent likelihood of complete pain relief. Overall, 90 percent of patients who undergo this procedure have at least some worthwhile pain improvement. Complications include lower extremity weakness due to lower motor neuron injury, and almost all patients develop dysesthesia.

DORSAL ROOT ENTRY-ZONE LESION

Ablative procedures are generally contraindicated in the setting of deafferentation pain. However, DREZ lesion is effective for a variety of deafferentation syndromes such as postherpetic neuralgia, traumatic brachial or lumbosacral root avulsion, phantom limb pain, and spinal cord injury pain. Either radio frequency or laser lesions are used to destroy Rexed layers I to V of the posterior horn of the spinal cord. It is important to distinguish between avulsion injuries and peripheral stretch injuries since DREZ is not effective in the latter. Electrophysiologic and imaging studies will help define the injury type. SCS or DBS may be useful for stretch injuries. DREZ is effective in over 80 percent of cases when used appropriately. It is the most effective treatment for deafferentation pain as a consequence of nerve-root avulsion. Also, DREZ is more effective than SCS for phantom limb pain.

There are two types of spinal cord pain. One type is end-zone pain, which is distributed to the dermatomes just caudal to the injury level and often triggered by local stimuli in the affected dermatomes. The second type is of a diffuse nondermatomal, constant, burning, non-paroxysmal variety. The former will be successfully treated with DREZ, whereas the latter may require cordectomy or stimulation procedures.

Phantom limb pain is pain perceived to be associated within an amputated extremity. This is distinguished from stump pain, which is located at the actual stump of the amputated limb. About 30 percent of true phantom limb pain patients will be effectively treated with DREZ lesions, whereas stump pain patients will not. Postherpetic neuralgia is effectively treated for prolonged periods in 25 percent of patients receiving DREZ lesions. Stimulation procedures may be more effective in the long term.

Sympathetic mediated pain, thought to be important in causalgia and RSD, may result from local sympathetic hyperactivity that releases humeral and intrinsic impulses to cause the painful response. It is believed to involve norepinephrine release with hypersensitivity of nerve terminals secondary to denervation and spasticity. It is distinguished by the triad of burning pain, autonomic dysfunction, and trophic skin changes. Typical findings associated with causalgia include burning pain with onset usually 24 h after the causal injury. RSD, in contrast, may take days or weeks to develop after an injury. The median, ulnar, and sciatic are the nerves most commonly involved with causalgia. The pain is often described as burning, but may be throbbing, aching, or stabbing as well. With time, this pain may spread proximally beyond its original distribution of the injured nerve. Also, non-noxious stimuli may trigger pain. Medical sympathectomy such as regional quanethidine blocks or alpha-adrenergic blocking agents like phenoxybenzane can be effective. In refractory cases, SCS has been successful.

SUGGESTED READINGS

Angel IF, Gould HJ III, Casey ME, et al: Intrathecal morphine pump as a treatment option in chronic pain of nonmalignant origin. *Surg Neurol* 1998; 49:92.

Bronec PR, Nashold BS: Dorsal root entry zone lesions for pain. In Youmans J ed. *Neurological Surgery,* 3d ed. Philadelphia: WB Saunders; 1988:4036.

Frank F, Fabrizi AP, Gaist G, et al: Stereotactic mesencephalotomy versus multiple thalamotomies in the treatment of chronic cancer pain syndromes. *Appl Neurophysiol* 1987; 50:314.

Friedman AH, Bullitt E: Dorsal root entry zone lesions in the treatment of pain following brachial plexus avulsion, spinal cord injury and herpes zoster. *Appl Neurophysiol* 1988; 51:164.

Kumar K, North R, Wyant GM: Treatment of chronic pain by epidural spinal cord stimulation. *J Neurosurg* 1991; 75:402.

Levy RM, Lamb S, Adams JE: Treatment of chronic pain by deep brain stimulation: Long-term follow-up and review of the literature. *Neurosurgery* 1987; 21:885.

Long DM: The current status of electrical stimulation of the nervous system for the relief of chronic pain. *Surg Neurol* 1998; 49:142.

Nashold BS Jr: Current status of the DREZ operation. *Neurosurgery* 1984; 15:942.

North RB, Ewend MG, Lawton MT, et al: Failed back surgery syndrome: 5-year follow-up after spinal cord stimulator implantation. *Neurosurgery* 1991; 28:692.

North RB, Kidd DH, Zahurak H, et al: Spinal cord stimulation for chronic, intractable pain: Experience over two decades. *Neurosurgery* 1993; 32:384.

Penn RD, Paice JA: Chronic intrathecal morphine for intractable pain. *J Neurosurg* 1987; 67:182.

Poletti CE: Open cordotomy medullary tractotomy. In: Schmidek HH, Sweet WH, (eds): *Operative Neurosurgical Techniques: Indications, Methods, Results,* 2d ed. New York: Grune and Stratton; 1989:1155.

Saris SC, Iacono RP, Nashold BS Jr: Dorsal root entry zone lesions for post-amputation pain. *J Neurosurg* 1985; 62:72.

Schwartz HG: High cervical cordotomy. *J Neurosurg* 1967; 26:452.

Shetter AG, Hadley MN, Wilkinson E: Administration of intraspinal morphine sulfate for the treatment of intractable cancer pain. *Neurosurgery* 1986; 18:740.

Tasker RR, DeCarvalho GTC: Intractable central pain of cord origin. *J Neurosurg* 1989; 70:316A (abstr).

Tasker RR: Percutaneous cordotomy: The lateral high cervical technique. In: Schmidek HH, Sweet WH, (eds): *Operative Neurosurgical Techniques: Indications, Methods, Results,* 2d ed. New York: Grune and Stratton; 1989:1196.

Young RF: Clinical experience with radio frequency and laser DREZ lesions. *J Neurosurg* 1990; 72:715.

Young RF, Kroening R, Fulton W, et al: Electrical stimulation of the brain in treatment of chronic pain: Experience over 5 years. *J Neurosurg* 1985; 62:389.

Chapter 157

REFLEX SYMPATHETIC DYSTROPHY

Brian Hainline

Reflex sympathetic dystrophy (RSD), or complex regional pain syndrome, is a syndrome of extremity pain and autonomic instability following soft tissue, peripheral nerve, or central nervous system injury. The pain of RSD is out of proportion to the injury. If untreated, RSD patients may develop a progressive pain syndrome accompanied by irreversible skin, soft tissue, and bone pathology. The cause of RSD is unknown, but involves perturbations in the peripheral and central mechanisms of pain control. Prompt recognition and treatment of this disorder are critical to a successful clinical outcome.

CLINICAL FEATURES

Pain is the outstanding feature of RSD. Typically, pain begins distally in the injured extremity. Patients with RSD usually complain of severe burning pain out of proportion to the injury, leading unsuspecting clinicians to search for other causes of pain, or to label a patient's pain as purely psychogenic in origin. Patients with RSD usually have extremity pain with some combination of the following: skin color and temperature changes; hyper- or hypohidrosis; trophic skin changes; edema; tremor or other movement disorder; and bone loss. When documented peripheral nerve injury occurs, RSD is referred to as causalgia.

A wide variety of precipitating factors and diseases are associated with RSD (Table 157-1). Trauma is the most common cause, but even seemingly trivial trauma, including arthroscopy, can be associated with severe RSD. This observation casts doubt on a purely peripheral pathophysiologic explanation for RSD.

RSD is divided clinically into three stages (Table 157-2). These stages are arbitrary and may overlap. Patients may remain in any stage for weeks or indefinitely.

Stage I RSD (acute stage) is characterized by pain that is out of proportion to the injury or insult. The pain may begin immediately or within days or weeks. Typically, the pain is intense, burning, and spontaneous, with associated hypersensitivity to touch. The affected limb may have associated edema, hyperthermia or hypothermia, increased hair and nail growth, and early bone demineralization.

In stage II RSD (dystrophic stage), the skin of the affected extremity often becomes indurated, cool, and hyperhidrotic. There is associated hair loss, and the nails become cracked and brittle. Pain remains severe and spontaneous and is worsened with limb movement. Roentgenograms may reveal osteoporosis of the affected distal extremity.

Stage III RSD (atrophic stage) is characterized by chronic pain and severe soft tissue damage. The skin is thin and shiny, the fascia is thickened, and flexion contractures may develop. Roentgenograms reveal marked demineralization. Pain often spreads proximally and even into other extremities.

Table 157-1

Causes of Reflex Sympathetic Dystrophy

Peripheral
  Soft tissue injury
  Surgical procedures
  Infection
  Connective tissue disease
  Vascular injury
  Peripheral nerve injury
  Burns
  Myocardial infarction
  Immobilization with cast or splint
  Myelography

Central
  Brain tumor
  Cerebrovascular accident
  Spinal cord injury

Idiopathic

Table 157-2

Stages of Reflex Sympathetic Dystrophy

Stage I
  Severe burning pain
  Extremity edema and hyper- or hypothermia
  Increased extremity hair and nail growth
  Early bone demineralization

Stage II
  Constant, severe pain
  Indurated, cold and hyperhidrotic skin
  Hair loss
  Cracked, ridged nails
  More diffuse osteoporosis

Stage III
  Proximal spread of severe extremity pain
  Thin, shiny skin
  Wasted digits
  Thickened fascia with flexion contractures
  Marked bony demineralization

The hallmark of all stages of RSD is unremitting pain with early autonomic instability progressing to profound metabolic changes if the syndrome progresses. Pain rarely follows a dermatomal or peripheral nerve distribution. Rather, pain typically begins in the distal extremity and may then progress proximally over time.

DIAGNOSIS

The key to diagnosing RSD successfully is a high clinical suspicion of this disorder. Patients commonly are misdiagnosed and have visited several physicians before being properly diagnosed. This causes considerable stress and emotional drain because the patient is suffering from a severe pain syndrome with no apparent help in sight. This may then lead to a worsening of the patient's condition, since fear and anxiety may cause increased sympathetic firing, thereby further perturbing the pain response and metabolic changes. Prompt diagnosis and patient reassurance are the first steps to successful treatment.

RSD is diagnosed clinically. Pain out of proportion to extremity injury or surgery is the hallmark of this disorder. The triad of severe pain, vasomotor instability, and extremity swelling strongly suggest RSD, but pain alone may be the only symptom. A careful clinical exam, possibly coupled with appropriate diagnostic tests, should exclude vascular disorders, peripheral nerve entrapment, other soft tissue lesions, and spinal cord pathology.

Roentgenographic studies may confirm the diagnosis, but are never pathognomonic. Patchy demineralization of the epiphyses may progress to subperiosteal bone resorption and to striating and tunneling in the cortices. Three-phase regional bone scan using ^{99m}Tc-methylene diphosphonate scintigraphy may help to confirm RSD. Most patients with stage I have normal bone scan findings, but the majority of stage II and stage III patients have abnormal findings, generally characterized by increased periarticular activity in both the blood pool and delayed images.

The best diagnostic test may also be therapeutic. Selective sympathetic blockade should lead to immediate pain relief in patients with stage I and early stage II RSD. Patients with stage III RSD have developed considerable soft tissue changes, and the pain is no longer sympathetically driven; therefore, sympathetic blockade is ineffective. If selective sympathetic blockade does not cause at least transient pain relief in early RSD, then another cause of pain must be considered.

PATHOPHYSIOLOGY

There is no single, satisfactory pathophysiologic explanation for RSD. It is noteworthy that the afferent C-fibers that are responsible for signaling deep, burning pain intertwine with sympathetic efferent fibers. Therefore, many believe that RSD results from artificial synapses (also known as *ephapses*, or sites of atypical synaptic contact where the potential for neural transmission has been suggested) between sensory afferent nerves and sympathetic efferent nerves following soft tissue trauma. This causes ephaptic transmission between sympathetic efferents and sensory afferents, which increases nociceptive input into the spinal cord. Alternatively, excessive peripheral firing may result from local demyelination or nerve sprout outgrowth following local injury. The injured nerve then incorporates excessive sodium, calcium, and alpha-adrenergic receptors with ectopic pacemaker activity and chemosensitivity. Increased spinal nociceptive input may cause changes in the dorsal horn neurons of the spinal cord.

Although peripheral pathophysiologic explanations make some sense, they do not account for the discrepancy between the severity and type of injury and the degree of pain coupled with progression of disease. It is conceivable that central control mechanisms play an important role in the genesis of RSD. Descending inhibition of pain is mediated by several areas of the limbic system, including the hypothalamus, brainstem, medial thalamic structures, and associated interconnections. Rather than RSD being considered a syndrome uniquely caused by peripheral nerve injury with subsequent central maladaptation, further work is needed to substantiate central mechanisms that may allow a vulnerability to the development of RSD.

Although no particular psychological profile has been identified as RSD substrate, many RSD patients harbor an intense emotional component of fear. Fear is a universal experience, but RSD patients typically have marked inner fear that may be the result of repetitive physical and psychic trauma, or that may be associated with a single traumatic event. When intense inner fear is not addressed, the sympathetic nervous system expression may be extreme. Furthermore, pain must be viewed as an emotional response as well as a physical nociceptive experience. As such, understanding the limbic contribution to pain becomes critical in meaningfully addressing the expression of pain in an individual.

The difficulty in trying to explain a painful disorder by central or limbic connections is that one risks labeling a pain disorder as psychogenic. The neurophysiologic reality is that there is no possible mind-body separation when explaining pain. Peripheral nociception influences central perception, and central perception influences the expression of peripheral nociception. Further research is needed to address both central and peripheral pain and nociceptive pathways in RSD patients.

TREATMENT

Early diagnosis and treatment are pivotal to a successful outcome in RSD (Table 157-3). Patients who progress to stage III suffer with profound soft tissue changes and perturbations in central modulation of sensory input. Pain control coupled with mobilization of the affected extremity is key; immobilization may exacerbate the problem.

Physical therapy, with attempts at improving mobility of the affected extremity, is necessary with all RSD patients. Physical therapy coupled with reassurance is critical in early RSD. However, both passive and active range of motion can be so painful that physical therapy can be counterproductive. When treating RSD patients, it is more important to focus on relaxation techniques, including massage therapy, myofascial release, craniosacral work, and visualization. Patients must take an active role in this process. Range-of-motion and strengthening exercises become incorporated as tolerated.

In more refractory cases, sympathetic blockade should be used. Selective sympathetic blockade enables patients to participate in physical therapy without pain, but with full sensory and motor control. In upper extremity RSD, the stellate ganglion is infused with procaine hydrochloride. In the lower extremity, epidural blocks are used. One method is to infuse 5 ml of 0.2 percent procaine hydrochloride; the other is to insert a catheter for continuous sympathetic blockade over 3 to 5 days. The advantage of the former technique is that physical therapy is unencumbered. Continuous blockade is more useful for patients with bilateral lower extremity symptoms, or for patients with more refractory pain.

Sympathetic blockade is typically performed consecutively over a period of 3 to 5 days. Alternatively, bier blocks may be employed. Bier block is a form of regional anesthesia using lidocaine, guanethidine, reserpine, or bretylium. Patients typically obtain pain relief for days to weeks, and sometimes even months. As with sympathetic blocks, bier blocks are coupled with physical therapy.

Table 157-3

Treatment of Reflex Sympathetic Dystrophy

Early mobilization with physical therapy

Sympathetic blockade
    Regional sympathetic blocks
    Bier blocks
    Sympatholytic medication
    Sympathectomy

Medication
    Tricyclic antidepressants
    Anticonvulsants
    Calcium channel blockers
    Corticosteroids
    Nonsteroidal anti-inflammatory drugs
    Narcotics

Introspective techniques
    Meditation
    Meditative exercises
        With physical therapy
        Yoga
        T'ai Chi
    Insight-oriented psychotherapy

Other
    TENS unit
    Biofeedback
    Inpatient multidisciplinary pain program
    Dorsal column spinal stimulation

Medications are often used to supplement sympathetic blockade. Tricyclic antidepressants modulate serotonergic and adrenergic descending pain inhibition and are successful not only in pain control, but also in helping to alleviate the depression that often accompanies the intense pain of RSD. Corticosteroids are variably successful, but should only be used for short-term treatment because of the risk of accelerating the osteopenia of RSD. Sympathetic blocking agents such as clonidine (including a regional clonidine patch) and phenoxybenzamine may be useful in some patients. Other drugs with variable success include nonsteroidal anti-inflammatories, anticonvulsants (phenytoin, carbamazepine, and gabapentin), and calcium channel blockers. The use of narcotics is controversial, but pain control is paramount and should override concerns about addiction. Alternative treatment strategies such as biofeedback and acupuncture have been successful with some patients.

Patients with chronic and refractory RSD may be candidates for surgical procedures. Sympathectomies play a role in some patients, but recurrent pain is common because of cross-innervation. Spinal cord stimulation may be of benefit if the pain is fairly well localized and patients are stable psychologically. Spinal cord stimulation requires placement of an indwelling electrode connected to a battery surgically implanted in the abdomen. The degree of stimulation is under external magnet control. Surgical techniques are not foolproof in RSD patients, and in some cases pain may worsen. All other treatment options should be tried before surgery.

Some patients develop severe pain coupled with depression and narcotic dependency. In such cases, an inpatient multidisciplinary pain program can be of tremendous benefit and should be considered before any surgical procedures are used.

Considerable clinical success may be achieved with a more introspective approach to working with RSD patients. This is in keeping with the hypothesis that RSD may represent a baseline or acute perturbation in the limbic control of pain perception and sympathetic outflow. Through a combination of physical and massage therapy, meditative techniques, and insight-oriented psychotherapy, many patients have become completely pain free without the use of sympathetic blockade. Such treatment requires close clinical supervision.

PROGNOSIS

The course of RSD is unpredictable. Patients treated early and successfully will generally do well, although recurrence is very possible. Patients refractory to early treatment should undergo other treatment strategies. Ultimately, any refractory patient should be referred to a specialty center for RSD. Once patients enter late stage II or stage III, the prognosis for recovery is poor, and patients require very intense treatment efforts in a specialty center.

SUGGESTED READINGS

Drucker WR, Hubay C, Holder WD: Pathogenesis of post-traumatic sympathetic dystrophy. *Am J Surg* 1959; 97:454.

Finsterbush A, Frankl U, Mann G, et al: Reflex sympathetic dystrophy of the patellofemoral joint. *Orthop Rev* 1991; 20:877.

Ogilvie-Harris DJ, Roscoe M: Reflex sympathetic dystrophy of the knee. *J Bone Joint Surg [Br]* 1987; 69:804.

Parkin A, Robinson PJ: Staging of reflex sympathetic dystrophy with ^{99}Tcm-HSA. *Nucl Med Commun* 1992; 13:292.

Schwartzman RJ, McLellan TL 1987: Reflex sympathetic dystrophy: A review. *Arch Neurol* 1987; 44:555.

Small NC: Complications in arthroscopic surgery performed by experienced arthroscopists. *Arthroscopy* 1988; 4:215.

Subbarao J, Stillwell GK: Reflex sympathetic dystrophy syndrome of the upper extremity: Analysis of total outcome of management of 125 cases. *Arch Phys Med Rehabil* 1981; 62:549.

Woolf CJ: Excitability changes in central neurons following peripheral damage: Role of central sensitization in the pathogenesis of pain. In Willis WD Jr (ed): *Bristol-Myers Squibb Symposium on Pain Research Series*, vol 19: *Hyperalgesia and Allodynia.* New York: Raven; 1992:221.

Chapter 158

EPIDEMIOLOGY AND OUTCOME MEASURES

Mary Louise Skovron, Gina B. Aharonoff, and Rudi N. Hiebert

Epidemiology is the study of the determinants and distribution of states of health and disease in populations. Clinical epidemiology is the study of the presentation, prognosis, diagnosis, and treatment of disease in groups of patients, as well as a developed methodology for testing scientific hypotheses in groups of individuals rather than in a laboratory setting.

There are two major categories of epidemiologic studies: *descriptive* and *analytic*. Descriptive epidemiology is used for identifying emerging health problems, describing and monitoring the health status of a population, and for developing causal hypotheses. Analytic epidemiology is used to test specific hypotheses regarding disease causality, treatment efficacy, effectiveness of prevention, treatment, and rehabilitation programs, and to test the validity of screening and diagnostic procedures.

Because it studies the health characteristics of *groups* of individuals, clinical epidemiology uses *statistics* to test hypotheses and draw conclusions. Much of clinical epidemiology is concerned with how clinical information is collected and analyzed.

BASIC MEASURES IN EPIDEMIOLOGY

Epidemiologic data are mainly relative and absolute measures of disease frequency and the characteristics of individuals with and without disease in the population of interest. The most obvious measures of frequency are *case counts* and their variations. The case count may be derived from cases of diseases reported to a health agency by office practitioners, from administrative records of hospital admissions or surgical procedures, or from insurance claim records. In clinical practice, the simple case count is usually derived by a review of charts (retrospectively) or by enrollment of patients seen during a given period (prospectively). The number of cases of a disorder can be a useful indicator of the demand placed by the disorder on the health care system.

Proportionate ratios (ratio of the number cases of a specific disease to total cases of all diseases) can give useful information about the importance of a particular disorder among all disorders of a particular type in the population. However, neither case counts nor proportionate ratios give reference to the underlying population at risk. Without that information there is not sufficient information to test hypotheses about disease causality. For instance, approximately 250,000 hip fractures occur annually in the United States. Without reference to the number of people at risk, it is not possible to estimate the risk of hip fracture in the population or to test hypotheses regarding risk factors for hip fracture. For this reason, rates are necessary to express disease frequency when the objective is to assess risk of disease or determinants of diseases or their outcomes.

Rates describe the frequency of a disease or disorder per unit size of the population per unit time of observation. The general form of a rate is:

$$\left(\frac{\textit{Number of cases}}{\textit{Number of persons at risk}}\right) \textit{per unit of time}$$

Everyone in the numerator is included in the denominator, and everyone in the denominator has a chance to get into the numerator.

Incidence and *prevalence* are special forms of rates. The incidence rate is the number of new cases that develop in a given population during a given time period. The denominator for an incidence rate is the population at risk of acquiring the disease (i.e., non-diseased at the start of the time interval).

The incidence rate can be quantified in a number of ways: as the number of new events per 1000 persons per year, when the population is stable and new events are counted each year, and alternatively, as the number of new events per 1000 person-years, as in prospective studies where a fixed population is followed until either disease occurs, the study ends, or subjects are lost to follow-up. Still another form of incidence rate is the cumulative probability of acquiring a disease, such as when a population of a particular age is followed through an older age, and the total frequency of new cases of the disease is expressed.

The *prevalence rate* is the number of existing cases of disease in a given population in a given time period. *Point prevalence* is the number of cases per unit population at one moment of counting. *Period prevalence* is the number of cases during a definable time interval such as 1-year, 5-year, or lifetime prevalence.

THE SCIENTIFIC METHOD IN EPIDEMIOLOGY

Causal hypotheses are developed by first observing and gathering information about patients; their physical environment and the temporal nature of the disease (descriptive epidemiology); and the anatomy, pathology, physiology, histology, etc. of the disease; and second, by applying inductive reasoning to that pool of knowledge to derive general principles from specific data. Specific hypotheses are then developed through deductive reasoning (deriving relevant particulars from general knowledge) and tested through analytic studies (analytic epidemiology). As the results of studies are reported, the accumulated data either do or do not support the causal hypothesis. Over time, the causal hypothesis may be supported, modified, or negated (see Table 158-1 for principles of causal inference).

DESCRIPTIVE EPIDEMIOLOGY

In descriptive epidemiology, the frequency of a disorder in the population is characterized in terms of person (e.g., age, sex, ethnicity-specific incidence rates, and economic, behavioral, occupational and other factors), place (e.g., rural vs. urban, type of housing, national variations, type of industry), and time (long-term trend, season, and occasionally day of week or time of day). Descriptive epidemiology supports the development of causal hypotheses but does not in itself support conclusions about disease causality or about any hypotheses.

Table 158-1

Principles of Causal Inference

1. Hypothesized cause must be demonstrated to have preceded the disease by a length of time sufficient to allow disease development and expression.

2. Disease should be more common in persons with the hypothesized cause than in those without it.

3. Frequency of the disorder should increase (dose-response relationship) with an increase in the intensity or duration of exposure to the hypothesized cause.

4. Association between the hypothesized causal factor and the disease should be consistently demonstrated in methodologically sound studies and should be biologically plausible.

5. The specificity of an association (degree that hypothesized cause is associated with only one disease or disorder) lends additional weight to a causal hypothesis, but is not necessary to causal inference; for example, cigarette smoking lacks a high degree of specificity as the causal hypothesis of lung cancer, because it is also associated with a variety of other disorders including obstructive pulmonary disease, heart disease, osteoporosis, and low back pain (particularly herniated intervertebral discs). Smoking is accepted as a nonspecific cause of lung cancer.

ANALYTIC EPIDEMIOLOGY

Analytic epidemiology relies on observational and interventional study designs. In observational studies, exposure to the hypothesized causal factor and development of the disease occur during the natural course of events. The study is designed to eliminate or minimize extraneous sources of variation to the extent possible. In interventional studies the investigator can control exposure to the factor of interest.

Observational studies are the first studies undertaken in analytic epidemiology. The interventional study is the final test of causality. However, it is often the case that once a substantial weight of observational evidence is accrued, causality is accepted, as in the case of smoking and lung cancer.

In general, the extent to which a specific study overcomes its intrinsic limitations and embodies the intrinsic strengths of its design, the more robust the evidence from that study. It is nevertheless, almost universally required in evaluations of treatment in clinical epidemiology that the final test of the hypothesis be an interventional, i.e., experimental study where conditions and confounding factors are controlled, such as a randomized controlled trial.

OBSERVATIONAL STUDY DESIGNS

There are three general types of observational studies: cohort, case-control, and cross-sectional.

Cohort Studies

In a cohort study a group of initially disease-free individuals is evaluated for the presence of a risk factor, and then followed over time (Fig. 158-1). At the end of the study period, some will have developed the disease of interest. The investigator then compares the incidence rate of the disease between those in whom exposure to the hypothesized risk factor was present and those in whom it was not.

Because it may take decades for disease to develop, cohort studies are often undertaken by identifying subjects based on existing

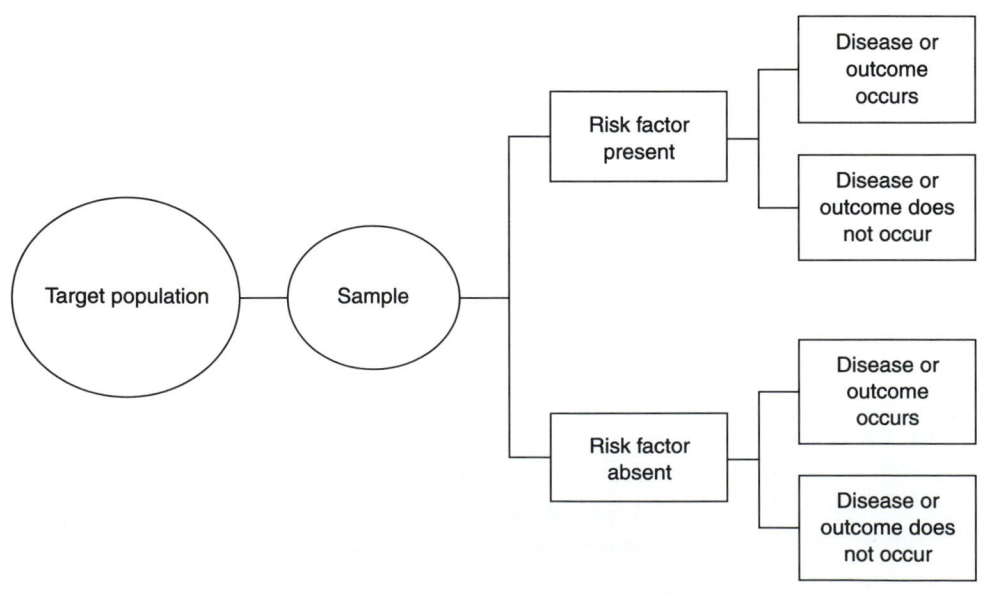

Figure 158-1

Cohort study. [Used with permission from Skovron ML: Epidemiology. In Nordin MN, Andersson GBJ. Pope MH (eds): *Musculoskeletal Disorders in the Workplace: Principles and Practice.* Philadelphia: Mosby-Year Book; 1997:6–15.]

records documenting their health status and exposure to the risk factor in the past and ascertaining subsequent development of disease in the more recent past or in the near future. This type of cohort study is called a *historical*, or *retrospective*, *cohort study*. When the subjects are enrolled at the time of onset of disease exposure and followed forward in time, the cohort study may be referred to as a *follow-up* or *prospective cohort study*.

A *prognostic* or *outcome study* is a special form of a cohort study. In an outcome study the population consists of people with the disease in question, and the exposure or prognostic factors of interest may be patient characteristics, signs and symptoms, treatments or other management strategies, or others.

Loss to follow-up is a potential problem in cohort studies. If a substantial proportion of subjects are lost to the study for any reason, it would be expected that fewer cases of the disease in question would arise in the study than originally planned. The number of study cases may ultimately be too small to yield stable estimates of the incidence rates and consequently of the relative risk.

Biased loss to follow-up occurs when people with the exposure or risk factors who develop the disease have a different probability of remaining in the study than do people without the exposure or risk factors who get the disease. This type of bias would yield a spuriously low estimate of disease incidence in those with the risk (or prognostic) factor.

Because most diseases or conditions are relatively uncommon or take a long time to develop, cohort studies or outcome studies of rare events require enrollment of a large number of subjects who may need years of follow-up. It can be more efficient to address the hypothesis by means of a case-control study, described below.

Case Control Studies

A case-control study compares exposure to a hypothesized causal or prognostic factor between a group of individuals with the disease of interest and another group of disease-free control subjects (Fig. 158-2). Although this appears on its face to be a simple undertaking, the case-control study presents a number of methodological challenges which must be solved in order for study results to be valid.

One of the principal problems occurs when cases and controls are not comparable on what is known as "exposure opportunity"; in other words, controls have been identified in such a way that one group was more or less likely to have been exposed to the risk factor for reasons other than the causal hypothesis being studied. In a case-control study of age as a predictor of spinal stenosis, where cases were identified from Medicare claims and controls were identified from workplace medical facility records, it is obvious that cases and controls would be of different ages because of the way they were selected. An observed association of age and spinal stenosis would therefore be due to selection bias.

Case-control studies can suffer from recall bias, in which a case subject is more or less likely to recall an event in the past than is a control subject. There is also the problem of recall failure, which can occur when subjects are asked to recall events or conditions which took place long ago. Establishing that the exposure to the factor of interest took place long enough before the outcome to be a biologically plausible determinant is difficult for certain types of hypotheses; for example, a case-control study examining degenerative disc disease as a determinant of chronicity (symptom duration greater than six months) in patients with whiplash injury could not establish that the disc problem predated chronicity, based on clinical or imaging examinations at the time of study. This type of problem can be avoided if the case-control study uses exposure or prognostic information which was recorded, in medical or prescription records, prior to the development of the disease.

Another potential problem of case-control studies is selective survival or selective attrition. This occurs when exposed cases have a different probability of being available for study than do exposed controls. One way to avoid this bias is to include only new, or incident, cases in the study.

Because of the difficulty in avoiding the problems described above, case-control studies can produce weaker causal evidence than do cohort studies. However, well-designed and well-executed case-control studies, which avoid the problems described above, can provide evidence as robust as that of cohort studies at considerably less cost and in considerably less time.

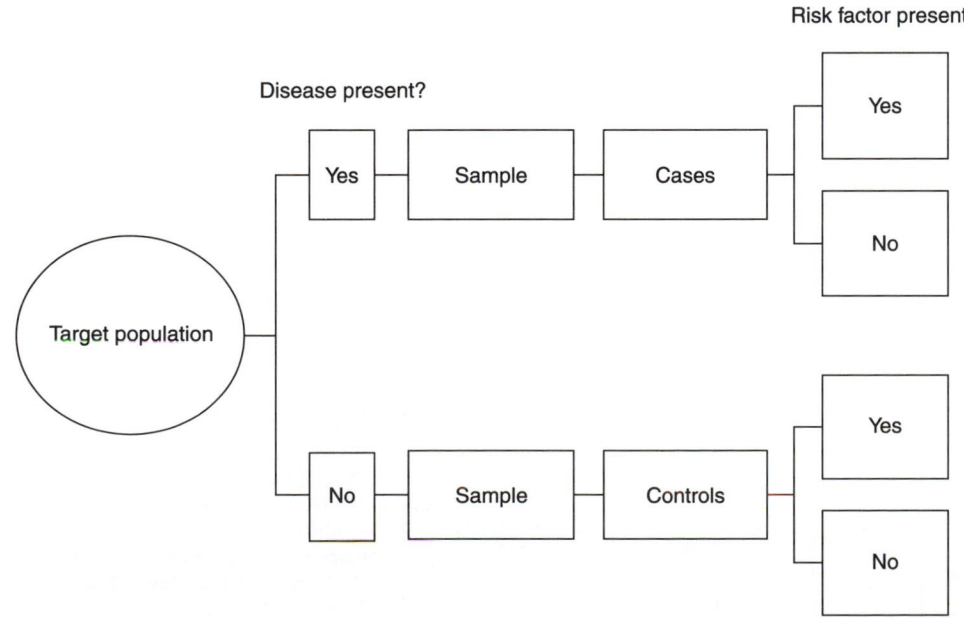

Figure 158-2

Case control study. [Used with permission from Skovron ML: Epidemiology. In Nordin MN, Andersson GBJ, Pope MH (eds): *Musculoskeletal Disorders in the Workplace: Principles and Practice*. Philadelphia: Mosby-Year Book; 1997:6–15.]

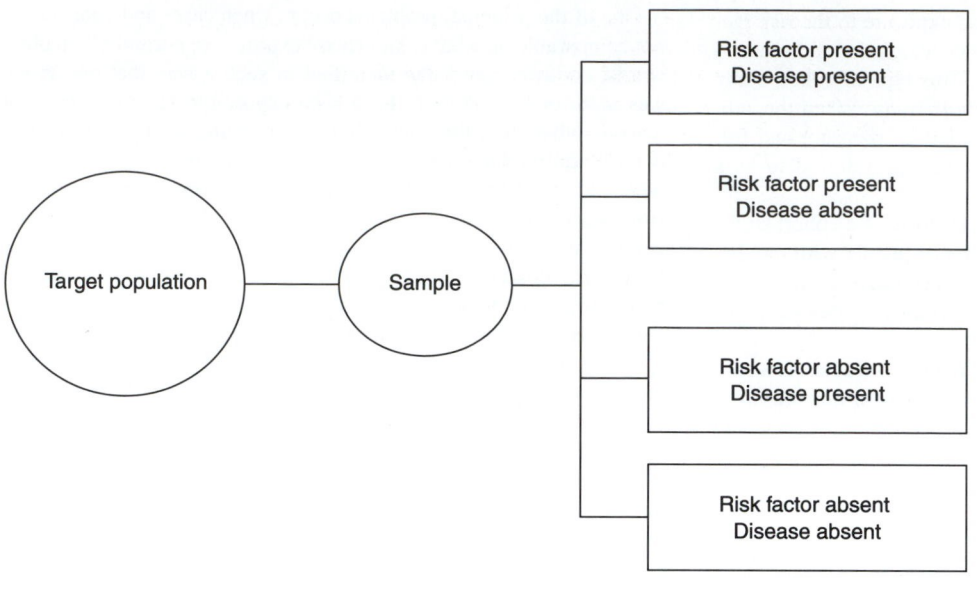

Figure 158-3
Cross-sectional study. [Used with permission from Skovron ML: Epidemiology. In Nordin MN, Andersson GBJ. Pope MH (eds): *Musculoskeletal Disorders in the Workplace: Principles and Practice.* Philadelphia: Mosby-Year Book; 1997:6–15.]

Cross-Sectional Studies

Cross-sectional studies evaluate the presence or absence of disease and hypothesized risk factors in a population of interest at a single point in time or during a specific period of time (Fig. 158-3). Cross-sectional studies require few a priori decisions regarding selection of subjects (unlike case control studies). Furthermore, cross-sectional studies do not require very long follow-up periods (unlike cohort studies). These advantages are, however, offset by a number of limitations. When rare diseases or exposures are being studied, a large number of people must be included. If information is collected at the time of the study rather than from previously existing records, there can be recall biases and recall failure. Selective survival or attrition also can affect these studies. In cross-sectional studies it is often not possible to establish that exposure to the hypothesized risk factor took place before disease developed. Because of these limitations cross-sectional studies cannot be used, by themselves, to establish disease causality. Nevertheless, for relatively common disorders and risk factors, cross-sectional studies may be a useful first step in exploring a hypothesis.

INTERVENTIONAL STUDY DESIGNS: RANDOMIZED CONTROLLED TRIALS

In a randomized controlled trial (RCT), participants are assigned to different treatment groups on a random basis and followed over time (Fig. 158-4). At the end of the study period outcome is compared between the treatment groups. At least one of the treatment groups serves as a control. Controls can receive no treatment, a placebo, or the currently accepted standard treatment.

The validity of RCTs depends on the methodological features described for the observational study designs and more. As in observational studies, the study data must be confined to those patients who have agreed to participate. Comparisons of treatment outcomes in patients who agree to participate with those in patients who refuse to participate are not valid.

The assignment of patients to treatments must use accepted methods of randomization, and the resulting comparability of the treatment groups on important covariates should be described, usually in a table summarizing baseline characteristics of the treatment groups. When randomization does not result in comparable groups, then potential confounding must be controlled for in the statistical analysis.

If surgeons strongly prefer or are more proficient in one surgical technique over another, it has been suggested to randomize patients to the different surgeons with their preferred technique. This can allow valid comparison of outcome by the different surgical methods, while avoiding confounding by surgeon's skills, and avoiding ethical dilemmas for the participating surgeons.

Independent assessment of baseline status and outcome is often necessary to minimize observer (treating surgeon) and participant (pa-

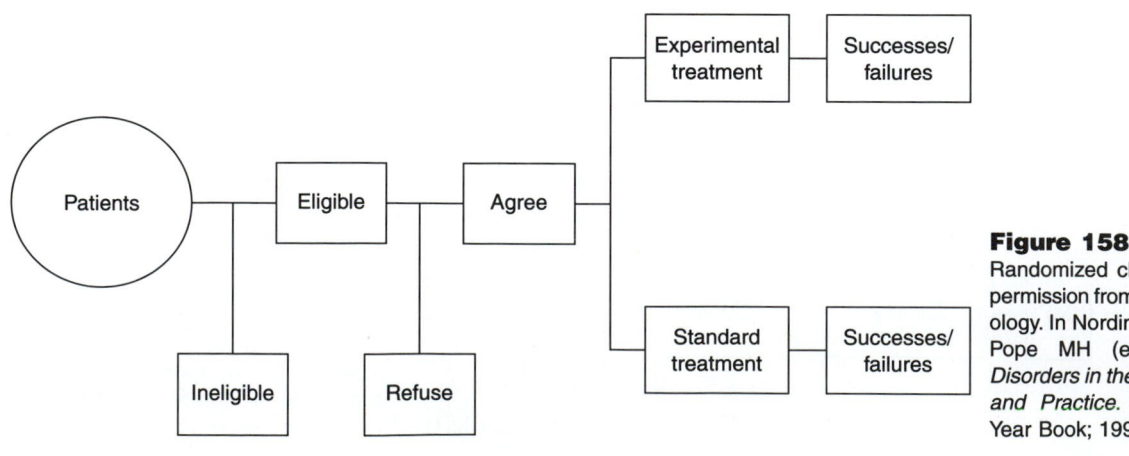

Figure 158-4
Randomized clinical trial. [Used with permission from Skovron ML: Epidemiology. In Nordin MN, Andersson GBJ. Pope MH (eds): *Musculoskeletal Disorders in the Workplace: Principles and Practice.* Philadelphia: Mosby-Year Book; 1997:6–15.]

--- Table 158-2 ---

Comparison of General Health Status Instruments

Instrument	No. Items	Application	Administered by (time)	Physical Functioning	Social Functioning	Role Functioning	Psychological	Pain	Energy/ Fatigue
SF-36	36	Survey	Self, interviewer (5–10 min)	*	*	*	*	*	*
SIP	136	Research, survey	Self, interviewer (20–30 min)	*	*	*	*	—	—
NHP	45	Clinical, survey	Self (10–15 min)	*	*	*	*	*	*
QWB	3	Clinical, survey	Interviewer (10–20 min)	*	*	*	—	—	*

NOTE: SF-36: MOS 36-Item Short-Form Health Survey (Ware JE, Jr, et al: *Medical Care* 1992; 30:473); SIP: Sickness Impact Profile (Bergner M, et al: *Medical Care*, 1981; 19:787); NHP: Nottingham Health Profile (Hunt SM, et al: *Soc Sci Med, Part A, Med Soc* 1981; 15 (3p+1):221); QWB: Quality of Well-Being Scale (Patrick DL, et al: *Health Serv Res* 1973; 8:228).

tient) biases. This is particularly important when the outcome being assessed is subjective. Information should be collected in the same way and with the same frequency in all treatment groups.

MEASURING OUTCOMES

Orthopaedic surgeons have focused in the past on indicators of immediate surgical success, such as rates of postoperative infection, nonunion, range of motion, and fatality. While these indicators are clinically important, the changing environment for medical practice and financing, including managed care, is a strong reason to expand the focus of study to longer-term outcomes and the functioning of the patient. For many orthopaedic procedures, it has been suggested that follow-up studies be conducted for a period of two years and that outcomes include overall health status, functional capacity (activities of daily living, or ADLs), general satisfaction, and quality of life.

There are two broad categories of standardized outcome measurement instruments which have been developed over the past thirty years: those which measure general health status and those which measure health status specific to a particular disease or condition. General health status assessments make possible the comparison of the health status of people with different diseases, thus supporting resource allocation. Disease-specific instruments, on the other hand, incorporate information which may not be included in generic measures and can thus give an enhanced understanding of outcomes of treatment for particular conditions. It is often advisable to use both when conducting outcome studies. Refer to Tables 158-2 and 158-3 for a summary of general and disease-specific health status measurement instruments useful for the orthopaedist.

ISSUES IN THE MEASUREMENT OF OUTCOME: VALIDITY AND RELIABILITY

The validity of a measurement instrument is its ability to measure accurately what it purports to measure. Validity can be expressed in a number of different ways. Several of these are described herein. *Content validity* refers to how completely a measurement instrument describes the different aspects of the characteristic or condition to be measured. For example, an outcome instrument which measures recovery from knee arthroplasty would have poor content validity if it failed to include a measure of range of motion. *Criterion validity* refers to how well a measurement instrument correlates with other, accepted measurements. *Construct validity* describes how well the measurement instrument represents the theoretical construct of the characteristic or condition measured. For example, an instrument which measures disability should produce poor scores for individuals unable to work because of impairment, who are in pain, or who are depressed, and good scores for individuals who are pain free, free from physical impairment, and so on.

The reliability or reproducibility of a measure is the extent to which it gives consistent results. *Test-retest reliability* is assessed by repeating measurements twice on the same subject and evaluating the degree of agreement. *Intra-rater reliability* is assessed when the same examiner conducts the assessment twice. When two or more persons conduct the repeat assessments on the same people and their measurements are compared, then *inter-rater reliability* is obtained.

Poor reliability reduces the *power* of the study (discussed below) to detect associations between the hypothesized factor and disease or outcome. More importantly, data collection instruments with poor reliability or validity can produce biased or misleading research results. For these reasons, published research reports should contain descriptions of the reliability or validity of the data collection instruments used.

SAMPLING

Because not every subject in a study population can be followed or identified, sampling is usually required. Care must be taken, however, since the manner in which study subjects are sampled can adversely affect conclusions drawn from the study. For example, studies which rely on volunteer participants may not be generalizable because the health behaviors and health status and prognosis of people who volunteer for research are well documented to be better than of those who refuse. The optimum method of sampling is a *probability* or *random* sample, in which only chance affects whether an individual is selected for study.

Table 158-3

Disease Specific Instruments

Instrument	Focus	Dimensions	Number of Components
Health Assessment Questionnaire (HAQ)	Arthritis	*Dressing and grooming, eating, walking, hygiene, reaching and bending, grip* (opening jars), *activities* (errands and chores), and *pain analog*	8
Arthritis Impact Measurement Scale (AIMS)	Arthritis	*Mobility, physical activity, dexterity, social role, social activity, activities of daily living, pain, depression, anxiety*	9
Harris	Hip arthroplasty	*Pain, function* [gait (limp, support), activities (stairs, shoes and socks, sitting, public transportation)], *absence of deformities, range of motion*	4
Hospital for Special Surgery (HSS)	Hip arthroplasty	*Pain, muscle power and motion, walking, function* (housework, shopping, etc.)	4
Iowa	Hip arthroplasty	*Pain, function* (housework, dressing, walking, sitting, bathing, use of stairs, carrying objects, getting in/out of car, driving), *gait* (limp, use of assistive devices), *absence of deformity, range of motion*	5
Mayo	Hip arthroplasty	Pain, function (distance walked, support aids), *mobility and muscle power* (car, footcare, limp, stairs), *roentogenographic examination*	4
Merle d'Aubigne	Hip arthroplasty	*Pain, mobility* (flexion and abduction), *ability to walk*	3

SOURCE: [Sources as follow: (HAQ: Fries JF, et al: *Arthritis Rheum*; 1980; 23:137) (AIMS: Meenan RF, et al: *Arthritis Rheum*; 1980; 23:146) (Harris: Harris WH, et al: *J Bone Joint Surg [Am]* 1969; 51:737) (HSS: Wilson PD Jr, et al: *J Bone Joint Surg [Am]* 1972; 54:207) (Iowa: Larson CB: *Clin Orthop* 1963; 31:85) (Mayo: Kavanagh BF, et al: *Clin Orthop* 1985; 193:133) (Merle d'Aubigne: D'Aubigne RM, et al: *J Bone Joint Surg [Am]* 1954; 36:451)]

METHODS OF ANALYSIS

The statistical analysis of any study data should be appropriate to the hypothesis and to the structure of the data collected. If it is necessary to control for pretreatment differences between the groups, the analysis will use multivariate methods, such as analysis of covariance or multiple regression. In cases where the outcome variable distribution or the conditions of the study do not conform to the requirements of commonly used statistical hypothesis tests (t-tests, analysis of covariance, regression analysis), a non-parametric method of statistical analysis is appropriate. Alternatively, the variable could be transformed for analysis (i.e., log or square root transformation).

When the hypothesis addresses the relative frequency of an event (e.g., a success rate or patient mortality rate), the relative incidence of disease in the subjects exposed to the risk factor and those not exposed is evaluated. A ratio of the incidence rates, called the relative risk, is used to express the association (Tables 158-4 and 158-5). A relative risk of one indicates no association. The further away from one, the stronger the observed association, and the stronger the evidence in favor of the research hypothesis.

In case-control studies, relative risks cannot be computed directly. Instead, an alternative measure of association, the odds ratio, is used to estimate the relative risk (Tables 158-4 and 158-5). The odds ratio is constructed by comparing the odds of exposure to the hypoth-

esized risk factor of interest between the diseased and the disease-free control groups. Like the relative risk, an odds ratio of one indicates no association. Divergence from one indicates a progressively stronger association between the hypothesized risk factor and disease or outcome. The odds ratio is a useful estimates of relative risk if the following conditions are met: (1) the cases are representative of all cases, (2) the controls are representative of the population at risk, and (3) the disease is uncommon.

PRECISION OF ESTIMATES

Because research is conducted on samples of the population, the results of any given study (such as the mean difference in Harris hip scores between two groups of patients), are estimates of the true population means (or proportions, relative risks, etc.) in the entire population. The precision of a study estimate of the population value (parameter) is described by the standard error of the estimate. The standard error is affected by the variability of the measurement and the number of subjects in the study. It is also useful to describe the precision of the estimates as a range within which the true population parameter probably lies. This is the confidence interval around the estimate, and is, by convention, expressed as the 95 percent confidence interval.

Table 158-4

Scheme for Classification of Patients in Observational Epidemiologic Studies

	Patients with Disease	Patients without Disease	
Exposed to risk factor	a	c	a + c
Not exposed to risk factor	b	d	b + d
	a + b	c + d	

STATISTICAL HYPOTHESIS TESTING

Clinical research is conducted on samples of patients, and the resulting observed relative risks (or differences between treatment groups) are estimates of the true magnitude of an association in the population. Because there is always a chance of sampling error, study results must be tested to determine the probability that the results could have occurred by chance alone.

The statistical hypothesis test evaluates whether the observed results could have occurred due to sampling error (the null hypothesis). If the observed association is large enough that sampling error probably does not explain it, the null hypothesis is rejected. The investigators then accept the alternative hypothesis—the observed estimates of relative risk or differences between treatments reflect the true situation in the population from which the samples were drawn. By convention, the cutoff (*alpha*) for rejecting the null hypothesis is usually set at .05. If the probability (*p* value) that the observed results of a particular study are due to sampling error is less than *alpha* (i.e., less than .05) the null hypothesis is rejected, and the results are declared statistically significant.

STATISTICAL POWER AND SAMPLE SIZE

Statistical hypothesis tests actually involve two possible types of error. In addition to incorrectly declaring an observed association statistically significant when in fact it is the result of sampling error (type I error, described above), there is also the possibility of declaring that the study results are due to sampling error (not statistically significant) when in fact they reflect a true association in the population from which the study subjects were drawn. This is the type II error and its probability is *beta*. The complementary probability that a study will be able to correctly detect an association when there is one in the population at large, is referred to as statistical power (1–*beta*).

In the planning phase of clinical research, the investigators should determine how strong an association (effect size), that is, how large an estimated relative risk or how big a difference between treatments, would be in order to be clinically important. The number of subjects to be studied is set to optimize the statistical power, that is, to have an acceptable probability of detecting a clinically important effect size. The larger the sample size, the more power the statistical test has to detect associations; in other words, as expected differences or relative risks get smaller, the number of subjects studied has to increase in order to have adequate power to test the hypothesis. Conversely, with very large numbers of study subjects, it is possible to declare trivial associations statistically significant. When studies with small sample sizes report results that were not statistically significant, they should comment on how strong the association would have had to be to have good power to detect it. The reader should evaluate whether the observed difference although not statistically significant, is clinically significant. When studies with very large numbers of subjects report statistically significant results, the reader should decide if the differences are clinically trivial, even though statistically significant.

CONFOUNDING

Confounding occurs when the study results (e.g., an increase in risk of the disease) can be explained by a factor extraneous to the hypothesis. By definition, a confounding factor is associated with both the disease in question and the hypothesized causal factor. Potential confounding factors can be eliminated in the design of the study (using restricted or

---

Table 158-5

Formulas Used in the Computation of Relative Risk and Odds Ratios

Quantity	Study Design	Expression
Relative risk	Population-based cohort and outcome studies, interventional studies	Risk of disease in exposed group $= \dfrac{a}{a+c}$ Risk of disease in unexposed group $= \dfrac{c}{c+d}$ $RR = \dfrac{\frac{a}{a+c}}{\frac{b}{b+d}}$
Odds ratio	Unmatched case-control studies	Exposed vs. unexposed in diseased group $= \dfrac{a}{b}$ Exposed vs. unexposed in disease-free group $= \dfrac{c}{d}$ $OR = \dfrac{\frac{a}{b}}{\frac{c}{d}} = \dfrac{ad}{bc}$

stratified or matched sampling) or in the data analysis phases (by performing stratified or multivariate analyses). In RCTs, potential confounding is controlled by random assignment of subjects to each treatment and by multivariate analysis if necessary. Identifying and controlling for potential confounders is very important, since confounders can distort relationships between hypothesized causal factors and disease or outcome, leading the investigator to incorrect conclusions.

CONCLUSION

The validity of clinical research relies on a number of factors. The hypothesis must be formulated specifically enough to be testable. The appropriate study subjects should be eligible, and there should not be differential participation. The information collected should be accurate and appropriate to the hypothesis. The study design and information sources should avoid potential information biases. Potential confounders should be eliminated in the study design or controlled in the statistical analysis. At the time the study is designed, a clinically significant result should be stated, the plan of statistical analysis determined, and the necessary number of study subjects defined. Study management should avoid the introduction of differential loss to follow-up, unblinding, and other potential problems. The statistical analysis should be appropriate to the structure of the data and to the hypothesis. Finally, although the discussion should place the study in the context of other work and what is already known about the question, the specific conclusions should not go beyond what was actually tested in the study.

SUGGESTED READINGS

Altman DC: Statistics and ethics in research. Part 1: Misuse of statistics is unethical. *BMJ* 1980;281:1182. Part 2: Study design, p. 1267. Part 3: How large a sample? p. 1336. Part 4: Collecting and screening data, p. 1399. Part 5: Analysing data, p. 1473. Part 6: Presentation of results, p. 1542. Part 7: Interpreting results, p. 1612. Part 8: Improving the quality of statistics in medical journals. *BMJ* 1981; 282:44.

AAOS Department of Research: *Fundamentals of Outcome Research.* Rosemont, IL: American Academy of Orthopaedic Surgeons; 1993.

Bailar JC III, Mosteller F: *Medical Uses of Statistics,* 2d ed. Waltham, MA: NEJM Books; 1992.

Deyo RA, Andersson G, Bombardier C, et al: Outcome measures for studying patients with low back pain. *Spine* 1994; 19:2032S.

Elston RC, Johnson WD: *Essentials of Biostatistics,* 2d ed. Philadelphia: FA Davis; 1994.

Fleiss JL: *The Design and Analysis of Clinical Experiments.* New York: John Wiley & Sons; 1986.

Friedman LM, Furberg C, DeMets, DL: *Fundamentals of Clinical Trials,* 3d ed. St. Louis, MO: Mosby-Year Book; 1996.

Gardner MJ, Altman DG: Confidence intervals rather than p values: Estimation rather than hypothesis testing. *BMJ* 1986; 292:746.

Hulley SB, Cummings SR: *Designing Clinical Research.* Baltimore: Williams & Wilkins; 1988.

McDowell I, Newell C: *Measuring Health: A Guide to Rating Scales and Questionnaires.* New York: Oxford University Press; 1996.

Morton RF, Hebel JR, McCarter RJ: *A Study Guide to Epidemiology and Biostatistics,* 4th ed. Gaithersburg, MD: Aspen Publishers; 1996.

Rudicel S, Esdaile J: The randomized clinical trial in orthopedics: Obligation or option? *J Bone Joint Surg [Am]* 1985; 67:1284.

Sackett DL: How to read clinical journals: Why to read them and how to start reading them critically. *CMAJ* 1981; 124:555 [Canada].

Shekelle PG, Andersson G, Bombardier C, et al: A brief introduction to critical reading of the clinical literature. *Spine* 1994; 19:2028S.

Troidl H, Spitzer WO, McPeek B, et al: *Principles and Practice of Research: Strategies for Surgical Investigators,* 3d ed. New York, NY: Springer-Verlag; 1997.

Weiss NS: *Clinical Epidemiology. The Study of the Outcome of Illness,* 2d ed. New York: Oxford University Press; 1996.

INDEX

Page numbers in italics indicate figures; those followed by t indicate tables.

ISBN 0-07-060355-3

90000

9 780070 603554

SPIVAK: ORTHOPAEDICS
A STUDY GUIDE